Pediatric
Hematology

Commissioning Editors: Gavin Smith and Maria Khan
Project Editor: Carol Parr
Project Controller: Mark Sanderson

Pediatric Hematology

EDITED BY

John S. Lilleyman
Consultant Haematologist and Professor of Paediatric Oncology,
The Royal London Hospital, London, UK

Ian M. Hann
Consultant Haematologist, Great Ormond Street Hospital for Sick Children, London, UK

Victor S. Blanchette
Professor of Paediatrics and Head, Division of Paediatric Haematology/Oncology,
The Hospital for Sick Children, Toronto, Canada

SECOND EDITION

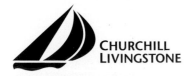

CHURCHILL
LIVINGSTONE

LONDON EDINBURGH NEW YORK PHILADELPHIA SYDNEY TORONTO

CHURCHILL LIVINGSTONE
An imprint of Harcourt Brace and Company Limited

© Harcourt Brace and Company 1999

First published 1992
Second edition 1999

ISBN 0–4430–5840–7

British Library Cataloguing in Publication Data
A catalogue record for this book is available from the British Library

Library of Congress Cataloging in Publication Data
A catalog record for this book is available from the Library of Congress

Note
Medical knowledge is constantly changing. As new information becomes available,
changes in treatment, procedures, equipment and the use of drugs become necessary.
The editors, the contributors and the publishers have, as far as it is possible, taken
care to ensure that the information given in the text is accurate and up-to-date.
However, readers are strongly advised to confirm that the information, especially
with regard to drug usage, complies with the latest legislation and standards of practice.

The
Publisher's
policy is to use
**paper manufactured
from sustainable forests**

Typeset by Paston PrePress Ltd, Beccles, Suffolk
Printed in China

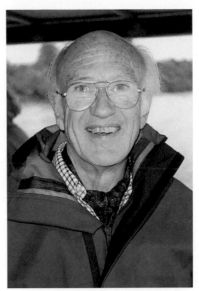

Photograph by John Stuart, 1992.

ROGER HARDISTY

Roger Hardisty died on 18 September 1997 at the age of 74 and shortly after completing his chapter on platelet functional disorders. The scholarship displayed there gives eloquent testimony to his undimmed scientific and journalistic skills, and the fact that he knew himself to be terminally ill while writing makes it a particularly poignant professional epitaph.

As mentioned in his obiturary in *The Times*, Roger was the first hematologist in the UK to devote himself entirely to the study of blood diseases in children and he founded an internationally renowned department for that purpose at The Hospital for Sick Children in Great Ormond Street. His many other professional achievements are well recorded and speak for themselves. Known throughout the world, he was mentor to many who followed in the specialty he helped to create, including several contributors to this book. His wise counsel and exacting professional standards will long be remembered.

A quiet, courteous and intellectual man, he had many friends as was evident at his memorial service. The editors are proud to dedicate this book to him.

Contents

Contributors

Maureen Andrew
Professor of Paediatrics
McMaster University and the University of Toronto

Director
Children's Thrombophilia Program
Hamilton Civic Hospitals Research Centre
Hamilton, Ontario, Canada

Sarah E Ball
Senior Lecturer in Haematology
St George's Hospital Medical School
London, UK

André Baruchel
Professor of Paediatric Haematology
Service d'Hématologie Pédiatrique
Hôpital Saint-Louis
Paris, France

Frederick G Behm
Director, Immunopathology and Flow Cytometry
Department of Pathology and Laboratory Medicine
St Jude Children's Research Hospital
Memphis, TN, USA

Alastair J Bellingham
Emeritus Professor of Haematology
King's College School of Medicine and Dentistry
London, UK

Victor S Blanchette
Chief and Professor of Paediatrics
Division of Haematology/Oncology
The Hospital for Sick Children
Toronto, Ontario, Canada

Lu Ann Brooker
Hamilton Civic Hospitals Research Centre
Hamilton, Ontario, Canada

Nancy J Bunin
Associate Professor of Pediatrics
The University of Pennsylvania School of Medicine

Director of Bone Marrow Transplant
Division of Oncology
The Children's Hospital of Philadelphia
Philadelphia, PA, USA

James B Bussel
Associate Professor of Pediatrics
The New York Hospital
Cornell University Medical Center
Department of Pediatrics
Division of Pediatric Hematology/Oncology
New York, NY, USA

Andrew Cant
Consultant in Paediatric Haematology & Infectious Diseases
Newcastle United Hospitals NHS Trust

Senior Lecturer in Child Health
University of Newcastle Medical School
Newcastle, UK

Elizabeth A Chalmers
Consultant Haematologist
Royal Hospital for Sick Children
Glasgow, Scotland, UK

Judith M Chessells
Leukaemia Research Fund Professor of Haematology and Oncology
Institute of Child Health
University College London Medical School

Honorary Consultant Physician
Great Ormond Street Hospital for Children NHS Trust
London, UK

Julie Dean
Clinical Associate Lecturer
Department of Paediatrics and Child Health
The New Children's Hospital
University of Sydney
Sydney, Australia

Inderjeet S Dokal
Consultant Paediatric Haematologist
Hammersmith Hospital
London, UK

John J Doyle
Assistant Professor
Division of Haematology/Oncology
The Hospital for Sick Children
University of Toronto
Toronto, Canada

OB Eden
Cancer Research Campaign Professor of Paediatric Oncology
Academic Unit of Paediatric Oncology
Christie Hospital and Manchester Children's Hospital Trusts
Manchester, UK

George H Elder
Professor and Head of Department of Medical Biochemistry
University of Wales College of Medicine
Cardiff, UK

Adam Finn
Senior Lecturer in Paediatric Immunology and Infectious Diseases
University of Sheffield Medical School

Honorary Consultant Paediatric Immunologist
Sheffield Children's Hospital
Sheffield, UK

Melvin H Freedman
Professor, Department of Paediatrics
University of Toronto Faculty of Medicine

Senior Associate Scientist, Research Institute
The Hospital for Sick Children
Toronto, Canada

Brenda ES Gibson
Consultant Haematologist
Royal Hospital for Sick Children
Glasgow, Scotland, UK

EC Gordon-Smith
Professor and Head of Department
Department of Cellular & Molecular Sciences
Division of Haematology
St George's Hospital Medical School
London, UK

Ian M Hann
Consultant Haematologist
Great Ormond Street Hospital for Children NHS Trust
London, UK

Roger M Hardisty (deceased)
Emeritus Professor of Haematology
University of London
Royal Free Hospital School of Medicine
London, UK

RF Hinchliffe
Senior Chief Medical Laboratory Scientific Officer
Roald Dahl Paediatric Haematology Centre
The Children's Hospital
Sheffield, UK

A Victor Hoffbrand
Emeritus Professor of Haematology
Royal Free Hospital School of Medicine
London, UK

Heather A Hume
Division of Haematology/Oncology
Hôpital Ste-Justine

Associate Professor
Université de Montréal
Montréal, Québec, Canada

Paul Imbach
Professor, Head of Pediatric Oncology/Hematology
Aarau/Basel Children's Hospital
Basel, Switzerland

Andreas E Kulozik
Professor of Pediatrics
Children's Hospital
Charité Virchow Medical Center
Humboldt University
Berlin, Germany

Beverly J Lange
Professor of Pediatrics
The University of Pennsylvania School of Medicine

Medical Director
Division of Oncology
The Children's Hospital of Philadelphia
Philadelphia, PA, USA

Brian D Lake
Emeritus Professor of Histochemistry
Department of Histopathology
Great Ormond Street Hospital for Children NHS Trust
London, UK

D Mark Layton
Senior Lecturer and Consultant Paediatric Haematologist
Department of Haematological Medicine
King's College School of Medicine and Dentistry
London, UK

Thierry Leblanc
Service d'Hématologie Pédiatrique
Hôpital Saint-Louis
Paris, France

RJ Liesner
Lecturer in Paediatric Haematology
Great Ormond Street Hospital for Children NHS Trust
London, UK

x

David Lillicrap
Professor
Departments of Pathology and Medicine
Queen's University
Kingston, Ontario, Canada

John S Lilleyman
Mark Ridgwell Professor
Department of Paediatric Oncology
St Bartholomew's and the Royal London School of Medicine and Dentistry

Honorary Consultant Haematologist
The Royal London Hospital
London, UK

Naomi LC Luban
Director of Transfusion Medicine
Children's National Medical Center
Department of Laboratory Medicine
Washington, DC, USA

Bertram H Lubin
Director of Medical Research
Children's Hospital Oakland

Adjunct Professor of Pediatrics
University of California San Francisco
San Francisco, CA, USA

Jeanne M Lusher
Marion I Barnhart Hemostasis Research Professor
Distinguished Professor of Pediatrics
Wayne State University School of Medicine

Co-Director, Division of Hematology–Oncology
Children's Hospital of Michigan
Detroit, MI, USA

Catherine Manno
Director of Transfusion Medicine
Children's Hospital of Philadelphia
Philadelphia, PA, USA

William C Mentzer
Professor and Director
Division of Hematology/Oncology
Department of Pediatrics
University of California San Francisco
San Francisco, CA, USA

Nancy F Olivieri
Department of Paediatrics
Division of Haematology
Hospital for Sick Children
Toronto, Ontario, Canada

Patricia Pisciotta
Director of Laboratories
University of Connecticut
School of Medicine
Department of Laboratory Medicine
Farmington, CT, USA

Ching-Hon Pui
Director, Leukemia/Lymphoma Division
Department of Hematology/Oncology
St Jude Children's Research Hospital

Professor of Pediatrics
University of Tennessee, College of Medicine
Memphis, TN, USA

Michael M Reid
Consultant Haematologist
Royal Victoria Infirmary

Honorary Senior Lecturer
University of Newcastle upon Tyne
Newcastle upon Tyne, UK

Jörg Ritter
Professor, University Children's Hospital
Münster, Germany

Irene AG Roberts
Senior Lecturer in Haematology
Imperial College School of Medicine

Honorary Consultant Paediatric Haematologist
Hammersmith Hospital
London, UK

David S Rosenblatt
Director, Division of Medical Genetics
Department of Medicine
McGill University Health Centre

Director, The Hess B and Diane Finestone Laboratory

Professor of Human Genetics, Medicine, Paediatrics and Biology
McGill University
Montreal, Quebec, Canada

Mark V Sapp
Fellow, Pediatric Hematology/Oncology
The New York Hospital
Cornell University Medical Center
Department of Pediatrics
Division of Pediatric Hematology/Oncology
New York, NY, USA

Gérard Schaison
Service d'Hématologie Pédiatrique
Hôpital Saint-Louis
Paris, France

Martin Schrappe
Senior Attending Pediatrician
Department of Pediatric Hematology and Oncology
Children's Hospital
Medical School Hannover
Hannover, Germany

Graham R Serjeant
Director, MRC Laboratories (Jamaica)
University of West Indies
Kingston, Jamaica

Owen P Smith
Consultant Paediatric Haematologist
National Children's Hospital
Dublin, Ireland

Richard F Stevens
Consultant Paediatric Haematologist
Royal Manchester Children's Hospital
Manchester, UK

Anton Heinz Sutor
Professor of Pediatric Hematology
Universitäts-Klinderklinik
Freiburg, Germany

David J Weatherall
Regius Professor of Medicine
Institute of Molecular Medicine
John Radcliffe Hospital
Oxford, UK

David KH Webb
Consultant Haematologist
Department of Haematology
Great Ormond Street Children's Hospital
London, UK

Brian A Wharton
Honorary Professor of University College, London
MRC Childhood Nutrition Centre
Institute of Child Health
London, UK

Andrew M Will
Consultant Paediatric Haematologist
Royal Manchester Children's Hospital
Manchester, UK

Preface to the Second Edition

An attempt by a small group of UK authors to write a long overdue replacement for Michael Willoughby's solo text on pediatric hematology resulted in the first edition of this book in 1992. Four years later the publishers persuaded the editors to contemplate a second edition, urging them to take the opportunity to expand the breadth and depth of the contents and to recruit an international authorship. A new co-editor, Victor Blanchette, was caught at a weak moment and persuaded to join the project. His wisdom and experience proved invaluable, and his influence will be obvious to anyone glancing beyond this page. An impressive list of international experts agreed to contribute (some for the second time, many for the first) and the editors are very grateful to them all. Particular mention must be made of Roger Hardisty who completed his chapter while terminally ill and whose chief concern was that he would not be able to read his own proofs. With much affection this book is dedicated to him.

The most obvious differences from the first edition are of size and scale. The number of contributors has increased from 17 to 57 and the number of chapters from 15 to 40. Also conspicuous is the more cosmopolitan nature of the author list with now less than half from the UK and the remainder coming from Canada, the US, Germany, Switzerland, France, Australia, Jamaica and Ireland. The pitch of the work has changed a little and it is now more of a fully fledged source of reference.

The larger number of individuals involved and the division of the book into many more self-contained chapters inevitably amplifies the two potential difficulties of all multi-author texts—heterogeneity of style and duplication of content. While these can be dealt with by stern editing up to a point, we have chosen to leave individual works of scholarship alone with as little tinkering as possible. We have simply cross-referenced duplication where a subject is covered from a different angle in more than one chapter. We have done so in the belief that books of this type are not read as a continuous narrative but rather as an occasional source of information on a single topic where more than one point of view can be an asset. We hope we are right and that the end result will prove useful to all pediatricians and hematologists.

As the book progressed there were several changes in personnel within Churchill Livingstone. Many people have therefore been involved in its gestation but we are particularly grateful to Gavin Smith who steered us through the first two trimesters and offer our special thanks to Maria Khan who took over the third. She had the difficult job of midwife and carried it out brilliantly.

John Lilleyman, Ian Hann and Victor Blanchette
London and Toronto, 1998

Reference values

RF HINCHLIFFE

The values of many hematologic variables change markedly in the first weeks and months of life and reference data are important to enable proper interpretation of laboratory results, both in infancy and until the age at which adult normal ranges can be applied.

Most reference data are affected to some degree by factors such as racial origin, diet, drug intake and the incidence of sub-clinical illness. Other variables include the methodology and instrumentation used to obtain the data and the method of statistical analysis. Ideally, each laboratory would generate its own reference ranges based on healthy individuals from the population it serves, but this is rarely if ever practical. The following data, selected to cover the commoner hematologic variables should, however, prove useful in most circumstances.

Contents

Acknowledgement

The author thanks Marie Elliott for expert secretarial assistance.

Table 1 Normal blood count values from birth to 18 years.

Age	Hb (g/dl)	RBC ($\times 10^{12}$/l)	Hct	MCV (fl)	WBC ($\times 10^9$/l)	Neutrophils ($\times 10^9$/l)	Lymphocytes ($\times 10^9$/l)	Monocytes ($\times 10^9$/l)	Eosinophils ($\times 10^9$/l)	Basophils ($\times 10^9$/l)	Platelets ($\times 10^9$/l)
Birth (term infants)	14.9–23.7	3.7–6.5	0.47–0.75	100–125	10–26	2.7–14.4	2.0–7.3	0–1.9	0–0.85	0–0.1	150–450
2 weeks	13.4–19.8	3.9–5.9	0.41–0.65	88–110	6–21	1.5–5.4	2.8–9.1	0.1–1.7	0–0.85	0–0.1	170–500
2 months	9.4–13.0	3.1–4.3	0.28–0.42	84–98	5–15	0.7–4.8	3.3–10.3	0.4–1.2	0.05–0.9	0.02–0.13	210–650
6 months	10.0–13.0	3.8–4.9	0.3–0.38	73–84	6–17	1–6	3.3–11.5	0.2–1.3	0.1–1.1	0.02–0.2	210–560
1 year	10.1–13.0	3.9–5.1	0.3–0.38	70–82	6–16	1–8	3.4–10.5	0.2–0.9	0.05–0.9	0.02–0.13	200–550
2–6 years	11.0–13.8	3.9–5.0	0.32–0.4	72–87	6–17	1.5–8.5	1.8–8.4	0.15–1.3	0.05–1.1	0.02–0.12	210–490
6–12 years	11.1–14.7	3.9–5.2	0.32–0.43	76–90	4.5–14.5	1.5–8.0	1.5–5.0	0.15–1.3	0.05–1.0	0.02–0.12	170–450
12–18 years											
Female	12.1–15.1	4.1–5.1	0.35–0.44	77–94	4.5–13	1.5–6	1.5–4.5	0.15–1.3	0.05–0.8	0.02–0.12	180–430
Male	12.1–16.6	4.2–5.6	0.35–0.49	77–92							

Compiled from various sources. Red cell values at birth derived from skin puncture blood; most other data from venous blood.

Table 2 Red cell values (mean ± 1 SD) on the first postnatal day from 24 weeks' gestational age.

Gestational age (weeks) (No. of infants)	24–25 (n = 7)	26–27 (n = 11)	28–29 (n = 7)	30–31 (n = 35)	32–33 (n = 23)	34–35 (n = 23)	36–37 (n = 20)	Term (n = 19)
RBC ($\times 10^{12}$/l)	4.65 ±0.43	4.73 ±0.45	4.62 ±0.75	4.79 ±0.74	5.0 ±0.76	5.09 ±0.5	5.27 ±0.68	5.14 ±0.7
Hb (g/dl)	19.4 ±1.5	19.0 ±2.5	19.3 ±1.8	19.1 ±2.2	18.5 ±2.0	19.6 ±2.1	19.2 ±1.7	19.3 ±2.2
Hematocrit	0.63 ±.04	0.62 ±.08	0.60 ±.07	0.60 ±.08	0.60 ±.08	0.61 ±.07	0.64 ±.07	0.61 ±.074
MCV (fl)	135 ±0.2	132 ±14.4	131 ±13.5	127 ±12.7	123 ±15.7	122 ±10.0	121 ±12.5	119 ±9.4
Reticulocytes (%)	6.0 ±0.5	9.6 ±3.2	7.5 ±2.5	5.8 ±2.0	5.0 ±1.9	3.9 ±1.6	4.2 ±1.8	3.2 ±1.4
Weight (g)	725 ±185	993 ±194	1174 ±128	1450 ±232	1816 ±192	1957 ±291	2245 ±213	

Counts performed on heel-prick blood. Reproduced with permission from Ref. 1.

Table 3 Hemoglobin values (median and 95% range) in the first 6 months of life in iron-sufficient (serum ferritin $\geqslant 10$ μg/l) preterm infants.

Age	Birth weight 1000–1500 g	Number tested	Birth weight 1501–2000 g	Number tested
2 weeks	16.3 (11.7–18.4)	17	14.8 (11.8–19.6)	39
1 month	10.9 (8.7–15.2)	15	11.5 (8.2–15.0)	42
2 months	8.8 (7.1–11.5)	17	9.4 (8.0–11.4)	47
3 months	9.8 (8.9–11.2)	16	10.2 (9.3–11.8)	41
4 months	11.3 (9.1–13.1)	13	11.3 (9.1–13.1)	37
5 months	11.6 (10.2–14.3)	8	11.8 (10.4–13.0)	21
6 months	12.0 (9.4–13.8)	9	11.8 (10.7–12.6)	21

All infants had an uncomplicated course in the first 2 weeks of life and none received exchange transfusion. Counts obtained from venous and skin-puncture blood. Reproduced with permission from Ref. 2.

Table 4 Values for mature and immature neutrophils and the immature:total neutrophil ratio in 24 infants of <33 weeks' gestation.

Age (hours)	Mature neutrophils ($\times 10^9$/l) Median (range)	Mean	Immature neutrophils ($\times 10^9$/l) Median (range)	Mean	Immature:total ratio Median (range)	Mean
1 (n = 10)	4.64 (2.20–8.18)	4.57	0.11 (0–1.5)	0.30	0.04 (0–0.35)	0.09
12 (n = 17)	6.80 (4.0–22.48)	8.61	0.27 (0–1.6)	0.48	0.04 0–0.21)	0.06
24 (n = 17)	5.60 (2.61–21.20)	7.64	0.14 (0–3.66)	0.47	0.03 (0–0.17)	0.05
48 (n = 20)	4.98 (1.02–14.43)	6.24	0.13 (0–2.15)	0.44	0.02 (0–0.17)	0.05
72 (n = 22)	3.19 (1.28–13.94)	4.63	0.16 (0–2.42)	0.38	0.3 (0–0.25)	0.05
96 (n = 21)	3.44 (1.37–16.56)	5.33	0.23) (0–3.95)	0.45	0.05 (0–0.37)	0.07
120 (n = 17)	3.46 (1.27–15.00)	4.98	0.25 (0–2.89)	0.44	0.05 (0–0.21)	0.07

Reproduced with permission from Ref. 3.

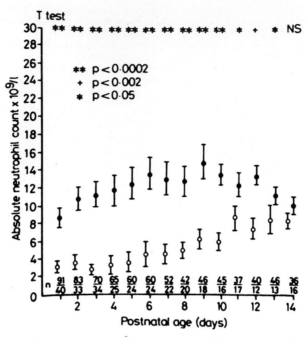

Fig. 1 Neutrophil count (×10⁹/l, bar indicates ±1 SD) during the first 14 days of life in babies of appropriate weight for gestational age (●) and those who were small for gestational age (○). Reproduced with permission from Ref. 4.

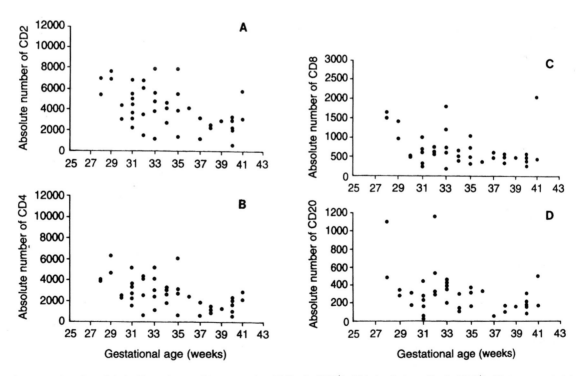

Fig. 2 Lymphocyte numbers (per μl) in healthy preterm and term neonates. (A) T cells (CD2⁺); (B) helper/inducer T cells (CD4⁺); (C) suppressor/cytotoxic T cells (CD8⁺); (D) B cells (CD20⁺). Reproduced with permission from Ref 5.

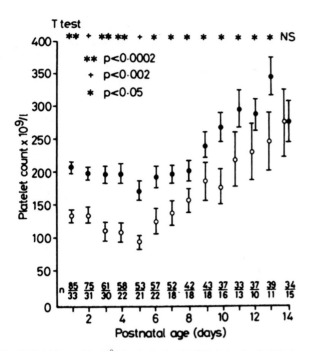

T test

** p<0.0002
+ p<0.002
* p<0.05

Fig. 3 Platelet count (× 10⁹/l, bar indicates ±1 SD) during the first 14 days of life in babies of appropriate weight for gestational age (●) and babies who were small for gestational age (○). Reproduced with permission from Ref. 4.

Table 5 Coagulation data (mean and 95% range) in 52 infants of 24–29 weeks' gestational age.

Birth weight (g)	992 (623–1489)
PT (s)	14.5 (11.7–21.6)
Adult mean PT (s)	11.6–12.1
PT ratio	1.2 (1–1.9)
APTT (s)	69.5 (40.6–101*)
Adult mean APTT (s)	30.5–32.5
APTT ratio	2.2 (1.3–3.3)
Fibrinogen (g/l)	1.35 (0.62–4.21)

PT = prothrombin time; APTT = activated partial thromboplastin time.
*6 values of >100 s recorded as 101 s.
Summarized from Ref. 6.

Table 6 Reference values for coagulation tests in healthy premature infants (30–36 weeks' gestation) during the first 6 months of life.

	Day 1		Day 5		Day 30		Day 90		Day 180		Adult	
	M	B	M	B	M	B	M	B	M	B	M	B
PT (s)	13.0	(10.6–16.2)**	12.5	(10.0–15.3)**¹	11.8	(10.0–13.6)**	12.3	(10.0–14.6)**	12.5	(10.0–15.0)**	12.4	(10.8–13.9)
APTT (s)	53.6	(27.5–79.4)⁺	50.5	(26.9–74.1)⁺	44.7	(26.9–62.5)	39.5	(28.3–50.7)	37.5	(21.7–53.3)**	33.5	(26.6–40.3)
TCT (s)	24.8	(19.2–30.4)**	24.1	(18.8–29.4)**	24.4	(18.8–29.9)**	25.1	(19.4–30.8)**	25.2	(18.9–31.5)**	25.0	(19.7–30.3)
Fibrinogen (g/l)	2.43	(1.50–3.73)**¹⁺	2.80	(1.60–4.18)**¹⁺	2.54	(1.50–4.14)**¹	2.46	(1.50–3.52)**¹	2.28	(1.50–3.60)¹	2.78	(1.56–4.00)
II (unit/ml)	0.45	(0.20–0.77)¹	0.57	(0.29–0.85)⁺	0.57	(0.36–0.95)¹⁺	0.68	(0.30–1.06)	0.87	(0.51–1.23)	1.08	(0.70–1.46)
V (unit/ml)	0.88	(0.41–1.44)**¹⁺	1.00	(0.46–1.54)	1.02	(0.48–1.56)	0.99	(0.59–1.39)	1.02	(0.58–1.46)	1.06	(0.62–1.50)
VII (unit/ml)	0.67	(0.21–1.13)	0.84	(0.30–1.38)	0.83	(0.21–1.45)	0.87	(0.31–1.43)	0.99	(0.47–1.51)**	1.05	(0.67–1.43)
VIII (unit/ml)	1.11	(0.50–2.13)**¹	1.15	(0.53–2.05)**¹⁺	1.11	(0.50–1.99)**¹⁺	1.06	(0.58–1.88)**¹⁺	0.99	(0.50–1.87)**¹⁺	0.99	(0.50–1.49)
VWF (unit/ml)	1.36	(0.78–2.10)¹	1.33	(0.72–2.19)¹	1.36	(0.66–2.16)¹	1.12	(0.75–1.84)**¹	0.98	(0.54–1.58)¹	0.92	(0.50–1.58)
IX (unit/ml)	0.35	(0.19–0.65)¹⁺	0.42	(0.14–0.74)¹⁺	0.44	(0.13–0.80)¹	0.59	(0.25–0.93)	0.81	(0.50–1.20)¹	1.09	(0.55–1.63)
X (unit/ml)	0.41	(0.11–0.71)	0.51	(0.19–0.83)	0.56	(0.20–0.92)	0.67	(0.35–0.99)	0.77	(0.35–1.19)	1.06	(0.70–1.52)
XI (unit/ml)	0.30	(0.08–0.52)¹	0.41	(0.13–0.69)⁺	0.43	(0.15–0.71)⁺	0.59	(0.25–0.93)⁺	0.78	(0.46–1.10)	0.97	(0.67–1.27)
XII (unit/ml)	0.38	(0.10–0.66)⁺	0.39	(0.09–0.69)⁺	0.43	(0.11–0.75)	0.61	(0.15–1.07)	0.82	(0.22–1.42)	1.08	(0.52–1.64)
PK (unit/ml)	0.33	(0.09–0.57)	0.45	(0.28–0.75)¹	0.59	(0.31–0.87)	0.79	(0.37–1.21)	0.78	(0.40–1.16)	1.12	(0.62–1.62)
HMWK (unit/ml)	0.49	(0.09–0.89)	0.62	(0.24–1.00)⁺	0.64	(0.16–1.12)⁺	0.78	(0.32–1.24)	0.83	(0.41–1.25)**	0.92	(0.50–1.36)
XIIIa (unit/ml)	0.70	(0.32–1.08)	1.01	(0.57–1.45)**	0.99	(0.51–1.47)**	1.13	(0.71–1.55)**	1.13	(0.65–1.61)**	1.05	(0.55–1.55)
XIIIb (unit/ml)	0.81	(0.35–1.27)	1.10	(0.68–1.58)**	1.07	(0.57–1.57)**	1.21	(0.75–1.67)	1.15	(0.67–1.63)	0.97	(0.57–1.37)
Plasminogen (CTA, unit/ml)	1.70	(1.12–2.48)¹⁺	1.91	(1.21–2.61)⁺	1.81	(1.09–2.53)	2.38	(1.58–3.18)	2.75	(1.91–3.59)⁺	3.36	(2.48–4.24)

All values are given as a mean (M) followed by lower and upper boundaries (B) encompassing 95% of the population. All factors except fibrinogen and plasminogen are expressed as unit/ml where pooled plasma contains 1.0 unit/ml. Plasminogen units are those recommended by the Committee on Thrombolytic Agents (CTA). Between 40 and 96 samples were assayed for each value for newborns.
**Values indistinguishable from those of adults.
¹Measurements are skewed owing to a disproportionate number of high values. Lower limit which excludes the lower 2.5% of the population is given (B).
⁺Values different from those of full-term infants.
PT = prothrombin time; APTT = activated partial thromboplastin time; TCT = thrombin clotting time; VWF = von Willebrand Factor; PK = prekallikrein; HMWK = high molecular weight kininogen.
Reproduced with permission from Ref 7.

Table 7 Reference values for inhibitors of coagulation in healthy premature infants (30–36 weeks' gestation) during the first 6 months of life.

	Day 1 M	Day 1 B	Day 5 M	Day 5 B	Day 30 M	Day 30 B	Day 90 M	Day 90 B	Day 180 M	Day 180 B	Adult M	Adult B
ATIII (unit/ml)	0.38	(0.14–0.62)[+]	0.56	(0.30–0.82)**	0.59	(0.37–0.81)[+]	0.83	(0.45–1.21)[+]	0.90	(0.52–1.28)[+]	1.05	(0.79–1.31)
α_2-M (unit/ml)	1.10	(0.56–1.82)[1+]	1.25	(0.71–1.77)**	1.38	(0.72–2.04)	1.80	(1.20–2.66)[1]	2.09	(1.10–3.21)[1]	0.86	(0.52–1.20)
α_2-AP (unit/ml)	0.78	(0.40–1.16)	0.81	(0.49–1.13)**	0.89	(0.55–1.23)[+]	1.06	(0.64–1.48)**	1.15	(0.77–1.53)	1.02	(0.68–1.36)
C_1E-INH (unit/ml)	0.65	(0.31–0.99)	0.83	(0.45–1.21)	0.74	(0.40–1.24)[1+]	1.14	(0.60–1.68)**	1.40	(0.96–2.04)[1]	1.01	(0.71–1.31)
α_1-AT (unit/ml)	0.90	(0.36–1.44)**	0.94	(0.42–1.46)[+]	0.76	(0.38–1.12)[+]	0.81	(0.49–1.13)**[+]	0.82	(0.48–1.16)**	0.93	(0.55–1.31)
HCII (unit/ml)	0.32	(0.00–0.60)[+]	0.34	(0.00–0.69)**	0.43	(0.15–0.71)	0.61	(0.20–1.11)[1]	0.89	(0.45–1.40)**[1+]	0.96	(0.66–1.26)
Protein C (unit/ml)	0.28	(0.12–0.44)**	0.31	(0.11–0.51)**	0.37	(0.15–0.59)[+]	0.45	(0.23–0.67)[+]	0.57	(0.31–0.83)	0.96	(0.64–1.28)
Protein S (unit/ml)	0.26	(0.14–0.38)[+]	0.37	(0.13–0.61)**	0.56	(0.22–0.90)	0.76	(0.40–1.12)[+]	0.82	(0.44–1.20)	0.92	(0.60–1.24)

All values are expressed in unit/ml, where pooled plasma contains 1.0 unit/ml. All values are given as a mean (M) followed by lower and upper boundaries (B) encompassing 95% of the population. Between 40 and 75 samples were assayed for each value for newborns.
**Values indistinguishable from those of adults.
[1]Measurements are skewed owing to a disproportionate number of high values. Lower limit which excludes the lower 2.5% of the population is given (B).
[+]Values different from those of full-term infants.
ATIII = antithrombin III; α_2-M = α_2-macroglobulin; α_2-AP = α_2-antiplasmin; C_1E-INH = C_1 esterase inhibitor; α_1-AT = α_1-antitrypsin; HCII = heparin cofactor II.
Reproduced with permission from Ref. 7.

Table 8 Normal hemoglobin (Hb) and red blood cell (RBC) values in the first year of life.

Hb/RBC value	Age (months) 0.5 (n = 232)	1 (n = 240)	2 (n = 241)	4 (n = 52)	6 (n = 52)	9 (n = 56)	12 (n = 56)
Hb (g/dl) (mean)	16.6	13.9	11.2	12.2	12.6	12.7	12.7
−2 SD	13.4	10.7	9.4	10.3	11.1	11.4	11.3
Hct (mean)	0.53	0.44	0.35	0.38	0.36	0.36	0.37
−2 SD	41	33	28	32	31	32	33
RBC ($\times 10^{12}$/l) (mean)	4.9	4.3	3.7	4.3	4.7	4.7	4.7
−2 SD, +2 SD	3.9–5.9	3.3–5.3	3.1–4.3	3.5–5.1	3.9–5.5	4.0–5.3	4.1–5.3
MCH (pg) (mean)	33.6	32.5	30.4	28.6	26.8	27.3	26.8
−2 SD	30	29	27	25	24	25	24
MCV (fl) (mean)	105.3	101.3	94.8	86.7	76.3	77.7	77.7
−2 SD	88	91	84	76	68	70	71
MCHC (g/dl) (mean)	31.4	31.8	31.8	32.7	35.0	34.9	34.3
−2 SD	28.1	28.1	28.3	28.8	32.7	32.4	32.1

Values after the age of 2 months were obtained from an iron-supplemented group in whom iron deficiency was excluded. Counts performed on venous blood.
Reproduced with permission from Ref. 8.

Table 9 Hemoglobin (Hb, g/dl), hematocrit (Hct) and red blood cell (RBC, $\times 10^{12}$/l) counts in term African neonates.

		Number tested	Mean ±1 SD Hb	Hct	RBC
Day	1	304	15.6 ± 2.0	0.450 ± 0.065	4.00 ± 0.67
	3	261	15.5 ± 2.1	0.442 ± 0.062	3.91 ± 0.61
	7	249	14.2 ± 2.3	0.413 ± 0.063	3.67 ± 0.55
Week	2	233	13.1 ± 1.9	0.391 ± 0.043	3.45 ± 0.56
	3	145	11.7 ± 1.8	0.356 ± 0.050	3.27 ± 0.47
	4	117	10.6 ± 1.6	0.325 ± 0.044	3.01 ± 0.48

Values are lower than those reported in neonates from Europe and North America, and may be intrinsic to this group. Other variables (RBC indices, reticulocytes) do not differ from those in other populations studied. Hb measured as oxyhemoglobin, Hct by centrifuged microhematocrit and RBC by hemocytometry, using venous blood.
Summarized from Ref. 9.

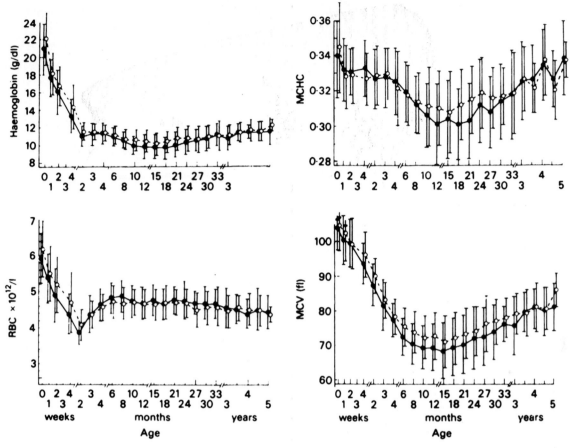

Fig. 4 Hemoglobin, MCHC, RBC and MCV values (mean ±1 SD) in Jamaican boys (●) and girls (○) aged from 1 day to 5 years. A cohort of 243 children was studied, although the data at each point are derived from varying numbers. Regular iron and folate supplements were not given. Both venous and skin puncture samples were used and counting was by a semi-automated method. Reproduced with permission from Ref. 10.

Table 10 Red cell values (3rd–97th centiles) derived from 2135 Irish school children.

Age (years)	Hb (g/dl)	RBC (×10¹²/l)	Hct	MCV (fl)	MCH (pg)	MCHC (g/dl)
Girls and boys						
4 + 5	11.0–13.6	3.93–4.99	0.32–0.40	75–87	25.4–29.6	32.9–35.7
6	11.1–13.8	3.93–4.98	0.32–0.40	76–87	25.6–30.7	32.9–35.6
7	11.3–14.2	3.98–5.05	0.33–0.41	75–87	25.4–30.7	33.2–35.7
8	11.5–14.2	4.00–5.11	0.33–0.41	77–89	26.3–31.7	33.1–36.4
9	11.9–14.5	4.08–5.04	0.34–0.41	76–89	26.2–31.2	33.3–35.8
10	11.9–14.5	4.12–5.06	0.34–0.42	77–90	26.5–30.9	33.2–35.7
11	12.1–14.5	4.13–5.19	0.35–0.42	78–89	25.9–31.2	33.1–35.7
12	12.1–14.7	4.16–5.17	0.35–0.43	77–90	26.3–30.9	32.7–35.7
Girls						
13 + 14	12.1–14.6	4.03–5.05	0.35–0.43	80–93	27.3–32.3	33.2–35.2
15–19	11.8–15.1	4.06–5.07	0.35–0.44	79–94	26.7–32.5	33.0–35.5
Boys						
13 + 14	12.4–15.6	4.33–5.42	0.36–0.45	79–91	26.9–31.8	33.4–35.4
15–18	13.2–16.6	4.46–5.61	0.38–0.49	79–92	26.9–31.9	33.5–35.2

Summarized from Ref. 11.

Table 11 Reticulocyte counts ($\times 10^9$/l) in the first year of life in term infants.

Age	Reticulocytes
1 day	110–450
7 days	10–80
1 month	10–65
2 months	35–200
5 months	15–110
12 months	30–130

Data from various sources, based on microscope and flow cytometric counts.

Table 12 Percentage of hemoglobin F in the first year of life.

Age	Number tested	Mean	2 SD	Range
1–7 days	10	74.7	5.4	61–79.6
2 weeks	13	74.9	5.7	66–88.5
1 month	11	60.2	6.3	45.7–67.3
2 months	10	45.6	10.1	29.4–60.8
3 months	10	26.6	14.5	14.8–55.9
4 months	10	17.7	6.1	9.4–28.5
5 months	10	10.4	6.7	2.3–22.4
6 months	15	6.5	3.0	2.7–13.0
8 months	11	5.1	3.6	2.3–11.9
10 months	10	2.1	0.7	1.5–3.5
12 months	10	2.6	1.5	1.3–5.0
1–14 years and adults	100	0.6	0.4	—

HbF measured by alkali denaturation.
Reproduced with permission from Ref. 12.

Table 13 Percentage of hemoglobin A_2 in the first 2 years of life.

Age (months)	A Number tested	Mean	SD	B Number tested	Mean	SD	Range
Birth	16	0.4	0.2				
1	6	0.8	0.3	5	0.8	0.4	0.4–1.3
2	7	1.3	0.7	9	1.3	0.5	0.4–1.9
3	8	1.7	0.3	8	2.2	0.6	1.0–3.0
4	9	2.1	0.3	3	2.4	0.4	2.0–2.8
5	8	2.3	0.2				
5–6				15	2.5	0.3	2.1–3.1
6	8	2.5	0.3				
7–8	6	2.5	0.4				
7–9				22	2.7	0.4	1.9–3.5
9–10	6	2.5	0.4				
10–12				14	2.7	0.4	2.0–3.3
12	5	2.5	0.3				
13–16				13	2.6	0.5	1.6–3.3
17–20				13	2.9	0.4	2.1–3.6
21–24				15	2.8	0.4	2.0–3.6

Data derived from 2 studies: A (Ref. 13) measured by microcolumn chromatography; B (Ref. 14) measured by elution following electrophoresis.

Table 14 Methemoglobin levels in children and adults.

Subjects	Methemoglobin (g/dl) Number	Mean	SD	Range	Methemoglobin (% of total Hb) Number	Mean	SD	Range
Prematures, birth–7 days	29	0.43	0.07	0.02–0.83	24	2.3	1.26	0.08–4.4
Prematures, 7–72 days	21	0.31	0.19	0.02–0.78	18	2.2	1.07	0.02–4.7
Newborns, 1–10 days	39	0.22	0.17	0–0.58	25	1.5	0.81	0–2.8
Infants, 1 month–1 year	8	0.14	0.09	0.02–0.29	8	1.2	0.78	0.17–2.4
Children, 1–14 years	35	0.11	0.09	0–0.33	35	0.79	0.62	0–2.4
Adults, 14–78 years	30	0.11	0.09	0–0.28	27	0.82	0.63	0–1.9

Summarized from Ref. 15.

Table 15 Comparison of enzyme activities and glutathione content in newborn and adult red blood cells.

Enzyme	Activity in normal adult RBC in IU/g Hb (mean ±1 SD at 37°C)	Mean activity in newborn RBC as percentage of mean (100%) activity in normal adult RBC
Aldolase	3.19 ± 0.86	140
Enolase	5.39 ± 0.83	250
Glucose phosphate isomerase	60.8 ± 11.0	162
Glucose-6-phosphate dehydrogenase	8.34 ± 1.59	174
WHO method	12.1 ± 2.09	
Glutathione peroxidase	30.82 ± 4.65	56
Glyceraldehyde phosphate dehydrogenase	226 ± 41.9	170
Hexokinase	1.78 ± 0.38	239
Lactate dehydrogenase	200 ± 26.5	132
NADH-methemoglobin reductase	19.2 ± 3.85 (at 30°C)	Increased
Phosphofructokinase	11.01 ± 2.33	97
Phosphoglycerate kinase	320 ± 36.1	165
Pyruvate kinase	15.0 ± 1.99	160
6-Phosphogluconate dehydrogenase	8.78 ± 0.78	150
Triose phosphate isomerase	211 ± 39.7	101
Glutathione	6570 ± 1040 nmol/g Hb	156

Percentage activity in newborn RBC compared to mean adult (100%) values is presented with quantitative data from studies on adult RBC. Newborn data from Ref. 16; quantitative date from Ref. 17. Reproduced with permission from Ref. 18.

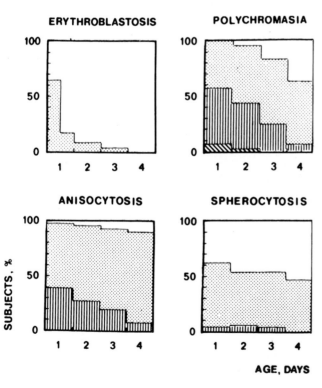

Fig. 5 RBC morphology in the first 4 days of life in 138 healthy term infants. Findings are graded from normal (white area) to mild, moderate and marked change (the last only in the case of polychromasia). Erythroblastosis: mild = 1-2 cells/10-15 fields; moderate = 1-5 cells/100 WBC. Polychromasia: mild = 1 cell in every or every other field; moderate = 1-3 cells/field; marked = >3 cells/field. Anisocytosis: mild = <5 cells/field differ in size from normal; moderate = the variation is more marked. Spherocytosis: mild = 1 spherocyte in every or every other field; moderate = on average >1 spherocyte/field. Reproduced with permission from Ref. 19.

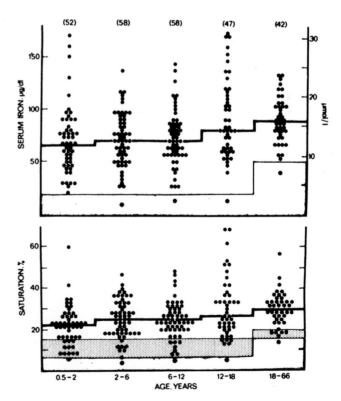

Fig. 6 Normal values for serum iron and transferrin saturation in individuals with normal levels of Hb, MCV, serum ferritin and free erythrocyte protoporphyrin. The heavy horizontal lines indicate the median values, the lower lines the lower limit of the 95% range, and the stippled area an intermediate zone of overlap between iron-deficient and normal subjects. Numbers of subjects are given in parentheses. Reproduced with permission from Ref. 20.

Table 16 Values of serum iron (SI), total iron-binding capacity (TIBC) and transferrin saturation (S%) from a group of 47 infants.

		Age (months)						
		0.5	1	2	4	6	9	12
SI (μmol/l)	Median	22	22	16	15	14	15	14
	(95% range)	11–36	10–31	3–29	3–29	5–24	6–24	6–28
(μg/dl)	Median	120	125	87	84	77	84	78
	(95% range)	(63–201)	(58–172)	(15–159)	(18–164)	(28–135)	(35–155)	(35–155)
TIBC (μmol/l)	Mean ± SD	34 ± 8	36 ± 8	44 ± 10	54 ± 7	58 ± 9	61 ± 7	64 ± 7
(μg/dl)	Mean ± SD	191 ± 43	199 ± 43	246 ± 55	300 ± 39	321 ± 51	341 ± 42	358 ± 38
S (%)	Median	68	63	34	27	23	25	23
	(95% range)	(30–99)	(35–94)	(21–63)	(7–53)	(10–43)	(10–39)	(10–47)

Not all infants were tested on each occasion, and those with Hb <11 g/dl, MCV <71 fl or serum ferritin <10 μg/l were excluded. Reproduced with permission from Ref. 21.

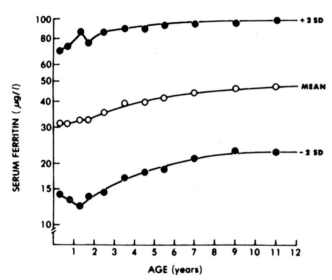

Fig. 7 Serum ferritin concentration (μg/l, mean ±2 SD) in 3819 children aged 6 months to 12 years. Subjects with low hematocrit and evidence of increased iron absorption were excluded. Mean values for boys and girls were similar in each age group and there was no significant difference between blacks, whites and American Indians in age-matched samples. Ferritin measured by a 2-site radioimmunometric assay. Reproduced with permission from Ref 22.

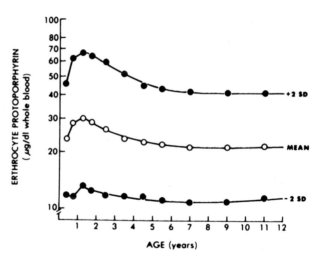

Fig. 8 Erythrocyte protoporphyrin concentration (μg/dl of whole blood, mean ±2 SD) measured in the same group of children as in Fig. 7. Mean values for boys and girls were similar in each age group and there was no significant difference between blacks, whites and American Indians in age-matched samples. Protoporphyrin measured as 'free' + zinc protoporphyrins. Reproduced with permission from Ref. 22.

Table 17 Zinc protoporphyrin values (μmol/mol heme, 95% range) in childhood.

Age	Number tested	Range
5 months	96	25–91
13 months	86	24–74
2–5 years	73	31–73
5–10 years	93	28–65
10–16 years	73	28–73

Data from the author's laboratory, obtained from children with no laboratory evidence of anemia or infection.

Table 18 Range of serum vitamin B$_{12}$ (pmol/l) and serum folate (nmol/l) levels in childhood.

| Age (years) | Vitamin B$_{12}$ | | Folate | |
	Male	Female	Male	Female
0–1	216–891	168–1117	16.3–50.8	14.3–51.5
2–3	195–897	307–892	5.7–34.0	3.9–35.6
4–6	181–795	231–1038	5.1–29.4	6.1–31.9
7–9	200–863	182–866	5.2–27.0	5.4–30.4
10–12	135–803	145–752	3.4–24.5	2.3–23.1
13–18	158–638	134–605	2.7–19.9	2.7–16.3

Measured by radioimmunoassay in 1486 children (vitamin B$_{12}$) and 1368 children (folate).
Summarized from Ref. 23.

Table 19 Red cell folate levels (μg/l, mean and range) in the first year of life.

Age	Term infants (n = 24)	Preterm infants (n = 20)
Birth	315 (100–960)	689 (88–1291)
2–3 months		164 (26–394)
3–4 months	283 (110–489)	
6–8 months	247 (100–466)	299 (139–558)
1 year	277 (74–995)	

Obtained by microbiologic assay.
Summarized from Refs 24 and 25.

Table 20 Range of erythropoietin values (mIU/ml) in childhood.

Age (years)	Male	Female
1–3	1.7–17.9	2.1–15.9
4–6	3.5–21.9	2.9–8.5
7–9	1.0–13.5	2.1–8.2
10–12	1.0–14.0	1.1–9.1
13–15	2.2–14.4	3.8–20.5
16–18	1.5–15.2	2.0–14.2

Measured by enzyme-linked immunosorbent assay (ELISA) in 1122 children.
Summarized from Ref. 26.

Table 21 Mean red cell, plasma and total blood volume (ml/kg) measurements in children.

Age	Red cell volume	Plasma volume	Total blood volume	Reference
Newborn	(43.4)	41.3	84.7	28
3 days	31**	51**	82**	29
	49^1	44^1	93^1	29
1–7 days	37.9	(39.8)	77.7	30
1 week–30 months	29.5	(48.5)	78.0	30
3 months–11 months	(32.7)	46.0	78.7	31
3 months–1 year	23.3	(45.4)	68.7	30
1–2 years	24.1	(43.6)	67.7	30
1–3 years	(34.9)	47.9	82.8	31
2–4 years	22.9	(40.0)	62.9	30
3–5 years	(36.0)	48.4	84.4	31
4–6 years	26.7	(42.9)	69.6	30
5–7 years	(34.9)	48.9	83.8	31
6–8 years	23.3	(42.8)	66.1	30
7–9 years	(35.9)	47.8	83.7	31
8–12 years	25.9	(40.8)	66.7	30
9–11 years	(38.0)	48.5	86.5	31
11–13 years	(37.4)	46.4	83.8	31

Data in parentheses calculated from the measured variables.
**No placental transfusion at birth.
^{1}Placental transfusion at birth.

Table 22 Red blood cell T$_{50}$ ^{51}Cr survival in term and premature infants.

	Number	Range (days)	Mean (days)
Term infants	10	17–25	22.8
	11	21–35	28.5
Premature infants	6	10–18	15.8
	6	9–20	15.2

Reproduced from Refs 32 and 33.

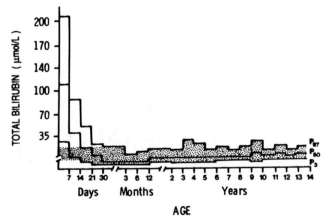

Fig. 9 Total bilirubin (μmol/l) measured in 2099 children. The 3rd, 50th and 97th percentiles and the adult normal range (stippled area) are shown. Reproduced with permission from Ref. 27.

Table 23 Serum haptoglobin (as hemoglobin-binding capacity in mg/dl) in term infants and children.

Age	Number tested	Mean	SD	Range
At delivery (cord blood)	21	0	0	0
1–7 days	24	10	11.7	0–41
1–4 weeks	23	28.2	15.7	0–45
1–3 months	8	59.4	16.9	41–95
3–6 months	13	91	21.1	64–134
6–12 months	17	114.9	33.5	43–160
1–5 years	28	108.7	25.5	51–160
5–10 years	37	107	25.5	62–186
Over 10 years	16	110	35.1	41–165

Measured as peroxidase activity of haptoglobin–hemoglobin complex. Summarized from Ref. 34.

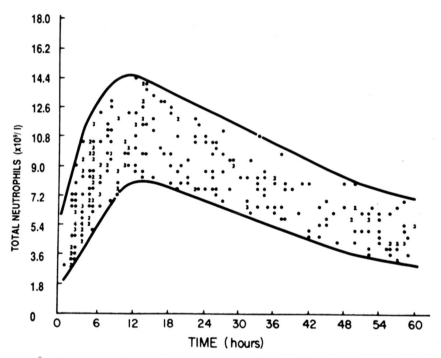

Fig. 10 Total neutrophil count ($\times 10^9$/l, including band cells and earlier forms) in the first 60 hours of life. Each dot represents a single value and numbers represent the number of values at the same point. Data based on automated leukocyte count and 100-cell differential. Reproduced with permission from Ref. 35.

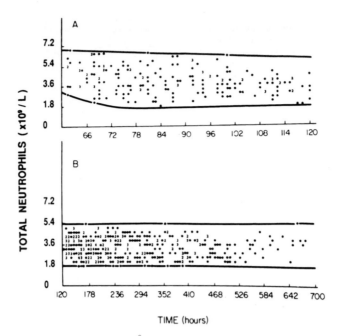

Fig. 11 Neutrophil count ($\times 10^9$/l) between (A) 60–120 hours and (B) 120 hours–28 days. Data obtained and expressed as in Fig. 10. Reproduced with permission from Ref. 35.

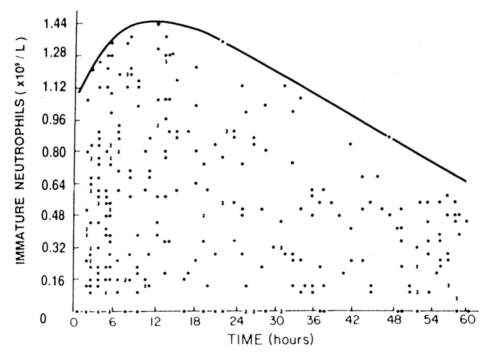

Fig. 12 Reference range for immature neutrophils ($\times 10^9$/l) in the first 60 hours of life. Data obtained and expressed as in Fig. 10. Reproduced with permission from Ref. 35.

Table 24 Normal values for lymphocytes, monocytes and eosinophils ($\times 10^9$/l) from birth to 28 days of age based on a study of 393 infants.

Cell	Percentile	Age (hours)		
		0–60	61–120	121–720
Lymphocytes	95	7.26	6.62	9.13
	50	4.19	8.66	5.62
	5	2.02	1.92	2.86
Monocytes	95	1.91	1.74	1.72
	50	0.6	0.53	0.67
	5	0	0	0.10
Eosinophils	95	0.84	0.81	0.84
	50	0.14	0.18	0.24
	5	0	0	0

Data based on 100-cell differential count.
Reproduced with permission from Ref. 36.

Table 25 Mean and range of values for neutrophils, band forms and lymphocytes ($\times 10^9$/l) in African neonates.

	Day 1	Day 7	Day 28
Neutrophils	5.67 (0.98–12.9)	2.01 (0.57–6.5)	1.67 (0.65–3.2)
Band forms	1.16 (0.16–2.3)	0.55 (0–1.5)	0.36 (0–0.39)
Lymphocytes	5.10 (1.4–8.0)	5.63 (2.2–15.5)	6.55 (3.2–9.9)

Data based on 100-cell differential count.
Summarized from Ref. 37.

Table 26 Normal limits of the immature:total and immature:segmented granulocyte ratios in healthy neonates.

	Day 1	Day 7	Day 28	Ref.
Immature:total	0.16	0.12	0.12	35
Immature:total (African)	0.22	0.21	0.18	37
Immature:segmented	0.3 (neonatal period)			38

Table 27 Total and differential white cell count ($\times 10^9$/l, mean and 95% range) from a cohort of children tested at 2, 5 and 13 months of age.

	Age (months)		
	2 (n = 100)	5 (n = 96)	13 (n = 86)
Total WBC	8.9 (5.1–15.3)	10.0 (5.9–17.0)	9.7 (5.8–16.2)
Neutrophils	1.8 (0.7–4.8)	2.5 (1.1–5.8)	2.7 (1.0–7.7)
Lymphocytes	5.8 (3.3–10.3)	6.2 (3.3–11.5)	6.0 (3.4–10.5)
Monocytes	0.7 (0.4–1.2)	0.56 (0.25–1.27)	0.5 (0.2–0.92)
Eosinophils	0.3 (0.09–0.8)	0.32 (0.1–1.1)	0.2 (0.05–0.9)
Basophils	0.05 (0.02–0.13)	0.07 (0.02–0.2)	0.06 (0.02–0.13)

Data from the author's laboratory obtained by automated differential counting.

Table 28 Differential leukocyte values ($\times 10^9$/l) in children 1–16 years old.

	Age in years															
	1	2	3	4	5	6	7	8	9	10	11	12	13	14	15	16
Neutrophils	1.5–6.9			1.8–7.7		1.5–5.9									1.7–5.7	
Lymphocytes	2.6–9.3	2.3–8.4	1.8–6.0		1.7–4.6		1.5–4.1									
Monocytes	0.15–1.28															
Eosinophils	0.06–0.62	0.04–1.19		0.09–1.04		0.08–1.01				0.04–0.76						
Basophils	0.02–0.12															

Data obtained by automated differential counting.
Summarized from Ref. 39.

Table 29 Numbers ($\times 10^9$/l, mean $\pm$ 1 SD) of T cell (CD3), helper/inducer T cell (CD4), suppressor/cytotoxic T cell (CD8) and B cell (CD20) lymphocytes in peripheral blood.

Age	Number	CD3	CD4	CD8	CD20
1–3 days	18	4.36 ± 1.22	3.31 ± 1.01	1.31 ± 0.46	1.01 ± 0.46
<6 months	23	3.64 ± 1.66	2.38 ± 0.87	1.07 ± 0.52	2.04 ± 0.89
>6–12 months	15	3.52 ± 0.99	2.31 ± 0.67	1.14 ± 0.36	1.79 ± 0.63
1–2 years	20	3.39 ± 1.11	1.88 ± 0.48	0.99 ± 0.19	1.59 ± 0.52
3–5 years	18	3.03 ± 0.92	1.51 ± 0.59	1.23 ± 0.42	1.02 ± 0.60
6–10 years	23	2.28 ± 0.91	1.08 ± 0.40	0.90 ± 0.40	0.50 ± 0.23
11–17 years (male)	23	2.12 ± 0.70	1.13 ± 0.45	0.88 ± 0.40	0.52 ± 0.23

Data obtained by flow cytometry.
Summarized from Ref. 40.

Table 30 Normal progenitor cell numbers during development.*

Age	PB BFU-E	BM BFU-E	BM CFU-E	PB CFU-GM	BM CFU-GM	PB CFU-Meg	BM CFU-Meg
Fetuses 18–20 weeks	75–1500			20–700		1–10	
Birth, term	40–100			10–200		5–20	
Adults	5–40	10–150	25–150	5–20	15–100	2–10	1–30

*Data are approximate ranges derived from various sources, and indicate numbers of progenitor cells per 10^5 mononuclear cells plated.
PB = peripheral blood; BM = bone marrow; BFU-E = erythroid burst-forming unit; CFU-E = erythroid colony-forming unit; CFU-GM = granulocyte-macrophage colony-forming unit; CFU-Meg = megakaryocyte colony-forming unit.
Reproduced with permission from Ref. 41.

Table 31 Reference values for coagulation tests in the healthy full-term infant during the first 6 months of life.

Tests	Day 1 (n)	Day 5 (n)	Day 30 (n)	Day 90 (n)	Day 180 (n)	Adult (n)
PT (s)	13.0 ± 1.43(61)**	12.4 ± 1.46(77)**[1]	11.8 ± 1.25(67)**[1]	11.9 ± 1.15(62)**	12.3 ± 0.79(47)**	12.4 ± 0.78(29)
APTT (s)	42.9 ± 5.80(61)	42.6 ± 8.62(76)	40.4 ± 7.42(67)	37.1 ± 6.52(62)**	35.5 ± 3.71(47)**	33.5 ± 3.44(29)
TCT (s)	23.5 ± 2.38(58)**	23.1 ± 3.07(64)[1]	24.3 ± 2.44(53)**	25.1 ± 2.32(52)**	25.5 ± 2.86(41)**	25.0 ± 2.66(19)
Fibrinogen (g/l)	2.83 ± 0.58(61)**	3.12 ± 0.75(77)**	2.70 ± 0.54(67)**	2.43 ± 0.68(60)**[1]	2.51 ± 0.68(47)**[1]	2.78 ± 0.61(29)
II (unit/ml)	0.48 ± 0.11(61)	0.63 ± 0.15(76)	0.68 ± 0.17(67)	0.75 ± 0.15(62)	0.88 ± 0.14(47)	1.08 ± 0.19(29)
V (unit/ml)	0.72 ± 0.18(61)	0.95 ± 0.25(76)	0.98 ± 0.18(67)	0.90 ± 0.21(62)	0.91 ± 0.18(47)	1.06 ± 0.22(29)
VII (unit/ml)	0.66 ± 0.19(60)	0.89 ± 0.27(75)	0.90 ± 0.24(67)	0.91 ± 0.26(62)	0.87 ± 0.20(47)	1.05 ± 0.19(29)
VIII (unit/ml)	1.00 ± 0.39(60)**[1]	0.88 ± 0.33(75)**[1]	0.91 ± 0.33(67)**[1]	0.79 ± 0.23(62)**[1]	0.73 ± 0.18(47)[1]	0.99 ± 0.25(29)
VWF (unit/ml)	1.53 ± 0.67(40)[1]	1.40 ± 0.57(43)	1.28 ± 0.59(40)[1]	1.18 ± 0.44(40)[1]	1.07 ± 0.45(46)[1]	0.92 ± 0.33(29)[1]
IX (unit/ml)	0.53 ± 0.19(59)	0.53 ± 0.19(75)	0.51 ± 0.15(67)	0.67 ± 0.23(62)	0.86 ± 0.25(47)	1.09 ± 0.27(29)
X (unit/ml)	0.40 ± 0.14(60)	0.49 ± 0.15(76)	0.59 ± 0.14(67)	0.71 ± 0.18(62)	0.78 ± 0.20(47)	1.06 ± 0.23(29)
XI (unit/ml)	0.38 ± 0.14(60)	0.55 ± 0.16(74)	0.53 ± 0.13(67)	0.69 ± 0.14(62)	0.86 ± 0.24(47)	0.97 ± 0.15(29)
XII (unit/ml)	0.53 ± 0.20(60)	0.47 ± 0.18(75)	0.49 ± 0.16(67)	0.67 ± 0.21(62)	0.77 ± 0.19(47)	1.08 ± 0.28(29)
PK (unit/ml)	0.37 ± 0.16(45)[1]	0.48 ± 0.14(51)	0.57 ± 0.17(48)	0.73 ± 0.16(46)	0.86 ± 0.15(43)	1.12 ± 0.25(29)
HMWK (unit/ml)	0.54 ± 0.24(47)	0.74 ± 0.28(63)	0.77 ± 0.22(50)**	0.82 ± 0.32(46)**	0.82 ± 0.32(48)**	0.92 ± 0.22(29)
XIIIa (unit/ml)	0.79 ± 0.26(44)	0.94 ± 0.25(49)**	0.93 ± 0.27(44)**	1.04 ± 0.34(44)**	1.04 ± 0.29(41)**	1.05 ± 0.25(29)
XIIIb (unit/ml)	0.76 ± 0.23(44)	1.06 ± 0.37(47)**	1.11 ± 0.36(45)**	1.16 ± 0.34(44)**	1.10 ± 0.30(41)**	0.97 ± 0.20(29)
Plasminogen (CTA, unit/ml)	1.95 ± 0.35(44)	2.17 ± 0.38(60)	1.98 ± 0.36(52)	2.48 ± 0.37(44)	3.01 ± 0.40(47)	3.36 ± 0.44(29)

All values expressed as mean ±1 SD. All factors except fibrinogen and plasminogen are expressed as unit/ml where pooled plasma contains 1.0 units/ml. Plasminogen units are those recommended by the Committee on Thrombolytic Agents (CTA). n = number studied.
**Values that do not differ statistically from adult values.
[1]These measurements are skewed because of a disproportionate number of high values.
PT = prothrombin time; APTT = activated partial thromboplastin time; TCT = thrombin clotting time; VWF = von Willebrand factor; PK = prekallikrein; HMWK = high molecular weight kininogen.
Note: Longer APTT and TCT values may be obtained in newborns and infants using reagent combinations other than those used in this study.
Reproduced with permission from Ref. 42.

Table 32 Reference values for the inhibitors of coagulation in the healthy full-term infant during the first 6 months of life.

Inhibitors	Day 1 (n)	Day 5 (n)	Day 30 (n)	Day 90 (n)	Day 180 (n)	Adult (n)
ATIII (unit/ml)	0.63 ± 0.12(58)	0.67 ± 0.13(74)	0.78 ± 0.15(66)	0.97 ± 0.12(60)**	1.04 ± 0.10(56)**	1.05 ± 0.13(28)
α_2-M (unit/ml)	1.39 ± 0.22(54)	1.48 ± 0.25(73)	1.50 ± 0.22(61)	1.76 ± 0.25(55)	1.91 ± 0.21(55)	0.86 ± 0.17(29)
α_2-AP (unit/ml)	0.85 ± 0.15(55)	1.00 ± 0.15(75)**	1.00 ± 0.12(62)**	1.08 ± 0.16(55)**	1.11 ± 0.14(53)**	1.02 ± 0.17(29)
C_1E-INH (unit/ml)	0.72 ± 0.18(59)	0.90 ± 0.15(76)**	0.89 ± 0.21(63)	1.15 ± 0.22(55)	1.41 ± 0.26(55)	1.01 ± 0.15(29)
α_1-AT (unit/ml)	0.93 ± 0.22(57)**	0.89 ± 0.20(75)**	0.62 ± 0.13(61)	0.72 ± 0.15(56)	0.77 ± 0.15(55)	0.93 ± 0.19(29)
HCII (unit/ml)	0.43 ± 0.25(56)	0.48 ± 0.24(72)	0.47 ± 0.20(58)	0.72 ± 0.37(58)	1.20 ± 0.35(55)	0.96 ± 0.15(29)
Protein C (unit/ml)	0.35 ± 0.09(41)	0.42 ± 0.11(44)	0.43 ± 0.11(43)	0.54 ± 0.13(44)	0.59 ± 0.11(52)	0.96 ± 0.16(28)
Protein S (unit/ml)	0.36 ± 0.12(40)	0.50 ± 0.14(48)	0.63 ± 0.15(41)	0.86 ± 0.16(46)**	0.87 ± 0.16(49)**	0.92 ± 0.16(29)

All values expressed in unit/ml as mean ±1 SD. n = number studied.
**Values indistinguishable from those of adults.
ATIII = antithrombin III; α_2-M = α_2-macroglobulin; α_2-AP = α_2-antiplasmin; C_1E-INH = C_1 esterase inhibitor; α_1-AT = α_1-antitrypsin; HCII = heparin cofactor II.
Reproduced with permission from Ref 42.

Table 33 Concentrations of D-dimers in blood from 15 preterm infants and 45 born at full term.

Concentration of D-dimers (mg/l)	Number (%) of infants		
	Full term (n = 45)	Preterm (n = 15)	Total (n = 60)
<0.25	24 (53)	7 (47)	31 (52)
0.25–0.5	14 (31)	2 (13)	16 (27)
0.5–1	6 (13)	2 (13)	8 (13)
1–2	1 (2)	2 (13)	3 (5)
2–4	0	2 (13)	2 (3)

All D-dimer concentrations in the pregnant mothers were <0.25 mg/l.
Reproduced with permission from Ref. 43.

Table 34 Vitamin $K_{1(20)}$ levels (pg/ml) in formula- and breast-fed infants with (K^+) and without (K^-) vitamin $K_{1(20)}$ prophylaxis.

	1–4 days				29–35 days			
	Mean	Median	Number	<DL[a]	Mean	Median	Number	<DL[a*]
Breast-fed (K^-)	280	249	12	2	913	646	10	1
Breast-fed (K^+)	32 711	24 446	13	—	697	535	9	—
Formula-fed	1900	1515	5	2	2890	2827	6	—

*<DL[a] = below detection limit of 60 pg/ml.
Reproduced with permission from Ref. 44.

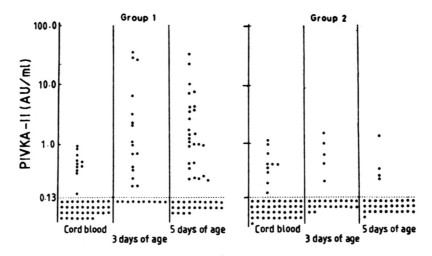

Fig. 13 Protein induced by vitamin K absence of antagonist-II (PIVKA-II) levels in cord blood and blood samples obtained at 3 or 5 days of age. Group 1 did not receive vitamin K and group 2 did. The dotted line indicates the lower limit of sensitivity of the assay. One arbitrary unit (AU) of PIVKA II corresponds to 1 μ of purified Factor II (prothrombin). Reproduced with permission from Ref. 45.

Table 35 Platelet count ($\times 10^9$/l) during childhood.

Age	Both sexes (n)	Girls (n)	Boys (n)
2 months	214–648 (119)		
5 months	210–560 (106)		
13 months	180–508 (101)		
1–3 years	207–558 (68)		
4–6 years		193–489 (118)	205–450 (159)
7–8 years		191–439 (155)	194–420 (202)
9–10 years		201–384 (182)	174–415 (258)
11–12 years		180–387 (206)	178–382 (274)
13–14 years		188–429 (129)	183–370 (157)
15–18 years		170–359 (151)	189–374 (116)

Data from the author's laboratory (2 months–3 years, 95% range) and Ref. 11 (3rd–97th centiles). Platelet counts are significantly lower at 5 months of age than at 2 months, and at 13 months than at 5 months (p < 0.001 for both). The fall in counts with age from 4 years is statistically significant, as are the overall higher values in girls than boys between 4 and 18 years (p < 0.0001 for both).

Table 36 Bleeding time (min) in newborns and children.

Subjects	Number	Sphygmomanometer pressure (mmHg)	Mean	Range
Term newborn	30	30	3.4	1.9–5.8
Preterm newborn:				
<1000 g	6	20	3.3	2.6–4.0
1000–2000 g	15	25	3.9	2.0–5.6
>2000 g	5	30	3.2	2.3–5.0
Children	17	30	3.4	1.0–5.5
Adults	20	30	2.8	0.5–5.5

Bleeding time performed using a template technique with incision 5 mm long and 0.5 mm deep. All subjects had normal platelet counts. Summarized from Ref. 46.

Table 37 Bleeding time (min) in children and adults.

Subjects	Number	Mean	SD	Range
Children	36	4.6	1.4	2.5–8.5
Adults	48	4.6	1.2	2.5–6.5

Bleeding time performed using a template technique with incision 6 mm long and 1 mm deep and sphygmomanometer pressure 40 mmHg.
Note: Using this technique, bleeding times up to 11.5 min have been observed in apparently healthy children tested in the author's laboratory.
Summarized from Ref. 47.

Table 38 Properties of cord blood platelets compared to mature platelets.

Parameter	Response compared to mature platelets	Ref.
Sensitive to ADP, collagen, epinephrine (adrenaline), thrombin	↓	48–50
Sensitivity to ristocetin	↑	49
Lag phase to collagen, ADP, thrombin	↑	48
Maximal aggregatory response	↓	48
Adhesives to glass fibers	↓	51
Content of ADP and ATP	↓	50
Release of ^{14}C-5 hydroxytryptamine	↓	49, 52
Lipid peroxidation	↓	53, 54
Availability of PF3	↓	51

Reproduced with permission from Ref. 18.

Table 39 Serum immunoglobulin levels in UK caucasians (−2 SD, meridian, +2 SD by log-Gaussian).

Age		IgG (g/l)	IgA (g/l)	IgM (g/l)
	Cord	10.8 (5.2–18.0)	<0.02	0.1 (0.02–0.2)
Weeks	0–2	9.4 (5.0–17.0)	0.02 (0.01–0.08)	0.1 (0.05–0.2)
	2–6	7.1 (3.9–13.0)	0.05 (0.02–0.15)	0.2 (0.08–0.4)
	6–12	3.9 (2.1–7.7)	0.15 (0.05–0.4)	0.4 (0.15–0.7)
Months	3–6	4.6 (2.4–8.8)	0.2 (0.1–0.5)	0.6 (0.2–1.0)
	6–9	5.2 (3.0–9.0)	0.3 (0.15–0.7)	0.8 (0.4–1.6)
	9–12	5.8 (3.0–10.9)	0.4 (0.2–0.7)	1.2 (0.6–2.1)
Years	1–2	6.4 (3.1–13.8)	0.7 (0.3–1.2)	1.3 (0.5–2.2)
	2–3	7.0 (3.7–15.8)	0.8 (0.3–1.3)	1.3 (0.5–2.2)
	3–6	9.9 (4.9–16.1)	1.0 (0.4–2.0)	1.3 (0.5–2.0)
	6–9	9.9 (5.4–16.1)	1.3 (0.5–2.4)	1.2 (0.5–1.8)
	9–12	9.9 (5.4–16.1)	1.4 (0.7–2.5)	1.1 (0.5–1.8)
	12–15	9.9 (5.4–16.1)	1.9 (0.8–2.8)	1.2 (0.5–1.9)
	15–45	9.9 (5.4–16.1)	1.9 (0.8–2.8)	1.2 (0.5–1.9)
	>45	9.9 (5.3–16.5)	1.9 (0.8–4.0)	1.2 (0.5–2.0)

Determined in 53 males and 54 females above 15 years and in groups of at least 30 subjects for the other age groups.
Reproduced with permission from Ref. 55.

Table 40 Mean and 5th–95th centile ranges (g/l) for IgG subclasses at various ages.

Age	IgG$_1$	IgG$_2$	IgG$_3$	IgG$_4$
Cord blood	4.7	2.1	0.6	0.2
	(3.6–8.4)	(1.2–4.0)	(0.3–1.5)	<0.5
6 months	2.3	0.4	0.3	<0.1
	(1.5–3.0)	(0.3–0.5)	(0.1–0.6)	
2 years	3.5	1.1	0.4	<0.1
	(2.3–5.8)	(0.3–2.9)	(0.1–0.8)	
5 years	3.7	2.0	0.5	0.3
	(2.3–6.4)	(0.7–4.5)	(0.1–1.1)	(<0.1–0.8)
10 years	5.2	2.6	0.7	0.4
	(3.6–7.3)	(1.4–4.5)	(0.3–1.1)	(<0.1–1.0)
15 years	5.4	2.6	0.7	0.4
	(3.8–7.7)	(1.3–4.6)	(0.2–1.2)	(<0.1–1.1)
Adult	5.9	3.0	0.7	0.5
	(3.2–10.2)	(1.2–6.6)	(0.2–1.9)	(<0.1–1.3)

In adults IgG$_3$ levels are higher in females than in males, and IgG$_4$ higher in males than females. No sex difference is seen before the age of 15 years.
Reproduced with permission from Ref. 55.

Table 41 Serum IgD levels (g/l).

Number	Age	IgD
23	6 weeks–19 months	<0.01–0.016
105	3–14 years	<0.01–0.036

Reproduced from Ref. 56.

Table 42 Total serum IgE levels.*

Age	Median	95th centile
Newborn	0.5	5
3 months	3	11
1 year	8	29
5 years	15	52
10 years	18	63
Adult	26	120

*Data expressed in units in relation to the first British Standard for human serum IgE 75/502.
Reproduced with permission from Ref. 55.

Table 43 Erythrocyte sedimentation rate (mm/h) in healthy children.

Method	Number	Age (years)	Mean	Range	% >20 mm/h
Wintrobe	245	4–11	12.0	1–41	9
	169	12–15	7.5	<1–34	7
Westergren	78	4–7	13	<1–55	
(read at 45 min)	153	8–14	10.5	1–62	

Summarized from Refs 57–59.

Table 44 Isohemagglutinin titer in relation to age.

Age	Mean (range)
Cord blood	0*
1–3 months	1:5[+] (0–1:10)
4–6 months	1:10[+] (0–1:160)
7–12 months	1:80** (0–1:640)
13–24 months	1:80** (0–1:640)
25–36 months	1:160[1] (1:10–1:640)
3–5 years	1:80 (1:5–1:640)
6–8 years	1:80 (1:5–1:640)
9–11 years	1:160 (1:20–1:640)
12–16 years	1:160 (1:10–1:320)
Adult	1:160 (1:10–1:640)

*Isohemagglutinin (IHA) activity is rarely detectable in cord blood.
[+]50% of normal infants will not have IHA at this age.
**10% of normal infants will not have IHA at this age.
[1]Beyond this age all normal individuals have IHA with the exception of those of blood group AB.
Summarized from Ref. 60.

REFERENCES

1. Zaisov R, Matoth Y. Red cell values on the first postnatal day during the last 16 weeks of gestation. *Am J Hematol* 1976; **1**: 272–278
2. Lundstrom U, Siimes MA, Dallman PR. At what age does iron supplementation become necessary in low-birth-weight infants? *J Pediatr* 1977; **91**: 878–883
3. Lloyd BW, Oto A. Normal values for mature and immature neutrophils in very preterm babies. *Arch Dis Child* 1982; **57**: 233–235
4. McIntosh N, Kempson C, Tyler RM. Blood counts in extremely low birthweight infants. *Arch Dis Child* 1988; **63**: 74–76
5. Sériès IM, Pichette J, Carrier C *et al*. Quantitative analysis of T and B cell subsets in healthy and sick premature infants. *Early Hum Dev* 1991; **26**: 143–154
6. Seguin JH, Topper WH. Coagulation studies in very low-birth-weight infants. *Am J Perinatol* 1994; **11**: 27–29
7. Andrew M, Paes B, Milner R *et al*. Development of the coagulation system in the healthy premature infant. *Blood* 1988; **72**: 1651–1657
8. Saarinen UM, Siimes MA. Developmental changes in red blood cell counts and indices of infants after exclusion of iron deficiency by laboratory criteria and continuous iron supplementation. *J Pediatr* 1978; **92**: 412–416
9. Scott-Emuakpor AB, Okola AA, Omene JA, Ukpe SI. Normal haematological values of the African neonate. *Blut* 1985; **51**: 11–18
10. Serjeant GR, Grandison Y, Mason K, Serjeant B, Sewell A, Vaidya S. Haematological indices in normal Negro children: a

Jamaican cohort from birth to five years. *Clin Lab Haematol* 1980; **2**: 169–178

11. Taylor MRH, Holland CV, Spencer R, Jackson JF, O'Connor GI, O'Donnell JR. Haematological reference ranges for schoolchildren. *Clin Lab Haematol* 1997; **19**: 1–15

12. Schröter W, Natz C. Diagnostic significance of hemoglobin F and A$_2$ levels in homo- and heterozygous β-thalassaemia during infancy. *Helv Paediatr Acta* 1981; **36**: 519–525

13. Galanello R, Melis MA, Ruggeri R, Cao A. Prospective study of red blood cell indices, hemoglobin A$_2$ and hemoglobin F in infants heterozygous for β-thalassaemia. *J Pediatr* 1981; **99**: 105–108

14. Metaxotou-Mavromati AD, Antonopoulo HK, Laskari SS, Tsiarta HK, Ladis VA, Kattamis CA. Developmental charges in hemoglobin F levels during the first two years of life in normal and heterozygous β-thalassaemia infants. *Pediatrics* 1982; **69**: 734–738

15. Kravitz H, Elegant LD, Kaiser E, Kagan BM. Methemoglobin values in premature and mature infants and children. *Am J Dis Child* 1956; **91**: 1–5

16. Konrad PM, Valentine WM, Paglia DE. Enzymatic activities and glutathione content of erythrocytes in the newborn: comparison of red cells of older normal subjects and those with comparable reticulocytosis. *Acta Haematol* 1972; **48**: 193–201

17. Beutler E. *Red Cell Metabolism*, 3rd edn. New York: Grune and Stratton, 1984

18. Hinchliffe RF, Lilleyman JS (eds). *Practical Paediatric Haematology*. Chichester: John Wiley and Sons, 1987

19. Hovi LM, Siimes MA. Red blood cell morphology in healthy full-term newborns. *Acta Paediatr Scand* 1983; **72**: 135–136

20. Koerper MA, Dallman PR. Serum iron concentration and transferrin saturation in the diagnosis of iron deficiency in children: normal developmental changes. *J Pediatr* 1977; **91**: 870–874

21. Saarinen UM, Siimes MA. Developmental changes in serum iron, total iron-binding capacity, and transferrin saturation in infancy. *J Pediatr* 1977; **91**: 875–877

22. Deinard AS, Schwartz S, Yip R. Developmental changes in serum ferritin and erythrocyte protoporphyrin in normal (non-anemic) children. *Am J Clin Nutr* 1983; **38**: 71–76

23. Hicks JM, Cook J, Godwin ID, Soldin SJ. Vitamin B$_{12}$ and folate. Pediatric Reference Ranges. *Arch Pathol Lab Med* 1993; **117**: 704–706

24. Vanier TM, Tyas JF. Folic acid status in newborn infants during the first year of life. *Arch Dis Child* 1966; **41**: 658–665

25. Vanier TM, Tyas JF. Folic acid status in premature infants. *Arch Dis Child* 1967; **42**: 57–61

26. Krafte-Jacobs B, Williams J, Soldin SJ. Plasma erythropoietin reference ranges in children. *J Pediatr* 1995; **126**: 601–603

27. Gomez P, Coca L, Vargas C, Acebillo J, Martinex A. Normal reference-intervals for 20 biochemical variables in healthy infants, children and adolescents. *Clin Chem* 1984; **30**: 407–412

28. Mollison PL, Veall N, Cutbush M. Red cell and plasma volume in newborn infants. *Arch Dis Child* 1950; **25**: 242–253

29. Usher R, Shephard M, Lind J. The blood volume of the newborn infant and placental transfusion. *Acta Paediatr Scand* 1963; **52**: 497–512

30. Sukarochana K, Parenzan L, Thalardas N, Kiesewelter WB. Red cell mass determinations in infancy and childhood, with the use of radioactive chromium. *J Pediatr* 1961; **59**: 903–908

31. Russell SJM. Blood volume studies in health children. *Arch Dis Child* 1949; **24**: 88–98

32. Foconi S, Sjolin S. Survival of Cr-labelled red cells from newborn infants. *Acta Paediatr* 1959; **48 (Suppl 117)**: 18–23

33. Kaplan E, Hsu KS. Determination of erythrocyte survival in newborn infants by means of Cr-labelled erythrocytes. *Pediatrics* 1961; **27**: 354–361

34. Khalil M, Badr-El-Din MK, Kassem AS. Haptoglobin level in normal infants and children. *Alexandria Med J* 1967; **13**: 1–9

35. Manroe BL, Weinberg AG, Rosenfeld CR, Browne R. The neonatal blood count in health and disease. 1: Reference values for neutrophilic cells. *J Pediatr* 1979; **95**: 89–98

36. Weinberg AG, Rosenfeld CR, Manroe BL, Browne R. Neonatal blood cell count in health and disease. II: Values for lymphocytes, monocytes, and eosinophils. *J Pediatr* 1985; **106**: 462–466

37. Scott-Emuakpor AB, Okolo AA, Omene JA, Ukpe SI. Pattern of leukocytes in blood of healthy African neonates. *Acta Haematol* 1985; **74**: 104–107

38. Zipursky A, Jaber HM. The haematology of bacterial infection in newborn infants. *Clin Haematol* 1978; **7**: 175–193

39. Cranendonk E, van Gennip AH, Abeling NGGM, Behrendt H, Hast AAM. Reference values for automated cytochemical differential count of leukocytes in children 0–16 years old: comparison with manually obtained counts from Wright-stained smears. *J Clin Chem Clin Biochem* 1985; **23**: 663–667

40. Panaro A, Amati A, di Loreto M *et al.* Lymphocyte subpopulations in pediatric age. Definition of reference values by flow cytometry. *Allergol Immunopathol* 1991; **19**: 109–112

41. Auerbach AD, Alter BP. Prenatal and postnatal diagnosis of aplastic anaemia. In: Alter BP (ed) *Perinatal Haematology. Methods in Haematology 19*. Edinburgh: Churchill Livingstone, 1989

42. Andrew M, Paes B, Milner R *et al.* Development of the human coagulation system in the full-term infant. *Blood* 1987; **70**: 165–172

43. Hudson IRB, Gibson BES, Brownlie J, Holland BM, Turner TL, Webber RG. Increased concentrations of D-dimers in newborn infants. *Arch Dis Child* 1990; **65**: 383–384

44. Lambert W, De Leenheer A, Tassaneeyakul W, Widdershoven J. Study of vitamin K$_1$ (20) in the newborn by HPLC with wet-chemical post-column reduction and fluorescence detection. In: Suttie JW (ed) *Current Advances in Vitamin K Research*. New York: Elsevier, 1987

45. Motohara K, Endo F, Matsuda I. Effect of vitamin K administration on acarboxy prothrombin (PIVKA-II) levels in newborns. *Lancet* 1985; **ii**: 242–244

46. Feusner JH. Normal and abnormal bleeding times in neonates and young children using a fully standardised template technique. *Am J Clin Pathol* 1980; **74**: 73–77

47. Buchanan GR, Holtkamp CA. Prolonged bleeding time in children and young adults with hemophilia. *Pediatrics* 1980; **66**: 951–955

48. Mull MM, Hathaway WE. Altered platelet function in newborns. *Pediatr Res* 1970; **4**: 229–237

49. Ts'ao C-H, Green D, Schultz K. Function and ultrastructure of platelets of neonates: enhanced ristocetin aggregation of neonatal platelets. *Br J Haematol* 1976; **32**: 225–233

50. Corby DG, Zuck TF. Newborn platelet dysfunction: a storage pool defect. *Thromb Haemostas* 1976; **36**: 200–207

51. Hrodek O. Les Fonctions des plaquettes sanguines chez le nouveau-né. *Hemostase* 1964; **4**: 55–62

52. Whaun JM. The platelet of the newborn infant. *Thromb Diath Haemorr* 1973; **30**: 327–333

53. Stuart MJ. The neonatal platelet: evaluation of platelet malonyl dialdehyde formation as an indicator of prostaglandin synthesis. *Br J Haematol* 1978; **39**: 83–90

54. Stuart MJ, Elrad H, Graeber JE, Hakanson DO, Sunderji SG, Barvinchak MK. Increased synthesis of prostaglandin endoperoxides and platelet hyperfunction in infants of mothers with diabetes mellitus. *J Clin Lab Med* 1979; **94**: 12–17

55. Ward AM (ed). *Protein Reference Unit Handbook of Clinical Immunochemistry*, 2nd edn. Sheffield: PRU Publications, 1988

56. Buckley RH, Fiscus SA. Serum IgD and IgE concentrations in immunodeficiency diseases. *J Clin Invest* 1975; **55**: 157–165

57. Hollinger N, Robinson SJ. A study of the erythrocyte sedimentation rate for well children. *J Pediatr* 1953; **42**: 304–319

58. Osgood EE, Baker RL, Brownlee IE, Osgood MW, Ellis M, Cohen W. Total, differential and absolute leukocyte counts and sedimentation rates of healthy children four to seven years of age. *Am J Dis Child* 1939; **58**: 61–70

59. Osgood EE, Baker RL, Brownlee IE, Osgood MW, Ellis M, Cohen W. Total, differential and absolute leukocyte counts and sedimentation rates for healthy children. Standards for children eight to fourteen years of age. *Am J Dis Child* 1939; **58**: 282–294

60. Ellis EF, Robbins JB. In: Johnson TR, Moore WH (eds) Children are different: developmental physiology. Columbus, Ohio: Ross Laboratories, 1978

Marrow failure syndromes

Inherited bone marrow failure syndromes

MELVIN H FREEDMAN AND JOHN J DOYLE

In the context of this chapter, bone marrow failure is defined as decreased production of one or more of the major hematopoietic lineages on an inherited basis (Table 1.1). The term 'constitutional' is often used interchangeably with 'inherited' and similarly implies that a genetic abnormality accounts for bone marrow dysfunction, especially when it occurs in 2 or more members of the same family or is associated with congenital physical abnormalities. The designation 'congenital' has a looser connotation and refers to conditions that manifest early in life, often at birth, but regardless of their causation. Thus, congenital marrow failure is not necessarily inherited or constitutional and may be due to acquired factors such as viruses and environmental toxins.

Because hematopoiesis is an orderly but complex interplay of stem and progenitor cells, marrow stromal elements, and positive and negative cellular and humoral regulators, marrow failure can potentially occur at a number of critical points in the hematopoietic lineage pathways. For the inherited marrow disorders, the notion is advanced that genetic mutations interfere with hematopoiesis and account for the marrow failure, although the specific molecular basis is not known for any of these conditions. Acquired factors may also be operative and may interact with the putative genetic mutations to produce overt disease with varying clinical expression. Hence, the conditions shown in Table 1.1 can be transmitted as a simple Mendelian disorder determined primarily by a single mutant gene with inheritance patterns of autosomal dominant, autosomal recessive or X-linked types. Alternatively, some or all of these can be multifactorial disorders caused by an interaction of multiple genes and multiple exogenous or environmental determinants.

The incidence of inherited marrow failure disorders can be roughly approximated from careful clinical observations compiled at large centers. For example, data from the Children's Hospital Medical Center, Boston, and the Prince of Wales Hospital, Australia, show that these syndromes comprise 30–35% of cases of pediatric marrow failure and Fanconi's anemia represents about two-thirds of the total.[1,2]

Table 1.1 Inherited bone marrow failure syndromes.

Pancytopenia
  Fanconi's anemia
  Shwachman–Diamond syndrome
  Dyskeratosis congenita
  Amegakaryocytic thrombocytopenia
  Other genetic syndromes:
    Down's syndrome
    Dubowitz's syndrome
    Seckel's syndrome
    Reticular dysgenesis
    Familial aplastic anemia (non-Fanconi's)

Unilineage cytopenia
  Diamond–Blackfan anemia (see Chapter 3)
  Kostmann's syndrome/congenital neutropenia
  Thrombocytopenia with absent radii

PANCYTOPENIA

FANCONI'S (APLASTIC) ANEMIA

This classical marrow failure disorder is inherited in an autosomal recessive manner with a heterozygote frequency of about 1 in 200. It is remarkable for its diversity in phenotype and occurs in all racial and ethnic groups. Although the original report by Professor Fanconi described pancytopenia combined with physical anomalies in 3 brothers,[3] a summary of the large body of published information on > 700 cases over the ensuing 70 years has underscored the clinical variability of the condition.[4] At presentation patients may have:

- typical physical anomalies but normal hematology;
- normal physical features but abnormal hematology; or

• physical anomalies and abnormal hematology, the so-called classic phenotype that fits the original description.

There can also be sibling heterogeneity in presentation with discordance in clinical and hematological findings, even in affected monozygotic twins.

About 75% of patients are between 3 and 14 years of age at the time of diagnosis with a mean age of about 8 years in males and 9 years in females.[4] It is noteworthy that 4% are diagnosed in the first year of life and 10% at 16 years of age or older.

Clinical features

The presence of one or more characteristic congenital physical anomalies in the setting of bone marrow failure makes a tentative diagnosis of Fanconi's anemia straightforward (Fig. 1.1). However, it is important to note that patients with Fanconi's anemia may lack anomalies. The older historical terms 'Estren-Dameshek aplastic anemia'[5] and 'constitutional aplastic anemia type II'[6] referred to such patients. With the introduction of clastogenic stress-induced chromosomal breakage analysis as a confirmatory test for Fanconi's anemia, data from the International Fanconi's Anemia Registry (IFAR) showed that of 202 patients tested, 39% had aplastic anemia and anomalies, 30% had aplastic anemia without anomalies, 24% had anomalies only and 7% had neither.[7] Hence, the Estren-Dameshek cases that lack anomalies should not be considered as a separate entity but as part of the pleiotropic continuum of Fanconi's anemia.

Table 1.2 shows the characteristic physical abnormalities and their approximate frequency. The commonest anomaly is skin hyperpigmentation, a generalized brown melanin-like splattering, which is most prominent on the trunk, neck and intertriginous areas and which becomes more obvious with age. Café-au-lait spots are common alone or combined with

Table 1.2 Characteristic physical anomalies in Fanconi's anemia. Modified from data compiled by Young and Alter.[4]

Anomaly	Approximate frequency (%)
Skin pigmentary changes	65
Short stature	60
Upper limb abnormalities (thumbs, hands, radii, ulnae)	50
Hypogonadal and genitalia changes (mostly male)	40
Other skeletal findings (head/face, neck, spine)	30
Eye/lid/epicanthal fold anomalies	25
Renal malformations	25
Ear anomalies (external and internal), deafness	10
Hip, leg, foot, toe abnormalities	10
Gastrointestinal/cardiopulmonary malformations	10

the generalized hyperpigmentation, and sometimes with vitiligo or hypopigmentation. The skin pigmentation should not be confused with hemosiderosis-induced bronzing in transfusion-dependent patients who have not been adequately chelated.

The majority of patients are small and have short stature. Of 19 published cases who had growth hormone assays performed, 14 showed a deficiency, but only about one-half of those treated with growth hormone showed a growth response.[4]

Malformations involving the upper limbs are common, especially hypoplastic, supernumerary, bifid or absent thumbs. Hypoplastic or absent radii are always associated with hypoplastic or absent thumbs in contrast to the thrombocytopenia with absent radii (TAR) syndrome in which thumbs are always present. Less often, anomalies of the feet are seen, including toe syndactyly, short toes, a supernumerary toe, clubfoot and flat feet. Congenital hip dislocation and leg abnormalities are occasionally seen.

Males often have gonadal and genitalia abnormalities, including an underdeveloped or micropenis, undescended, atrophic or absent testes, hypospadias, phimosis and an abnormal urethra. Female patients occasionally have malformations or atresia of the vagina, uterus and ovary.

Many patients have a Fanconi 'facies' and unrelated patients can resemble each other almost as closely as siblings. The head and facial changes vary but commonly consist of microcephaly, small eyes, epicanthal folds, and abnormal shape, size or positioning of the ears. About 10% of Fanconi's patients are mentally retarded.

Renal anomalies occur but require imaging for documentation. Ectopic, pelvic or horseshoe kidneys are detected often as well as duplicated, hypoplastic, dysplastic or absent organs. Occasionally, hydronephrosis or hydroureter is present.

Auerbach et al[7] developed a scoring system for the probability of an accurate diagnosis of Fanconi's anemia using discriminating clinical and laboratory variables in patients enrolled in the IFAR whose diagnosis was confirmed by clastogenic stress-induced chromosomal breakage analysis (Table 1.3a). One point is added or subtracted for each

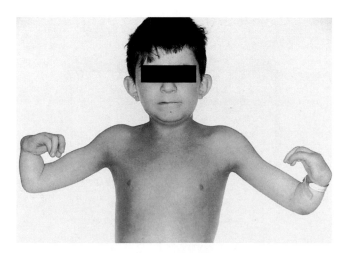

Fig. 1.1 Classical phenotype of Fanconi's anemia. Patient has pigmentary changes around the neck, shoulders and trunk, short stature, absent radii and thumbs bilaterally, microcephaly and low-set ears.

Table 1.3a Discriminating clinical and laboratory variables in Fanconi's anemia (FA). Modified from Auerbach et al.[7]

Variable	Frequency (%)			
	FA	Non-FA	Coefficient	Contribution
Growth retardation	60.9	24.1	0.70	38.47
Skin pigmentation	58.4	22.2	0.78	27.09
Kidney, urinary	35.1	9.3	0.71	17.56
Thumb, radius	51.0	21.3	0.85	15.24
Micro-ophthalmia	44.1	13.9	0.81	12.80
Learning disability	15.8	18.5	−0.66	11.62
Other skeletal anomaly	30.2	26.9	−0.57	8.47
Thrombocytopenia	80.2	61.1	0.73	7.43

Table 1.3b Probability of having Fanconi's anemia (FA) based on simplified score. Modified from Auerbach et al.[7]

Simplified score	Number		Probability
	FA (n)	Non-FA (n)	
−1	0	5	0.00
0	5	20	0.20
1	27	59	0.31
2	53	18	0.75
3	59	5	0.92
≥4	58	1	0.98
Total	202	108	

variable with a positive or negative coefficient, respectively. A patient with a score of 4+ or greater has a 98% probability of having Fanconi's anemia (Table 1.3b).

Hematologic features

A cardinal feature is the gradual onset of bone marrow failure with declining values in one or more hematopoietic lineages. Thrombocytopenia usually develops initially (see Chapter 21) with subsequent onset of granulocytopenia and then anemia. Severe aplasia eventually develops in most cases but the full expression of pancytopenia is variable and ensues over a period of months to years. The development of aplastic anemia can be accelerated by intercurrent infections or by drugs such as chloramphenicol. Within families, there is a tendency for the hematologic changes to occur at about the same age in affected siblings.[8] Data from 388 patients reported to the IFAR showed that 332 developed hematologic abnormalities at a median of 7 years (range: birth to 31 years).[9] The actuarial risk of developing hematologic abnormalities rose progressively with age and was 98% by 40 years.

The red blood cells are macrocytic with mean cell volumes often >100 fl even before the onset of significant anemia. Erythropoiesis is characterized by increased fetal hemoglobin (HbF) and increased expression of i antigen, but not necessarily both features in individual cells. The increased

HbF production is not clonal and has an heterogeneous distribution. Ferrokinetic studies indicate that most patients have an element of ineffective erythropoiesis as part of the marrow failure. Red blood cell life-span may be slightly shortened but this is a minor component, if any, of the anemia.

In the early stages of the disease, the bone marrow can show erythroid hyperplasia, sometimes with dyserythropoiesis and even megaloblastic-appearing cells. As the disease progresses, the marrow becomes hypocellular and fatty, but this is sometimes patchy, and shows a relative increase in lymphocytes, plasma cells, reticulum cells and mast cells. With full-blown marrow failure, the morphology on biopsy is identical to that seen in severe acquired aplastic anemia.

Chromosome breakage studies

A major finding is abnormal chromosome fragility; this is seen readily in metaphase preparations of peripheral blood lymphocytes cultured with phytohemagglutinin. The karyotype shows 'spontaneously' occurring chromatid breaks, rearrangements, gaps, endoreduplications and chromatid exchanges in cells from homozygous patients with Fanconi's anemia. Cultured skin fibroblasts also show the abnormal karyotype underscoring the constitutional basis for the disorder. The abnormal lymphocyte chromosome pattern, number of breaks/cell and variations in proportion of abnormal cells have no direct correlation with the hematologic or clinical course of individual patients.

'Spontaneous' chromosomal breaks are occasionally absent in true cases of homozygote Fanconi's anemia.[7] The clastogenic stress-induced chromosomal breakage analysis was introduced, in part, to circumvent this problem and to bring specificity to testing for Fanconi's anemia.[10] Chromosomal breakage is strikingly enhanced compared with controls if clastogenic agents such as diepoxybutane (DEB) are added to the cultures.[7,10] Indeed, homozygote Fanconi cells are hypersensitive to many oncogenic and mutagenic inducers, such as ionizing radiation, SV40 viral transformation, and alkylating and chemical agents including mitomycin C, cyclophosphamide, nitrogen mustard and platinum compounds.[4] For definitive diagnostic purposes, the IFAR has defined Fanconi's anemia as increased numbers of chromosome breaks/cell after exposure to DEB[7,11] with a mean of 8.96 (range: 1.3–23.9) compared to normal controls of 0.06 (range: 0–0.36).

The abnormal chromosome picture can be used to make a prenatal diagnosis of Fanconi's anemia.[11,12] Diagnostic testing can be performed on fetal amniotic fluid cells obtained at 16 weeks' gestation or on chorionic villus biopsy specimens at 9–12 weeks. A very high degree of prenatal diagnostic accuracy has been documented by looking at both spontaneous and DEB-induced breaks.[11,12]

Biologic and molecular aspects

A breakthrough in the search for the defective genes in Fanconi's anemia evolved from the important observation that hybrid cells formed from Fanconi's anemia and normal cells resulted in correction of the abnormal chromosome fragility, a process known as complementation.[13–17] It was further demonstrated that fusion of cells from several unrelated Fanconi's patients could also produce the corrective effect on chromosomal fragility by complementation.[15–17] Currently, 8 complementation groups and hence 8 separate genes (termed types A, B, C, D, E, F, G and H) have been distinguished on the basis of these somatic cell hybridization experiments,[14,18,19] with Fanconi's anemia type A (FA-A) accounting for over 65% of the cases analyzed.[20,21] A cDNA for the group C gene was identified in 1992 and localized to chromosome 9q22.3.[22] Using the same successful expression cloning method, a cDNA representing the group A gene on chromosome 16q24.3 has also been reported.[23] Even though the precise functions of the FA-C and FA-A proteins are unclear, complementation analysis suggests that they operate in concert with at least 6 additional proteins—the products from the other Fanconi genes. Although FA-D has not been cloned, genetic mapping localizes it to 3p22–26. The FA-A protein localizes primarily to the cell nucleus, whereas the FA-C gene product is located in both the nucleus and cytoplasm. All of the FA proteins may thus control or participate in a conceptually novel biochemical process which must play an important role in the various physiologic and cellular processes implicated in the Fanconi phenotype such as skeletal development, blood-cell formation and maintenance of genomic integrity. Cloning the remaining genes should help to elucidate this process at the molecular level.

A knock-out mouse model of FA-C has provided some insight into the role of this gene.[24] When mice were generated with targeted inactivation of the FA-C gene, the nullizygous genotype did not exhibit developmental abnormalities or gross hematologic defects for up to 9 months of age. Spleen cells from the knock-out mice had increased numbers of chromosomal aberrations in response to 2 agents that enhance fragility—mitomycin C and DEB. Homozygous male and female mice also had compromised gametogenesis and markedly impaired fertility, mimicking some of the features of the human disease. Although the mice did not exhibit gross hematologic defects, FA-C nullizygous mouse hematopoietic progenitors were markedly sensitive to γ-interferon, a cytokine implicated in growth arrest and apoptosis.

Further information regarding the importance of FA-C in hematopoiesis was provided by experiments in which normal human lymphocytes and bone marrow cells were exposed to an antisense oligodeoxynucleotide (ODN) complementary to bases -4 to $+14$ of FA-C mRNA.[25] The mitomycin C assay showed that the antisense ODN repressed FA-C gene expression in lymphocytes. Escalating doses of antisense ODN increasingly inhibited clonal growth of erythroid and granulocyte–macrophage progenitors, thereby demonstrating a seemingly important role for the gene in sustaining normal hematopoiesis.

A recent study[26] examined the phenotypic consequences of mutations of FA-C in patients. Kaplan–Meier analysis showed that IVS4 or exon 14 mutations define poor risk subgroups clinically as they are associated with earlier onset of hematologic abnormalities and poorer survival compared to patients with the exon 1 mutation and the non-FA-C population.

Etiology and pathogenesis

There are two theories of pathogenesis of Fanconi's anemia: one relates to defective DNA repair and the other to an inability of Fanconi's cells to remove oxygen-free radicals that damage cells. Despite an extensive body of published data, neither theory has prevailed. The strongest evidence supporting an oxygen metabolism deficiency is the G_2-phase cell cycle defect of Fanconi's cells, consisting of both a phase transit delay and/or a complete arrest.[27,28] This effect is reduced when Fanconi's cells are grown in low oxygen levels, and a similar defect can be induced in normal cells grown at high oxygen levels.[29,30] This phenotype cannot be induced by treatment with DNA cross-linking agents, suggesting that it is not related to a DNA repair defect.

The best evidence supporting the theory that the primary defect is in DNA repair comes from experiments in which the frequency of mutations induced by 8-methoxy psoralen (8-MOP) plus near ultraviolet light (320–360 mm; UVA) at the hypoxanthine phosphoribosyl transferase and $Na^+ + K^+$-ATPase loci was lower in FA-A and FA-D cells than in controls.[31,32] These results could indicate that Fanconi's cells cannot repair cross-links through the normal pathway involving either mismatch repair or recombinational repair following bypass of the lesion, or both. Similar studies that assayed the repair of cross-linked herpes simplex virus DNA following transfection found that Fanconi's cells, unlike controls, could repair cross-linked DNA only under conditions of multiple infection.[33] Since multiplicity reactivation is dependent on recombinational repair, it can be inferred that Fanconi's cells are defective in an excision repair pathway.

To reconcile the evidence of defective oxygen metabolism with the data demonstrating the involvement of the DNA repair system in the pathology of Fanconi's cells a hypothesis is advanced that in Fanconi's anemia a set of proteins, closely involved in DNA repair, is particularly sensitive to oxidative damage. The Fanconi's anemia mutation could either make the repair pathway sensitive to oxidative damage or cause a transient increase of oxidative damage to which the repair machinery is particularly sensitive.

The bone marrow dysfunction in Fanconi's anemia is evident at the hematopoietic progenitor level in bone marrow and peripheral blood. The frequencies of erythroid colony-forming unit (CFU-E), erythroid burst-forming unit (BFU-E) and granulocyte-macrophage colony-forming unit (CFU-GM) cells are reduced fairly consistently in almost all patients after aplastic anemia ensues,[34-42] as well as in a few patients prior to the onset of aplastic anemia.[43] Although marrow cells from Fanconi's patients show normal transcripts for the α- and β-chains of the GM-CSF/interleukin (IL)-3 receptor and for c-kit protein, there is a deficient growth response in the majority of patients of colony-forming unit granulocyte, erythyroid, monocyte, megakaryocyte (CFU-GEMM), BFU-E and CFU-GM progenitors to granulocyte-macrophage colony-stimulating factor (GM-CSF) plus stem cell factor (c-kit ligand) or IL-3 plus stem cell factor, a finding not seen in controls.[44] Because all hematopoietic lineages are affected in these studies, the basic defect is likely to involve the pluripotent stem cell compartment. Confirmatory data for this hypothesis using long-term bone marrow cultures were reported by one group,[45] but contradicted by another.[46] Decreased colony numbers in these studies can be interpreted as being due to an absolute decrease in progenitors, or alternatively due to adequate numbers of progenitors that have faulty proliferative properties and cannot form colonies *in vitro*. Both interpretations may be true.

Cytokine studies in Fanconi's patients have shown varied abnormalities. Whereas Fanconi's fibroblasts showed no deficiencies in stem cell factor or macrophage colony-stimulating factor (M-CSF) production, variability ranging from diminished production to augmentation of production of IL-6, GM-CSF and G-CSF was seen in different patients.[47] A fairly consistent finding that may relate directly to pathogenesis is diminished IL-6 production in Fanconi's patients and markedly heightened abnormal tumor necrosis factor (TNF)-α generation.[48]

Predisposition to malignancy

The karyotype data, the defects in DNA repair, and the cellular damage that occur in Fanconi's patients translate into an enormous predisposition for malignancy. More than 60 patients have been reported with leukemia, about 30 with liver tumors and 30 with other cancers, giving an overall incidence of malignant transformation of about 20%.[49] Fanconi's patients may also develop myelodysplastic syndromes (MDS) (see Chapter 4). These are traditionally defined as clonal refractory cytopenias with characteristic dysplastic changes in marrow cells and a propensity to evolve into acute myelogenous leukemia (AML). Some patients also have clonal cytogenetic findings in marrow cells without overt MDS/AML. The clonal findings of deletions, translocations and marker chromosomes often involve chromosomes 1 and 7.

To determine the risk of malignant myeloid transformation in patients with Fanconi's anemia, Butturini et al[9] used the observational database of the IFAR in which most patients' diagnoses were confirmed by DEB testing. They defined MDS as 5–30% myeloblasts in marrow or 5–20% myeloblasts in blood. AML was defined as >30% marrow blasts or >20% blasts in blood. Marrow dysplastic morphology was not used as a criterion. Of 332 patients in the IFAR who developed varying hematologic abnormalities, 59 (18%) developed MDS or AML with a median interval of observation prior to the transformation of 13 years (range: 1 month to 32 years). Using the authors' strict disease definitions, 34 patients had MDS and 25 had AML. It is noteworthy that 20 of these 59 patients initially presented at diagnosis with established MDS or AML and the diagnosis of Fanconi's anemia was made secondarily. Using the same IFAR data, the actuarial risk of MDS or AML developing over time could be determined. At 5, 10, 20 and 40 years of age, the probability of malignant transformation escalates from <5% to approximately 8%, 25% and 52%, respectively. The risk of MDS/AML was higher for patients in whom a prior clonal marrow cytogenetic abnormality had been detected. Loss of chromosome 7 (monosomy 7) or rearrangement or partial loss of 7q, rearrangements of 1p36 and 1q24–34, and rearrangements of 11q22–25 were the most frequently recurring cytogenetic changes.

Young and Alter[4] compiled published data on 42 patients who developed one or more malignancies other than leukemia or liver tumors. Almost all patients were at least 10 years old when the tumors presented; the average age was 23 years. Most of the tumors were squamous cell carcinomas involving the gastrointestinal tract at any site from the oropharynx to the anorectal-colonic area. Less frequently, gynecologic malignancies were also described with primaries arising in the vulva, cervix and breast. Unusual combinations were occasionally described such as Wilms' tumor with medulloblastoma, cancer of the vulva and tongue, hepatic carcinoma and cancer of the tongue, and hepatic carcinoma and esophageal carcinoma.

Liver tumors, benign and malignant, as well as peliosis hepatis consisting of blood-filled empty spaces in liver, occur at increased frequency in Fanconi's anemia.[4] The commonest tumors reported were hepatocellular carcinoma followed by hepatomas and adenomas. Since almost all patients were taking androgen therapy at the time the liver disease presented, androgens have been implicated as having a direct relationship in pathogenesis. Indeed, peliosis hepatis is reversible when androgens are stopped, and in 3 patients with tumors, discontinuation of androgens alone or coupled with bone marrow transplantation effected a regression of the tumors.

Differential diagnosis

Patients with abnormal hematology and characteristic physical anomalies pose little problem for making a tentative diagnosis, especially if there are previously affected siblings. Distinguishing Fanconi's anemia from *acquired aplastic anemia* on clinical grounds can be difficult if the Fanconi's patient lacks physical anomalies. In this situation, the clastogenic stress-induced chromosomal breakage analysis using DEB will specifically identify Fanconi's anemia and lead to the correct diagnosis.

Although neutropenia is the consistent feature of *Shwachman–Diamond syndrome*, anemia and/or thrombocytopenia is seen in more than half of these patients and can be confused with Fanconi's anemia. Since growth failure is also a manifestation of Shwachman–Diamond, differentiating between the 2 disorders can initially be problematic. The major difference between them is that Shwachman–Diamond syndrome is a disorder of exocrine pancreatic dysfunction which produces gut malabsorption. This can be confirmed by fecal fat analysis and by pancreatic function studies using intravenous secretin and cholecytokinin which confirm markedly impaired enzyme secretion. Computed tomography (CT) of the pancreas may also demonstrate fatty changes within the body of the pancreas. Other skeletal distinguishing features found in some Shwachman–Diamond patients are short, flared ribs, thoracic dystrophy at birth, and metaphyseal dysostosis of the long bones. Finally, chromosomes are normal in Shwachman–Diamond syndrome and no increased breakage is seen after clastogenic stress.

Dyskeratosis congenita shares some features with Fanconi's anemia, including development of pancytopenia, a predisposition to cancer, and skin pigmentary changes. However, the pigmentation pattern is somewhat different and manifests with a lacy reticulated pattern affecting the face, neck, chest and arms, often with a telangiectatic component. At some point, usually in the first decade, dyskeratosis congenita patients also develop dystrophic nails of the hands and feet, and, somewhat later, leukoplakia involving the oral mucosa, especially the tongue. Other findings seen in dyskeratosis congenita but not Fanconi's anemia are teeth abnormalities with dental decay and early tooth loss, hair loss, and hyperhidrosis of the palms and soles. Although there are contradictory data regarding chromosomal fragility in dyskeratosis congenita, DEB testing has not shown any difference between patients and controls which contrasts sharply with Fanconi's patients.

Amegakaryocytic thrombocytopenia and *TAR syndrome* both present in the neonatal period with an isolated decrease of platelets. A neonatal hematologic presentation is very atypical for Fanconi's anemia since <5% of patients are diagnosed in the first year of life. Neither of the thrombocytopenic syndromes shows chromosome fragility, which readily distinguishes them from Fanconi's anemia. In the TAR syndrome, thumbs are always preserved and intact despite the absence of radii, whereas in Fanconi's anemia the thumbs are hypoplastic or absent when the radii are absent.

Therapy and prognosis

Because of their clinical complexity, patients with Fanconi's anemia should be supervised at a tertiary care center using a comprehensive and multidisciplinary approach. On the initial visit, the following should be performed:

- a careful physical examination with emphasis on physical anomalies;
- complete blood counts and chemistries, DEB (and/or mitomycin C) chromosome fragility testing on peripheral blood lymphocytes on patient and siblings;
- HLA tissue typing on patient and family members.

Arrangements should then be made for diagnostic studies to search for any internal anomalies. When all the results have been catalogued, a follow-up visit with the family should be arranged to discuss management options and prognosis.

It is important to emphasize that the prognosis is improving. The older literature describing an early demise of Fanconi's patients is flawed because it does not take into account the diversity in clinical and hematologic phenotype. Diagnosis can now be made before the onset of serious marrow failure or malignant transformation and survival from the time of diagnosis is longer. Also, the newer forms of management, especially marrow transplantation, have dramatically changed the prognosis. Data from the IFAR for the 1980s indicate that Fanconi's patients have a median survival of 25 years of age.[50] Indeed, older female Fanconi's patients can be sexually active; at least 17 patients have become pregnant resulting in 19 births and 18 surviving children.[51]

If the patient is stable and has only minimal to moderate hematologic changes and no transfusion requirements, a period of observation is indicated. Blood counts should be monitored every 1–3 months and bone marrow aspirates and biopsies performed annually for morphology and cancer cytogenetics to identify the emergence of a malignant clone or overt transformation to MDS/AML. Depending on the types of congenital anomalies, subspecialty consultations, e.g. with orthopedic surgeons, can be arranged during this interval.

Bone marrow transplantation

Bone marrow transplantation (BMT) is currently the only curative therapy for the hematologic abnormalities of Fanconi's anemia and the best donor source is an HLA-matched sibling. Initial efforts to transplant Fanconi's patients using standard preparative regimens and graft-versus-host prophylaxis were plagued by 2 serious and often lethal problems—severe cytotoxicity to chemotherapy and exaggerated graft-versus-host disease (GVHD). BMT protocols were subsequently modified for Fanconi's patients and the outcomes improved substantially.

Gluckman *et al*[52] analyzed the data of HLA-identical sibling BMT performed on 151 Fanconi's patients from 42 institutions. The 2-year survival rate was 66%. Factors associated with a favorable outcome were a younger patient age, higher pre-BMT platelet count, use of antithymocyte globulin (ATG), use of low-dose cyclophosphamide (15–25 mg/kg) plus limited field irradiation for pre-BMT conditioning, and cyclosporine for GVHD prophylaxis.

At the Children's Hospital Medical Center, Cincinnati, 30 Fanconi's patients received matched sibling donor BMT and the survival rate with normal blood counts was about 85% with a median follow-up of >3 years.[53] The successful Cincinnati protocol comprises cyclophosphamide 5 mg/kg/day for 4 days (days −5 to −2) followed by thoracoabdominal irradiation 400 cGy (day−1), ATG (40 mg/kg days−6, −4, −2, and 20 mg/kg days +2, +4, +6, +8, +10, +12), and cyclosporine for 6 months after transplantion for GVHD prophylaxis. If a cytogenetic clone or MDS/AML is identified pre-BMT, the preparative therapy is escalated to cyclophosphamide 10 mg/kg/day for 4 days followed by total body irradiation 450 cGy. Methylprednisolone is also added post-BMT, 1 mg/kg/day for 33 days.

Excellent results can also be achieved with conditioning regimens that use a reduced dosage of cyclophosphamide but which omit radiation and ATG.[54] The Kaplan–Meier survival estimate with this Seattle protocol was 89% with a median follow-up of 285 days.

Despite the clear-cut success in correcting the marrow failure of Fanconi's anemia with BMT, data from a joint Paris and Seattle study of 79 patients indicate that a subset of survivors will develop secondary cancers, particularly of the head and neck.[55] The occurrence of cancer of the tongue in 1 such patient illustrates the problem.[56] These malignancies reflect the ongoing genetic susceptibility of host non-hematopoietic tissue to cancer despite successful BMT for marrow failure.

For patients who do not have a matched sibling donor for BMT, a search for a matched unrelated donor can be initiated. Because of the heightened graft-versus-host response observed in Fanconi's patients, survival and cure rates have not been as good compared to matched sibling donor BMT. Even when matched unrelated marrow is fully compatible with the recipient at the DNA level ('molecular match'), these transplants are still very problematic. In the analysis by Gluckman et al,[52] the 2-year probability of survival for 48 Fanconi's patients transplanted with donor marrow comprised of matched unrelated or alternative related sources was only 29%. In another multicenter report of 49 cases of Fanconi's anemia who received unrelated stem-cell transplants, survival was only 43% in those using HLA-matched marrow and 32% in mismatched recipients.[57] Because of the increased risks associated with alternative donor marrow, it is not recommended that Fanconi's patients undergo this type of BMT if the clinical and hematologic picture is stable. Criteria to proceed with an alternative donor BMT include:

- failure to respond adequately to androgen therapy and/or cytokine treatment resulting in an impending need for chronic transfusional support;

- presence of a persistent cytogenetic clone in bone marrow cells, e.g. monosomy 7;
- overt malignant transformation to MDS/AML.

Cord blood cells, naturally enriched with hematopoietic stem and progenitor cells, are being used increasingly as a donor source. The first cord blood transplantation was performed in 1988 for a patient with Fanconi's anemia using a matched sibling donor.[58] Since then, cord blood collections and transplants have increased quickly for a variety of indications,[59–63] including Fanconi's anemia.[63] Using cord cells from related donors, engraftment in Fanconi's patients was about 78% and the incidence of GVHD was reported to be lower than in allogeneic BMT.[63] Recently, cord cells from unrelated donors were transplanted into 5 Fanconi's patients.[64] Some of the donor specimens were mismatched at 1 or 2 loci yet graft failure was only seen in 1 of the 5 cases, there were no instances of lethal GVHD, and event-free-survival beyond day 60 post-transplantation was 80% (4 of the 5 cases). To date, of 17 patients with Fanconi's anemia who have received unrelated cord blood transplants in the United States, 10 are alive.[53]

Hematopoietic growth factors

The potential for recombinant growth factor (cytokine) therapy for Fanconi's anemia has not been fully explored but short-term data are encouraging. An important multicenter clinical trial[65] examined the effect of prolonged administration of G-CSF in 12 Fanconi's patients with neutropenia. The patients were treated with varying subcutaneous dosages daily or every other day for 40 weeks. By week 8 of the study, all patients showed an increase in absolute neutrophil numbers and 4 an increase in platelet counts. Additionally, 4 patients who were not being transfused had a significant increment in hemoglobin levels and a fifth patient no longer required transfusion. Concurrent with the impressive improvements in hematology, 8 of 10 patients who completed 40 weeks of G-CSF treatment showed increases in the percentage of marrow and peripheral blood CD34$^+$ cells.

Since genomic instability and a marked predisposition to leukemia and cancer are features of Fanconi's anemia, the wisdom of using a growth-promoting cytokine on a long-term basis for this disorder is a central issue. In the G-CSF study, 1 patient had a marrow clonal cytogenetic abnormality (48 XXY, +14) without MDS or AML at week 40 of treatment. Therapy was stopped and within 3 months the +X, +14 clone disappeared but monosomy 7 appeared in 11% of metaphases and increased over the ensuing months, prompting a BMT. Since monosomy 7 manifested and progressed after G-CSF was stopped, it seems unlikely that G-CSF was involved in the transformation event in this case. Also, the appearance of the +X, +14 clone while receiving G-CSF treatment and its disappearance on discontinuing the cytokine must be viewed in the context of Fanconi's anemia *per se*, in which clones, seemingly unstable, are known to manifest and disappear spontaneously.[66] Thus, this pilot study showed overall that G-CSF is probably a safe and effective form of treatment for Fanconi's anemia. One patient had a low-grade fever that resolved with dosage modification, and no other untoward clinical effects were noted in any patients.

At one institution, patients without a matched sibling donor who did not have a marrow cytogenetic clone were given combination cytokine therapy consisting of G-CSF 5 μg/kg with erythropoietin 50 units/kg administered subcutaneously or intravenously 3 times a week.[53] Androgen therapy was added if the response was inadequate. Of 20 patients treated, all but 1 showed improved neutrophil numbers, 20% achieved a sustained rise in platelets, and 33% showed an increase in hemoglobin levels. Although more than one-half of the responders lost the response after 1 year due to progression of marrow failure, the requirement for androgen therapy could be delayed by about a year.

Androgens

Androgen therapy has been used to treat Fanconi's anemia for almost 4 decades. The overall response rate in the literature is about 50%[4] heralded by reticulocytosis and a rise in hemoglobin within 1–2 months. If the other lineages respond, white cells increase next and finally platelets, but it may take many months to achieve the maximum response. When the response is deemed maximal, the androgens should be slowly tapered but not stopped entirely.

Oxymetholone, an oral 17-α alkylated androgen, is used most frequently at 2–5 mg/kg/day with preference for the lowest dose initially. Corticosteroids are commonly added to 'counter the androgen-induced growth acceleration' and to prevent thrombocytopenic bleeding by 'promoting vascular stability'. For this purpose, prednisone 5–10 mg is given orally every second day. If an injectable androgen is preferred to decrease the risk of liver toxicity, nandrolone decanoate 1–2 mg/kg/week is given intramuscularly followed by suitable pressure and ice packs to prevent hematomas.

Almost all patients relapse when androgens are stopped. Those few who successfully discontinue treatment are often in the puberty age range when temporary 'spontaneous hematologic remissions' have been observed to occur. Many patients on long-term androgens eventually become refractory to therapy as marrow failure progresses. Potential side-effects include masculinization, which is especially troublesome in female patients, and elevated hepatic enzymes, cholestasis, peliosis hepatis and liver tumors. Those receiving androgens should be evaluated serially with liver chemistry profiles and ultrasonography and/or CT scan of liver.

Future directions

The premise for gene therapy in Fanconi's anemia is based on the presumption that corrected hematopoietic cells have a growth advantage. Strengthening this supposition are recent descriptions of rare patients with Fanconi's anemia who show spontaneous disappearance of cells with the Fanconi's phenotype. These so-called 'mosaic' patients appear to have two populations of leukocytes, one sensitive to mitomycin C and the other with normal resistance to mitomycin C. The phenotypically normal cells appear to have undergone an intragenic mitotic recombination generating one allele with both Fanconi's anemia mutations, whereas the other allele has none (equivalent to a heterozygous carrier). These 'mosaic' patients go into hematologic remission suggesting that hematopoiesis derived from progenitor cells spontaneously revert to a normal phenotype.

Pre-clinical studies using retroviral vectors showed that the FA-C gene can be successfully integrated into normal and Fanconi's anemia cells.[67–69] This prompted a clinical trial in 3 FA-C patients.[70] The patients underwent peripheral blood stem cell harvesting and CD34$^+$ cell fractionation following G-CSF administration. The CD34$^+$ cells were admixed with a retrovirus containing the corrected copy of the FA-C gene and the cells were reintroduced into each patient intravenously. The stem cell harvesting and virus transduction were repeated every 3 months for a total of 4 procedures. Analysis of the peripheral blood and bone marrow cells demonstrated that the FA-C gene was transferred to a small percentage (0.1%) of the total cells but that various lineages expressed the FA-C gene. Clinically, 1 patient showed improvement in hemoglobin which increased from a pre-treatment level of 8–9 g/dl to 12 g/dl post-treatment. Although that patient received androgens and G-CSF during the initial period of the trial, both these medications were reduced without affecting blood counts. The other 2 patients demonstrated variable cell marking at lower levels without significant changes in blood counts.

SHWACHMAN–DIAMOND SYNDROME

This is an inherited disorder of exocrine pancreatic dysfunction with additional features of short stature, variable hematologic abnormalities and radiological skeletal changes.[71–73] The gene responsible for this complex, pleiotropic phenotype is not known and no unifying pathogenesis has been confirmed that can account for all the multisystem features of Shwachman–Diamond syndrome. Chromosomes are normal and no increased breakage is seen after clastogenic stress. None of these patients has cystic fibrosis and sweat chloride levels are normal. Many families have been identified with at least 2 affected children and published studies of segregation ratios and family pedigrees support an autosomal recessive mode of inheritance.

Table 1.4 Clinical features of Shwachman–Diamond syndrome.

Pancreatic	Exocrine pancreatic hypoplasia
Hematologic	Neutropenia (persistent or intermittent)
	Red cell hypoplasia
	Thrombocytopenia
	Pancytopenia
	Elevated fetal hemoglobin
	Myelolymphoproliferative diseases
Skeletal	Metaphyseal dysplasia
	Long bone tubulation
	Short or flared ribs
	Thoracic dystrophy
	Clinodactyly
Growth	Short stature (normal growth velocity)
Other	Psychomotor delay
	Renal tubular dysfunction
	Diabetes mellitus
	Dental abnormalities
	Ichthyosis
	Hepatomegaly
	Hirschsprung's disease

Clinical features

The many manifestations that occur in varying combinations are shown in Table 1.4. Pancreatic dysfunction of variable severity is a consistent feature. The pancreatic lesion appears to be due to failure of pancreatic acinar development. Pathologically, there is extensive fatty replacement of pancreatic acinar tissue and normal ductular architecture. Pancreatic function studies using intravenous secretin and cholecystokinin confirm the presence of markedly impaired enzyme secretion averaging 10–14% of normal, but with preserved ductal function.[74,75]

The vast majority of patients have symptoms of maldigestion from birth due to the pancreatic insufficiency. The absence of steatorrhea, however, does not exclude a diagnosis of Shwachman–Diamond syndrome. If the syndrome is suspected, a quantitative pancreatic function test should be performed. Alternatively, CT of the pancreas may demonstrate fatty changes within the body of the pancreas. A low serum immunoreactive trypsinogen concentration is highly suggestive of severe pancreatic exocrine deficiency.[76] Approximately 50% of patients appear to exhibit a modest improvement in enzyme secretion with advancing age.[75] Consequently, a number of older patients with Shwachman–Diamond syndrome actually develop pancreatic sufficiency with normal fat absorption when assessed by 72-hour fecal fat balance studies.

The most conspicuous physical findings relate to the pancreatic insufficiency and malabsorption, especially short stature which is another consistent feature of the syndrome. Most patients when treated show a normal growth velocity, yet remain consistently below the third percentile for height and weight. Some patients have evidence of delayed puberty. The occasional adult achieves the 25th percentile for height.

Skeletal abnormalities are quite variable. Some patients present at birth with thoracic dystrophy, while others have short flared ribs. Metaphyseal dysostosis of the long bones is a common radiologic abnormality and is thought to be quite specific, particularly in the femoral head and proximal tibia. These changes may not be detectable until after 12 months of age. The etiology of the metaphyseal changes is unclear. In the majority of patients these bony lesions fail to produce any symptoms. However, the integrity of the growth plate may be affected, which in turn may result in skeletal growth disturbances and joint deformities, particularly in the knees and hips.

Additional, less frequent, manifestations thought to be associated with Shwachman–Diamond syndrome include psychomotor delay, hypotonia, massive hepatomegaly, elevated transaminase levels in the absence of hepatomegaly, dental abnormalities, endocardial fibrosis, renal tubular acidosis and diabetes mellitus.

Hematologic features

Published data from 2 large institutions probably represent the spectrum of hematologic findings fairly accurately.[75,77] The combined data from 25 patients in the Toronto series and 21 patients in the London series confirmed that neutropenia is present in virtually all patients on at least one occasion and can be chronic, cyclic or intermittent. It has been identified early in some patients in the neonatal period during an episode of sepsis. Anemia, usually normochromic-normocytic, was recorded in up to 66% of patients,[77] and thrombocytopenia in up to 60%.[75] HbF was elevated in 80% of patients at some stage during the disease course.[77] Whether this reflects 'stress' hematopoiesis and/or ineffective erythropoiesis concomitant with chronic infections, or reflects MDS in transformation has not been clarified. Reticulocyte responses were inappropriately low for the levels of hemoglobin in 75% of patients.[77]

More than one lineage can be affected, and pancytopenia was observed in up to 44% of cases.[75] The pancytopenia can be severe due to full-blown aplastic anemia. However, bone marrow biopsies and aspirates vary widely with respect to cellularity; varying degrees of marrow hypoplasia and fat infiltration are the usual findings, but marrows showing normal or even increased cellularity have also been observed.[76] The severity of neutropenia does not always correlate with bone marrow cellularity, nor is the severity of the pancreatic insufficiency concordant with the hematologic abnormalities.

Patients with Shwachman–Diamond syndrome are particularly susceptible to severe infections, including otitis media, bronchopneumonia, osteomyelitis, septicemia and recurrent furuncles. Overwhelming sepsis is a well recognized fatal complication, particularly early in life. Shwachman–Diamond neutrophils may have a defect in mobility, migration and chemotaxis that does not appear to be caused by malnutrition.[78–80] In the London series, all 13 patients

31

tested showed defective chemotaxis.[77] Lithium in some manner appears to restore chemotaxis when used *in vitro*[81] and *in vivo*.[82] Alterations in neutrophil cytoskeletal/microtubular function may play a prominent role in causing the defective chemotaxis.[80]

Etiology and pathogenesis

Until the molecular genetics for this syndrome are defined, the pathophysiologic link between exocrine pancreatic dysfunction, physical anomalies and partial-to-complete marrow failure remains speculative. Copper deficiency *in utero* provides one hypothetical unifying etiology for the various phenotypic manifestations of Shwachman–Diamond syndrome, but has not been confirmed.[83]

Regarding the neutropenia, an early but still informative study of marrow function was performed in which granulopoiesis was analyzed in 10 children from the Toronto series.[84] Marrow proliferative activity was normal as assessed by determination of mitotic indices and tritiated thymidine uptake into granulocytic cells. Assay of bone marrow CFU-GM progenitors demonstrated normal numbers in 4 patients and reduced numbers in 5. The granulocyte colonies were indistinguishable from normal colonies morphologically. Production of 'colony-stimulating activity' from patients' peripheral blood leukocytes appeared normal when tested on control marrow. No serum inhibitors against CFU-GM or 'colony-stimulating activity' could be demonstrated using both control and autologous marrow, and co-culture of patients' peripheral blood lymphocytes with control marrow did not inhibit CFU-GM growth. Thus, in Shwachman–Diamond syndrome, committed granulocytic progenitors were proliferative and their frequency *in vitro* varied widely, as did the clinical neutropenia. The proliferative activity of mitotic granulocytic cells was normal, and neither a deficiency of humoral stimulators nor the presence of serum or cellular inhibitors of granulopoiesis could be demonstrated. Other investigators[85–88] showed decreased CFU-GM and CFU-E compatible with a defective stem cell origin for the marrow failure in Shwachman–Diamond syndrome.

Predisposition to leukemia

Similar to some other inherited bone marrow failure disorders, Shwachman–Diamond syndrome shares a predilection for MDS and leukemic transformation.[75,77,89–93] In the London series,[77] MDS developed in 7 cases (33%). Five of these patients ultimately evolved into AML (M6 in 2, M5 in 2 and M2 in 1) following a period of MDS (RAEBT in 2, RA in 2 and RAEB in 1). During the MDS phase, 5 cases had clonal marrow cytogenetic abnormalities, mostly structural changes involving chromosome 7. In the Toronto series,[75] 11 of the 25 patients had pancytopenia and 3 of these developed AML (12%). In published literature of 165 patients,[49] 9 (5%) developed leukemia (3 cases of acute

lymphoid leukemia [ALL], 2 of AML [M2], 1 M4, 1 M5, 1 M6 and 1 juvenile chronic myeloid leukemia [JCML]). These sporadic reports in the literature probably represent a gross underestimate of the true incidence of malignant transformation judging from the London and Toronto data. Clearly, the propensity for leukemic conversion in Shwachman–Diamond syndrome is extremely high compared with the general population but is probably not as high as in Fanconi's anemia.

A new issue is the occurrence of MDS/AML in Shwachman–Diamond patients while receiving G-CSF therapy for severe neutropenia. In a report of 14 patients with congenital disorders of myelopoiesis who developed MDS/AML (n = 13) or a clonal cytogenetic abnormality (n = 1) while receiving G-CSF, 2 of the study group had Shwachman–Diamond syndrome.[93] The concern is that G-CSF therapy may have played a role in the malignant transformation. To date, there is no strong evidence to incriminate the cytokine directly in leukemogenesis (see below).

Differential diagnosis

The syndrome of *refractory sideroblastic anemia with vacuolization of bone marrow precursors*, or 'Pearson's syndrome', is clinically similar to Shwachman–Diamond syndrome but very different in bone marrow morphology.[94–103] Severe anemia requiring transfusions rather than neutropenia is often present at birth and by 1 year of age occurs in all cases. In contrast to Shwachman–Diamond syndrome, the major marrow morphologic findings are ringed sideroblasts with decreased erythroblasts, and prominent vacuolation of erythroid and myeloid precursors. The disorder shares clinical similarities with Shwachman–Diamond syndrome because there is exocrine pancreatic dysfunction in both. Malabsorption and resultant severe failure to thrive occurs in about 50% of cases within the first 12 months of life. Qualitative pancreatic function tests show depressed acinar function and reduced fluid and electrolyte secretion. About 50% of reported cases die early in life from sepsis, acidosis and liver failure; the others appear to improve spontaneously with reduced transfusion requirements. At autopsy, the pancreas shows acinar cell atrophy and fibrosis; fatty infiltration as seen in Shwachman–Diamond syndrome is not a prominent feature. The need for long-term pancreatic enzyme replacement is unclear. These patients have abnormalities of mitochondrial DNA (mtDNA),[99] which encodes enzymes in the mitochondrial respiratory chain that are relevant to oxidative phosphorylation, including the reduced form of nicotinamide-adenine dinucleotide dehydrogenase (NADH), cytochrome oxidase, and adenosine triphosphatase (ATPase), as well as transfer and ribosomal RNAs.

Shwachman–Diamond syndrome shares some manifestations with *Fanconi's anemia* such as marrow dysfunction and growth failure, but Shwachman–Diamond patients are readily distinguished because of pancreatic insufficiency with a resultant malabsorption syndrome, fatty changes within the pancreatic body visualized on CT, characteristic skeletal abnormalities not seen in Fanconi's patients, and no increase in chromosome breakage after clastogenic stress testing (see above).

Therapy and prognosis

Patient management is ideally shared by a hematologist and gastroenterologist. The malabsorption component of Shwachman–Diamond syndrome responds to treatment with oral pancreatic enzyme replacement. When monitored over time, about 50% of patients convert from pancreatic insufficiency to sufficiency due to spontaneous improvement in pancreatic enzyme secretion.[75] This improvement is particularly evident after 4 years of age.

Growth factors and other strategies

G-CSF has been given for profound neutropenia and is very effective in inducing a clinically beneficial neutrophil response.[93,104–107] In 1 patient, cross-over treatment using G-CSF initially, followed later by GM-CSF, demonstrated that both cytokines can effect a neutrophil response.[107] Three Shwachman–Diamond patients enrolled in the Severe Chronic Neutropenia International Registry in Seattle have received G-CSF with good responses lasting from 6 months to >6 years (David Dale, personal communication).

Hematologic improvement has been noted in 6 of 12 patients treated with corticosteroids.[4] A smaller number have received androgens plus steroids as in the treatment of Fanconi's anemia and improved marrow function was noted. One patient improved on cyclosporine therapy.[108]

Bone marrow transplantation

The only definitive therapy for severe marrow failure in Shwachman–Diamond syndrome is allogeneic BMT, although the experience with this is very limited. As of 1996, only 5 patients with this disorder had been reported to have received a marrow allograft.[109–113] The small number of transplanted patients is partly explained by the fact that the usual clinical presentation is isolated neutropenia, and if severe this can be successfully managed with antibiotics and growth factor therapy such as G-CSF. Transfusional management can also be applied effectively on a long-term basis for patients with advanced bi- and trilineage marrow failure.

A note of caution should be sounded regarding BMT for Shwachman–Diamond syndrome. Left ventricular fibrosis and necrosis without coronary arterial lesions have been reported in 50% of Shwachman–Diamond patients at autopsy,[114] suggesting that there may be an increased risk of cardiotoxicity with the intensive preparatory chemotherapy used in BMT. Indeed, of 2 patients who underwent BMT, 1 died from cardiotoxicity ascribed to cyclophospha-mide[110] and the other had significant left ventricular dysfunction throughout the pre-BMT clinical course.[111] A third patient[109] and 2 others transplanted in London[77] showed no cardiac dysfunction or cardiotoxicity using comparable conditioning protocols. Although these data are limited, it is recommended that cardiac function is carefully assessed prior to starting chemotherapy for BMT.

DYSKERATOSIS CONGENITA

This is an inherited disorder of the mucocutaneous and hematopoietic systems. The diagnostic ectodermal component consists invariably of the triad of reticulate skin pigmentation of the upper body, mucosal leukoplakia and nail dystrophy.[115–117] Dyskeratosis congenita is also an inherited bone marrow failure syndrome in which aplastic anemia occurs in about 50% of cases, usually in the second decade of life. There is also a predisposition to cancer. Because of the cluster of abnormalities involving skin and bone marrow and the predilection to cancer, dyskeratosis congenita resembles Fanconi's anemia, but the genetics and physical abnormalities of the two conditions are quite different and they should be considered as totally discrete entities. Two recent reviews highlight the salient features of dyskeratosis congenita.[118,119]

The inheritance pattern is somewhat complicated. There are about 200 published cases of dyskeratosis congenita of whom about 85% are male, which is compatible with an X-linked recessive trait. Linkage studies in 1 large family[120] using X chromosome-specific restriction fragment length polymorphism markers have assigned a gene for the syndrome to Xq28, a finding confirmed in 3 additional families.[121] In X-linked families it is possible to identify female carriers using informative Xq28-specific polymorphic probes. Approximately 15% of cases appear to have another mode of inheritance. Sporadic female cases, familial cases with affected male and female siblings in one generation, and cases with known parental consanguinity fit an autosomal recessive inheritance pattern. An autosomal dominant mode best fits other cases in families with affected male and female members in consecutive generations. Clinically, the autosomal dominant group seems to be milder in its manifestations, and the autosomal recessive group appears to have more physical anomalies and a higher incidence of aplastic anemia and cancer.[118] It seems likely that the dyskeratosis congenita phenotype is due to more than 1 gene.

Clinical features

Clinical manifestations in dyskeratosis congenita often appear during childhood. The skin pigmentation and nail changes typically appear in the first 10 years of life, mucosal leukoplakia and excessive ocular tearing appear later, and by the mid-teens the serious complications of bone marrow failure and malignancy begin to develop. In rare cases the marrow abnormalities may appear before the skin manifes-

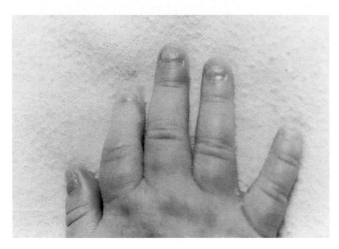

Fig. 1.2 Dystrophic nails in dyskeratosis congenita.

tations. The main causes of death relate to either bone marrow failure or malignancy. The mean age of death is approximately 30 years.

Cutaneous findings are the most consistent feature of the syndrome. Lacy reticulated skin pigmentation affecting the face, neck, chest and arms is a common finding. The degree of pigmentation increases with age and can involve the entire skin surface. There may also be a telangiectatic erythematous component. Nail dystrophy of the hands and feet is the next commonest finding (Fig. 1.2). It usually starts with longitudinal ridging, splitting or pterygium formation and may progress to complete nail loss. Leukoplakia usually involves the oral mucosa, especially the tongue (Fig. 1.3) but can also be seen in the conjunctiva, anal, urethral or genital mucosa. Hyperhidrosis of the palms and soles is common, and hair loss is sometimes seen. Eye abnormalities are observed in approximately 50% of cases.[122] Excessive tearing (epiphora) secondary to nasolacrimal duct obstruction is common. Other ophthalmologic manifestations include conjunctivitis, blepharitis, loss of eyelashes, strabismus, cataracts and optic atrophy. Abnormalities of the teeth, particularly an increased rate of dental decay and early loss

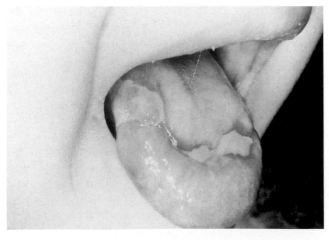

Fig. 1.3 Leukoplakia of the tongue in dyskeratosis congenita.

of teeth, are common. Skeletal abnormalities such as osteoporosis, avascular necrosis, abnormal bone trabeculation, scoliosis and mandibular hypoplasia are seen in approximately 20% of cases.[123,124] Genitourinary abnormalities include hypoplastic testes, hypospadias, phimosis, urethral stenosis and horseshoe kidney. Gastrointestinal findings, such as esophageal strictures, hepatomegaly or cirrhosis, are seen in 10% of cases.[125]

Several physical findings can be used to distinguish Fanconi's anemia from dyskeratosis congenita clinically. The following abnormalities are seen only in dyskeratosis congenita: nail dystrophy, leukoplakia, teeth abnormalities, hyperhidrosis of palms and soles and hair loss.[49]

Hematologic features

About 50% of X-linked male patients with dyskeratosis congenita and 70% of autosomal recessive patients develop aplastic anemia, usually in the teenage years. It occurs much less frequently in autosomal dominant patients. Most of these cases already have manifestations of dyskeratosis congenita, but some younger patients can develop marrow failure prior to the clinical onset of the mucocutaneous manifestations. The initial hematologic change is usually thrombocytopenia, anemia or both, followed by full-blown pancytopenia due to aplastic anemia. The red cells are often macrocytic and the HbF can be elevated. Oddly, early bone marrow aspirations and biopsies may be hypercellular; however, with time the cellular elements decline with a symmetrical decrease in all hematopoietic lineages. Ferrokinetic studies at this point are consistent with aplastic anemia.

Chromosome instability data

As summarized by Dokal,[119] there is a large body of contradictory information regarding chromosomal fragility and instability in dyskeratosis congenita. Spontaneous chromosome breaks in patients' lymphocytes were reported in some studies but not confirmed in others. Similarly, excessive spontaneous and clastogenic-induced sister chromatid exchange in patients' lymphocytes were observed by some investigators but not others. Standard clastogenic stress studies, however, of dyskeratosis congenita cells using the DNA alkylating agents mitomycin C and DEB in several laboratories clearly have not shown any difference in chromosome breakage between patients and controls.[126–131] This contrasts sharply with Fanconi's anemia cells and distinguishes one disorder from the other.

However, Dokal et al[132,133] argue strongly that dyskeratosis congenita is, indeed, a chromosome 'instability' disorder of a somewhat different type from Fanconi's anemia. They found that primary skin fibroblasts in culture were not only abnormal in morphology and doubling rate, but in some patients metaphases in peripheral blood cells, marrow cells and fibroblasts in culture showed numerous unbalanced chromosome rearrangements such as dicentrics, tricentrics and translocations in the absence of clastogenic agents. These findings were confirmed by other investigators[119] and provide evidence for a defect that predisposes patient cells to developing chromosomal rearrangements.

Etiology and pathogenesis

Most studies of the pathogenesis of aplastic anemia in dyskeratosis congenita have been limited to clonogenic assays. A marked reduction or absence of CFU-GEMM, BFU-E, CFU-E and CFU-GM progenitors has been consistently reported.[34,35,134–136] The absence of a serum inhibitor of CFU-GM was documented in 1 case, and the absence of T-cell-mediated hematopoietic suppression in another case. Although Hanada *et al*[137] reported 1 case of T-cell-mediated suppression of CFU-GM, but not of CFU-E, this effect was not seen after splenectomy or after recurrence of the pancytopenia.

Marsh *et al*[136] used long-term bone marrow cultures to study hematopoiesis in 3 patients with dyskeratosis congenita. Two had aplastic anemia and the third had normal blood counts and normal marrow cellularity. Hematopoiesis was severely defective in all 3 patients with a low frequency of colony-forming cells and a low level of hematopoiesis in long-term cultures. Marrow stromal cells showed a normal ability to support growth of hematopoietic progenitors from normal marrow seeded onto them in all 3 cases, but generation of progenitors from patient marrow cells inoculated onto normal stroma was reduced, strongly suggesting that the defect in dyskeratosis congenita is of stem cell origin.

Thus, marrow failure in this disorder may be due to a progressive attrition and depletion of hematopoietic stem cells which manifests as pancytopenia in the mid-teens. Alternatively, marrow dysfunction may not be a simple consequence of a limited stem cell pool but may represent a failure of replication and/or maturation.

Predisposition to cancer

Cancer develops in about 10% of patients, usually in the third or fourth decades of life. In contrast to Fanconi's anemia in which malignant tumours and MDS/AML are both seen, patients with dyskeratosis congenita are not predisposed to leukemia but only to solid tumours. Young and Alter[4] have summarized the literature on cancers in 20 patients—15 X-linked males, 4 autosomal recessive cases and 1 autosomal dominant patient. Most of the cancers were squamous cell carcinoma or adenocarcinomas, and the oropharynx and gastrointestinal tract were involved most frequently. One patient had 3 separate primaries in the tongue, nasopharynx and rectum, 1 had esophageal and cheek carcinomas, and 1 had separate nasal and tongue malignancies. Thus, the sites of most of the cancers involve areas known to be abnormal in dyskeratosis congenita such as mucous membranes and the gastrointestinal tract.

Therapy and prognosis

Management of aplastic anemia is similar to that for Fanconi's anemia. Androgens, usually combined with low-dose prednisone, can be expected to induce improved marrow function in about 50% of patients. If a response is seen and deemed to be maximal, the androgen dose can be slowly tapered but not stopped. As in Fanconi's anemia, patients can become refractory to androgens as the aplastic anemia progresses. There is no published information on the use of immunosuppressive therapy for this disorder.

Bone marrow transplantation

As recently summarized,[138] 16 patients with dyskeratosis congenita worldwide have been reported to have received allogeneic BMT for marrow failure.[138–145] Eight were <11 years of age at the time of the procedure; the others were in their 20s and 30s. All received cyclophosphamide-based preparative regimens with or without irradiation. The results were remarkably poor; only 3 of the 16 survived and appeared cured by BMT, but 1 of these was only 8 months post-BMT at the time of the report. The others died of early, transplant-related complications or, notably, of very late complications. Of concern, lethal pulmonary fibrosis or renal failure occurred years after BMT. Gluckman *et al*[146] suggested that the epithelial and endothelial cells of these patients might be abnormally sensitive to the preconditioning agents without any relation to chromosomal fragility. This sensitivity may be reflected by raised von Willebrand factor levels in patients' plasma.[119] Gluckman *et al*[146] reported 2 patients with dyskeratosis congenita treated with BMT who developed diffuse vasculitis caused by endothelial activation several years after BMT. Their renal histology at post-mortem showed similar lesions characterized by alteration of the capillary walls of glomeruli, mesangiolysis, arteriolonecrosis and occasional arteriolar luminal fibrosis.

Thus, judging from available information, strong endorsement cannot be made for BMT in dyskeratosis congenita, although there usually is no other recourse for life-threatening aplastic anemia. Perhaps modified conditioning similar to Fanconi's anemia will ensure a safer procedure and a more optimistic outcome.

Growth factors

Three patients were reported who responded to G-CSF therapy with significant increases in absolute neutrophil counts.[147–149] Similarly, GM-CSF therapy in 2 other patients resulted in improved neutrophil numbers.[150,151] Stem cell factor increased the *in vitro* growth of erythroid progenitors in some patients with dyskeratosis congenita[152] but it has not yet been used clinically. Although the reports are scanty, there appears to be potential benefit from cytokine therapy, at least in the short-term, especially for improving granulopoiesis.

Gene therapy

In the X-linked form of dyskeratosis congenita, the assignment of a gene to Xq28 and the availability of most of this region as contiguous yeast artificial chromosomes may facilitate positional cloning of the gene. Although this raises hope for gene therapy in the future, the prospects are not imminent.

AMEGAKARYOCYTIC THROMBOCYTOPENIA

Amegakaryocytic thrombocytopenia, or congenital amegakaryocytic thrombocytopenia (CAT), is a varied syndrome that presents in infancy with isolated thrombocytopenia due to reduced or absent marrow megakaryocytes with preservation initially of granulopoietic and erythroid lineages. Aplastic anemia subsequently ensues in about 45% of patients, usually in the first few years of life. The diagnosis depends on the exclusion of all other specific causes for thrombocytopenia in early life (see Chapter 21). Although most cases are sporadic, familial cases also occur and the syndrome is felt to be an inherited bone marrow failure disorder. Peripheral blood chromosomes do not show increased fragility and this distinguishes CAT from Fanconi's anemia. Male cases outnumber females, suggesting that some cases may be X-linked and that others may have an autosomal recessive mode of inheritance. Examples of male-only affected sibships as well as mixed male-female affected sibships are reviewed by Young and Alter.[4]

Clinical and hematologic features

Almost all patients present with a petechial rash, bruising or bleeding in the first year of life. Most cases are obvious at birth or within the first 2 months. Roughly half of patients have characteristic physical anomalies, whereas the others have normal physical and imaging features. Some affected sibships manifest both normal and abnormal physical findings in the same family. Similar to Fanconi's anemia, CAT patients with and without anomalies should be considered as part of the clinical spectrum of one entity.

The commonest manifestations in those with anomalies are neurologic and cardiac. Findings relating to cerebellar and cerebral atrophy are a recurrent theme and developmental delay is a prominent feature in this group. Patients may also have microcephaly and an abnormal facies. Congenital heart disease with a variety of malformations can be detected, including atrial and ventricular septal defects, patent ductus arteriosus, tetralogy of Fallot and coarctation of the aorta. Some of these can occur in combinations. Other anomalies include abnormal hips or feet, kidney malformations, eye anomalies and cleft or high-arched palate.

Thrombocytopenia is the major laboratory finding with normal hemoglobin levels and white blood cell counts initially. Although there are usually measurable numbers of platelets, albeit reduced, peripheral blood platelets may be

totally absent. Similar to other inherited bone marrow failure syndromes, red cells may be macrocytic. HbF can be increased and there may be increased expression of i antigen. Bone marrow specimens show normal cellularity with markedly reduced or absent megakaryocytes. In patients who develop aplastic anemia, marrow cellularity is decreased with fatty replacement; the erythroid and granulopoietic lineages are also symmetrically reduced.

Etiology and pathogenesis

Serial studies of bone marrow hematopoiesis using clonogenic assays were performed in an infant from Toronto with CAT.[153] Initially, when the only hematologic abnormality was isolated thrombocytopenia, the number of clonogenic hematopoietic progenitors was comparable to controls, including the number of megakaryocyte precursors (CFU-Meg). As the disease evolved into aplastic anemia over an 11-month period, the peripheral blood counts declined, and colony numbers from 4 classes of progenitors also declined in parallel. When added to the marrow cultures, the patient's plasma was not inhibitory to control or patient's colony growth. Similarly, no cellular inhibition of hematopoiesis was observed when the patient's marrow was cultured after depleting the sample of T lymphocytes or after adding them back. Furthermore, stromal cells established in short- and long-term cultures of the patient's marrow showed normal proliferative activity and yielded a 'fertile' marrow microenvironment for patient's and control colony growth. The data suggest that the central problem in CAT is an intrinsic hematopoietic stem cell defect rather than an abnormality of the marrow milieu. The findings are consistent with either a progressive, quantitative attrition of progenitors or their inability to proliferate into colonies *in vitro* and into differentiated, functional cells *in vivo*.

Guinan *et al*[154] reported assayable numbers of CFU-Meg progenitors *in vitro* from 5 patients with CAT in response to IL-3, GM-CSF or a combination of both. The presence of megakaryocyte progenitors in these patients fits with the data from the Toronto patient when studied early in the course of the disease.[153] When studied by PCR, marrow cells from a Japanese patient with CAT had no detectable *c-mpl* mRNA compared to controls, suggesting that impaired *c-mpl* expression may account for a defective response to thrombopoietin in this disorder.[155]

Predisposition to leukemia

Alter[49] described 2 patients with CAT who developed leukemia. One male with a normal physical appearance had amegakaryocytic thrombocytopenia from day 1 of life, developed aplastic anemia at 5 years of age, responded poorly to androgens and steroids, and then developed acute myelomonocytic leukemia (AMML) at age 16, with death at 17. A female had thrombocytopenia at 2 months of age, pancytopenia at 5 months, and thereafter developed a pre-leukemic picture with abnormalities involving chromosome 19. The Toronto patient described above had thrombocytopenia at 6 months of age, progressive aplastic anemia over the next 2 years, acquired monosomy 7 in marrow cells at 5 years and then developed MDS with an activating *ras* oncogene mutation in hematopoietic cells. Hence, evidence shows that CAT is another inherited marrow failure disorder that is pre-leukemic. The risk or incidence of malignant conversion is difficult to determine because of the rarity of the disease and paucity of published data dealing with this issue.

Therapy and prognosis

Historically, treatment has been unsatisfactory and the mortality rate from thrombocytopenic bleeding, complications of aplastic anemia, or malignant myeloid transformation has been very close to 100%. For this reason, HLA typing of family members should be performed as soon as the diagnosis is confirmed to see if a matched related donor for BMT exists. If not, a search for a matched unrelated donor should ensue as soon as the seriousness of the clinical picture dictates. The need for transfusional support is a cogent indication.

Platelet transfusions should be used discretely. Platelet numbers should not be a sole indication; clinical bleeding is the more appropriate trigger for the use of platelets. Single donor platelets are preferred to multiple unfiltered random donors to minimize sensitization, and if BMT is a realistic possibility all blood products should test negative for cytomegalovirus.

Corticosteroids have been used for thrombocytopenia with no apparent efficacy. For aplastic anemia, androgens in combination with corticosteroids may induce a temporary partial response but the effect is short-lived and does not prevent mortality.

Based on the *in vitro* augmentation of megakaryocyte progenitor colony growth in response to IL-3, GM-CSF or both, a phase I/II clinical trial was initiated for 5 patients with CAT.[154] IL-3 but not GM-CSF resulted in improved platelet counts in 2 patients, and decreased bleeding and transfusion requirements in the other 3. GM-CSF had no observable benefit when given after IL-3 pre-treatment. Prolonged IL-3 administration in 2 additional patients also resulted in platelet increments. This pilot study illustrates that IL-3 may be an important adjunct to the medical management of CAT.

There is curative potential using BMT. In the original Toronto series of patients with inherited marrow failure studied by clonogenic assays,[34,35,156] a case of familial CAT in the aplastic anemia phase received a BMT from his sister in 1974 and is currently alive and cured. More recently, 2 infants of 22 and 42 months of age, respectively, underwent allogeneic BMT, 1 of them with an unrelated donor marrow.[157] Both patients were well with good engraftment of donor marrow and normal blood counts at 12 and 31

months after BMT, respectively. An additional male patient with familial CAT who had a robust response to IL-3 initially and then later to the IL-3:GM-CSF fusion product underwent a matched unrelated BMT when he became refractory to cytokine therapy. He appeared cured 1 year post-BMT (Laurence Boxer, personal communication).

The Toronto patient described above received a 1-antigen mismatched T-cell depleted unrelated donor BMT in desperation because of clinical deterioration. Engraftment ensued readily but the patient died several months post-BMT from complications of grade IV GVHD (unpublished data). Despite this negative experience, the other successful BMTs illustrate the potential for cure by this procedure.

OTHER GENETIC SYNDROMES

Bone marrow failure can occur in the context of several, specific non-hematologic syndromes, and also in familial settings that do not exactly correspond with the entities described above.

Down's syndrome

Down's syndrome, or trisomy 21, has a unique association with aberrant hematology. Three seemingly related events can occur.[158]

1. In the neonatal period, a myeloproliferative blood picture with large numbers of circulating blast cells has been observed in many of these infants. The blasts apparently are clonal but, remarkably, disappear spontaneously over several weeks in most cases. The term 'transient leukemia' is often used to reflect this unusual natural history.
2. In about 20% of cases, 'true' leukemia recurs and requires oncologic management. Acute lymphoblastic and myeloblastic leukemias are both seen in Down's syndrome, and acute megakaryoblastic leukemia (M7) is the commonest form of the myeloblastic leukemias. It has been estimated that the incidence of M7 is 500 times greater in children with Down's syndrome than in normal children.[158]
3. The onset of M7 is frequently preceded by an interval of MDS characterized by thrombocytopenia, abnormal megakaryocytopoiesis, megakaryoblasts in the marrow, and an abnormal karyotype, commonly trisomy 8.[159]

In addition to the propensity for leukemia, a few patients have been reported with aplastic anemia. Alter[49] summarized 5 of these cases, 3 of whom died of marrow failure and 2 who responded to androgen therapy.

Dubowitz's syndrome

This is an autosomal recessive disorder characterized by a peculiar facies, infantile eczema, small stature and mild microcephaly. The face is small with a shallow supraorbital ridge, a nasal bridge at the same level as the forehead, short palpebral fissures, variable ptosis and micrognathia.[160] This is a rare disorder and incidence rates are difficult to establish; however, as reviewed recently, there appears to be a predilection to cancer as well as to bone marrow dysfunction.[161] Patients have developed ALL, AML, neuroblastoma, and lymphoma.[161–163] About 10% of cases also develop hematopoietic disorders varying from hypoplastic anemia, moderate pancytopenia and full-blown aplastic anemia.[161,164]

Seckel's syndrome

Sometimes called 'bird-headed dwarfs', patients with this autosomal recessive developmental disorder have marked growth and mental deficiency, microcephaly, a hypoplastic face with a prominent nose, and low-set and/or malformed ears.[165] These patients can be distinguished from Fanconi's anemia on the basis of a negative DEB clastogenic chromosome stress test. About 10% of cases develop aplastic anemia, usually severe.[166–168]

Reticular dysgenesis

This is an immunologic deficiency syndrome coupled with congenital agranulocytosis.[169] The mode of inheritance is probably autosomal recessive but an X-linked mode is also possible in some cases. The disorder is a variant of severe combined immune deficiency (SCID) in which cellular and humoral immunity are absent and patients additionally have severe lymphopenia and neutropenia. Because of profoundly compromised immunity, the syndrome presents early with severe infection at birth or shortly thereafter. A striking feature is absent lymph nodes and tonsils, and an absent thymic shadow on chest film. In addition to lymphopenia and neutropenia, anemia and thrombocytopenia may also be present. Bone marrow specimens are hypocellular with markedly reduced myeloid and lymphoid elements. Clonogenic assays of hematopoietic progenitors consistently show reduced to absent colony growth indicating that the disorder has its origins at the pluripotential lympho-hematopoietic stem cell level.[170–173] The only curative therapy is BMT.[172]

Familial aplastic anemia

Bone marrow failure can cluster in families but many of these cases cannot be readily classified into discrete diagnostic entities such as Fanconi's anemia. The phenotype of these conditions can be complex with varying combinations of hematologic abnormalities, immunologic deficiency, physical malformations and development of leukemia. One approach to nosology is to divide the disorders into inheritance patterns, and then subdivide them into those with and without physical anomalies.[4]

Some families show an autosomal dominant mode of inheritance of marrow dysfunction associated with physical anomalies. The *WT syndrome* is characterized by successive generations of affected family members who have radial-ulnar hypoplasia, abnormal thumbs, short fingers, and fifth finger clinodactyly.[174] Pancytopenia or thrombocytopenia, sometimes with leukemia, occurs in some of the affecteds. The *IVIC syndrome*[175] or *oculo-otoradial syndrome*[176] manifests with radial ray hypoplasia, absent thumbs or hypoplastic radial carpal bones, impaired hearing, strabismus and sometimes imperforate anus. Mild thrombocytopenia is seen in about 50% of cases. The *ataxia-pancytopenia syndrome* is a combination of cerebellar atrophy and ataxia associated in affected family members with varied manifestations of anemia, aplastic anemia, MDS, AML, monosomy 7 in marrow cells and immune deficiency.[177,178] Other autosomal dominant syndromes with anomalies include:

- a family with marrow failure, ALL, skin pigmentation, warts, immune dysfunction and multiple spontaneous abortions;[179]
- successive generations of family members with unilineage cytopenia or pancytopenia with vascular occlusions;[180]
- proximal fusion of the radius and ulna, and aplastic anemia or leukemia.[181]

Autosomal recessive inheritance of anomalies and marrow dysfunction also occurs. Consanguinity can result in a syndrome of microcephaly, mental retardation, skin pigmentation, short stature and pancytopenia, possibly with a clonal cytogenetic marker in bone marrow cells.[182] A second example of this inheritance mode presents with central nervous system anomalies, such as the Dandy-Walker syndrome or ventricular dilatation and asymmetry, and aplastic anemia.[183]

Autosomal dominant inheritance of a wide-ranging pattern of disordered marrow function can be seen without physical anomalies. Successive generations have been described with the following:

- 'acquired' aplastic anemia in 4 families comprising 9 patients, with an affected parent, aunt or uncle;[184]
- aplastic anemia in a mother and neutropenia and thrombocytopenia in her offspring;[185]
- aplastic anemia, AML and monosomy 7 in various family members;[186]
- hypoplastic anemia in a parent and offspring with either myelofibrosis, AML, MDS, or pancytopenia, all associated with the acquired Pelger-Huet anomaly.[187]

Marrow dysfunction can also be inherited without anomalies in an autosomal recessive pattern. One example encompasses pancytopenia, immune deficiency, multiple cutaneous basal cell and squamous cell carcinomas, oral telangiectasias and neck and chest poikiloderma.[188] Another pattern comprises immune deficiency, pure red cell aplasia and/or neutropenia, and unusual crystalloid structures seen on electron microscopy in neutrophils.[189]

An X-linked inheritance is suggested by a syndrome affecting males in successive generations with one or more of pancytopenia, AML, ALL and light chain disease but with no physical anomalies.[190]

Etiology and pathogenesis

These genetic disorders are very heterogeneous clinically and hematologically and only generic descriptives can be used in their characterization. Patients have variable manifestations of cytopenia involving one or more hematopoietic lineages, usually with hypocellular marrows. In the familial syndromes, additional findings such as physical malformations, immunologic deficiency and marrow cytogenetic markers such as monosomy 7 distinguish them from cases of sporadic acquired bone marrow failure. Patients' marrows generally show reduced numbers of hematopoietic progenitors in clonogenic assays but this is common to almost all marrow failure disorders and does not distinguish genetic and familial cases from acquired aplastic anemia.

Therapy

Because these disorders are rare, broad conclusions about management are difficult to formulate. For full-blown aplastic anemia with a hypocellular, fatty marrow, curative therapy with BMT remains the first choice if a matched donor is identified. In familial cases, potential marrow donors must be thoroughly assessed clinically, hematologically and by marrow morphology, clonogenic activity and cytogenetics to ensure that latent or masked marrow dysfunction is not present. If a matched donor is not available, the same principles of medical management as used for Fanconi's anemia and acquired aplastic anemia should be used.

UNILINEAGE CYTOPENIA

DIAMOND–BLACKFAN ANEMIA

Diamond–Blackfan anemia (DBA), or congenital hypoplastic anemia, is a constitutional form of pure red cell aplasia.[191] The syndrome is heterogeneous with respect to inheritance patterns, clinical and laboratory findings, in vitro data, and therapeutic outcome. About 80% of cases are sporadic, suggesting new mutations or acquired disease, but there are examples of recessive inheritance (autosomal and possibly X-linked), as well as autosomal dominant patterns.[192] There is suspicion that DBA represents a family of disorders with different etiologies that share the common hematologic phenotype of pure red cell aplasia. Using data from the DBA registries in France[193] and the UK,[194] the incidence of the disorder in Europe is 5–7 cases/million live births. Further details of this disorder are given in Chapter 3.

KOSTMANN'S SYNDROME/CONGENITAL NEUTROPENIA

Severe chronic neutropenia (SCN) and recurrent serious infections are features of an heterogeneous group of disorders of myelopoiesis including congenital neutropenia, cyclic neutropenia, and idiopathic neutropenia. Kostmann's syndrome (KS) is a subtype of congenital neutropenia inherited in an autosomal recessive manner with onset in early childhood of profound neutropenia (absolute neutrophil count < 200/ml), recurrent life-threatening infections, and a maturation arrest of myeloid precursors at the promyelocyte-myelocyte stage of differentiation. Congenital neutropenia and KS have the same hematologic phenotype and clinical presentation. The recessive inheritance of KS is deduced by inference when there is > 1 affected child in a family. Congenital neutropenia is the proper designation used for a single 'sporadic' case in a family, and hence may or may not be inherited in an autosomal recessive manner like KS. Since the molecular defect is not known for either diagnostic category, the option to 'lump' or 'split' the two disorders remains a subject of argument. Here, the terms 'KS' and 'congenital neutropenia' are used interchangably.

The Severe Chronic Neutropenia International Registry (SCNIR) was established in 1994 to catalog the clinical features and to monitor the clinical course, treatment, and disease outcomes in patients with SCN.[195–204] The Registry is a valuable resource for clinical data because of the large numbers of patients entered into its worldwide database. Patient data are submitted internationally to the co-ordinating centers at the University of Washington, Seattle and the Medizinische Hochschule, Hannover. In late 1996, short- and long-term information dating back to 1987 on a total of 506 patients was available for analysis. Of these, 249 patients were classified as congenital neutropenia including KS.

Clinical features

KS, or 'infantile genetic agranulocytosis', as described in 1956,[205] comprised an original 14 cases and a subsequent 10 patients[206] belonging to a large intermarried kinship in northern Sweden. The mode of inheritance in these patients was clearly autosomal recessive. Subsequently, the disorder has been recognized widely, despite its rarity, and in various ethnic groups including Asians, American Indians and blacks. Consanguinity is not a uniform finding in cases enrolled in the SCNIR.

About half the patients develop clinically impressive infections within the first month of life and almost all do by 6 months. Skin abscesses are common but deep-seated tissue infections and blood-borne septicemia also occur. SCNIR data illustrate examples of every conceivable form of bacterial and sometimes fungal infection in the pre-cytokine era. Especially troublesome in survivors were recurrent episodes of otitis media and pneumonia, advanced gingival-stomatitis, and, in the extreme case, gut bacterial flora overgrowth leading to malabsorption requiring total parenteral nutritional therapy. In contrast to some of the other inherited bone marrow failure syndromes, physical malformations are not a feature. Birth weights are generally unremarkable and physical examinations are normal. There are a small number of reports of short stature, microcephaly, mental retardation and cataracts but the association with KS does not appear to be strong. Data from the SCNIR indicate that some patients with KS develop bone demineralization before and during G-CSF therapy. The underlying pathogenesis is unclear but patients can develop bone pain and unusual fractures.

Laboratory features

Neutropenia is profound in KS (usually $<200/\mu l$ but often absolute). Compensatory monocytosis and sometimes eosinophilia is seen. At diagnosis, platelet numbers and hemoglobin values are normal. In survivors in the pre-cytokine era, anemia of chronic disease associated with recurrent infections and inflammation was common. Aside from neutropenia, humoral and cellular immunology is completely normal.

Bone marrow specimens are usually normocellular. The striking classical finding is a maturation arrest at the promyelocyte or myelocyte stage of granulocytic differentiation. Cellular elements beyond are markedly reduced or totally absent. The other hematopoietic lineages are normal, active and undisturbed.

Etiology and pathogenesis

Initial studies of KS CFU-GM progenitor growth *in vitro* yielded variable data.[207–229] CFU-GM numbers can be decreased or increased, but are usually normal, and the colonies are comprised of myeloid elements arrested in differentiation, thereby mimicking the disease *in vitro*. Some patients, however, yield CFU-GM colonies with mature neutrophils.[213,216] KS serum is not inhibitory to CFU-GM growth. Long-term cultures from some patients also show decreased myeloid differentiation.[219]

More recent studies of stromal and marrow mononuclear cells from patients with KS suggest that the primary defect is at the level of the myeloid progenitor. In particular, these experiments have shown normal serum G-CSF levels, normal G-CSF production by marrow stromal cells *ex vivo*, a normal or increased number of G-CSF receptors on hematopoietic cells and defective myeloid colony growth.[224,227–229] The G-CSF receptor contains discrete cytoplasmic domains that transduce proliferative and differentiating signals.[230–232] Dong et al[233] found a mutation that removed the carboxy tail of the G-CSF receptor in a congenital neutropenia patient after developing MDS (see below). This truncated receptor retained the ability to stimulate cell growth, but deleted the differentiation domain. The G-CSF receptor mutation was restricted to

the myeloid lineage and was not detected in DNA extracted from other tissues. The absence of germ-line mutations of the G-CSF receptor gene is consistent with the concept that the neutropenia of KS is not caused by this mechanism.

Predisposition to leukemia

There is concern regarding the phenomenon of malignant myeloid transformation in KS patients receiving G-CSF therapy. Of 249 patients in the SCNIR in late 1996 classified as congenital neutropenia, including KS, 24 developed MDS/AML yielding an overall incidence or crude rate of about 10% with an average follow-up of 5 years. No cases of MDS/AML occurred in the subgroup of congenital neutropenia patients with glycogen storage disease type 1b nor with cyclic or idiopathic neutropenia.

Conversion to MDS/AML in the KS patients was associated with one or more cellular genetic abnormalities which may identify a subgroup of patients at high risk.[234] Of 24 who transformed in the SCNIR series, 14 developed partial or complete loss of chromosome 7 (7q- or monosomy 7) in marrow cells; none of the patients who was tested prior to G-CSF therapy had loss of chromosome 7. Activating *ras* oncogene mutations were discovered in 5 of 10 patients from the series of 24 after the transformation to MDS/AML but not before. Four of these also had monosomy 7. The mutated fragments were cloned and sequenced and showed GGT (glycine) to GAT (aspartic acid) substitutions at codon 12 in all 5 (K12ASP in 2 patients and N12ASP in 3 patients). Marrow cells from 5 transformed patients also showed point mutations in the gene for G-CSF receptor resulting in a truncated C-terminal cytoplasmic region of the receptor that is crucial for maturation signaling.[235,236] Twenty patients without receptor mutations showed no evidence of progression to MDS/AML; however, 4 additional patients have been identified with mutations but without MDS/AML[235] and are currently being closely monitored.

Can G-CSF be implicated in the malignant conversion of congenital neutropenic patients? Development of MDS/AML must be viewed in the context of the underlying primary problem. Prior to the availability of G-CSF therapy, it was recognized that leukemic transformation occurs occasionally in patients with KS/congenital neutropenia.[237–240] However, in the pre-cytokine era, many KS/congenital neutropenia patients died in the first years of life from other causes. Of published cases, 42% of patients died at a mean age of 2 years secondary to sepsis and pneumonia.[49] Thus, the true risk of congenital neutropenia patients developing MDS/AML was not defined. Currently, with G-CSF therapy, most patients do not develop life-threatening infections and survive, but it is not known if longer survival will allow for the natural expression of leukemogenesis in this population. Moreover, since the long-term effects of G-CSF are barely known beyond 10 years of observation, it is still unclear whether MDS or AML will occur with increased frequency in patients who receive prolonged therapy with G-CSF to correct the neutropenia.

Differential diagnosis

The commonest cause of isolated neutropenia in very young children is *viral-induced marrow suppression*. An antecedent history of good health, the occurrence of a viral illness, and the transient nature of the neutropenia distinguishes this disorder from KS/congenital neutropenia. Autoimmune neutropenia of infancy is being recognized more frequently as a fairly specific syndrome of early childhood. Low neutrophil numbers are often discovered during the course of routine investigation for a benign febrile illness. The illness abates but the neutropenia persists, sometimes for months and occasionally longer than a year. A marrow biopsy is normocellular and an aspirate shows active granulopoiesis up to the band stage; neutrophils may be normally represented or reduced. The neutropenia is due to increased peripheral destruction and the diagnosis is confirmed serologically by demonstrating antigranulocyte antibodies. The prognosis is good, the neutropenia is self-limiting albeit protracted, and patients seldom develop serious bacterial infections due to it. Other infrequent acquired causes of severe, isolated neutropenia in this age group include marrow suppression from a drug or toxin, and neutrophil sequestration as part of a hypersplenism syndrome.

Of the inherited forms of neutropenia, *Shwachman–Diamond syndrome* can also manifest as isolated neutropenia but can be identified because of growth failure, the malabsorption component due to pancreatic insufficiency, fatty changes in the pancreas seen on CT scanning, and characteristic skeletal abnormalities (see above). Neutropenia can also be a prominent part of antibody deficiency syndromes, dysgammaglobulinemia and agammaglobulinemia; investigation of chronic neutropenia of childhood should include an immunoglobulin electrophoresis. Cyclic neutropenia is distinguished by predictable symptomatology, especially mouth sores every 21 days in classic cases, often associated with chronic gingivitis. A complete blood count 3 times a week for a month will demonstrate the diagnostic oscillation pattern with the 21-day nadir. Familial cases of neutropenia with an autosomal dominant mode of inheritance are also described; parents of all cases should be screened with a complete blood count.

Therapy and prognosis

Prior to the introduction of G-CSF as a specific therapy of KS and other forms of severe chronic neutropenia, there was limited treatment. Antibiotics were the mainstay of management for active infection and for prophylaxis. Attempts to mobilize neutrophils in KS with lithium had narrow application.[241,242]

Cytokines

G-CSF has supplanted all other forms of management and should be initiated as front-line treatment when the diagnosis is established.[243] GM-CSF in cross-over trials with G-CSF for KS is not as effective and does not induce a neutrophil response consistently. The starting dose of G-CSF is 5 μg/kg/day subcutaneously and can be escalated until the desired neutrophil number is achieved. Neutrophils $>500/\mu l$ generally afford some protection from infection but counts $>1000/\mu l$ are clearly safer.

Documentation of the efficacy of G-CSF for SCN is described in a definitive phase III randomized controlled trial.[244] The trial enrolled 123 patients (60 congenital, 21 cyclic and 42 idiopathic) of whom 120 had evaluable responses. Defining a complete response over the 4-month treatment period and beyond as the maintenance of median neutrophil numbers $>1500/\mu l$, 90% of patients showed a complete response to G-CSF therapy, and infection-related events and antibiotic use were significantly decreased. Safety data were analyzed[245] and events related to the treatment were generally mild and consisted of headache, general musculoskeletal pain, transient bone pain and rash. None of these required the discontinuation of G-CSF. Thus, the vast majority of patients benefited substantially from G-CSF therapy with minimal adverse or toxic effects and almost all of the originally treated patients entered a long-term G-CSF maintenance program. The reduction in fevers, infections and inflammation translated into a well-documented improvement in the quality of life for these patients.

In the SCNIR 1996 annual report (on file at Clinical Safety, AMGEN Boulder Inc, 3200 Walnut Street, Boulder, CO, 80301, USA), the consistent sustained hematologic response in patients treated with G-CSF for >8 years was confirmed. With therapy, neutrophil counts rose in $>90\%$ of SCN patients and were maintained at a plateau for protracted periods, resulting in vast clinical benefits. In no instance has there been marrow or hematopoietic lineage 'exhaustion' or depletion with G-CSF therapy. The overall safety of long-term administration of G-CSF is reviewed in detail by Freedman.[243]

Bone marrow transplantation

Prior to the use of G-CSF, BMT was tried in a small number of KS patients with mixed success. Data from the International Bone Marrow Transplantation Registry are limited; the small series is heterogeneous with regard to donor source and clinical status of patients at the time of the procedure. In the SCNIR database, 13 KS patients who developed MDS/AML were transplanted after the transformation. Only 3 appeared to be cured of MDS/AML and KS. Results may have been better but 9 of the procedures were from matched unrelated donors or were performed in desperation using mismatched donors. One of the 3 who appeared cured by

BMT died of liver failure secondary to chronic hepatitis from type C virus infection.

THROMBOCYTOPENIA WITH ABSENT RADII

TAR syndrome was first described in 1929,[246] defined by Hall et al[247] in 1969, and subsequently reviewed.[248] The two essential features of TAR syndrome are hypomegakaryocytic thrombocytopenia (see Chapter 21) and bilateral radial aplasia. The rest of the phenotype varies widely and can manifest with abnormalities involving skeletal, skin, gastrointestinal and cardiac systems.

Most of the genetic evidence supports an autosomal recessive mode of inheritance for TAR syndrome since many families have been observed with >1 affected sibling. The possibility of other modes of inheritance has been raised however.[248] Almost always, parents of TAR patients are phenotypically normal. Females with TAR syndrome can conceive and give birth to hematologically and phenotypically normal offspring.

Aside from the occurrence of 1 case of ALL in a child with TAR syndrome,[249] there is no predisposition to leukemia nor to other bone marrow dysfunction or cancer.

Clinical features

The diagnosis is made in the newborn period because of the absent radii, and in about half of patients because of a petechial rash and overt hemorrhage such as bloody diarrhea. Patients have bilateral radial aplasia (Fig. 1.4) with preservation of thumbs and fingers on both sides. Additional upper extremity deformities include radial club hands,

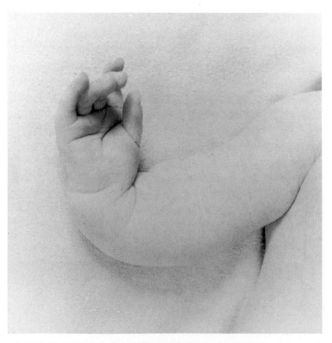

Fig. 1.4 Radial aplasia with preservation of the thumb in a newborn with TAR syndrome.

hypoplastic carpals and phalanges, and hypoplastic ulnae, humeri and shoulder girdles. Syndactyly and clinodactyly of toes and fingers are also seen. Characteristic findings include a selective hypoplasia of the middle phalanx of the fifth finger and altered palmar contours. Upper extremity involvement ranges from isolated absent radii to true phocomelia, often asymmetric. The lower extremities are involved in about half of cases. Malformations include hip dislocation, coxa valga, femoral torsion, tibial torsion, abnormal tibiofibular joints, small feet and valgus and varus foot deformities. Abnormal toe placement is commonly seen, especially the fifth toe overlapping the fourth. Like upper limb involvement, lower extremity deformities range from minimal involvement to complete phocomelia. An asymmetric first rib, cervical rib, cervical spina bifida and fused cervical spine can occur, but trunk involvement is usually minimal. Micrognathia has been associated with the TAR syndrome in up to 65% of cases.

Cardiac abnormalities occur in one-third of patients. The commonest are atrial septal defect, tetralogy of Fallot and ventricular septal defect. Facial hemangiomas are common, as well as redundant nuchal folds. Hays et al[250] described 3 additional findings in TAR syndrome: dorsal pedal edema, hyperhidrosis and gastrointestinal disturbances such as diarrhea and feeding intolerance.

There are important clinical differences that distinguish TAR syndrome from *Fanconi's anemia*. In Fanconi's patients, when radii are absent thumbs are hypoplastic or absent. Fanconi's patients do not have skin hemangiomas like some TAR patients, whereas TAR patients do not show abnormal skin pigmentation like 65% of Fanconi's patients. Confirmation of Fanconi's anemia is made by the clastogenic chromosome stress test showing increased fragility (see above); TAR patients do not have increased chromosomal breakage.

Prenatal diagnosis has been demonstrated readily both by quantitating platelet numbers obtained by fetoscopy or cordocentesis, and by imaging. In 1 confirmed case, a prenatal *in utero* platelet transfusion was given to effect a safe delivery.[251]

Laboratory features

Thrombocytopenia due to bone marrow underproduction is a consistent finding. Marrow specimens show normal to increased cellularity with decreased to absent megakaryocytes. The erythroid and myeloid lineages are normally represented. When a few megakaryocytes can be identified in biopsies they are small, contain few nuclear segments and show immature non-granular cytoplasm. If platelet counts increase spontaneously in patients after the first year of life, megakaryocytes increase in parallel and appear more mature morphologically. At diagnosis, leukocytosis is seen in the majority of patients and is sometimes extreme (>100 × 10^9/l) with a 'left shift' to immature myeloid forms. The cause of this leukemoid reaction is unclear but it is usually transient and subsides spontaneously. If anemia is present, the likeliest etiology is blood loss due to thrombocytopenia. When platelet numbers are adequate for study, their size is generally normal, with rare exception,[252] and function is unremarkable,[253-255] although some patients may show abnormal platelet aggregation and storage pool defects.[256-258] Unlike some of the other inherited marrow failure syndromes, red cell size and fetal hemoglobin levels are normal. Studies of spontaneous and clastogenic-induced chromosome breakage are also normal.

Etiology and pathogenesis

Thrombocytopenia in TAR syndrome is due to a defect in megakaryocytopoiesis/thrombocytopoiesis.[259,260] Initial contradictory data claiming either high levels of 'megakaryocyte-CSA' in sera of TAR patients,[259,261] or normal levels,[260] have been resolved. Thrombopoietin levels in serum are consistently elevated in TAR syndrome, thereby excluding a cytokine production defect as a cause for thrombocytopenia in this disorder.[262] Also, expression studies of the thrombopoietin receptor, c-mpl, on the surface of platelets from TAR patients is normal and has a similar molecular weight to that from controls.[262] Marrow CFU-Meg progenitors are either absent,[259,261] or are present in normal frequencies, but are comprised of colonies in vitro with abnormal morphology.[260] Cells within these colonies are smaller and the number of cells per colony is much higher than in normal CFU-Meg colonies. CFU-GM and BFU-E colony growth is often increased.

Platelet response to adenosine diphosphate (ADP) or the thrombin receptor agonist peptide SFLLRN (TRAP) is normal in TAR patients.[262] However, in contrast to controls there is no in vitro reactivity of platelets from TAR patients to recombinant thrombopoietin as measured by testing thrombopoietin synergism to ADP and TRAP in platelet activation.[262] Thrombopoietin-induced tyrosine phosphorylation of platelet proteins in this setting is completely absent or markedly decreased. The results indicate that defective megakaryocytopoiesis/thrombocytopoiesis in TAR syndrome is due to a lack of response to thrombopoietin in the signal transduction pathway of c-mpl.

Therapy and prognosis

The risk of hemorrhage is greatest in the first year of life. Deaths are usually due to intracranial or gastrointestinal bleeding. If patients survive the first year of life, platelet counts spontaneously increase inexplicably to levels that are hemostatically safe and which do not require platelet transfusional support. A minority of patients have sustained, profound thrombocytopenia that does not improve spontaneously.

Similar to other inherited marrow failure disorders associated with thrombocytopenia, platelet transfusions should be used judiciously. Clinical bleeding or prophylaxis for orthopedic surgical procedures are appropriate indications.

Persistent platelet counts $<10 \times 10^9/l$ may require preventative platelet transfusions on a regular basis, especially in the first year of life when the expectation is that a spontaneous improvement in platelet numbers will ensue with time in most infants. Single donor platelets are preferred to multiple random donors to minimize the risk of alloimmunization. HLA partially-matched donors for platelets may be required if patients become refractory to transfusions.

As the overall prognosis for survival is good and because patients do not develop aplastic anemia, or leukemia with rare exception,[249] supportive management is the mainstay. In exceptional situations, profound persistent life-threatening thrombocytopenia can be successfully treated by BMT.[263] The role of thrombopoietin in the management of TAR patients is unclear. Elevated serum thrombopoietin levels at baseline[342] may predict a poor response to cytokine therapy. IL-11, another thrombopoietic cytokine, has yet to be studied in clinical trials; however, endogenous IL-11 serum levels in TAR patients are also elevated.[342] Androgens, corticosteroids and splenectomy are ineffective therapies for TAR syndrome.

INHERITED MARROW FAILURE AND MALIGNANT HEMATOPOIETIC TRANSFORMATION

Historically, the inherited marrow failure syndromes were classified as 'benign' hematology, which contrasted sharply with the malignant myeloid disorders. Patients with KS/congenital neutropenia, Shwachman–Diamond syndrome, Fanconi's anemia, CAT and Diamond–Blackfan anemia often died early in life from complications of their disorders. However, in the current era of advanced supportive care and availability of recombinant cytokines and other effective therapeutics, patients with these conditions usually survive the early years of life and beyond. With the extended lifespan of patients, a new natural history for some of these disorders is evident. As recently reviewed,[264] one of the most sobering observations is that most of these 'benign' disorders confer an inordinately high predisposition to MDS/AML. Thus, the distinction between 'benign' and 'malignant' hematology in the context of the inherited marrow failure disorders has become blurred, and a new clinical and hematologic continuum is evident.

Carcinogenesis occurs as a sequence of events driven by genetic damage and epigenetic changes. In the traditional view, the initiation of cancer starts in a normal cell through mutations from exposure to carcinogens. In the promotion phase that follows, the genetically altered, initiated cell undergoes selective clonal expansion that enhances the probability of additional genetic damage from endogenous mutations or DNA-damaging agents. Finally, during cancer progression, malignant cells show phenotypic changes, gene amplification, chromosomal alterations and altered gene expression.

In the inherited marrow failure syndromes described above, the first 'hit' or cancer-initiating step may be the constitutional genetic abnormality itself that initially manifests as the single- or multiple-lineage myelopathy. The 'predisposed' progenitor, already initiated, could conceptually show decreased responsiveness to the signals that regulate homeostatic growth, terminal cell differentiation or programmed cell death. The leukemic promotion and progression steps leading to MDS/AML could then ensue readily in the initiated pool of progenitors or stem cells. Discovery of the molecular defects that produce the marrow failure syndromes should elucidate the nature of the leukemogenic-initiating events in these conditions.

REFERENCES

1. Alter BP, Potter NU, Li FP. Classification and aetiology of the aplastic anaemias. *Clin Haematol* 1978; **7**: 431–465

2. Windass B, Vowels MR, O'Gorman Hughes D, White L. Aplastic anaemia in childhood: prognosis and approach to therapy. *Med J Aust* 1987; **146**: 15–19

3. Fanconi G. Familiäre infantile perniziosaartige Anämie (perniziöses Blutbild und Konstitution). *Jahrbuch Kinder* 1927; **117**: 257

4. Young NS, Alter BP. Clinical features of Fanconi's anemia. In: *Aplastic Anemia, Acquired and Inherited*. Philadelphia, PA: WB Saunders, 1994, pp 275–309

5. Estren S, Dameshek W. Familial hypoplastic anemia of childhood: report of eight cases in two families with beneficial effect of splenectomy in one case. *Am J Dis Child* 1947; **73**: 671–687

6. O'Gorman Hughes DW. The varied pattern of aplastic anaemia in childhood. *Aust Paediatr J* 1966; **2**: 228–236

7. Auerbach AD, Rogatko A, Schroeder-Kurth TM. International Fanconi Anemia Registry: relation of clinical symptoms to diepoxybutane sensitivity. *Blood* 1989; **73**: 391–396

8. Fanconi G. Familial constitutional panmyelocytopathy, Fanconi's anemia (F.A.) I. Clinical aspects. *Semin Hematol* 1967; **4**: 233–240

9. Butturini A, Gale RP, Verlander PC *et al*. Hematologic abnormalities in Fanconi Anemia: An international Fanconi Anemia Registry study. *Blood* 1994; **84**: 1650–1655

10. Auerbach AD. Fanconi anemia diagnosis and the diepoxybutane (DEB) test. *Exp Hematol* 1993; **21**: 731–733

11. Auerbach AD, Ghosh R, Pollio PC, Zhang M. Diepoxybutane test for prenatal and postnatal diagnosis of Fanconi anemia. In: Schroeder-Kurth TM, Auerbach AD, Obe G (eds) *Fanconi Anemia: Clinical, Cytogenetic and Experimental Aspects*. Berlin: Springer-Verlag, 1989, p 71

12. Auerbach AD, Alter BP. Prenatal and postnatal diagnosis of aplastic anemia. In: Alter BP (ed) *Methods in Hematology: Perinatal Hematology*. Edinburgh: Churchill Livingstone, 1989, p 225

13. Yoshida MC. Suppression of spontaneous and mitomycin C-induced chromosome aberrations in Fanconi's anemia by cell fusion with normal human fibroblasts. *Hum Genet* 1980; **55**: 223–226

14. Duckworth-Rysiecki G, Cornish K, Clarke CA, Buchwald M. Identification of two complementation groups in Fanconi anemia. *Somatic Cell Mol Genet* 1985; **11**: 335–341

15. Zakrzewski S, Sperling K. Genetic heterogeneity of Fanconi's anemia demonstrated by somatic cell hybrids. *Hum Genet* 1980; **56**: 81–84

16. Zakrzewski S, Sperling K. Analysis of heterogeneity in Fanconi's anemia patients of different ethnic origin. *Hum Genet* 1982; **62**: 321–323

17. Zakrzewski S, Koch M, Sperling K. Complementation studies between Fanconi's anemia cells with different DNA repair characteristics. *Hum Genet* 1983; **64**: 55–57

18. Strathdee CA, Duncan AMV, Buchwald M. Evidence for at least four Fanconi anemia genes including FACC on chromosome 9. *Nature Genet* 1992; **1**: 196–198

19. Joenje H, Lo Ten Foe JR, Oostra AB *et al*. Classification of Fanconi anemia patients by complementation analysis: evidence for a fifth genetic subtype. *Blood* 1995; **86**: 2156–2160

20. Buchwald M. Complementation groups: one or more per gene? *Nature Genet* 1995; **11**: 228–230

21. Joenje H. Fanconi anemia complementation groups in Germany and The Netherlands. *Hum Genet* 1996; **97**: 280–282

22. Strathdee CA, Gavish H, Shannon WR *et al*. Cloning of Fanconi anemia cDNAs through functional complementation. *Nature* 1992; **356**: 763–767

23. Lo Ten Foe JR, Rooimans MA, Bosnoyan-Collins L *et al*. Expression cloning of a cDNA for the major Fanconi anemia gene, FAA. *Nature Genet* 1996; **14**: 320–323

24. Chen M, Tomkins DJ, Auerbach AD *et al*. Chromosomal instability induced by bifunctional alkylating agents and severely reduced fertility in mice with a defective Fac gene. *Nature Genet* 1996; **12**: 448–451

25. Segal GM, Magenis RE, Brown M *et al*. Repression of Fanconi anemia gene (FACC) expression inhibits growth of hematopoietic progenitor cells. *J Clin Invest* 1994; **94**: 846–852

26. Gillio AP, Verlander PC, Batish SD *et al*. Phenotypic consequences of mutations in the Fanconi anemia FAC gene: an International Fanconi Anemia Registry study. *Blood* 1997; **90**: 105–110

27. Dutrillaux B, Dutrillaux AM, Buriot D, Prier M. The cell cycle in Fanconi anaemia. *Hum Genet* 1982; **62**: 327–332

28. Sabatier L, Dutrillaux B. Effect of caffeine in Fanconi anaemia: restoration of a normal duration of G_2 phase. *Hum Genet* 1988; **79**: 242–244

29. Hoehne H, Kubbies M, Schindler D, Poot M, Rabinovitch PS. BrdU-Hoechst flow cytometry links the cell kinetic defect of Fanconi anaemia to oxygen hypersensitivity. In: Schroeder-Kurth TM, Auerbach AD, Obe G (eds) *Fanconi Anaemia: Clinical, Cytogenetic and Experimental Aspects*. Berlin: Springer-Verlag, 1989, pp 174–182

30. Schindler D, Hoehn H. Fanconi anaemia mutation causes cellular susceptibility to ambient oxygen. *Am J Hum Genet* 1988; **43**: 429–435

31. Moustacchi E, Diatloff-Zito C. DNA semi-conservative synthesis is normal in Fanconi's anaemia fibroblasts following treatment with 8-methoxypsoralen and ultraviolet light or with X-rays. *Hum Genet* 1985; **70**: 236–242

32. Papadopoulo D, Guilouf C, Mohrenweiser H, Moustacchi E. Hypomutability in Fanconi anemia cells is associated with increased deletion frequency at the HPRT locus. *Proc Natl Acad Sci USA* 1990; **87**: 8383–8387

33. Coppey J, Sala-Trepat M, Lopez B. Multiplicity reactivation and mutagenesis of trimethylpsoralens-damaged herpes virus in normal and Fanconi anaemia cells. *Mutagenesis* 1989; **4**: 67–71

34. Freedman MH, Saunders EF. Hematopoietic stem cell failure of constitutional aplastic anemia. In: Hibino S, Takaku F and Shahidi NT (eds) *Aplastic Anemia*. Baltimore: University Park Press, 1978, pp 133–140

35. Saunders EF, Freedman MH. Constitutional aplastic anaemia: defective haematopoietic stem cell growth *in vitro*. *Br J Haematol* 1978; **40**: 277–287

36. Mera CL, Freedman MH. Clostridium abscess and massive hemolysis: unique demise in Fanconi's aplastic anemia. *Clin Pediatr* 1984; **23**: 126–127

37. Barton JC, Parmley RT, Carroll AJ *et al*. Preleukemia in Fanconi's anemia: hematopoietic cell multinuclearity, membrane duplication, and dysgranulogenesis. *J Submicrosc Cytol* 1987; **19**: 355–364

38. Shihab-el-Deen A, Guevara C, Prchal JF. Bone marrow cultures in dysmyelopoietic syndrome: diagnostic and prognostic evaluation. *Acta Haematol* 1987; **78**: 17–22

39. Lui VK, Ragab AH, Findley HS, Frauen BJ. Bone marrow cultures in children with Fanconi anemia and the TAR syndrome. *J Pediatr* 1977; **91**: 952–954

40. Chu JY. Granulopoiesis in Fanconi's aplastic anemia. *Proc Soc Exp Biol Med* 1979; **161**: 609–612

41. Greenberg BR, Wilson FD, Woo L *et al*. Cytogenetics and granulopoietic effects of bone marrow fibroblastic cells in Fanconi's anaemia. *Br J Haematol* 1981; **48**: 85–93

42. Auerbach AD, Weiner M, Warburton D *et al*. Acute myeloid leukemia as the first hematologic manifestation of Fanconi anemia. *Am J Hematol* 1982; **12**: 289–300

43. Daneshbod-Skibba G, Martin J, Shahidi NT. Myeloid and erythroid colony growth in non-anemic patients with Fanconi's anaemia. *Br J Haematol* 1980; **44**: 33–38

44. Bagnara GP, Strippoli P, Bonsi L *et al*. Effect of stem cell factor on colony growth from acquired and consitutional (Fanconi) aplastic anemia. *Blood* 1992; **80**: 382–387

45. Stark R, Thierry D, Richard P, Gluckman E. Long-term bone marrow culture in Fanconi's anaemia. *Br J Haematol* 1993; **83**: 554–559

46. Butturini A, Gale RP. Long-term bone marrow culture in persons with Fanconi anemia and bone marrow failure. *Blood* 1994; **83**: 336–339

47. Bagby GC Jr, Segal GM, Auerbach AD *et al*. Constitutive and induced expression of hematopoietic growth factor genes by fibroblasts from children with Fanconi anemia. *Exp Hematol* 1993; **21**: 1419–1426

48. Rosselli F, Sanceau J, Gluckman E, Wietzerbin J, Moustacchi E. Abnormal lymphokine production: a novel feature of the genetic disease Fanconi anemia. II. *In vitro* and *in vivo* spontaneous overproduction of tumor necrosis factor alpha. *Blood* 1994; **83**: 1216–1225

49. Alter BP. Inherited bone marrow failure syndromes. In: Handin RI, Stossel TP, Lux SE (eds) *Blood: Principles and Practice of Hematology*. Philadelphia: Lippincott, 1995, pp 227–291

50. Auerbach AD, Frissora CL, Rogatko A. International Fanconi anemia registry (IFAR): survival and prognostic factors. *Blood* 1989; **74**: 43A

51. Alter BP, Frissora CL, Halperin DS *et al*. Fanconi's anaemia and pregnancy. *Br J Haematol* 1991; **77**: 410–418

52. Gluckman E, Auerbach AD, Horowitz MM *et al*. Bone marrow transplantation for Fanconi anemia. *Blood* 1995; **86**: 2856–2862

53. Harris RE. The unified approach to the care of FA patients. *Fanconi Anemia Research Fund Inc Sci Lett* 1997; **27**: 9–16

54. Flowers ME, Zanis J, Pasquini R *et al*. Marrow transplantation for Fanconi anaemia: conditioning with reduced doses of cyclophosphamide without radiation. *Br J Haematol* 1996; **92**: 699–706

55. Deeg HJ, Socie G, Schoch G *et al*. Malignancies after marrow transplantation for aplastic anemia and Fanconi anemia: a joint Seattle and Paris analysis of results in 700 patients. *Blood* 1996; **87**: 386–392

56. Hamre MR, Kirkpatrick DV, Humbert JR. Squamous cell carcinoma of the tongue in a patient with Fanconi anemia post bone marrow transplant. *Pediatr Res* 1989; **25**: 151A

57. Davies SM, Harris RE, van Weel-Sipman MH *et al*. Unrelated stem cell transplant for Fanconi anemia. Fanconi Anemia Research Fund, Inc. *Sci Lett* 1998; **23**: 22

58. Gluckman E, Broxmeyer HE, Auerbach AD. Hematopoietic reconstitution in a patient with Fanconi's anemia by means of umbilical cord blood from an HLA-identical sibling. *N Engl J Med* 1989; **321**: 1174–1178

59. Wagner JE, Broxmeyer HE, Byrd RL *et al*. Transplantation of umbilical cord blood after myeloablative therapy: Analysis of engraftment. *Blood* 1992; **79**: 1874–1881

60. Bogdanic V, Nemet D, Kastelal A *et al*. Umbilical cord blood transplantation in a patient with Philadelphia-chromosome positive chronic myeloid leukemia. *Transplantation* 1993; **56**: 477–479

61. Vowels MR, Lam-Po-Tang R, Berdoukas V *et al*. Brief report: Correction of X-linked lymphoproliferative disease by transplantation of cord-blood stem cells. *N Engl J Med* 1993; **329**: 1623–1625

62. Issaragrassil S, Visuthisakchai S, Suvatte V *et al*. Brief report: Transplantation of cord-blood stem cells into a patient with severe thalassemia. *N Engl J Med* 1995; **332**: 367–369

63. Wagner JE, Kernan NA, Steinbuch M *et al*. Allogeneic sibling cord blood transplantation in forty-four children with malignant and non malignant disease. *Lancet* 1995; **346**: 214–219

64. Hashmi R, Sambrano JE, Morris JD *et al*. Unrelated stem cell transplant for Fanconi anemia. *Blood* 1996; **88 (Suppl 1)**: 267A

65. Rackoff WR, Orazi A, Robinson CA *et al*. Prolonged administration of granulocyte colony-stimulating factor (Filgrastim) to patients with Fanconi anemia: a pilot study. *Blood* 1996; **88**: 1588–1593

66. Alter BP, Scalise A, McCombs J, Najfeld V. Clonal chromosomal abnormalities in Fanconi's anemia: what do they really mean? *Br J Haematol* 1993; **85**: 627–630

67. Freie BW, Dutt P, Clapp DW. Correction of Fanconi anemia type C phenotypic abnormalities using a clinically suitable retroviral vector infection protocol. *Cell Transplant* 1996; **5**: 385–393

68. Lu L, Ge Y, Li ZH *et al*. CD34 stem/progenitor cells purified from cryopreserved normal cord blood can be transduced with high efficiency by a retroviral vector and expanded *ex vivo* with stable integration and expression of Fanconi anemia complementation C gene. *Cell Transplant* 1995; **4**: 493–503

69. Walsh CE, Grompe M, Vanin E *et al*. A functionally active retrovirus vector for gene therapy in Fanconi anemia group C. *Blood* 1994; **84**: 453–459

70. Walsh C. Gene therapy trial for Fanconi anemia: An update. *Fanconi Anemia Research Fund Inc Sci Lett* 1997; **21**: 11

71. Shwachman H, Diamond LK, Oski FA, Khaw K-T. The syndrome of pancreatic insufficiency and bone marrow dysfunction. *J Pediatr* 1964; **65**: 645–663

72. Bodian M, Sheldon W, Lightwood R. Congenital hypoplasia of the exocrine pancreas. *Acta Paediatr* 1964; **53**: 282–293

73. Aggett PJ, Cavanagh NPC, Matthew DJ *et al*. Shwachman's syndrome: a review of 21 cases. *Arch Dis Child* 1980; **55**: 331–347

74. Kopelman H, Corey M, Gaskin K *et al*. Impaired chloride secretion as well as bicarbonate secretion, underlies the fluid secretory defect in the cystic fibrosis pancreas. *Gastroenterology* 1988; **95**: 349–355

75. Mack DR, Forstner GG, Wilschanik M, Freedman MH, Durie PR. Shwachman syndrome: Exocrine pancreatic dysfunction and variable phenotypic expression. *Gastroenterology* 1996; **111**: 1593–1602

76. Moore DJ, Forstner GG, Largman C *et al*. Serum immunoreactive trypsinogen: a useful indicator of severe exocrine pancreatic dysfunction in the pediatric patient without cystic fibrosis. *Gut* 1986; **27**: 1362–1368

77. Smith OP, Hann IM, Chessels JM *et al*. Haematological abnormalities in Shwachman–Diamond syndrome. *Br J Haematol* 1996; **94**: 279–284

78. Thong YH. Impaired neutrophil kinesis in a patient with Shwachman–Diamond syndrome. *Aust Paediatr J* 1978; **14**: 34–37

79. Aggett PJ, Harries JT, Harvey BAM, Soothill JF. An inherited defect of neutrophil mobility in Shwachman syndrome. *J Pediatr* 1979; **94**: 391–394

80. Ruutu P, Savilhati E, Repo H, Kosunen TU. Constant defect in neutrophil locomotion but with age decreasing susceptibility to infection in Shwachman syndrome. *Clin Exp Immunol* 1984; **57**: 249–255

81. Azzara A, Carulli G, Polidori R *et al*. *In vitro* restoration by lithium of defective chemotaxis in Shwachman–Diamond syndrome. *Br J Haematol* 1988; **70**: 502

82. Azzara A, Carulli G, Ceccarelli M *et al*. *In vivo* effectiveness of lithium on impaired neutrophil chemotaxis in Shwachman–Diamond syndrome. *Acta Haematol* 1991; **85**: 100–102

83. Paterson CR, Wormsley KG. Hypothesis: Shwachman's syndrome of exocrine pancreatic insufficiency may be caused by neonatal copper deficiency. *Ann Nutr Metab* 1988; **32**: 127–132

84. Saunders EF, Gall G, Freedman MH. Granulopoiesis in Shwachman's syndrome (pancreatic insufficiency and bone marrow dysfunction). *Pediatrics* 1979; **64**: 515–519

85. Ikuta K, Sasaki H, Koiso Y *et al*. A case of Shwachman's syndrome (pancreatic insufficiency and bone marrow dysfunction): evaluation of hemopoietic disorder by *in vitro* culture technique. *Jpn J Clin Hematol* 1980; **21**: 1989–1991

86. Woods WG, Krivit W, Lubin BH, Ramsay NKC. Aplastic anemia associated with the Shwachman syndrome: *in vivo* and *in vitro* observations. *Am J Pediatr Hematol Oncol* 1981; **3**: 347–355

87 Woods WG, Roloff JS, Lukens JN, Krivit W. The occurrence of leukemia in patients with the Shwachman syndrome. *J Pediatr* 1981; **99**: 425–428

88. Suda T, Mizoguchi H, Miura Y *et al*. Hemopoietic colony-forming cells in Shwachman's syndrome. *Am J Pediatr Hematol Oncol* 1982; **4**: 129–133

89. Nezeloff C, Watchi M. L'hypoplasie congénitale lipomateuse du pancréas exocrin chez l'enfant (deux observations et revue de la littérature). *Arch Françaises Pediatr* 1961; **18**: 20–24

90. Stevens MJ, Lilleyman JS, Williams RB. Shwachman's syndrome and acute lymphoblastic leukaemia. *Br Med J* 1978; **ii**: 18–20

91. Caselitz J, Kloppel G, Delling G *et al*. Shwachman's syndrome and leukaemia. *Virchows Arch (A)* 1979; **385**: 109–112

92. Gretillat F, Delepine N, Taillard F *et al*. Shwachman's syndrome transformed into leukaemia. *Presse Médicale* 1985; **14**: 45–48

93. Kalra R, Dale D, Freedman MH *et al*. Monosomy 7 and activating ras mutations accompany malignant transformation in patients with congenital neutropenia. *Blood* 1995; **86**: 4579–4586

94. Pearson HA, Lobel JS, Kocoshis SA *et al*. A new syndrome of refractory sideroblastic anemia with vacuolization of marrow precursors and exocrine pancreatic dysfunction. *J Pediatr* 1979; **95**: 976–984

95. Stoddard RA, McCurnin DC, Shultenover SJ, Wright JE, DeLemos RA. Syndrome of refractory sideroblastic anemia with vacuolization of marrow precursors and exocrine pancreatic dysfunction presenting in the neonate. *J Pediatr* 1981; **99**: 259–261

96. Demeocq F, Storme G, Schaison G *et al*. Anémie refractaire sideroblastique avec vacuolisation des precurseurs medullaires et défficit de la fonction exocrine du pancreas. Etude d'une nouvelle observation. *Arch Française Pediatr* 1983; **40**: 631–635

97. Favaretto F, Caprino D, Micalizzi C *et al*. New clinical aspects of Pearson's syndrome. Report of three cases. *Haematologica* 1989; **74**: 591–594

98. Larsson N-G, Holme E, Kristiansson B, Oldfors A, Tulinius M. Progressive increase of the mutated mitochondrial DNA fraction in Kearns-Sayre syndrome. *Pediatr Res* 1990; **28**: 131–136

99. Rotig A, Cormier V, Blanche S *et al*. Pearson's marrow-pancreas syndrome. A multisystem mitochondrial disorder in infancy. *J Clin Invest* 1990; **86**: 1601–1608

100. Majander A, Suomalainen A, Vettenranta K *et al*. Congenital hypoplastic anemia, diabetes, and severe renal tubular dysfunction associated with a mitochondrial DNA deletion. *Pediatr Res* 1991; **30**: 327–330

101. McShane MA, Hammans SR, Sweeney M *et al*. Pearson syndrome and mitochondrial encephalomyopathy in a patient with a deletion of mtDNA. *Am J Hum Genet* 1991; **48**: 39–42

102. Jakobs C, Danse P, Veerman AJP. Organic aciduria in Pearson syndrome. *Eur J Pediatr* 1991; **150**: 684

103. Cormier V, Rotig A, Bonnefont JP *et al*. Pearson's syndrome. *Arch Française Pediatr* 1991; **48**: 171–178

104. Bonilla MA, Gilmore B, Gillio A *et al*. *In vivo* administration of recombinant G-CSF corrects the neutropenia associated with Shwachman–Diamond syndrome. *Blood* 1989; **74**: 324A

105. Adachi N, Tsuchiya H, Nunoi H *et al*. rhG-CSF for Shwachman's syndrome. *Lancet* 1990; **336**: 1136

106. Grill J, Bernaudin F, Dresch C, Lumerie S, Reinert P. Traitement de la neutropenie du syndrome de Shwachman par le facteur de croissance des granuleux (G-CSF). *Arch Françaises Pediatr* 1993; **50**: 331–333

107. Vic PH, Nelken B, Mazingue F *et al*. Effect of recombinant human granulocyte and granulocyte-macrophage colony-stimulating factor in Shwachman's syndrome. *Int J Pediatr Hematol Oncol* 1996; **3**: 463–466

108. Barrios NJ, Kirkpatrick DV. Successful cyclosporin A treatment of aplastic anaemia in Shwachman–Diamond syndrome. *Br J Haematol* 1990; **74**: 540–541

109. Barrios NJ, Kirkpatrick DV. Bone marrow transplant in Shwachman–Diamond syndrome. *Br J Haematol* 1991; **79**: 337–338

110. Tsai PH, Sahdev I, Herry A, Lipton JM. Fatal cyclophosphamide-induced congestive heart failure in a 10-year-old boy with Shwachman–Diamond syndrome and severe bone marrow failure treated with allogeneic bone marrow transplantation. *Am J Pediatr Hematol Oncol* 1990; **12**: 472–476

111. Seymour JF, Escudier SM. Acute leukaemia complicating bone marrow hypoplasia in an adult with Shwachman's syndrome. *Leukaemia Lymphoma* 1993; **12**: 131–135

112. Smith OP, Chan MY, Evans JP, Veys P. Shwachman–Diamond syndrome and matched unrelated donor BMT. *Bone Marrow Transplant* 1995; **16**: 717–718

113. Arseniev L, Diedrich H, Link H. Allogeneic bone marrow transplantation in a patient with Shwachman–Diamond syndrome. *Ann Hematol* 1996; **72**: 83–84

114. Savilahti E, Rapola J. Frequent myocardial lesions in Shwachman's syndrome: eight fatal cases among 16 Finnish patients. *Acta Paediatr Scand* 1984; **73**: 642–651

115. Zinsser F. Atrophia cutis reticularis cum pigmentatione, dystrophia unguium et leukoplakia oris. *Ikonogr Dermatol (Hyoto)* 1906; **5**: 219–223

116. Engmann MF. A unique case of reticular pigmentation of the skin with atrophy. *Arch Dermatol Syphiligraph* 1926; **13**: 685–687

117. Cole HN, Rauschkolb JC, Toomey J. Dyskeratosis congenita with pigmentation, dystrophia unguis and leukokeratosis oris. *Arch Dermatol Syphiligraph* 1930; **21**: 71–95

118. Drachtman RA, Alter BP. Dyskeratosis congenita. *Dermatol Clin* 1995; **13**: 33–39

119. Dokal I. Dyskeratosis congenita: an inherited bone marrow failure syndrome. *Br J Haematol* 1996; **92**: 775–779

120. Connor JM, Gatherer D, Gray FC, Pirrit LA, Affara NA. Assignment of the gene for dyskeratosis congenita to Xq28. *Hum Genet* 1986; **72**: 348–351

121. Arngrimsson R, Dokal I, Luzzatto L, Connor JM. Dyskeratosis congenita: three additional families show linkage to a locus in Xq28. *J Med Genet* 1993; **30**: 618–619

122. Chambers JK, Salinas CF. Ocular findings in dyskeratosis congenita. *Birth Defects* 1982; **18**: 167–174

123. Kelly TE, Stelling CB. Dyskeratosis congenita: radiological features. *Paediatr Radiol* 1982; **12**: 31–36

124. Kalb RE, Grossman ME, Hutt C. Avascular necrosis of bone in dyskeratosis congenita. *Am J Med* 1986; **80**: 511–513

125. Berezin S, Schwarz SM, Slim MS *et al*. Gastrointestinal problems in a child with dyskeratosis congenita. *Am J Gastroenterol* 1996; **91**: 1271–1272

126. Auerbach AD, Adler B, Chaganti RSK. Prenatal and postnatal diagnosis and carrier detection of Fanconi anemia by a cytogenetic method. *Pediatrics* 1981; **67**: 128–135

127. Womer R, Clark JE, Wood P, Sabio H, Kelley TE. Dyskeratosis congenita: two examples of this multisystem disorder. *Pediatrics* 1983; **71**: 603–609

128. Pai GS, Yan Y, DeBauche DM, Stanley WS, Paul SR. Bleomycin hypersensitivity in dyskeratosis congenita fibroblasts, lymphocytes, and transformed lymphoblasts. *Cytogenet Cell Genet* 1989; **52**: 186–189

129. Drachtman RA, Alter BP. Dyskeratosis congenita: clinical and genetic heterogeneity. *Am J Pediatr Hematol Oncol* 1992; **14**: 297–304

130. Philips RJ, Judge M, Webb D, Harper JI. Dyskeratosis congenita: delay in diagnosis and successful treatment of pancytopenia by bone marrow transplantation. *Br J Dermatol* 1992; **127**: 278–280

131. Forni GL, Melevendi C, Jappelli S, Rasore-Quartino A. Dyskeratosis congenita: unusual presenting features within a kindred. *Pediatr Hematol Oncol* 1993; **10**: 145–149

132. Dokal I, Bungey J, Williamson P *et al*. Dyskeratosis congenita fibroblasts are abnormal and have unbalanced chromosomal rearrangements. *Blood* 1992; **80**: 3090–3096

133. Dokal I, Luzzatto L. Dyskeratosis congenita is a chromosomal instability disorder. *Leukemia Lymphoma* 1994; **15**: 1–7

134. Colvin BT, Baker H, Hibbin JA *et al*. Hematopoietic progenitor cells in dyskeratosis congenita. *Br J Haematol* 1984; **56**: 513–517

135. Friedland M, Lutton JD, Spitzer R, Levere RD. Dyskeratosis congenita with hypoplastic anemia: a stem cell defect. *Am J Hematol* 1985; **20**: 85–87

136. Marsh JCW, Will AJ, Hows JH *et al*. 'Stem cell' origin of the hematopoietic defect in dyskeratosis congenita. *Blood* 1992; **79**: 3138–3144

137. Hanada T, Abe T, Nakazawa M *et al*. Bone marrow failure in dyskeratosis congenita. *Scand J Hematol* 1984; **32**: 496–500

138. Yabe M, Yabe H, Hattori K *et al*. Fatal interstitial pulmonary disease in a patient with dyskeratosis congenita after allogeneic bone marrow transplantation. *Bone Marrow Transplant* 1997; **19**: 389–392

139. Conter V, Johnson FL, Paoluccy P *et al*. Bone marrow transplantation for aplastic anemia associated with dyskeratosis congenita. *Am J Pediatr Hematol Oncol* 1988; **10**: 99–102

140. Berthou C, Devergie A, D'Agay MF *et al*. Late vascular complications after bone marrow transplantation for dyskeratosis congenita. *Br J Haematol* 1991; **79**: 335–336

141. Ling NS, Fenske NA, Julius RL *et al*. Dyskeratosis congenita in a girl simulating chronic graft-versus-host disease. *Arch Dermatol* 1985; **121**: 1424–1428

142. Langston AA, Sanders JE, Deeg HJ *et al*. Allogeneic marrow transplantation for aplastic anemia associated with dyskeratosis congenita. *Br J Haematol* 1996; **92**: 758–765

143. Mahmoud HK, Schaefer UW, Schmidt CG *et al*. Marrow transplantation for pancytopenia in dyskeratosis congenita. *Blut* 1985; **51**: 57–60

144. Phillips RJ, Judge M, Webb D, Harper JI. Dyskeratosis congenita: delay in diagnosis and successful treatment of pancytopenia by bone marrow transplantation. *Br J Dermatol* 1992; **127**: 278–280

145. Storb R, Sanders JE, Pepe M *et al*. Graft-versus-host disease prophylaxis with methotrexate/cyclosporine in children with severe aplastic anemia treated with cyclophosphamide and HLA-identical marrow grafts. *Blood* 1991; **78**: 1144–1145

146. Gluckman E, Devergie A, Dutreix J. Bone marrow transplantation for Fanconi anemia. In: Schroeder-Kurth TM (ed) *Fanconi Anemia*. Berlin: Springer-Verlag, 1989, pp 60–68

147. Yel L, Tezcan I, Sanal O, Ersoy F, Berkel AI. Dyskeratosis congenita: unsual onset with isolated neutropenia at an early age. *Acta Paediatr Jpn* 1996; **38**: 288–290

148. Oehler L, Reiter E, Friedl J *et al*. Effective stimulation of neutropoiesis with rh G-CSF in dyskeratosis congenita: a case report. *Ann Hematol* 1994; **69**: 325–327

149. Pritchard SL, Junker AK. Positive response to granulocyte-colony-stimulating factor in dyskeratosis congenita before matched unrelated bone marrow transplantation. *Am J Pediatr Hematol Oncol* 1994; **16**: 186–187

150. Putterman C. Safadi R, Zlotogora J *et al*. Treatment of the hematological manifestations of dyskeratosis congenita. *Ann Hematol* 1993; **66**: 209–212

151. Russo C, Glader B, Israel R, Galasso F. Treatment of neutropenia associated with dyskeratosis congenita with granulocyte-macrophage colony stimulating factor. *Lancet* 1990; **336**: 751–752

152. Alter BP, Knobloch ME, He L et al. Effect of stem cell factor on in vitro erythropoiesis in patients with bone marrow failure syndromes. *Blood* 1992; **80**: 3000–3008

153. Freedman MH, Estrov Z. Congenital amegakaryocytic thrombocytopenia: an intrinsic hematopoietic stem cell defect. *Am J Pediatr Hematol Oncol* 1990; **12**: 225–230

154. Guinan EC, Lee YS, Lopez KD *et al*. Effects of interleukin-3 and granulocyte-macrophage colony-stimulating factor on thrombopoiesis in congenital amegakaryocytic thrombocytopenia. *Blood* 1993; **81**: 1691–1698

155. Muraoka K, Ishii E, Tsuji K *et al*. Defective response thrombopoietin and impaired expression of c-mpl mRNA of the marrow cells in congenital megakaryocytic thrombocytopenia. *Br J Haematol* 1997; **96**: 287–292

156. Freedman MH. Congenital failure of hematopoiesis in the newborn infant. *Clin Perinatol* 1984; **11**: 417–431

157. Henter JI, Winiarski J, Ljungman P *et al*. Bone marrow transplantation in two children with congenital amegakaryocytic thrombocytopenia. *Bone Marrow Transplant* 1995; **15**: 799–801

158. Zipursky A, Poon A, Doyle J. Leukemia in Down's syndrome. A review. *Pediatr Hematol Oncol* 1993; **9**: 139–149

159. Zipursky A, Thorner P, De Harven E, Christensen H, Doyle J. Myelodysplasia and acute megakaryoblastic leukemia in Down's syndrome. *Leukemia Res* 1994; **18**: 163–171

160. Wilroy RS, Tipton RE, Summitt RD. The Dubowitz's syndrome. *Am J Med Genet* 1978; **2**: 275–284

161. Emami A, Vats TS, Schmike RN, Trueworthy RC. Bone marrow failure followed by acute myelocytic leukemia in patient with Dubowitz syndrome. *Int J Pediatr Hematol Oncol* 1997; **4**: 187–191

162. Grobe H. Dubowitz syndrome and acute lymphatic leukemia. *Monatsschr Kinderheilkd* 1983; **131**: 467–468

163. Sauer O, Spelger G. Dubowitz syndrome with immunodeficiency and solid malignant tumor in two siblings. *Monatsschr Kinderheilkd* 1977; **125**: 885–887

164. Walters TR, Desposito F. Aplastic anemia in Dubowitz syndrome. *J Pediatr* 1985; **106**: 622–623

165. McKusick VA, Mahloudji M, Abbott MH *et al*. Seckel's bird-headed dwarfism. *N Engl J Med* 1967; **277**: 279–286

166. Upjohn C. Familial dwarfism associated with microcephaly, mental retardation and anemia. *Proc R Soc Med* 1955; **48**: 334–335

167. Lilleyman JS. Constitutional hypoplastic anemia associated with familial "bird-headed" dwarfism (Seckel syndrome). *Am J Pediatr Hematol Oncol* 1984; **6**: 207–209

168. Butler MG, Hall BD, Maclean RN, Lozzio CB. Do some patients with Seckel syndrome have hematological problems and/or chromosome breakage? *Am J Med Genet* 1987; **27**: 645–649

169. Gitlin D, Vawter G, Craig JM. Thymic alymphoplasia and congenital aleukocytosis. *Pediatrics* 1964; **33**: 184–192

170. Bujan W, Ferster A, Azzi N *et al*. Use of recombinant human granulocyte colony stimulating factor in reticular dysgenesis. *Br J Haematol* 1992; **81**: 128–130

171. Haas RJ, Niethammer D, Goldmann SF, Heit W, Bienzle U, Kleihauer E. Congenital immunodeficiency and agranulocytosis (reticular dysgenesis). *Acta Paediatr Scand* 1977; **66**: 279–283

172. Levinsky RJ, Tiedeman K. Successful bone-marrow transplantation for reticular dysgenesis. *Lancet* 1983; **1**: 671–673

173. Roper M, Parmley RT, Crist WM, Kelly DR, Cooper MD. Severe congenital leukopenia (reticular dysgenesis). *Am J Dis Child* 1985; **139**: 832–835

174. Gonzalez CH, Durkin-Stamm MV, Geimer NF *et al*. The WT syndrome: a "new" autosomal dominant pleiotropic trait of radial/ulnar hypoplasia with high risk of bone marrow failure and/or leukemia. *Birth Defects* 1977; **13**: 31–38

175. Arias S, Penchaszadeh VB, Pinto-Cisternas J, Larrauri S. The IVIC syndrome: a new autosomal dominant complex pleiotropic syndrome with radial ray hypoplasia, hearing impairment, external ophthalmoplegia, and thrombocytopenia. *Am J Med Genet* 1980; **6**: 25–59

176. Neri G, Sammito V. Re: IVIC syndrome report by Czeizel et al. *Am J Med Genet* 1989; **33**: 284–285

177. Li FP, Potter NU, Buchanan GR *et al*. A family with acute leukemia, hypoplastic anemia and cerebellar ataxia: association with bone marrow C-monosomy. *Am J Med* 1978; **65**: 933–940

178. Li FP, Hecht F, Kaiser-McCaw B, Barankoo PV, Potter NU. Ataxia-pancytopenia: syndrome of cerebellar ataxia, hypoplastic anemia, monosomy 7, and acute myelogenous leukemia. *Cancer Genet Cytogenet* 1981; **4**: 189–196

179. Alter CL, Levine PH, Bennett J *et al*. Dominantly transmitted hematologic dysfunction clinically similar to Fanconi's anemia. *Am J Hematol* 1989; **32**: 241–247

180. Aufderheide AC. Familial cytopenia and vascular disease: a newly recognized autosomal dominant condition. *Birth Defects* 1972; **8**: 63–68

181. Dokal I, Ganly P, Riebero I *et al.* Late onset bone marrow failure associated with proximal fusion of radius and ulna: a new syndrome. *Br J Haematol* 1989; **71**: 277–280

182. Yanabe Y, Nunoi H, Tsuchiya *et al.* A disease with immune deficiency, skin abscesses, pancytopenia, abnormal bone marrow karyotype, and increased sister chromatid exchanges: An autosomal recessive chromosome instability syndrome? *Jpn J Hum Genet* 1990; **35**: 263–269

183. Drachtman R, Weinblatt M, Sitarz A *et al.* Marrow hypoplasia associated with congenital neurologic anomalies in two siblings. *Acta Paediatr Scan* 1990; **79**: 990–993

184. Sleijfer DT, Mulder NH, Niewig HO *et al.* Acquired pancytopenia in relatives of patients with aplastic anemia. *Acta Med Scand* 1980; **207**: 397–402

185. Kato J, Niitsu Y, Ishigaki S *et al.* Chronic hypoplastic neutropenia. A case of familial occurrence of chronic hypoplastic neutropenia and aplastic anemia. *Rinsho Ketsueki* 1986; **27**: 407–411

186. Chitambar CR, Robinson WA, Glode LM. Familial leukemia and aplastic anemia associated with monosomy 7. *Am J Med* 1983; **75**: 756–762

187. Kaur J, Catovsky D, Valdimarsson H *et al.* Familial acute myeloid leukaemia with acquired Pelger-Huet anomaly and aneuploidy of C group. *Br Med J* 1972; **4**: 327–331

188. Abels D, Reed WB. Fanconi-like syndrome. Immunologic deficiency, pancytopenia, and cutaneous malignancies. *Arch Dermatol* 1973; **107**: 419–423

189. Linsk JA, Khoory MS, Meyers KR. Myeloid, erythroid, and immune system defects in a family. A new stem-cell disorder? *Ann Intern Med* 1975; **82**: 659–662

190. Li FP, Marchetto DJ, Vawter GR. Acute leukemia and preleukemia in eight males in a family: An X-linked disorder? *Am J Hematol* 1979; **6**: 61–69

191. Diamond LK, Blackfan KD. Hypoplastic anemia. *Am J Dis Child* 1938; **56**: 464–467

192. Halperin DS, Freedman MH. Diamond–Blackfan anemia: etiology, pathophysiology, and treatment. *Am J Pediatr Hematol Oncol* 1989; **11**: 380–394

193. Willig IN, Croisille L, Leblanc T *et al.* French register of Diamond–Blackfan anemia. Preliminary results. *Blood* 1996; **88 (Suppl 1)**:143A

194. Ball SE, McGuckin CP, Jenkins G *et al.* Diamond–Blackfan anaemia in the United Kingdom: analysis of 80 cases from a 20-year birth cohort. *Br J Haematol* 1996; **94**: 645–653

195. Dale D, Bonilla MA, Boxer L *et al.* Development of AML/MDS in a subset of patients (PTS) with severe chronic neutropenia (SCN) [abstract]. *Blood* 1994; **84 (Suppl 1)**: 518A

196. Dale DC, Cottle T, Bolyard AA *et al.* Severe chronic neutropenia: Report on treatment and outcome from a new international registry. *Blood* 1995; **86 (Suppl 1)**: 425A

197. Boxer L, Dale D, Bonilla MA *et al.* Administration of r-met-HuG-CSF during pregnancy in patients with severe chronic neutropenia (SCN) [abstract]. *Blood* 1995; **86 (Suppl 1)**: 508A

198. Boxer L, Bonilla MA, Cham B *et al.* Severe chronic neutropenia: from the laboratory to the clinic. *Int J Hematol* 1996; **64 (Suppl 1):** 59

199. Kannourakis G, Kurtzberg J, Bonilla MA *et al.* Report on patients with glycogen storage disease 1b with severe chronic neutropenia treated with filgrastim. *Blood* 1996; **88 (Suppl 1)**: 349A

200. Zeidler C, Bonilla MA, Boxer L *et al.* Report on patients with severe chronic neutropenia refractory to G-CSF. *Blood* 1996; **88 (Suppl 1)**: 349A

201. Freedman MH, Bonilla MA, Boxer L *et al.* MDS/AML in patients with severe chronic neutropenia receiving G-CSF. *Blood* 1996; **88 (Suppl 1)**: 448A

202. Bonilla MA, Dale DD, Zeidler C *et al.* Long-term safety of treatment with recombinant human granulocyte colony-stimulating factor (r-metHuG-CSF) in patients with severe congenital neutropenias. *Br J Haematol* 1994; **88**: 723–730

203. Heussner P, Haase D, Kanz L *et al.* G-CSF in the long-term treatment of cyclic neutropenia and chronic idiopathic neutropenia in adult patients. *Int J Hematol* 1995; **62**: 225–234

204. Zeidler C, Reiter A, Yakisan E *et al.* Langzeitbehandlung mit rekombinantem humanen Granulozyten-Kolonien stimulierenden Faktor bei Patienten mit schwerer kongenitaler Neutropenie. *Klin-Padiatr* 1993; **205**; 264–271

205. Kostmann R. Infantile genetic agranulocytosis: a new recessive lethal disease in man. *Acta Paediatr Scand* 1956; **45 (Suppl 105)**: 1–368

206. Kostmann R. Infantile genetic agranulocytosis. A review with presentation of ten new cases. *Acta Paediatr Scand* 1975; **64**: 362–368

207. Falk PM, Rich K, Feig S *et al.* Evaluation of congenital neutropenic disorders by *in vitro* bone marrow culture. *Pediatrics* 1977; **59**: 739–748

208. Daghistani D, Jimenez JJ, Toledano SR *et al.* Congenital neutropenia: A case study. *Am J Pediatr Hematol Oncol* 1990; **12**: 210–214

209. Chusid MJ, Pisciotta AV, Duquesnoy RJ *et al.* Congenital neutropenia: Studies of pathogenesis. *Am J Hematol* 1980; **8**: 315–324

210. Barak Y, Paran M, Levin S, Sachs L. *In vitro* induction of myeloid proliferation and maturation in infantile genetic agranulocytosis. *Blood* 1971; **38**: 74–80

211. Parmley RT, Ogawa M, Darby CP Jr, Spicer SS. Congenital neutropenia: Neutrophil proliferation with abnormal maturation. *Blood* 1975; **46**: 723–734

212. Olofsson T, Olsson I, Kostmann R, Malmstrom S, Thilen A. Granulopoiesis in infantile genetic agranulocytosis. *In vitro* cloning of marrow cells in agar culture. *Scand J Haematol* 1976; **16**: 18–24

213. Amato D, Freedman MH, Saunders EF. Granulopoiesis in severe congenital neutropenia. *Blood* 1976; **47**: 531–538

214. Zucker-Franklin D, L'Esperance P, Good RA. Congenital neutropenia: An intrinsic cell defect demonstrated by electron microscopy of soft agar colonies. *Blood* 1977; **49**: 425–436

215. Nishihira H, Nakahata T, Terauchi A, Akabane T. Congenital neutropenia with a decrease in neutrophilic colony forming cells and with an abnormal colony stimulating activity. *Acta Haematol Jpn* 1977; **40**; 52–61

216. Komiyama A, Yamazaki M, Yoda S *et al.* Morphologic and functional heterogeneity of chronic neutropenia of childhood with normal neutrophil colony formation *in vitro*. *Am J Hematol* 1981; **11**: 175–182

217. Kawaguchi Y, Kobayashi M, Tanabe A *et al.* Granulopoiesis in patients with congenital neutropenia. *Am J Hematol* 1985; **20**: 223–234

218. Ishiguro A. Complement-mediated cytotoxicity against marrow late neutrophilic cells in Kostmann's syndrome. *Acta Haematol Jpn* 1987; **50**: 1196–1209

219. Coulombel L, Morardet N, Veber F *et al.* Granulopoietic differentiation in long-term bone marrow cultures from children with congenital neutropenia. *Am J Hematol* 1988; **27**: 93–98

220. Chang J, Craft AW, Reid MM *et al.* Lack of response of bone marrow, *in vitro*, to growth factors in congenital neutropenia. *Am J Hematol* 1990; **35**: 125–126

221. Bonilla MA, Gillio AP, Ruggiero M *et al.* Effects of recombinant human granulocyte colony-stimulating factor on neutropenia in patients with congenital agranulocytosis. *N Engl J Med* 1989; **320**: 1574–1580

222. Kobayashi M, Yumiba C, Kawaguchi Y *et al.* Abnormal responses of myeloid progenitor cells to recombinant human colony-stimulating factors in congenital neutropenia. *Blood* 1990; **75**: 2143–2149

223. Vadhan-Raj S, Jeha SS, Buescher S *et al.* Stimulation of myelopoiesis in a patient with congenital neutropenia; Biology and nature of response to recombinant human granulocyte-macrophage colony-stimulating factor. *Blood* 1990; **75**: 858–864

224. Glasser L, Duncan BR, Corrigan JJ Jr. Measurement of serum granulocyte colony-stimulating factor in a patient with congenital agranulocytosis (Kostmann's syndrome). *Am J Dis Child* 1991; **145**: 925–928

225. L'Esperance P, Brunning R, Good RA. Congenital neutropenia: *In vitro* growth of colonies mimicking the disease. *Proc Natl Acad Sci USA* 1973; **70**: 669–672

226. Parmentier C, Maraninchi D, Teillet F. Granulocytic progenitor cells

(CFC*) in a child with infantile genetic agranulocytosis (IGA) and in phenotypically normal parents. *Nouv Rev Française Hematol* 1980; **22**: 217–222

227. Kyas U, Pietsch T, Welte K. Expression of receptors for granulocyte colony-stimulating factor on neutrophils from patients with severe congenital neutropenia and cyclic neutropenia. *Blood* 1992; **79**: 1144–1147

228. Hammond WP, Chatta GS, Andrews RG, Dale DC. Abnormal responsiveness of granulocyte-committed progenitor cells in cyclic neutropenia. *Blood* 1992; **79**: 2536–2539

229. Hestdal K, Welte K, Lie SO *et al.* Severe congenital neutropenia: Abnormal growth and differentiation of myeloid progenitors to granulocyte colony-stimulating factor (G-CSF) but normal responses to G-CSF plus stem cell factor. *Blood* 1993; **82**: 2991–2997

230. Fukunaga R, Ishizaka-Ikeda E, Nagata S. Growth and differentiation signals mediated by different regions in the cytoplasmic domain of granulocyte colony-stimulating factor receptor. *Cell* 1993; **74**: 1079–1087

231. Dong F, van Buitenen C, Pouwels K *et al.* Distinct cytoplasmic regions of the human granulocyte colony-stimulating factor receptor involved in induction of proliferation and maturation. *Mol Cell Biol* 1993; **13**: 7774–7781

232. Bashey A, Healy L, Marshall CJ. Proliferative but not nonproliferative responses to granulocyte colony-stimulating factor are associated with rapid activation of the p21ras/MAP kinase signalling pathway. *Blood* 1994; **83**: 949–957

233. Dong F, Brynes RK, Tidow N *et al.* Mutations in the gene for the granulocyte colony-stimulating-factor receptor in patients with acute myeloid leukemia preceded by severe congenital neutropenia. *N Engl J Med* 1995; **333**: 487–492

234. Kalra R, Dale D, Freedman M *et al.* Monosomy 7 and activating ras mutations accompany malignant transformation in patients with congenital neutropenia. *Blood* 1995; **86**: 4579–4586

235. Tidow N, Pilz C, Teichmann B *et al.* Clinical relevance of point mutations in the cytoplasmic domain of the granulocyte colony-stimulating factor (G-CSF) receptor gene in patients with severe congenital neutropenia. *Blood* 1997; **89**: 2369–2375

236. Dong F, Dale DC, Bonilla MA *et al.* Mutations in the granulocyte-colony stimulating factor receptor gene in patients with severe congenital neutropenia. *Leukemia* 1997; **11**: 120–125

237. De Vries A, Peketh L, Joshua H. Leukemia and agranulocytosis in a family with hereditary leukopenia. *Acta Med Orientalia* 1958; **17**: 26–32

238. Gilman PA, Jackson DP, Guild HG. Congenital agranulocytosis: prolonged survival and terminal acute leukemia. *Blood* 1970; **36**: 576–585

239. Wong W, Williams D, Slovak ML *et al.* Terminal acute myelogenous leukemia in a patient with congenital agranulocytosis. *Am J Hematol* 1993; **43**: 133–138

240. Rosen RB, Kang SJ. Congenital agranulocytosis terminating in acute myelomonocytic leukemia. *J Pediat* 1979; **94**: 406–408

241. Barrett AJ. Clinical experience with lithium in aplastic anemia and congenital neutropenia. *Adv Exp Med Biol* 1980; **127**: 305–320

242. Chan HSL, Freedman MH, Saunders EF. Lithium therapy of children with chronic neutropenia. *Am J Med* 1981; **70**: 1073–1077

243. Freedman MH. The safety of long-term administration of G-CSF for severe chronic neutropenia. *Curr Opin Hematol* 1997; **4**: 217–224

244. Dale DC, Bonilla MA, Davis MW *et al.* A randomized controlled phase III trial of recombinant human granulocyte colony-stimulating factor (Filgrastim) for treatment of severe chronic neutropenia. *Blood* 1993; **81**: 2496–2502

245. Decoster G, Rich W, Brown SL. Safety profile of filgrastim (r-metHuG-CSF). In: Morstyn G, Dexter TM (eds) *Filgrastim (r-metHuG-CSF) in Clinical Practice.* New York: Marcel Dekker, 1994, p 267

246. Greenwald HM, Sherman I. Congenital essential thrombocytopenia. *Am J Dis Child* 1929; **38**: 1245–1251

247. Hall JG, Levin J, Kuhn JP *et al.* Thrombocytopenia with absent radius (TAR). *Medicine* 1969; **48**: 411–439

248. Hedberg VA, Lipton JM. Thrombocytopenia with absent radii. A review of 100 cases. *Am J Pediat Hematol Oncol* 1988; **10**: 51–64

249. Camitta BM, Rock A. Acute lymphoidic leukemia in a patient with thrombocytopenia/absent radii (TAR) syndrome. *Am J Pediat Hematol Oncol* 1993; **15**: 335–337

250. Hays RM, Bartoshesky LE, Feingold M. New features of thrombocytopenia and absent radius syndrome. *Birth Defects* 1982; **18**: 115–121

251. Weinblatt M, Petrikovsky B, Bialer M, Kochen J, Harper R. Prenatal evaluation and in utero platelet transfusion for thrombocytopenia absent radii syndrome. *Prenat Diagn* 1994; **14**: 892–896

252. Bessman JD, Harrison RL, Howard LC, Peterson D. The megakaryocyte abnormality in thrombocytopenia-absent radius syndrome. *Blood* 1983; **62 (Suppl 1)**: 143A

253. Thevenieau D, Mattei JF, Juhan I *et al.* Anomalies du membre superieur, thrombopénie et thrombopathie. A propos de trois observations. *Arch Française Pediatr* 1978; **35**: 631–640

254. Giuffre L, Cammarata M, Corsello G, Vitaliti SM. Two new cases of thrombocytopenia absent radius (TAR) syndrome: Clinical, genetic and nosologic features. *Klin Pediatr* 1988; **200**: 10–14

255. Armitage JO, Hoak JC, Elliott TE, Fry GL. Syndrome of thrombocytopenia and absent radii. Qualitatively normal platelets with remission following splenectomy. *Scand J Haematol* 1978; **20**: 25–28

256. Sultan Y, Scrobohaci ML, Rendu F *et al.* Abnormal platelet function, population, and survival-time in a boy with congenital absent radii and thrombocytopenia. *Lancet* 1972; **2**: 653

257. Day HJ, Holmsen H. Platelet adenine nucleotide "storage pool deficiency" in thrombocytopenic absent radii syndrome. *JAMA* 1972; **221**: 1053–1054

258. O'Flanagan SJ, Cunningham JM, McManus S, Otridge BW, McManus F. Thrombocytopenia-radial aplasia (TAR) syndrome with associated immune thrombocytopenia. *Postgrad Med J* 1989; **65**: 485–487

259. Homans AC, Cohen JL, Mazur EM. Defective megakaryocytopoiesis in the syndrome of thrombocytopenia with absent radii. *Br J Haematol* 1988; **70**: 205–210

260. de Alarcon PA, Graeve JA, Levine RF, McDonald TP, Beal DW. Thrombocytopenia and absent radii syndrome: defective megakaryo-cytopoiesis-thrombocytopoiesis. *Am J Pediat Hematol Oncol* 1991; **13**: 77–83

261. Kanz L, Kostielniak E, Welte K. Colony-stimulating activity (CSA) unique for the megakaryocytic hemopoietic cell lineage, present in the plasma of a patient with the syndrome of thrombocytopenia with absent radii (TAR). *Blood* 1989; **74 (Suppl 1)**: 248A

262. Ballmaier M, Schulze H, Strauss *et al.* Thrombopoietin in patients with congenital thrombocytopenia and absent radii: Elevated serum levels, normal receptor expression, but defective reactivity to thrombopoietin. *Blood* 1997; **90**: 612–619

263. Brochstein J, Shank B, Kerman N *et al.* Marrow transplantation for thrombocytopenia-absent radii syndrome. *J Pediatr* 1992; **121**: 587–589

264. Freedman MH. Congenital bone marrow failure syndromes and malignant hematopoietic transformation. *Oncologist* 1996; **1**: 354–360

Acquired aplastic anemia

JOHN J DOYLE AND MELVIN H FREEDMAN

Acquired aplastic anemia is an hematologic disorder characterized by peripheral blood cytopenias, reduced bone marrow cellularity and the absence of an underlying myeloproliferative disorder or malignancy.[1] In the absence of a definable syndrome or familial tendency, the disorder is considered to be acquired. The International Agranulocytosis and Aplastic Anemia Study (IAAAS)[2] defined aplastic anemia as:

- hemoglobin $\leqslant 100$ g/dl or hematocrit $\leqslant 0.30$;
- platelet count $\leqslant 50 \times 10^9$/l;
- white blood cell count $\leqslant 3.5 \times 10^9$/l or granulocytes $\leqslant 1.5 \times 10^9$/l.

Bone marrow biopsy must show a decrease in cellularity and the absence of significant fibrosis or neoplastic infiltration.

Severe aplastic anemia (SAA) is generally defined as either marked ($<25\%$) or moderate (25–50% with $<30\%$ of cells being hematopoietic) hypocellularity as estimated from a bone marrow biopsy and two of the following peripheral blood findings:

- granulocytes $<0.5 \times 10^9$/l;
- platelets $<20 \times 10^9$/l; or
- reticulocyte count $<1\%$ (corrected for hematocrit).[3]

Aplasia is categorized as very severe (vSAA) when the above criteria are met and the granulocyte count is $<0.2 \times 10^9$/l.[4]

EPIDEMIOLOGY

Reported incidence figures for aplastic anemia are influenced by numerous factors. Case ascertainment techniques have varied from retrospective chart reviews and audits of autopsy figures[5,6] to the more recent advent of prospective registry data.[2,7,8] Clustering of cases in areas with a relatively small population base can lead to higher estimates.[5] The current best data suggest that the incidence rate of aplastic anemia in childhood (<15 years) is 1–3/million children/

year (Table 2.1). A high proportion ($>70\%$) of children have severe disease at the time of presentation.[7] The sex incidence is roughly equal with no statistically significant difference in any single study; however, it is striking that there appears to be a slightly higher incidence in males in each study. Given the limitations of these studies (potential for incomplete patient accrual, differences in diagnostic criteria and assumptions regarding population at risk), there has been surprisingly little variation between regions over the last 2 decades. Most reports from Asia cite a relatively high incidence of aplastic anemia, possibly due to environmental or genetic differences.[9,10]

ETIOLOGY

Identified causes of aplastic anemia include:

- viral infections, notably hepatitis;
- drugs and toxins;
- immune disorders;
- thymoma.

However, the large majority of cases remain unexplained or idiopathic. In most series 70–80% of cases are idiopathic.[4,7,11,12] In a large prospective study by the French Cooperative Group,[7] the suspected etiology was recorded for 243 cases of aplastic anemia in children and adults diagnosed over a 3-year period (May 1984 to April 1987); 74% were idiopathic, 13% were associated with drugs, 5% with hepatitis, 5% with toxins and the rest were categorized as miscellaneous including 2 cases that were pregnancy related. Of the drug exposures, only 1 was associated with chloramphenicol, highlighting the largely historic nature of this drug as an etiologic agent of aplastic anemia in the western world.

Many case reports and series implicate a multitude of different drugs in the etiology of aplastic anemia (e.g. antimalarials,[13] chloramphenicol[14,15] and anticonvulsants[16,17]). Such reports are often confounded by patient

Table 2.1 Incidence of aplastic anemia in children in different regions of the world.

Region	Year	Age (years)	Male		Female		Reference
			Number	(/10^6/year)	Number	(/10^6/year)	
Baltimore	1970–78	<20	9	3.7	4	1.7	6
South Carolina	1970–81	<20	4	9.7	1	2.5	5
Israel and Europe	1980–84	<15	12	1.7	5	0.7	2
France	1984–87	<15	24	1.34 (87% SAA)	17	1.00 (73% SAA)	7
Bangkok	1989	<15	5	3.8	1	0.8	10
Nordic countries (used SAA criteria)	1982–93	<15	64	2.42	37	1.47	8

factors underlying illness and use of other medications. Despite these limitations such reports have been clear enough convincingly to implicate certain medications such as chloramphenicol,[14,15] gold compounds[18] and butazones;[19] however, for others the association may be nothing more than one of chance. Several larger-scale epidemiologic investigations have attempted to clarify the risk of aplastic anemia associated with medication use.

The IAAAS reported on the recent (preceding 6 months) medication history of 113 patients with aplastic anemia.[2] Comparisons were made with 1724 sex- and age-matched controls enlisted from patients admitted to the same hospitals for management of an acute illness or an elective procedure; a history of use of butazones (phenbutazone, oxyphenbutazone), indomethacin and diclofenac was more common in patients with aplastic anemia. For both the phenbutazones and indomethacin the risk was shown to be greater for chronic repeated use of the drug. The repeated use of salicylates tended toward an association with aplastic anemia but did not reach statistical significance. This study presumed that important drug exposures were confined to the preceding 6 months and that hospitalized controls reflect the pattern of use of these various medications in the local community.

The French Cooperative Group reported on 147 patients with aplastic anemia compared to 287 hospitalized controls and 108 neighbours.[20] Drug histories for the preceding 5 years were collected. These results implicated gold salts, D-penicillamine, salicylates (therapeutic use) and colchicine as causes of aplastic anemia. Statistically, the use of fenamates, indolic derivatives (indomethacin), propionic and carboxylic acids (diclofenac), allo/thiopurinol and sulfonamides could not be linked to aplastic anemia. An association between rheumatoid arthritis and aplastic anemia was noted which confounded the ability clearly to link anti-inflammatory agents with the disease. Similarly, the use of non-phenicol antibiotics appeared to be linked to aplastic anemia; however, the relationship to a recent history of an infectious episode confounded the interpretation of this result. The use of chloramphenicol and thiamphenicol was too limited to allow any conclusions.

Hepatitis-associated aplastic anemia is defined as the occurrence of aplastic anemia several weeks to months after the onset of what is usually an unremarkable hepatitis.[5–8,10,20,21] Most commonly, the hepatitis is not associated with any specific serologic marker, i.e. A–G.[21–23] It appears to be more common in males.

Exposure to different toxins (pesticides,[24–26] paints,[27] etc.) has often been implicated as a cause of aplastic anemia. Current industrial standards appear to have reduced this risk to the point that it is difficult to demonstrate clearly. Benzene and its metabolites have been implicated as a cause of aplasia.[28] For other compounds there is less certainty. In a large-scale epidemiologic investigation, the French Cooperative Group reported on the results of detailed interviews from 98 patients with aplastic anemia, 181 hospitalized controls and 72 neighbour controls matched for sex and age.[27] Occupational histories were grouped into several categories. Only exposures to glue and possibly paints (not statistically significant) were associated with aplastic anemia. The trend towards an association between aplastic anemia and paints supports the previous investigation of Linet et al.[29] There was no increased incidence in farmers despite their exposure to insecticides.

PATHOPHYSIOLOGY

The phenotype of aplastic anemia reflects the ultimate failure of hematopoietic progenitors to differentiate into erythroid, megakaryocytic or myeloid elements. This is the result of injury either to the stem cells themselves or the microenvironment or stroma that supports them within the bone marrow. Failure of the stem cells seems more probable, as borne out by studies that have demonstrated reduced numbers of CD34$^+$ peripheral blood and marrow cells,[30] reduced colony-forming cells (CFC), reduced long-term culture-initiating cells (LTC-IC),[31] poor colony growth in long-term marrow cultures (LTMC)[32] and a decrease in cobblestone area-forming cells.[33] Cross-over experiments, in which adherent cell-depleted marrow cells were inoculated onto preformed irradiated stroma, demonstrated that marrow cells from patients with aplastic anemia grew poorly on normal stroma while normal marrows grew well on the stroma layers prepared from patients with aplastic anemia.[32,34] None of these changes is predictive of the severity or duration of aplastic anemia or of the response to immunosuppressive therapy.

Support for microenvironment or stromal injury as a cause of aplastic anemia comes from the observations that some patients with aplastic anemia do not form a confluent stromal layer in LTMC, and that morphologic differences can be seen in the stroma.[32] These changes include a reduced number and shorter survival of hematopoietic foci, late or absent fat cells in some patients and early appearance in others, and in some a high level of CFU-F (fibroblast colony-forming unit). In one of the cross-over cultures, it was observed that the stromal layer of an aplastic anemia patient supported significantly reduced numbers of CFU-GM (granulocyte–macrophage CFU) from the marrow of a normal subject. Holmberg et al[35] analyzed the stromal cell function of 89 patients with aplastic anemia; 6 showed no stromal cell growth, 37 failed either to produce a confluent fibroblastoid layer and/or had deficient numbers of adipocytes or macrophages and the remaining 46 developed morphologically normal appearing stroma cell layers. Those patients with no stromal cell growth had a longer duration of aplasia and tended towards a poorer outcome; otherwise, there was no difference in disease severity or outcome between groups.

A proposed mechanism for microenvironmental injury leading to pancytopenia is through disruption of the cytokine networks that regulate hematopoietic differentiation. In a large study of children and adults, the Seattle group[35] demonstrated differences in basal and interleukin (IL)-1α-stimulated cytokine release from stromal cell layers of patients with aplastic anemia compared with normal controls. Some of the differences in cytokines, such as the increase in granulocyte colony-stimulating factor (G-CSF) and granulocyte–macrophage CSF (GM-CSF), constitute the expected humoral response of trying to stimulate marrow growth. Others, such as the elevation of macrophage inflammatory protein (MIP)-1α and the increase in leukemia-inhibitory factor (LIF) as well as the decrease in IL-1 receptor antagonist (IL-1ra), are uncertain in origin and effect. No differences in IL-6 were seen either basally or following stimulation with IL-1α. The latter is in contrast to the results of Dilloo et al[36] who studied 3 children with aplastic anemia and reported decreased IL-6 production when compared to controls following challenge with IL-1, tumor necrosis factor (TNF)-α and cytomegalovirus (CMV). Recently, significantly increased amounts of fetal liver tyrosine 3 (flt3) ligand in patients with aplastic anemia which return to normal following successful therapy have been reported.[37,38] This suggests that elevation of the flt3 ligand is a physiologic response to the cytopenias rather than an etiologic event.

Injury to either stem cells or stroma may occur in a number of ways, although at present immune mechanisms are favored as a common pathway for much of the damage.[39] Toxins and drugs may be directly injurious,

resulting in reduced number or function of stem or stromal cells. Certain persons may be genetically more susceptible to the actions of such compounds through variations in different metabolic pathways. Different compounds or metabolites may bind to macromolecules leading to an immune hapten-directed response against stem or stromal cells. In a similar way, viruses could directly infect stem or stromal cells leading to cell death and pancytopenia. Infection of progenitor cells could lead to cytokine-mediated destruction of the progenitor cells by cytotoxic lymphocytes. Expression of viral particles on the surface of infected cells could also lead to immune-mediated attack (Fig. 2.1).[40] These mechanisms can lead either directly to stem cell loss through direct toxicity or microenvironmental failure, or to immune suppression of marrow elements by an activated immune system.[41] Much of the support for immune-mediated injury is inferred from the successful use of immunosuppressive therapy (see below).

Analyses of T cells from patients with SAA have shown them to have predominantly a CD8+ phenotype, which provides further evidence for the importance of the immune system as a cause of aplasia.[42] Co-culture experiments have shown that T cells elaborate suppressive factors, most notably γ-interferon and TNF, that interfere with the

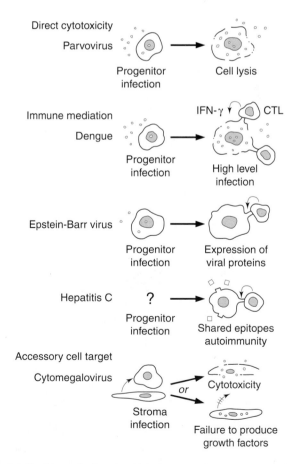

Fig. 2.1 Possible mechanisms by which viruses may induce hematopoietic failure. Reproduced with permission from Ref. 40.

mitotic cycle of hematopoietic precursors as well as causing apoptosis.[43-45] Interferon-γ and TNF induce expression of Fas receptors on CD34$^+$ hematopoietic stem cells, activation of which causes the cell to undergo apoptosis.[46-49]

DIAGNOSIS, CLINICAL PRESENTATION AND NATURAL HISTORY

Most children with aplastic anemia present with increased bruising or other bleeding manifestations, fatigue or infection.[8,50,51] Apart from these presenting signs and symptoms, they have generally been previously well and have normal physical examinations with no dysmorphic features. Family history is often unremarkable; however, one study found an over-representation of bone marrow hypoplasia and hematologic malignancies in first-degree relatives.[8] Most children will have had symptoms for <1 month and >80% for <3 months.[7,8] Three-quarters of children meet the criteria for SAA at first presentation, while the remainder evolve to SAA over the next few years (median of 2 months). Thrombocytopenia is the commonest initial presenting cytopenia.[8]

Laboratory investigation shows anemia, leukopenia and/or thrombocytopenia conforming to the definition of aplastic anemia.

- Reticulocyte counts are reduced and the mean corpuscular volume (MCV) is increased.
- Bone marrow aspirate and biopsy are important morphologically to confirm the hypoplasia and to rule out malignant disease. Bone marrow cytogenetics should be done to look for evidence of a clonal disorder suggesting either a myelodysplastic or myeloproliferative process. Rarely, an acute leukemia presents initially with a period of hypoplastic anemia.[52] Examination of the bone marrow is also helpful to exclude megaloblastic anemia.
- Measurement of vitamin B$_{12}$ and red blood cell folate should also be made to exclude dietary deficiency as a cause of pancytopenia.
- A limited immune work-up (quantitative immunoglobulins, antinuclear factor, direct antiglobulin test, antineutrophil and antiplatelet antibody measurements) may implicate other etiologies and direct therapy differently.
- Liver function tests, viral serology (CMV, Epstein-Barr virus [EBV], parvovirus and hepatitis serology) and directed viral cultures are also of value in diagnosis and later management.
- Either a sugar water test or a Ham's acid serum test should be performed to look for evidence of paroxysmal nocturnal hemoglobinuria (PNH), although this is a very uncommon finding in childhood aplastic anemia.
- Chromosome fragility (breakage frequency) must be measured using a clastogenic agent to rule out Fanconi's anemia (see Chapter 1), a proportion of which patients will not have a dysmorphic appearance.[53]

- In some circumstances (short stature, nutritional deficit, history suggesting steatorrhea) it may be important to test pancreatic function to exclude Shwachman–Diamond syndrome (see Chapter 1).

Untreated aplastic anemia has a high fatality with early death occurring as a result of either an infectious episode or hemorrhagic event. Supportive modalities (transfusion and antibiotic therapy) have substantially improved survival. Specific therapy (immunosuppression or bone marrow transplantation [BMT]) has dramatically changed the outlook for children diagnosed with aplastic anemia. Clausen et al.[8] in a study of Nordic children under 15 years of age reported an actuarial survival at 1 year of 79%, and at 5 years of 68%. Median survival of those children who died was 8 months and the causes of death included infection (about one-third were fungal infections), complications of the BMT, intracranial bleeding and other bleeding.

TREATMENT

Supportive modalities should be used to treat infection and to prevent bleeding.

- Use of blood products must be judicious to minimize donor exposure.
- For CMV-negative recipients, the blood products should either be CMV negative or filtered.
- Whenever possible, single donor platelets should be used as opposed to pooled random donor product.
- HLA typing of the patient and family should be done on an urgent basis to facilitate early BMT or the searching of unrelated donor registries.

A decision on how to proceed with therapy should be made as quickly as possible for patients with SAA. Patients with moderate disease need the same work-up and careful follow-up. The approach to patients with moderate disease is less clear than for those with severe disease but appropriate steps should be taken to set the stage for early therapy should progression occur.

BONE MARROW TRANSPLANTATION

BMT as therapy for SAA has been investigated for almost 3 decades with successful transplantation being reported as early as 1970.[54] During the 1970s, BMT was established as the best therapy for aplastic anemia.[3] At that time, alternative therapy consisted of transfusion support with or without androgens. Subsequent investigators have explored the optimal conditioning regimen and means of graft-versus-host disease (GVHD) prophylaxis to overcome the problems of failure to engraft and significant GVHD. As results have improved, investigators have begun to evaluate the use of donors other than HLA-matched siblings. This is increasingly important as family donors are found for only a fraction of patients.

Matched sibling donor BMT

For children and young adults afflicted with SAA, early BMT from a fully HLA-matched sibling donor is considered best therapy. Several recent trials are reporting overall survivals of 79–100% following matched sibling donor BMT.[55–58] Cyclophosphamide (200 mg/kg over 4 days) is the most commonly used conditioning agent in BMT for SAA. Various groups have used cyclophosphamide on its own, with limited field irradiation (total lymphoid [TLI] or thoraco-abdominal [TAI]) and total body irradiation (TBI).[59] Following a report from the Seattle group,[57] there has been increasing enthusiasm for the use of cyclophosphamide with antithymocyte globulin (ATG).[55,60] The use of cyclophosphamide is associated with high rates of long-term survival when accompanied by the use of cyclosporine A as GVHD prophylaxis.[56,58,59] The need for conditioning therapy is borne out by the high incidence of graft failure seen with syngeneic (identical twin) BMT. In the largest report, 16 of 23 patients given syngeneic marrow without first receiving conditioning therapy of some kind failed to engraft.[61]

Failed engraftment has been a significant problem in matched sibling BMT for SAA. Data from the European Bone Marrow Transplant (EBMT) registry[62] showed a graft rejection rate of 32% prior to 1980, 8.8% between 1980 and 1984, and 7.6% after 1984. The Seattle group reported no change in the incidence of graft rejection in children transplanted prior to or following 1980,[56] but the pattern of graft loss changed from early to late rejection. They attributed the latter to the increased use of cyclosporine A GVHD prophylactic regimens during the 1980s. Early transplantation in patients who are minimally transfused is associated with a lower incidence of graft rejection,[56,59,62,63] as is the addition of irradiation,[59,62,63] and use of higher marrow doses ($>3 \times 10^8$ cells/kg).[56] Post-transplant immunosuppression is also a factor in decreasing the incidence of graft rejection. The use of cyclosporine A GVHD prophylactic regimens is associated with lower rates of graft failure,[58,59,62,63] and cyclophosphamide and ATG conditioning with cyclosporine A with or without short-course methotrexate results in an engraftment failure rate of 0–5%.[55,57,60]

GVHD is a significant problem for children undergoing matched sibling BMT. The probability of acute GVHD (grades II–IV) in children undergoing matched sibling BMT and receiving only methotrexate for GVHD prophylaxis was about 27%.[64] The use of cyclosporine with methotrexate reduced acute GVHD to about 11%.[65] The incidence of chronic GVHD has not been influenced by cyclosporine A and occurs in about 30% of patients.[56,57] Approximately one-fifth of patients who develop chronic GVHD die of associated complications.[56]

Long-term sequelae on growth and endocrine function have been minimal. The use of only chemotherapeutic agents and relatively low-dose radiation therapy spares the thyroid gland. Secondary sexual characteristics develop at an appropriate age and the frequency of impairment to ovarian or testicular endocrine function is low. Many of these children are able to have children.[56]

Second malignant tumors are a further consequence of successful therapy. Although leukemias are sometimes seen post-BMT for aplastic anemia, more commonly the problem is solid tumors, particularly epidermoid carcinomas. In a combined long-term follow-up of patients treated in Seattle and Paris, the incidence of any second malignancy at 10 years is 14% (95% CI 4–24%) and for solid tumors 13% (95% CI 3–23%).[66] In univariate analysis, the use of irradiation in the conditioning regimen, development of acute or chronic GVHD, treatment of GVHD with azathioprine, male sex and patient age were significant risk factors for the development of a second tumour; in multivariate analysis, only treatment of GVHD with azathioprine, age and irradiation retained their significance. The European BMT–SAA working party in a review of their registry data noted a lower incidence of second tumors with an overall rate of 3.1% (95% CI 1.6–6.2%), leukemia of 0.4% (95% CI 0.1–1.8%), and solid tumors of 2.9% (1.3–6.2%).[67] Male sex, age at diagnosis and the use of a radiation-based conditioning regimen emerged as significant predictors of second cancers in their multivariate analysis.

The role of irradiation requires further consideration. The Paris group noted that patients from within a cohort treated with TAI-based regimens who developed second solid malignancies did so within the penumbra of the radiation field.[68] The same group reported an 8-year cumulative incidence of second solid malignancies of 22% (1 SE = 11%).[69] The outcome of these patients was poor and subsequent therapy difficult.[70] The Seattle group reported a much lower incidence of second solid tumors from a group treated without irradiation, with a 10-year incidence of 1.4% (95% CI 0–3.4%).[71] The solid second tumors were primarily epidermoid carcinomas of the head and neck for both groups.

Alternative donor BMT

For the majority of children with aplastic anemia, matched sibling donors will not be available for BMT. Amongst available options under these circumstances is the use of alternative donors for BMT. In general, this requires a greater intensity of conditioning therapy to overcome the problem of failure to engraft and greater post-infusion immunosuppression to prevent GVHD.

The use of phenotypic HLA-matched family donors appears to give outcomes similar to the use of matched sibling donors. The EBMT working group reported 6 survivors among 9 such transplants.[72] Most of these patients had been previously treated with immunosuppressive therapy and/or androgens and underwent BMT as a last effort. Conditioning regimens were variable as was GVHD prophylaxis. The Seattle group reported on 9 patients transplanted from phenotypic family matches;[73,74] most underwent early transplantion with minimal pretreatment, although 8 were previously transfused. Eight were conditioned with cyclophosphamide alone. Two patients ultimately failed to engraft and required a second transplant from the same donor. All 9 are survivors, although 3 developed significant acute GVHD and 6 chronic GVHD. Karnofsky scores were 100% for 8 and 70% for 1 recipient who developed bronchiolitis obliterans. Their overall outcome is not that different from matched sibling donors.

BMTs from mismatched family member donors have been reported in several small series.[72,73,75] Hows et al[75] reported 3 mismatched family donor transplants performed between 1981 and 1986. The 1-antigen mismatch transplant (conditioned with cyclophosphamide and ATG) was a long-term survivor with successful engraftment and no significant GVHD. Two patients who received 2-antigen disparate transplants showed early toxic deaths, 1 from GVHD and the other from hemorrhage. The EBMT group[72] reported 3 survivors among 7 patients transplanted prior to 1988 from 1-antigen mismatched family members. Only 1 of 17 patients who received transplants from 2- or 3-antigen mismatched family members survived. There high rate of graft rejection and acute GVHD led to the observed mortality. The Seattle group[73] reported a series of patients grafted between 1970 and 1993 from mismatched family donors (mostly 1 antigen). Fifteen were conditioned using cyclophosphamide-based regimens with or without ATG. Ten failed to sustain first engraftment; 5 had second transplants but were not salvaged. At least 9 had acute GVHD of grade II or higher. All 15 died with infection being the ultimate cause of death in most. Eight of 16 patients transplanted under the same circumstances but having TBI in their conditioning survived; 12 engrafted successfully, at least 11 developed acute GVHD of grade II or higher and 6 of the survivors have chronic GVHD. Karnofsky scores for survivors range from 70 to 100% with a median of 90%. Infection was the leading cause of death.

Data regarding the outcome of unrelated donor BMT for SAA are limited. Margolis et al[76] presented current representative data on children (median age 8.5 years, range 9 months to 24 years) conditioned with cyclophosphamide, cytosine arabinoside and TBI. The grafts came from unrelated donors and were T-cell depleted. Four of 8 recipients of fully matched transplants survived compared with 6 of 11 patients who received 1-antigen mismatched marrows (class-1 mismatch) and 5 of 9 who received marrows that were class 2 mismatches or mismatched for >1 antigen. Regimen-related toxicity was high with interstitial pneumonia, adult respiratory distress syndrome (ARDS) and lymphoproliferative disorders. Severe infection was also common. Only 7 patients developed grade II or higher acute GVHD; 8 developed limited chronic GVHD and 2 extensive chronic GVHD. Overall survival for the group is 54%.

Recently, several groups have begun to use umbilical cord blood as a source of stem cells for BMT. Reports of the use of such cells for children with SAA are limited but it is clear that similar problems exist for this stem cell source. Of 6 pediatric patients transplanted from HLA-matched sibling placental blood, 3 failed to engraft and died despite attempts at rescue with allogeneic donor marrow.[77,78] Matched and mismatched unrelated cord-blood transplants have been done for the management of malignant diseases with reportedly low rates of acute GVHD.[79] Others have reported GVHD rates comparable to the use of bone marrow from matched unrelated donors.[80] The use of umbilical cord-blood transplants holds promise but more data are needed before any recommendation regarding its usefulness in the therapy of SAA can be made.

IMMUNOSUPPRESSIVE THERAPY

Based on reports implicating immune mechanisms as a cause of aplasia, attempts were made to treat aplastic anemia with immunosuppressive regimens.[81–85] ATG with or without other agents (androgens, haploidentical bone marrow and/or steroids) emerged as clearly more effective than supportive care alone.[11,86–88] Survivals ranged from 30 to 70%, with responses typically occurring within the first 3 months following therapy. Cyclosporine A was also shown to be effective.[89,90] In a randomized comparison of ATG with methylprednisolone versus cyclopsorine A using a cross-over design at 3 months for those with no or minimal response to first therapy, Gluckman et al[91] showed that the two therapies had equivalent responses with an overall survival of about 66% at 2 years. Notably, survival for patients under 10 years of age was 72% and for children between 10 and 18 years old was 60%. Patients with vSAA did significantly worse with a survival of 41.3% versus 65.5% for the others.

Other trials have focussed on the use of combination immunosuppressive therapy for aplastic anemia. The German group compared ATG and methylprednisolone versus ATG, methylprednisolone and cyclosporine A.[92] A cross-over design was used for patients who had not responded by 3 months. The response rate at 3 months was significantly higher in the group receiving cyclosporine A (65 versus 39%, p <0.03), primarily because of an increased response rate in patients with severe disease. Those with less severe disease had equivalent responses in both arms of the study. The improvement in outcome persisted at 6 months but the statistical significance was lost by 12 months due to patients having been crossed over to the other arm of the trial.

The Seattle group studied ATG, oxymethalone and low-dose steroids versus ATG, oxymethalone and high-dose steroids.[93] The latter component was based on the earlier work of Bacigalupo et al.[83,84] The outcome and response rates were similar in both the severe and moderate aplastic groups, with a 36% response rate in the low-dose steroid arm versus a 48% response in the high-dose arm. Response rates in this trial were lower than those these investigators had seen previously in a non-randomized trial of the high-dose therapy, which was accounted for by a higher early mortality across both of the study arms.

The EBMT compared ATG and methylprednisolone with or without androgens (oxymethalone).[94] Overall survival at 3 years was similar between groups (71% with androgens versus 65% without). For the entire group, survival was influenced by the severity of the aplasia with the very severe group having a 43% 3-year survival compared to 78% for severe disease and 83% for moderate disease. Despite the apparent lack of difference in survival, there was a significantly greater frequency of response in the androgen arm at 120 days (68% versus 48%, p = 0.02). This was particularly pronounced in females with severe aplasia. The failure of this to impact on overall survival probably reflects the censure of patients subsequently undergoing BMT as well as the success of different salvage regimens.

A common problem in the above investigations is recurrence of aplasia. Patients treated with immunosuppressive therapy regain apparently normal hematopoiesis but when more detailed studies are performed defects in the number and quality of progenitor cells are easily found.[31–34] A new but still tenuous balance in hematopoiesis is the result of successful immunosuppressive therapy. In the German study,[92] 10 of 52 responders had recurrent aplasia from 4 to 37 months after treatment. Of those treated with cyclosporine A, virtually all relapses occurred after withdrawal of the cyclosporine A. Seven of the 10 with recurrent aplasia responded to further immunosuppressive therapy. In the Seattle study,[93] 6 of 27 evaluable responders developed recurrent aplasia at a median of 8.6 months after therapy (range: 3.6–35.5 months). In a large study from the EBMT–SAA registry,[95] 74 of 358 patients treated with immunosuppressive therapy relapsed at a mean of 778 days from first immunosuppressive therapy. Thirty-nine showed a second response with further therapy. Those who responded most quickly to the original immunosuppressive therapy were at the highest risk of relapse. It should be noted that very few of these patients received cyclosporine A as part of their original immunosuppressive therapy. Rosenfeld et al[96] reported an 18% relapse rate at 1 year and 36% at 2 years following therapy with ATG and 6 months of cyclosporine A. Most of the relapsers responded to subsequent therapies.

The other manifestation of the tenuous balance in hematopoiesis attained by the use of immunosuppressive therapy is the development of clonal disorders characterized by the problems of myelodysplasia (MDS) and paroxysmal nocturnal hemoglobinuria (PNH) (Fig. 2.2). The use of X-linked restriction fragment length polymorphisms (RFLPs) has shown some cases of aplastic anemia to have clonal X-inactivation both at diagnosis and at later follow-up after immunosuppressive therapy.[97,98] Similar findings have been seen in children, although the frequency of clonal hematopoiesis was low.[99] Estimates of the frequency of clonal hematopoiesis range from only a few percent to 72%. Accumulated injury to clonal hematopoietic precursors may ultimately lead to the development of PNH or MDS and leukemia.[100]

Myelodysplasia

Several large studies have demonstrated the risk of MDS and/or leukemia in survivors of aplastic anemia.[93,101–104] Most commonly, MDS is diagnosed and then progresses to leukemia, although occasionally patients present with overt leukemia. In a long-term follow-up of patients surviving for more >5 years after the original diagnosis of aplastic anemia and treated primarily with androgens, 5 of 156 developed MDS.[103] All 5 cases occurred in adult patients (median age 52, range: 39–67) and all 5 died. In the EBMT experience of patients surviving for >2 years from initial immunosuppressive therapy with ATG regimens, 11 of 223 and 1 of 223 patients developed MDS and acute leukemia respectively, and 4 of these 12 died.[101] Five of the 11 who developed MDS had progressed to acute leukemia by the time of the report. MDS occurred at a median of 4.6 years (range: 2.5–7.5) post immunosuppressive therapy and acute leukemia by 5.0 years (range: 2.8–7.6). The median age of these patients at the time of diagnosis of aplastic anemia was 21 years (range: 9–56). The actuarial risk of MDS/leukemia at 7 years was 15% for these long-term survivors. Doney et al[102] reported that 20 of 227 patients with aplastic anemia treated with immunosuppressive therapy developed MDS/leukemia.

It is clear from the aggregate data that patients of any age diagnosed with aplastic anemia and treated with immunosuppressive therapy are at risk of the development of MDS and that the MDS will progress to an acute non-lymphoid leukemia. Treatment of these leukemias is associated with poor survival.

Paroxysmal nocturnal hemoglobinuria (see also Chapter 10)

PNH is an acquired clonal hematopoietic disorder characterized by hemolytic anemia, thrombosis and progression to pancytopenia. At the molecular level it is the result of mutations in the phosphatidyl glycan class A (PIGA) gene on the short arm of the X chromosome. The mutation leads to a defect in the glycosylphosphatidynylinositol (GPI) anchor and the loss of several of the normal membrane proteins that are usually fixed to the membrane via this anchor. Chief among these are CD55 (decay accelerating factor) and CD59 (membrane inhibitor of reactive lysis).

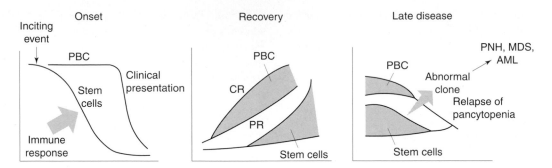

Fig. 2.2 Stem cell counts and peripheral blood counts (PBC) during the course of immune-mediated aplastic anemia. The left-hand panel shows the onset of disease. After an inciting event, such as drug exposure or viral infection, the hematopoietic compartment is destroyed by the immune system. Small numbers of surviving stem cells support adequate hematopoiesis for some time but eventually the cell counts become very low and symptoms appear. The middle panel shows the recovery of blood counts. Either a partial response (PR) or a complete response (CR) can occur, at least initially, without increased numbers of stem cells. The right-hand panel shows late disease. Years after recovery, blood counts may fall as a relapse of pancytopenia occurs, or an abnormal clone of stem cells may emerge, leading to a new diagnosis of paroxysmal nocturnal hemoglobinuria (PNH), myelodysplasia (MDS) or acute myelogenous leukemia (AML). CTL = cytotoxic lymphocyte. Reproduced with permission from Ref. 39.

These proteins protect the surface of the erythrocyte membrane from naturally occurring attack by the complement system and their absence leaves the erythrocyte prone to hemolysis in acidified serum, which is the basis of the Ham's test.[105] A small percentage of patients with PNH progress to leukemia. Fifty percent of children given a diagnosis of PNH present initially with aplastic anemia.[106]

Several groups have reported PNH following immunosuppressive therapy for aplastic anemia,[101,103,104] but it has not been reported as a significant complication following BMT. Tichelli *et al*[104] reported PNH diagnosed in 17 of 117 immunosuppression-treated patients a median of 30 months after therapy (range: 12–97 months). Najean *et al*[103] reported PNH in 13 of 156 immunosuppression-treated patients; this group included several pediatric patients none of whom had progressed to MDS/ANLL prior to publication and several of whom resolved spontaneously. In the report by de Planque *et al*,[101] an actuarial incidence of PNH of 13% was calculated at 7 years follow-up. Most cases were diagnosed a median of 3 years after immunosuppressive therapy (range: 0.5 to 7.5 years). In most reports, those patients who developed PNH had significantly poorer survivals than those who did not. The PNH seen following immunosuppressive therapy for aplastic anemia is the same as the naturally occurring disease.[107–109]

The high incidence of PNH in patients treated for SAA with immunosuppressive therapy is difficult to understand and a number of theories have been proposed. The current prevailing hypothesis is that the somatic mutation of the PIGA gene is a common occurrence but because these stem cells proliferate poorly when compared to normal stem cells, the PNH clone remains small.[105] The suppressive influence that leads to aplastic anemia spares the PNH cells (possibly because of the absence of a GPI-anchored protein) giving them a relative proliferative advantage and in this way, the PNH clone emerges and causes clinical disease.

BONE MARROW TRANSPLANTATION VERSUS IMMUNOSUPPRESSION

There are few direct comparisons of the two modalities. Those that do exist are either collected from large registries[4] or are single institution studies of patients treated synchronously with one or the other option.[102,110–114] None of the studies is randomized and they generally compare patients with an HLA-matched sibling treated with BMT to patients without a suitable donor who are treated with immunosuppression. For single centers to accumulate a sufficient number of patients for a meaningful analysis, a long period of time must be reviewed, during which supportive modalities and immunosuppressive regimens will have changed; BMT results have also improved substantially over the decades.[4]

The EBMT reported registry data comparing BMT to various ATG protocols between 1970 and 1986.[4] Cyclosporine A was not part of the immunosuppressive regimens. One hundred and thirty-four children (aged 0–20 years) were treated with BMT (cyclophosphamide $\pm$ irradiation $\pm$ buffy coat) and compared with 115 treated with immunosuppression. Survival in the BMT group was 66% versus 56% in the immunosuppression group (p = 0.01). When stratified for neutrophil counts, children with vSAA did much better with BMT, having a 64% versus a 38% survival in the immunosuppression group (p = 0.01). Children with moderate SAA (absolute neutrophil count $>0.2 \times 10^9$/l) showed no difference in outcome regardless of therapy (58% versus 62%; p = 0.1).

The Seattle experience between 1978 and 1991 compared BMT (numerous cyclophosphamide-based regimens) to immunosuppressive treatment and ATG, corticosteroids and androgens.[102] Of patients under 6 years old, all 12 of those treated with BMT survived as compared to 51% of the 25 treated with immunosuppression (p = 0.006). For patients between the ages of 6 and 19 years, survival was again significantly better following BMT. Several earlier papers demonstrated a similar benefit for children receiving BMT rather than immunosuppressive therapy.[110,111,114]

ANDROGENS AND GROWTH FACTORS

The role of androgens as part of multiagent immunosuppressive protocols has been alluded to above. Bacigalupo *et al*[94] demonstrated an increased rate of response in females with severe aplasia but were unable to demonstrate an improved survival. Androgens have no role as a single agent for the treatment of SAA. In the landmark paper of Camitta *et al*,[12] patients were randomized to intramuscular, oral or no androgens. There was no difference in survival in any of the 3 arms. In patients with non-SAA, responses to androgen therapy have been seen but the relative merit of this form of therapy compared to other immunosuppressive drugs has not been explored.

Several growth factors have been used in the therapy of aplastic anemia. As a supportive therapy, both G-CSF and GM-CSF can improve neutrophil counts in some patients. GM-CSF has been used both with and without other therapies. Hord *et al*[115] treated 7 children with ATG, steroid, cyclosporine A and subcutaneous GM-CSF at 5 μg/kg/day. In comparison to historic controls, treated patients spent fewer days in hospital and were less likely to develop infection. Guinan *et al*[116] used continuous infusion GM-CSF to treat 9 children with aplastic anemia; 6 showed a rise in neutrophil numbers, but only 1 showed improvement in the

other cell lines. The latter patient ultimately showed a sustained improvement in all 3 cell lines, while all others lost their response following cessation of the drug. G-CSF has been shown to increase neutrophil numbers in some children with aplastic anemia, although very high doses are sometimes necessary for this.[117–120] The effect is transient and sustained responses are not seen unless the therapy is accompanied by immunosuppressive agents such as cyclosporine A.[118,120] IL-3 has been tried in some adult patients with aplastic anemia and although transient responses were seen, none was sustained.[121]

Available growth factors are little more than adjuncts to other therapies and it is important that their use does not obscure the need to pursue other therapies, particularly BMT, on an urgent basis.[122]

SUMMARY

Aplastic anemia is an immune disorder that results in irreparable damage to the hematopoietic stem cell population. In some instances, the injury may involve stromal cells or the microenvironment. The resulting hematopoietic failure leads to death from either bleeding or infection.

The different therapeutic modalities have been reviewed and the following recommendations can be made (Fig. 2.3):

- For children diagnosed with vSAA or SAA and having either a matched sibling donor or a phenotypic matched

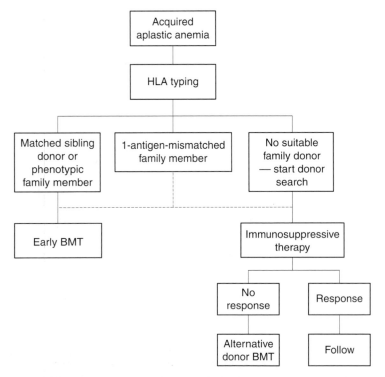

Fig. 2.3 Algorithm for the therapeutic approach to a pediatric patient with acquired aplastic anemia. The dotted line indicates the uncertainty of how to proceed when the best available donor is a 1-antigen mismatched family member.

family donor, early BMT should be the treatment of first choice. The optimal conditioning regimen is unknown but either cyclophosphamide alone or cyclophosphamide with ATG (particularly if there is a phenotypic match) appear to give the best outcomes. BMT from a 1-antigen mismatched family member may be considered at this juncture but the increased problems of graft rejection and GVHD reduce the outcomes to levels either inferior or equal to those obtained from immunosuppressive therapy.

- For children lacking an appropriate donor, immunosuppressive therapy with a combination of ATG, cyclosporine A and steroids yields survivals of about 70%. During the time that such therapy is given and while waiting for a positive result, a search of the different BMT volunteer donor registries should be undertaken. If the immunosuppressive therapy succeeds, then patients should be followed carefully for the development of clonal disorders. If the patients do not respond to immunosuppressive therapy, the outlook is poor. This group should then undergo BMT from either a mismatched (1- or 2-antigen) family member or a matched unrelated donor. If a donor is not readily found, then mismatched cord blood or unrelated donor transplant become possible options, although at this time they are still investigative treatments.

REFERENCES

1. Camitta BM, Storb R, Thomas ED. Aplastic anemia: pathogenesis, diagnosis, treatment and prognosis. *N Engl J Med* 1982; **306**: 645–652

2. The International Agranulocytosis and Aplastic Anemia Study. Incidence of aplastic anemia: the relevance of diagnostic criteria. *Blood* 1987; **70**: 1718–1721

3. Camitta BM, Thomas ED, Nathan DG *et al.* Severe aplastic anemia: a prospective study of the effect of early marrow transplantation on acute mortality. *Blood* 1976; **48**: 63–70

4. Bacigalupo A, Hows J, Gluckman E *et al.* Bone marrow transplantation (BMT) versus immunosuppression for the treatment of severe aplastic anaemia (SAA): a report of the EBMT SAA Working Party. *Br J Haematol* 1988; **70**: 177–182

5. Linet MS, McCaffrey LD, Morgan WF *et al.* Incidence of aplastic anemia in a three county area in South Carolina. *Cancer Res* 1986; **46**: 426–429

6. Szklo M, Sensenbrenner L, Markowitz J, Weida S, Warm S, Linet M. Incidence of aplastic anemia in metropolitan Baltimore: a population-based study. *Blood* 1985; **66**: 115–119

7. Mary JY, Baumelou E, Guiget M, The French Cooperative Group for Epidemiologic Study of Aplastic Anemia.. Epidemiology of aplastic anemia in France: a prospective multicentric study. *Blood* 1990; **75**: 1646–1653

8. Clausen N, Kreuger A, Salmi T, Storm-Mathisen I, Johanneson G. Severe aplastic anaemia in the Nordic countries: a population based study of incidence, presentation, course, and outcome. *Arch Dis Child* 1996; **74**: 319–322

9. Young NS, Issaragrasil S, Chieh CeW, Takaku F. Aplastic anaemia in the Orient. *Br J Haematol* 1986; **62**: 1–6

10. Issaragrisil S, Sriratanasatavorn C, Piankijagum A *et al.* Incidence of aplastic anemia in Bangkok. *Blood* 1991; **77**: 2166–2168

11. Camitta B, O'Reilly RJ, Sensenbrenner L *et al.* Antithoracic duct lymphocyte globulin therapy of severe aplastic anemia. *Blood* 1983; **62**: 883–888

12. Camitta BM, Thomas ED, Nathan DG *et al.* A prospective study of

13. Custer RP. Aplastic anemia in soldiers treated with atabrine (quinacrine). *Am J Med Sci* 1946; **212**: 211–224

14. Plaut ME, Best WR. Aplastic anemia after parenteral chloramphenicol: warning renewed. *N Engl J Med* 1982; **306**: 1486

15. Wallerstein RO, Condit PK, Kasper CK. Statewide study of chloramphenicol therapy and fatal aplastic anemia. *JAMA* 1969; **208**: 2045–2050

16. Pennell PB, Ogaily MS, Macdonald RL. Aplastic anemia in a patient receiving felbamate for complex partial seizures. *Neurology* 1995; **45**: 456–460

17. Gerson WT, Fine DG, Spielberg SP, Sensenbrenner LL. Anticonvulsant-induced aplastic anemia: increased susceptibility to toxic metabolites in vitro. *Blood* 1983; **61**: 889–893

18. Hansen RM, Csuka ME, McCarty DJ, Saryan LA. Gold induced aplastic anemia. Complete response to corticosteroids, plasmapheresis, and N-acetylcysteine infusion. *J Rheumatol* 1985; **12**: 794–797

19. Cunningham JL, Leyland MJ, Delamore IW, Price Evans DA. Acetanilide oxidation in phenylbutazone-associated hypoplastic anaemia. *Br Med J* 1974; **3**: 313–317

20. Baumelou E, Guiget M, Mary JY, The French Cooperative Group for Epidemiological Study of Aplastic Anemia. Epidemiology of aplastic anemia in France: a case-control study. I. Medical history and medication use. *Blood* 1993; **81**: 1471–1478

21. Brown KE, Tisdale J, Barrett J, Dunbar CE, Young NS. Hepatitis-associated aplastic anemia. *N Engl J Med* 1997; **336**: 1059–1064

22. Pol S, Thiers V, Driss F *et al.* Lack of evidence for a role of HCV in hepatitis-associated aplastic anemia. *Br J Haematol* 1993; **85**: 808–810

23. Hibbs JR, Frickhofen N, Rosenfeld SJ *et al.* Aplastic anemia and viral hepatitis. Non-A, non-B, non-C? *JAMA* 1992; **267**: 2051–2054

24. Roberts HJ. Pentacholorophenol-associated aplastic anemia, red cell aplasia, leukemia and other blood disorders. *J Florida Med Assoc* 1990; **77**: 86–90

25. Rugman FP, Cosstick R. Aplastic anaemia associated with organochlorine pesticides: case reports and review of evidence. *J Clin Pathol* 1990; **43**: 98–101

26. Sánchez-Medal L, Castanedo JP, García-Rojas F. Insecticides and aplastic anemia. *N Engl J Med* 1963; **269**: 1365–1367

27. Guiguet M, Baumelou E, Mary JY, French Cooperative Group for Epidemiological Study of Aplastic Anaemia. A case-control study of aplastic anaemia: occupational exposures. *Int J Epidemiol* 1995; **24**: 993–999

28. Yardley-Jones A, Anderson D, Parke DV. The toxicity of benzene and its metabolism and molecular pathology in human risk assessment. *Br J Ind Med* 1991; **48**: 437–444

29. Linet MS, Markowitz JA, Sensenbrenner LL *et al.* A case-control study of aplastic anemia. *Leukemia Res* 1989; **13**: 3–11

30. Scopes J, Daly S, Atkinson R, Ball SE, Gordon-Smith EC, Gibson FM. Aplastic anemia: evidence for dysfunctional bone marrow progenitor cells and the corrective effect of granulocyte colony-stimulating factor *in vitro*. *Blood* 1996; **87**: 3179–3185

31. Maciejewski JP, Selleri C, Sato T, Anderson S, Young NS. A severe and consistent deficit in marrow and circulating primitive hematopoietic cells (long-term culture-initiating cells) in acquired aplastic anemia. *Blood* 1996; **88**: 1983–1991

32. Marsh JCW, Chang J, Testa NG, Hows JM, Dexter TM. The hematopoietic defect in aplastic anemia assessed by long-term marrow culture. *Blood* 1990; **76**: 1748–1757

33. Schrezenmeier H, Jenai M, Herrmann F, Heimpel H, Raghavachar A. Quantitative analysis of cobblestone area-forming cells in bone marrow of patients with aplastic anemia by limiting dilution assay. *Blood* 1996; **88**: 4474–4480

34. Novitzky N, Jacobs P. Immunosuppressive therapy in bone marrow aplasia: the stroma functions normally to support hematopoiesis. *Exp Hematol* 1995; **23**: 1472–1477

35. Holmberg LA, Seidel K, Leisenring W, Torok-Storb B. Aplastic

anemia: analysis of stromal cell function in long-term marrow cultures. *Blood* 1994; **84**: 3685–3690

36. Dilloo D, Vöhringer R, Josting A, Habersang K, Scheidt A, Burdach S. Bone marrow fibroblasts from children with aplastic anemia exhibit reduced interleukin-6 production in response to cytokines and viral challenge. *Pediatr Res* 1995; **38**: 716–721

37. Wodnar-Filipowicz A, Lyman SD, Gratwohl A, Tichelli A, Speck B, Nissen C. Flt3 ligand level reflects hematopoietic progenitor cell function in aplastic anemia and chemotherapy-induced bone marrow aplasia. *Blood* 1996; **88**: 4493–4499

38. Lyman SD, Seaberg M, Hanna R *et al*. Plasma/serum levels of flt3 ligand are low in normal individuals and highly elevated in patients with Fanconi anemia and acquired aplastic anemia. *Blood* 1995; **86**: 4091–4096

39. Young NS, Maciejewski J. The pathophysiology of acquired aplastic anemia. *N Engl J Med* 1997; **336**: 1365–1372

40. Frickhofen N, Liu JM, Young NS. Etiologic mehanisms of hematopoietic failure. *Am J Pediatr Hematol Oncol* 1990; **12**: 385–395

41. Torok-Storb B. Etiologic mechanisms in immune-mediated aplastic anemia. *Am J Pediatr Hematol Oncol* 1990; **12**: 396–401

42. Viale M, Merli A, Bacigalupo A. Analysis at the clonal level of T-cell phenotype and functions in severe aplastic anemia patients. *Blood* 1991; **78**: 1268–1274

43. Selleri C, Sato T, Anderson S, Young NS, Maciejewski JP. Interferon-γ and tumor necrosis factor-α suppress both early and late stages of hematopoiesis and induce programmed cell death. *J Cell Physiol* 1995; **165**: 538–546

44. Tong J, Bacigalupo A, Piaggio G, Figari O, Sogno G, Marmont A. *In vitro* response of T cells from aplastic anemia patients to antilymphocyte globulin and phytohemagglutinin: colony-stimulating activity and lymphokine production. *Exp Hematol* 1991; **19**: 312–316

45. Zoumbos NC, Gascon P, Djeu JY, Young NS. Interferon is a mediator of hematopietic suppression in aplastic anemia *in vitro* and possibly *in vivo*. *Proc Natl Acad Sci USA* 1985; **82**: 188–192

46. Philpott NJ, Scopes J, Marsh JCW, Gordon-Smith EC, Gibson FM. Increased apoptosis in aplastic anemia bone marrow progenitor cells: possible pathophysiologic significance. *Exp Hematol* 1995; **23**: 1642–1648

47. Maciejewski JP, Selleri C, Sato T, Anderson S, Young NS. Increased expression of Fas antigen on bone marrow CD34$^+$ cells of patients with aplastic anaemia. *Br J Haematol* 1995; **91**: 245–252

48. Nagafuji K, Shibuya T, Harada M *et al*. Functional expression of Fas antigen (CD95) on hematopoietic progenitor cells. *Blood* 1995; **86**: 883–889

49. Maciejewski J, Selleri C, Anderson S, Young NS. Fas antigen expression on CD34$^+$ human marrow cells is induced by interferon γ and tumor necrosis factor α and potentiates cytokine-mediated hematopoietic suppression *in vitro*. *Blood* 1995; **85**: 3183–3190

50. Davies SM, Walker DJ. Aplastic anaemia in the northern region 1971–1978 and follow-up of long term survivors. *Clin Lab Haematol* 1986; **8**: 307–313

51. Alter BP. Aplastic anemia in children: diagnosis and management. *Pediatr Rev* 1984; **6**: 46–54

52. Liang R, Cheng G, Wat MS, Ha SY, Chan LC. Childhood acute lymphoblastic leukaemia presenting with relapsing hypoplastic anaemia: progression of the same abnormal clone. *Br J Haematol* 1993; **83**: 340–342

53. Giampietro PF, Verlander PC, Davis JG, Auerbach AD. Diagnosis of Fanconi anemia in patients without congenital malformations: an International Fanconi Anemia Registry study. *Am J Med Genet* 1997; **68**: 58–61

54. Mathé G, Amiel JL, Schwarzenberg L *et al*. Bone marrow graft in man after conditioning by antilymphocyte serum. *Br Med J* 1970; **2**: 131–136

55. Bunin N, Leahey A, Kamani N, August C. Bone marrow transplantation in pediatric patients with severe aplastic anemia: cyclophosphamide and anti-thymocyte globulin conditioning followed by

56. Sanders JE, Storb R, Anasetti C *et al*. Marrow transplanrt experience for children with severe aplastic anemia. *Am J Pediatr Hematol Oncol* 1994; **16**: 43–49

57. Storb R, Etzioni R, Anasetti C *et al*. Cyclophosphamide combined with antithymocyte globulin in preparation for allogeneic marrow transplants in patients with aplastic anemia. *Blood* 1994; **84**: 941–949

58. May WS, Sensenbrenner LL, Burns WH *et al*. BMT for severe aplastic anemia using cyclosporine. *Bone Marrow Transplant* 1993; **11**: 459–464

59. Gluckman E, Horowitz MM, Champlin RE *et al*. Bone marrow transplantation for severe aplastic anemia: influence of conditioning and graft-versus-host disease prophylaxis regimens on outcome. *Blood* 1992; **79**: 269–275

60. Horstmann M, Stockschläder M, Kabisch H, Zander A. Cyclophosphamide/antithymocyte globulin conditioning of patients with severe aplastic anemia transplanted with bone marrow from HLA-identical related donors. *Blood* 1995; **85**: 1404–1405

61. Hinterberger W, Rowlings PA, Hinterberger-Fischer M *et al*. Results of transplanting bone marrow from genetically identical twins into patients with aplastic anemia. *Ann Intern Med* 1997; **126**: 116–122

62. McCann SR, Bacigalupo A, Gluckman E *et al*. Graft rejection and second bone marrow transplants for acquired aplastic anaemia: a report from the aplastic anaemia working party of the European Bone Marrow Transplant group. *Bone Marrow Transplant* 1994; **13**: 233–237

63. Champlin RE, Horowitz MM, van Bekkum DW *et al*. Graft failure following bone marrow transplantation for severe aplastic anemia: risk factors and treatment results. *Blood* 1989; **73**: 606–613

64. Sanders JE, Whitehead J, Storb R *et al*. Bone marrow transplantation experience for children with aplastic anemia. *Pediatrics* 1986; **77**: 179–186

65. Storb R, Sanders JE, Pepe M *et al*. Graft-versus-host disease prophylaxis with methotrexate/cyclosporine in children with severe aplastic anemia treated with cyclophosphamide and HLA-identical marrow grafts. *Blood* 1991; 78: 1144–1145

66. Deeg HJ, Socié G, Schoch G *et al*. Malignancies after marrow transplantation for aplastic anemia and Fanconi anemia: a joint Seattle and Paris analysis of results in 700 patients. *Blood* 1996; **87**: 386–392

67. Socié G, Henry-Amar M, Bacigalupo A *et al*. Malignant tumours occurring after treatment of aplastic anemia. *N Engl J Med* 1993; **329**: 1152–1157

68. Pierga J-Y, Socie G, Gluckman E *et al*. Secondary solid malignant tumours occurring after bone marrow transplantation for severe aplastic anemia given thoraco-abdominal irradiation. *Radiother Oncol* 1994; **30**: 55–58

69. Socié G, Henry-Amar M, Cossett JM, Devergie A, Girinsky T, Gluckman E. Increased incidence of solid malignant tumors after bone marrow transplantation for severe aplastic anemia. *Blood* 1991; **78**: 277–279

70. Socié G, Henry-Amar M, Devergie A *et al*. Poor clinical outcome of patients developing malignant solid tumors after bone marrow transplantation for severe aplastic anemia. *Leukemia Lymphoma* 1992; **7**: 419–423

71. Witherspoon RP, Storb R, Pepe M, Longton G, Sullivan KM. Cumulative incidence of secondary solid malignant tumors in aplastic anemia patients given marrow grafts after conditioning with chemotherapy alone. *Blood* 1992; **79**: 289–292

72. Bacigalupo A, Hows J, Gordon-Smith EC *et al*. Bone marrow transplantation for severe aplastic anemia from donors other than HLA identical siblings: a report of the BMT working party. *Bone Marrow Transplant* 1988; **3**: 531–535

73. Wagner JL, Deeg HJ, Seidel K *et al*. Bone marrow transplantation for severe aplastic anemia from genotypically HLA-nonidentical relatives. *Transplantation* 1996; **61**: 54–61

74. Beatty PG, Di Bartolomeo P, Storb R *et al*. Treatment of aplastic

anemia with marrow grafts from related donors other than HLA genotypically-matched siblings. *Clin Transplant* 1987; **1**: 117–124

75. Hows JM, Yin JL, Marsh J *et al.* Histocompatible unrelated volunteer donors compared with HLA nonidentical family donors in marrow transplantation for aplastic anemia and leukemia. *Blood* 1986; **68**: 1322–1328

76. Margolis D, Camitta B, Pietryga D *et al.* Unrelated donor bone marrow transplantation to treat severe aplastic anaemia in children and young adults. *Br J Haematol* 1996; **94**: 65–72

77. Wagner JE, Kernan N, Steinbuch M, Broxmeyer HE, Gluckman E. Allogeneic sibling umbilical-cord-blood transplantation in children with malignant and non-malignant disease. *Lancet* 1995; **346**: 214–219

78. Neudorf SML, Blatt J, Corey S *et al.* Graft failure after an umbilical blood transplant in a patient with severe aplastic anemia. *Blood* 1995; **85**: 2291–2292

79. Wagner JE, Rosenthal J, Sweetman R *et al.* Successful transplantation of HLA-matched and HLA-mismatched umbilical cord blood from unrelated donors: analysis of engraftment and acute graft-versus-host disease. *Blood* 1996; **88**: 795–802

80. Goldman S, Sweetman R, Suen Y *et al.* A high incidence of severe (grade > III) acute graft vs host disease (aGvHD) following unrelated cord blood transplants (UCBT): HLA mismatching but not serum soluble IL-2 receptor levels are predictive of aGvHD following UCBT. *Blood* 1996; **88 (Suppl 1)**: 422A

81. Griner PF. A survey of the effectiveness of cyclophosphamide in patients with severe aplastic anemia. *Am J Hematol* 1980; **8**: 55–60

82. Speck B, Gluckman E, Haak HL, Van Rood JJ. Treatment of aplastic anaemia by anti-lymphocyte globulin with and without allogeneic bone marrow infusions. *Lancet* 1977; **ii**: 1145–1148

83. Bacigalupo A, Giordano D, Van Lint MT, Vimercati R, Marmont AM. Bolus methylprednisolone in severe aplastic anemia. *N Engl J Med* 1979; **300**: 501–502

84. Bacigalupo A, Podesta M, Van Lint MT *et al.* Severe aplastic anaemia: correlation of *in vitro* tests with clinical response to immunosuppression in 20 patients. *Br J Haematol* 1981; **47**: 423–433

85. Torok-Storb B, Doney K, Sale G, Thomas ED, Storb R. Subsets of patients with aplastic anemia identified by flow microfluorometry. *N Engl J Med* 1985; **312**: 1015–1022

86. Young N, Griffith P, Brittain E *et al.* A multicentre trial of antithymocyte globulin in aplastic anaemia and related diseases. *Blood* 1988; **72**: 1861–1869

87. Marsh JCW, Hows JM, Bryett KA, Al-Hashimi S, Fairhead SM, Gordon-Smith EC. Survival after antilymphocyte globulin therapy for aplastic anaemia depends on disease severity. *Blood* 1987; **70**: 1046–1052

88. Champlin R, Ho W, Gale RP. Antithymocyte globulin treatment in patients with aplastic anemia. A prospective randomized trial. *N Engl J Med* 1983; **308**: 113–118

89. Hinterberger-Fischer M, Höcker P, Lechner K, Seewann H, Hinterberger W. Oral cyclosporin-A is effective treatment for untreated and also for previously immunosuppressed patients with severe bone marrow failure. *Eur J Haematol* 1989; **43**: 136–142

90. Leonard EM, Raefsky E, Griffith P, Kimball J, Nienhuis AW, Young NS. Cyclosporine therapy of aplastic anaemia, congenital and acquired red cell aplasia. *Br J Haematol* 1989; **72**: 278–284

91. Gluckman E, Esperou-Bourdeau H, Baruchel A *et al.* Multicenter randomized study comparing cyclosporine-A alone and antithymocyte globulin with prednisone for treatment of severe aplastic anemia. *Blood* 1992; **79**: 2540–2546

92. Frickhofen N, Kaltwasser JP, Schrezenmeier H *et al.* Treatment of aplastic anemia with antilymphocyte globulin and methylprednisolone with or without cyclosporine. *N Engl J Med* 1991; **324**: 1297–1304

93. Doney K, Pepe M, Storb R *et al.* Immunosuppressive therapy of aplastic anemia: results of a prospective, randomized trial of antithymocyte globulin (ATG), methylprednisolone, and oxymethalone to ATG, very high-dose methylprednisolone, and oxymethalone. *Blood* 1992; **79**: 2566–2571

94. Bacigalupo A, Chaple M, Hows J *et al.* Treatment of aplastic anaemia (AA) with antilymphocyte globulin (ALG) and methylprednisolone (MPred) with or without androgens: a randomized trial from the EBMT SAA working party. *Br J Haematol* 1993; **83**: 145–151

95. Schrezenmeier H, Marin P, Raghavachar A *et al.* Relapse of aplastic anaemia after immunosuppressive treatment: a report from the European Bone Marrow Transplantation Group SAA Working Party. *Br J Haematol* 1993; **85**: 371–377

96. Rosenfeld SJ, Kimball J, Vining D, Young NS. Intensive immunosuppression with antithymocyte globulin and cyclosporine as treatment for severe acquired aplastic anemia. *Blood* 1995; **85**: 3058–3065

97. van Kamp H, Landegent JE, Jansen RPM, Willemze R, Fibbe WE. Clonal hematopoiesis in patients with acquired aplastic anemia. *Blood* 1991; **78**: 3209–3214

98. Raghavachar A, Jansen JWG, Schrezenmeier H *et al.* Clonal hematopoiesis as defined by polymorphic X-linked loci occurs infrequently in aplastic anemia. *Blood* 1995; **86**: 2938–2947

99. Tsuge I, Kojima S, Matsuoka H *et al.* Clonal hematopoiesis in children with acquired aplastic anaemia. *Br J Haematol* 1993; **84**: 137–143

100. Young NS. The problem of clonality in aplastic anemia: Dr. Dameshek's riddle restated. *Blood* 1992; **79**: 1385–1392

101. de Planque MM, Bacigalupo A, Würsch A *et al.* Long-term follow-up of severe aplastic anaemia patients treated with antithymocyte globulin. *Br J Haematol* 1989; **73**: 121–126

102. Doney K, Leisenring W, Storb R, Appelbaum FR, the Seattle Bone Marrow Transplant Team. Primary treatment of acquired aplastic anemia: outcomes with bone marrow transplantation and immunosuppressive therapy. *Ann Intern Med* 1997; **126**: 107–115

103. Najean Y, Haguenauer O, the Cooperative Group for the Study of Aplastic and Refractory Anemias. Long-term (5 to 20 years) evolution of nongrafted aplastic anemias. *Blood* 1990; **76**: 2222–2228

104. Tichelli A, Gratwohl A, Nissen C, Signer E, Gysi CS, Speck B. Morphology in patients with severe aplastic anemia treated with antilymphocyte globulin. *Blood* 1992; **80**: 337–345

105. Rosse WF. Paroxysmal nocturnal hemoglobinuria as a molecular disease. *Medicine* 1997; **76**: 63–93

106. Ware RE, Hall SE, Rosse WF. Paroxysmal nocturnal hemoglobinuria with onset in childhood and adolescence. *N Engl J Med* 1991; **325**: 991–996

107. Nagarajan S, Brodsky RA, Young NS, Medof ME. Genetic defects underlying paroxysmal nocturnal hemoglobinuria that arises out of aplastic anemia. *Blood* 1995; **86**: 4656–4661

108. Nakakuma H, Nagakura S, Iwamoto N *et al.* Poroxysmal nocturnal hemoglobinuria clone in bone marrow of patients with pancytopenia. *Blood* 1995; **85**: 1371–1376

109. Griscelli-Bennaceur A, Gluckman E, Scrobohaci ML *et al.* Aplastic anemia and paroxysmal nocturnal hemoglobinuria: search for a pathogenetic link. *Blood* 1995; **85**: 1354–1363

110. Champlin R, Ho W, Winston DJ, Feig SA, Gale RP. Antithymocyte globulin treatment for aplastic anemia: a controlled randomized trial and comparison with marrow transplantation. *Transplant Proc* 1983; **XV**: 595–598

111. Bayever E, Champlin R, Ho W *et al.* Comparison between bone marrow transplantation and antithymocyte globulin in treatment of young patients with severe aplastic anemia. *J Pediatr* 1984; **105**: 920–925

112. Arranz R, Otero MJ, Ramos R *et al.* Clinical results in 50 multiply transfused patients with severe aplastic anemia treated with bone marrow transplantation or immunosuppressive therapy. *Bone Marrow Transplant* 1994; **13**: 383–387

113. Werner EJ, Stout RD, Valdez LP, Harris RE. Immunosuppressive therapy versus bone marrow transplantation for children with aplastic anemia. *Pediatrics* 1989; **83**: 61–65

114. Halpérin DS, Grisaru D, Freedman MH, Saunders EF. Severe acquired aplastic anemia in children: 11-year experience with bone marrow transplantation and immunosuppressive therapy. *Am J Pediatr Hematol Oncol* 1989; **11**: 304–309

115. Hord JD, Gay JC, Whitlock JA *et al.* Long-term granulocyte-macrophage stimulating factor and immunosuppression in the treatment of acquired severe aplastic anemia. *J Pediatr Hematol Oncol* 1995; **17**: 140–144

116. Guinan EC, Sieff CA, Oette DH, Nathan DG. A phase I/II trial of recombinant granulocyte-macrophage colony-stimulating factor for children with aplastic anemia. *Blood* 1990; **76**: 1077–1082

117. Kojima S, Fukuda M, Miyajima Y, Matsuyama T, Horibe K. Treatment of aplastic anemia in children with recombinant human granulocyte colony-stimulating factor. *Blood* 1991; **77**: 937–941

118. Kojima S, Matsuyama T. Stimulation of granulopoiesis by high-dose recombinant human granulocyte colony-stimulating factor in children with aplastic anemia and very severe neutropenia. *Blood* 1994; **83**: 1474–1478

119. Hibi S, Yoshihara T, Nakajima F, Misu H, Mabuchi O, Imashuku S. Effect of recombinant human granulocyte-colony stimulation factor (rhG-CSF) on immune system in pediatric patients with aplastic anemia. *Pediatr Hematol Oncol* 1994; **11**: 319–323

120. Nawata J, Toyoda Y, Nisihira H, Honda K, Kigasawa H, Nagao T. Haematological improvement by long-term administration of recombinant human granulocyte-colony stimulating factor and recombinant human erythropoietin in a patient with severe aplastic anaemia. *Eur J Pediatr* 1994; **153**: 325–327

121. Ganser A, Lindemann A, Seipelt G *et al.* Effects of recombinant human interleukin-3 in aplastic anemia. *Blood* 1990; **76**: 1287–1292

122. Marsh JCW, Socie G, Schrezenmeier H *et al.* Haemopoietic growth factors in aplastic anaemia: a cautionary note. *Lancet* 1994; **344**: 172–173

Failure of red cell production

SARAH E BALL AND EC GORDON-SMITH

RED CELL APLASIA

The 3 major causes of pure red cell aplasia in childhood are:

- Diamond–Blackfan anemia (DBA);
- transient erythroblastopenia of childhood (TEC);
- an acute aplastic crisis on the background of a chronic hemolytic anemia.

Of these disorders, the chronic red cell aplasia of DBA and the self-limiting red cell aplasia of TEC are unique to early childhood, while an aplastic crisis may occur at any age. Acquired chronic pure red cell aplasia, more common in adults, may also be seen in children, especially in an older age group.

DIAMOND–BLACKFAN ANEMIA

Incidence and inheritance

DBA, a congenital pure red cell aplasia presenting early in infancy, was first described in the 1930s.[1,2] The results of national registries have now put its incidence at 4–7/million live births,[3–5] higher than the more traditional figure of 1/million. There is no apparent ethnic predominance, and both sexes are equally affected.

Familial DBA accounts for 10–20% of newly diagnosed cases,[4–6] and is usually characterized by an autosomal dominant pattern of inheritance,[4,7–10] although, in some cases, autosomal recessive inheritance has been inferred from parental consanguinity; DBA is apparently sporadic in the remaining cases. However, the finding of raised red cell adenosine deaminase (ADA) in first-degree relatives of some children with apparently non-familial DBA[11–13] probably reflects an inherited disorder in these families. In addition, a high incidence of miscarriages has been reported in some mothers of affected children.[4,14]

When familial DBA affects 2 or more generations, the older members of the family may appear to be relatively mildly affected and may present at an older age.[4,15,16] However, in individual cases presenting in infancy, it is not usually possible to distinguish between familial and sporadic DBA on clinical grounds. There is also increasing evidence that at least a proportion of cases of sporadic DBA arise from a germline mutation, thus becoming familial DBA in subsequent generations. In one report,[17] 8 adults with apparently sporadic DBA had a total of 13 children, of whom 3 were found to be affected. Adults with DBA should therefore be advised that there is a risk that their offspring may also be affected, even if there is no positive family history of DBA, and offered genetic counselling, although no prenatal diagnostic test is currently available.

Clinical features

Age at presentation

Infants most commonly present at 2–3 months of age (Fig. 3.1) with symptoms of anemia, such as pallor or poor feeding. Anemia is evident at birth in 25% of cases,[4,6] but fetal anemia leading to hydrops has only rarely been reported.[18–20] In the absence of associated physical anomalies or an unequivocal family history, the diagnosis of DBA should be accepted with caution in children over the age of 1 year. However, mildly affected individuals may be diagnosed as adults, for example through family studies, or when anemia is exacerbated during pregnancy.[21,22]

Associated physical anomalies

These are present in approximately 50% of children with DBA (Table 3.1)[4,5,17,23] and have a wide range of severity. Craniofacial abnormalities are the commonest, with cleft or high arched palate, hypertelorism and flat nasal bridge contributing to the typical DBA facies described by Cathie (Fig. 3.2).[24] Thumb abnormalities are present in 10–20% of affected children, ranging in severity from a flat thenar eminence to absent radii, including the classic triphalangeal

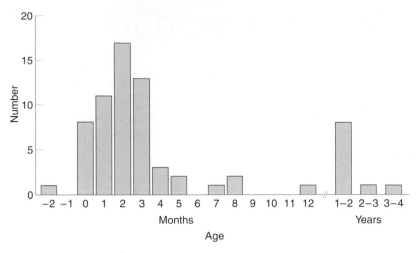

Fig. 3.1 Age at presentation of children with Diamond–Blackfan anemia born in the UK over the 20-year period 1975–1994.[4]

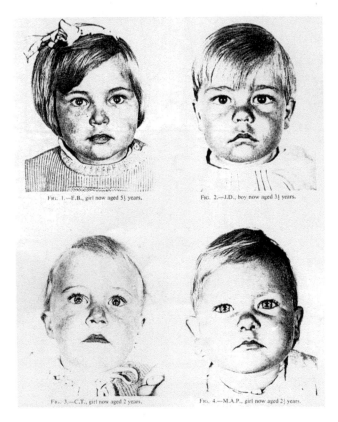

Fig. 3.2 Diamond–Blackfan anemia (DBA) facies: similarity in appearance between unrelated children with DBA. Reproduced with permission from Ref. 24.

Table 3.1 Prevalence and pattern of physical anomalies in children with Diamond–Blackfan anemia born in the UK over the 20-year period 1975–1994.[4]

	Number (%)
Physical anomalies	
Any abnormality	38 (58)
Any craniofacial anomaly	34 (52)
Eyes	22 (34)
Palate/jaw	19 (29)
Thumbs	12 (18)
Total evaluable	65
Growth retardation	
Height below 3rd centile	18 (27)
With associated anomalies	11 (17)
Isolated growth retardation	7 (10)
Total evaluable	66

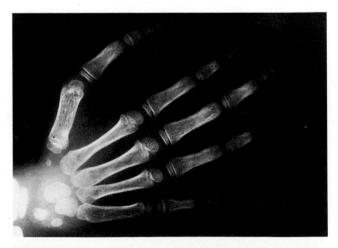

Fig. 3.3 Radiograph of triphalangeal thumb. Kindly supplied by Dr M Freedman.

thumb described by Aase and Smith (Fig. 3.3).[25] Deafness is a relatively common feature, and musculoskeletal, renal and cardiac abnormalities may also occur. Some affected children have learning difficulties of varying severity. An influence of gender on associated physical anomalies is apparent from UK registry data, which show that anomalies tend to be more severe in affected boys than girls, in both sporadic and familial cases.[4]

Growth retardation

Over 60% of children reported in the UK DBA registry were below the 25th centile for height at the time of study, 28% being below the 3rd centile.[4] Of affected children, 10–30% have low birth weight prior to the onset of anemia or starting steroid therapy,[4,5,26] and short stature is then likely to persist.[4] Short stature can therefore be considered to be part of the spectrum of physical anomalies, although the final height achieved by each affected individual will be influenced by other factors, particularly anemia, steroids and iron overload.

Hematologic findings

Red cell indices

The anemia at presentation may be normocytic or macrocytic. The mean corpuscular volume (MCV) is usually within the normal range for neonates,[17] while infants presenting after the first few months are more likely to have macrocytosis. The anemia is, by definition, associated with reticulocytopenia. The white blood cell count is usually normal at presentation, and platelets are normal or raised.

Fetal characteristics of red cells frequently persist after response to therapy, in the form of raised MCV, high levels of fetal hemoglobin (HbF) and increased expression of i antigen.[27] These may be useful in the diagnosis of difficult cases, but are relatively non-specific, and notably can occur during the recovery phase of TEC,[28] as discussed below.

Bone marrow aspirate

This reveals a cellular marrow, with an isolated reduction in erythroid precursors (Plate 1) and normal myeloid and megakaryocytic differentiation. In some cases there may be an apparent maturation arrest at the proerythroblast stage. Bone marrow erythroid culture is seldom helpful in making the diagnosis, but has been an important tool in the investigation of the pathogenesis of the erythroid defect in DBA.

Erythrocyte adenosine deaminase

Raised levels of red cell ADA have been described in a high proportion of patients with DBA.[11,12,29,30] Red cell ADA is not raised in normal cord blood[29] or in juvenile chronic myeloid leukemia[11] despite the fetal pattern of erythropoiesis characteristic of that disorder.[31] However, red cell ADA may also be high in other disorders, including leukemia and myelodysplastic syndromes,[32,33] and so cannot be considered a specific marker for DBA. Its measurement, however, may be useful in establishing family phenotypes for genetic studies.

Pathogenesis

The typical age at onset of anemia, the apparent sparing of fetal erythropoiesis and the persistence of fetal erythroid characteristics during transfusion independence form a pattern which suggests that the normal switch from fetal to adult erythropoiesis may be disrupted in DBA. Identification of the gene or genes involved in DBA may therefore help to elucidate the fetal-adult switch, as well as suggesting new therapeutic approaches.

DBA is heterogenous with respect to pattern of inheritance, clinical presentation, associated anomalies and response to therapy. In the absence of a definitive diagnostic test it is not clear whether it represents a single or an overlapping group of disorders. The pattern of inheritance of familial DBA is consistent with a single gene defect, although the affected gene may not necessarily be the same in all families, by analogy with Fanconi's anemia in which at least 5 genetic complementation groups can be distinguished (see Chapter 1).[34]

Sporadic cases might arise as a result of damage to the developing embryo early in gestation at the stage of craniofacial development[35] which coincides with the first appearance of definitive hemopoietic stem cells.[36] However, the description of DBA in the offspring of some individuals with apparently sporadic disease is consistent with a germline mutation, presumably affecting the same gene or genes as in familial DBA.

There is no specific karyotype associated with DBA, although abnormalities affecting chromosomes 1 and 16 have been reported.[37,38] Recently, a translocation involving the long arm of chromosome 19 was described in a sporadic case of DBA,[39] and significant linkage to 19q13 has been established in familial DBA.[39] In addition, a further patient with sporadic DBA has been found to have a 3.3-Mb deletion within the same region.[39] When the gene underlying this linkage is identified it will be possible to study sporadic cases and families who are non-informative for linkage analysis, and to answer such questions as whether or not DBA is truly monogenic, and whether all sporadic cases are associated with germline mutations.

In vitro *erythroid defect*

Short-term clonogenic assays reveal markedly reduced erythroid colony formation in most, but not all, cases of DBA. However, the profound red cell aplasia observed *in vivo* is not always mirrored by *in vitro* culture results; near normal erythroid colony formation *in vitro* can be observed in some cases who are totally transfusion dependent. In addition, the observed *in vitro* response to interleukin (IL)-3[40] did not correlate with clinical efficacy in subsequent trials of recombinant IL-3;[41–44] it may therefore be unwise to extrapolate directly from *in vitro* observations.

The typical clinical response to steroids in DBA was initially interpreted as reflecting an immune-mediated suppression of erythropoiesis, despite the general lack of efficacy of other immunosuppressive agents. However, there is no consistent *in vitro* evidence to support the existence of an humoral inhibitory agent,[45] or of cell-mediated inhibition of erythropoiesis.[46] Reports suggesting immune suppression of erythropoiesis in DBA[47–49] may in fact be attributable to transfusion-related alloimmunization.

Culture results are generally more consistent with an intrinsic defect in erythroid differentiation. The clinical response to steroids could then be attributable to a direct effect on erythroid progenitor cells,[50–52] or possibly to the stimulation of bone marrow stromal cells to enhance production of stimulatory cytokines.

DBA erythroid progenitors are relatively insensitive to erythropoietin in clonogenic assays.[53] This is reflected by the failure of erythropoietin to induce a clinical response,[54,55] and the finding of increased apoptosis of erythroid progenitor cells from DBA patients in the presence of erythropoietin.[56] These findings are consistent with a defect in erythropoietin receptor (epoR) activation or signal transduction. However, this erythropoietin insensitivity cannot be localized to the epoR molecule itself; polymorphisms affecting the *epoR* gene do not co-segregate with familial DBA, and direct analysis of the *epoR*-coding sequence has revealed no abnormalities.[57] The abnormality resulting in impaired erythropoietin response may still be located downstream of the receptor at some point within the signal transduction cascade.

The availability of recombinant cytokines and advances in marrow culture and cell sorting techniques have allowed more detailed study of *in vitro* erythroid differentiation in DBA. The inability of sorted CD34+ marrow cells from DBA patients to undergo erythroid maturation *in vitro*,[58] despite achieving normal granulocytic maturation, provides powerful supporting evidence for an intrinsic progenitor defect, primarily affecting erythroid differentiation.

The addition of stem cell factor to erythroid colony assays significantly increases DBA marrow erythroid burst-forming unit (BFU-E) in response to erythropoietin, often to within normal levels.[59–63] However, family studies and direct searches for mutations do not directly implicate the genes encoding stem cell factor and its receptor (*c-kit*) in DBA,[64–66] despite the apparent similarities between DBA and the macrocytic anemia observed in Steel or White Spotted mice, which are deficient in stem cell factor and its receptor, respectively.

Erythroid transcription factors represent another possible site at which erythroid differentiation may be disrupted in DBA. Preliminary *in vitro* studies have revealed no apparent differences in the expression of erythroid transcription factors between normal and DBA CD34+ marrow progenitor cells during erythroid differentiation.[67]

Treatment

Steroids

These remain the mainstay of treatment in DBA nearly half a century after the original reports of their efficacy.[68] Prednisolone is usually started at a dose of 2 mg/kg, to which up to 70% of patients show a good initial response (Fig. 3.4).[3–6] An increase in reticulocytes is usually seen within 2 weeks, but a rise in hemoglobin may take up to 1 month. The dose may then be gradually tapered to determine the minimum alternate-day dosage required for continuing transfusion independence. Hemoglobin levels of 8–9 g/dl are often the highest that can be achieved, but should be acceptable provided that growth and normal activity are not compromised. Macrocytosis and markers of fetal erythropoiesis generally persist during response to treatment.

The maintenance dose of prednisolone in steroid responders is highly variable, some children requiring extremely small doses. Sometimes steroids may be stopped completely, although in some cases steroid-independent remission with completely normal hematologic parameters suggest the original diagnosis may have been TEC rather than DBA.

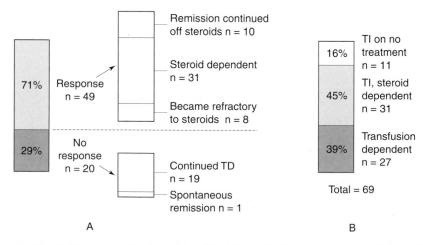

Fig. 3.4 (A) Initial response to steroids and (B) subsequent treatment status of 69 children with Diamond–Blackfan anemia born in the UK over the 20-year period 1975–1994. TI = transfusion independence; TD = transfusion dependence.[4]

However, true spontaneous remission can undoubtedly occur, often after many years of transfusion dependence. An accurate estimate of DBA's real incidence is difficult in the absence of agreed criteria in the literature for diagnosis and response to therapy, as well as whether the definition of spontaneous remission should include a return to normal of all hematologic parameters.

Steroid therapy may have to be discontinued in responders in the presence of unacceptable side-effects, including growth suppression. Growth curves should be closely monitored, especially during periods of high growth velocity in infants and at puberty. A growth plateau may indicate that steroids should be interrupted and substituted with a short-term transfusion program. Pregnancy or the oral contraceptive pill may exacerbate the anemia of DBA,[21,22] and transfusions may be required during pregnancy in women who are normally steroid responsive.

Chicken pox carries a high risk of serious and potentially fatal complications in DBA as a consequence of long-term steroid therapy, which is often started at a very young age before natural immunity can develop. Families should be advised to seek urgent medical attention following exposure to chicken pox, for treatment with acyclovir and/or varicella-zoster immunoglobulin. Active immunization with attenuated varicella vaccine may be considered,[69] although varicella vaccine is not currently licensed in the UK.

High-dose methylprednisolone

This has been reported to be effective in some cases of DBA.[70–73] In one study, 3 of 8 patients refractory to conventional prednisolone therapy achieved a sustained response to 100 mg/kg methylprednisolone, having failed to respond to 30 mg/kg.[73] All 3 responders were treated with high-dose methylprednisolone within 6 months of diagnosis, including 2 under the age of 1 year.[73] There is a significant risk of side-effects, including growth suppression and infection, which will have to be taken into account in the evaluation of high-dose methylprednisolone as second-line therapy in DBA. Further trials are warranted, using consensus diagnostic criteria and common protocols to ensure that results are comparable between centers.

Transfusion program

Of children with DBA, 40–50% are ultimately dependent on long-term transfusion (Fig. 3.4), having failed to respond to steroids, or because of unacceptable steroid side-effects.[3–6] Others may require intermittent transfusions and a hepatitis B immunization program should be initiated as soon as possible after diagnosis. Chelation therapy forms an essential part of a long-term transfusion program as iron overload contributes significantly to morbidity and mortality in this patient group (see Chapter 5).[5,17] Transfusion programs may also be associated with problems of venous access; 2 deaths reported by the French registry,[5] and 1 in the UK,[4] have been attributed to sepsis of indwelling central venous lines.

Interleukin-3

Clinical trials of IL-3[41–44] were prompted by the finding that IL-3 can enhance *in vitro* erythropoiesis in some cases.[40] Combined results from 77 patients reported in the literature revealed a disappointingly low response rate of only 11%,[44] although IL-3 and steroid-independent remission persisted for >3 years in at least 2 patients.[41,44] Further trials of IL-3 have not been attempted in view of the low chance of response, difficulties in obtaining recombinant IL-3 for clinical use, and increasing recognition of the long-term risk of acute myeloid leukemia (AML) in DBA.[17,74,75]

Recombinant stem cell factor may in due course be found to be useful in the treatment of steroid-refractory patients, but it must be remembered that the *in vitro* stimulation of erythroid activity may not translate into clinical response, on the basis of IL-3 experience. The possible risk of exacerbating a long-term risk of leukemia would also be relevant to the use of stem cell factor in DBA.

Alternative therapies

Cyclosporin A,[76] erythropoietin,[54,55] intravenous immunoglobulin,[77] androgens or splenectomy have been used with some reports of success in anecdotal cases, but without consistent evidence of benefit. Prior splenectomy or androgen therapy were in fact associated with significantly worse survival in a follow-up study of patients treated at a single center over a 60-year period.[17] Splenectomy may still be indicated in the event of an increased transfusion requirement secondary to hypersplenism.

Bone marrow transplantation

Bone marrow transplantation (BMT) is potentially curative in DBA,[78–80] with 75–80% long-term survival reported following matched sibling donor BMT,[81] including a successful outcome from a cord-blood transplant.[82] BMT can therefore be considered an option for transfusion-dependent patients where there is a suitable donor. Risk stratification for BMT in thalassemia, which is significantly influenced by the degree of iron overload,[83] is probably equally applicable to DBA. The chance that a spontaneous remission may occur in DBA often influences the decision to undertake BMT in an individual case, but against this must be balanced the increased long-term risk of AML,[17,74,75] which is still apparent after spontaneous remission.[17]

Prognosis

Many adults with DBA who are stable on small doses of steroids or who achieve spontaneous remission are often lost to follow-up, and representative data on long-term prognosis are hard to collate.

Janov *et al*[17] analyzed 76 patients with DBA seen at Boston Children's Hospital over a 60-year period. The median survival for the entire group was 38 years, with a significantly worse prognosis for those treated before the routine use of steroids in 1960. Many deaths were directly or indirectly attributable to iron overload, a finding echoed in the data from the French DBA registry,[5] underscoring the need for adequate chelation in this group. AML developed in 4 of 76 of the Boston patients, 1 of whom had previously received radiotherapy, and a further patient developed aplastic anemia.[17] Aplastic anemia has also been reported in 2 of 132 French patients,[5] and neutropenia and thrombocytopenia are relatively common after the first decade. There is thus evidence for progressive hemopoietic stem cell dysfunction, which is also reflected in the reduced *in vitro* cloning efficiency of myeloid progenitors in DBA with increasing patient age.[84]

TRANSIENT ERYTHROBLASTOPENIA OF CHILDHOOD

TEC is an acquired, self-limiting red cell aplasia unique to childhood, which was recognized as a clinical entity in 1970.[85,86] One regional study in the UK of red cell aplasia in childhood over a 7-year period suggests an incidence of 5/million/year.[87] In another study, >25% of children with TEC were already in the recovery phase at the time of presentation.[88] The true incidence of TEC may therefore be higher as many episodes of transient anemia may go unrecognized.

Clinical features

The usual presentation is a previously fit child up to the age of 5 years, with gradual onset of symptoms of anemia. The commonest age at presentation is 2 years, but TEC has also been described in infants under the age of 6 months.[89,90] TEC thus tends to present in an older age group than DBA, although there is some overlap. Boys and girls are equally affected, and there is no ethnic predominance. Unlike DBA, there are no associated physical anomalies, and affected children are generally of normal stature.[91]

Transient neurologic abnormalities, including seizures and hemiparesis, have occasionally been described in association with otherwise typical TEC.[92–94]

Hematologic findings

The anemia of TEC is normochromic and normocytic and is characterized by reticulocytopenia, although macrocytosis may occur during recovery, and reticulocytosis may be noted if recovery has already started by the time of presentation. Raised levels of HbF and expression of i antigen have been reported during recovery, but red cell ADA levels should be normal.[28]

There is a high incidence of neutropenia in TEC. In one study of 50 patients, 64% had a neutrophil count below $1.5 \times 10^9/l$, and in 28% this was below $1.0 \times 10^9/l$.[88] The platelet count is usually normal, although thrombocytopenia has been documented in some cases of TEC following parvovirus infection.[95,96]

Bone marrow examination reveals a normocellular marrow with erythroid hypoplasia; the presence of left-shifted erythropoiesis with apparent maturation arrest suggests early recovery. Myeloid maturation appears normal, despite the frequent association with neutropenia.

Serum lactate dehydrogenase, bilirubin and serum haptoglobin levels are normal in TEC. If there is evidence of hemolysis, the alternative diagnosis of an acute aplastic crisis on the background of a previously unrecognized hemolytic anemia should be considered.

Red cell enzyme activities tend to be low at the nadir of TEC,[97,98] consistent with an older red cell population in the absence of new red cell production. Similarly, glycosylated hemoglobin (HbA1c) is likely to be raised.[99] Although these tests might theoretically aid discrimination between acute erythroblastopenia and chronic hypoplastic anemia, in practice it is seldom necessary to do more than the basic investigations.

Etiology and pathophysiology

Many children give a history of antecedent viral infection, and there have been several reports of clustering of cases of TEC.[91,100,101] Occasionally, siblings may also be affected,[91,102] which may lead to the erroneous diagnosis of familial DBA. There have been varying reports of seasonality in TEC, but no consistent pattern has emerged. Although viral serology may reveal evidence of recent infection, for example echovirus,[103] adenovirus or parainfluenza,[87] no specific candidate agent has been implicated.

These findings do not suggest a direct viral etiology for TEC and are more consistent with a post-viral process, presumably immune-mediated, analogous to childhood idiopathic thrombocytopenic purpura (ITP). This is supported by *in vitro* culture results. Erythroid colony numbers may be normal or reduced, and serum inhibitors of erythroid colony formation have been detected in a high proportion of cases of TEC.[104–106] Cell-mediated suppression of erythroid colony formation has also been reported.[106,107]

There is usually no serological evidence of recent infection with parvovirus B19.[88] However, occasional cases of a TEC-like hypoplastic anemia have been reported following parvovirus infection. These tend to differ a little from typical TEC in that both thrombocytopenia and neutropenia may occur and the marrow may be hypocellular.[95,95] The pathogenesis of parvovirus-associated TEC might reflect direct marrow suppression, equivalent to the acute aplastic crisis of chronic hemolytic anemias, rather than sharing the probable immune-mediated process underlying TEC which follows other viral infections. Certainly, parvoviral infection of hematologically normal volunteers causes reticulocytopenia, neutropenia and thrombocytopenia.[108]

Treatment and prognosis

Spontaneous, complete recovery of TEC usually occurs within 4–8 weeks of presentation and recurrence is rare.[109] A peak reticulocyte response is usually seen within a month of presentation, and some children will already have entered the recovery phase at the time of diagnosis.[88] A raised MCV and increased red cell distribution width (RDW) accompany the reticulocytosis, but after recovery the steady-state hemoglobin and red cell indices are normal. Any associated neutropenia also resolves and no complications due to infection have been reported. All reported cases with neurologic abnormalities recovered fully, with no neurologic sequelae.

Transfusion may be necessary at the nadir of TEC, but the decision to transfuse should be made on clinical grounds, rather than the hemoglobin level, given the gradual onset of anemia and predicted early recovery. There is no indication to treat TEC with steroids or intravenous immunoglobulin.

ACUTE ACQUIRED RED CELL APLASIA

Clinical features

Transient erythroid hypoplasia underlies the aplastic crisis which may occur in hemolytic anemias, first recognized in association with hereditary spherocytosis (HS).[110] Any event leading to an interruption of erythropoiesis, however short, is likely to cause profound anemia in the presence of a shortened red cell life-span. Thus a precipitous, potentially fatal fall in hemoglobin may be sustained by children with a severe underlying hemolytic process, such as homozygous sickle cell disease, in which the steady-state hemoglobin may be as low as 6–7 g/dl despite massive erythroid expansion. Alternatively, a period of erythroid hypoplasia may induce anemia on a background of otherwise well compensated hemolysis, as in mild HS, and can be the event leading to the diagnosis of the hematologic disorder. Interestingly, a parvovirus-induced acute exacerbation of anemia has also been described in a patient with DBA.[111]

The presentation is usually that of an acute onset of symptoms of anemia in a child with a pre-existing hemolytic anemia, often with a febrile illness during the preceding week, but without exacerbation of jaundice. The duration of reticulocytopenia is generally 7–10 days, and this resolves with the emergence of an antibody response. Children are infectious during this time and therefore represent a risk to other children with hematologic or immunologic abnormalities. The risk to staff, especially early in pregnancy, should also be considered.[112]

Hematologic features

The aplastic crisis is characterized by a decrease in hemoglobin in association with reticulocytopenia, but neutropenia and thrombocytopenia may also occur. Bone marrow aspirate, although rarely required for diagnosis, shows erythroid hypoplasia, often with the giant basophilic proerythroblasts, which are up to 100 μm in diameter with prominent nucleoli and are characteristic of parvoviral infection (Plate 2).

Etiology and pathogenesis

An infectious etiology for the aplastic crisis in patients with an underlying hemolytic process was inferred from clustering of cases. The realization that the illness has a relatively well-defined pattern and usually occurs only once in each individual, suggested that a single infectious agent was largely responsible. Parvovirus B19 was first discovered in the serum of normal blood donors,[113] and was subsequently linked to aplastic crisis in sickle cell anemia.[114,115]

The tropism of parvovirus B19 for erythroid progenitor cells, at all stages of maturation,[116] is explained by the identification of the erythrocyte P antigen (globoside) as the parvovirus receptor.[117] The virus inhibits erythroid colony formation,[118] and is cytotoxic for erythroid progenitor cells at the erythroid colony-forming unit (CFU-E) stage *in vitro*.[119]

Although the majority of aplastic crises are attributable to parvovirus, in a small percentage of cases there is no evidence of B19 infection[120] and other infections may be responsible.

Chronic parvovirus B19 infection

Parvovirus B19 infection in the absence of an effective antiviral immune response may cause prolonged rather than transient red cell aplasia.[121–123] This has been described in association with AIDS,[124] as well as in children with congenital immune deficiency disorders.[125] Hemophiliacs who are HIV-positive may be particularly vulnerable as parvovirus can persist in factor concentrates despite solvent-detergent treatment.[126] Severe chronic anemia may also result from parvovirus infection in children receiving chronic immune suppressive therapy, including chemotherapy for acute lymphoblastic leukemia (ALL).[127] Chronic parvovirus infection may occur in the absence of other evidence for an immunocompromised state,[128] and should be considered as a cause of chronic acquired red cell aplasia even in the absence of other evidence for immune deficiency. Bone marrow aspirate may reveal the giant typical pronormoblasts (Plate 2). Viral serology is unreliable in the diagnosis of parvovirus-induced chronic red cell aplasia, as affected patients often fail to mount an antibody response.[123] The diagnosis may be confirmed by direct detection of parvovirus DNA in serum or bone marrow.[129]

Intravenous immunoglobulin can be effective in decreasing parvoviremia and restoring bone marrow erythroid activity,[130] although repeated courses may be necessary.

CHRONIC ACQUIRED RED CELL APLASIA

Although DBA represents the likeliest cause of chronic red cell aplasia in infants and young children, in older age groups there is a clear overlap with the spectrum of adult acquired red cell aplasia (PRCA). It is however rare; in a regional study of 33 children with red cell aplasia, none had 'adult-type' PRCA.[87]

Chronic PRCA may be idiopathic in both children and adults, or associated with autoimmune, viral and neoplastic disorders, including acute lymphoblastic leukemia[131] and juvenile chronic arthritis.[132] Despite the classical association,[133] thymoma is relatively rare.[134] Many drugs have been associated with PRCA;[135] amongst those with particular relevance to pediatric practice are carbamazepine,[136,137] phenytoin[138] and sodium valproate.[139] Resolution of the anemia usually follows withdrawal of the relevant drug.

Pathophysiology

While the chronic red cell aplasia associated with chronic parvovirus infection is probably directly attributable to infection of erythroid progenitor cells,[118,119] the pathogenesis of other subtypes of PRCA is by contrast more likely to be autoimmune. Both antibody-[140,141] and cell-mediated[142–144] mechanisms of erythroid suppression have been demonstrated.[145]

Treatment

Treatment is directed at the underlying cause and immunosuppression is used where appropriate. The remission rate with steroids is of the order of 40%,[134] and other forms of immunosuppressive therapy[134,146] may be effective in patients who fail to respond to steroids. The demonstration of normal colonies in clonogenic assays *in vitro* may be predictive of clinical response.[147,148] Plasmapheresis has been found to be effective in some cases,[149] providing further evidence for humoral-mediated suppression of erythropoiesis.

DIFFERENTIAL DIAGNOSIS

Although the major cause of chronic red cell aplasia in infancy is DBA, other differential diagnoses should be considered, especially in the absence of dysmorphic features or a positive family history, to reduce the risk of inappropriate treatment with steroids or misleading counselling of parents. Only the main features allowing differentiation between DBA and other causes of red cell aplasia in infancy are considered here. TEC and parvovirus B19-associated red cell aplasia are discussed in fuller detail above.

Diamond–Blackfan anemia versus transient erythroblastopenia of childhood

Both may present in infancy[89,90] and TEC represents the major differential diagnosis in DBA. The distinction between TEC and sporadic DBA may be difficult unless physical anomalies are present, and a diagnosis of TEC is often made retrospectively after recovery.[87] Neutropenia at presentation is more consistent with a diagnosis of TEC.[88] Red cell ADA levels may be helpful, and persistence of anemia and macrocytosis in remission also favor the diagnosis of DBA,[97] although fetal characteristics of erythropoiesis in the form of raised MCV, high HbF and i antigen expression may also occur during the recovery phase of TEC.[28] When there is doubt it may be appropriate simply to observe the patient for a few months, rather than starting steroids immediately, as an apparent response to steroids may be coincidental with the recovery of TEC.

Diamond–Blackfan anemia versus parvovirus B19 infection

Parvovirus infection during pregnancy is associated with hydrops fetalis at all gestational ages,[150] while hydrops is a very rare presentation of DBA.[18–20] In addition, physical anomalies are an unlikely consequence of intrauterine parvovirus infection.[151] However, parvovirus infection should be excluded in a new case of presumed DBA by viral serology (IgM and IgG) in both mother and infant. As chronic red cell aplasia is more likely in the absence of an effective immune response to parvovirus,[123] polymerase chain reaction (PCR) amplification of viral nucleic acid from presentation bone marrow should also be performed.

Alloimmune erythroid hypoplasia

Maternal anti-Kell alloimmunization may result in profound fetal anemia, but with relative reticulocytopenia,[152] consistent with erythroid progenitor suppression.[153,154] This is analogous to the pure red cell aplasia which may occur after ABO incompatible bone marrow transplantion, and which is probably mediated by residual recipient isohemagglutinins.[145,155] Maternal and infant blood group serology should therefore be included in the investigation of babies with presumed DBA who are anemic at birth.

Fanconi's anemia

DBA and Fanconi's anemia have an overlapping spectrum of physical anomalies,[156] and macrocytic anemia may be an early hematologic manifestation of Fanconi's anemia (see Chapter 1).[157] In practice, the distinction is rarely difficult and is resolved by the demonstration of increased chromosome breakages in response to clastogenic agents in Fanconi's anemia.[158]

CONGENITAL DYSERYTHROPOIETIC ANEMIAS

The congenital dyserythropoietic anemias (CDAs) are uncommon, inherited disorders of erythropoiesis characterized by chronic mild-to-moderate anemia associated with distinct morphologic changes in the bone marrow, coupled to ineffective erythropoiesis with or without significant hemolysis.[159–161] The most striking changes are seen in the red cell precursors in the marrow which show some degree of multinuclearity with changes in nuclear structure. The CDAs have been classified into three types (Table 3.2) based on morphologic and serologic findings, but there is clearly heterogeneity within the types and many individual cases of CDA have been reported which do not fit into this classification.[162]

Apart from chronic anemia, most CDAs are associated with some intramedullary destruction of red cell precursors with elevation of the serum bilirubin and lactic dehydrogenase (LDH), shortening of the red cell survival with mild splenomegaly and a marked tendency to increased iron absorption, sometimes leading to hemosiderosis and organ damage from iron overload. The mildness of the anemia may delay diagnosis until adolescence or adulthood when additional demands on hemopoiesis may produce symptomatic anemia. Rarely, CDA may present with severe neonatal jaundice and anemia and even occasionally with hydrops fetalis. Skeletal anomalies are not a consistent feature of CDA, although some dysmorphisms have been reported, particularly in CDA type I. The genetic defects which

underlie the CDAs appear to affect cell membranes, including nuclear membranes, plasma membranes and probably those of organelles, but only in the CDA type II have biochemical defects and enzyme deficiencies been identified.

The CDAs need to be distinguished from congenital hemolytic anemias, β-thalassemia intermedia and erythroleukemia (FAB M6). The prognosis for most CDAs is excellent providing the problem of iron overload is addressed when necessary by chelation therapy or venesection.

CONGENITAL DYSERYTHROPOIETIC ANEMIA TYPE I

The 80 or more cases of CDA type I reported in the literature indicate that it is inherited as an autosomal recessive disorder.[163,164] No method exists to identify heterozygotes and hence sporadic cases cannot be ruled out. The diagnostic phenotype is probably produced by genetic heterogeneity.

Clinical features

Typically, there is mild anemia with slight icterus and the spleen is palpable although not usually markedly enlarged.[163,164] The spleen may slowly enlarge with increasing age. Skeletal abnormalities are not usual, although they have been described in 2 unrelated patients.[165] In 1 of these there were no distal phalanges on the third and fourth fingers and complex malformations in the feet with syndactyly and lack of distal phalanges and nails. The diagnosis of CDA

Table 3.2 Comparison of the 3 types of congenital dyserythropoietic anemia (CDA).

	CDA I	CDA II (HEMPAS)	CDA III
Inheritance	Autosomal recessive	Autosomal recessive	Autosomal dominant
Clinical	Splenomegaly	Splenomegaly, hepatomegaly, jaundice	Occasional splenomegaly
Anemia	Mild to moderate	Mild to moderate	Mild
MCV	Increased	Slight increase	Normal or mild increase
Reticulocytes	Normal	Normal	Normal
Platelets	Normal	Normal	Normal
Bilirubin	Increased	Increased	Normal or mild increase
Lactic dehydrogenase	Increased	Increased	Mild increase
Bone marrow	Mainly affecting early erythroblasts: Megaloblastic changes Internuclear bridging Few binucleate cells	Mainly affecting late erythroblasts: Binuclearity Multinuclearity Pluripolar mitosis Karyorrhexis	Gigantoblasts Multinuclearity (up to 12 nuclei) Macrocytosis
Electron microscopy	Spongy nuclei Invasion of nuclear region by cytoplasm	Cisternae and 'double membrane'	Nuclear clefts Spongy nuclei Autolytic areas in cytoplasm
Serology			
Acidified serum test	Negative	Positive (selected sera)	Negative
Sucrose lysis	Negative	Negative	Negative
Anti-i lysis/agglutination	Negative	+ +	+ +
Anti-I lysis/agglutination	±	+ +	+ +

type I was made when both patients were young adults, although the second patient had had severe neonatal jaundice requiring exchange transfusion. There have been other reports of growth retardation, membranous syndactyly of the toes and brown pigmentation of the skin in patients with CDA type I,[166,167] but the similarity of the skeletal abnormalities in the 2 patients described above is such as to make it probable that they represent a true subtype of the condition.

A major study of CDA type I in Bedouin patients from the Negev, Israel[164] revealed no skeletal abnormalities, only 4 of 20 patients were below 2 standard deviations of the mean height for their age and mild splenomegaly was found in 11 of the 20 patients. Fourteen of the 20 were the product of consanguineous marriages and all came from the same Bedouin tribe. It is likely therefore that they represent a uniform homozygous genotype producing the CDA type I phenotype, although there was some heterogeneity in the severity between individuals. The age at diagnosis in this group varied from birth to 23 years. In 6 patients anemia became severe enough to require blood transfusion but the remainder were clinically unaffected by anemia.

Laboratory findings

The hemoglobin is usually between 8 and 11 g/dl but milder or more anemic cases may be seen. There is macrocytosis (MCV 92–107 fl) and considerable anisocytosis and poikilocytosis. Reticulocytes are slightly reduced in number for the degree of anemia. Cabot rings, a thin circle of nuclear remnant within the circulating red cells which stains purple with Romanowsky stains, may be seen in CDA type I and most conspicuously in splenectomized patients.[166,167] White cells and platelets are normal in number, morphology and function. Unconjugated bilirubin is elevated, usually 2–3 times normal, and serum LDH is raised. Serum ferritin was moderately elevated in the Bedouin study, mean level 385 ± 293 µg/l (normal range 10–300 µg/l; highest value 1245 µg/l). The acidified serum lysis test is negative and the expression of i and I antigens on the red cell surface is within the normal adult range. HbF levels are usually within the normal range or only slightly raised (0.5–2.0%), although occasional individuals with higher levels (up to 6.0%) may be found. Hemoglobin A_2 levels are usually high normal or slightly raised. Serum folate and vitamin B_{12} levels are normal.

The characteristic features of CDA type I are seen on the bone marrow, which is generally hypercellular with a reversal of the M:E ratio. Early red cell precursors appear normal but a small proportion, 5–10%, of basophilic and polychromatophilic erythroblasts have anomalies of nuclear division with binucleate forms and, most characteristically, incompletely separated normoblasts connected by an internuclear bridge.[168] Abnormalities of nuclear chromatin condensation make the erythropoiesis appear megaloblastic.[163]

Electron microscopy

Electron microscopy of erythroblasts typically shows a spongy appearance of heterochromatin (so-called 'Swiss cheese' appearance), increased nuclear pore size and invaginations of the nucleus resulting in cytoplasm with some hemoglobin, intruding into the nuclear region. Mitochondria usually show iron loading.[168–170]

Pathogenesis

The molecular defects which underlie CDA type I are unknown. They seem to affect only erythroid precursors; colony-forming units—erythroid (CFU-E) and burst-forming units—erythroid (BFU-E) are increased in both the marrow and peripheral blood, although typical abnormalities in the cells of the colonies are present.[164] Colony-forming units in culture (CFU-C) are normal. Abnormalities of membrane which produce secondary changes in nuclear membranes, the presence of abnormal histones[171] and abnormalities of early polychromatophilic erythroblasts[172] have been described. Tamary et al[164] found an increased arrest of erythroid cells in S phase in CDA type I compared to normal and suggested that increased apoptosis might be a consequence of premature activation of the cell cycle, although no direct evidence of increased apoptosis could be found.

Treatment

The majority of patients require no treatment, merely needing reassurance that the anemia is benign and life expectancy is normal. As mentioned above, iron overload may produce clinical problems and it is important that these patients are not given iron and that ferritin levels are monitored at least until adulthood. An exception to this was appropriate in one patient with morphologic features of CDA type I who had intravascular hemolysis, hemosiderinuria and iron deficiency.[173]

Occasionally, patients may become more anemic as they get older, possibly because of progressive enlargement of the spleen and pooling of red cells. Splenectomy has been successful in ameliorating the anemia in some of these patients,[163] but it carries the problems of infections and thrombotic tendency common to all splenectomized patients.

By chance, α-interferon has been found to have a beneficial effect on hemoglobin levels in some patients with CDA type I.[174] A 28-year-old patient with CDA type I who required monthly transfusions became infected with hepatitic C virus. She was given α-interferon 3 million units 3 times weekly for 24 weeks. The MCV was unaffected but the hemoglobin rose to 13.0 g/dl after 4 weeks and remained above 11.5 g/dl until α-interferon was stopped. The hemoglobin then fell to pre-treatment levels until α-interferon was re-introduced 6 months later when it again rose to normal levels. Erythrokinetic studies demonstrated correction of the ineffective erythropoiesis by showing increased iron utilization. In a second case, where α-interferon was given as therapy for the CDA Type I,[175] a response was achieved with 3 million units twice weekly but not when the dose was reduced to once weekly. The bone marrow changes of CDA type I remained whilst on treatment but the M:E ratio reverted to normal as the ineffective erythropoiesis recovered. Life-long α-interferon therapy does not seem to be an ideal type of management, particularly as the long-term effects of starting therapy in childhood are unknown. Furthermore, α-interferon is not a recognized treatment for this condition. However, it may be that such treatment could be considered as a way of raising the hemoglobin to allow venesection to reduce iron overload.

CONGENITAL DYSERYTHROPOIETIC ANEMIA TYPE II

CDA type II is often referred to by the acronym HEMPAS which stands for Hereditary Erythroblastic Multinuclearity with a Positive Acidified Serum test.[176] The condition has also been called familial benign erythroblastic polyploidy and hemolytic-splenomegalitic erythropolydyskaryosis.[177] CDA type II is commoner than type I and has been described in most ethnic groups. It is inherited as an autosomal recessive disorder with wide variability in severity. The characteristic serologic abnormalities are the consequence of abnormal glycosylation of membrane proteins; minor serologic changes from normal may be found in heterozygotes.

Clinical features

There is a broad spectrum in the clinical presentation of CDA type II. The majority of patients have mild-to-moderate anemia with jaundice and splenomegaly. In some patients jaundice may be the only clinical finding and the increased red cell destruction be fully compensated. As with other CDAs, type II may lead to iron overload with liver cirrhosis, diabetes and cardiac failure in later life.[178,179] In severe cases, anemia is present from birth with considerable medullary hyperplasia leading to widening of the diploe and facial deformities similar to those seen in β-thalassemia.[180] A number of conditions have been reported in association with CDA Type II, although they are probably coincidental and not part of the same genetic defect. They include mental retardation, Sweet's syndrome,[181] ectodermal dysplasia,[182] Dubin–Johnson syndrome[183] and von Willebrand's disease.[184]

Hematologic findings

There is wide variation in the degree of anemia, both between different families and between siblings. The MCV is normal or slightly increased and the reticulocyte count normal. The circulating red cells may be irregularly contracted (acanthocytes) and show bizarre forms. Both I and i antigens are expressed on CDA type II cells and may be detected by anti-i antibodies.[176] The i antigen is expressed on normal fetal cells but becomes weak or negative on normal adult cells. Heterozygotes also show increased expression of i antigens.[180]

The characteristic feature of the red cells, which give the syndrome its acronym, is their lysis by acidified serum; serum from about one-third of normal individuals will lyse CDA type II red cells when acidified. The patient's own serum will not produce lysis which helps to distinguish the syndrome from paroxysmal nocturnal hemoglobinuria (PNH). It is thought that CDA type II cells express an abnormal antigen to which 30% of normal sera contain a complement fixing (IgM) antibody, but the nature of this antigen has not been determined. CDA type II red cells may also have abnormal complement activation control.[185]

Bone marrow aspirate provides the characteristic morphologic features of CDA type II. There is erythroid hyperplasia. Abnormalities are seen in the late stages of erythroid differentiation with polychromatophilic erythroblasts and late normoblasts showing binuclearity (and sometimes multinuclearity).

Electron microscopy

Electron microscopy reveals some similarities to CDA type I but in addition there is a characteristic linear structure running parallel to the plasma membrane, cisternal in appearance which seems to be continuous with the endoplasmic reticulum.[186] Such changes are not unique to CDA type II and may be seen to a lesser extent in other hemoglobinopathies.[187]

Pathogenesis

The underlying defect in CDA type II is a failure of normal glycosylation of membrane proteins, particularly band 3, the anion channel of the red cell.[188] Polyacrylamide gel electrophoresis has shown that band 3 protein from CDA Type II patients migrated faster than normal,[189–191] the reduction in molecular weight being the result of loss of glycosyl residues rather than an abnormal protein.[192] Other membrane proteins, including band 4.5, and some plasma proteins, e.g. transferrin, are also underglycosylated.[188] In the glycosylation of membrane proteins, a mannose-rich core structure is enzymatically added to the protein via an asparagine residue and is then progressively modified by other reactions which remove mannose and add N-acetyl glucosamine.[160,188] These enzymes are present in the endoplasmic reticulum. Two separate enzyme deficiencies in the pathway have been described by Fukuda et al, α-mannosidase II deficiency[193] and N-acetylglucosaminyl transferase II deficiency.[194]

Band 3 is not only the anion channel but also makes contact with the membrane cytoskeleton through ankyrin. In CDA type II there is a clustering of band 3 compared to the normal even distribution of the fully glycosylated protein.[195] It is thought that this may alter in some way cell division in the stages of erythroblast differentiation where polylactosaminoglycans become fully expressed, i.e. at the erythroblast stage and subsequently. Evidence in favor of α-mannosidase II producing the defect in this way comes from the observation that inhibition of the enzyme by swainsonine[196] in *in vitro* culture of normal erythroblasts produces binucleate forms similar to those seen in CDA type II.[188] Excessive removal of abnormally glycosylated glycoproteins by the liver may contribute to the tendency of CDA type II patients to develop cirrhosis and may even increase the risk of gallstones and possibly diabetes.[188]

Treatment

Management depends upon the degree of symptomatic anemia, the presence or absence of iron overload and biliary problems. Splenectomy may raise the hematocrit in patients with symptomatic anemia and enlarged spleens. Deferoxamine (desferrioxamine) therapy should be considered in patients who demonstrate increasing ferritin levels or progressive liver damage. Once a patient has been identified, siblings should be checked and advice given concerning the risks of iron overload and liver damage.

CONGENITAL DYSERYTHROPOIETIC ANEMIA TYPE III

CDA type III is the rarest of the classified syndromes, although the striking bone marrow abnormalities meant that it was the first to be recognized.[196] It is mainly inherited as an autosomal dominant disorder although there may be families with recessive inheritance.[197] The abnormal gene has been located to 15q21–q25 in a Swedish family with dominant inheritance.[198]

Clinical features

Anemia is usually mild and is accompanied by slight icterus. Splenomegaly may occur but is absent in a substantial proportion of reported cases. The condition is usually discovered in young adult life unless there is a known family history.

Hematologic findings

There is mild macrocytic anemia with anisocytosis and poikilocytosis of the red cells. There may be evidence of intravascular hemolysis with hemosiderinuria and iron deficiency rather than the usual iron overload of other CDAs.[199] The acidified serum lysis test is negative and there is variable expression of I and i antigens.

The bone marrow shows erythroid hyperplasia with striking multinuclearity of the erythroblasts (up to 12 nuclei) in a single cell producing so-called 'gigantoblasts'.

The nuclei may be of the same or different maturity. Similar appearances may occur in erythroleukemia from which CDA type III should be differentiated.

Electron microscopy

Electron microscopy reveals nuclear clefts and autolytic areas within the cytoplasm[197] with multiple nuclei within the cell.

Management

Patients do not usually present a clinical problem other than differentiating the condition from other causes of macrocytosis and excluding erythroleukemia. Advice on the genetic features of the condition should be given.

UNCLASSIFIED CONGENITAL DYSERYTHROPOIETIC ANEMIAS

A number of cases of CDA have been reported which do not fit the above classification. In one family, a proband with mild anemia and multinucleated cells at all stages of erythroid differentiation had an affected child who died with hydrops fetalis.[200] Four other infants with hydrops fetalis and unusual types of CDA have been identified;[201–204] in most cases there was a history of previous neonatal deaths with hydrops or multiple abortions.[201]

CONGENITAL DYSERYTHROPOIETIC ANEMIA AND GLOBIN CHAIN SYNTHESIS

Ineffective erythropoiesis due to inclusions of excess α chain plays an important role in the symptomatology of β-thalassemia.[205] There has been some suggestion that there may be cases of CDA where imbalance of globin chain synthesis produces features of both disorders.[206] Inclusions found in CDA type III react with monoclonal antibody against β-globin chains but not α — findings similar to those in hemoglobin H disease.[207] In 2 other patients with severe transfusion-dependent anemia due to unclassified CDA, nuclear inclusions resembling those of CDA type III by electron microscopy did not react with antibodies against either α or β chains.[208] In most patients with CDA type I there is some imbalance of globin chain synthesis but this is not sufficient to add to the ineffective erythropoiesis of the underlying disorder.[164,208]

SUMMARY

CDA is a rare group of disorders characterized by the morphology of erythropoietic progenitor cells and ineffective erythropoiesis with some degree of intramedullary destruction of mature cells. The majority of cases have a benign course but severe variants present as hydrops fetalis or neonatal jaundice and require exchange transfusions. The conditions need to be distinguished from other causes of megaloblastic anemia, de Guglielmos's disease and erythroleukemia (AML FAB type M6).

REFERENCES

1. Josephs HW. Anemia of infancy and early childhood. *Medicine* 1936; **15**: 307–451

2. Diamond LK, Blackfan KD. Hypoplastic anemia. *Am J Dis Child* 1938; **56**: 464–467

3. Bresters D, Bruin MCA, Van Dijken PJ. Congenitale hypoplastische anemie in Nederland (1963–1989). *Tijdschrift Kindergeneeskunde* 1991; **59**: 203–210

4. Ball SE, McGuckin CP, Jenkins G *et al*. Diamond–Blackfan anemia in the U.K.: analysis of 80 cases from a 20-year birth cohort. *Br J Haematol* 1996; **94**: 645–653

5. Willig IN, Croisille L, Leblanc T *et al*. French register of Diamond–Blackfan anemia. Preliminary results. *Blood* 1996; **88 (Suppl 1)**: 143A

6. Vlachos A, Alter B, Buchanan G, Freedman M, Glader B, Lipton JM. The Diamond Blackfan Anemia Registry (DBAR): preliminary data. *Blood* 1993; **82**: 88A

7. Hunter RE, Hakami N. The occurrence of congenital hypoplastic anemia in half brothers. *J Pediatr* 1972; **81**: 346–348

8. Gojic V, Van't Veer-Korthof ET, Bosch LJ, Puyn WH, Van Haeringen A. Congenital hypoplastic anemia: another example of autosomal dominant transmission. *Am J Med Genet* 1994; **50**: 87–89

9. Altman AC, Gross S. Severe congenital hypoplastic anemia: transmission from a healthy female to opposite sex step-siblings. *Am J Pediatr Hematol Oncol* 1983; **5**: 99–101

10. Lawton JWM, Aldrich JE, Turner TL. Congenital erythroid hypoplastic anaemia: autosomal dominant transmission. *Scand J Haematol* 1974; **13**: 276–280

11. Glader BE, Backer K. Elevated red cell adenosine deaminase activity: a marker of disordered erythropoiesis in Diamond–Blackfan anaemia and other haematologic diseases. *Br J Haematol* 1988; **68**: 165–168

12. Whitehouse DB, Hopkinson DA, Evans DIK. Adenosine deaminase activity in Diamond–Blackfan syndrome. *Lancet* 1984; **ii**: 1398–1399

13. Filanovskaya LI, Nikitin DO, Togo AV, Blinov MN, Gavrilova LV. The activity of purine nucleotide degradation enzymes and lymphoid cell subpopulation in children with Diamond–Blackfan syndrome. *Gematologiia Transfuziologiia* 1993; **38**: 19–22

14. Janov A, Leong T, Nathan D, Guinan E. Natural history and sequelae of treatment in patients (pts) with Diamond–Blackfan Anemia. *Blood* 1993; **82**: 311A

15. Greenbaum BH, Reid CS, Donaldson MH. Congenital hypoplastic anemia in multiple generations. *Pediatr Res Commun* 1987; **2**: 65–74

16. Gray PH. Pure red cell aplasia: occurrence in three generations. *Med J Aust* 1982; **1**: 519–521

17. Janov AJ, Leong T, Nathan DG *et al*. Diamond Blackfan anemia. Natural history and sequelae of treatment. *Medicine* 1996; **75**: 77–78

18. Van Hook JW, Gill P, Cyr D *et al*. Diamond–Blackfan anemia as an unusual cause of nonimmune hydrops fetalis: A case report. *J Reprod Med Obstet Gynecol* 1995; **40**: 850–854

19. Scimeca PG, Weinblatt ME, Slepowitz G, Harper RG, Kochen JA. Diamond–Blackfan syndrome: an unusual cause of hydrops fetalis. *Am J Pediatr Hematol Oncol* 1988; **10**: 241–243

20. McLennan AC, Chitty LS, Rissik J, Maxwell DJ. Prenatal diagnosis of Blackfan–Diamond syndrome; case report and review of the literature. *Prenat Diagn* 1996; **16**: 349–353

21. Rijhsinghani A, Wiechert RJ. Diamond–Blackfan anemia in pregnancy. *Obstet Gynecol* 1994; **83 (Suppl)**: 827–829

22. Balaban EP, Buchanan GR, Graham M, Frenkel EP. Diamond–Blackfan syndrome in adult patients. *Am J Med* 1985; **78**: 533–538

23. Alter BP. Childhood red cell aplasia. *Am J Pediatr Hematol Oncol* 1980: **2**: 121–139

24. Cathie IAB. Erythrogenesis imperfecta. *Arch Dis Child* 1950; **25**: 313–324

25. Aase JM, Smith DW. Congenital anemia and triphalyngeal thumbs: a new syndrome. *J Pediatr* 1969; **74**: 471–474

26. Halperin DS, Freedman MH. Diamond–Blackfan anemia: Etiology, pathophysiology, and treatment. *Am J Pediatr Hematol Oncol* 1989; **11**: 380–394

27. Diamond LK, Wang WC, Alter BP. Congenital hypoplastic anemia. *Adv Pediatr* 1976; **22**: 349–378

28. Link MP, Alter BP. Fetal-like erythropoiesis during recovery from transient erythroblastopenia of childhood (TEC). *Pediatr Res* 1981; **15**: 1036–1039

29. Glader BE, Backer K, Diamond LK. Elevated erythrocyte adenosine deaminase activity in congenital hypoplastic anemia. *N Engl J Med* 1983; **309**: 1486–1490

30. Whitehouse DB, Hopkinson DA, Pilz AJ, Arredondo FX. Adenosine deaminase activity in a series of 19 patients with the Diamond–Blackfan syndrome. *Adv Exp Med Biol* 1986; **195**: 85–92

31. Gahr M, Scgroter W. The pattern of reactivated fetal erythropoiesis in bone marrow disorders of childhood. *Acta Paediatr Scand* 1982; **71**: 1013–1018

32. Van der Weyden MB, Harrison C, Hallam L, McVeigh D, Gan TE, Taaffe LM. Elevated red cell adenosine deaminase and haemolysis in a patient with a myelodysplastic syndrome. *Br J Haematol* 1989; **73**: 129–131

33. Tani K, Fujii H, Takahashi K, Kodo H, Asano S, Takaku F, Miwa S. Erythroyte enzyme activities in myelodysplastic syndromes: elevated pyruvate kinase activity. *Am J Hematol* 1989; **30**: 97–103

34. Joenje H, Lo ten Foe JR, Oostra AB *et al*. Classification of Fanconi anemia patients by complementation analysis: evidence for a fifth genetic subtype. *Blood* 1995; **86**: 2156–2160

35. Moore GE. Molecular genetic approaches to the study of human craniofacial dysmorphologies. *Int Rev Cytol* 1995; **158**: 215–277

36. Zon LI. Developmental biology of hematopoiesis. *Blood* 1995; **86**: 2876–2891

37. Tartaglia AP, Propp S, Amarose AP *et al*. Chromosome abnormality and hypocalcemia in congenital erythroid hypoplasia (Blackfan–Diamond syndrome). *Am J Med* 1966; **41**: 990–999

38. Heyn R, Kurczynski E, Schmickel R. The association of Blackfan–Diamond syndrome, physical abnormalities and an abnormality of chromosome 1. *J Pediatr* 1974; **85**: 531–533

39. Gustavsson P, Willig TN, van Haeringen A *et al*. Diamond–Blackfan anemia: genetic homogeneity for a gene on chromosome 19q13 restricted to 1.8 Mb. *Nature Genet* 1997; **16**: 368–371

40. Halperin DS, Estrov Z, Freedman MH. Diamond–Blackfan anemia: promotion of marrow erythropoiesis *in vitro* by recombinant interleukin-3. *Blood* 1989; **73**: 1168–1174

41. Dunbar CE, Smith DA, Kimball J, Garrison L, Nienhuis AW, Young NS. Treatment of Diamond Blackfan anemia with haematopoietic growth factors, granulocyte-macrophage colony stimulating factor and interleukin 3: sustained remissions following IL-3. *Br J Haematol* 1991; **79**: 316–321

42. Gillio AP, Faulkner LB, Alter BP *et al*. Treatment of Diamond–Blackfan anemia with recombinant human interleukin-3. *Blood* 1993; **82**: 744–751

43. Olivieri NF, Feig SA, Valentino L, Berriman AM, Shore R, Freedman MH. Failure of recombinant human interleukin-3 therapy to induce erythropoiesis in patients with refractory Diamond–Blackfan anemia. *Blood* 1994; **83**: 2444–2450

44. Ball SE, Tchernia G, Wranne L *et al*. Is there a role for interleukin-3 in Diamond–Blackfan anaemia? Results of a European multicentre study. *Br J Haematol* 1995; **91**: 313–318

45. Freedman MH, Amato D, Saunders EF. Erythroid colony growth in congenital hypoplastic anemia. *J Clin Invest* 1976; **57**: 673–677

46. Freedman MH, Saunders EF. Diamond–Blackfan syndrome: evidence against cell-mediated erythropoietic suppression. *Blood* 1978; **51**: 1125–1128

47. Hoffman R, Zanjani ED, Vila J, Zaluky R, Lutton JD, Wasserman LR. Diamond–Blackfan syndrome: lymphocyte-mediated suppression of erythropoiesis. *Science* 1976; **193**: 899–900

48. Steinberg MH, Colemen MF, Pennebaker JN. Diamond–Blackfan syndrome: evidence for T-cell mediated suppression of erythroid development and a serum blocking factor associated with remission. *Br J Haematol* 1979; **41**: 57–68

49. Ershler WB, Ross J, Finlay JL, Shaidi NT. Bone marrow microenvironment defect in congenital hypoplastic anemia. *N Engl J Med* 1980; **302**: 1321–1327

50. Chan HS, Saunders EF, Freedman MH. Diamond–Blackfan syndrome I. Erythropoiesis in prednisone responsive and resistant disease. *Pediatr Res* 1982; **16**: 474–476

51. Chan HS, Saunders EF, Freedman MH. Diamond–Blackfan syndrome II. *In vitro* corticosteroid effect on erythropoiesis. *Pediatr Res* 1982; **16**: 477–478

52. Kalmanti M, Kalmantis T, Dimitriou H, Kattamis C. Correlation of in vitro enhancement of erythropoiesis and clinical response to steroids in Diamond–Blackfan anaemia. *Haematologia* 1993; **25**: 263–269

53. Lipton JM, Kudisch M, Gross R, Nathan DG. Defective erythroid progenitor differentiation system in congenital hypoplastic (Diamond–Blackfan) anemia. *Blood* 1986; **67**: 962–968

54. Niemeyer CM, Baumgarten E, Holldack J *et al*. Treatment trial with recombinant human erythropoietin in children with congenital hypoplastic anemia. *Contrib Nephrol* 1991; **88**: 276–281

55. Fiorillo A, Poggi V, Migliorati R, Parasole R, Selleri C, Rotoli B. Unresponsiveness to erythropoietin therapy in a case of Blackfan Diamond anemia. *Am J Hematol* 1991; **37**: 61

56. Perdahl EB, Naprstek BL, Wallace WC, Lipton JM. Erythroid failure in Diamond–Blackfan anemia is characterized by apoptosis. *Blood* 1994; **83**: 645–650

57. Dianzani I, Garelli E, Dompe C *et al*. Mutations in the erythropoietin receptor gene are not a common cause of Diamond–Blackfan anemia. *Blood* 1996; **87**: 2568–2572

58. Bagnara GP, Zauli G, Vitale L *et al*. *In vitro* growth and regulation of bone marrow enriched CD34$^+$ hematopoietic progenitors in Diamond–Blackfan anemia. *Blood* 1991; **78**: 2203–2210

59. Olivieri NF, Grunberger T, Ben-David Y *et al*. Diamond Blackfan anemia: heterogeneous response of hematopoietic progenitor cells *in vitro* to the protein prduct of the Steel locus. *Blood* 1991; **78**: 2211–2215

60. Abkowitz JL, Sabo KM, Nakamoto B *et al*. Diamond–Blackfan anemia: *in vitro* response of erythroid progenitors to the ligand for c-kit. *Blood* 1991; **78**: 2198–2202

61. Sieff CA, Yokoyama CT, Zsebo KM *et al*. The production of Steel factor mRNA in Diamond–Blackfan anaemia long-term cultures and interactions of Steel factor with erythropoietin and interleukin-3. *Br J Haematol* 1992; **82**: 640–647

62. Alter BP, Knobloch ME, He L *et al*. Effect of stem cell factor on *in vitro* erythropoiesis in patients wih bone marrow failure syndromes. *Blood* 1992; **80**: 3000–3008

63. McGuckin CP, Ball SE, Gordon-Smith EC. Diamond–Blackfan anemia: Three patterns of *in vitro* response to haemopoietic growth factors. *Br J Haematol* 1995; **89**: 457–464

64. Drachtman RA, Geissler EN, Alter BP. The *SCF* and *c-kit* genes in Diamond–Blackfan anemia. *Blood* 1992; **79**: 2177–2178

65. Abkowitz JL, Broudy VC, Bennett LG, Zsebo KM, Martin FH. Absence of abnormalities of c-kit or its ligand in two patients with Diamond–Blackfan anemia. *Blood* 1992; **79**: 25–28

66. Paquette RL, Hsu NC, Koeffler HP. Analysis of c-*kit* gene integrity in aplastic anemia. *Blood Cell Mol Dis* 1996; **22**: 159–168

67. Rath A, Schmal G, Niemeyer C. Diamond–Blackfan anemia patients express normal levels of erythroid transcription factors during erythroid differentiation *in vitro*. *Blood* 1996; **88 (Suppl 1)**:143A

68. Gasser C. Aplastische anamia (chronische Erythroblastophtise) und Cortison. *Schweiz Med Wochenschr* 1951; **81**: 1241–1242

69. Krause PR, Klinman DM. Efficacy, immunogenicity, safety and use of live attenuated chickenpox vaccine. *J Pediatr* 1995; **127**: 518–525

70. Ozsoylu S: High-dose intravenous corticosteroid for a patient with Diamond–Blackfan syndrome refractory to classical prednisone treatment. *Acta Haematol* 1984; **71**: 207–210

71. Ozsoylu S. High-dose intravenous corticosteroid treatment for patients with Diamond–Blackfan syndrome resistant or refractory to conventional treatment. *Am J Pediatr Hematol Oncol* 1988; **10**: 210–217

72. Ozsoylu S. Oral megadose methylprednisolone for treatment of Diamond Blackfan anaemia. *Br J Haematol* 1992; **81**: 135–136

73. Bernini JC, Carillo JM, Buchanan GR. High-dose intravenous methylprednisolone therapy for patients with Diamond–Blackfan anemia refractory to conventional doses of prednisone. *J Pediatr* 1995: **127**: 654–659

74. Wasser JS, Yolken R, Miller DR, Diamond L. Congenital hypoplastic anemia (Diamond–Blackfan syndrome) terminating in acute myelogenous leukemia. *Blood* 1978; **51**: 991–995

75. Glader BE, Flam MS, Dahl GV, Hyman CB. Hematologic malignancies in Diamond–Blackfan anemia. *Pediatr Res* 1990; **27**: 142A

76. Splain J, Berman BW. Cyclosporin A treatment for Diamond–Blackfan anemia. *Am J Hematol* 1992; **39**: 208–211

77. Bejaoui M, Fitouri Z. Failure of immunosuppressive therapy and high-dose intravenous immunoglobulins in four transfusion-dependent, steroid-unresponsive Blackfan–Diamond anemia patients. *Haematologica* 1993; **78**: 38–39

78. August CS, King E, Gihens JH *et al*. Establishment of erythropoieis following bone marrow transplantation in a patient with congenital hypoplastic anemia (Diamond–Blackfan syndrome). *Blood* 1976; **48**: 491–498

79. Iriondo A. Garijo J, Baro J *et al*. Complete recovery of hemopoiesis following bone marrow transplant in a patient with unresponsive congenital hypoplastic anemia (Blackfan–Diamond syndrome). Blood 1984; **64**: 348–351

80. Wiktor-Jedrzejczak W, Szczylik C, Pojda Z *et al*. Success of bone marrow transplantation in congenital Diamond–Blackfan anaemia: a case report. *Eur J Haematol* 1987; **38**: 204–206

81. Mugishima H, Gale RP, Rowlings PA *et al*. Bone marrow transplantation for Diamond–Blackfan anemia. Bone Marrow Transplant 1995; **15**: 55–58

82. Bonno M, Azuma E, Nakano T *et al*. Successful hematopoietic reconstitution by transplantation with umbilical cord blood cells in a patient with Diamond–Blackfan anemia. *Blood* 1995; **86**: 938A

83. Giardini C, Galimberti M, Lucarelli G. Bone marrow transplantation in thalassemia. *Ann Rev Med* 1995; **46**: 319–330

84. Casadevall N, Croisille L, Auffray I, Tchernia G, Coulombel L. Age-related alterations in erythroid and granulopoietic progenitors in Diamond–Blackfan anaemia. *Br J Haematol* 1994; **87**: 369–375

85. Wranne L. Transient erythroblastopenia in infancy and childhood. *Scand J Haematol* 1970; **7**: 76–81

86. Lovric VA. Anemia and temporary erythroblastopenia in children. *Aust Ann Med* 1970; **1**: 34–39

87. Kynaston JA, West NC, Reid MM. A regional experience of red cell aplasia. *Eur J Pediatr* 1993; **152**: 306–308

88. Cherrick I, Karayalcin G, Landzowsky P. Transient erythroblastopenia of childhood: prospective study of fifty patients. *Am J Pediatr Hematol Oncol* 1994; **16**: 320–324

89. Ware RE, Kinney TR. Transient erythroblastopenia in the first year of life. *Am J Hematol* 1991; **37**: 156–158

90. Miller R, Berman B. Transient erythroblastopenia of childhood in infants <6 months of age. *Am J Pediatr Hematol Oncol* 1994; **16**: 246–248

91. Labotka RJ, MaurerMS, Honig GR. Transient erythroblastopenia of childhood: review of 17 cases including a pair of identical twins. *Am J Dis Child* 1981; **135**: 937–940

92. Young RSR, Rannels DE, Hilmo A, Gerson JM, Goodrich D. Severe anemia in childhood presenting as transient ischemic attacks. *Stroke* 1983; **14**: 622–623

93. Green N, Garvin J, Chutorian A. Transient erythroblastopenia of childhood presenting with papilledema. *Clin Ped* 1986; **25**: 278–279

94. Michelson A, Marshall P. Transient neurological disorder associated with transient erythroblastopenia of childhood. *Am J Pediatr Hematol Oncol* 1987; **9**: 161–163

95. Hanada T, Koike K, Hirano C *et al*. Childhood transient erythroblastopenia complicated by thrombocytopenia and neutropenia. *Eur J Haematol* 1989; **42**: 77–80

96. Wodzinski MA, Lilleyman JS. Transient erythroblastopenia of childhood due to human parvovirus B19 infection. *Br J Haematol* 1989; **73**: 127–131

97. Wang WC, Mentzer WC. Differentiation of transient erythroblastopenia of childhood from congenital hypoplastic anemia. *J Pediatr* 1976; **88**: 784–789

98. Paglia D, Renner S, Valentine W, Nakatani M, Brockway R. The significance of distinctive enzyme profiles in transient erythroblastopenia of childhood and congenital hypoplastic anemia. *Blood* 1991; **78**: 98A

99. Karsten J, Anker AP, Odink RJ. Glycosylated haemoglobin and transient erythroblastopenia of childhood. *Lancet* 1996; **347**: 273

100. Bhambhani K, Inoue S, Sanaik SA. Seasonal clustering of transient erythroblastopenia of childhood. *Am J Dis Child* 1988; **142**: 175–177

101. Kubic PT, Warkentin PI, Levitt CJ, Coccia PF. Transient erythroblastopenia of childhood (TEC) occurring in clusters. *Pediatr Res* 1979; **13**: 435

102. Seip M. Transient erythroblastopenia in siblings. *Acta Paediatr Scand* 1982; **71**: 689–690

103. Elian JC, Frappaz D, Pozzetto B, Freycon F. Transient erythroblastopenia of childhood presenting with echovirus 11 infection. *Acta Paediatr* 1993; **82**: 492–494

104. Koenig HM, Lightsey AL, Nelson DP, Diamond LK. Immune suppression of erythropoiesis in transient erythroblastopenia of childhood. *Blood* 1979; **54**: 742–746

105. Dessypris EN, Krantz SB, Roloff JS, Lukens JN. Mode of action of the IgG inhibitor of erythropoiesis in transient erythroblastopenia of childhood. *Blood* 1982; **59**: 114–123

106. Freedman M, Saunders EF. Transient erythroblastopenia of childhood: varied pathogenesis. *Am J Hematol* 1983; **14**: 247–254

107. Hanada T, Abe T, Takita H. T-cell-mediated inhibition of erythropoiesis in transient erythroblastopenia of childhood. *Br J Haematol* 1985; **59**: 391–392

108. Anderson MJ, Higgins PG, Davis LR *et al*. Experimental parvoviral infection in humans. *J Infect Dis* 1985; **152**: 257–265

109. Freedman MH. "Recurrent" erythroblastopenia of childhood. *Am J Dis Child* 1983; **137**: 458–460

110. Owren PA. Congenital hemolytic jaundice. The pathogenesis of the 'hemolytic crisis'. *Blood* 1948; **3**: 231–248

111. Tchernia G, Morinet F, Congard B, Croisille L. Diamond Blackfan anemia: apparent relapse due to B19 parvovirus. *Eur J Pediatr* 1993; **152**: 209–210

112. Bell LM, Naides SJ, Stoffman P, Hodinka RL, Plotkin SA. Human parvovirus B19 infection among hospital staff members after contact with infected patients. *N Engl J Med* 1989; **321**: 485–491

113. Cossart YE, Cant B, Field AM, Widdows D. Parvovirus-like particles in human sera. *Lancet* 1975; **i**: 72–73

114. Pattison JR, Jones SE, Hodgson J *et al*. Parvovirus infections and hypoplastic crisis in sickle cell anemia *Lancet* 1981; **i**: 664–665

115. Serjeant GR, Topley JM, Mason K *et al*. Outbreak of aplastic crises in sickle cell anaemia associated with parvovirus-like agent. *Lancet* 1981; **ii**: 595–597

116. Harris JW. Parvovirus B19 for the hematologist. *Am J Hematol* 1992; **39**: 119–130

117. Brown KE, Anderson SM, Young NS. Erythrocyte P antigen: cellular receptor for B19 parvovirus. *Science* 1993; **262**: 114–117

118. Mortimer PP, Humphries RK, Moore JG *et al*. A human parvovirus-like virus inhibits haematopoietic colony formation *in vitro*. Nature 1983; **302**: 426–429

119. Young NS, Mortimer PP, Moore JG, Humphries RK. Characteriza-

tion of a virus that causes transient aplastic crisis. *J Clin Invest* 1984; **73**: 224–230

120. Brownell AI, McSwiggan DA, Cubitt WD, Anderson MJ. Aplastic and hypoplastic episodes in sickle cell disease and thalassaemia intermedia. *J Clin Path* 1986; **39**: 121–124

121. Kurtzman GJ, Ozawa K, Cohen B, Hanson G, Oseas R, Young NS. Chronic bone marrow failure due to persistent parvovirus B19 infection. *N Engl J Med* 1987; **317**: 287–294

122. Frickhofen N, Young NS. Persistent parvovirus B19 infections in humans. *Microbial Pathogen* 1989; **7**: 319–327

123. Kurtzman GJ, Cohen BJ, Field AM, Oseas R, Blaese RM, Young NS. Immune response to B19 parvovirus and an antibody defect in persistent viral infection. *J Clin Invest* 1989; **84**: 1114–1123

124. Nigro G, Gattinara GC, Mattia S, Caniglia M, Fridell E. Parvovirus B19-related pancytopenia in children with HIV infection. *Lancet* 1992; **340**: 145

125. Gahr M, Pekrun A, Eiffert H. Persistence of parvovirus B19-DNA in blood of a child with severe combined immunodeficiency associated with pure red cell aplasia. *Eur J Pediatr* 1991; **150** :470–472

126. Lefrere J-J, Mariotti M, Thauvin M. B19 parvovirus DNA in solvent/detergent-treated anti-haemophilia concentrates. *Lancet* 1994; **343**: 211–212

127. Kurtzman GJ, Cohen B, Meyers P, Amunullah A, Young NS. Persistent B19 parvovirus infection as a cause of severe chronic anaemia in children with acute lymphocytic leukaemia. Lancet 1988; **ii**: 1159–1162

128. Murray JC, Greisik MV, Leger F, McClain KL. B19 parvovirus-induced anemia in a normal child. *Am J Ped Hematol Oncol* 1993; **15**: 420–423

129. Salimans MM, Holsappel S, van de Rijke FM, Jiwa NM, Raap AK, Weiland HT. Rapid detection of human parvovirus B19 DNA by dot-hybridization and the polymerase chain reaction. *J Virol Methods* 1989; **23**: 19–28

130. Kurtzman GK, Frickhofen N, Kimball J, Jenkins DW, Nienhuis AW, Young NS. Pure red cell aplasia of 100 years' duration due to persistent parvovirus B19 infection and its cure with immunoglobulin therapy. *N Engl J Med* 1989; **321**: 519–525

131. Imamura N, Kuramoto A, Morimoto T, Ihara A. Pure red cell aplasia associated with acute lymphoblastic leukemia of pre-T-cell origin. Med J Aust 1986; **144**: 724

132. Rubin RN, Walker BK, Ballas SK, Travis SF. Erythroid aplasia in juvenile rheumatoid arthritis. *Am J Dis Child* 1978; **132**: 760–762

133. Schmid JR, Kiely JM, Harrison EG Jr *et al*. Thymoma associated with red cell agenesis: review of literature and report of cases. Cancer 1965; **18**: 216–230

134. Clark DA, Dessypris EN, Krantz SB. Studies on pure red cell aplasia. XI. Results of immunosuppressive treatment of 37 patients. *Blood* 1984; **63**: 277–286

135. Thompson DF, Gales MA. Drug-induced pure red cell aplasia. *Pharmacotherapy* 1996; **16**: 1002–1008

136. Hirai H. Two cases of erythroid hypoplasia caused by carbamazepine. *Jpn J Clin Hematol* 1977; **18**: 33–38

137. Medberry CA, Pappas AA, Ackerman BH. Carbamazepine and erythroid arrest. *Drug Intell Clin Pharm* 1987; **21**: 439–442

138. Dessypris EN, Redline S, Harris JW, Krantz SB. Diphenylhydantoin-induced pure red cell aplasia. *Blood* 1985; **65**: 789–794

139. MacDougall LG. Pure red cell aplasia associated with sodium valproate therapy. *JAMA* 1982; **247**: 53–54

140. Krantz SB, Kao V. Studies on red cell aplasia. I. Demonstration of a plasma inhibitor to heme synthesis and an antibody to erythroblastic nuclei. *Proc Natl Acad Sci USA* 1967; **58**: 493–500

141. Nagasawa M, Okawa H, Yata J. A B cell line from a patient with pure red cell aplasia produces an immunoglobulin that suppresses erythropoiesis. *Clin Immunol Immunopathol* 1991; **61**: 18–28

142. Abkowitz JL, Kadin ME, Powell JS, Adamson JW. Pure red cell aplasia:lymphocyte inhibition of erythropoiesis. *Br J Haematol* 1986; **63**: 59–67

143. Hanada T, Abe T, Nakamura H, Aoki Y. Pure red cell aplasia: relationship between inhibitory activity of T cells to CFU-E and erythropoiesis. *Br J Haematol* 1984; **58**: 107–113

144. Corcione A, Pasino M, Claudio-Molinari AC, Acquila M, Marchese P, Mori PG. A paediatric case of pure red cell aplasia: successful treatment with anti-lymphocyte globulin and correlation with *in vitro* T cell-mediated inhibition of erythropoiesis. *Br J Haematol* 1991; **79**: 129–130

145. Krantz SB. Pure red cell aplasia: biology and treatment. In: Feig SA, Freedman MH (eds) *Clinical Disorders and Experimental Models of Erythropoetic Failure*. Boca Raton, FL: CRC Press, 1993, pp 85–124

146. Abkowitz JL, Powell JS, Nakamura JM, Kadin ME, Adamson JW. Pure red cell aplasia: response to therapy with antilymphocyte globulin. *Am J Hematol* 1986; **28**: 363–371

147. Lacombe C, Casadevall N, Muller O, Varet B. Erythroid progenitors in adult chronic pure red cell aplasia: relationship of *in vitro* erythroid colonies to therapeutic response. *Blood* 1984; **64**: 71–77

148. Charles RJ, Sabo KM, Kidd PG, Abkowitz JL. The pathophysiology of pure red cell aplasia: implications for therapy. *Blood* 1996; **87**: 4831–4838

149. Messner HA, Fauser AA, Curtis JE, Dotten D. Control of antibody-mediated pure red-cell aplasia by plasmapheresis. *N Engl J Med* 1981; **304**: 1334–1338

150. Public Health Laboratory Service Working Party on Fifth Disease. Prospective study of human parvovirus (B19) infection in pregnancy. *Br Med J* 1990; **33**: 1166–1170

151. Young NS. B19 parvovirus. *Baillière's Clin Haematol* 1995; **8**: 25–56

152. Vaughan JL, Warwick R, Letsky E, Nicolini U, Rodeck CH, Fisk NM. Erythropoietic suppression in fetal anemia because of Kell alloimmunization. *Am J Obstet Gynecol* 1994; **171**: 247–252

153. Weiner CP, Widness JA. Decreased fetal erythropoiesis and hemolysis in Kell hemolytic anemia. *Am J Obstet Gynecol* 1996; **174**: 547–551

154. Manning M, Warwick R, Vaughan J, Roberts IAG. Inhibition of erythroid progenitor cell growth by anti-Kell: a mechanism for fetal anaemia in Kell-immunized pregnancies. *Br J Haematol* 1996; **93 (Suppl 1)**: 13

155. Sahovic EA, Flick J, Graham CD, Stuart RK. Case report: isoimmune inhibition of erythropoiesis following ABO-incompatible bone marrow transplantation. *Am J Med Sci* 1991; **302**: 369–373

156. Nilsson LR. Chronic pancytopenia with multiple congenital abnormalities (Fanconi's anemia). *Acta Paediatr* 1960; **49**: 519–529

157. Butturini A, Gale RP, Verlander PC, Adler-Brecher B, Gillio AP, Auerbach AD. Hematologic abnormalities in Fanconi anemia: an International Fanconi Anemia Registry study. *Blood* 1994; **84**: 1650–1655

158. German J, Schonberg S, Caskie S, Warburton D, Falk C, Ray JH. A test for Fanconi's anemia. *Blood* 1987; **69**: 1637–1641

159. *Ciba Foundation Symposium 37 (New Series) Congenital Disorders of Erythropoiesis*. Amsterdam: Elsevier, 1976, pp 135–203

160. Marks PW, Mitus AJ. Congenital dyserythropoietic anemias. *Am J Hematol* 1996; **51**: 55–63

161. Lewis SM, Verwilghen RN (eds). *Dyserythropoiesis*. London: Academic Press, 1977, p 350

162. Heimpel H, Wendt F. Congenital dyserythropoietic anemia with karyorrhexis and multinuclearity of erythroblasts. *Helv Med Acta* 1968; **34**: 103–115

163. Heimpel H. Congenital dyserythropoietic anemia Type I. In: Lewis SM, Verwilghen RL (eds) *Dyserythropoiesis*. London: Academic Press, 1977, pp 55–70

164. Tamary H, Shalev H, Luria D *et al.* Clinical features and studies of erythropoiesis in Israeli Bedouins with congenital dyserythropoietic anemia type I. *Blood* 1996; **87**: 1763–1770

165. Brichard B, Vermylen C, Scheiff JM, Muichanze JL, Ninane J, Cornu G. Two cases of congenital dyserythropoietic anaemia type I associated with unusual skeletal abnormalities of the limbs. *Br J Haematol* 1994; **86**: 201–202

166. Clauvel JP, Cosson A, Breton-Gorius J *et al.* Dysérythropoïèse con-

génitale (étude de 6 observations). *Nouv Rev Française Hématol* 1972; **12**; 653–652

167. Heimpel H, Wendt F, Klemm D, Schubothe H, Heilmeyer L. Kongenitale Dyserythropoietsche Anämie. *Archiv Klin Med* 1968; **215**: 174–194

168. Heimpel H, Forteza-Vila J, Queisser W, Spiertz E. Electron and light microscopic study of the erythroblasts of patients with congenital dyserythropoietic anemia. *Blood* 1971; **37**: 299–310

169. Londe E, Mazo E, Baro J *et al.* Transmission and scanning electron microscopy study on congenital dyserythropoietic anaemia type I. *Acta Haematol* 1983; **70**: 243–249

170. Lewis SM, Frische B. Congenital dyserythropoietic anaemias: electron microscopy. In: *Ciba Foundation Symposium 37 (New Series) Congenital Disorders of Erythropoiesis*. Amsterdam: Elsevier, 1976, pp 171–203

171. Meuret G, Taschan P, Schulter G, Eyerlingk DG, Boll I. DNA, histone, RNA, hemoglobin-content and DNA synthesis in erythroblasts in a case of congenital dyserythropoietic anemia type I. *Blut* 1972; **24**: 32–41

172. Wickramasinghe S, Pippard MJ. Studies of erythroblast function in congenital dyserythropoietic anaemia, type I: evidence of impaired DNA, RNA and protein synthesis and unbalanced globin chain synthesis in ultrastructurally abnormal cells. *J Clin Pathol* 1986; **39**: 881–890

173. Hewitt PE, Win AA, Davies SC. CDA type I with persistent haemosideriunuria: absence of iron loading. *Br J Haematol* 1984; **56**: 682–684

174. Lavabre-Bartrand T, Blanc P, Navarro R *et al.* Alpha-interferon therapy for congenital dyserythropoiesis type I. *Br J Haematol* 1995; **89**: 929–932

175. Virjee S, Hatton C. Congenital dyserythropoiesis type I and alpha-interferon therapy. *Br J Haematol* 1996; **94**: 581–582

176. Crookston JH, Crookston MC, Burnie KL *et al.* Hereditary erythroblastic multinuclearity associated with a positive acidified serum lysis test: a type of congenital dyserythropoietic anaemia. *Br J Haematol* 1969; **17**: 11–26

177. Verwilghen RL, Lewis SM, Dacie JV, Crookston JH, Crookston MC. HEMPAS: Congenital dyserythropoietic anaemia type II. *Q J Med* 1973; **42**: 257–278

178. Faruqui S, Abraham A, Berenfeld MR, Galenzda TG. Normal serum ferritin in a patient with HEMPAS syndrome and iron overload. *Am J Clin Pathol* 1982; **78**: 97–101

179. Halpern Z, Rahman R, Levo Y. Severe haemochromatosis: the predominant clinical manifestation of congenital dyserythropoietic anaemia type II. *Acta Haematol* 1985; **74**: 178–180

180. Verwilghen RL. Congenital dyserythropoietic anaemia type II (Hempas). In: *Ciba Foundation Symposium 37 (New Series) Congenital Disorders of Erythropoiesis*. Amsterdam: Elsevier, 1976, pp 151–170

181. Majeed HA, Kalaawi M, Mohanty D *et al.* Congenital dyserythropoietic anemia and chronic multifocal osteomyelitis in three related children and the association with Sweet syndrome in two siblings. *J Pediatr* 1989; **115**: 730–734

182. Sykora KW, Niedich J, Price J, Bussel J. Type II congenital dyserythropoietic anemia in a patient with ectodermal dysplasia. Distinction from dyskeratosis congenita. *Am J Pediatr Hematol Oncol* 1994; **16**: 173–176

183. Clauvel JP, Erlinger S. Congenital dyserythropoietic anemia and the Dublin–Johnson syndrome. A case report. *Gastroenterology* 1974; **67**: 686–690

184. Hernandez P, Almagro D, Corral JF, Opolski A, Sanchez JA, Rodriguez N. Association of type II congenital dyserythropoietic anaemia and von Willebrand's disease. *Br J Haematol* 1974; **27**: 453–462

185. Tomita A, Parker CJ. Aberrant regulation of complement by the erythrocytes of hereditary erythroblastic multinuclearity with a positive acidified serum lysis test (HEMPAS). *Blood* 1994; **83**: 250–259

186. Alloisio N, Texier P, Denoroy L *et al.* The cisternae decorating the red blood cell membrane in congenital dyserythropoietic anemia (type

II) originate from the endoplasmic reticulum. *Blood* 1996; **87**: 4433–4439

187. Frische B, Lewis SM, Sherman D, White JM, Gordon-Smith EC. The ultrastructure of erythropoiesis in two haemoglobinopathies. *Br J Haematol* 1974; **28**: 109–117

188. Fukuda MN. Congenital dyserythropoietic anaemia type II (HEMPAS) and its molecular basis. *Baillière's Clin Haematol* 1993; **6**: 493–511

189. Anselstetter V, Horstmann H-J, Heimpel H. Congenital dyserythropoietic anamia type I and II: aberrant pattern of erythrocyte membrane proteins in CDA II, as revealed by two-dimensional polyacrylamide gel electrophoresis. *Br J Haematol* 1977; **35**: 209–215

190. Baines AJ, Banga JPS, Gratzer WB, Linch DC, Huehns ER. Red cell membrane protein anomalies in congenital dyserythropoietic anaemia type II (HEMPAS). *Br J Haematol* 1982; **50**: 563–574

191. Harlow RWH, Lowenthal RM. Erythrocyte membrane proteins in an unusual case of congenital dyserythropoitic anaemia type II (CDA II). *Br J Haematol* 1982; **50**: 35–41

192. Fukuda MN, Papayannopoulou T, Gordon-Smith EC, Rochant H, Testa U. Defect on glycosylation of erythrocyte membrane proteins in congenital dyserythropoietic anaemia type II (HEMPAS). *Br J Haematol* 1984; **56**: 55–68

193. Fukuda MN, Masri KA, Dell A, Luzzatto L, Moreman KW. Incomplete synthesis of N-glycans in congenital dyserytrhopoietic anemia type II (HEMPAS) caused by a gene defect encoding a-mannosidase II. *Proc Natl Acad Sci USA* 1990; **87**: 7443–7557

194. Fukuda MN, Dell A, Scartezzini P. Primary defect of congenital dyserythropoietic anemia type II: Failure in glycosylation of erythrocyte lactosaminoglycan proteins caused by lowered N-acetylglucosaminyltransferase II. *J Biol Chem* 1987; **67**: 95–101

195. Fukuda MN, Klier G, Scartezzini P. Anomalous clustering of underglycosylated band 3 in erythrocytes and their precursor cells in congenital dyserythropoietic anemia type II. *Blood* 1986; **68**: 521–529

196. Wolff JA, von Hofe FH. Familial erythroid multinuclearity. *Blood* 1951; **6**: 1274–1283

197. Goudsmit R. Congenital dyserythropoietic anaemia, type III. In: Lewis SM, Berwilghen RL (eds) *Dyserythropoiesis*. London: Academic Press, 1977, pp 83–92

198. Lind L, Sandström H, Whalin A *et al*. Localization of the gene for congenital dyserythropoietic anemia type II, CDA N23, to chromosome 15q21-q25. *Hum Mol Genet* 1995; **4**: 109–112

199. Sandström H, Wahlin A, Eriksson M, Bergström I, Wickramasinghe SN. Intravascular haemolysis and increased prevalence of myeloma and monoclonal gammopathy in congenital dyserythropoietic anaemia type III. *Eur J Haematol* 1994; **52**: 42–46

200. Roberts DJ, Nadel A, Lage J, Rutherford CJ. An unusual variant of congenital dyserythropoietic anaemia with mild maternal and lethal fetal disease. *Br J Haematol* 1993; **84**: 549–551

201. Cantu-Rajinoldi A, Zanella Z, Couter U *et al*. A severe transfusion-dependent congenital dyserythropoietic anaemia presenting as hydrops fetalis. *Br J Haematol* 1997; **96**: 530–533

202. Carter C, Darbyshire PJ, Wickramasinghe SN. A congenital dyserythropoietic anaemia presenting as hydrops foetalis. *Br J Haematol* 1989; **72**: 289–290

203. Williams G, Lorimer S, Merry CC, Greenberg CR, Bishop AJ. A variant congenital dyserythropoietic anaemia presented as a fatal hydrops foetalis. *Br J Haematol* 1990; **76**: 438–439

204. Sansone G, Masera G, Cantu-Rajnoldi A, Terzoli S. An unclassified case of congenital dyserythropoietic anaemia with a severe neonatal onset. *Acta Haematol* 1992; **88**: 41–45

205. Fessas Ph. Inclusions of hemoglobin in erythroblasts and erythrocytes of thalassaemias. *Blood* 1973; **21**: 21–32

206. Weatherall DJ, Clegg JB, Knox-Macaulay HHM, Bunch C, Hopkins CR, Temperley IJ. A genetically determined disorder with features both of thalassaemia and congenital dyserythropoietic anaemia. *Br J Haematol* 1973; **24**: 681–702

207. Wickramasinghe SN, Goudsmit R. Precipitation of β-globin chains within the erythropoietic cells of a patient with congenital dyserythropoietic anaemia, type III. *Br J Haematol* 1987; **65**: 250–251

208. Wickramasinghe SN, Lee MJ, Furukawa T, Eguchi M, Reid CDL. Composition of the intra-erythroblastic precipitates in thalassaemia and congenital dyserthropoietic anaemia (CDA): identification of a new type of CDA with intra-erythroblastic precipitates not reacting with monoclonal antibodies to α and β-globin chains. *Br J Haematol* 1996; **93**: 570–585

Myelodysplastic syndromes

JUDITH M CHESSELLS

Over 95% of children with leukemia have acute myeloid leukemia (AML) or acute lymphoblastic leukemia (ALL); the others have more chronic disorders, either myeloproliferative or myelodysplastic. Chronic lymphocytosis in childhood is usually a response to an infection or an immunoregulatory disorder (see Chapter 25); there have only been a handful of reports of apparent chronic lymphocytic leukemia in childhood.

The term chronic myeloproliferative disorder, denoting an abnormal proliferation of the bone marrow with, usually, a correspondingly raised blood count, was coined in the 1950s by Dameshek to describe a spectrum of diseases that included chronic granulocytic leukemia, polycythemia rubra vera, essential thrombocythemia and myelofibrosis. The myelodysplastic syndromes (MDSs) were historically characterized by a cellular marrow with peripheral pancytopenia, but the distinction between the two groups is really an artificial one, since both myeloproliferative and myelodysplastic disorders arise from an abnormal clone of cells and carry a risk of progression to acute leukemia, albeit at a variable pace. The MDSs were first described as smouldering leukemia or pre-leukemia and, being largely a disease of the elderly, have been well classified in the extensive adult literature.

Early reports of chronic leukemias in childhood[1,2] make no distinction between chronic myeloid leukemia (CML) and what would now be deemed MDS and only in the last few years have any serious attempts been made to classify pediatric MDS, which differs in many important respects from the disease in adults.[3–10] The advent of more effective treatment, in particular bone marrow transplantation (BMT), has made a rational approach to diagnosis and management of increasing importance. The myeloproliferative syndromes, save chronic granulocytic leukemia (see Chapter 20), are exceptionally rare. This chapter reviews the MDSs.

HISTORICAL PERSPECTIVE

Thirty-five years ago Hardisty et al[11] distinguished two types of what they called chronic granulocytic leukemia in childhood. The so-called adult type, with a relatively long survival, was associated with the then newly described Philadelphia chromosome, and juvenile chronic myeloid leukemia, subsequently called, at least by the French, juvenile chronic myelomonocytic leukemia,[12] was associated with suppurative infections, severe thrombocytopenia, a non-specific but very characteristic skin rash and a very poor prognosis. Further interest in this rare disorder was awakened by the reports of a consistently raised fetal hemoglobin (HbF) level and fetal red cell characteristics.[13] A third chronic disorder was described in young infants with a missing C group chromosome,[14] which was subsequently identified as a number 7.[15] These three conditions, dependent in part on clinical features for diagnosis, comprised the most clinically distinct myeloproliferative or myelodysplastic disorders in childhood but there was no systematic review of the associated blood and marrow morphology. At the same time, retrospective and more stringent analysis of cases of pediatric AML showed that a proportion of cases, perhaps 17%, had a more indolent prodrome and might be called pre-leukemic or myelodysplastic.[16]

Meanwhile, the morphologic classification of MDS in adults was rationalized by the efforts of the French-American-British (FAB) group (see below),[17] and terms such as pre-leukemia tended to be abandoned in favor of the appropriate FAB type of MDS. Until recently, pediatricians have tended to pay scant attention to these morphologic niceties, have continued to classify patients according to the various clinical features outlined above and have only recently recognized that a proportion of children entered onto protocols for AML, could, on morphologic review, be more accurately classified as having MDS.

INCIDENCE AND EPIDEMIOLOGY

MDS is largely a disease of the elderly and the incidence rises dramatically with increasing age.[18,19] There have been a number of recent attempts to estimate its incidence in childhood, but these have been derived from relatively small populations and it seems probable that the incidence of the more indolent forms of MDS has been underestimated. A population-based study in Denmark estimated that the incidence of MDS approximated that of AML at 4.0 new cases/million children/year, thus representing 9% of all hematologic malignancies,[20] whereas in the northern region in England the estimated incidence was 0.53/million or 1% of malignancies.[21] These discrepancies could be due in part to the inclusion or exclusion of more aggressive forms (e.g. refractory anemia with excess of blasts in transformation) as either MDS or AML rather than any true variation in incidence. Larger studies in progress should put these estimates on a firmer footing.

A characteristic feature of MDS in childhood is its frequent association with other conditions (Table 4.1); in recent non-population-based reports between one-quarter and one-half of patients[8,9] have shown some phenotypic abnormality. Some of these are non-specific such as mental retardation or small stature but others are recognized genetic conditions. Children with Down's syndrome have a 10–20-fold increased risk of development of leukemia, usually the early pre-B or common type of lymphoblastic leukemia or the megakaryoblastic (M7) subtype of AML. Patients with megakaryoblastic leukemia often have a preceding phase of MDS which may last some weeks or months. This evolving myeloid leukemia, which is fatal if untreated,[22] should not be confused with the transient abnormal myelopoiesis (TAM) seen in some newborn babies with Down's syndrome and in occasional normal neonates; a condition resembling acute leukemia but which usually resolves without specific treatment.[23] Constitutional trisomy 8 usually occurs in mosaic form and is associated with facial dysmorphism, skeletal abnormalities and mild-to-moderate mental retardation.[24]

Table 4.1 Conditions associated with the development of myelodysplasia in childhood.

Congenital disorders
Down's syndrome
Trisomy 8
Neurofibromatosis type 1
Congenital bone marrow disorders
   Fanconi's anemia
   Congenital neutropenia including Kostmann's syndrome
   Diamond–Blackfan anemia
   Shwachman–Diamond syndrome

Familial MDS

Acquired disorders
Aplastic anemia with previous immunosuppressive therapy
Previous cytotoxic or radiation therapy

Trisomy 8 is a common cytogenetic finding in myeloid malignancies but there are a number of patients with constitutional trisomy 8 who have developed hematologic disorders including MDS.[25,26] The author has seen 3 such cases but the precise frequency is unknown.

There is an increased risk of chronic myelomonocytic leukemia (CMML) in the common autosomal dominant form of neurofibromatosis[27,28] and MDS in infants with monosomy 7[29] is also associated with this disorder. A number of congenital bone marrow disorders predispose to the development of AML and MDS, including congenital neutropenia, in particular Kostmann's syndrome (see Chapters 1 and 16), where treatment with granulocyte colony-stimulating factor (G-CSF) may improve symptoms and obviate the need for BMT, but has been associated with an increased risk of development of monosomy 7 and MDS.[30] Patients with the Shwachman–Diamond syndrome of pancreatic exocrine insufficiency and neutropenia have generalized abnormalities of hematopoiesis and are at increased risk of AML, ALL and MDS.[31,32] Patients with Fanconi's anemia are at significant risk of the development of AML but may also present with MDS.[33]

There are a number of families described in the literature with no apparent congenital or genetic abnormality in whom >1 member has developed MDS or AML. MDS with monosomy 7 has been described in infant siblings,[3,34] but in other families >1 member has developed AML or MDS in later childhood or adult life, sometimes in association with a familial platelet storage pool disorder.[35] In several instances, the development of MDS has been associated with evolution of a cytogenetic abnormality in the bone marrow, most often monosomy 7 or 5.

Immunosuppressive therapy with antilymphocyte globulin, cyclosporin A and other agents, often with the addition of G-CSF has improved survival in patients with acquired aplastic anemia, particularly those without a histocompatible sibling donor (see Chapter 2). However, there is now increasing evidence that patients surviving immunosuppressive treatment are at increased risk of MDS.[36]

Secondary MDS with a predilection to development of AML was first described in patients treated for Hodgkin's disease, multiple myeloma and ovarian cancer and more recently after high-dose chemoradiotherapy and infusion of autologous bone marrow.[37,38] By contrast, secondary acute leukemia in patients who have been treated with topoisomerase II inhibitors usually occurs without any dysplastic prodrome.

CLINICAL FEATURES

The symptoms and signs of MDS are more insidious than those of acute leukemia, and the diagnosis may even be made incidentally. Pallor is common, bacterial infections may be a consequence of neutropenia or defective neutrophil function and bruising may be due to thrombocytopenia or defective platelet function. Patients may also present with a prolonged history of repeated infections which is suggestive of congenital immune deficiency. Lymph node enlargement is unusual except in CMML. The liver and spleen may be enlarged or impalpable. A characteristic skin rash, mimicking Langerhan's cell histiocytosis, may occur on the face or trunk in CMML, and occasionally in infants with other types of MDS in association with monosomy 7 (Plate 3).

INVESTIGATIONS

BLOOD AND BONE MARROW EXAMINATION

Table 4.2 lists the recommended investigations in children with suspected MDS. The blood and bone marrow appearances are extremely variable and a list of noteworthy features is given in Table 4.3. It is essential to examine the blood film and bone marrow in tandem and *the blood film is often more informative in reaching a diagnosis*. A trephine biopsy of the bone marrow should be obtained in all cases and important observations include:

- overall cellularity of the bone marrow;
- relative proportions and morphology of the three cell lines, especially the megakaryocytes;

Table 4.2 Evaluation of suspected myelodysplastic syndrome.

History
Family history of leukemia or genetic disorders
History of previous cytotoxic therapy

Examination
Associated clinical disorders:
 Neurofibromatosis*
 Down's syndrome
 Fanconi's anemia
 Shwachman–Diamond syndrome
 Other congenital abnormalities

Blood samples
Full blood count and differential
Well stained blood film
Absolute count, monocytes, basophils, eosinophils
HbF level before blood transfusion
Virology, especially parvovirus, CMV and EBV*

Bone marrow aspiration
Morphology including iron stain
Cytogenetics including FISH
In vitro cultures of CFU-GM*

Bone marrow trephine biopsy
Morphology, especially of megakaryocytes
Cellularity and fibrosis
Presence of ALIP

Observation
Consistent hematologic abnormalities over 2 months

*Investigations indicated in *all* cases of chronic myelomonocytic leukemia (CMML).

Table 4.3 Common morphologic abnormalities in myelodysplasia. Based on Bennett et al.[17]

Cell lineage	Blood film	Bone marrow
Erythroid	Macrocytes Punctate basophilia Poikilocytes Normoblasts	Dyserythropoiesis Multinucleate normoblasts Cytoplasmic vacuolation Ringed sideroblasts
Megakaryocytic	Giant platelets Megakaryocyte fragments	Small megakaryocytes Abnormal nuclear morphology
Granulocytes	Hypogranular Agranular Hypersegmentation Pelger forms	Promyelocytes with sparse granules Hypogranular precursors
Monocytes	Elongated lobes Azurophilic granules	Promonocytes sometimes present
Blasts	Usually small mononuclear blasts with scanty agranular (Type I) or sparsely granular (Type II) blasts	

- presence of fibrosis and reticulin and of abnormally-localized immature precursor cells (ALIP). These are aggregates of myeloblasts and promyelocytes in the intertrabecular region in the bone marrow biopsy.

Immunohistochemical staining of bone marrow biopsies facilitates the identification of these immature precursors[39] and deserves further systematic study in children.

Other investigations, such as measurement of HbF, neutrophil function and platelet function may serve to confirm abnormalities of development of the 3 cell lines. Measurement of the HbF before any transfusions of red cells, may be helpful in evaluating prognosis (see below). Immunologic abnormalities may include low immunoglobulins, autoantibodies or even abnormalities of lymphocyte subsets. It may be necessary to exclude congenital viral infections. The hematologic appearances of HIV infection in adults may mimic MDS but this presentation has not been described in children.

Lastly, the diagnosis of MDS implies the finding of *consistent* hematologic abnormalities over a period of time, thus excluding patients with morphologic abnormalities in association with infection which may resolve spontaneously or patients whose abnormalities progress to frank AML within weeks.

Morphologic classification: The French-American-British (FAB) classification

The FAB classification[17] remains the gold standard for diagnosis and classification of MDS and every effort should

Table 4.4 FAB classification of myelodysplastic syndromes.[17]

Type	Blood film	Bone marrow
Refractory anemia (RA)	Blasts <1%	Blasts <5%
RA with ringed sideroblasts (RARS)	As in RA	As in RA but >15% of erythroblasts as ringed sideroblasts
RA with excess of blasts (RAEB)	Blasts <5%	Blasts 5–20%
RAEB in transformation (RAEBt)	Blasts >5% Auer rods	As RAEB but 20–30% blasts Auer rods
Chronic myelomonocytic leukemia (CMML)	Monocytes >1 × 10⁹/l Blasts <5%*	Blasts <20%

*CMML in children is often associated with a higher blast count in the blood, but marrow blasts should not exceed 20% and Auer rods should not be present.

be made to assign an FAB subtype to all suspected cases. The original FAB classification (Table 4.4) has recently been modified to take account of the overlap between some cases of apparent atypical Ph-negative CML and classic CMML with the suggestion that some CMML should be classed as a myeloproliferative disorder.[40] This modification is probably more confusing than helpful in pediatric practice. There have also been concerns that the FAB classification does not address the distinction between refractory cytopenia with multilineage dysplasia and aplastic anemia,[41] and this issue remains unresolved.

The FAB classification has a number of limitations in childhood.

- Many children with MDS have a monocytosis which thus automatically classes them as having CMML. However, in many such cases there may be >5% blasts in the blood without an excess of blasts in the marrow. This finding should in theory mean reclassification as RAEB in transformation but in most pediatric studies such cases have been included in the category of CMML.
- There are a number of patients, e.g. those with eosinophilia and dysplastic blood and bone marrows, for whom it is impossible to assign an FAB type.
- Both therapy-induced MDS and MDS occurring in association with congenital bone marrow disorders may defy classification by the scheme, the bone marrow showing hyoplasia and/or fibrosis in addition to dysplasia.

Despite these limitations, systematic morphologic classification is important to facilitate the increasing number of collaborative studies and to assess prognosis and response to treatment. There have been a number of recent reports where the FAB classification has been applied to pediatric MDS.[3,6,8,9,20,42] The relative frequencies of the various subtypes of MDS in children and adults, as determined by ongoing studies in the UK, are illustrated in Table 4.5 with the *caveat* that the results are not strictly population based.

Table 4.5 Relative frequency of FAB types in children and adults; based on personal and UK experience for children and the Third MIC for adults.[49]

Type of MDS	Percentage	
	Adults	Children
RA	28	24
RARS	24	<1
RAEB	23	16
RAEBt	9	5
CMML	16	50
Other/unclassified		4

Pitfalls in morphologic diagnosis of refractory anemias

Refractory anemia must be distinguished from congenital dyserythropoietic anemias (see Chapter 3) and megaloblastic anemia (see Chapter 8) and the presence of clonal cytogenetic abnormalities is helpful in confirming the diagnosis; without such abnormalities the diagnosis should be entertained with caution.

Refractory anemia with ringed sideroblasts (RARS) as a true MDS is exceptionally rare in pediatrics and can only be diagnosed with confidence in the presence of a cytogenetic abnormality. Congenital sideroblastic anemia, due to abnormalities of heme synthesis, is usually associated with a dimorphic blood film; abnormalities of megakaryocytes and granulocytes are not seen. Sideroblastic anemia is also a feature of mitochondrial cytopathies, a group of disorders characterized by cortical neurologic impairment, metabolic acidosis and multiorgan involvement. The most typical of these is Pearson's syndrome of pancreatic insufficiency, neutropenia and a bone marrow showing vacuolated precursors and ringed sideroblasts.[43] Hematologic abnormalities may be the dominant and indeed the only clinical feature of mitochondrial cytopathies at presentation and thus the distinction from MDS may be difficult.[9,44] Mitochondrial cytopathies should be excluded in any patient with apparent sideroblastic anemia and it may be necessary to look for abnormal mitochondrial DNA on several occasions and to perform a muscle biopsy to confirm the diagnosis.

MDS or AML?

The distinction between refractory anemia with an excess of blasts with or without transformation and AML is an arbitrary one since patients may present with an abnormal count but a low percentage of blasts in the marrow and develop overt AML within weeks or even days (see Chapter 19). A classical presentation of this type is the extramedullary leukemic deposit (sometimes called a chloroma) found in patients with t(8;21) and M2 AML. The diagnosis of true MDS implies a more indolent course and in a recent French review an essential feature for the diagnosis was the presence of consistent hematologic abnormalities without evolution to AML over a 2-month period.[9] The distinction between a MDS and typical acute leukemia presenting with a low blast count is potentially important since the latter may respond more favorably to chemotherapy. The distinction is helped by careful review of morphology since patients with true MDS will exhibit multilineage dysplasia and also by the cytogenetic findings; t(8;21), t(15;17), t(9;11) and inv (16) all being associated with *de novo* AML.[45]

MDS or hypoplastic anemia?

A degree of dysplasia, particularly in the red cell series, is not unusual in chronic aplastic anemia, but the hypoplastic trephine appearances, absence of ALIP and absence of cytogenetic abnormalities in aplasia should help to make the distinction apparent.

Diagnosis of chronic myelomonocytic leukemia

There have been recent attempts by the FAB group to reclassify CMML in adults into classic CMML and a more proliferative form resembling older descriptions of Ph-negative CML, a distinction which is of no established value in pediatrics. There can be occasional problems in distinguishing pediatric CMML from acute monoblastic or myelomonocytic leukemia but dysplasia in the granulocyte series is marked in CMML and the bone marrow appearances do not show such a predominance of early monocytic precursors.

CMML in pediatrics is an extremely heterogeneous disease (see below) and in order to define prognosis and improve management there is a need for a systematic attempt at investigation. Additional investigations recommended in these patients, such as *in vitro* bone marrow cultures, are listed in Table 4.2 and are discussed further below. Cytomegalovirus,[46] parvovirus[47] and Epstein–Barr virus infections,[48] particularly in infants, may mimic

CMML and should be excluded by appropriate virologic investigations.

CYTOGENETICS

Investigation of bone marrow cytogenetics, supplemented when possible by fluorescent *in situ* hybridization (FISH) (Plate 4), is essential in the evaluation of MDS. Cytogenetic abnormalities are found in about 50% of cases of primary MDS in both children and adults and in >90% of patients with therapy-induced MDS.[49,50] Some of the commoner findings are listed in Table 4.6. This list is not exhaustive and is based on the adult literature. The most notable distinction between the cytogenetic findings in MDS and those in AML is the predominance of whole chromosome losses or partial deletions and the relative infrequency of translocations in MDS. There are some differences in the incidence of cytogenetic abnormalities in children and adults, most notably the marked predominance of monosomy 7 in pediatric MDS.[51] Monosomy 7 is also the commonest cytogenetic finding in leukemia or MDS occurring in patients with congenital bone marrow disorders. Deletions of chromosome 5q, so common in adult practice, are rare in childhood. Cytogenetic abnormalities in MDS, unlike those in AML, are not usually associated with any specific morphologic subtype. The adult exception to this is the association of loss of part of the long arm of chromosome 5 (5q-syndrome) in elderly women with macrocytic anemia, a normal or raised platelet count and relatively prolonged survival,[52] and the pediatric exception, the infantile monosomy 7 syndrome (see below).

Cytogenetic findings have been incorporated into several scoring systems to assess prognosis and, in general, the development of more complex abnormalities is associated with a worse prognosis and/or progression to AML. Cyto-

Table 4.6 Examples of some of the more common cytogenetic findings in MDS.[49,50]

Primary MDS	Secondary MDS
Chromosome loss	
Monosomy 7	Monosomy 7
Loss of Y chromosome	Loss of Y chromosome
Monosomy 17	Monosomy 17
Chromosome gain	
Trisomy 8	Trisomy 8
Partial chromosome deletion	
del 5q	del 5q
del 20q	del 7q
del 11q	del 12p
del 7q	
Translocations	
	t(1;7)(p11;p11)
	t(5;17) (p11;p11)
	t(3;3)(q21:q26)

genetic abnormalities are almost invariably found in patients with therapy-related MDS or leukemia and the type of abnormality is related to preceding treatment (see below).

BIOLOGY AND PATHOGENESIS

Studies of variants of glucose-6-phosphate dehydrogenase and other X-linked restriction fragment length polymorphisms[53] confirm that MDS is a clonal disorder. The use of FISH in combination with cytology and immunophenotyping[54] shows that in some cases the disease arises in progenitor cells restricted to myelopoiesis and erythropoiesis while in others the lymphoid series is involved as well, thus indicating malignant transformation in a more primitive hematopoietic cell. The event(s) initiating this change remain unknown.

Many of the chromosomal abnormalities in MDS involve the loss of genetic material, particularly from the long arm of chromosomes 5q and 7q.[55] The regions involved in these cytogenetic changes are rich in genes with a role in hematopoiesis and it has been postulated that both 5q and 7q may be the site of tumor-suppressor genes. Intensive investigation of the critical region 5q31–q33 is underway to try and identify a tumor suppressor gene associated with the development of the 5q-syndrome,[52] and similar critical regions have been identified on chromosome 7.[55] A recent excellent review of the significance of the cytogenetic finding of monosomy 7 in pediatric AML and MDS emphasizes its frequent occurrence in many conditions with a predisposition to leukemia, including most of the congenital bone marrow disorders.[51] The authors postulate that loss of a gene(s) located on chromosome 7 may contribute to leukemogenesis as part of a final common pathway following a number of genetic events. It remains unclear if inactivation of both alleles is essential for disease progression, i.e. a tumor suppressor gene is involved, or there is a gene dosage effect associated with deletion of one gene only.

The literature on MDS in adults is full of reports of mutations in various proto-oncogenes, including p53 mutations associated with a deletion in the short arm of chromosome 17,[56] in FMS in association with deletions in the FMS locus at chromosome 5q33 and mutations in the genes of the *ras* family.[57] *Ras* mutations have been most extensively investigated in CMML in adults, and more recently in children. It seems probable that such genetic changes are part of a final common pathway in the development of disease rather than initiating events in MDS.[58]

The search to identify critical genetic changes has been accompanied by many investigations of cellular biology and cell culture in MDS. The paradox of cytopenias in the blood despite a cellular bone marrow has been debated for many years. However, recent investigations have shown that while cell proliferation in the bone marrow in MDS is high with large numbers of cells entering S phase;[59] these cells rapidly undergo programed cell death (apoptosis) and thus never enter the circulation. Both proliferation and apoptosis are influenced by the complex cytokine network in the hematopoietic microenvironment, including tumor necrosis factor (TNF)-α, transforming growth factor (TGF)-β and interleukin-1β. Increased levels of these cytokines have been demonstrated in biopsies of patients with MDS.

FACTORS INFLUENCING PROGNOSIS

Treatment of MDS, particularly when involving BMT, carries a significant risk of morbidity and mortality and it is thus important to determine which patients are at early risk of death from leukemia or pancytopenia and in which patients a more conservative approach might be appropriate. This search for prognostic factors has been energetically pursued in adult MDS, a disease of the elderly, where the approach to management may be justifiably conservative. Numerous attempts to assess factors influencing both survival and progression to leukemia have been made. The original Bournemouth score[60] and subsequent modifications[61,62] used the presence of cytopenias, bone marrow blasts and ALIP. Other scores have also incorporated cytogenetics.[63] Most recently, an international scoring system has been developed using cytopenias, the percentage of blasts in the bone marrow and cytogenetics to predict evolution of AML and, in addition to these variables, age and sex for survival.[64] There have been few attempts to apply such systems in children and attempts have been hampered by the dominance and clinical heterogeneity of CMML and the fact that these scores do not afford sufficient discrimination between morphologic subtypes of pediatric MDS.[8]

There is little information about the risk of transformation of MDS to acute leukemia in childhood; in the author's experience, transformation to AML is confined to patients with RA and RAEB with or without transformation. The deterioration in CMML is associated with increasing requirement for blood products and systemic symptoms (see below), rather than development of a frank new acute leukemia. Analysis of prognostic factors in a retrospective review of 68 cases showed that age and sex were not significant prognostic factors,[8] except that in CMML as previously reported,[12] younger children had a better prognosis. Both the unmodified FAB classification and the degree of cytogenetic complexity were also of some prognostic significance. A score was developed based on objective criteria which could be measured at diagnosis; each of the following scores 1 point if present:

- platelets $< 40 \times 10^9$/l;
- cytogenetic complexity score of 2 (i.e. cases with no clonal abnormalities scoring 0, those with a single simple abnormality 1 and complex abnormalities 2);
- HbF $> 10\%$.

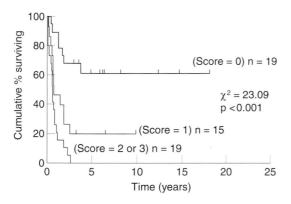

Fig. 4.1 Actuarial survival curve for 68 children with myelodysplasia based on the objective criteria scoring system described in the text. Reproduced with permission from Ref. 8.

The results of this scoring system in a cohort of children are shown in Fig. 4.1. In practice, most patients with a score of 0 have refractory anemia or RAEB with or without a simple cytogenetic abnormality such as monosomy 7, whereas those with a score of 2 or 3 tend to have either CMML with a low platelet count and raised HbF level or thrombocytopenia and complex cytogenetic abnormalities.

TREATMENT

This section contains a general review of the methods of treatment available for patients with MDS; more specific recommendations about treatment are given in the individual subtype sections. There are no systematic prospective studies of treatment of pediatric MDS and most of the information about chemotherapy is derived from studies of AML where patients with MDS have been identified retrospectively. Optimum supportive care with blood products (see Chapter 35) and appropriate management of infection (see Chapter 38) are essential for all patients.

CHEMOTHERAPY

There is relatively little information about the role of intensive cytotoxic chemotherapy in adult MDS and most studies have been retrospective and involve small numbers of patients. There is a widespread clinical impression that treatment of MDS is associated with more toxicity than that for AML, remission rates are lower and remissions are of shorter duration. Reported complete remission rates in adults vary from 15% to 64%.[65] Factors predictive of successful treatment are:

- younger age;
- normal karyotype;
- RAEBt at diagnosis;
- presence of Auer rods.

A recent European protocol has given somewhat encouraging results with an overall remission rate of 54%, again favoring younger patients and those without cytogenetic abnormalities. However, remissions were poorly sustained unless patients proceeded to BMT.[66]

There is of course even less information about chemotherapy in children but it appears that response rates are inferior to those achieved in AML.[67] A comparison of 20 children treated for MDS with 31 who had AML showed that the remission rate was lower at 35% (74% in AML), resistant disease was more common occurring in 25% (10% in AML) and 3-year survival was 15% (35% in AML); however, 8 of the patients with MDS had CMML, a subtype which in general responds poorly to chemotherapy (see below).[68] Comparison of outcome in children with classical dysplasia and those with AML with a low blast count showed that the remission rate was 30% for those with unequivocal MDS and 88% for the small number who had more typical AML; the latter group largely consisted of children with M2 or M4 AML and several had chloromas. The 4-year event-free survival was 50% for the AML patients compared with 23% in those with MDS.[45]

Low-dose cytarabine was originally used in adults with MDS in the belief that it was a differentiating agent, but it probably acts as a cytotoxic drug. Few children have been treated with low-dose cytarabine and there is no evidence that it is effective.[67]

Oral cytotoxic drugs such as mercaptopurine or hydroxyurea have been used to reduce the leukemic burden in MDS but, as expected, they do not achieve remission. It is perhaps of interest that etoposide, a drug with a reputation for efficacy in monocytic leukemias, was inferior to hydroxyurea in a randomized trial in adults with CMML.[69] More recently, topotecan, a topoisomerase inhibitor, has shown some activity in adult patients with all types of MDS.[70]

CYTOKINES AND DIFFERENTIATING AGENTS

There is understandable interest in whether or not these agents can reduce the consequences of pancytopenia in older patients with MDS where intensive chemotherapy or BMT may not be feasible. Clinical trials are in progress to evaluate various combinations of G-CSF, granulocyte-macrophage CSF (GM-CSF), IL-3,[71] and eythropoietin sometimes in combination with low-dose cytosine arabinoside. The growth factors may improve neutropenia,[72] but there are concerns that they may accelerate progression to AML. The newly available human megakaryocyte growth and development factor or thrombopoietin will no doubt be evaluated in the same way.[73–75] A number of differentiating agents such as all-*trans* retinoic acid[76] have also been used in adults with little clinical benefit. There is some interest in these agents in CMML (see below), but no justification for their routine use in children where the aim of management is not palliation but cure.

BONE MARROW TRANSPLANTATION

High-dose chemotherapy and/or radiotherapy with BMT is the only curative treatment for most patients with MDS. The first successful reports from BMT centers treating mainly adult patients showed a 3-year disease-free survival of about 40% for patients transplanted from a histocompatible sibling.[77,78] Children tolerate BMT better than adults, but only about 1 in 3 children in the UK have a histocompatible sibling. However, in the last few years the potential role for BMT in treatment has been expanded by the increased availability of volunteer unrelated donors and the start of programs for the use of cord blood. There is an increasing tendency to use peripheral blood stem cells (PBSC) rather than bone marrow, particularly in the context of autologous rescue from high-dose chemotherapy, and studies are in progress to evaluate allogeneic PBSC as a substitute for bone marrow.[79,80]

Complications

Infection

Allogeneic transplantation from a histocompatible sibling carries a 5–15% risk of early death from bacterial or fungal infection during the immediate period of pancytopenia and mucositis[81] and a subsequent risk for the development of non-bacterial infections. Herpes simplex infection is an important factor in causing or exacerbating mucositis and delaying engraftment. Common viral infections after engraftment include varicella zoster, adenoviruses and most importantly cytomegalovirus (CMV). The management of CMV has been facilitated by improved methods of early diagnosis and the chances of infection have been significantly reduced by the use of CMV-negative blood products where appropriate, leukocyte filtration and judicious and early use of immunoglobulin and ganciclovir,[82–84] but infection still remains a significant problem. Other important infections are *Pneumocystis carinii* pneumonitis and pneumococcal sepsis, the risk of which is increased by chronic graft-versus-host disease (GVHD).

Graft-versus-host disease

Even when there is full HLA compatibility between donor and sibling recipient, GVHD is an important and potentially lethal complication of BMT and measures to prevent it are essential. GVHD is mediated by immunocompetent T cells infused with the bone marrow which react against minor antigens in the recipient. The symptoms of acute GVHD, usually developing up to 5–6 weeks after the infusion of bone marrow, are skin rash, diarrhea and abnormal liver function. A scoring system for GVHD has been developed based on the number and extent of organ involvement; the severity varies from a maculopapular skin rash to exfoliation, severe jaundice, severe abdominal pain and the passage of liters of diarrhea.

There are two approaches to the prevention of GVHD:

1. *Immunosuppression of the recipient.* There are a number of protocols for immunosuppression but the most widely used in the context of sibling transplants is a combination of short-term methotrexate and cyclosporin therapy for about 6 months. Cyclosporin is nephrotoxic and tends to cause weight gain and hypertension so careful monitoring of the level is essential. Other agents and regimens are being evaluated for prevention of GVHD including tacrolimus.[85]

2. *Depletion of T cells in the bone marrow.* This can be accomplished by a variety of techniques, most commonly incubation of the marrow with monoclonal antibodies and complement before reinfusion, and can be accompanied by the use of monoclonal antibodies *in vivo*. It has been convincingly shown in chronic granulocytic leukemia that T-cell depletion reduces the risk of GVHD at the expense of a greater risk of graft rejection and leukemic relapse,[86] and the balance between successful engraftment, prevention of relapse and prevention of serious GVHD is even more difficult to maintain in the context of volunteer unrelated or haploidentical donors.

Acute GVHD is treated with steroids, and often with other agents such as monoclonal antibodies. Chronic GVHD is an extremely unpleasant complication which may follow acute GVHD or arise *de novo*. It is characterized by chronic changes in the skin and mucous membranes which can resemble scleroderma, contractures and immunodeficiency. Other features may include hepatic fibrosis, cholestasis, myositis and chronic pulmonary disease. Treatment is unsatisfactory and it is usual to give steroid therapy, sometimes in conjunction with azathioprine or thalidomide.[87] The risk of GVHD is in general increased by the use of donors who are not HLA identical.

Veno-occlusive disease of the liver

The other major specific complication of BMT is veno-occlusive disease of the liver, a complication which usually ensues within the first month after BMT with hyperbilirubinemia, hepatomegaly and fluid retention.[88]

Choice of regimen

The choice of a preparative regimen for BMT depends on the age of the child, the diagnosis and the type of transplant. The most widely used regimen involves various combinations of total body irradiation (TBI) and cyclophosphamide, sometimes with the addition of other drugs such as cytarabine and etoposide. TBI is used in various schedules, sometimes as a single dose but more usually fractionated over 3–4 days. The most widely used chemotherapy regimen is a combination of busulfan and cyclophosphamide which was developed originally for CML and AML.[89,90]

The choice between chemotherapy alone and regimens including TBI is in part dictated by consideration of the potential late effects of treatment, naturally an issue of extreme concern in the growing child. Although intensive chemotherapy carries the risk of significant late effects, including cardiotoxicity after anthracyline therapy, nephrotoxicity and potential sterility,[91] TBI is associated with additional complications and younger children are most vulnerable. Children who have received TBI have growth failure which is in part due to spinal shortening and partly to hypothalamic–pituitary failure; this will be exacerbated if there is chronic GVHD. Delayed puberty and gonadal failure are common and there is a variable risk of hypothyroidism, cataracts and learning problems. The combination of busulfan and cyclophosphamide has not been subjected to such rigorous long-term follow-up studies as TBI and it may induce sterility, but it is unlikely to have such a significant effect on skeletal growth and neuropsychologic development.

Randomized comparisons of chemotherapy and TBI have been performed in adults with CML[92] and AML[93] with conflicting results, but in a recent comparative study of adults with refractory anemia the combination of busulfan and cyclophosphamide was as satisfactory as cyclophosphamide and TBI.[94] There are no randomized pediatric trials but the combination of busulfan and cyclophosphamide has been used in children with AML[95,96] and the 2 drugs in combination with melphalan are undergoing assessment in pediatric MDS.[97] Currently, therefore, it seems appropriate to use chemotherapy alone as a preparative regimen, at least in standard transplants from an HLA-identical sibling.

Type of transplant

The number of reports confined to BMT in children with MDS is small, with the exception of CMML (see below) but overall results, as for other hematologic malignancies, show that younger patients and those with less advanced disease do better.[98,99] For the many children with MDS who do not have a histocompatible sibling donor and for whom the only chance of cure may lie in BMT, it is reasonable to consider the use of alternative donors.[100] Most studies have involved the use of volunteer unrelated donors and availability has increased significantly in recent years.[101] The chances of finding a donor depend on the patient's haplotype and ethnic group. In the last few years, cord blood has been used as a source of stem cells[102] but uncertainties remain about the risk of relapse and the stability of engraftment with this source.

Prognosis

There is a risk of relapse after BMT as after all other forms of treatment for MDS. This varies with the type and stage of

MDS and the type of donor and the results of treatment after relapse are unsatisfactory. Donor leukocyte infusions have shown some promise in the management of relapse in CML,[103,104] presumably by induction of a graft-versus-leukemia effect. The use of such infusions is limited by the ethical issues involved in leukaphoresis of young siblings but is feasible in consenting older siblings and volunteer unrelated donors. This treatment is being evaluated in other hematologic malignancies and may play a role in the management of relapsed MDS.

An alternative form of high-dose therapy in MDS is the use of autologous rescue with bone marrow or blood stem cells. There have been several recent randomized trials of the use of autologous BMT in AML (see Chapter 20) and this form of treatment is being systematically evaluated in adults with MDS who achieve a stable remission. There are a few anecdotal reports of long-term remission after ABMT in children with MDS,[8] but the value of this form of treatment has not been established and it cannot be recommended outside a clinical trial.

It is clear that BMT is the most encouraging form of treatment for MDS, and while the choice between TBI- and chemotherapy-based regimens will depend on the age of the patient and type of transplant, it would seem possible to avoid TBI in many instances. The results from donors other than histocompatible siblings leave room for improvement but consideration of this approach is justified in children with a poor prognosis.

DIAGNOSIS AND MANAGEMENT OF MDS SUBTYPES

REFRACTORY ANEMIA

The diagnosis of refractory anemia is easier in the presence of a cytogenetic abnormality in the bone marrow. An expectant approach is reasonable if the patient is well, not blood product dependent, and has no evidence of disease progression, and is recommended particularly in the absence of any cytogenetic abnormality. The risk of such a policy is of course that the patient may develop acute leukemia which is likely to be less responsive to chemotherapy than *de novo* AML. There is very little published information about the use of chemotherapy, as for AML, in refractory anemia and BMT is the treatment of choice.[94]

It is reasonable to consider early BMT in patients with a histocompatible sibling donor; in others the potential risks and benefits of an unrelated donor transplant must be carefully evaluated.

REFRACTORY ANEMIA WITH EXCESS OF BLASTS AND RAEB IN TRANSFORMATION

This category of patients includes both those with stable disease over months or years and those where the distinction from AML is a semantic one. In many national studies these patients are eligible for treatment with chemotherapy as if they had frank AML and this approach is recommended for patients with significant numbers of blasts in the marrow. In the absence of favorable cytogenetics such as t(8;21), such patients would in most centers be deemed eligible for BMT after initial chemotherapy, at least if they have a histocompatible sibling donor. The role of unrelated donor BMT for patients with advanced MDS who have a good response to chemotherapy remains unclear.

CHRONIC MYELOMONOCYTIC LEUKEMIA (JUVENILE CHRONIC MYELOMONOCYTIC LEUKEMIA, JUVENILE MYELOMONOCYTIC LEUKEMIA)

Clinical features and diagnosis

CMML in children, as reflected in the confusion about its nomenclature, is an extremely heterogeneous disease. It was first described as juvenile chronic myeloid leukemia (JCML) as a contrast to adult (i.e. Ph-positive) chronic myeloid or granulocytic leukemia, a disease to which it bears virtually no clinical or morphologic resemblance. While the morphologic appearances of this uniquely pediatric disease most comfortably conform to CMML in the FAB classification, it bears little resemblance to its adult counterpart, a condition with a median age of onset of 70 years.[49]

CMML is more common in boys[8,12] and in the under-2s and occurs in association with neurofibromatosis,[27,105] which may be found in 14% of patients.[106]

The clinical spectrum varies from a relatively benign disease in infants with hepatosplenomegaly and monocytosis to the classical disease usually in older children with bleeding, thrombocytopenia, enlarged lymph nodes and splenomegaly. Progression of the disease is accompanied by wasting, fever, infections, bleeding and pulmonary infiltrations. The typical skin rash, which may precede other symptoms by months, is classically of a butterfly distribution but may be more extensive, and on biopsy shows a nonspecific infiltration with lymphocytes and histiocytes.

Hematologic findings

While the morphologic features are consistent with the FAB description of CMML and monocytosis is always present, the blood count may also show eosinophilia, basophilia and a higher number of blasts than would be acceptable for strict diagnosis of CMML on the FAB criteria. The appearance of the blood film is more diagnostic than that of the bone marrow, where abnormal monocytes and blast cells may be increased with, usually, dysplasia in all cell lines.

The original detailed hematologic description of CMML[12] has been complemented by a recent retrospective review of 110 cases strictly classified by the FAB criteria, except that >5% blasts were allowed in the blood.[106] The median leukocyte count was $35 \times 10^9/l$ and exceeded $100 \times 10^9/l$ in only 7% of cases, eosinophilia was present in 8% of cases and basophilia in 28% while over half the patients had thrombocytopenia of $<50 \times 10^9/l$.

A characteristic feature of CMML is an increase in the HbF level,[13,107] which may increase progressively as the disease progresses, and a fetal pattern of γ-globin chain synthesis.[108] This is accompanied by a raised mean corpuscular volume (MCV), fetal pattern of 2,3-DPG and red cell enzyme production, red cell i/I antigen and carbonic anhydrase.[12] There may also be a number of immunologic abnormalities such as antinuclear antibodies and anti-IgG antibodies.[12,109]

While the diagnosis of CMML usually presents little difficulty, some patients with classical clinical features, including a grossly raised HbF, have a blood film with dominant normoblasts, almost suggestive of erythroleukemia, while in others the distinction from AMML may be a fine one. Cytogenetic analysis in classical CMML with a grossly raised HbF is classically normal, but monosomy 7 may be found in some cases (see below).

Biology

The assumption that CMML is a clonal disorder, which is difficult to establish in the absence of cytogenetic abnormalities, has been confirmed by X-chromosome inactivation studies[110] and by the demonstration that transplantation of cells from CMML patients can induce a CMML-like disease in irradiated severe combined immune-deficient mice.[111] The laboratory hallmark of the disease is spontaneous *in vitro* proliferation of granulocyte-macrophage colony-forming units (CFU-GM) which are formed at low cell densities and without the addition of exogenous growth factors.[112] This phenomenon has been the subject of intense study over many years and has prompted investigation of the role of a number of cytokines, including IL-1, TNF-α and GM-CSF in CMML.[113] Cells from patients with CMML cultured *in vitro* exhibit profound hypersensitivity to GM-CSF as compared to those from normal controls. This appears to be a selective effect since responsiveness to other cytokines is normal and it is postulated that the other cytokines such as TNF-α, responsible for some of the clinical features in advanced disease, are produced as a secondary response by hyperactivated monocytes.[114] Investigations are in progress to determine whether a growth factor hypersensitivity assay, which is claimed to be both sensitive and specific for pediatric CMML, can be used in the diagnosis and monitoring of treatment.

The precise mechanism for growth factor hypersensitivity in CMML remains unknown and there is no evidence that it is associated with mutations in the GM-CSF receptor,[115] but it has been attributed to abnormalities in the GM-CSF signal transduction pathway. The proteins encoded by the *ras* family of proto-oncogenes play a central role in this pathway and *ras* mutations have been demonstrated in

20–30% of patients with CMML. It is of great interest, in view of the clinical association with neurofibromatosis, that neurofibromin, the protein encoded by the NF type 1 gene, also plays a role in the *ras* signalling pathway and *NF1* may function as a tumor suppressor gene in hematopoietic cells. Inactivation of neurofibromin may provide an alternative means of deregulation of the *ras* signalling pathway. Recent investigations have shown that hematopoietic cells from so-called 'knock-out' mice, which are homozygous for the *NF1* mutation, exhibit marked hypersensitivity to GM-CSF[116] and that transplantation of such *NF1*-deficient hemopoietic liver cells induces a disease resembling CMML in irradiated mice.[117] The net result of this deregulated pathway is an hypersensitivity of cells to GM-CSF with proliferation of monocytes and myeloid cells which infiltrate tissues, causing bone marrow failure, and produce TNF-α and other cytokines, thus accounting for the fever, wasting and inanition so characteristic of advanced CMML.

CMML, JCML and infantile monosomy 7: How many diseases?

Monosomy 7 is the commonest cytogenetic finding in pediatric MDS but there have been many descriptions of a specific syndrome associated with monosomy 7 in young infants,[15,118–121] a constellation of features which shares many characteristics with CMML including a male prevalence and an association with neurofibromatosis.[29] The disorder may occur in siblings,[3,34] characteristically in early childhood. Unlike patients with aggressive CMML, these young children may have a long preceding history of infections associated with defective granulocyte function in relation to the loss of gene(s) on chromosome 7,[122] hematologic features of other FAB subtypes, usually RA or RAEB, and may develop either massive splenomegaly associated with bone marrow fibrosis, or, more commonly a frank AML. Some patients with the infantile monosomy 7 syndrome remain in a stable state for many years without specific treatment and some, unlike children with aggressive CMML, achieve remission and long-term disease-free survival with intensive chemotherapy alone.[120]

These distinctive features have lead some workers, including the author, to suggest that infantile monosomy 7 syndrome should be considered as a distinctive subclass of MDS,[8] but there is no doubt that there is considerable overlap between this condition and CMML. At a molecular level, investigation of patients with CMML who do not have monosomy 7 has failed to demonstrate submicroscopic loss of segments of chromosome 7.[123] It is probable that a number of distinct molecular events contribute to leukemogenesis in this group of diseases and a multistep model has been proposed to explain the similarities and differences between the monosomy 7 syndrome and other categories of CMML.

A recent clinical review of children with a morphologic diagnosis of CMML, which thus does not necessarily include

all cases which can be classified as infantile monosomy 7 syndrome,[106] showed no difference in clinical features between the patients with monosomy 7 cytogenetically and the others. However, patients with monosomy 7 tended to have normal or only moderately elevated HbF levels and a lower leukocyte count than other cases of CMML.

Despite this ongoing debate about classification, it is clear that older children with CMML and those with a high HbF and a low platelet count have a worse prognosis. In all reports involving significant numbers of patients, there is a small number of children who may survive for many years with minimal or no treatment; these tend to be under 2 years of age at diagnosis, with higher platelet counts and without gross elevation of HbF.

Management

The essential investigations are shown in Table 4.2 and, particularly in the younger child with normal cytogenetics, appropriate investigations to exclude a viral infection are essential. If there is any doubt about the diagnosis of CMML, particularly in young infants, a period of observation is recommended, and there is no evidence that this will prejudice the efficacy of any subsequent treatment.

While intensive chemotherapy, as given for AML, has achieved remission and even long-term survival in a small number of children with 'infantile monosomy 7', there is no real information about remission or survival rates, although this should come from current AML trials in Europe and America. Monosomy 7 in *de novo* AML is associated with a poor response to treatment,[124] but it is unknown whether primary MDS with monosomy 7 in childhood is similarly resistant to chemotherapy.

Intensive chemotherapy has been notably unsuccessful in patients with aggressive CMML with high HbF and rapidly progressive disease. Despite some reports of response,[125,126] true remission does not seem to be achievable and the survival in a group of 72 children with CMML who did not receive a BMT was 6%, with no difference between those patients who did and did not receive intensive treatment.[106]

BMT is the only curative treatment for CMML and if the patient has no histocompatible sibling a search for an alternative donor is justified in all children, save the small minority of infants with indolent disease; the disease is difficult to eradicate by BMT,[127,128] and there is evidence that a graft-versus-leukemia effect plays an important role in cure.[129] The results of transplants from both siblings and alternative donors leave much room for improvement.[127,128,130] The first report of successful BMT in CMML from Seattle used a preparative regimen of TBI and cyclophosphamide[131] and in view of the difficulties in eradicating the disease there have been concerns that a chemotherapy-based protocol such as busulfan and cyclophosphamide would prove insufficient to eradicate the malignant clone.[132] Survival in the largest case series to date of 43 children with CMML treated by BMT was 38%

at 5 years for the 25 children with a sibling donor and 18% for those with an unrelated donor. The actuarial probability of relapse was 58% and survival was superior for children whose preparative regimen did not include TBI.[133] The combination of busulfan, cyclophosphamide and melphalan appears promising for both sibling and alternative transplants[134] and is undergoing further assessment. The role of intensive chemotherapy and/or splenectomy to reduce the burden of disease before transplantation remains unclear but either form of treatment may be indicated in some patients.

The refractory nature and unique biologic features of CMML have prompted the investigation of various differentiating agents and cytokines. The most widely used has been 13–*cis*-retinoic acid, reported as producing complete or partial response in 5 of 10 children[135] and, with other retinoids, is undergoing further study. Alternative approaches being studied *in vitro* include the use of antagonists to the GM-CSF receptor[136] and the IL-1 receptor.[137]

DOWN'S SYNDROME AND ABNORMAL MYELOPOIESIS

Clinical and laboratory features of transient abnormal myelopoiesis

Transient abnormal myelopoiesis (TAM)[23,138,139] is usually discovered as an incidental finding on routine blood count in babies with Down's syndrome, but has also rarely been described in normal non-mosaic infants. The precise incidence of TAM is unknown but preliminary reports from a screening program suggested that it might be found in up to 1 in 10 neonates with Down's syndrome. TAM has also been diagnosed in hydropic fetuses *in utero*. Affected infants may have no associated clinical features but there is often enlargement of the liver and spleen with significant numbers of blasts in the blood, but a lesser degree of bone marrow infiltration. There is usually persistent evidence of hematopoietic maturation, with maintenance of hemoglobin, neutrophils and normal or raised platelet count in many patients. The maturing blood cells may show a degree of dysplasia.

Morphologically, cytochemically and on immunophenotyping the blast cells resemble those of acute megakaryoblastic leukemia and may exhibit clonal cytogenetic abnormalities; there are no real distinctions between these blasts and those of patients with unequivocal leukemia.

Prognosis and management

The majority of patients with TAM show spontaneous improvement which usually occurs over weeks to months but may take longer. This condition is benign in the majority of patients, but there have been a number of reports of death in the neonatal period associated with TAM; a characteristic finding at post-mortem is extensive visceral fibrosis.[139] In general, however, supportive care is all that is needed in the

majority of patients and cytotoxic treatment should be avoided; if indicated it would be appropriate to use low-dose cytarabine in the first instance. The risks of subsequent development of myeloid leukemia after TAM has been estimated at 20–30% but these proportions need confirmation from larger prospective studies.

The post-neonatal period

Virtually all cases of myeloid leukemia in Down's syndrome are megakaryoblastic or erythroblastic leukemia, subtypes which are exceptionally rare in other children and usually occur in the first 4 years of life. Many cases have a long prodrome of MDS with low platelets, dysplastic cells in the blood and a low proportion of blast cells in the marrow; thus cases may be classified at various stages as having RAEB or REABt or AML.[140] The cytogenetic findings are also distinctive with very few instances of the typical translocations t(8;21) or t(15;17); the commonest finding is trisomy 8.[138] The patients may remain well without treatment for weeks or months, but in contrast to TAM deterioration is inevitable and patients die if untreated.[22] There is good evidence that children with Down's syndrome and AML respond very well to chemotherapy, although they exhibit more toxicity than others,[67,141–143] and this may be related to enhanced sensitivity to cytarabine.[144] The event-free survival for such patients is, in several series, superior to that for other children without recourse to high-dose therapy and BMT. It has been suggested that a regimen of low-dose cytarabine may afford adequate treatment,[145,146] but this approach has only been used in small numbers of patients, several of whom relapsed, and it cannot be recommended in view of the excellent results from conventional intensive therapy. There is no indication that early treatment during the prodrome of AML offers any advantage in these children and it is usually appropriate to instigate treatment once symptoms develop.

FAMILIAL MDS AND CONGENITAL BONE MARROW DISORDERS

AML/MDS

There are a number of case reports from the older literature, usually reports of single families with a myelo-proliferative or -dysplastic disorder, which are imperfectly investigated compared with modern techniques, such as the large kindred described by Randall *et al.*[147] More recently a number of families have been described in whom >1 member has developed AML or MDS; this may be associated with emergence of a cytogenetic abnormality in the marrow, usually involving chromosomes 7[148] or 5[149] and in some cases with platelet storage pool deficiency.[35,150] From the practical point of view, it is important when examining families for suitable donors to exclude the presence of familial or genetically determined MDS.

Fanconi's anemia

Patients with Fanconi's anemia (see Chapter 1) have an estimated actuarial risk of development of a myeloid malignancy of 52% by the age of 40 years[151] and may present with AML or MDS.[33] The risk is higher in patients with clonal cytogenetic abnormalities which most often involve chromosome 7;[152] however, clonal cytogenetic abnormalities are of little value for prediction of leukemic change in the individual patient.[152,153] Treatment of Fanconi's anemia by BMT[154] is likely to be more effective when undertaken early and should reduce the risk of leukemic transformation, although not of solid tumors.[155] Treatment after transformation is associated with a high risk of relapse. The results of unrelated donor transplants for patients without an HLA-compatible sibling are improving but all transplants will be more effective before development of MDS or leukemia.

Shwachman–Diamond syndrome

The Shwachman–Diamond syndrome of exocrine pancreatic insufficiency and neutropenia is a rare autosomal recessive disorder (see Chapter 1) characterized hematologically by variable neutropenia, thrombocytopenia and a raised HbF and has been known for many years to predispose to the development of leukemia.[31] In a recent review of 21 patients, MDS developed in 7 and was associated in 5 with clonal cytogenetic abnormalities in the bone marrow; 5 patients progressed to AML.[32] While BMT could in theory correct the hematologic deficiency in Shwachman's syndrome there have been no reports of successful BMT and both patients in the series quoted died after transplantation.

Congenital neutropenia: Kostmann's syndrome

In the last few years the use of cytokines, in particular G-CSF, has reduced the incidence of infections and improved quality of life for patients with a variety of neutropenias (see Chapter 37) and for those with severe congenital neutropenia (SCN). Treatment with G-CSF has been preferred to BMT, particularly in cases who lack a histocompatible sibling donor. Patients with SCN have previously been recognized as having a predisposition to the development of leukemia, but since the introduction of treatment with G-CSF the number of reports has increased. It is not known, however, whether this is a direct consequence of G-CSF treatment or a reflection of improved survival. Monosomy 7 and *ras* mutations have developed in the bone marrow of patients with severe congenital neutropenia undergoing malignant transformation during G-CSF therapy.[30] Mutations in the G-CSF receptor gene have been demonstrated in some patients with SCN during development of AML/MDS.[156,157] Patients treated with growth factors for SCN should be monitored with regular bone marrow examinations including cytogenetics.

MDS WITH EOSINOPHILIA

A raised eosinophil count is characteristic of chronic myeloproliferative disorders, CMML and the idiopathic hypereosinophilic syndrome[158] and, of course, may be secondary to infections or infestation. There are a few reports of patients with marked eosinophilia and dysplastic blood and bone marrow whose hematologic features cannot readily be assigned to a FAB subtype; the author has arbitrarily classed such patients as having eosinophilic MDS.[4] Two such infants had hepatosplenomegaly and leukocytosis in association with t(1;5), 1 of whom rapidly deteriorated and the other was a long-term survivor.[159] Another 8-year-old girl recently described with t(5;12) (q31;p12–13) had stable eosinophilia for 7 years[160] while the author has seen translocation t(5;12)q(31;q13) in association with marked skin infiltration in a 7-year-old boy whose clinical condition has remained essentially unchanged for over 5 years.[161] Although both hydroxyurea and interferon therapy have been recommended in eosinophilic MDS, both have proved ineffective in the author's experience, and BMT would appear to be the most appropriate form of treatment provided that there is strong evidence of a clonal disorder.

THERAPY-RELATED MDS

Clinical and laboratory features

Secondary MDS and AML were first reported in adults treated for Hodgkin's disease, but also after non-Hodgkin's lymphoma, myeloma and a variety of non-hematologic solid tumors.[162] An associated genetic disease predisposing to malignancies such as a Li-Fraumeni syndrome cannot be confidently excluded in all cases but preliminary investigation of the frequency of p53 mutations in 19 pediatric secondary malignancies showed a germline mutation in only 1 child who had a family history of cancer.[163]

Two main types of secondary AML/MDS are associated with cancer treatment and each is associated with development of a characteristic pattern of cytogenetic change.[56] Alkylating agent-induced MDS/AML tends to occur after 4–5 years, is associated with a preceding phase of MDS and is characterized by deletions from chromosomes 5 and 7.[164] This disease is refractory to chemotherapy. The second, more recently described type of acute leukemia is related to treatment with topoisomerase II inhibitors and is associated with a shorter induction period and presentation as acute leukemia without a preceding MDS. Although secondary AML/MDS is rarer in children than adults, the correlation between type of previous therapy and clinical and chromosomal abnormalities is similar.[165]

Alkylating agent-induced AML/MDS is typified by patients treated for Hodgkin's disease and the drugs implicated include cyclophosphamide, chlorambucil, procarbazine and nitrosoureas. The risk is highest with increasing numbers of treatment cycles containing alkylating agents, prolonged chemotherapy and splenectomy; it does not appear to be increased further by radiotherapy.[166] Alkylating agents are also the major risk factor in patients with other tumor types such as non-Hodgkin lymphoma: a high rate of secondary AML/MDS was observed in the first UK Children's Cancer Study Group protocol for non-Hodgkin's lymphoma in which the protocol contained nitrosoureas in addition to cyclophosphamide and epipodophyllotoxins.[167]

Most recently, high-dose therapy with autologous BMT (ABMT), usually performed for patients with high-risk Hodgkin's disease or non-Hodgkin's lymphoma has been recognized to be associated with subsequent development of MDS, but it is difficult to dissociate the risks of the ABMT from the preceding chemotherapy which such patients have almost inevitably received.[37,38] Secondary MDS/AML has also recently been described in patients with aplastic anemia who have been treated with intensive immunosuppressive therapy.[36]

Patients with secondary MDS may be asymptomatic initially when an abnormal film or blood count may prompt investigation; subsequently, as in primary MDS, symptoms of bone marrow failure develop with a mean duration of the pre-leukemic phase of about 11 months.

Alkylating agent-induced MDS does not always conform to the FAB subtypes. There is often a relatively low proportion of blasts at the time of diagnosis but this is accompanied by marked morphologic changes in all cell lines. There may be basophilia in both blood and bone marrow and cellularity is variable, with fibrosis in some cases producing a dilute aspirate.[49] Clonal cytogenetic abnormalities are found in >90% of cases and the majority involve chromosomes 5 and 7.[164,168] Topoisomerase inhibitor-related leukemia, which may be lymphoblastic or myeloblastic, has been more systematically studied in children because of its increased incidence in children with ALL receiving intensive epipodophyllotoxin treatment.[169] Secondary AML was diagnosed in 21 of 734 patients treated for ALL; the overall cumulative risk was 3.8% at 6 years, but in a subgroup of children receiving drugs weekly or twice weekly the risk was >12%. The scheduling of drug administration influenced the development of AML; the total dose, type of leukemia and radiotherapy had no influence on the risk of AML. More detailed study showed that the majority of patients had myeloid or myelomonocytic leukemia and that chromosomal translocations predominantly involved the 11q23 region, most commonly as t(9;11) or t(11;19).[170]

More recently, another group of therapy-related leukemias has been described in association with t(8;21), inv(16) and t(8;16) after topoisomerase inhibitor therapy, alkylating agent therapy or anthracycline therapy.[171] These do not usually have a dysplastic prodrome and the risk factors have not been so precisely defined, but there is a similar correlation between the cytogenetic findings, morphology and response to treatment, as in *de novo* AML, so that patients may respond to chemotherapy.

Management

The advent of a second cancer in a highly curable condition is, of course, a tragedy to be avoided if at all possible and the identification of such cancers emphasizes the importance of morphology review and karyotyping in all cases of relapsed leukemia. Ideally, it is desirable to avoid this disastrous complication and this is sometimes possible by alterations in choice of drug or scheduling, always bearing in mind that such changes must not prejudice the chance of cure.

There is relatively little reported pediatric experience in the management of secondary malignancies. It appears that the response to treatment can be predicted by the biology of the leukemia, but any remissions achieved tend to be short lived. Thus, secondary AML with chromosome 5 and 7 abnormalities is highly resistant to chemotherapy and while remissions can be achieved with combination chemotherapy in children with 11q23 leukemia, and even in half those receiving 2-chlorodeoxyadenosine as a single agent, the long-term survival rate is extremely poor. The only exception to this poor prognosis is the small group of patients with more favorable translocations such as t(8;21), who, as do those with AML, tend to have a better response to treatment.

A recent study of intensive chemotherapy for secondary AML showed a 2-year disease-free survival of only 8% for patients with abnormal cytogenetics;[66] thus confirming the dismal prognosis. It would appear that BMT affords the only chance of cure[78] and in such circumstances the use of unrelated donors is justifiable.

CONCLUSIONS

Pediatric myelodysplasias are a rare but challenging group of diseases, which have only recently attracted systematic study. They frequently occur in association with other genetically determined disorders. A methodical approach to investigation and differential diagnosis is essential. The FAB classification can be applied to most cases but CMML in children is an heterogeneous disorder with unique clinical and biologic features, is resistant to chemotherapy and has a high relapse risk after BMT. A 'wait and see' approach to treatment may be appropriate for children with refractory anemia or younger children with CMML, particularly in the absence of cytogenetic abnormalities. Children with MDS with an excess of blasts are eligible in many countries for inclusion in AML trials and the role of intensive chemotherapy should thus become apparent within the next few years. BMT, the most effective treatment for MDS, should be considered in most children with an histocompatible sibling donor. The results from unrelated donor transplants still leave much room for improvement but these and other types of transplant should be considered in high-risk patients, particularly those with aggressive CMML and secondary leukemias. National and international collaboration is essential to afford a better understanding of these rare diseases.

REFERENCES

1. Nix WL, Fernbach DJ. Myeloproliferative diseases in childhood. *Am J Pediatr Hematol Oncol* 1981; **3**: 397–407

2. Smith KL, Johnson W. Classification of chronic myelocytic leukemia in children. *Cancer* 1974; **34**: 670–679

3. Brandwein JM, Horsman DE, Eaves AC *et al*. Childhood myelodysplasia: Suggested classification as myelodysplastic syndromes based on laboratory and clinical Findings. *Am J Pediatr Hematol Oncol* 1990; **12**: 63–70

4. Chessells JM. Myelodysplasia. *Baillière's Clin Haematol* 1991; **4**: 459–482

5. Gadner H, Haas OA. Experience in pediatric myelodysplastic syndromes. *Hematol Oncol Clin North Am* 1992; **6**: 655–672.

6. Tuncer MA, Pagliuca A, Hicsonmez G, Yetgin S, Ozsoylu S, Mufti GJ. Primary myelodysplastic syndrome in children: the clinical experience in 33 cases. *Br J Haematol* 1992; **82**: 347–353

7. Hasle H. Myelodysplastic syndromes in childhood – classification, epidemiology and treatment. *Leukemia Lymphoma* 1994; **13**: 11–26

8. Passmore SJ, Hann IM, Stiller CA *et al*. Pediatric myelodysplasia: a study of 68 children and a new prognostic scoring system. *Blood* 1995; **85**: 1742–1750

9. Bader-Meunier B, Mielot F, Tchernia G *et al*. Myelodysplastic syndromes in childhood: report of 49 patients from a French multi-centre study. *Br J Haematol* 1996; **92**: 344–350

10. Haas OA, Gadner H. Pathogenesis, biology, and management of myelodysplastic syndromes in children. *Semin Hematol* 1996; **33**: 225–235

11. Hardisty RM, Speed DE, Till M. Granulocytic leukaemia in childhood. *Br J Haematol* 1964; **10**: 551–566

12. Castro-Malaspina H, Schaison G, Passe S *et al*. Subacute and chronic myelomonocytic leukemia in children (juvenile CML). *Cancer* 1984; **54**: 675–686

13. Weatherall DJ, Edwards JA, Donohoe WTA. Haemoglobin and red cell enzyme changes in juvenile chronic myeloid leukaemia. *Br Med J* 1968; **1**: 679–681

14. Teasdale JM, Worth AJ, Corey MJ. A missing group C chromosome in the bone marrow cells of three children with myeloproliferative disease. *Cancer* 1970; **25**: 1468–1477

15. Sieff CA, Chessells JM, Harvey BAM, Pickthall VJ, Lawler SD. Monosomy 7 in childhood: A myeloproliferative disorder. *Br J Haematol* 1981; **49**: 235–249.

16. Blank J, Lange B. Preleukemia in children. *J Pediatr* 1981; **98**: 565–568

17. Bennett JM, Catovsky D, Daniel MT *et al*. Proposals for the classification of the myelodysplastic syndromes. *Br J Haematol* 1982 ;51: 189–199

18. Williamson PJ, Kruger AR, Reynolds PJ, Hamblin TJ, Oscier DG. Establishing the incidence of myelodysplastic syndrome. *Br J Haematol* 1994; **87**: 743–745

19. Aul C, Gattermann N, Schneider W. Age-related incidence and other epidemiological aspects of myelosdysplastic syndromes. *Br J Haematol* 1992; **82**: 358–367

20. Hasle H, Kerndrup G, Jacobsen BB. Childhood myelodysplastic syndrome in Denmark: incidence and predisposing conditions. *Leukemia* 1995; **9**: 1569–1572

21. Jackson GH, Carey PJ, Cant AJ, Bown NP, Reid MM. Myelodysplastic syndromes in children. *Br J Haematol* 1993; **84**: 185–186

22. Levitt GA, Stiller CA, Chessells JM. Prognosis of Down's syndrome with acute leukaemia. *Arch Dis Child* 1990; **65**: 212–216

23. Bain B. Down's syndrome – Transient abnormal myelopoiesis and acute leukaemia. *Leukemia Lymphoma* 1991; **3**: 309–317

24. Secker-Walker LM, Fitchett M. Consititutional and acquired trisomy 8. *Leukemia Res* 1995; **19**: 737–740

25. Seghezzi L, Maserati E, Minelli A *et al*. Constitutional trisomy 8 as first mutation in multistep carcinogenesis: clinical, cytogenetic, and molecular data on three cases. *Genes Chromosomes Cancer* 1996; **17**: 94–101

26. Hasle H, Clausen N, Pedersen B, Bendix-Hansen K. Myelodysplastic syndrome in a child with constitional trisomy 8 mosaicism and normal phenotype. *Cancer Genet Cytogenet* 1995; **79**: 79–81

27. Bader JL, Miller RW. Neurofibromatosis and childhood leukemia. *J Pediatr* 1978; **92**: 925–929

28. Stiller CA, Chessells JM, Fitchett M. Neurofibromatosis and childhood leukaemia/lymphoma: a population-based UKCCSG study. *Br J Cancer* 1994; **70**: 969–972

29. Shannon KM, Watterson J, Johnson P *et al*. Monosomy 7 myeloproliferative disease in children with neurofibromatosis, Type 1: Epidemiology and molecular analysis. *Blood* 1992; **79**: 1311–1318

30. Kalra R, Dale D, Freedman M *et al*. Monosomy 7 and activating *RAS* mutations accompany malignant transformation in patients with congenital neutropenia. *Blood* 1995; **86**: 4579–4586

31. Woods WG, Roloff JS, Lukens JN, Krivit W. The occurrence of leukemia in patients with the Shwachman syndrome. *J Pediatr* 1981; **99**: 425–428

32. Smith OP, Hann IM, Chessells JM, Reeves BR, Milla P. Haematologic abnormalities in Shwachman–Diamond Syndrome. *Br J Haematol* 1996; **94**: 279–284.

33. Auerbach AD, Weiner MA, Warburton D. Acute myeloid leukemia as the first hematologic manifestation of Fanconi anemia. *Am J Hematol* 1982; **12**: 289

34. Carroll WL, Morgan R, Glader BE. Childhood bone marrow monosomy 7 syndrome: A familial disorder? *J Pediatr* 1985; **107**: 578–580

35. Gerrard JM, McNicol A. Platelet storage pool deficiency, leukemia, and myelodysplastic syndromes. *Leukemia Lymphma* 1992; **8**: 277–281

36. Socie G, Henry-Amar M, Bacigalupo A *et al*. Malignant tumors occurring after treatment of aplastic anemia. *N Engl J Med* 1993; **329**: 1152–1157

37. Stone RM, Neuberg D, Soiffer R *et al*. Myelodysplastic syndrome as a late complication following autologous bone marrow transplantation for non-Hodgkin's lymphoma. *J Clin Oncol* 1994; **12**: 2535–2542

38. Darrington DL, Vose JM, Anderson JR *et al*. Incidence and characterization of secondary myelodysplastic syndrome and acute myelogenous leukemia following high-dose chemoradiotherapy and autologous stem-cell transplantation for lymphoid malignancies. *J Clin Oncol* 1994; **12**: 2527–2534.

39. Mangi MH, Mufti GJ. Primary myelodysplastic syndromes: Diagnostic and prognostic significance of immunohistochemical assessment of bone marrow biopsies. *Blood* 1992; **79**: 198–205.

40. Bennett JM, Catovsky D, Daniel MT *et al*. The chronic myeloid leukaemias: guidelines for distinguishing chronic granulocytic, atypical chronic myeloid, and chronic myelomonocytic leukaemia. *Br J Haematol* 1994; **87**: 746–754

41. Rosati S, Mick R, Xu F *et al*. Refractory cytopenia with multilineage dysplasia: further characterization of an 'unclassifiable' myelodysplastic syndrome. *Leukemia* 1996; **10**: 20–25

42. Barnard DR, Kalousek DK, Wiersma SR *et al*. Morphologic, immunologic, and cytogenetic classification of acute myeloid leukemia and myelodysplastic syndrome in childhood: a report from the Children's Cancer Group. *Leukemia* 1996; **10**: 5–12

43. Smith OP, Hann IM, Woodward CE, Brockington M. Pearson's marrow/pancreas syndrome: haematological features associated with deletion and duplication of mitochondrial DNA. *Br J Haematol* 1995; **90**: 469–472

44. Bader-Meunier B, Rotig A, Mielot F *et al*. Refractory anaemia and mitochondrial cytopathy in childhood. *Br J Haematol* 1994; **87**: 381–385

45. Chan GC, Wang WC, Raimondi SC *et al*. Myelodysplastic syndrome in children: differentiation from acute myeloid leukemia with a low blast count. *Leukemia* 1997; **11**: 206–211

46. Kirby MA, Weitzman S, Freedman M. Juvenile chronic myelogenous leukaemia; differentiation from cytomegalovirus infection. *Am J Pediatr Hematol Oncol* 1990; **12**: 292–296

47. Hasle H, Kerndrup G, Jacobsen BB, Heergaard ED, Hornsleth A, Lillevang ST. Chronic parvovirus infection mimicking myelodysplasia syndrome in a child with subclinical immunodeficiency. *Am J Pediatr Hematol Oncol* 1994; **16**: 329–333

48. Herrod HG, Dow LW, Sullivan JL. Persistent Epstein–Barr virus infection mimicking juvenile chronic myelogenous leukemia: Immunologic and hematologic studies. *Blood* 1983; **61**: 1098–1104

49. Third MIC Cooperative Study Group. Recommendations for a Morphologic, Immunologic, and Cytogenetic (MIC) Working Classification of the Primary and Therapy-Related Myelodysplastic Disorders. A Report of the Workshop held in Scottsdale, Arizona, USA, on February 23-25 1987. *Cancer Genet Cytogenet* 1988; **32**: 1–10

50. Fenaux P, Morel P, Lai JL. Cytogenetics of myelodysplastic syndromes. *Semin Hematol* 1996; **33**: 127–138

51. Luna-Fineman S, Shannon KM, Lange BJ. Childhood monosomy 7: epidemiology, biology and mechanistic implications. *Blood* 1995; **85**: 1985–1999

52. Boultwood J, Lewis S, Wainscoat JS. The 5q-syndrome. *Blood* 1994; **84**: 3253–3260

53. Tefferi A, Thibodeau SN, Solberg LAJ. Clonal studies in the myelodysplastic syndrome using X-linked restriction fragment length polymorphisms. *Blood* 1990; **75**: 1770–1773

54. van Lom K, Hagemeijer A, Smit EME, Hahlen K, Groeneveld K, Lowenberg B. Cytogenetic clonal analysis in myelodysplastic syndrome: monosomy 7 can be demonstrated in the myeloid and in the lymphoid lineage. *Leukemia* 1995; **9**: 1818–1821

55. Johnson EJ, Scherer SW, Osborne L *et al*. Molecular definition of a narrow interval at 7q22.1 associated with myelodysplasia. *Blood* 1996; **87**: 3579–3586

56. Pedersen-Bjergaard J, Pedersen M, Roulston D, Philip P. Different genetic pathways in leukemogenesis for patients presenting with therapy-related myelodysplasia and therapy-related acute myeloid leukemia. *Blood* 1995; **9**: 3542–3552

57. Bartram CR. Molecular genetic aspects of myelodysplastic syndromes. *Semin Hematol* 1996; **33**: 139–149

58. Paquette RL, Landaw EM, Pierre RV *et al*. N-*ras* mutations are associated with poor prognosis and increased risk of leukemia in myelodysplastic syndrome. *Blood* 1993; **82**: 590–599

59. Raza A, Gregory SA, Preisler HD. The myelodysplastic syndromes in 1996: complex stem cell disorders confounded by dual actions of cytokines. *Leukemia Res* 1996; **20**: 881–890

60. Mufti GJ, Stevens JR, Oscier DG, Hamblin TJ, Machin D. Myelodysplastic syndromes: A scoring system with prognostic significance. *Br J Haematol* 1985; **59**: 425–433

61. Goasguen JE, Garand R, Bizet M *et al*. Prognostic factors of myelodysplastic syndromes – A simplified 3-D scoring system. *Leukemia Res* 1990; **14**: 255–262

62. Mufti GJ, Galton DAG. Myelodysplastic syndromes: Natural history and features of prognostic importance. *Clinic Haematol* 1986; **15**: 953–971

63. Morel P, Hebbar M, Lai J *et al*. Cytogenetic analysis has strong independent prognostic value in de *novo* myelodysplastic syndromes and can be incorporated in a new scoring system: a report on 408 cases. *Leukemia* 1993; **7**: 1315–1323

64. Greenberg P, Cox C, LeBeau MM *et al*. International scoring system for evaluating prognosis in myelodysplastic syndromes. *Blood* 1997; **89**: 2079–2088

65. Hirst WJR, Mufti GJ. Management of myelodysplastic syndromes. *Br J Haematol* 1993; **84**: 191–196

66. De Witte T, Suciu S, Peetermans M *et al*. Intensive chemotherapy for poor prognosis myelodysplasia (MDS) and secondary acute myeloid leukemia (sAML) following MDS of more than 6 months duration. A pilot study by the Leukemia Cooperative Group of the European Organisation for Research and Treatment in Cancer (EORTC-LCG). *Leukemia* 1995; **9**: 1805–1811

67. Creutzig U, Cantu-Rajnoldi A, Ritter J *et al*. Myelodysplastic syndromes in childhood. Report of 21 patients from Italy and West Germany. *Am J Pediatr Hematol Oncol* 1987; **9**: 324–330

68. Hasle H, Kerndrup G, Yssing M *et al*. Intensive chemotherapy in childhood myelodysplastic syndrome. A comparison with results in acute myeloid leukemia. *Leukemia* 1996; **10**: 1269–1273

69. Wattel E, Hecquet GB, Economopoulos T *et al*. A randomized trial of hydroxyurea versus VP16 in adult chronic myelomonocytic leukemia. *Blood* 1996; **88**: 2480–2487

70. Beran M, Kantarjian H, O'Brien S *et al*. Topotecan, a topoisomerase I inhibitor, is active in the treatment of myelodysplastic syndrome and chronic myelomonocytic leukemia. *Blood* 1996; **88**: 2473–2479

71. Nand S, Sosman J, Godwin JE, Fisher RI. A PhaseI/II study of sequential interleukin-3 and granulodyte-macrophage colony-stimulating factor in myelodysplastic syndromes. *Blood* 1994; **83**: 357–360

72. Negrin RS, Stein R, Doherty K *et al*. Maintenance treatment of the anemia of myelodysplastic syndromes with recombinant human granulocyte colony-stimulating factor and erythropoietin: evidence for *in vivo* synergy. *Blood* 1996; **87**: 4076–4081

73. Fanucchi M, Glaspy J, Crawford J *et al*. Effects of polyethylene glycol-conjugated recombinant human megakaryocyte growth and development factor on platelet counts after chemotherapy for lung cancer. *N Engl J Med* 1997; **336**: 404–409

74. Molineux G, Hartley C, McElroy P, McCrea C, McNiece IK. Megakaryocyte growth and development factor accelerates platelet recovery in peripheral blood progenitor cell transplant recipients. *Blood* 1996; **88**: 366–376

75. Basser RL, Rasko JEJ, Clarke K *et al*. Thrombopoietic effects of pegylated recombinant human megakaryocyte growth and development factor (PEG-rHuMGDF) in patients with advanced cancer. *Lancet* 1996; **348**: 1279–1281

76. Ohno R, Naoe T, Hirano M *et al*. Treatment of myelodysplastic syndromes with all-trans retinoic acid. Leukemia Study Group of the Ministry of Health and Welfare. *Blood* 1993; **81**: 1152–1154

77. Appelbaum FR, Barrall J, Storb R *et al*. Bone Marrow transplantation for patients with myelodysplasia. Pretreatment variables and outcome. *Ann Intern Med* 1990; **112**: 590–597

78. De Witte T, Zwaan F, Hermans J *et al*. Allogeneic bone marrow transplantation for secondary leukaemia and myelodysplastic syndrome: a survey by the Leukaemia Working Party of the European Bone Marrow Transplantation Group (EBMTG). *Br J Haematol* 1990; **74**: 151–157

79. Bensinger WI, Clift R, Martin P *et al*. Allogeneic peripheral blood stem cell transplantation in patients with advanced hematologic malignancies: a retrospective comparison with marrow transplantation. *Blood* 1996; **88**: 2794–2800

80. Ottinger HD, Beelan DW, Scheulen B, Schaefer UW, Grosse-Wilde H. Improved immune reconstitution after allotransplantation of peripheral blood stem cells instead of bone marrow. *Blood* 1996; **88**: 2775–2779

81. Psiachou H, Hann IM, Chessells JM. Early deaths in children following bone marrow transplantation. *Bone Marrow Transplant* 1994; **14**: 975–980

82. Forman SJ, Zaia JA. Treatment and prevention of cytomegalovirus pneumonia after bone marrow transplantation: where do we stand? *Blood* 1994; **83**: 2392–2398

83. Boeckh M, Gooley TA, Myerson D, Cunningham T, Schoch G, Bowden RA. Cytomegalovirus pp65 antigenemia-guided early treatment with Ganciclovir versus Ganciclovir at engraftment after allogeneic marrow transplantation: a randomized double-blind study. *Blood* 1996; **88**: 4063–4071

84. Bowden RA, Slichter SJ, Sayers *et al*. A comparison of filtered leucocyte-reduced and cytomegalovirus (CMV) seronegative blood products for the prevention of transfusion-associated CMV infection after marrow transplant. *Blood* 1995; **86**: 3598–3603

85. Fay JW, Wingard JR, Antin JH *et al*. FK506 (Tacrolimus) monotherapy for prevention of graft-versus-host disease after histocompatible sibling allogeneic bone marrow transplantation. *Blood* 1996; 87: 3514–3519

86. Goldman JM, Glae RP, Horowitz MM *et al*. Bone marrow transplantation for chronic myelogenous leukemia in chronic phase. *Ann Intern Med* 1988; **108**: 806–814

87. Parker P, Chao N, Nademanee A *et al*. Thalidomide as salvage therapy for chronic graft-versus-host disease. *Blood* 1995; **86**: 3604–3609

88. Bearman SI. The syndrome of hepatic veno-occlusive disease after marrow transplantation. *Blood* 1995; **85**: 3005–3020

89. Copelan EA, Grever MR, Kapoor N, Tutschka PJ. Marrow transplantation following busulphan and cyclophosphamide for CML. *Br J Haematol* 1989; **71**: 487–491

90. Santos GW, Tutschka PJ, Brookmeyer R *et al*. Marrow transplantation for acute nonlymphocytic leukemia after treatment with busulfan and cyclophosphamide. *N Engl J Med* 1983; **309**: 1347–1353

91. Leisner RJ, Leiper AD, Hann IM, Chessells JM. Late effects of intensive treatment for acute myeloid leukemia and myelodysplasia in childhood. *J Clin Oncol* 1994; **12**: 916–924

92. Clift RA, Buckner CD, Thomas ED *et al*. Marrow transplantation for chronic myeloid leukemia: a randomized study comparing cyclophosphamide and total body irradiation with busulfan and cyclophosphamide. *Blood* 1994; **84**: 2036–2043

93. Blaise D, Maraninchi D, Archimbaud E *et al*. Allogeneic bone marrow transplantation for acute myeloid leukemia in first remission: A randomized trial of a busulfan-cytozan versus cytoxan-total body irradiation as preparative regimen: A report from the Groupe d'Etudes de la Greffe de Moelle Osseuse. *Blood* 1992; **79**: 2578–2582

94. Anderson JE, Appelbaum FR, Schoch G *et al*. Allogeneic marrow transplantation for refractory anemia: A comparison of two preparative regimens and analysis of prognostic factors. *Blood* 1996; **87**: 51–58

95. Michel G, Gluckman GME, Esperou-Bourdeau H *et al*. Allogeneic bone marrow transplantation for children with acute myeloblastic leukemia in first complete remission: impact of conditioning regimen without total-body irradiation – A report from the Societe Francaise de Greffe de Moelle. *J Clin Oncol* 1994; **12**: 1217–1222

96. Woods WG, Kobrinsky N, Buckley JD *et al*. Timed-sequential induction therapy improves postremission outcome in acute myeloid leukemia: A report from the Children's Cancer Group. *Blood* 1996; **87**: 4979–4989

97. Locatelli F, Pession A, Bonetti F *et al*. Busulfan, cyclophosphamide and melphalan as conditioning regimen for bone marrow transplantation in children with myelodysplastic syndromes. *Leukemia* 1994; **8**: 844–849

98. Anderson JE, Appelbaum FR, Fisher LD *et al*. Allogeneic bone marrow transplantation for 93 patients with myelodysplastic syndrome. *Blood* 1993; **82**: 677–681

99. Sutton L, Chastang C, Ribaud P *et al*. Factors influencing outcome in de novo myelodysplastic syndromes treated by allogeneic bone marrow transplantation: A long-term study of 71 patients. *Blood* 1996; **88**: 358–365

100. Anderson JE, Anasetti C, Appelbaum FR *et al*. Unrelated donor marrow transplantation for myelodysplasia (MDS) and MDS-related acute myeloid leukaemia. *Br J Haematol* 1996; **93**: 59–67

101. Kernan NA, Bartsch G, Ash RC *et al*. Analysis of 462 transplantations from unrelated donors facilitated by the national marrow donor program. *N Engl J Med* 1993; **328**: 593–602

102. Kurtzberg J, Laughlin M, Graham ML *et al*. Placental blood as a source of hematopoietic stem cells for transplantation into unrelated recipients. *N Engl J Med* 1996; **335**: 157–166

103. Kolb H-J, Schattenberg A, Goldman JM *et al*. Graft-versus-leukemia effect of donor lymphocyte transfusions in marrow grafted patients. *Blood* 1995; **86**: 2041–2050

104. Collins RH, Shpilberg O, Droyski WR *et al*. Donor leukocyte infusions in 140 patients with relapsed malignancy after allogeneic bone marrow transplantation. *J Clin Oncol* 1997; **15**: 433–444

105. Mays JA, Neerhout RC, Bagby GC, Koler RD. Juvenile chronic granulocytic leukemia. *Am J Dis Child* 1980; **134**: 654–658

106. Niemeyer CM, Arico M, Basso A *et al*. Chronic myelomonocytic leukemia in childhood: a retrospective analysis of 110 cases. *Blood* 1997; **89**: 3534–3543

107. Sheridan BL, Weatherall DJ, Clegg JB *et al*. The patterns of fetal haemoglobin production in leukaemia. *Br J Haematol* 1976; **32**: 487–506

108. Weinberg RS, Leibowitz D, Weinblatt ME, Kochen J, Alter BP. Juvenile chronic myelogenous leukaemia: The only example of truly fetal (not fetal-like) erythropoiesis. *Br J Haematol* 1990; **76**: 307–310

109. Cannat A, Seligmann M. Immunological abnormalities in juvenile myelomonocytic leukaemia. *Br Med J* 1973; **1**: 71–74

110. Busque L, Gilliland DG, Prchal JT, Sieff CA, Weinstein HJ, Sokol JM, Belickova M *et al*. Clonality in juvenile chronic myelogenous leukemia. *Blood* 1995; **1**: 21–30

111. Lapidot T, Grunberger T, Vormoor J *et al*. Indentification of human juvenile chronic myelogenous leukemia stem cells capable of initiating the disease in primary and secondary SCID mice. *Blood* 1996; **88**: 2655–2664

112. Gualtieri RJ, Emanuel PD, Zuckerman KS *et al*. Granulocyte-macrophage colony-stimulating factor is an endogenous regulator of cell proliferation in juvenile chronic myelogenous leukaemia. *Blood* 1989; **74**: 2360–2367

113. Freedman MH, Cohen A, Grunberger T *et al*. Central role of tumour necrosis factor, GM-CSF, and interleukin 1 in the pathogenesis of juvenile chronic myelogenous leukaemia. *Br J Haematol* 1992; **80**: 40–48

114. Emanuel PD, Shannon KM, Castleberry RP. Juvenile myelononocytic leukemia: molecular understanding and prospects for therapy. *Mol Med Today* 1996; **November**: 468–475

115. Freeburn RW, Gale RE, Wagner HM, Linch DC. Analysis of the coding sequence for the GM-CSF receptor a and b chains in patients with juvenile chronic myeloid leukemia (JCML). *Exp Hematol* 1997; **25**: 306–311

116. Bollag G, Clapp D, Shih S *et al*. Loss of *NF1* results in activation of the Ras signaling pathway and leads to aberrant growth in haematopoietic cells. *Nature Genet* 1996; **12**: 144–148

117. Largaespada DA, Brannan CI, Jenkins NA, Copeland NG. *Nf1* deficiency causes Ras-mediated granulocyte/macrophage colony stimulating factor hypersensitivity and chronic myeloid leukaemia. *Nature Genet* 1996; **12**: 137–143

118. Baranger L, Baruchel A, Leverger G, Schaison G, Berger R. Monosomy-7 in childhood hemopoietic disorders. *Leukemia* 1990; **4**: 345–349

119. Weiss K, Stass S, Williams D *et al*. Childhood monosomy 7 syndrome: Clinical and *in vitro* studies. *Leukemia* 1987; **1**: 97–104

120. Evans JPM, Czepulkowski B, Gibbons B, Swansbury GJ, Chessells JM. Childhood monosomy 7 revisited. *Br J Haematol* 1988; **69**: 41–45

121. Gyger M, Bonny Y, Forest L. Childhood monosomy 7 syndrome. *Am J Hematol* 1982; **13**: 329–334

122. Kere J, Ruutu T, de la Chapelle A. Monosomy 7 in granulocytes and monocytes in myelodysplastic syndrome. *N Engl J Med* 1987; **316**: 499–503

123. Butcher M, Frenck R, Emperor J *et al*. Molecular evidence that childhood Monosomy 7 syndrome is distinct from juvenile chronic myelogenous leukemia and other childhood myeloproliferative disorders. *Genes Chromosomes Cancer* 1995; **12**: 50–57

124. Woods WG, Nesbit ME, Buckley J *et al*. Correlation of chromosome abnormalities with patient characteristics, histologic subtype, and induction success in children with acute nonlymphocytic leukemia. *J Clin Oncol* 1985; **3**: 3–11

125. Chan HSL, Estrov Z, Weitzman SS, Freedman MH. The value of intensive combination chemotherapy for juvenile chronic myelogenous leukemia. *J Clin Oncol* 1987; **5**: 1960–1967

126. Festa RS, Shende A, Lanzkowsky P. Juvenile chronic myelocytic leukemia: experience with intensive combination chemotherapy. *Med Pediatr Oncol* 1990; **18**: 311–316

127. Chown SR, Potter MN, Cornish J *et al*. Matched and mismatched unrelated donor bone marrow transplantation for juvenile chronic meyloid leukaemia. *Br J Haematol* 1996; **93**: 674–676

128. Donadieu J, Stephan JL, Blanche S *et al*. Treatment of juvenile chronic myelomonocytic leukemia by allogeneic bone marrow transplantation. *Bone Marrow Transplant* 1994; **13**: 777–782

129. Rassam SMB, Katz F, Chessells JM, Morgan G. Successful allogeneic bone marrow transplantation in juvenile CML: conditioning or graft-versus-leukaemia effect? *Bone Marrow Transplant* 1993; **11**: 247–250

130. Bunin NJ, Casper JT, Lawton C *et al*. Allogeneic marrow transplantation using T cell depletion for patients with juvenile chronic myelogenous leukemia without HLA-identical siblings. *Bone Marrow Transplant* 1992; **9**: 119–122

131. Sanders JE, Buckner CD, Thomas ED *et al*. Allogeneic marrow transplantation for children with juvenile chronic myelogenous leukemia. *Blood* 1988; **71**: 1144–1146

132. Urban C, Schwinger W, Slavc I *et al*. Busulfan/cyclophosphamide plus bone marrow transplantation is not sufficient to eradicate the malignant clone in juvenile chronic myelogenous leukemia. *Bone Marrow Transplant* 1990; **5**: 353–356

133. Locatelli F, Niemeyer C, Angelucci E *et al*. Allogenic bone marrow transplantation for chronic myelomonocytic leukemia in childhood: a report from the European Working Group on Myelodysplastic Syndrome in childhood. *J Clin Oncol* 1997; **15**: 566–573

134. Locatelli F, Pession A, Comoli P *et al*. Role of allogeneic bone marrow transplantation from an HLA-identical sibling or a matched unrelated donor in the treatment of children with juvenile chronic myeloid leukaemia. *Br J Haematol* 1996; **92**: 49–54

135. Castleberry RP, Emanuel PD, Zuckerman KS *et al*. A pilot study of isotretinoin in the treatment of juvenile chronic myelogenous leukaemia. *N Engl J Med* 1994; **331**: 1680–1684

136. Iverson PO, Rodwell RL, Pitcher L, Taylor KM, Lopez AF. Inhibition of proliferation and induction of apoptosis in juvenile myelomonocytic leukemic cells by the granulocyte-macrophage colony-stimulating factor analogue E21R. *Blood* 1996; **88**: 2634–2639

137. Schiro R, Longoni D, Rossi V *et al*. Suppression of juvenile chronic myelogenous leukemia colony growth by interleukin-1 receptor antagonist. *Blood* 1994; **83**: 460–465

138. Avet-Loiseau H, Mechinaud F, Harousseau J. Clonal heamatologic disorders in Down syndrome. *J Pediatr Hematol Oncol* 1995; **17**: 19–24

139. Zipursky A, Poon A, Doyle J. Leukemia in Down syndrome: a review. *J Pediatr Hematol Oncol* 1992; **9**: 139–149

140. Zipursky A, Thorner P, De Harven E, Christensen H, Doyle J. Myelodysplasia and acute megakaryoblastic leukemia in Down's syndrome. *Leukemia Res* 1994; **18**: 163–171

141. Creutzig U, Ritter J, Vormoor J *et al*. Myelodysplasia and acute myelogenous leukemia in Down's syndrome. A report of 40 children of the AML-BFM study Group. *Leukemia* 1996; **10**: 1677–1686

142. Ravindranath Y, Abella E, Krischer JP *et al*. Acute myeloid leukemia (AML) in Down's syndrome is highly responsive to chemotherapy: experience of Pediatric Oncology Group AML study 8498. *Blood* 1992; **80**: 2210–2214

143. Lie SO, Jonmundsson G, Mellander L, Siimes MA, Yssing M, Gustafsson G. A population-based study of 272 children with acute myeloid leukaemia treated on two consecutive protocols with different intensity: best outcome in girls, infants, and children with Down's syndrome. *Br J Haematol* 1996; **94**: 82–88

144. Taub JW, Matherly LH, Stout ML, Buck SA, Gurney JG, Ravindranath Y. Enhanced metabolism of 1-b-D-Arabinofuranosylcytosine in Down syndrome cells: A contributing factor to the superior event free survival of Down syndrome children with acute myeloid leukemia. *Blood* 1996; **87**: 3395–3403

145. Zipursky A. The treatment of children with acute megakaryoblastic leukemia who have Down syndrome. *J Pediatr Hematol Oncol* 1996; **18**: 10–12

146. Tchernia G, Lejeune F, Boccara J, Denavit M, Dommergues J, Bernaudin F. Erythroblastic and/or megakaryoblastic leukemia in Down syndrome: Treatment with low-dose arabinosyl cytosine. *J Pediatr Hematol Oncol* 1996; 18: 59–62

147. Randall DL, Reiquam CW, Githens JH, Robinson A. Familial myeloproliferative disease. *Am J Dis Child* 1965; **110**: 479–490

148. Paul B, Reid MM, Davison EV, Abela M, Hamilton PJ. Familial myelodysplasia: progressive disease associated with emergence of monosomy 7. *Br J Haematol* 1987; **65**: 321–323

149. Olopade O, Roulston D, Baker T *et al*. Familial myeloid leukemia associated with loss of the long arm of chromosome 5. *Leukemia* 1996; **10**: 669–674

150. Gerrard JM, Israels ED, Bishop AJ *et al*. Inherited platelet-storage pool deficiency associated with a high incidence of acute myeloid leukaemia. *Br J Haematol* 1991; **79**: 246–255

151. Butturini A, Gale RP, Verlander PC, Adler-Brecher B, Gillio AP, Auerbach AD. Hematologic abnormalities in Fanconi anemia: an International Fanconi Anemia Registry study. *Blood* 1994; **84**: 1650–1655

152. Maaarek O, Jonveaux P, Le Coniat M, Derre J, Berger R. Fanconi anemia and bone marrow clonal chromosome abnormalities. *Leukemia* 1996; **10**: 1700–1704

153. Alter BP, Scalise A, MCombs J, Najfeld V. Clonal chromosomal abnormalities in Fanconi's anaemia: what do they really mean? *Br J Haematol* 1993; **85**: 627–630

154. Gluckman E, Auerbach AD, Horowitz MM *et al*. Bone marrow transplantation for Fanconi anemia. *Blood* 1995; **86**: 2856–2862

155. Alter BP. Fanconi's anemia and malignancies. *Am J Hematol* 1996; **53**: 99–110

156. Dong F, Brynes RK, Tidow N, Welte K, Lowenberg B, Touw IP. Mutations in the gene for the granulocyte colony-stimulating-factor receptor in patients with acute myeloid leukemia preceded by severe congenital neutropenia. *N Engl J Med* 1995; **333**: 487–493

157. Dong F, Dale DC, Bonilla MA *et al*. Mutations in the granulocyte colony-stimulating factor receptor gene in patients with severe congenital neutropenia. *Leukemia* 1997; **11**: 120–125

158. Bain BJ. Eosinophilic leukaemias and the idiopathic hypereosinophilic syndrome. *Br J Haematol* 1996; **95**: 2–9

159. Darbyshire PJ, Shortland D, Swansbury GJ, Sadler J, Lawler SD, Chessells JM. A myeloproliferative disease in two infants associated with eosinophilia and chromosome t(1;5) translocation. *Br J Haematol* 1987; **66**: 483–486

160. Pellier I, Le Moine PJ, Rialland X *et al*. Myelodysplastic syndrome with t(5;12)(q31;p12-p13) and eosinophilia: a pediatric case with review of literature. *J Pediatr Hematol Oncol* 1996; **18**: 285–288

161. Jani K, Kempski HM, Reeves BR. A case of myelodysplasia with eosinophilia having a translocation t(5;12)(q31;q13) restricted to myeloid cells but not involving eosinophils. *Br J Haematol* 1994; **87**: 57–60

162. Park DJ, Koeffler HP. Therapy-related myelodysplastic syndromes. *Semin Hematol* 1996; **33**: 256–273

163. Felix CA, Hosler MR, Provisor D *et al*. The p53 gene in pediatric therapy-related leukemia and myelodysplasia. *Blood* 1996; **87**: 4376–4381

164. Le Beau MM, Albain KS, Larson RA *et al*. Clinical and cytogenetic correlations in 63 patients with therapy related myelodysplastic syndromes and acute non lymphocytic leukemias: Further evidence for characteristic abnormalities of chromosome nos. 5 and 7. *J Clin Oncol* 1986; **4**: 325–345

165. Rubin CM, Arthur DC, Woods WG *et al*. Therapy-related myelodysplastic syndrome and acute myeloid leukemia in children: Correlation between chromosomal abnormalities and prior therapy. *Blood* 1991; **78**: 2982–2988

166. Kaldor JM, Day NE, Clarke A *et al*. Leukemia following Hodgkin's disease. *N Engl J Med* 1990; **322**: 7–13

167. Ingram L, Mott MG, Mann JR, Raafat F, Darbyshire PJ, Morris Jones PH. Second malignancies in children treated for non-Hodgkin's

lymphoma and T-cell leukaemia with the UKCCSG regimens. *Br J Cancer* 1987; **55**: 463–466

168. Michels SD, McKenna RW, Arthur DC, Brunning RD. Therapy-related acute myeloid leukemia and myelodysplastic syndrome: A clinical and morphologic study of 65 cases. *Blood* 1985; **65**: 1364–1372.

169. Pui C, Ribeiro RC, Hancock MI *et al*. Acute myeloid leukemia in children treated with epipodophyllotoxins for acute lymphoblastic leukemia. *N Engl J Med* 1991; **325**: 1682–1687

170. Pui C, Relling MV, Rivera GK *et al*. Epipodophyllotoxin-related acute myeloid leukemia: a study of 35 cases. *Leukemia* 1995; **9**: 1990–1996

171. Quesnel B, Kantarjian H, Bjergaard JP *et al*. Therapy-related acute myeloid leukemia with t(8;21), inv(16), and t(8;16): a report on 25 cases and review of the literature. *J Clin Oncol* 1993; **11**: 2370–2379

Red cell disorders

Iron metabolism, sideroblastic anemia and iron overload

ANDREW M WILL

Despite being one of the commonest substances in the natural world, iron is treated by the body as if it were a trace element. Iron is efficiently recycled and excretion is limited. In part, at least, this is because most naturally occurring iron is in the ferric (Fe^{3+}) form which is highly insoluble and therefore relatively unavailable for absorption from the diet. Complex mechanisms to facilitate iron absorption have had to develop.

Iron's importance in biochemistry lies in its ability to exist in 2 stable forms: the relatively inactive ferric (Fe^{3+}) and biochemically active ferrous (Fe^{2+}) state. This property makes it an ideal atom to be involved in electron transfer, which forms the basis of many enzyme-controlled biochemical reactions. Iron is therefore not just important as heme iron to carry oxygen but is also essential to the working of many of the body's enzyme systems (Table 5.1). Approximately half the enzymes of the Krebs cycle contain iron or require it as a cofactor. Therefore, although most of the iron metabolized each day is used to synthesize hemoglobin, chronic iron deficiency may produce a wide variety of effects other than anemia.

The potential reactivity of iron has led to the evolution of a group of specialized proteins to transport and store iron and regulate the iron-dependent synthetic pathways. Providing the ability of these proteins to contain ionic iron is maintained, iron can be safely stored and metabolized. In iron overload these systems become overwhelmed and the uncontrolled reactivity of ionic iron causes life-threatening tissue damage.

IRON METABOLISM

Humans appear to be unique in their inability to excrete excess iron.[1] Iron loss (about 1–1.5 mg/day) is achieved almost exclusively in the male by desquamation of skin and loss of mucosal cells from the gastrointestinal and urinary tracts.[2] In the female, iron is also lost through menstruation and during pregnancy. Iron loss by any of these means is relatively constant and cannot be altered in response to changes in body iron status. In the absence of a physiologic mechanism for the excretion of excess iron, iron balance is achieved by control of iron absorption.[3]

IRON ABSORPTION

Three factors are important in determining the amount of iron absorbed from the diet: total iron content of the diet, bioavailability of the iron in the diet and control of iron absorption by the intestinal mucosal cells. Only the latter is responsive to body iron status and requirements.

Dietary iron content

Total iron content is probably the single most important dietary factor in determining the amount of iron that is absorbed from the gut. A mixed western diet contains about 6 mg iron/1000 kcal.[4] An adult male will absorb about 10% of this (0.5–1 mg/day). In iron deficiency, the amount of iron absorbed can be increased to a maximum of 3.5 mg/day.[5] Large amounts of dietary iron do not block iron absorption but as the amount in the diet increases, the percentage absorbed decreases. Different foodstuffs contain different proportions of iron (Table 5.2); vegetarian diets are more likely to have an inadequate iron content than mixed diets.

Table 5.1 Iron-containing enzymes.

Cytochromes a, b and c
Succinate dehydrogenase
Cytochrome c oxidase
Cytochrome P450
Catalase
Myeloperoxidase
Tryptophan pyrrolase
Xanthine oxidase
NADH dehydrogenase
Ribonucleotide reductase

Table 5.2 Iron content of foodstuffs.

Foodstuff	Iron/100 g	% Available for absorption
Rice flour	0.9	1
Bread	2.0	5
Wheat flour	2.3	5
Cod	0.9	10
Mackerel	1.0	10
Sardines in oil	1.5	10
Oysters	7.1	10
Beef sausages	2.4	
Chicken	3.0	> 10
Pork chops	3.0	> 10
Bacon (cooked)	3.3	
Beef (rump)	2.4	> 10
(kidney)	6.5	
(liver)	12.1	

Table 5.3 Factors affecting iron absorption of non-heme iron from the gastrointestinal tract.

Increased absorption	Decreased absorption
Acids	Alkalis
Vitamin C	Antacids
Hydrochloric acid	Pancreatic secretions
	Hypochlorhydria
Solutes	Precipitating agents (vegetables)
Sugars	Phytates
Amino acids (meats)	Phosphates

Details of dietary iron intake at different ages are given in Chapter 6.

Bioavailability of dietary iron

The bioavailability of dietary iron is also important in determining the amount of iron absorbed from the diet.[6] Dietary iron is in 2 forms: organic or heme iron derived from hemoglobin and myoglobin, and inorganic or non-heme iron. There is a different absorptive pathways by which iron can enter the gut mucosal cells for each of the 2 types of dietary iron:[3,7]

1. Heme iron is taken up directly by specialized receptors in the mucosal membrane[8] and passes unchanged into the cytoplasm where the porphyrin ring is cleaved and the iron released.[9] The heme iron pathway is relatively efficient and unlike non-heme iron, absorption is little affected by the intraluminal factors discussed below. Although heme iron only accounts for about 10% of the total iron in a mixed diet, it accounts for up to 25% of the total iron absorbed.
2. Non-heme iron exists almost exclusively as insoluble ferric salts. To be absorbed the ferric salts must first be converted to the ferrous form and are then bound to the intestinal iron transport protein, mucosal apotransferrin. Bound to apotransferrin, the non-heme iron can enter the gut mucosal cell. Within the cell, iron is cleaved from the mucosal transferrin and joins the same pool as heme-derived iron.

The uptake of non-heme iron by the gastrointestinal mucosal cells is affected by factors that enhance and inhibit absorption:[10,11]

- Foodstuffs vary in their ability to give up iron for absorption (Table 5.2).[12] Rice, for example, is not only poor in total iron content but only 1–2% of this is available for absorption. Even relatively iron-rich vegetables such as spinach and wheat have only a small percentage of their total iron content available for absorption (1–2% and 5%, respectively). By contrast, heme-rich, animal-derived foodstuffs not only contain more iron/g but a much higher percentage is available for absorption.
- Different foods can interact either to increase or decrease the absorption of iron from them (Table 5.3). Meat in the diet increases the absorption of even the non-heme iron from the gut lumen. The addition of veal to a meal of maize can double the amount of iron absorbed from the cereal.[13] On the other hand, tannates in tea or coffee[14] and substances such as egg yolk have the opposite effect and reduce non-heme iron absorption.[15]
- Intraluminal factors can influence the percentage of non-heme iron that can be reduced from the insoluble ferric to the soluble, absorbable ferrous form.[16] Acids such as hydrochloric acid and vitamin C promote the production of ferrous iron, enhancing absorption, whereas antacids and hypochlorhydria reduce the amount of ferrous iron available from the diet. Phosphates and phytates, which are common in vegetables, also prevent the reduction of ferric to ferrous salts, thereby inhibiting iron absorption by forming insoluble complexes with iron salts.

The bioavailability of iron is clinically important. Vegans are at risk of iron deficiency even if their total dietary iron content appears satisfactory because the assimilation of iron from vegetable sources is inefficient. Moreover, the absorption of the non-heme-derived iron is reduced by the absence of heme iron and the increased intake of phytates and phosphates further reduces the availability of absorbable iron. In contrast, human milk has a low total iron content but the iron is in a form which is highly bioavailable[17] and which is also able directly to enhance the amount of iron absorbed from other foodstuffs in the early weaning diet.[18] Therefore, the vegan even with an apparently adequate total dietary iron content is at risk of iron deficiency but the breast-fed infant is less so.

Mucosal cell control

Gut mucosal cell control of iron absorption is not well defined but the amount of iron absorbed via the mucosa is responsive to body iron stores[19] and the erythropoietic activity of the bone marrow.[20] Increases in body iron lead to a reduction in iron absorbed from the gastrointestinal tract and when body iron stores are reduced, more iron is absorbed. Erythropoietic activity has the opposite effect—in conditions associated with high levels of erythropoietic activity, iron absorption is increased, but in disorders such as hypoplastic anemia where erythropoietic activity is reduced, iron absorption is reduced.

The amount of dietary iron absorbed can be controlled at both phases of mucosal cell absorption:

1. *At the uptake of iron from the gut lumen into the mucosal cells.* For non-heme iron to be absorbed from the gut lumen across the brush border of the intestinal mucosal cells, iron must first be attached to the mucosal cell transport protein, apotransferrin.[21] The transferrin-iron complex produced is internalized by the small intestine, mainly in the duodenum and jejenum. Control of the uptake of dietary iron can be achieved during this phase of absorption because the amount of apotransferrin secreted by the liver into the bile is inversely proportional to hepatic iron stores. Increased hepatic storage reduces the synthesis of apotransferrin by the liver, hence reducing the gut mucosal cell iron uptake. A reduction in hepatic iron stores has the opposite effect.[22]

2. *During the transfer of iron to the portal blood.* Once inside the mucosal cells the iron released from the transferrin-iron complex joins with heme-derived iron. Iron from this combined intracellular pool has 2 possible fates. It is either transferred to the portal blood for further metabolism within the body or combined with the mucosal cell storage protein, apoferritin.[23] If the latter, the iron becomes trapped in the mucosal cell as storage ferritin. After 3–4 days the cell and any ferritin it contains is sloughed off into the intestinal lumen as the villus mucosal cell completes its life-span. Control of absorption is achieved because the amount of apoferritin produced by the mucosal cells is dependent on body iron stores. When body iron stores are low, little is produced by the gut mucosal cells and a high percentage of the absorbed dietary iron can pass into the portal venous system. Conversely, when body iron stores are replete, the gut mucosal cells produce more apoferritin which traps absorbed dietary iron in the intestinal villus cells and this is later excreted in the feces.

BODY IRON DISTRIBUTION AND TURNOVER

The adult contains about 55 mg/kg of iron[4] and an adult male will have 3.5–4 g of iron in his body. The majority of that iron, about 70%, is carried in red blood cells as hemoglobin and most of the rest is stored as ferritin and hemosiderin with approximately two-thirds within macrophages and one-third in hepatocytes. Small amounts of iron are present in myoglobin and traces in cellular enzymes (Fig. 5.1).

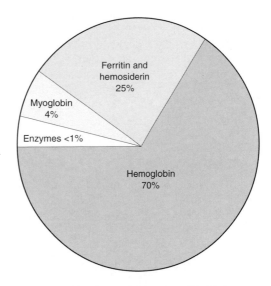

Fig. 5.1 Distribution of iron in man (adult male = 3.5–4.0 g).

Although the distribution of iron in the body is fairly constant, the iron in the different compartments is continually being recycled. Each day about 25 ml of red blood cells need to be replaced. This represents a need for 25 mg of iron but only about 1 mg/day is absorbed from the diet. The other 24 mg required for red cell replacement alone needs to be recycled from senescent red cells and tissue stores. This daily iron cycle (Fig. 5.2) is reliant upon plasma transferrin (TF), cell surface transferrin receptors (TFRs) and the storage protein ferritin. Intracellular control, in the erythroid cell at least, is dependent upon the interaction of an iron-responsive binding protein (IRE-BP) with iron-responsive elements (IRE) present on the TFR, ferritin and also erythroid cell-specific δ-aminolevulinic acid synthetase (ALAS) which is the initial enzyme involved in the production of heme from glycine and succinyl CoA in mitochondria (Fig. 5.3).

Transferrin

TF is the specialized plasma transport protein for iron.[24] It is a single polypeptide β-globulin of 679 amino acids and a molecular weight of 79 570 kDa, which is mainly synthesized

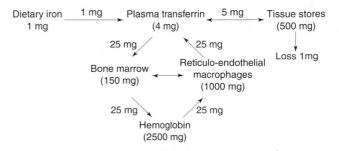

Fig. 5.2 Daily iron cycle. Values in parentheses represent average quantities of stored iron in a normal male adult. Other values represent average daily turnover in mg.

in the liver. Unusually for a transport protein, TF can be recycled after intracellular delivery of iron and it has a half-life of 8–10 days.[25] TF is produced from a single gene q21-qter on chromosome 3[26] near the gene for its receptor.[27] Normally active structural variants have been described.

TF has 2 iron-binding sites, 1 at the N- and 1 at the C-terminal domain.[28] Therefore, it can exist in 4 states: apotransferrin with no bound iron, as 2 different monoferric transferrases and as diferric transferrase. At neutral pH, TF has a high affinity for binding ferric iron and when fully iron saturated, undergoes a conformational change making the diferric molecule more soluble and and more resistant to enzymatic degradation. Diffferic TF has about 3.5 times the affinity for TFR than either of the monoferric transferrins[29] and because of this the diferric form is preferentially bound to cells for intracellular iron delivery. At neutral pH, apoferritin binds poorly to TFR.

Production of transferrin by the liver is inversely related to hepatocyte ferritin concentration, being increased when hepatic stores of iron are low and reduced when stores are increased.[30] Plasma TF concentration, usually measured as total iron binding capacity, is therefore a convenient assessment of iron stores.

Plasma TF is crucial for the daily iron cycle (Fig. 5.2). At any one time, only about 4 mg of body iron is present bound to TF, yet every 24 hours >30 mg of iron is transported throughout the body. Therefore, every day each molecule of TF carries several molecules of ferric iron between cells and >80% of this iron is transported to or reutilized in the bone marrow to make heme. The bulk of other daily iron turnover involves iron exchange with hepatocytes. There appears to be no alternative pathway for the iron to enter the red cell precursors. Congenital absence of TF is associated with severe iron deficiency anemia but uptake by non-erythropoietic tissues continues even in the absence of TF.[31]

Transferrin receptor

The TFR is a transmembrane glycoprotein which exists as a dimer of 2 subunits joined by a disulfide bond.[32] Each TFR can bind 2 TF molecules. At the neutral pH of the cell surface, TFR has an increased affinity for diferric TF compared to monoferric TF and this in turn is greater than the affinity of TFR for apotransferrin.

Each TFR can therefore bind up to 4 ferric ions and because the efficiency of TFR binding to TF is dependent on the degree of TF iron saturation, the plasma transferrin saturation (or total iron-binding capacity [TIBC]) directly affects the availability of iron for intracellular metabolism. In adults, a TIBC of >16% is needed to maintain normal erythropoiesis. Lower levels of about 7% are adequate to maintain red cell production in children.[33,34]

The number of TFRs present on a cell's surface reflects the ability of that cell to accept iron from circulating TF. TFRs are particularly numerous on cells that metabolize a large amount of iron, such as erythroid precursors, reticulocytes and placental trophoblasts.[35]

Ferritin and hemosiderin

Iron can be stored either as ferritin or hemosiderin.[36] Ferritin is a water-soluble protein whose iron stores are relatively available for iron metabolism as and when required. In sudden hemorrhage, for example, iron loss can temporarily exceed supply. However, the extra blood cells required can be produced without interruption by using iron supplies mobilized from stored ferritin.

Hemosiderin in an insoluble protein-iron complex whose iron is less available, in the short term at least, for metabolic requirements. Unlike ferritin, hemosiderin is visible on light microscopy and stains deep blue with Perl's (Prussian Blue) reagent. It is found primarily in the Kupffer cells of the liver and the macrophages of the spleen and bone marrow. In iron overload, hemosiderin begins to be deposited in the parenchymal cells of the liver and other organs.

Ferritin is produced as a hollow spherical protein with 22–24 apoferritin subunits.[37] It has a molecular weight of 468 000 kDa. Six channels penetrate the spherical shell through which iron passes into the core. Up to about 4500 iron atoms can be contained in 1 ferritin molecule, mostly as ferric hydroxide with some ferric phosphate. Ferritin is usually about 50% saturated.

Two types of apoferritin subunits have been identified: L (light) and H (heavy).[38] In different tissues, different proportions of L and H chains are found in their respective ferritin molecules. Liver, a site of iron storage, contains ferritin consisting of a preponderance of L chains but the heart, not normally a site of iron storage, has mainly H chains in its ferritin molecules. Ferritin with an excess of L chains may well be essentially for long-term storage and those mostly consisting of H chains may be more active in iron metabolism.[39]

Although different tissues may produce differing apoferritin spheres, all tissues need to be able to assemble the spheres quickly to protect themselves from the potential toxicity of free iron. As ferritin is produced, a small amount proportional to the intracellular ferritin concentration leaks into the plasma. Thus plasma ferritin concentration is related to cellular iron stores.[40]

ASSESSMENT OF BODY IRON STORES

Reduced iron store

Detectable abnormalities occur in sequence as the magnitude of iron deficiency worsens (Table 5.4).[41] The eventual changes in red cell morphology are non-specific and occur late. Of more importance, and usually the first indication of iron deficiency, are changes in red cell indices. Most modern automated instruments measure red blood cells, hemoglobin and mean cell corpuscular volume (MCV) directly. The

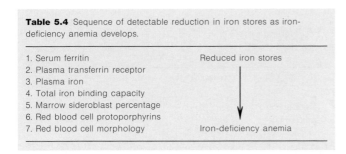

Table 5.4 Sequence of detectable reduction in iron stores as iron-deficiency anemia develops.

1. Serum ferritin   Reduced iron stores
2. Plasma transferrin receptor
3. Plasma iron
4. Total iron binding capacity
5. Marrow sideroblast percentage
6. Red blood cell protoporphyrins
7. Red blood cell morphology   Iron-deficiency anemia

direct measurement of MCV has made this a sensitive parameter of red cell changes and it has overtaken the more traditional measurements of mean corpuscular hemoglobin concentration (MCHC) and mean corpuscular hemoglobin (MCH) as the primary indication of possible iron deficiency. Many modern blood counters produce 2-dimensional red cell maps which can often demonstrate the presence of iron-deficient red cells.

No single confirmatory test is appropriate in all situations:

- *Serum ferritin* is a sensitive measurement of iron deficiency[40] but is an 'acute phase reactant' whose synthesis increases non-specifically in response to inflammation, infection or malignancy. Liver cell damage also raises the serum ferritin independently of body iron status.
- The increasing availability of *radioimmunoassays of plasma TFRs* will provide a new method of diagnosing iron deficiency.[42] Plasma TFR concentration is proportional to marrow red cell turnover: erythroid hypoplasia (hypoplastic anemia, chronic renal failure) reduces it and erythroid hyperplasia (chronic hemolytic anemia) increases levels. TFR levels are also increased in iron deficiency and in the absence of other conditions causing erythroid hyperplasia plasma TFR is a sensitive indicator of iron deficiency.[43] Unlike serum ferritin, plasma TFR is not affected by chronic inflammation or liver disease.
- *Plasma iron and transferrin saturation* (ratio of plasma iron: TIBC) provide a measure of current iron supply to the tissues. These tests are widely used but are strongly influenced by physiologic variation, concurrent inflammatory disease and recent prior ingestion of iron.
- *Free erythrocyte zinc protoporphyrin (ZPP)* is a simple test which can be performed on a drop of EDTA blood. This makes ZPP a convenient adjunct to MCV estimation and red cell mapping as it is immediately available from the same blood sample that went through the blood count analyzer. In iron deficiency, protoporphyrin IX cannot combine with iron to form heme in the final step of heme synthesis. In the absence of iron, protoporphyrin combines with zinc to form ZPPs, which are stable and persist throughout the life-span of the red cell. Estimation of red cell ZPP provides an indication of iron supply to the red cell over a longer period than serum ferritin or plasma iron.[44] ZPP therefore can be used to confirm iron deficiency in a patient who has recently been started on iron

supplements. ZPP may be affected by chronic inflammation but less so by acute infections of recent onset than the more traditional measurements of body iron.

- In difficult cases, *bone marrow examination* after staining with Perl's reagent will clarify the situation. In iron deficiency, neither the marrow macrophages nor erythroblasts contain iron. In the anemia of chronic disease there is plenty of iron present in the macrophages but none is present in the red cell precursors. Normally, about 20% of erythroblasts contain iron (sideroblasts).

Increased iron stores

In practice, assessment of increased iron stores relies on repeated serum ferritin estimations and if definitive diagnosis is required on liver biopsy.

Plasma iron and transferrin saturation are poor indicators of reticuloendothelial iron overload. They are not reliably elevated by increased macrophage iron as occurs during the early stages of transfusional hemosiderosis. Serum ferritin on the other hand is elevated early even in macrophage iron deposition. As mentioned above, serum ferritin is influenced by several factors other than body iron status. Repeated measurements give a more reliable estimation of body iron stores than a single result.

Although marrow biopsy can give a subjective assessment of iron overload, liver biopsy provides much more useful information, including histologic assessment of the degree and distribution of hepatic iron stores and quantification of hepatic iron concentrations in μmol iron/g dry weight of liver tissue.[45] Liver biopsy is not to be undertaken lightly and is not practicable for regular assessment of body iron stores. Currently, repeat serum ferritin estimations have to be undertaken but non-invasive radiologic approaches are being developed and evaluated. Magnetic susceptometry using a Superconducting Quantum Interference Device (SQUID)[46] and dual energy computed tomography[47] have both been developed but are not available for routine clinical use. Techniques using magnetic resonance imaging (MRI) are not yet fully developed but may in the future offer a repeatable and non-invasive quantitative assessment of body iron stores.[48]

CONTROL OF HEME SYNTHESIS WITHIN THE ERYTHROBLAST (Fig. 5.3)

In plasma, iron binds to apotransferrin to form mono and differic TFs. At the neutral pH on the outside of the cell membrane, differic TF preferentially binds to TFRs on the cell surface.[49] The iron-bearing TF-TFR complex rapidly clusters with other similar complexes and is internalized. Here, the clusters of iron-TF-TFR complexes coalesce with other similar clusters to form endosomes. Once within the cytosol, the pH within the endosome is lowered permitting release of iron into the cytosol. The apoTF-TFR complex remains tightly bound until it reaches the cell surface. Under

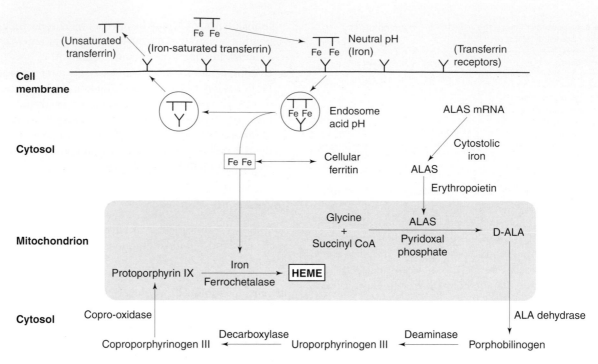

Fig. 5.3 Heme synthesis. Binding of iron-saturated transferrin to cell membrane transferrin receptors, endosome formation, release of iron into the cytosol and the role of mitochondrial and cytosolic enzymes in the production of heme. ALAS = δ-aminolevulinic acid synthase.

the neutral pH conditions at the cell surface, the unsaturated apoTF is released to be recycled and bind with more iron. The TFRs remain at the cell surface ready to bind more differic transferrin.[50]

Control of intracellular iron metabolism is mediated at the mRNA level by the iron-responsive binding protein (IRE-BP).[51] The IRE-BP appears to be structurally identical to cytosolic aconitase, an iron–sulfur enzyme active in the Krebs cycle.[52] Evidence suggests that the IRE-BP and cytosolic aconitase can reversibly convert from one form to another in response to alterations in intracellular iron availability.[53] This is mediated by changes in the molecular iron content of the aconitase/IRE-BP internal iron–sulfur cluster.[54] Where intracellular iron is readily available, the aconitase enzymatic activity predominates, whereas low intracellular iron promotes the mRNA-binding activity of IRE-BP.

In the erythroid progenitors, IRE-BP acts by binding to iron-responsive elements (IRE) present on the mRNA of TFR, ferritin and ALAS, the first enzyme in the pathway for the formation of heme from glycine and succinyl co-enzyme A.

IRE-BP binding to TFR IRE stabilizes TFR mRNA, reducing its cytoplasmic degradation and hence increasing the amount of cytoplasmic mRNA and the rate of TFR synthesis. More TFRs become available on the cell surface to bind differic transferrins.[55] IRE-BP binding to ferritin and ALAS mRNA has the opposite effect of reducing translation of both ferritin and ALAS,[39,56] and thus reducing intracellular iron metabolism.

The effects of increased IRE-BP binding in the presence of low cytosolic iron and reduced IRE-BP binding in the presence of high cytosolic iron are summarized in Fig. 5.4. When cytosolic iron is low, more TFRs are produced which in turn increases the amount of iron-saturated TF taken into the cell. Storage and metabolism of iron by ferritin and ALAS are reduced, which again will tend to increase the iron content of the cytosol. The situation is reversed in the presence of high cytosolic iron levels. In

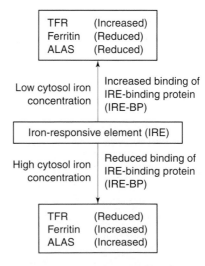

Fig. 5.4 Effect of cytosol iron content on the intracellular synthesis of transferrin receptors (TFR), ferritin and δ-aminolevulinic acid synthase (ALAS) mediated via the iron responsive element (IRE).

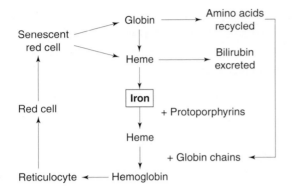

Fig. 5.5 Red cell cycle.

consequence, iron uptake by erythroid cells has a positive effect promoting ALAS activity. Increased ALAS activity increases protoporphyrin synthesis, thus coupling protoporphyrin production to iron availability within the erythroblast.[57] Under physiologic conditions, the IRE-BP controls intracellular iron homeostasis.

THE RED CELL CYCLE (Fig. 5.5)

Each day 25 ml of senescent red cells are destroyed. The globin chains are broken down into amino acids which are then recycled to make more globin chains. The heme groups are split into iron and porphyrins. The porphyrins are metabolized and excreted as bilirubin. The iron is recycled into the production of more red cell heme and combined with globin chains to form hemoglobin in erythroblasts and reticulocytes. The mature red blood cells survive 120 days on average before expressing red cell senescent antigen on their cell surface. This signals their imminent destruction and the initiation of the recycling process.

DEVELOPMENTAL ASPECTS

Fetus and neonate

The developing fetus is little affected by maternal iron stores. Only in extreme maternal iron deficiency is any degree of anemia seen in the fetus.[58] In general, the fetus acts as a parasite receiving maternal iron at the expense of the mother. In the vast majority of cases, babies of iron-deficient mothers are born with normal hemoglobin concentrations. Infant serum iron and TIBC are also usually normal in the presence of maternal iron deficiency.[59–61] At the same time as being able to sequester iron from the mother into the fetus, the placenta also acts as a barrier excluding excess iron and preventing fetal iron overload. Consequently, maternal iron supplementation does not influence fetal iron status.[62]

A full-term infant at birth is iron replete with about 80 mg/kg of body weight of iron as compared with 55 mg/kg of body weight for an adult male;[63] 50 mg/kg is as red blood cell iron, 25 ml/kg as storage iron and 5 ml/kg as myoglobin.[64]

The extra iron is needed to cope with the additional requirements of the accelerated rate of growth which takes place in the first few months of life.

Iron stores at birth may be almost completely independent of maternal iron status but they are dependent on 2 other factors: birth weight and neonatal red cell mass.

Placental iron transport is insignificant until the third trimester when iron transport increases dramatically to as much as 4 mg/day. Infants born before 26 weeks' gestation have very low iron stores; in those born in the third trimester, iron stores are proportional to birth weight. A 1-kg preterm infant will have about 50 mg of total body iron compared to the 320 mg of a 4-kg full-term baby. The effect of this reduction is accentuated by the greater relative growth potential of the 1-kg preterm infant.

Red cell mass is determined by hemoglobin concentration and red cell volume. Although red cell volume is more or less uniform at 80–90 ml/kg, hemoglobin concentration at birth can vary from 13.5 g/dl to 21 g/dl in normal infants. The timing of umbilical cord clamping influences birth hemoglobin concentration (see also Chapter 9). At delivery, two-thirds of the red cells in the fetal circulation are in the infant and one-third in the placenta and cord. In the 3 min immediately following birth, uterine contractions will increase the amount of blood cells in the fetus to >85%,[65] so early clamping of the cord can reduce the infant's iron content by between 15 and 30%.[66]

Infancy

During the first few weeks of life, erythropoiesis almost stops as the infant's red cell mass drops to a level appropriate for the oxygen-rich extrauterine environment.[67] Iron is stored until erythropoiesis resumes, usually when the infant's hemoglobin concentration has dropped to 11–12 g/dl.[68] In the normal, term infant, the iron stored during this time is adequate to cope with the expected doubling of body weight that takes place in the first 5 months of life. After this time, iron absorption from the diet becomes critical to the maintenance of normal iron balance. It has been estimated that a term infant needs 100 mg of iron in the first year of life from the diet to maintain a hemoglobin level of 11 g/dl but a preterm infant may require 2–4 times as much.[69]

As stated above, newly born infants are iron replete. This is reflected by laboratory findings. Cord blood iron levels are high at 150–250 μg/dl, dropping to 130 μg/dl after 24 hours. Following resumption of erythropoiesis at 8 weeks, iron levels drop further to 80 μg/dl.[33] Serum ferritin is also raised at birth with levels between 100 and 200 μg/l; it then increases further over the first 8 weeks of life but then begins to drop following resumption of erythropoiesis.[37] At 1 year, the mean serum ferritin is usually 30 μg/l. Serum transferrin levels are proportional to gestational age. This is a developmental phenomenon and in the preterm infant, at least, is not related to iron status.[70]

Early childhood

During childhood total body iron increases in proportion to body weight. After 6 months of age, growth slows and the diet becomes more varied. As long as the diet has an adequate iron content, iron deficiency anemia is unusual. Even so, measured parameters of serum iron and transferrin saturation remain persistently low. Transferrin saturations of 10% are not uncommon during early childhood but despite this erythropoiesis continues satisfactorily. Serum ferritin also remains low but levels below 10 μg/l indicate depletion of iron stores.

Puberty

At puberty the secondary growth spurt increases iron requirements to allow for the increase in red cell and muscle mass. Another 80–90 ml of blood alone are required for every extra kilogram of lean body weight. This need for more iron is particularly marked in boys whose increase in lean body mass is on average double that seen in girls. In girls, however, as the growth spurt ends menstruation begins and there is a need for extra iron to compensate for menstrual blood loss. Pregnancy can further increase the iron intake requirement of fertile females.

INHERITED DISORDERS

Inherited disorders of iron metabolism are extremely rare. They are usually characterized by iron-deficient erythropoiesis despite the absorption of excessive quantities of iron.

Congenital atransferrinemia[31]

Congenital absence of TF is an autosomal recessive disorder. Affected infants present at birth with a severe microcytic hypochromic anemia with a low serum iron and TIBC. Plasma TF is absent. The anemia does not respond to iron but transfusion with plasma can induce a reticulocyte response. Treatment is with blood transfusion and TF.[71]

Although bone marrow iron is absent, iron is absorbed from the gastrointestinal tract and deposited in the liver, pancreas, heart and kidneys. One affected child died from the effects of myocardial hemosiderosis. Therefore, TF does not appear to be required for the release and transport of iron from the intestinal mucosal cells. However, the absence of TF prevents iron transport to the erythron.

Congenital microcytic hypochromic anemia with iron overload

Two sets of siblings have been described with a severe microcytic hypochromic anemia despite fully saturated TIBC and an increased serum iron.[72,73] Liver parenchymal cells contained excess iron and there was associated fibrosis. No iron was present in liver macrophages or the bone marrow, suggesting a functional defect of the transfer of iron to red cell precursors and macrophages.

Other syndromes

Three siblings have been described with a microcytic hypochromic anemia apparently due to an isolated abnormality of malabsorption and defective utilization of iron.[74] A single patient has also been described as having reduced iron incorporation into red cell precursors in the presence of a raised serum iron caused by an IgM autoantibody to the TF receptor.[75]

SIDEROBLASTIC ANEMIAS

The sideroblastic anemias are an heterogeneous group of disorders characterized by variable red cell hypochromia, anemia and the presence of a significant number of ringed sideroblasts in the marrow. By definition, the ringed sideroblasts should total 10% or more of the nucleated red cell precursors.[76] Diagnostic ringed sideroblasts contain 6 or more siderotic granules arranged in a perinuclear collar around one-third or more of the erythroblast nucleus. These perinuclear granules consist of iron-laden mitochondria.[77]

All forms are characterized by failure to utilize iron properly during heme synthesis in the mitochondria. Iron accumulates within the mitochondria and eventually adversely affects mitochondrial function. Premature erythroblast cell death follows, resulting in ineffective erythropoiesis.

CLASSIFICATION (Table 5.5)

All forms of sideroblastic anemia are rare in childhood. The congenital forms are occasionally encountered but the

---

Table 5.5 Classification of the sideroblastic anemias.

Congenital
  Primary X-linked
  Primary autosomal
  Pearson's syndrome
  Stoddart variant
  DIDMOAD or Wolfram syndrome
  Syndromes of increased erythropoietic protoporphyrins

Acquired
  Primary idiopathic also called refractory anemia with excess ringed sideroblasts (RARS; one of the myelodysplasias)
  Secondary acquired:
    Drugs: isoniazid, chloramphenicol
    Toxins: alcohol (chronic abuse), lead
    Copper deficiency
    Zinc excess
  Diseases sometimes associated with an excess of ringed sideroblasts:
    Hemolytic anemias
    Megaloblastic anemias
    Myeloid malignancies
    Autoimmune disorders

aquired forms are much less commonly seen in children than in adults.

CONGENITAL SIDEROBLASTIC ANEMIAS

Etiology

In most families affected by sideroblastic anemia inheritance is X-linked and may be associated with the co-inheritance of other X-linked traits such as glucose-6-phosphate dehydrogenase deficiency[79] or ataxia.[80] Female carriers may show minor changes with a variable population of circulating hypochromic red cells, the size of the hypochromic population in female carriers is probably dependent on random X chromosome inactivation (Lyon hypothesis). In some cases where lyonization is extreme, females are more severely affected.[81] In other families, females are affected because the sideroblastic anemia is inherited as an autosomal trait.[82,83]

Molecular basis (Fig. 5.3)

The first step in the synthesis of heme from glycine and succinyl co-enzyme A is catalyzed by ALAS in the presence of pyridoxal phosphate. Two types of ALAS exist in the body: one is an ubiquitous enzyme found in all tissues and is coded for by a gene on chromosome 3; the other is expressed by a gene on the X chromosome and is specific to erythroid cells.[84] This explains why most cases of inherited sideroblastic anemia are X-linked and why the synthesis of heme proteins other than hemoglobin is unaffected.

ALAS requires the presence of pyridoxal phosphate as a co-enzyme to initiate mitochondrial heme production efficiently. In some cases of inherited X-linked sideroblastic anemia, mutant ALAS enzymes have been demonstrated.[85] Theoretically, pyridoxine in pharmacologic doses could act to improve the enzyme activity of a mutant ALAS in several ways and thereby improve the production of heme. It could stabilize the quaternary structure of mutant ALAS and thereby improve enzyme activity.[85] In other situations, pyridoxine might protect mutant ALAS from premature degradation by mitochondrial proteases.[86] Finally, the mutant enzyme might require a higher concentration of pyridoxal phosphate than is usually necessary to promote normal activity.[87]

In other families with sideroblastic anemia, defects of ferrochelatase and COPRO-oxidase have been described.[88,89] COPRO-oxidase does not have pyridoxal phosphate as a cofactor, so these patients would not be expected to respond to pyridoxine therapy. In other patients, multiple or ill-defined enzyme deficiencies interfere with mitochondrial function and heme synthesis.[90] Some of these patients may respond to pyridoxine, others will not. Nevertheless. in all cases of inherited sideroblastic anemia a trial of pyridoxine therapy is indicated.[91]

Diagnosis

Most cases present in infancy or early childhood but less severe forms may pass unnoticed until adulthood. Some patients are discovered during routine testing of close relatives of a suspected patient. Others present late with the clinical effects of iron overload–liver disease, diabetes mellitus or heart failure. Late presentation with iron overload most often occurs in cases where anemia is mild or occasionally in female carriers. Examination is usually normal except for pallor but splenomegaly or hepatomegaly may be present.

Investigation reveals microcytosis with a variable degree of anemia. The microcytosis can be severe and an MCV of 50 fl can be seen in the more anemic patients. A novel form of macrocytic hereditary sideroblastic anemia was recently described.[92] The characteristic red cell dimorphism is most marked in cases with milder anemia and in female carriers. This can be detected by microscopic examination of the blood film or mechanically from erythrocyte volume distribution curves or red cell maps depending on the type of blood counter technology used. Serum iron and ferritin are elevated and TIBC reduced.

The dimorphic blood picture, raised serum iron, raised serum ferritin and reduced iron-binding capacity may be confused with partially treated iron-deficiency anemia, particularly as many patients will have already received iron, blood transfusions or both. Free erythrocyte porphyrins, however, are normal and help to distinguish partially treated iron deficiency. Levels of protoporphyrin are reduced and coproporphyrin levels remain normal.

Other non-specific abnormalities are often present, i.e. mild hyperbilirubinemia and reduced haptoglobins in the presence of a normal or only slightly increased reticulocytosis. Iron staining of peripheral blood will demonstrate circulating red cells which contain iron-laden mitochondrial remnants (Pappenheimer bodies). However, definitive diagnosis is most often made following microscopic examination of a bone marrow aspirate. Iron staining reveals the presence of large numbers of pathologic ringed sideroblasts. In inherited sideroblastic anemia, the ringed sideroblasts are predominantly seen in the late erythroblast population.

Differential diagnosis

Initial confusion with *partially treated treated iron-deficiency anemia* will be clarified following iron staining of a bone marrow aspirate. It is important to consider performing a bone marrow aspirate in infants, especially males with an unexplained iron-deficiency anemia, or where investigation of microcytosis fails to elucidate a cause for the reduction in red cell size, particularly if the MCV has remained low despite iron therapy.

Once significant (> 10%) numbers of ringed sideroblasts have been demonstrated, inherited sideroblastic anemia has to be differentiated from *acquired disorders* associated with the

Table 5.6 Differentiation of hereditary from primary acquired sideroblastic anemia.

	Hereditary	Acquired
Red blood cell size	Microcytic	Macro- or normo-cytic
Ringed sideroblasts	Late erythroblasts	Early erythroblasts
Free red blood cell porphyrins	Normal	Increased
Red blood cell coproporphyrins	Normal	Increased
Marrow chromosomes	Normal	Abnormal in 60%
Relatives	Often abnormal	Normal

presence of excess ringed sideroblasts in the marrow (Table 5.5). It is usually possible to differentiate inherited sideroblastic anemia from the primary acquired form on clinical grounds alone. In cases where there is uncertainty, laboratory findings will allow differentiation (Table 5.6). Red cell macrocytosis, raised red cell porphyrins and the presence of marrow chromosomal abnormalities are particularly helpful. Investigation of close relatives is important as it helps to identify cases of inherited sideroblastic anemia and at the same time permits quantification of iron loading in asymptomatic siblings and carriers.

Other *rare inherited disorders* presenting in childhood can be associated with the presence of significant numbers of ringed sideroblasts in the marrow. Pearson et al[93] described a syndrome of refractory anemia presenting in early childhood as a severe transfusion-dependent normocytic or macrocytic anemia with reticulocytopenia. Neutropenia is usually present and a variable thrombocytopenia is common. Examination of the marrow reveals prominent degenerative cytoplasmic vacuolation in both erythroid and granulocytic precursors. Iron stores are markedly increased and ringed sideroblasts are prominent. The disease is not limited to the bone marrow; marked fibrosis of the exocrine pancreas was found at post-mortem examination of 2 children with the syndrome who died in the first 3 years of life, and 3 less severely affected children also showed *in vivo* evidence of abnormal pancreatic function. *Pearson's anemia* probably represents a disorder of multiorgan cellular mitochondrial dysfunction. A possible variant of Pearson's anemia with early onset of severe pancytopaenia and thyroid fibrosis has been described.[94]

Two children with *DIDMOAD syndrome* (Wolfram syndrome)[95] have been described as having a megaloblastic and sideroblastic anemia.[96] The patients were first cousins and both demonstrated a response to thiamine with improvement in anemia and associated neutropenia and thrombocytopenia. Insulin requirements also reduced significantly following the introduction of thiamine therapy. The authors speculated that DIDMOAD syndrome may be a multisystem degenerative disorder caused by an inherited abnormality of thiamine metabolism.

Three reports have been published describing sideroblastic anemia in the presence of excess erythrocyte protoporphyrins.[97–99] These cases share some similarities with erythropoietic porphyria; 2 patients had skin photosensitivity and 1 developed liver disease with increased hepatic protoporphyrins.

Although primary acquired sideroblastic anemia is very unusual in childhood, secondary acquired cases do occur (Table 5.5). A full *drug history* needs to be taken. Some drugs like isoniazid act as pyridoxine inhibitors, others like chloramphenicol may inhibit mitochondrial protein synthesis by interfering with ferrochelatase activity.

Lead toxicity is not uncommon in pre-school children[100] and it can be associated with anemia and ringed sideroblasts in the marrow. Acute lead intoxication usually presents as lead encephalopathy with anemia as a late manifestation. However, chronic lead poisoning often co-exists with iron deficiency and consequent microcytic anemia. Basophilic stippling, a precipitation of RNA and mitochondrial fragments, is often prominent on the blood film.[101] Lead binds to the red blood cell membrane and is absorbed into the red cell, interfering with several enzymes including ferrochelatase which are involved with heme synthesis.[102] Iron, heme intermediates and zinc protoporphyrins accumulate inside the red cells. An increase in free erythrocyte protoporphyrins is a useful screening test for lead poisoning and also helps to differentiate lead toxicity from sideroblastic anemia.[103] Diagnosis is confirmed by estimation of blood lead concentration. Treatment is based on the removal of the sources of lead ingestion and dual chelation therapy with dimercaprol (BAL) and calcium EDTA.[104]

Ringed sideroblasts may also be seen with abnormalities of other metals and occur in *copper deficiency* and *zinc overload*. Copper deficiency is only seen in malnourished premature babies[105] and in patients receiving long-term parenteral nutrition with inadequate copper supplementation.[106] Copper is absorbed almost exclusively during the last trimester and deficiency in a premature infant may be accentuated if the child is put onto copper-deficient feeds such as cows' milk at an early age. Early severe copper deficiency presents as a hypochromic anemia and neutropenia. Examination of the marrow reveals ringed sideroblasts, vacuolation of erythroid and granulocytic precursors and granulocytic maturation arrest. More chronic cases produce osteoporosis, depigmentation of the skin and hair and central nervous system changes. Diagnosis is made by demonstrating a low serum copper and ceruloplasmin. The effects of copper deficiency are quickly reversed by treatment with 2–5 mg/day of copper sulfate orally or by the addition of 100–500 μg/day of copper to intravenous feeds. In excess, zinc interferes with copper absorption and can cause a secondary copper deficiency.[107] A high serum zinc is associated with low serum copper and ceruloplasmin levels. Discontinuation of zinc ingestion will reverse the changes over 2–3 months.

Other causes of secondary sideroblastic anemia are much commoner in adults than children. Ringed sideroblasts are only occasionally found in the marrows of children with myelodysplastic syndromes other than primary acquired sideroblastic anemia (refractory anemia with ringed sideroblasts). They can also be rarely seen in cases of acute myeloid leukemias. Careful examination of the marrow will distinguish these from primary inherited sideroblastic anemia. Significant numbers of ringed sideroblasts can sometimes be seen in juvenile rheumatoid arthritis[108] and 1 case of an antibody-mediated acquired sideroblastic anemia has been reported.[109]

Management

Between 25% and 50% of patients with hereditary sideroblastic anemia show some response to oral pyridoxine. A trial of pyridoxine 25–100 mg 3 times a day for 3 months is indicated in all patients. Response is variable and in many cases the MCV remains abnormal and residual microcytic, hypochromic cells can be seen on the blood film. Responders should continue pyridoxine for life but because pyridoxine can produce a peripheral neuropathy, the dose should be titrated to the lowest daily dose that maintains response.[110] In one report a patient who had not responded to oral pyridoxine responded to parenteral pyridoxal-5′-phosphate.[111] Folic acid supplements should also be given.

The majority of patients do not respond to pyridoxine and require regular blood transfusions which further increase iron overload. Strict adherence to chelation therapy with deferoxamine (desferrioxamine) is essential for long-term survival.

Mildly affected patients and even some female carriers may eventually develop symptoms of iron toxicity as a result of excess absorption from the diet.[112] These patients should be carefully monitored for excess iron deposition. If this is detected, most patients will tolerate therapeutic venesection to remove iron from the body.[113]

Splenectomy should be avoided as it is associated with a high incidence of thromboembolism and persistent post-operative thrombocytosis.

ACQUIRED SIDEROBLASTIC ANEMIAS

Those occurring in childhood have been described above in the differential diagnosis of the inherited sideroblastic anemias.

Primary acquired idiopathic sideroblastic anemia/refractory anemia

Primary acquired idiopathic sideroblastic anemias is one the myelodysplastic syndromes, refractory anemia with ringed sideroblasts (RARS).[114] RARS is usually a disease of the elderly and is seen only rarely in childhood. However, with the increasingly successful use of powerful chemotherapy and radiotherapy to treat pediatric malignancies, secondary forms of RARS may begin to be seen in pediatric practice.

In adults, RARS has a relatively benign course with a 50-month median survival and about a 10% incidence of leukemic progression.[115] The more malignant forms are associated with marrow clonal chromosomal abnormalities other than trisomy 8 which has no adverse prognostic significance. Monosomy 7 or partial deletion of the long arm of chromosome 7, in particular, have a poor prognosis with an increased risk of leukemic transformation. Other factors associated with a poorer outcome are anemia requiring regular transfusions and hence early iron overload and the presence of associated neutropenia and/or thrombocytopenia. It is likely that the same factors are relevant to children as well.

In general, myelodysplasias occurring in children should be treated aggressively (see Chapter 4). If differentiation from inherited sideroblastic anemia is certain and particularly in the presence of poor prognostic indicators, bone marrow transplantation should be considered early in the course of the disease. If a conservative approach is taken, patients must be closely monitored for iron overload and progression to more advanced types of myelodysplasia or frank leukemia.

IRON OVERLOAD

ACUTE OVERDOSE

Accidental overdose is not uncommon, particularly in pre-school children. A 1990 study of 339 cases found that 83.9% occurred in children under 6 years old.[116] This is because iron tablets look like sweets and are often available in the home because the child's mother is pregnant and has been prescribed iron supplements. Toxicity is directly related to the dose ingested. Doses of >60 mg/kg are likely to induce serious toxicity and ingestion of >180 mg/kg may prove fatal.

Acute iron poisoning can be divided into four phases:

1. The patient experiences nausea and vomiting, abdominal pain and diarrhea due to irritation of the gastrointestinal tract. In some cases, ulceration can occur in the upper gastrointestinal tract during this phase with hematemesis and melena.
2. The patient appears to be well. Most recover at this stage but a minority progress into the third phase.
3. The patient develops iron encephalopathy with fits and fluctuating conscious level, shock, metabolic acidosis and acute renal tubular and hepatic necrosis.
4. Those that recover may go on to develop high intestinal obstruction with strictures, usually in the pyloric region. This fourth phase most often occurs in children 2–6 weeks after apparent recovery.

Treatment is also dependent on the amount of iron ingested. Where there is doubt about how many tablets if any have been taken, a plain abdominal X-ray may help to confirm significant overdose because iron tablets are radio-opaque.

Serious toxicity occurs when the ability of TF and apoferritin to mop up the excess iron is exceeded. This is usually seen when serum iron is >90 μmol/l and the TIBC is overwhelmed and toxic free iron oxyradicals are generated. Guidelines suggest that when >20 mg/kg has been ingested, gastric lavage should be performed.[116] If the patient is too young or cannot tolerate this procedure, an emetic should be administered. Patients who have taken >40 mg/kg or an intentional overdose should be admitted for observation following lavage. In cases of significant overdose, deferoxamine (desferrioxamine) should be given orally to prevent further absorption from the gastrointestinal tract and parenterally to remove iron already absorbed.

CHRONIC IRON OVERLOAD

The effects of chronic iron overload are most often seen in patients who have increased dietary iron absorption and/or are receiving regular blood transfusions. The extent of tissue damage is related to the total amount of iron absorbed, the speed of iron accumulation and the distribution of iron in the body tissues. Iron stored in tissue macrophages appears to be relatively innocuous whereas deposits in parenchymal cells are often associated with extensive tissue damage.

The mechanism producing cellular damage appears to be the same irrespective of the underlying cause of the iron overload. As tissue stores build up, the protective iron-binding proteins TF and ferritin become overwhelmed by the excess iron. This allows increasing amounts of free non-TF-bound iron to exist as ionic iron in the plasma and tissues,[117] which promotes the production of free hydroxyl radicals. These oxyradicals damage intracellular lipids, nucleic acids and proteins, disrupting intracellular organelles and breaking down intracellular lysozymes which release hydrolytic enzymes into the cytosol and thereby cause further intracellular destruction. Cell death follows accompanied by pericellular necrosis and fibrosis.[118,119]

Etiology and distribution of abnormal iron deposition in the body

The clinical manifestations of iron overload differ according to the underlying disease process (Table 5.7).

In *hereditary hemochromatosis*, increased oral absorption causes a gradual increase in tissue iron and symptoms usually do not develop until middle age or later when total body iron stores have increased by 15–20 g.[120] Iron deposition is predominantly in parenchymal cells, initially in the liver but eventually affecting other organs.[121] In the rare cases presenting in childhood, the pattern of iron deposition is often more marked in the heart and thyroid.[122] In both the adult and pediatric forms, bone marrow macrophage iron deposition is unimpressive and may be absent.[123]

Excessive oral absorption of iron is also seen in the *iron-loading anemias*. These are the group of anemias associated with erythroid hyperplasia and ineffective erythropoiesis

Table 5.7 Etiology of iron overload.

Increased gastrointestinal absorption
  Hereditary hemochromatosis
  Erythroid hyperplasia with ineffective erythropoiesis:
    β-Thalassemia major
    β-Thalassemia intermedia
    Hemoglobin E/β-thalassemia
    Congenital dyserythropoietic anemias
    Pyruvate kinase deficiency
    Sideroblastic anemias
  Atransferrinemias and other rare disorders of iron transport

Repeated red cell transfusions

Perinatal iron overload
  Hereditary tyrosinemia (hypermethioninemia)
  Zellweger syndrome (cerebrohepatorenal syndrome)
  Neonatal hemochromatosis

Focal iron sequestration
  Idiopathic hemochromatosis
  Hallervorden–Spatz syndrome
  Chronic hemoglobinuria

and include β-thalassaemia major and intermedia, the congenital dyserythropoietic anemias, chronic hemolytic anemias and some of the sideroblastic anemias. The iron distribution is similar to that seen in hereditary hemochromatosis and is predominately in the parenchymal cells of the liver, spreading later to other organs. In some conditions such as β-thalassemia major the increase in dietary iron absorption is of secondary importance to the iron deposition caused by the need for regular blood transfusions. In those conditions not requiring regular blood transfusions, increased oral iron absorption is the primary mechanism of iron overload. Although occurring more slowly than transfusion-related siderosis, this will eventually cause clinically significant tissue damage. Even patients with mild anemia can develop significant iron overload because the rate of iron deposition is not related to the severity of the underlying anemia.[112]

In *transfusional iron overload*, iron deposition occurs more quickly. Each unit of blood contains 200–250 mg of iron and most patients require >200 ml/kg/year of blood, equivalent to about 200 mg/kg iron/year.[124] Clinical symptoms usually appear when >15 g of excess iron has been transfused. Initially, iron is stored in the marrow and reticuloendothelial macrophages which have a storage capacity of about 10–15 g. When this storage capacity has been exceeded, parenchymal iron deposition occurs and tissue damage follows. Transfusional iron toxicity occurs relatively quickly. Iron-induced hepatic fibrosis has been detected in children under 3 years old.[123]

In the early stages of iron accumulation, histologic assessment of the pattern of iron deposition in the liver and bone marrow can help in differentiating the underlying cause. In advanced iron overload, however, the differences in tissue distribution disappear as iron deposition becomes more widespread.

Perinatal iron overload

Perinatal iron overload is rare and presumably occurs where the normal but poorly understood mechanisms for transferring iron from the maternal blood to the fetus via the trophoblast, basement membrane and fetal endothelium fail to control entry of iron into the fetus.[126] Two distinct inherited disorders have been described. In *hereditary tyrosinemia* (hypermethioninemia) iron deposition is restricted to the liver which is usually cirrhotic.[127] Pancreatic islet cell hyperplasia and renal abnormalities are also present. In *Zellweger syndrome* (cerebro-hepato-renal syndrome) iron is deposited in the parenchymal cells of the liver, spleen, kidney and lungs.[128]

The syndrome of *neonatal hemochromatosis* is less well defined and the underlying defect has not been identified.[129] In affected infants, iron is deposited in the parenchymal cells of the liver, heart and endocrine organs but not in the bone marrow or spleen. Death usually occurs in the neonatal period from liver disease which in some cases may precede widespread iron deposition.[130] The disorder may represent the common end stage of a group of disorders with different etiologies. In some cases an infective agent may be responsible; in others there is evidence of abnormal feto-maternal iron transport.

Focal iron overload

Focal sequestration of iron into the pulmonary alveolar macrophages occurs in idiopathic pulmonary hemosiderosis and in the basal ganglia of patients with the rare neurodegenerative disorder Hallervorden–Spatz syndrome.[131] In idiopathic pulmonary hemosiderosis, the iron sequestered in the pulmonary macrophages is unavailable for iron metabolism and eventually iron-deficiency anemia develops. The pathogenic role of the iron deposited in the central nervous system in Hallervorden–Spatz syndrome is uncertain. Renal hemosiderosis can occur in patients with chronic hemoglobinuria but is not associated *per se* with any renal dysfunction.

Clinical effects

Prior to the introduction of chelation therapy the clinical effects of iron overload presented in late childhood and the early teenage years in most regularly transfused patients. In hereditary hemochromatosis the slow rate of tissue iron overload usually delayed significant tissue damage until middle age or later. Generally, children developed normally during the first decade of life as long as adequate amounts of blood were transfused. In the second decade, patients often presented with growth failure and delayed or absent pubertal development. In the early teenage years, heart disease and abnormalities of liver function were commonly seen and a minority of patients developed hypothyroidism.[132] In the late teenage years, abnormalities of glucose tolerance and even diabetes mellitus occurred but the clinical picture was

most often dominated by deteriorating heart disease which was frequently fatal before the age of 20.[133]

Iron chelation therapy has dramatically altered the clinical picture of iron overload. However, chelation regimens need to be strictly adhered to if they are to be effective but unfortunately many patients fail to do so. In a study following variably chelated but regularly transfused thalassemic patients over a period of 21 years, the incidence of iron-overload complications was still significant at 20 years of age; 30% had heart disease, 43% diabetes mellitus, 28% hypothyroidism and 22% hypoparathyroidism. In patients older than 20, 60% had one or more iron-related, life-threatening complications.[134] The consequences of iron overload and the potential benefits of chelation therapy are shown in Table 5.8.

Heart

When total body iron is > 1 g/kg significant amounts begin to be deposited in the myocardium and the conducting system of the heart.[124] In transfusional iron overload, the ECG changes of left ventricular hypertrophy and conduction defects may be detected by 10–12 years of age. Echocardiographic changes occur late in the disease process.[135] In inadequately chelated patients, cardiac disease is the commonest cause of death and may occur in the late teens.[133] Except in the rare childhood forms of hereditary hemochromatosis,[120] the cardiac effects of excessive iron deposition are only seen at a late stage of the illness in about 10–15% of the most seriously affected patients.

Liver

In hereditary hemochromatosis iron is primarily deposited in the parenchymal cells and so liver cell damage is initiated early and becomes clinically significant when the liver

Table 5.8 Complications of iron overload and the effect of chelation therapy.

Complication	Effect of chelation therapy	
	Protection	Reversibility of established disease
Liver	Yes	Yes
Heart	Yes	Yes
Endocrine:		
Growth	Yes	Yes
Hypogonadism	Yes	No
Diabetes mellitus	Yes	No
Hypothyroidism	Yes	No
Hypoparathyroidism	Yes	No
Arthropathy	Unknown	
Infections	No (Yersinia seen with chelation therapy)	

contains about 5000 μg iron/g dry weight of liver.[136] However, because the development of iron overload in hemochromatosis is slow, liver disease usually takes decades to develop. In transfusional iron overload, iron is first deposited in the protective liver reticulo-endothelial storage cells and about twice as much iron needs to be deposited in transfusional iron overload as in herediary hemochromatosis before clinical problems develop.[137] Nevertheless, the rate of iron deposition in transfusional siderosis is so rapid that liver abnormalities can be detected within 2 years of initiating transfusion therapy.[138]

Hepatomegaly is detectable early followed by abnormal liver function tests. With further deposition parenchymal damage induces fibrosis which may be present before 3 years of age.[125] Eventually macronodular or mixed macro-micronodular cirrhosis develops . In adults with hemochromatosis the incidence of development of hepatoma in the cirrhotic liver is high.

In transfusional siderosis liver disease was often multifactorial due to a high incidence of hepatitis B and C. Immunization of patients against hepatitis B and the introduction of effective screening tests for hepatitis B and C by the blood transfusion services have greatly reduced the incidence of viral hepatitis in these patients.

Endocrine system

Even well transfused patients develop growth failure and hypogonadism in the second decade of life.[139] Poor pubertal growth in unchelated patients is probably caused by a combination of central hypogonadism[140] and reduced production of insulin-like growth factor (IGF)-1.[141] Failure or delay of sexual development remains a problem for patients who do not fully comply with chelation regimes.

There was a high incidence of abnormalities of glucose tolerance but frank diabetes mellitus only occurred in 6.5% of transfused unchelated thalassemics and usually not before 17 years of age. The incidence was higher in patients with a family history of diabetes.[142]

Hypothyroidism occurs in about 6% of non-chelated thalassemics[132] and hypoparathyroidism in a similar number. Minor abnormalities of adrenal androgen secretion have also been described.

Joints

Arthropathy, particularly of large joints, is relatively common in older patients with hemochromatosis. It can also be seen at a younger age in a minority of patients with transfusional siderosis.[143]

Infections

The increased availability of iron may predispose to infection with a variety of bacteria and fungi, particularly *Yersinia* *enterocolitica* but also *Listeria monocytogenes*, *Escherichia coli*, *Vibrio vilnificus* and some Candida species.[144]

Iron chelation therapy

The introduction of effective iron chelation therapy has revolutionized the management of patients with iron-overload disorders and the problems of management of multiply transfused patients have shifted from detection and treatment of iron-induced organ damage to early detection and control of the unwanted effects of chelation. Modern pediatric practice is increasingly involved with the prevention rather than the management of iron overload.

Although great advances are being made towards a safe, cheap and effective oral chelator, parenteral deferoxamine remains the only effective iron chelator in routine clinical use. Its use in the management of regularly transfused thalassemic patients has recently been extensively reviewed and the potential benefits of deferoxamine are summarized in Table 5.8.[145,146]

Deferoxamine (desferrioxamine)

Deferoxamine acts by binding to available ferric iron in a 1:1 molecular ratio to form feroxamine which can be excreted in the urine and feces.[147] It is poorly absorbed orally, is cleared rapidly from the plasma and has an half-life of 5–10 min; to be effective deferoxamine has to be given parenterally by slow infusion.[148]

The first reports of the effective promotion of iron excretion by intramuscular or intravenous deferoxamine were published in the early 1960s.[149,150] The modern self-administered 12-h subcutaneous regimens using portable pumps were not developed until the mid 1970s.[150,152] Deferoxamine is undoubtedly effective in ameliorating the clinical effects of iron overload. If complied with, modern regimens can achieve negative iron balance in nearly all patients. Two early studies of the long-term effects of parenteral deferoxamine, including a controlled UK study, demonstrated that even pre-existing liver and heart abnormalities could potentially be reversed.[153,154]

More recent studies confirm the early findings. The most recent studies have a higher percentage of long-term chelated patients who started therapy at early age. There is increasing evidence that when chelation is introduced at an early stage, cardiac disease,[155] liver disease[156] and the endocrine consequences of iron overload can be prevented.[156] Even the effects of iron overload on fertility can be prevented in some male and female patients.[158] One study reported the results of iron chelation with subcutaneous deferoxamine in a group of 57 patients in whom treatment had been life-long and initiated at the start of transfusion therapy.[145] Adequate compliance was assessed by mean serum ferritins of 1000–1600 $\mu g/l$ (never > 2000 $\mu g/l$) and serial liver biopsies which confirmed that hepatic liver stores remained in an acceptable range. The mean follow-up was 14.5 ± 3.6 years. There

Table 5.9 Deferoxamine toxicity.

Local reactions
Anaphylaxis
Growth failure
Neurotoxicity:
  Optic
  Auditory
Renal toxicity
Pulmonary toxicity
Infection (Yersinia)

was a complete absence of life-threatening complications and a marked improvement in hypogonadism with normal pubertal development in 73% of females and 58% of males. However, 70% of patients showed reduced growth requiring reduction of the dose of deferoxamine which was probably due to premature introduction of the chelation therapy (see below).

The commonest difficulty with deferoxamine therapy is non-compliance. However, patients who do comply with modern chelation regimens can often experience side-effects (Table 5.9). At particular risk of serious toxicity are young patients receiving high doses of deferoxamine in the presence of only modestly increased iron stores. The actual mechanisms of toxicity are unclear but may be related to the excess chelation of iron which could adversely affect iron-dependent enzyme systems. Alternatively, the unwanted chelation of other metals such as zinc or copper may interfere with their normal metabolic activities.

Local reactions are common and are important because they can reduce compliance. Adequate training in the correct techniques to self-administer the infusion is essential and the addition of 5–10 mg of hydrocortisone to the deferoxamine solution is often helpful. *Generalized anaphylaxis* can occur and rapid infusion of high doses intravenously can also cause a serious systemic reaction.[160]

Deferoxamine can induce *growth failure* in children undergoing chelation therapy. This is due to cartilaginous dysplasia of the long bones and spine. There is a disproportional reduction of truncal growth with early loss of sitting height.[161,162] This toxicity is most marked when the drug is administered in high doses of >50 mg/kg/day and particularly when given from the inception of a regular transfusion regimen.[163,164] Doses of 15–35 mg/kg/day do not appear to induce any abnormality of sitting or standing height and spinal X-rays remain normal. Established growth failure is usually not reversible.

Neurotoxicity is not uncommon and can affect the vision and/or hearing. Patients receiving relatively high doses of subcutaneous deferoxamine (>40 mg/kg/day) may complain of reduced visual acuity accompanied by subjective hearing loss. Symptoms are usually acute in onset.[165] On these high-dose regimens many more patients on laboratory testing in the absence of subjective symptoms are found to have significantly reduced visually evoked responses (VER). Regimens using very high-dose intravenous deferoxamine

can induce other visual problems including night blindness and visual field defects.[166] Ototoxicity is not infrequent in younger patients receiving high doses in the presence of only limited increases in iron stores.[160] Ototoxicity presents as subjective loss of hearing due to high frequency deafness and using audiometry, this too can be detected at an early stage before symptoms appear. Neurotoxicity usually responds to prompt withdrawal of deferoxamine at the onset of symptoms or at the first detection of abnormalities on VER or audiogram.

Other toxicities are uncommon. *Pulmonary*[167] and *renal toxicity*[168] can occur but are nearly always associated with very high-dose regimens. *Yersinia infection* has been described during deferoxamine therapy in the absence of significant iron overload. Yersinia can metabolize ferrioxamine, the product of combination of iron and deferoxamine.

Management of deferoxamine therapy. The timing of initiation of therapy needs careful consideration. High-dose therapy begun at the time of the first transfusion is associated with reduced growth[163] but on the other hand significant changes in liver histology have been described before the age of 3 in unchelated children.[125] To prevent deferoxamine-associated toxicity and at the same time avoid the irreversible tissue damage caused by iron overload, it is probably best to start therapy when iron stores are moderately increased. Therapy should be introduced using a low dose of deferoxamine. It has recently been suggested that significant iron overload should be confirmed by liver biopsy before starting chelation,[146] but it would seem more practicable to use a sustained increase in serum ferritin with a level of about 1000 μg/l triggering deferoxamine therapy.

The association of toxicity with relatively high doses of deferoxamine has led to the development of lower dose regimens; doses of 25–35 mg/kg/day are safer than those using >50 mg/kg/day. Toxicity is also related to the degree of iron overload. During therapy it is necessary to compensate for reducing iron stores. Serum ferritin should be measured regularly and estimation of the ratio of daily mean deferoxamine dose in mg/kg to serum ferritin in μg/l can then be made. To avoid toxicity the ratio should not exceed 0.025.[160]

Ascorbic acid deficiency is sometimes seen in thalassemic patients and this reduces the availability of iron for chelation.[169] Supplementary vitamin C in this situation can significantly increase deferoxamine iron excretion.[170] However, increasing the chelatable iron pool is associated with an increase in iron-induced free radical formation and increased tissue damage.[171] It is probably not advisable to give vitamin C routinely to patients with iron overload. However, if there is a reduction in the efficacy of chelation therapy despite apparently good compliance, ascorbic acid levels should be determined. If found to be low, vitamin C (100 mg orally 30–60 min into the infusion) should be given in a therapeutic trial on days when deferoxamine is being administered.[146]

Non-compliance. This is a major problem. A recent UK study demonstrated good compliance in only 36% of children with thalassemia. Up to 70% of older patients may have prolonged periods of non-compliance.[172] Survival in poorly chelated patients is much reduced with a median survival of 17.5 years compared to 31 years in well chelated patients.[173]

Non-compliance should be approached aggressively. Vitamin C levels and if necessary liver biopsy should be performed to confirm failure to comply with treatment. Socio-psychologic support may be helpful as might changes in the method of administration of chelation therapy. Continuous ambulatory intravenous administration is very effective and is associated with better compliance, although this requires insertion of an indwelling catheter.[174] Catheter sepsis does occur but is usually easily dealt with.[175] Intermittent bolus injections have been used.[176] More recently regimens with continuous ambulatory infusions of subcutaneous deferoxamine using a gravity balloon pump system have been developed and are well tolerated by older patients.

Alternative iron chelators

The development of successful chelation with deferoxamine has been a major medical advance. A high percentage of transfusion-dependent patients are now reaching adolescence and adulthood.[177] However, its cost and the need for accessory delivery systems have to a large extent precluded its use in the poorer countries where transfusion-dependent anemias such as β-thalassemia major are particularly common. This has prompted research into the development of a less expensive, non-toxic, orally active alternative to deferoxamine.

A handful of alternative chelators have been assessed. 2.3-dihydrobenzoic acid (2.3-DHB) does increase iron excretion when given orally but was not found to be effective in clinical practice.[178]

The relatively inexpensive plant maltose derivative 1,2-dimethyl-3-hydroxypyrid-4-one (L1) is under extensive evaluation in several centers throughout the world. At doses of 75 mg/kg it produces urinary iron losses equivalent to those seen with 30–40 mg/kg deferoxamine.[179] However, fecal iron excretion is less than with deferoxamine. Therefore, in the short term at least, L1 is less effective than deferoxamine in its ability to reduce body iron stores. Also, toxicity has been a problem with reversible agranulocytosis that recurs on re-challenge seen in 4% of patients.[180] Abnormalities of liver function occur in 44% of patients and arthropathy in 25%. Severe nausea which can necessitate withdrawal of the drug occurs in 8%. Most recently, a suspected but infrequent alteration in immune function has been confirmed with the occurrence of agranulocytosis, arthritis and systemic vasculitis in a 24-year-old thalassemic patient.[181] Disappointingly, two trials have been terminated prematurely; hepatic iron concentrations in L1-treated patients were at above safe levels in 33% of patients in one study and in the other a mean 50% increase in baseline hepatic iron concentration compared to 0% for those receiving deferoxamine was seen. Therefore, in the long term L1 may not provide adequate control of body iron stores in a significant minority of patients.[146]

Management of iron overload

Iron-loading anemias

Any condition associated with erythroid hyperplasia and ineffective erythropoiesis can be complicated by significant iron overload caused by increased gastrointestinal absorption. The degree of iron overload is not related to the degree of anemia and can occur even in those patients with little or no reduction in their hemoglobin concentrations. The excess iron tends to be deposited in the parenchymal cells and so as in hereditary hemochromatosis tissue iron damage is initiated at an early stage of iron overload. Therefore, any patient with an iron-loading anemia needs to be monitored throughout life with intermittent estimations of serum ferritin. Any patient with a sustained, significant rise in serum ferritin, especially if levels are continuing to increase, needs to be considered for treatment with therapeutic phlebotomy. Once significant iron overload has been confirmed, treatment should begin promptly as delay will only increase parenchymal tissue damage. For every 2 ml of blood venesected, approximately 1 mg of iron is removed from the body.

Despite being well tolerated by most patients with absent or mild anemia, phlebotomy should be initiated carefully. Five to 10 ml/kg up to a maximum of 500 ml should be withdrawn per week with the hemoglobin concentration and hematocrit checked prior to each venesection. As therapy continues there should be a progressive fall in serum ferritin. Eventually, serum iron and iron-binding capacity will return to normal when body iron stores become nearly depleted. Occasionally, serum iron may fall and anemia worsen in the presence of a persistently high serum ferritin. In this situation, suspending phlebotomy for a few weeks may allow iron to be mobilized from long-term iron stores, and then re-introduction of phlebotomy will be followed by further reductions in the serum ferritin. When the serum ferritin has become normal, weekly therapeutic phlebotomy should be discontinued. Thereafter, maintenance phlebotomy will be required every few weeks with the aim of keeping serum ferritin < 50 μg/l and TIBC normal.

Patients requiring regular blood transfusions

A minority of patients cannot tolerate regular venesection usually because of worsening anemia. They require regular transfusion to suppress erythropoiesis and hence reduce dietary iron absorption to normal and regular chelation therapy to remove the excess iron introduced by the transfused blood.

A regular transfusion regimen should not be introduced without proper consideration of the potential benefits for the patient and the risks involved. Iron chelation therapy is the crucial factor. Parents and patients must be educated about the effects of iron overload and the critical need for compliance with chelation. The physician in charge needs to have a comprehensive plan for the management of regular transfusion therapy and be able carefully to monitor the patient for the effects of iron overload and deferoxamine toxicity.

Pre-transfusion considerations (Table 5.10). In all patients, the ultimate goal of transfusion therapy is to ensure normal growth and development and promote well-being.

In the hypoerythroblastic anemias, such as Diamond–Blackfan anemia, the only aim of therapy is to achieve the minimum hemoglobin concentration that ensures normal growth and development whilst preventing dyspnea and the other symptoms of clinical anemia. The appropriate level of pre-transfusion hemoglobin will vary from patient to patient but in most at least 8 g/dl is necessary.

Those patients with anemias associated with erythroid hyperplasia and concomitant increase in iron absorption from the gastrointestinal tract also need regimens which promote normal growth and development. However, the regimen chosen for these patients must also adequately suppress marrow expansion and hypersplenism in order to prevent skeletal deformity and extramedullary hemopoiesis and at the same time reduce the excess absorption of dietary iron. In rare conditions such as pyruvate kinase deficiency in which the oxygen dissociation curve is shifted to the right relatively low levels of post-transfusion hemoglobin concentration may be adequate.[182] However, in the majority of patients, maintenance of a near normal mean hemoglobin concentration is required.

Table 5.10 Preparation for the introduction of regular transfusion therapy.

State clinical aims

Plan regimen
   Type of red cells to be used
   Pre-transfusion hemoglobin level
   Frequency of transfusion
   Logistics: who, when and where?
   Deferoxamine:
      Initiation of therapy
      Initial dose
      Patient/parent training

Investigations
   Red cell antigen studies
   Baseline virology

Immunize against hepatitis B

Hypertransfusion regimens which aim for a trough hemoglobin of 9–10 g/dl are undoubtably effective in preventing the physical effects of anemia and at the same time adequately suppress dietary iron absorption.[183] Supertransfusion regimens that aim for a higher pre-transfusion hemoglobin of >11 g/dl have been developed[184] but have not proven to be any more effective than hypertransfusion.[185]

Transfusions should aim to raise the patient's hemoglobin by about 4 g/dl and are given at 3 or 4 weekly intervals. Appropriately matched packed red cells with as long an expiry date as possible should be transfused. Attempts to improve the life-span of transfused blood and hence increase the interval between transfusions by selecting out younger red cells from blood donations have been developed,[184] but in clinical practice these 'neocytes' have been shown to prolong transfusion interval by only 13–16%.[186,187] Neocytes are about 3 times more expensive per unit and they increase donor exposure considerably. Leukocyte-depleted blood should be transfused to reduce the incidence of nonfebrile transfusion reactions and to prevent the production of HLA antibodies, which is particularly important in patients who may at a later date be considered for bone marrow transplantation.

Logistic considerations are particularly important in pediatric patients. Children tolerate regular transfusion regimens better if they are treated in familiar surroundings by medical and nursing staff well known to them who are skilled in the insertion of intravenous cannulas and the management of blood transfusions. Much of the pain associated with cannula insertion can be avoided by the use of topical anesthetic cream. Interference with schooling can be minimized with appropriate timing of outpatient appointments and by planning hospital visits well in advance. School work can be performed during hospitalization for transfusions.

As discussed above, the timing of the introduction of deferoxamine and the dose used is important. The side-effects of chelation therapy are most often seen when high doses are given before iron stores have significantly increased. A practical approach is to introduce deferoxamine when the serum ferritin is confirmed to be >1000 μg/l. The serum ferritin should be maintained between 1000 and 2000 μg/l. The ratio of daily deferoxamine dose to serum ferritin should be assessed 3–4/year and should not exceed 0.025.

Prior to first transfusion, the patient's own red cell antigens should be identified, including full Rhesus genotype and Kell, Ss, Kidd and Duffy types. It is not possible to transfuse fully matched red cells but units with the appropriate Rhesus and Kell type should be selected for routine use. If at a later date red cell antibodies develop, prior knowledge of the patient's own red cell antigens makes their identification much easier. Antibodies to these blood groups are particularly likely to complicate regular red cell transfusions in patients with sickle cell disease or β-thalassemia.[188]

Table 5.11 Monitoring of regular red cell transfusion.

Effect of transfusions
 Pre- and post-hemoglobin levels
 Growth
 Development
 Regression of hepatosplenomegaly
 Volume of blood transfused/year/kg

Deferoxamine

Serum ferritin	(3 monthly)
Deferoxamine:ferritin ratio	(3 monthly)
Liver function tests	(6 monthly)
Audiogram	(6 monthly)
Visual evoked responses	(6 monthly)
Sitting and standing heights	(12 monthly)
Spinal X-rays	(12 monthly; particularly early life)
Calcium/phosphate/alkaline phosphatase	(12 monthly when over 10 years old)
ECG ± echocardiography	(12 monthly when over 10 years old)
Glucose tolerance test	(12 monthly when over 10 years old)
Thyroid function test	(12 monthly when over 10 years old)

Regular assessment by a pediatric endocrinologist

Baseline virology studies should be performed before transfusion to determine antibody status to hepatitis B and C, human immunodeficiency viruses I and II and cytomegalovirus. As long as there has been no proven infection with hepatitis B, the patient should be immunized.

Assessment during transfusion therapy. Patients receiving regular blood transfusions need to be assessed at intervals to ensure that the aims of transfusion are being met and that the side-effects of iron overload or deferoxamine toxicity have not developed. A suitable scheme for monitoring patients is outlined on Table 5.11. The calculation of annual total red cell/kg is important. An increase in transfusion requirement significantly more than that expected for growth suggests that splenectomy may be indicated. In this situation, splenectomy significantly reduces the red cell requirement and thus helps to maintain control of body iron balance. The operation is best avoided until after 5 years of age and should be preceded by antipneumococcal and anti-haemophilus immunizations. Parents and patients need to be made aware of the dangers of infections post splenectomy and a patient-held card warning that the patient has had a splenectomy should be issued. Prophylactic penicillin is necessary postoperatively and pneumococcal immunization must be repeated at appropriate intervals.

Hereditary hemochromatosis

The pediatrician is mainly involved with the screening of children for the possible inheritance of hemochromatosis rather than in treating established cases. However, hereditary hemochromatosis can in rare instances present in childhood, even in those as young as 2 years old.[122,189] Males and females are equally affected. The illness has a different clinical pattern in childhood from that seen in adults; the cardiac and gonadal consequences of iron overload predominate rather than the hepatic and pancreatic effects seen in adults.

Screening is best carried out using a combination of serum ferritin and transferrin saturation. If either or both of these are elevated, a confirmatory liver biopsy should be performed. Children presenting with idiopathic cardiomyopathy, hypogonadism, amenorrhea, diabetes mellitus or arthritis should be tested to exclude hereditary hemochromatosis. Screening may need to be repeated at intervals in children at risk as initial results may be normal in early childhood because the rate of iron overload occurs so slowly in most cases. Most often screening will be initiated following the diagnosis of hemochromatosis in an older relative. The gene for hereditary hemochromatosis has been mapped to the HLA class I region on chromosome 6,[190] and homozygotes and heterozygotes can be confidently diagnosed from HLA class I typing. Recently, a candidate gene, HFE (or HLA-H), has been identified and two HFE mutations described.[191,192]

The treatment of iron overload in hereditary hemochromatosis is similar to that described above for the iron-loading anemias. The introduction of phlebotomy should not be delayed once diagnosis has been made. In cases where significant organ damage has occurred, iron chelation therapy may be required as well. When treatment is instituted at an early stage before significant organ damage has taken place, patients should have a normal life expectancy.[120]

REFERENCES

1. Finch CA, Ragan HA, Dyer IA *et al*. Body iron loss in animals. *Proc Soc Exp Biol Med* 1986; **159**: 335
2. Green R, Charlton R, Seftel H *et al*. Body iron excretion in man. *Am J Med* 1968; **45**: 336
3. Finch CA, Huebers HA. Iron metabolism. *Clin Physiol Biochem* 1986; **4**: 5
4. Committee on Iron Deficiency. Report of the American Medical Association Council on Foods and Nutrition. *JAMA* 1968; **203**: 407
5. Finch CA, Cook JD, Labbe RF *et al*. Effect of blood donation on iron stores as evaluated by serum ferritin. *Blood* 1977; **50**: 441
6. Cook JD, Lipschitz DA. Clinical measurements of iron absorption. *Clin Haematol* 1977; **6**: 567
7. Turnbull AL, Cleton F, Finch CA. Iron absorption. IV. The absorption of hemoglobin iron. *J Clin Invest* 1962; **41**: 1898
8. Finch CA, Huebers HA. Perspectives in iron metabolism. *N Engl J Med* 1982; **306**: 1520
9. Weintraub LR, Weinstein MB, Huser HJ. Absorption of hemoglobin iron: the role of a heme-splitting substance in the intestinal mucosa. *J Clin Invest* 1968; **47**: 531
10. Cook JD, Layrisse M, Martinez-Torres C *et al*. Food iron absorption measured by an extrinsic tag. *J Clin Invest* 1972; **51**: 805
11. Hallberg L, Bjorn-Rasmussen E. Determination of iron absorption from whole diet: a new two-pool model using two radio-iron isotopes given as haem and and non-haem iron. *Scand J Haematol* 1972; **9**: 193

12. Martinez-Torres C, Layrisse M. Nutritional factors in iron deficiency: food iron absorption. *Clin Haematol* 1973; **2**: 339

13. Layrisse M, Martinez-Torres C, Roche M. The effect of interactions of various foods on iron absorption. *Am J Clin Nutr* 1968; **21**: 1175

14. Disler PB, Lynch SR, Charlton RW *et al*. The effect of tea on iron absorption. *Gut* 1975; **16**: 193

15. Callender ST, Marney SR, Warner GT. Eggs and iron absorption. *Br J Haematol* 1970; **19**: 657

16. Crosby WH. Control of iron absorption by intestinal luminal factors. *Am J Clin Nutr* 1968; **21**: 1189

17. McMillan JA, Oski FA, Lourie G *et al*. Iron absorption from human milk, simulated human milk and proprietary formulas. *Pediatrics* 1977; **60**: 896

18. Saarinen UM, Siimes MA, Dallman PR. Iron absorption in infants: high bioavailability of breast milk iron is indicated by the extrinsic tag method of iron absorption and by the concentration of serum ferritin. *J Pediatr* 1977; **91**: 36

19. Cook JD, Skikne BS. Intestinal regulation of body iron. *Blood Rev* 1987; **1**: 267

20. Pootrakul P, Kitcharoen K, Yansukon P *et al*. The effect of erythroid hyperplasia on iron balance. *Blood* 1988; **71**: 1124

21. Huebers HA, Huebers E, Csiba E *et al*. The significance of transferrin for intestinal iron absorption. *Blood* 1983; **61**: 283

22. Idzerda RL, Huebers H, Finch CA, McKnight GS. Rat transferrin gene expression: tissue-specific regulation by iron deficiency. *Proc Natl Acad Sci USA* 1986; **83**: 3723

23. Crosby WH. The control of iron balance by the intestinal mucosa. *Blood* 1963; **22**: 441

24. Huebers HA, Finch CA. Transferrin: physiological behaviour and clinical implications. *Blood* 1984; **64**: 743

25. Awai M, Brown EB. Clinical and experimental studies of the metabolism of I131-labled human transferrin. *J Lab Clin Med* 1963; **61**: 363

26. Huerre C, Uzan G, Grzeschik K *et al*. The structural gene for transferrin (TF) maps to 3q21-qter. *Ann Genet* **27**: 5

27. Rabin M, McClelland A, Kuhn L *et al*. Regional localisation of the human transferrin receptor gene to 3q26-qter. Am J Hum Genet 1985; **37**: 1112

28. Bailey S, Evans RW, Garratt RC *et al*. Molecular structure of serum transferrin at 3.3-A resolution. *Biochemistry* 1988; **27**: 5804

29. Huebers J, Csiba E, Josephson B *et al*. Interaction of human diferric transferrin with reticulocytes. *Proc Natl Acad Sci USA* 1981; **78**: 621

30. Morton AG, Tavill AS. The role of iron in the regulation of hepatic transferrin sysnthesis. *Br J Haematol* 1977; **36**: 383

31. Goya N, Miyazaki S, Kodate S, Ushio B. A family of congenital atransferrinaemia. *Blood* 1972; **40**: 239

32. McClelland A, Kuhn LC, Ruddle FH. The human transferrin receptor gene: genomic organisation and the complete primary structure of the receptor deduced from a cDNA sequence. *Cell* 1984; **39**: 267

33. Saarinen UM, Siimes MA. Developmental changes in serum iron, total iron binding capacity, and transferrin saturation in infancy. *J Pediatr* 1977; **91**: 875

34. Koeper MA, Dallman PR. Serum iron concentration and transferrin saturation in the diagnosis of iron deficiency in children: normal developmental changes. *J Pediatr* 1979; **91**: 870

35. Iacopetta BJ, Morgan EH, Yeoh G. Transferrin receptors and iron uptake during erythroid cell development. *Biochim Biophys Acta* 1982; **687**: 204

36. Aisen P, Listowski I. Iron transport and storage proteins. *Ann Rev Biochem* 1980; **49**: 357

37. Worwood M. Ferritin in human tissues and serum. *Clin Haematol* 1982; **11**: 275

38. Harrison PM, Andrews SC, Artymiuk PJ *et al*. Ferritin p.81. In:

39. Ponka P, Schulman HM, Woodworth RC (eds) *Iron Transport and Storage*. Boca Raton, FL: CRC Press, 1990

39. Munro H. The ferritin genes: their response to iron status. *Nutr Rev* 1993; **51**: 65

40. Jacobs A, Worwood M. Ferritin in serum. Clinical and biochemical implications. *N Engl J Med* 1975; **292**: 951

41. Herbert V. Anaemias p.593. In: Paige DM (ed) *Clinical Nutrition*, 2nd edn. St Louis: CV Mosby, 1988

42. Flowers CH, Skikne BS, Covell AM *et al*. The clinical measurement of serum transferrin receptor. *J Lab Clin Med* 1989; **114**: 368

43. Skikne BS, Flowers CH, Cook JD. Serum transferrin receptor: a quantitative measure of tissue iron deficiency. *Blood* 1990; **75**: 1870

44. Labbe RF, Rettmer RL. Zinc protoporphyrin. *Semin Hematol* 1989; **26**: 40

45. Brittenham GM, Danish EH, Harris JW. Assessment of bone marrow and body iron stores. *Semin Hematol* 1981; **18**: 194

46. Brittenham GM, Farrell DE, Harris J *et al*. Magnetic susceptibility measurement of human iron stores. *N Engl J Med* 1982; **307**: 1671

47. Leighton DM, Matthews R *et al*. Dual energy CT estimation of liver iron content in thalassaemic children. *Aust Radiol* 1988; **32**: 214

48. Kaltwasser JP, Schalk KP, Werner E. Juvenile hemochromatosis. *Ann NY Acad Sci* 1988; **526**: 339

49. Pippard MJ, Hoffbrand AV. Iron. In: Hoffbrand AV, Lewis SM (eds) *Postgraduate Haematology*, 3rd edn. London: Heinemann, 1989

50. Irie S, Tavasolli M. Transferrin-mediated cellular iron uptake. *Am J Med Sci* 1987; **293**: 103

51. Theil EC. The IRE (iron regulatory element) family: structures which regulate mRNA translation or stability. *Biofactors* 1993; **4**: 87

52. Kennedy MC, Mende-Mueller L, Blondin GA *et al*. Purification and characterization of cytosolic aconitase from beef liver and its relationship to the iron responsive element binding protein. *Proc Natl Acad Sci USA* 1992; **89**: 11730

53. Klausner RD, Rouault TA. A double life: cytosolic aconitase as a regulatory RNA binding protein. *Mol Biol Cell* 1993; **4**: 1

54. Constable A, Quick S, Gray NK *et al*. Modulation of thre RNA-binding activity of a regulatory protein by iron *in-vitro*: switching between enzymatic and genetic function. *Proc Natl Acad Sci USA* 1992; **89**: 4554

55. Leibold EA, Guo B. Iron-dependent regulation of ferritin and transferrin receptor expression by the iron-responsive element binding protein. *Annu Rev Nutr* 1992; **12**: 345

56. Bhasker CR, Gurgeil G, Neupert B *et al*. The putative iron-responsive element in the human erythroid 5-aminolevulinate synthase mRNA mediates translational control. *J Biol Chem* 192; **268**: 12699

57. May BK, Bhasker CR, Bawden MJ, Cox TC. Molecular regulation of 5-animolevulinate synthase. Diseases related to heme synthesis. *Mol Biol Med* 1990; **7**: 405

58. Singla PN, Chand S, Khanna S, Agarwal KN. Effect of maternal anaemia on the placenta and the newborn infant. *Acta Paediatr Scand* 1978; **67**: 645

59. Lanzkowsky P. The influence of maternal iron-deficiency anaemia on the haemoglobin of the infant. *Arch Dis Child* 1961; **36**: 205

60. Shott RJ, Andrews BF. Iron status of a medical high-risk populaton at delivery. *Am J Dis Child* 1972; **124**: 369

61. Murray MJ, Murray AB, Murray NJ, Murray MB. The effect of iron status of Nigerian mothers on that of their infants at birth and 6 months, and on the concentration of iron in the breast milk. *Br J Nutr* 1978; **39**: 627

62. Sturgeon P. Studies of iron requirements in infants. III. Influence of supplemental iron during normal pregnancy on mother and infant. B. The infant. *Br J Haematol* 1959; **5**: 45

63. Rios E, Lipschitz DA, Cook JD, Smith NJ. Relationship of maternal and infant iron stores as assessed by determination of plasma ferritin. *Pediatrics* 1975; **55**: 694

64. Widdowson EM, Spray CM. Chemical development *in utero*. *Arch Dis Child* 1951; **26**: 205

65. Yao AC, Moinian M, Lind J. Distribution of blood between infant and placenta after birth. *Lancet* 1969; **2**: 871

66. Burman D. Iron requirements in infancy. *Br J Haematol*,1971;**19**: 657

67. Finne PH, Halvorsen S. Regulation of erythropoiesis in the fetus and newborn. *Arch Dis Child* 1972; **47**: 683

68. O'Brien RT, Pearson HA. Physiologic anemia of the newborn infant. *J Pediatr* 1971; **79**: 132

69. Gorten MK. Iron metabolism in premature infants. III. Utilisation of iron as related to growth in infants with low birth weights. *Am J Clin Nutr* 1965; **17**: 322

70. Galet S, Schulman HM, Bard H.The postnatal hypotransferrinemia of early preterm newborn infants. *Pediatr Res* 1976; **10**: 118

71. Schwick HG, Cap J Goya N. Therapy of atransferrinaemia with transferrin. *J Clin Chem* 1978; **16**: 75

72. Shahidi NT, Nathan DG, Diamond LK. Iron deficiency anaemia associated with an error of iron metabolism in two siblings. *J Clin Invest* 1964; **43**: 510

73. Stavem P, Saltvedt E. Elgjo K, Rootwelt K. Congenital hypochromic microcytic anaemia with iron overload of the liver and hyperferraemia. *Scand J Haematol* 1973; **10**: 153

74. Buchanan GR, Sheehan RG. Malabsorption and defective utilisation of iron in three siblings. *J Pediatr* 1981; **98**: 723

75. Larrick JW, Hyman E. Acquired iron deficiency anemia caused by an antibody against the transferrin receptor. *N Engl J Med* 1984; **311**: 214

76. Bottomley S. Sideroblastic anaemia. *Clin Haematol* 1982; **11**: 389

77. Cartwright GE, Deiss A. Sideroblasts, siderocytes and sideroblastic anemia. *N Engl J Med* 1975; **292**: 185

78. MacGibbon BH, Mollen DL. Sideroblastic anaemia in man; observation on seventy cases. *Br J Haematol* 1965; 11: 59

79. Prasad AS, Tranchida L, Konno AT et al. Hereditary sideroblastic anaemia and glucose-6-phosphate dehydrogenase deficiency in a negro family. *J Clin Invest* 1968; **47**: 1415

80. Pagon RA, Bird TD, Detter JC, Pierce I. Hereditary sideroblastic anaemia and ataxia: an X-linked recessive disorder. *J Med Genet* 1985; **22**: 267

81. Weatherall DJ, Pembrey ME, Hall EG, Sanger R et al. Familial sideroblastic anaemia: problem of Xg and X chromosome inactivation. *Lancet* 1970; **ii**: 744

82. Soslan G, Brodsky I. Hereditary sideroblastic anemia with associated platelet abnormalities. *Am J Hematol* 1989; **32**: 298

83. van Waveran Hogervorst GD, van Roermund HPC, Snijders PJ. Hereditary sideroblastic anaemia and autosomal inheritance of erythrocyte dimorphism in a Dutch family. *Eur J Haematol* 1987; **38**: 405

84. Bishop DF, Henderson AS, Astrin KH. Human delta-aminolevulinate synthase: assignment of the housekeeping gene to 3p21 and the erthroid-specific gene to X chromosome. *Genomics* 1990; **7**: 207

85. Cox TC, Bottomley SS, Wiley JS et al. X-linked pyridoxine-responsive sideroblastic anemia due to a THR388-SER substitution in erythroid 5-aminolevulinate synthase. *N Engl J Med* 1994; **330**: 675

86. Aoki Y, Muranaka S, Nakabayashi K, Ueda Y. Delta-aminolevulinic synthetase in erythroblasts of patients with pyridoxine-responsive.anaemia. *J Clin Invest* 1979; **64**: 119

87. Konopa L, Hoffbrand AV. Haem synthesis in sideroblastic anaemia. *Br J Haematol* 1979; **42**: 73

88. Garby L. Chronic refractory hypochromic anaemia with disturbed haem-metabolism. *Br J Haematol* 1957; **3**: 55

89. Stavem P, Romslo I, Rootwelt K, Emblem R. Ferrochelatase deficiency in the bone marrow in a syndrome of congenital hypochromic microcytic anaemia, hyperferraemia and iron overload of the liver. *Scand J Gastroenterol* 1985; **20 (Suppl 107)**: 73

90. Aoki Y. Multiple enzymatic defects in mitochondria of haemato-logical cells of patients with primary sideroblastic anaemia. *J Clin Invest* 1980; **66**: 43

91. Raab SO. Pyridoxine responsive anaemia. *Blood* 1961;**18**: 285

92. Tuckfield A, Ratnaike S, Hussein S, Metz J. A novel form of hereditary sideroblastic anaemia with macrocytosis. *Br J Haematol* 1997; **97**: 279

93. Pearson HA, Lobel JS, Kocoshis SA et al. A new syndrome of refractory sideroblastic anemia with vacuolization of marrow precursors and exocrine pancreatic dysfunction. *J Pediatr* 1979; **95**: 976

94. Stoddard RA, McCurnin Dc, Shultenover SJ et al. Syndrome of refractory sideroblastic anemia with vacuolization of marrow precursors in the neonate. *J Pediatr* 1981; **99**: 259

95. Anon. DIDMOAD (Wolfram) syndrome (Editorial). *Lancet* 1986; **1**: 1075–1076

96. Borgna-Pignatti C, Marradi P, Monetti N, Patrini C. Thiamine-responsive anemia in DIDMOAD syndrome. *J Pediatr* 1989; **114**: 405–410

97. Rothstein G, Lee R, Cartwright GE. Sideroblastic anaemia with dermal photosensitivity and greatly increased erythrocyte proto-porphyrin. *N Engl J Med* 1969; **280**: 587

98. Romslo I, Brun A, Sandberg S et al. Sideroblastic anaemia with markedly increased free erythrocyte porphyrin without dermal sensitivity. *Blood* 1982; **59**: 628

99. Scott AJ, Ansford AJ, Webster BH, Stringer HCW. Erythropoietic protoporphyria with features of a sideroblastic anemia terminating in liver failure. *Am J Med* 1973; **54**: 251

100. Lin-Fu JS. Vulnerability of children to lead exposure and toxicity. *N Engl J Med* 1973; **289**: 1289

101. Paglia DE, Valentine WN, Dalgren JG et al. Effects of low-level lead exposure on pyrimidine-5-nucleotidase and other erythrocyte enzymes. Possible role of pyrimidine-5-nucleotidase in the patho-genesis of lead-induced anaemia. *J Clin Invest* 1975; **56**: 1164

102. Goldberg A. Lead poisoning as a disorder of heme synthesis. *Semin Hematol* 1968; **5**: 424

103. Piomelli S, Davidow B, Guinee VF et al. The FEP (free erythrocyte porphyrins) test: a screening micromethod for lead poisoning. *Pediatrics* 1973; **51**: 254

104. Piomelli S, Rosen JF, Chisolm JJ, Graef JW. Management of childhood lead poisoning. *Pediatrics* 1984; **105**: 523

105. Askenazi A, Levin S, Djaldetti M et al. The syndrome of neonatal copper deficiency. *Pediatrics* 1973; **52**: 525

106. Zidar BL, Shadduck RK, Zeigler Z, Winklestein A. Observations on the anemia and neutropenia caused by copper deficiency. *Am J Hematol* 1977; **3**: 177

107. Ramadurai J, Shapiro C, Kozloff M, Telfer M. Zinc abuse and sideroblastic anemia. *Am J Hematol* 1993; **42**: 227

108. Harvey AR, Pippard MJ, Ansell BM. Microcytic anaemia in juvenile chronic arthritis. *Scand J Rheumatol* 1987; **16**: 53

109. Ritchie AK, Hoffman R, Dainiak N et al. Antibody-mediated sideroblastic anaemia: response to cytotoxic therapy. *Blood* 1979; **54**: 734

110. Parry GJ, Bredesen DE. Sensory neuropathy with low-dose pyr-idoxine. *Neurology* 1985; **35**: 1466

111. Mason DY, Emerson PM. Primary acquired sideroblastic anaemia: response to treatment with pyridoxal-5-phosphate. *Br Med J* 1973; **1**: 389

112. Peto TEA, Pippard MJ, Weatherall DJ. Iron overload in mild sideroblastic anaemias. *Lancet* 1983; **i**: 375

113. Weintraub LR, Conrad ME, Crosby WH. Iron loading anemia. Treatment with repeated phlebotomies and pyridoxine. *N Engl J Med* 1966; **275**: 169

114. Bennett JM, Catovsky D, Daniel MT et al. Proposals for the classification of the myelodysplastic syndromes. *Br J Haematol* 1982; **51**: 189

115. Third MIC Cooperative Study Group. Recomendations for a morphologic, immunological and cytogenetics (MIC) working

classification of the primary and therapy-related myelodysplastic disorders. *Cancer Genet Cytogenet* 1988; **32**: 1

116. Klein-Schwartz W, Odeka GM, Gorman RL *et al*. Assessment and management guidelines for acute iron ingestion. *Clin Pediatr* 1990; **29**: 316

117. Hershko C, Peto TEA. Annotation: Non-transferrin plasma iron. *Br J Haematol* 1987; **66**: 149

118. Halliwell B, Gutteridge JMC. Oxygen toxicity, oxygen radicals, transitional metals and disease. *Biochemistry* 1984; *219*: 1

119. Slater TF. Free radical mechanisms in tissue injury. *Biochemistry* 1984; **222**: 1

120. Niederau CR, Fisher R, Sonnenberg A *et al*. Survival and causes of death in cirrhotic and non-cirrhotic patients with primary hemochromatosis. *N Engl J Med* 1985; **313**: 1256

121. Cartwright GE, Edwards CQ, Kravitz K *et al*. Hereditary hemochromatosis: phenotypic expression of the disease. *N Engl J Med* 1979; **301**: 175

122. Haddy TB, Castro OL, Rana SR. Hereditary hemochromatosis in children, adolescents and young adults. *Am J Pediatr Hematol Oncol* 1988; **10**: 23

123. Brink B, Disler P, Lynch S *et al*. Patterns of iron storage in dietary iron overload and idiopathic haemochromatosis. *J Lab Clin Med* 1977; **88**: 725

124. Model B, Berdoukas V. *The Clinical Approach to Thalassaemia*. London: Grune & Stratton, 1984

125. Iancu TC, Neustein HB. Ferritin in human liver cells of homozygous beta thalassaemia: ultrastructural observations. *Br J Haematol* 1977; **37**: 527

126. Knisley AS, Grady RW, Kramer EE, Jones RL. Cytoferrin, maternal iron transport, and neonatal Hemochromatosis. *Am J Pathol* 1989; **92**: 755

127. Perry TL, Hardwick DF, Dixon G *et al*. Hypermethioninemia. *Pediatrics* 1965; **36**: 236

128. Volpe JJ, Adams RD. Cerebro-hepato-renal syndrome of Zellweger. *Acta Neuropathol* 1972; **20**: 175

129. Knisley AS, Harford JB, Klausner RD, Taylor SR. Neonatal hemochromatosis. *Am J Pathol* 1989; **134**: 439

130. Hoogstraten J, Derek J de SA, Knisley AS. Fetal liver disease may precede extrahepatic siderosis in neonatal hemochromatosis. *Gastroenterology* 1990; **98**: 1699

131. Dooling EC, Schoene WC, Richardson EP. Hallervorden-Spatz syndrome. *Arch Neurol* 1974; **30**: 70

132. De Sanctis V, Pintor C, AliquO MC. Prevalence of endocrine complications in patients with beta thalassaemia major: An Italian multicentre study. In: Pintor C, Muller EE, Loche S, New MI (eds) *Advances in Pediatric Endocrinology*. Berlin: Springer, 1992, pp 127–133

133. Zurlo MG, DE Stephano P, Borgna-Pignatti C *et al*. Survival and causes of death in thalassaemia. *Lancet* 1989; **i**: 27

134. Gabutti V, Piga A, Sachetti L *et al*. Quality of life and life expectancy in thalassaemic patients with complications. In: Buckner CD, Gale RP, Lucarelli G (eds) *Advances and Controversies in Thalassaemia Therapy: Bone Marrow Transplantation and Other Approaches*. New York: Liss, 1989, pp 35–41

135. Ley TJ, Griffith P, Nienhuis AW. Transfusion haemosiderosis and chelation therapy. *Clin Haematol* 1982; **11**: 437

136. Bassett ML, Halliday JW, Powell LW. Value of hepatic iron measurements in early haemochromatosis and determination of the critical iron level associated with fibrosis. *Hepatology* 1986; **6**: 24

137. Risdon RA, Barry M, Flynn DM. Transfusional iron overload: the relationship between tissue iron concentration and hepatic fibrosis in thalassaemia. *J Pathol* 1975; **116**: 83

138. Cohen AR. Management of iron overload in the pediatric patient. *Hematol Oncol Clin North Am* 1987; **1**: 521

139. Borgna-Pignetti C, De Stephano P, Zonta L *et al*. Growth and sexual maturation in thalasssemia major. *J Pediatr* 1985; **106**: 150

140. Kletzky OA, Costin G, Marrs RP *et al*. Gonadotrophin insuffi-

141. Herington AC, Wertha GA, Matthews RN, Gurger HG. Studies on the possible mechanism for deficiency of nonsuppressible insulin-like activity in thalassaemia major. *J Clin Endocrinol Metab* 1981; **12**: 293

142. De Sanctis V, Zurlo MG, Senesi E *et al*. Insulin dependent diabetes in thalassaemia. *Arch Dis Child* 1988; **63**: 58

143. Abbott DF, Gresham GA. Arthropathy in transfusional siderosis. *Br Med J* 1972; **1**: 1418

144. Hershko C, Peto T, Wetherall DJ. Iron and infection. *Br Med J* 1987; **296**: 660

145. Gabutti V, Piga A. Results of long-term iron-chelating therapy. *Acta Haematol* 1996; **95**: 26

146. Olivieri NF, Brittenham GM. Iron-chelating therapy and the treatment of thalassaemia. *Blood* 1997; **89**: 739

147. Pippard MJ, Johnson DK, Finch CA. Hepatocyte iron kinetics in the rat explored with an iron chelator. *Br J Haematol* 1982; **52**: 211

148. Summers MR, Jacob A, Tudway D *et al*. Studies in desferrioxamine anf ferrioxamine metabolism in normal and iron-loaded subjects. *Br J Haematol* 1979; **42**: 547

149. Sephton-Smith R. Iron excretion in thalassaemia major after administration of chelating agents. *Br Med J* 1962; **2**: 1577

150. Bannerman RM, Callender ST, Williams DL. Effect of desferrioxamine and DTPA in iron overload. *Br Med J* 1962; **2**: 1577

151. Hussain MAM, Fltnn DM, Green N, Hoffbrand AV. Effect of dose, time, and ascorbate on iron excretion after subcutaneous desferrioxamine. *Lancet* 1977; **i**: 977

152. Propper RL, Cooper B, Rufo RR *et al*. Continuous subcutaneous administration of of deferoxamine in patients with iron overload. *N Engl J Med* 1977; **297**: 418

153. Barry M, Flynn DM, Letsky EA, Rison RA. Long-term chelation therapy in thalassaemia: effect on iron concentration, liver histology and clinical progress. *Br Med J* 1974; **2**: 16

154. Seshadri R, Colebatch JH, Gordon P. Long-term administration of desferrioxamine in thalassaemia major. *Arch Dis Child* 1974; **49**: 8

155. Olivieri NF, Nathan DJ, MacMillan JH *et al*. Survival of medically treated patients with homozygous beta thalassemia major. *N Engl J Med* 1994; **331**: 574

156. Hoffbrand AV, Gorman A, Laulicht M *et al*. Improvement in iron status and liver function in patients with transfusional iron overload.with long-term subcutaneous desferrioxamine. *Lancet* 1979; **i**: 946

157. Brittenham GM, Griffith PM, Nienhuis AW *et al*. Efficacy of deferoxamine in preventing complications of iron overload in patients with thalassemia major. *N Engl J Med* 1994; **331**: 567

158. Jensen CE, Tuck SM, Wonke B. Fertility in thalassaemia major: A report of 16 pregnancies, preconceptual evaluation and a review ofthe literature. *Br J Obstet Gynaecol* 1995; **102**: 625

159. Roberts IAG, Derbyshire PJ, Will AM. Bone marrow transplantation for children with beta thalassaemia major in the UK. *Bone Marrow Transplant* 1997; **19 (Suppl 2)**: 60

160. Porter JB, Jaswon MS, Huehns ER *et al*. Desferrioxamine ototoxicity: Evaluation of risk factors in thalassaemic patients and guidelines for safe dosage. *Br J Haematol* 1989; **73**: 403

161. Rodda CP, Reid ED, Johnson S *et al*. Short stature in homozygous beta thalassaemia is due to disproportionate truncal shortening. *Clin Endocrinol* 1995; **42**: 587

162. Piga A, Luzzatto L, Capalbo P *et al*. High-dose desferrioxamine as a cause of growth failure in thalassaemic patients. *Eur J Haematol* 1988; **40**: 380

163. De Virgilis S, Congia M, Frau F *et al*. Deferoxamine-induced growth retardation in patients with thalassaemia major. *J Pediatr* 1982; **113**: 661

164. Olivieri NF, Basran RK, Talbot AL *et al*. Abnormal growth in thalassaemia major associated with deferoxamine-induced destruc-

ciency in patients with thalassaemia major. *J Clin Endocrinol Metab* 1979; **48**: 901

tion of spinal cartilage and compromise of sitting height. *Blood* 1995; **86 (Suppl 1)**: 482A

165. Olivieri NF, Buncic R, Chew E. Visual and auditory toxicity in patients receiving subcutaneous deferrioxamine infusions. *N Engl J Med* 1986; **314**: 869

166. Davies SC, Hungerford JL, Arden GB *et al*. Ocular toxicity of high-dose intravenous desferrioxamine. *Lancet* 1983; **ii**: 181

167. Freedman MH, Olivieri NF, Grisaru D *et al*. Pulmonary syndrome in patients receiving intravenous deferoxamine infusions. *Am J Dis Child* 1990;**144**: 565

168. Koren G, Bentur Y, Strong D *et al*. Acute changes in renal function associated with deferoxamine therapy. *Am J Dis Child* 1989; **143**: 1077

169. Cohen AR, Cohen IJ, Schwartz E. Scurvy and altered iron stores in thalassemia major. *N Engl J Med* 1981; **304**: 158

170. Hussain MAM, Flynn DM, Green N *et al*. Subcutaneous infusion and intramiscular injection of desferrioxamine in patients with transfusional iron overload. *Lancet* 1976; **ii**:1278

171. Nienhuis AW. Vitamin C and iron. *N Engl J Med* 1981; **304**: 170

172. Piga A, Magliano M, Bianco L *et al*. Compliance with chelation therapy in Torino. In: Sirchia G, Zanella A (eds) *Thalassaemia Today: Second Mediterranean Meeting on Thalassaemia*. Milan: Policlinico di Milano, 1987, p 141

173. Ehlers KH, Giardina PJ, Lesser ML *et al*. Prolonged survival in patients with beta thalassemia major treated with deferoxamine. *J Pediatr* 1991; **118**: 540

174. Olivieri NF, Berriman AM, Davies SA *et al*. Continuous intravenous administration of deferoxamine in adults with severe iron overload. *Am J Hematol* 1992; **41**: 61

175. Cohen AR, Mizanin J, Schwartz E. Rapid removal of excessive iron with daily, high-dose intravenous chelation therapy. *J Pediatr* 1989; **115**: 151

176. Borgna-Pignatti C, Cohen AR. An alternative method of subcutaneous deferoxamine administration. *Blood* 1995; **86 (Suppl 1)**: 483A

177. Pearson HA, Guiliotis DK, Rink L *et al*. Patient age distribution in thalassaemia major: Changes from 1973 to 1985. *Pediatrics* 1987; **80**: 53

178. Peterson CM, Graziano JH, Grady RW *et al*. Chelation studies with 2,3-dihydrobenzoic acid in patients with beta thalassaemia major. *Br J Haematol* 1976; **33**: 477

179. Olivieri NF, Koren G, Hermann C *et al*. Comparison of oral iron chelator L1 and desferrioxamine in iron-loaded patients. *Lancet* 1990; **336**: 1275

180. Hoffbrand AV. Oral iron chelators. *Semin Hematol* 1996; **33**: 1

181. Castriota-Scanderbeg A, Sacco M. Agranulocytosis, arthritis and systemic vasculitis in a patient receiving the oral iron chelator L1 (deferiprone). *Br J Haematol* 1997; 96: 254

182. Oski FA, Marshall BE, Delivoria-Papdopoulos M *et al*. Exercise with anemia: the role of the left-shifted or right-shifted oxygen hemoglobin equilibrium curve. *Ann Intern Med* 1971; **74**: 44

183. Piomelli S, Danoff S, Becker M *et al*. Prevention of bone malformations and cardiomegaly in Cooley's anemia by early hypertransfusion regimen. *Ann NY Acad Sci* 1969; **165**: 427

184. Propper RL, Button LN, Nathan DJ. New approaches to the transfusion management of thalassaemia. *Blood* 1980; **55**: 55

185. Cazzola M, De Stefano P, Ponchio L *et al*. Relationship between transfusion regimen and suppression of erythropoiesis in beta thalassaemia major. *Br J Haematol* 1995; **89**: 473

186. Cohen AR, Martin M, Schwartz E. A clinical trial of young red cell transfusions. *Pediatr Res* 1983; **17**: 231A

187. Marcus RE, Wonke B, Bantock HM *et al*. A prospective trial of young red cells in 48 patients with transfusion dependent thalassaemia. *Br J Haematol* 1985; **60**: 153

188. Coles SM, Klein HG, Holland PV. Alloimmunisation in two multitransfused populations. *Transfusion* 1981; **21**: 462

189. Kaltwasser JP, Gottschalk R, Schalk KP *et al*. Non-invasive quantitation of liver iron-overload by magnetic resonance imaging. *Br J Haematol*,1990; **74**: 360

190. Totaro A, Rommens JM, Grifa A *et al*. Hereditary hemochromatosis: Generation of a transcription map within a refined and extended map of the HLA class 1 region. *Genomics* 1996; **31**: 319

191. Feder JN, Gnirke A, Thomas W *et al*. A novel MHC class 1-like gene is mutated in patients with hereditary haemochromatosis. *Nature Genet* 1996; **13**: 399

192. Bodmer JG, Parham P, Albert ED, Marsh SG on behalf of the WHO Nomenclature Committee for Factors of the HLA System. Putting a hold on HLA-H. *Nature Genet* 1997; **15**: 234

Iron deficiency

BRIAN A WHARTON

CLASSIFICATION AND DIAGNOSIS

Iron nutrition deficiency can be divided into 4 progressive stages:

1. *Iron sufficiency*: no anemia, red blood cells normal in number, appearance, size and biochemistry, adequate iron stores.
2. *Iron deficiency*: no anemia, red blood cells normal, but iron stores are depleted (usually indicated by a low plasma ferritin).
3. *Iron-deficient erythropoiesis*: no anemia, iron stores depleted, red blood cells have abnormal biochemistry (erythrocyte protoporphyrin [EPP] raised) and on average are smaller (mean corpuscular volume [MCV] reduced) but vary considerably in size (red cell distribution width [RDW]% increased).
4. *Iron-deficiency anemia*: as for iron-deficient erythropoiesis

but anemia is defined by a low blood concentration of hemoglobin.

Table 6.1 gives cut-off points suggested by Oski *et al*[1] for differing iron statuses in young children and cut-off points suggested by the British Nutrition Foundation for adults,[2] which broadly may be applied to teenagers. Other cut-off points are often used so that comparison of individual studies can be difficult.

The assays used in the classification and diagnosis of iron nutrition status vary in methodologic and biologic stability. Hemoglobin and red cell measurements by automated cell counters (analysis of at least 10 000 cells) show little day-to-day variation in individuals, as long as the blood sample itself is adequate. Biochemical measurements show greater coefficients of variation—15–26% for serum ferritin, 27–33% for serum iron, 11% for total iron binding capacity (TIBC) and 12% for EPP in adults. Additionally, different methods of analysis give differing results and external reference standards should be used, particularly for plasma ferritin—for

Table 6.1 Suggested cut-off points defining iron status.[1,2]

Factor	Iron sufficient	Iron-depleted non-anemic	Iron-deficient erythropoiesis	Iron-deficient anemia
Children				
Hb(g/l)	⩾110	⩾110	⩾110	<110
Ferritin (µg/l)[a]	⩾12	<12	<12	<12
Transferrin saturation (%)	⩾10	⩾10	<10	<10
EPP (µmol/mol heme)	<100	<100	⩾100	⩾100
Adults (> 17 years)				
Hb (g/l): men	⩾130	⩾130	⩾130	<130
women	⩾120	⩾120	⩾120	<120
Ferritin (µg/l)[b]	⩾13	<13	<13	<13
Transferrin saturation (%)	>16	⩾16	<16	<16
EPP (µmol/mol heme)[c]	<80	<80	⩾80	⩾80
Transferrin receptor (mg/l)	<8.5	<8.5	>8.5	>8.5

[a]Others have adopted more stringent criteria, e.g. ferritin of 7 µg/l[3] or 10 µg/l.[4]
[b]13–25 µg/l sometimes referred to as low iron stores.
[c]Erythrocyte protoporphyrin (EPP) is usually measured as zinc protoporphyrin (ZPP). If washed cells are used, the cut-off value should be 40 µmol/mol heme.

Table 6.2 Suggested indications for determination of blood hemoglobin concentration.

Any child with symptoms or signs suggesting anemia
Any child referred for a pediatric opinion by a family practitioner[a]
Any child admitted to hospital[a]

Preterm infants (whatever the feeding regimen) at 3-monthly intervals during infancy
Exclusively breast-fed children at age 10 months
All toddlers around the time of the MMR immunization (14 months) unless they have received an iron-containing infant formula for 8 or more months previously
Children living in deprived circumstances whose main drink is not iron fortified, e.g. cows' milk, at 18 months
Adolescents: girls who are athletic, menstruating, dieting, eating lunch out of school

[a]Misleading results are common following infection; a reassessment after the illness may save the need for more extensive investigation.

fuller discussion of variation see Worwood.[5] Physiologic variations in healthy subjects are also induced by conditions other than iron deficiency, e.g. altitude. The ultimate gold standard for iron-deficiency anemia is an increase in hemoglobin concentration following iron therapy but while this is a simple maneuvre in an individual and is part of routine clinical management, it can rarely be applied to epidemiologic studies.

INDICATIONS FOR INVESTIGATION

Table 6.2 suggests indications for a determination of hemoglobin—based on the author's experience and moderated by the views of Dallman et al[4] and James et al.[6] These are wider indications than many pediatricians would agree with and may be modified after a careful clinical and dietetic history. Routine screening of adolescents is not included but there may be arguments for doing so in girls who are athletic, menstruating, aiming to lose weight or eating 'lunch' out of school. This might be achieved at a logistically convenient time, such as the adolescent BCG and/or rubella immunization.

If a reduced hemoglobin concentration is found which persists after the disappearance of any intercurrent infection, then further investigation is indicated.

DIFFERENTIAL DIAGNOSIS

The main differential diagnoses are the other causes of hypochromic microcytic red cells. Particular problems are thalassemia and the anemia of infection (Table 6.3), but there are other rarer possibilities.

Anemia and infection

Perhaps the most frequent practical problem is the child with true iron deficiency who because of an intercurrent infection (often mild) has a normal plasma ferritin. If everything else (clinical picture and laboratory investigations) points to dietary iron deficiency, it is reasonable to give iron supplements with appropriate follow-up to make the diagnosis.

The anemia of infection and chronic disease is often normochromic and normocytic but hypochromia and microcytosis occur in about a third of affected children (see Chapter 38). Despite moderately raised levels of erythropoietin, erythropoiesis is inhibited by cytokines, particularly tumor necrosis factor and γ-interferon, released from activation of the immune system. Mild infections (even from measles immunization) lead to a slight fall in hemoglobin, serum iron and transferrin saturation, and a rise in plasma

Table 6.3 Interpretation of red cell indices and iron biochemistry in the differential diagnosis of iron deficiency.

Factor	Iron-deficiency anemia	Thalassemia	Infection and chronic disease[d]
Mean corpuscular volume (MCV)	Low	Low	Normal
MCH	Low	Low	Low
RDW	High	Normal	Normal
Iron	Low	Normal[c]	Low
Transferrin or iron-binding capacity	High	Normal[c]	Low
Transferrin saturation	Low	Normal or High[c]	Normal
Ferritin	Low[a]	Normal or High[c]	Low, Normal or High[e]
Erythrocyte protoporphyrin (EPP)	High[b]	Normal[c]	High
Transferrin receptor	High	High	Normal
Other	Confirm by response to iron therapy	Confirm by Hb studies	ESR or CRP may be raised

[a]If reduced, iron deficiency is established. Normal or increased ferritin may be found in iron-deficient children with an infection.
[b]If normal iron deficiency is very unlikely. Increased also in infection and lead poisoning.
[c]Below the age of 2 years children with thalassemia are not infrequently also iron deficient.
[d]Many children with true iron deficiency may also have an intercurrent infection.
[e]Moderately reduced plasma ferritin with a reduced hemoglobin may occur in chronic disease but some patients with no stainable iron in the bone marrow nevertheless have normal plasma ferritin; infection/inflammation leads to increased ferritin via action of cytokines; particularly in hepatitis.

ferritin and EPP, while serum transferrin receptor concentration remains normal.[7,8] The relationships of infection and chronic disease to measurements of iron status are reviewed by Worwood[5] and Walter et al.[9]

Genetic disorders

There are rare hereditary disorders which result in hypochromic anemia. Most are associated with iron overload in various tissues rather than deficiency. Atransferrinemia is a rare autosomal recessive disorder which results in a severe hypochromic anemia but there is excessive deposition of iron in various organs, including the heart (see Chapter 5).[10] It seems that transferrin is not essential for absorption of iron but it is essential for delivery of iron to the red cell precursors in the bone marrow.

The combination of hypochromic anemia and iron overload is described in a variety of disorders where plasma concentrations of plasma transferrin are normal. Clearly, some of these conditions are due to an intrinsic abnormality of hemoglobin synthesis such as in the thalassemias with secondary changes in iron metabolism. It may be that other hereditary disorders where hypochromic anemia and iron overload occur together are also due to abnormalities in the synthesis of iron-associated proteins but their molecular basis has not been determined. Shahidi et al[11] described an hypochromic microcytic anemia in 2 siblings with excessive deposition of iron in whom the plasma transferrin concentration was normal, and Cooley[12] an X-linked recessive hypochromic anemia in childhood followed by death due to hemoglobinochromatosis at a relatively early age. Sideroblastic anemias may also cause confusion and these are described in Chapter 5.

Genetic defects resulting in microcytic hypochromic anemia without accompanying iron overload in other tissues are rare. Three such siblings have been described in whom some evidence of specific iron malabsorption was found.[13] The condition has some similarities to the recessively inherited microcytic anemia of the mk-mk mouse which may be due to a defective transferrin receptor leading to a generalized impairment of iron uptake into cells.[14]

It is perhaps surprising that genetic disorders affecting iron nutrition are more ones of overload than deficiency. It may be, however, that any defect resulting in a substantial reduction in iron uptake by cells would not allow a fetus to survive.

ETIOLOGY

There are 4 contributory causes of iron deficiency which are not, of course, mutually exclusive:

1. Stores of iron may be abnormally low if, for example, a baby was born preterm, or because the hemoglobin concentration immediately after birth was lower than normal (e.g. due to hemorrhage) so that iron stores derived from postnatal physiologic hemolysis are much less.
2. Growth velocity may be very rapid so that the demands for iron are unusually high, e.g. in low-birth-weight babies experiencing rapid catch-up growth, older infants and adolescents.
3. Iron in the diet may be too low, is not easily available, or there is malabsorption (see Chapter 5).
4. Increased losses may occur in many disease processes, in menstruating girls and in endurance athletes.

DETERMINATION OF PREVALENCE

The prevalence of iron deficiency can be determined by applying multiple tests of iron status. It might be presumed if anemia exists with 2 or more other indicators of deficiency. This approach is often used in ad hoc field surveys and was applied nationally in the USA during the National Health Nutrition Examination Survey (NHANES) conducted between 1988 and 1994. In this survey, iron deficiency was defined in 2 'models' as 2 or more of the following 3 tests being abnormal: transferrin saturation and EPP plus either MCV or plasma ferritin determination.[4]

Multiple tests are not always easy to apply and Yip et al[15] have argued that a considerable amount can be learned about the prevalence and possible cause of iron deficiency in a population from hemoglobin distributions at different ages (and not just cut-off points). This point is illustrated by the observations that:

- Palestinian women and children have a lower distribution of hemoglobin than the 'reference population' (from the NHANES study excluding those with iron-deficiency anemia) but the distribution in Palestinian men is similar to the reference. This suggests that extra demands for iron in children and women result in the anemia, whereas the lower demands in men are met by the diet. Iron is the potential (and actual) culprit although on this model alone other dietary deficiencies such as folic acid could not be excluded.
- In Zanzibar, children, women and men all have a lower hemoglobin distribution than the reference. This suggests some cause affecting the whole population, e.g. hookworm.

EFFECTS OF IRON DEFICIENCY

Apart from its hematologic effects, iron deficiency also affects the immunologic system, gut and brain.

Table 6.4 Prospective studies of infection in children receiving extra iron.

Study	Country	Age (months)	Number	Type of control	Vehicle for iron	Reduction in respiratory infection	Reduction in intestinal infection
Mackay 1928[18]	UK	2–12	154	Historical	Supplement	Yes (50%)	Yes (50%)
Andelman and Sered 1966[19]	USA	6–9	1048	Concurrent	Formula	Yes, self-reported	No
Tunessen and Oski[20]	USA	6–12	167	Concurrent but self selection of formula or cows' milk	Formula	No	Yes
Walter et al 1997[9]	Chile	4–15	252	Almost concurrent	Acidified formula; iron-free formula not acidified	No	Yes, during summer months
Burman 1972[21]	UK	3–24	190	Concurrent	Supplement	No, self-reported	No
Stekel et al 1988[22]	Chile	3–15	382	Concurrent	As for study[9]	No	No
Heresi et al 1995[23]	Chile	4–12	200	Concurrent	Heme iron fortified cereal formula as in study[9]	No	No

IMMUNOLOGIC SYSTEM

Once infection is established there are secondary changes in measurements of iron nutrition (see above) and this confounds attempts to relate apparent iron deficiency to infection. The reported higher prevalence of meningitis, pneumonia[16] or gastroenteritis[17] in iron deficiency and anemic children are therefore difficult to interpret.

To avoid this problem of interpretation, prospective studies in which dietary iron regimens and or measurements of iron nutrition are established before infection occurs have been attempted (Table 6.4). The very much higher prevalence of infection reported in the East End of London by Mackay in 1928[18] has not been found in subsequent studies. There is a suggestion of increased intestinal infection (3 studies) but this is not consistent.

With the possible exception of an increased malaria risk,[9,24] against this background it is necessary to question the clinical importance of the reported abnormalities of immunologic function in iron deficiency. Some aspects of T-cell and neutrophil function seem to be impaired, although humoral immunity is little affected. The abnormalities are reviewed by Brock,[25] Farthing,[26] and Walter et al.[9]

These abnormalities of immune function in iron-deficient children are in no way as severe as those arising in hereditary or acquired immune deficiency syndromes, and the lack of a consistently apparent increased susceptibility to infection may reflect varying degrees of iron deficiency.

INTESTINE

It is difficult to separate the effects on the gut of iron deficiency *per se* from those of the underlying disease which has caused the iron deficiency. This is particularly so in hookworm infection.

Malabsorption and varying degrees of partial villous atrophy are well documented in children with hookworm infection. Hookworm infection occurs commonly in bare-footed children of humid regions (see also Chapter 38). The adult worms, *Ankylostoma duodenale* and *Necator americanus*, attach to the mucosa of the duodenum where they feed on the blood of the individual. Steatorrhoea, xylose absorption and the partial villous atrophy all revert to normal after the worms have been expelled and the nutritional deficiencies corrected. It is uncertain whether the structural and functional abnormalities are due to the hookworms *per se* or whether they are secondary to the altered nutritonal state of the host. However, gastrointestinal changes do not seem to be directly related to the size of the worm load, the variety of worm or the length of stay in the gut, and significant changes in structure and function are found only in those children who have very low serum iron levels. Children with low albumin levels but normal serum iron have normal gastrointestinal tracts. This, and the observation that changes in jejunal appearance and function, including an increased permeability, occur in children with iron deficiency not due to parasitic disease[27–29] suggest that the malabsorption of hookworm disease is secondary to the associated iron deficiency.[27,30,31]

Other enteropathies are associated with iron deficiency, particularly celiac disease or allergic enteropathy with protein and iron loss, but in these disorders, while iron deficiency may contribute to the continuation of the lesion, there is little doubt that the enteropathy has caused the iron deficiency and not vice versa.

BRAIN

There is ample evidence of an association between iron-deficiency anemia and impaired performance in various assessments of psychomotor function in young children and with scholastic impairment in school children. While not all studies confirm this association, by far the majority do in children aged from 9 months to 11 years.[2,32,33]

While there is no doubt about the association, this does not automatically infer cause and effect. Confounding factors abound and iron-deficiency anemia might be merely a marker for a generally poorer environment both nutritionally and psychosocially. Moreover, in human studies it is difficult to control for genetic factors—no twin studies of iron deficiency and development have been reported.

Intervention studies are the only way to assess cause and effect. Does giving iron to treat (or prevent) iron-deficiency anemia also lead to an improvement in psychomotor development? Some trials have described a surprisingly quick response after only a few days of oral or intramuscular iron therapy. This may be due to a 'training effect', i.e. most children will do better in a test of cerebral function if they have recently done it before. On the other hand, changes in neurotransmitter metabolism which can occur in response to iron could explain rapid changes particularly in 'responsiveness' of the children. Longer-term controlled intervention studies of treatment or prevention have mostly shown a higher developmental performance in those receiving iron.[2]

The evidence for mechanisms relating iron deficiency to brain function is circumstantial and derives from studies of brain iron, brain lipids, neurotransmitter metabolism and behavioral processes, chiefly in rodents.

Brain iron

In the rat, iron deficiency occurring during a period of rapid development (10–28 days of life) causes a permanent decrease in brain iron concentration despite adaptive increases in transferrin uptake rate and later iron supplementation.[34,35]

Neural lipids

Iron deficiency in young rats is associated with changes in the fatty acid composition of myelin lipids. The n9 series of fatty acids proceed from stearic acid (C18:0; not an essential fatty acid) by desaturation to oleic acid (C18:1;n9) and then via chain elongation and desaturation steps to lignoceric (C24:0) and nervonic acid (C24:1;n9). Desaturation at the n9 position seems to be less effective in iron-deficient rats so that the proportions of oleic and nervonic acid (a major component of myelin) are reduced.[36] The significance of this in humans is unknown.

Neurotransmitter metabolism

In the iron-deficient rat, 2 abnormalities have been detected in the catecholamine pathway from tyrosine to epinephrine (adrenaline): dopamine D_2 binding sites are reduced;[37] and reduced monoamine oxidase activity. Norepinephrine (noradrenaline) excretion is increased in rats and children.[38,39] Also, in the pathway from tryptophan to serotonin (5-OH

tryptamine), aldehyde oxidase activity is reduced so that serotonin is increased in brain tissue. These abnormalities are reversed within 1 week of starting iron.[40]

Behavioral processes

A feature of the response to iron in some studies is the speed with which children become more alert and active. The changes are very similar to those seen shortly after starting appropriate treatment for celiac disease or kwashiorkor. In rats, severe iron deficiency may have a profound effect on behavior in that the diurnal pattern of activity (normally active at night, quiet in the day) is completely reversed,[41,42] although this has not been a universal finding.[43,44] Preliminary electrophysiologic observation in iron-deficient infants shows some alteration in sleep-wake patterns and there is a greater latency in audio-evoked potentials.[33]

These observations suggest that iron deficiency primarily has an effect on behavior patterns (possibly via the rapid changes in neurotransmitter metabolism) so that a listless apathetic child is less able to appreciate stimuli from the environment and falls behind in performance, while changes in structure (e.g. in lipids or total brain iron) occur only with prolonged severe deficiency.

PREVENTION

Prevention of iron deficiency is the same as for any other nutrient and the principles are shown in Table 6.5.

Screening represents secondary prevention in that it detects an abnormality early before it has caused much or any harm. Suggested indications for hemoglobin determination are presented in Table 6.2 and include some indications for targeted screening where the child is apparently well but is at a high risk of iron deficiency, such as toddlers who have not received an iron-supplemented formula throughout infancy or teenage girls who are menstruating, trying to lose weight and not eating school dinners.

Other methods are true or primary prevention, i.e. aiming to prevent the disorder altogether, not just to detect it early.

Table 6.5 Methods for preventing a nutrient deficiency.

Secondary prevention
Screening to detect an abnormality before it is severe in order to initiate treatment early

Primary prevention
Health education: on diet and feeding practices
Fiscal measures: e.g. to promote use of certain foods by providing them more cheaply or free of charge
Supplements: 'medicines' given in addition to the normal diet
Food fortification: addition of a nutrient to a food commonly eaten by the target population

Table 6.6 Food fortification: choice of food vehicle.[46]

Steps in developing an iron-fortification strategy:

1. Determine the iron status of the population
2. Choose an appropriate iron compound and food vehicle combination
3. Establish the acceptability and stability of the fortified vehicle
4. Assess the bioavailability of iron from the vehicle in the appropriate dietary setting
5. Carry out a controlled field trial
6. Implement a regional or national fortification program

Considerations in the choice of a food vehicle

Consumption	Technical
High proportion of population	Centrally processed
Minimal regional variation	Few production facilities
Unrelated to socio-economic status	Minimal segregation of fortificant
Minimal individual variation	Good masking qualities
Low potential for excess intake	Low cost
Contained in all meals	Limited storage
Linked to caloric intake	High bioavailability

The choice of strategies for prevention varies according to age and geographic location and examples are considered below. There are some general principles which apply to all ages, however.

Iron supplements

In normal children on an adequate diet, including the use of iron-fortified foods where appropriate, iron supplementation should not be necessary.

Opinion varies as to whether vulnerable groups such as vegetarians or dieting, menstruating girls should receive supplements. Hemoglobin monitoring is a more desirable strategy but the cost may be greater and compliance less than for the use of an iron supplement. Numerous supplements are available without prescription, some of them combined with other micronutrients. For prophylaxis, the dose would be around the Reference Nutrient Intake (RNI).[45]

Food fortification

Fortification of a food with nutrients is a frequent administrative strategy because it reaches all sectors of the population. Fortification with iron should be introduced only after careful consideration and trials. MacPhail and Bothwell[46] discuss this in detail and, although their work has been mainly concerned with adults, their general conclusions (Table 6.6) apply to all ages.

POSSIBLE ADVERSE EFFECTS OF PREVENTION PROGRAMS

There has been concern that prevention policies could result in:

- *A high intake*: more than that necessary to prevent iron deficiency. Successful examples of primary prevention have usually brought the average iron intake of a population into an accepted range at or near the RNI so that the distribution is about the same (not higher) as that in an iron-replete population.
- *Pre-absorption*: more gastrointestinal upsets. Extra iron has been implicated as a cause of regurgitation, colic, constipation or loose stools, but controlled trials do not support this suspicion in infants.[47–49] Exclusion of fortification iron from a formula compared with an iron-fortified formula, does shift the fecal flora a little towards that seen in breast-fed infants (e.g. more lactobacilli and fewer enterococci) but the patterns are still very different from that in breast-fed babies.[50,51] Whatever the exact reason for the different fecal flora and the greater resistance to intestinal infection of breast-fed infants, the addition or exclusion of iron to an infant formula does not seem to be an important factor in the pathogenesis of intestinal infection in bottle-fed infants.
- *During absorption*: interference with absorption of other nutrients. While there are interactions between iron and zinc, and manganese and copper absorption, these seem to occur only when there are high ratios of iron to other metals or when other factors are present in the diet, e.g. phytate.
- *Following absorption*: impaired resistance to infection. There are a few reports describing increased infection rates in association with oral iron therapy in children with kwashiorkor[52] and in adult Somali nomads.[53] Generally, however, there is little convincing evidence of increased susceptibility to infection following oral iron. Prevention programs using parenteral iron are best avoided although even here evidence is conflicting,[54–57] apart from in malaria (see below).

TREATMENT

Iron deficiency is a laboratory sign not a disease. Treatment is by attention to the underlying cause and supplementation with oral iron.

ORAL IRON

Standard oral treatment of iron deficiency is 3 mg iron/kg body weight/day up to a maximum of 180 mg daily. In young children (below 2 years) it may be given in one dose and preferably at least half an hour before a meal to avoid interference with absorption.

Three milligrams of iron is provided by:

- 15 mg ferrous sulfate;
- 9 mg ferrous fumarate;
- 26 mg ferrous gluconate;

Table 6.7 Liquid preparations of iron.

Preparation	Preparation (ml)	Amount of iron in preparation (mg)	Amount of preparation to provide 3 mg (ml)
Ferrous sulfate oral solution (Paediatric 'BP')	5	12	1.25
Ferrous fumarate BP (Fersamal [Forley], Galfer [Galen])	5	45	0.3
Ferrous succinate elixir	5	37	0.4
Ferrous glycine sulfate (Plesmet [Link])	5	25	0.6
Sodium iron edetate (Sytron [Link])	5	28	0.5
Polysaccharide iron complex (Niferex [Tillomed] drops)*	5	100	0.15

*Available in 'drop' presentation for use in low-birth-weight babies.

- 9 mg ferrous succinate;
- 17 mg ferrous glycine sulfate;
- 21 mg sodium iron edetate;
- 9 mg ferrous sulfate dried.

Ferrous sulfate is most commonly used. Available preparations provide 60–100 mg iron/tablet or capsule. Ferrous fumarate (65 mg/tablet), glycine sulfate (100 mg) and gluconate (35 mg) are also available as tablets/capsules.

For children unable to swallow tablets or where the total daily dose to be prescribed is less than these amounts, a number of liquid preparations are available (Table 6.7). 'Ferrous Sulphate Oral Solution Paediatric BP' is cheap but its disadvantages are the volume necessary, its taste and its deterioration within 3–4 weeks of dispensing. Various proprietary preparations are available which though more expensive have fewer problems and so encourage compliance. Many children's hospitals have their own formulations for iron therapy, usually using sulfate or fumarate.

The optimum frequency of oral iron supplementation is uncertain. It is conceivable that treatment on one day 'saturates' or 'blocks' the intestinal absorption processes so that doses for the next day or so are much less well absorbed. Consequently, oral iron given once or twice weekly might be more effective than daily doses. There is some support for this approach in adults and animals,[54–58] but the situation in children is not known.

Follow-up is necessary to show an adequate response (an hemoglobin rise of 10 g/l or more in 1 month) and if there has been a response, treatment should be continued for 3 months to replenish stores. If there has been no response, poor compliance and other causes of anemia should be considered.

Iron medication should be kept in child-resistant containers and out of the reach of young children.

PARENTERAL IRON

It is doubtful whether there are any routine indications for giving parenteral iron to children except as part of a full parenteral nutrition regimen. However, it may be indicated in exceptional circumstances if compliance is likely to be poor and follow-up impossible.

Parenteral iron should always be avoided in:

- the newborn—where there is some evidence of an associated increase in Gram-negative infections;[59–61]
- geographic areas where systemic parasites are endemic; there is evidence of increased susceptibility to malaria;[62]
- conditions where the plasma transferrin is reduced, e.g. kwashiorkor,[63] non-selective nephrotic syndrome, concurrent infection.

If a clinician decides parenteral iron therapy is unavoidable, e.g. because of poor compliance with oral therapy, Iron Sorbitol Citric Acid Complex BP ('Jectofer' Astra), which contains 50 mg of elemental iron/ml, can be used. The manufacturers do not recommend its use in infants < 3 kg in weight. The suggested dose is intramuscular 1.5 mg of iron (i.e. 0.03 ml)/kg body weight; approximately 3 doses at daily or alternate-day intervals will result in an hemoglobin rise of 10 g/l and begin to replenish iron stores. The prescriber should consult the manufacturer's literature. Preventative strategies have included 150 mg of elemental iron (as iron dextran 3 ml) given at birth or within 2 months as 1 dose (i.e. about 50 mg/kg).[59–61,63]

Iron in an intravenous nutrition regimen for smaller children (up to 15 kg body weight) may be given as an individual additive to the dextrose/amino acid solution, e.g. 1.8 μmol iron (100 μg)/kg/day. In larger children (15–40 kg body weight) iron is often given as part of a multi trace element additive, e.g. Additrace 0.1 ml/kg/day, containing iron 0.2 μmol (11 μg); for children > 40 kg body weight, the recommended dose of Additrace is 10 ml daily total, containing 20 μmol iron (1100 μg). A typical USA regimen recommends that after 4 weeks' total parenteral nutrition iron should be added: in infants 100 μg (1.8 μmol)/kg; in children: 1–2 mg (18–36 μmol) total/day.[64,65]

PROBLEMS AT DIFFERENT AGES

YOUNG INFANTS (0–4 MONTHS)

Effects of maternal iron deficiency

Measurements of iron status (plasma ferritin, EPP) in mothers have been compared with the same measurements

133

in their newborn babies. Most studies from developed countries have shown little or no relationship between the iron status of the mother and that of her baby.[66-76] A few, from both developed and developing countries, have found a relationship.[77-83]

Whatever the exact relationship between the iron status of the mother and 'stored' iron in the newborn, the net effect on total body iron will be small since stored iron accounts for only a quarter of the total body iron, the majority being in hemoglobin.

Hemoglobin in later infancy

Most studies have compared maternal iron status with the iron status of the baby at birth or shortly afterwards; only a few have followed infants for longer and have shown that maternal iron status in pregnancy is a predictor of iron status at 12 months.[84,85] This could be the effect of low maternal stores or a sign that both mother and child are living in an iron-deprived environment.

Reduced hemoglobin mass at birth

A reduction in the initial mass of hemoglobin may be due to reduced production or perinatal blood loss. Reduced production occurs in preterm deliveries. The average blood hemoglobin concentration at 28 weeks' gestation is 145 g/l compared with 180 g/l on day 1 in term babies. Consequently, there is less iron to call on for subsequent growth. These deficiencies, however, are small compared with those that can occur from blood loss.

Perinatal blood loss may be due to feto-maternal transfusion (the Kleihauer test will indicate the size of the bleed), twin-to-twin transfusion (a discrepancy of at least 20 g/l in the cord hemoglobin concentrations) or external loss such as from a cord accident. External blood loss, if not treated, may contribute to iron deficiency in infancy. Blood loss internally into the baby's tissues (e.g. in a subaponeurotic hematoma or around a fractured bone) may be large enough to cause neonatal anemia but will not contribute to later iron deficiency since the iron remains within the body and is available for hemoglobin synthesis later.

Growth and iron balance

Following a normal pregnancy and delivery, the circulating hemoglobin on day 1 (mean 180 g/l) acts as the main store of iron. As physiologic hemolysis occurs, the released iron is stored in the reticuloendothelial system and this is called on as the baby begins to grow. Normally there is no increase in total body iron during the first 4 months of life. The total iron present in hemoglobin at 4 months is about 10% higher than at birth. This small increase is easily met from other stores.

This balance will be distorted, however, if the initial mass of hemoglobin is reduced, or if the increase in weight is much

faster. A smaller amount of storage iron at birth will also distort the balance but this makes only a small contribution (60 mg) to the total body iron (265 mg).

Rapid growth rate

A rapid growth rate relative to initial size is seen in preterm babies, small-for-gestational-age babies, and in twins (many of whom are preterm or small for gestational age).

The preterm baby has a lower absolute endowment of iron at birth than his term counterpart mainly because of his smaller size, but also partly because of the lower hemoglobin concentration. The demands of growth are about the same as in the term child however—in 4 months he will gain 3 kg or more in weight yet the initial stores of iron to meet this growth are much less. There is a 150% increase in hemoglobin iron.

The small-for-gestational-age baby has a lower absolute endowment of iron at birth mainly because of his smaller size. This deficit is offset a little by the increased concentration of circulating hemoglobin which many of these babies have (probably reflecting a mild hypoxia while *in utero*). If they remain well, many will grow more rapidly (catch-up growth) so their demands for iron are also greater than in the term baby. There is an 80% increase in hemoglobin iron.

Preterm babies

Compared with term babies, preterm babies:

- show a greater fall in hemoglobin concentration in the first 2 months of life;
- reach their hemoglobin nadir a little (2 months) earlier;
- have much greater need for extra iron (+70 mg compared with +20 mg);
- reach the iron-dependent stage of erythropoiesis earlier (2–3 months compared with 4 months);
- are much more likely to have raised external losses mostly from diagnostic blood sampling and are also much more likely to have a blood transfusion.

As described in Chapter 10, early anemia may be treated/prevented by red blood cell transfusion and/or erythropoietin therapy. Smaller doses of iron or postponement of therapy should be considered if blood transfusions are given.[88,89] Larger doses should be considered during erythropoietin treatment, e.g. 6 mg/kg/day.[90,91] Both methods have implications for iron and nutrition. Later anemia can be prevented by an adequate intake of iron. An intake of 2.0–2.5 mg/kg/day is sufficient and can be achieved with a formula containing 1.5–1.7 mg iron/100 kcal, or by giving a supplement. It should be maintained until the age of 1 year.[86,87]

Iron is often omitted from parenteral nutrition regimens in the first 2 or 3 weeks of life. If included, an intake of up to 200 mg/kg/day is recommended.[92]

Term babies

Iron deficiency due to dietary lack should not occur in the first 4 months of life. If an anemia suggesting iron deficiency is apparent (e.g. microcytosis and hypochromia), other diagnoses should be considered. If there is biochemical evidence of iron deficiency, then the likely cause is blood loss. This may have occurred around birth or there may be a continuing occult loss, usually from the gastrointestinal tract. Meckel's diverticulum may present at any time in childhood, usually as an intestinal torsion or as a diverticulitis. Bleeding may occur from ectopic gastric mucosa and present as anemia or frank rectal bleeding.

Symptoms due to cows' milk allergy mostly present within 3 months of exposure and so may not be apparent at this age. Anemia is an unusual presentation (about 2% of cases with proven milk allergy in an Australian series).[93]

OLDER INFANTS (4–12 MONTHS)

The proportional daily increases in hemoglobin iron during the later part of infancy are greater than at any other time in life. From 4 to 12 months the increment in total body iron is from about 270 mg to 440 mg.

The changes in hemoglobin iron are given in Table 6.8 for term, preterm and small-for-gestational-age infants in later infancy. In *term babies*, total hemoglobin iron, having increased by only 10% in months 0–4, increases by 50% in months 4–12. Some *small-for-gestational-age babies* will have shown catch-up growth to near normal weight; their hemoglobin mass, having doubled in the first 4 months, will just as in term babies increase by 50% in months 4–12. The *very preterm baby*, having more than doubled his hemoglobin concentration in the first 4 months, continues to grow rapidly in proportion to body size and his hemoglobin concentrations are normal for age, so the amount of hemoglobin iron trebles from month 4 to the first birthday. The demands for extra iron in all older infants are considerable; the legacy of preterm birth reaches throughout infancy.

Causes of iron deficiency

Various factors occur at this age which contribute to iron deficiency:

- The preterm baby continues to have a much greater increase in hemoglobin iron than a term baby.
- An 'early anemia' (e.g. due to blood loss around birth or in the early months) may have been missed and the extra requirement for iron to achieve 'catch-up in hemoglobin' is not met from the diet.
- Rapid growth rates may occur in normal-sized infants, more often in boys than girls and in children of tall than short parents.
- Diet changes from a single food (breast milk or an infant formula) to a variety of foods (the weaning diet) and so the opportunity for significant inhibition of iron absorption and of increased iron loss from the gut increases.

Prevalence of iron deficiency

Table 6.9 shows the prevalence of anemia in various countries. The criteria for anemia and iron deficiency (use of cut-off points) vary and so direct comparison of results between studies is difficult. However, various points can be made:

- Many anemic children do not have low plasma ferritin concentrations. Perhaps this implies too high a cut-off point for diagnosis of anemia, some other cause of anemia or anemia due to iron deficiency but in the presence of an infection.
- Iron-deficiency anemia is more common in less developed countries, in underprivileged communities (e.g. Asians in the UK, although the mechanism responsible for the difference is not clear) and in those receiving non-iron-fortified formula or cows' milk.
- Exclusively breast-fed (i.e. no other foods) infants in developed countries do not become iron deficient during the first 6 months of life and not many are deficient at 9 months.

It is interesting that at the age of 12 months those who have been exclusively breast fed for 7 months or more have a

Table 6.8 Changes in hemoglobin iron during later infancy in a normal term, preterm and small-for-gestational-age infant.

Infant	Weight (kg)	Blood volume (ml)	Hb concentration (g/l)	Total Hb mass (g)	Hb iron (mg)
Normal term					
4 months	6.6	530	115	61	211
12 months	10.2	816	120	98	340
Preterm					
4 months	4.0	320	100	32	110
12 months	9.0	720	120	86	300
Small for gestational age					
4 months	6.0	480	115	55	192
12 months	10.0	800	120	96	333

Table 6.9 Prevalence of anemia and iron deficiency in late infancy.

Study and age at study	Diet	Hemoglobin (% below 110 g/l)	Ferritin (% below 10–12 µg/l)
Europe[94]			
12 months	Exclusive breast feeding		
	> 7 months	0	22
	< 7 months	9	52
Chile[95]			
9 months	Breast fed	27	15
	Formula without iron	37	20
	Formula with added iron	8	1
USA[96]			
9 months	Whole cows' milk and fortified cereals		17
	Formula with iron	2	7
12 months	Whole cows' milk and fortified cereals	4	29
	Formula with iron	0	1
Argentina[97]			
6 months	Exclusive breast feeding	44	7
	Iron-fortified formula	14	4
9 months	Exclusive breast feeding to 6 months	28	28
	Iron-fortified formula	7	Nil
UK[98]			
6 months	Asian	12	40
	Non-Asian	4	36
12 months	Asian	26	37
	Non-Asian	12	21
UK[99]			
6 months	Whole cows' milk recently commenced	13	10
12 months	Whole cows' milk from 6 months	31	
12 months	Iron-fortified formula from 6 months	3	
UK[100]			
6 months	Whole cows' milk recently commenced	28	3
9 months	Iron-fortified formula from 6 months	20	14
	Non-iron-fortified formula from 6 months	23	2
12 months	Iron-fortified formula from 6 months	21	8
	Non-iron-fortified formula from 6 months	17	14

'better' iron status than those who have started a mixed diet earlier.[94]

Iron intake

Liquid part of the diet

If exclusive breast feeding continues, iron deficiency will be present in a few infants by 9 months of age. Eventually, some extra dietary source of iron will be necessary.

Bottle-fed babies will usually (if current policies are followed) receive an iron-fortified product. Cows' milk without iron fortification is unsuitable for babies of this age.[101–103]

Solid (weaning) foods

Cereal-based weaning foods are most commonly used in the developed world and many of these are iron fortified. Initial weaning foods elsewhere may be unfortified, cereal-based (e.g. gruels of maize, sorghum and millet flours) dishes or very low iron-containing (and low fat and protein) carbohydrate-rich foods such as plantain (steamed banana), cassava and taro.

The mother in the developed world often next introduces 'baby meals', many of which are fortified with iron, and also family foods. Generally, mothers who choose to feed their older infants mainly commercially-available foods achieve a greater iron intake than those giving 'family' foods.[104,105]

The child in the developing world commonly continues on a low-iron diet. Lamb is acceptable in many communities (but not pork in Moslems or beef in Hindus). However, the lamb and lamb-based sauce is often served at the side of a plate of a staple food and so may be difficult for an older infant to retrieve with his fingers.

Absorption

As a weaning diet of many different foods is introduced, the various factors modifying the absorption of non-heme iron become operative, such as the enhancing effect of ascorbic acid, organic acids and animal protein and the inhibiting effects of phytate, calcium, tea and eggs (see Chapter 5).

Iron losses

The unresolved question at this age is whether the use of cows' milk (where pasteurization is the only form of processing) leads to increased iron losses from the intestine when compared to the use of an infant formula. While iron loss from the intestine in young infants (0–4 months) who consume cows' milk is well established, this is less certain in older infants.[106] A study in Iowa found that significant blood loss, calculated as equivalent to about a quarter of the iron absorbed, occurred in about a third of infants who had changed to whole cows' milk from the age of 6 months. Blood loss was less frequent in those given an infant formula.[107] In a similar study in New Orleans, infants received cows' milk and iron-fortified cereal, iron-fortified infant formula or follow-on formula. The mean ferritin and MCV were lower at 12 months of age in the group receiving whole cows' milk and the proportion of children with very low plasma ferritin (<12 g/l) was much higher in the whole cows' milk group (28%) than in those receiving an infant formula or follow-on milk ($<1\%$). This was ascribed to the low availability of iron in the diet as a whole, which consisted mainly of cereals, rather than to blood loss.[96,108] The validity of methods used to assess fecal blood loss has been questioned.[106]

It seems that while the association of iron-deficiency anemia with the early introduction of cows' milk ('cows' milk anemia') is well founded, the exact pathologic mechanisms behind the observations are unclear.

Prevention

Screening

Some pediatricians screen for a low hemoglobin concentration at around 10 months in breast-fed infants but this is not a widespread practice. If the infant is exclusively breast fed after the age of 6 months (i.e. receiving no weaning foods), the risk of iron deficiency is higher and there is a much stronger case for screening.

Health education

There are good examples of how education can reduce the prevalence of iron-deficiency anemia in a small community.[5] However, attempts to apply this to larger populations (e.g. a British inner city health district population of 250 000) have not been successful.[109]

Fiscal measures

In Britain certain groups of families receive infant formula and cows' milk at a reduced price or free of charge. It is unfortunate that the choice of an iron-fortified product (i.e.

an infant formula) or a non-fortified one (i.e. cows' milk) is left to the mother's discretion. Follow-on formulas are not included in the scheme. The efficiency of the scheme in preventing iron or other deficiencies has not been studied.

The 'Special Supplemental Food Program for Women, Infants and Children' (WIC) in the USA is aimed at low income families. About a quarter of all US infants are enrolled in the program which provides infant formula and iron-fortified cereal weaning foods. The introduction of this program has been followed by a substantial reduction in the prevalence of anemia[110] but other factors may also have contributed to the secular improvement. One analysis of the scheme showed that at enrolment in 1973 the prevalence of anemia was 12% in 6–11-month olds and at subsequent visits after receiving the iron-fortified foods the prevalence was 6%. By 1984 the figures were 5% and 4%, respectively. It seems that being enrolled in the scheme is followed by a fall in the number who remain anemic. The fall in the prevalence of anemia at enrolment, however—from 12% to 5% between 1973 and 1984—cannot be explained by the effects of the scheme because treatment had not yet commenced. This might be explained by the use of iron-fortified formula in early infancy prior to enrolment (non-fortified formulas were often used in the US in 1973) but without a controlled trial the reason for it is not known.

Food fortification

Infant formulas. In Europe the iron concentration of fortified formulas is set at 0.5–1.5 mg/100 kcal for an infant formula and 1–2 mg/100 kcal for a follow-on formula. In the USA, the concentration is around 1.8 mg/100 kcal for most infant formulas (some low iron formulas are available); follow-on formulas are little used and instead infant formulas are continued throughout infancy.

As the amount of fortification iron is increased, the proportion absorbed falls so that the increase in the absolute amount of iron absorbed is modest, and a larger amount of unabsorbed iron is left in the intestine. The European rationale was that this was undesirable in a young infant and so lower limits of iron were set.[111,112]

Until recently it was common practice for infants to receive whole cows' milk from about the age of 6 months. However, various trials have shown a reduced prevalence of anemia at the age of 12 months in those receiving iron-fortified formulas throughout infancy rather than changing to cows' milk (see Table 6.9).

Solid (weaning) foods. Cereal flours may be fortified during the manufacture of cereal dishes designed specifically for the older infant. There is a problem that iron which is freely soluble and well absorbed, such as ferrous sulfate and gluconate, is also very reactive and catalyzes the oxidation of unsaturated fats in the cereal causing rancidity (a pro-oxidant effect of iron). One answer is to pack such products in nitrogen. An easier and cheaper alternative is to add heme iron (in effect to add red cells or concentrated blood). This approach has been successful in Chile, reducing iron-deficiency anemia at 12 months of age from 17% to 10%.[113]

Iron salts which are not reactive are often used but absorption from them is poor. Ground powders of elemental iron have variable absorption and reactivity; the more finely ground, the greater the absorption (around that for ferrous sulfate) but the greater is the pro-oxidant reactivity.[114,115] Baby meals are also fortified with ferrous sulfate and ascorbic acid and many contain meat.

TODDLERS (1–4 YEARS)

Growth and iron balance

At this stage the very rapid growth rates of infancy are over and both height and weight velocity continue at steady rates until the pre-pubertal acceleration from the age of 10 years. The daily increments in body iron are modest compared to other age periods. Nevertheless, iron deficiency is most prevalent at this stage of development, particularly between the first and second birthdays. This is probably due not only to limited intake of iron but is also the legacy of poor intake in late infancy. Many children pass their first birthday with vulnerable iron status and this incipient iron deficiency was recognized by Moe 30 years ago.[116]

Prevalence of iron deficiency

Table 6.10 shows the prevalence of toddler anemia and iron deficiency in various studies. The varying age divisions of the different studies and the dissimilar socio-economic and ethnic backgrounds make comparisons difficult, but some general conclusions can be reached. Iron deficiency and iron-deficiency anemia:

- are common but there are notable geographic exceptions, e.g. Hong Kong, USA;
- are more common in certain ethnic/immigrant groups (e.g. children in Britain whose parents came from the Indian subcontinent);
- are more common in 'deprived' communities such as inner city areas;
- reach a peak between 18 and 24 months and then the prevalence declines.

Iron uptake

Many children have low iron stores early in the toddler years, particularly those who have received whole cows' milk throughout many months of infancy. The average intake of iron in toddlers is low compared with the RNI—mean intake was about three-quarters of the RNI in children up

Table 6.10 Prevalence of anemia and iron deficiency in toddlers.

Study	Age (months)	Subjects/detail	Reduced hemoglobin concentration (% <110 g/l)	Reduced ferritin concentration (% <10 μg/l)
UK[117]	22	Asian	31	57
UK[118]	18	Inner city	26	47% <7 μg/l
UK[98]	12	Asian	26	37
	12	Non-Asian	12	21
UK[3]	12–24	Mixed inner city	25% <105 g/l	
UK[119]	15	Asian	39	
		White	16	
		Afro-Caribbean	20	
UK[120]	8–24	Asian	16	
		White	9	
UK[121]	18–29	National sample	12	28
	30–41		6	18
UK[99]	18	Iron-fortified formula	2	Nil
		Cows' milk	33	34
UK[100]	15	Iron-fortified formula	0	5
		Non-iron-fortified formula	9	9
	18	Iron-fortified formula	0	16
		Non-iron-fortified formula	15	26
UK[122]	15	Iron-fortified formula	11	6
		Non-iron-fortified formula	13	22
		Cow's milk	33	43
Argentina[123]	9–24	Buenos Aires	48	60
Argentina[124]	9–24	Tierra del Fuego	24	52
	9–24	Missiones	55	55
Venezuela[125]	12–36	Ferritin <10 and/or Trans stn <16%		35
USA[126]	9–26	National sample 1982–1986	3	
	24–47		2	
Canada[127]	12	Disadvantaged, Montreal	25	37
Hong Kong[128]	18	Shatin area	2	1% <7 μg/l

to the age of 3.5 years in the British surveys; half the average intake was non-heme iron in cereals.

Absorption

Tea is an adverse factor in some young children (a third drank tea in one British survey).[122] Celiac disease should also be considered.

Iron losses

While insufficient stores and poor dietary intake are common causes of iron deficiency at this age, it is unwise to accept them uncritically as the cause of anemia after the age of 3 years. Further investigation should aim to exclude malabsorption, bleeding, or chronic disease with true or apparent iron deficiency.

Inflammatory bowel disease may occasionally present in toddlers. Ulcerative colitis presents as bloody diarrhea with incidental anemia. Crohn's disease is often more insidious; sometimes only vague ill health and anemia are found. Hematologic investigations may reflect iron deficiency and/or a chronic inflammatory response. Although disease of the terminal ileum causes B_{12} malabsorption, B_{12} deficiency does not occur until the stores of B_{12} are exhausted as the child enters the pre-pubertal growth spurt.

Prevention

In view of the high prevalence of iron-deficiency anemia at this age and its association with delayed psychomotor development, prevention programs are common.

Screening

The MMR (measles, mumps, rubella) vaccination (at about 14 months) provides a convenient time for screening children for anemia. Another opportunity is the routine check of psychomotor development, e.g. at 18 months.[109] The ideal time for a screen in the toddler years is unclear because the natural history of iron deficiency during this period is not fully understood. Many children not anemic at 14 months have become so before their second birthday. Iron deficiency is more common between the ages of 1 and 2 years and declines thereafter, but the picture may be complicated by inappropriate reference values rather than true pathology.

Fortification

Solid (weaning) foods have been replaced by family foods at this age. Some 'adult foods' consumed by the toddler are iron fortified, such as bread and breakfast cereals and these sources (all non-heme iron) contribute about a third of the total iron intake in Britain.

Toddlers in the tropics

There are special considerations for toddlers living in the tropics.

Food and absorption

Fortified foods are less commonly available or are too expensive for widespread use in developing countries. The common staple foods such as rice, maize and plantain contain about 0.3 mg iron/100 kcal. (In comparison, unfortified bread in Britain provides 0.8 mg/100 kcal and fortified breakfast cereals provide up to 5 mg/100 kcal.)

Heme iron from meat is eaten with variable frequency and predominantly vegetarian meals have low iron bioavailability. However, fish and chicken may be eaten with them (so enhancing absorption) and some cooking is performed in iron pots which adds iron to the meal.

Other nutrient deficiencies

Other nutrient deficiencies often co-exist with iron deficiency such as protein-energy malnutrition, vitamin A and riboflavin deficiency.

Treatment of protein-energy deficiency stimulates catch-up growth and so the iron requirements are increased. Children with kwashiorkor who have very low plasma transferrin have a higher infection-associated mortality rate than those with higher concentrations. It has been suggested that oral iron given during treatment saturates the available plasma transferrin and this predisposes to overwhelming infection. It is equally likely that low plasma transferrin is a marker for the severity of kwashiorkor just as many other plasma proteins are.[52,129]

In susceptible populations of children and pregnant women, vitamin A supplementation by itself may improve the hemoglobin concentration. Iron alone also improves the concentration and the 2 given together have a synergistic effect.[130,131] Correcting riboflavin deficiency has also been shown to improve the hematologic response to iron.[132]

Tropical parasites

Blood loss due to hookworm infection is common in tropical toddlers. They sit on the ground and do not wear shoes, giving plenty of opportunity for skin puncture by the parasite. The concentration of hookworm ova in the stool can give a broad indication of the number of hookworms in the duodenum and from this the potential daily blood loss.[133] Infection with *Helicobacter pylori* is also common, leading to gastritis and mild blood loss.[134]

Malaria is a common cause of anemia in most tropical countries and in many areas of Africa the differential diagnosis of severe anemia is primarily malaria, hookworm or sickle cell disease. There is good evidence that parenteral iron given for prophylaxis of iron deficiency at 2 months of age results in a greater incidence of malaria (as judged from blood smears and spleen rates) at 6 and 12 months of age,[63] so such therapy should be avoided.

PRE-PUBERTAL SCHOOL CHILDREN (5–10 YEARS)

These are 'quiet years' in terms of iron nutrition. In Britain, one study showed the mean intake of 10-year olds was similar to the RNI.[135] Iron deficiency at this age nearly always has some non-nutritional cause and always warrants detailed investigation. Possibilities to consider are:

- gut disorders, including Meckel's diverticulum, reflux esophagitis, peptic ulceration, celiac disease and inflammatory bowel disease;
- extremely reduced intake due to an almost exclusive cows' milk diet in a disturbed child or due to 'therapeutic accidents' where iron has been excluded in error from a tube feed.
- regurgitation and esophagitis in children with cerebral palsy in whom regurgitation and feeding difficulties are common.
- bilharzia with losses from the urinary and/or gastrointestinal tract.

Peptic ulceration and bilharzia are new diagnoses to be considered at this age. Gastritis associated with *Helicobacter pylori* infection is more common than frank ulceration but if an ulcer is diagnosed, the agent should be sought by endoscopy and biopsy or by the urea breath test.[134,136]

Bilharzia (schistosomiasis) in certain areas becomes more common once children are able to paddle or swim in infected water. The disease presents with symptoms such as bloody stools or hematuria rather than anemia. Portal hypertension due to pre-sinusoidal extrahepatic obstruction from schistosomal granulomata in the liver may contribute to the anemia, partly due to iron loss from esophageal and large bowel varices but mostly due to the associated 'hypersplenism' of the condition.[137]

ADOLESCENTS (10–18 YEARS)

The adolescent years are defined here as from the beginning of the pre-pubertal growth spurt (10 years for girls, 12 years for boys) to maturity (18 years). This is a period of great physiologic change and demand for iron. Growth velocity accelerates to reach levels almost as high as those seen in infancy (e.g. 97th centile: for boys 12 kg/year at 14 years; for girls 10 kg/year at 12 years). This is associated with a greater blood volume and greater circulating hemoglobin mass.

In girls:

- peak growth velocity is earlier (on average at 12 years) so demands for iron for growth increments are earlier;
- once peak growth velocity is achieved, growth demands

diminish but shortly afterwards menstruation begins with increased physiologic losses;

- extra requirements for menstrual losses continue after the extra demands of growth have subsided.

In boys:

- peak growth velocity is later than in girls (on average 14 years) so demands for growth increments are later but continue to a later age;
- the increase in muscle bulk increases the demands for iron in myoglobin, but it is difficult to put a figure on this extra demand and it will be related to the amount of exercise which the boy does, which is a stimulus to muscle development.
- testosterone leads to an increase in circulating hemoglobin mass so that iron requirements to sustain this are increased;
- the overall increase in body weight, blood volume, hemoglobin and myoglobin add up to a substantial increase in body iron during the adolescent years;
- the extra requirements for iron are considerably reduced when growth velocity decelerates and stops at maturity.

A longitudinal study in 60 pubertal boys followed from the age of 11.7 years for 2 years found that the concentration of hemoglobin was related more to the stage of puberty reached rather than chronological age. The mean hemoglobin concentration at genital stage 1 of puberty was 129.1 g/l and 141.9 g/l at genital stage 5.[138]

Hemoglobin and plasma ferritin concentrations

Table 6.11 shows the prevalence in various studies. Again, different age divisions and different cut-off points make comparisons difficult but it seems that the prevalence of low hemoglobin and/or ferritin concentrations is greater in girls than boys, in the older boys and girls, and in certain ethnic groups.

Dietary intake

In a nutritionally representative sample of British children,[147] the mean intake of iron in girls aged 10–15 years was less than two-thirds of the RNI (8–9 mg). Older girls who were on slimming diets or choosing to eat out of school at lunch time had the lowest intakes. More recent studies in smaller British populations have recorded slightly higher intakes (10–11 mg)[139,140,148] with similar findings in France.[149] Swedish girls also had slightly higher intakes (13 mg).[144]

Mean intakes in boys in all studies have been above the RNI.

Anorexia nervosa will include an inadequate intake of iron as well as other nutrients. Anemia may not be an outstanding feature because growth slows. With successful

Table 6.11 Prevalence of anemia and iron deficiency in adolescents.

Study	Sex	Age (years)	Number	Anemia/iron deficiency cut-off	Prevalence (%)
Nelson et al (1993) (London)[139]	M	12–14	202	Hb <122/126 g/l	4
				Serum ferritin <12 μg/l	1
				Serum ferritin 12–20 μg/l	14
	F	12–14	197	Hb <120 mg/l	11
				Serum ferritin <12 μg/l	4
				Serum ferritin 12–20 μg/l	16
Doyle et al (1994) (London)[140]	M	12–13	34	Serum ferritin <10 μg/l	8
				Serum ferritin <20 μg/l	33
	F	12–13	32	Serum ferritin <10 μg/l	28
				Serum ferritin <20 μg/l	64
Nelson et al (1994) (London)[141]	F	11–14	114	Hb <120 g/l	20
Southon et al (1994) (Norwich)[142]	M	13–14	19	Hb <120 g/l	5
				Serum ferritin <10 μg/l	11
	F	13–14	35	Hb <110 g/l	0
				Serum ferritin <10 μg/l	21
Armstrong 1989 (Ireland)[143]	M	14.5–18.4	86	Hb <130 g/l	13
				Serum ferritin <10 μg/l	32
	F		148	Hb <120 g/l	7
				Serum ferritin <10 μg/l	43
Hallberg et al (Sweden)[144]	M	15–16	207	Serum ferritin <15 μg/l	15
	F		220		40
	M	15–16	620		25
	F		624		40
Bergstrom et al (Sweden)[145]	M	14	201	Serum ferritin <12 μg/l	10
	M	17	271		4
	F	14	197		17
	F	17	198		10
Anttila et al (Finland)[138,146]	M	11.7	60	Serum ferritin <10 μg/l (<15 μg/l)	2 (3)
		12.2			0 (5)
		12.7			0 (7)
		13.2			8 (33)
		13.7			12 (27)
	after iron	13.9			2 (9)

treatment catch-up growth occurs and then requirements will be greater.

Vegetarians

Many teenagers pass through a phase of temporary but inexpert vegetarianism, mainly in support of animal rights. If there is no tradition of safe vegetarianism in the family from which to learn, the chosen diet is often capricious and deficient in iron. Management is to encourage the consumption of vegetable sources of iron accompanied by absorption enhancers, such as fruit and/or juices containing vitamin C, together with fish or chicken if these are acceptable. Supplements, as medication, may be indicated.

REFERENCES

1. Oski FA. Iron deficiency in infancy and childhood. *N Engl J Med* 1993; **329**: 190–193

2. British Nutrition Foundation. *Iron: Nutritional and Physiological Significance.* London: Chapman and Hall, 1995, pp 1–186

3. Saarinen UM, Siimes MA. Serum ferritin in assessment of iron nutrition in healthy infants. *Acta Paediatr Scand* 1978; **67**: 741–751

4. Dallman PR, Looker AC, Johnson CL, Carroll M. Influence of age on laboratory criteria for the diagnosis of iron deficiency in infants and children. In: Halberg L, Asp NG (eds) *Iron Nutrition in Health and Disease.* London: John Libbey, 1996, pp 65–74

5. Worwood M. Influence of disease on iron status. *Proc Nutr Sci* 1997; **56**: 409–419

6. James J, Lawson P, Male P, Oakhill A. Preventing iron deficiency in preschool children by implementing an educational and screening programme in an inner city practice. *Br Med J* 1989; **299**: 838–840

7. Olivares M, Walter T, Osorio M et al. Anemia of a mild viral infection: the measles vaccine as a model. *Pediatrics* 1989; **84**: 851–855

8. Olivares M, Walter T, Cook JD, Llaguno S. Effect of acute infection on measurement of iron status: usefulness of the serum transferrin receptor. *Int J Pediatr Hematol Oncol* 1995; **2**: 31–33

9. Walter T, Olivares MO, Pizarro F, Munoz C. Iron, anaemia and infection. *Nutr Rev* 1997; **55**: 111–124

10. Goya M, Miyazaki S, Kodate S, Ushio B. A family of congenital atransferrinaemia. *Blood* 1972; **40**: 239–245

11. Shahidi NT, Nathan DE, Diamond LK. Iron deficiency anaemia associated with an error or iron metabolism in two siblings. *J Clin Invest* 1964; **43**: 510–521

12. Cooley TB. A severe form of hereditary anaemia with elliptocytosis: interesting sequence of splenectomy. *Am J Med Sci* 1945; **209**: 561–568

13. Buchanan GR, Sheehan RG. Malabsorption and defective utilisation of iron in three siblings. *J Pediatr* 1981; **98**: 725–728

14. Bannerman RF. Of mice and men and microcytes. *J Pediatr* 1981; **98**: 760–762

15. Yip R, Stoltzfus RJ, Simmons WK. Assessment of the prevalence and the nature of iron deficiency for populations: the utility of comparing haemoglobin distributions. In: Hallberg L, Asp NG (eds) *Iron Nutrition in Health and Disease*. London: John Libbey, 1996, pp 31–48

16. Oppenheimer SJ, MacFarlane SBJ, Moody JB *et al*. Effect of iron prophylaxis on morbidity due to infectious disease. *Trans R Soc Trop Med Hygiene* 1986; **80**; 596–602

17. Lovrie VA. Normal haematologic values in children aged 6 to 36 months and socio-medical implications. *Med J Aust* 1970; **2**: 366–377

18. Mackay HNM. Anaemia in infancy: its prevalence and prevention. *Arch Dis Child* 1928; **3**: 117–146

19. Andelman MB, Sered BR. Utilization of dietary iron by term infants. *Arch Dis Child* 1966; **111**: 45–55

20. Tunnessen WW, Oski FA. Consequences of starting whole cow milk at 6 months of age. *J Pediatr* 1987; **111**: 813–816

21. Burman D. Haemoglobin levels in normal infants aged 3 to 24 months, and the effect of iron. *Arch Dis Child* 1972; **47**: 261

22. Stekel A, Olivares M, Cayazzo M *et al*. Prevention of iron deficiency by milk fortification. II. A field trial with a full fat acidified milk. *Am J Clin Nutr* 1988; **47**: 265–269

23. Heresi G, Pizarro F, Olivares M *et al*. Effect of supplementation with an iron-fortified milk on incidence of diarrhea and respiratory disease in urban resident infants. *Scand J Infect Dis* 1995; **27**: 358–389

24. Oppenheimer SJ. Iron and infection: the clinical evidence. *Acta Paediatr Scand* 1989; **361 (Suppl)**: 53–62

25. Brock JH. Iron and immunity. *J Nutr Immunol* 1993; **2**: 47–106

26. Farthing MJG. Iron and immunity. *Acta Paediatr Scand* 1989; **361 (Suppl)**: 44–52

27. Berant M, Kourie M, Menzies I. Effect of iron deficiency on small intestinal permeability in infants and young children. J *Pediatr Gastroenterol Nutr* 1992; **14**: 17–20

28. Naiman JL, Oski FA, Dramion LK *et al*. The gastrointestinal effects of iron deficiency. *Pediatrics* 1964; **33**: 83–99

29. Ghosh S, Daga S, Kasthuri D, Misra RC, Chuttani HK. Gastrointestinal function in iron deficiency states in children. *Am J Dis Child* 1972; **123**: 14–17

30. Tandon BN, Kohli RK, Saraya AK *et al*. Role of parasites in the pathogenesis of intestinal malabsorption in hookworm disease. *Gut* 1969; **10**: 293–298

31. Ghai DK, Walia BNS, Tandon BN, Ghai OP. Functional and structural changes in the small intestine of children with hookworm infection. *Arch Dis Child* 1968; **43**: 235–238

32. Parks YA, Wharton BA. Iron deficiency and the brain. *Acta Paediatr Scand* 1989; **361 (Suppl)**: 71–77

33. de Andraca I, Castillo M, Walter T. Psychomotor development and behaviour in iron deficient anaemic infants. *Nutr Rev* 1997; **55**: 125–132

34. Taylor EM, Crowe A, Morgan EH. Transferrin and iron intake by the brain: effects of altered iron status. *J Neurochem* 1991; **57**: 1584–1592

35. Dallman PR. Biochemical basis for the manifestations of iron deficiency. *Ann Rev Nutr* 1986; **6**: 13–40

36. Larkin EC, Garratt BA, Rao GA. Relation of relative levels of nervonic to lignoceric acid in the brain of rat pups due to iron deficiency. *Nutr Rev* 1986; **6**: 309–317

37. Ben-Shachar D, Ashkerrazi R, Youdim MBH. Long term consequences of early iron deficiency on dopaminergic neurotransmission. *Int J Dev Neurosci* 1986; **6**: 309–317

38. Voorhess ML, Stuart MJ, Stockman JA, Oski FA. Iron deficiency anemia and increased urinary norepinephrine excretion. *J Pediatr* 1975; **86**: 542–547

39. Symes AL, Missala K, Sourkes TL. Iron and riboflavin metabolism of a monoamine in the rat *in vivo*. *Science* 1971; **174**: 153–155

40. Mackler B, Person R, Miller LR *et al*. Iron deficiency in the rat: Biochemical studies of brain metabolism. *Pediatr Res* 1978; **12**: 217–220

41. Glover J, Jacobs A. Activity pattern in iron deficient rats. *Br Med J* 1972; **2**: 627–628

42. Youdim MBH, Yohuda S, Ben-Uriah Y. Iron deficiency induced circadian rhythm reversal of dopaminergic-mediated behaviours and thermoregulation in rats. *Eur J Pharmacol* 1981; **74**: 295–301

43. Dallman PR, Refino CA, Dallman MF. The pituitary-adrenal response to stress in the iron-deficient rat. *J Nutr* 1984; **114**: 1747–1753

44. Edgerton VR, Bryant SL, Gillespie CA, Gardner GW. Iron deficiency and physical performance and activity of rats. *J Nutr* 1972; **102**: 381–400

45. Department of Health. *Dietary Reference Values for Food Energy and Nutrients for the United Kingdom*. London: HMSA, 1991, pp 1–120

46. MacPhail AP, Bothwell TH. Fortification of the diet as a strategy for preventing iron deficiency. *Acta Paediatr Scand* 1989; **361 (Suppl)**: 114–124

47. Nelson SE, Ziegler EE, Copeland AM *et al*. Gain in weight and length during early infancy. *Early Hum Dev* 1989; **19**: 223–239

48. Nelson SE, Rogers RR, Copeland AM *et al*. Lack of adverse reactions in iron-fortified formula. *Pediatrics* 1988; **81**: 360–364

49. Oski FA. Iron-fortified formulas and gastrointestinal symptoms in infants: a controlled study. *Pediatrics* 1980; **66**: 168–170

50. Balmer SE, Wharton BA. Diet and faecal flora in the newborn: iron. *Arch Dis Child* 1991; **66**: 1390–1394

51. Mevissen-Verhage EAE, Marcelis JH, Harmsen-Van Amerongen WCM *et al*. Effect of iron on neonal gut flora during the first three months of life. *Eur J Clin Microbiol* 1985; **4**: 273–278

52. McFarlane H, Reddy S, Adcock KJ *et al*. Immunity transferrin and survival in kwashiorkor. Br Med J 1970: 4: 268–270

53. Murray MJ, Murray AB, Murray MB, Murray Q. The adverse effect of iron repletion on the course of certain infections. *Br Med J* 1978; **11**: 113–115

54. Cook JD, Reddy M. Efficacy of weekly compared to daily iron supplementation. *Am J Clin Nutr* 1995; **62**: 117–120

55. Wright AJA, Southon S. The effectiveness of various iron-supplementation regimens in improving the iron status in anaemic rats. *Br J Nutr* 1990; **63**: 579–585

56. Viteri FE, Liu X-N, Tolomei K, Martin A. True absorption and retention of supplemental iron is more efficient when administered every three days rather than daily to iron-normal and iron-deficient rats. *J Nutr* 1995; **125**: 82–91

57. Solomons NW. Weekly versus daily oral iron administration: are we asking the right questions? *Nutr Rev* 1997; **55**: 141–142

58. Fairweather-Tait SJ. Iron availability – the implications of short-term regulation. *BNF Nutr Bull* 1986; **11**: 174–180

59. Barry DMJ, Reeve AW. Increased incidence of Gram-negative neonatal sepsis with intramuscular iron administration. *Pediatrics* 1977; **60**: 908–912

60. Leikin SL. The use of intramuscular iron in the prophylaxis of the iron deficiency anemia of prematurity. *Am J Dis Child* 1960; **99**: 739–745

61. Salmi T, Hanninen P, Peltonen T. Applicability of chelated iron in the care of prematures. *Acta Paediatr Scand* 1963; **140**: 114–115

62. Blacklock NJ. Bladder trauma in the long distance runner – 10,000 meter haematuria. *Br J Chol* 1977; **49**: 129–132

63. Oppenheimer SJ, Gibson FD, McFarlane SB *et al*. Iron supplementation increasesx prevalence and effects of malaria: report on clinical studies in Papua New Guinea. *Trans R Soc Trop Med Hygiene* 1986; **80**: 603–612

64. Ball PA, Booth IW, Holden CE, Puntis JWL. *Paediatric Parenteral Nutrition*. Milton Keynes: Pharmacia, 1995, pp 15–29

65. Noel RA, Udall JN. In: Walker WA, Watkins JB (eds) *Nutrition in Pediatrics*, 2nd edn. Ontario: Decker, 1996, pp737–740

66. Ajayi OA. Iron stores in pregnant Nigerians and their infants at term. *Eur J Clin Nutr* 1988; **42**: 23–28

67. Zittoun J, Blot I, Hill C *et al*. Iron supplements versus placebo during

pregnancy: its effects on iron and folate status of mothers and newborn. *Ann Nutr Metab* 1983; **27**: 320–327

68. Rios E, Lipschitz DA, Cook JD *et al*. Relationship of maternal and infant iron stores as assessed by determination of plasma ferritin. *Pediatrics* 1975; **55**: 694–699

69. Okuyama T, Tawada T, Furuya H, Villee CA. The role of transferrin and ferritin in the fetal-maternal-placental unit. *Am J Obstet Gynecol* 1985; **152**: 344–350

70. Lao TT, Loong EPL, Chin RKH, Lam CWK, Lam YM. Relationship between newborn and maternal iron status and haematological indices. *Biol Neonate* 1991; **60**: 30–37

71. Hussain MAM, Gaafar TH, Laulicht M, Hoffbrand AV. Relation of maternal and cord blood serum ferritin. *Arch Dis Child* 1977; **52**: 782–784

72. Bratlid D, Moe PJ. Hemoglobin and serum ferritin levels in mothers and infants at birth. *Eur J Pediatr* 1980; **134**: 125–27

73. Celada A, Busset R, Gutierrez J, Herreros V. Maternal and cord blood ferritin. *Helv Paediatr Acta* 1982; **37**: 239–244

74. Chong SKF, Thompson MJ, Shaw JEH, Barltrop D. Free erythrocyte protoprophyrin as an index of perinatal iron status. *J Pediatr Gastroenterol Nutr* 1984; **3**: 224–229

75. Wong C-T, Saha N. Inter-relationships of storage iron in the mother, the placenta and the newborn. *Acta Obstet Gynaecol Scand* 1990; **69**: 613–616

76. Blot I, Tehernia G, Chenayer M *et al*. La carence martiale chez la femme enceinte. *J Gynecol Obstet Biol Reprod* 1980; **9**: 489–495

77. Agrawal RMD, Tripathi AM, Agrawal KN. Cord blood haemoglobin, iron and ferritin status in maternal anaemia. *Acta Paediatr Scand* 1983; **72**: 545–548

78. Milman N, Agger AO, Nielsen OJ. Iron status markers and serum erythropoietin in 120 mothers and newborn infants. *Acta Obstet Gynecol Scand* 1994; **73**: 200–204

79. De Benaze C, Galan P, Wainer R, Hercberg S. Prevention de l'anemie ferroprive au cours de la grassesse par un supplementation martiale precoce: un essaie controle. *Rev Epidemiol Sante Publique* 1989; **27**: 109–119

80. Kelly AM, MacDonald DJ, McDougall AN. Observations on maternal and fetal ferritin concentrations at term. *Br J Obstet Gynaecol* 1978; **85**: 338–343

81. McPhail AP, Charlton RW, Bothwell TH, Torrance JD, The relationship between maternal and infant iron stores. *Scand J Haematol* 1989; **25**: 141–150

82. Puolakka J, Jann O, Vihko R. Evaluation by serum ferritin assay of the influence of maternal iron stores on the iron status of newborns and infants. *Acta Obstet Gynaecol Scand* 1980; **95 (Suppl)**: 53–56

83. Kaneshige E. Serum ferritin as an assessment of iron stores and other hematologic parameters during pregnancy. *Obstet Gynecol* 1980; **57**: 238–242

84. Strauss MB. Anemia of infancy from maternal iron deficiency in pregnancy. *Clin Invest* 1993; **12**: 345–353

85. Colomer J, Colomer C, Guttierez D *et al*. Anaemia during pregnancy as a risk factor for infant iron deficiency: report from the Valencia Infant Anaemia Cohort (VIAC) study. *Paediatr Perinat Epidemiol* 1990; **4**: 196–204

86. Wharton BA. *Nutrition and Feeding of Preterm Infants*. Oxford: Blackwell Scientific Publications, 1987, pp 1–238

87. Tsang RC, Lucas A, Uauy R, Zlotkin S. *Nutritional Needs of the Preterm Infant*. Baltimore: Williams & Wilkins, 1993, pp 177–194

88. Dauncey MJ, Davies CG, Shaw JCL, Urman J. The effect of iron supplements and blood transfusion on iron absorption by low birth weight infants fed pasteurised human breast milk. *Pediatr Res* 1978; **12**: 899–904

89. Shaw JCL. Iron absorption by the premature infant: the effect of iron supplements on serum ferritin levels. *Acta Paediatr Scand* 1982; **299 (Suppl)**: 83–89

90. Meyer MP, Meyer JH, Commerford A *et al*. Recombinant human erythropoietin in the treatment of the anemia of prematurity: Results of a double-blind, placebo-controlled study. *Pediatrics* 1994: **93**: 918–923

91. Kivivuori SM, Heikiheimo M, Siimes MA. Early rise in serum concentrations of transferrin receptor is induced by recombinant human erythropoietin in very low-birth-weight infants. *Pediatr Res* 1994; **36**: 85–80

92. Green HL, Hambidge KM, Shanler R *et al*. Guidelines for the use of vitamins, trace elements, calcium, magnesium and phosphorus in infants receiving total parenteral nutrition. *Am J Clin Nutr* 1988; **48**: 1324–1342

93. Hill DJ, Hosking GS. The cow's milk allergy complex: overlapping disease profiles in infancy. *Eur J Clin Nutr* 1995; **49 (Suppl 1)**: S1–S12

94. Pisacane A, De Vizia B, Valiante A *et al*. Iron status in breast fed infants. *J Pediatr* 1995; **127**: 429–431

95. Pizarro F, Yip R, Dallman PR *et al*. Iron status with different infant feeding regimens: relevance to screening and prevention of iron deficiency. *J Pediatr* 1991; **118**: 687–692

96. Fuchs GJ, Farris RP, DeWier M *et al*. Iron status and intake of older infants fed formula vs cow milk with cereal. *Am J Clin Nutr* 1993; **58**: 343–348

97. Calvo EB, Galindo A, Aspres NB. Iron status in exclusively breast fed infants. *Pediatrics* 1992; **90**: 375–379

98. Morton RE, Nysenbaum A, Price K. Iron status in the first year of life. *J Pediatr Gastroenterol Nutr* 1988; **7**: 707–712

99. Daly A, MacDonald A, Aukett A *et al*. Prevention of anaemia in inner city toddlers by an iron supplemented cows' milk formula. *Arch Dis Child* 1996; **75**: 9–16

100. Stevens D, Nelson A. The effect of iron in formula milk after 6 months of age. *Arch Dis Child* 1995; **73**: 216–220

101. Wharton BA. Milk for babies and children: no ordinary cows' milk before 1 year. *Br Med J* 1990; **301**: 774–775

102. American Academy of Pediatrics. The use of whole cows' milk in infancy. *Pediatrics* 1992; **89**: 1105–1106

103. Department of Health. *Weaning and Weaning Diet*. Report on Health and Social Subjects, No 45. London: HMSO, 1994, pp 1–114

104. Mills A, Tyler H. *Food and Nutrient Intakes of British Infants Aged 6–12 Months*. London: HMSO, 1992, pp 1–98

105. Stordy BJ, Redfern AM, Morgan JB. Healthy eating for infants – mothers' action. *Acta Paediatr* 1995; **84**: 733–741

106. Sullivan PB. Cows' milk induced intestinal bleeding in infancy. *Arch Dis Child* 1993; **68**: 240–245

107. Ziegler EE, Fomon SH, Nelson SE *et al*. Cow milk feeding in infancy: Further observations on blood loss from gastrointestinal tract. *J Pediatr* 1990; **116**: 11–18

108. Fuchs GJ, De Wier M, Hutchinson S, Sundeen M, Schwartz S, Suskind R. Gastrointestinal blood loss in older infants: impact on cow milk versus formula. *J Pediatr Gastroenterol Nutr* 1993; **16**: 4–9

109. Childs F, Aukett MA, Darbyshire P *et al*. Does nutritional education work in preventing iron deficiency in the inner city? *Arch Dis Child* 1997; **76**: 144–147

110. Dallman PR. Iron deficiency in the weanling. *Acta Paediatr Scand* 1986; **323 (Suppl)**: 59–67

111. Brennan RE, Kohrs MB, Nordstrom JW, Sauvage JP, Shank RE. Composition of diets of low income pregnant women: Comparison of analysed and calculated values. *J Am Diet Assoc* 1983; **83**: 538–545

112. Department of Health and Social Security. *Artificial Feeds for the Young Infant*. Report on Health and Social Subjects, No 18. London: HMSO, 1984, pp 1–104

113. Hertramph F, Olivares O, Pizarro F *et al*. Haemoglobin fortified cereal: a source of available iron in breast fed infants. *Eur J Clin Nutr* 1990; **44**: 793–798

114. Hurrell RF. Preventing iron deficiency through food fortification. *Nutr Rev* 1997; **55**: 210–222

115. Rios E, Hunter RE, Cook JD, Smith NJ, Finch CA. The absorption of iron as supplements in infant cereal and infant formulas. *Pediatrics* 1975; **55**: 686–693

116. Moe PJ. Iron requirements in infancy. II. The influence of iron

fortified cereals during the first year of life on the red blood cell picture of children at 1.5–3 yrs of age. *Acta Paediatr* 1964; **53**: 422–432

117. Grindulis H, Scott PH, Belton NR, Wharton BA. Combined deficiency of iron and vitamin D in Asian toddlers. *Arch Dis Child* 1986; **61**: 843–848

118. Aukett MA, Parks YA, Scott PH, Wharton BA. Treatment with iron increases weight gain and psychomotor development. *Arch Dis Child* 1986; **61**: 849–857

119. Marder E, Nicoll A, Polnay L, Shulman CE. Discovering anaemia at child health clinics. *Arch Dis Child* 1990; **65**: 892–894

120. Mills AF. Surveillance for anaemia: risk factors in pattern of milk intake. *Arch Dis Child* 1990; **65**: 428–432

121. Gregory JR, Collins DL, Davies PSW *et al*. *National Diet and Nutrition Survey: Children aged $1\frac{1}{2}$ and $4\frac{1}{2}$ years*. Volume 1. Report of the Diet and Nutrition Survey. London: HMSO, 1995, pp 1–391

122. Gill DG, Vincent S, Segal DS. Follow on formula in the prevention of iron deficiency: a multicentre study. *Acta Paediatr* 1997; **86**: 683–689

123. Calvo EB, Gnazzo N. Prevalence of iron deficiency in children aged 9–24 mo from a large urban area in Argentina. *Am J Clin Nutr* 1990; **52**: 534–540

124. O'Donnell AM, Carmuega ES, Duran P. Preventing iron deficiency in infants and preschool children in Argentina. *Nutr Rev* 1997; **55**: 189–194

125. Taylor PG, Martinez-Torres C, Mendez-Castellano H *et al*. The relationship between iron deficiency and anaemia in Venezualan children. *Am J clin Nutr* 1993; **53**: 215–218

126. Yip R, Walsh KM, Goldfarb MG, Binkin NJ. Declining prevalence of anaemia in childhood in a middle-class setting: a pediatric success story? *Pediatrics* 1987; **80**: 330–334

127. Lehmann F, Gray-Donald K, Mongeon M *et al*. Iron deficiency anemia in 1-year-old children of disadvantaged families in Montreal. *Can Med Assoc J* 1992; **146**: 1571–1577

128. Leung SSF, Davies DP, Lui S *et al*. Iron deficiency in healthy Hong Kong infants at 18 months. *J Trop Pediatr* 1988; **34**: 100–103

129. Wharton BA. Protein-energy malnutrition. *Acta Paediatr Scand* 1991; **374 (Suppl)**: 5–14

130. Mejia LA, Chew F. Hematological effect of supplementing anemic children with vitamin A alone and in combination with iron. *Am J Clin Nutr* 1988; **48**: 595–600

131. Suharno D, West CE, Muhilal *et al*. Supplementation with vitamin A and iron for nutritional anaemia in pregnant women in West Java, Indonesia. *Lancet* 1993; **342**: 1325–1328

132. Powers HJ. Riboflavin iron interaction with particular emphasis on the gastrointestinal tract. *Proc Nutr Soc* 1995; **54**: 509–571

133. Stoltzfus RJ, Dreyfus ML, Hababuu M *et al*. Hookworm control as a strategy to prevent iron deficiency. *Nutr Rev* 1997; **55**: 195–209

134. De Giacomoa C, Fiocca R, Villani L *et al*. *Helicobacter pylori* infection and chronic gastritis. *J Pediatr Gastroenterol Nutr* 1990; **11**: 310–316

135. Nelson M, Naismith DJ, Burley V. Nutrient intakes, vitamin-mineral supplementation and intelligence in British schoolchildren. *Br J Nutr* 1990; 64: 13–22

136. Vandenplas Y, Blecker U, Devreker T *et al*. Contribution of the 13C urea breath test to the detection of *Helicobacter pylori* gastritis in children. *Pediatrics* 1992; **90**: 608–611

137. Andrade ZA, Peixoto E, Guerret S, Grimaud JA. Hepatic connective tissue changes in hepatosplexic schistosomiasis. *Hum Pathol* 1992; **23**: 566–573

138. Anttila R, Siimes MA. Development of iron status and response to iron medication in pubertal boys. *J Pediatr Gastroenterol Nutr* 1996; **22**: 312–317

139. Nelson M, White J, Rhodes C. Haemoglobin, ferritin and iron intakes in British schoolchildren. *Br J Nutr* 1993; **70**: 147–155

140. Doyle W, Jenkins S, Crawford MA, Puvandendran K. Nutritional status of schoolchildren in an inner city area. *Arch Dis Child* 1994; **70**: 376–381

141. Nelson M, Bakaliou F, Trivedi A. Iron-deficiency anaemia and physical performance in adolescent girls from different ethnic backgrounds. *Br J Nutr* 1994; **72**: 427–433

142. Southen S, Wright AJA, Finglas PM *et al*. Dietary intake and micronutrient status of adolescents: effect of vitamin and trace element supplementation on indices of status and performance in tests of verbal and non-verbal intelligence. *Br J Nutr* 1994; **71**: 897–918

143. Armstrong PL. Iron deficiency in adolescents. *Br Med J* 1989; **298**: 499

144. Hallberg L, Hulten L, Lindstedt G *et al*. Prevalence of iron deficiency in Swedish adolescents. *Pediatr Res* 1993; **34**: 680–687

145. Bergstrom E, Hernell O, Lonnerdal B, Persson LA. Sex differences in iron stores of adolescents: what is normal? *J Pediatr Gastroenterol Nutr* 1995; **20**: 215–224

146. Antilla R, Koistinen R, Seppala M, Koistinen H, Siimes MA. Insulin-like growth factor I and insulin-like growth factor binding protein 3 as determinants of blood haemoglobin concentration in healthy subjects. *Pediatr Res* 1994; **36**: 754–758

147. Department of Health. *The Diets of British School Children*. Report on Health and Social Subjects, No 36. London: HMSO, PP 1–293

148. Moynihan PJ, Anderson C, Adamson AJ *et al*. Dietary sources of iron in English adolescents. *J Hum Nutr Diet* 1994; **7**: 225–230

149. Preziosi P, Hercbert S, Galan P *et al*. Iron status of a healthy French population: factors determining biochemical markers. *Ann Nutr Metab* 1994; **38**: 192–202

Porphyria

GEORGE H ELDER

The porphyrias are a group of metabolic disorders that result from partial deficiencies of the enzymes of heme biosynthesis.[1,2] All are inherited in monogenic patterns, apart from some forms of porphyria cutanea tarda (PCT). Each of the main types is defined by the association of characteristic clinical features with a specific pattern of overproduction of heme precursors that reflects increased formation of the substrate of the enzyme that is deficient in that particular type of porphyria. Increased substrate concentration compensates the enzyme deficiencies and maintains normal or near normal rates of heme formation. Thus, heme deficiency is not prominent in the porphyrias—a feature that is in marked contrast to the anemia of acquired disorders of heme synthesis such as iron deficiency, lead poisoning and certain types of sideroblastic anemia. The porphyrias are characterized clinically by 2 types of illness:

- skin lesions caused by photosensitization by porphyrins;
- acute neurovisceral crises that are always associated with overproduction of the porphyrin precursor, 5-aminolevulinate (ALA).[1,2]

Symptoms never occur in the absence of demonstrable overproduction of heme precursors and may be regarded as the price paid to maintain the vital function of heme synthesis.

Porphyrias are uncommon in pediatric practice and rarely present as hematologic problems. However, hematologists may become involved in the clinical management of children with porphyria and their families. For some porphyrias, specialized hematologic procedures are required for treatment and, in future, therapy by gene transfer into erythroid stem cells may be introduced for some disorders. This chapter focuses on those porphyrias that normally present during childhood and aspects of other porphyrias, such as screening for latent disease, that particularly concern children.

CLASSIFICATION

Table 7.1 shows the classification of the porphyrias that is followed in this chapter and the main clinical features of each disorder. Each of the 7 main types of porphyria (ADP, AIP, CEP, PCT, HCP, VP, EPP) results from partial deficiency of a different enzyme of heme biosynthesis; other disorders listed in Table 7.1 are subtypes or variants of these main types. The main types of porphyria may be subdivided into acute porphyrias (AIP, HCP, VP, ADP) and purely cutaneous porphyrias (CEP, EPP, PCT) or according to the main site of overproduction of heme precursors: erythropoietic (CEP, EPP) and hepatic (AIP, HCP, VP, PCT) porphyrias.[1,2] Individuals and families with more than one type of porphyria have been reported.[1,2]

HEME BIOSYNTHESIS

Heme (ferroprotoporphyrin IX) is synthesized by all mammalian cells, although erythroid cells lose this capacity as mitochondria disappear during the later stages of differentiation. It functions as an essential catalyst for oxygen transport, oxygen activation and electron transfer. These catalytic properties are conferred by combination with specific apoproteins such as globin and apocytochromes to form hemoproteins. Iron supply, heme biosynthesis and apoprotein formation are closely co-ordinated in mammalian cells by interacting regulatory processes that are tissue specific.[3] Thus, in mature erythrocytes, heme bound to globin is in 26 000-fold molar excess of porphyrin.

Normal adults synthesize about 7 μmol heme/kg body weight/day. About 80–85% is produced within the bone marrow for hemoglobin formation; most of the rest is synthesized in the liver where at least 50% is incorporated into microsomal hemoproteins of the CYP (cytochrome P450) family.[1] Heme is catabolized to biliverdin, with

Table 7.1 Classification of the porphyrias.

Disorder	Clinical features		Age at presentation
	Neurovisceral crises	Skin lesions	
Autosomal recessive porphyrias			
Aminolaevulinate dehydratase deficiency porphyria (ADP)	+[a]	−	Any age
Congenital erythropoietic porphyria (CEP)	−	+	Usually before age of 1 year; rare adult onset form
Autosomal dominant acute porphyrias			
Acute intermittent porphyria (AIP)	+	−	Usually second to
Hereditary coproporphyria (HCP)	+	+[b]	fifth decade; very rare
Variegate porphyria (VP)	+[c]	+[c]	before puberty
Homozygous variants of the autosomal dominant acute hepatic porphyrias			
Homozygous AIP	+[d]	−	Infancy
Homozygous HCP	+[e]	+	Early childhood
Harderoporphyria	−	+	Infancy
Homozygous VP	−	+	Early childhood
Uroporphyrinogen decarboxylase deficiency disorders			
Porphyria cutanea tarda (PCT)			
sporadic (type I) PCT	−	+	20–80+ years; rare before 20 years
familial (type II) PCT	−	+	Early childhood to 80+ years
familial (type III) PCT	−	+	Adults
toxic PCT	−	+	Any age
Hepatoerythropoietic porphyria (HEP)	−	+	Early childhood
Erythropoietic protoporphyria (EPP)	−	+	Childhood, usually before 4 years old

[a]Chronic neuropathy without acute crises in some patients; [b]Usually associated with neurovisceral crises; [c]May present with skin lesions alone, an acute neurovisceral attack alone or with both together; [d] No acute crises: progressive neurologic disorder; [e]At or after puberty.

release of iron and carbon monoxide, by the heme oxygenase isoenzymes, H0–1 (HSP32) and H0–2, which are encoded by different genes and differ markedly in their properties, tissue distribution and regulation.[4]

ENZYMES AND PATHWAY

Formation of 5-aminolevulinate

ALA is the first of 4 intermediates that are common to the biosynthetic pathways that lead to heme, chlorophylls, phycobilins, corrinoids (vitamin B_{12}) and other metal-containing tetrapyrrolic pigments that are essential for life. In animals, yeast and some bacteria, ALA is formed by the pyridoxal 5′-phosphate (PLP)-dependent condensation of succinyl CoA and glycine which is catalyzed by ALA synthase (ALAS) (Fig. 7.1). In plants, algae and most bacteria, glutamate is converted to ALA via glutamyl-tRNA and glutamate-1-semialdehyde (GSA) with the final reaction being catalyzed by another PLP-enzyme, GSA aminotransferase.[5]

Mammals and birds have separate housekeeping and erythroid isoenzymes of ALAS.[6] In humans, the gene for the housekeeping isoenzyme (ALAS-1), which is expressed in all tissues, is on chromosome 3 (3p21.1), while the erythroid isoenzyme (ALAS-2) is encoded by a gene on the X chromosome at Xp11.21. The structural organization of both genes is similar and conserved between species, suggesting that they may have evolved from a common ancestor. The human ALAS-2 gene contains 11 exons spread over 22 kb. Exons 5–11 encode a highly conserved, catalytic domain that is similar in both isoenzymes. Exon 2 encodes a 49 amino acid pre-sequence that directs the enzyme to the mitochondrial matrix space; exon 1 is not translated. The human ALAS-1 gene has not been characterized but it is likely to have a similar structure.

Processing of the 65 kDa precursor form of ALAS-2 during mitochondrial import leads to the formation of a catalytically active homo-dimer containing 59.5 kDa subunits that lack the pre-sequence. The PLP cofactor is bound through a Schiff's base linkage to a lysine residue at position 391;[7] mutations that cause X-linked sideroblastic anemia show some clustering in this region which is encoded by exon 9 (see Chapter 5). Another highly conserved region contains a glycine-rich sequence (GXGXXG), which is present in other PLP enzymes and phosphate-binding nucleoproteins, and may interact with the phosphate moiety of PLP.[7]

Conversion of ALA to uroporphyrinogen III

The reactions that convert ALA to uroporphyrinogen III take place in the cytosol (Fig. 7.1).

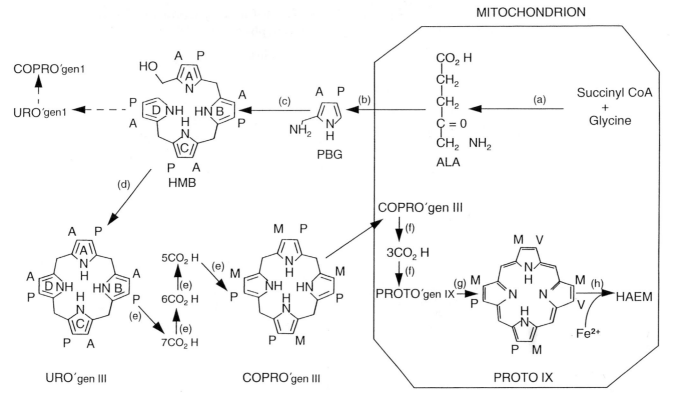

Fig. 7.1 Heme biosynthesis. Reactions are catalyzed by 5-aminolevulinate (ALA) synthase (a), ALA dehydratase (b), porphobilinogen (PBG) deaminase (c), uroporphyrinogen (URO'gen) III synthase (d), URO'gen decarboxylase (e), coproporphyrinogen (COPRO'gen) oxidase (f), protoporphyrinogen (PROTO'gen) oxidase (g) and ferrochelatase (h).

5-Aminolevulinate dehydratase

ALA dehydratase (porphobilinogen synthase) (ALAD) catalyzes the asymmetric condensation of 2 molecules of ALA to form the colorless monopyrrole, porphobilinogen (PBG). The enzyme is an octamer containing identical 35-kDa subunits whose primary sequence is highly conserved between species.[8,9] Mammalian ALAD contains 8 Zn^{2+} molecules/octamer, 4 of which are essential for catalytic activity. Each active site appears to involve 2 adjacent monomers that interact in a way that allows 2 ALA molecules and 2 Zn^{2+} atoms to be bound in different environments to enable a sequential, asymmetric condensation reaction to proceed. In the human enzyme, the lysine residue at position 252 forms a Schiff's base with the first ALA molecule that binds during catalysis and a cysteine and histidine-rich region (residues 119–133) forms a probable zinc-binding site.[9]

ALAD is inhibited by compounds of clinical importance—heavy metals, especially lead, and succinylacetone, an intermediate that accumulates in hereditary tyrosinemia and acts as a potent competitive inhibitor of the enzyme.[10] Lead inhibits ALAD by competitive displacement of the 4 tightly-bound Zn^{2+} atoms that are essential for catalytic activity; an action that is readily reversed by sulfhydryl-group reagents. It can also bind at the lower affinity Zn^{2+}

sites without inhibiting enzyme activity.[8] In addition to its catalytic activity, ALAD also acts as the 240-kDa proteosome inhibitor (CF-2) of proteosome-mediated, ubiquitin-dependent protein degradation; an action that is not inhibited by lead.[8,11]

Human ALAD is encoded by a single 13-kb gene on chromosome 9 (9q34) that contains 13 exons.[9] Exons 2–12 encode the enzyme monomer. Exons 1A and 1B undergo tissue-specific alternative splicing to exon 2.[9,12] ALAD mRNA containing exon 1B is found only in erythroid cells while exon 1A is present in mRNA from all tissues. Alternative splicing is determined by the presence of separate ubiquitous and erythroid-specific promoter regions 5′ to exons 1A and 1B.

Porphobilinogen deaminase

PBG deaminase (hydroxymethylbilane synthase) catalyzes the head-to-tail polymerization of 4 PBG molecules to form the linear tetrapyrrole, hydroxymethylbilane (pre-uroporphyrinogen). The discovery by ^{13}C NMR spectroscopy of the extremely unstable product of this reaction initiated a series of investigations that have produced an almost complete picture of the mechanism of this fascinating and unique enzyme.[13–15] The structure of the enzyme from *Escherichia coli* has been determined by X-ray crystallography at 1.76Å resolution.[13] It contains 3 domains of similar size with a deep catalytic cleft between domains 1 and 2. The shape of these 2 domains resembles transferrin and the periplasmic binding proteins, proteins that undergo marked conformational change on interaction with their ligands.

The primary structures of PBG deaminases are highly conserved. Alignment of amino acid sequences shows 70% similarity and 46% identity between the *E. coli* and human enzymes. Thus, the *E. coli* enzyme is a good model for its human counterpart; the main difference being an additional loop of 14 amino acids (residues 270–283) of unknown function in the human enzyme.[14] PBG deaminase contains a dipyrromethane cofactor which is covalently bound by a thioether link to a cysteine residue (C242) on a loop of domain 3 which projects into the base of the catalytic cleft. PBG residues are added stepwise to the cofactor by condensation reactions to form a growing polymer. Once 4 residues have been added, the hydroxymethylbilane product is released. Arginine residues projecting into the catalytic cleft interact with the side chains of the cofactor, substrate and growing polymer and are essential for the reaction. Polymerization may be facilitated by movements of the domains that draw the growing chain into the catalytic cleft; the maximum dimensions of the cleft appear to allow addition of only 4 PBG molecules, a factor that may be important in initiating release of the product.[13–15] An aspartate residue (D84) in domain 1 is essential for catalysis of the condensation reactions.[14,15]

Human PBG deaminase exists in 2 forms: a 40-kDa erythroid isoenzyme and a housekeeping (or ubiquitous) isoenzyme which contains an additional 17 amino acids at its NH$_2$-terminus and is expressed in all tissues. Both are encoded by a single 10-kb gene on chromosome 11 (11q24.1–24.2) containing 15 exons. Tissue-specific expression is determined by separate erythroid and ubiquitous promoters 5′ to exons 2 and 1 with translation initiation codons in exons 3 and 1, respectively.[16]

Uroporphyrinogen III synthase

In the absence of uroporphyrinogen III synthase (UROS), hydroxymethylbilane rapidly cyclizes to the symmetrical hexahydroporphyrin, uroporphyrinogen I (Fig. 7.1) which has no physiologic function. UROS catalyzes both cyclization and reversal of the orientation of ring D of hydroxymethylbilane to give the III isomer (Fig. 7.1) which is the common precursor of all tetrapyrrolic pigments. Several mechanisms for this unique reaction have been suggested; current evidence favors the formation of a spiro-intermediate.[17] The enzyme is unstable, shows little sequence similarity between species and has proved difficult to study directly. The human UROS gene on chromosome 10 (10q25.2–26.3) covers 45 kb and contains 9 exons that encode a 29-kDa protein.[18]

Conversion of uroporphyrinogen III to protoporphyrinogen IX

Protoporphyrinogen IX is formed from uroporphyrinogen III by sequential modification of 4 acetic and 2 propionic acid substituents (Fig. 7.1). The cytosolic enzyme, uroporphyrinogen decarboxylase (UROD), catalyzes the decarboxylation of uroporphyrinogens I and III to the corresponding coproporphyrinogens.[19] Under physiologic conditions, the acetic acid substituents are decarboxylated in a clockwise order around the porphyrinogen macrocycle, starting at ring D, with the formation of 7-, 6- and 5- carboxyl intermediates (Fig. 7.1). As substrate concentrations increase, this specificity is lost and mixtures of all possible isomeric intermediates are produced. All URODs are inhibited by sulfhydryl group reagents, including heavy metals, and most require reducing agents for full activity *in vitro*. Evidence from study of natural mutants and from site-directed mutagenesis experiments is consistent with the hypothesis that each side chain is decarboxylated at the same catalytic site,[19,20] but the mechanism by which the substrate rotates remains obscure. Human UROD is an 82-kDa homodimer[21] encoded by a gene on chromosome 1 (1p34) which contains 10 exons spread over 3 kb.[22]

Sequential hydrogenation and decarboxylation of the 2- and 4-proprionate side chains of coproporphyringen III to protoporphyrinogen IX, with formation of the tricarboxylic intermediate, harderoporphyrinogen, is catalyzed by coproporphyrinogen oxidase (CPGOX) (Fig. 7.1). Coproporphyrinogen I is not metabolized so it is at this stage that the pathway becomes specific for the asymmetric series III isomers. Mammalian CPGOXs have an absolute requirement for molecular oxygen; no cofactors have been identified. Human CPGOX is a metal-free 74-kDa homodimer[23] situated in the mitochondrial intermembrane space, possibly loosely attached to the outer surface of the inner membrane.[24] It is synthesized as a precursor with a 110 amino acid pre-sequence that directs it to the intermembrane space.[25] Human CPGOX is encoded by a single 14-kb gene on chromosome 3 (3q12) that contains 7 exons.[25] There is no evidence for tissue-specific isoenzymes; the gene contains 2 polyadenylation signals but it is not certain that these have any regulatory function.

Formation of heme from protoporphyrinogen IX

The terminal stages of heme biosynthesis are all associated with the inner mitochondrial membrane (Fig. 7.1).[24] The insertion of Fe^{2+} into protoporphyrin IX to form heme, the reaction catalyzed by ferrochelatase (FC), takes place at the inner face of this membrane. Delivery of the 2 substrates to this site requires aromatization of protoporphyrinogen IX to protoporphyrin IX by protoporphyrinogen oxidase (PPOX), transport of protoporphyrin(ogen) and iron across the membrane and reduction of Fe^{3+} to Fe^{2+}.

Most attention has focused on the enzymatic reactions and relatively little is known about the other processes, all of which are potential sites for inhibition of heme biosynthesis.

Protoporphyrinogen oxidase

PPOX is a flavoprotein with an absolute requirement for molecular oxygen.[26] Little is known about its mechanism of action. Mammalian, plant and some bacterial enzymes are competitively inhibited by diphenyl ether herbicides.[26] Human PPOX is encoded by a gene on chromosome 1 (1q21–23) which contains 13 introns spread over 5.5 kb.[27–29] Unusually for a mitochondrial enzyme, there is no pre-sequence; the import signal is presumably contained within the mature protein but has not been identified.

Ferrochelatase

FCs from different species and tissues have been extensively studied.[30] In addition to protoporphyrin IX and Fe^{2+}, other dicarboxylic porphyrins (mesoporphyrin, deuteroporphyrin) and metals (Zn^{2+}, Co^{2+}) serve as substrates. Eukaryotic FCs are activated by lipids and inhibited by sulfhydryl group reagents and heme;[30,31] it is unclear whether inhibition by the latter is significant at physiological concentrations. Mechanistic studies using N-alkylporphyrins as inhibitors suggest that the porphyrin ring becomes distorted during the reaction in order to facilitate Fe^{2+} insertion; precise identification of the residues involved in binding porphyrin substrates is likely to require knowledge of the 3-dimensional structure of the enzyme. The residues that bind Fe^{2+} have not been unequivocally identified. Biochemical evidence for utilization of cysteine residues is not supported by sequence comparisons that show no conservation of cysteines between species.[30] More recent site–directed mutagenesis experiments implicate histidine residues, particularly H263 in the human enzyme.[30]

Newly synthesized FC contains a pre-sequence, which directs transport into the mitochondrion and is cleaved to form the mature 40-kDa protein. FC functions *in vitro* as a monomer,[30] but radiation inactivation experiments suggest that it may be present in the mitochondrial membrane as a dimer.[32] Mammalian but not bacterial FCs have a carboxy-terminal extension which contains an [2Fe–2S] cluster.[33] Removal of this extension inactivates the enzyme—an unexpected finding in view of the similarity of the remaining sequence with those of active bacterial enzymes.[30] The functional significance of this cluster has yet to be determined.

Human FC is encoded by a single 45-kb gene on chromosome 18 (18q21.3) that contains 11 exons.[34] The gene contains 2 polyadenylation sites; the upstream site producing a 2.2-kb transcript that may be used preferentially in erythroid cells.[3,34]

Transport of substrates and reduction of iron

Intact mitochondria are impermeable to protoporphyrin. It has been suggested that the 3 terminal enzymes form a complex that spans the inner membrane and that substrate channeling between PPOX and FC transfers protoporphyrin.[24] However, subsequent cloning and sequence analysis of PPOX and FC showed no recognizable membrane-spanning domains. Thus, both the mechanism of substrate transfer and the precise orientation of PPOX and FC remain unresolved problems.

The mechanism of transport of iron across the mammalian inner mitochondrial membrane is also unknown. There may be a specific mitochondrial iron-transport protein. Abnormalities of iron metabolism in the Belgrade rat and *hgd* strain of mouse are consistent with defective mitochondrial iron uptake; identification of the genetic defect in these animals may help to explain how iron enters mitochondria.[35] Reduction and, possibly, transport of iron may be linked to oxidation of NADH by complex I of the mitochondrial electron transport chain which co-purifies with FC from membranes.[36] Heteroplasmic mutations in erythroid mitochondrial DNA encoding components of this complex have been identified in anemias associated with accumulation of ferric iron in mitochondria.[37] Lead poisoning, like iron deficiency, leads to accumulation of zinc-protoporphyrin in erythrocytes, whereas FC defects are characterized by accumulation of metal-free protoporphyrin. Lead may inhibit delivery of Fe^{2+} to FC rather than inhibit the enzyme directly.

REGULATION

The rate of heme formation is determined by the activity of the first committed enzyme of the pathway, ALAS.[1–3,6] The basal activity of ALAS is substantially lower than the activities of subsequent enzymes with the exception of PBG deaminase in non-erythroid cells.[1,2] PBG deaminase limits the rate of heme synthesis in human liver once basal ALAS activity increases more than a few fold. ALAS-1 and ALAS-2 activities are regulated by separate mechanisms and there are tissue-specific differences in the regulation of ALAS-1.[6]

Regulation of ALAS-1 in liver and other tissues

A large number of lipophilic compounds of diverse structure, including many drugs and some steroid hormones, induce ALAS-1 in mammalian and avian liver and, to a lesser extent, kidney and small intestine but not in other tissues. Induction is repressed by heme.[1–3,6] Because the turnover of mitochondrial ALAS-1 is rapid, with a half-life of 70 min in rat liver, repression of the formation of mitochondrial ALAS-1 by heme provides an effective mechanism for rapidly decreasing hepatic ALAS activity. Since the discovery of this effect of heme by Granick in 1966,[38] the concept that hepatocytes contain an as yet unidentified regulatory heme pool that both supplies heme for hemoprotein synthesis and acts to repress induction of ALAS-1 has been supported by a large number of experiments in animals and cell culture systems.[6] Depletion of this pool by hemoprotein assembly would then lead to increased ALAS-1 activity and restoration of the heme pool to equilibrium.

Three mechanisms by which heme prevents induction of hepatic ALAS-1 activity have been identified: inhibition of translocation to the mitochondrial matrix, destabilization of mRNA and inhibition of transcription. In 1972 Kikuchi and colleagues discovered that heme blocks the import of ALAS-1 into mitochondria.[39] Pre-ALAS-1 contains 3 copies of a conserved heme regulatory motif (HRM) that is also present in heme oxygenase-2, heme lyase, catalase, the reticulocyte kinase HRI and the yeast transcriptional activator HAP1, all of which interact with heme.[40,41] Mutation of the cysteine residues to serine in all 3 HRMs abolishes heme inhibition of ALAS-1 import.[42] Heme probably binds to the HRMs while pre-ALAS-1 is in the cytoplasm, thus preventing unfolding and translocation across the mitochondrial membranes. Heme also decreases the increase in ALAS-1 mRNA concentrations that accompany induction of ALAS-1 activity by drugs in avian and mammalian hepatocytes.[6] At least part of this effect is caused by destabilization of ALAS-1 mRNA. In avian hepatocytes, this appears to be the only mechanism and the heme effect may be mediated by a labile protein.[43] In mammals, inhibition of transcription of the ALAS-1 gene may also contribute to the decrease in mRNA levels.[6]

Many lipophilic drugs that induce ALAS-1 also induce specific CYPs.[1,6] In theory, induction of ALAS-1 could be entirely a secondary effect, mediated through depletion of the regulatory heme pool in response to increased synthesis of apocytochrome P450. In avian hepatocytes, drugs increase transcription; induction induces mRNAs for ALAS-1 and cytochrome P450 simultaneously and the transcription rate is not altered by heme.[43] In rats, there is evidence to suggest that transcription is increased both by a direct action and by derepression by heme,[6] but the relative contributions of these two mechanisms remain undetermined.

Little is known about the regulation of transcription of the ALAS-1 gene. Analysis of the rat gene promoter has identified 2 nuclear respiratory factor-1 (NRF-1) binding sites that together are essential for basal expression, and are likely to be involved in co-ordination of synthesis of respiratory chain subunits.[44] Other regions necessary for basal expression have been identified by deletion analysis but the molecular basis of tissue-specific induction is unknown.[6]

Regulation of ALAS-2 in erythroid cells

Initiation of erythroid differentiation by erythropoietin is accompanied by activation of transcription of erythroid-specific genes. The promoter regions of ALAS-2,[6] CPGOX,[25] PPOX,[27] FC[34] and the erythroid promoters of ALAD[9] and PBG deaminase[16] contain putative or func-

tional binding sites for GATA-1, NFE-2 and other erythroid-specific transcription factors that are also present in the globin and transferrin genes. Induction of enzyme activities in differentiating mouse erythroleukemia (MEL) cells was reported to be sequential, starting with ALAS.[45] However, more recent measurements of mRNA levels and enzyme activities suggest that late induction of the terminal enzymes does not limit heme synthesis during differentiation.[46,47] In human erythroblasts, FC activity exceeds ALAS activity throughout differentiation.[48]

In erythroid cells, the rate of heme formation is determined by iron supply.[3,49] The activity of ALAS-2 is regulated by iron and, in contrast to ALAS-1 in liver, is unaffected by drugs. The 5' untranslated region of mRNA for ALAS-2, encoded by exon 1, contains a stem-loop iron-responsive element (IRE) similar to the IREs of mRNAs for other iron-regulated proteins. Binding of the iron-regulatory proteins, IRP-1 and IRP-2, to the IRE blocks translation of ALAS-2. IRP-1 is a [4Fe-4S] iron-sulfur protein; when iron replete, it has aconitase but not IRE-binding activity. As cellular iron levels fall, iron is lost from the iron-sulfur cluster, aconitase activity declines and IRE-binding increases. Thus, lack of iron prevents synthesis of ALAS-2. IRP-2 concentrations are regulated by iron-dependent proteolysis.[49]

Heme at physiologic concentrations[3,6] does not repress or inhibit ALAS-2; indeed, heme concentrations increase during erythroid differentiation of MEL cells.[50] Experiments previously interpreted as showing feedback inhibition of ALAS by heme in reticulocytes[46] and MEL cells did not take account of probable changes in intracellular iron levels.[3] In addition, there is now evidence that the HRMs in pre-ALAS-2 may not function under physiologic conditions.[42]

However, heme has a central role in co-ordinating iron supply and globin synthesis with heme formation. It inhibits acquisition of iron from transferrin by erythroid cells,[3] thus decreasing its own synthesis. Heme also controls globin synthesis at the translation level by inactivating an erythroid-specific eIF-2α protein kinase (heme-regulated inhibitor kinase, HRI) which, in the absence of heme, catalyzes phosphorylation of the α subunit of the initiation factor eIF-2, thus inhibiting translation of erythroid mRNAs, including globin mRNA.[6]

METABOLISM AND EXCRETION OF HEME PRECURSORS

There is little alternative metabolism of heme precursors so the quantities that are excreted reflect the extent of loss of intermediates from the pathway. In normal circumstances, the total daily excretion of heme precursors represents <2.5% of the amount of ALA used for heme synthesis. Table 7.2 shows reference ranges for heme precursors in urine, feces, plasma and erythrocytes from normal adults. Ranges for children are similar,[51–53] although urinary porphyrin excretion expressed per mmol creatinine tends to be

Table 7.2 Heme precursors in normal adult urine, feces and blood.

	Urine*	Feces*	Plasma	Erythrocytes
Porphobilinogen (PBG) (μmol/day)	0–11			
5-Aminolevulinic acid (ALA) (μmol/day)	0–46			
Total porphyrin (nmol/1)	40–320	0–200 (nmol/g dry weight)	0.5–10.5	90–1700
Porphyrins (mean % of total)				
Proto-	—	72.5		>90 (>80% zinc-protoporphyrin)
Copro- (% isomer Type III)	76.8 (50–60)	23.5 (5–15)		<10
Isocopro-	—	0.03		—
Pentacarboxylic (5CO$_2$H)	2.3	1.7		—
Hexacarboxylic (6CO$_2$H)	0.8	0.6		—
Heptacarboxylic (7CO$_2$H)	4.5	0.2		—
Uro-	15.3	1.0		—

*Figures for porphyrins in urine and feces include porphyrins derived from porphyrinogens by oxidation during analysis.

highest in infants and to decline with increasing age. Non-enzymatic oxidation of porphyrinogen occurs within the body and during excretion, so that urine contains variable proportions of porphyrins and porphyrinogens.

ALA and PBG are excreted exclusively in the urine while porphyrins and porphyrinogens are excreted in the urine and bile. Hydrophilic porphyrin(ogen)s with >4 acidic side chains are preferentially excreted in the urine while the less water-soluble compounds, such as protoporphyrin, are restricted to the bile (Table 7.2). Coproporphyrins I and III are excreted by both routes with preferential excretion of the I isomer in the bile. This isomer is a substrate for the canalicular multispecific organic anion transporter (cMOAT),[54] encoded by the MRP2 gene.[55] Mutations in this gene cause the anion transport defect in Dubin-Johnson syndrome,[55] which shows a characteristic increase in the proportion of coproporphyrin I in urine.[57] Much more commonly, even mild cholestasis from any cause diverts sufficient coproporphyrin I from the bile to cause coproporphyrinuria.[57,58] Other causes of coproporphyrinuria include alcoholism, drugs that induce hepatic CYPs and lead poisoning.[58]

The main porphyrin in human bile is coproporphyrin; relatively little protoporphyrin is present. This pattern is reversed in feces (Table 7.2). Much of the protoporphyrin and related dicarboxylic porphyrin in normal feces is formed within the colon by the action of anaerobic micro-organisms on heme from the diet, minor gastrointestinal bleeding and other sources.[59]

BIOCHEMICAL AND MOLECULAR GENETICS

The enzymatic and molecular basis of the porphyrias has been extensively investigated since the discovery in 1970 by Marver and colleagues that AIP is caused by an enzyme deficiency and not by primary overproduction of ALA.[60] All enzyme deficiencies in the porphyrias are inherited (Table 7.3), apart from the hepatic UROD defect in sporadic (type I) PCT. The enzyme defect in each inherited porphyria is present in all tissues; the only exception being the uncommon form of acute intermittent porphyria (AIP) in which mutations are located in the section of the gene that encodes only the ubiquitous isoenzyme.[16]

Mutational analysis has revealed extensive allelic heterogeneity in all the porphyrias;[61] >120 mutations of the PBG deaminase gene that cause AIP have been identified.[61,62] Outside geographic areas where founder effects occur, most mutations are restricted to one or a few families and patients with autosomal recessive or homozygous variant porphyrias are often heteroallelic. In the autosomal dominant porphyrias, mutations cause complete or near complete loss of function; enzyme activities are therefore close to 50% of normal in those who inherit the enzyme deficiencies that underly these disorders.[1,2,63] Not unexpectedly, those mutations that have been characterized in the much rarer autosomal recessive and homozygous variant porphyrias preserve some activity from at least one allele.[61]

The kinetics of the heme biosynthetic pathway allow increases in substrate concentrations to compensate for the enzyme deficiencies and maintain normal or near normal rates of heme formation. These compensatory changes are brought about through operation of the regulatory mechanisms described above. The reason why compensatory changes should be more marked in either the liver or bone marrow, according to the particular enzyme that is defective (Table 7.3), remains an intriguing and largely unexplained phenomenon.

In the autosomal recessive and homozygous variant porphyrias, enzyme activities are usually <20% of normal (Table 7.3), heme precursor overproduction is persistent and symptoms are usually present from an early age. In contrast, low penetrance is a striking and important clinical feature of the autosomal dominant porphyrias. In AIP, variegate porphyria (VP) and hereditary porphyria (HCP) >80% of

Table 7.3 Inherited enzyme defects in the porphyrias.[1,2,63,131]

Mode of inheritance	Disorder	Deficient enzyme	Enzyme activity (% mean normal)	Clinical penetrance (%)	Main site of heme precursor overproduction
Autosomal dominant	AIP	PBG deaminase	40–64	<20	Liver
	PCT (type II)	UROD	41–57	<20	Liver
	HCP	CPGOX	50	<20	Liver
	VP	PPOX	4–20	<20	Liver
	EPP	FC	19–37[b], 32–49[c]	<20	Bone marrow
Homozygous variants	Homozygous AIP	PBG deaminase	1–17	100	Liver
	HEP	UROD	3–25	100	Liver
	Homozygous HCP	CPGOX	10	100	Liver
	Harderoporphyria	CPGOX	10	100	Liver
	Homozygous VP	PPOX		100	Liver
Autosomal recessive	ADP	ALAD	2–12	100	Liver
	CEP	UROS	2–27	100	Bone marrow
	EPP[a]	FC	6	100	Bone marrow

[a]Uncommon form of EPP; clinical phenotype indistinguishable from autosomal dominant EPP; [b]Clinically overt; [c]Asymptomatic individuals.

affected individuals never develop symptoms; most of these have no detectable overproduction of heme precursors (latent porphyria) while others have heme precursor overproduction without symptoms (subclinical or latent porphyria). Symptomatic and latent porphyria often co-exist in the same family and neither enzyme activities nor types of mutation differ between unrelated individuals with overt or latent disease. The explanation for the low penetrance of the autosomal dominant acute porphyrias is uncertain. Although environmental and endocrine factors are undoubtedly important, they do not appear to provide the whole explanation.[64] Inherited factors determined by distant loci may also contribute. In erythropoietic protoporphyria (EPP) and type II PCT, enzyme activities are lower in those with overt disease.[63,65] Mechanisms determining penetrance in these disorders are discussed below.

PATHOGENESIS OF CLINICAL MANIFESTATIONS

The metabolic disturbances of porphyria are associated with two distinct types of clinical manifestation: skin lesions and acute neurovisceral cases (Table 7.1). The former result from photosensitization of the skin by porphyrins; their pathogenesis is well understood and they can readily be reproduced experimentally. In contrast, the mechanism of the neurologic manifestations remains uncertain.

CUTANEOUS MANIFESTATIONS

Patients with cutaneous porphyria present clinically in 1 of 2 ways:

- acute photosensitivity without skin fragility, a reaction which is seen only in EPP;
- skin fragility and subepidermal bullae, often associated

with hypertrichosis and patchy pigmentation, features which characterize all other cutaneous porphyrias.

In spite of these differences, the histopathologic changes in light-exposed skin are qualitatively similar in all porphyrias. The characteristic finding is the presence of amorphous, hyaline, PAS-positive material in and around the walls of small blood vessels in the dermis and, often, also at the dermo-epidermal junction.[66,67] This material is derived from the walls and contents of blood vessels and represents the cumulative, reparative response to repeated cycles of endothelial cell injury with local leakage of vascular contents.[68] Bullae are formed by a split in the lamina lucida of the basement membrane;[69] dermal papillae, stiffened by hyaline deposits, project into the floor and there is no surrounding inflammatory infiltrate.

These changes are provoked by the oxygen-dependent action of light at wavelengths around 400 nm on porphyrins in the dermis. Light at this wavelength is strongly absorbed by porphyrins (Soret absorption peak), penetrates the deeper layers of the dermis and passes through window glass. Absorption of light energy converts a porphyrin to a singlet excited state which either returns rapidly to the ground state with emission of red light (fluorescence) or undergoes intersystem crossing to the longer-lived triplet state. Triplet-state porphyrins react with molecular oxygen by energy transfer to give singlet oxygen or, less efficiently, by electron transfer to form superoxide anion. They may also directly initiate other free radical reactions.

Singlet oxygen is the most important mediator of photodamage to the skin. Since it is short-lived, the site of photodamage is determined largely by the distribution of porphyrins within the cell. Protoporphyrin has particular affinity for membrane lipids while more hydrophilic porphyrins preferentially accumulate in the lower dermis and cells of the basement membrane zone. These differences in distribution may explain the clinical differences between

EPP and the bullous porphyrias. Porphyrin-catalyzed, photodynamic reactions damage proteins, lipids and DNA[70] and may activate complement,[71] degranulate mast cells[72] and enhance degradation of dermal components by metalloproteinases.[73]

NEUROLOGIC MANIFESTATIONS

Abdominal pain, mental confusion and peripheral neuropathy typify acute neurovisceral attacks of porphyria. All 3 features are believed to be neurologic in origin and to be caused by a transient metabolic disturbance that affects the peripheral, autonomic and central nervous systems.[74,75] Associated histopathologic lesions include axonal degeneration and chromatolysis, particularly of the anterior horn cells of the spinal cord and brain stem nuclei, with some secondary demyelination. During recovery, axon regeneration progresses from the extremities.

Acute attacks of porphyria are always associated with induction of hepatic ALAS-1 activity and a marked increase in production of ALA over the basal level for that patient. These changes are often provoked by drugs, particularly those that induce CYP proteins. Numerous hypotheses have attempted to relate them to neuronal dysfunction. Attention has focused on 3 putative mechanisms that are not mutually exclusive:

- neurotoxicity of ALA;
- neurotransmitter abnormalities secondary to hepatic heme deficiency;
- neuronal heme deficiency.[75]

Neurovisceral attacks are *always* associated with overproduction of ALA. They do not occur in porphyrias in which ALA excretion is normal and do occur in hereditary tyrosinemia when ALA accumulates secondary to inhibition of ALAD by succinylacetone.[10] However, there is no clear dose-response relationship between ALA concentrations and neuronal dysfunction; asymptomatic patients often excrete excess ALA.

Various effects of ALA on neuronal function have been demonstrated in animal experiments and *in vitro* preparations, but their physiologic relevance is uncertain. Administration of ALA to normal subjects has no discernible effects at plasma concentrations similar to those during acute attacks.[76] The blood-brain barrier is relatively impermeable to ALA; concentrations in CSF (usually <12 nmol/l) are about 10-fold lower than in plasma.[77] At these concentrations, ALA which is structurally similar to γ-aminobutyric acid (GABA) acts as a partial GABA antagonist *in vitro*.[78,79] The low plasma metalonin concentrations found in acute porphyria have been attributed to an effect of ALA on pineal GABA receptors.[80] Direct evidence is required for other postulated actions of ALA on neuronal function in acute porphyria.

There is evidence for heme deficiency in the liver in acute porphyria. Administration of heme reverses the metabolic abnormalities,[81] enhances CYP function[82] and reactivates tryptophan dioxygenase.[83] Decreased tryptophan dioxygenase activity in the liver leads to increased delivery of tryptophan to the brain and formation of serotonin (5-HT). Plasma 5-HT concentrations are increased in acute porphyria[83] and serotonergic effects may underlie some clinical symptoms, particularly those ascribed to the autonomic nervous system.[75] There is little evidence for heme deficiency in the nervous system itself. Exogenous heme does not appear to enter the CNS.[75] Neuronal ALAS-1 is not induced by drugs that provoke acute porphyria.[84] Nevertheless, the possibility of impaired function of mitochondrial cytochromes, nitric oxide synthase and other hemoproteins within the nervous system requires further investigation.

Although the metabolic abnormalities of acute porphyria can readily be reproduced in animals given chemicals that inhibit heme synthesis,[1] the neurologic disorder has not been reproduced. Transgenic mice with 30% of normal PBG deaminase activity have recently been produced.[85] In these animals, barbiturates provoke overproduction of ALA but not acute neuronal dysfunction. However, the mice have chronic ataxia and poor agility and the histology of peripheral nerves shows an axonal neuropathy, even in mice who have never received drugs.[75] These changes may resemble homozygous AIP (see below) more than acute porphyria.

AUTOSOMAL RECESSIVE PORPHYRIAS

5-AMINOLEVULINATE DEHYDRATASE DEFICIENCY PORPHYRIA

This very rare autosomal recessive disorder was described in 1979 by Doss *et al*.[86] The variable clinical features include attacks of acute porphyria after puberty,[86,87] persistent hypotonia from birth with intermittent episodes of anorexia, muscle pain and polyneuropathy,[88] and mild, predominantly motor polyneuropathy (described in a previously asymptomatic 63-year-old man with a myeloproliferative disorder).[89] Erythrocyte ALAD activities were <5% of normal in all patients and all had markedly increased urinary ALA, coproporphyrin III and erythrocyte zinc protoporphyrin concentrations (Table 7.4). Mutations in the ALAD gene have been identified in 2 patients; both were compound heterozygotes.[90,91] One inactivating mutation (R240W) lies in the substrate-binding site close to the active-site lysine (K252) while another (G133R) disrupts the highly conserved zinc-binding site. Enzyme activities in carrier relatives were close to half of normal. Such carriers are more susceptible to the effects of lead intoxication than normal individuals.[92] ADP itself does not produce significant hematologic abnormalities.

ADP is differentiated from other porphyrias by the characteristic pattern of urinary and erythrocyte abnormalities (Table 7.4). This pattern is identical to that of lead

Table 7.4 Patterns of overproduction of heme precursors in the porphyrias.

Disorder	Urine		Feces porphyrins	Erythrocyte porphyrins	Plasma fluorescence emission peak (nm)
	PBG/ALA	Porphyrins			
ALA dehydratase deficiency	ALA	Copro III	Not increased	Zn-proto	—
Acute intermittent porphyria	PBG > ALA	(Porphyrin mainly from PBG)	Not increased	Not increased	615
Congenital erythropoietic porphyria	Not increased	Uro I Copro I	Copro I	Zn-proto, proto Copro I, Uro I	615
Porphyria cutanea tarda	Not increased	Uro Hepta[b]	Isocopro, Hepta[b]	Not increased	615
Hereditary coproporphyria	PBG > ALA[a]	Copro III (Porphyrin from PBG)	Copro III	Not increased	615
Variegate porphyria	PBG > ALA[a]	Copro III (Porphyrin from PBG)	Proto IX > Copro III, X-porphyrin	Not increased	624–626
Protoporphyria	Not increased	Not increased	± Protoporphyrin	Protoporphyrin	632

[a]PBG and ALA excretion may be normal when only skin lesions are present.
[b]Hexa- and penta-carboxylic porphyrins and coproporphyrin are increased to a smaller extent. Uroporphyrin is a mixture of type I and III isomers; heptacarboxylic porphyrin is mainly type III.
ALA = 5-aminolevulinate; PBG = porphobilinogen

poisoning which needs to be excluded by blood lead measurement and demonstration that the decreased ALAD activity is not reversed by sulfhydryl-group reagents. Treatment is as for other acute porphyrias (see below). Neither carbohydrate loading nor hematin had any noticeable clinical effect on the child with ADP.[88]

CONGENITAL ERYTHROPOIETIC PORPHYIA

Congenital erythropoietic porphyria (CEP; Gunther's disease; hereditary erythropoietic porphyria) is by far the most severe cutaneous porphyria. Since the first description by Schultz in 1874 of a patient with the striking photomutilation that is characteristic of this condition, about 130 cases have been reported.[93] The disease occurs worldwide in all races; its prevalence in the UK is about 2–3×10^6 live births.

Inheritance and molecular pathology

CEP is inherited in an autosomal recessive fashion. Erythrocyte UROS activities are decreased to <20% in patients and to around 50% in carriers who are always asymptomatic. This defect leads to massive overproduction of hydroxymethylbilane, mainly in erythroid cells in the bone marrow. At least 22 mutations in the UROS gene that cause CEP in homozygotes or compound heterozygotes have been characterized.[18,94] One mutation (C73R) is present on about 40% of alleles from European patients; the others are restricted to one or a few families. The C73R mutation decreases UROS activity by >98%,[18] and C73R homozygotes have particularly severe disease. The effect of other mutations on enzyme activity varies; some of the least severe

have been identified only in the mild, late-onset form of CEP.[18,94]

Clinical features

CEP ranges in severity from fatal hydrops fetalis,[95] through severe disease starting in infancy, to milder forms that start in later childhood or in adulthood. Most patients have the severe, infantile-onset form.[93] Common early signs are blisters and erosions on light-exposed skin and reddish-brown staining of diapers by urinary porphyrins. Porphyrins accumulate in amniotic fluid throughout pregnancy and the mother may notice brown liquor at the onset of labour. The severe and persistent skin lesions resemble those of other bullous porphyrias: subepidermal bullae, skin fragility with erosions, milia, hypertrichosis, particularly of the face, and patchy pigmentation are all common. Bullae and erosions may become infected and heal with scarring; repetitive cycles lead to photomutilation with erosion and resorption of the terminal phalanges, contractures, destruction of the ears, nose and eyelids, and scarring alopecia. Ocular complications may lead to blindness.[93]

Clinical manifestations are not confined to the skin. Hemolytic anemia and splenomegaly are common. Thrombocytopenia secondary to hypersplenism may cause purpura, bruising and hemorrhagic blisters; extensive bruising and anemia with hepatosplenomegaly may be present at birth. Porphyrin is deposited in growing bones; the teeth are brown (erythrodontia) and fluoresce red in ultraviolet (UVA) light. Other skeletal changes include resorption secondary to photomutilation, expansion of the bone marrow with osteopenia and decreased bone density with pathologic fractures. Vitamin D metabolism may be impaired by avoidance of sunlight.

Late onset forms are milder. Skin lesions are often similar to PCT. Erythrodontia is absent if tooth development ceased before the onset of porphyrin overproduction. However, in contrast to PCT, most patients have mild hemolysis, which may be fully compensated, and splenomegaly. Occasionally, skin lesions are mild enough to be overlooked until patients present with thrombocytopenia or their discolored urine leads to investigation for hematuria.

Metabolic abnormalities and diagnosis

Accumulated hydroxymethylbilane rapidly cyclizes to uroporphyrinogen I, some of which is metabolized to coproporphyrinogen I, before oxidation to the corresponding porphyrins. Large amounts of these porphyrins are excreted in the urine and feces, and accumulate in erythrocytes and plasma to give the diagnostic pattern shown in Table 7.4. Erythrocyte protoporphyrin may also be increased as in other hemolytic anemias.

The diagnosis is established by demonstrating massive overproduction of isomer type I porphyrins; UROS assay is not essential for this purpose.[96] Reliable prenatal diagnosis can be made by measuring uroporphyrin I in amniotic fluid together with DNA mutation analysis.[97]

Hematologic abnormalities

Abnormalities within the red cell series are well documented but less attention has been given to thrombocytopenia and leukopenia, both of which may be present at birth.[93,98,99] Most patients have an hemolytic anemia with normochromic, normocytic erythrocytes, reticulocytosis, unconjugated hyperbilirubinemia and increased urobilinogen excretion. Increased erythrocyte PBG deaminase activity reflects the increased proportion of young erythrocytes in the circulation.[98] The degree of anemia varies both between patients and with time in individuals. Some patients require regular transfusion; in others there may be complete compensation. Bone marrow examination shows normoblastic hyperplasia; most normoblasts and reticulocytes contain sufficient porphyrin to fluorescence red in UVA light. Fluorescence is mainly associated with the nucleus; fluorescent normoblasts, but not non-fluorescent cells, are morphologically abnormal with heme-containing nuclear inclusion bodies.

The mechanism of the hemolysis is uncertain.[98] Hemolysis is not a feature of EPP, where protoporphyrin accumulates in erythrocytes, so it is presumably related to accumulation of hydrophilic porphyrins, such as uroporphyrin I. Uroporphyrin-containing cells have an intrinsic membrane defect,[98,99] which may result from oxidative photodamage in the superficial circulation. However, this is unlikely to be the only explanation; hemolysis is not related to light exposure[98] and may occur *in utero*. Defective erythrocytes are removed by the spleen; there is little evidence for direct photolysis in the circulation, although this can readily be produced *in vitro*.

Erythroid cells are the main source of porphyrins in CEP. Successful transplantation reduces porphyrin formation by >95%.[100] Most of the porphyrin probably comes from destruction of cells within the bone marrow or soon after their release into the circulation.[99] Ineffective erythropoiesis is markedly increased in CEP and ablation of cells prior to transplantation reduces plasma porphyrin concentrations to normal within a few days.

Treatment and prognosis

Allogeneic bone marrow transplantation (BMT) is the only curative treatment for children with severe CEP.[100,101] When bone marrow or umbilical cord blood is not available from an HLA–compatible sibling donor, gene transfer therapy remains a potential future alternative. The enzyme defect has been corrected *in vitro* by retroviral gene transfer to bone marrow cells.[102]

Other treatments are palliative. Prevention of severe skin damage requires strict avoidance of sunlight[93] and good skin care with prompt treatment of secondary infections. Reflectant sunscreen ointments rarely provide sufficient protection by themselves; β-carotene is similarly ineffective in most patients. Suppression of erythropoiesis by hypertransfusion[103] or hematin[104] may temporarily decrease porphyrin formation but long-term use is not practical. Interruption of the enterohepatic circulation by trapping porphyrins in the gut with activated charcoal is ineffective.[105] Hemolytic anemia may require repeated transfusion with appropriate measures to prevent iron overload. Splenectomy may decrease the need for transfusion but often has only a temporary effect. The antioxidants, α-tecopherol and ascorbic acid, may diminish hemolysis in some patients.[93] Although often socially and physically disabled, most patients with severe, infantile-onset CEP survive to at least the age of 40 years; modern supportive care should improve their life expectancy.

AUTOSOMAL DOMINANT ACUTE HEPATIC PORPHYRIAS

The life-threatening acute neurovisceral attacks that characterize the three autosomal dominant acute hepatic porphyrias, AIP, HCP and VP (Table 7.1), are the most important clinical manifestation of the porphyrias. They are rare in children; it is usual for all 3 conditions to be clinically and biochemically latent before puberty. In pediatric practice, identification and management of latent AIP, HCP or VP is a much commoner problem than diagnosis and treatment of the acute attack.

AIP is the commonest of the acute hepatic porphyrias. It occurs in all races. The estimated prevalence of clinically overt AIP in western Europe is about 1–2/100 000 population.[106] Since at least 80% of those who inherit AIP are asymptomatic throughout life, the gene frequency is higher;

recent surveys of blood donors suggest about 1/1500 population.[107] VP is less common; about 1.3/100 000 population in Finland[108] and probably elsewhere in Europe. In South Africa, about 10 000–20 000 of the Afrikaans population have inherited VP from a single ancestor.[109] HCP, with an estimated prevalence of 2/1 000 000 population, is rare.

The acute neurovisceral attacks are identical in AIP, HCP and VP and are the only clinical manifestation of AIP. In adults, 60–70% of patients with VP present with skin lesions, clinically indistinguishable from PCT, while the rest have either acute attacks alone (15–20%) or an acute attack combined with skin lesions (15–20%).[108,110,111] Acute attacks are the main clinical feature of HCP; about one-third of cases also have mild skin lesions.[112]

Molecular pathology

Acute intermittent porphyria

Over 120 mutations that cause acute intermittent porphyria (AIP) have been identified in the PBG deaminase gene.[61,62] Four are located in or around exon 1 and cause an uncommon variant of AIP that involves only the ubiquitous isoenzyme, leaving erythroid PBG deaminase activity unimpaired. Systematic surveys of the molecular epidemiology of AIP in France (121 families) and Finland (39 families) have revealed similar patterns of mutation.[62,113] About half the mutations were clustered in exons 10, 12 and 14 and about half were missense mutations. Most mutations were restricted to one or a few families; prevalence rates for the commonest were <5% in France and 11% in Finland. A single mutation (W198X) is common in northern Sweden, where the high prevalence of AIP, about 1/1500 population, is explained by a founder effect.[114] Three *de novo* mutations have been reported and the mutation rate has been estimated as about 3%.[62,113,115] In the 20% of patients who present without a family history, investigation usually reveals latent porphyria in preceding generations.

The availability of a 3-dimensional model of human PBG

deaminase derived from the structure of the *E. coli* enzyme, together with site-directed mutagenesis and *in vitro* expression of mutants, has provided insights into the mechanisms by which AIP mutations affect enzyme function.[13,14] This approach has been particularly informative for the <40% of missense mutations that alter catalytic activity without destabilizing the enzyme. Most mutations appear to decrease activity by at least 95%. In view of this rather uniform effect and the extensive allelic heterogeneity, the apparent lack of any correlation between disease severity or penetrance and type of mutation is perhaps not surprising.

Variegate porphyria and hereditary coproporphyria

Genealogic studies indicate that the 10 000–20 000 individuals with variegate porphyria (VP) in South Africa are all descended from a couple from the Netherlands who married at the Cape in 1688.[109] Molecular investigations have confirmed this hypothesis by showing that >95% of South African VP families share the same mutation (R59W) in the PPOX gene.[116] This mutation has been identified in the Netherlands[117] but not elsewhere in Europe (unpublished information). Outside South Africa and Finland, where founder effects operate,[116] VP shows extensive allelic heterogeneity. Over 60 mutations, mostly restricted to one or a few families, have been identified (unpublished information).[118,119] Hereditary coproporphyria (HCP) is also heterogeneous at the DNA level.[120]

Clinical features

Acute neurovisceral attacks may occur as children, particularly girls, enter puberty but symptoms at a younger age are extremely rare. A few cases have been reported, including 1 infant aged 4 months.[121,122] Most children with acute porphyria have AIP. As in adults, attacks almost invariably start with severe abdominal pain in any quadrant and often radiating to the back, thighs or buttocks (Table 7.5).[1,2,111] Physical signs are often absent; there may occasionally be

Table 7.5 Clinical features of acute porphyria.[111]

Symptom/sign	Percentages of number of acute attacks			
	Goldberg 1959 (n = 50)	Stein and Tschudy 1970 (n = 46)	Mustajoki and Nordmann 1993 (n = 51)	Hift 1986–1995 (n = 92)
Abdominal pain	94	95	96	98
Non-abdominal pain	52	50	25	
Vomiting	88	43	84	85
Constipation	84	48	78	28
Psychologic symptoms	58	40	19	2
Convulsions	16	20		5
Muscle weakness	68	60	8	7
Sensory loss	38	26		2
Hypertension (diastolic blood pressure >85 mmHg)	54	36	57	68
Tachycardia (>80/min)	64	80	79	57
Hyponatremia (<135 nmol/l)			32	39

some guarding but no true peritonism. Anorexia, vomiting and constipation are common. Central nervous symptoms include mental confusion and convulsions. The latter may be provoked by hyponatremia, caused in some patients by inappropriate secretion of vasopressin, or result from metabolic affects on the CNS.[75] Severe attacks may progress within days to a predominantly motor neuropathy which may remain peripheral or become generalized with respiratory paralysis. Moderate tachycardia and hypertension are common; patients with fluctuating blood pressure and/or arrhythmias are at particular risk from cardiac arrest.

Most patients have only one severe attack; a minority suffer from repeated attacks over several years. Regular premenstrual attacks may occur in young women and may be initiated by the return of menstruation after pregnancy. The prognosis for most patients is good; few attacks now end fatally, particularly if the diagnosis is made early.[64,123] The neuropathy reverses slowly as axons grow back towards the periphery. Long-term complications include physical disability, hypertension, chronic renal failure and an increased risk of hepatocellular carcinoma.[1,2,111] There is little evidence that acute porphyria causes long-term psychiatric illness, apart from generalized anxiety.[124]

In adults, drugs, particularly those that induce CYPs, and menstruation provoke most attacks.[1,2,64,106,111] Other precipitants include alcohol, calorie restriction, infection and stress. In the past, both pregnancy and general surgery have been hazardous but the dangers seem largely to be related to use of inappropriate drugs and anesthetic agents. Provided the diagnosis of porphyria is known in advance and the patient is managed accordingly, neither need now be discouraged.[111]

Diagnosis

The diagnosis of an acute attack of AIP, HCP or VP is established by demonstrating increased excretion of PBG in urine (Table 7.4). There are 2 main reasons for delay in diagnosis. The more important is failing to consider the possibility and therefore not asking for the appropriate investigations. This is particularly a problem when there is no family history of porphyria, when the clinical presentation is atypical or the disease unexpected, as in a young child. The second reason is inappropriate laboratory investigation.

The method of choice for measurement of PBG in urine is ion exchange chromatography followed by reaction with Ehrlich's aldehyde reagent (p-aminodimethylbenzaldehyde in HCl) to give a red compound.[96,125] Screening tests, such as the Watson-Schwartz test, are less sensitive and less specific.[96,125] Positive screening tests should always be confirmed by a specific, quantitative method. In AIP, PBG and ALA excretion usually remains increased for many weeks after the onset of an acute attack. In VP and HCP, excretion falls rapidly and may be normal within a week. Thus, fecal and plasma porphyrin analyses, in addition to quantitative determination of PBG and ALA, are essential investigations

if either of these disorders is suspected (Table 7.4). Once the diagnosis of acute porphyria has been established, AIP, HCP and VP are differentiated by measuring fecal and plasma porphyrins (Table 7.4). Enzyme assays are less reliable and rarely necessary for this purpose. The plasma in VP contains an unique protein-bound porphyrin with a fluorescence emission peak at 624–626 nm.[126]

Treatment

The treatment of acute porphyria in children and adults is similar.[1,2,81,106,111] Any precipitating agents should be withdrawn. Supportive measures include analgesia, which is likely to require opiates; sedation with promazine or chlorpromazine, which may reduce the requirement for analgesics; suppression of vomiting with prochlorperazine; and correction of any dehydration. Maintenance of an adequate calorie intake is important and may require nasogastric feeding.

Two maneuvres reverse the metabolic defect in the liver by decreasing ALAS-1 activity and consequent ALA and PBG formation: carbohydrate loading[127] and intravenous administration of hematin.[81,128] The latter has now largely replaced the former as the treatment of choice. If carbohydrate is used, the large amounts recommended (400 g glucose or fructose/day) are more easily and safely given through a nasogastric tube than intravenously. Intravenous administration of 5% or 10% dextrose may provoke hyponatremia and should be avoided. Uncontrolled data suggest that intravenous heme arginate (Normosang) is highly effective.[81] If given early in an acute attack, it decreases analgesic requirement and reduces length of stay in hospital, and the use of hematin is probably responsible for the decrease in the frequency of severe neuropathy in recent years.[111] However, it will not reverse an established neuropathy. The effectiveness of hematin may be limited by induction of hepatic heme oxygenase (HO-1) if repeated doses are given at short intervals; co-administration of inhibitors of HO-1 may prolong its action.[128]

Repeated acute attacks may be difficult to control. When these are regularly pre-menstrual, suppresion of menstruation with GnRH agonists is often effective.[2,111] Estrogen replacement therapy, under regular gynecologic monitoring, to prevent osteoporosis and other side-effects appears to be safe and is necessary if GnRH agonists are continued for 2–3 years as is usual. In other cases, repeated administration of heme arginate, particularly as a single dose (3 mg/kg) to abort an attack, may be required but is not always successful.

LATENT ACUTE PORPHYRIA

Identification

Identification of asymptomatic, affected individuals, so that they can be advised to avoid agents that provoke acute attacks, is an essential part of the management of families

Table 7.6 Identification of latent acute autosomal dominant porphyrias.[63,129,130]

Disease	Test	Limitations	Sensitivity	Specificity
AIP	Urinary PBG	Normal before puberty	Low	High
	Erythrocyte PBG deaminase	Not before age of 8 months	Overlap between AIP and normal ranges contains 10–20% of asymptomatic relatives	
HCP	Fecal coproporphyrin (isomer III/I ratio)	Sensitivity in children not established	High[a]	High[a]
	CPGOX measurement	Requires fresh lymphocytes or cell culture; technically complex	ND	ND
VP	Fecal porphyrins; copro isomer ratio	Normal before puberty	36% at age 15 or over	
	Fluorescence emission spectroscopy of plasma	Normal before puberty	86% at age 15 or over	100%[b]
	PPOX measurement	Requires fresh lymphocytes or cell culture; technically complex	ND	ND

[a]For adults; [b]When erythrocyte free protoporphyrin concentration is normal.
AIP = acute intermittent porphyria; HCP = hereditary coproporphyria; VP = variegate porphyria; PBG = porphobilinogen; CPGOX = coprophorphyrinogen; PPOX = protoporphyrinogen oxidase; ND = not determined; overlap between activities for affected and unaffected individuals small.

with AIP, HCP or VP. Detection of latent porphyria during childhood before there is any real risk of acute porphyria is useful.

Metabolite and enzymatic methods for the identification of latent porphyria are summarized in Table 7.6. Metabolite measurements are normal before puberty with the possible exception of the fecal coproporphyrin isomer ratio in some children with latent HCP.[129] Assay of PBG deaminase activity in erythrocytes is currently the most widely used method for detection of latent AIP. Enzyme activity decreases markedly as erythrocytes age and is therefore dependent on the age distribution of the circulating cells. Its use should be restricted to hematologically normal, healthy individuals over the age of 8 months. Interpretation is also complicated by the overlap between the upper range of AIP activities and the lower range of normal[1,2,63] and by the uncommon variant of AIP in which the erythroid isoenzyme is unaffected. For these reasons, DNA methods are likely to become the method of choice.[62,113]

Enzyme methods for the detection of latent HCP and VP require nucleated cells and are technically more complex than PBG deaminase assay. As for AIP, DNA methods are more accurate and, once the mutation has been identified in the family, technically straightforward.[118,120] The mutation responsible for most VP in South Africa can now be detected by a simple *Ava I* digest of PCR-amplified genomic DNA.[116]

Prevention

Individuals with latent AIP, HCP or VP should be advised to avoid drugs that are known or, on experimental grounds, believed to provoke acute porphyria. Lists of safe and unsafe drugs have been published.[1,2,106] Prescribing for individuals with latent porphyria may be difficult. Outside those drugs that have repeatedly been associated with acute attacks, the choice often depends on assessing the benefit of using a drug against an uncertain risk; individuals vary unpredictably in their likelihood of developing acute porphyria both over time and in comparison with others. Previous use of a drug is no guarantee that a repeated course will be safe. In general, risks are greatest for those who have shown symptoms, particularly if recently, or have persistently high excretion of metabolites.[64] Daily monitoring of PBG excretion may help to predict an adverse reaction. Although the risks are far lower, prescribing policy for children should be as for adults.

Other measures to decrease the likelihood of acute porphyria include avoidance of alcohol, maintenance of a normal calorie intake with regular meals and wearing warning jewellery in case of an accident. There is little evidence to suggest that a high carbohydrate diet is necessary between attacks; the drawbacks of obesity are the same in porphyria as in other individuals. Patient support groups exist in several countries.

HOMOZYGOUS VARIANTS

This group of rare porphyrias is characterized by onset during childhood and severe enzyme deficiency (Table 7.3) with both parents showing biochemical features of the corresponding autosomal dominant porphyria, although there is only rarely a family history of overt porphyria in preceding generations. Clinical features are variable. In addition to those typical of adult porphyrias, there may be skeletal abnormalities, growth retardation and CNS dysfunction, suggesting that some of these enzyme defects impair intrauterine and later development. In spite of the severity of the enzyme defects, anemia is not a feature of this group of porphyrias, although erythrocyte zinc, and to a lesser extent free, protoporphyrin concentrations are increased. This erythrocyte abnormality is a constant, but unexplained, feature of homozygous variant and autosomal recessive porphyrias.

Homozygous acute intermittent porphyria

Homozygous AIP has the poorest prognosis of all porphyrias. Four children with this disorder have been described;[131] a fifth who had convulsions and bilateral cataracts probably also had homozygous AIP.[132] Psychomotor deterioration is progressive from birth with convulsions, ataxia, leukodystrophy and bilateral cataracts.[131,132] Three of the 5 affected children died by the age of 8 years. Attacks typical of acute porphyria have not been reported.

PBG and ALA excretion is markedly increased. Erythrocyte PBG deaminase activities range from 1 to 17% of normal.[131] All patients have been homo- or hetero-allelic for mutations at arginine codons in exon 10 of the PBG deaminase gene (R167Q; R167W; R173W). *In vitro* expression of these mutations shows 5% or less residual activity. All are known to cause clinically overt AIP in heterozygotes.

Homozygous hereditary coproporphyria

Severe deficiency of CPGOX is associated with 2 distinct syndromes. The first resembles HCP, except that skin lesions appear in childhood and growth is retarded.[63,133] CPGOX activity is < 10% of normal and coproporphyrin III excretion is markedly increased. One patient has been shown to be homoallelic for a mutation (R231W) that decreases both GPGOX activity and stability.[134]

The second syndrome, known as harderoporphyria, is characterized by markedly increased fecal excretion of harderoporphyrin, derived from the tricarboxylic intermediate of the CPGOX reaction (Fig. 7.1). Three families have been described.[135] Infants present with neonatal hyperbilirubinemia, hemolysis and blisters typical of porphyria. Progress after the neonatal period is uneventful although mild photosensitivity and compensated hemolytic anemia may persist. Mutations in exon 6 of the CPGOX gene, which alter substrate affinity, have been identified in 2 families.[135] The distinctive porphyrin excretory abnormality of harderoporphyria has not been identified in adults with overt porphyria and harderoporphyria may be a true autosomal recessive condition.

Homozygous variegate porphyria

At least 12 unrelated patients with homozygous VP have been described.[136,137] Apart from a 12-year-old girl with acute porphyria, who had no skin lesions and later died, all have developed skin fragility, subepidermal bullae and hypertrichosis before the age of 2 years. Other clinical manifestations include growth retardation, clinodactyly and flexion deformities of the fingers, mental retardation, convulsions and nystagmus; not all features are present in all patients.[138] Acute porphyria has been reported only in the one atypical patient without skin lesions. Several others are now adults and the continuing absence of acute attacks is a puzzling and unexplained feature.

The pattern of overproduction of heme precursors resembles VP (Table 7.4) both quantitatively and qualitatively. Increased PBG and ALA excretion has only been reported in the one atypical case. PPOX activities are < 20% of normal in patients[136,137] and 50–70% of normal in their parents who may have other biochemical features of VP, although they and their relatives only rarely have overt VP.[116] Patients are homoallelic for mutations that preserve some PPOX activity or heteroallelic for mutations, at least 1 of which preserves residual activity.[116,137]

UROPORPHYRINOGEN DECARBOXYLASE DEFICIENCY DISORDERS

Two cutaneous porphyrias result from decreased activity of UROD in the liver:

- porphyria cutanea tarda (PCT);
- hepatoerythropoietic porphyria (HEP).

PCT, the commonest of all porphyrias, with an incidence in the UK of about 2–5/1 000 000 population/year,[65] is mainly a disease of adults. The very much rarer HEP normally presents in early childhood.[138]

PORPHYRIA CUTANEA TARDA

Classification

About 80% of patients have sporadic or type I PCT (Table 7.1) in which UROD deficiency is restricted to the liver and there is no family history of overt PCT.[65] Another 20% have familial or type II PCT in which half the normal UROD activity is inherited in an autosomal dominant fashion and the deficiency is present in all tissues. Clinical penetrance is low; < 10% of affected individuals become symptomatic. In addition, there is an uncommon form of PCT (type III) which is familial but otherwise biochemically indistinguishable from type I.[65] PCT may also be caused by chemicals that decrease hepatic UROD activity.[1,2,19,65] In the late 1950s, a large number of children and adults in south-eastern Turkey became affected after consuming wheat contaminated with hexachlorobenzene.

Clinical features

Skin lesions are the only consistent clinical feature of PCT. Sun-exposed skin, particularly on the face and backs of the hands, becomes fragile, and develops subepidermal bullae, erosions and milia, often with hypertrichosis and patchy pigmentation. Healed lesions may leave scars but the skin changes are usually mild; photomutilation is uncommon, even in sunny climates. Patchy scleroderma and other less common lesions have been described.[139] Acute photosensitivity is uncommon and acute neurovisceral attacks do not occur. Skin lesions usually start in middle-age with almost as many women being affected as men in most countries.[65,139] Onset during childhood is uncommon but has been reported before the age of 2 years.[138] Almost all cases below the age of 20 years have the familial (type II) form.

Most patients show some evidence of liver dysfunction and abnormal biochemical tests of liver function are common,[140] although this is not usually apparent clinically. The liver contains large amounts of uroporphyrin; needle biopsy samples fluoresce red in UVA light. Histopathologic examination in most cases shows mild fatty infiltration, focal necrosis and inflammation of portal tracts.[140] Cirrhosis is present in <15% of patients and carries a greater risk of hepatocellular carcinoma than other types of cirrhosis. The risk may be decreased by early, effective treatment of the metabolic abnormality.[141]

Associated conditions

All types of PCT usually occur in association with other conditions that appear important for its pathogenesis.[65,139] These include alcohol, administration of natural or synthetic estrogens and hepatotropic viruses, particularly hepatitis C[65,142] and HIV.[143] PCT has also been reported in association with many other conditions, most of which affect the liver or iron metabolism: chronic renal failure and long-term hemodialysis, systemic lupus erythrematosus, hematologic malignancies, sideroblastic anemia, thalassemia and adult-onset diabetes.[1,2,65,143]

Evidence of mild-to-moderate iron overload is common. Most patients have hepatic siderosis; hepatic non-heme iron concentrations and total body iron stores are increased in about 65% of patients.[144,145] Less than 20% have biochemical evidence of hemochromatosis and clinically overt hemochromatosis is unusual. PCT in black South Africans is associated with hepatic siderosis caused by consumption of alcoholic beverages and food with a high iron content.[146] About 45% of patients of northern European descent are heterozygous or homozygous for the C282Y mutation in the hemochromatosis (*HFE*) gene, irrespective of the type of PCT.[147]

Diagnosis

Hepatic UROD deficiency produces a characteristic pattern of increased excretion and accumulation of acetic acid-substituted porphyrins (Table 7.4). In an adult, demonstration of this pattern is sufficient to confirm PCT. It is essential to investigate both urine and feces, or urine and plasma, to differentiate PCT unequivocally from VP because urinary porphyrin excretion may occasionally be similar in both conditions.[65,96] Sporadic and familial (type II) PCT can be distinguished by measuring erythrocyte UROD activities.[148]

In children, measurement of erythrocyte UROD activity and protoporphyrin concentration is required to distinguish HEP from type II PCT. Other bullous porphyrias of childhood should not cause confusion, provided individual porphyrins are measured in urine and feces.

Treatment

PCT responds to two specific treatments: depletion of body iron stores[149] and low-dose chloroquine.[150,151] Body iron stores are most easily depleted by phlebotomy. One unit of blood is removed every 1 or 2 weeks until the transferrin saturation reaches 16% or the hemoglobin concentration falls to 11–12 g/dl. Serum ferritin may also be used to monitor treatment but co-existing liver disease may complicate determination of the end-point. Iron depletion usually requires removal of 2.5–7.0 l of blood and may precede clinical improvement or any substantial fall in porphyrin excretion by 2 months or more. Full remission usually follows in about 6 months. Deferoxamine (desferrioxamine) infusion is useful when venesection is contraindicated.[149] In patients with chronic renal failure, hepatic iron stores can be depleted by giving erythropoietin without iron supplements.[152]

Chloroquine releases uroporphyrin from the liver, probably by an effect on lysosomes.[150] Antimalarial doses cause an acute hepatotoxic reaction but, at the lower doses used for PCT (125 mg twice weekly for adults; less for children),[2,150] uroporphyrin is released with only minor increases in serum transaminase activities. Chloroquine should be continued until urinary uroporphyrin concentrations fall to around 100 nmol/l, which may take 10 months or more.[151]

In addition to these specific measures, patients should abstain from alcohol. Estrogens should also be withdrawn, unless their continued use is strongly indicated. Associated conditions often determine prognosis and should be managed as in the absence of PCT. There is no need to avoid the drugs and other factors that provoke acute neurovisceral attacks in the acute porphyrias. The type of porphyria does not alter management and screening families for type II PCT brings little benefit.[65]

Molecular pathology and pathogenesis

PCT is not a simple monogenic disorder. Patients appear to be predisposed to develop hepatic UROD deficiency as a reaction to hepatocyte damage by various common agents, particularly alcohol, hepatotropic viruses and estrogens, that do not normally provoke this response. Several different genes may interact to determine this predisposition.[19,65,153]

Measurements of UROD activity in the liver in clinically overt PCT and in HEP suggest that accumulation of substrate sufficient to cause symptoms does not occur until activities are at least 20% of normal.[65] In PCT, this decrease appears to be caused by catalytic site-directed inactivation of

UROD; enzyme concentration remains at least normal in sporadic PCT and half normal in familial PCT.[154] Inactivation is reversed by iron depletion which, together with clinical evidence that PCT is an iron-dependent disease,[144–146] suggests that iron is required for the inactivation process. The process has been extensively studied in animal models of PCT.[155] These experiments suggest that a heme precursor, iron and CYPIA2 are required for the inactivation process. Iron may act by promoting the oxidative conversion of uroporphyrinogen to a specific inhibitor of UROD in the liver. Polymorphic variation or mutation in genes whose products contribute to this process may underlie any inherited predisposition to PCT. One such susceptibility gene, that for hemochromatosis, has recently been identified.[147]

Inherited defects in UROD, the target of inactivation, would be expected to predispose to PCT. Individuals who inherit type II PCT have a greatly increased risk of developing overt porphyria; at half the normal UROD concentration, less inactivation is required to decrease activity to 20% or less. At least 14 mutations causing type II PCT have now been identified in the UROD gene.[61] In sporadic (type I) PCT, mutations at the UROD locus have been excluded.[153] It thus seems unlikely that abnormalities in the structure of the target enzyme, as opposed to variations in its concentration, predispose to PCT.

HEPATOERYTHROPOIETIC PORPHYRIA

About 30 cases of HEP have been reported.[22,138,156] One patient developed skin lesions during the third decade;[22] in all others they appeared before the age of 6 years. These are similar to those of PCT but are more persistent and may lead to severe scarring, sclerodermatous changes, photomutilation and deformities of the hand. The most severely affected patients resemble CEP but erythrodontia is usually absent. HEP is usually a purely cutaneous disorder but mild hemolytic anemia has been reported in 2 patients and 1 other developed a hemiparesis.

Erythrocyte UROD activities are usually <10% of normal, ranging from 3 to 25% in patients[157] and close to 50% of normal in their parents who are biochemically indistinguishable from latent cases of familial (type II) PCT. Molecular investigations have provided insights into the relationship between the 2 disorders. Eight missense mutations and 1 large deletion of the UROD gene have been identified in HEP.[22,61] One of these mutations (G281E) is present in 9 families from Spain and north Africa. It produces an unstable enzyme and almost complete loss of activity. Homozygotes develop severe skin lesions at an early age. It is the only HEP mutation to have been shown to cause overt PCT in heterozygotes.[22] Some of the other mutations are associated with milder disease;[22] these might be expected to have a very low penetrance in heterozygotes or only cause disease in homozygotes or compound heterozygotes. It seems likely that severe UROD mutations cause type II PCT and mild ones cause HEP, while mutations of intermediate severity which preserve some activity may cause both disorders.

ERYTHROPOIETIC PROTOPORPHYRIA

Erythropoietic protoporphyria (EPP) was first identified as a porphyria in 1961.[158] It presents during childhood with acute photosensitivity unaccompanied by the skin fragility and bullae that occur in all other cutaneous porphyrias. Estimates of its prevalence in western Europe range from 1/75 000 to 1/130 000 of the general population.[159]

Molecular pathology and inheritance

EPP results from decreased activity of FC (Table 7.3). Although this defect is present in all tissues, FC becomes rate-limiting for heme synthesis only in erythroid cells which are the main site of overproduction of protoporphyrin IX.[160,161] Protoporphyrin accumulates in the liver when its rate of formation exceeds the capacity for biliary excretion.[160]

FC deficiency in EPP is inherited in either an autosomal dominant or autosomal recessive pattern.[161,162] Most families show autosomal dominant inheritance with low clinical penetrance. In these families, FC activity in overt EPP is about 10–30% of normal, less than the 50% predicted by haplodeficiency and reported for their asymptomatic relatives.[63] In one autosomal dominant-type family, clinical expression of EPP (and FC activities of 10–30%) required coinheritance of 2 defective FC alleles; 1 contained a mutation that abolished FC activity while the other was associated with a low level of expression of structurally normal enzyme.[163] The 'low expression' allele appears to be in linkage disequilibrium with a polymorphism of the FC gene[164] and may be relatively common in the normal population. These molecular studies provide support for the hypothesis, suggested by Went and Klasen in 1984,[165] that the low clinical penetrance of EPP could be explained if clinical expression required co-inheritance of a rare FC allele with a marked effect on activity and a commoner allele with less effect. Over 20 mutations that alter or disrupt the coding sequence for FC have been identified in this type of EPP,[16,166] but the molecular basis of the 'low expression' allele has not been defined.

Autosomal recessive EPP, unlike homozygous variants of the other autosomal dominant porphyrias, is not phenotypically distinct. Mutations on both alleles of the FC gene have been identified in 2 families.[161,167] In 1 of these families, the presence of severe splice-defective mutations on both alleles was associated with liver failure, an uncommon complication of EPP;[161] exon deletions have also been identified in a high proportion of autosomal dominant-type patients with liver disease.[168] These observations suggest that the presence of severe mutations on both alleles or, possibly, exon deletions on 1 allele may predispose to liver disease in EPP but further studies of patients with this complication are required.

Clinical features

Most patients develop acute photosensitivity between the ages of 1 and 6 years.[159,169] Although the diagnosis may not be made until much later, onset of symptoms during adult life is very rare. Patients experience an intense burning, pricking, itching sensation, particularly of the hands and face, usually with 30 min of exposure to sunlight. The intensely painful, burning sensation persists for hours or, occasionally, days and is not relieved by darkness or covering the skin. Exposed skin may show erythema followed by edematous swelling and crusting; occasionally, it may look normal throughout. Recurrent episodes may lead to chronic lesions but these are often minor and may be difficult to detect. Shallow linear scars over the bridge of the nose, puckering around the mouth, small pit-like scars elsewhere on the face, with thickened, waxy skin, especially over the knuckles, are common. Photosensitivity persists throughout life although its severity may vary.

Progressive hepatic failure is an uncommon but serious complication of EPP.[159–161] Jaundice is usually the first clinical sign and may occur at any age, although most patients have been older than 30 years. Biochemical tests of liver function are abnormal in up to 35% of patients but few of these progress to liver failure,[159] which probably affects no more than 2–5% of patients.[159] Liver damage is caused by accumulation of protoporphyrin in hepatocytes.[159,160] EPP may increase the risk of chilelithiasis with high concentrations of protoporphyrin in bile promoting stone formation.[169]

Hematologic abnormalities

About 25% of EPP patients have a mild, hypochromic, microcytic anemia with, in some patients, biochemical evidence of iron deficiency,[159,169,170] the cause of which is unknown.[170] Ultrastructural examination of erythroblasts shows iron deposits in mitochondria in about 30% of patients, irrespective of their iron status, indicating impaired iron utilization secondary to FC deficiency.[170] Very rarely, patients with acquired sideroblastic anemia develop the clinical and biochemical features of EPP,[171] which may be caused by clonal proliferation of erythroid cells with 18q deletions that include the FC gene.

Fluorescence microscopy of bone marrow cells shows that protoporphyrin accumulates in erythroid cells from just before the loss of nuclei from normoblasts until mitochondria are extruded from reticulocytes.[172] Reticulocytes and erythrocytes in peripheral blood contain variable amounts of porphyrin which is released into plasma with a half-life for protoporphyrin in erythrocytes of 12–14 days.[173] Erythrocytes can also take up protoporphyrin from plasma but most intracellular porphyrin appears to be produced within the cell during differentiation. Peripheral blood reticulocytes can be divided into two populations: one of cells containing varying amounts of porphyrin and the other of cells without porphyrin,[173] suggesting that the reaction to FC deficiency during erythroid differentiation varies between cells.

Diagnosis

The diagnosis of EPP is established by demonstrating an increased concentration of free protoporphyrin in erythrocytes and plasma.[96,159] In iron deficiency, lead poisoning and hemolytic and other anemias in which total erythrocyte protoporphyrins concentrations are increased,[96,125] most protoporphyrin is present as the zinc-chelate, whereas in EPP >80% is in the free, unchelated form. Zinc is an effective substrate for FC; the absence of zinc-protoporphyrin indicates FC deficiency. Screening tests for EPP, with the exception of fluorescence microscopy in expert centers,[174] are unreliable and should be replaced by measurement of total erythrocyte porphyrin followed by determination of the proportions of free and zinc-chelated compounds.[96] Other porphyrin measurements are not essential for diagnosis. Fecal protoporphyrin excretion is increased in about 60% of patients; urinary porphyrin excretion is normal except when cholestasis and liver disease lead to coproporphyrinuria.

Some asymptomatic relatives may have minor increases in free erythrocyte protoporphyrin, suggesting FC deficiency. Measurement of FC activity in nucleated cells[63] or mutational analysis[166] are more certain methods for detecting individuals with FC deficiency. Methods for identifying the 'low expression' allele, and thus predicting overt disease, may soon become available.

Treatment

Avoidance of sunlight prevents photosensitivity. Many patients develop a style of clothing that provides protection. Reflectant sunscreen ointments, photoprotective tanning with dihydroxyacetone or by gradual exposure to sunlight, and desensitization by narrow-band UVB phototherapy may be helpful.[159,175]

Oral β-carotene, which acts as a singlet oxygen quencher, is effective for some patients.[176] The dose ranges from 30 to 90 mg/day for children to 100–300 mg/day for adults.[159] It should be adjusted to maintain a plasma concentration of 6–8 mg/l for 3 months and then discontinued if ineffective. Other treatments, such as oral cysteine, are under evaluation.[177]

There is no reliable method for prediction of liver disease. Patients should have at least annual biochemical tests of liver function with investigation of persistent abnormalities by liver biopsy. Progression of liver disease may be slowed by interrupting the enterohepatic circulation of protoporphyrin with cholestyramine or activated charcoal or, as a short-term measure, by suppression of erythropoiesis by hypertransfusion or hematin.[159–161,178] Once liver failure develops, liver transplantation is the only treatment.[164,166] Protoporphyrin may reaccumulate in the transplanted liver.

EPP, like CEP, is primarily a bone marrow disorder and is therefore a good candidate for treatment by bone marrow transplantation or gene transfer therapy.[161] Any future use of such hazardous and complex procedures is likely to require an accurate method for selecting those patients who have a high risk of developing the one life-threatening complication, liver failure.

REFERENCES

1. Kappas A, Sassa S, Galbraith RA *et al.* The porphyrias. In: Scriver CR, Beaudet al, Sly WS, Valle D (eds) *The Metabolic and Molecular Bases of Inherited Disease.* New York: McGraw-Hill, 1995, pp 2103–2159
2. Anderson K. The porphyrias. In: Zakim D, Boyer TD (eds) *Hepatology: A Textbook of Liver Disease.* Philadelphia: WB Saunders, 1995, pp 417–463
3. Ponka P. Tissue-specific regulation of iron metabolism and heme synthesis: distinct control mechanism in erythroid cells. *Blood* 1997; **89**: 1–25
4. Maines MD. The heme oxygenase system: a regulator of second messenger gases. *Annu Rev Pharmacol Toxicol* 1997; **37**: 517–554
5. Hennig M, Grimm B, Contestabile R, John RA, Jansonius N. Crystal structure of glutamate-1-semialdehyde aminomutase: An α_2-dimeric vitamin B_6-dependent enzyme with asymmetry in structure and active site reactivity. *Proc Natl Acad Sci USA* 1997; **94**: 4866–4871
6. May BK, Dogra SC, Sadlon TJ *et al.* Molecular regulation of haem biosynthesis in higher vertebrates. *Prog Nucl Acids Res Mol Biol* 1995; **51**: 1–51
7. Ferreira GC, Goag J. 5-Aminolevulinate synthase and the first step of heme biosynthesis. *J Bioenerg Biomembr* 1995; **27**: 151–160
8. Jaffe E. Porphobilinongen synthase, the first source of heme's asymmetry. J Bioenerg Biomembr 1995; **27**: 169–180
9. Kaya AH, Plewinska M, Wong DM, Desnick RJ, Wetmur JG. Human δ-aminolevulinate dehydratase (ALAD) gene: Structure and alternative splicing of the erythroid and housekeeping mRNAs. *Genomics* 1994; **19**: 242
10. Mitchell G, Larochelle J, Lambert M *et al.* Neurologic crises in hereditary tyrosinaemia. *N Engl J Med* 1990; **322**: 432–437
11. Guo GG, Gu M, Etlinger JD. 240-kDa proteasome inhibitor (CF-2) is identical to δ-aminolevulinic dehydratase. *J Biol Chem* 1994; **269**: 12399
12. Bishop TR, Milles MW, Beall J, Zon LI, Dierks P. Genetic regulation of δ-aminolevulinic dehydratase during erythropoiesis. *Nucleic Acids Res* 1996; **24**: 2511
13. Louie GV, Browlie PD, Lambert R *et al.* The three-dimensional structures of mutants of porphobilinogen deaminase: a flexible multidomain polymerase with a single catalytic site. *Nature* 1992; **359**: 33–39
14. Brownlie PD, Lambert R, Louie GV *et al.* The three-dimensional structures of mutants of porphobilinogen deaminase: toward an understanding of the structural basis of acute intermittent porphyria. *Protein Sci* 1994; **3**: 1644–1650
15. Jordan PM. Porphobilinogen deaminase: mechanism of action and role in the biosynthesis of uroporphyrinogen III. In: *The Biosynthesis of the Tetrapyrole Pigments, Ciba Foundation Symposium 180.* Chichester John Wiley, 1994, pp 70–96
16. Chretien S, Dubart A, Beaupain D *et al.* Alternative transcription and splicing of the human porphobilinogen deaminase gene result either in tissue-specific or in housekeeping expression. *Proc Natl Acad Sci USA* 1988; **85**: 6–10
17. Shoolingin-Jordan, PM. Porphobilinogen deaminase and uroporphyrinogen III synthase. *J Bioenerg Biomembr* 1995; **27**: 181–196
18. Tsai SF, Bishop DF, Desnick RJ. Human uroporphyrinogen III synthase: Molecular cloning, nucleotide sequence, and expression of a full-length cDNA. *Proc Natl Acad Sci USA* 1988; **85**: 7049
19. Elder GH, Roberts AG. Uroporphyrinogen decarboxylase. *J Bioenerg Biomembr* 1995; **27**: 207–214
20. Wyckoff EE, Phillips JD, Sowa AM, Franklin MR, Kushner JK. Mutational analysis of human uroporphyrinogen decarboxylase. *Biochim Biophys Acta* 1996; **1298**: 294–304
21. Phillips JD, Whitby FG, Kushner JP, Hill CP. Characterization and crystallization of human uroporphyrinogen decarboxylase. *Protein Sci* 1997; **6**: 1343–1346
22. Moran-Jimenez, MJ, Ged C, Romana M *et al.* Uroporphyrinogen decarboxylase complete gene sequence and molecular study of three families with hepatoerythropoietic porphyria. *Am J Hum Genet* 1996; **58**: 712–721
23. Medlock AE, Dailey HA. Human coproporphyrinogen oxidase is not a metalloprotein. *J Biol Chem* 1996; **271**: 32507–32510
24. Dailey HA. Conversion of coproporphyrinogen to protoheme in higher eukaryotes and bacteria: Terminal three enzymes. In: Dailey HA (ed) *Biosynthesis of Heme and Chlorophylls.* New York: McGraw-Hill, 1990, p 123
25. Belfau-Larue M-H, Martasek P, Grandchamp B. Coproporphyrinogen oxidase: Gene organisation and description of a mutation leading to exon 6 skipping. *Hum Mol Genet* 1994; **3**: 1325
26. Dailey TA, Dailey HA. Expression, purification and characteristics of mammalian protoporphyrinogen oxidase. *Methods Enzymol* 1997; **281**: 340–349
27. Taketani S, Inazawa J, Abe T *et al.* The human protoporphyrinogen oxidase gene (PPOX) – Organization and location to chromosome 1. *Genomics* 1995; **29**: 698
28. Roberts AG, Whatley SD, Daniels J *et al.* Partial characterization and assignment of the gene for protoporphyrinogen oxidase and variegate porphyria to human chromosome 1q23. *Hum Mol Genet* 1995; **4**: 2387
29. Puy H, Robréau A-M, Rosipal R, Nordmann, Y, Deybach J-C. Protoporphyrinogen oxidase: complete genomic sequence and polymorphisms in the human gene. *Biochem Biophys Res Commun* 1996; **226**: 227–230
30. Ferreira GC, Ricardo F, Lloyd SG, Moura I, Moura JJG, Huynh BH. Structure and function of ferrochelatase. *J Bioenerg Biomembr* 1995; **27**: 221–230
31. Dailey HA, Finnegan MG, Johnson MK. Human ferrochelatase is an iron sulfur protein. *Biochemistry* 1994; **33**: 403
32. Straka JG, Bloomer JR, Kempner ES. The functional size of ferrochelatase determined *in situ* by radiation inactivation. *J Biol Chem* 1991; **266**: 24637–24641
33. Franco R, Moura, JJG, Moura I *et al.* Characterization of the iron-binding site in mammalian ferrochelatase by kinetic and Mössbauer methods. *J Biol Chem* 1995; **270**: 26352
34. Taketani S, Inazawa J, Nakahashi Y, Abe T, Tokunaga R. Structure of the human ferrochelatase gene. *Eur J Biochem* 1992; **205**: 217
35. Vulpe C, Gitschier J. Ironing out anaemia. *Nature Genet* 1997; **16**: 319–320
36. Taketani S, Tanaka-Yoshioka A, Masaki R, Tashiro Y, Tokunaga R. Association of ferrochelatase with complex I in bovine heart mitochondria. *Biochim Biophys Acta* 1986; **883**: 277
37. Bridges KR. Sideroblastic anemia: a mitochondrial disorder. *J Pediatr Hematol Oncol* 1997; **19**: 274–278
38. Granick S. The induction *in vitro* of the synthesis of δ-aminolevulinic acid synthetase in chemical porphyria: a response to certain drugs, sex hormones and foreign chemicals. *J Biol Chem* 1966; **241**: 1359–1375

39. Hayashi N, Kurashima Y, Kikuchi G. Mechanisms of allylisopropyl-acetamide-induced increase of δ-aminolevulinate synthetase in liver mitochondria. *Arch Biochem Biophys* 1972; **148**: 10–21

40. Lathorp JT, Timko MP. Regulation by heme of mitochondrial protein transport through a conserved amino acid motif. *Science* 1993; **259**: 522

41. Zhang L, Guarente L. Heme binds to a short sequence that serves a regulatory function in diverse proteins. *EMBO J* 1995; **14**: 313

42. Munakata H, Furuyama K, Hayashi N. Regulation by the heme regulatory motif of mitochondrial import of 5-aminolevulinate synthase in intact cells. *Acta Hematol* 1997; **98 (Suppl 1)**: 107

43. Hamilton JW, Bement WJ, Sinclair PR, Sinclair JF, Alcedo JA, Wetterhahn KE. Heme regulates hepatic 5-aminolevulinate synthase mRNA expression by decreasing mRNA half-life and not by altering its rate of transcription. *Arch Biochem Biophys* 1991; **289**: 387–392

44. Braidotti G, Borthwick IA, May BK. Identification of regulatory sequences in the gene for 5-aminolevulinate synthase from rat. *J Biol Chem* 1993; **268**: 1109–1117

45. Sassa S. Sequential induction of heme pathway enzymes during erythroid differentiation of mouse Friend leukemia virus-infected cells. *J Exp Med* 1976; **143**: 305

46. Beaumont C, Deybach J-C, Grandchamp B, da Silva V, de Verneuil H, Nordman Y. Effects of succinylacetone on dimethylsulfoxide-mediated induction of heme pathway enzymes in mouse Friend virus-transformed erythroleukemia cells. *Exp Cell Res* 1984; **154**: 474

47. Taketani S, Yoshinaga T, Furukawa T *et al*. Induction of terminal enzymes for heme biosynthesis during differentiation of mouse erythroleukemia cells. *Eur J Biochem* 1995; **230**: 760

48. Houston T, Moore MR, McColl KEL, Fitzsimons EJ. Regulation of haem biosynthesis in normoblastic erythropoiesis: Role of 5-aminolaevulinic acid synthase and ferrochelatase. *Biochim Biophys Acta* 1994; **1201**: 85

49. Hentze MW, Kuhn CL. Molecular control of vertebrate iron metabolism: mRNA-based regulatory circuits operated by iron, nitric oxide, and oxidative stress. *Proc Natl Acad Sci USA* 1996; **93**: 8175–8182

50. Granick JL, Sassa S. Hemin control of heme biosynthesis in mouse Friend virus-transformed erythroleukemia cells in culture. *J Biol Chem* 1978; **253**: 5402

51. Bloom KE, Zaider EF, Morledge LJ, Poh-Fitzpatrick MB. Urinary porphyrin excretion in normal children and adults. *Am J Kidney Dis* 1991; **18**: 483–489

52. Badcock NR, Szep DA. Diagnosis of erythropoietic protoporphyria using cord blood. *Ann Clin Biochem* 1996; **33**: 73–74

53. Rocchi E, Balli F, Gibertini P *et al*. Coproporphyrin excretion in healthy newborn babies. *J Pediatr Gastroenterol Nutr* 1984; **3**: 402–407

54. Elferink RPJO, Meijer DFK, Folkert K, Janse PLM, Groen AK, Groothuis GMM. Hepatobiliary secretion of organic compounds; molecular mechanisms of membrane transport. *Biochim Biophys Acta* 1995; **1241**: 215–268

55. Keppler D, Konig J. Expression and localization of the conjugate export pump encoded by the *MRP2* (c*MRP*/c*MOAT*) gene in liver. *Faseb J* 1997; **11**: 509–516

56. Paulusma CC, Kool M, Bosma PJ *et al*. A mutation in the human canalicular multispecific organic anion transporter gene causes the Dubin-Johnson syndrome. *Hepatology* 1997; **25**: 1539–1542

57. Frank M, Doss MO. Relevance of urinary coproporphyrin isomers in hereditary hyperbilirubinemias. *Clin Biochem* 1989; **22**: 221–222

58. Bonkovsky H, Barnard G. Diagnosis of porphyric syndromes. *Semin Liver Dis* 1998; **18**: 57–65

59. Beukeveld GJJ, Wolthers BG, van Saen JJM *et al*. Patterns of porphyrin excretion in feces as determined by liquid chromatography; reference values and the effect of flora suppression. *Clin Chem* 1987; **33**: 2164–2170

60. Strand LJ, Felsher BW, Redeker AJ, Marver HS. Enzymatic abnormalities in heme biosynthesis in intermittent acute porphyria: decreased hepatic conversion of porphobilinogen to porphyrins and increased δ-

61. Elder GH. Genetic defects in the porphyrias: types and significance. *Clin Dermatol* 1998; **16**: 225–234

62. Puy H, Deybach JC, Lamoril J *et al*. Molecular epidemiology and diagnosis of PBG deaminase gene defects in acute intermittent porphyria. *Am J Hum Genet* 1997; **60**: 1373–1383

63. Nordmann Y, Deybach JC. Human hereditary porphyrias. In: Dailey HA (ed) *Biosynthesis of Heme and Chlorophylls*. New York: McGraw-Hill, 1990, pp 491–542

64. Kauppinen R, Mustajoki P. Prognosis of acute porphyria: occurrence of acute attacks, precipitating factors and associated diseases. *Medicine* 1992; **71**: 1–13

65. Elder GH. Porphyria cutanea tarda. *Semin Liver Dis* 1998; **18**: 67–75

66. Epstein JH, Tuffanelli DL, Epstein WL. Cutaneous changes in the porphyrias – a microscopic study. *Arch Dermatol* 1973; **107**: 689–698

67. Wolff K, Honigsmann H, Rauschmeier W *et al*. Microscopic and fine structural aspects of porphyrias. *Acta Dermatol Venereoligica* 1982; **100 (Suppl)**: 17–28

68. Wick G, Hönigsmann H, Timpl R. Immunofluorescence demonstration of type IV collagen and a noncollagenous glycoprotein in thickened vascular basal membranes in protoporphyria. *J Invest Dermatol* 1979; **73**: 335–338

69. Dabski C, Beutner EH. Studies of laminin and type IV collagen in blisters of porphyria cutanea tarda and drug-induced pseudoporphyria. *J Am Acad Dermatol* 1991; **25**: 28–32

70. Spikes JD. Photobiology of porphyrins. In: Doiron DR, Gomer CF (eds) *Porphyrin Localization and Treatment of Tumors*. New York: Liss, 1984, pp 19–39

71. Lim HW, Poh-Fitzpatrick MB, Gigli I. Activation of the complement system in patients with porphyrias after irradiation *in vivo*. *J Clin Invest* 1984; **74**: 1961–196

72. Glover RA, Bailey CS, Barrett KE *et al*. Histamine release from rodent and human mast cells induced by protoporphyrin and ultraviolet light: studies of the mechanism of mast-cell activation in erythropoietic protoporphyria. *Br J Dermatol* 1996; **134**: 880–885

73. Herrmann G, Wlaschek M, Bolsen K *et al*. Photosensitization of uroporphyrin augments the ultraviolet A-induced synthesis of matrix metalloproteinases in human dermal fibroblasts. *J Invest Dermatol* 1996; **107**: 398–403

74. Laiwah ACY, Moore MR, Goldberg A. Pathogenesis of acute porphyria. *Q J Med* 1987; **63**: 377–392

75. Meyer UA, Schuurmans MM, Pindberg RLP. Acute porphyrias: Pathogenesis of neurological manifestations. *Semin Liver Dis* 1998; **18**: 43–52

76. Mustajoki P, Himberg JJ, Tokola O *et al*. Rapid normalization of antipyrine oxidation by heme in variegate porphyria. *Clin Pharmacol Ther* 1992; **51**: 320–324

77. Gorchein A, Webber R. δ-Aminolevulinic acid in plasma, cerebrospinal fluid, saliva and erythrocytes: studies in normal, uraemic and porphyric subjects. *Clin Sci* 1987; **72**: 103–112

78. Müller WE, Snyder SH. δ-Aminolevulinic acid: influences on synaptic GABA receptor binding may explain CNS symptoms of porphyria. *Ann Neurol* 1977; **2**: 340–342

79. Brennan MJW, Cantrill RC. δ-Aminolevulinic acid and amino acid neurotransmitters. *Mol Cell Biochem* 1981; **38**: 49–58

80. Puy H, Deybach J-C, Nogdan A *et al*. Increased δ aminolevulinic acid and decreased pineal melatonin production. *J Clin Invest* 1996; **97**: 104–110

81. Mustajoki P, Nordmann Y. Early administration of heme arginate for acute porphyric attacks. *Arch Intem Med* 1993; **153**: 2004–2008

82. Mustajoki P, Mustajoki S, Rautio A, Arvela P, Peklonen O. Effects of heme arginate on cytochrome P450-mediated metabolism of drugs in patients with variegate porphyria and in healthy men. *Clin Pharmacol Ther* 1994; **56**: 9–13

83. Puy H, Deybach J-C, Baudry P *et al*. Decreased nocturnal plasma

melatonin levels in patients with recurrent acute intermittent porphyria attacks. *Life Sci* 1993; **53**: 621–627

84. De Matteis F, Ray RE. Studies on cerebellar haem metabolism in the rat *in vivo*. *J Neurochem* 1982; **39**: 551–556

85. Lindberg RLP, Porcher C, Grandchamp B *et al*. Porphobilinogen deaminase deficiency in mice causes a neuropathy resembling that of human hepatic porphyria. *Nature Genet* 1996; **12**: 195–199

86. Doss M, von Tiepermann R, Schneider J, Schmid H. New type of hepatic porphyria with porphobilinogen synthase defect and intermittent acute clinical manifestations. *Lin Wochenschr* 1979; **57**: 1123–1127

87. McKusick VA, Francomano CA, Antonarakis SE. *Mendelian Inheritance in Man—Catalogues of Autosomal Dominant, Autosomal Recessive and X-linked Phenotypes*, 11th edn. Baltimore: Johns Hopkins University Press, 1994

88. Thunell S, Holmberg L, Lundgren J. Aminolaevulinate dehydratase porphyria in infancy. *J Clin Chem Clin Biochem* 1987; **25**: 5–14

89. Mercelis R, Hassoun A, Verstraeten L, De Bock R, Martin J-J. Porphyric neuropathy and hereditary δ-aminolevulinic acid dehydratase deficiency in an adult. *J Neurol Sci* 1990; **95**: 39

90. Plewinska M, Thunell S, Holmberg L *et al*. δ-Aminolevulinic dehydratase deficient porphyria: identification of the molecular lesions in a severely affected homozygote. *Am J Hum Genet* 1991; **49**: 167–174

91. Ishida N, Fujita H, Fukuda Y *et al*. Cloning and expression of the defective genes from a patient with δ-aminolevulinate dehydratase porphyria. *J Clin Invest* 1992; **89**: 1431–1437

92. Dyer J, Garrick DP, Inglis A, Pye IF. Plumboporphyria (ALAD deficiency) in a lead worker: a scenario for potential diagnostic confusion. *Br J Ind Med* 1993; **50**: 1119–1121

93. Fritsch C, Bolsen K, Ruzicka T, Günter G. Congenital erythropoietic porphyria. *J Am Acad Dermatol* 1997; **36**: 594–610

94. Fontanellas A, Bensidhoum M, De Salamanca RE *et al*. A systematic analysis of the mutations of the uroporphyrinogen III synthase gene in congenital erythropoietic porphyria. *Eur J Hum Genet* 1996; **4**: 272–282

95. Verstraeten L, Regemorter NV, Pardon A *et al*. Biochemical diagnosis of a fatal case of Gunther's disease in a newborn with hydrops foetalis. *Eur J Clin Chem Clin Biochem* 1993; **31**: 121–128

96. Elder GH, Smith SG, Smyth SJ. Laboratory investigation of the porphyrias. *Ann Clin Biochem* 1990; **27**: 395–412

97. Ged C, Moreau-Gaudry F, Taine L *et al*. Prenatal diagnosis in congenital erythropoietic porphyria by metabolite measurement and DNA mutation analysis. *Prenat Diagn* 1996; **16**: 83–86

98. Nordmann Y, Deybach JC. Congenital erythropoietic porphyria. *Semin Dermatol* 1986; **5**: 106–114

99. Marver HS, Scmid R. The porphyrias. In: Stanbury JB, Wyngaarden JB, Fredrickson DS (eds) *The Metabolic Basis of Inherited Disease*, 3rd edn. New York: McGraw-Hill, 1972, pp 1087–1140

100. Zix-Kieffer I, Langer B, Eyer D *et al*. Successful cord blood stem cell transplantation for congenital erythropoietic porphyria (Gunther's disease). *Bone Marrow Transplant* 1996; **18**: 217–220

101. Thomas C, Ged C, Nordmann Y *et al*. Correction of congenital erythropoietic porphyria by bone-marrow transplantation. *J Pediatr* 1996; **129**: 453–456

102. Mazurier F, Moreau-Gaudry F, Salesse S *et al*. Gene transfer of the uroporphyrinogen III synthase cDNA into haematopoietic progenitor cells in view of a future gene therapy in congenital erythropoietic porphyria. *J Inherit Metab Dis* 1997; **20**: 247–257

103. Guarini L, Piomelli S, Poh-Fitzpatrick. Hydroxyurea in congenital erythropoietic porphyria. *N Engl J Med* 1994; **331**: 1091–1092

104. Rank JM, Straba JG, Weimer MK *et al*. Hematin therapy in late onset congenital erythropoietic porphyria. *Br J Haematol* 1990; **75**: 617–622

105. Minder EI, Schneider-Yin X, Moll F. Lack of effect of oral charcoal in congenital erythropoietic porphyria. *N Engl J Med* 1994; **331**: 1092–1093

106. Moore MR, McColl KEL, Rimington C, Goldberg A. *Disorders of Porphyrin Metabolism*. New York: Plenum, 1987

107. Nordmann Y, Puy H, DaSilva V *et al*. Acute intermittent porphyria: prevalence of mutations in the porphobilinogen deaminase gene in blood donors in France. *J Int Med* 1997; **242**; 213–217.

108. Mustajoki P. Variegate porphyria. *Q J Med* 1980; **49**: 191–203

109. Dean G. *The Porphyrias*, 2nd edn. London: Pitman Medical, 1971

110. Eales L, Day RS, Blekkenhorst GH. The clinical and biochemical features of variegate porphyria: an analysis of 300 cases studied at Groote Schuur Hospital, Cape Town. *Int J Biochem* 1980; **12**: 837–854

111. Elder GH, Hift R, Meissner PN. The acute porphyrias. *Lancet* 1997; **349**: 1613–1617

112. Goldberg A, Smith JA, Lockhead A. Hereditary coproporphyria. *Br Med J* 1963; **2**: 1270–1275.

113. Kauppinen R, Mustajoki S, Phihlaja H *et al*. Acute intermittent porphyria in Finland: 19 mutations in the porphobilinogen deaminase gene. *Hum Mol Genet* 1995; **4**: 215–222

114. Lee JS, Anvret M. Identification of the most common mutation within the porphobilinogen deaminase gene in Swedish patients with acute intermittent porphyria. *Proc Natl Acad Sci USA* 1991; **88**: 10912–10915

115. Whatley SD, Roberts AG, Elder GH. *De-novo* mutation and sporadic presentation of acute intermittent porphyria. *Lancet* 1995; **346**: 1007–1008

116. Meissner PN, Dailey TA, Hift RJ *et al*. A R59W mutation in human protoporphyrinogen oxidase results in decreased enzyme activity and is prevalent in South Africans with variegate porphyria. *Nature Genet* 1996; **13**: 95–97

117. De Rooij FWM, Minderman G, De Baar E *et al*. Six new protoporphyrinogen oxidase mutation in Dutch variegate porphyria patients and the R59W mutation in historical perspective. *Acta Hematol* 1997; **98 (Suppl 1)**: 103.

118. Frank J, Lam HM, Zaider E *et al*. Molecular basis of variegate porphyria: a missense mutation in the protoporphyrinogen oxidase gene. *J Med Genet* 1998; **35**: 244–247

119. Kauppinen R, Timonen K, Laitinen E *et al*. Molecular genetics and clinical characteristics of variegate porphyria. *Acta Hematol* 1997; **98 (Suppl 1):** 96

120. Rosipal R, Lamoril J, Puy H *et al*. Systematic analysis of coproporphyrinogen oxidase gene defects in hereditary coproporphyria and mutation update. *Hum Mutat* 1998; **13**

121. Barclay N. Acute intermittent porphyria in childhood: a neglected diagnosis? *Arch Dis Child* 1974; **49**: 404–405

122. Beauvais P, Klein M-L, Denave L *et al*. Porphyria ague intermittente a l'age de quatre mois. *Arch Franc Pediatr* 1976; **33**: 987–992

123. Jeans JB, Savik K, Gross CR *et al*. Mortality in patients with acute intermittent porphyria requiring hospitalization: a United States case series. *Am J Med Genet* 1996; **65**: 269–273

124. Crimlisk HL. The little imitator – porphyria: a neuropsychiatric disorder. *J Neurol Neurosurg Psych* 1997; **62**: 319–328

125. Bonkovsky H, Barnard G. Diagnosis of porphyric syndromes. *Semin Liver Dis* (in press)

126. Poh-Fitzpatrick MB. A plasma porphyrin fluorescence marker for variegate porphyria. *Arch Dermatol* 1980; **116**: 543–547

127. Brodie MJ, Moore MR, Thompson GG, Goldberg A. The treatment of acute intermittent porphyria with laevulose. *Clin Sci Mol Med* 1977; **53**: 365–371

128. Bonkovsky HL. Advances in understanding and treating 'The little imitator,' acute porphyria. *Gastroenterology* 1993; **105**: 2

129. Blake D, McManus J, Cronin V *et al*. Fecal coproporphyrin isomers in hereditary coproporphyria. *Clin Chem* 1992; **38**: 96–100

130. Long C, Smyth SJ, Woolf J *et al*. Detection of latent variegate porphyria by fluorescence emission spectroscopy of plasma. *Br J Dermatol* 1993; **129**: 9–13

131. Elder GH. Hepatic porphyrias in children. *J Inherit Metab Dis* 1997; **20**: 237–246

132. Gregor A, Kostrzweska E, Prokurat H, Pucek Z, Torbicka E. Increased protoporphyrin in erythrocytes in a child with acute intermittent porphyria. *Arch Dis Child* 1977; **52**: 945–950

133. Grandchamp B, Phung N, Nordmann Y. Homozygous case of hereditary coproporphyria. *Lancet* 1977; **ii**: 1348–1349

134. Grandchamp B, Lamoril J, Puy H. Molecular abnormalities of coproporphyrinogen oxidase in patients with hereditary coproporphyria. *J Bioenerg Biomembr* 1995; **27**: 215–220.

135. Lamoril J, Puy H, Gouya L *et al*. Neonatal haemolytic anaemia due to inherited harderoporphyria: clinical characteristics and molecular basis. *Blood* 1998; **91**: 1–6

136. Hift R, Meissner PN, Todd G *et al*. Homozygous variegate porphyria: an evolving clinical syndrome. *Postgrad Med J* 1993; **69**: 781–786

137. Roberts AG, Whatley SD, Dailey TA *et al*. Molecular characterization of homozygous variegate porphyria. *J Inherit Metab Dis* 1996; **19 (Suppl 1)**: 17

138. Hift R, Meissner PN, Todd G. Hepatoerythropoietic porphyria precipitated by viral hepatitis. *Gut* 1993; **34**: 1632–1634

139. Grossman ME, Bickers DR, Poh-Fitzpatrick MB *et al*. Porphyria cutanea tarda. Clinical features and laboratory findings in 40 patients. *Am J Med* 1979; **67**: 277

140. Bruguera M. Liver involvement in porphyria. *Semin Dermatol* 1986; **5**: 178–185

141. Siersema PD, ten Kate FJW, Mulder PGH *et al*. Hepatocellular carcinoma in porphyria cutanea tarda: frequency and factors related to its occurrence. *Liver* 1992; **12**: 56–61

142. Fargion S, Piperno A, Cappellini MD *et al*. Hepatitis C virus and porphyria cutanea tarda: evidence of strong association. *Hepatology* 1992; **16**: 1322–1326

143. Castanet J, Lacour JP, Bodokh I *et al*. Porphyria cutanea tarda in association with human immunodeficiency virus infection: is it related to hepatitis C virus infection? *Arch Dermatol* 1994; **130**: 664–665

144. Lundvall O, Weinfeld A, Lundin P. Iron storage in porphyria cutanea tarda. *Acta Med Scand* 1970; **188**: 37–53

145. Edwards CQ, Griffen LM, Goldgar DE *et al*. HLA-linked hemochromatosis alleles in sporadic porphyria cutanea tarda. *Gastroenterology* 1989; **97**: 972–981

146. Sweeney GD. Porphyria cutanea tarda, or the uroporphyrinogen decarboxylase deficiency diseases. *Clin Biochem* 1986; **19**: 3–14

147. Elder GH, Worwood M. Mutations in the hemochromatous gene, porphyria cutanea tarda, and iron overload. *Hepatology* 1998; **27**: 289–291

148. Held JL, Sassa S, Kappas A *et al*. Erythrocyte uroporphyrinogen decarboxylase activity in porphyria cutanea tarda: A study of 40 consecutive patients. *J Invest Dermatol* 1989; **93**: 332–334

149. Rocchi E, Gibertini P, Cassanelli M *et al*. Iron removal therapy in porphyria cutanea tarda: phlebotomy versus slow subcutaneous desferrioxamine infusion. *Br J Dermatol* 1986; **114**: 621–629

150. Kordac V, Jirsa M, Kotal P *et al*. Agents affecting porphyrin formation and secretion: implications for porphyria cutanea tarda. *Semin Hematol* 1989; **26**: 16–23

151. Ashton RE, Hawk JLM, Magnus IA. Low-dose oral chloroquine in the treatment of porphyria cutanea tarda. *Br J Dermatol* 1981; **111**: 609–613

152. Sarkell B, Patterson JW. Treatment of porphyria cutanea tarda of end-stage renal disease with erythropoietin. *J Am Acad Dermatol* 1993; **29**: 499–500

153. Garey JR, Franklin KF, Brown AD *et al*. Analysis of uroporphyrinogen decarboxylase complementary DNAs in sporadic porphyria cutanea tarda. *Gastroenterology* 1993; **105**: 165–169

154. Elder GH, Urquhart AJ, De Salamanea R *et al*. Immunoreactive uroporphyrinogen decarboxylase in the liver in porphyria cutanea tarda. *Lancet* 1985; **i**: 229–232

155. Constantin D, Francis JE, Akhtar A *et al*. Uroporphyria induced by 5-aminolevulinic acid in *Ahr^d* SWR mice. *Biochem Pharmacol* 1996; **52**: 1407–1413

156. Parsons JL, Sahn EE, Holden KR *et al*. Neurologic disease in a child with hepatoerythropoietic porphyria. *Pediatr Dermatol* 1994; **11**: 216–221

157. Koszo F, Morvay M, Dobozy A *et al*. Erythrocyte uroporphyrinogen decarboxylase activity in 80 unrelated patients with porphyria cutanea tarda. *Br J Dermatol* 1992; **126**: 446–449

158. Magnus IA, Jarrett A, Prankerd TAJ *et al*. Erythropoietic protoporphyria: a new porphyria syndrome with solar urticaria due to protoporphyrinaemia. *Lancet* 1961; **ii**: 448–445

159. Todd DJ. Erythropoietic protoporphyria. *Br J Dermatol* 1994; **131**: 751–766

160. Bloomer JR. The liver in protoporphyria. *Hepatology* 1988; **8**: 402–407

161. Cox TM. Erythropoietic protoporphyria. *J Inherit Metab Dis* 1997; **20**: 258–269

162. Goerz G, Bunselmeyer S, Bolsen K *et al*. Ferrochelatase activities in patients with erythropoietic protoporphyria and their families. *Br J Dermatol* 1996; **134**: 880–885

163. Gouya L, Deybach J-C, Lamoril J *et al*. Modulation of the phenotype in dominant erythropoietic protoporphyria by a low expression of the normal ferrochelatase allele. *Am J Hum Genet* 1996; **58**: 292–299

164. Poh-Fitzpatrick MB, Piomelli S, Deybach J-C *et al*. Erythropoietic protoporphyria: a triallelic inheritance model. *J Invest Dermatol* 1997; **108**: 598

165. Went LN, Klasen EC. Genetic aspects of erythropoietic protoporphyria. *Ann Hum Genet* 1984; **48**: 105–117

166. Wang X, Piomelli S, Peacocke M *et al*. Erythropoietic protoporphyria: four novel frameshift mutations in the ferrochelatase gene. *J Invest Dermatol* 1997; **109**: 688–691

167. Lamoril J, Boulechfar S, De Verneuil H *et al*. Human erythropoietic protoporphyria: two point mutations in the ferrochelatase gene. *Biochem Biophys Res Commun* 1991; **181**: 594–599

168. Bloomer J Bruzzone C, Zhu L *et al*. Molecular defects in ferrochelatase in patients with protoporphyria requiring liver transplantation. *Hepatology* 1996; **24**: 199A

169. De Leo VA, Poh-Fitzpatrick M, Mathews-Roth M *et al*. Erythropoietic protoporphyria: 10 years experience. *Am J Med* 1976; **60**: 8–22

170. Rademakers LHPM, Koningsberger JC, Sorber CWJ *et al*. Accumulation of iron in erythroblasts of patients with erythropoietic protoporphyria. *Eur J Clin Invest* 1993; **23**: 130–138

171. Lim HW, Cooper D, Sassa S *et al*. Photosensitivity, abnormal porphyrin profile and sideroblastic anemia. *J Am Acad Dermatol* 1992; **27**: 287–292

172. Clark K, Nicholson D. Erythrocyte protoporphyrin and iron uptake in erythropoietic protoporphyria. *Clin Sci* 1971; **41**: 363–370

173. Brun A, Steen H, Sandberg S. Erythropoietic protoporphyria: two populations of reticulocytes, with and without protoporphyrin. *Eur J Clin Invest* 1996; **26**: 270–278

174. Rimington C, Cripps DJ. Biochemical and fluorescence-microscopy screening tests for erythropoietic protoporphyria. *Lancet* 1965; **i**: 624–646

175. Collins P, Ferguson J. Narrow-band UVB (TL-01) phototherapy: an effective preventative treatment for the photodermatoses. *Br J Dermatol* 1995; **132**: 956–963

176. Mathews-Roth MM. Beta-carotene therapy for erythropoietic protoporphyria and other photosensitivity diseases. *Biochimie* 1986; **68**: 875–884

177. Mathews-Roth MM, Rosner B, Benfell K, Roberts JE. A double-blind study of cysteine photoprotection in erythropoietic protoporphyria. *Photodermatol Photoimmunol Photomed* 1994; **10**: 244–248

178. Potter C, Tolaymat N, Bobo R *et al*. Hematin therapy in children with protoporphyric liver disease. *J Pediatr Gastroenterol Nutr* 1996; **23**: 402–407

Megaloblastic anemia and disorders of cobalamin and folate metabolism

DAVID S ROSENBLATT AND A VICTOR HOFFBRAND

Megaloblastic anemia in childhood, as in adults, is most frequently due to deficiency of vitamin B_{12} (cobalamin) or folate. In children, however, and especially in neonates, inborn errors of cobalamin or folate metabolism or of absorption or transport of the 2 vitamins, although rare, are relatively more frequent causes. Moreover, defects of DNA synthesis not involving cobalamin or folate may also cause megaloblastic anemia in infants. Some of the errors of cobalamin metabolism are not associated with megaloblastic anemia, but for the sake of completeness, these are also described here. In this chapter, therefore, only a brief description of the nutritional and metabolic aspects of cobalamin and folate is given and the reader is referred to a recent major review of various aspects of cobalamin and folate.[1] The inherited and acquired causes of megaloblastic anemia relevant to neonates and children are then described.

COBALAMIN (VITAMIN B_{12})

The cobalamins share the same structure, a planar corrin ring with a central cobalt atom, attached to a nucleotide structure, 5,6-dimethyl benziminazole, attached to ribose-3 phosphate (Fig. 8.1). The 2 main natural compounds have a methyl (CH_3-) or a 5-deoxyadenosyl group attached to the cobalt atom but both are rapidly converted by light to hydroxocobalamin. Cyanocobalamin was the form in which the vitamin was first isolated and this is the form radioactively labeled with Co^{57} or Co^{58} for diagnostic uses. Hydroxocobalamin, which has the cobalt atom in the oxidized stable Cob(III) state, is used in therapy.

In nature, cobalamin is synthesized by micro-organisms and is only present in foods of animal origin. It is absorbed through the ileum after combination with a glycoprotein, intrinsic factor (IF) of MW 45 000 Da synthesized by the parietal cells in the stomach. Cobalamin is first released by enzymatic digestion from protein complexes in food and from a glycoprotein 'R' binder present in saliva and gastric juice. This binder is closely related to transcobalamin (TC)I present in plasma, and is similar to a binder in milk and

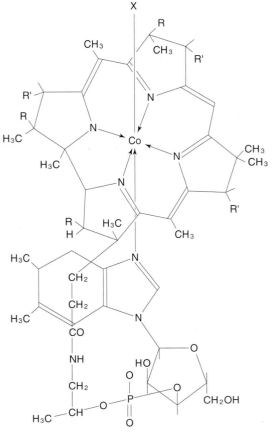

Fig. 8.1 Structure of cobalamin. A cobalt atom is at the center of a planar, corrin ring. This is attached to a nucleotide, 5,6-dimethyl benziminazole ribose 3-phosphate. Attached to the cobalt atom at 'X' may be a methyl-deoxyadenosyl-, hydroxo- or cyano-moiety.

other body secretions. Cobalamin in bile is also attached to IF for reabsorption in the ileum. The IF-cobalamin complex attaches to a specific receptor (cubilin, see p. 170) on the ileal brush border, the number of receptors limiting absorption of cobalamin by the IF mechanism in adults to 2–3 μg from a single oral dose, however large. A small fraction (<1%) of a large oral dose can be absorbed passively through the buccal, gastric and small intestine mucosae.

Within the enterocyte, the IF-cobalamin complex is digested, probably within lysosomes, and the cobalamin appears in portal blood attached to TCII, a polypeptide MW 38 000 Da, synthesized by the liver, macrophages and ileum. TCII binds cobalamin (1:1) and carries it to tissues with TCII receptors, e.g. bone marrow and placenta. TCII is not reutilized.

FOLATE

Folic acid (Fig. 8.2) is the parent compound of natural folates with the same vitamin activity, which are:

- reduced to tetrahydrofolate (THF) forms at positions 5, 6, 7 and 8;
- have single carbon units: methyl (CH_3-), formyl ($CHO-$), methylene ($CH_2=$), methenyl $CH\equiv$, or formimino ($CHNO-$) attached to nitrogens N_5, N_{10} or both;
- have a chain of 4–6 glutamate moieties attached by γ-peptide bonds (polyglutamates) These are the active folate coenzymes whereas the monoglutamates are transport forms.

Folates are present in most foods, the highest content being in liver, leafy vegetables, fruits and yeast. Cows' and human milk contain about 50 $\mu g/l$. Cooking, especially in large volumes of water for prolonged periods, destroys folates, especially if vitamin C and other reducing agents which protect folates are first destroyed. Absorption of folates is through the upper small intestine and involves digestion of polyglutamates to monoglutamates and conversion of these to a single compound, 5-methyl THF which appears in portal blood. The enterocyte is the main site of the reactions

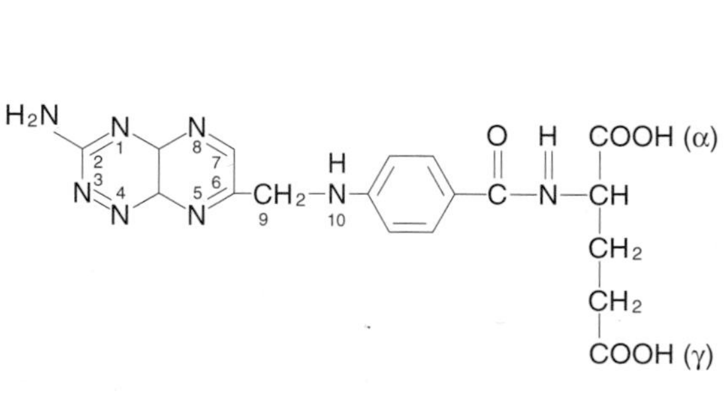

Fig. 8.2 Structure of folic acid. Natural folates may contain a single carbon unit (methyl [CH_3-], methylene [$CH_2=$], methenyl [$CH\equiv$], formyl [$CHO-$], formimino [$CHNO-$] attached at the N_5 or N_{10} position. A chain of glutamic acid residues attached by peptide bond linkage are reduced to dihydro (DH) or tetrahydro (TH) forms at positions 7, 8 or 5, 6, 7, 8 in the pteridine portion respectively.

involved, although some hydrolysis of polyglutamates may occur in the small intestinal lumen. Folic acid (pteroylglutamic acid) is absorbed largely unchanged, especially when given in large, pharmacologic doses, since it is a poor substrate for dihydrofolate reductase and so enters portal blood largely unchanged and is converted to natural folates in the liver. Bile contains 4–5 $\mu g/l$ folate or about 60–90 $\mu g/$day and interruption of the enterohepatic circulation leads to a fall in serum folate within 6 hours. Folate stores in adults are sufficient for about 4 months. Absence of dietary intake also leads to a fall in serum folate within 2–3 weeks.

Folate in plasma is about one-third free and the rest loosely and non-specifically bound to proteins such as albumin. Specific folate binding proteins occur in trace amounts of plasma but more substantially in milk. Their exact function is unclear (see below).

COBALAMIN AND FOLATE METABOLISM

Cobalamin is involved in 2 biochemical reactions in human tissues:

- as methylcobalamin in methionine synthase, a reaction in which 5-methyl tetrahydrofolate acts as methyl donor (Fig. 8.3);
- as deoxyadenosylcobalamin in isomerization of methylmalonyl coenzyme A to succinyl coenzyme A.

Folate in cells takes part in intracellular biochemical reactions in its polyglutamate forms. These coenzymes are involved in 3 amino-acid interconversions: homocysteine to methionine, serine to glycine and forminino glutamic acid to glutamic acid; and in 3 reactions in DNA synthesis: formylation of the purines glycine amidoribotide (GAR) and of aminoimidazolecarboxamideribotide (AICAR) and methylation of the pyrimidine deoxyuridine monophosphate (dUMP) to deoxythymidine monophosphate (dTMP, thymidylate). This last reaction is rate limiting for DNA synthesis, involves degradation of a minor fraction of the folate coenzyme at the C_a-N_{10} bond so that folate is utilized excessively when cell turnover and hence DNA synthesis is increased. Thymidylate synthesis also causes oxidation of the folate coenzyme from the THF to dihydrofolate (DHF) state. The enzyme DHF reductase, inhibited by, for example, methotrexate is required to return folate to the active THF state. Deficiency of folate reduces DNA replication by inhibiting thymidylate synthesis. The mechanism by which deficiency of cobalamin reduces DNA synthesis and causes megaloblastic anemia is also probably a result of reduced thymidylate synthesis. Plasma folate (5-methyl THF) entering cells is first 'demethylated' to THF through the homocysteine methionine reaction. Cobalamin deficiency is considered to reduce this reaction and so reduces cell THF concentration. Folate polyglutamate synthase, the intracellular enzyme needed to synthesize folate polyglutamates, the intracellular folate coenzymes, requires THF (or formyl THF) as substrate but cannot use methyl THF as

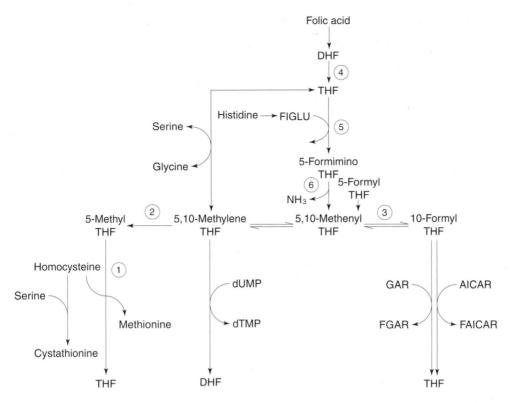

Fig. 8.3 Folate biochemical reactions: (1) Methionine synthase; (2) methylene-THF reductase; (3) methenyl-THF cyclohydrolase; (4) DHF reductase; (5) glutamate formiminotransferase; (6) formimino-THF cyclodeaminase. DHF = dihydrofolate; THF = tetrahydrofolate; FIGLU = formiminoglutamate; dUMP = deoxyuridine monophosphate; dTMP = deoxythymidine monophosphate; GAR = glycinamide ribotide; AICAR = aminoimadazole carboxamide ribotide; FGAR = formylglycinamide ribotide; FAICAR = formyl iminoimidazole carboxamide ribotide. Reproduced with permission from Ref. 197.

substrate. Thus, cobalamin deficiency results in reduction in synthesis of all intracellular folate (polyglutamate) co-enzymes. Total cell folate is reduced, plasma folate (methyl THF) rises, and the intracellular folate reactions in DNA synthesis and amino acid conversion are impaired.

The detailed mechanisms by which inhibition of DNA synthesis leads to the morphologic and biochemical features of megaloblastic anemia are unclear. Commencement of DNA replication at multiple replication origins along the chromosomes with failure to join up these replicating segments because of starvation of thymidine triphosphate is likely to lead to fragmentation of replicating DNA. Misincorporation of uracil instead of thymine because of an intracellular pile up of deoxyuridine monophosphate has also been postulated.

The neuropathy associated in some patients with cobalamin deficiency is considered to be a result of reduced methionine synthesis because of disordered methionine synthase. This results in an increased ratio of homocysteine: methionine, and of S-adenosyl homocysteine (SAH):S-adenosyl methionine (SAM). The change in relative concentrations of SAM to SAH may cause reduced methylation of myelin, resulting in degeneration of the lateral and posterior columns of the spinal cord and peripheral nerves.

INBORN ERRORS OF VITAMIN B$_{12}$ TRANSPORT AND METABOLISM

TRANSPORT DISORDERS

Intrinsic factor deficiency

This inherited form of pernicious anemia results from an absence of effective IF. Evidence of vitamin B$_{12}$ deficiency usually appears in early childhood after the first year of life, but may not appear until adolescence or adulthood. Patients typically show megaloblastic anemia, developmental delay and myelopathy.[2-4] They have normal gastric acid secretion and gastric cytology. In some cases, immunologically active but non-functional IF is produced, whereas in others none is found. An IF, labile to destruction by acid and pepsin and with a low affinity for vitamin B$_{12}$, has also been reported.[5] Absorption of cobalamin is abnormal in children with IF deficiency, but is normalized when the vitamin is mixed with a source of normal IF. Inheritance is autosomal recessive and the gene for human IF has been localized to chromosome 11. Southern analysis of DNA from patients with inherited IF deficiency has not revealed any large deletions.[6]

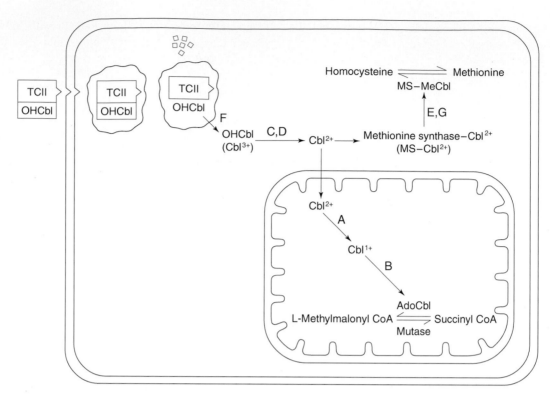

Fig. 8.4 Intracellular cobalamin metabolism. Cbl^{1+}, Cbl^{2+}, Cbl^{3+} refer to the oxidation state of the central cobalt atom of cobalamin. A–G refer to the sites of blocks that have been identified by complementation analysis. AdoCbl = adenosylcobalamin; MeCbl = methylcobalamin; TC = transcobalamin. The mitochondrial lysosomal and cytoplasmic compartments are indicated. Reproduced with permission from Ref. 198.

Defective vitamin B$_{12}$ transport by enterocytes

Also known as the Imerslund–Gräsbeck syndrome, this disease presents with clinical manifestations of vitamin B$_{12}$ deficiency in childhood, usually within the first 2 years.[7–10] Findings include pallor, weakness, anorexia, failure to thrive, recurrent infections and gastrointestinal symptoms.[10] About 180 cases have been described and are more common in Norway, Finland, among Sephardic Jews in Israel, and in Saudi Arabia.[10] All investigated patients had normal IF, no evidence of antibodies to IF, and normal intestinal morphology. They had a selective defect in vitamin B$_{12}$ absorption that was not corrected by treatment with IF. In some patients, proteinuria of the tubular type was found. Systemic vitamin B$_{12}$ corrects the anemia but not the proteinuria.

Normal quantities of IF-vitamin B$_{12}$ receptor were found in ileal biopsies in one sibship.[11] Ileal homogenates bound IF-vitamin B$_{12}$ normally, suggesting that the basic defect is not an absence of receptors. There has been an apparent absence of the ileal receptor in other patients.[12] A model for this disorder has been described in dogs.[13,14]

Linkage studies had assigned the gene locus for this autosomal recessive disorder to chromosome 10 using multiplex families from Finland and Norway.[10] Complete cDNA cloning of the receptor, cubilin, has shown a 3597 amino acid membrane protein, mapped to chromosome 10p.[14a] The cDNA encodes a precursor protein which undergoes cleavage at a recognition site for the trans-Golgi proteinase, furin. The gene is within the 6-cM region harboring the locus for

the recessive syndrome. In rodents it is expressed in the epithelia of the intestine, yolk sac and renal proximal tubules. Presumably impaired synthesis, processing or ligand binding of cubilin is responsible for Imerslund–Gräsbeck syndrome. The recent substantial decrease in the number of new cases diagnosed in these countries[10] has led to the suggestion that dietary or other factors may influence the expression of disease.

Transcobalamin (haptocorrin, R binder) deficiency

A deficiency or complete absence of TCI has been found in the plasma, saliva and leukocytes of 6 individuals, but it is not clear if this deficiency is the cause of disease in any of these patients.[15–20] Serum cobalamin levels are low, but TCII-vitamin B$_{12}$ levels are normal, and the patients are not clinically cobalamin deficient.

In the first report, 1 of 2 brothers with TCI deficiency had optic atrophy, ataxia, long tract signs and dementia.[18] In a more recent report, the patient had findings resembling those seen in subacute combined degeneration of the spinal cord.[20] A role for TCI has been proposed as a scavenger of cobalamin analogs that may be toxic.[21]

Transcobalamin II deficiency

There are at least 30 known patients with autosomal recessive TCII deficiency.[15,22–25] Because TCI binds larger amounts of cobalamin in blood than TCII, serum cobalamin levels will be normal in TCII-deficient patients. Even though TCII in cord blood is of fetal origin,[26] infants with undetectable TCII in their plasma are born healthy and do not demonstrate cobalamin deficiency until several days after birth. Usually, patients develop severe megaloblastic anemia in the first few months of life, but others present with pancytopenia or even isolated erythroid hypoplasia.[27] The presence of immature white cell precursors in an otherwise hypocellular marrow can result in the misdiagnosis of leukemia. Other symptoms include failure to thrive, weakness, and diarrhea; neurologic disease has appeared from 6–30 months following the onset of symptoms.[28–31] Severe immunologic deficiency with defective cellular and humoral immunity has been seen, as has defective granulocyte function. Homocystinuria has been detected in at least 2 patients prior to vitamin B_{12} therapy; in 3 of 5 patients[15] who were tested before the initiation of therapy, methylmalonic aciduria was found.

Usually, no TCII able to bind cobalamin is detected; however, immunologically reactive TCII was found in 3 patients. In a 43-year-old woman, TCII was able to bind cobalamin, but the complex did not mediate vitamin uptake into cells.[32] An abnormal Schilling test was usually found in TCII deficiency (5 of 5 patients), and in 2 patients in which the absorption of cobalamin was normal, immunoreactive TCII was present. This suggests that the TCII molecule may play a role in the IF-mediated transport of cobalamin across the ileal cell.

On the basis of electrophoretic polymorphisms,[33,34] the TCII gene was originally linked to the P blood group on chromosome 22.[35] The cDNA for TCII has been cloned[36] and the molecular basis of some of the variants defined.[37] The first mutant alleles in TCII deficiency have included deletions[22] and nonsense mutations.[38] TCII is synthesized by amniocytes and prenatal diagnosis is possible even in the absence of known mutations in a family at risk.[39,40]

Serum cobalamin levels must be kept very high (1000–10 000 pg/ml) in order to treat TCII-deficient patients successfully and are achieved with twice weekly doses of hydroxocobalamin orally (500–1000 μg) or of systemic hydroxocobalamin (1000 μg) weekly or more often. Folate in the form of folic acid or folinic acid in milligram doses has been successful in reversing the hematologic findings in most patients. However, folate should not be given alone to patients with TCII deficiency as hematologic relapse and neurologic damage can occur when folate supplementation is given without cobalamin.[15,41]

DISORDERS OF UTILIZATION

Methylmalonic acidurias

Disorders causing methylmalonic aciduria (MMA)[42] are characterized by severe metabolic acidosis and the accumulation of large amounts of methylmalonic acid in blood,

urine and cerebrospinal fluid. Patients with MMA have a defect in the nuclear-encoded mitochondrial matrix protein L-methylmalonyl CoA mutase (MCM), which requires adenosylcobalamin (AdoCbl) as a cofactor, and catalyzes the conversion of L-methylmalonyl CoA to succinyl CoA. The incidence of all forms of MMA in Massachusetts is about 1 in 48 000.[43] Classification of the MMAs has been largely on the basis of somatic cell complementation studies in cultured fibroblasts. All the MMAs due to functional methylmalonyl CoA mutase (MCM) deficiency are inherited as autosomal recessive diseases and prenatal diagnosis is possible.

Deficiency of methylmalonyl CoA mutase (mut⁰, mut⁻)

Mutations in the MCM apoenzyme result in MMA, which is not responsive to cobalamin therapy.[44,45] Mature mutase purified from human liver is an homodimer of 710 amino-acid (78 489 Da) subunits produced from a 742 amino-acid (82 145 Da) precursor.[44] There are at least 2 types of MCM deficiency as defined in cultured fibroblasts from patients with MMA. Cell lines having no detectable MCM activity are designated *mut⁰*; those with residual activity that can be stimulated by high concentrations of cobalamin are called *mut⁻*. Some cell lines synthesize no detectable protein, whereas others synthesize unstable proteins, and at least one has a mutation that interferes with transfer of the mutase to the mitochondria.[46,47] Similarly, variable levels of mRNA have been demonstrated in different *mut⁰* lines. Although *mut⁰* and *mut⁻* define a single complementation class, intragenic (interallelic) complementation has been seen between some *mut* lines.[48,49]

Patients with MCM deficiency rapidly become symptomatic with protein feeding. Major clinical findings include lethargy, vomiting, failure to thrive, muscular hypotonia, respiratory distress and recurrent vomiting and dehydration. In normal children, methylmalonic acid is usually <15–20 μg/g of creatinine, whereas in MMA excretion is usually >100 mg and as much as several grams per day. Patients with MMA may have ketones and glycine in both blood and urine, as well as elevated levels of ammonia. Many also have hypoglycemia, leukopenia and thrombocytopenia and methylmalonic acid has been shown to inhibit bone marrow stem cells in a concentration-dependent manner.[50] Follow-up of children identified by newborn screening[51] has identified a number of individuals who excrete methylmalonic acid, have mutase deficiency by complementation analysis, and yet are clinically well and have never developed acidosis.

A single locus encodes MCM on chromosome 6p21. The gene spans 40 kb and consists of 13 exons.[52–55] At least 30 mutations and 2 benign sequence changes have been found, including a large number near the carboxyl terminus which appear to alter AdoCbl binding to the enzyme.[49,56,57] There is a premature stop codon in the mitochondrial leader sequence.[47] A common mutation (G717V) was found in 5 black patients who had a similar phenotype; of these, 4 were Afro-American and 1 was from Ghana.[58,59] In Japan, 6 of 16 patients studied shared one mutation (E117X).[60]

Treatment consists of protein restriction using a formula deficient in valine, isoleucine, methionine and threonine, with the goal of limiting the amino acids that use the propionate pathway. Patients in the *mut* complementation class are not responsive to vitamin B_{12}. Therapy with carnitine has been advocated in patients who are deficient.[61,62] Lincomycin and metronidazole have been used to reduce enteric propionate production by anaerobic bacteria.[63-65] Glutathione deficiency has been recently described.[66] Even with therapy, prognosis is guarded, with reports of brain infarcts and renal dysfunction as late complications.[42]

Adenosylcobalamin deficiency (cblA, cblB)

Vitamin B_{12}-responsive MMA is caused by an intracellular deficiency in AdoCbl in both *cblA* and *cblB*. These 2 disorders are distinguished by complementation analysis. Cell extracts but not intact cells from patients are capable of AdoCbl synthesis; neither cell extracts nor intact cells from *cblB* patients are capable of AdoCbl synthesis. Recent evidence suggests that the defect in *cblA* is in a mitochondrial NADPH-linked aquacobalamin reductase.[67] The defect in *cblB* lies in the adenosyltransferase, which is the final step in the synthesis of AdoCbl.[68] In a single patient, fibroblasts behaved like those from *cblA* patients, but complementation was seen with *cblA* cells.[69]

Most *cblA* and *cblB* patients become sick early in the first year of life with symptoms that are similar to those seen in MCM deficiency.[70] Ninety percent of *cblA* patients respond to vitamin B_{12}, and almost 70% are well up to 14 years of age. Forty percent of *cblB* patients respond to therapy and only 30% show long-term survival. Therapy has been with systemic OHCbl or CNCbl. It is uncertain whether AdoCbl offers any therapeutic advantage.[71,72]

Both *cblA* and *cblB* are presumed to be inherited as autosomal recessive diseases. Roughly equal numbers of patients of both sexes have been reported, and obligate heterozygotes of *cblB* patients show decreased adenosyltransferase activity.[33] Although prenatal therapy with vitamin B_{12} has good therapeutic result, it is not certain whether therapy from birth would be equally effective.[73,74]

Combined deficiencies of adenosylcobalamin and methylcobalamin (cblC, cblD, cblF)

These 3 disorders result in failure of the cell to *synthesize* both methylcobalamin (MeCbl) and AdoCbl.[33] Patients have a functional deficiency in both methionine synthase and MCM, leading to homocystinuria and hypomethioninemia along with MMA. The defects occur after both the endocytosis of TCII-vitamin B_{12} and the hydrolysis of the TCII-vitamin B_{12} complex in the lysosome. In *cblF* disease, the defect appears to block the exit of vitamin B_{12} from the lysosome. In *cblC* and *cblD* disease, the defect is presumed to be in a cytosolic cob(III)alamin reductase or reductases.[75] Partial deficiencies of cyanocobalamin β-ligand transferase and microsomal cob(III)alamin reductase in *cblC* and *cblD* fibroblasts have been described.[76,77] When incubated with labeled CNCbl, fibroblasts from *cblC* and *cblD* accumulate very little intracellular vitamin B_{12} and virtually no AdoCbl or MeCbl. In contrast, *cblF* fibroblasts accumulate excess vitamin B_{12}, but it is all unmetabolized, non-protein bound, and localized to lysosomes.[78,79]

There are > 100 patients with *cblC* disease,[24,80] 2 patients in 1 sibship with *cblD* disease, and 5 unrelated patients with *cblF* disease. Most *cblC* disease presents in the first month or before the end of the first year of life with poor feeding, failure to thrive and lethargy.[81] Most, but not all, have macrocytic megaloblastic anemia, and some have hypersegmented neutrophils and thrombocytopenia. Others have onset later in childhood or adolescence with spasticity, delirium and psychosis.[82] A pigmentary retinopathy with perimacular degeneration has been described,[15,81-84] as have hydrocephalus, cor pulmonare and hepatic failure.[80,85,86] Methylmalonic acid levels are lower than those seen in MCM deficiency but higher than those reported for the defects in vitamin B_{12} transport.

The *cblD* sibship was not as severely affected as most *cblC* patients, coming to attention because of mild mental retardation and behavioral problems.[87] In 1 of the brothers, cerebrovascular disease due to thromboemboli was found at age 18.[33]

The first 2 *cblF* patients, both female, were small for gestational age and had poor feeding, growth retardation and persistent stomatitis.[88,89] The first had glossitis and an abnormal Schilling test,[90] and the second had a persistent skin rash. The first also had dextrocardia and both had minor facial abnormalities. Only the second patient had macrocytosis and homocystinemia as reflected by elevated total blood homocysteine.[88] The second patient died suddenly despite an apparent clinical response to vitamin B_{12}. The next *cblF* patient, a boy, had recurrent stomatitis in infancy, arthritis at age 4 years, and confusion, disorientation and a pigmentary skin abnormality at age 10 years. He was subsequently found to have pancytopenia, an increased corpuscular cell volume (MCV), low serum vitamin B_{12} and abnormal vitamin B_{12} absorption.[91] The fourth patient, also a boy, had aspiration pneumonia at birth and developed hypotonia, lethargy, hepatomegaly, hypoglycemia, neutropenia and thrombocytopenia.[92] Both boys responded to vitamin B_{12}. The fifth *cblF* patient, a native Canadian girl, was diagnosed at age 6 months with anemia, failure to thrive, developmental delay, and recurrent infections. Her serum vitamin B_{12} and vitamin B_{12} absorption were low.[92]

There are roughly equal numbers of male and female patients with *cblC* which is inherited as an autosomal recessive disease, as is *cblF*. Since both known siblings with *cblD* disease are males, the possibility of X linkage cannot be formally excluded.

The *cbl* disorders can be differentiated by studies in cultured fibroblasts. Reduced uptake of labeled CNCbl distinguishes *cblC* and *cblD* from all other *cbl* mutations. The incorporation of the substrates propionate and methyltetrahydrofolate into macromolecules is reduced in all 3 disorders, as is synthesis of AdoCbl and MeCbl. Complementation analysis between an unknown cell line and previously defined groups will provide the specific diagnosis.[78] Prenatal diagnosis has been successfully accomplished in *cblC* disease, using amniocytes, and the diagnosis has been ruled out using chorionic villus biopsy material and cells.[93,94]

Treatment in *cblC* disease can be difficult, particularly in cases with early onset. Many patients with onset in the first month of life die[33,95] and many improve with systemic OHCbl therapy, 1 mg/day, by reducing methylmalonic acid and homocystine excretion. Results from cultured cells and clinical studies suggest that OHCbl rather than CNCbl should be used. Therapy with MeCbl and AdoCbl has been used, but it is unclear whether they offer a therapeutic advantage. In a detailed study of therapy,[96] the effectiveness of oral as opposed to systemic OHCbl was compared along with the effect of carnitine, folinic acid and betaine (250 mg/kg/day). Systemic OHCbl was much more effective than oral therapy; betaine appeared to be helpful in combination with OHCbl. Neither folinic acid nor carnitine had any effect. The result of therapy with daily oral betaine and twice weekly injections of OHCbl was reduced methylmalonic acid, normal serum methionine and homocysteine concentration, and resolution of lethargy, irritability and failure to thrive. However, complete reversal of the neurologic and retinal findings did not occur. Even with good metabolic control, surviving patients usually have moderate-to-severe developmental delay.[15,33] The prognosis appears to be better in patients with onset at a later age.

The patients with *cblF* disease responded to systemic therapy with OHCbl, the first patient responded to oral cobalamin.[89,91,92,97] The disease has been excluded in twins and in a single pregnancy by studies on amniocytes.

Methylcobalamin deficiency (cblE, cblG)

Functional methionine synthase (MS) deficiency is characterized by homocystinuria and hypomethioninemia without MMA. One *cblE* patient had transient MMA.[98] On the basis of complementation analysis, 2 distinct groups have been identified, *cblE* and *cblG*.

Although patients usually come to medical attention in the first 2 years of life, in 1 case the patient was diagnosed at age 21 years and she had findings resembling multiple sclerosis. In both *cblE* and *cblG*, males and females have been described, although there is an excess of males with *cblE*.[80] The commonest findings in both *cblE* and *cblG* include megaloblastic anemia and various neurologic problems, particularly developmental delay and cerebral atrophy.[99] Other findings include electroencephalographic abnormalities, nystagmus, hypotonia, hypertonia, seizures, blindness and ataxia.

Following incubation in labeled CNCbl, fibroblasts from both *cblE* and *cblG* patients show decreased intracellular levels of MeCbl in the presence of normal levels of AdoCbl.[100] There is normal total CNCbl uptake and binding to MCM and MS in *cblE* fibroblasts and in fibroblasts from most *cblG* patients. In fibroblasts from a minority of *cblG* patients, there is no binding of labeled Cbl to MS.[101] In both *cblE* and *cblG*, there is decreased incorporation of methyltetrahydrofolate, reflecting the functional MS deficiency. The standard assay for MS gives activities within the range of controls in *cblE* fibroblast extracts, but most *cblG* extracts have low MS activity. In *cblE* extracts, a relative deficiency in MS activity can be seen when the assay is performed under suboptimal reducing conditions, suggesting that the defect lies in a reducing system associated with the enzyme.[102,103] This has recently been confirmed by the cloning of a cDNA for human methionine synthase reductase and the identification of mutations in the *cblE* gene.[104] In some *cblG* patients it has been suggested that the defect may lie in the interaction of methionine synthase with *S*-adenosylmethionine.[105] With the cloning of the gene for MS,[106,107] the first mutations in this gene in *cblG* patients have been described.[106,108]

Both *cblE* and *cblG* are inherited in an autosomal recessive pattern. Decreased MeCbl levels have been seen in obligate heterozygotes for *cblE*.[109]

OHCbl systemically, first daily and then once or twice weekly, is the commonest treatment. Usually, this results in correction of the anemia and metabolic abnormalities. The neurologic findings have been difficult to reverse once established, particularly in *cblG* disease.

There has been successful prenatal diagnosis of *cblE* disease in amniocytes, and the mother carrying an affected fetus was treated with twice weekly OHCbl from the second trimester.[109] The baby continued to be treated after birth and has subsequently done very well through the first decade of life.

INBORN ERRORS OF FOLATE METABOLISM AND TRANSPORT

Methylenetetrahydrofolate reductase deficiency

Methylenetetrahydrofolate reductase (MTHFR) deficiency is the commonest inborn error of folate metabolism and >40 cases are known.[110,111] It is not usually associated with megaloblastic anemia because reduced folates are still available for purine and pyrimidine metabolism. Since methyltetrahydrofolate serves as 1 of 3 methyl donors for the conversion of homocysteine to methionine, MTHFR deficiency results in elevated homocysteine levels and decreased levels of methionine.

MTHFR deficiency may be diagnosed at any time from

infancy to adulthood and clinically asymptomatic but bio-chemically affected individuals have been reported.[111,112] In general, clinical severity is related to the proportion of methyltetrahydrofolate in cells.[113] Most of the patients have been diagnosed in the first year of life and developmental delay is the commonest clinical manifestation. Breathing disorders, seizures and microcephaly are often present along with motor and gait abnormalities. The report of patients with schizophrenia leads to speculation on the role of MTHFR deficiency in psychiatric disease.[114,115]

MTHFR-deficient patients have homocystinuria, with a mean homocysteine excretion of 130 nmol/24 h and a range of 15–667 nmol/24 h,[110] values which are much lower than those seen in classic homocystinuria due to cystathionine synthase deficiency. More than one determination of homocystine excretion may be needed to eliminate the possibility of a false negative value. Plasma methionine levels are low and values have ranged from 0 to 18 nM (mean 12 nM);[110] normal fasting plasma methionine levels are usually in the range of 23–35 nM. Neurotransmitter levels have been measured in the cerebrospinal fluid of only a few patients, and they have usually been low.[110]

The diagnosis of severe MTHFR deficiency has been made by direct measurement of enzyme activity in liver, leukocytes and cultured fibroblasts and lymphocytes. The specific activity of MTHFR in cultured fibroblasts is depen-dent on the stage of the culture cycle, being several fold higher in confluent cells than in cells in logarithmic growth. Therefore, it is important to compare activities of unknown samples and control cell lines in confluent cells. There is a rough correlation between residual enzyme activity and clinical severity.[116] In cultured fibroblasts, the proportion of total folate that is methyltetrahydrofolate and the extent of labeled formate incorporated into methionine provide better correlations with clinical severity.[116,117] Cultured fibroblasts from patients with MTHFR deficiency do not grow on tissue culture medium in which homocysteine replaces methio-nine.[114,118] This methionine auxotrophy is shared by a number of inborn errors of cobalamin metabolism that affect methionine synthesis (cblC, cblD, cblE, cblF and cblG). The clinical heterogeneity in MTHFR deficiency is reflected at the biochemical level. The enzyme from fibroblasts of the first reported case of MTHFR deficiency had increased thermolability compared to control fibroblasts, especially when the assay was performed in the presence of the cofactor FAD.[118]

The findings at autopsy in severe MTHFR deficiency include dilated cerebral vessels, internal hydrocephalus, microgyria, perivascular changes, demyelination, macro-phage infiltration, gliosis and astrocytosis.[119–126] The major factor in the death of some patients was thrombosis of arteries and cerebral veins.[119] The neurovascular findings in MTHFR deficiency are similar to those seen in classic homocystinuria due to cystathionine synthase deficiency. There have been 2 reports[125,126] of patients with classic findings of subacute combined degeneration of the spinal cord similar to those described for vitamin B_{12} deficiency. Methionine deficiency may cause demyelination by interfer-ing with methylation. Since MTHFR is present in the mammalian brain and only methyltetrahydrofolate can cross the blood–brain barrier, MTHFR deficiency may result in functionally low levels of folate in the brain. It is not clear whether most of the neuropathology in MTHFR deficiency arises from decreased methionine, elevated homo-cysteine or effects of low folate.

There has been increasing interest in the measurements of total homocysteine (tHcy) in serum or plasma. This is performed by treatment of samples with reducing agents to free homocysteine from the proteins to which it is bound. These measurements have defined patients[127] with elevated levels of tHcy and an increased risk for cardiovascular disease.[128–130] Measurement of MTHFR in cell extracts has revealed thermolability of specific activity in some of these patients, and the term 'intermediate homocystinuria' was coined by Kang et al.[128] These patients were adults without the usual manifestations of MTHFR deficiency, in particu-lar the absence of neurologic manifestations. In addition, the specific activity of MTHFR is much higher in these indivi-duals than in patients with severe MTHFR deficiency. An alanine to valine substitution in a conserved residue of the MTHFR gene on chromosome 1 has been identified as the polymorphism associated with both thermolability and elevated tHcy.[131–133]

The prognosis is poor in severe MTHFR deficiency once there is evidence of neurologic involvement. The following treatments have been used: folates to maximize residual enzyme activity; methyltetrahydrofolate to replace the missing product of MTHFR; methionine to correct the deficiency of this amino acid; pyridoxine, which is a cofactor for cystathionine synthase and therefore may lower homo-cysteine levels; vitamin B_{12}, because MeCbl is a cofactor for MS; carnitine, because of its requirement for adenosyl-methionine; and betaine, because along with homocysteine it is a substrate for betaine methyltransferase, an enzyme that also converts homocysteine to methionine.

Betaine will both raise methionine levels and decrease homocysteine levels. Because betaine methyltransferase is a liver enzyme, the effects of betaine on the brain are thought to be mediated through changes in circulating levels of metabolites. A summary has been published of the treatment protocols for a number of patients with MTHFR defi-ciency.[110] Treatment with either methionine alone or with methyltetrahydrofolate has not been effective, and was largely unsuccessful until the introduction of betaine. Betaine following prenatal diagnosis has resulted in the best outcome to date.[134–137]

More than 1 case has been described in several families, both affected males and females have been born to unaf-fected parents, and consanguinity has been reported, fea-tures which are all consistent with autosomal recessive inheritance. Phenotypic heterogeneity is reflected by geno-typic heterogeneity, and 14 different mutations are known.[137–140] Prenatal diagnosis has been reported using amniocytes,[141] and the diagnosis has been excluded using amniocytes or chorionic villus cells.[111,142]

Glutamate formiminotransferase deficiency

Histidine catabolism is associated with the transfer of a formimino group to tetrahydrofolate, followed by the release of ammonia and the formation of 5,10-methenyl-tetrahydrofolate. Glutamate formiminotransferase and formiminotetrahydrofolate cyclodeaminase, two activities that share a single octameric enzyme, are involved in these reactions. These activities are found only in the liver and kidneys, and defects in them result in the excretion of formiminoglutamate (FIGLU). It is not clear that gluta-mate formiminotransferase deficiency (GFD) is associated with a consistent clinical picture. FIGLU excretion is the one constant finding. Patients with GFD range in age from 3 months to 42 years at diagnosis and 13 patients have been described. Several had macrocytosis and hypersegmentation of neutrophils. Three had speech delay, 2 seizures and 2 mental retardation on clinical presentation. Two individuals were studied because they were siblings of known patients. Although mental retardation was described in most of the original patients from Japan,[143] many of the subsequently described patients did not have this finding.

Both mild and severe phenotypes have been described. In the mild form, mental retardation is not seen but there is greater excretion of FIGLU. In the severe form, mental and physical retardation, abnormal electroencephalographic activity, and dilatation of the cerebral ventricles with corti-cal atrophy are seen. It has been proposed, without direct enzyme measurements, that the mild form is due to a defect in the formiminotransferase enzyme, and that the severe form results from one in the cyclodeaminase enzyme.[144]

In most cases in which enzyme activity in the liver has been examined, it has been higher than might be expected. Activity in 5 patients, ranged from 14 to 54% of control values. The enzyme activity is only expressed in the liver and it has not been possible to confirm the diagnosis of GFD using cultured cells. There has also been debate as to whether the enzyme is expressed in erythrocytes.[110,145]

Elevated FIGLU in the blood and urine following histi-dine load, and high to normal serum folate levels, have been reported in GFD. Amino acid levels, including that of histidine, were usually normal in the plasma. Hyperhistidi-nemia and hyperhistidinuria have been found on occasion, as has low plasma methionine levels. The excretion of 2 other metabolites, hydantoin-5-propionate, the stable oxidation product of the FIGLU precursor, 4-imidazolone-5-propio-nate, and 4-amino-5-imidazolecarboxamide, an intermedi-ate in purine synthesis has also reported.

Autosomal recessive inheritance is the probable means of transmission. Affected individuals of both sexes with unaf-fected parents have been reported. There have been no reported enzyme levels in the livers of the parents or reports of consanguinity. Definitive understanding of the genetics of this disorder awaits the cloning of the gene and the localiza-tion of the molecular defect.

Two patients in 1 family[146] responded with decreased FIGLU excretion to therapy with folates; 6 other patients did not.[110] One of 2 patients responded to methionine supplementation.[147,148] As the relationship between clinical expression and FIGLU excretion is unclear, it is uncertain that reducing FIGLU excretion has clinical utility.

Hereditary folate malabsorption

Hereditary folate malabsorption (HFM), also called con-genital malabsorption of folate, is characterized by megalo-blastic anemia, diarrhea, mouth ulcers, failure to thrive, and usually progressive neurologic deterioration. Eighteen patients with HFM have been reported, of whom 13 were female.[149–151] The most important diagnostic feature is megaloblastic anemia in the first few months of life associ-ated with low serum, red blood cell and cerebrospinal fluid folate levels.

Excretion of FIGLU and orotic acid may be found in patients with HFM. All patients have a severe abnormality in the absorption of oral folic acid or reduced folates. HFM provides the best evidence for a specific transport system of folates across both the intestine and choroid plexus and that the carrier system in both the intestine and brain is coded by a single gene product. Even when blood folate levels are raised sufficiently to correct anemia, levels in the cerebro-spinal fluid (CSF) remain low.[152] The uptake of folate into other cells is probably not defective in HFM, and uptake of folate into cultured cells is not abnormal.

Oral folic acid in doses of 5–40 mg and lower parenteral doses do effect a therapeutic response in some patients through correction of the hematologic abnormality. CSF folate levels remain low. Oral methyltetrahydrofolate and folinic acid raise CSF folate levels only slightly.[153] Folinic acid or methyltetrahydrofolic acid given systemically may be more effective in getting into the CSF in HFM; however, even with these agents, it is difficult to achieve normal concentrations of CSF folates.

Seizures in some HFM patients improved and in others deteriorated with folate therapy.[149,154] In treating these patients, it is essential to maintain levels of folate in the blood and CSF in the range that is associated with folate sufficiency. Oral doses of folates may be increased to 100 mg or more daily if necessary; if oral therapy is not effective, systemic therapy with reduced folates should be instituted. It may be necessary to give intrathecal reduced folates if CSF levels cannot be normalized.

All but 5 of the 18 HFM patients have been female. One male had atypical clinical findings, including a lack of mental retardation and correction of CSF folate levels in conjunction with correction of serum folate levels.[155] There may be unrecognized cases of HFM as several of the patients had siblings who died. Consanguinity has been reported in 4 families, and the father of 1 patient has intermediate levels of folate absorption. These findings make autosomal recessive inheritance probable.

CELLULAR UPTAKE DEFECTS

Although patients have been described with well-characterized abnormalities of folate uptake into cells, it is not clear that any of these represent primary defects.

There was a very high prevalence of severe hematologic disease, including anemia, pancytopenia and leukemia in 34 individuals in 1 family, resulting in the death of 18.[156,157] A marked reduction was seen in the uptake of methyltetrahydrofolate despite normal uptake of folic acid in stimulated lymphocytes from the proband and 4 family members. The proband and his son also had a less severe reduction of methyltetrahydrofolate uptake in bone marrow cells. One son only developed the transport defect after becoming neutropenic, suggesting that the abnormality may not be the primary defect. In another family, the proband and 3 daughters had dyserythropoiesis without anemia.[158] There was abnormal methyltetrahydrofolate uptake in red blood cells and bone marrow cells but not in lymphocytes. There was no clear correlation in the family between clinical findings and the disorder of cellular uptake.

An 18-year-old man was described as having a defect in a folate-binding protein in the CSF leading to an isolated defect in the choroid plexus transport of folate. He had neurologic but no hematologic findings.[153,159]

OTHER INHERITED DISORDERS ASSOCIATED WITH MEGALOBLASTIC ANEMIA

Thiamine-responsive megaloblastic anemia

About a dozen patients have been described with an autosomal recessive disorder characterized by megaloblastic anemia that is responsive to treatment with thiamine.[160–168] Diabetes mellitus and sensineural deafness are additional features; although the anemia responds to thiamine therapy, the diabetes requires insulin. The defect is in phosphorylation of thiamine.

Hereditary orotic aciduria

Hereditary orotic aciduria is an autosomal recessive disease due to a defect in the last 2 activities of the pyrimidine *de novo* synthetic pathway: orotate phosphoribosyltransferase (OPRT) and orotidine-5′-monophosphate decarboxylase (ODC).[169] These 2 enzyme activities reside in a single bifunctional polypeptide, uridine-5′-monophosphate synthase (UMPS), which is coded for by a single gene. There have been 15 patients described with hereditary orotic aciduria and laboratory findings have included elevated excretion of orotic acid and a macrocytic hypochromic

megaloblastic anemia. Renal tract obstruction by crystals, cardiac malformation, strabismus, infection and mild intellectual impairment have been described. There has been 1 reported patient with ODC deficiency and elevated OPRT activity but all others have had a reduction in both activities. Most patients have responded to treatment with uridine in doses ranging from 100 to 200 mg/kg/day.

The UMP synthase gene on chromosome 3q13 comprises 6 exons over approximately 15 kb; the first mutations causing hereditary orotic aciduria have been reported.[170]

ACQUIRED DISORDERS OF COBALAMIN METABOLISM

Nitrous oxide

Nitrous oxide (N_2O) is well established reversibly to oxidize body cobalamin from the cob(I) to cob(III) state. Methionine synthase requires cobalamin in the fully reduced cob(I) state and is therefore rapidly inactivated by N_2O, whereas methylmalonyl CoA mutase is spared until inhibited by cobalamin analogs produced by chronic exposure.[171] Megaloblastosis may occur within 24 hours of a single exposure and lasts < 1 week. After prolonged exposure to N_2O, as in intensive care units, pancytopenia with megaloblastic hemopoiesis may occur; after prolonged intermittent exposure as in anesthesiology or dentistry, a neuropathy resembling that of cobalamin deficiency has been described. Since recognition of this syndrome, its incidence has fallen with the use of alternative forms of anesthesia.

COBALAMIN DEFICIENCY (Table 8.1)

Nutrition

An average adult western diet contains 5–7 μg cobalamin/day and there is an obligatory loss of about 0.1% of body

Table 8.1 Acquired causes of cobalamin deficiency.

Nutritional
  Maternal deficiency
  Vegan

Malabsorption
Gastric
  Pernicious anemia
  Total or subtotal gastrectomy
Intestinal
  Stagnant-loop syndrome
  Ileal resection
  Fish tapeworm
  Chronic tropical sprue

Malabsorption of cobalamin occurs in the following conditions but the deficiency is not usually sufficiently severe to cause megaloblastic anemia:
  Gluten-induced enteropathy
  Cystic fibrosis and chronic pancreatitis
  Crohn's disease uncomplicated by resection or stagnant loop
  Drugs—slow K, colchicine, PAS, phenformin, metformin, cholestyramine

stores/day. Recommended intakes are 0.3 μg in the first year, 0.9 μg between 1 and 3 years, 1.5 μg between 4 and 9 years, 2.0 μg over the age of 10, 3.0 μg during pregnancy and 2.5 μg during lactation.[172] Infants born to cobalamin-deficient mothers may become cobalamin deficient because of reduced placental transfer of cobalamin and, if breast fed, because of cobalamin-deficient milk (normal values 0.01–0.15 μg/100ml). Most frequently, the mother is a vegan and does not eat meat, fish, eggs or cheese (milk cobalamin content: 0.003–0.07 μg/100 ml),[173] but the syndrome also occurs if the mother has unrecognized pernicious anemia (PA).[174] This is extremely rare because untreated PA usually causes sterility. The mother may or may not complete the pregnancy without megaloblastic anemia or neuropathy. Infants present with irritability, anorexia, failure to thrive, late, slow development and megaloblastic anemia within the first 18 months of life. Neurologic abnormalities may occur with poor brain growth and poor intellectual development.[175] Veganism can also cause cobalamin deficiency in children. As in adults, serum cobalamin levels are frequently low with megaloblastic anemia developing only in a small minority. There may be homocystinuria and methylmalonic aciduria. The enterohepatic circulation, accounting for a turnover of 5–10 μg/day in adults, for cobablamin is intact and helps to preserve body cobalamin.

Malabsorption

Pernicious anemia

Autoimmune gastritis leading to achloryhyria and reduced or absent intrinsic factor production with severe malabsorption of cobalamin is rare in childhood. As in adults, it may occur in any ethnic group and affects both sexes. Typically, juvenile PA presents in the first or second decade of life and is associated with the polyendocrinopathy syndrome affecting the adrenals, parathyroids, ovaries and thyroid. Mucocutaneous candidiasis, vitiligo, alopecia areata, diabetes mellitus and hypogammaglobulinemia are also frequent features.[176] A primary T-cell disorder with failure of self-recognition appears to underlie the syndrome. Children or teenagers with PA usually show 2 types of intrinsic factor (IF) antibodies in the serum: Type I or blocking antibody inhibiting IF attachment to cobalamin while Type II or binding antibody inhibits IF-cobalamin complex binding to ileal receptors. Parietal cell antibodies are usually absent in juvenile PA.

Other causes

Total or subtotal gastrectomy, intestinal stagnant loop syndrome and ileal resection may all cause severe cobalamin deficiency with megaloblastic anemia or neuropathy in children as in adults. Malabsorption of sufficient severity to cause clinical features is rare in other syndromes. Thus, children with megaloblastic anemia or neuropathy due to

cobalamin deficiency are rare in cystic fibrosis[177] or in children with *Diphyllobothrium latum* infestation.[178] A number of drugs—slow K, cholestyramine, biguanides, neomycin, para-aminosalicylate, colchicine—have been reported to cause cobalamin malabsorption but only metformin and phenformin have been described to cause megaloblastic anemia.

FOLATE DEFICIENCY (Table 8.2)

Nutrition

Folate deficiency arises when dietary supplies are insufficient to meet requirements, either because dietary intake is subnormal or folate malabsorption occurs, or because requirements are increased, as in pregnancy, in the face of suboptimal intake. Dietary folate consists largely of folate polyglutamates. The daily requirement in adults is about 100 μg, increased to 400–500 μg during pregnancy and 300 μg during lactation. A normal adult western diet contains about 250–300 μg/day (recommended intake 3 μg/kg).

Malnutrition is a frequent cause of folate deficiency in children in underdeveloped countries. This may occur with protein-calorie malnutrition and multiple vitamin deficiencies. It is more common in the winter months and where cooking techniques destroy folates and infections are frequent. Conditions of increased folate need, e.g sickle cell anemia, HIV infection, hepatitis and malaria increase the risk of the deficiency.

Newborn infants have higher serum and red cell folate levels than adults but these fall in the first few weeks of life. In premature infants the fall is steeper, folate reaches lower levels and folate deficiency with megaloblastic anemia may develop, especially if there are feeding difficulties, hemolytic disease, exchange transfusion or infection. Special artificial diets, unless folate is added, can lead to deficiency. Goats' milk has only 6 μg/l and infants fed only on this may develop significant deficiency. Folate-binding proteins are considered to reduce the bioavailability of milk folate to the neonate by reducing duodenal and jejunal transport, but they may allow ileal transfer of folate.[179] The binding proteins may also reduce folate availability to folate-requiring intestinal bacteria.

Pregnancy

Folate requirements are increased in pregnancy by about 300–400 μg/day due to increased folate breakdown and transfer of folate to the fetus. Mutilple pregnancy also increases the demand. Megaloblastic anemia may develop if the diet is inadequate and prophylactic folic acid is not given, and deficiency can also lead to premature low-birth-weight infants. Folate supplements of 400 μg/day at the time of conception reduces the incidence of neural tube defects (NTDs) (spina bifida, meningocele, anencephaly) by

177

75%,[180] and may also reduce the incidence of hare lip and cleft palate.[181] A defect of folate metabolism, a mutation (677C→T) in the gene coding for the enzyme MTHFR, changing alanine for valine, may underlie the defect in some cases, since the incidence of the mutation has been found to be higher in the mothers (and fathers) of affected fetuses than controls.[182,183] This mutation alone, however, can only account for about 15% of cases prevented by folic acid supplements. Red cell folate levels are lower in clinically normal subjects with the mutation than in controls.[184] The lower the maternal folate and cobalamin levels, even in the normal range, the more likely is an NTD.[185] The mechanism by which the deficiency affects the fetus is not clear but raised homocysteine levels have been postulated to affect the methylation ratio (S-adenosyl methionine: S-adenosyl homocysteine ratio) resulting in defects of methylation in various tissues (see above).[186]

Malabsorption

Gluten-induced enteropathy (celiac disease), in a minority of cases associated with dermatitis herpetiformis, is the most frequent cause of folate deficiency due to malabsorption in Western countries. Virtually all affected children have subnormal serum and red cell folate levels. Most of them are also iron deficient so anemia is often dimorphic. Malabsorption of cobalamin is frequent but cobalamin deficiency is never sufficiently severe to be the main cause of megaloblastic anemia.[187] Antigliadin and antiendomysial antibodies are usually present in plasma and the diagnosis is made by endoscopy and duodenal biopsy. Splenic atrophy, which occurs in 15% of adults with the disease, is less frequent in children. The intestinal lesion responds to withdrawal of gluten (glutamine-rich protein) from the diet. This also reduces the risk of subsequent development of gastointestinal lymphoma or carcinoma (especially of the esophagus).

Tropical sprue occurs in the local population and visitors to areas in the tropics where the condition is endemic. Generalized small intestinal malabsorption occurs and in the acute phase may lead to folate deficiency. In the chronic disease, cobalamin deficiency may become severe and cause megaloblastic anemia or a neuropathy. The cause of tropical sprue is likely to be an infection and the response to antibiotics supports this. About 60% of cases respond to folic acid in the first year of the illness, possibly due to a beneficial effect on the small intestinal mucosa.

Other acquired causes of folate malabsorption are rare in childhood. These include extensive Crohn's disease affecting the upper small intestine, HIV infection, systemic bacterial infections and the drugs salazopyrine, cholestyramine and triamterene. Deficiency only occurs in these situations if folate intake is suboptimal. In the intestinal stagnant-loop syndrome, folate excess occurs due to synthesis of folate by intestinal bacteria which is then absorbed from the upper small intestine.

Table 8.2 Acquired causes of folate deficiency.

Nutritional
  Inadequate, poor quality diet, goats' milk, special diets, scurvy

Malabsorption
  Gluten-induced enteropathy
  Tropical sprue
  Jejunal resection
  Systemic infections

Increased requirements
Pregnancy, pre-maturity
Conditions with increased cell turnover:
  Hemolytic anemias
  Widespread skin and other inflammatory diseases, e.g. tuberculosis, malaria
  Malignant diseases

Excess loss
  Chronic dialysis
  Liver disease
  Congestive heart failure

Drugs
  Anticonvulsants, triamterene, sulfasalazine

Liver diseases

Excess utilization

In a wide range of inflammatory and malignant diseases, folate requirements are increased (Table 8.2). These include chronic hemolytic anemias, severe chronic infections and widespread skin diseases. Folate may also be lost by dialysis, and is also lost excessively in the urine in congestive heart failure.

Antifolate drugs

Inhibitors of human dihydrofolate reductase (DHFR) include methotrexate, pyrimethamine and, to a much lesser degree, trimethoprim. Methotrexate causes megaloblastosis in humans whereas the main action of pyrimethamine is against malarial parasite DHFR. Trimethoprim acts against the bacterial enzyme and is at least 1000-fold less active than methotrexate against the human enzyme. Methotrexate is converted to polyglutamate forms in cells and this may result in prolonged inhibition of DNA synthesis. In the case of red cells, the polyglutamates remain in the cells until they die.

Recently, prostate-specific membrane (PSM) antigen has been shown to be a folate hydrolase-carboxypeptidase which can release glutamates with either γ or α linkages.[188] The physiologic importance of this is unclear.

Anticonvulsants (barbiturates, primidone) may also be associated with folate deficiency but the mechanism is uncertain. Induction of enzymes concerned with folate metabolism seems most likely. Alcohol, which may be the commonest cause of folate deficiency in the US, has a variety of effects on folate metabolism, as well as a direct effect on the bone marrow causing vacuolated normoblasts or megaloblasts. Inadequate folate intake is present in those who drink excessive alcohol and develop megaloblastic anemia due to folate deficiency.

TISSUE EFFECTS OF COBALAMIN AND FOLATE DEFICIENCIES

The characteristic abnormality is megaloblastic anemia and infants may present with failure to thrive, vomiting, anorexia and diarrhea. The blood film shows oval macrocytes and hypersegmented neutrophils (>5 nuclear lobes) and the marrow shows megaloblastic erythroblasts and giant metamyelocytes. The MCV is raised and in severe cases, leukopenia and thrombocytopenia accompany the anemia. Neuropathy due to cobalamin deficiency presents in infants and children with failure to reach milestones, and slow mental development. Permanent mental retardation may result if treatment is delayed.[41,175] In older children, features of a peripheral neuropathy mainly affecting the legs with, in severe cases, posterior column and pyramidal features are characteristic. Paraesthesiae, loss of sensation in the feet and unsteadiness in the dark are typical symptoms. Psychiatric and ophthalmic features may be present.

The deficiencies affect epithelial surfaces and sore tongue may be a presenting feature. Other epithelia, e.g. buccal, bladder, bronchial and cervical, show dysplastic features on cytology.

Serum bone alkaline phosphatase is reduced due to an effect on osteoblasts.[189] Widespread melanin pigmentation, reversible by treatment with the appropriate vitamin, may occur. The biochemical basis for this is unclear. Cobalamin deficiency has also been found to impair neutrophil function.[190] The deficiencies are associated with raised serum homocysteine levels. The role this may play in NTD is discussed above. Raised serum homocysteine levels are also associated with vascular damage (see above).

DIAGNOSIS

Measurement of serum cobalamin and serum and/or red cell folate are the standard techniques. Except in rare cases with increased transcobalamin I (haptocorrin) levels due to a myeloproliferative disease, the serum cobalamin level is reduced in cobalamin deficiency. It may also be subnormal in about a third of cases of megaloblastic anemia due to folate deficiency. Serum folate is low in folate deficiency and normal or raised in cobalamin deficiency. Red cell folate may be reduced in cobalamin deficiency, becoming subnormal in a proportion of cases, particularly the most anemic.

Other tests for the deficiencies include measurement of serum methylmalonic acid (MMA) (raised in cobalamin deficiency) and serum homocysteine (raised in either deficiency). Although some groups have suggested that measurement of these metabolites is more sensitive than assay of the serum levels of the vitamins,[191–194] this has been questioned.[195] Also, the specificity of the metabolite assays, particularly of serum homocysteine, has been questioned.

The deoxyuridine (dU) suppression test is an indirect test of thymidylate synthesis. dU does not suppress uptake of radioactively-labeled thymidine into DNA in cells deficient in cobalamin or folate as much as it suppresses thymidine uptake into DNA in normal marrow. The test is corrected in cobalamin deficiency by cobalamin or 5-formyl THF, but not by 5-methyl THF. In folate deficiency 5-formyl THF and 5-methyl THF both correct the test but cobalamin does not.[196] The test is only performed in specialized laboratories.

TREATMENT

Cobalamin deficiency is first treated by a series of intramuscular or subcutaneous injections of hydroxocobalamin (1000 μg in adults); usually 6 are given over a few weeks at intervals of a few days. Maintenance is 1000 μg hydroxocobalamin every 3 months. Vegans with cobalamin deficiency are also initially loaded with cobalamin and they may then be advised to eat food supplemented with cobalamin, e.g. certain breads, cereals and biscuits. Prophylactic cobalamin therapy is given to patients with an ileal resection or total gastrectomy.

Folate deficiency is initially corrected by giving folic acid 5 mg daily for 4 months. The treatment is continued if the underlying condition causing folate deficiency cannot be reversed and daily folate dietary intake is not improved. Folinic acid (5-formyl THF) is used to reverse the effect of methotrexate. Prophylactic folic acid is usually given to children with severe hemolytic anemias, e.g. sickle cell anemia, thalassemia major and severe autoimmune hemolytic anemia; 5 mg once weekly is probably sufficient. Annual check of serum cobalamin levels is advisable to avoid masking of unsuspected cobalamin deficiency. It is unnecessary in mild hemolytic anemia, particularly where hemopoiesis is effective, e.g the majority of cases of hereditary splerocytosis and pyruvate kinase deficiency, particularly if the diet is normal. Prophylactic folic acid 1 mg daily is also given to premature babies, particularly those weighing <1500 g, in order to reduce the incidence of anemia. In 1996, the US Food and Drug Administration announced that specified grain products, including most enriched breads, flours, cornmeal, rice noodles, and macaroni are required to be fortified with folic acid to levels ranging from 0.43 to 1.5 mg/lb (453 g) of product and consideration is being given to fortifying the British diet with folate. An extra intake of 400 μg/day is recommended before conception and during pregnancy in females, 5 mg/day if there has been a previous NTD infant. Currently, this is achieved with folic acid supplements.

OTHER ACQUIRED CAUSES OF MEGALOBLASTIC ANEMIA

Drugs inhibiting synthesis of purine or pyrimidine DNA precursors at various points in DNA synthesis cause megaloblastic anemia. These drugs include hydroxyurea, mercaptopurine, 5-fluorouracil and cytosine arabinoside. Erythropoiesis may also be megaloblastic in acute myeloid leukemia and myelodysplasia but the site of the presumed block in DNA synthesis is unknown.

REFERENCES

1. Wickramasinghe SN (ed). Megaloblastic anaemia. *Baillière's Clin Haematol* 1995; **8**

2. Katz M, Lee SK, Cooper BA. Vitamin B$_{12}$ malabsorption due to a biologically inert intrinsic factor. *N Engl J Med* 1972; **287**: 425–429

3. Carmel R. Gastric juice in congenital pernicious anemia contains no immunoreactive intrinsic factor molecule: study of three kindreds with variable ages of presentation including a patient in adulthood. *Am J Hum Genet* 1983; **35**: 67–77

4. Remacha AF, Sambeat MA, Barcelo MJ, Mones J, Garcia-Die J, Gimferrer E. Congenital intrinsic factor deficiency in a Spanish patient. *Ann Hematol* 1992; **64**: 202–204

5. Yang Y-M, Ducos R, Rosenberg AJ *et al*. Cobalamin malabsorption in three siblings due to abnormal intrinsic factor that is markedly susceptible to acid and proteolysis. *J Clin Invest* 1985; **76**: 2057–2065

6. Hewitt JE, Gordon MM, Taggart RT, Mohandas TK, Alpers DH. Human gastric intrinsic factor: characterization of cDNA and genomic clones and localization to human chromosome 11. *Genomics* 1991; **10**: 432–440

7. Chanarin I. *The Megaloblastic Anaemias*. London: Blackwell Scientific Publications, 1979, pp 144–146

8. Gräsbeck R. Familial selective vitamin B$_{12}$ malabsorption (letter). *N Engl J Med* 1972; **287**: 358

9. Wulffraat NM, De Schryver J, Bruin M, Pinxteren-Nagler E, Van Dijken PJ. Failure to thrive is an early symptom of the Imerslund–Gräsbeck syndrome. *Am J Hematol Oncol* 1994; **16**: 177–180

10. Arminoff M, Tahvanainen E, Gräsbeck R, Weissenbach J, Broch H, de la Chapelle A. Selective intestinal malabsorption of vitamin B$_{12}$ displays recessive Mendelian inheritance: assignment of a locus to chromosome 10 by linkage. *Am J Hum Genet* 1995; **57**: 824–831

11. Mackenzie IL, Donaldson RMJr, Trier JS, Mathan VI. Ileal mucosa in familial selective vitamin B$_{12}$ malabsorption. *N Engl J Med* 1972; **286**: 1021–1025

12. Burman JF, Walker WJ, Smith JA *et al*. Absent ileal uptake of IF-bound-vitamin B$_{12}$ in the Imerslund–Gräsbeck syndrome (familial vitamin B$_{12}$ malabsorption with proteinuria). *Gut* 1985; **26**: 311–314

13. Fyfe JC, Ramanujam KS, Ramaswamy K, Patterson DF, Seetharam B. Defective brush-border expression of intrinsic factor-cobalamin receptor in canine inherited intestinal cobalamin malabsorption. *J Biol Chem* 1991; **266**: 4489–4494

14. Fyfe JC, Giger U, Hall CA *et al*. Inherited selective intestinal cobalamin malabsorption and cobalamin deficiency in dogs. *Pediatr Res* 1991; **29**: 24–31

14a. Kozyraki R, Kristiansen M, Silahtaroglu A, Hansen C, Jacobsen C, Tommerup N, Verroust PJ, Moestrup SK. The human intrinsic factor—vitamin B$_{12}$ receptor, cubilin: molecular characterization and chromosomal mapping of the gene to 10p within the autosomal recessive megaloblastic anemia (MGA1) region. *Blood* 1998; **91**: 3593–3600

15. Cooper BA, Rosenblatt DS. Inherited defects of vitamin B$_{12}$ metabolism. *Ann Rev Nutr* 1987; **7**: 291–320

16. Carmel R. A new case of deficiency of the R binder for cobalamin, with observations on minor cobalamin binding proteins in serum and saliva. *Blood* 1982; **59**: 152–156

17. Carmel R. R-binder deficiency. A clinically benign cause of cobalamin pseudodeficiency. *JAMA* 1983; **250**: 1886–1890

18. Carmel R, Herbert V. Deficiency of vitamin B$_{12}$ alpha globulin in two brothers. *Blood* 1969; **33**: 1–12

19. Jenks J, Begley J, Howard L. Cobalamin-R binder deficiency in a woman with thalassemia. *Nutr Rev* 1983; **41**: 277–280

20. Sigal SH, Hall CA, Antel JP. Plasma R binder deficiency and neurologic disease. *N Engl J Med* 1988; **317**: 1330–1332

21. Kolhouse JF, Kondo H, Allen NC, Podell ER, Allen RH. Cobalamin analogues are present in human plasma and can mask cobalamin deficiency because current radioisotope dilution assays are not specific for true cobalamin. *N Engl J Med* 1978; **299**: 785–792

22. Li N, Rosenblatt DS, Kamen BA, Seetharam S, Seetharam B. Identification of two mutant alleles of transcobalamin II in an affected family. *Hum Mol Genet* 1994; **3**: 1835–1840

23. Kaikov Y, Wadsworth LD, Hall CA, Rogers PC. Transcobalamin II deficiency: case report and review of the literature. *Eur J Pediatr* 1991; **150**: 841–843

24. Linnell JC, Bhatt HR. Inherited errors of cobalamin metabolism and their management. *Baillière's Clin Haematol* 1995; **8**: 567–601

25. Rothenberg SP, Quadros EV. Transcobalamin II and the membrane receptor for the transcobalmin II-cobalamin complex. *Baillière's Clin Haematol* 1995; **8**: 499–514

26. Porck HJ, Frater-Schroder M, Frants KI *et al*. Genetic evidence for fetal origin of transcobalamin II in human cord blood. *Blood* 1983; **62**: 234

27. Nierbrugge DJ, Benjamin DR, Christie D, Scott CR. Hereditary transcobalamin II deficiency presenting as red cell hypoplasia. *J Pediatr* 1982; **101**: 732–735

28. Burman JF, Mollin DL, Sourial NA, Sladden RA. Inherited lack of transcobalamin II in serum and megaloblastic anemia: a further patient. *Br J Haematol* 1979; **43**: 27–38

29. Meyers PA, Carmel R. Hereditary transcobalamin II deficiency with subnormal serum cobalamin levels. *Pediatrics* 1984; **74**: 866–871

30. Thomas PK, Hoffbrand AV, Smith IS. Neurological involvement in hereditary transcobalamin II deficiency. *J Neurol Neurosurg Psychiat* 1982; **45**: 74–77

31. Zeitlin HC, Sheppard K, Bolton FG, Hall CA. Homozygous transcobalamin II deficiency maintained on oral hydroxocobalamin. *Blood* 1985; **66**: 1022–1027

32. Haurani FI, Hall CA, Rubin R. Megaloblastic anemia as a result of an abnormal transcobalamin II. *J Clin Invest* 1979; **64**: 1253–1259

33. Fenton W, Rosenberg LE. Inherited disorders of cobalamin transport and metabolism. In: Scriver CR, Beaudet AL, Sly WS, Valle D (eds) *The Metabolic and Molecular Bases of Inherited Disease*. New York: McGraw-Hill, 1995, pp 3129–3149

34. Daiger SP, Labowe ML, Parsons M, Wang L, Cavalli-Sforza LL. Detection of genetic variation with radioactive ligands. III. Genetic polymorphism of transcobalamin II in human plasma. *Am J Hum Genet* 1989; **30**: 202–214

35. Eiberg H, Moller N, Mohr J, Nielsen LS. Linkage of transcobalamin II (TC2) to the P blood group system and assignment to chromosome 22. *Clin Genet* 1986; **29**: 354

36. Platica O, Janeczko R, Quadros EV, Regec A, Romain R, Rothenberg SP. The cDNA sequence and the deduced amino acid sequence of human transcobalamin II show homology with rat intrinsic factor and human transcobalamin I. *J Biol Chem* 1991; **266**: 7860–7863

37. Li N, Seetharam S, Lindemans J, Alpers DH, Arwert F, Seetharam B. Isolation and sequence analysis of variant forms of human transcobalamin II. *Biochim Biophys Acta Gene Struct Expression* 1993; **1172**: 21–30

38. Li N, Rosenblatt DS, Seetharam B. Nonsense mutations in human transcobalamin II deficiency. *Biochem Biophys Res Commun* 1994; **204**: 1111–1118

39. Rosenblatt DS, Hosack A, Matiaszuk N. Expression of transcobalamin II by amniocytes. *Prenat Diagn* 1987; **7**: 35–39

40. Mayes JS, Say B, Marcus DL. Prenatal diagnosis in a family with transcobalamin II deficiency. *Am J Hum Genet* 1987; **41**: 686

41. Thomas PK, Hoffbrand AV. Hereditary transcobalamin II deficiency: a 22 year follow up. *J Neurol Neurosurg Psychiat* 1997; **62**: 197

42. Mahoney MJ, Bick D. Recent advances in the inherited methylmalonic acidemias. *Acta Paediatr Scand* 1987; **76**: 689–696

43. Coulombe JT, Shih VE, Levy HL. Massachusetts metabolic disorders screening program. II Methylmalonic aciduria. *Pediatrics* 1981; **67**: 26–31

44. Fenton WA, Hack AM, Helfgott D, Rosenberg LE. Biogenesis of the mitochondrial enzyme methylmalonyl-CoA mutase: synthesis and processing of a precursor in a cell-free system and in cultured cells. *J Biol Chem* 1984; **259**: 6616–6621

45. Ledley FD, Rosenblatt DS. Mutations in mut methylmalonic acidemia: clinical and enzymatic correlations. *Hum Mutat* 1997; **98**: 1–6

46. Fenton WA, Hack AM, Kraus JP, Rosenberg LE. Immunochemical studies of fibroblasts from patients with methylmalonyl-CoA mutase apoenzyme deficiency: detection of a mutation interfering with mitochondrial import. *Proc Natl Acad Sci USA* 1987; **84**: 1421–1424

47. Ledley FD, Jansen R, Nham SU, Fenton WA, Rosenberg LE. Mutation eliminating mitochondrial leader sequence of methylmalonyl CoA mutase causes mut0 methylmalonic aciduria. *Proc Natl Acad Sci USA* 1990; **87**: 3147–3150

48. Raff ML, Crane AM, Jansen R, Ledley FD, Rosenblatt DS. Genetic characterization of a MUT locus mutatation discriminating heterogeneity in *mut0* and *mut−* methymalonic aciduria by interallelic complementation. *J Clin Invest* 1991; **87**: 203–207

49. Qureshi AA, Crane AM, Matiaszuk NV, Rezvani I, Ledley FD, Rosenblatt DS. Cloning and expression of mutations demonstrating intragenic complementation in mut0 methylmalonic aciduria. *J Clin Invest* 1994; **93**: 1812–1819

50. Inque S, Kreiger I, Sarnaik A, Ravindranath Y, Fracassa M, Ottenbreit MJ. Inhibition of bone marow stem cell growth in vitro by methylmalonic acid: a mechanism for pancytopenia in a patient with methylmalonic acidemia. *Pediatr Res* 1981; **15**: 95

51. Ledley FD, Levy HL, Shih VE, Benjamin R, Mahoney MJ. Benign methylmalonic aciduria. *N Engl J Med* 1984; **311**: 1015–1018

52. Ledley FD, Lumetta M, Nguyen PN, Kolhouse JF, Allen RH. Molecular cloning of L-methylmalonyl CoA mutase: gene transfer and analysis of *mut* cell lines. *Proc Natl Acad Sci USA* 1988; **85**: 3518–3521

53. Ledley FD, Lumetta MR, Zoghbi HY, VanTuinen P, Ledbetter DH. Mapping of human methylmalonyl CoA mutase (MUT) locus on chromosome 6. *Am J Hum Genet* 1988; **42**: 839–856

54. Zoghbi HY, O'Brien WE, Ledley FD. Linkage relationships of the human methylmalonyl CoA mutase to the HLA and D6S4 loci on chromosome 6. *Genomics* 1988; **3**: 396–398

55. Jansen R, Kalousek F, Fenton WA, Rosenberg LE, Ledley FD. Cloning of full-length methylmalonyl CoA mutase from a cDNA library using the polymerase chain reaction. *Genomics* 1989; **4**: 198–205

56. Crane AM, Ledley FD. Clustering of mutations in methylmalonyl CoA mutase associated with *mut−* methylmalonic acidemia. *Am J Hum Genet* 1994; **55**: 42–50

57. Adjalla CE, Hosack AR, Gilfix BM *et al.* Seven novel mutations in *mut−* methylmalonic aciduria. *Hum Mutat* 1998; **11**: 270–274

58. Crane AM, Martin LS, Valle D, Ledley FD. Phenotype of disease in three patients with identical mutations in methylmalonyl CoA mutase. *Hum Genet* 1992; **89**: 259–264

59. Adjalla CE, Hosack AR, Matiaszuk NV, Rosenblatt DS. A common mutation among blacks with *mut−* methylmalonic aciduria. *Hum Mutat* 1998; **Suppl 1**: S248–S250

60. Ogasawara M, Matsubara Y, Mikami H, Narisawa KK. Identification of two novel mutations in the methylmalonyl-CoA mutase gene with decreased levels of mutant mRNA in methylmalonic acidemia. *Hum Mol Genet* 1994; **3**: 867–872

61. Chalmers RA, Stacey TE, Tracey BM *et al.* L-Carnitine insufficiency in disorders of organic acid metabolism: response to L-carnitine by patients with methylmalonic aciduria and 3- hydroxy-3-methylglutaric aciduria. *J Inherit Metab Dis* 1984; **7**: 109–110

62. Wolff JA, Carroll JE, Le Phuc Thuy, Prodanos C, Haas R, Nyhan WL. Carnitine reduces fasting ketogenesis in patients with disorders of propionate metabolism. *Lancet* 1986; **i**: 289–291

63. Bain MD, Jones M, Borriello SP *et al.* Contribution of gut bacterial metabolism to human metabolic disease. *Lancet* 1988; **i**: 1078–1079

64. Snyderman SE, Sansaricq C, Norton P, Phansalkr SV. The use of neomycin in the treatment of methylmalonic aciduria. *Pediatrics* 1972; **50**: 925–927

65. Koletzko B, Bachmann C, Wendel U. Antibiotic treatment for improvement of metabolic control in methylmalonic aciduria. *J Pediatr* 1990; **117**: 99–101

66. Treacy E, Arbour L, Chessex P *et al.* Glutathione deficiency as a complication of methylmalonic acidemia, response to high ascorbate. *J Pediatr* 1996; **129**: 445–448

67. Watanabe F, Saido H, Yamaji R *et al.* Mitochondrial NADH- or NADP-Linked Aquacobalamin reductase activity is low in human skin fibroblasts with defects in synthesis of cobalamin coenzymes. *J Nutr* 1996; **126**: 2947–2951

68. Fenton WA, Rosenberg LE. The defect in the cblB class of human methylmalonic acidemia: deficiency of cob(I)alamin adenosyltransferase activity in extracts of cultured fibroblasts. *Biochem Biophys Res Commun* 1981; **98**: 283–289

69. Cooper BA, Rosenblatt DS, Watkins D. Methylmalonic aciduria due to a new defect in adenosylcobalamin accumulation by cells. *Am J Hematol* 1990; **34**: 115–120

70. Matsui SM, Mahoney MJ, Rosenberg LE. The natural history of the inherited methylmalonic acidemias. *N Engl J Med* 1983; **308**: 857–861

71. Batshaw ML, Thomas GH, Cohen SR, Matalon R, Mahoney MJ. Treatment of the cblB form of methylmalonic acidaemia with adenosylcobalamin. *J Inherit Metab Dis* 1984; **7**: 65–68

72. Bhatt HR, Linnell JC, Barltrop D. Treatment of hydroxocobalamin-resistant methylmalonic acidaemia with adenosylcobalamin (letter). *Lancet* 1986; **ii**: 465

73. Ampola MG, Mahoney MJ, Nakamura E, Tanaka K. Prenatal therapy of a patient with vitamin B12 responsive methylmalonic acidemia. *N Engl J Med* 1975; **293**: 313–317

74. Zass R, Leupold MA, Fernandez MA, Wendel U. Evaluation of prenatal treatment in newborns with cobalamin-responsive methylmalonic acidaemia. *J Inherit Metab Dis* 1995; **18**: 100–101

75. Mellman I, Willard HF, Youngdahl-Turner P, Rosenberg LE. Cobalamin coenzyme synthesis in normal and mutant fibroblasts: evidence for a processing enzyme activity deficient in *cblC* cells. *J Biol Chem* 1979; **254**: 11847

76. Pezacka EH, Rosenblatt DS. Intracellular metabolism of cobalamin. Altered activities of β-axial-ligand transferase and microsomal cob(III)alamin reducatase in *cblC* and *cblD* fibroblasts. In: Bhatt HR, James VHT, Besser GM, Bottazzo GF, Keen H. (eds) *Advances in Thomas Addison's Diseases.* Bristol: Journal of Endocrinology Press, 1994, pp 315–323

77. Pezacka EH. Identification and characterization of two enzymes involved in the intracellular metabolism of cobalamin. Cyanocobalamin β-ligand transferase and microsomal cob(III)alamin reductase. *Biochim Biophys Acta* 1993; **1157**: 167–177

78. Rosenblatt DS, Cooper BA. Inherited disorders of vitamin B12 metabolism. *Blood Rev* 1987; **1**: 177–182

79. Vassiliadis A, Rosenblatt DS, Cooper BA, Bergeron JJ. Lysosomal cobalamin accumulation in fibroblasts from a patient with an inborn error of cobalamin metabolism (*cblF* complementation group): visualization by electron microscope radioautography. *Exp Cell Res* 1991; **195**: 295–302

80. Rosenblatt DS. Inherited errors of cobalamin metabolism: an overview. In: Bhatt HR, James VHT, Besser GM, Bottazzo GF, Keen H (eds) *Advances in Thomas Addison's Diseases.* Bristol, Journal of Endocrinology Press, 1994, pp 303–313

81. Mitchell GA, Watkins D, Melancon SB *et al.* Clinical heterogeneity in cobalamin C variant of combined homocystinuria and methylmalonic aciduria. *J Pediatr* 1986; **108**: 410–415

82. Shinnar S, Singer HS. Cobalamin C mutation (methylmalonic

aciduria and homocystinuria) in adolescence. A treatable cause of dementia and myelopathy. *N Engl J Med* 1984; **311**: 451–454

83. Robb RM, Dowton SB, Fulton AB, Levy HL. Retinal degeneration in vitamin B$_{12}$ disorder associated with methylmalonic aciduria and sulfur amino acid abnormalities. *Am J Ophthalmol* 1984; **97**: 691–696

84. Traboulsi EI, Silva JC, Geraghty MT, Maumenes IH, Valle D, Green WR. Ocular histopathologic characteristics of cobalamin C complementation type vitamin B$_{12}$ defect with methylmalonic aciduria and homocystinuria. *Am J Ophthalmol* 1992; **113**: 269–280

85. Weintraub L, Tardo C, Rosenblatt DS, Shapira E. Hydrocephalus as a possible complication of the *cblC* type of methylmalonic aciduria. *Am J Hum Genet* 1991; **49**: 108A

86. Caouette G, Rosenblatt D, Laframboise R. Hepatic dysfunction in a neonate with combined methylmalonic aciduria and homocystinuria. *Clin Invest Med* 1992; **15**: A112

87. Goodman SI, Moe PG, Hammond KB, Mudd SH, Uhlendorff BW. Homocystinuria with methylmalonic aciduria: two cases in a sibship. *Biochem Med* 1970; **4**: 500–515

88. Shih VE, Axel SM, Tewksbury JC, Watkins D, Cooper BA, Rosenblatt DS. Defective lysosomal release of vitamin B$_{12}$ (*cblF*): a hereditary cobalamin metabolic disorder associated with sudden death. *Am J Med Genet* 1989; **33**: 555–563

89. Rosenblatt DS, Laframboise R, Pichette J, Langevin P, Cooper BA, Costa T. New disorder of vitamin B$_{12}$ metabolism (cobalamin F) presenting as methylmalonic aciduria. *Pediatrics* 1986; **78**: 51–54

90. Laframboise R, Cooper BA, Rosenblatt DS. Malabsorption of vitamin B$_{12}$ from the intestine in a child with *cblF* disease: evidence for lysosomal-mediated absorption (letter). *Blood* 1992; **80**: 291–292

91. MacDonald MR, Wiltse HE, Bever JL, Rosenblatt DS. Clinical heterogeneity in two patients with *cblF* disease. *Am J Hum Genet* 1992; **15**: A353

92. Wong LTK, Rosenblatt DS, Applegarth DA, Davidson AGF. Diagnosis and treatment of a child with *cblF* disease. *Clin Invest Med* 1992; **15**: A111

93. Zammarchi E, Lippi A, Falorni S, Pasquini E, Cooper BA, Rosenblatt DS. *cblC* Disease: case report and monitoring of a pregnancy at risk by chorionic villus sampling. *Clin Invest Med* 1990; **13**: 139–142

94. Chadefaux-Vekemans B, Rolland MO, Lyonet S, Rabier D, Divry P, Kamoun P. Prenatal diagnosis of combined methylmalonic aciduria and homocystinuria (cobalamin *CblC* or *CblD* mutant) (letter). *Prenat Diagn* 1994; **14**: 417–418

95. Rosenblatt DS, Aspler AL, Shevell MI, Pletcher BA, Fenton WA, Seashore MR. Clinical heterogeneity and prognosis in combined methylmalonic aciduria and homocystinuria (*cblC*). *J Inherit Metab Dis* 1997; **20**: 528–538

96. Bartholomew DW, Batshaw ML, Allen RH *et al.* Therapeutic approaches to cobalamin-C methylmalonic acidemia and homocystinuria. *J Pediatr* 1988; **112**: 32–39

97. Shih VE, Axel SM, Tewksbury JC, Watkins D, Cooper BA, Rosenblatt DS. Defective lysosomal release of vitamin B$_{12}$ (*cblF*) a hereditary metabolic disorder associated with sudden death. *Am J Med Genet* 1989; **33**: 555–563

98. Tuchman M, Kelly P, Watkins D, Rosenblatt DS. Vitamin B$_{12}$-responsive megaloblastic anemia, homocystinuria, and transient methylmalonic aciduria in *cblE* disease. *J Pediatr* 1988; **113**: 1052–1056

99. Watkins D, Rosenblatt DS. Functional methionine synthase deficiency (*cblE* and *cblG*): clinical and biochemical heterogeneity. *Am J Med Genet* 1989; **34**: 427–434

100. Watkins D, Rosenblatt DS. Genetic heterogeneity among patients with methylcobalamin deficiency. *J Clin Invest* 1988; **81**: 1690–1694

101. Sillaots SL, Hall CA, Hurteloup V, Rosenblatt DS. Heterogeneity in *cblG*: differential retention of cobalamin on methionine synthase. *Biochem Med Meta Biol* 1992; **47**: 242–249

102. Rosenblatt DS, Cooper BA, Pottier A, Lue-Shing H, Matiaszuk N, Grauer K. Altered vitamin B$_{12}$ metabolism in fibroblasts from a patient with megaloblastic anemia and homocystinuria due to a new defect in methionine biosynthesis. *J Clin Invest* 1984; **74**: 2149–2156

103. Rosenblatt DS, Cooper BA. Selective deficiencies of methyl B$_{12}$ (*cblE* and *cblG*). *Clin Invest Med* 1989; **12**: 270–271

104. Leclerc D, Wilson A, Dumas R *et al.* Cloning and mapping of a cDNA for methionine synthase reductase, a flavoprotein defective in patients with homocystinuria. *Proc Natl Acad Sci USA* 1998; **95**: 3059–3064

105. Hall CA, Lindenbaum RH, Arenson E, Begley JA, Chu RC. The nature of the defect in cobalamin G mutation. *Clin Invest Med* 1989; **12**: 262–269

106. Leclerc D, Campeau E, Goyette P *et al.* Human methionine synthase: cDNA cloning and identification of mutations in patients of the *cblG* complementation group of folate/cobalamin disorders. *Hum Mol Genet* 1996; **5**: 1867–1874

107. Li YN, Gulati S, Baker PJ, Brody LC, Banerjee R, Kruger WD. Cloning, mapping and RNA analysis of the human methionine synthase gene. *Hum Mol Genet* 1996; **5**: 1851–1858

108. Gulati S, Baker P, Li YN, Fowler B, Kruger WD, Brody LC, Banerjee R. Defects in human methionine synthase in *cblG* patients. *Hum Mol Genet* 1996; **5**: 1859–1865

109. Rosenblatt DS, Cooper BA, Schmutz SM, Zaleski WA, Casey RE. Prenatal vitamin B$_{12}$ therapy of a fetus with methylcobalamin deficiency (cobalamin E disease). *Lancet* 1985; **i**: 1127–1129

110. Erbe RW. Inborn errors of folate metabolism. In: Blakley RL, Whitehead VM (eds). *Folates and Pterins, vol 3. Nutritional, Pharmacological and Physiological Aspects.* New York: John Wiley 1986, pp 413–466

111. Marquet J, Chadefaux B, Bonnefont JP, Saudubray JM, Zittoun J. Methylenetetrahydrofolate reductase deficiency: prenatal diagnosis and family studies. *Prenat Diagn* 1994; **14**: 29–33

112. Haworth JC, Dilling LA, Surtees RAH *et al.* Symptomatic and asymptomatic methylenetetrahydrofolate reductase deficiency in two adult brothers. *Am J Med Genet* 1993; **45**: 572–576

113. Rosenblatt DS, Cooper BA, Lue-Shing S *et al.* Folate distribution in cultured human cells: studies on 5,10-CH$_2$-H4PteGlu reductase deficiency. J Clin Invest 1979; 63: 1019–1025

114. Mudd SH, Uhlendorf BW, Freeman JM, Finkelstein JD, Shih VE. Homocysteinuria associated with decreased methylenetetrahydrofolate reducatase activity. *Biochem Biophys Res Commun* 1972; **46**: 905

115. Pasquier F, Lebert F, Petit H, Zittoun J, Marquet J. Methylenetetrahydrofolate reductase deficiency revealed by a neuropathy in a psychotic adult (letter). *J Neurol Neurosurg Psychiat* 1994; **57**: 765–766

116. Rosenblatt DS, Cooper BA, Lue-Shing S *et al.* Folate distribution in cultured human cells: studies on 5,10-CH2-H4PteGlu reductase deficiency. *J Clin Invest* 1979; **63**: 1019–1025

117. Boss GR, Erbe RW. Decreased rates of methionine synthesis by methylenetetrahydrofolate reductase-deficient fibroblasts and lymphoblasts. *J Clin Invest* 1981; **67**: 1659

118. Rosenblatt DS, Erbe RW. Methylenetetrahydrofolate reductase in cultured human cells. II Genetic and biochemical studies of methylenetetrahydrofolate reductase deficiency. *Pediatr Res* 1977; **11**: 1141–1143

119. Kanwar YS, Manaligod JR, Wong PWK. Morphologic studies in a patient with homocystinuria due to 5,10-methylenetetrahydrofolate reductase deficiency. *Pediatr Res* 1976; **10**: 598

120. Wong PWK, Justice P, Hruby M, Weiss EB, Diamond E. Folic acid non-responsive homocystinuria due to methylenetetrahydrofolate reductase deficiency. *Pediatrics* 1977; **59**: 749–756

121. Baumgartner ER, Schweizer K, Wick H. Different congenital forms of defective remethylation in homocystinuria. Clinical, biochemical, and morphological studies. *Pediatr Res* 1977; **11**: 1015

122. Haan EA, Rogers JG, Lewis GP, Rowe PB. 5,10-methylenetetrahydrofolate reductase deficiency: clinical and biochemical features of a further case. *J Inherit Metab Dis* 1985; **8**: 53

123. Hyland K, Smith I, Howell DW, Clayton PT, Leonard JV. The determination of pterins, biogenic amino metabolites, and aromatic amino acids in cerebrospinal fluid using isocratic reverse phase liquid chromatography within series dual cell coulometric electrochemical and fluorescence determinations (use in the study of inborn errors of

dihydropteridine reductase and 5,10-methylenetetrahydrofolate reductase. In: Wachter H, Curtius H, Pfleiderer W (eds) *Biochemical and Clinical Aspects of Pteridines, Vol 4.* Berlin: de Gruyter, 1985, pp 85–89

124. Baumgartner ER, Stokstad ELR, Wick H, Watson JE, Kusano G. Comparison of folic acid coenzyme distribution patterns in patients with methylenetetrahydrofolate reductase and methionine synthetase deficiencies. *Pediatr Res* 1985; **19**: 1288

125. Clayton PT, Smith I, Harding B *et al.* Subacute combined degeneration of the cord, dementia and Parkinsonian due to an inborn error of folate metabolism. *J Neurol Neurosurg Psychiat* 1986; **49**: 920–927

126. Beckman DR, Hoganson G, Berlow S, Gilbert EF. Pathological findings in 5,10-methylenetetrahydrofolate reductase deficiency. *Birth Defects* 1987; **23**: 47

127. Kang SS, Zhou J, Wong PWK, Kowalisyn J, Strokosch G. Intermediate homocysteinemia: a thermolabile variant of methylenetetrahydrofolate reductase. *Am J Hum Genet* 1988; **43**: 414–421

128. Kang S-S, Wong PWK, Susmano A, Sora J, Norusis M, Ruggie N. Thermolabile methylenetetrahydrofolate reductase: an inherited risk factor for coronary artery disease. *Am J Hum Genet* 1991; **48**: 536–545

129. Engbersen AMT, Franken DG, Boers GHJ, Stevens EMB. Thermolabile 5, 10-methylenetetrahydrofolate reductase as a cause of mild hyperhomocysteinemia. *Am J Hum Genet* 1995; **56**: 142–150

130. Boushey CJ, Beresford SAA, Omenn GS, Motulsky AG. A quantitative assessment of plasma homocysteine as a risk factor for vascular disease: probable benefits of increasing folic acid intakes. *JAMA* 1995; **274**: 1049–1057

131. Frosst P, Blom HJ, Milos R *et al.* A candidate genetic risk factor for vascular disease: a common methylenetetrahydrofolate reductase mutation causes thermoinstability. *Nature Genet* 1995; **10**: 111–113

132. Christensen B, Frosst P, Lussier-Cacan S *et al.* Correlation of a common mutation in the methylenetetrahydrofolate reductase (MTHFR) gene with plasma homocysteine in patients with premature coronary artery disease. *Arter Thromb Vasc Biol* 1997; **17**: 569–573

133. Brugada R, Marian AJ. A common mutation in methylenetetrahydrofolate reductase gene is not a major risk of coronary artery disease or myocardial infarction. *Atherosclerosis* 1997; **128**: 107–112

134. Kang SS. Treatment of hyperhomocyst(e)inemia: physiological basis. *J Nutr* 1996; **126 (Suppl 4)**: 1273S–1275S

135. Wendel U, Bremer HJ. Betaine in the treatment of homocystinuria due to 5,10-methylenetetrahydrofolate reductase deficiency. *Eur J Pediatr* 1984; **142**: 147

136. Brandt NJ, Christensen E, Skovby F, Djernes B. *Treatment of Methylenetetrahydrofolate Reductase Deficiency from the Neonatal Period.* Amersfoort: The Society for the Study of Inborn Errors of Metabolism, 1986, p23

137. Ronge E, Kjellman B. Long term treatment with betaine in methylenetetrahydrofolate reductase deficiency. *Arch Dis Child* 1996; **74**: 239–241

138. Goyette P, Frosst P, Rosenblatt DS, Rozen R. Seven novel mutations in the methylenetetrahydrofolate reductase gene and genotype/phenotype correlations in severe methylenetetrahydrofolate reductase deficiency. *Am J Hum Genet* 1995; **56**: 1052–1059

139. Goyette P, Milos R, Ducan AM, Rosenblatt DS, Matthews RG, Rozen R. Human methylenetetrahydrofolate reductase: isolation of cDNA, mapping and mutation identification. *Nature Genet* 1994; **7**: 195–200

140. Goyette P, Christensen B, Rosenblatt DS, Rozen R. Severe and mild mutations in cis for the methylenetetrahydrofolate (MTHFR) gene, and description of 5 novel mutations in MTHFR. *Am J Hum Genet* 1996; **59**: 1268–1275

141. Christensen E, Brandt NJ. Prenatal diagnosis of 5,10-methylenetetrahydrofolate reductase deficiency. *N Engl J Med* 1985; **313**: 50

142. Wendel U, Claussen U, Dickmann E. Prenatal diagnosis for methylenetetrahydrofolate reductase deficiency. *J Pediatr* 1983; **102**: 938

143. Arakawa T. Congenital defects in folate utilization. *Am J Med* 1970; **48**: 594–598

144. Rowe PB. Inherited disorders of folate metabolism. In: Stanbury JB,

Wyngaarden JB, Frederickson DS, Goldstein JL, Brown MS (eds) *The Metabolic Basis of Inherited Diseases.* New York: McGraw-Hill, 1983, p 498

145. Shin YS, Reiter S, Zelger O, Brunstler I, Vrucker A. Orotic aciduria, homocystinuria, formiminoglutamic aciduria and megaloblastosis associated with the formiminotransferase/cyclodeaminase deficiency. In: Nyhan WL, Thompson LF, Watts RWE (eds) *Purine and Pyrimidine Metabolism in Man.* New York: Plenum, 1986, p 71

146. Perry TL, Applegarth DA, Evans ME, Hansen S. Metabolic studies of a family with massive formiminoglutamic aciduria. *Pediatr Res* 1975; **9**: 117

147. Russel A, Statter M, Abzug S. Methionine-dependent formiminoglutamic acid transferase deficiency: human and experimental studies in its therapy. *Hum Hered* 1977; **27**: 205

148. Duran M, Ketting D, deBree PK *et al.* A case of formiminoglutamic aciduria. *Eur J Pediatr* 1981; **136**: 319

149. Rosenblatt DS. Inherited disorders of folate transport and metabolism. In: Scriver CR, Beaudet al, Sly WS, Valle D (eds) *The Metabolic and Molecular Bases of Inherited Disease.* New York: McGraw-Hill, 1995, pp 3111–3128

150. Lankowsky P. Congenital malabsorption of folate. *Am J Med* 1970; **48**: 580

151. Corbeel L, Van Den Berghe G, Jaeken J, Vantornout J, Eeckels R. Congenital folate malabsorption. *Eur J Pediatr* 1985; **143**: 284–290

152. Steinschneider M, Sherbany A, Pavlakis S, Emerson R, Lovelace R, De Vivo DC. Congenital folate malabsorption: reversible clinical neurophysiological abnormalities. *Neurology* 1990; **40**: 1315

153. Zittoun J. Congenital errors of folate metabolism. *Bailliere's Clin Haematol* 1995; **8**: 603–616

154. Buchanan JA. *Fibroblast Plasma Membrane Vesicles to Study Inborn Errors of Transport.* PhD Thesis, McGill University, 1984

155. Urbach J, Abrahamov A, Grossowicz N. Congenital isolated folate acid malabsorption. *Arch Dis Child* 1987; **62**: 78–80

156. Branda RF, Moldow CF, MacArthur JR, Wintrobe MM, Anthony BK, Jacob HS. Folate-induced remission in aplastic anemia with familial defect of cellular folate uptake. *N Engl J Med* 1978; **298**: 469–475

157. Arthur DC, Danzyl TJ, Branda FR. Cytogenetic studies of a family with a hereditary defect of cellular folate uptake and high incidence of hematologic disease. In: *Nutritional Factors in the Induction and Maintenance of Malignancy.* New York: Academic Press, 1983, pp 101–111

158. Howe RB, Branda RF, Douglas SD, Brunning RD. Hereditary dyserythropoiesis with abnormal membrane folate transport. *Blood* 1979; **54**: 1080

159. Wevers RA, Hansen SI, van Hellenberg Hubar JLM, Holm J, Hoier-Madsen M, Jongen PJH. Folate deficiency in cerebrospinal fluid associated with a defect in folate binding protein in the central nervous system. *J Neurol Neurosurg Psychiat* 1994; **57**: 223–226

160. Abboud MR, Alexander D, Najjar SS. Diabetes mellitus, thiamine-dependent megaloblastic anemia, and sensorineural deafness associated with deficient alpha-ketoglutarate dehydrogenase activity. *J Pediatr* 1985; **107**: 537–541

161. Duran M, Wadman SK. Thiamine-responsive inborn errors of metabolism. *J Inherit Metab Dis* 1985; **8**: 70–75

162. Haworth C, Evans DIK, Mitra J, Wickramasinghe SN. Thiamine responsive anemia: a study of two further cases. *Br J Haematol* 1982; **50**: 549–561

163. Mandel H, Berant M, Hazani A, Naveh Y. Thiamine-dependent beriberi in the "thiamine-responsive anemia syndrome". *N Engl J Med* 1984; **311**: 836–838

164. Poggi V, Longo G, DeVizia B *et al.* Thiamine-responsive megaloblastic anaemia: a disorder of thiamine transport? *J Inherit Metab Dis* 1984; **7 (Suppl 2)**: 153–154

165. Poggi V, Rindi G, Patrini C, DeVizia B, Longo G, Andria G. Studies on thiamine metabolism in thiamine-responsive megaloblastic anaemia. *Eur J Pediatr* 1989; **148**: 307–311

166. Rindi G, Casirola D, Poggi V, De Vizia B, Patrini C, Laforenza U.

Thiamine transport by erythrocytes and ghosts in thiamine-responsive megaloblastic anaemia. *J Inherit Metab Dis* 1992; **15**: 231–242

167. Rogers LE, Porter FS, Sidbury JBJr. Thiamine-responsive megaloblastic anemia. *J Pediatr* 1969; **74**: 494–504

168. Viana MB, Carvalho RI. Thiamine-responsive megaloblastic anemia, sensineural deafness, and diabetes mellitus: a new syndrome? *J Pediatr* 1978; **93**: 235–238

169. Webster DR, Becroft DMO, Suttle DP. Hereditary orotic aciduria. In: Scriver CR, Beaudet AL, Sly WS, Valle D (eds) *The Metabolic and Molecular Bases of Inherited Disease*. New York: McGraw Hill, 1995, pp 1799–1837

170. Suchi M, Mizuno H, Kawai Y *et al*. Molecular cloning of human UMP synthase gene and characterization of point mutations in two hereditary orotic aciduria families. *Am J Hum Genet* 1997; **60**: 525–539

171. Weir DG, Scott JM. The biochemical basis of the neuropathy in cobalamin deficiency. *Clin Haematol* 1995; **8**: 479–498

172. WHO. *Requirements of Ascorbic Acid, Vitamin D, Vitamin B_{12}, Folate and Iron. WHO Technical Report Series No.452*. Geneva, WHO, 1970

173. Jathar VS, Kamath SA, Parikh MN *et al*. Material milk and serum vitamin B_{12}, folic acid and protein levels in India subjects. *Arch Dis Child* 1970; **45**: 236–241

174. Lampkin BC, Shore NA, Chadwick D. Megaloblastic anemia of infancy secondary to material pernicious anemia. *N Engl J Med* 1966; **274**; 1168–1171

175. Graham S, Aruela OM, Wise GA. Long term consequences of nutritional vitamin B_{12} deficiency in infants. *J Pediatr* 1992; **121**: 10–14

176. McIntyre OR, Sullivan LW, Jeffries GJ, Silver RH. Pernicious anemia in childhood. *N Engl J Med* 1965; **272**: 981–986

177. Rucker RW, Harrison GM.Vitamin B_{12} deficiency in cystic fibrosis. *N Engl J Med* 1973; **289**: 329

178. Tötterman G, Ahrenberg P. The age distribution in pernicious tapeworm anaemia and Addisonian pernicious anaemia. *Acta Medica Scand* 1956; **153**; 421–426

179. Antony AC. The biological chemistry of folate receptors. Blood 1992; 79: 2807–2820

180. MRC Vitamin Study Research Group. Prevention of neural tube defects: results of the Medical Research Council vitamin study. *Lancet* 1991; **338**: 131–137

181. Shaw GM, Hammer EJ, Wasserman CR *et al*. Risks of facial clefts in children born to women using multivitamins containing folic acid periconceptionally. *Lancet* 1995; **346**; 393–396

182. Van der Put NIYJ, Steegers-Theunissen RPM, Frosst P *et al*. Mutated methylenetetrahydrofolate reductase as a risk factor for spina bifida. *Lancet* 1995; **346**: 1070–1071

183. Whitehead AS, Gallagher P, Mills JL *et al*. A genetic defect in 5, 10-methylenetetrahydrofolate reductase in neural tube defects. *Q J Med* 1995; **88**: 763–766

184. Molloy AM, Daly S, Mills JL *et al*. Thermolabile variant of 5, 10-methylenetetrahydrofolate reductase associated with low red cell folates: implications for folate intake recommendations. *Lancet* 1997; **349**: 1591–1593

185. Kirke PN, Molloy AM, Daley LE *et al*. Maternal plasma folate and vitamin B_{12} are independent risk factors for neural tube defects. *Q J Med* 1993; **86**: 703–708

186. Mills JL, McFarlin JM, Kirke PN *et al*. Homocysteine metabolism in pregnancies complicated by neural-tube defects. *Lancet* 1995; **345**: 149–151

187. Hoffbrand AV. Anaemia in adult coeliac disease. *Clin Gastroenterol* 1974; **3**: 71–89

188. Heston WD. Characterization and glutamyl preferring carboxypeptidase function of prostate specific membrane antigen: a novel folate hydrolase. *Urology* 1997; **49 (Suppl 3A)**: 104–112

189. Carmel R, Hau KHW, Baylink DJ *et al*. Cobalamin and osteoblast-specific proteins. *N Engl J Med* 1988; **319**: 70–75

190. Skacel PO, Chanarin I. Impaired chemiluminescence and bacterial killing of neutrophils from patients with severe cobalamin deficiency. *Br J Haematol* 1983; **55**: 203–215

191. Savage DG, Lindenbaum J, Stabler SP, Allen RH. Sensitivity of serum methylmalonic acid and total homocysteine determinations for diagnosing cobalamin and folate deficiencies. *Am J Med* 1994; **96**: 239–246

192. Lindenbaum J, Savage DG, Stabler SP, Allen RH. Diagnosis of cobalamin deficiency. II Relative sensitivities of serum cobalamin, methylmalonic acid and total homocysteine concentrations. *Am J Hematol* 1990; **34**: 99–107

193. Green R. Metabolite assays in cobalamin and folate deficiency. *Clin Haematol* 1995; **8**: 533–566

194. Carmel R. Subtle and atypical cobalamin deficiency states. *Am J Hematol* 1990; **34**: 108–114

195. Chanarin I, Metz J. Diagnosis of cobalamin deficiency: the old and the new. *Br J Haematol* 1997; **97**: 695–700

196. Wickramasinghe SN. Morphology, biology and biochemistry of cobalamin and folate-deficient bone marrow cells. *Clin Haematol* 1995; **8**: 441–460

197. Rosenblatt DS, Shevell MI. Inherited disorders of cobalamin and folate absorption and metabolism. In: Fernandes J, Sandubray JM, Vanden Berghe G (eds) *Inborn Metabolic Diseases: Diagnosis and Treatment*. Berlin: Springer-Verlag, 1995, pp 239–258

198. Rosenblatt DS, Cooper BA. Inherited disorders of vitamin B_{12} utilisation. *Bioassays* 1990; **12**: 331–334

Non-immune neonatal anemias

RJ LIESNER

During fetal life and in the first weeks postnatally many dynamic changes occur in the composition of the blood and it is not until the age of 6 months that an established population of 'adult'-like red cells exists in the circulation. Fetal and 'adult' red cells have different metabolic and antigenic properties, different hemoglobins and fetal red cells have a much shorter life-span. The red cells can also be influenced by inherited genetic disease, acquired perinatal problems and maternal conditions. Interpretation of any hematologic abnormality in the neonate must therefore take all these confounding factors into consideration.

ERYTHROPOIESIS AFTER BIRTH

To understand fully the complex physiologic causes and effects of anemia in the term and preterm infant it is advisable to have some knowledge of the hematologic changes that occur around the time and in the weeks following birth. In the third trimester of gestation, the rate of red cell production is very high – about 3–5 times that of a normal adult and hence cord blood contains 12–16 times more erythroid progenitors than adult blood.[1] In the first few days after delivery, the rates of hemoglobin synthesis and red cell production fall dramatically to about a tenth of the rate pre-birth by 1 week of age and erythropoietin levels in the plasma reach almost 0. This suppression of erythropoiesis is most likely related to improved oxygenation, decreased erythropoietin production and a decreased response of erythropoietin production to available oxygen.[2,3] However, all healthy infants initially experience a rise in hemoglobin immediately after birth due to placental transfusion (see below) and in term infants the hemoglobin does not start to fall until after the first week of life.

The rate of hemoglobin and red cell production is lowest in the second week of life, after which it again very slowly begins to increase until about 12 weeks of age; during this time of diminished hemopoietic activity, red cell survival is reduced to 60–80 days in term infants or 35–50 in preterm infants.[4] The infant remains reticulocytopenic from 1–6 weeks as the erythroid activity in the bone marrow does not start to increase until at least 3–4 weeks. Despite this and despite detectable and increasing erythropoietin levels, there is a delay in hemoglobin recovery because the rate of red cell destruction exceeds production and continued rapid growth results in expansion of the blood volume and hemodilution. The mean hemoglobin nadir of 10.7 g/dl is reached at about 8–9 weeks[5] and by 6 months of age a mean level of 12.5 g/dl is achieved in the normal healthy infant.

In contrast, the anemic or hypoxic neonate responds to increased demand by not producing the same dramatic decrease in erythroid activity but instead continues to produce erythropoietin levels in the first few weeks.

HEMATOLOGIC VALUES AT BIRTH

These are shown in detail in the Reference values at the front of this book, but as there are important variables than can influence the apparent 'normal' values of hemoglobin and other red cell indices at birth, such as gestational age, management of labor and cord clamping and site and time of sampling of blood postnatally, these aspects are discussed here.

Blood volume and placental transfusion

The average blood volume at birth in normal full-term infants is 86 ml/kg with a range of 69–107 ml/kg but is higher in small-for-gestational age and preterm infants (see below).[6] The placental vessels contain approximately 150 ml of blood, with a range of 50–200 ml. A delay in cord clamping increases the blood volume and by allowing complete emptying of the placental vessels before clamping, it can be increased by 50–60%.[7,8] Therefore, an increase in hemoglobin concentration in the first few hours after birth is

Table 9.1 Effect of cord clamping on blood volume, hematocrit (Hct) and hemoglobin concentration (Hb).

	Early clamping	Late clamping
Blood volume at birth (ml/kg)[9]	82	93
Hct (l/l) at 2 hours of age[8]	0.47	0.63
Hct (l/l) at 24 hours of age[8]	0.43	0.59
Hct (l/l) at 120 hours of age[8]	0.44	0.59
Hb (g/dl) at 20–30 hours[9]	15.6	19.3
Hb (g/dl) at 72–96 hours[10]	18.1	19.7
Hb (g/dl) at 3 months[11]	11.1	11.1

a uniform phenomenon in all healthy newborns, even in infants in whom the cord has been clamped quickly because about a quarter of the placental blood volume transfuses into the infant in the first 15 s after birth and 50% by 1 min. The rate of placental transfusion is increased in women who receive ergotamine derivatives at the onset of the third stage of labor and decreased in placenta praevia, multiple gestation and caesarian section. Examples of how the variable management of the umbilical cord at birth can result in different blood volumes, hematocrit and hemoglobin concentrations are shown in Table 9.1. These differences can take up to 3 months to equalize.

Gestational age

There appears to be little difference in the hemoglobin level of the premature compared to the term infant at birth,[12] assuming all other factors such as time of cord clamping are equal. However, unlike term infants in whom the hemoglobin value remains stable until after the first week of life, in premature infants the decline is more rapid for increasing degrees of immaturity. This is related to the shorter red cell survival of the extremely premature infant and is exacerbated in the sick infant who requires multiple blood sampling. Therefore, the advantages of late clamping of the umbilical cord may be important to the premature infant in whom red cell mass and total iron stores are decreased and a hemoglobin concentration of < 15 g/dl in the first week of life has been found to be a significant predictor of severe refractory anemia of prematurity.[13] The placental transfusion in the premature infant may also facilitate postnatal lung adaptation.[14]

Blood volumes in small-for-gestational age and preterm infants are higher than in the well grown term infant due to an increased plasma volume but comparable red cell volume. The average is 106 ml/kg, range 85–143 ml/kg.[6,15] The exception is premature infants with hyaline membrane disease who have a reduced blood volume and red cell mass.[16]

Site of sampling

The site of sampling of blood in the neonate can have an important impact on hematologic values and this must be taken into consideration in the interpretation of abnormal values. The quality of the sample can affect the results considerably but good capillary flow from a deep stick in a well-warmed heel will minimize the capillary-to-venous or arterial differences in values. Skin puncture or capillary samples have a consistently higher hemoglobin level than those collected simultaneously by a venous or arterial route.[17] During the first few hours after birth capillary samples have an average hemoglobin 3.5 g/dl higher than venous samples,[18] and in a study on premature infants born at 24–32 weeks' gestation the mean capillary hemoglobin was 2.6 g/dl higher than venous and 2.3 g/dl higher than arterial samples.[19]

The capillary:venous hematocrit ratio is > 1.0 in all infants and in sick premature infants, in whom differences tend to be most marked, the ratio can be as high as 1.2[20] although the hematocrit has been found to correlate poorly with red cell mass in preterm and mature infants.[21]

Table 9.2 Causes of anemia in the neonate.

Anemia secondary to blood loss (see Table 9.4)
  Concealed hemorrhage prior to birth or during delivery
    Feto-maternal
    Feto-placental
    Twin-to-twin
  Obstetric accidents, malformations of the cord or placenta
  Internal hemorrhage
    Extracranial
    Intracranial
    Intra-abdominal
    Pulmonary
  Iatrogenic blood loss

Anemia as a result of a hemolytic process (see Table 9.7)
  Immune
    Alloimmune
    Autoimmune (passively acquired)
    Drug-induced
  Infection
    Acquired (bacterial sepsis)
    Congenital infection—rubella, cytomegalovirus, etc.
  Macro- and micro-angiopathic hemolytic anemias
  Hereditary disorders of the red cell membrane
    Hereditary spherocytosis
    Hereditary elliptocytosis
    Other rare membrane disorders
  Red cell enzyme deficiencies
    Glucose-6-phosphate dehydrogenase deficiency
    Pyruvate kinase deficiency
    Glucose phosphate isomerase deficiency
    Other rare enzyme deficiencies
  Abnormal/unstable hemoglobins

Anemia due to impaired red cell production
  Congenital red cell aplasia—Diamond–Blackfan anemia
  Anemia of the preterm infant
  Infection
    Bacterial sepsis
    Congenital infections
    Parvovirus B19 infection
  Nutritional deficiencies
  Congenital leukemia (see Chapter 21)
  Osteopetrosis (see Chapter 21)

Table 9.3 Expected results of investigations into the cause of neonatal anemia.

Cause of anemia	Reticulocyte count	Bilirubin	DAT	MCV	Red cell morphology
Acute blood loss	N	N	Neg	N	Normal
Chronic blood loss	↑	N/↑	Neg	↓	Microcytic, hypochromic, NRBCs
Immune hemolysis	↑	↑	Pos/neg	N/↑	NRBCs ± spherocytes
Infection with hemolysis	↑	N/↑	Neg	N/↑	Normal or NRBCs, poikilocytes
MAHA	↑	N	Neg	N/↑	Fragmented RBCs
Red cell membrane disorder	↑	↑	Neg	N/↑	Abnormal depending on disorder
Red cell enzyme disorder	↑	↑	Neg	N/↑	Normal or abnormal
α-Thalassemia	↑	N	Neg	↓	Microcytic, NRBCs
Impaired red cell production	↓	N	Neg	N/↑	Normal or abnormal

DAT = Direct antiglobulin test; MCV = mean corpuscular volume; MAHA = microangiopathic hemolytic anemia; Pos = positive; Neg = Negative; NRBC = nucleated red blood cell.

CLASSIFICATION OF NEONATAL ANEMIA

Anemia is defined as a condition in which the concentration of hemoglobin, or the number of red blood cells, or both, is reduced below the age-corrected value. The physiologic defect caused is a decrease in the oxygen-carrying capacity of blood and a reduction in the oxygen available to tissues. When anemia is present at birth or appears during the first 6 weeks of life the causes can be broadly classified into 3 major categories (Table 9.2).

Severe anemia present at birth (i.e. hemoglobin level <8.0 g/dl) is usually due to immune hemolysis or hemorrhage. If either process has been chronic, 'hydrops fetalis' can result. This condition has hematologic and non-hematologic causes but is characterized in the fetus and neonate by gross edema and effusions, cardiac failure and profound anemia. Anemia that becomes apparent after 24 hours is most often due to internal or external hemorrhage or non-immune hemolytic disorders. Infants with impaired red cell production as a cause do not generally develop anemia until after 3 weeks. Table 9.3 outlines the expected results in the investigation of neonatal anemias.

ANEMIA SECONDARY TO BLOOD LOSS

Anemia in the newborn period due to blood loss can result from bleeding prenatally, at the time of delivery or in the first few hours or days after birth. The newborn has limited capacity to tolerate acute hemorrhage and prompt diagnosis and therapy are therefore essential for survival. The causes can be divided into the following categories (Table 9.4):

- concealed or occult hemorrhage prior to or during delivery;
- internal hemorrhage in the fetus or neonate;
- obstetric accidents;

- bleeding due to umbilical cord or placenta malformations;
- iatrogenic blood loss due to excessive sampling.

The clinical manifestations of hemorrhage are dependent upon the site of bleeding, extent of the hemorrhage and whether the blood loss was acute and chronic (Table 9.5). In some situations the hemoglobin can be normal initially, even in severe hemorrhage, but it falls rapidly within hours of birth.

Table 9.4 Causes of blood loss resulting in anemia in the neonate.

Concealed hemorrhage prior to birth or during delivery
  Feto-maternal
    Spontaneous
    Traumatic amniocentesis
    Following external cephalic version
  Feto-placental
  Twin-to-twin

Obstetric accidents
  Rupture of normal cord during normal, precipitous or forceps delivery
  Hematoma of cord or placenta
  Incision of placenta at caesarian section
  Placenta praevia
  Placental abruption

Malformations of the umbilical cord or placenta
  Abnormally short cord
  Venous tortuosities of varices of cord
  Aneurysm of cord
  Velamentous insertion of cord into placenta
  Vasa praevia
  Multilobed placenta

Internal hemorrhage
  Extracranial—cephalohematoma, subgaleal hemorrhage
  Intracranial—intraventricular, subarachnoid
  Retroperitoneal
  Ruptured liver
  Ruptured spleen
  Pulmonary
  Hemangiomas of skin or gastrointestinal tract

Iatrogenic blood loss

Table 9.5 Characteristics of acute and chronic blood loss in the neonate.

Acute blood loss	Chronic blood loss
Pallor	Pallor
Shallow tachypnea	Signs of cardiac failure:
Tachycardia	Cardiac enlargement
Poor peripheral perfusion	Tachypnea
Hypotension	Hepatomegaly
No organomegaly	Ascites
Normochromic, macrocytic anemia	Hypochromic, microcytic anemia
(may have normal hemoglobin initially)	Reticulocytosis

CONCEALED HEMORRHAGE IN THE FETUS PRIOR TO OR DURING DELIVERY

The causes of concealed or occult hemorrhage can be divided into feto-maternal, feto-placental or twin-to-twin.

Feto-maternal hemorrhage

Spontaneous leakage of fetal erythrocytes into the maternal circulation was first demonstrated by differential agglutination in the 1950s[22,23] and it is now well recognized that small numbers of fetal red cells (0.01 ml or more) pass through the placental trophoblastic lining and enter the maternal circulation in >75% of normal pregnancies. These cells have been detected using sensitive Kleihauer-Betke[24,25] or fluorescence-activated cell sorter techniques[26] (see below) from as early as 4–8 weeks' gestation,[23] but most spontaneous feto-maternal bleeding occurs in the third trimester and during labor and delivery. The frequency and magnitude of feto-maternal hemorrhage is increased by invasive procedures in pregnancy and by many maternal conditions (Table 9.6).[26–33]

If there are differences between fetal and maternal antigens, a feto-maternal transfusion can sensitize the mother. An example of this is Rh(D) incompatibility where the mother can be given a dose of anti-D immune globulin to 'mop-up' fetal D^+ cells to prevent sensitization (see Chapter 10).

Table 9.6 Conditions associated with increased risk and magnitude of feto-maternal hemorrhage.

Amniocentesis
Termination of pregnancy
Abdominal trauma
Chorioangioma or choriocarcinoma of placenta
Fetal blood sampling
Intrauterine transfusions
External cephalic version
Antepartum hemorrhage
Obstetric instrumentation
Manual removal of the placenta
Caesarian section
Pregnancy-induced hypertension

Clinical manifestations

These vary with the magnitude of the hemorrhage, rapidity and chronicity of the bleeding and time at which the bleeding occurs with respect to delivery. Normally, the volume transfused does not exceed 0.5 ml but in 1–6% of pregnancies the volume is >3 ml and in 0.3% of normal deliveries is >10 ml.[29,34–36] If the fetus suffers an acute loss of >20% of blood volume, hydrops fetalis and stillbirth can result if no intrauterine transfusion is instigated. If born alive, the infant will have clinical shock, apnea and severe anemia.[29,36,37] If the same degree of blood loss occurs over a more prolonged period of time, then the fetus is more likely to compensate hemodynamically. Otherwise, the degree of anemia is variable; if mild it may go undetected by the clinician but if the hemoglobin is <12.0 g/dl the infant may display some signs of anemia such as pallor, tachypnea or poor feeding. Infants with severe anemia and hemoglobin levels <4.0 g/dl have been reported and although this is a well recognized cause of late stillbirth or neonatal death, there are reports of surviving infants. Perinatal morbidity rates associated with occult feto-maternal hemorrhage range from 1 in 1000 to 1500 (0.1–0.7%) deliveries to 3% of all fetal deaths.[36,38]

Laboratory diagnosis

Once a low hemoglobin value has been recorded, a blood film examination will appear normochromic and normocytic in acute blood loss and the reticulocyte count is likely to be normal initially but increases after a few hours with a concomitant increase in nucleated red cells in the peripheral blood. The direct antiglobulin test is negative and these infants are not usually jaundiced initially but may become so over subsequent days. If the transfusion has been more chronic, the neonatal film may indicate iron deficiency with hypochromia, microcytosis, anisocytosis and poikilocytosis. However, the diagnosis can only be made with certainty by demonstrating the presence of fetal red cells in the maternal circulation. In the past agglutination techniques were used but nowadays the most widely used method is the Kleihauer and Betke technique of acid elution,[24,25,39] although flow cytometer methods using fluorescent antibodies are increasingly employed.[26,40]

The Kleihauer test is based on the fact that at low pH fetal hemoglobin resists acid elution, whereas adult cells lose their hemoglobin and can be differentiated by visual counting from the fetal cells once they have been appropriately stained. This technique is not reliable when maternal fetal hemoglobin levels are increased such as in some hemoglobinopathies, in hereditary persistence of fetal hemoglobin and in some normal women in whom a pregnancy-induced rise in fetal hemoglobin occurs, particularly in the first and second trimester.[34]

Flow cytometric analysis permits the rapid, objective and

reproducible evaluation of 50 000 to 100 000 red blood cells and is able to detect as little as 0.03 ml of fetal red cells.

If ABO incompatibility exists between maternal and fetal cells, the latter may be agglutinated and removed within hours from the circulation by maternal antibody, and a blood sample should be taken as soon as a feto-maternal hemorrhage is suspected.

Feto-placental hemorrhage

Rarely a transfusion of blood from the fetal circulation can accumulate within placental tissue or retroplacentally rather than passing to the maternal circulation and this is exacerbated by a tight nuchal cord.[41,42] If the infant is inadvertently held above the level of the placenta before the umbilical cord is cut at delivery, this can result in direct transfusion from the fetus into the placenta.

Twin-to-twin transfusion

This occurs in monozygotic multiple pregnancies in the 70% of cases in whom there is a monochorial placenta.[43] A degree of transfusion probably occurs in all such pregnancies but is thought to cause significant morbidity and mortality from anemia in the donor twin and polycythemia in the recipient twin in only 15–30%.[44,45] It is probably more common when there is an abnormality of the umbilical cord, such as a single umbilical artery or a velamentous cord insertion (see below). Acute bleeding occurs when there is rapid transfer of blood from one twin to the other via the placental anastamoses, usually in the second stage of labor as a result of a sudden relative rise of blood pressure in one of the fetal circulations. The condition should be suspected if there is a difference in hemoglobin of >5.0 g/dl between the twins.

Typically, the anemic infant has pallor, lethargy and cardiac failure and his hemoglobin ranges from 3.5 to 18.0 g/dl, whereas the polycythemic twin is plethoric with an hemoglobin of between 20.0 and 30.0 g/dl and develops the hyperviscosity syndrome, and hyperbilirubinemia and disseminated intravascular coagulation (DIC) can be a further complication.[46] If the transfusion has been chronic over several weeks or months there can be marked difference in birth weight, organ size and amniotic fluid volume with severe growth retardation and oligohydramnios in the anemic twin and polyhydramnios in the polycythemic twin; this chronic twin-to-twin transfusion has been shown to be a major contributing factor in weight-discordant twins.[47]

OBSTETRIC ACCIDENTS AND MALFORMATIONS OF THE UMBILICAL CORD OR PLACENTA

Umbilical cord

In precipitous unattended deliveries or traumatic forceps deliveries a normal umbilical cord can rupture and result in fetal hemorrhage and anemia. In normal deliveries rupture can occur if the cord is abnormally short, entangled around the fetus or has vascular abnormalities such as venous tortuosity or an aneurysm.[48] Inflammation of the cord by meconium can weaken the vessels within it and predispose to rupture. If the hemorrhage is contained within the cord, a hematoma can form which can contain a large proportion of the fetal blood volume. In 1% of pregnancies there is a 'velamentous' insertion of the cord into the edge of the placenta. This is more common in twin pregnancies and in pregnancies in which the placenta is low-lying (see below) and in an estimated 1–2% of these pregnancies there is significant fetal blood loss[49,50] with a fresh stillbirth rate of >60%.

Placenta

Abnormally-implanted placentae or malformations of the placenta can cause fetal as well as maternal hemorrhage. Vasa praevia is present when fetal vessels cross the internal os as a velamentous insertion of the umbilical cord with or without a succenturiate lobe or an abnormal multilobed placenta. There appears to be an increased risk of this occurring in *in vitro* fertilization pregnancies.[51] If labor is allowed to continue vaginally, these vessels can become compressed and/or lacerated and there is high chance of fetal death perinatally.[52] Doppler ultrasound examinations antenatally should diagnose this condition so that the baby can be delivered by elective caesarian section.

Placenta praevia and large placental abruptions can also both result in hemorrhage from the fetal as well as the maternal side of the placenta and can cause neonatal anemia if the fetus survives.[53]

Massive fetal hemorrhage can be associated with accidental incision of the placenta at caesarian section; this complication is more likely if the placenta is anterior and low-lying.

INTERNAL HEMORRHAGE

Internal hemorrhage following a traumatic delivery is a well-recognized cause of neonatal anemia, although trends in modern obstetric care and the increase in caesarian section rates for potentially difficult deliveries has resulted in a considerable fall in the incidence of these birth injuries. Nevertheless, there remains a risk of fetal hemorrhage with all deliveries, particularly if the fetus is large, small or abnormal, during instrumental deliveries, and in situations where there has been poor antenatal care. The sites most affected are listed in Table 9.4. The presence of a coagulopathy in the neonate, such as vitamin K deficiency or hemophilia, is likely to worsen the extent of any hemorrhage.

Signs of anemia due to internal hemorrhage often present within 24–72 hours after birth, although when the hemorrhage is brisk the newborn may have poor Apgar scores and shock at delivery.[54]

Extracranial bleeds

Bleeds involving the cranium can be extra- or intra-cranial. Extracranial hemorrhages are most common following difficult deliveries or vacuum extraction and include a subgaleal hemorrhage in which there is blood loss into the subaponeurotic area of the scalp where there are no periosteal attachments to limit the hemorrhage and hence the entire calvarium can be involved.[55–57] The infant develops a boggy, blue, edematous swelling extending from orbital ridges to the nape of the neck. Although approximately 50% of these hemorrhages are due to vacuum-assisted delivery, a quarter follow spontaneous vaginal delivery and 9% caesarian section.[58] Hemorrhage under the periosteum, however, tends to be limited to the area over one skull bone but nevertheless the resulting cephalohematoma can contain a significant volume of blood and both cephalohematomata and subaponeurotic bleeds can cause severe anemia.[59,60] The latter have also been reported to cause neonatal exsanguination and death.[61,62] Once the acute phase of these bleeds has been appropriately managed, with resuscitation and blood transfusion if required, then recovery is usually complete but in the days following birth the absorption of the products of red cell breakdown can cause neonatal hyperbilirubinemia for which exchange transfusion is occasionally required.

Intracranial bleeds

Intracranial hemorrhage is usually either intraventricular or subarachnoid. Intraventricular hemorrhage can occur in up to 50% of premature infants weighing < 1500 g at birth,[63] and when extensive it can be associated with long-term neurologic sequelae.[64] The infant may be asymptomatic or may develop a bulging fontanelle, apnea, seizures or hypothermia. It can be a cause of anemia at birth or a sudden drop in hemoglobin in the first days of life. Tentorial tears can follow vacuum-assisted deliveries. These are often mild and may be diagnosed if signs of hemorrhage are noted in the cerebrospinal fluid.

Intra-abdominal hemorrhage

Breech deliveries of infants who are large-for-gestational age are particularly associated with intra-abdominal hemorrhage, although these have also been described in normal deliveries. Organs involved include adrenals, kidneys, liver and spleen or the hemorrhage can be into the retroperitoneal space. Adrenal hemorrhage can cause sudden collapse and cyanosis and this and a retroperitoneal hemorrhage can present with bluish discoloration of the skin of the flank and sometimes a palpable mass. Retroperitoneal hemorrhage has also been described following perforation or rupture of an umbilical artery by catheterization.[65]

In the past, rupture of the liver was found at 1.2–9.6% of post-mortems for stillbirth or neonatal death[66,67] and even though obstetric care has improved over the last few decades, small subcapsular hemorrhages probably occur more frequently after traumatic births than is clinically appreciated, particularly in low-birth-weight infants.[68] The severity of the clinical picture depends on whether the hemorrhage is confined within the capsule of the liver, when the infant may develop abdominal swelling and anemia but can recover without complications, or whether the capsule ruptures. This usually occurs 24–48 hours after delivery, resulting in free blood in the peritoneal cavity and rapid onset of shock. X-rays of the abdomen reveal free fluid and paracentesis can confirm the presence of blood in the peritoneum. The prognosis is typically poor but infants do survive with prompt resuscitation, blood transfusion and surgical repair.

Hemorrhage due to a ruptured spleen has been reported in the past following extreme distension of the spleen in severe hemolytic disease of the newborn, usually due to Rh(D) incompatibility between mother and infant.[69] This is an exceedingly rare event nowadays in countries with anti-D prophylactic programs but splenic rupture can occur after apparently normal deliveries, most often in large-for-dates infants.[70,71]

Other sites

Another site for neonatal bleeding resulting in anemia is hemorrhage into the lungs which can occur in infants on ventilatory support, particularly in those born prematurely.[72] If severe, the lungs become impossible to perfuse and ventilate and unless extracorporeal membrane oxygenation (ECMO) is urgently available the prognosis is extremely poor. Rarely, hemangiomas of the skin,[73] gastrointestinal tract[74] and thymus[75] can present with significant neonatal hemorrhage.

IATROGENIC BLOOD LOSS

In modern neonatal practice, despite the use of micromethods, sampling losses in preterm babies have become a common cause of neonatal anemia.[76]

THERAPY

Therapy for blood loss in the neonate is dictated by the infant's clinical condition. If the infant is in shock from acute massive hemorrhage, rapid transfusion of group-matched, cytomegalovirus-negative packed red cells is mandatory, aiming to get the hemoglobin level up to 13–14 g/dl. If necessary, the 'flying squad' O negative blood can be used but this carries a risk of hemolysis if maternally-derived antibodies to some Rh antigens (e.g. anti-c or anti-e) are present in the infant's serum. If red cells are not immediately available, plasma expanders should be given until the blood is available.

Mildly anemic infants require early iron therapy.

ANEMIA AS A RESULT OF A HEMOLYTIC PROCESS

A hemolytic process is defined as a pathologic state that results in shortening of the normal red cell life-span (100–120 days in the adult, 60–80 days in the term infant, 30–50 in the preterm infant). This reduction in red cell survival can be caused by acquired or congenital defects which affect the red cell membrane, hemoglobin or intracellular metabolism. In the steady-state, hemolytic anemia is characterized by both increased red cell destruction and production, producing 2 of the 'triad' of features that occur with hemorrhage: reticulocytosis and hyperbilirubinemia. If the extent of the destruction cannot be compensated for by the capability of the marrow reserve, then anemia also occurs.

In the neonate the features of hemolysis can be variable but the extent of the anemia will depend on the marrow reserve for stress erythropoiesis and the degree of hemolysis. Hyperbilirubinemia is the most constant feature but this also occurs in neonates who are not hemolyzing but have 'physiologic' jaundice due to transient impaired hepatic bilirubin conjugation. However, physiologic jaundice is not usually detected until the infant is at least 36–48 hours old, and the bilirubin level does not usually exceed 300 μmol/l. In the presence of hemolysis these levels are exceeded and clinical jaundice usually appears on the first day of life.

Anemia is not a universal feature of neonatal hemolysis but, if present, it can develop rapidly and become severe, particularly if there is no prompt reticulocyte response. In other cases, there can be a persistent increase in reticulocyte count with a normal hemoglobin or mild anemia only. Although the reticulocyte count is normally elevated at birth, it should be normal by the third day.

Evaluation of a case of neonatal hemolysis requires attention to the family history and any history of consanguinity, as well as maternal factors such as infections and medications during pregnancy and assessment of maternal hematology and serology.

The major causes of a shortened red cell life-span in the neonatal period are listed in Table 9.7. Only the features of those non-immune hemolytic anemias that manifest in the neonatal period are discussed in this chapter.

INFECTION

Both intrauterine and postnatally acquired infections are associated with anemia and other hematologic abnormalities in the neonatal period. Although these changes are sometimes produced by marrow suppression and a decrease in red cell production, severe neonatal infection is also usually accompanied by hemolysis. In severe bacterial sepsis, the hemolysis develops because of infection-induced small vessel damage and fibrin deposition which can damage red cells. This is one of the neonatal causes of DIC (see below).

Table 9.7 Causes of hemolysis in the first 6 weeks of life.

Immune
 Hemolytic disease of the newborn due to Rh or ABO or minor blood group incompatibility
 Maternal autoimmune hemolytic anemia
 Drug-induced hemolytic anemia

Infection
 Bacterial sepsis
 Congenital infection
  Cytomegalovirus
  Rubella
  Toxoplasmosis
  Herpes simplex
  Malaria
  Syphilis

Macro- and micro-angiopathic hemolytic anemias
 Disseminated intravascular coagulation
 Cavernous hemangioma
 Severe coarctation of the aorta
 Renal artery stenosis
 Large vessel thrombi

Hereditary disorders of the red cell membrane
 Hereditary spherocytosis
 Hereditary elliptocytosis
  With infantile poikilocytosis
  Homozygous hereditary elliptocytosis
  Hereditary pyropoikilocytosis
  Hereditary spherocytic-elliptocytosis
 Other rare membrane disorders

Red cell enzyme deficiencies
 Glucose-6-phosphate dehydrogenase deficiency
 Pyruvate kinase deficiency
 Glucose phosphate isomerase deficiency
 Other rare enzyme deficiencies

Abnormal hemoglobins
 α-Thalassemia syndromes or α-chain structural abnormalities
 γ-Thalassemia syndromes or γ-chain structural abnormalities

Infections acquired by hematogenous spread *in utero* that can cause hemolysis include toxoplasmosis, cytomegalovirus, congenital syphilis and rubella (Table 9.8).[77] Herpes simplex infections are generally acquired from the cervix and vagina during delivery. The hemolytic process in these cases is thought to arise from direct injury to the red cell membrane or reticuloendothelial hyperplasia and occasionally an antibody produced in response to the infection can cross-react with an antigen on the surface of the red cell and give a positive direct antiglobulin test.

Clinical suspicion of intrauterine infection in the neonate with hemolysis is supported by associated findings of jaundice, chorioretinitis, pneumonitis, central nervous system abnormalities, growth retardation, skin lesions or hepatosplenomegaly.[78] If the spleen is enlarged, hypersplenism can increase the rate of red cell destruction. Laboratory features include thrombocytopenia, leukocytosis with immature forms, reticulocytosis, large numbers of circulating erythroblasts as well as high antibody titers against the infecting organism and direct harvesting of the infective agent from

Table 9.8 Congenital infections that may be complicated by anemia in the neonatal period.

Infection	Proportion of babies with any symptom of stated infection (%)	Features of the anemia
Cytomegalovirus	<10	Hb 8.0–12.0 g/dl in 1st week Hb 5–10 g/dl at 3–6 weeks with reticulocytosis Blood film—poikilocytes, NRBCs
Herpes simplex	>90 have generalized disease	Mild microangiopathic changes
Rubella	>90 if infected in first trimester, less in 2nd	Mild anemia in 15–30% of infected infants Exaggerated postnatal decline in Hb
Toxoplasmosis	30–50	Anemia in 40–50% of infected infants. Can be severe (Hb < 8.0 g/dl) and cause hydrops. Reticulocytosis NRBCs on blood film
Syphilis	15 if mother untreated	>90% infected infants are anemic. Can be severe (Hb < 8.0 g/dl) Reticulocytosis NRBCs on blood film
Malaria	10 in endemic areas	Can be severe and life-threatening Reticulocytosis Parasitemia on blood film
Parvovirus	<10	Reticulocytopenic anemia which can be mild → severe and can cause hydrops Giant pro-normoblasts in bone marrow with general erythroid hypoplasia

NRBCs = nucleated red blood cells

the urine or blood.[78] Hyperbilirubinemia may be conjugated and unconjugated due to co-existent hepatitis with hemolysis.

Although malaria remains a major health hazard in many parts of the world, vertical transmission appears to be rare; when it does occur it can cause severe fetal infection and stillbirth, more commonly when infection occurs in women who are travelling to endemic from non-endemic areas.[79] The placenta is a preferential site for reproduction and growth of the malarial parasite but also acts as a relative barrier to infection of the fetus. Maternal immunoglobulins and fetal hemoglobin also protect the fetus to a certain extent and if the parasites are not eradicated they may enter a latent phase which can delay presentation of malaria in the infected neonate for several weeks. Features of malaria in the newborn include fever, irritability and hepatosplenomegaly, as well as anemia which is usually severe and reticulocytosis. In 1 reported case the neonate had an hematocrit of 12% and a reticulocyte count of 10%.[80]

The diagnosis of congenital malaria requires a high index of clinical suspicion. The blood film should be carefully examined following suitable staining and blood should be sent for serologic testing to laboratories that specialize in tropical diseases. If the diagnosis is a possibility at birth, usually because the mother has been treated for malaria in pregnancy, the placental bed can also be examined for the parasite and treatment instituted in the first days of life to prevent severe sequelae later on.

MACRO- AND MICRO-ANGIOPATHIC NEONATAL ANEMIAS

Severe cardiac defects and large vessel thrombi have been described to cause hemolysis in the newborn by a process involving shear-related disruption to the red cell membrane and/or interaction of red cells with abnormal surfaces within the heart. A microangiopathic process results from red cell damage in partially occluded small blood vessels where red blood cells can be damaged by fibrin strands or trapped by the damaged endothelium.

Disseminated intravascular coagulation

This is a common complication of neonatal infection, particularly bacterial infection. It can also be associated with severe birth asphyxia, respiratory distress syndrome, hypovolemia and hypothermia. Anemia is only one of the hematologic problems associated with DIC (see Chapter 33).

Hemangiomas

Microangiopathic hemolytic anemia can occur in association with a giant hemangioma—the Kasabach–Merritt syndrome. This can present at birth or in the neonatal period.[81]

HEREDITARY DISORDERS OF THE RED CELL MEMBRANE

A number of the hereditary red cell membrane disorders present in the neonatal period (see also Chapter 13). All are associated with morphologic abnormalities of the red cell, which presumably reflect abnormalities of the cell membrane and function. In many instances the primary molecular defects have still to be identified.

Hereditary spherocytosis

This is the commonest inherited red cell membrane defect. The inheritance pattern is autosomal dominant in 75% of cases and the remainder are either due to spontaneous mutation, incomplete penetrance or an autosomal recessive form of the disease. The primary membrane defect in hereditary spherocytosis (HS) involves deficiencies or defects of spectrin, the major skeletal structural protein in the red cell membrane, ankyrin, protein 4.2 or the anion exchange protein (protein 3). This causes the red cell to lose surface area and results in the decreased surface area-to-volume characteristics of HS, although much of the mechanism of this is not understood. The red cell loses its biconcave disc shape and appears to lose its central pallor under light microscopy. The cells are abnormally fragile under osmotic stress and susceptible to extravascular hemolysis in the spleen.

HS is commonly symptomatic in the neonatal period. In published series, 20–50% of affected patients present with a history of jaundice with or without moderate hemolysis and mild splenomegaly in the newborn period,[82,83] usually in the first 48 hours of life, but in 20% onset is delayed until after the first week of life. However, unless there is a family history of HS the diagnosis is made infrequently at this time. Severe anemia as a manifestation of neonatal HS is rare, but mild anemia is not uncommon.[84] As the spectrin content in the red cell membrane correlates well with the degree of hemolysis,[85] it is likely that the increased content of membrane lipids in the neonatal red cell stabilizes to a certain extent the defect due to decreased spectrin in HS.

The diagnosis of HS is often more difficult in the neonatal period than later in life; the reticulocytosis and splenomegaly can be variable and the number of spherocytes in the peripheral blood may not be significantly increased until the infant is 2–3 months of age. The haptoglobin level is also not a reliable indicator of hemolysis during the first months of life.

The osmotic fragility test is used most often to diagnose HS, but in the newborn, as the increased lipid content of neonatal red cells makes them osmotically resistant, it is important to do an incubated osmotic fragility test and to use a control neonatal sample.[82,86] Protein electrophoresis of the membrane proteins can also yield additional diagnostic information although this method is not widely available.

The major differential diagnosis is ABO incompatibility, although spherocytes can also be present on the blood film in bacterial sepsis, hemolytic transfusion reactions and oxidative injury. Symptomatic ABO incompatibility is about 40–50 times as common as HS and presents with jaundice, anemia and spherocytosis, with a negative or weakly positive direct antiglobulin test. Maternal serology and sometimes elution of the anti-A or -B antibody from the red cells will differentiate the two diagnoses. If not, differentiation of HS from acquired conditions is aided by family studies, or the diagnosis becomes clear with time.

Neonates with hemolysis due to HS are managed in a similar way to other babies with hyperbilirubinemia. In most, the jaundice can be controlled with phototherapy but kernicterus is a risk and exchange transfusion or packed red cell transfusion for anemia may be required. Supplementary dietary folic acid is recommended. There is no evidence that children with HS who are symptomatic as neonates have a more severe form of the disease.

Hereditary elliptocytosis

This condition is a clinically and genetically heterogeneous disorder characterized by the presence of elliptically-shaped cells in the peripheral blood. An abnormality in the lateral association of skeletal proteins is responsible for the elongated red cell morphology. The commonest form of this condition, *mild hereditary elliptocytosis (HE)*, is inherited in an autosomal dominant manner and apart from an abnormal blood film with 25–75% elliptocytes, it is generally a benign condition and does not cause problems in the first weeks of life.

In contrast, *HE with infantile poikilocytosis* is a cause of moderately severe hemolytic anemia and jaundice characterized by marked red cell budding, fragmentation and poikilocytosis usually in black infants.[87] In most cases there are enough elliptocytes to suggest the diagnosis but sometimes this condition can be confused with infantile pyknocytosis, hereditary pyropoikilocytosis or a microangiopathic hemolytic disorder. The correct diagnosis is easily made if the parents' smears are examined because one will have classical mild HE. With time, fragmentation and hemolysis in the infant decline and the benign clinical picture of mild HE emerges by 6 months to 2 years.

The underlying cause of poikilocytosis in some infants with HE is not known but it has been suggested that the elevated free 2,3-DPG levels in fetal cells may weaken spectrin-actin bonds and lead to increased fragility.[88]

Homozygote or double heterozygote inheritance of HE causes a severe transfusion-dependent hemolytic anemia from birth with marked red cell fragmentation, poikilocytosis and elliptocytosis.[89] Clinically, the disease is indistinguishable from hereditary pyropoikilocytosis and patients respond to splenectomy.

Hereditary spherocytic-elliptocytosis

This condition is a phenotypic hybrid of mild HE and HS and is characterized by the presence of elliptocytes and spherocytes on the blood film. It is inherited in a dominant fashion and primarily affects European populations. The osmotic fragility pattern and the clinical manifestations are similar to HS.[90]

Hereditary pyropoikilocytosis

This occurs primarily in Afro-American newborns and is inherited as a recessive disorder or represents double heterozygosity for 2 spectrin mutations.[91–93] Like HE with infantile poikilocytosis, hereditary pyropoikilocytosis (HPP) presents early in life. It is characterized by severe hemolytic anemia and extreme poikilocytosis with budding red cells, fragments, spherocytes, elliptocytes and marked thermal instability of the red cells. However, these abnormalities do not improve with time and after the newborn period subjects continue to have problems secondary to severe hemolytic anemia with splenomegaly, frontal bossing and early gallbladder disease[91] and require splenectomy to improve the hemolysis.

Osmotic fragility tests are very abnormal, particularly after incubation, and autohemolysis is greatly elevated. The mean corpuscular volume (MCV) of the red cells is low due to the large number of red cell fragments.

Parental studies show that in many cases one or both parents have HE; in cases where this is not so, it is postulated that they have a silent carrier state for HE, which, although the red cell morphology is normal, is associated with subtle changes in the membrane skeleton and decreased red cell thermal stability.[94]

RED CELL ENZYME DEFICIENCIES

Inherited disorders of red cell metabolism are an important cause of hemolytic anemia early in life (see also Chapter 14). Although some of these metabolic defects are associated with characteristic morphologic changes, most have no distinct morphology. Thus, the diagnosis of an enzyme defect as a cause of hemolytic anemia in the newborn can only be made if the clinician considers the possibility and performs the essential steps in evaluation; the family history and ethnic background are important initial considerations. Clinically, jaundice is again the prominent clinical finding but anemia can arise if the hemolysis is severe.

Glucose-6-phosphate dehydrogenase (G6PD) deficiency

This is the commonest of the red cell enzyme deficiencies. It is an X-linked disorder common in some ethnic groups, mainly from the Mediterranean, Africa and China, and over 150 variants have been identified based on molecular and biochemical studies.[95,96] Female carriers are affected only if the normal gene on one X chromosome is inactivated by extreme lyonization.

G6PD is an enzyme in the hexose-monophosphate shunt and is important in NADPH generation and in the regeneration of reduced glutathione which protects the red cell from oxidative damage. In the G6PD-deficient cell, oxidative injury from oxidant drugs, infection, acidosis or following ingestion of fava beans can lead to denaturation of hemoglobin which precipitates as intracellular inclusions called Heinz bodies. These attach to the cell membrane and are removed with a portion of the cell membrane as the cell passes through the reticuloendothelial system, resulting in a characteristic 'bite' cell.[97]

G6PD in the Afro-American population, the A variant, is often clinically mild because the defect causes enzyme instability rather than deficiency. Young red cells contain a normal amount of enzyme but this becomes unstable as the red cells age. Thus, the A variant does not typically cause hemolysis and hyperbilirubinemia in the newborn, although it has been reported in black premature infants.

In contrast, the Mediterranean and Asian forms of the disease can present early, first because the enzyme deficiency is present in cells of all ages.[98] Secondly, the neonatal red cells have a high ascorbic acid content, which has been shown to shorten survival of G6PD-deficient erythrocytes, and thirdly, vitamin E levels and catalase activity are often low which can predispose the red cell to hydrogen peroxide hemolysis. Therefore, spontaneous hemolysis in full-term male or female infants can cause severe hyperbilirubinemia with mild anemia.[99, 100] In global terms G6PD deficiency is probably the commonest cause of severe neonatal jaundice.

The onset of jaundice is often not until day 2–3, in contrast to that due to hemolytic disease of the newborn, but it can be confused with 'physiologic' jaundice. However, the family history, ethnic origin or history of maternal drug exposure that could cross the placenta may suggest the diagnosis and the level of hyperbilirubinemia is often much higher than that seen in physiologic jaundice and may be severe enough to require an exchange transfusion. The blood film may have microspherocytes in severe cases but often there are no specific morphologic findings. Enzyme assay may confirm the diagnosis but if the result is within normal limits in the presence of a reticulocytosis the assay should be repeated when the acute episode has subsided as the level can be falsely elevated by the presence of large numbers of immature red cells.

Pyruvate kinase (PK) deficiency

This is the second commonest red cell enzyme deficiency causing neonatal hemolysis and the commonest red cell enzyme deficiency of the Embden–Meyerhof pathway, but overall is relatively uncommon.[101] It is autosomal recessive in inheritance, and is primarily seen in northern Europeans, in whom there is wide variety in expression of the disorder although the severity remains fairly constant within a family. Because of the position of the block caused in the glycolytic pathway by PK deficiency, 2,3-DPG levels are increased. This improves oxygen delivery to the tissues and helps alleviate the clinical and biochemical effects of the anemia. However, in the neonate the hemolysis can be particularly severe with jaundice developing within the first 24 hours of life, associated with anemia, reticulocytosis and splenomegaly, and hydrops fetalis has also been reported in severely affected families.[102] Exchange transfusion is frequently required to avoid the risks of kernicterus. Infants who present at birth appear to be have more severe hemolysis in later life. Red cell morphology reveals a small number of spherocytes, oval cells, an occasional poikilocyte, irregularly contracted cells as well as normoblastosis. Diagnosis can be made by demonstrating the carrier state in both parents, who are otherwise hematologically normal, as heterozygotes can be detected by enzyme assay in 90% of cases. In later life, if multiple transfusions are required, splenectomy may lessen the transfusion requirement.

Glucose phosphate isomerase deficiency

This is the third commonest red cell enzymopathy after G6PD and PK deficiencies and one-third of affected individuals develop symptoms as a neonate.[98] Hydrops fetalis has also been described.[103] Inheritance is autosomal recessive and the clinical manifestations and morphologic features are similar to those of the other congenital non-spherocytic anemias.

ABNORMAL HEMOGLOBINS (see also chapters 11, 12 and 15)

Abnormalities in synthesis, structure and function of hemoglobin can cause hemolytic anemia in the newborn. At birth the red blood cells contain approximately 80% fetal hemoglobin (HbF), and 20% hemoglobin A (HbA), which is the predominant hemoglobin over the age of 6 months. HbF is composed of 2 α and 2 γ chains and HbA, 2 α and 2 β chains. Therefore, owing to the relationship between gestational age and globin synthesis, abnormalities in the neonate must involve either α- or γ-globin molecules. In the case of abnormalities affecting γ globin, clinical manifestations may be severe at birth and subside as the switch from fetal to adult hemoglobin occurs. As β-globin synthesis is limited in the newborn, defects involving the β-globin gene rarely manifest in the first weeks of life. Other defects that might be thought to be similar in their clinical manifestations throughout life, such as α-chain defects, may act differently in the newborn period when paired with a γ chain rather than a β chain.

In the premature infant, HbF can persist for longer and in children with congenital hemolytic anemias there is a delayed γ to β switch, resulting in increased HbF levels throughout life.

Globin-chain structural abnormalities

When α-chain variants of hemoglobin occur they are present at birth, since all forms of hemoglobin at birth contain α-chains. However, it is likely that most α-chain structural abnormalities are not associated with clinical consequences in neonates or adults and most infants with these mutations are detected only during routine neonatal screening programs. Occasionally, an α-chain variant may be clinically significant in the neonate, but not in the adult. An example is the infant with Hb Hasheron ($\alpha_2^{14 \, Asp} \rightarrow {}^{His} \beta_2$),[104] who can present with a transient hemolytic anemia in the newborn period as this α-chain variant is unstable when it associates with γ- but not β-globin chains. The hemolysis in the neonate resolves with transition from the fetal to the adult form of Hb Hasheron trait.[104]

γ-Chain structural variants also rarely cause clinical problems and if they do, they resolve as the γ to β switch occurs. HbF-Poole is a γ-chain variant that is sufficiently unstable in the newborn to cause a significant hemolytic anemia.[105]

Although β-chain abnormalities can be detected at birth using sensitive electrophoretic techniques, they do not usually cause clinical problems. The newborn with the commonest β-chain variant, sickle cell disease, is usually asymptomatic until the age of 4–6 months due to the presence of HbF in each red cell. However, hyperbilirubinemia appears to be more common in newborns with sickle cell disease[106] and there has been a report of lethal sickling in a 5-day-old infant.[107]

Defective hemoglobin synthesis: the thalassemia syndromes (see also Chapter 15)

The thalassemia syndromes collectively are probably the commonest single gene disorders worldwide. A reduced rate of α-globin chain synthesis characterizes the α-thalassemias, which are usually due to deletions of one or more of the 4 α-globin genes. This produces a common hemoglobin abnormality that primarily affects Asian and Afro-American races.

The clinical and laboratory manifestations vary depending on the number of genes affected.[108]

α-Thalassemias

In the presence of α-globin gene deletions, excess γ chain accumulates inside the cell and forms a tetramer called Hb-Barts (γ^4). The amount of this form of hemoglobin present in the newborn is dependent on the number of genes deleted. Silent carrier α-thalassemia (α^+ thalassemia) occurs when one gene is deleted and is associated with slight elevations of Hb-Barts at birth ($<2\%$) but no clinical manifestations. α-Thalassemia trait (α^0-thalassemia) occurs when 2 genes are deleted and, although older children and adults may demonstrate only a mild anemia and microcytosis and normal hemoglobin electrophoresis, the diagnosis is easy to make in the newborn. It causes microcytic red cell indices (MCV <95 fl) and a mild anemia and as microcytosis is rare at this age, α-thalassemia trait is the commonest cause. Also, the level of Hb-Barts is detectable at 3–10% at birth but not by 3 months of age. This disorder is common in Orientals, with an incidence of about 20% in south-east Asia and 2–5% in blacks. In the latter, the α-thalassemia gene mutations are almost invariably on different chromosomes, i.e. the abnormal gene is always linked to a normal gene. Consequently, offspring from 2 black α-thalassemia trait individuals will not inherit >2 α-thalassemia genes.[109] In south-east Asians, the 2 gene mutations are usually on 1 chromosome and if both parents pass on their affected chromosome, then a 4-gene deletion results (see below).

If 3 α genes are deleted, HbH disease results. HbH is unstable and precipitates within the red cell and can be demonstrated by incubation of the blood with supravital oxidizing stains. HbH disease presents in the neonatal period with a significant microcytic, hemolytic anemia[110] and a level of Hb-Barts ranging from 15 to 25%, as well as detectable HbH—a tetramer of 4 β chains. By 3 months of age, as the γ to β globin switch occurs, the Hb-Barts disappears and is replaced by HbH. Infants with HbH disease may require transfusion for severe anemia at birth but beyond this time the severity of the anemia is very variable.

When all 4 α genes are deleted, no α-chain synthesis occurs, no HbF or HbA are produced and homozygous α-thalassemia results.[111] This is a common cause of fetal death throughout south-east Asia. These fetuses invariably become severely hydropic in the second or third trimester, virtually all of the hemoglobin at birth is Hb-Barts, and the hemoglobin is usually 3–10 g/dl with microcytosis and normoblastosis in the blood film. The infants are stillborn or die soon after birth, although intrauterine transfusions and a post-delivery transfusion program have been reported to result in occasional survivors.[112,113] The peripheral blood film demonstrates marked hypochromia, poikilocytosis and target cells. This disorder must be distinguished from other causes of hydrops fetalis with severe anemia. In future, it is possible that *in utero* stem cell transplantation or gene therapy may cure this disease.

β-Thalassemias

Homozygous β-thalassemia does not cause problems in the newborn but as the γ to β globin switch occurs, a microcytic anemia develops, nucleated red cells appear on the blood film and HbF levels are maintained. Any disorder that significantly alters the survival of fetal red cells, such as intrauterine blood loss or blood group incompatibility, can make the β-thalassemia clinically obvious at a younger age.[114]

γ-Thalassaemias

γ-Thalassaemia syndromes, if significant, are probably lethal *in utero*, although the severity depends on the extent to which the γ genes are involved.[115] If only 1 or 2 are affected, only slight anemia and microcytosis ensues and these are probably not detected in the neonatal period and disappear as β-chain synthesis begins.

γβ-Thalassemia

There have been reports of γβ-thalassemia as a cause of severe anemia, erythroblastosis fetalis and hydrops in the newborn.[116] Globin-chain analysis has shown a reduction in the synthesis of both γ and β chains. The severe anemia seems to be self-limiting and surviving children have progressed to a mild hypochromic, microcytic anemia with normal levels of HbF and HbA$_2$.

ANEMIA DUE TO IMPAIRED RED CELL PRODUCTION

Impaired red cell production is a relatively unusual cause of anemia in the newborn, with the exception of the 'physiologic' anemias of both the term and preterm infant (see below). Of the inherited causes of impaired red cell production, Diamond–Blackfan anemia (DBA) is the most likely to present in the first 6 weeks of life.

CONGENITAL PURE RED CELL APLASIA: DIAMOND–BLACKFAN ANEMIA

DBA is an uncommon condition characterized by a life-long failure of erythropoiesis, with normal production of white cells and platelets. It is discussed in full in Chapter 3. The majority of cases are sporadic and the remainder are familial, with either autosomal dominant or recessive inheritance.

Up to a quarter of patients can present with anemia and reticulocytopenia in the newborn period[117,118] and there have been reports of the condition presenting as hydrops fetalis.[119] Even at this early stage, the bone marrow shows an absence or marked reduction of erythroid precursors. The anemia is normochromic and usually macrocytic. Physical anomalies are present in up to 30% of these babies. The commonest of these is short stature which will not be evident in the neonate, but other frequent abnormalities include microcephaly, cleft palate, eye anomalies and deformed thumbs. The birth weight is low (<2500 g) in 10%.

The differential diagnosis includes human parvovirus infection (see below) and transient erythroblastopenia of childhood (TEC). The former can be differentiated by the bone marrow, which in parvovirus typically shows abnormal giant pronormoblasts, serology and by looking for viral DNA. TEC does not usually present until later in infancy and rarely has the extreme erythroid hypoplasia seen in DBA.

Once the definitive diagnosis of DBA has been made, steroids should be instituted and the majority of cases will respond.

ANEMIA OF PREMATURITY

All newborns experience a fall in hemoglobin in the first few weeks of life but in premature infants the fall often starts from birth and its rapidity and magnitude vary directly with the degree of immaturity of the newborn. In term infants, the nadir of hemoglobin concentration is not usually reached until 8–12 weeks of age and can fall to 11.4 ± 0.9 g/dl but in premature infants weighing <1500 g the hemoglobin can fall as low as 8.0 g/dl by 4–8 weeks of age.[120] This fall in hemoglobin concentration results primarily from a reduction in red cell mass, due to shortened red cell survival, reticulocytopenia and a decrease in marrow erythroid elements, although an expanding plasma volume may also contribute.[121] Clinically, these infants have tachycardia, tachypnea, feeding problems, decreased activity and apneic attacks.

Pathophysiology

Factors which contribute to the pathophysiology and severity of the anemia of prematurity of small preterm infants are listed in Table 9.9.

There has been enormous interest over the last decade in the role of erythropoietin in the pathophysiology of anemia of prematurity, largely because of the availability of recombinant human erythropoietin (r-Hu Epo) as an option for treatment. Erythropoietin production in the fetus is well established as maternal erythropoietin does not cross the placenta and is measurable in increasing amounts with increasing gestational age.[122,123] The level of hormone in cord blood and amniotic fluid is higher in anemic fetuses than normal and also in the offspring of anemic mothers. It is also elevated in infants with fetal distress, severe respiratory distress and in children with cyanotic congenital heart disease.[124] Thus, the fetus is capable of responding to

Table 9.9 Factors which contribute to the pathophysiology and severity of the anemia of prematurity.

Reduced erythropoietin response to anemia or hypoxia
Hepatic synthesis of erythropoietin
Reduced life-span of neonatal erythrocytes
Neonatal reticulocytopenia
Rapid growth rate and increase in blood volume
Frequent blood sampling
Reduced tissue oxygen availability
Low levels of other hemopoietic growth factors
Nutritional deficiencies

hypoxemia whether the cause is fetal, placental or maternal. However, the response to hypoxia or anemia in the preterm infant is poor compared to that in the mature infant or adult and the preterm infant retains his *in utero* hyporesponsiveness *ex utero*.[125] The effects of this are greatest in the most immature infants.[3]

Recent clinical and laboratory investigations have shown that although there is a diminished erythropoietin response in anemia of prematurity, the progenitor cells committed to erythroid differentiation are present and the intrinsic responsiveness of the burst-forming unit erythroid pool (BFU-E) to erythropoietin is normal or increased.[126,127] This has established that inadequate production of erythropoietin is the cause of quantitatively insufficient erythropoiesis in affected infants. Other hemopoietic growth factors such as insulin-like growth factors I and II may also play a role.[128] It is unclear why plasma erythropoietin levels are low in newborn infants, but one reason is that during the first weeks of life the liver is the chief site of erythropoietin production, rather than the kidney, and the liver is less sensitive than the kidney to tissue hypoxia.

Treatment

Following the research that established insufficient erythropoietin production in preterm infants there have been numerous clinical trials, starting in the late 1980s, of r-Hu Epo in anemia of prematurity, since prior to this the standard therapy was red cell transfusion with its associated risks. r-Hu Epo had already been shown to stimulate erythroid proliferation in progenitors from preterm infants *in vitro*[127,129,130] and had been used successfully to treat the anemia of chronic renal failure. The early clinical trials in infants involved few subjects and varied in the dose of r-Hu Epo given and the use of concurrent iron. In general, they did show that r-Hu Epo at a weekly dose of 300–1200 U/kg consistently stimulated erythropoiesis and was not associated with any adverse effects,[131–133] although the studies using lower doses (<300 U/kg/week) reported no improvements in red cell levels or reduced need for transfusions.[134]

Three large randomized trials from Europe, South Africa and the US have been reported and confirm that r-Hu Epo has a predictable and impressive biologic effect on erythropoiesis in preterm infants.[135–137] These are reviewed in detail in a recent publication.[138]

In the European trial,[135] 241 preterm infants were randomized to receive either 750 unit/kg/week of r-Hu Epo from day 3 of life with 2 mg/kg/day of supplemental iron from day 14 or no treatment. The authors found no significant differences between the 2 groups in the use of transfusions or maintenance of the hematocrit above 32% during the first 2 weeks of treatment. However, the groups diverged in the following weeks with the r-Hu Epo-treated infants showing overall reductions in the cumulative volume of blood transfused and in the number of transfusions per infant, and a higher number maintained their hematocrit.

The South African trial[136] was double blinded; r-Hu Epo at 600 unit/kg/week with supplemental iron in low dose escalating to high dose if the ferritin fell below 65 $\mu g/dl$, versus placebo. In this trial also, the investigators saw a significant enhancement in erythropoietic activity among infants who received r-Hu Epo; they had increased reticulocyte counts and a stable hematocrit. They also received fewer and smaller volume red cell transfusions.

The United States Multicenter trial[137] was also double blinded and placebo controlled and the dose used was 500 unit/kg/week with iron at 3–6 mg/kg/day. The results mirrored those of the other 2 studies.

Side-effects of treatment included neutropenia in pilot studies but this complication was not substantiated in the above 3 studies. The European study[135] was the only one to report any side-effects, namely an increase in serious infections and a decrease in median weight gain in the study group compared to controls. However, there were no differences in the blood counts. Supplemental iron administration has emerged as an important consideration in the management of infants treated with r-Hu Epo and doses of at least 3–6 mg/kg/day are required with doses of r-Hu Epo of 500–750 unit/kg/week. Intravenous iron preparations have also been used for infants not on enteral feeds.[139]

Despite the conclusions of these trials, r-Hu Epo therapy is unlikely to be cost-effective if prescribed indiscriminately for most premature infants with low birth weights, largely because improvements in neonatal practice over the last decade have meant that there has been a significant drop in transfusion of neonates for anemia of prematurity and the factors that limit transfusion also limit the need for r-Hu Epo. The contributing factors have included treatment with surfactant, the use of modern ventilators and smaller blood losses during phlebotomy. Therefore, the greatest benefit from r-Hu Epo probably lies in averting transfusion in infants weighing < 1000 g but the studies to date have not addressed its use in large numbers of such infants.

INFECTION

The placenta, fetal membranes and fetus himself may become infected with agents that injure the fetal hematopoietic system or infections can be acquired from the cervix and vagina during delivery. Anemia is a frequent symptom of all the most significant intrauterine infections: toxoplasmosis, rubella, cytomegalovirus (CMV), herpes simplex and syphilis (see Table 9.8 and Chapter 38) and, although there may be some marrow suppression contributing to the anemia, there is usually significant hemolysis as well (see above). Severe bacterial sepsis in the neonate with pathogens such as Group B streptococcus can also cause marrow suppression and anemia.

In the last decade, maternal infection with *human parvovirus B19* has been recognized as a cause of intrauterine infection and fetal damage, particularly anemia and non-immune hydrops fetalis, as it appears to have a direct effect on hematopoiesis by infecting fetal erythroid precursors.[140–143] It is the causative agent of a common exanthematous disease which occurs in outbreaks in winter and spring, predominantly in young children when the infection is known as erythema infectiosum, fifth disease or slapped cheek syndrome. Infection can also be asymptomatic in children and particularly in adults, although in the latter it can cause polyarthralgia. In subjects suffering from a chronic hemolytic condition, such as sickle cell disease, it can cause an aplastic crisis, which when severe can be precipitous and life-threatening.[144]

Prospective studies on parvovirus B19 infection in pregnancy suggest that the majority of maternal infections cause no significant harm to mother or fetus.[145–147] However, infection early in gestation can result in spontaneous fetal loss in the first or second trimester and there have been rare cases of B19-associated birth defects[140,148,149] although no epidemiologic studies exist to support a definite correlation between maternal B19 infection and an increased risk of birth defects in infants.[150]

Infection during the second trimester can cause hydrops and fetal loss or premature delivery when the fetus can be born with severe anemia, with or without leukopenia and thrombocytopenia, requiring urgent blood product support. Studies on fetuses with apparently idiopathic non-immune hydrops fetalis suggest that parvovirus B19 infection may be the cause in 10–13% of cases,[151,152] and there have been reports of intrauterine transfusion successfully to treat mid-trimester hydrops due to B19 infection.[153,154] Although the B19 virions have been demonstrated in the erythroid precursors of hydropic fetuses,[155] B19 DNA has also been found by hybridization studies in practically every fetal organ, demonstrating widespread infection.[156] Maternal infection acquired late in gestation is rarely associated with fetal damage, possibly because this virus has a predilection for actively dividing cells and the relative reduction in cell turnover that occurs in the third trimester may protect the fetus.

The laboratory findings of parvovirus B19 infection are anemia, reticulocytopenia and giant pronormoblasts in the bone marrow in which readily identified amphophilic intranuclear inclusions can be seen and electron microscopy can identify viral particles. Antibodies to B19 may be detected serologically but will not always be positive, particularly in cases of immunodeficiency, and it may be necessary to examine the serum for viral DNA using gene amplification and the polymerase chain reaction.

The anemia in parvovirus infection is usually transient and the neonate is likely to require only 1 or 2 supportive transfusions. However, in cases of immunodeficiency, the anemia can persist for months or years and therapy with intravenous immunoglobulin may be required. This appears to break the cycle of viral replication in the erythron and has been shown to be of use in chronic parvoviremia.[157]

NUTRITIONAL DEFICIENCIES

Nutritional deficiencies are the commonest cause of anemia in the first year of life (see Chapter 6), yet they are an uncommon cause of anemia in the neonatal period. However, when they do occur early in life they can cause significant sequelae if left untreated.

Vitamin B$_{12}$ deficiency

This has been reported in infants of mothers with pernicious anemia and in some cases the maternal deficiency was diagnosed only after the infant presented.[158–160] Anemia is more likely to develop if the infant is exclusively breast fed[160] and he can develop neurologic as well as hematologic abnormalities if not treated promptly.

Folate deficiency (see also Chapter 8)

This is a common problem in rapidly growing preterm infants at 1–3 months of age and it contributes towards the anemia of prematurity. It is common therefore to give folate supplements to all preterm infants. Other conditions associated with folic acid deficiency include congenital folate malabsorption, defective cellular folate uptake and inborn errors of folate metabolism.[161]

Iron deficiency

During pregnancy the fetus is a very successful parasite in terms of securing iron stores and the fetal stores can be adequate at birth even in mothers with low ferritin levels in the third trimester. There is no consistent correlation between fetal and maternal ferritin levels.[162,163] In the newborn infant, there is a huge individual variation in iron stores and the quantity of placental blood transfused perinatally can have a significant impact on circulating hemoglobin and therefore total body iron content.

Iron deficiency in infancy is rare in the first 2 months of life, except in preterm infants, and when it occurs it is usually due to inadequate iron intake combined with rapid growth and dilution of body iron. Breast milk is a relatively poor source of iron but the iron that is present is very efficiently absorbed.

In preterm infants, iron supplementation from shortly after birth does not prevent the physiologic anemia of prematurity experienced by healthy growing infants, but it does reduce the incidence of it, and is therefore recommended for all premature infants. In the infant receiving erythropoietin, supplemental iron is essential to prevent significant iron deficiency.[139]

Blood loss is another cause of iron deficiency in infancy. This can be due to placentally related conditions or gastrointestinal blood loss in the infant or it can be iatrogenic as a result of frequent blood sampling (see above).

Vitamin E deficiency

This is now primarily of historic interest. It was described in the 1960s in preterm infants who presented with a complex of symptoms between 4 and 12 weeks of life which included hemolytic anemia, reticulocytosis and pretibial edema. The infants were fed on low vitamin E-containing formula feeds which were high in polyunsaturates. All symptoms resolved when they were treated with vitamin E. Today this deficiency is only seen in infants with prolonged fat malabsorption.[164]

Deficiencies of vitamins A, B$_6$ and C

These do not cause neonatal anemias except for scanty case reports of vitamin B$_6$ deficiency in young infants.

REFERENCES

1. Issaragrisil S. Correlation between hematopoietic progenitors and erythroblasts in cord blood. *Am J Clin Pathol* 1983; **80**: 865–867

2. Hellebostad M, Haga P, Mary Cotes P. Serum immunoreactive erythropoietin in healthy normal children. *Br J Haematol* 1988; **70**: 247–250

3. Brown MS, Garcia JF, Phibbs RH, Dallman PR. Decreased response of plasma immunoreactive erythropoietin to 'available oxygen' in anaemia of prematurity. *J Pediatr* 1984; **105**: 793–798

4. Pearson HA. Life span of the fetal red blood cell. *J Pediatr* 1967; **70**: 166–171

5. Matoth Y, Zaizov R, Varsano I. Postnatal changes in some red cell parameters. *Acta Paediatr Scand* 1971; **60**: 317–323.

6. Maertzdorf WJ, Aldenhuyzen-Dorland W, Slaaf DW, Tangelder GJ, Blanco CE. Circulating blood volume in appropriate and small for gestational age full term and preterm polycythaemic infants. *Acta Paediatr Scand* 1991; **80**: 620–627

7. Yao AC, Moinian M, Lind J. Distribution of blood between infant and placenta after birth. *Lancet* 1969; **2**: 871–873

8. Linderkamp O, Nelle M, Kraus M, Zilow EP. The effect of early and late cord-clamping on blood viscosity and other hemorheological parameters in full-term infants. *Acta Pediatr* 1992; **81**: 745–750

9. Usher R, Shephard M, Lind J. The blood volume of the newborn infant and placental transfusion. *Acta Paediatr Scand* 1963; **52**: 497–512

10. Colozzi AE. Clamping the umbilical cord: its effect on the placental transfusion. *N Engl J Med* 1954; **250**: 629–631

11. Lanzkowsky P. Effects of early and late clamping of umbilical cord on infant's haemoglobin level. *Br Med J* 1960; **2**: 1777–1782

12. Zaizov R, Mathoth Y. Red cell values on the first postnatal day during the last 16 weeks of gestation. *Am J Hematol* 1976; **1**: 276–280

13. Holland BM, Jones JG, Wardrop CAJ. Lessons from the anemia of prematurity. *Hematol Oncol Clin North Am* 1987; **1**: 355–366

14. Wardrop CA, Holland BM. The roles and vital importance of placental blood to the newborn infant. *J Perinat Med* 1995; **23**: 139–143

15. Usher R, Lind J. Blood volume of the newborn premature infant. *Acta Paediatr Scand* 1965; **54**: 419–431

16. Brown EG, Krouskop RW, McDonnell FE, Sweet AY. Blood volume and blood pressure in infants with respiratory distress. *J Pediatr* 1975; **87**: 1133–1138

17. Moe PJ. Umbilical cord blood and capillary blood in the evaluation of anaemia in erythroblastosis fetalis. *Acta Paediatr Scand* 1967; **56**: 391–394

18. Oettinger L Jnr, Mills WB. Simultaneous capillary and venous haemoglobin determinations in newborn infants. *J Pediatr* 1949; **35**: 362–365

19. Thurlbeck SM, McIntosh N. Preterm blood counts vary with sampling site. *Arch Dis Child* 1987; **62**: 74–87

20. Linderkamp O, Versmold HT, Strohhacker I, Messow-Zahn K, Riegel KP, Betke K. Capillary-venous hematocrit differences in newborn infants. Relationship to blood volume, peripheral blood flow, and acid-base parameters. *Eur J Pediatr* 1977; **127**: 9–14

21. Phillips H, Holland BM, Jones JG *et al.* Determination of red cell mass in assessment and management of anaemia in babies needing blood transfusion. *Lancet* 1986; **i**: 882–884

22. Chown B. Anaemia from bleeding of the fetus into the mother's circulation. *Lancet* 1954; **i**: 1213–1215

23. Zipursky A, Hull A, White FD, Israels LG. Foetal erythrocytes in the maternal circulation. *Lancet* 1959; **i**: 451–452

24. Kleihauer E, Hildegard B. Demonstration von fetalem Hamoglobin in den Erythrocyten eines Blutausstrichs. *Klin Wochenschr* 1957; **35**: 637–638

25. Bowman JM, Pollock JM, Penston LE. Fetomaternal transplacental haemorrhage during pregnancy and after delivery. *Vox Sanguis* 1986; **51**: 117–121

26. Nance SJ, Nelson JM, Arndt PA, Lam HC, Garratty G. Quantitation of feto-maternal hemorrhage by flow cytometry. A simple and accurate method. *Am J Clin Pathol* 1989; **91**: 288–292

27. Bowman JM, Pollock JM. Transplacental fetal hemorrhage after amniocentesis. *Obstet Gynecol* 1985; **66**: 749–754

28. Brambati B, Guercilena S, Bonacchi I, Oldrini A, Lanzani A, Piceni L. Fetomaternal transfusion after chorionic villus sampling: clinical implications. *Hum Reprod* 1986; **1**: 37–40

29. Flieghner JR, Fortune DW, Barrie JU. Occult fetomaternal hemorrhage as a cause of fetal morbidity and mortality. *Aust NZ J Obstet Gynecol* 1987; 27: 158–161

30. Lipitz S, Achiron R, Horoshovski D, Rotstein Z, Sherman D, Schiff E. Fetomaternal hemorrhage discovered after trauma and treated by fetal intravascular transfusion. *Eur J Obstset Gynecol Reprod Biol* 1997; **71**: 21–22

31. Marcus RG, Crewe-Brown H, Krawitz S, Katz J. Feto-maternal haemorrhage following successful and unsuccessful attempts at external cephalic version. *Br J Obstet Gynaecol* 1975; **82**: 578–580.

32. Stiller AG, Skafish PR. Placental chorioangioma; a rare cause of feto-maternal transfusion with maternal hemolysis and fetal distress. *Obstet Gynecol* 1986; **67**: 296–298

33. Tabor A, Bang J, Norgaard-Pedersen B. Feto-maternal haemorrhage is associated with genetic amniocentesis: results of a randomized trial. *Br J Obstet Gynaecol* 1987; **94**: 528–534.

34. Mollison PL. Quantitation of transplacental haemorrhage. *Br Med J* 1972; **3**: 31–34

35. Cohen F, Zuelzer WW, Gustafson DC, Evans MM. Mechanism of isoimmunisation. I The transplacental passage of fetal erythrocytes in homospecific pregnancies. *Blood* 1964; **23**: 621–646.

36. Renaer M, Van de Putte I, Vermylen C. Massive feto-maternal hemorrhage as a cause for perinatal mortality and morbidity. *Eur J Obstet Gyaecol Reprod Biol* 1976; **6**: 125–140.

37. Fay RA. Feto-maternal haemorrhage as a cause of fetal morbidity and mortality. *Br J Obstet Gynaecol* 1983; **90**: 443–446.

38. Laube DW, Schauberger CW. Feto-maternal bleeding as a cause for "unexplained" fetal death. *Obstet Gynecol* 1982; **60**: 649–651

39. Bayliss KM, Kueck BD, Johnson ST *et al.* Detecting fetomaternal haemorrhage; a comparison of five methods. *Transfusion* 1991; **31**: 303–307

40. Medearis AL, Hensleigh PA, Parks DR, Herzenberg CA. Detection of fetal erythrocytes in maternal blood post-partum with the fluorescence-activated cell sorter. *Am J Obstet Gynecol* 1984; 148: 290–295

41. Chown B. The fetus can bleed. *Am J Obstet Gynecol* 1955; **70**: 1298–1308.

42. Cashore WJ, Usher RH. Hypovolemia resulting from a tight nuchal cord at birth. *Pediatr Res* 1973; **7**: 399

43. Becker AH, Glass H. Twin to twin transfusion syndrome. *Am J Dis Child* 1963; **106**: 624–629

44. Fisk NM, Borrell A, Hubinont C, Tannirandorn Y, Nicolini U, Rodeck CH. Fetofetal transfusion syndrome: do the neonatal criteria apply *in utero*? *Arch Dis Child* 1990; **65**: 657–661

45. Rausen R, Seki M, Strauss L. Twin transfusion syndrome. A review of 19 cases studied at one institution. *J Pediatr* 1965; **66**: 613–628.

46. Pochedly C, Musiker S. Twin-to-twin transfusion syndrome. *Postgrad Med* 1970; **47**: 172–176

47. Sonntag J, Waltz S, Schollmeyer T, Schuppler U, Schroder H, Weisner D. Morbidity and mortality of discordant twins up to 34 weeks of gestational age. *Eur J Pediatr* 1996; **155**: 224–229

48. Benirschke K. Obstetrically important lesions of the umbilical cord. *J Reprod Med* 1994; **39**: 262–272

49. Kirkman HN, Riley HD. Posthemorrhagic anemia and shock in the newborn. A review. *Pediatrics* 1959; **24**: 97–105

50. Vestermark V, Christensen I, Kay L, Windfeldt M. Spontaneous rupture of a velamentous umbilical cord; a case report. *Eur J Obstet Gynecol Reprod Biol* 1990; **35**: 279–281.

51. Englert Y, Imbert MC, Van-Rosendael E *et al.* Morphological anomalies in the placentae of IVF pregnancies: report of a multicentre study. *Hum Reprod* 1987; **2**: 155–157

52. Kouyoumjian A. Velamentous insertion of the umbilical cord. *Obstet Gynecol* 1980; **56**: 737–742

53. McShane PM, Heyl PS, Epstein MF. Maternal and perinatal morbidity resulting from placenta praevia. *Obstet Gynecol* 1985; **65**: 176–182

54. Lubin BH. Neonatal anaemia secondary to blood loss. *Clin Haematol* 1978; **7**: 19–34

55. Benaron DA. Subgaleal hematoma causing hypovolaemic shock during delivery after failed vacuum extraction. *J Perinatol* 1993; **13**: 228–231

56. Florentino-Pineda I, Ezhuthachan SG, Sineni LG, Kumar SP. Subgaleal haemorrhage in the newborn infant associated with silicone elastomer vacuum extractor. *J Perinatol* 1994; **14**: 95–100

57. Hall SL. Simultaneous occurrence of intracranial and subgaleal haemorrhages complicating vacuum extraction delivery. *J Perinatol* 1992; **12**: 185–187

58. Plauché WC. Subgaleal hematoma. A complication of instrumental delivery. *JAMA* 1980; **244**: 1597–1598

59. Leonard S, Anthony B. Giant cephalohaematoma of the newborn in an infant with haemorrhagic disease and hyperbilirubinaemia. *Am J Dis Child* 1961; **101**: 170–173

60. Pachman DJ. Massive hemorrhage into the scalp of a newborn infant. Hemorrhagic caput succedaneum. *Pediatrics* 1962; **29**: 907–910

61. Ng PC, Siu YK, Lewindon PJ. Subaponeurotic haemorrhage in the 1990s: a 3 year surveillance. *Acta Paediatr* 1995; **84**: 1065–1069

62. Robinson RJ, Rossiter MA. Massive subaponeurotic haemorrhage in babies of African origin. *Arch Dis Child* 1968; **43**: 684–687

63. Trounce JQ, Rutter N, Levene MI. Periventricular leucomalacia and intraventricular haemorrhage in the preterm neonate. *Arch Dis Child* 1986; **61**: 1196–1202

64. Stewart AL, Thorburn RJ, Hope PL, Goldsmith M, Lipscombe AP, Reynolds EOR. Ultrasound appearance of the brain in very preterm infants and neurodevelopmental outcome at 18 months of age. *Arch Dis Child* 1983; **58**: 598–604

65. Van Leewen G, Patney M. Complications of umbilical vessel catheterisation: peritoneal perforation. *Pediatrics* 1969; **44**: 1028–1030

66. Potter EL. Fetal and neonatal deaths: a statistical analysis of 2000 autopsies. *JAMA* 1940; **115**: 996–999

67. Brown JJM. Hepatic haemorrhage in the newborn. *Arch Dis Child* 1957; **32**: 480–483.

68. Shankaran S, Elias E, Ilagan N. Subcapsular haemorrhage of the liver in the very low birthweight infant. *Acta Paediatr Scand* 1991; **80**: 616–619

69. Philipsborn HF Jr, Traisman HS, Greer D Jr. Rupture of the spleen: a complication of erythroblastosis fetalis. *N Engl J Med* 1955; **252**: 159–162

70. Delta BG, Eisenstein EM, Rothenberg AM. Rupture of a normal

spleen in the newborn: a report of a survival and review of the literature. *Clin Pediatr* 1968; **7**: 373–376

71. Leape LL, Bordy MD. Neonatal rupture of the spleen. Report of a case successfully treated after spontaneous cessation of hemorrhage. *Pediatrics* 1971; **47**: 101–104

72. Cole VA, Norman ICS, Reynolds EOR, Rivers RPA. Pathogenesis of hemorrhagic pulmonary edema and massive pulmonary hemorrhage in the newborn. *Pediatrics* 1973; **51**: 175–187

73. Svane S. Foetal exsanguination from haemangioendothelioma of the skin. *Acta Paediatr Scand* 1966; **55**: 536–539

74. Nader PR, Margolin F. Hemangioma causing gastrointestinal bleeding. Case report and review of the literature. *Am J Dis Child* 1966; **111**: 215–222

75. Walsh SV, Cooke R, Mortimer G, Loftus BG. Massive thymic hemorrhage in a neonate: an entity revisited. *J Pediatr Surg* 1996; **31**: 1315–1317

76. Obladen M, Sachsenweger M, Stahnke M. Blood sampling in very low birth weight infants on different intensive care levels. *Eur J Pediatr* 1988; **147**: 399–404

77. Plotkin SA. Routes of fetal infection and mechanisms of fetal damage. *Am J Dis Child* 1975; **129**: 444–448

78. Klein JO, Remington JS. Current concepts of infections of the fetus and newborn infant. In: Remington JS, Klein JO (eds) *Infectious Diseases of the Fetus and Newborn Infant*. Philadelphia: WB Saunders, 1991

79. Meerstadt PW. Congenital malaria. *Clin Exp Obstet Gynaecol* 1986; **13**: 78–82

80. Malviya S, Shurin SJB. Congenital malaria. Case report and review. *Clin Pediatr* 1984; **23**: 516–517

81. Currie BG, Schell D, Bowring AC. Giant hemangioma of the arm associated with cardiac failure and the Kasabach–Merritt syndrome in a neonate. *J Pediatr Surg* 1991; **26**: 734–737.

82. Stamey CC, Diamond LK. Congenital hemolytic anemia in the newborn. *Am J Dis Child* 1957; **94**: 616–622

83. Burman D. Congenital spherocytosis in infancy. *Arch Dis Child* 1958; **33**: 335–341

84. Trucco JL, Brown AK. Neonatal manifestations of hereditary spherocytosis. *Am J Dis Child* 1967; **113**: 263–270

85. Agre P, Asimos A, Casella JF, Mc Millan C. Inheritance pattern and clinical response to splenectomy as a reflection of erythrocyte spectrin deficiency in hereditary spherocytosis. *N Engl J Med* 1986; **315**: 1579–1583

86. Schröter W, Kahsnitz E. Diagnosis of hereditary spherocytosis in newborn infants. *J Pediatr* 1983; **103**: 460–463

87. Austin RF, DesForges JF. Hereditary elliptocytosis: an unusual presentation of hemolysis in the newborn associated with transient morphologic abnormalities. *Pediatrics* 1969; **44**: 196–200

88. Mentzer WC, Iarocci TA, Narla M. Modulation of erythrocyte membrane mechanical stability by 2,3-DPG in the neonatal poikilocytosis/elliptocytosis syndrome. *J Clin Invest* 1987; **79**: 943–949

89. Garbarz M, Lecomte MC, Dhermy D *et al*. Double inheritance of an $\alpha^{1/65}$ spectrin variant in a child with homozygous elliptocytosis. *Blood* 1986; **67**: 1661–1667

90. Cutting HO, McHugh WJ, Conrad FG. Autosomal dominant hemolytic anaemia characterised by ovalocytosis: a family study of seven involved members. *Am J Med* 1965; **39**: 21–34

91. Zarkowsky HS, Mohandas N, Speaker CB, Shohet SB. A congenital haemolytic anaemia with thermal sensitivity of the erythrocyte membrane. *Br J Haematol* 1975; **29**: 537–543

92. Iarocci TH, Wagner GM, Mohandas N, Lane PA, Mentzer WC. Hereditary poikilocytic anemia associated with coinheritance of two α spectrin abnormalities. *Blood* 1988; **71**: 1390–1396

93. Coetzer T, Palek J, Lawler J *et al*. Structural and functional heterogeneity of α spectrin mutations involving the spectrin heterodimer self-association site: relationships to haematologic expression of homozygous hereditary elliptocytosis and hereditary pyropoikilocytosis. *Blood* 1990; **75**: 2235–2244

94. Mentzer WC, Turetsky T, Mohandas N, Schrier S, Wu C-S C, Koenig H. Identification of the hereditary pyropoikilocytosis carrier state. *Blood* 1984; **63**: 1439–1446

95. Luzzatto L. Inherited hemolytic states: Glucose-6-phosphate dehydrogenase deficiency. *Clin Hematol* 1975; **4**: 83–108

96. Sodeinde O. Glucose-6-phosphate dehydrogenase deficiency. *Baillière's Clin Haematol* 1992; **5**: 367–382

97. Johnson GJ, Allen DW, Cadman S *et al*. Red-cell membrane polypeptide aggregates in glucose-6-phosphate dehydrogenase mutants with chronic hemolytic diseases. *N Engl J Med* 1979; **301**: 522–527

98. Matthay KK, Mentzer WC. Erythrocyte enzymopathies in the newborn. *Clin Haematol* 1981; 10: 31–55

99. Doxiades SA, Valaes T. The clinical picture of glucose-6-phosphate dehydrogenase deficiency in early childhood. *Arch Dis Child* 1964; **39**: 545–553

100. Mallouh AA, Imseeh G, Abu-Osba YK Hamdan JA. Screening for glucose-6-phosphate dehydrogenase deficiency can prevent neonatal jaundice. *Ann Trop Paediatr* 1992; **12**: 391–395

101. Nathan DG, Oski FA, Miller DR, Gardner FH. Life span and organ sequestration of the red cells in pyruvate kinase deficiency. *N Engl J Med* 1968; **278**: 73–81

102. Gisanz F, Vega MA, Gomez-Castillo E, Ruiz-Balda JA, Omenaca F. Fetal anaemia due to pyruvate kinase deficiency. *Arch Dis Child* 1993; **69**: 523–524

103. Ravindranath Y, Paglia DE, Warrier I, Valentine W, Nakatani M, Brockway RA. Glucose phosphate isomerase deficiency as a cause for hydrops fetalis. *N Engl J Med* 1987; **316**: 258–261

104. Levine RL, Lincoln DR, Buchholz T, Gribble J, Schwarz HC. Hemoglobin Hasheron in a premature infant with hemolytic anemia. *Pediatr Res* 1975; **9**: 7–11

105. Lee-Potter JP, Deacon-Smith RA, Simkiss MJ, Kamuzora H, Lehmann H. A new cause of haemolytic anaemia in the newborn: A description of an unstable fetal haemoglobin F-Poole a2Gg2 Tryptophan-Glycine. *J Clin Pathol* 1975; **28**: 317–320

106. Van-Wijgerden JA. Clinical expression of sickle cell anemia in the newborn. *South Med J* 1983; **76**: 477–480

107. Hegyi T, Delphin ES, Bank A, Polin RA, Blanc WA. Sickle cell anemia in the newborn. *Pediatrics* 1977; **60**: 213–216

108. Weatherall DJ. The thalassaemias. In: Stamatoyannopoulos G, Nienhuis A, Majerus PW, Varmus H (eds) *Molecular Basis of Blood Diseases*. Philadelphia: WB Saunders, 1993

109. Dozy AM, Kan YW, Emberg SH *et al*. Alpha-globin gene organisation in blacks precludes the severe form of alpha-thalassaemia. *Nature* 1979; **280**: 605–607

110. Koenig HM, Vedvick TS, Dozy AM, Golbus MS, Kan YW. Prenatal diagnosis of hemoglobin H disease. *J Pediatr* 1978; **92**: 278–281

111. Taylor JM, Dozy A, Kan YW *et al*. Genetic lesion in homozygous alpha-thalassaemia (hydrops fetalis). *Nature* 1974; **251**: 392–393

112. Beaudry MA, Ferguson DJ, Pearse K, Yanofsky RA, Rubin EM, Kan YW. Survival of a hydropic infant with homozygous α-thalassemia-1. *J Pediatr* 1986; **108**: 713–716

113. Bianchi DW, Beyer EC, Stark AR, Saffan D, Sachs BP, Wolfe L. Normal long-term survival with alpha-thalassemia. *J Pediatr* 1986; **108**: 716–8

114. Erlandson ME, Hilgartner M. Hemolytic disease in the neonatal period. *J Pediatr* 1959; **54**: 566–585

115. Stamatoyannopoulos G. Gamma thalassaemia. *Lancet* 1971; **2**: 192–193

116. Kan YW, Forget BG, Nathan DG. Gamma-beta thalassemia: A cause of hemolytic disease of the newborn. *N Engl J Med* 1972; **286**: 129–134

117. Alter BP, Nathan DG. Red cell aplasia in children. *Arch Dis Child* 1979; **54**: 263–267

118. Diamond LK, Allen DM. Congenital (erythroid) hypoplastic anemia. *Am J Dis Child* 1961; **102**: 403–415

119. Scimeca PG, Weinblatt ME, Slepowitz G, Harper RG, Kochen JA. Diamond–Blackfan syndrome: an unusual cause of hydrops fetalis. *Am J Pediatr Hematol Oncol* 1988; **10**: 241–243

120. Schulman J. The anemia of prematurity. *J Pediatr* 1959; **54**: 663–672
121. Bratteby LE. Studies on erythrokinetics in infancy. XI. The change in circulating red cell volume during the first five months of life. *Acta Paediatr Scand* 1968; **57**: 215–224
122. Finne PH. Erythropoietin levels in cord blood as an indicator of intrauterine hypoxia. *Acta Paediatr Scand* 1966; **55**: 478–489
123. Finne PH, Halvorsen S. Regulation of erythropoiesis in the fetus and newborn. *Arch Dis Child* 1972; **47**: 683–687
124. Eckhart K-U, Hartmann W, Vetter U, Pohlandt F, Burghardt R, Kurtz A. Serum erythropoietin levels in health and disease. *Eur J Pediatr* 1990; **149**: 459–464
125. Stockman JA III. Erythropoietin: off again, on again. *J Pediatr* 1988; **112**: 906–908
126. Emmerson AJ, Westwood NB, Rackham RA, Stern CM, Pearson TC. Erythropoietin responsive progenitors in anaemia of prematurity. *Arch Dis Child* 1991; **66**: 810–811
127. Shannon KM, Naylor GS, Torkildson JC et al. Circulating erythroid progenitors in the anemia of prematurity. *N Engl J Med* 1987; **317**: 728–733
128. Han P, Stacy D, Story C, Owens PC. The role of haemopoietic growth factors in the pathogenesis of the early anaemia of prematurity. *Br J Haematol* 1995; **91**: 327–329.
129. Sieff CA, Emerson SJG, Mufson A, Gesner TG, Nathan DG. Dependence of highly enriched human bone marrow progenitors on hemopoietic growth factors and their response to recombinant erythropoietin. *J Clin Invest* 1986; **77**: 74–81
130. Rhondeau SM, Christensen RD, Ross MP, Rothstein G, Simmons MA. Responsiveness to recombinant human erythropoietin of marrow erythroid progenitors from infants with the 'anemia of prematurity'. *J Pediatr* 1988; **112**: 935–940
131. Beck D, Masserey E, Meyer M, Calame A. Weekly intravenous administration of recombinant human erythropoietin in infants with the anemia of prematurity. *Eur J Pediatr* 1991; **150**: 767–772
132. Carnielli V, Montini G, Da-Riol R, Dall'Amico R, Cantarutti F. Effect of high doses of human recombinant erythropoietin on the need for blood transfusions in preterm infants. *J Pediatr* 1992; **121**: 98–102
133. Halperin DS, Wacker P, Lacourt G et al. Effects of recombinant human erythropoietin in infants with the anemia of prematurity: a pilot study. *J Pediatr* 1990; **116**: 779–785
134. Shannon KM, Mentzer WC, Abels RI et al. Recombinant human erythropoietin in the anemia of prematurity: results of a placebo-controlled pilot study. *J Pediatr* 1991; **118**: 949–955
135. Maier R, Obladen M, Scigalla P et al. The effect of epoietin beta (recombinant human erythropoietin) on the need for transfusion in very low birth weight infants. *N Engl J Med* 1994; **330**: 1173–1178
136. Meyer MP, Meyer JH, Commerford A et al. Recombinant human erythropoietin in the treatment of the anemia of prematurity: results of a double-blind, placebo-controlled study. *Pediatrics* 1994; **93**: 918–923
137. Shannon KM, Keith JF, Mentzer WC et al. Recombinant human erythropoietin stimulates erythropoiesis and reduces erythrocyte transfusions in very-low-birthweight preterm infants. *Pediatrics* 1995; **95**: 1–8
138. Shannon KM. Recombinant human erythropoietin in neonatal anaemia. *Clin Perinatol* 1995; **22**: 627–640
139. Meyer MP, Haworth C, Meyer JH, Commerford A. A comparison of oral and intravenous iron supplementation in preterm infants receiving recombinant erythropoietin. *J Pediatr* 1996; **129**: 258–263
140. Anand A, Gray ES, Thomas Brown Ch B, Clewley JP, Cohen BJ. Human parvovirus in pregnancy and hydrops fetalis. *N Engl J Med* 1987; **316**: 183–186
141. Anderson LJ, Hurwitz ES. Human parvovirus B19 and pregnancy. *Clin Perinatol* 1988; **15**: 273–286
142. Brown KE. What threat is human parvovirus B19 to the fetus? A review. *Br J Obstet Gynaecol* 1989; **96**: 764–767
143. Samra JS, Obhrai MS, Constantine G. Parvovirus infection in pregnancy. *Obstet Gynecol* 1989; **73**: 832–834
144. Smith MA, Ryan ME. Parvovirus infections. From benign to life-threatening. *Postgrad Med* 1988; **84**: 127–134.
145. Gratacós E, Torres P-J, Vidal J et al. The incidence of human parvovirus B19 infection during pregnancy and its impact on perinatal outcome. *J Infect Dis* 1995; **171**: 1360–1363
146. Guidozzi F, Ballot D, Rothberg AD. Human B19 parvovirus infection in an obstetric population. A prospective study determining fetal outcome. *J Reprod Med* 1994; **39**: 36–38
147. Public Health Laboratory Service Working Party on Fifth Disease. Prospective study of human parvovirus (B19) infection in pregnancy. *Br Med J* 1990; **300**: 1166–1170
148. Katz VL, Chescheir NC, Bethea M. Hydrops fetalis from B19 parvovirus infection. *J Perinatol* 1990; **10**: 366–368
149. Weiland HT, Vermey-Keers C, Salimans MMM, Fleuren GJ, Verwey RA, Anderson MJ. Parvovirus B19 associated with fetal abnormality. *Lancet* 1987; **i**: 682–683
150. Mortimer PP, Cohen BJ, Buckley MM et al. Human parvovirus and the fetus. *Lancet* 1985; **ii**: 1012
151. Jordan JA. Identification of human parvovirus B19 infection in non-immune hydrops fetalis. *Am J Obstet Gynecol* 1996; **174**: 37–42
152. Yaegashi N, Okamura K, Yajima A, Murai C, Sugamura K. The frequency of human parvovirus B19 infection in nonimmune hydrops fetalis. *J Perinat Med* 1994; **22**: 159–163
153. Fairley CK, Smoleniec JS, Caul OE, Miller E. Observational study of effect of intrauterine transfusions on outcome of fetal hydrops after parvovirus B19 infection. *Lancet* 1995; **346**: 1335–1337
154. Schwarz TF, Roggendorf M, Hottentrager B et al. Human parvovirus B19 infection in pregnancy. *Lancet* 1988; **ii**: 566–567
155. Knisely AS, O'Shea PA, McMillan P, Singer DB, Magid MS. Electron microscopic identification of parvovirus virions in erythroid-line cells in fetal hydrops fetalis. *Pediatr Pathol* 1988; **8**: 163–170
156. Van-Elsacker-Niele AMW, Salimans MMM, Weiland HT, Vermey-Kreers C, Anderson MJ, Versteeg J. Fetal pathology in human parvovirus B19 infection. *Br J Obstet Gynaecol* 1989; **96**: 768–775
157. Kurtzman G, Frickhofen N, Kimball J, Jenkins DW, Nienhuis AW, Young NS. Pure red cell aplasia of 10 years' duration due to persistent parvovirus B19 infection and its cure with immunoglobulin therapy. *N Engl J Med* 1989; **321**: 519–523
158. Lampkin BC, Shore NA, Chadwick D. Megaloblastic anaemia of infancy secondary to maternal pernicious anaemia. *N Engl J Med* 1966; **274**: 1168–1171
159. Michaud JL, Lemieux B, Ogier H, Lambert MA. Nutritional vitamin B12 deficiency: two cases detected by routine newborn urinary screening. *Eur J Pediatr* 1992; **151**: 218–220
160. Johnson PR, Rolof JS. Vitamin B_{12} deficiency in an infant strictly breast-fed by a mother with latent pernicious anemia. *J Pediatr* 1982; **100**: 917–919
161. Rosenblatt DS. Inherited disorders of folate transport and metabolism. In: Scriver CR, Stanbury JB, Wyngaarden JB et al (eds) *The Metabolic and Molecular Basis of Inherited Disease.* New York: McGraw-Hill, 1995
162. Van Eijk HG, Kroos MJ, Hoogendoorn GA, Wallenberg HC. Serum ferritin and iron stores during pregnancy. *Clin Chim Acta* 1978; **83**: 81–91
163. Worwood M. Ferritin in human tissues and serum. *Clin Haematol* 1982; **11**: 275–307
164. Williams, ML, Shoot RJ, O'Neal PL et al. Role of dietary iron and fat on vitamin E deficiency of infancy. *N Engl J Med* 1975; **292**: 887–890

Immune hemolytic anemias

MARK V SAPP AND JAMES B BUSSEL

Immune hemolytic anemia (IHA) in both the pediatric and adult population is mediated through the recognition of red blood cell (RBC) antigens by either auto- or allo-immune antibodies. Alloimmunization may result from either the passive transplacental passage of antibody (IgG), or through an active process such as the transfusion of incompatible red blood cells. Autoimmune hemolytic anemia (AIHA) is a relatively rare condition in childhood, affecting approximately 1/million children, and it manifests primarily as an extravascular process. An individual with AIHA produces antibodies capable of either opsonization and phagocytosis, or complement-mediated lysis of his own red blood cells.

Autoimmune diseases affect 5–7% of the general population and may cause chronic debilitating illness.[1] Over the past 20 years the role of immune mechanisms in the pathophysiology of human tissue and cell damage has emerged as a major field of both clinical and basic science research. Immunologic disorders comprise a clinically heterogeneous group of diseases which can be classified as either systemic, such as rheumatoid arthritis, or organ specific, such as AIHA. The two principal factors which determine the clinical and pathologic manifestations of such disease are:

1. type of immune response that leads to tissue injury;
2. nature and location of antigen that initiates or is the target of this immune response.[2] These antigens may be intinsic to the RBC membrane or foreign antigens acquired by the RBC.

This chapter discusses the underlying mechanisms of the immune response and on the clinical syndromes associated with AIHA.

IMMUNE MECHANISMS

A variety of factors are known to determine the nature and severity of immunologically-mediated RBC destruction:

- Red cell antigens;
- anti-red-cell antibodies;
- non-immunoglobulin components such as serum complement proteins;
- mononuclear phagocytic system, especially the Fc receptors on splenic macrophages.

The erythrocyte membrane contains structural and contractile proteins in conjunction with numerous enzymes and surface antigens. The two major membrane proteins are spectrin and glycophorin. It is believed that glycophorin, an 'intrinsic' membrane protein, carries the A-, B-, M- and N-specific blood group antigens, as well as receptors for viruses and other surface-reactive substances.[3]

RED BLOOD CELL ANTIGENS

The structure and function of surface proteins, their density and topography, as well as the distribution of antigenic sites, all play a role in cell lysis and destruction. The chemical composition of red blood antigens may be of several basic biochemical structures, e.g. the polysaccharide-determined antigens of the ABO blood group system, the proteins or lipoproteins of the Rh system, the MNS glycoprotein antigens and glycosphingolipids comprising the P system surface antigens. Approximately 600 antigenic specificities have been recognized on RBCs, comprising almost 20 different blood group systems.[4] Estimates of the number of antigen receptors on erythrocytes can be obtained by immuno-electron microscopy in which antibody molecules are coupled covalently to electron-dense markers, or by measuring the uptake of antibody labeled with radioactive iodine. Single-group A1 cells have 810 000–1 170 000 A-specific sites;[5] Rh on the other hand has 6800–19 600 D sites[6] and Kell only 2100–5400 K sites.[7]

ABO blood group system

The ABO blood group is the most clinically significant blood group system and is composed of 2 antigens, A and B.

Two independent loci, ABO and H, are involved in determining the expression of ABO. Whereas the ABO loci is known to be near the end of the long arm of chromosome 9,[8] the loci for the H antigen has been mapped to chromosome 19. O group individuals have the H antigenic determinant that is not readily detectable on A and B cell types. A precursor molecule with H specificity is modified through a glycosidic linkage with specific transferase molecules subsequently determining A and B antigenicity on respective RBCs. The ABH antigens occur frequently in other species, including perhaps half of the bacterial flora of the gut. This widespread occurrence may account for the ubiquitous anti-AB reactivity of human sera (isohemagglutinins) even in persons never previously exposed to human blood groups through transfusion or pregnancy.[9] The Bombay phenotype is a rare genetic trait whereby no H gene is inherited (L/L), leading to a total absence of the H gene-specific transferase and subsequent H chain formation. A and B gene-specific transferase add their sugars to this H chain, creating both A and B antigens. Thus the inability to synthesize this H chain will result in the inability to synthesize both A and B surface antigens.[10] A and B subgroups differ in the amount of antigen carried on the RBC membrane. The 2 principal subgroups of A are A_1 and A_2. Red cells, however, from both A_1 and A_2 individuals react strongly with reagent anti-A in the direct agglutination test. Approximately 80% of group A or AB individuals can be classified as A_1 and the remaining 20% as A_2. Anti-A_1 occurs as an alloantibody in 1–8% of A_2 individuals and in 22–35% of A_2B persons. However, anti-A_1 is clinically insignificant unless ABO discrepancies arise while cross-matching for incompatible blood.

Rhesus system

The Rh system is second only to the ABO blood group system in terms of clinical significance; its importance lies in the ease with which an Rh-negative person will form anti-Rh antibodies following transfusion with incompatible Rh-positive blood. Approximately 55% of incompatible blood transfusions which involve the D antigen result in the formation of anti-D, followed in frequency by Kell (approximately 20%) and A-antigen discrepancies. Whereas antibodies to ABO tend to be of the IgM class, anti-Rh antibodies are IgG. Such antibodies can cross the placenta and thus can cause significant morbidity and mortality, as in erythroblastosis fetalis (see below).

Unlike the ABO-H system, the Rh blood type system is restricted to the erythrocyte. The blood group is a complex system of multiple alleles at closely linked genetic loci, resulting in the expression of over 30 antigenic variants. Clinically, an Rh-positive individual is defined here as one whose RBCs possess an immunogenic Rh antigen (Rh[D]) and an Rh-negative person as one who lacks such an antigen (Rh[d]). Of all the Rh notation systems, the simplest denotes antigens generated by 3 closely linked

genetic loci, C, D and E, and their principal allelic counterparts c, d and e. Rh(D) and Rh(CE) are proteins comprised of 416 amino acids which traverse the RBC membrane creating short loops capable of extending to the exterior of the membrane. Structural differences between D an d are seen in the extension of the final loop of D into the membrane exterior, whereas the entire amino acid structure of d remains hidden within the membrane structure.[11] An Rh-negative individual must be d/d, although he is most likely to be not only d/d but also cde/cde; the ce component can be simply tested serologically while the d component cannot. Multiple allelic combinations are possible, accounting for the variability in gene patterns with regard to race and geography. The frequency of the d/d genotype ranges from a high of 40% in the Basque population to approximately 15% in caucasians, 5% in Afro-Americans and 1% in the Asian population.

Approximately 400 human blood groups are known; however, mechanisms to explain associations between major and minor blood group systems and disease are not completely understood (Table 10.1). Group A individuals are known to have a 20% greater chance of developing stomach cancer compared to those with group O blood type.[12] A strong correlation between the presence of the I adult phenotype and the development of early childhood cataracts has been noted in some Japanese families.[13,14] This phenomenon is best explained by the close linkage between the gene coding for I type and a gene associated with the early onset of cataracts. Ii is also the membrane antigen system implicated in most cold hemagglutinin diseases including infectious mononucleosis and chronic hemagglutinin disease.

Table 10.1 Association between implicated blood group and human disease.

Disease	Blood group system
Hemolytic disease of the fetus and newborn	ABO Rh Kell Duffy Kidd Lutheran
Malaria (*Plasmodium vivax*)	Duffy
Infectious mononucleosis Chronic cold hemagglutinin disease	Ii
Familial cataracts (in Japan)	I
Escherichia coli urinary tract infection	P Dr^a
Haemophilus influenza infection	AnWj
Chronic granulomatous disease	Kell (McLeod type)

IMMUNOGLOBULINS

Structural similarities among all antibodies explain certain common chemical and physical features, such as charge and solubility. All immunoglobulins have a common core structure consisting of 2 identical light chains (approximately 24 kDa) as well as 2 identical heavy chains (approximately 55 or 70 kDa). The sequence of amino acids in these immmunoglobulin polypeptide chains is regulated by the genes of the antibody-producing B cells. The antibody is constructed such that 1 light chain is attracted to each heavy chain and the 2 heavy chains are attached to each other. The heavy and light chains are comprised of a series of domains, each consisting of approximately 110 amino acids. Both types of light chain, κ and λ, consist of 2 domains. The immunoglobulin heavy chains are of serveral types and their designation denotes the class of antibody—IgA, IgD, IgE, IgG and IgM. IgA and IgG are further classified into subclasses IgA_1, IgA_2 and IgG_1, IgG_2, IgG_3 and IgG_4.

The ability of an immunoglobulin to combine with an antigen is dependent on only a few amino acid residues at the end of each heavy chain. This region of the immunoglobulin which retains the antigen-binding capability is termed the Fab piece or fragment. The remainder of the antibody structure is called the Fc region because it can be crystallized. The Fc piece is responsible for other functions such as complement fixation and placental transport.

The IgG molecule is made up of 1220–1500 amino acid residues with a molecular weight of approximately 160 kDa. There are 4 IgG subclasses numbered according to decreasing serum concentration: IgG_1 (9 mg/ml), IgG_2 (3 mg/ml), IgG_3 (1 mg/ml), IgG_4 (0.5 mg/ml). Each IgG molecule possesses 2 antigen-binding sites, usually binding to the protein structure of the RBC membrane in diseases such as AIHA and hemolytic disease of the newborn. The IgG molecule formed in AIHA reacts primarily at 37°C; however, it may also react at lower temperatures. Thus, IgG is termed warm reacting. The hallmark of IgG-mediated AIHA is the opsonization or clearance of autoantibodies via the macrophage Fc receptor located in the spleen.[15] IgG, on the other hand, fixes complement inefficiently; thus, intravascular hemolysis is unusual.

IgM has a pentameric structure with 10 antigen-binding sites and a molecular weight of approximately 900 kDa. IgM clearance is characterized by efficient C1 fixation, complement binding and sequestration by the liver. Intravascular hemolysis may occur along with agglutination of red cells secondary to the multiple binding sites on the IgM molecule. In AIHA, IgM molecules are usually temperature restricted with optimum activity in the range of 4–22°C. Thus, these molecules are termed cold reactive or cold agglutinins. Anti-red cell antibodies without activity at 37°C are not uncommon but are usually clinically insignificant.

For an anti-RBC antibody to agglutinate RBCs, they must either overcome the net repulsive force (zeta potential) or be structurally large enough to avoid this repellent force.

Table 10.2 Characteristics of IgG and IgM.

	IgG	IgM
Geometric configuration	Monomer	Pentamer
Heavy chain isotype	Gamma	Mu
Molecular weight (Da)	150 000	900 000
Antigen-binding sites	2	10
Serum concentration (mg/dl)	1000–1500	85–205
Subclasses	IgG_1, IgG_2, IgG_3, IgG_4	None
Present in secretions	No	Yes
Complement fixation	Occasionally	Yes
Fc-receptor binding	Yes	No
Agglutinates red blood cells	Rare	Yes
Crosses placenta	Yes	No

The zeta potential stipulates that RBCs will naturally remain 30 nm apart while free floating in circulation secondary to the cells net negative membrane charge. If, however, the density of antigenic sites on the red blood cell is high, this distance restriction may be overcome. For example, where IgG anti-Rh antibodies cannot agglutinate Rh-positive cells (a maximum of 30 000 D sites/RBC), IgG anti-A is effective at causing agglutinatin (up to 1 000 000 A sites/cell).

Although AHIA is mediated primarily by 2 distinct classes of anti-RBC antibodies, IgG and IgM, in approximately 1% of AIHA, the direct agglutination test will be positive with polyspecific antihuman globulin, while negative for both IgG and C3-specific globulin. This is due to the presence of IgA on the cell alone. IgA-mediated red cell destruction is very rare and can be treated like primary idiopathic warm AIHA (IgG mediated). Futher discussions pertain to IgG and IgM only and their characteristics are listed in Table 10.2.

In the early 1970s, Schreiber and Frank[16] developed an experimental mouse model of immune clearance in which they demonstrated the principal differences between IgG and IgM AIHA. They showed that 103 molecules of IgM were needed for 117 complement-fixing sites, suggesting that every IgM molecule was capable of fixing C1. An average of 2012 IgG antibody molecules on the other hand were required to form 1.4 IgG complement-fixing sites on the erythrocyte surface.

COMPLEMENT SYSTEM

The complement system is comprised of a series of plasma proteins which exist naturally in an inactive form. Upon stimulation by an antigen-antibody complex or a bacterial polysaccharide, for example, they become activated and cleaved, generating fragments capable of initiating and propagating immune effector functions. Two groups of proteins, the classical and alternate pathways, are can trigger this proteolytic cascade.

The *classical pathway* is initiated by fixation of C1 to an antibody (IgM and IgG) combined to a cell-surface antigen.

205

This reaction requires 2 Fc complement receptor sites on an antibody molecule to be 25–40 nm apart. Thus, the IgM molecule is efficient at C1-complement fixation when bound to the RBC membrane as compared to the smaller, monomeric IgG structure. The C1-Ag-Ab complex then effects the binding and activation of C4 and C2, respectively. The C142 complex has enzymatic activity which in turn cleaves C3, resulting in fragments of C3a and C3b. The *alternate pathway*, of less significance in AIHA, leads to the same activation and cleavage of C3 but without an Ag-Ab binding requirement. Once C3b is generated, it possesses proteolytic activity which promotes fixation of C5. A common final effector sequence utilizing C5 though C9 leads to the generation of the membrane attack complex (MAC). This attack complex (C5–9) mediates cell lysis by creating a lesion in the antibody-coated cell membrane, increasing ionic permeability and thus causing osmotic lysis of the cell. C3b can also act as an opsonin favoring phagocytosis by neutrophils and macrophages which bear cell-surface receptors for C3b. Other enzymatic byproducts such as C3a and C5a are anaphylotoxins which increase vasodilation by release of histamines from mast cells. C5 fixation is a relatively inefficient system in humans, which might explain why so many RBC immune reactions result in C3 binding and hemolysis by sequestration in the mononuclear-phagocytic system (MPS) rather than intravascularly.[17] This inefficiency is in part explained by the existence of mechanisms to inactivate C3b before it can trigger C5 fixation.

MONONUCLEAR PHAGOCYTIC SYSTEM

AIHA may also be further classified based on the actual location of RBC destruction. Processes such as an ABO-incompatible blood transfusion reaction is termed intravascular because the immune-mediated destruction occurs within the circulation. However, in the pediatric population, IHAs are mostly extravascular, primarily in the MPS. The erythrocytes are destroyed via direct contact with the monocytes and macrophages of the reticulo-endotheial organs through phagocytosis. Several important biologic functions of the MPS include:

- involvement in antigen presentation and the generation of immune responses;
- clearance of circulating cells sensitized to antibody, primarily IgG;
- removal of senescent RBCs;
- removal of structurally abnormal erythrocytes created secondary to disorders of erythropoiesis.

The monocyte/macrophage is responsible for these functions.

Serving dual roles as both an organ of clearance and an organ important in the generation of an immune response, the spleen is widely accepted as the major organ of the MPS; 50% of all T cells and 10% of all B cells are located within the spleen.[18] All circulating cells traverse the spleen with a disproprotionately large 6% of cardiac output pumped to this organ with a transit time in the circulation of 13 s. The spleen is important for generating primary IgM responses to antigen and this might help to explain why IgM levels fall after splenectomy.[19–21] Hemoconcentration of blood flow through the splenic cords allows for greater contact time between sensitized or abnormal RBCs and the reticulo-endothelial macrophages.[22] The unique physical property of the spleen thus enables a greater degree of efficiency in phagocytosis and clearance of defective erythrocytes.

Membrane Fc receptors on the spleen macrophage allow for IgG-mediated phagocytosis. This process involves the binding of the Fc receptor on the macrophage to the Fc portion of the IgG molecule. Most cells sensitized by (multiple molecules of) IgG can bind to the reticuloendothelial macrophage with subsequent phagocytosis and RBC clearance.[22] The filtering of abnormally-shaped RBCs or the removal of cellular elements such as inclusions or microorganisms is maximized by the immense vascular nature of the splenic red pulp.[24,25] A decrease in deformability is seen when a RBC loses a portion of its membrane, resulting in spherocyte formation. The affected cells are unable to pass through the interendothelial slits, become trapped and subsequently phagocytosed by the mononuclear phagocyte.

The second major organ of the reticuloendothelial system is the liver. Where the spleen is crucial in the clearance of injured cells sensitized to IgG, the liver is capable of rapid sequenstration and clearance of C3b-expressing cells sensitized by complement-binding IgM anti-RBC antibodies. Studies have shown that a greater number of IgG molecules/RBC are required for phagocytosis by the liver in a splenectomized animal.[16]

AUTOIMMUNE HEMOLYTIC ANEMIA

CLINICAL PATTERNS

AIHA has been estimated to have an annual incidence of approximately 1/100 000 persons in the general population.[26] It may be organized into clinical patterns based on the properties of the specific autoantibodies (Table 10.3): warm versus cold reactive. Warm-type antibodies precipitate a clinical syndrome characterized by pallor, jaundice, splenomegaly and severe anemia. In over two-thirds of the cases attributed to IgG warm type, the antibody is directed against an erythrocyte antigen of the Rh group based on lack of reactivity with Rh null cells.[27] Clearance of RBCs coated with IgG warm-reactive antibodies is primarily extravascular via interaction with splenic Fc receptors.

Unlike IgG autoantibodies, IgM cold-reactive antibodies do not react directly with the destructive reticuloendothelial cells of the immune system. The degree of clinically significant hemolysis is dependent on several factors including the cold agglutinin titer, the thermal amplitude of the antibody,

Table 10.3 Classification of autoimmune hemolytic anemia.

Warm-reactive autoantibodies
  Primary (idiopathic)
  Secondary
    Lymphoproliferative disorders
    Autoimmune disorders (SLE)
    Infectious mononucleosis
  Evans' syndrome
  HIV associated

Cold-reactive autoantibodies
  Idiopathic (cold agglutinin disease)
  Secondary
    Atypical or mycoplasma pneumonia
    Infectious mononucleosis
    Lymphoproliferative disorders

Paroxysmal cold hemoglobinuria (PCH)
  Tertiary syphilis
  Post-viral infection

Drug-induced hemolytic anemia
  Hapten mediated (PCN)
  Immune complex type (quinidine, quinine)
  True autoimmune anti-RBC type (methyldopa)
  Metabolite driven

the level of circulating complement in the vasculature, and exposure to external cold. Clinical symptoms associated with agglutination of red blood cells secondary to IgM cold antibodies include stasis, cyanosis and a Raynaud's-like phenomenon. IgM-mediated hemolytic syndromes occurring secondary to infectious agents are generally acute and self-limiting.

Few large series of pediatric AIHA have been described in the recent literature. Discordance regarding clinical syndromes and related morbidity and mortality is noted among earlier reports (Table 10.4).[28–33]

In a study of 80 pediatric patients <16 years of age, Habibi et al[28] identified 2 categories of pediatric AIHA. Forty-two percent of these children were characterized as younger (80% <4 years) with acute or hyperacute onset, rare association with an underlying chronic disease, efficient response to steroid therapy and rapid and complete resolution of clinical symptoms in <3 months. Prodromal infections were reported in 70% of this group and no significant mortality was noted. The remaining 58% included those patients with a chronic and more insidious onset and a greater degree of variability in age at onset. On average, these patients were older, rarely reported a prodromal infection, and often had associated, concomitant underlying chronic disorders such as systemic lupus erythematosus (SLE) or chronic lymphadenitis. A variable response to steroids was noted, often necessitating further treatment measures such as splenectomy or immunosuppressive therapy. The overall mortality for children in this series was 11%, restricted entirely to the more chronic AIHA pattern of disease. In this 'chronic' clinical pattern, serologic testing revealed an 87% IgG or mixed IgG/C3 positive Coombs'

test while 67.7% of the patients with an acute or transient clinical pattern were only C3 positive in the Coombs' test. Upper respiratory tract infections were the most frequent prodromal-associated illness but other syndromes, including influenza, measles, mumps, scarlet fever, varicella, pneumonia and otitis were also noted.

In contrast, Zupanska et al[30] reported that a majority of children (77%) had AIHA with an acute transient clinical course. This series classified patients according to specific immunologic mechanisms of cellular destruction, primarily the presence of either warm- or cold-reactive autoantibodies. Seventy percent of the patients were IgG warm reactive with the remaining 30% IgM cold reactive. Of the 31 warm-reactive individuals, 81% had an acute or subacute clinical presentation. In general, the warm-antibody patients were found to have a good prognosis despite a sudden onset of severe anemia associated with an infectious prodrome. The 30% of patients who were cold reactive were found more often to have a milder form of AIHA, rarely having severe anemia and often displaying full recovery within 1 month. Irrespective of serologic findings, patients with acute disease had an increased association with infections and those with a chronic clinical course had a stronger correlation with concurrent chronic disease.

Both Zupanska et al[30] and Zuelzer et al[29] reported an association between older children and the occurrence of a chronic disease pattern. Heisel and Ortega[33] not only noted an increased association of chronic AIHA with children >12 years of age, but also in children <2 years. A 16% overall association with an accompanying chronic disease was noted compared to an observed acute infectious process occurring within 2 weeks prior to the onset of AIHA symptoms in 50%.

Although death never resulted directly from severe anemia, Zupanska et al[30] reported a 10% mortality rate. Death was noted as secondary to treatment complications or uncontrollable bleeding secondary to thrombocytopenia (see below). The majority of all published series, including Habibi et al[28] and Buchanan et al[31], found a male predominance in the acute clinical pattern, whereas Heisel and Ortega[33] reported more females in the transient acute type. The smaller pediatric AIHA series reported by Buchanan et al[31] included 22 children of whom 77% had an acute self-limiting course unassociated with any recognizable underlying disease, although an association of AIHA with immune deficiency, SLE and malignant lymphomas was made. A mortality rate of 18% was noted, although again death was not directly caused by severe anemia but rather resulted from complications of the therapy employed in attempts to eradicate the hemolytic process. Mortality secondary to sepsis in the post-splenectomized young child, renal failure in the patient with SLE and uncontrollable bleeding secondary to associated immune thrombocytopenia were reported causes of death, the latter presumably connected with Evans' syndrome.

The large study population of Habibi et al[28] allowed

Table 10.4 Findings from studies of large series of AIHA.

	Habibi et al[28]	Zupanska et al[30]	Carapella de Luca[32]	Heisel and Ortega[33]	Buchanan et al[31]	Comments
Number	80	44	29	25	22	
Sex						
Male	53	25	18	14	12	Male predominance
Female	27	19	11	11	10	
Age (years)						
0–2	37	—	14	10		>50% <4 years at
2–12	32	—	15	12		presentation
>12	11	—	0	3		
		0–1 10			<1 2	
		1–5 11			1–3 8	
		6–10 15			3–6 3	
		11–14 8			6–10 4	
					>10 5	
Acute (Ac)	34	34	15	9	17	Ac:Ch
Chronic (Ch)	46	10	14	16	5	1.2:1.0
Blood count at diagnosis	RBC<2×10⁶/mm³ Ch 17/36	<6 g/dl 21/44 >6 g/dl 23/44	RBC<2×10⁶ mm³ Ac 10/15 Ch 8/14	Mean Hgb Ac 4.3 g/dl Ch 5.3 g/dl	Hct >20% 1/22 15–19% 8/22 10–14% 9/22 <10% 4/22	No consensus between studies
Reticulocyte count	Ch 4/46 <50 000/mm³; 18/46 100 000–200 000/mm³ Ac range up to 700 000/mm³		<5% Ch 3/14 Ac 4/15	(mean) Ch 34.6% Ac 9.4%	<5% 11/22	
Hepatomegaly						Hepato-
Ac	8/34			5/9	Common	splenomegaly
Ch	16/46			11/16		present in >50% Chronic AIHA; less frequent in acute cases
Splenomegaly						
Ac	10/34		6/15	4/9	Common	
Ch	34/46		9/14	14/16		
Viral prodrome						
Ac	70%	39%	53%	78		Association with
Ch	4%	77%	57%	62		both acute and chronic
Associated diseases						3/5 chronic series
Ac	5.8%	13%	27%	11%	Overall 18%	with >50%
Ch	58%	23%	50%	50%		association
Serology DAT						
IgG						
Ac	7/34			13/25	2/17	
Ch	13/46				0/5	
C3						
Ac	18/34			15/25	6/17	
Ch	4/46				1/5	
Mixed						
Ac	4/34				4/17	
Ch	26/46				3/5	
Cold agglutination						
Ac	1/34				5/17	
Ch	3/46				1/5	
Warm Ab	72/80	31/44	26/29	17/25		>2/3 warm Ab in
Cold Ab	8/80	13/44	3/29	6/25		each study
Treatment prednisone						
Ac	31/34		4/29	23/25	3/22	
Ch	46/46					
	1.5–3 mg/kg		2/5 mg/kg	2 mg/kg	1–2 mg/kg	
Transfusion						
Ac	23/34		1/29	21/25	3/22	
Ch	0/46					
Steroids + transfusion			15/29		16/22	
Splenectomy						
Ac	0/34		2/29	5/25	4/22	
Ch	16/46					
Immunosupressives						
Ac	0/34			7/25	2/22	
Ch	13/46			7/16		
Miscellaneous*			7/29			
Mortality	11%	9%	28%	16%	23	

*Various combinations of steroids, transfusion, immunosuppressive agents and radiation.
Ac = acute, Ch = chronic.

striking differences to be observed between AIHA in the adult and pediatric populations. Of the total 767 patients, 42.5% of the children and only 4.5% of the adults had a transient acute clinical pattern of disease. Adult AIHA does not have the strong association with an infectious prodromal state, but does have a greater correlation with a concurrent chronic illness. The adult mortality rate was also signficantly higher at 28.7% compared to the corresponding pediatric rate of 11%.

Overall AIHA is associated with greater morbidity on average than idiopathic thrombocytopenic purpura in childhood. The spontaneous remission rate is lower, it takes longer to increase the hemoglobin with acute therapy, more adolescents are affected, and a higher percentage of patients have other disease including Evans' syndrome.

CLINICAL AND LABORATORY EVALUATION

The patient with AIHA frequently seeks medical attention because of generalized symptoms such as fatigue, weakness, malaise and fever. Jaundice and change in color of the urine may also be noted. The clinical picture may be more complicated and characterized by not only hyperbilirubinemia, but also abdominal pain and signs of impending cardiorespiratory collapse. Splenomegaly and hepatomegaly are common. The child's presentation is dependent not only upon the severity of the anemia but also upon the rapidity of onset of the hemolytic process. Additional physical findings may be present in the patient whose hemolytic process is secondary to an underlying disorder such as lupus or chronic glomerulonephritis.

Peripheral blood smear

An evaluation of the peripheral blood smear may reveal generalized signs of hemolysis, such as spherocyte formation, polychromasia and poikilocytosis. Occasionally, the smear may be remarkably normal. Evidence of increased RBC production is usually noted with polychromatophilic macrocytes consistent with an elevated reticulocyte count and the presence of nucleated RBCs. At the time of diagnosis, all patients with either acute or chronic disease have the unifying characteristic of a decreased hemoglobin, on average ranging from 3.0 to 9.0 g/dl. There is considerable variation in the degree of reticulocytosis and the number of nucleated RBCs seen on the blood smear. Patients with acute AIHA have a mean reticulocyte count of 9.4% (range: 0.1–79.7%).[33] From the same study population, 66% of the children with acute AIHA compared to 20% of those with chronic disease were found to have reticulocyte counts <6% at the time of diagnosis. Reticulocytopenia may be common in the early phase of the disease, in part because of the physiologic time requirement before there can be an increase in new RBC production if the hemolysis is hyperacute. However, a small percentage of patients may continue such a trend for days or weeks, presumably because their anti-

RBC antibodies also recognize the identical antigen present on RBC precursors, resulting in intramedullary red cell destruction and 'ineffective erythropoiesis'.[34,35] Buchanan et al[31] found that most children with moderate-to-severe anemia had inappropriately low reticulocyte counts, with 50% of patients having values of 5% or less. Bone marrow aspirations usually reveal normoblastic erythroid hyperplasia even in those patients who are reticulocytopenic.[31] Nucleated red blood cells are more commonly seen in patients with chronic AIHA.

White blood cell counts may vary from normal to elevated with only very infrequent cases showing white cell precursors (metamyelocytes, myelocytes, promyelocytes) on peripheral smear. Platelet counts in patients with AIHA are highly variable. Normal or elevated levels are typically seen, the high counts being consistent with the homology between erythropoietin and thrombopoietin. Conversely, there are infrequent thrombocytopenic patients who may present with both immune thrombocyptopenia and immune-mediated RBC hemolysis, as in Evans' syndrome.

Coombs' test

The ability to detect autoantibodies and determine the quantity of antibody present and the characteristics of the autoantibody are crucial steps in the diagnosis and treatment of AIHA. In 1954 Coombs et al[36] described a method to detect free (unbound) antibodies in serum. This discovery later lead to the demonstration and detection in vivo of RBCs coated with antibody and/or components of complement. This test is termed the antiglobulin test (Coombs' test) and is used to generate visible agglutination of sensitized red cells. The Coombs' reagent for the antiglobulin test (DAT or direct Coombs') is produced by the injection of human globulin into a heterologous species, e.g. rabbit. Upon mixing the antiglobulin antibodies produced in the animal with the Fc portion of the antibody molecules on the human red cells, the 2 Fab sites of the antiglobulin molecule form a bridge between adjacent sensitized red cells and a lattice network of cells, thus leading to agglutination. The strength of the observed agglutination is dependent on the amount of bound globulin coating the cell. The direct Coombs' test is used to detect RBCs coated with globulins, primarily IgG or C3, and is useful in the diagnosis of disease processes such as AIHA, hemolytic disease of the newborn and alloimmune reactions secondary to incompatible red cell transfusions.

The indirect Coombs' or antiglobulin test is a two-step process which identifies unbound (free) antibodies in the serum. This test is useful, for example, in blood-group compatibility testing and for cross-matching for transfusion. Patient serum is incubated with normal red cells. These cells are then washed to remove unbound globulin. Antiglobulin antibody is then added to the washed red blood cells. Any agglutination that occurs indicates a reaction between an antibody in the patient's serum and an antigen present on the RBC.

The antiglobulin or Coombs' test may detect immunoglobulins both alone or in conjunction with complement, and also detects complement components in the absence of any immunoglobulin. The great advantage of this test is that it has been standardized and simplified such that it can be reliably performed by the great majority, if not virtually all, blood banks. Furthermore, a Coombs' test may be reliably performed 24 hours a day as an antiglobulin test is a manual technique capable of being performed without the need of specialized equipment; thus a diagnosis of AIHA can be readily made at essentially any time of day or night. Different patterns of AIHA may be seen. Immune complexes unrelated to RBC antigens may activate complement which may in turn adhere to RBCs in a non-specific manner. Such attachment irrespective of an antigen-antibody complex is referred to as 'innocent bystander' complement coating and is seen in some drug-induced hemolytic reactions. Sokol et al[37] reported a 10–20% incidence of patients with warm IgG AIHA, non-drug induced, whose RBCs were positive for C3 coating alone. In cold hemagglutinin disease, the cold-reactive autoantibodies can react with RBCs at temperatures below 37°C, for example, as the RBCs pass through vessels of the skin and extremities. These autoantibodies are highly capable of activating complement. If the cells escape intravascular hemolysis, upon returning to more central regions of the body where the temperature is 37°C the IgM autoantibodies will dissociate from the cell leaving a cell coated by complement only.

Other methods of detecting antigen-antibody reactions are the inhibition of agglutination test, radioimmunoassay, enzyme-linked immunosorbent assay (ELISA), and solid-phase red cell adherence test. These may convey greater sensitivity, i.e. for careful titration of the strength of antibody, in some clinical settings, but are not as useful for routine clinical screening.

Two special settings exist for consideration. The first is the so-called 'Coombs' negative' immune hemolytic anemia. It is hard to define these cases since the Coombs' test is negative by definition. One form of testing relies on overcoming the zeta potential to allow the Coombs' test to become positive; substances such as polybrene have been used. The problem is that the number of false positives increases as well. The second setting is commonest in either the post-therapy patient or when multiple serum antibodies are detected. In either of these situations, elution of antibody from the RBC by one or more techniques such as acid elution followed by testing of the specificity of the eluate will usually allow determination of the specificity of the antibody bound to the RBC.

In summary, the clinical picture of AIHA may be either mild with generalized symptoms attributable to a minor degree of anemia or more complicated and severe. RBCs may be coated with IgG in the presence or absence of complement or with complement alone (IgM-mediated hemolysis and cold hemagglutinin disease). At onset,

however, it is neither possible to predict the chronicity of the disease based on the serologic results nor to establish the exact immunologic basis mediating the destruction of the RBC based on the degree of severity noted at the onset of the disease. The Coombs' test (DAT) is useful and reliable in confirming the diagnosis of AIHA and can be performed routinely at any time.

TREATMENT

Many patients with AIHA, whether IgG or IgM mediated, require no therapeutic intervention because of the mild character of the disease process. Other patients may present as a medical emergency with severe hemolysis necessitating immediate medical management. In general, the goal of therapy is to return hematologic values to normal, reducing the hemolytic process to a clinically asymptomatic state with minimal medical side-effects. Close attention should always be paid to supportive care issues such as hydration status, urine output and cardiac status.

Steroids

The therapeutic approach in the pediatric population usually begins with the institution of glucocorticoid therapy. More than three-quarters of all children with IgG autoantibodies show an initial response to high-dose steroids (2–10 mg/kg/day of prednisone). Cases of cold hemagglutinin disease, primarily an IgM mediated process, as well as other IgM mediated AIHA, are relatively refractory to corticosteroid therapy. Explanation for this might lie in part with the large number of IgM and especially C3b molecules present on the RBC surface.[38–40] Glucocorticoids have 2 well established mechanisms of action in the treatment of immune hemolysis. A rapid clinical response is attributed to the suppression of macrophage Fc and C3b receptors with a resultant decrease in the rate of phagocytosis of the RBC. A rise in the hemoglobin level may be noticed within 1–4 days. The RBC remains coated with IgG and C3b and thus will continue to give a positive direct antiglobulin test. The second mechanism involves the actual suppression of antibody production and a fall in the level of circulating autoantibody. This effect will produce a delayed increase in the hemoglobin level over a 4–5-week period. As hemolysis decreases (as monitored by both the hemoglobin and reticulocyte count), doses of steroids should be tapered. If a relapse occurs, escalation to the initial therapeutic dose may be required. Risks and benefits of long-term steroid use must be weighed against changing to an alternative treatment modality. Administered in high doses or for prolonged periods, steroids have a number of well described toxicities: electrolyte imbalance, exacerbation of diabetes, increased appetite and weight gain, increased risk of infection and adverse effects on growth. Patients who are steroid unresponsive or who require large daily or alternate-day dosing of maintenance therapy should be considered for alternative therapy.

Intravenous gammaglobulin

In children intravenous gammaglobulin (IVIG) may be helpful in conjunction with steroids. While rarely effective as sole therapy, IVIG seems to confer an adjunctive benefit and may help to support intravascular volume. Treatment in conjunction with steroids at doses of $\geqslant 2$ g/kg at onset is probably warranted when there is severe anemia.[40]

Transfusions

RBC transfusions should be avoided whenever possible. The benefits are very transient as a result of typically rapid destruction of the transfused cells by the autoantibodies and alloantibodies. Indications should be based more upon clinical condition, i.e. signs of heart failure and measurements of pulse and respiration, rather than on absolute hemoglobin level. It is generally considered, based on anecdotal clinical experience, especially in the setting of chronic anemia, that transfusion, if attempted, should be slow, i.e. 5 ml/kg over 3–4 hours. The blood bank can attempt to find the least incompatible unit but the value of this in most cases is uncertain as well.

Other therapies

Considerations for splenectomy include:

- safety (primarily age of patient, ideally >5 years);
- response to other therapy (usually persistent unremitting disease beyond 6–12 months from diagnosis);
- nature of the disease (warm-reactive antibody, Coombs' test not only complement positive);
- other considerations specific to the individual such as compliance, severity of disease and toxicity of other therapy.

Immunodeficiency, especially hypogammaglobulinemia, is also a reason to postpone splenectomy because of the greater risk of post-splenectomy sepsis. Concurrent disease (see below), including SLE, reduces the favorability of splenectomy because of apparently lower cure rates.

Other therapies run the gamut of those used in chronic refractory immune thrombocytopenic purpura (ITP): danazol, vinca alkaloids, azathioprine, cyclophosphamide and others. In view of the greater rarity of AIHA as compared to ITP, insufficient evidence exists to be conclusive about the use of any of these. It should be recognized that only vinca alkaloids, or perhaps IV cyclophosphamide, have the potential to demonstrate any effect within 1 week. Only danazol (in adult patients) has been reported to be effective in as many as 10 patients. If danazol or azathioprine were to be used, at least 4 months would need to elapse before it could be certain that they were *ineffective* in view of their long time to onset, presumably as a result of inhibiting and decreasing (auto)antibody production.

EVANS' SYNDROME

Evans' syndrome refers to a major disorder in immunoregulation characterized by AIHA accompanied by immune thrombocytopenia. Both cytopenias do not have to be present simultaneously and in fact more commonly occur at different times. This disorder results from the development of multiple autoantibodies targeting at least RBCs and platelets. In approximately 50% of cases, neutropenia is also transiently present.[41] Kakaiya et al[42] demonstrated that the antibodies targeting RBCs are different from those directed against platelets. IgG antiplatelet antibodies can be demonstrated on platelet membranes as can both IgG and C3d be found on the surface of RBCs in Evans' patients. These autoantibodies are directed against specific antigens on erythrocytes and platelets and appear not to cross-react.[43] Although a variety of defects in cellular immunity have also been proposed, including decreased serum immunoglobulins, decreased T-helper (CD4) function and increased T-suppressor (CD8) cell function, a distinct pattern of immunoregulatory disturbance has not yet been characterized. Evans' syndrome has been associated with many autoimmune and hemolytic conditions such as SLE, other collagen vascular diseases, malignancies and paroxysmal nocturnal hemoglobinuria (PNH). An association with pregnancy and hyperthyroidism has also been reported.[44,45]

Management

Treatment of Evans' syndrome is complicated by its poor prognosis. If a patient has ITP and a positive direct Coombs' test even in the absence of hemolysis, Evans' syndrome can be recognized at the time of identification of ITP. However, the converse is not possible. The current lack of a diagnostic platelet antibody test does not allow distinction of 'routine' AIHA from AIHA associated with Evans' syndrome if the platelet count is normal.

Once the diagnosis of Evans' syndrome is made, management remains highly debated because of the lack of a universally effective regimen. The pattern is either non-response or tachyphylaxis to the common therapies such as corticosteroids and IVIG. Splenectomy is unfortunately curative in only a minority of cases. The authors have proposed a multi-agent treatment protocol but its efficacy remains to be confirmed, especially with a view to retreatment in the future. Despite the tendency to relapse and the lower rate of response to splenectomy, initial management at least can be similar to that of uncomplicated AIHA of childhood.

HIV-ASSOCIATED AIHA

Peripheral blood and bone marrow abnormalities are common in patients with AIDS and HIV infection, especially in the setting of other complications of HIV. The etiology of such hematopoietic disturbances is, however, multifactorial, in part secondary to immune mechanisms, drug therapy, opportunistic infections and the HIV itself. In both HIV infected as well as uninfected individuals, the incidence of ITP appears to be more common than that of AIHA. Mild-to-profound anemia along with thrombocytopenia and granulocytopenia have been reported in many studies of AIDS patients.[46,47] Multiple centers have retrospectively looked at the transfusion records for incidence of positive direct antiglobulin tests and RBC antibodies in AIDS pateints prior to blood transfusions. McGinniss et al[48] evaluated blood samples from 28 hospitalized AIDS patients and found 18 (64%) positive for anti-I, 9 (32%) positive for autoanti-U and 12 (43%) with a positive direct antiglobulin test. Thirty patients with diseases other than AIDS and 60 healthy blood donors were also tested for the presence of RBC antibodies; none had autoanti-U antibodies or a positive DAT test.

In another study of adults, Toy et al[49] looked at both the prevalence and clinical significance of a positive direct antiglobulin test in 55 HIV patients. Ten patients (18%) had a positive DAT compared to 0.6% of the general hospital patient population. Four had mixed IgG and complement DAT patterns, 4 IgG alone and 2 complement only. None of the patients, however, had clinically detectable hemolysis or any association with an AIHA process. Therefore, the bottom line appears to be that despite these relatively frequent findings of positive DATs (which appear to be less common in children), clinically evident AIHA remains a rare entity in AIDS patients.[50] This may or may not be a result of the reported lower rates of Fc receptor-mediated clearance of sensitized RBCs.[51]

Management

The authors have managed 2 such patients and the precepts followed those of AIHA in the non-HIV-infected patient. The potential for important complications as a result of prolonged high-dose steroid use is high in the HIV-infected patient and therefore other modes of therapy would be desirable. However, unlike ITP in which AZT has been shown to increase the platelet count, antiviral medications have as yet shown no proven efficacy in increasing the hemoglobin. In one small report where antiviral therapy was administered to 5 patients, plus the addition of cyclosporin to 2 of these individuals, no consistent alteration in blood counts was noted. Fortunately, these cases have remained rare; however, such small series makes statistical analysis and interpretation of data difficult, resulting in a lack of more useful scientific information.

PAROXYSMAL NOCTURNAL HEMOGLOBINURIA (see also Chapter 2)

PNH is an acquired defect in myeloid, megakaryocytic and erythroid progenitor cells that produces granulocytes, erythrocytes and platelets with membrane defects rendering them highly susceptible to complement-mediated lysis. The defect has been found in the phosphatidyl inositol glucosamine linkage of a number of glycoproteins attached to the cell membrane. Although a variety of biochemical abnormalities (> 10 missing proteins have been identified) have been ascribed to PNH erythrocytes, the membrane glycoprotein decay accelerating factor (DAF), along with other complement regulatory proteins and the membrane inhibitor of reactive lysis (MIRL) have been identified as the most important surface molecules in the pathogenesis of PNH. These surface molecules can limit complement expression and activation and/or cell binding, and have been found to be either decreased or absent in patients with PNH.[52,53] DAF was first recognized in normal stromal cells by its ability to inhibit both classic and alternate pathways of complement through accelerating the intrinsic decay of C3 convertase.[54]

PNH erythrocytes have been classified into subpopulations according to their in vitro sensitivity to complement. Type I PNH-erythrocytes behave like normal erythrocytes and are thought to arise from normal progenitor cells. Type II PNH red cells are 3–5-fold and type III PNH-erythrocytes 15–25-fold more sensitive to complement-mediated lysis than normal red blood cells. This classification system inversely correlates with the presence or absence of DAF on the surface membrane of PNH-affected erythrocytes. PNH-erythrocytes also have an increased ratio of C3/C4b compared with normal erythrocytes.[55] This ratio correlates with a prolonged decay of the C4b2a convertase allowing augmented deposition of C3b on the cell surface. Enhanced membrane binding of C3b would serve to facilitate the conversion of C3 convertases to C5 convertase, facilitating the formation of the C5–C9 lytic complex (membrane attack complex—MAC).[54]

PNH is a stem cell disorder of clonal nature which affects not only erythrocytes but also platelets, monocytes, granulocytes and pluripotent hematopoietic stem cells.[56] PNH may evolve out of other bone marrow dyscrasias such as aplastic anemia and myelofibrosis or it may itself transform into such hematologic disorders. Although rarely, PNH has also been reported to evolve into acute leukemia.

Clinical presentation

Clinically, PNH is characterized by chronic intravascular hemolysis and a propensity toward venous thrombosis.[57] The disorder was first described more than 100 years ago, depicted as a paroxysmal hemolytic process which was often more frequent at night.[58] The classical picture of PNH is paroxysmal episodes of hemolysis, hemoglobinuria and abdominal and back pain. Patients may also present with generalized musculoskeletal discomfort or intermittent glove-stocking anesthesia. Pain may be attributed to the intravascular hemolytic process, hemoglobinuria or thrombus formation (? in small vessels), which is seen in PNH patients. Vessels such as the hepatic and portal veins as well as the cerebral and mesenteric veins may develop clinically overt thrombi and potentially contribute to the patient's demise. While early treatment with tissue plasminogen activator (tPA) or urokinase may be useful, patients will also require long-term anticoagulant therapy.[59–61] The exact etiology of the thrombus formation is unknown; platelet activation by complement fixation is well described although it may also be related in some part to the presence of pro-coagulant elements, i.e. ADP, released during hemolysis.[62]

Although rare in the pediatric population, PNH should be considered in any child who presents with an history of anemia and dark urine on early morning voiding. It should be considered in patients with complement-mediated hemolytic anemia, as well as cases of pancytopenia or aplastic anemia when no etiology or mechanism of cell destruction is obvious.[63] Also common to the picture of PNH is iron deficiency, which occurs secondary to iron losses in urine as hemoglobinuria.

Diagnosis

Diagnosis of PNH is made from both the clinical picture and by laboratory testing specifically designed to show increased sensitivity of RBCs to complement lysis. The acid hemolysis or Ham test takes normal serum of a compatible blood type and acidifies that medium to a pH of 6.4. This serum is then combined with PNH cells. The acidified medium will preferentially lyse the membrane-defective cells of a PNH patient. The sugar-water test lyses cells by lowering the ionic strength of the medium without changing the pH. Both these laboratory tests create an environment which promotes the activation of complement and selectively lyses PNH without disturbing healthy cells.

Treatment

Goals of therapy range from attempts to replace abnormal stem cells through bone marrow transplantation (BMT), to pharmacologic methods of limiting hemolysis, treating and preventing iron deficiency or overload, and the treatment and prevention of venous thrombosis. Considerable iron, as much as 22 g of hemoglobin and 20 mg of hemosiderin, may be lost in a single 24-h period.[60] Iron losses usually cannot be replenished simply from dietary sources and concern exists over both oral and parenteral iron therapy regarding the further potentiation of hemolysis and an exacerbation of existing hemoglobinuria. This concern is founded on the knowledge that iron supplementation in the iron-deficient patient results in a burst of erythropoiesis which in turn may increase the number of PNH cells in the circulation with the subsequent hemolysis of these newly formed cells.[64] Most clinicians, however, treat with iron therapy since it is essential and once iron has been repleted, no more hemolysis should occur.

Possibly by inhibiting the alternate pathway of complement, prednisone has been thought to be successful in treating adult patients. Doses of 15–40 mg of prednisone (as low as possible) on an alternate day schedule are recommended. Higher doses given daily were found to be beneficial in decreasing hemolysis; however, side-effects, especially the increased incidence of infection, were intolerable for patients requiring long-term therapy. Danazol has been used in anecdotal cases with some benefit. The ideal treatment for a disorder which originates at the stem cell level would be the replacement of such progenitor cells with donor unaffected stem cells. BMT remains controversial in the treatment of PNH, although it does appear to serve a role in the treatment of patients with markedly hypoplastic marrows.[65]

PAROXYSMAL COLD HEMOGLOBINURIA

Cold hemagglutinin diseases are generally characterized by high titers of cold-reactive antibodies, usually IgM-specific for I/i erythrocyte antigens, in association with hemolytic disease and intolerance to the cold.[66] Paroxysmal cold hemoglobinuria (PCH), the cold-reactive autoantibody, unlike other cold hemolytic syndromes, is a complement-fixing IgG with specificity for the P antigen on the RBC membrane. This biphasic antibody (Donath Landsteiner) fixes on the cell in the cold extremities and causes lysis when the cell is warmed later. PCH, a possible post viral sequelae or association with tertiary syphilis, is typically an acute, self-limiting disease characterized by leg and back pain, abdominal pain with cramps, nausea/vomiting/diarrhea and dark brown urine following exposure to the cold. Episodes of hemoglobinuria are usually preceded by fever and chills and may follow infectious disease such as upper respiratory infection, measles, mumps, chicken pox and influenza.[67–69] Episodes of PCH usually resolve over a few weeks and protection from the cold is usually the only prophylactic (treatment) measure needed.

DRUG-INDUCED AIHA

Although rare in the pediatric population, immune-mediated hemolysis may occur secondary to the administration of certain medications. Implicated drugs include: methyldopa, quinidine, quinine, sulfonamides, phenacetin, α-aminobenzoic acid and high-dose penicillin. Mechanisms of destruction may include antibody formation (both IgG and IgM) directed against the medication or one of its metabolites. Although IgM may be produced in large quantities, it rarely causes significant clinically apparent hemolysis. True drug-induced AIHA is most commonly associated with the use of methyldopa—10–20% of patients given methyldopa will develop a positive response to the direct agglutination test (DAT), although many of these patients will not hemolyze. Other drugs may induce antigen-antibody complexes which are adsorbed to the RBC membrane promoting complement fixation and hemolysis. The rare occurrence of drug-induced hemolysis may simply represent the minimal use of many of these medications within the pediatric population. However, close attention should be paid to any child receiving medications which may be implicated in the induction of an hemolytic state.

NEONATAL IMMUNE HEMOLYTIC ANEMIA

Anemia in the newborn infant develops secondary to a variety of both intra- and extra-uterine factors which may manifest at birth with pallor, congestive heart failure, hydrops fetalis or shock. At term gestation, fetal hemoglobin has risen to a cord blood value of 16.8 g/dl (14–20 g/dl) with an expected physiologic decrease in hemoglobin at 8–12 weeks of life of approximately 4–6 g/dl. A similar physiologic anemia is seen in the premature infant at roughly the sixth week of life. Anemia at birth may result from delivery trauma, with tearing or cutting of the cord, from placenta previa or abruption, or from organ-specific hemorrhage such as in the liver, spleen or cranium (see Chapter 9). However, a relatively common cause of anemia at birth and soon thereafter is immune hemolytic disease of the fetus and newborn. This condition arises when maternal IgG antibodies specific for fetal RBC antigens inherited solely from the father cross the placenta and enter the fetal circulation with subsequent destruction of fetal and neonatal red cells bearing these specific antigens.

One form of hemolysis is extravascular, mediated through the mononuclear phagocytic system via the spleen. Certainly in the past, the great majority of these cases of hemolytic disease of the newborn resulted secondary to the transplacental passage of anti-D (Rh$_0$) antibodies from an Rh-negative mother to her Rh-positive fetus. Clinical manifestations associated with hemolytic disease of the fetus and newborn may range from mild anemia requiring no treatment to the catastrophic *in utero* hydrops fetalis or the postnatal neurologic damage caused by hyperbilirubinemia (kernicterus). Rh disease used to affect as many as 1 in 100 live births until prophylaxis was instituted (see below). It is still the commonest cause in most series of significant fetal anemia.

Although ABO incompatiblity may be present in up to 20–25% of all pregnancies, actual hemolytic anemia is less common although not rare. Unlike Rh antigens which are specific to the RBC, A and B antigens are located on many cells in many organ systems throughout the body. A possible explanation for the low frequency of hemolytic disease may be due in part to the low antigenicity of the A and B antigens and the fact that these antigens are not fully developed (glycosylated) in the fetus and infant. With such a wide dispersal of antigens in a wide variety of tissues/organs, maternal antibodies reaching the fetus may be neutralized by large pools of non-erythroid antigens.[70] The majority of cases are mild, necessitating either no therapy or phototherapy alone. If the hemolytic process becomes severe enough,

the same indications for exchange transfusion apply here as in the case of Rh hemolytic disease.[70] ABO hemolysis is characterized by the peak bilirubin at 24–48 hours and the absence of a positive direct Coombs' test if performed after the first day and sometimes only on cord blood. While late anemia may occur, it is not usually severe enough to require transfusion.

Rarely, hemolytic disease may arise secondary to C and E antigens as well as other red cell antigens such as Kell, M, Kidd and Duffy. Many of these resulted from sensitization via a prior incompatible transfusion. Over the past 20–30 years, major advances have been made not only in the ante- and post-natal management of such infants, but also in the astoundingly successful use of Rh immune globulin to prevent maternal sensitization to fetal Rh antigens. Amniotic fluid analysis, fetal blood sampling with intrauterine transfusion as needed, and improved postnatal nursery management have all contributed to better outcome for these fetuses, but programs for maternal prevention have been the primary contributor to the sharp reduction in perinatal mortality from Rh fetal-maternal incompatibility.[71]

RHESUS HEMOLYTIC DISEASE OF THE NEWBORN

A mentioned above, Rh hemolytic disease of the newborn develops secondary to the transplacental passage of anti-D (Rh$_0$) antibodies from an Rh-negative mother to her Rh-positive fetus. The D antigen is the most immunogenic of the Rh antigens and, unlike the ABO-H group, the Rh blood type system is lineage restricted to the erythrocytes. The incidence of Rh disease is dependent on the prevalence of the Rh-negative genotype within the population.[72] With a 0% Rh-negative prevalence, Rh disease in Japan and China is very rare. Caucasians have a prevalence of approximately 15% and the Irish population, 20%.

Recent studies suggest an improved prognosis and survival in Rh disease. In one study of Rh-sensitized pregnancies, 51% required no therapy, 31% required treatment after full-term delivery and 10% required induced early delivery and exchange transfusion. Only 9% of the study patients required intrauterine transfusion and the overall mortality rate was 1.5%.[71]

Unlike ABO incompatiblity which is thought to occur because of naturally occurring isohemagglutinins, Rh-negative mothers do not have natural antibodies to Rh antigens. Immunization occurs almost exclusively during pregnancy as Rh-positive erythrocytes cross the placenta to enter the maternal circulation. Fetal erythrocytes can be found in the maternal circulation as early as 4–8 weeks' gestation.[73] Only a small volume, 0.5–1.0 ml, is needed to induce a primary immune response. Once maternal antibodies are formed, their transfer into the fetal circulation of an Rh-positive fetus is responsible for the basic pathogenic mechanism of Rh hemolytic disease. Radiolabeled studies of Rh-sensitized cells demonstrate an extravascular pattern of cellular destruction.

IgG-sensitized cells are preferentially sequestered and destroyed in the reticuloendothelial system, primarily in the spleen.[74] The rate of hemolysis is directly proportional to the number of anti-D molecules present on the RBC membrane.[75] The accumulation of hemosiderin in splenic macrophages seen in infants with Rh disease provides further evidence in support of this extravascular pattern of cell sequestration and death.[76]

Clinical manifestations

Clinical manifestations of Rh hemolytic disease represent a wide spectrum of maladies ranging from those infants born with only laboratory abnormalities and mild hemolysis (15%), to the fetus with severe anemia and subsequent hydrops. In the fetus, the pathogenesis of hydrops fetalis in Rh disease is founded on the principal of increased erythrocyte destruction which exceeds the compensatory capabilities of fetal erythropoiesis with resultant anemia. As the anemia progresses, cardiac failure ensues with circulatory collapse, shock, resultant tissue hypoxia, acidosis and often death.[77] The severity of the hydrops is aggravated by a concurrent reduction in oncotic pressure secondary to hepatic dysfunction which in turn results from conversion of the liver into a predominant organ of extramedullary hematopoiesis. Massive edema and generalized anasarca result from decreased serum albumin and further decrease in the intravascular volume of the already anemic fetus. As a consequence, severe respiratory distress develops with pulmonary edema and bilateral pleural effusions. Even following resuscitation, these infants remain in severe respiratory distress requiring mechanical ventilatory support.[78] In severe cases, petechia, purpura and thrombocytopenia may develop, either representing a decrease in platelet number or frank disseminated intravascular coagulation (DIC). Hypoglycemia has also been seen in severe cases of isoimmune hemolytic disease reflecting hyperinsulinism and hyperplasia of pancreatic islet cells as well as possible liver failure.

In the newborn, jaundice and hyperbilirubinemia can cause devastating sequelae of neonatal hemolytic disease. While *in utero*, the placenta clears the lipid-soluble unconjugated bilirubin. Thus, in severe hemolysis, both the amniotic fluid and cord may be stained with bilirubin pigments, while the fetus remains essentially unharmed. However, following delivery, jaundice may appear as early as day 1 and close monitoring of blood bilirubin levels is crucial in the prevention of possible morbidity secondary to a rapidly rising bilirubin with potential neurologic side-effects (kernicterus). As hemolysis continues, the unconjugated bilirubin accumulates due to the immature state of liver enzymes which are incapble of conjugating and excreting bilirubin load.

Diagnosis

The possibility of Rh hemolytic disease is of great concern for any Rh-negative woman, especially one with a history of a previous abortion or delivery. Maternal IgG anti-D titers should be determined at 12–16 weeks' gestation (first prenatal visit) and then at 28–32 weeks and 36 weeks in the completely asymptomatic case with no evident risk other than being Rh negative. Titer determination every 4 weeks is advisable in women who have received previous obstetric care without appropriate monitoring and prophylaxis. Prenatal counseling involves typing of both parents for the presence of ABO and Rh blood group incompatibilities; paternal zygosity determination requires DNA-based testing. Significant hemolytic disease may be indicated by the presence of measurable titers at the beginning of the pregnancy, a rapid rise in the titer, or a titer $\geq 1:64$. A history of a previously affected infant suggests a very high likelihood for similar or greater morbidity in association with subsequent Rh-positive pregnancies unless the fetus can be shown to be Rh negative.

Fetal assessment may be obtained through amniocentesis, ultrasound or percutaneous umbilical blood sampling (PUBS). Ultrasound may be used to detect the presence and severity of hemolysis from mild to hydropic. Evaluation of skin and scalp edema, cardiac and pleural effusions as well as hepatosplenomegaly, ascites and placental thickening may all be used to assess the severity of the immune destructive process. However, there is no reliable means to diagnose anemia prior to the development of hydrops so this is not an optimal method.

Amniocentesis provides a means of evaluating hemolysis though spectrophotometric analysis of bilirubin content in amniotic fluid ($\Delta OD450$). Indications for amniocentesis include a maternal IgG anti-D titer of $\geq 1:16$ or ultrasonographic evidence of hydrops. PUBS with transfusion should be instituted immediately. Amniocentesis may be performed as early as 14–16 weeks' gestation. If testing or history indicate a high likelihood of fetal anemia with risk of death, PUBS may be performed to determine the fetal hemoglobin level with potential subsequent intrauterine transfusion of packed red blood cells.

Immediately following delivery of all infants to an Rh-negative mother, blood should be evaluated for the presence of direct Coombs' and blood typing, including ABO and Rh antigen screens, as well as hemoglobin and hematocrit values with reticulocyte count should be performed. If the Coombs' test is positive, further evaluation is indicated to determine specific antibody identity and to prevent any delay in obtaining compatible blood should exchange or straight transfusion be necessary.

Prevention of Rh immunization in the mother

The major advance in management of Rh disease has been the prevention of immunization of Rh-negative women. This goal has been the subject of much work by many groups over the past several decades, all focusing on the administration of anti-D gammaglobulin. Anti-D gammaglobulin acts by two mechanisms to prevent maternal sensitization. First, the gammaglobulin serves to divert the erythrocyte from the antigen-reactive areas and secondly, directly interferes with the direct immunogenicity of the Rh antigen.[80] A number of guidelines exist from the American College of Obstetrics and Gynecology and through blood banks.

Treatment

Therapeutic goals for Rh hemolytic disease are directed not only at preventing intra- and extra-uterine death from severe anemia and tissue hypoxia but also avoiding the neurotoxic side-effects of hyperbilirubinemia. For the unborn fetus who has been diagnosed with severe hemolytic disease by ultrasound or amniocentesis, intrauterine transfusion is the treatment of choice until early delivery can be safely performed. Direct fetal intravenous transfusion of packed RBCs has replaced the original method of intraperitoneal infusion of RBCs. In cases of fetal anemia in an infant with pulmonary immaturity, a hemoglobin of <10 g/dl is a sufficient indication to proceed with transfusion. Cytomegalovirus (CMV)-negative, irradiated packed RBCs should be transfused, generally to attain a target post-transfusion hematocrit of 40–50%. Until lung maturity is attained, allowing safe induction of the fetus, transfusions may be performed ever 2 and then every 3–4 weeks depending upon the volume to be transfused.

Treatment of the live-born infant with Rh disease requires that at delivery, low titer, group O Rh-negative blood, crossmatched with the mother's serum should be available for emergent use if dictated by the infant's clincial status. Depending on the severity of the hemolytic process, the infant will require varying degrees of medical management and stabilization such as correction of acidosis, mechanical ventilation and circulatory support through fluids and pressors. Indications for exchange transfusion are not absolute and are dependent on the level of bilirubin in the blood as well as the degree of ongoing hemolysis dictating the rate of rise of the bilirubin content. According to reference charts, a cord hemoglobin of ≤10 g/dl and bilirubin of ≥5 mg/dl suggest the need for immediate transfusion. Other physicians consider past kernicterus, or severe erythroblastosis in a sibling, reticulocyte count >15%, and prematurity to be important factors in indicating exchange transfusions soon after birth. The decision to perform an exchange transfusion should be governed by the likelihood that the serum bilirubin will reach a level that has a substantial risk for inducing kernicterus. Whether transfusions are initiated immediately or whether the decision is made to wait, extremely close monitoring of bilirubin and hemoglobin is warranted. Symptoms suggestive of kernicterus are mandatory indicators for exchange transfusion. The majority of infants born with Rh disease will have mild-to-moderate hemolysis and hyperbilirubin states can be controlled by phototherapy alone. One study attempted to modify the course of Rh hemolytic disease by the administration of high-dose IVIG to the neonate;[81] results revealed a decrease in the need for exchange transfusion from 69% in those not receiving IVIG to only 12.5% in the group receiving IVIG. Postnatal IVIG therapy may be a valuable supplement to the standard treatment regimen of Rh hemolytic disease.

As suggested by Millard et al[82] and confirmed by Scaradovou et al,[83] intrauterine transfusion may cause postnatal suppression of erythropoiesis. This demonstrates the potential for severe postnatal anemia in the infant of 4–8 weeks of age. Therefore, selected neonates who have received intrauterine transfusions may benefit from postnatal erythropoietin in order to prevent late anemia and avoid the need for postnatal transfusions.

SUMMARY

AIHA is an uncommon clinical disease. None the less, because of the widespread availability and reproducibility of the Coombs' test, it is far better understood than other commoner entities. Treatment is not easy if there is no spontaneous remission and depends at least in part upon the type of antibody identified. Recognition of Evans' syndrome as a form of AIHA with a uniquely adverse prognosis is important for modifying treatment accordingly. PNH is a complex and fascinating, very rare form of AIHA in children.

Rh disease provides a model story for the study and understanding of a disease leading to its prevention. It is sufficiently infrequent currently that materno-fetal medicine specialists and neonatologists may never see a severely-affected case. ABO incompatibility is clinically distinct, presumably because of intravascular as compared to extravascular hemolysis in Rh disease.

REFERENCES

1. Kuby J. *Autoimmunity in Immunology*, 2nd edn. New York: WH Freeman and Company, 1991, p 446
2. Abbas AK. Diseases caused by humoral and cellular-mediated immune reactions. In: *Cellular and Molecular Immunology*. Philadelphia: WB Saunders, 1991, p 369
3. Marchesi VT. Recent membrane research and its implications for clinical medicine. *Ann Rev Med* 1978; **29**: 593
4. Marsh WL. Blood groups of human red cells. In: Petz LD, Swisher SN (ed) *Clinical Practice of Blood Transfusion*. New York: Churchill Livingstone, 1981, p 8
5. Economidou L, Hughes-Jones NC et al. Quantitative measurements concerning A and B antigen sites. *Vox Sang* 1967; **12**: 321
6. Hughes-Jones NC, Gardner B et al. Observations of the number of available C, D and E antigen sites on red cells. *Vox Sang* 1971; **21**: 210
7. Masouredis SP. Red cell membrane blood group antigens. In: *Membrane Structure and Function of Human Blood Cells*. San Francisco: American Association of Blood Banks Symposium, 1976, p 43
8. Westerveld A, Jongsma APM et al. Assignment of the Ak₁: Np:ABO linkage group to chromosome 9. *Proc Natl Acad Sci* USA 1976; **73**: 895
9. Springer GF. Blood group and Forssman antigenic determinants shared

between microbes and mammalian cells. In: Kallus P, Wakesman BH (Eds) *Progress in Allergy*, vol 15. Basel: Karger, 1971, pp 9–77

10. Watkins W. Relationship between structure, specificity and genes within the ABO and Lewis blood group systems. *Proceedings of the 10th Congress of the International Society Blood Transfusion*, Stockholm, 1964, p 443

11. Tippett P, Lomas-Francis C, Wallace M. The Rh antigen D; Partial D antigens and associated low incidence antigens. *Vox Sang* 1996; **70**: 123–131

12. Aird I, Bentall HH *et al.* A relationship between cancer of the stomach and the ABO blood groups. *Br Med J* 1953; **1**: 799

13. Yamaguchi H, Okubu Y *et al.* A note on the possible close linkage between the Ii blood group locus and a congenital cataract locus. *Proc Jpn Acad* 1972; **48**: 625

14. Ogata H, Okubu Y *et al.* Phenotype I associated with congenital cataracts in Japan. *Transfusion* 1979; **19**: 166

15. Engelfriet CP, Overbeeke MAM, Vondemborne AEGK. Autoimmune hemolytic anemia. *Semin Hematol* 1992; **29**: 3–12

16. Schreiber AD, Frank MM. Role of antibody and complement in the immune clearance and destruction of erythrocytes. II: Molecular nature of IgG and IgM complement fixing sites and effects of their interactions with serum. *J Clin Invest* 1972; **51**: 583

17. Muller-Eberhard HJ. Complement. *Ann Rev Biochem* 1975; **44**: 697

18. Christensen BE, Jonsson V *et al.* Traffic of T and B lymphocytes in the normal spleen. *Scand J Haematol* 1978; **20**: 246

19. Sullivan JL, Ochs HD *et al.* Immune responses after splenectomy. *Lancet* 1978; **i**: 178

20. Rowlay DA. The effect of splenectomy on the formation of circulating antibody in the adult male albino rat. *J Immunol* 1959; **64**: 189

21. Rowlay DA. The formation of circulating antibody in the splenecto-mized human being following the intravenous injection of heterologous erythrocytes. *J Immunol* 1950; **65**: 515

22. Lockwood CM. Immunologic functions of the spleen. *Clin Haematol* 1983; **12**: 449

24. Rifkind RA. Destruction of injured red cells *in vivo. Am J Med* 1966; **41**: 721

25. Weed RI, Weiss L. The relationship of red cell fragmentation occurring within the spleen to cell destruction. *Trans Assoc Am Physicians* 1966; **179**: 426

26. Flores G, Cunningham-Rundles C, Newland AC, Bussel JB. Efficacy of intravenous immunoglobulin in the treatment of autoimmune hemo-lytic anemia: results in 73 patients. *Am J Hematol* 1993; **44**: 237

27. Vos GH, Petz LH, Fudenberg HH. Specificity and immunoglobulin characteristics of autoantibodies in acquired hemolytic anemia. *J Immunol* 1971; **106**: 1172

28. Habibi B, Homberg JC, Schaison G, Salmon C. Autoimmune hemo-lytic anemia in children. A review of 80 cases. *Am J Med* 1974; **56**: 61

29. Zuelzer WW, Mastrangelo R, Stulberg CS, Poulik MD, Page RH, Thompson RI. Autoimmune hemolytic anemia. Natural history and viral-immunologic interactions in childhood. *Am J Med* 1970; **49**: 80

30. Zupanska B, Lawkowicz W, Gorska B *et al.* Autoimmune hemolytic anaemia in children. *Br J Haematol* 1976; **34**: 511

31. Buchanan GR, Boxer LA, Nathan DG. The acute and transient nature of idiopathic immune hemolytic anemia in childhood. *J Pediatr* 1976; **88**: 780

32. Carapella de Luca, Casadei AM, di Piero G, Midulla M, Bisdomini C, Purpura M. Auto-immune haemolytic anaemia in childhood: follow-up in 29 cases. *Vox Sang* 1979; **36**: 13–20

33. Heisel MA, Ortega JA. Factors influencing prognosis in childhood autoimmune hemolytic anemia. *Am J Pediatr Hematol Oncol* 1983; **52**: 147–152

34. Conley CL, Lipman SM *et al.* Autoimmune hemolytic anemia with reticulocytopenia and erythroid marrow. *N Engl J Med* 1982; **306**: 281

35. Greenberg J, Curtis-Cohen M *et al.* Prolonged reticulocytopenia in autoimmune hemolytic anemia in childhood. *J Pediatr* 1980; **97**: 784

36. Coombs RRA, Mourant AE, Race RR. A new test for the detection of weak and "incomplete" Rh agglutinins. *Br J Exp Pathol* 1945; **26**: 255–266

37. Sokol RJ, Hewitt S, Stamps BK. Autoimmune haemolysis: An 18-year study of 865 cases referred to a regional transfusion centre. *Br Med J* 1981; **282**: 2023–2027

38. Schreiber AD. Clinical immunology of corticosteroids. *Prog Clin Immunol* 1977; **3**: 103

39. Schreiber AD, Herskvitz B, Bolwein M. Low-titer cold hemagglutinin disease: mechanism of hemolysis and response to corticosteroids. *N Engl J Med* 1977; **296**: 1490

40. Meyetes D, Adler M *et al.* High-dose methylprednisolone in acute immune cold hemolysis. *N Engl J Med* 1985; **312**: 318c

41. Evans RS, Takahasi K *et al.* Primary thrombocytopenia purpura and acquired hemolytic anemia: evidence for a common etiology. *Arch Intern Med* 1951; **87**: 48

42. Kakaiya RM, Sherman LA, Miller WV *et al.* Nature of platelet antibody in Evans's syndrome: A case report. *Ann Clin Lab Sci* 1981; **11**: 511

43. Wang WC. Evans' syndrome in childhood: Pathophysiology, clinical course and treatment. *Am J Pediatr Hematol Oncol* 1988; **10**: 330

44. Silverstein MN, Aaro LA, Kempers RD. Evans' syndrome and pregnancy. *Am J Med Sci* 1966; **252**: 206–211

45. Lee F-Y, Ho C-H, Chong L-L. Hyperthyroidism and Evans' syndrome. A case report. *J Formosan Med Assoc* 1985; **84**: 256

46. Spivak JL, Bender BS, Quinn TC. Hematologic abnormalties in the acquired immune deficiency syndrome. *Am J Med* 1984; **77**: 224

47. Berner YN, Berrebi A, Green L, Handzel ZT, Bentwich Z. Erythro-blastopenia in acquired immunodeficiency syndrome. *Acta Haematol* 1983; **70**: 273

48. McGinniss MH, Macher AM, Rook AH, Alter HJ. Red cell auto-antibodies with acquired immune deficiency syndrome. *Transfusion* 1986; **26**: 405

49. Toy PTCY, Reid ME, Burns M. Positive antiglobulin test associated with hyperglobulinemia in acquired immunodeficiency syndrome (AIDS). *Am J Hematol* 1985; **19**: 145

50. Simpson MB, Delong N. Autoimmune hemolytic anemia in a patient with acquired immunodeficiency syndrome. *Blood* 1987; **705**: 127

51. Scadden DT, Zon LI, Groopman JE. Pathophysiology and manage-ment of HIV-associated hematologic disorders. *Blood* 1989; **74**: 1455

52. Nicholson-Weller A, Burge J, Fearon DT, Weller PF, Austin KF. Isolation of a human erythrocyte membrane glycoprotein with decay accelerating activity for C3 convertases of the complement system. *Immunology* 1982; **129**: 184

53. Fearon DT. Regulation of the amplification of C3m convertases of human complement by an inhibitory protein isolated from human erythrocyte membrane. *Proc Natl Acad Sci USA* 1979; **76**: 5867

54. Nicholson-Weller A. Affected erythrocytes of patients with paroxysmal nocturnal hemoglobinuria are deficient in the complement regulatory protein, decay accelerating factor. *Proc Natl Acad Sci USA* 1983; **80**: 5066

55. Rosse W, Logue GL, Adams J, Crookston JH. *Clin Invest* 1974; **53**: 31

56. Dessyis EN, Clark DA *et al.* Increased sensitivity to complement erythroid and myeloid progenitors in paroxysmal nocturnal hemoglo-binuria. *N Engl J Med* 1983; **309**: 690

57. Rosse WF. Paroxysmal nocturnal hemoglobinuria. The biochemical defects and the clinical syndrome. *Blood* 1989; **3**: 192

58. Crosby WH. *Blood* 1951; **6**: 270–284

59. Sholar PW, Bell WR. Thrombolytic therapy for inferior vena cava thrombosis in paroxysmal nocturnal hemoglobinuria. *Ann Intern Med* 1985; **103**: 539

60. Rosse WF. Treatment of paroxysmal nocturnal hemoglobinuria. *Blood* 1982; **60**: 20

61. Valla D, Dhumeaux D *et al.* Hepatic vein thrombosis in paroxysmal nocturnal hemoglobinuria. *Gastroenterology* 1987; **93**: 569

62. Dixon RH, Rosse WF. Mechanism of complement-mediated activation of human blood platelet *in vitro*: Comparison of paroxysmal nocturnal hemoglobinuric platelet. *J Clin Invest* 1977; **59**: 360

63. Conrad ME, Barton JC. The aplastic anemia–paroxysmal nocturnal hemoglobinuria syndrome. *Am J Hematol* 1979; **7**: 61

64. Rosse WF, Gutterman LA. The effect of iron therapy in paroxysmal nocturnal hemoglobinuria. *Blood* 1970; **36**: 559

65. Storb R, Thomas ED, Weiden PL *et al.* Aplastic anemia treated by allogeneic bone marrow transplantation: A report of 49 new cases from Seattle. *Blood* 1976; **49**: 817

66. Silberstein LE, Berkman EM, Schreiber AD. Cold hemagglutinin disease associated with IgG cold-reactive antibody. *Ann Intern Med* 1987; **106**: 238

67. Colley EW. Paroxysmal cold haemoglobinuria after mumps. *Br Med J* 1964; **1**: 1552

68. Nordhagen R *et al.* Paroxysmal haemoglobinuria: the most frequent autoimmune haemolytic anemia in children. *Acta Paediatr Scand* 1984; **73**: 258

69. O'Neill J, Marshall WC. Paroxysmal cold haemoglobinuria and measles. *Arch Dis Child* 1967; **42**: 183

70. Rifkind RA. Hemolytic anemias: injury at the red cell membrane. *Fundamentals of Hematology*. Chicago: Year Book Medical Publishers, 1986, p 55

71. Bowman JM, Pollock J. Rh immunization in Manitoba: Progress in prevention and management. *Can Med Assoc* 1983; **129**: 343–345

72. Prokop O, Uhlenbruck G. *Human Blood and Serum Groups*. New York: Wiley Interscience, 1969

73. Zipursky A, Pollack J *et al.* The transplacental passage of foetal red blood cells and the pathogenesis of Rh immunization during pregnancy. *Lancet* 1963; **ii**: 489

74. Jandl JH, Jones AR *et al.* The destruction of red cells by antibodies in man. I. Observations on the sequestration and lysis of red cells altered by immune mechanisms. *Clin Invest* 1957; **36**: 1428

75. Mollison PL, Crome P *et al.* Rate of removal from the circulation of red cells sensitized with different amounts of antibody. *Br J Haematol* 1965; **11**: 461

76. Linsay S. Hemolytic disease of the newborn infant (erythroblastosis fetalis). *J Pediatr* 1950; **37**: 582

77. Phibbs RH, Johnson P *et al.* Circulatory changes in newborns with erythroblastosis fetalis. *Pediatr Res* 1967; **1**: 321

78. Baum JD, Harris D. Circulatory pressure in erythroblastic fetalis. *Br Med J* 1972; **1**: 601

79. Parer JT. Severe Rh isoimmunization—current methods of *in utero* diagnosis and treatment. *Am J Obstet Gynecol* 1988; **158**: 1323

80. Zipursky A. Rh hemolytic disease of the newborn—the disease eradicated by immunology. *Clin Obstet Gynecol* 1977; **20**: 759

81. Wahn V *et al.* High-dose intravenous immune globulin therapy for hyperbilirubinemia caused by Rh hemolytic disease. *J Pediatr* 1992; **121**: 93

82. Ney JA, Socol ML, Dooley SL, MacGregor SN, Silver RK, Millard DD. Perinatal outcome following intravascular transfusion in severely isoimmunized fetuses. *Int J Gynaecol Obstet* 1991; **35(1)**: 41–46

83. Scaravadon A, Inglis S, Peterson P, Dunne J, Chevenak F, Bussel J. Suppression of erythropoiesis by intrauterine transfusions in hemolytic disease of the newborn: use of erythropoietin to treat the late anemia. *J Pediatr* 1993; **123(2)**: 279–284

Sickle cell disease

GRAHAM R SERJEANT

The sickle cell (HbS) gene has arisen as a spontaneous mutation in the DNA nucleotide triplet coding for the sixth amino acid from the N-terminus of the β-globin chain. The insertion of valine in place of glutamic acid changes the charge (resulting in the electrophoretic difference used in the detection of sickle hemoglobin) and characteristics of the molecule; it tends to polymerize with adjacent molecules on deoxygenation, deforming the cell into the characteristic sickle cell shape. Inheritance of the HbS gene from 1 parent and a normal gene for adult hemoglobin (HbA) from the other results in the sickle cell trait. This condition is usually harmless because the amount of HbS (20–45%) is not enough to cause polymerization and its sequelae under normal conditions of oxygenation. However, the trait has an important survival advantage in areas of *Falciparum malaria*, where carriers are less likely to die from malaria than normal persons and the sickle cell trait has consequently achieved high frequencies.

GEOGRAPHIC DISTRIBUTION

The initial worldwide distribution of the HbS gene has been determined by 2 factors: the occurrence of the HbS mutation and its selection by *Falciparum malaria*.

The most malarious area of the world is equatorial Africa and studies in Africa of the DNA structure surrounding the β-globin locus have identified at least 3 patterns of DNA upon which the HbS mutation has been superimposed relatively recently. These DNA polymorphisms or haplotypes are named after the areas where they were first described—Senegal, Benin and Bantu (or Central African Republic [CAR]) haplotypes.[1] They are of interest not only as genetic markers but also as a research tool since differences in the clinical or hematologic picture between the haplotypes may identify areas of the DNA remote from the β-globin locus which influence its expression. Another DNA structure associated with the HbS gene occurs in the eastern Province

of Saudi Arabia and throughout central India[2] and this appears to represent a fourth independent occurrence of the HbS gene (Asian haplotype).

This primary distribution of the HbS gene has been modified by subsequent gene movement. From equatorial Africa, the gene was carried to North America, South America, the Caribbean and latterly Europe, so persons with the sickle cell genes in these areas are predominantly of West African origin. In North America, the Caribbean and the UK, the haplotype is predominantly Benin, with <10% having the Senegal or Bantu haplotypes. In Brazil, the Benin and Bantu haplotypes are equally frequent, reflecting the origin of the African population from areas currently known as Zaire and Angola. The Benin haplotype also accounts for the distribution of HbS gene in Sicily, northern Greece, southern Turkey, the Middle East and south-west Saudi Arabia. In the eastern Province of Saudi Arabia and throughout central India, especially the states of Orissa, Madhya Pradesh and Maharastra, the HbS gene is entirely of the Asian haplotype.

NOMENCLATURE

Sickle cell trait

The sickle cell trait is not a form of sickle cell disease, HbS levels being too low to cause problems under normal oxygen conditions, with the exception of the renal medulla. At this site, conditions of low oxygen tension, acidity and high tonicity are uniquely conducive to sickling, and vascular and functional changes may occur even in the trait, resulting in an inability to concentrate urine normally and an increased risk of hematuria. Hypoxia associated with conditions of low ambient oxygen levels at high altitude, cyanotic congenital heart disease and respiratory depression from anesthesia or drugs, may rarely precipitate problems in the trait. However, the great majority of subjects with the sickle cell trait living under normal conditions do not encounter such problems and the trait should be firmly excluded from the definition of sickle cell disease.

Sickle cell disease

Sickle cell disease is an 'umbrella' term useful if the genotype is unknown, but much more information is conveyed by the use of the exact genotype. This condition contains several genotypes, all manifesting higher levels of HbS than the sickle cell trait but displaying marked clinical variability between genotypes.

- Most common at birth and generally most severe is *homozygous sickle cell (SS) disease* where the sickle cell gene is inherited from both parents. In Jamaica, where 10% of the population have sickle cell trait, SS disease affects 1 in every 300 births, this frequency falling at older ages because of the greater mortality of this genotype.
- Inheritance of the sickle cell gene with that for HbC results in *sickle cell-hemoglobin C (SC) disease*. HbC trait (the second commonest abnormal hemoglobin among people of West African ancestry) occurs in 3.5% of Jamaicans and SC disease affects 1 in 500 births, this condition generally being mild and frequently undiagnosed.
- Two conditions result from the inheritance of the sickle cell gene with a gene for β-thalassemia. β^0-Thalassemia is a severe gene associated with total suppression of β-chain synthesis and *sickle cell–β^0 thalassemia*, which occurs in 1 in 7000 Jamaican births, is a generally severe condition similar to SS disease. The β^+-thalassemia gene, on the other hand, is associated with some normal β-chain synthesis and hence HbA (usually 20–30%), which inhibits sickling. *Sickle cell-β^+-thalassemia*, which occurs in 1 in 3000 Jamaican births, is therefore a mild condition similar to SC disease.

PATHOPHYSIOLOGY

HbS molecules polymerize on deoxygenation and therefore increase the internal viscosity of the red cell, causing secondary membrane changes and deforming the red cells into the sickled shape. Such cells have difficulty negotiating the capillary beds and are destroyed prematurely (hemolysis) and block flow in blood vessels (vaso-occlusion). Generally, the consequences of rapid hemolysis are well tolerated, but those of capillary or arteriolar occlusion cause more severe symptoms, the nature of which are determined by the site of vessel occlusion.

Rapid red cell destruction in SS disease (mean red cell survival of 10–15 days compared to 120 days in a normal individual) is associated with anemia (Hb 6–9 g/dl) and jaundice. Consequent clinical complications include pigment gallstone formation, markedly expanded bone marrow activity with increased demands for proteins, calories and specific vitamins such as folic acid, and the aplastic crisis (a sudden cessation of this increased activity).

The spleen is central to much of the early serious pathology of sickle cell disease. This organ acts as a filter in the blood stream removing intravascular bacteria and processing damaged red cells. The excess of damaged or deformed red cells in SS disease compromises this function of bacterial filtration leading to a susceptibility to encapsulated organisms, especially pneumococcus, and also causing acute enlargement (acute splenic sequestration), chronic enlargement (hypersplenism) and in most patients, a progressive splenic fibrosis. The active bone marrow is also susceptible to necrosis affecting the small bones of the hands and feet (dactylitis or hand–foot syndrome) in early childhood and the juxta-articular areas of the long bones, spine and pelvis (the painful crisis) and femoral head (femoral head necrosis) at later ages. Avascular necrotic bone is also susceptible to secondary infection, especially by Salmonella organisms causing osteomyelitis. Involvement of the pulmonary capillary bed in sickle cell disease by a spectrum of infection, infarction and pulmonary sequestration is common and is known as the acute chest syndrome. Vessel occlusion may also affect the skin, especially around the malleoli causing chronic leg ulcers in adolescents, the corpora cavernosa causing priapism, the retina causing proliferative retinopathy, and the brain causing strokes. Growth and development are usually retarded.

DIAGNOSIS

Diagnosis is based on the demonstration of HbS and hemoglobin electrophoresis to distinguish the sickle cell trait from the genotypes of sickle cell disease. In screening, HbS may be detected by the slide sickle test or solubility test. The former mixes a reducing agent such as 2% sodium metabisulfite with a drop of blood sealed between a microscope slide and a coverslip and sickling of the red cells occurs within 24 h. The solubility test is based on the precipitation of HbS in hypermolar phosphate buffer which causes a cloudy suspension within minutes. These tests confirm the presence of HbS but hemoglobin electrophoresis (under alkaline conditions on cellulose acetate or under acid conditions on agar gel) is necessary to distinguish the genotypes. The differential diagnosis of the genotypes of sickle cell disease is summarized in Table 11.1.

The many ways in which early morbidity and mortality may be ameliorated in SS disease (see below) imply that early diagnosis is essential in order to implement education and preventive programs. Diagnosis at birth is a simple cost-effective exercise and should be the objective in all communities. Only then can penicillin prophylaxis, parental education on acute splenic sequestration, complete immunization, better management of the aplastic crisis, and general

Table 11.1 Differential diagnosis of major genotypes of sickle cell disease.

Genotype	Sickle test	Electrophoresis		HbA$_2$ (%)	MCV (fl)	Family studies
		Alkali	Agar			
Homozygous sickle cell disease	+	FSA$_2$	SF	1.5–4.0	80–100	Both parents S gene
Sickle cell-hemoglobin C disease	+	SC	CS	*	70–90	One parent has HbC gene
Sickle cell-β^0-thalassemia	+	FSA$_2$	SF	>5.0	60–80	One parent has β^0-thalassemia gene
Sickle cell-β^+-thalassemia	+	AFSA$_2$	SAF	>4.0	70–82	One parent has β^+-thalassemia gene

*HbA$_2$ in SC disease is obscured by HbC which travels in the same position.
F, S, A$_2$ refer to hemoglobin bands visible on electrophoresis: F, HbF (fetal hemoglobin); A, HbA (normal adult hemoglobin; S, HbS (sickle hemoglobin); C, HbC; A$_2$, HbA$_2$ (normal minor hemoglobin component).
MCV = mean corpuscular volume.

education on disease management have their full potential impact in improving survival from the disease.

Counseling services should explain the basic genetics of the disease and the chances of further affected children. Prenatal diagnosis should be available for couples who wish to make informed decisions on whether to complete an affected pregnancy. Social and general support services can help patients and their families find solutions to social and other problems which so often manifest in symptoms of the disease.

The following description of hematologic and clinical features applies to all genotypes of sickle cell disease, although generally the features are more marked and frequent in SS disease and sickle cell-β^0-thalassemia than in SC disease and sickle cell-β^+-thalassemia.

Oxygen affinity

HbS, at the high intracellular concentrations occurring in SS disease, behaves as a low-affinity hemoglobin becoming nearly fully saturated in the lungs but releasing more oxygen in the periphery than HbA. Furthermore, the degree of shift in the oxygen dissociation curve varies inversely with the total hemoglobin level, implying that patients with low steady-state hemoglobin levels have near normal peripheral oxygen delivery. The bone marrow is capable of a greater response, but is switched off at sub-maximal levels because of a lack of erythropoietic drive. This implies that transfusing patients at their steady-state hemoglobin level, although increasing the hematocrit, will shift the oxygen dissociation curve back towards normal and the higher oxygen affinity of stored HbA blood may achieve little or nothing in terms of oxygen delivery.

HEMATOLOGY

The hematology is characteristic for the individual in the clinically well 'steady-state' but may vary markedly between individuals and between genotypes. Some hematologic indices in the major genotypes are summarized in Table 11.2.

CLINICAL FEATURES AND THEIR MANAGEMENT

ACUTE ANEMIA

A sudden lowering of hemoglobin to life-threatening levels may occur with acute splenic sequestration (ASS) and the aplastic crisis.

Table 11.2 Range of steady-state hematologic indices in major genotypes of sickle cell disease.[42]

Genotype	HbA$_2$ (%)	HbF (%)	Hb (g/dl)	MCV (fl)	Reticulocytes (%)	Red blood cell morphology
SS disease**	2.8 (1.5–4.0)	5.5 (0.1–25.0)	7.8 (6–9)	90 (80–100)	11 (5–15)	ISC + +, very variable morphology
SC disease	*	2.5 (0.1–6.0)	12.4 (9–15)	78 (70–85)	6 (3–10)	Target cells
Sβ^0-thalassemia	5.5 (5.0–7.0)	7.0 (0.1–25.0)	8.9 (7–10)	66 (60–75)	7 (5–15)	ISC +, microcytosis + +
Sβ^+-thalassemia	4.7 (4.0–6.0)	5.1 (0.1–15.0)	11.6 (9–15)	76 (70–82)	3 (3–8)	Target cells, microcytosis +

*HbA$_2$ in SC disease is obscured by HbC which travels to the same position.
**Interaction with α-thalassemia increases HbA$_2$ range to 4.8%, does not change HbF, increases hemoglobin to 9.5 g/dl, lowers mean corpuscular volume (MCV) to 65 fl, and lowers reticulocyte count to 5%.
ISC, irreversibly sickled cells.

Acute splenic sequestration

This condition is a common cause of death in SS children and occurs most frequently between 4 months and 5 years of age; it affected 30% of Jamaican Cohort Study children by 5 years.[3] Acute splenic enlargement of unknown etiology traps circulating red cells and the hemoglobin may fall by 2–6 g/dl within as little as 3 hours. There is usually a reticulocytosis, although some cases may be so acute that there is only an outpouring of nucleated red cells. Diagnosis is based on the low hemoglobin, high reticulocyte or nucleated red cell count, and splenic enlargement which is usually 3–6 cm below the costal margin. Blood transfusion may be life saving in the acute episode and the hemoglobin may rise higher than calculated because red cells may also be released from the spleen which shrinks. Teaching parents to palpate the spleen daily and to bring the affected child immediately to clinic if they suspect ASS has led to an apparent increase in incidence (implying that parents can detect this complication) and to a 90% reduction in mortality from this complication (since early detection of ASS allows urgent transfusion).[3] After 2 attacks, events tend to recur at shorter intervals and prophylactic splenectomy is usually recommended.

Aplastic crisis

In the aplastic crisis, bone marrow activity suddenly ceases, reticulocytes disappear from the peripheral blood and hemoglobin falls at the rate of red cell destruction (usually 1 g/dl/day). These events are commonest before the age of 15 years, occur in epidemics, and cluster in families, and this complication is now known to be due to human parvovirus infection.[4] Diagnosis is based on anemia, usually 3–4 g/dl by the time of presentation, and the absence of reticulocytes from the peripheral blood. Occasionally, reticulocytes may be present but, if so, they should show a daily dramatic increase consistent with the recovery phase of the aplastic crisis. Treatment is by transfusion and bone marrow activity is usually restored after 7–10 days of aplasia. The outcome is so predictable that in Jamaica transfusion is usually performed at a day-care center with outpatient monitoring to ensure that the reticulocytosis of bone marrow recovery occurs. Siblings with SS disease living in the same house as an affected patient should be closely monitored since there is a 50% chance of their being affected within 3 weeks of the initial aplastic crisis. After an aplastic crisis, immunity is lifelong and recurrent aplasias have never been described. A human parvovirus vaccine has been developed and is awaiting clinical trial.

CHRONIC ANEMIA

A more gradual lowering of hemoglobin level may occur in chronic hypersplenism, in megaloblastic change, in iron deficiency and in chronic renal failure in which low hemo-

globin levels may be tolerated with surprisingly mild symptoms.

Chronic hypersplenism

Sustained marked splenomegaly (usually 8–15 cm below the left costal margin) may be associated with sustained expansion of bone marrow activity and a new hematologic equilibrium with hemoglobin levels of 3–5 g/dl, reticulocytosis of 20–30% and a red cell survival of 2–3 days. Platelet counts are usually reduced ($<250 \times 10^9$/l). The metabolic demands of the grossly expanded bone marrow for proteins and calories compete with those for growth which may cease, and a growth spurt follows the greater availability of protein and calories after splenectomy. The cause of hypersplenism is not well understood but the risks of superimposed ASS or aplastic crisis, the dangers of thrombocytopenia, and the metabolic demands of the grossly expanded bone marrow cause morbidity and occasionally mortality. The condition may be treated by chronic transfusion or splenectomy, the latter being preferred in Jamaica if there is no evidence of spontaneous resolution after an observation period of 6 months.

Megaloblastic change

The greatly expanded bone marrow activity increases requirements for folic acid which, if deficient, may result in megaloblastic change, signaled by a gradual lowering of hemoglobin level to 2–3 g/dl, lower reticulocyte counts of 2–3%, macrocytosis (an increase in mean corpuscular volume [MCV] of approximately 20 fl and usually exceeding 100 fl) and occasionally megaloblasts in the peripheral blood. This complication is commonest in the first 3 years, especially in West Africa where dietary folate content appears to be low. In Jamaica, megaloblastic change is uncommon and a trial of folate supplementation showed no difference in hematology, clinical features or growth from children receiving a placebo control.[5] However, folic acid is cheap and harmless and has become routine in the management of sickle cell disease elsewhere, although care should be taken to avoid psychologic dependency. If supplementation is considered necessary, one tablet weekly or twice weekly is probably adequate.

Iron deficiency

Iron released by hemolysis is usually available for reutilization and iron deficiency has been considered unusual. However, low dietary iron intakes and losses from infestation may cause an iron-deficient erythropoiesis with lowered hemoglobin, low reticulocyte counts and microcytosis. Short-term iron supplementation may be beneficial in such cases. Occasionally, a combined deficiency of iron and folic acid may lead to diagnostic confusion and an hypoplastic picture with low hemoglobin and low reticulocytes occurring without change in MCV. Such cases may show biochemical evidence of both iron and folate deficiency and treatment with one agent reveals erythropoiesis limited by the other. Thus, treatment with folate reveals iron-limited erythropoiesis and the MCV falls, whereas treatment with iron unmasks folate-limited erythropoiesis and the MCV rises.

Renal failure

Although uncommon in childhood, chronic renal failure is common in older patients with SS disease and may occur as early as adolescence. Usually attributed to a progressive glomerular sclerosis from damage by sustained hyperfiltration, lower erythropoietin levels result in falling hemoglobin levels and a symptomatic anemia. Treatment requires maintenance of hemoglobin by chronic transfusion and renal replacement may be considered (see below).

GALLSTONES

A consequence of chronic hemolysis is the formation of pigment gallstones. These are usually small and multiple and reach an incidence of 40% in SS patients aged 20 years in the Jamaican Cohort Study, a group of 315 SS children followed from birth in whom annual gallbladder ultrasound examinations are performed. These gallstones may cause specific symptoms by obstructing the cystic duct or common bile duct, or by acute or chronic cholecystitis. Most stones remain asymptomatic, specific symptoms developing in only 5 of 81 patients known to have gallstones for 1–10 years in the Jamaican Cohort Study. Gallstones are associated with non-specific abdominal pain but further analysis suggests that both abdominal pain and gallstones are independent associates of severity and are not causally related.[6] Cholecystectomy is justified in patients with specific symptoms but does not appear to be justified for asymptomatic gallstones.

FEVER AND INFECTION

The loss of normal splenic function renders SS patients particularly prone to overwhelming blood-borne infections, especially pneumococcal, *Haemophilus influenzae* type b and salmonella septicemias.

Pneumococcal septicemia

The risk of pneumococcal septicemia is greatly increased and maximal during the first 3 years of life; age-specific incidence rates fall sharply after 5 years.[7] It presents with high fever in a seriously sick 'septic' child and, in the past, has had a mortality rate approaching 50%. Prevention is essential and this may be achieved by prophylactic penicillin,[8,9] which should be started at age 4 months and continued until at least 4 years. Effective prophylaxis prevents the development

of acquired immunity and penicillin should not be stopped without administering pneumococcal vaccine. Current vaccines do not work well at the age when they are most needed (first 2 years) and the Jamaican protocol uses monthly injections of depot penicillin from 4 months to 4 years with pneumococcal vaccine given with the last month of penicillin cover. Penicillin-sensitive children may be given oral prophylaxis with erythromycin. The emergence of penicillin-resistant pneumococci may compromise the effectiveness of penicillin prophylaxis and makes urgent the need for trials of the new conjugated pneumococcal vaccines.

Haemophilus influenzae type b septicemia

The risk of *Haemophilus influenzae* type b (Hib) septicemia is also increased and, although less frequent than pneumococcal disease prior to penicillin prophylaxis, it is now emerging more frequently.[10] Prophylaxis is recommended and based on conjugated Hib vaccines given with normal immunization schedules between 2 and 6 months.

Salmonella septicemia

The susceptibility of avascular bone marrow to secondary infection by salmonella species is well established but salmonella septicemia in the absence of localized bone lesions is less well recognized. In Jamaica, half the salmonella isolations over a 20-year period occurred in the absence of obvious bone involvement, in a seriously sick child presenting with high fever ($\geqslant 40°C$), and often jaundice. There was no mortality among the osteomyelitis group who were given specific antisalmonella treatment early but 22% of those with salmonella septicemia died.[11] A case can be made for salmonella prophylaxis in any febrile, septic child, pending the results of blood culture.

BONE AND ABDOMINAL PAINS

Dactylitis and the painful crisis result from avascular necrosis of bone marrow but the etiology of the abdominal painful crisis is still unclear.

Dactylitis (hand–foot syndrome)

Painful swelling of the small bones of the hands and feet is such a characteristic early manifestation of sickle cell disease that it should lead to the underlying diagnosis if this has not been made at birth. Episodes are frequently recurrent, commencing as early as 3–4 months of age and becoming rare after the age of 5 years when active bone marrow has usually disappeared from these small bones. In the Jamaican Cohort Study, dactylitis affected 45% of children by the age of 2 years. Clinical involvement may be limited to a single phalanx or metacarpal or may involve all small bones of all 4 extremities. Radiologic changes become apparent after a few days and include patchy areas of osteoporosis and sclerosis,

223

periosteal new bone formation, and occasionally apparent disappearance of a bone. Resolution is usually complete both clinically and radiologically although occasionally premature epiphyseal fusion occurs and causes permanently shortened, deformed small bones. This is believed to be the sequel of infection superimposed on the necrotic bone marrow and should be suspected if there is marked swelling over the affected bones, when surgical drainage may be necessary. Parents need reassurance that this manifestation is not serious and treatment of uncomplicated cases requires pain relief and hydration if necessary.

Painful crisis

The painful crisis is the later counterpart of dactylitis and represents avascular necrosis of the bone marrow in the juxta-articular areas of the long bones, sternum, spine and pelvis. In limb pains there is a high frequency of bilateral symmetrical involvement.[12] Pain is often interpreted as joint pain because it usually affects the juxta-articular bones of the knee, elbows, ankles, shoulders and wrists but palpation reveals maximal tenderness over the bones adjacent to the joints. Occasionally, 'sympathetic' effusions may occur but aspiration reveals a clear, straw-colored and sterile fluid. Involvement of the shaft of the long bones also occurs, especially of the humerus, radius, femur and tibia or fibula. There is often associated fever and the passage of dark or reddish-brown urine, possibly associated with increased urinary excretion of porphyrins.[13] Duration of symptoms also varies markedly between and within patients, some events being limited to mild transient bone pain and others experiencing severe debilitating pain for days or weeks. After a severe attack, there may be residual bone tenderness or ache persisting for weeks. Painful crises are commonly recurrent but their frequency and severity vary markedly between individual patients.

Precipitating factors for painful crises include skin cooling, infection, dehydration and emotional stress. In Jamaica, skin cooling is the commonest precipitating event and may result from seasonal change, getting caught in the rain, taking cold baths—especially at cold times of day, swimming in the river or sea, and even limited cold exposure such as washing cars or doing laundry. The mechanism leading to avascular necrosis of bone marrow is not completely understood but the common symmetrical and peripheral bone pain and the relationship with skin cooling has led to the hypothesis of a centrally-mediated reflex shunting of blood away from the bone marrow.[14] Recent physiologic studies of the blood-flow response to mild skin cooling has identified subgroups of patients responding differently and the signficant relationship between their vascular response and painful crisis experience is consistent with this hypothesis.[15]

Risk factors include high total hemoglobin level, low fetal hemoglobin (HbF) levels and pregnancy, especially the last trimester and early post-partum period.[16,17] There is a dramatic increase in painful crises in males between 15 and 25 years and evidence that this is attributable to the increasing hemoglobin level associated with puberty,[16] raises the interesting speculation that lowering the hemoglobin by venesection may be effective prophylaxis. A high HbF level appears to protect some patients from painful crises, although there is no simple relationship between pain frequency and HbF. In Jamaica, some patients with HbF levels >15% have frequent bone pains and others with HbF levels <1% never have pains. In the eastern Province of Saudi Arabia where adults have a mean HbF of 16%, painful crises continue to be a major manifestation of the disease. However, the extensive data from the Cooperative Study of Sickle Cell Disease in the US[17] and the reduction in painful crises in adults with hydroxyurea-induced elevation of HbF levels[18] are consistent with a protective effect of HbF levels in some patients.

Pain relief is a challenging clinical problem and the response to pain is markedly influenced by social and cultural factors. The patient's ability to cope may be greatly enhanced by a supportive environment and the reassurance that the pain is not life-threatening. Precipitating factors should be sought and, if identified, avoided. Simple measures such as avoiding cold exposure by bathing at warm times of the day or by heating water may avoid many painful crises. Patients should be taught to keep mild analgesics at home and early in episodes of bone pain, to rest, keep warm, drink plenty and take analgesia. A knowledgeable, confident family can do much to reassure patients and increase their ability to cope. Distracting activities such as watching television or playing video games may also reduce the awareness of pain. If simple measures are ineffective, patients should be encouraged to attend clinic early for assessment to exclude underlying infection and for treatment with stronger analgesia. The latter is usually achieved by oral codeine but occasionally parenteral Sosegon (pentazocine) or pethidine may be necessary. If vomiting, dehydrated or unable to co-operate with drinking plenty, intravenous fluid should be given. In Jamaica, most cases are monitored at a day-care center and the patient chooses to return to the supportive environment of home in the evening.

Avascular necrosis of the femoral head

Avascular necrosis of the bone marrow of the femoral head has particular implications because of its specialized function. Continued weight bearing on a softened femoral head may lead to fractures of the femoral articular surface and depression of the avascular area. The consequent irregularity of the joint surface leads to a painful limitation of movement of the hip and secondary osteoarthritic changes of the femoral and acetabular surfaces may increase the functional limitation. Clinically, the patient complains of persistent pain on walking, usually localized to one hip, and particularly marked on climbing steps, and there may be a limp. Examination shows painful limitation of passive movement of the affected hip, especially on internal or external rotation. This complication occurs most commonly in late adolescence and early adult life, although it may be seen as early as 8–10 years of age.

Early diagnosis is essential to avoid the destruction caused by continued weight-bearing, the most sensitive diagnostic procedure probably being magnetic resonance imaging (MRI) of the femoral head. Changes on conventional bone radiology are relatively late and are most apparent when articular surface disruption has already occurred. Treatment focuses on avoidance of weight-bearing which may be achieved by plaster casts maintaining flexion of either the hip or knee alternately every 6 weeks for 6 months with crutches. This approach has the advantage of allowing the child to remain at school and participate in many normal activities. Occasionally, traction in hospital may be necessary for a period. If weight-bearing and consequent damage to the joint surface can be avoided, the femoral head may heal without deformity. If permanent damage occurs, limited remodelling surgery may be necessary and persistent symptoms and functional limitation may require total hip replacement, but this is rarely indicated before young adult life.

Abdominal painful crisis

Episodes of abdominal pain are common, especially in children, and result from a variety of mechanisms. Pain may be referred from the spine or lower ribs when these are affected by avascular necrosis and the acute chest syndrome, especially when involving the lower lobes, may cause abdominal pain. Right upper quadrant or epigastric pain may be associated with symptomatic gallstones, although it should be recalled that non-specific central abdominal pain which is more common in children with gallstones, does not appear to be etiologically related. This implies that symptoms may persist and recur following cholecystectomy. Some cases of recurrent abdominal pain in children with sickle cell disease do not have a clear etiology and may reflect the well recognized concept of 'little belly-achers' among otherwise normal children.

A particularly characteristic form of the abdominal painful crisis is associated with pain, generalized abdominal distension and tenderness. There may be vomiting and diminished or absent bowel sounds, and ileus manifest on erect radiologic films of the abdomen by distended loops of bowel with fluid levels. These findings are consistent with an acute loss of function of a discrete loop of bowel with distension of loops proximal to the functional obstruction. The etiology of this syndrome is unclear but there are features consistent with a transient autonomic neuropathy. Clearly, this syndrome can mimic an acute surgical abdomen but laparotomy has usually revealed nothing except occasional 'mesenteric adenitis'. Unless there are compelling features suggestive of a ruptured appendix or other surgical condition, treatment should be conservative, and with parenteral fluids and nasoesophageal aspiration,

restoration of normal gut activity usually occurs after 2–3 days.

ACUTE CHEST SYNDROME

The acute chest syndrome (ACS) is a major cause of morbidity and mortality in SS disease at all ages and is the largest single contributor to death after the age of 2 years. This syndrome represents a spectrum of pulmonary pathology which includes elements of infection, infarction, embolism and pulmonary sequestration. Presenting clinically like pneumonia with fever, cough, dyspnea and pleuritic pain, these events may resolve promptly with antibiotic therapy but more commonly run complicated clinical courses. Some patients manifest a severe, rapidly progressive course with marked dyspnea and high mortality unless treated by emergency exchange transfusion.

The etiology of ACS is complex and probably multifactorial. The role of infection is controversial, bacterial agents rarely being isolated from adult cases but commoner in children,[19] although more recent studies yielded evidence of bacterial infection in only 4–14% of children.[20-22] It is usual to cover patients with broad-spectrum antibiotics since these may also serve the purpose of preventing secondary infection of infarcted areas.

Fat embolism secondary to bone marrow infarction has long been recognized as an occasional cause of a severe progressive course, the diagnosis usually being made at autopsy when fat globules, necrotic bone marrow and even spicules of bone have been observed in the pulmonary capillaries. The clinical course frequently commences with a typical bone pain crisis which deteriorates with severe back pain, chest tightness, dsypnea, falling arterial oxygen tension and signs of systemic embolism with respiratory, renal and cerebral involvement and occasionally skin petechiae. It is presumed that the emboli gain access to the arterial circulation by traversing intrapulmonary shunts. Fat embolism, diagnosed by fat-laden pulmonary macrophages from bronchoalveolar fluid, was seen in 12 of 27 patients with ACS investigated in the Cooperative Study of Sickle Cell Disease, and was significantly associated with preceding bone and chest pain and neurologic symptoms.[23] Diagnosis is suggested by the clinical course and there is often laboratory evidence of disseminated intravascular coagulation (DIC). Treatment involves exchange transfusion, antibiotics, oxygen and heparin.

Another pathologic process contributing to ACS is acute pulmonary sequestration, in which stasis in the pulmonary capillaries impairs gas exchange, promoting a vicious cycle of deoxygenation, sickling and further stasis. Patients deteriorate rapidly with extensive radiologic opacities ('whiteout') and progressive dyspnea. This is a life-threatening emergency which may respond to an emergency exchange transfusion repeated if necessary after 4–6 hours. In successful cases, dyspnea and radiologic pulmonary white-out may be reversed within 48 hours, indicating this to be an acutely reversible vascular pathology. Because of the rapid deterioration that may occur in some patients with ACS, it is good clinical practice to monitor all severe cases by pulse oximetry and to utilize emergency exchange transfusion early if such deterioration occurs.[22,24,25]

Avascular necrosis of the ribs or sternum may also cause a pleuritic type of pain because of their movement on respiration. Diagnosed initially by localized tenderness and sometimes swelling of the affected bones,[26] the lungs are clinically unaffected, although lung involvement may develop secondary to splinting and reduced movement of the affected ribs. A trial of incentive spirometry (deep breathing encouraged by an instrument that draws a ball into the air with sharp inspiration) in patients with rib necrosis significantly reduced the risk of secondary ACS.[27]

STROKE

Stroke affected 8% of the Jamaican Cohort Study group by 14 years and occurred at a median age of 8 years.[28] There is a high risk of recurrence, 50–70% of affected patients developing further episodes within 3 years of the first attack.[29] The clinical picture is usually that of an hemiplegia and the pathology is predominantly infarctive secondary to occlusion of major cerebral vessels. This is an unexplained and surprising finding in a condition characterized by small vessel vaso-occlusion. Involvement of the internal carotid, anterior or middle cerebral arteries occurred in 71% of one series.[30] Diagnosis is made on the clinical picture and the extent of damage assessed by MRI. Examination of the cerebral vasculature by angiography or magnetic resonance arteriography is of interest but of limited relevance to treatment. Cerebral hemorrhage becomes a more important pathology at later ages, although hemorrhage into infarcted areas or rupture of aneurysms and subarachnoid hemorrhage has been described as early as 4 years of age.

The risk factors for initial stroke are largely unknown so prevention is not possible and treatment is currently based on preventing recurrent events by chronic transfusion programs aimed at maintaining HbS levels below 30%. There are many problems with such programs including the development of alloimmunization, iron overload, maintaining venous access, transfusion-acquired infections, duration of the necessary transfusion and most appropriate methods of monitoring. Stroke has recurred with 'successful' programs maintaining HbS levels below 25%. Transfusion reactions continue to occur despite leukocyte- and platelet-depleted blood and some patients develop so many antibodies as to be untransfusable. Iron overload may be prevented by subcutaneous chelation with deferoxamine (desferrioxamine) (see Chapter 5) and the use of syringe-driving pumps for at least 5 nights each week; this treatment is expensive and commonly fails because of lack of compliance in adolescence. Many patients lose peripheral veins and require permanent ports such as Portacaths or Hickman lines, which are both subject to infection and thrombosis. Transfusion-acquired

infections have been reduced with screening of transfused blood but there remains a window when HIV may be undetectable. Cessation of transfusion programs after periods of up to 12 years was associated with stroke recurrence rates higher than if transfusion had never been commenced, resulting in a policy of transfusion for life.[31] The enormous cost and logistical difficulties with such treatment places it beyond the resources of most developing countries, although exchange transfusion may be offered at the acute event. A final disadvantage of current therapy is that it cannot be commenced until the child develops his initial stroke.

Understanding the risk factors for initial stroke is essential if this is to be prevented. This is currently being addressed by two initiatives. The first is a trial of transcranial Doppler (TCD) to detect cerebral vessel stenoses predictive of stroke. A controlled trial randomizing patients with TCD evidence of stenosis to prophylactic transfusion or conservative therapy was prematurely stopped because one stroke occurred in the treatment group compared with 11 among the controls.[32] The other initiative is to assess the predictive role of upper airway obstruction by overnight oximetry recordings to detect episodic hypoxemia. The coincidence of stroke with a history of snoring has been reported several times and this study plans to assess the relationships between tonsillar size, snoring history, episodic hypoxemia and subsequent stroke. If snoring can be identified as a risk factor for stroke, a more aggressive surgical approach may be recommended for even mild degrees of tonsillar enlargement. The high recurrence rate and predictability of further strokes provides a basis for discussing bone marrow transplantation (BMT) as a potential therapy.

EYES

Retinal vaso-occlusion, which affects predominantly the peripheral retina, may result in the development of fragile new vessel systems. These proliferative sickle retinopathy (PSR) lesions may bleed causing vitreous hemorrhage with transient blurring of vision and large lesions with associated fibrosis may cause retinal detachment and permanent visual loss. Symptoms are commonest in late adolescence and early adult life and are much commoner in the relatively benign syndromes of SC disease and sickle cell-β^+-thalassemia than in SS disease and sickle cell -β^0-thalassemia. In the Jamaican Cohort Study, annual ocular assessments have detected PSR as early as 8 years of age and the greatest incidence is in late adolescence.

Prevention of these symptoms has led to attempts to render PSR lesions avascular by coagulation of the feeding arterioles by xenon arc or argon laser and also ablation of the ischemic retina by argon laser. Three trials involving much effort, expense and potential complications confirmed a significant decrease in the risk of vitreous hemorrhage,[33,34] but it was clear that although PSR was common (70% of adult SC patients), visual loss was relatively rare.

Spontaneous non-perfusion (autoinfarction) of these lesions is now realized to be common and there is a moratorium on treatment in Jamaica until the risk factors for autoinfarction are better understood. It is then hoped to focus treatment on patients unlikely spontaneously to autoinfarct PSR lesions and in whom the risks of visual loss justify the potential complications of treatment.

GENITOURINARY PROBLEMS

Priapism

Involuntary painful erection of the penis affects approximately 30–40% of postpubertal Jamaican male patients with SS disease and may occur in early adolescence. In adults, it is under-reported because of embarrassment or lack of realization that it is related to sickle cell disease but occurrence in childhood is usually reported by a concerned mother. There are two clinical patterns:[35] stuttering priapism which is generally nocturnal, lasts 3–4 hours, is relieved by simple physical measures such as exercise, and is associated with normal intervening sexual function; and major attacks lasting >24 hours, with extreme pain, often penile edema, and usually followed by irreversible damage to the vascular erectile system and impotence.

Stuttering attacks are commonly a prodrome for a major attack, although some major attacks occur *de novo*. If stuttering attacks occur on >2 nights/week, they may be stopped by stilboestrol,[36] after which the dose is rapidly decreased to the minimal amount required to prevent stuttering priapism but allow normal erections and avoid gynecomastia. The usual regimen is 5 mg daily for 3 days to stop the attacks, then decreasing to 5 mg twice weekly for 2 weeks, 2.5 mg twice weekly for 2 weeks, 2.5 mg weekly for 2 weeks, 2.5 mg alternate weeks for 2 weeks, and then stopping stilboestrol to see if attacks return. Patients vary in the dosage required, some being controlled by almost homeopathic doses of 1 mg every 3 weeks but attacks recurring if this is stopped or replaced by a placebo. An alternative but more expensive approach is the injection of luteinizing hormone releasing hormone (LHRH) but this has not been tested in controlled trials.

Major attacks do not respond to stilboestrol but require surgical relief which should be minimal. Aspiration and irrigation of the corpora by wide-bore needles allow detumescence and a spongioso-cavernosal shunt is a simple procedure giving more permanent relief. In the past, surgical drainage was avoided in the belief that the procedure induced impotence but this is now recognized to result from permanent damage to the erectile vascular system. Vascular function may recover in patients sustaining major attacks before the age of 15 years and occasionally other patients recover some erectile function over 1–2 years following a major attack, but usually impotence results. Ejaculation is normal and the mechanical problems of impotence may be treated by penile prostheses. The dense fibrosis of the corpora render insertion of even simple rigid prostheses such as the Small–Carrion prosthesis difficult and there is no place for the more sophisticated pneumatic penile prostheses.

Enuresis

Nocturnal enuresis, defined as bed wetting on at least 2 nights/week, occurred in 52% of boys and 38% of girls by the age of 8 years in the Jamaican Cohort Study.[37] The mechanism may be related to high urinary volumes and lower functional bladder capacities. Treatment is unsatisfactory, relying on conservative measures such as limiting late fluid intake and waking the child to empty the bladder during the night. Enuresis always resolves spontaneously.

Renal disease

Renal tubular damage impairing the ability to concentrate urine is common in SS disease and demonstrable from early childhood. However, it is the glomerular disease that has more serious significance and may result in chronic renal failure. The glomerular filtration rate is supranormal in young children and this hyperfiltration is believed to lead to progressive glomerular damage and glomerulosclerosis with a falling glomerular filtration rare and elevation of serum creatinine. Reduced erythropoietin production by the kidney leads to an increased anemia which is initially well tolerated, although later may compromise cardiac function requiring simple top-up transfusion. The anemia of renal failure has been treated with recombinant human erythropoietin, but the most appropriate dose is not known and with this there is the potential disadvantage of increasing circulating HbS compared to the alternative treatment of transfusion. Where renal replacement therapy is an option, early referral to a renal physician is recommended. The severity of renal impairment in SS disease may be underestimated since patients generally run lower serum creatinine and levels exceeding 60 μmol/l probably reflect significant impairment. Impaired cardiac or respiratory function may necessitate early entry into a dialysis program. Renal transplantation has been successful in SS disease although sickle-induced damage may occur in the transplanted kidney.

LEG ULCERS

Chronic leg ulcers around the ankles affect 75% of Jamaican SS adults and develop most frequently between the ages of 15 and 20 years. Their cause is believed to be multifactorial but trauma is a common initiating factor and minor traumatic lesions around the ankles should be taken seriously and treated intensively. Ulcers develop at a critical time for education and there is a direct relationship between age at ulceration and educational attainment. In the absence of a reliable way to heal ulcers quickly, this secondary educational deprivation must be avoided by persuading teachers and parents to allow children to continue attending school

227

while dressing their ulcers at home at the beginning and end of the day.

Healing is generally slow and ulcers are prone spontaneously to relapse. Standard treatment includes regular dressing at home twice daily with mild antiseptic agents such as half-strength Eusol or 0.01% potassium permanganate. Debridement is achieved where necessary by crushed papaya which has a proteolytic enzyme. Oral zinc sulfate (200 mg 3 times daily) significantly improved healing in a controlled trial. Skin grafting (only pinch grafts and not split skin or full thickness) may be used in clean vascular ulcers but ambulation before complete healing commonly leads to failure of pinch grafts. Complete bed rest in hospital for periods of 2–4 months always improves ulcer healing and there is no evidence for a beneficial effect of transfusion or hyperbaric oxygen. The recurrence rate following complete healing is 80–90% within 2 years.

GROWTH

Physical development is generally delayed in SS disease, the mechanism possibly related to the increased metabolic rate and metabolic demands of the greatly expanded bone marrow. Weight is usually subnormal throughout life, this difference emerging in the first year, and being associated with lack of body fat and thinner skin folds.[38] Height also lags behind by the first year, the difference increasing with age, especially when normal children enter the puberty-associated growth spurt. Puberty is delayed but with onset of puberty, the height velocity increases, and final height is similar to or exceeds that in the normal population. It is important to explain these growth differences to parents, so that they are reassured and avoid spending resources on tonics to promote growth.

PREGNANCY AND CONTRACEPTION

Sexual development is retarded with a mean delay in menarche in girls of 2.5 years in the Jamaican Cohort Study. The interval between first unprotected sexual exposure and pregancy is similar in SS disease and normal controls,[39] contrary to the view of relative infertility.

There is an increased risk of painful crises and ACS during pregnancy, especially in the third trimester and immediate post-partum period. Fetal loss is increased at every stage of pregnancy and the baby is usually of low birth weight. Delivery should be by the vaginal route unless there are obstetric contraindications. All mothers should receive regular antenatal care with daily supplementation for iron and folic acid and be booked for delivery in hospital. There is no evidence that prophylactic transfusion improves fetal outcome and this is not performed in the Jamaican management of pregnancy. Many pregnant women with SS disease continue in good health throughout pregnancy and have normal deliveries but some are seriously ill and the maternal mortality in Jamaica is 1%.

Contraception

Patients requesting contraception should be given the best methods available. The frequent assumption of serious risks of contraception in SS disease is unjustified and the risks of pregnancy, although small, far outweigh the theoretical risk of contraception. The injectable contraceptive medroxyprogesterone (Depoprovera) is an effective contraceptive agent and it also increases red cell survival and decreases bone pain in SS disease, and is the method of choice. Many Jamaican patients prefer to have regular menstruation and choose the low estrogen pill. An intrauterine device is offered to patients requiring longer-lasting methods, or tubal ligation if a permanent method is requested.

Antenatal diagnosis

Analysis of DNA isolated from amniotic fluid or chorionic villus sampling can detect the presence of SS disease in a fetus at 12–14 weeks' gestation. Early diagnosis offers parents several options, one of which is to make an informed decision on completion of an affected pregnancy. The information requested by such patients is the likely clinical course that their children will follow but such prediction is impossible with current knowledge. Parents who are more likely to act on antenatal information are those who already have a child with sickle cell disease and therefore have enough information for self-counseling. The inability to predict the clinical course is a major limitation to the take-up of antenatal diagnosis and also to defining the role of BMT in the treatment of SS disease.

SURGERY AND ANESTHESIA

Surgery is performed as infrequently as possible, conservative management being preferred for asymptomatic gallstones and non-specific abdominal pain. Common reasons for surgery are splenectomy, orthopedic procedures, and operations unassociated with sickle cell disease such as tonsillectomy and adenoidectomy. Elective surgery should only be performed with the patient clinically well and at steady-state hemoglobin levels. Preoperative transfusion is not routine in Jamaica but blood is cross-matched to replace that lost at surgery. Most patients are pre-oxygenated before induction and close monitoring is essential in the immediate postoperative period when anesthesia-induced respiratory depression is common. Continued oxygenation and physiotherapy is important following upper abdominal surgery to prevent post-operative ACS. The randomized study of transfusion in the Cooperative Study in the US[40] found no benefit of aggressive transfusion programmes over more conservative transfusion but did not assess a group without transfusion. Jamaican experience of no transfusion has a similar morbidity to that observed in transfused groups elsewhere, casting doubt on the value of routine preoperative transfusion.

NEW APPROACHES TO TREATMENT

There have been many attempts to find effective antisickling agents on the assumption that inhibiting sickling may ameliorate manifestations of the disease. Higher levels of HbF have been induced by hydroxyurea with significant reductions in the prevalence of painful crises and transfusion requirements in a selected group of severely affected adults.[18] Chronic transfusion programs have been overutilized and, although giving some short-term benefits, have often induced serious iatrogenic pathology. In Jamaica, no patients receive regular transfusion with the exception of a small group with chronic renal failure and no patients are receiving hydroxyurea for prevention of painful crises. There seem to be other more appropriate ways of preventing and managing painful crises and since a high hemoglobin is a clearly documented risk factor, venesection is currently under controlled assessment. Currently, knowledge of the natural history of the disease is not sufficiently detailed to be able to predict the most appropriate forms of intervention. BMT may represent a treatment option in the prevention of stroke recurrence.[41] However, the cost, short-term mortality of 10%, limited availability of suitable compatible donors and long-term risks of sterility limit the application of this procedure.

OPTIMAL CARE

Care is best provided in specialized centers with extensive experience of the disease and familiar, competent staff in whom the patient has confidence. Patients should be regularly reviewed at 3–6-month intervals when clinically well and encouraged to attend at any time they feel unwell. Steady-state hematologic assessments are performed in Jamaica every 2 years or more frequently if clinically indicated and these allow earlier detection of problems such as chronic renal failure. Counseling and other support services should be available within the center. A day-care approach to pain management of the painful crisis may provide a more acceptable alternative to frequent emergency room attendances or hospital admissions. The average survival of patients with SS disease in developed countries is currently approximately 50 years and will continue to improve with better medical and social care.

REFERENCES

1. Chebloune Y, Pagnier J, Trabuchet G et al. Structural analysis of the 5'-flanking region of the β-globin gene in African sickle cell anemia patients: further evidence for three origins of the sickle cell mutation in Africa. Proc Natl Acad Sci USA 1988; 85: 4431–4435

2. Kulozik AE, Wainscoat JS, Serjeant GR et al. Geographical survey of β^s-globin gene haplotypes: Evidence for an independent Asian origin of the sickle-cell mutation. Am J Hum Genet 1986; 39: 239–244

3. Emond AM, Collis R, Darvill D, Higgs DR, Maude GH, Serjeant GR. Acute splenic sequestration in homozygous sickle cell disease: natural history and management. J Pediatr 1985; 107: 201–206

4. Serjeant GR, Topley JM, Mason K et al. Outbreak of aplastic crises in sickle cell anaemia associated with parvovirus-like agent. Lancet 1981; ii: 595–597

5. Rabb LM, Grandison Y, Mason K, Hayes RJ, Serjeant BE, Serjeant GR. A trial of folate supplementation in children with homozygous sickle cell disease. Br J Haematol 1983; 54: 589–594

6. Webb DKH, Darby JS, Dunn DT, Terry SI, Serjeant GR. Gallstones in Jamaican children with homozygous sickle cell disease. Arch Dis Child 1989; 64: 693–696

7. Zarkowsky HS, Gallagher D, Gill FM et al. Bacteremia in sickle hemoglobinopathies. J Pediatr 1986; 109: 579–585

8. John AB, Ramlal A, Jackson H, Maude GH, Waight-Sharma A, Serjeant GR. Prevention of pneumococcal infection in children with homozygous sickle cell disease. Br Med J 1984; 288: 1567–1570

9. Gaston MH, Verter JI, Woods G et al. Prophylaxis with oral penicillin in children with sickle cell anemia. N Engl J Med 1986; 314: 1593–1599

10. Lee A, Thomas P, Cupidore L, Serjeant B, Serjeant G. Improved survival in homozygous sickle cell disease: lessons from a cohort study. Br Med J 1995; 311: 160–162

11. Wright J, Thomas P, Serjeant GR. Septicemia caused by salmonella infection: an overlooked complication of sickle cell disease. J Pediatr 1997; 130: 394–399

12. Serjeant GR, De Ceulaer C, Lethbridge R, Morris JS, Singhal A, Thomas PW. The painful crisis of homozygous sickle cell disease—clinical features. Br J Haematol 1994; 87: 586–591

13. Naumann HN, Diggs LW, Schlenker FS, Barreras L. Increased urinary porphyrin excretion in sickle cell crisis. Proc Soc Exp Biol Med 1966; 123: 1–4

14. Serjeant GR, Chalmers RM. Is the painful crisis of sickle cell disease a "steal" syndrome? J Clin Pathol 1990; 43: 789–791

15. Mohan JS, Marshall JM, Reid HL, Thomas PW, Hambleton I, Serjeant GR. Peripheral vascular response to mild indirect cooling in patients with homozygous sickle cell (SS) disease and the frequency of painful crisis. Clin Sci 1998; 94: 111–120

16. Baum KF, Dunn DT, Maude GH, Serjeant GR. The painful crisis of homozygous sickle cell disease: a study of risk factors. Arch Int Med 1987; 147: 1231–1234

17. Platt OS, Thorington BD, Brambilla DJ et al. Pain in sickle cell disease. Rates and risk factors. N Engl J Med 1991; 325: 11–16

18. Charache S, Terrin ML, Moore RD et al. Effect of hydroxyurea on the frequency of painful crises in sickle cell anemia. N Engl J Med 1995; 332: 1317–1322

19. Barrett-Connor E. Acute pulmonary disease and sickle cell anemia. Am Rev Resp Dis Assoc 1971; 224: 997–1000

20. Poncz M, Kane E, Gill FM. Acute chest syndrome in sickle cell disease: etiology and clinical correlates. J Pediatr 1985; 107: 861–866

21. Sprinkle RH, Cole T, Smith S, Buchanan GR. Acute chest syndrome in children with sickle cell disease. A retrospective analysis of 100 hospitalized cases. Am J Pediatr Hematol Oncol 1986; 8: 105–110

22. Mallouh AA, Asha MI. Beneficial effect of blood transfusion in children with sickle cell chest syndrome. Am J Dis Child 1988; 142: 178–182

23. Vichinsky E, Williams R, Das M et al. Pulmonary fat embolism: a distinct cause of severe acute chest syndrome in sickle cell anemia. Blood 1994; 83: 3107–3112

24. Lanzkowsky P, Shende A, Karayalcin G, Kim YJ, Aballi AJ. Partial exchange transfusion in sickle cell anemia. Am J Dis Child 1978; 132: 1206–1208

25. Davies SC, Luce PJ, Win AA, Riordan JF, Brozovic M. Acute chest syndrome in sickle-cell disease. Lancet 1984; i: 36–38

26. Rucknagel DL, Kalinyak KA, Gelfand MJ. Rib infarcts and acute chest syndrome in sickle cell diseases. Lancet 1991; 337: 831–833

27. Bellet PS, Kalinyak KA, Shukla R, Gelfand MJ, Rucknagel DL.

229

Incentive spirometry to prevent acute pulmonary complications in sickle cell disease. *N Engl J Med* 1995; **333**: 699–703

28. Balkaran B, Char G, Morris JS, Serjeant BE, Serjeant GR. Stroke in a cohort study of patients with homozygous sickle cell disease. *J Pediatr* 1992; **120**: 360–366

29. Powars D, Wilson B, Imbus C, Pegelow C, Allen J. The natural history of stroke in sickle cell disease. *Am J Med* 1978; **65**: 461–471

30. Gerald B, Sebes JI, Langston JW. Cerebral infarction secondary to sickle cell disease: arteriographic findings. *AJR* 1980; **134**: 1209–1212

31. Wang WC, Kovnar EH, Tonkin IL *et al*. High risk of recurrent stroke after discontinuance of five to twelve years of transfusion therapy in patients with sickle cell disease. *J Pediatr* 1991; **118**: 377–382

32. Adams RJ, McKie VC, Hsu L *et al*. Prevention of a first stroke by transfusions in children with sickle cell anemia and abnormal results on transcranial Doppler ultrasonography. *N Engl J Med* 1998; **339**: 5–11

33. Jampol LM, Condon P, Farber M, Rabb M, Ford S, Serjeant GR. A randomised clinical trial of feeder vessel photocoagulation of proliferative sickle cell retinopathy. I. Preliminary results. *Ophthalmology* 1983; **90**: 540–545

34. Farber MD, Jampol LM, Fox PD *et al*. A randomized clinical trial of scatter photocoagulation of proliferative sickle cell retinopathy. *Arch Ophthalmol* 1991; **109**: 363–367

35. Emond A, Holman R, Hayes RJ, Serjeant GR. Priapism and impotence in homozygous sickle cell disease. *Arch Intern Med* 1980; **140**: 1434–1437

36. Serjeant GR, De Ceulaer K, Maude GH. Stilboestrol and stuttering priapism in homozygous sickle cell disease. *Lancet* 1985; **ii**: 1274–1276

37. Readett DRJ, Morris JS, Serjeant GR. Nocturnal enuresis in sickle haemoglobinopathies. *Arch Dis Child* 1990; **65**: 290–293

38. Stevens MCG, Maude GH, Cupidore L, Jackson H, Hayes RJ, Serjeant GR. Prepubertal growth and skeletal maturation in sickle cell disease. *Pediatrics* 1986; **78**: 124–132

39. Alleyne SI, D'Hereux Rauseo R, Serjeant GR. Sexual development and fertility of Jamaican female patients with homozygous sickle cell disease. *Arch Intern Med* 1981; **141**: 1295–1297

40. Vichinsky EP, Haberkern CM, Naumayr L *et al*. A comparison of conservative and aggressive transfusion regimens in the perioperative management of sickle cell disease. *N Engl J Med* 1995; **333**: 206–213

41. Walters MC, Patience M, Leisenring W *et al*. Bone marrow transplantation for sickle cell disease. *N Engl J Med* 1996; **335**: 369–376

42. Serjeant GR, Serjeant BE. Comparison of sickle cell-β^0 thalassemia and sickle cell-β^+ thalassemia in black populations. In *Birth Defects*; Original Article Series, vol 18, 1982, Alan R Liss Inc., New York, pp 223–229

Hemoglobin variants and the rarer hemoglobin disorders

ANDREAS E KULOZIK

Hemoglobin is a tetrameric protein complex consisting of 2 pairs of globin chains with a combined molecular weight of 64 400 Da. One type of globin chain is coded at the tip of the short arm of chromosome 16 where the α-globin gene cluster containing the embryonic ζ- and the adult $\alpha2$ and $\alpha1$ genes is located.[1] The other type is coded on the short arm of chromosome 11 (11p14) by the β-globin gene cluster with the embryonic ε-, fetal $^{G}\gamma$- and $^{A}\gamma$-, and adult δ- and β-genes.[1] Each of the 4 subunits is covalently bound to the ferroprotoporphyrin heme as a ligand. The structure and function of hemoglobin enable it to be soluble and stable in the erythrocyte, and to allow uptake, transport and release of large quantities of oxygen under physiologic conditions.

As of January 1996, 693 hemoglobin variants had been described, most of which are of no functional significance.[2] This chapter reviews aspects of normal hemoglobin structure and function and describes the less common pathologic hemoglobin anomalies.

HEMOGLOBIN STRUCTURE

PRIMARY STRUCTURE

The globin chains are coded in the α- and β-gene cluster (Fig. 12.1) and contain 141 and 146 amino acids, respectively.[3] The strong evolutionary and functional kinship of these proteins is reflected by the high degree of sequence homology. The α- and ζ-chains show identity at 84 of 141 residues (60%). The homology of the ε-, γ, δ-, and β genes is even more striking with an identity of 94 of 146 residues (64%). The heme is bound covalently between the iron and the proximal F8 His at position 87 in the α chain and at position 92 in the β chain. The functionally important residues such as those at the α–β interfaces or at the heme-binding sites are especially highly conserved.

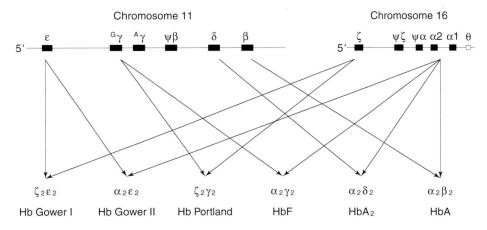

Fig. 12.1 The α- and β-globin gene clusters on chromosomes 11 and 16. The β-globin gene cluster contains the embryonic ε-, fetal γ- and adult δ- and β-globin genes. In addition, there is a non-expressed pseudogene ($\psi\beta$) with significant sequence homology to the β gene. The α-globin gene cluster contains the embryonic ζ- and adult α-globin genes. In addition, there are various pseudogenes ($\psi\zeta$, $\psi\alpha1$, θ). Different hemoglobins are produced in the course of ontogeny. All contain 2 α- or ζ-chains and 2 β- or β-like chains (Embryonic stage: Hb Gower I, Hb Gower II, Hb Portland; fetal stage: HbF; postnatal and adult stage: HbA$_2$, HbA).

SECONDARY STRUCTURE

The globin chains are wound up into segments of α helices which are interrupted by non-helical configurations where the polypeptide chains bend.[3] The helices with 3.6 amino acids per turn are stabilized by H-bonds between the carbonyl and amino groups of residues 4 positions apart. The β chain consists of 8 helical segments (designated A–H). The α chain is similar, although the D helix has been deleted in the course of evolution by a functionally neutral mutation.[4] The residues can be assigned to their position in the helices and the degree of homology between globin chains is particularly striking when the alignment is oriented at the secondary structure. For example, the heme-binding histidines at positions 87 in the α and 92 in the β chain are at position 8 in the F helix (F8) in both globin chains. Homologous positions in the globins are therefore best represented by the helical designation rather than by their numerical position in the primary structure.

TERTIARY AND QUATERNARY STRUCTURE

Much of the information available about the 3D structure and the function of hemoglobin has been obtained by X-ray crystallography.[5–10] Tertiary structure refers to the steric relationship of residues within the individual globin chain, whereas quaternary structure refers to subunit interactions. Both determine the functionally important 3D structure of the entire tetrameric protein–heme complex and are therefore dealt with together.

The helices of the individual globin chains form a compact spherical structure (Fig. 12.2). The residues facing outward are mainly polar, whereas those facing inwards are mainly non-polar. This distribution is responsible for both the excellent solubility of hemoglobin and its high degree of stability by blocking the influx of water into the central part of the complex.

Near to the surface, the heme molecule is suspended between the proximal and distal histidines at position F8 and E7. The 6 electrons in the outermost orbital of the ferrous iron (Fe^{2+}) co-ordinate with the 4 nitrogens of the pyrrole molecule, the imidazole nitrogen of His F8 and the oxygen. Additionally, there are multiple contacts to mainly non-polar residues of the heme pocket between the E and F helices, but also to residues of the C, G and H helices. The porphyrin ring is held in this pocket by 60 hydrophobic bonds conferring a high degree of stability. The functional importance of these contact points is highlighted by their strong evolutionary conservation and by the effect of amino-acid substitutions that result in unstable hemoglobin variants.

The 4 subunits are assembled to form an ellipsoid measuring $64 \times 55 \times 50\,\text{Å}$. In the center of the tetrameric complex runs a 2-fold, dyad axis of symmetry, which means that any

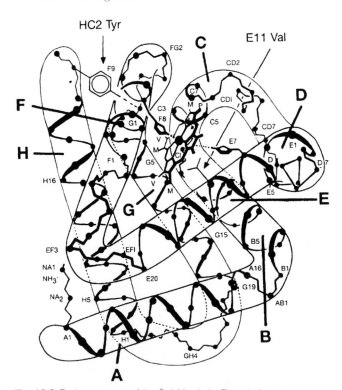

Fig. 12.2 Tertiary structure of the β-globin chain. The α-helices are designated A–F from the N- to the C-terminal. Modified with permission from Ref. 84.

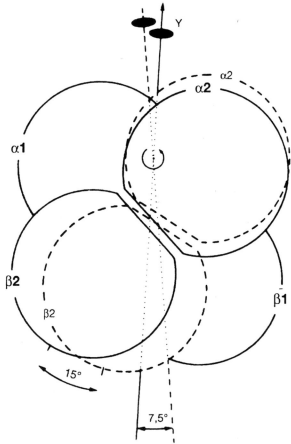

Fig. 12.3 Quaternary structure of hemoglobin in the T- (solid line) and R- (dotted line) quaternary conformations. The $\alpha_1\beta_1$ contact remains unchanged, whereas the $\alpha_1\beta_2$ contact rotates by about 15°, when the allosteric switch occurs. Modified with permission from Ref. 11.

Table 12.1 $\alpha_1\beta_1$ ($\alpha_2\beta_2$) Subunit contacts in deoxyhemoglobin.

α_1 residues	β_1 residues	Type of contact
31 B12 Arg	127 H5 Gln	Polar
31 B12 Arg	124 H2 Pro	Hydrophobic
31 B12 Arg	123 H1 Phe	Hydrophobic
31 B12 Arg	122 GH5 Phe	Hydrophobic
34 B15 Leu	128 H6 Ala	Hydrophobic
34 B15 Leu	125 H3 Pro	Hydrophobic
34 B15 Leu	124 H2 Pro	Hydrophobic
35 B16 Ser	131 H9 Gln	Hydrophobic
35 B16 Ser	128 H6 Ala	Hydrophobic
35 B16 Ser	127 H5 Gln	Hydrophobic
36 C1 Phe	131 H9 Gln	Hydrophobic
103 G10 His	131 H9 Gln	Polar
103 G10 His	108 G10 Asn	Hydrophobic
106 G13 Leu	35 C1 Tyr	Polar
107 G14 Val	127 H5 Gln	Hydrophobic
107 G14 Val	115 G17 Ala	Hydrophobic
107 G14 Val	112 G14 Cys	Hydrophobic
110 G17 Ala	116 G18 His	Hydrophobic
110 G17 Ala	115 G17 Ala	Hydrophobic
110 G17 Ala	112 G14 Cys	Polar
111 G18 Ala	119 GH2 Gly	Hydrophobic
111 G18 Ala	115 G17 Ala	Hydrophobic
114 GH2 Pro	116 G18 His	Polar
117 GH5 Phe	116 G18 His	Hydrophobic
117 GH5 Phe	30 B12 Arg	Polar
118 H1 Thr	30 B12 Arg	Hydrophobic
119 H2 Pro	55 D6 Met	Hydrophobic
119 H2 Pro	33 B15 Val	Hydrophobic
119 H2 Pro	30 B12 Arg	Hydrophobic
122 H5 His	112 G14 Cys	Hydrophobic
122 H5 His	35 C1 Tyr	Polar
122 H5 His	34 B16 Val	Hydrophobic
122 H5 His	30 B12 Arg	Polar
123 H6 Ala	34 B16 Val	Hydrophobic
126 H9 Asp	35 C1 Tyr	Polar
126 H9 Asp	34 B16 Val	Hydrophobic

Table 12.2 $\alpha_1\beta_2$ ($\alpha_2\beta_1$) Subunit contacts in deoxyhemoglobin.

α_1 residues	β_2 residues	Type of contact
37 C2 Pro	146 HC3 His	Hydrophobic
38 C3 Thr	99 G1 Asp	2 Polar, 1 hydrophobic
38 C3 Thr	100 G2 Pro	Hydrophobic
40 C5 Lys	146 HC3 His	Polar
41 C6 Thr	145 HC2 Tyr	Hydrophobic
41 C6 Thr	99 G1 Asp	1 Polar, 1 hydrophobic
41 C6 Thr	98 FG5 Val	Hydrophobic
41 C6 Thr	97 FG4 His	1 Polar, 1 hydrophobic
41 C6 Thr	41 C7 Phe	Hydrophobic
41 C6 Thr	40 C6 Arg	2 Polar
42 C7 Tyr	99 G1 Asp	Polar
42 C7 Tyr	98 FG5 Val	Hydrophobic
42 C7 Tyr	40 C6 Arg	1 Polar, 1 hydrophobic
44 CD2 Pro	97 FG4 His	Hydrophobic
88 F9 Ala	37 C3 Trp	Polar
88 F9 Ala	36 C2 Pro	Polar
91 FG3 Leu	40 C6 Arg	Polar
92 FG4 Arg	105 G7 Leu	Polar
92 FG4 Arg	43 CD2 Glu	Polar
92 FG4 Arg	40 C6 Arg	Hydrophobic
92 FG4 Arg	37 C3 Trp	Hydrophobic
94 G1 Asp	105 G7 Leu	Hydrophobic
94 G1 Asp	101 G3 Glu	Polar
94 G1 Asp	99 G1 Asp	Hydrophobic
94 G1 Asp	37 C3 Trp	Polar
95 G2 Pro	37 C3 Trp	Hydrophobic
96 G3 Val	101 G3 Glu	Hydrophobic
97 G4 Asn	99 G1 Asp	2 Polar
140 HC2 Tyr	37 C3 Trp	Hydrophobic
140 HC2 Tyr	36 C2 Pro	Hydrophobic
141 HC3 Arg	36 C2 Pro	Hydrophobic
141 HC3 Arg	35 C1 Tyr	Hydrophobic
141 HC3 Arg	34 B16 Val	Polar

part of the molecule will superimpose on an identical counterpart if rotated by 180° around this axis (Fig. 12.3).[11] The α and β chains have 2 interfaces between each other, 1 between the α_1 (α_2) and β_1 (β_2) and the other between the α_1 (α_2) and β_2 (β_1) chains. The $\alpha_1\beta_1$ ($\alpha_2\beta_2$) contact is established by about 40 van der Waals and H-bonds involving 16 α- and 17 β-chain residues (Table 12.1).[3] The characteristic of the $\alpha_1\beta_2$ contact is that there are 2 possible conformations that are assumed while oxygenated or deoxygenated. The deoxy-form is tight (T-form) with about 40 van der Waals and H-bonds (Table 12.2),[3] whereas the oxy-form is relaxed by about 7Å and established by only 22 van der Waals and H-bonds (R-form). Consequently, oxyhemoglobin is less stable than deoxyhemoglobin. This allosteric movement at the $\alpha_1\beta_2$ interface is also paramount to the co-operative effect of oxygen binding. Calculations of conformational energies and direct structural analyses suggest that oxygen binding to the T-form puts an increased strain on the $\alpha_1\beta_2$ ($\alpha_2\beta_1$) interface that can be relieved by the conformational change to the R-form which can then more readily accept more oxygen at the other hemes in the complex. Mechanistically, the transition from the T- to the R-form requires oxygen binding according to a 'symmetry rule', i.e. whenever oxygen binding creates a tetramer with at least 1 ligated subunit on each dimeric half-molecule ($\alpha_1\beta_1$ or $\alpha_2\beta_2$), quaternary switching occurs.[12]

The T-form is further stabilized by chloride and 2,3-diphosphoglycerate (2,3-DPG) which confer intra- and inter-subunit salt bonds. Cl^- establishes 2 bonds between the N-terminal Val of α_2 to α_2 131 Ser and α_1 141 Arg and also neutralizes repulsive forces of positively charged residues in the central cavity.[13] 2,3-DPG is a polyanion that associates with the positive charges of the N-terminal amino groups of lysine 82 and of the histidines 2 and 143 of the β chains. When 2,3-DPG is lost during oxygenation, Cl^- and H^+ ions are ejected from the central cavity.

HEMOGLOBIN FUNCTION

The chief function of hemoglobin is to take up oxygen in the lungs and transport it to the peripheral tissues, where it is unloaded in exchange for CO_2. The quantities of oxygen transported are enormous. One mole of hemoglobin can bind 4 moles of O_2. As 1 mole of a gas at standard temperature and pressure is 22.4 liters, 1 g of Hb can bind

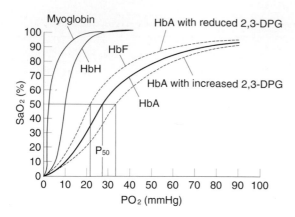

Fig. 12.4 Sigmoid binding curve of HbF and HbA at high and low 2,3-DPG concentrations. The hyperbolic binding curves of myoglobin and HbH which do not show a co-operative effect on oxygen binding are shown for comparison. Modified with permission from Ref. 84.

1.39 ml of O_2. At a hemoglobin concentration of 15 g/dl, 100 ml of blood can thus transport $\sim$20 ml of O_2.

The basic mechanism is the co-operative effect of the subunits which is structurally based on the allosterism of the R- and T-forms. This means that binding of oxygen induces allosteric changes in particular at the the $\alpha_1\beta_2$ contact which facilitates the uptake of the further oxygen molecules (homotropism). This co-operative effect is modified by the influence of other molecules, such as 2,3-DPG, H^+, Cl^- and CO_2 (heterotropism). The physiologic corollary of this co-operative effect is the sigmoid binding curve of hemoglobin, i.e. oxygen is rapidly loaded and unloaded at physiologic oxygen tensions (Fig. 12.4).

HOMOTROPIC INTERACTIONS OF OXYGEN BINDING

A powerful model of oxygen binding was proposed by Monod et al,[14] which has recently been modified.[12] According to this model, the R- and the T-forms are in equilibrium and differ in their oxygen affinity. The binding of the ligand to the individual subunit causes the tertiary structure to relax. When 1 subunit of each $\alpha_1\beta_1$ and $\alpha_2\beta_2$ dimer is oxygenated, the quaternary switch to the R conformation occurs facilitating oxygen loading of the remaining 2 subunits. This basic shift of the equilibrium induced by the ligand itself is modified heterotropically by CO_2, 2,3-DPG and chloride as detailed below.

HETEROTROPIC INTERACTIONS OF OXYGEN BINDING

Bohr effect

Bohr, Hasselbalch and Krogh showed in 1904 that oxygen affinity is reduced by CO_2. The major mechanism of the Bohr effect is the formation of carbonic acid from CO_2 and H_2O by catalysis of carbonic anhydrase ($CO_2 + H_2O \rightleftharpoons$

H_2CO_3), which readily dissociates into HCO_3^- and H^+. HCO_3^- is rapidly exported into the plasma in exchange for Cl^-, thus decreasing intracellular pH. The protons stabilize the T-form by forming H-bonds predominantly at β 146 His, but also at β 94 Asp, α 122 His and the N-terminal amino groups.[15–18] On oxygenation these protons are extruded, breaking the salt bonds and changing the pK_a from 8.0 in deoxy- to 7.1 in oxy-hemoglobin.[8,19–21] The Bohr effect therefore facilitates gas exchange, because oxygen affinity is decreased and oxygen unloaded at high concentrations of CO_2, i.e. in the peripheral tissues. Conversely, when CO_2 is exhaled in the lungs and intracellular pH rises, oxygen affinity is increased, which favors oxygen uptake.

A smaller portion of the CO_2 is directly bound to reactive amino groups to form carbamino complexes that also stabilize the T-form. However, in comparison to the Bohr effect, carbamino formation is probably of much less significance in terms of controlling allosterism and co-operative oxygen binding.[22]

Interaction with chloride

Chloride is transported into the red cell when bicarbonate is exported during protonation and deoxygenation (see above). Chloride reinforces the stabilization of the T-form by neutralizing electrostatic repulsion by an excess of positive charges in the central cavity of the molecule.[13,23,24] Additionally, Cl-binding at the N-terminus of the α chains appears to stabilize protonation and the T-form thus modulating allosterism. Upon oxygenation, chloride is released together with the protons that are required for the reverse carbonic anhydrase reaction. The efficiency of the Bohr effect is reduced to about half in a chloride-depleted system demonstrating the physiologic importance of the chloride interaction.[25] Clinically, the importance of the interaction of chloride with positively-charged residues is demonstrated by the variants with altered oxygen affinity and additional or missing positive charges in the central cavity of the molecule.[13]

Interaction with 2,3-diphosphoglycerate

2,3-DPG is a polyanion with a high affinity for positively-charged residues in the hemoglobin complex. It is a potent modifier of oxygen affinity[26,27] and forms H-bonds with the N-terminal amino groups, the imidazole of β 143 His, and the amino groups of β 82 Lys in the T-conformation. In the R-conformation, these interactions are much weaker.[28,29] 2,3-DPG thus stabilizes deoxyhemoglobin and reduces O_2 affinity. The higher O_2 affinity of HbF in comparison to HbA is due to a sequence difference between the γ and β chains. β 143 His corresponds to γ 143 Ser, which is an uncharged amino acid that does not bind to 2,3-DPG.

The concentration of intracellular 2,3-DPG can be upregulated in conditions of chronic hypoxia, thus reducing O_2 affinity and increasing O_2 availability in peripheral tissues.

This is also one of the compensatory mechanisms of chronic anemia.

HEMOGLOBIN VARIANTS

ADULT HEMOGLOBINS

HbA

After completion of the fetal to adult switch (see below), HbA ($\alpha_2\beta_2$) is the predominant hemoglobin. HbA is post-translationally glycosylated at the N-terminal valine and at internal lysine residues. This is a 2-step reaction, first quickly and reversibly transforming the Hb–NH$_2$ group to an aldimine and then slowly and irreversibly to a ketoamine. The post-translational modifications can be identified as fast eluting fractions (HbA$_{Ia-c}$) of a column chromatography (Fig. 12.5). One of these fractions (HbA$_{Ic}$) can be readily quantified and is a useful marker for the long-term metabolic control of patients with diabetes mellitus. In rare cases of substitutions of the N-terminal Val residue, HbA can be acetylated, in this respect resembling HbF. In cation exchange chromatography, these variants may be mistakenly identified as raised HbA$_{Ic}$.[30–32]

HbA$_2$

About 2.5% of adult hemoglobin is HbA$_2$ ($\beta_2\delta_2$). Functionally, HbA$_2$ is identical to HbA, although due to its low level of expression it is physiologically irrelevant and total lack of its synthesis has no clinical effect.

The δ chain is highly homologous to the β chain and differs by only 10 amino acids. Because of the difference in charge, HbA$_2$ can be easily separated from HbA by electrophoresis or chromatography. The δ globin gene is located immediately 5′ of the β-gene (Fig. 12.1) and switched on roughly in parallel to the β gene. The much lower level of δ globin expression results from:

1. reduced transcriptional activity of the δ-globin gene, which is caused by the relative inefficiency of its promoter[33] and probably by the lack of or a less efficiently functioning enhancer in the second intron;[34]
2. reduced δ-globin mRNA stability;[35]
3. a lesser affinity of δ- for α-globin chains.[36] This characteristic is exploited for the diagnosis of heterozygous β-thalassemia. When β-globin chains are present in low concentrations, δ-globin chains are able to form tetramers with α-chains and HbA$_2$ levels thus increase.

FETAL HEMOGLOBIN

Structure and function

Structurally and functionally, fetal hemoglobin (HbF; $\alpha_2\gamma_2$) is similar to HbA. However, there are some significant differences. The amino acid sequence of the γ-chain differs from the β-chain at 39 residues. Twenty-two of these occur at the external surface, explaining the different electrophoretic/ chromatographic behavior and the increased solubility of HbF. Four substitutions are located at the $\alpha_1\beta_1$ ($\alpha_1\gamma_1$) interface which results in the increased stability of HbF. The $\alpha_1\beta_2$ ($\alpha_1\gamma_2$) contacts are identical in both HbA and HbF, which is reflected by similar co-operative effects of oxygen binding in both hemoglobins. The substitution β 143 His → γ 143 Ser causes a diminished interaction of HbF with 2,3-DPG, thus increasing oxygen affinity of fetal red cells.[37] The diagnostically important increased resistance of HbF to alkali (see below) can be explained by the β 112 Cys → γ 112 Thr and β 130 Tyr → γ 130 Trp substitutions.[38]

HbF is structurally heterogeneous. The γ-globin chains are coded for by 2 closely linked genes that are located between the ε and the δ genes within the β-globin gene cluster (Fig. 12.1). The amino acid sequence that is coded for by the more 5′ gene differs from that of the 3′ gene at position 136, where the 5′ gene codes for a glycine ($^G\gamma$) and the 3′ gene for an alanine ($^A\gamma$) residue.[39] During fetal life, about 75% of the HbF contains $^G\gamma$ chains, whereas the small amounts of HbF present in adult life contain predominantly $^A\gamma$ chains.[40] In addition to these allelic differences, the $^A\gamma$ gene contains a common polymorphism coding either for Ile ($^A\gamma^I$) or Thr ($^A\gamma^T$) at position 75.[41] The major post-translational modification of HbF is by acetylation at the N-terminal Gly, which results in a more negatively charged component (HbF$_I$).

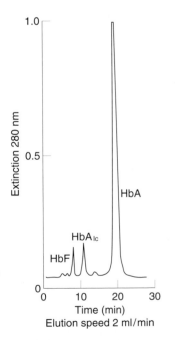

Fig. 12.5 Quantitation of HbF and HbA$_{Ic}$ by FPLC (Mono S® HR 5/5, Pharmacia). Modified with permission from Ref. 84.

235

Diagnostic and therapeutic relevance

Following the fetal to adult hemoglobin switch during the first 6 months of life there are only trace amounts of HbF in the peripheral blood.[42] The discovery of a method to differentiate fetal from adult red cells by acid HbA elution[43] and the identification of fetal red cells in the maternal circulation post-partum was part of the logical foundation for anti-D prophylaxis in Rh⁻ mothers (see Chapter 10). Practically, this method is useful for the estimation of feto-maternal blood transfusion.[44]

Increased HbF levels occur both in hemoglobin disorders and in acquired hematopoietic diseases. In *sickle cell disease* (see Chapter 11), HbF is raised as a result of selective survival of F cells. In patients from Saudi Arabia and India HbF synthesis is increased and associated with a milder clinical phenotype.[45,46] The sickle cell mutation in Asia occurred on a different genetic background from that in African patients.[47] There is probably more than one genetic factor responsible for the raised HbF levels, which are probably both linked and not linked to the β-globin gene cluster.[48–51] The clinical benefit of hydroxyurea in the treatment of sickle cell disease is related to an increase of HbF, although HbF-independent factors probably play an additional important role.[52]

In patients with *homozygous β-thalassemia*, the increase of the relative HbF is pathognomonic (see Chapter 15). While HbF synthesis per cell is not increased in most patients, in absolute terms F cells are produced in larger numbers than normal by the greatly expanded bone marrow. These cells subsequently survive selectively, because the α/non-α chain synthesis imbalance is less marked in F cells than in cells not expressing γ globin.[53] If genetic determinants that increase γ-globin gene expression per cell are present, such as point mutations of the γ-globin gene promoters or deletions of the β-globin gene cluster,[54] the clinical and hematologic manifestations of homozygous β-thalassemia can be considerably ameliorated and adult individuals with hereditary persis-

tence of HbF (HPFH) and 100% HbF can be perfectly healthy (see Chapter 15). Therapeutic attempts pharmacologically to reactivate HbF synthesis have been promising but have not been shown to be applicable to most patients in large-scale trials.[55,56]

There is a multitude of acquired conditions that are associated with an increase of HbF.[57] This is invariably so and is a diagnostic feature of juvenile chronic myeloid leukemia (JCML), Fanconi's anemia and erythroleukemia.[58–62] Raised HbF levels can be commonly seen but are not of specific diagnostic value in other myeloproliferative disorders and during the hematologic recovery following bone marrow transplantation or intensive chemotherapy.[63]

EMBRYONIC HEMOGLOBINS

During the second to fourteenth week of embryonic life the yolk sac produces 3 different hemoglobins: $\zeta_2\varepsilon_2$ (Hb Gower I), $\alpha_2\varepsilon_2$ (Hb Gower II), and $\zeta_2\gamma_2$ (Hb Portland).[64–66] The ε chains are homologous to the β and γ chains and are coded for by a single gene at the 5' end of the β-globin gene cluster (Fig. 12.1). The ζ chain is homologous to the α-chain and is coded for by a single gene at the 5' end of the α-globin gene cluster (Fig. 12.1). All 3 embryonic hemoglobins show allosterism, a co-operative effect on oxygen binding, and sensitivity to 2,3-DPG, but they exhibit a higher oxygen affinity than HbA and a decreased Bohr effect.[67] Under normal conditions these hemoglobins are not detectable during fetal or postnatal life. However, in deletional α°-thalassemia embryonic hemoglobins can be found at later stages of development.[68–70]

DEVELOPMENTAL CHANGES

The individual globin genes are activated to high levels of expression selectively in erythroid cells and programed to be

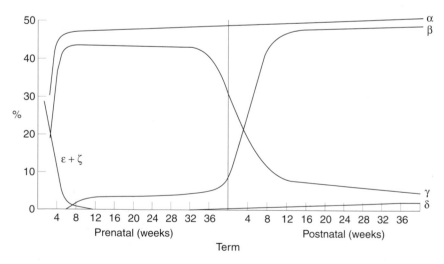

Fig. 12.6 Developmental changes in globin synthesis.

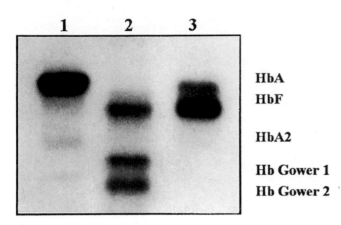

1   2   3

HbA
HbF

HbA2

Hb Gower 1
Hb Gower 2

Fig. 12.7 Starch bloc electrophoresis of hemoglobins at the adult (lane 1), embryonic (lane 2) and fetal (lane 3) stages of development.

predominantly expressed at specific developmental stages. In both clusters on chromosome 11 and 16 the globin genes are arranged in the order of their expression during development (Fig. 12.1). About 14 days following conception, Hbs Gower I and II, Hb Portland, and a little later HbF, begin to be synthesized in the yolk sac. By about 8 weeks the embryonic genes are silenced and HbF becomes the predominant hemoglobin and is synthesized in the fetal liver and spleen, and increasingly also in the bone marrow. HbA is made in small amounts during this period. At around birth, γ-globin chain and HbF synthesis are substituted by β-globin chain and HbA synthesis. Postnatally, the bone marrow becomes the only site of normal erythropoiesis (Figs 12.6 and 12.7).[71]

In the α-globin gene cluster there is a genetic embryonic (ζ) to fetal/adult (α) switch, whereas the β-globin gene cluster performs an embryonic (ε) to fetal (γ) and a fetal to adult (β) switch in gene expression. These switches are important paradigms of ontogenetic gene regulation and have therefore been the subject of intense study by biologists. The motivation for the medical sciences to study the fetal to adult hemoglobin switch results from the interest in reactivating γ-globin gene expression as a therapeutic option for the hemoglobinopathies.

The mechanisms responsible for the developmental specificity of hemoglobin synthesis are dependent on specific sequences within both the promoters and remote regulatory sequences.[72–75] These DNA sequences interact with erythroid specific and ubiquitous transcription factors, which results in the activation or silencing of the individual genes. Experiments in transgenic mice and the analysis of naturally occurring mutants suggest that the individual genes can be either autonomously regulated or require competition with other genes of the cluster.[54,76–81]

METHODS OF HEMOGLOBIN IDENTIFICATION

The practical approach to hemoglobin analysis is summarized in Fig. 12.8. The laboratory hematologist needs to be informed about relevant clinical details, in particular any recent erythrocyte transfusions, results of routine hematology and iron status. The blood needs to be anticoagulated with EDTA or citrate and, except for the analysis of highly unstable variants or HbH to diagnose α-thalassemia, can be stored for a few days. Generally, a blood volume of 5 ml is sufficient to perform all necessary analyses.

Routine hematology

This should include a complete blood count, including erythrocyte indices and reticulocytes, and a careful examination of a blood film.

Cytologic tests

These tests are valuable, simple and reproducible but are relatively labor intensive as they are not automated.

HbF cells (Kleihauer technique)

This technique is based on the acid elution of HbA but not HbF from single cells.[43] The thin film is fixed and dried in 80% ethanol and then incubated for 5 min in a citrate-phosphate buffer at pH 3.2 and 37°. The slide is then rinsed and H&E-stained. HbA cells appear as empty ghosts, whereas HbF cells are stained (Fig. 12.9). If HbF cells are not present there is no need to quantitate HbF by more sensitive techniques such as alkali denaturation or chromatography.

Inclusion bodies

HbH cells and Heinz bodies that reflect denatured hemoglobin can be identified by incubation for 30 min at room temperature of a drop of blood with a drop of brilliant cresyl blue or New methylene blue.[82] Microscopically, Heinz bodies are coarse and rather plump and located peripherally against the membrane, whereas HbH inclusions are smaller and more evenly distributed within the cell. The Kleihauer technique (see above) is also useful for the demonstration of inclusion bodies (Fig. 12.10).

Sickle test

This can be used to demonstrate HbS in blood films, although hemoglobin electrophoresis or chromatography are more useful quantitative methods as in addition they can distinguish heterozygotes, homozygotes and compound heterozygotes.[82]

Technically, a small amount of blood is diluted with NaCl 0.9% containing Na-dithionite 2% and cover slipped. After 15–30 min all erythrocytes assume the characteristic sickled form.

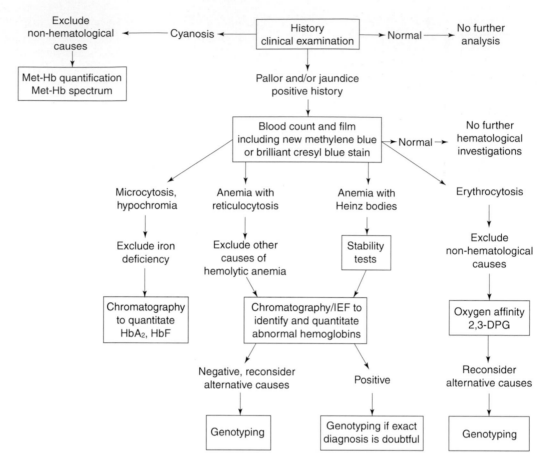

Fig. 12.8 Strategy for the analysis of the hemoglobinopathies.

Denaturation tests

HbF

Denaturation by alkali is the classic technique to determine HbF quantitatively.[83] In principle, this is based on the increased stability of HbF than HbA in the presence of alkali due to the amino acid substitutions at positions 112 (β Cys $\to$ γ Thr) and 130 (β Tyr $\to$ γ Trp). The detailed protocol of alkali denaturation of a cyanmethemoglobin solution has to be followed accurately with respect to the concentrations of hemoglobin solution, NaOH and ammonium sulfate, as well as to the timing and temperature. The method is reliable for low HbF concentrations. At higher concentrations ($>20\%$) the alkali denaturation method tends to underestimate, because some of the HbF is co-precipitated with the HbA.

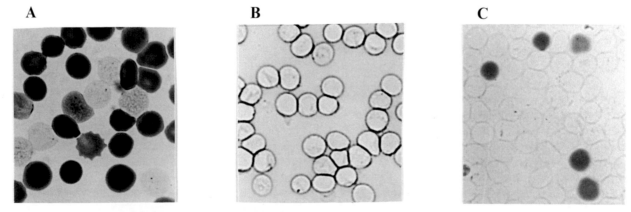

Fig. 12.9 The Kleihauer technique. Acid elution of HbA and demonstration of HbF in single red cells. (A) Cord blood; (B) Normal adult blood; (C) Maternal blood after feto-maternal transfusion. Modified with permission from Ref. 84.

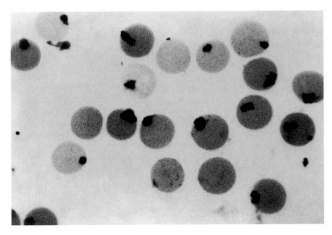

Fig. 12.10 Heinz bodies in a brilliant cresyl blue-stained film of a patient with Hb Köln.

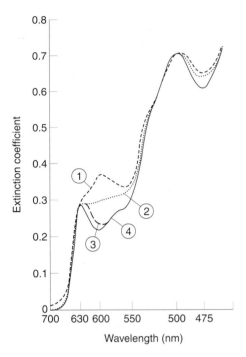

Fig. 12.11 Methemoglobin spectrum of HbM Saskatoon (curve 1), HbM Boston (curve 2), and HbM Milwaukee (curve 3) in comparison to normal methemoglobin (curve 4). Modified with permission from Ref. 84.

Unstable variants

If an unstable variant cannot be specifically identified by electrophoretic, chromatographic or isoelectric focusing techniques, its presence may be demonstrated as Heinz bodies or by an increased denaturation by heat or isopropanol.[82] For the heat denaturation test a buffered cyanmethemoglobin solution is incubated at 69.5° for 6 min, which results in the precipitation of unstable variants. For the isopropanol test the hemolysate is incubated with 17% buffered isopropanol at 37°, which also results in the precipitation of unstable hemoglobins. If the specific identification of the variant is not possible by standard techniques, DNA analysis is probably the most economical diagnostic procedure to be employed next.

Solubility test

This method is still used by some laboratories to discriminate HbS from other rarer variants with the same electrophoretic behavior. The hemoglobin solution is deoxygenated by incubation with dithionite, which results in the precipitation of HbS. Disadvantages of the solubility test are the low sensitivity which precludes its use in neonatal screening, the inability to discriminate hetero- from homo-zygotes, and that other pathological hemoglobins are not detected.

Spectral analysis

This is an important method to identify HbM anomalies that show a characteristic 450–650 nm methemoglobin spectrum (Fig. 12.11). The hemolysate is transformed completely into methemoglobin by K-ferricyanide and the absorption compared to a normal control with an identical concentration and pH.[84]

Oxygen affinity

The oxygen dissociation curve can be measured by using commercially available tonometers. In principle, red cells are deoxygenated and suspended at a low concentration at a defined temperature and pH. Oxygen at known pO$_2$ is then added stepwise and the amount of oxyhemoglobin measured by spectrometry (Fig. 12.4).

Hb electrophoresis

The identification of hemoglobin variants by electrophoretic techniques depends on the introduction of a charge difference by the amino acid substitution. Commonly used routine methods are alkaline cellulose acetate and acid agar-gel electrophoresis of hemolysates.[82] Although the commoner variants are detected with these methods, 45% of all pathologic hemoglobin variants are not associated with a charge difference and are therefore electrophoretically silent. Furthermore, electrophoretic methods are generally unreliable for the quantitation of hemoglobin variants. An exception is the technically difficult and laborious starch bloc electrophoresis that results in particularly sharp bands that allow reproducible quantitative measurements (Fig. 12.7).[84]

Isoelectric focusing

A pH gradient is generated in a polyacrylamide gel separating the loaded hemoglobins by their pK$_a$. In contrast to hemoglobin electrophoresis, this method does not rely on the charge and many variants not detectable by electrophoretic

239

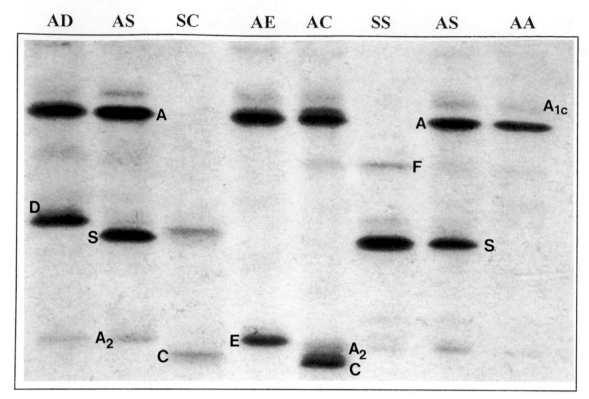

Fig. 12.12 Immobilized pH gradient (IPG) of common hemoglobin variants. Kindly provided by Dr P Sinha.

methods can be identified by isoelectric focusing (IEF).[85] The technical effort associated with IEF can be much reduced by using immobilized pH gradients in polyacrylamide gels, which can be used to detect common (Fig. 12.12) and rare variants (Fig. 12.13) with a high degree of sensitivity and specificity.[86]

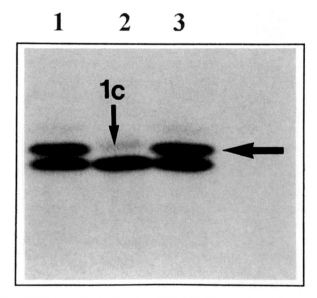

Fig. 12.13 Immobilized pH gradient (IPG) of Hb Okayama (arrow) (lanes 1 and 3) and a normal control with HbA[1c] in the same position (lane 2). Kindly provided by Dr P Sinha.

Chromatography

With these methods, hemoglobin variants can be reliably identified and quantitated. Recently, in larger laboratories HPLC and FPLC techniques have largely superceded the formerly used DEAE-Sephadex chromatography (Fig. 12.5). Apart from their high degree of accuracy and reproducibility, chromatographic methods can also be used to prepare samples for further biochemical and biophysical analysis.

Electro-spray-mass spectrometry

This method has recently been introduced accurately to determine the molecular weight of globin chains. The likely amino acid substitution can thus be predicted without protein sequencing. This method complements DNA sequencing in that it detects post-translational modifications.[87] However, the immense cost of the equipment and the special expertise required limit this technique to specialized laboratories.

DNA analysis

The invention of the polymerase chain reaction (PCR)[88,89] caused a revolution in clinically applied molecular biology. PCR-amplified DNA can be subjected to various diagnostic procedures such as allele-specific oligonucleotide hybridization, restriction enzyme analysis[90,91] or even direct

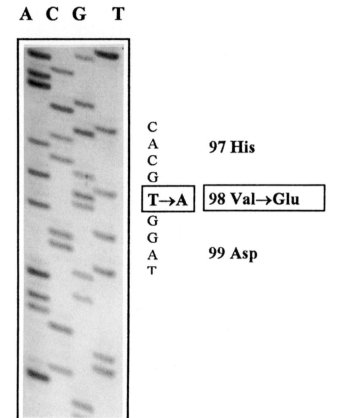

A C G T

C
A
C
G
        97 His
T→A   98 Val→Glu
G
G
A   99 Asp
T

Fig. 12.14 Characterization of an unstable variant by DNA sequence analysis. The G*T*G→G*A*G mutation in codon 98 can be demonstrated directly and the Val→Glu amino acid substitution of Hb Mainz deduced according to the genetic code.

sequencing.[92] The structure of variant hemoglobins and the amino acid substitution can thus be indirectly determined (Fig. 12.14), although post-translational modifications detectable by biochemical analysis do, of course, remain unidentified.[87, 93–96] Molecular genetic techniques are particularly useful in prenatal diagnosis.[97]

RARE HEMOGLOBIN DISORDERS

UNSTABLE VARIANTS (CONGENITAL HEINZ BODY HEMOLYTIC ANEMIA)

Hemoglobin is a highly organized complex whose function and stability is dependent on the subtle arrangement of the various structural features described above. Many mutations thus lead to some degree of instability that can be recognized by *in vitro* testing but do not result in significant clinical consequences. The clinical definition of unstable hemoglobinopathies therefore refers to congenital Heinz-body hemolytic anemia (CHBA) only.[98,99]

Pathogenesis

The common pathway for unstable hemoglobin denaturation is the relaxation of the strict steric organization, which then favors the R configuration and thus the oxygenated state. In oxyhemoglobin, ferrous iron is more likely to be oxidized to the ferric form (Hb Fe^{2+} + O_2 → Hb Fe^{3+} + O_2^-). Both the superoxide anion and hydrogen peroxide can induce the generation of more methemoglobin. As ferriheme has a lower affiniy for globin, this in itself may lead to heme loss and rapid denaturation.[100,101] Additionally, the distortion of the quaternary configuration allows the E7 histidine directly but reversibly to bind to the oxidized heme (reversible hemichrome). If on further distortion other residues bind to the oxidized heme, this is irreversible and results in denaturation and finally precipitation as a Heinz body. These become attached to the inner surface of the red cell membrane and cause trapping in the spleen where the inclusions are removed or hemolysis occurs. In addition to this rather mechanical view of splenic hemolysis, autologous antibodies were reported to bind to modified membrane constituents.[102,103]

Many unstable variants can be detected electrophoretically (Fig. 12.14). However, if instability is severe in the so-called hyperunstable hemoglobins, protein-based analytical techniques are not sufficient (see below). In some such variants the clinical features are remarkably mild.[104] In others, there is marked ineffective erythropoiesis with low reticulocyte counts for the degree of anemia and unbalanced α/non-α-globin chain synthesis suggesting that an early step of complex formation such as dimerization may be affected.[105–110]

There are 5 different and not mutually exclusive molecular mechanisms destabilizing the 3D structure of the complex. In some variants the mechanism for instability cannot be predicted from the amino acid substitution and X-ray crystallography data are not available.

Destabilization of the globin–heme interaction

Heme is bound to the heme pocket at the surface of the complex where non-polar residues in the CD, E, F and FG regions interact hydrophobically with the porphyrin ring. Many of the clinically relevant unstable variants, including the most common Hb Köln (β 98 [FG5] Val→Met), affect these residues resulting in a weaker globin to heme link.[111,112]

If the F8 histidine is substituted in Hbs Istanbul (β 92 His→Gln),[113] Mozhaisk (β 92 His→Arg)[114] and Newcastle (β 92 His→Pro),[115] heme cannot be bound to globin which results in instability.

The E7 histidine binds directly to molecular oxygen and, together with E11 Val, produces a steric configuration that prevents access of larger molecules to the heme pocket. If E7 His is substituted by Arg in Hb Zürich (β 63 His→Arg), a molecular gap is opened that allows oxidant substances, such

241

as sulfonamide drugs, to attack the ferrous iron, resulting in methemoglobin formation which triggers denaturation. In Hb Zürich, ferrous iron oxidation can be inhibited by CO (e.g. in smokers) resulting in a decrease of Heinz bodies.

A substitution of E11 Val was the first unstable hemoglobin to be characterized at the molecular level.[116] This rare variant has been described in 4 families from the UK, Japan and Russia, and results in considerable anemia (Hb 5–8 g/dl) with regular transfusion requirements.[87] In the initial protein analysis, E11 Val was found to be substituted by Asp and was designated Hb Bristol. Subsequent DNA analysis showed a GTG→ATG mutation of codon 67, thus replacing the codon of Val with Met, not Asp. Met has therefore been post-translationally modified to Asp. Post-translational modifications have also been observed in Hb Redondo (β 92 His → Asn → Asp), Hb La Roche-sur-Yon (β 81 Leu→His → β 80 Asn→Asp) and Hb Atlanta-Coventry (β 75 Leu → Pro → β 141 Leu deleted).[87,93–96]

Disruption of secondary structure

The predominant secondary structure of globin chains is the α helix which is crucial for the tight assembly of the tertiary and quaternary structure. Any substitution that inhibits α-helix formation is therefore likely to be associated with clinical manifestations. Proline cannot participate in helix formation and variants introducing this residue are almost always unstable. An exception is the stable variant Hb Singapore (α 141 Arg → Pro) which is located at the C-terminal end of the chain which does not participate in helix formation.[117]

Substitutions at the hydrophobic core

The interior of the complex is highly hydrophobic. A common mechanism of destabilization is a substitution of a charged for an uncharged amino acid, thus allowing water to enter into the tightly fitting core.[118] Similarly, the tight steric fit may be disturbed by the replacement of one hydrophobic residue with another. Finally, if the strong $\alpha_1\beta_1$ interface is relaxed the internal SH-groups may become highly reactive as is the case in Hb Tacoma and Hb Philly.[119,120]

Amino acid deletions

Deletions of amino acids can have a serious effect on the conformation of the entire complex, which may be so severe that a thalassemic phenotype develops.

Elongation of a subunit

These variants are caused by DNA insertions, by mutations of the translation termination codon (Ter), or by a frame-shift in the third exon putting Ter out of frame. If translation is continued into the 3′ UTR of the α-globin gene, the mRNA becomes unstable and this is associated with a thalassemic phenotype.[121,122]

Genetics

Unstable hemoglobins are inherited as an autosomal dominant trait with CHBA in the heterozygote. As the clinical consequences are part of the definition of unstable hemoglobinopathies, it is not surprising that β variants (Table 12.3) are more common than α variants (Table 12.4). Each of the 2 β-globin alleles directs 50% of the total β-globin chain synthesis, whereas there are 2 α2- and 2 α1-globin alleles of which α2 is expressed at about twice the level of α1.[123,124] Each α2 allele thus accounts for ~30–35% and each α1 allele for about 15–20% of the total α-chain synthesis. α1-variants are therefore mildly expressed phenotypically even when present homozygously.[125] Also, analogous amino acid substitutions lead to clinically milder presentations in the α- than in the β-globin chains. Thus, α-chain variants are less likely to be identified than β-chain variants (e.g. Hb Iwata α F8 His→Arg, no anemia, 5% abnormal hemoglobin[126] versus Hb Mozhaisk β F8 His→Arg, Hb 7g/dl, 32% abnormal hemoglobin and CHBA).[114]

γ-Chain variants are rare. In Hb F-Poole ($^G\gamma$ 130 Trp → Gly) there is neonatal (and presumably fetal) hemolytic anemia that disappears with the fetal to adult hemoglobin switch after the first few months of life.[127] More severe γ-chain variants are not known which is probably due to the duplication of the γ genes and to the negative selection bias presumably operating in fetal hemoglobinopathies.

No selective pressure seems to have favored unstable hemoglobins in the course of evolution. Therefore, these variants are generally rare and have often been described in single families only. Spontaneous mutations are not uncommon.

There are single reports of patients who are compound heterozygotes for an unstable variant and a thalassemia mutation. The clinical picture of these cases depends on the degree of instability of the abnormal variant; some are mildly affected,[128,129] whereas others exhibit severe hemolytic disease.[130] Homozygotes are also exceedingly rare. A patient with homozygous Hb Bushwick (β74 (E18) Gly→Val) was reported to suffer from chronic anemia caused by a combination of hemolysis and ineffective erythropoiesis which was severely exacerbated at times of infection.[131]

Clinical features

The age at presentation and the severity of CHBA depends on the degree of instability and on the type of chain affected. For the reasons discussed above, β- tend to be more severe than α-chain variants. In severe CHBA, patients may become symptomatic in early childhood. They present either with chronic anemia, a hemolytic crisis associated with fever and/or oxidant stress of sulfonamide medication,

Table 12.3 β-Chain substitutions causing congenital Heinz body hemolytic anemia (CHBA).

Reference	Amino acid substitution	Mutation	Variant name	Mechanism
161	6(A3) or 7(A4)	Glu→0	Leiden	Deletion
162	11(A8)	Val→Asp	Windsor	Internal, heme contact
163	24(B6)	Gly→Val	Savannah	Internal, close contact to E helix
164	24(B6)	Gly→Asp	Moscva	Internal, close contact to E helix
165	28(B10)	Leu→Gln	St. Louis	Internal, spontaneous met-Hb formation
166	28(B10)	Leu→Pro	Genova	Helix disruption
167	31(B13)	Leu→Pro	Yokohama	Helix disruption
168	31(B13)	Leu→Arg	Hakkari	Heme contact
134	32(B14)	Leu→Pro	Perth	Helix disruption
169	32(B14)	Leu→Arg	Castilla	Internal
120	35(C1)	Tyr→Phe	Philly	$\alpha_1\beta_1$ Contact
170	41(C7)	Phe→Tyr	Mequon	Heme contact
171	41(C7) or 42(CD1)	Phe→0	Bruxelles	Deletion
172	42(CD1)	Phe→Ser	Hammersmith	Heme contact
173	54(D5)	Val→Asp	Jacksonville	Internal
174	56(D7)-59(E3)	Gly-Asn-Pro-Lys→0	Tochigi	Deletion
175	63(E7)	His→Arg	Zürich	Heme binding; distal histidine
176, 177	63(E7)	His→Pro	Bicêtre	Heme binding; distal histidine
87, 116, 178	67(E11)	Val→Met→Asp	Bristol/Alesha	Heme contact
179	67(E11)	Val→Ala	Sydney	
180	68(E12)	Leu→Pro	Mizuho	Internal
181	71(E15)	Phe→Ser	Christchurch	Internal; heme
182	74(E18)	Gly→Val	Bushwick	Internal
183	74(E18)	Gly→Asp	Shepherds Bush	Internal
184	91(F7)	Leu→Pro	Sabine	Helix disruption
185	91(F7)-95(FG1)	Leu-His-Cys-Asp-Lys→0	Gun Hill	Deletion of heme contact, including proximal histidine
114	92(F8)	His→Arg	Mozhaisk	Heme contact; proximal histidine
94	92(F8)	His→Asn→Asp	Redondo	Heme contact; proximal histidine
186	95(FG2)-96(FG3)	Leu-His-Asp-Lys insertion	Koriyama	Anti Gun Hill insertion; heme contact; including proximal histidine
187	97(FG4)	His→Pro	Nagoya	$\alpha_1\beta_2$ Contact; Helix disruption
112	98(FG5)	Val→Met	Köln	$\alpha_1\beta_2$ Contact; heme contact
188	98(FG5)	Val→Gly	Nottingham	$\alpha_1\beta_2$ Contact; heme contact
Fig. 12.14	98(FG5)	Val→Glu	Mainz	$\alpha_1\beta_2$ Contact; heme contact
189	97(FG4)-98(FG5)	His-Val deletion; Leu insertion	Galicia	$\alpha_1\beta_2$ contact; haem contact
190	106(G8)	Leu→Pro	Southampton	Helix disruption
191	115(G17)	Ala→Pro	Madrid	$\alpha_1\beta_1$ Contact; helix disruption
192	115(G17)	Ala→Asp	Hradec Kralove	$\alpha_1\beta_1$ Contact
193	117(G19)	His→Pro	Saitama	External
194	127(H5)	Gln→Lys	Brest	$\alpha_1\beta_1$ Contact
195	130(H8)	Tyr→Asp	Wien	Internal
189	141–144	Leu-Ala-His-Lys deletion; Gln insertion	Birmingham	Deletion

Table 12.4 α-Chain substitutions causing severe congenital Heinz body hemolytic anemia (CHBA).

Reference	Amino acid substitution	Mutation	Variant name	Mechanism
154,155	43(CE1)	Phe→Val	Torino	Heme contact
156,157	43(CE1)	Phe→Leu	Hirosaki	Heme contact
158	130(H13)	Ala→Pro	Sun Prairie	Helix disruption
159	131(H14)	Ser→Pro	Questembert	Helix disruption
160	136(H19)	Leu→Pro	Bibba	Heme contact, helix disruption

or an aplastic crisis usually following parvovirus infection.[132] The urine is often dark due to the presence of bilirubin degradation products (mesobilifuscinuria). Pigment gallstones are also common and may cause colic. Milder unstable variants may not be associated with any clinical symptoms and may only be detected fortuitously.

The findings on clinical examination depend on the severity of the hemolysis. Jaundice and splenomegaly are common. In some, this may be associated with hypersplenism. Cyanosis may be noted in those with a significant methemoglobin concentration (e.g. Hb Freiburg).[133] Occasionally, leg ulcers have been described.[134,135]

The hyperunstable and thalassemic variants can be mild but often cause severe anemia and may present as thalassemia intermedia or even major (see below). They differ from other types of CHBA in that Heinz bodies are not necessarily seen, the abnormal hemoglobin cannot be identified by hemoglobin analysis, and the α/non-α ratio is often unbalanced. Ineffective erythropoiesis may be suggested by low reticulocyte counts for the degree of anemia and the degree of plasma transferrin receptor elevation, and by inclusion bodies in the erythroblasts in the bone marrow (see Table 12.5).

243

Table 12.5 Thalassemic hemoglobin variants.

Reference	Variant type and name	Mutation	Mechanism
Reduced transcriptional activity			
196–200	Hb Lepore Boston	$\delta\beta$-Globin gene fusion	Transcriptional control by δ-globin gene promoter
	Hb Lepore Hollandia		
	Hb Lepore Baltimore		
Impaired mRNA processing efficiency			
204	HbE	β 26 Glu→Lys	Activation of a cryptic splice site
205	Hb Knossos	β 27 Ala→Ser	Activation of a cryptic splice site
211	Hb Monroe	β 30 Arg→Thr	Mutation of the splice donor consensus sequence
Reduced mRNA stability			
121,122,212,213	Hb Constant Spring	α 142 Ter→Gln	Associated with translational readthrough into the 5'-UTR
214	Hb Icaria	α 142 Ter→Lys	See Hb Constant Spring
215	Hb Koya Dora	α 142 Ter→Ser	See Hb Constant Spring
216	Hb Seal Rock	α 142 Ter→Glu	See Hb Constant Spring
Reduced post-translational stability			
219,220	Hb Suan Dok	α 109 Leu→Arg	Hyperunstable
221	Hb Quong Sze	α 125 Leu→Pro	Hyperunstable
222	Hb Toyama	α 136 Leu→Arg	Hyperunstable
110	Hb Chesterfield	β 28 Leu→Arg	Hyperunstable
104	No name	β 30–31 +Arg	Hyperunstable
223	Hb Korea	β 33–34 Val-Val→0–0	Hyperunstable
Figs 12.16 and 12.17	Hb Dresden	β 33–35 Val-Val-Tyr→0–0-Asp	Hyperunstable
224	Hb Cagliari	β 60 Val→Glu	Hyperunstable
225	Hb Agnana	β 94 +TG	
107	Hb Terre Haute	β 106 Leu→Arg	Hyperunstable
108	Hb Manhattan	β 109 ΔG	Extended hyperunstable β chain of 156 amino acids
226	Hb Showa-Yakushiji	β 110 Leu→Pro	Hyperunstable
227,228	Hb Brescia/Durham-NC	β 114 Leu→Pro	Hyperunstable
229	Hb Geneva	β 114 ΔCT, +G	Hyperunstable
192	Hb Hradec Kralove (HK)	β 115 Ala→Asp	Hyperunstable
230	FS 123 ΔA (β chain Makabe)	β 123 ACC→-CC	Extended hyperunstable β chain of 156 amino acids
231	FS 124 ΔA	β 124 CCA→CC-	Extended unstable β chain of 156 amino acids
231	No name	β 124–125 +Pro	?
232	Hb Vercelli	β 126 GTG→G-G	Extended unstable β chain of 156 amino acids
233	Hb Neapolis	β 126 Val→Gly	Hyperunstable
108	Hb Houston	β 127 Ala→Pro	Hyperunstable
234,235	β-chain Gunma	β 127–128 Gln-Ala→Pro	Hyperunstable, shortened by 1 residue
105	No name	β 128–135 rearrangement (4 bp 128/129 deleted, 11 bp 132–135 deleted, CCACA inserted)	
236	No name	β 134–137 Val-Ala-Gly-Val→Gly-Arg	Hyperunstable, shortened by 2 residues
Premature translational termination			
237	NS 121	β 121 Glu→Ter	Premature termination of translation
238	NS 127	β 127 Gln→Ter	Premature termination of translation

Laboratory diagnosis

Routine hematology shows signs of hemolytic anemia with reticulocytosis, indirect hyperbilirubinemia, and decreased haptoglobin. New methylene blue- or brilliant cresyl blue-stained blood films show Heinz bodies (Fig. 12.10). The heat and/or isopropanol denaturation tests are positive. Hemoglobin analysis often demonstrates characteristic findings allowing the identification of the abnormal variant (Fig. 12.15). In cases of hyperunstable variants, the biochemical methods may remain inconclusive and DNA analysis need to be performed to establish the diagnosis (Fig. 12.14).

Treatment

Most CHBA patients do not require specific treatment. If severe hemolysis is present, folic acid should be supplemented, oxidant drugs avoided and increased awareness exercised at times of pyrexia. Paracetamol or acetylsalicylic acid are generally safe. Sulfonamides should be avoided.

Splenectomy

This is clearly indicated in cases with hypersplenism but has been tried in other patients with varied success. Generally,

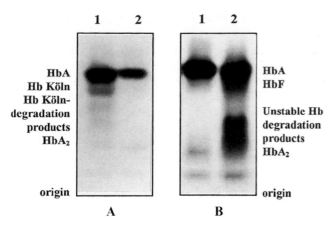

Fig. 12.15 Characterization of unstable variants by starch bloc electrophoresis. (A) Hemolysate of a patient with Hb Köln (A, lane 1) and another with an unidentified unstable hemoglobin (B, lane 2) is compared to a normal control (A, lane 2 and B, lane 1). Modified with permission from Ref. 84.

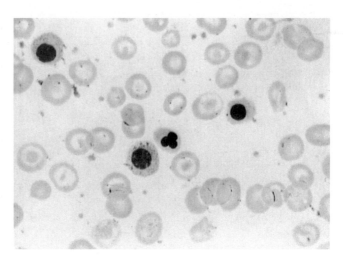

Fig. 12.16 Peripheral blood film of a splenectomized patient with the highly unstable and thalassemic variant Hb Dresden (β 33–35 Val-Val-Tyr→0–0-Asp) showing marked hypochromia, target cells and dysplastic normoblasts. Hemoglobin electrophoresis and immobilized pH gradient (IPG) showed high levels of HbF. The abnormal hemoglobin could not be identified by these methods.

caution is adequate because of the danger of post-splenectomy septicemia, particularly in young children, and because of post-splenectomy thromboembolism.[136–138] Penicillin prophylaxis is mandatory and vaccination against *Streptococcus pneumoniae* and possibly *Neisseria meningitidis* is indicated and should ideally be performed 3 months before the operation.[139,140] The duration of penicillin prophylaxis is controversial and recommendations are often based on anecdotal reports. Controlled studies are difficult because of the rarity of this complication and the uncertain long-term compliance of patients. However, there are numerous reports of post-splenectomy septicemia occurring many years after the operation and the risk probably depends on the underlying disorder. There are also reports of post-splenectomy pulmonary embolism following the development of polycythemia and pulmonary hypertension in unstable hemoglobinopathies.[141,142] Recently, priapism following splenectomy in a patient with the hyperunstable Hb Olmsted (β 141 [H19] Leu → Arg) has been reported,[143] which is also a well recognized complication of splenectomy in thalassemia intermedia.[144–146]

Cholecystectomy

Gallstones are often asymptomatic and do not generally require treatment. However, in patients with colic or stones in the bile duct, surgical treatment may be warranted.

Hydroxyurea

This drug has a definite place in the therapy of adults and children with sickle cell disease[52,147–150] and possibly in thalassemia intermedia.[51,152] Recently, there has been a report of 2 adult patients with severe CHBA who benefited from hydroxyurea treatment.[153]

THALASSEMIC VARIANTS

In these variants there is, in addition to the structural abnormality, a net decrease in globin chain synthesis which may be caused by reduced transcriptional activity, a decrease in mRNA processing efficiency or mRNA stability, or increased post-translational degradation (Table 12.5). There are clinical and hematologic characteristics of thalassemia (Fig. 12.16), such as hypochromia, microcytosis, splenomegaly and anemia due to ineffective erythropoiesis and dyserythropoiesis in the β-chain variants or signs of hemolysis in the α-chain variants.

Pathogenesis and clinical features

The paradigm of this type of hemoglobin variant is Hb Lepore which contains a $\delta\beta$ fusion chain. This is coded for by a $\delta\beta$-globin fusion gene that is the result of an unequal cross-over event between the highly homologous δ- and β-globin genes. The cross-over has occurred at 3 different points: Hb Lepore Boston ($\delta87\beta116$),[196,197] Hollandia ($\delta22\beta50$)[198] and Baltimore ($\delta50\beta86$).[199,200] These variants do not differ in their pathogenetic or clinical effect. The transcriptional activity of these fusion genes is controlled by the δ-globin gene promoter containing only a single CACCC-box and is thus much reduced compared to the β-globin gene that contains this regulatory element in duplicate. Heterozygotes for the Hb Lepore anomaly are hypochromic with about 7–15% of the variant and 2–3% HbF. Compound heterozygotes with a β°- or a severe β^+ allele on the other chromosome are usually transfusion dependent, as are the rare cases of homozygotes.[201–203]

The commonest thalassemic hemoglobin variant is HbE (β 26 Glu→Lys), which reaches extraordinarily high gene frequencies in south-east Asia. Both the β^E mutation and the much rarer variant Hb Knossos (β 27 Ala→Ser) cause activation of a cryptic splice site in exon 1 of the β-globin gene and thus defective mRNA processing.[204,205] In addition, HbE is mildly unstable which contributes to the reduced availability of these globin chains. HbE causes hemolysis in the homozygote and thalassemia major when in compound with a β° thalassemia mutation.[206,207] Hb Knossos/β° thalassemia compound heterozygotes have been described to exhibit the phenotype of thalassemia intermedia[208,209] or major.[210]

Another example of a variant with impaired splice efficiency is Hb Monroe (β 30 Arg→Thr). The G→C mutation affects the last nucleotide of the first exon, which is part of the consensus sequence of the splice donor site surrounding the invariant GT dinucleotide.[211] Hb Monroe is a severe β^+ thalassemia mutation with <1% residual activity.

mRNA stability and globin chain synthesis and stability is reduced in termination codon mutations that cause ribosomal readthrough into the 3′-UTR and an elongation of the α-globin chain (Hb Constant Spring, Hb Icaria, Hb Koya Dora, Hb Seal Rock). Clinically, these defects are typical thalassemia mutations and the variants are detectable in small amounts.[121,122,212–216]

Finally, a thalassemic phenotype of hemoglobin variants may be caused post-translationally. In some of these variants the globin chains are markedly unstable and degraded before they can be incorporated into the tetramer. Others cause hyperinstability of the complete hemoglobin molecule. In either case, protein-based analytical techniques are unlikely to be informative and DNA analysis has to be employed (Fig. 12.17). A special type of abnormality that may be classified with this group of variants is characterized by premature translational stop codons in the third β-globin exon, which results in the synthesis of C-terminally truncated and non-functional globin chains. In all of these mutations, the erythropoietic precursor in the bone marrow has to degrade α- and β-globin chains, which overloads the proteolytic capacity of the system and causes ineffective erythropoiesis.[105,217,218] The clinical hallmark of these abnormalities is the dominant mode of inheritance of the thalassemic phenotype which may be mild or severe with chronic transfusion requirements.

Genetics

In these variants typical features of thalassemia are seen in the heterozygote. If expressed in sufficient amounts, the diagnosis may be made by hemoglobin analysis. Otherwise, DNA analysis will identify the gene mutation enabling the deduction of the amino acid substitution in most cases.

Treatment

Treatment guidelines for thalassemia intermedia and major are decribed in Chapter 15.

VARIANTS WITH INCREASED OXYGEN AFFINITY

In these variants the equilibrium between the R- and the T-quaternary conformation is disturbed and the R-form is more readily assumed. The sigmoid oxygen binding curve is shifted to the left, i.e. oxygen uptake in the lungs is facilitated and oxygen release in the peripheral tissues impeded. Many variants with altered oxygen affinity are also unstable to some degree. In contrast to CHBA, the clinical hallmark of variants with altered oxygen affinity is erythrocytosis/polycythemia but not hemolysis.

Pathogenesis

The more the oxygen binding curve is shifted to the left, the more difficult it is for the tetramer to change its quaternary conformation. Generally, this loss of allosterism results in loss of the co-operative and Bohr effects. These variants thus resemble other hemoproteins such as myoglobin and with an increasing degree of oxygen affinity tend not to function as oxygen carriers. Although there is no hypoxemia, oxygen availability is decreased. This results in erythropoietin production and erythrocytosis as a compensatory mechanism. Most patients with high-affinity variants show normal exercise tolerance, although blood loss or venesection to a numerically normal Hb may result in clinically relevant hypoxia.[239–242]

Many high affinity variants have substitutions at the $\alpha_1\beta_2$ interface, where most of the allosteric changes occur (Tables 12.6 and 12.7). The C-terminal ends of the subunits are also

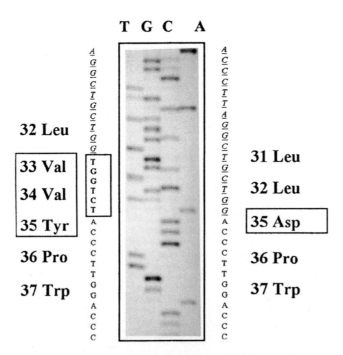

Fig.12.17 Sequence analysis of the β-globin gene in Hb Dresden. The TGGTCT deletion of a hexanucleotide within the codons 33–35 can be readily identified and the structure of the abnormal globin deduced.

Table 12.6 α-Globin variants with increased oxygen affinity.

Affected residue	Mutation	Variant name	Mechanism	Clinical characteristic
41 (C6)	Thr→Ser	Miyano	$\alpha_1\beta_2$ Contact	Erythrocytosis
44 (CE2)	Pro→Leu	Milledgeville	$\alpha_1\beta_2$ Contact	Mild erythrocytosis
88 (F9)	Ala→Val	Columbia-Missouri	$\alpha_1\beta_2$ Contact	Erythrocytosis
89 (FG1)	His→Leu	Luton	?	Erythrocytosis
92 (FG4)	Arg→Gln	J-Cape Town	$\alpha_1\beta_2$ Contact	Mild erythrocytosis
92 (FG4)	Arg→Leu	Chesapeake	$\alpha_1\beta_2$ Contact	Mild erythrocytosis
97 (G4)	Asn→Lys	Dallas	$\alpha_1\beta_2$ Contact	Mild erythrocytosis
126 (H9)	Asp→Asn	Tarrant	$\alpha_1\beta_1$ Contact	Mild erythrocytosis
126 (H9)	Asp→Val	Fukutomi	$\alpha_1\beta_1$ Contact	Mild erythrocytosis
139 (HC1)	Lys→Glu	Hanamaki	?	Mild erythrocytosis
140 (HC2)	Tyr→His	Ethiopia	$\alpha_1\beta_2$ Contact	Erythrocytosis
141 (HC3)	Arg→Leu	Legnano	$\alpha_1\beta_2$ Contact	Erythrocytosis
141 (HC3)	Arg→Cys	Nunobiki	$\alpha_1\beta_2$ Contact	Mild erythrocytosis

important sites for high-affinity variants because they greatly contribute to the stabilization of the T-conformation forming salt bonds (α141 Arg,[243,244] β 146 His[245–248]) and to the anchoring of the loose end in a pouch between the F and H helices (α140 Tyr, β 145 Tyr).[15] In addition, 2,3-DPG binding can be affected by changes of β 143 His[249–251] or β 82 Lys.[252–254]

Genetics

High-affinity traits are autosomal dominant. α Variants (Table 12.6) are usually less apparent than β variants (Table 12.7) for the reasons discussed above. Homozygotes or compound heterozygotes with β-thalassemia mutations are rare and expected to be viable only in variants with a moderate increase in oxygen affinity and preserved functional properties. For example, the high-affinity variant Hb Headington (β 72 (E16) Ser→Arg) exhibits a moderate decrease in co-operativity and a normal Bohr effect. In compound with $\delta\beta°$-thalassemia, a 62-year-old male has been reported to have erythrocytosis but no symptoms related to this abnormality.[255] Rather more severely, a patient with thalassemia intermedia has been reported to be compound heterozygous for $\delta\beta°$-thalassemia and Hb Crete (β 129 (H7) Ala→Pro), which is an unstable variant with a high oxygen affinity but normal Bohr effect.[256]

Clinical features

Most patients are asymptomatic but may present with a violaceous complexion or peripheral cyanosis. Splenomegaly occurs in some patients but is not common. Most commonly, high-affinity variants are detected on a routine blood count showing erythrocytosis. Hyperviscosity-related symptoms do not usually occur although there are anecdotal reports of exceptions.[257] In theory, oxygen delivery to the fetus will be affected if the mother's blood contains a high-affinity hemoglobin. In practice, however, this is not the case and for mothers with an exclusive or predominant occurrence of HbF, fetal outcome is normal.[258–260]

Laboratory diagnosis

The blood count shows erythrocytosis to be the commonest abnormality. The Hb ranges between 17 and 22 g/dl. In some patients, leukocytosis has been reported and Polycythemia vera must be carefully excluded in these cases.

Only about 50% of all high-affinity variants are detectable electrophoretically. The diagnosis can be established by measuring the oxygen dissociation curve of the hemolysate.[261] Additionally, PCR-amplified α- and β-globin genes can be sequenced directly.

Treatment

Variants with high oxygen affinity cause benign changes in the hematologic parameters. Erythrocytosis is the mode of compensation for decreased oxygen availability. Phlebotomy should not, therefore, generally be performed but exceptions may be the rare cases with symptoms related to hyperviscosity. It is important to establish the correct diagnosis in order to avoid inappropriate therapy.[262]

VARIANTS WITH DECREASED OXYGEN AFFINITY

Pathogenesis

In these rare variants the T conformation is stabilized, thus impeding oxygen uptake and facilitating oxygen unloading. This right shift of the oxygen binding curve leads to good oxygen availability to the peripheral tissues but a less active hematopoietic stimulus, and slight anemia is a possible feature.

Clinical features

Heterozygous individuals are healthy but may have slight anemia without functional consequences. Cyanosis due to incomplete oxygen loading is a feature of some low-affinity variants such as Hb Kansas (β 102 Asn → Thr), Hb Beth

247

Table 12.7 β-Globin variants with increased oxygen affinity.

Affected residue	Mutation	Variant name	Mechanism	Clinical characteristic
20(B2)	Val→Met	Olympia	?	Erythrocytosis
20(B2)	Val→Gly	Trollhättan	?	Mild erythrocytosis
23(B5)	Val→Phe	Palmerston North	?	Erythrocytosis
27(B9)	Ala→Val	Grange-Blanche	?	Erythrocytosis
34(B16)	Val→Phe	Pitie-Salpetriere	$\alpha_1\beta_2$ Contact	Erythrocytosis
36(C2)	Pro→Thr	Linköping	$\alpha_1\beta_2$ Contact	Erythrocytosis
36(C2)	Pro→Ser	North Chicago	$\alpha_1\beta_2$ Contact	Erythrocytosis
36(C2)	Pro→Arg	Sunnybrook	$\alpha_1\beta_2$ Contact	Mild erythrocytosis
37(C3)	Trp→Gly	Howick	$\alpha_1\beta_2$ Contact	Mild erythrocytosis
68(E12)	Leu→His	Brisbane	$\alpha_1\beta_2$ Contact	Mild erythrocytosis
72(E16)	Ser→Arg	Headington	?	Mild erythrocytosis
81(EF5)	Leu→Arg	Baylor	DPG binding	Erythrocytosis; hemolysis
82(EF6)	Lys→Thr	Rahere	DPG binding	Mild erythrocytosis
82(EF6)	Lys→Met	Helsinki	DPG binding	Erythrocytosis
86(F2)	Ala→Asp	Olomouc	DPG binding	Mild erythrocytosis
89(F5)	Ser→Asn	Creteil	?	Mild erythrocytosis
89(F5)	Ser→Arg	Vanderbilt	?	Mild erythrocytosis
89(F5)	Ser→Thr	Villaverde	?	Mild erythrocytosis
90(F6)	Glu→Asp	Pierre Benite	?	Erythrocytosis
94(FG1)	Asp→His	Barcelona	?	Mild erythrocytosis
94(FG1)	Asp→Asn	Bunbury	?	Mild erythrocytosis
96(FG3)	Leu→Val	Regina	?	Mild erythrocytosis
97(FG4)	His→Gln	Malmö	$\alpha_1\beta_2$ Contact	Erythrocytosis
97(FG4)	His→Leu	Wood	$\alpha_1\beta_2$ Contact	Erythrocytosis
99(G1)	Asp→Asn	Kempsey	$\alpha_1\beta_2$ Contact	Erythrocytosis
99(G1)	Asp→His	Yakima	$\alpha_1\beta_2$ Contact	Erythrocytosis
99(G1)	Asp→Ala	Radcliffe	$\alpha_1\beta_2$ Contact	Erythrocytosis
99(G1)	Asp→Tyr	Ypsilanti	$\alpha_1\beta_2$ Contact	Erythrocytosis
99(G1)	Asp→Gly	Hotel Dieu	$\alpha_1\beta_2$ Contact	Erythrocytosis
99(G1)	Asp→Val	Chemilly	$\alpha_1\beta_2$ Contact	Erythrocytosis
99(G1)	Asp→Glu	Coimbra	$\alpha_1\beta_2$ Contact	Erythrocytosis
100(G2)	Pro→Leu	Brigham	$\alpha_1\beta_2$ Contact	Erythrocytosis
100(G2)	Pro→Arg	New Mexico	$\alpha_1\beta_2$ Contact	Erythrocytosis
101(G3)	Glu→Lys	British Columbia	$\alpha_1\beta_2$ Contact	Mild erythrocytosis
101(G3)	Glu→Gly	Alberta	$\alpha_1\beta_2$ Contact	Erythrocytosis
101(G3)	Glu→Asp	Potomac	$\alpha_1\beta_2$ Contact	Erythrocytosis
103(G5)	Phe→Leu	Heathrow	?	Erythrocytosis
103(G5)	Phe→Ile	Saint Nazaire	?	Erythrocytosis
105(G7)	Leu→Phe	South Milwaukee	?	Erythrocytosis
109(G11)	Val→Met	San Diego	$\alpha_1\beta_2$ Contact	Erythrocytosis
109(G11)	Val→Leu	Johnstown	$\alpha_1\beta_2$ Contact	Mild erythrocytosis
124(H2)	Pro→Gln	Ty Gard	$\alpha_1\beta_2$ Contact	Erythrocytosis
130(H8)	Tyr→Ser	Nevers	?	Mild erythrocytosis
135(H13)	Ala→Pro	Altdorf	?	Mild erythrocytosis
139(H17)	Asn→Tyr	Aurora	?	Mild erythrocytosis
140(H18)	Ala→Thr	Saint-Jacques	?	Erythrocytosis
140(H18)	Ala→Val	Puttelange	?	Erythrocytosis
142(H20)	Ala→Asp	Ohio	?	Erythrocytosis
143(H21)	His→Arg	Abruzzo	DPG contact	Erythrocytosis
143(H21)	His→Glu	Little Rock	DPG contact	Erythrocytosis
143(H21)	His→Pro	Syracuse	DPG contact	Erythrocytosis
144(HC1)	Lys→Asn	Andrew-Minneapolis	$\beta\beta$ Contact	Erythrocytosis
144(HC1)	Lys→Glu	Mito	$\beta\beta$ Contact	Mild erythrocytosis
145(HC2)	Tyr→His	Bethesda	$\beta\beta$ Contact	Erythrocytosis
145(HC2)	Tyr→Cys	Rainier	$\beta\beta$ Contact	Erythrocytosis
145(HC2)	Tyr→Term	Osler	$\beta\beta$ Contact	Erythrocytosis
145(HC2)	Tyr→Term	McKees Rocks	$\beta\beta$ Contact	Erythrocytosis
146(HC3)	His→Asp	Hiroshima	$\beta\beta$ Contact	Mild erythrocytosis
146(HC3)	His→Pro	York	$\beta\beta$ Contact	Erythrocytosis
146(HC3)	His→Leu	Cowtown	$\beta\beta$ Contact	Erythrocytosis

Israel (β 102 Asn→Ser) and Hb St. Mande (β 102 Asn→Tyr). Exercise tolerance, however, is not affected, because of the facilitated oxygen delivery.[263–266] As there are no functionally significant clinical symptoms, treatment is not required.

HbM ANOMALIES

The HbM anomalies are rare variants that occur throughout the world. They are characterized by amino acid substitutions of the heme-iron binding region that cause permanent and virtually complete oxidation of the heme iron to the ferric (Fe^{3+}) form. HbMs are therefore unable to carry oxygen and have a typical methemoglobin absorption spectrum. Instability is not a prominent feature of the M-hemoglobins which also differentiates M hemoglobins from the unstable variants with a high rate of spontaneous oxidation such as Hb Freiburg, Hb Tübingen and Hb St. Louis. Heterozygotes are cyanotic without any other clinical symptoms.

Pathogenesis

Normal hemoglobin is slowly oxidized to methemoglobin at a calculated rate of $\approx 3\%$ daily. There are 5 known adult and 2 fetal HbM variants (Table 12.8). Six of these are His→Tyr substitutions of the the proximal (F8) or the distal (E7) heme-binding site. Tyr forms a covalent bond with ferric iron which is thus stabilized.[267] In HbM Milwaukee, the hydrophobic Val at position β 67 is substituted by the polar Glu which binds covalently to the ferric heme iron exactly one helical winding carboxy-terminal of His E7.[268] Methemoglobin formation stabilizes the R-quaternary conformation, which obliterates hemoglobin function both directly by blocking oxygen loading of the affected subunits and indirectly by increasing oxygen affinity of the normal subunits, thus impeding oxygen delivery.[269,270]

Normally, methemoglobin is efficiently reduced to ferrohemoglobin by the NADH-dependent cytochrome b_5 reductase and to a much lesser extent by the NADPH-dependent flavin reductase.[271–276] The normal methemoglobin concentration is <1%. Three of the 5 known adult M hemoglobins cannot be enzymatically reduced and the other 2 are oxidized too fast for the enzyme to be effective.[277] Clinical tolerance of methemoglobin depends on the acuteness of its formation which is very much analogous to the tolerance of anemia. In chronic cases such as those with M hemoglobins or those with cytochrome b_5 reductase deficiency,[278] Met-Hb concentrations of up to 40% are well tolerated. In contrast, when methemoglobinemia develops suddenly following intoxication with oxidant drugs or chemicals, symptoms of hypoxia may start at levels of 20%.[279] Toxic methemoglobinemia is most likely to occur in infants, whose cytochrome b_5 reductase is only about half as active as that of adults.[280]

Genetics and clinical features

M hemoglobins are inherited in an autosomal dominant fashion, although spontaneous mutations are common. Heterozygotes are cyanotic without impairment of physical abilities. The lower α- than β-M hemoglobin levels can be explained by the presence of 4 α- but only 2 β-globin genes in the genome (see above). Homozygotes have not yet been described. Newborns with HbFM variants present with transient cyanosis which disappears with the fetal to adult hemoglobin switch.

Laboratory diagnosis

In alkaline hemoglobin electrophoresis, M hemoglobins may be detected as a grayish-green band that migrates slightly more slowly than HbA. At pH 7.0, HbM can be separated from normal methemoglobin following ferricyanide oxidation. The absorption spectrum of HbM at pH 6.8–7.0 is characteristically changed in comparison to normal methemoglobin, although the spectrum of Hb Milwaukee is difficult to differentiate (Fig. 12.11). The globin gene mutation can be detected by DNA analysis.

For routine hematologic analysis, the reduced reactivity of HbM with KCN must be considered. The total hemoglobin level may be underestimated if the commonly used conversion to cyanmethemoglobin with Drabkin's solution is employed. Incubation times must be prolonged up to 1 h.

Treatment

The most important treatment is to establish the diagnosis (Table 12.9) and to reassure the patient and parents of the normal physical prognosis. Unnecessary and possibly

Table 12.8 HbM anomalies.

	Structure	Hb (g/dl)	Variant (%)	Hematology
HbM Boston[267]	α58 (E7) His→Tyr	15	25–32	Cyanosis
HbM Iwate[281]	α87 (F8) His→Tyr	17	20–27	Cyanosis
HbM Saskatoon[282]	β63 (E7) His→Tyr	13–16	35–40	Cyanosis and some degree of haemolysis
HbM Hyde Park[283]	β92 (F8) His→Tyr	10–12.5	25–40	Cyanosis and some degree of haemolysis
HbM Milwaukee[284]	β67 (E11) Val→Glu	14–15	26–40	Cyanosis
HbFM Osaka[285]	γ63 (E7) His→Tyr			Cyanosis of the newborn
HbFM Fort Ripley[286,287]	γ92 (F8) His→Tyr			Cyanosis of the newborn

Table 12.9 Differential diagnosis of cyanosis.

Inadequate oxygenation
  Pulmonary disease
  Cardiac disease with right to left shunting
  Congestive heart failure and shock
  Hb variants with decreased oxygen affinity

Methemoglobinemia
  Inherited
  ● Cytochrome b_5 reductase deficiency
  ● M hemoglobins
  ● Unstable hemoglobins with a high rate of spontaneous oxidation
    (Hb Freiburg, Hb Tübingen, Hb St. Louis)

  Acquired
  ● Drugs
  ● Toxins
  ● Cows' milk protein intolerance
  ● *Helicobacter pylori* infection in infancy

Sulfhemoglobinemia
  Acquired
  ● Toxins
  ● Drugs

dangerous diagnostic procedures to exclude heart and lung disease must be avoided. Redox agents such as methylene-blue or ascorbic acid have no effect.

Cyanosis occurs at levels of normal deoxyhemoglobin >5 g/dl. It follows that acquired conditions that result in inadaequate oxygenation are the commonest causes of cyanosis. In severe polycythemia, cyanosis may occur in the absence of hypoxemia. Methemoglobinemia or sulfhemo-globinemia are rare causes of cyanosis (>1.5 g/dl Met-Hb; >0.5 g/dl Sulf-Hb) and may be inherited or acquired.

Acknowledgement

I am grateful to Profesor Kleihauer for his critical advice on the manuscript.

REFERENCES

1. Weatherall DJ, Clegg JB. *The Thalassaemia Syndromes*. Oxford: Blackwell Scientific Publications, 1981
2. Huisman THJ, Carver MFH, Efremov GD. *A Syllabus of Human Hemoglobin Variants (1996)*. Augusta, Georgia: The Sickle Cell Anemia Foundation, 1996
3. Bunn HF, Forget BG. *Hemoglobin: Molecular, Genetic and Clinical Aspects*. Philadelphia: WB Saunders, 1986
4. Komiyama NH, Shih DT, Looker D, Tame J, Nagai K. Was the loss of the D helix in α globin a functionally neutral mutation? *Nature* 1991; **352**: 349–351
5. Perutz MF, Lehmann H. Molecular pathology of human haemoglobin. *Nature* 1968; **219**: 902–909
6. Perutz MF, Muirhead H, Cox JM, Goaman LC. Three-dimensional Fourier synthesis of horse oxyhaemoglobin at 2.8 A resolution: the atomic model. *Nature* 1968; **219**: 131–139
7. Perutz MF, Miurhead H, Cox JM *et al*. Three-dimensional Fourier synthesis of horse oxyhaemoglobin at 2.8 A resolution: (1) X-ray analysis. *Nature* 1968; **219**: 29–32
8. Fermi G, Perutz MF, Shaanan B, Fourme R. The crystal structure of human deoxyhaemoglobin at 1.74 A resolution. *J Mol Biol* 1984; **175**: 159–174
9. Liddington R, Derewenda Z, Dodson E, Hubbard R, Dodson G. High resolution crystal structures and comparisons of T-state deoxyhaemo-globin and two liganded T-state haemoglobins: T(α-oxy)haemoglobin and T(met)haemoglobin. *J Mol Biol* 1992; **228**: 551–579
10. Paoli M, Liddington R, Tame J, Wilkinson A, Dodson G. Crystal structure of T state haemoglobin with oxygen bound at all four haems. *J Mol Biol* 1996; **256**: 775–792
11. Fermi G, Perutz M. Hemoglobin and myoglobin. In: Philipps DC, Richards FM (eds) *Atlas of Molecular Structures in Biology*. Oxford: Clarendon Press, 1981
12. Ackers GK, Doyle ML, Myers D, Daugherty MA. Molecular code for cooperativity in hemoglobin. *Science* 1992; **255**: 54–63
13. Perutz MF, Shih DT, Williamson D. The chloride effect in human haemoglobin. A new kind of allosteric mechanism. *J Mol Biol* 1994; **239**: 555–560
14. Monod J, Wyman J, Changeux JP. On the nature of allosteric transtions: A plausible model. *J Mol Biol* 1965; **12**: 88–95
15. Perutz MF. Stereochemistry of cooperative effects in haemoglobin. *Nature* 1970; **228**: 726–739
16. Perutz MF, Kilmartin JV, Nishikura K, Fogg JH, Butler PJ, Rollema HS. Identification of residues contributing to the Bohr effect of human haemoglobin. *J Mol Biol* 1980; **138**: 649–668
17. Kilmartin JV, Fogg JH, Perutz MF. Role of C-terminal histidine in the alkaline Bohr effect of human haemoglobin. *Biochemistry* 1980; **19**: 3189–3183
18. Nishikura K. Identification of histidine-122α in human haemoglobin as one of the unknown alkaline Bohr groups by hydrogen-tritium exchange. *Biochem J* 1978; **173**: 651–657
19. Shih DT, Luisi BF, Miyazaki G, Perutz MF, Nagai K. A mutagenic study of the allosteric linkage of His (HC3) 146β in haemoglobin. *J Mol Biol* 1993; **230**: 1291–1296
20. Perutz MF, Muirhead H, Mazzarella L, Crowther RA, Greer J, Kilmartin JV. Identification of residues responsible for the alkaline Bohr effect in haemoglobin. Nature 1969; **222**: 1240–1243
21. Kilmartin JV, Breen JJ, Roberts GC, Ho C. Direct measurement of the pK values of an alkaline Bohr group in human hemoglobin. *Proc Natl Acad Sci USA* 1973; **70**: 1246–1249
22. Bauer C, Schroder E. Carbamino compounds of haemoglobin in human adult and foetal blood. *J Physiol Lond* 1972; **227**: 457–471
23. Kelly RM, Hui HL, Noble RW. Chloride acts as a novel negative heterotropic effector of hemoglobin Rothschild (β 37 Trp→Arg) in solution. *Biochemistry* 1994; **33**: 4363–4367
24. Bonaventura C, Arumugam M, Cashon R, Bonaventura J, Moo Penn WF. Chloride masks effects of opposing positive charges in Hb A and Hb Hinsdale (β 139 Asn→Lys) that can modulate cooperativity as well as oxygen affinity. *J Mol Biol* 1994; **239**: 561–568
25. Rollema HS, de Bruin SH, Janssen LH, van Os GA. The effect of potassium chloride on the Bohr effect of human haemoglobin. *J Biol Chem* 1975; **250**: 1333–1339
26. Chanutin A, Curnish RR. Effect of organic and inorganic phosphates on the oxygen equilibrium of human erythrocytes. *Arch Biochem Biophys* 1967; **121**: 96–102
27. Benesch R, Benesch RE. The effect of organic phosphates from the human erythrocyte on the allosteric properties of hemoglobin. *Biochem Biophys Res Commun* 1967; **26**: 162–167
28. Gupta RK, Benovic JL, Rose ZB. Location of the allosteric site for 2,3-bisphosphoglycerate on human oxy- and deoxyhemoglobin as observed by magnetic resonance spectroscopy. *J Biol Chem* 1979; **254**: 8250–8255
29. Arnone A. X-ray diffraction study of binding of 2,3-diphospho-glycerate to human deoxyhemoglobin. *Nature* 1972; **237**: 146–149
30. Boissel JP, Kasper TJ, Shah SC, Malone JI, Bunn HF. Amino-terminal processing of proteins: hemoglobin South Florida, a variant

with retention of initiator methionine and N α-acetylation. *Proc Natl Acad Sci USA* 1985; **82**: 8448–8452

31. Vasseur C, Blouquit Y, Kister J *et al*. Hemoglobin Thionville. An α-chain variant with a substitution of a glutamate for valine at NA-1 and having an acetylated methionine NH2 terminus. *J Biol Chem* 1992; **267**: 12682–12691

32. Boissel JP, Kasper TJ, Bunn HF. Cotranslational amino-terminal processing of cytosolic proteins. Cell-free expression of site-directed mutants of human hemoglobin. *J Biol Chem* 1988; **263**: 8443–8449

33. Humphries RK, Ley T, Turner P, Moulton AD, Nienhuis AW. Differences in human α-, β- and δ-globin gene expression in monkey kidney cells. *Cell* 1982; **30**: 173–183

34. LaFlamme S, Acuto S, Markowitz D, Vick L, Landschultz W, Bank A. Expression of chimeric human β- and δ-globin genes during erythroid differentiation. *J Biol Chem* 1987; **262**: 4819–4826

35. Ross J, Pizarro A. Human β and δ globin messenger RNAs turn over at different rates. *J Mol Biol* 1983; **167**: 607–617

36. Bunn HF, Forget BG. *Hemoglobin: Molecular, Genetic and Clinical Aspects*. Philadelphia: WB Saunders, 1986, pp 417–421

37. Frier JA, Perutz MF. Structure of human foetal deoxyhaemoglobin. *J Mol Biol* 1977; **112**: 97–112

38. Perutz MF. Mechanism of denaturation of haemoglobin by alkali. *Nature* 1974; **247**: 341–344

39. Schroeder WA, Huisman TH, Shelton JR *et al*. Evidence for multiple structural genes for the γ chain of human fetal hemoglobin. *Proc Natl Acad Sci USA* 1968; **60**: 537–544

40. Schroeder WA. The synthesis and chemical heterogeneity of human fetal hemoglobin: overview and present concepts. *Hemoglobin* 1980; **4**: 431–446

41. Ricco G, Mazza U, Turi RM *et al*. Significance of a new type of human fetal hemoglobin carrying a replacement isoleucine replaced by threonine at position 75 (E 19) of the γ chain. *Hum Genet* 1976; **32**: 305–313

42. Bard H. The postnatal decline of hemoglobin F synthesis in normal full-term infants. *J Clin Invest* 1975; **55**: 395–398

43. Kleihauer E, Braun HKB. Demonstration von fetalem Hämoglobin in den Erythrocyten eines Blutausstrichs. *Klinische Wochenschrift* 1957; **35**: 637–638

44. Kleihauer E, Hötzel U, Betke K. Die materno-fetale Transfusion. *Monatschrift Kinderheilkunde* 1967; **115**: 145–146

45. Kar BC, Satapathy RK, Kulozik AE *et al*. Sickle cell disease in Orissa State, India. *Lancet* 1986; **2**: 1198–1201

46. Padmos MA, Roberts GT, Sackey K *et al*. Two different forms of homozygous sickle cell disease occur in Saudi Arabia. *Br J Haematol* 1991; **79**: 93–98

47. Kulozik AE, Wainscoat JS, Serjeant GR *et al*. Geographical survey of βˢ-globin gene haplotypes: evidence for an independent Asian origin of the sickle-cell mutation. *Am J Hum Genet* 1986; **39**: 239–244

48. Kulozik AE, Kar BC, Satapathy RK, Serjeant BE, Serjeant GR, Weatherall DJ. Fetal hemoglobin levels and βˢ-globin haplotypes in an Indian population with sickle cell disease. *Blood* 1987; **69**: 1742–1746

49. Thein SL, Sampietro M, Rohde K *et al*. Detection of a major gene for heterocellular hereditary persistence of fetal hemoglobin after accounting for genetic modifiers. *Am J Hum Genet* 1994; **54**: 214–228

50. Chang YC, Smith KD, Moore RD, Serjeant GR, Dover GJ. An analysis of fetal hemoglobin variation in sickle cell disease: the relative contributions of the X-linked factor, β-globin haplotypes, α-globin gene number, gender, and age. *Blood* 1995; **85**: 1111–1117

51. Craig JE, Rochette J, Fisher CA *et al*. Dissecting the loci controlling fetal hemoglobin production on chromosomes 11p and 6q by the regressive approach. *Nature Genet* 1996; **12**: 58–64

52. Charache S, Terrin ML, Moore RD *et al*. Effect of hydroxyurea on the frequency of painful crises in sickle cell anemia. Investigators of the Multicenter Study of Hydroxyurea in Sickle Cell Anemia [see comments]. *N Engl J Med* 1995; **332**: 1317–1322

53. Weatherall DJ, Clegg JB, Wood WG. A model for the persistence or reactivation of fetal hemoglobin production. *Lancet* 1976; **ii**: 660–663

54. Wood WG. Increased HbF in adult life. *Baillière's Clin Haematol* 1993; **6**: 177–213

55. Perrine SP, Ginder GD, Faller DV *et al*. A short-term trial of butyrate to stimulate fetal-globin-gene expression in the β-globin disorders [see comments]. *N Engl J Med* 1993; **328**: 81–86

56. Sher GD, Ginder GD, Little J, Yang S, Dover GJ, Olivieri NF. Extended therapy with intravenous arginine butyrate in patients with β-hemoglobinopathies. *N Engl J Med* 1995; **332**: 1606–1610

57. Bunn HF, Forget BG. *Hemoglobin: Molecular, Genetic and Clinical Aspects*. Philadelphia: WB Saunders, 1986, p 74

58. Weatherall DJ, Brown MJ. Juvenile chronic myeloid leukaemia. *Lancet* 1970; **1**: 526

59. Maurer HS, Vida LN, Honig GR. Similarities of the erythrocytes in juvenile chronic myelogenous leukemia to fetal erythrocytes. *Blood* 1972; **39**: 778–784

60. Pagnier J, Lopez M, Mathiot C *et al*. An unusual case of leukemia with high fetal hemoglobin: demonstration of abnormal hemoglobin synthesis localized in a red cell clone. *Blood* 1977; **50**: 249–258

61. Krauss JS, Rodriguez AR, Milner PF. Erythroleukemia with high fetal hemoglobin after therapy for ovarian carcinoma. *Am J Clin Pathol* 1981; **76**: 721–722

62. Miniero R, David O, Saglio G, Paschero C, Nicola P. The Hbf in Fanconi's anemia (author's transl). *Pediatr Med Chir* 1981; **3**: 167–170

63. Alter BP, Rappeport JM, Huisman TH, Schroeder WA, Nathan DG. Fetal erythropoiesis following bone marrow transplantation. *Blood* 1976; **48**: 843–853

64. Huehns ER, Flynn FV, Butler EA, Beaven GH. Two new haemoglobin variants in a young human embryo. *Nature* 1961; **189**: 1877–1879

65. Capp GL, Rigas DA, Jones RT. Evidence for a new haemoglobin chain (ζ-chain). *Nature* 1970; **228**: 278–280

66. Capp GL, Rigas DA, Jones RT. Hemoglobin Portland 1: a new human hemoglobin unique in structure. *Science* 1967; **157**: 65–66

67. Hofmann O, Mould R, Brittain T. Allosteric modulation of oxygen binding to the three human embryonic haemoglobins. *Biochem J* 1995; **306**: 367–370

68. Todd D, Lai MC, Beaven GH, Huehns ER. The abnormal haemoglobins in homozygous α-thalassaemia. *Br J Haematol* 1970; **19**: 27–31

69. Chui DH, Wong SC, Chung SW, Patterson M, Bhargava S, Poon MC. Embryonic ζ-globin chains in adults: a marker for α-thalassemia-1 haplotype due to a greater than 17.5-kb deletion. *N Engl J Med* 1986; **314**: 76–79

70. Chung SW, Wong SC, Clarke BJ, Patterson M, Walker WH, Chui DH. Human embryonic ζ-globin chains in adult patients with α-thalassemias. *Proc Natl Acad Sci USA* 1984; **81**: 6188–6191

71. Weatherall DJ, Clegg JB. *The Thalassaemia Syndromes*. Oxford: Blackwell Scientific, 1981, pp 58–70

72. Grosveld F, van Assendelft GB, Greaves DR, Kollias G. Position-independent, high-level expression of the human β-globin gene in transgenic mice. *Cell* 1987; **51**: 975–985

73. Tuan D, Solomon W, Li Q, London IM. The "β-like-globin" gene domain in human erythroid cells. *Proc Natl Acad Sci USA* 1985; **82**: 6384–6388

74. Sharpe JA, Chan Thomas PS, Lida J, Ayyub H, Wood WG, Higgs DR. Analysis of the human α globin upstream regulatory element (HS-40) in transgenic mice. *Embo J* 1992; **11**: 4565–4572

75. Vyas P, Vickers MA, Simmons DL, Ayyub H, Craddock CF, Higgs DR. Cis-acting sequences regulating expression of the human α-globin cluster lie within constitutively open chromatin. *Cell* 1992; **69**: 781–793

76. Amrolia PJ, Cunningham JM, Ney P, Nienhuis AW, Jane SM. Identification of two novel regulatory elements within the 5'-untranslated region of the human A γ-globin gene. *J Biol Chem* 1995; **270**: 12892–12898

77. Jane SM, Ney PA, Vanin EF, Gumucio DL, Nienhuis AW. Identification of a stage selector element in the human γ-globin gene promoter that fosters preferential interaction with the 5' HS2 enhancer when in competition with the β-promoter. *Embo J* 1992; **11**: 2961–2969

78. Raich N, Enver T, Nakamoto B, Josephson B, Papayannopoulou T, Stamatoyannopoulos G. Autonomous developmental control of human embryonic globin gene switching in transgenic mice. *Science* 1990; **250**: 1147–1149

79. Raich N, Clegg CH, Grofti J, Romeo PH, Stamatoyannopoulos G. GATA1 and YY1 are developmental repressors of the human ε-globin gene. *Embo J* 1995; **14**: 801–809

80. Orkin SH. Globin gene regulation and switching: circa 1990. *Cell* 1990; **63**: 665–672

81. Orkin SH. Regulation of globin gene expression in erythroid cells. *Eur J Biochem* 1995; **231**: 271–281

82. Dacie JV, Lewis SM. *Practical Haematology*. Edinburgh: Churchill Livingstone, 1984, pp 179–199

83. Betke K, Marti HR, Schlicht I. Estimation of small percentages of foetal hemoglobin. *Nature* 1959; **184**: 1877–1878

84. Kleihauer E, Kohne E, Kulozik AE. *Anomale Hämoglobine und Thalassämiesyndrome*. Landsberg: Ecomed, 1996, pp 57–67

85. Monte M, Beuzard Y, Rosa J. Mapping of several abnormal hemoglobins by horizontal polyacrylamide gel isoelectric focusing. *Am J Clin Pathol* 1976; **66**: 753–759

86. Sinha P, Galacteros F, Righetti PG, Kohlmeier M, Kottgen E. Analysis of hemoglobin variants using immobilized pH gradients. *Eur J Clin Chem Clin Biochem* 1993; **31**: 91–96

87. Rees DC, Rochette J, Schofield C et al. A novel silent posttranslational mechanism converts methionine to aspartate in hemoglobin Bristol (β 67 [E11] Val-Met→Asp). *Blood* 1996; **88**: 341–348

88. Mullis KB, Faloona FA. Specific synthesis of DNA *in vitro* via a polymerase-catalyzed chain reaction. *Methods Enzymol* 1987; **155**: 335–350

89. Mullis K, Faloona F, Scharf S, Saiki R, Horn G, Erlich H. Specific enzymatic amplification of DNA *in vitro*: the polymerase chain reaction. *Cold Spring Harb Symp Quant Biol* 1986; **51**: 263–273

90. Chehab FF, Doherty M, Cai SP, Kan YW, Cooper S, Rubin EM. Detection of sickle cell anemia and thalassaemias [letter]. *Nature* 1987; **329**: 293–294 [published erratum appears in *Nature* 1987; **329**: 678]

91. Kulozik AE, Lyons J, Kohne E, Bartram CR, Kleihauer E. Rapid and non-radioactive prenatal diagnosis of β thalassaemia and sickle cell disease: application of the polymerase chain reaction (PCR). *Br J Haematol* 1988; **70**: 455–458

92. Thein SL, Hinton J. A simple and rapid method of direct sequencing using Dynabeads. *Br J Haematol* 1991; **79**: 113–115

93. George PM, Myles T, Williamson D, Higuchi R, Symmans WA, Brennan SO. A family with haemolytic anaemia and three β-globins: the deletion in haemoglobin Atlanta-Coventry (β 75 Leu→Pro, 141 Leu deleted) is not present at the nucleotide level. *Br J Haematol* 1992; **81**: 93–98

94. Wajcman H, Vasseur C, Blouquit Y et al. Hemoglobin Redondo [β 92 (F8) His→Asn]: an unstable hemoglobin variant associated with heme loss which occurs in two forms. *Am J Hematol* 1991; **38**: 194–200

95. Brennan SO, Shaw J, Allen J, George PM. β 141 Leu is not deleted in the unstable haemoglobin Atlanta-Coventry but is replaced by a novel amino acid of mass 129 daltons. *Br J Haematol* 1992; **81**: 99–103

96. Wajcman H, Kister J, Vasseur C et al. Structure of the EF corner favors deamidation of asparaginyl residues in hemoglobin: the example of Hb La Roche-sur-Yon [β 81 (EF5) Leu→His]. *Biochim Biophys Acta* 1992; **1138**: 127–132

97. Old JM, Fitches A, Heath C et al. First-trimester fetal diagnosis for hemoglobinopathies: report on 200 cases. *Lancet* 1986; **2**: 763–767

98. Rieder RF. Human hemoglobin stability and instability: molecular mechanisms and some clinical correlations. *Semin Hematol* 1974; **11**: 423–440

99. Williamson D. The unstable hemoglobins. *Blood Rev* 1993; **7**: 146–163

100. Jacob H, Winterhalter K. Unstable hemoglobins: the role of heme loss in Heinz body formation. *Proc Natl Acad Sci USA* 1970; **65**: 697–701

101. Jacob HS, Winterhalter KH. The role of hemoglobin heme loss in Heinz body formation: studies with a partially heme-deficient hemo-

102. Low PS, Waugh SM, Zinke K, Drenckhahn D. The role of hemoglobin denaturation and band 3 clustering in red blood cell aging. *Science* 1985; 227: 531–533

103. Waugh SM, Willardson BM, Kannan R et al. Heinz bodies induce clustering of band 3, glycophorin, and ankyrin in sickle cell erythrocytes. The role of hemoglobin denaturation and band 3 clustering in red blood cell aging. *J Clin Invest* 1986; **78**: 1155–1160

104. Arjona SN, Eloy Garcia JM, Gu LH, Smetanina NS, Huisman TH. The dominant β-thalassaemia in a Spanish family is due to a frameshift that introduces an extra CGG codon (=arginine) at the 5' end of the second exon. *Br J Haematol* 1996; **93**: 841–844

105. Thein SL, Hesketh C, Taylor P et al. Molecular basis for dominantly inherited inclusion body β-thalassemia. *Proc Natl Acad Sci USA* 1990; **87**: 3924–3928

106. Girodon E, Ghanem N, Vidaud M et al. Rapid molecular characterization of mutations leading to unstable hemoglobin β-chain variants. *Ann Hematol* 1992; **65**: 188–192

107. Coleman MB, Steinberg MH, Adams JGd. Hemoglobin Terre Haute arginine β 106. A posthumous correction to the original structure of hemoglobin Indianapolis. *J Biol Chem* 1991; **266**: 5798–5800

108. Kazazian HH Jr, Dowling CE, Hurwitz RL, Coleman M, Stopeck A, Adams JGD. Dominant thalassemia-like phenotypes associated with mutations in exon 3 of the β-globin gene. *Blood* 1992; **79**: 3014–3018

109. Thein SL, Wood WG, Wickramasinghe SN, Galvin MC. β-thalassemia unlinked to the β-globin gene in an English family. *Blood* 1993; **82**: 961–967

110. Thein SL, Best S, Sharpe J, Paul B, Clark DJ, Brown MJ. Hemoglobin Chesterfield (β 28 Leu→Arg) produces the phenotype of inclusion body β thalassemia [letter]. *Blood* 1991; **77**: 2791–2793

111. Jones RV, Grimes AJ, Carrell RW, Lehmann H. Koln haemoglobinopathy. Further data and a comparison with other hereditary Heinz body anemias. *Br J Haematol* 1967; **13**: 394–408

112. Carrell RW, Lehmann H, Hutchison HE. Haemoglobin Koln (β-98 valine→methionine): an unstable protein causing inclusion-body anaemia. *Nature* 1966; 210: 915–916

113. Aksoy M, Erdem S, Efremov GD et al. Hemoglobin Istanbul: substitution of glutamine for histidine in a proximal histidine (F8(92)). *J Clin Invest* 1972; **51**: 2380–2387

114. Spivak VA, Molchanova TP, Postnikov Yu V, Aseeva EA, Lutsenko IN, Tokarev Yu N. A new abnormal hemoglobin: Hb Mozhaisk β 92 (F8) His leads to Arg. *Hemoglobin* 1982; **6**: 169–181

115. Finney R, Casey R, Lehmann H, Walker W. Hb Newcastle: β92 (F8) His replaced by Pro. *FEBS Lett* 1975; **60**: 435–438

116. Steadman JH, Yates A, Huehns ER. Idiopathic Heinz body anaemia: Hb-Bristol (β 67 (E11) Val to Asp). *Br J Haematol* 1970; **18**: 435–446

117. Clegg JB, Weatherall DJ, Boon WH, Mustafa D. Two new haemoglobin variants involving proline substitutions. *Nature* 1969; **222**: 379–380

118. Perutz MF, Kendrew JC, Watson HC. Structure and function of haemoglobin. II. Some relations between polypeptide chain configuration and amino acid sequence. *J Mol Biol* 1965; **13**: 669–678

119. Brimhall B, Jones RT, Baur EW, Motulsky AG. Structural characterization of hemoglobin Tacoma. *Biochemistry* 1969; **8**: 2125–2129

120. Rieder RF, Oski FA, Clegg JB. Hemoglobin Philly (β 35 tyrosine phenylalanine): studies in the molecular pathology of hemoglobin. *J Clin Invest* 1969; **48**: 1627–1642

121. Weiss IM, Liebhaber SA. Erythroid cell-specific determinants of α-globin mRNA stability. *Mol Cell Biol* 1994; **14**: 8123–8132

122. Weiss IM, Liebhaber SA. Erythroid cell-specific mRNA stability elements in the α 2-globin 3' nontranslated region. *Mol Cell Biol* 1995; **15**: 2457–2465

123. Liebhaber SA, Kan YW. Differentiation of the mRNA transcripts originating from the α1- and α2-globin loci in normals and α-thalassemics. *J Clin Invest* 1981; **68**: 439–446

124. Liebhaber SA, Cash FE, Ballas SK. Human α-globin gene expression.

The dominant role of the α2-locus in mRNA and protein synthesis. *J Biol Chem* 1986; **261**: 15327–15333

125. Darbellay R, Mach Pascual S, Rose K, Graf J, Beris P. Haemoglobin Tunis-Bizerte: a new α1 globin 129 Leu→Pro unstable variant with thalassaemic phenotype. *Br J Haematol* 1995; **90**: 71–76

126. Ohba Y, Miyaji T, Hattori Y, Fuyuno K, Matsuoka M. Unstable hemoglobins in Japan. *Hemoglobin* 1980; **4**: 307–312

127. Lee Potter JP, Deacon Smith RA, Simpkiss MJ, Kamuzora H, Lehmann H. A new cause of haemolytic anemia in the newborn. A description of an unstable fetal hemoglobin: F Poole, α2-G-γ2 130 trptophan yields glycine. *J Clin Pathol* 1975; **28**: 317–320

128. Galacteros F, Loukopoulos D, Fessas P *et al*. Hemoglobin Koln occurring in association with a β zero thalassemia: hematologic and functional consequences. *Blood* 1989; **74**: 496–500

129. Vassilopoulos G, Papassotiriou I, Voskaridou E *et al*. Hb Arta [β45 (CD4) Phe→Cys]: a new unstable haemoglobin with reduced oxygen affinity in trans with β-thalassaemia. *Br J Haematol* 1995; **91**: 595–601

130. Curuk MA, Dimovski AJ, Baysal E *et al*. Hb Adana or α 2 (59) (E8) Gly→Asp β2, a severely unstable α1-globin variant, observed in combination with the -(α)20.5 Kb α-thal-1 deletion in two Turkish patients. *Am J Hematol* 1993; **44**: 270–275

131. Srivastava P, Kaeda JS, Roper D, Vulliamy TJ, Buckley M, Luzzatto L. Severe hemolytic anemia associated with the homozygous state for an unstable hemoglobin variant (Hb Bushwick). *Blood* 1995; **86**: 1977–1982

132. Serjeant GR, Serjeant BE, Thomas PW, Anderson MJ, Patou G, Pattison JR. Human parvovirus infection in homozygous sickle cell disease [see comments]. *Lancet* 1993; **341**: 1237–1240

133. Jones RT, Brimhall B, Huisman TH, Kleihauer E, Betke K. Hemoglobin Freiburg: abnormal hemoglobin due to deletion of a single amino acid residue. *Science* 1966; **154**: 1024–1027

134. Jackson JM, Yates A, Huehns ER. Haemoglobin Perth: β-32 (B14) Leu leads to Pro, an unstable haemoglobin causing haemolysis. *Br J Haematol* 1973; **25**: 607–610

135. Dianzani I, Ramus S, Cotton RG, Camaschella C. A spontaneous mutation causing unstable Hb Hammersmith: detection of the β42 TTT—TCT change by CCM and direct sequencing. *Br J Haematol* 1991; **79**: 127–129

136. Linet MS, Nyren O, Gridley G *et al*. Causes of death among patients surviving at least one year following splenectomy. *Am J Surg* 1996; **172**: 320–323

137. Lehne G, Hannisdal E, Langholm R, Nome O. A 10-year experience with splenectomy in patients with malignant non-Hodgkin's lymphoma at the Norwegian Radium Hospital. *Cancer* 1994; **74**: 933–939

138. Cullingford GL, Watkins DN, Watts AD, Mallon DF. Severe late postsplenectomy infection. *Br J Surg* 1991; **78**: 716–721

139. Lane PA. The spleen in children. *Curr Opin Pediatr* 1995; **7**: 36–41

140. Reid MM. Splenectomy, sepsis, immunisation, and guidelines [see comments]. *Lancet* 1994; **344**: 970–971

141. Egan EL, Fairbanks VF. Postsplenectomy erythrocytosis in hemoglobin Koln disease. *N Engl J Med* 1973; **288**: 929–931

142. Beutler E, Lang A, Lehmann H. Hemoglobin Duarte: (α2 β2 62 (E6) Ala leads to Pro): a new unstable hemoglobin with increased oxygen affinity. *Blood* 1974; **43**: 527–535

143. Thuret I, Bardakdjian J, Badens C *et al*. Priapism following splenectomy in an unstable hemoglobin: hemoglobin Olmsted β141 (H19) Leu→Arg. *Am J Hematol* 1996; **51**: 133–136

144. Rao KR, Patel AR. Priapism and thalassaemia intermedia [letter]. *Br J Surg* 1986; **73**: 1048

145. Jackson N, Franklin IM, Hughes MA. Recurrent priapism following splenectomy for thalassaemia intermedia. *Br J Surg* 1986; **73**: 678

146. Macchia P, Massei F, Nardi M, Favre C, Brunori E, Barba V. Thalassaemia intermedia and recurrent priapism following splenectomy [letter] [see comments]. *Haematologica* 1990; **75**: 486–487

147. Jayabose S, Tugal O, Sandoval C *et al*. Clinical and hematologic effects of hydroxyurea in children with sickle cell anemia. *J Pediatr* 1996; **129**: 559–565

148. Scott JP, Hillery CA, Brown ER, Misiewicz V, Labotka RJ. Hydroxyurea therapy in children severely affected with sickle cell disease. *J Pediatr* 1996; **128**: 820–828

149. Ferster A, Vermylen C, Cornu G *et al*. Hydroxyurea for treatment of severe sickle cell anemia: a pediatric clinical trial. *Blood* 1996; **88**: 1960–1964

150. Claster S, Vichinsky E. First report of reversal of organ dysfunction in sickle cell anemia by the use of hydroxyurea: splenic regeneration. *Blood* 1996; **88**: 1951–1953

151. Zeng YT, Huang SZ, Ren ZR *et al*. Hydroxyurea therapy in β-thalassaemia intermedia: improvement in haematological parameters due to enhanced β-globin synthesis. *Br J Haematol* 1995; **90**: 557–563

152. Hajjar FM, Pearson HA. Pharmacologic treatment of thalassemia intermedia with hydroxyurea. *J Pediatr* 1994; **125**: 490–492

153. Rose C, Bauters F, Galacteros F. Hydroxyurea therapy in highly unstable hemoglobin carriers [letter]. *Blood* 1996; **88**: 2807–2808

154. Beretta A, Prato V, Gallo E, Lehmann H. Haemoglobin Torino–α-43 (CD1) phenylalanine replaced by valine. *Nature* 1968; **217**: 1016–1018

155. Prato V, Gallo E, Ricco G, Mazza U, Bianco G, Lehmann H. Haemolytic anaemia due to haemoglobin Torino. *Br J Haematol* 1970; **19**: 105–115

156. Ohba Y, Miyaji T, Matsuoka M, Yokoyama M, Numakura H. Hemoglobin Hirosaki (α43 [CE 1] Phe replaced by Leu), a new unstable variant. *Biochim Biophys Acta* 1975; **405**: 155–160

157. Ohba Y, Miyaji T, Matsuoka M, Yokoyama M. Further studies on hemoglobin Hirosaki: demonstration of its presence at low concentration. *Hemoglobin* 1978; **2**: 281–286

158. Harkness M, Harkness DR, Kutlar F *et al*. Hb Sun Prairie or α (2) 130 (H13) Ala→Pro β2, a new unstable variant occurring in low quantities [see comments]. *Hemoglobin* 1990; **14**: 479–489

159. Wajcman H, Vasseur C, Blouquit Y *et al*. Unstable α-chain hemoglobin variants with factitious β-thalassemia biosynthetic ratio: Hb Questembert (α131 [H14] Ser→Pro) and Hb Caen (α132 [H15] Val→Gly). *Am J Hematol* 1993; **42**: 367–374

160. Kleihauer EF, Reynolds CA, Dozy AM *et al*. Hemoglobin-Bibba or α-2–136 Pro-β 2, an unstable α chain abnormal hemoglobin. *Biochim Biophys Acta* 1968; **154**: 220–222

161. De Jong WW, Went LN, Bernini LF. Haemoglobin Leiden: deletion of β-6 or 7 glutamic acid. *Nature* 1968; **220**: 788–790

162. Gilbert AT, Fleming PJ, Sumner DR, Hughes WG, Holland RA, Tibben EA. Hemoglobin Windsor or β11 (A8) Val→Asp: a new unstable β-chain hemoglobin variant producing a hemolytic anemia. *Hemoglobin* 1989; **13**: 437–453

163. Huisman TH, Brown AK, Efremov GD *et al*. Hemoglobin Savannah (B6 (24) β-glycine is greater than valine): an unstable variant causing anemia with inclusion bodies. *J Clin Invest* 1971; **50**: 650–659

164. Idelson LI, Didkowsky NA, Casey R, Lorkin PA, Lehmann H. New unstable hemoglobin (Hb Moscva, β24 (B4) Gly leads to Asp) found in the USSR. *Nature* 1974; **249**: 768–770

165. Thillet J, Cohen Solal M, Seligmann M, Rosa J. Functional and physicochemical studies of hemoglobin St. Louis β28 (B10) Leu replaced by Gln: a variant with ferric β heme iron. *J Clin Invest* 1976; **58**: 1098–1106

166. Sansone G, Carrell RW, Lehmann H. Haemoglobin Genova: β-28 (B10) leucine replaced by proline. *Nature* 1967; **214**: 877–879

167. Nakatsuji T, Miwa S, Ohba Y *et al*. A new unstable hemoglobin, Hb Yokohama β 31 (B13) Leu substituting for Pro, causing hemolytic anemia. *Hemoglobin* 1981; **5**: 667–678

168. Gurgey A, Altay C, Gu LH *et al*. Hb Hakkari or α 2 β 2 31 (B13) Leu→Arg, a severely unstable hemoglobin variant associated with numerous intra-erythroblastic inclusions and erythroid hyperplasia of the bone marrow. *Hemoglobin* 1995; **19**: 165–172

169. Garel MC, Blouquit Y, Rosa J, Arous N, Romero Garcia C. Hemoglobin Castilla β32 (B14) Leu leads to Arg; a new unstable variant producing severe hemolytic disease. *FEBS Lett* 1975; **58**: 144–148

170. Burkert LB, Sharma VS, Pisciotta AV, Ranney HM, Bruckheimer S.

Hemoglobin M equon β 41 (C7) phenylalanine leads to tyrosine. *Blood* 1976; **48**: 645–651

171. Blouquit Y, Bardakdjian J, Lena Russo D *et al*. Hb Bruxelles: α2Aβ (2) 41 or 42 (C7 or CD1) Phe deleted. *Hemoglobin* 1989; **13**: 465–474

172. Dacie JV, Shinton NK, Gaffney PJ Jr, Lehmann H. Haemoglobin Hammersmith (β-42 (CDI) Phe replaced by ser). *Nature* 1967; **216**: 663–665

173. Gaudry CL Jr, Pitel PA, Jue DL, Hine TK, Johnson MH, Moo Penn WF. Hb Jacksonville [α2 β2 (54) (D5) Val→Asp]: a new unstable variant found in a patient with hemolytic anemia. *Hemoglobin* 1990; **14**: 653–659

174. Yamada K, Shinkai N, Nakazawa S, Yamada Z, Saito K. Hemoglobin Tochigi disease, a new unstable hemoglobin hemolytic anemia found in a Japanese family. *Nippon Ketsueki Gakkai Zasshi* 1971; **34**: 484–497

175. Müller CJ, Kingma S. Hemoglobin Zürich α2 β63 Arg. *Biochimica Biophysica Acta* 1961; **50**: 595–597

176. Allard C, Mohandas N, Wacjman H, Krisnnamoorthy R. A case of great instability of the hemoglobin: hemoglobin bicetre (author's translation). *Nouv Rev Française Hematol* 1976; **16**: 23–35

177. Miller DR, Wilson JB, Kutlar A, Huisman TH. Hb Bicetre or α2 β(2) 63 (E7) His→Pro in a white male: clinical observations over a period of 25 years. *Am J Hematol* 1986; **21**: 209–214

178. Molchanova TP, Postnikov Yu V, Pobedimskaya DD *et al*. Hb Alesha or α 2 β (2) 67 (E11) Val→Met: a new unstable hemoglobin variant identified through sequencing of amplified DNA. *Hemoglobin* 1993; **17**: 217–225

179. Carrell RW, Lehmann H, Lorkin PA, Raik E, Hunter E. Haemoglobin sydney: β-67 (E11) valine modified to alanine: an emerging pattern of unstable hemoglobins. *Nature* 1967; **215**: 626–628

180. Ohba Y, Miyaji T, Matsuoka M, Sugiyama K, Suzuki T, Sugiura T. Hemoglobin Mizuho or β 68 (E 12) leucine leads to proline, a new unstable variant associated with severe hemolytic anemia. *Hemoglobin* 1977; **1**: 467–477

181. Carrell RW, Owen MC. A new approach to hemoglobin variant identification. Hemoglobin Christchurch β-71 (E15) phenylalanine leads to serine. *Biochim Biophys Acta* 1971; **236**: 507–511

182. Rieder RF, Wolf DJ, Clegg JB, Lee SL. Rapid postsynthetic destruction of unstable haemoglobin Bushwick. *Nature* 1975; **254**: 725–727

183. White JM, Brain MC, Lorkin PA, Lehmann H, Smith M. Mild "unstable haemoglobin haemolytic anemia" caused by haemoglobin Shepherds Bush (B74 (E18) Gly→Asp). *Nature* 1970; **225**: 939–941

184. Schneider RG, Ueda S, Alperin JB, Brimhall B, Jones RT. Hemoglobin sabine β 91 (F7) Leu to Pro. An unstable variant causing severe anemia with inclusion bodies. *N Engl J Med* 1969; **280**: 739–745

185. Bradley TB Jr, Wohl RC, Rieder RF. Hemoglobin Gun Hill: deletion of five amino acid residues and impaired heme-globin binding. *Science* 1967; **157**: 1581–1583

186. Kawata R, Ohba Y, Yamamoto K *et al*. Hyperunstable hemoglobin Koriyama anti-Hb Gun Hill insertion of five residues in the β chain. *Hemoglobin* 1988; **12**: 311–321

187. Ohba Y, Imanaka M, Matsuoka M *et al*. A new unstable, high oxygen affinity hemoglobin: Hb Nagoya or β97 (FG4) His—Pro. *Hemoglobin* 1985; **9**: 11–24

188. Gordon Smith EC, Dacie JV, Blecher TE, French EA, Wiltshirre BG, Lehmann H. Haemoglobin Nottingham, β FG 5 (98) Val—Gly: a new unstable haemoglobin producing severe haemolysis. *Proc R Soc Med* 1973; **66**: 507–508

189. Wilson JB, Webber BB, Hu H *et al*. Hemoglobin Birmingham and hemoglobin Galicia: two unstable β chain variants characterized by small deletions and insertions. *Blood* 1990; **75**: 1883–1887

190. Hyde RD, Hall MD, Wiltshire BG, Lehmann H. Haemoglobin Southampton, 106 (G8) Leu leads to Pro: an unstable variant producing severe haemolysis. *Lancet* 1972; **i**: 1170–1172

191. Outeirino J, Casey R, White JM, Lehmann H. Haemoglobin Madrid β 115 (G17) alanine–proline: an unstable variant associated with haemolytic anemia. *Acta Haematol* 1974; **52**: 53–60

192. Divoky V, Svobodova M, Indrak K, Chrobak L, Molchanova TP, Huisman TH. Hb Hradec Kralove (Hb HK) or α2 β2 115 (G17) Ala→Asp, a severely unstable hemoglobin variant resulting in a dominant β-thalassemia trait in a Czech family. *Hemoglobin* 1993; **17**: 319–328

193. Ohba Y, Hasegawa Y, Amino H *et al*. Hemoglobin saitama or β117 (G19) His leads to Pro, a new variant causing hemolytic disease. *Hemoglobin* 1983; **7**: 47–56

194. Baudin Chich V, Wajcman H, Gombaud Saintonge G *et al*. Hemoglobin Brest [β127 (H5) Gln→Lys] a new unstable human hemoglobin variant located at the α1 β1 interface with specific electrophoretic behavior. *Hemoglobin* 1988; **12**: 179–188

195. Kleihauer E, Betke K. Properties of the unstable Hb Wien. *Klin Wochenschr* 1972; **50**: 907–909

196. Baird M, Schreiner H, Driscoll C, Bank A. Localization of the site of recombination in formation of the Lepore Boston globin gene. *J Clin Invest* 1981; **68**: 560–564

197. Mavilio F, Giampaolo A, Care A, Sposi NM, Marinucci M. The δ β crossover region in Lepore boston hemoglobinopathy is restricted to a 59 base pairs region around the 5′ splice junction of the large globin gene intervening sequence. *Blood* 1983; **62**: 230–233

198. McDonald MJ, Noble RW, Sharma VS, Ranney HM, Crookston JH, Schwartz JM. A comparison of the functional properties of two lepore haemoglobins with those of haemoglobin A1. *J Mol Biol* 1975; **94**: 305–310

199. Metzenberg AB, Wurzer G, Huisman TH, Smithies O. Homology requirements for unequal crossing over in humans. *Genetics* 1991; **128**: 143–161

200. Ostertag W, Smith EW. Hemoglobin-Lepore-Baltimore, a third type of a δ, β crossover (δ 50, β 86). *Eur J Biochem* 1969; **10**: 371–376

201. Camaschella C, Serra A, Bertero MT *et al*. Molecular characterization of Italian chromosomes carrying the Lepore Boston gene. *Acta Haematol* 1989; **81**: 136–139

202. Efremov DG, Efremov GD, Zisovski N *et al*. Variation in clinical severity among patients with Hb Lepore-Boston-β-thalassaemia is related to the type of β-thalassaemia. *Br J Haematol* 1988; **68**: 351–355

203. Quattrin N, Luzzatto L, Quattrin S Jr. New clinical and biochemical findings from 235 patients with hemoglobin Lepore. *Ann NY Acad Sci* 1980; **344**: 364–374

204. Orkin SH, Kazazian HH Jr, Antonarakis SE, Ostrer H, Goff SC, Sexton JP. Abnormal RNA processing due to the exon mutation of β E-globin gene. *Nature* 1982; **300**: 768–769

205. Orkin SH, Antonarakis SE, Loukopoulos D. Abnormal processing of β Knossos RNA. *Blood* 1984; **64**: 311–313

206. Wong SC, Ali MA. Hemoglobin E diseases: hematological, analytical, and biosynthetic studies in homozygotes and double heterozygotes for α-thalassemia. *Am J Hematol* 1982; **13**: 15–21

207. Fairbanks VF, Oliveros R, Brandabur JH, Willis RR, Fiester RF. Homozygous hemoglobin E mimics β-thalassemia minor without anemia or hemolysis: hematologic, functional, and biosynthetic studies of first North American cases. *Am J Hematol* 1980; **8**: 109–121

208. Arous N, Galacteros F, Fessas P *et al*. Structural study of hemoglobin Knossos, β27 (B9) Ala leads to Ser. A new abnormal hemoglobin present as a silent β-thalassemia. *FEBS Lett* 1982; **147**: 247–250

209. Fessas P, Loukopoulos D, Loutradi Anagnostou A, Komis G. 'Silent' β-thalassaemia caused by a 'silent' β-chain mutant: the pathogenesis of a syndrome of thalassaemia intermedia. *Br J Haematol* 1982; **51**: 577–583

210. Vetter B, Schwarz C, Kohne E, Kulozik AE. β-thalassemia in the immigrant and non-immigrant German populations. *Br J Haematol* 1997; **97**: 266–277

211. Vidaud M, Gattoni R, Stevenin J *et al*. A 5′ splice-region G—C mutation in exon 1 of the human β-globin gene inhibits pre-mRNA splicing: a mechanism for β+-thalassaemia. *Proc Natl Acad Sci USA* 1989; **86**: 1041–1045

212. Milner PF, Clegg JB, Weatherall DJ. Haemoglobin-H disease due to a

unique haemoglobin variant with an elongated α-chain. *Lancet* 1971; **1**: 729–732

213. Clegg JB, Weatherall DJ, Milner PF. Hemoglobin Constant Spring— a chain termination mutant? *Nature* 1971; **234**: 337–340

214. Clegg JB, Weatherall DJ, Contopolou Griva I, Caroutsos K, Poungouras P, Tsevrenis H. Hemoglobin Icaria, a new chain-termination mutant with causes α thalassaemia. *Nature* 1974; **251**: 245–247

215. De Jong WW, Meera Khan P, Bernini LF. Hemoglobin Koya Dora: high frequency of a chain termination mutant. *Am J Hum Genet* 1975; **27**: 81–90

216. Merritt D, Jones RT, Head C *et al*. Hemoglobin Seal Rock [(α2) 142 Term-Glu, codon 142 TAA-GAA] an extended α chain variant associated with anemia, microcytosis and α-thalassemia-2 (−3.7 kb). *Hemoglobin* 1997; **21**: 331–344

217. Hanash SM, Rucknagel DL. Proteolytic activity in erythrocyte precursors. *Proc Natl Acad Sci USA* 1978; **75**: 3427–3431

218. Kugler W, Enssle J, Hentze MW, Kulozik AE. Nuclear degradation of nonsense mutated β-globin mRNA: a post-transcriptional mechanism to protect heterozygotes from severe clinical manifestations of β-thalassaemia? *Nucleic Acids Res* 1995; **23**: 413–418

219. Sanguansermsri T, Matragoon S, Changloah L, Flatz G. Hemoglobin Suan-Dok (α2 109 (G16) Leu replaced by Arg β2): an unstable variant associated with α-thalassaemia. *Hemoglobin* 1979; **3**: 161–174

220. Weiss I, Cash FE, Coleman MB *et al*. Molecular basis for α-thalassemia associated with the structural mutant hemoglobin Suan-Dok (α2 109 Leu→Arg). *Blood* 1990; **76**: 2630–2636. [Published erratum appears in *Blood* 1991; **77**: 1404]

221. Goossens M, Lee KY, Liebhaber SA, Kan YW. Globin structural mutant α125 Leu leads to Pro is a novel cause of α-thalassaemia. *Nature* 1982; **296**: 864–865

222. Ohba Y, Yamamoto K, Hattori Y, Kawata R, Miyaji T. Hyperunstable hemoglobin Toyama [α2 136 (H19) Leu→Arg β2]: detection and identification by in vitro biosynthesis with radioactive amino acids. *Hemoglobin* 1987; **11**: 539–556

223. Park SS, Barnetson R, Kim SW, Weatherall DJ, Thein SL. A spontaneous deletion of β 33/34 Val in exon 2 of the β globin gene (Hb Korea) produces the phenotype of dominant β thalassaemia. *Br J Haematol* 1991; **78**: 581–582

224. Podda A, Galanello R, Maccioni L *et al*. Hemoglobin Cagliari (β 60 [E4] Val→Glu): a novel unstable thalassemic hemoglobinopathy. *Blood* 1991; **77**: 371–375

225. Ristaldi MS, Pirastu M, Murru S *et al*. A spontaneous mutation produced a novel elongated β-globin chain structural variant (Hb Agnana) with a thalassemia-like phenotype [letter]. *Blood* 1990; **75**: 1378–1379

226. Kobayashi Y, Fukumaki Y, Komatsu N, Ohba Y, Miyaji T, Miura Y. A novel globin structural mutant, Showa-Yakushiji (β110 Leu→Pro) causing a β-thalassaemia phenotype. *Blood* 1987; **70**: 1688–1691

227. Murru S, Poddie D, Sciarratta GV *et al*. A novel β-globin structural mutant, Hb Brescia (β114 Leu→Pro), causing a severe β-thalassaemia intermedia phenotype. *Hum Mutat* 1992; **1**: 124–128

228. de Castro CM, Devlin B, Fleenor DE, Lee ME, Kaufman RE. A novel β-globin mutation, β Durham-NC [β114 Leu→Pro], produces a dominant thalassemia-like phenotype. *Blood* 1994; **83**: 1109–1116

229. Beris P, Miescher PA, Diaz Chico JC *et al*. Inclusion body β-thalassemia trait in a Swiss family is caused by an abnormal hemoglobin (Geneva) with an altered and extended β chain carboxy-terminus due to a modification in codon β114. *Blood* 1988; **72**: 801–805

230. Fucharoen S, Kobayashi Y, Fucharoen G *et al*. A single nucleotide deletion in codon 123 of the β-globin gene causes an inclusion body β-thalassaemia trait: a novel elongated globin chain β Makabe. *Br J Haematol* 1990; **75**: 393–399

231. Curuk MA, Molchanova TP, Postnikov Yu V *et al*. β-thalassemia alleles and unstable hemoglobin types among Russian pediatric patients. *Am J Hematol* 1994; **46**: 329–332

232. Murru S, Loudianos G, Deiana M *et al*. Molecular characterization of β-thalassemia intermedia in patients of Italian descent and

identification of three novel β-thalassemia mutations. *Blood* 1991; **77**: 1342–1347

233. Pagano L, Lacerra G, Camardella L *et al*. Hemoglobin Neapolis, β126 (H4) Val→Gly: a novel β-chain variant associated with a mild β-thalassemia phenotype and displaying anomalous stability features. *Blood* 1991; **78**: 3070–3075

234. Hattori Y, Yamane A, Yamashiro Y *et al*. Characterization of β-thalassemia mutations among the Japanese. *Hemoglobin* 1989; **13**: 657–670

235. Fucharoen S, Fucharoen G, Fukumaki Y *et al*. Three-base deletion in exon 3 of the β-globin gene produced a novel variant (β gunma) with a thalassemia-like phenotype [letter]. *Blood* 1990; **76**: 1894–1896

236. Oner R, Oner C, Wilson JB, Tamagnini GP, Ribeiro LM, Huisman TH. Dominant β-thalassaemia trait in a Portuguese family is caused by a deletion of (G)TGGCTGGTGT(G) and an insertion of (G)GCAG(G) in codons 134, 135, 136 and 137 of the β-globin gene. *Br J Haematol* 1991; **79**: 306–310

237. Fei YJ, Stoming TA, Kutlar A, Huisman TH, Stamatoyannopoulos G. One form of inclusion body β-thalassemia is due to a GAA—TAA mutation at codon 121 of the β chain [letter]. *Blood* 1989; **73**: 1075–1077

238. Hall GW, Franklin IM, Sura T, Thein SL. A novel mutation (nonsense β 127) in exon 3 of the β globin gene produces a variable thalassaemic phenotype. *Br J Haematol* 1991; **79**: 342–344

239. Butler WM, Spratling L, Kark JA, Schoomaker EB. Hemoglobin Osler: report of a new family with exercise studies before and after phlebotomy. *Am J Hematol* 1982; **13**: 293–301

240. Winslow RM, Butler WM, Kark JA, Klein HG, Moo Penn W. The effect of bloodletting on exercise performance in a subject with a high-affinity hemoglobin variant. *Blood* 1983; **62**: 1159–1164

241. Wranne B, Berlin G, Jorfeldt L, Lund N. Tissue oxygenation and muscular substrate turnover in two subjects with high hemoglobin oxygen affinity. *J Clin Invest* 1983; **72**: 1376–1384

242. Wranne B, Jorfeldt L, Berlin G *et al*. Effect of haemodilution on maximal oxygen consumption, blood lactate response to exercise and cerebral blood flow in subjects with a high-affinity haemoglobin. *Eur J Haematol* 1991; **47**: 268–276

243. Mavilio F, Marinucci M, Tentori L, Fontanarosa PP, Rossi U, Biagiotti S. Hemoglobin Legnano (α2 141 (HC3) Arg replaced by Leu β2): a new abnormal human hemoglobin with high oxygen affinity. *Hemoglobin* 1978; **2**: 249–259

244. Shimasaki S. A new hemoglobin variant, hemoglobin Nunobiki [α 141 (HC3) Arg→Cys]. Notable influence of the carboxy-terminal cysteine upon various physico-chemical characteristics of hemoglobin. *J Clin Invest* 1985; **75**: 695–701

245. Kosugi H, Weinstein AS, Kikugawa K, Asakura T, Schroeder WA. Characterization and properties of Hb York (β146 His leads to Pro). *Hemoglobin* 1983; **7**: 205–226

246. Schneider RG, Bremner JE, Brimhall B, Jones RT, Shih TB. Hemoglobin Cowtown (β146 HC3 His→Leu): a mutant with high oxygen affinity and erythrocytosis. *Am J Clin Pathol* 1979; **72**: 1028–1032

247. Shih T, Jones RT, Bonaventura J, Bonaventura C, Schneider RG. Involvement of His HC3 (146) β in the Bohr effect of human hemoglobin. Studies of native and N-ethylmaleimide-treated hemoglobin A and hemoglobin Cowtown (β146 His replaced by Leu). *J Biol Chem* 1984; **259**: 967–974

248. Nagel RL, Gibson QH, Hamilton HB. Ligand kinetics in hemoglobin Hiroshima. *J Clin Invest* 1971; **50**: 1772–1775

249. Bonaventura C, Bonaventura J, Amiconi G, Tentori L, Brunori M, Antonini E. Hemoglobin Abruzzo (β143 (H21) His replaced by Arg). Consequences of altering the 2,3-diphosphoglycerate binding site. *J Biol Chem* 1975; **250**: 6273–6277

250. Perutz MF. Stereochemical interpretation of high oxygen affinity of haemoglobin Little Rock (α2 β2 143 His leads to Gln). *Nature New Biol* 1973; **243**: 180

251. Jensen M, Oski FA, Nathan DG, Bunn HF. Hemoglobin Syracuse (α 2 β 2–143(H21) His leads to Pro), a new high-affinity variant detected

by special electrophoretic methods. Observations on the auto-oxidation of normal and variant hemoglobins. *J Clin Invest* 1975; **55**: 469–477

252. Bonaventura J, Bonaventura C, Sullivan B *et al*. Hemoglobin providence. Functional consequences of two alterations of the 2,3-diphosphoglycerate binding site at position β82. *J Biol Chem* 1976; **251**: 7563–7571

253. Sugihara J, Imamura T, Nagafuchi S, Bonaventura J, Bonaventura C, Cashon R. Hemoglobin Rahere, a human hemoglobin variant with amino acid substitution at the 2,3-diphosphoglycerate binding site. Functional consequences of the alteration and effects of bezafibrate on the oxygen bindings. *J Clin Invest* 1985; **76**: 1169–1173

254. Ikkala E, Koskela J, Pikkarainen P *et al*. Hb Helsinki: a variant with a high oxygen affinity and a substitution at a 2,3-DPG binding site (β82[EF6] Lys replaced by Met). *Acta Haematol* 1976; **56**: 257–275

255. Rochette J, Barnetson R, Kiger L *et al*. Association of a novel high oxygen affinity haemoglobin variant with δ β thalassaemia. *Br J Haematol* 1994; **86**: 118–124

256. Maniatis A, Bousios T, Nagel RL *et al*. Hemoglobin Crete (β129 ala leads to pro): a new high-affinity variant interacting with β^0—and $\delta\beta^0$—thalassemia. *Blood* 1979; **54**: 54–63

257. Charache S, Weatherall DJ, Clegg JB. Polycythemia associated with a hemoglobinopathy. *J Clin Invest* 1966; **45**: 813–822

258. Charache S, Catalano P, Burns S *et al*. Pregnancy in carriers of high-affinity hemoglobins. *Blood* 1985; **65**: 713–718

259. Kulozik AE, Bellan Koch A, Kohne E, Kleihauer E. A deletion/inversion rearrangement of the β-globin gene cluster in a Turkish family with $\delta\beta^0$-thalassemia intermedia. *Blood* 1992; **79**: 2455–2459

260. Kaeda JS, Prasad K, Howard RJ, Mehta A, Vulliamy T, Luzzatto L. Management of pregnancy when maternal blood has a very high level of fetal haemoglobin. *Br J Haematol* 1994; **88**: 432–434

261. Lichtman MA, Murphy MS, Adamson JW. Detection of mutant hemoglobins with altered affinity for oxygen. A simplified technique. *Ann Intern Med* 1976; **84**: 517–520

262. Bagby GC Jr, Richert Boe K, Koler RD. 32P and acute leukemia: development of leukemia in a patient with hemoglobin Yakima. *Blood* 1978; **52**: 350–354

263. Bunn HF. Subunit dissociation of certain abnormal human hemoglobins. *J Clin Invest* 1969; **48**: 126–138

264. Gibson QH, Riggs A, Imamura T. Kinetic and equilibrium properties of hemoglobin Kansas. *J Biol Chem* 1973; **248**: 5976–5986

265. Nagel RL, Lynfield J, Johnson J, Landau L, Bookchin RM, Harris MB. Hemoglobin Beth Israel. A mutant causing clinically apparent cyanosis. *N Engl J Med* 1976; **295**: 125–130

266. Arous N, Braconnier F, Thillet J *et al*. Hemoglobin Saint Mande β102 (G4) Asn replaced by Tyr: a new low oxygen affinity variant. *FEBS Lett* 1981; **126**: 114–116

267. Pulsinelli PD, Perutz MF, Nagel RL. Structure of hemoglobin M Boston, a variant with a five-coordinated ferric heme. *Proc Natl Acad Sci USA* 1973; **70**: 3870–3874

268. Perutz MF, Pulsinelli PD, Ranney HM. Structure and subunit interaction of haemoglobin M Milwaukee. *Nature New Biol* 1972; **237**: 259–263

269. Nagai M, Takama S, Yoneyama Y. Reduction and spectroscopic properties of haemoglobins M. *Acta Haematol* 1987; **78**: 95–98

270. Nagai M, Yoneyama Y, Kitagawa T. Characteristics in tyrosine coordinations of four hemoglobins M probed by resonance Raman spectroscopy. *Biochemistry* 1989; **28**: 2418–2422

271. Passon PG, Reed DW, Hultquist DE. Soluble cytochrome b 5 from human erythrocytes. *Biochim Biophys Acta* 1972; **275**: 51–61

272. Kuma F, Ishizawa S, Hirayama K, Nakajima H. Studies on methemoglobin reductase. I. Comparative studies of diaphorases from normal and methemoglobinemic erythrocytes. *J Biol Chem* 1972; **247**: 550–555

273. Kuma F, Inomata H. Studies on methemoglobin reductase. II. The purification and molecular properties of reduced nicotinamide adenine dinucleotide-dependent methemoglobin reductase. *J Biol Chem* 1972; **247**: 556–560

274. Choury D, Leroux A, Kaplan JC. Membrane-bound cytochrome b5 reductase (methemoglobin reductase) in human erythrocytes. Study in normal and methemoglobinemic subjects. *J Clin Invest* 1981; **67**: 149–155

275. Yubisui T, Matsuki T, Tanishima K, Takeshita M, Yoneyama Y. NADPH-flavin reductase in human erythrocytes and the reduction of methemoglobin through flavin by the enzyme. *Biochem Biophys Res Commun* 1977; **76**: 174–182

276. Tomoda A, Yubisui T, Tsuji A, Yoneyama Y. Changes in intermediate haemoglobins during methaemoglobin reduction by NADPH-flavin reductase. *Biochem J* 1979; **179**: 227–231

277. Nagai M, Yubisui T, Yoneyama Y. Enzymatic reduction of hemoglobins M Milwaukee-1 and M Saskatoon by NADH-cytochrome b5 reductase and NADPH-flavin reductase purified from human erythrocytes. *J Biol Chem* 1980; **255**: 4599–4602.

278. Jaffe ER, Hsieh HS. DPNH-methemoglobin reductase deficiency and hereditary methemoglobinemia. *Semin Hematol* 1971; **8**: 417–437

279. Mansouri A, Lurie AA. Concise review: methemoglobinemia. *Am J Hematol* 1993; **42**: 7–12

280. Bartos HR, Desforges JF. Erythrocyte DPNH dependent diaphorase levels in infants. *Pediatrics* 1966; **37**: 991–993

281. Sick H, Gersonde K. Co-binding studies on Hb M Iwate. Allostery of a T state hemoglobin. *Biochim Biophys Acta* 1979; **581**: 34–43

282. Nagai M, Kitagawa T, Yoneyama Y. Molecular pathology of hemoglobin M Saskatoon disease. *Biomed Biochem Acta* 1990; **49**: S317–322

283. Ranney HM, Nagel RL, Heller P, Udem L. Oxygen equilibrium of hemoglobin M-Hyde Park. *Biochim Biophys Acta* 1968; **160**: 112–115

284. Udem L, Ranney HM, Bunn HF, Pisciotta A. Some observations on the properties of haemoglobin M Milwaukee-1. *J Mol Biol* 1970; **48**: 489–498

285. Hayashi A, Fujita T, Fujimura M, Titani K. A new abnormal fetal hemoglobin, Hb FM-Osaka (α2 γ2 63 His replaced by Tyr). *Hemoglobin* 1980; **4**: 447–448

286. Glader BE. Hemoglobin FM-Fort Ripley: another lesson from the neonate. *Pediatrics* 1989; **83**: 792–793

287. Hain RD, Chitayat D, Cooper R *et al*. Hb FM-Fort Ripley: confirmation of autosomal dominant inheritance and diagnosis by PCR and direct nucleotide sequencing. *Hum Mutat* 1994; **3**: 239–342

Red cell membrane abnormalities

WILLIAM C MENTZER AND BERTRAM H LUBIN

The red cell membrane provides a protective layer between hemoglobin and other intracellular components and the extracellular environment. It facilitates the transport of cations, anions, urea, water and other small molecules in and out of the cell but denies entry to most larger molecules, particularly if they are charged. It is a sturdy yet flexible container, consisting of a lipid bilayer studded with numerous integral proteins and an underlying proteinaceous membrane skeleton. With only a limited capacity for repair or self renewal, it lasts the entire 120-day life-span of the normal red cell. This chapter summarizes the structure and functions of the normal red cell membrane and then gives a more detailed account of the major red cell membrane abnormalities that cause human disease. Several excellent extensive reviews of this topic are available to the interested reader.[1–4]

LIPID BILAYER

The average human red cell contains about 455 million lipid molecules, all found within the lipid bilayer of the plasma membrane. Phospholipids (250 million) and unesterified cholesterol (195 million) molecules are present in nearly equimolar concentrations but there is a lower amount of glycolipid (10 million molecules).[5–8] The major phospholipids are phosphatidyl choline, phosphatidyl ethanolamine, sphingomyelin and phosphatidyl serine. Small quantities of phosphatidic acid, phosphatidyl inositol and lyso-phosphatidyl choline are also found. The usual phospholipid structure (with the exception of sphingomyelin and lyso-phosphatidyl choline) is that of a glycerol backbone with 2 attached medium chain fatty acids which may be saturated or unsaturated. Attachment is via an ester or vinyl (in the case of plasmalogens) linkage. The particular composition of fatty acids partially determines the properties of the various phospholipids and can affect various membrane properties.[8,9] A family of red cell enzymes with specificity for each phospholipid class is thought to maintain the precise fatty acyl composition characteristic of that class.[10] Lysophospholipids, the precursors of phospholipids, have a single fatty acid attached to the first position of the glycerol backbone. Echinocyte formation and cell lysis may follow accumulation of lysophospholipids in the red cell membrane.

The shape of the lipid bilayer is responsive to slight variations in the surface area of either the inner or outer leaflet.[11,12] Increasing the surface area of the inner leaflet produces a stomatocytic change in shape while increasing that of the outer leaflet transforms the cell into an echinocyte. These observations have generated a bilayer couple hypothesis which predicts that red cell membrane changes in shape are the result of expansion of one lipid leaflet compared to the other and that commensurate alteration of the unperturbed leaflet can compensate for such expansion, restoring the normal biconcave shape. Supporting this hypothesis are experiments in which chlorpromazine, a cationic amphipath which preferentially localizes to the inner leaflet of the membrane lipid bilayer, is added to acanthocytes and transforms their shape to that of biconcave discs.[13]

PHOSPHOLIPID ORGANIZATION AND DYNAMICS

Individual phospholipid molecules are aligned in the lipid bilayer with their polar head groups exposed at one or another surface and their hydrophobic fatty acyl side chains buried in the bilayer core. Hexagonal phospholipid

257

structures are occasionally also present and influence the functional properties of the bilayer. Glycolipids and cholesterol are intercalated between the phospholipids with their long axes perpendicular to the bilayer plane. Cholesterol molecules are distributed evenly across the bilayer but glycolipids are localized to the outer leaflet where they contribute to the structure of the blood group antigens. Some membrane proteins require phospholipids, particularly aminophospholipids, in order to function properly. As techniques to evaluate specific lipid domains within the membrane become available, it is likely that other membrane-bound or associated proteins will be found to have specific phospholipid requirements for biologic activity.

There is an increasing realization that lipids are important for normal membrane function as well as structure, and that they are in dynamic flux rather than static. For example, unesterified cholesterol molecules in the bilayer exchange with those in the plasma,[14] and also move back and forth across the bilayer,[15] often in a matter of seconds. The entire cholesterol content of the membrane can be exchanged with the plasma within 24 hours. Since most plasma cholesterol is esterified by the action of plasma lecithin cholesterol acyl transferase, the major pool of unesterified cholesterol is in the red cell. The half-life for the exchange between red cell and plasma unesterified cholesterol is 7 hours. If plasma unesterified cholesterol levels are elevated, as may occur in obstructive liver disease, red cell cholesterol content increases. The resulting increased membrane surface area, unmatched by a concomitant increase in cell volume, leads to formation of target cells, which only disappear when plasma cholesterol levels fall upon resolution of the obstructive liver disease. In the case of phospholipids, movement of phospholipids across the bilayer and within the plane of the bilayer, as well as the remodeling of acyl side chains within each phospholipid class has been observed.[16] Exchange of phospholipids within the plane of the bilayer is rapid, occurring almost 10^7 times/s.

Transbilayer movements of phospholipids are also rapid, vary according to phospholipid class,[16,17] and for aminophospholipids are mediated by aminophospholipid translocase or 'flippase'.[18,19] This adenosine triphosphate-dependent enzyme translocates phosphatidyl serine (PS) and, to a lesser extent, phosphatidyl ethanoamine (PE) from the outer to the inner leaflet with a half-life of 5 and 60 min, repectively at 37°C.[20,21] 'Flippase' is inhibited by sulfhydryl-modifying reagents, vanadate and elevated levels of free intracellular calcium. A 'floppase' may also exist to facilitate the movement of phospholipids from the inner to the outer leaflet. Finally, slow bidirectional passive diffusion of all phospholipids occurs throughout the life-span of the red cell.[19] The combined impact of passive diffusion and flippase and floppase activities determines the equilibrium distribution of phospholipids in the bilayer and leads to the asymmetric distribution of aminophospholipids.[22,23] At equilibrium, although the amount of phospholipid in both leaflets is equal, the outer leaflet is rich in sphingomyelin and

phosphatidyl choline and also contains a small amount of phosphatidyl ethanoamine.[8] In contrast, the inner leaflet contains all of the phosphatidyl serine, most of the phosphatidyl ethanoamine, and a small amount of phosphatidyl choline. The absence of phosphatidyl serine on the outer leaflet is important because this phospholipid can activate coagulation, contribute to cell–cell interactions,[24,25] and participate in membrane fusion events.[26] The basis for phospholipid asymmetry does not appear to be strongly related to abnormalities in membrane skeletal protein function, since asymmetry is maintained in hereditary spherocytosis.[27,28]

Alterations in lipid asymmetry have been reported in several pathologic states. In sickle cell disease, the sickling of red cells under hypoxic conditions leads to translocation of aminophospholipids from the inner to the outer leaflet.[29,31] The most deformed domains of the membrane, areas where the sickle hemoglobin polymer has dramatically distorted and stretched the membrane, appear to be the sites where asymmetry is lost.[32] In these domains, dissociation of lipids from proteins may contribute to loss of asymmetry. Red cells that have lost phospholipid asymmetry have been detected in the circulation of sickle cell anemia patients.[33] The presence of phosphatidyl serine on the surface of these cells confers pro-coagulant activity,[34,35] raising the possibility that they may be involved in some of the pathophysiologic events found in sickle cell anemia. In fact, a positive association between the number of cells that have lost asymmetry and stroke in sickle cell disease has been reported.[35] Loss of asymmetry has also been described in red cells from patients with diabetes.[37]

An interesting class of phospholipids in the membrane are the phosphoinositides. These phospholipids have a phosphoinositol-containing polar head group, which may be mono- (PIP or PI-4-monophosphate) or bi-phosphorylated (PIP2 or PI-4,5-biphosphate).[38] Although representing only 2–5% of membrane phospholipids, phosphoinositides have considerable biologic activity and are involved in maintaining red cell shape and deformability. Phosphoinositides reside in the inner leaflet of the bilayer, undergo rapid phosphorylation and dephosphorylation, help regulate Ca^{2+} transport, interact with membrane proteins and influence membrane shape.

Some membrane proteins, including one involved in complement regulation, are anchored to the red cell membrane through a phosphoinositol lipid domain.[39] The advantage of the lipid footing is that it allows these proteins to move laterally in the membrane and in this way to prevent complement-mediated membrane damage. Phosphoinositol-anchored proteins are lost through the release of lipid-enriched vesicles from the cell during the membrane remodeling that accompanies reticulocyte maturation or cell aging. This process of vesiculation and loss of complement regulatory proteins is accelerated in sickle cell anemia by repeated cycles of sickling, making these cells sensitive to complement-mediated lysis.[40]

LIPID RENEWAL PATHWAYS

Although considerable lipid synthesis takes place during red cell development, mature erythrocytes are unable to synthesize fatty acids, phospholipids or cholesterol. However, in the circulation, cholesterol molecules are constantly being exchanged with plasma cholesterol and membrane phospholipids, especially those in which fatty acid side chains have been oxidized, are renewed as well.[41] The outer bilayer phospholipids, phosphatidyl choline and sphingomyelin, are slowly exchanged with plasma lipids. Interestingly, the molecular species composition of red cell phospholipids is quite distinct from that of plasma phospholipids, suggesting that specific pathways exist in red cells to remodel phospholipids to optimize their function. Plasma-free fatty acids and lysophospholipids provide the substrates for phospholipid renewal. ATP-requiring metabolic pathways to synthesize phospholipids and phospholipases that can remove unwanted fatty acids are found in red cells.[10] Dietary changes have only a minimal effect on the molecular species composition of red cell membrane phospholipids.[42] In contrast, it is likely that oxidant damage, particularly to unsaturated fatty acid groups, can alter membrane structure and function. Removal of oxidized fatty acids and replacement by normal fatty acids appears to be essential for red cell survival.

MEMBRANE PROTEINS

The major red cell membrane proteins, particularly those associated with the hemolytic anemias, are listed in Table 13.1. They were originally named on the basis of their migration on electrophoresis in sodium dodecyl sulfate (SDS)-polyacrylamide gels as Band 1, Band 2, etc. More recently, many of have been given names that evoke their function in the membrane.

STRUCTURE AND BIOSYNTHESIS

A number of proteins important for the interaction of the red cell with its external environment are attached to the lipid bilayer through a glycosyl-phosphatidylinositol anchor. These include enzymes (i.e. acetylcholinesterase), receptors, cell adhesion proteins and several components of the complement system.[43] In addition, embedded in the lipid bilayer are numerous transmembrane integral proteins that mediate transport, bear receptors or blood group antigens, or serve a structural role. Chief among these is the anion exchanger, Band 3, which regulates chloride bicarbonate exchange.[43] Band 3 is a 100 kDa protein which spans the membrane 14 times. It is assembled in the membrane as a dimer or, less frequently, as a tetramer. The portion of Band 3 that is exposed on the outer surface of the cell membrane bears the Ii blood group antigens while the cytoplasmic tail of the molecule serves as an attachment site for the cytoskeleton, hemoglobin and several glycolytic enzymes. A second major integral membrane protein is glycophorin A, a sialated glycoprotein which confers the negative charge on the cell.[45] It bears the MNSs antigen systems. Two closely related proteins, glycophorins C and D, carry the Gerbich blood groups and serve as the other major anchoring site for the cytoskeleton to the lipid bilayer through binding of their cytoplasmic tails to protein 4.1.[46] Among the many other

Table 13.1 Properties of red cell membrane proteins.[1,2,48,49,284]

Band	Protein	Mol Wt (kDa)*	Copies per cell ($\times 10^{-3}$)**	Chromosomal localization	Associated red cell diseases
1	α spectrin	240	240	1q22→q23	HS, HE, HPP
2	β spectrin	220	240	14q23→q24.2	HS, HE, HPP
2.1	Ankyrin	210	120	8p11.2	HS
3	Anion exchanger	90–100	1200	17q21→qter	HS, SAO
4.1	Protein 4.1	78–80	200	1p33→p34.2	HE
4.2	Pallidin	72	250	15q15→q21	HS
5	β actin	43	500	7pter→q22	
	Urea transporter	36		18q12→q21	
6	G3PD	35	500	12q13	
7	Stomatin	31	200	9q34.1	HST
7	Aquaporin				
	CHIP	28		7p14	
PAS 1	Glycophorin A	36	1000	4q31	
PAS 2	Glycophorin C	32	200	2q14→q21	HE
PAS 3	Glycophorin D	23	200	2q14→q21	HE
	Glycophorin B	20	200	4q31	

*Molecular weights estimated on SDS PAGE.
**Approximate.
HS = hereditary spherocytosis; HE = hereditary elliptocytosis; HPP = hereditary pyropoikilocytosis; HST = hereditary stomatocytosis; SAO = south-east Asian ovalocytosis.

intrinsic membrane proteins are several that are involved in transport: Band 7.2b, a phosphorylated molecule that is thought to play a role in the regulation of monovalent cation transport;[47] the urea transport protein which carries the Kidd blood group antigen;[48] and aquaporin CHIP, a water channel protein that also bears the Colton blood group antigen.[49]

An intricately interwoven meshwork of proteins forms the cytoskeleton, which underlies the lipid bilayer and is largely responsible for the biconcave disc shape of the red cell. Spectrin, the major component of the cytoskeletal meshwork, is a long, rod-shaped molecule present in two structurally distinct species, α and β spectrin.[50] The basic spectrin structural unit is a heterodimer of α and β spectrin molecules, linked along their length to form a hairpin-like structure. Dimers are associated head-to-head with other dimers to form tetramers and high molecular weight oligomers. Midway along the length of β spectrin is an attachment site for another membrane protein, ankyrin or Band 2.1, which also binds to the cytoplasmic tail of Band 3, thus providing the major linkage between the lipid bilayer and the cytoskeleton.[51] Strengthening this linkage is a third protein, pallidin or Band 4.2, which binds to both Band 3 and to ankyrin.[52] Near the tail end (N-terminus) of β spectrin is an attachment site for another important cytoskeletal protein, protein 4.1, which, through its association with glycophorin C, provides a second anchoring point connecting the lipid bilayer and the cytoskeleton.[53] Numerous short actin filaments also bind to the N-terminal region of β spectrin as well as to protein 4.1, forming a junctional complex easily seen on electron microscopy of spread membrane skeleton preparations.[54] Other proteins associated with the junctional complex are adducin (Band 2.9), dematin (Band 4.9), p55, tropomyosin, tropomodulin, and heavy and light chain myosin heterodimers.

The membrane proteins are synthesized beginning early in the differentiation of erythroid progenitor cells. Large excesses of protein 4.1 are generated relative to the amount actually incorporated into the cytoskeleton. Several isoforms of protein 4.1 are produced in a developmentally regulated sequence during the maturation of erythroid precursors; only the function of the form found in mature red cells has been established.[55] There is asymmetric synthesis of α and β spectrin, the former exceeding the latter by several fold. Proteins not incorporated into the membrane are rapidly degraded and lost. Thus, overall, membrane protein biosynthesis and incorporation can be viewed as a somewhat inefficient process. There is considerable experimental evidence *in vitro* suggesting that spectrin and ankyrin are assembled onto the membrane in only small amounts until Band 3 is synthesized and introduced into the bilayer, providing an attachment site for ankyrin, spectrin and the other skeletal proteins in sequence.[56] However, creation of a Band 3 null phenotype in mice by targeted disruption has called the pivotal role of Band 3 in membrane protein assembly into question, since relatively normal amounts of skeletal proteins are present despite the total absence of Band 3.[57]

MEMBRANE DEFORMABILITY

The normal red cell has a biconcave disc shape in the resting state, but in circulation it assumes elliptical, parachute-like, or other shapes in response to circulatory shear forces. Its ability to deform is determined by the surface area:volume ratio, cytoplasmic viscosity and membrane material properties. A decrease in the surface area:volume ratio, such as is seen in spherocytes, reduces deformability and may impede passage of the red cell through constricted areas of the microcirculation such as are found in the spleen. Changes in cytoplasmic viscosity are usually the result of osmotic movement of water into or out of the red cell. Movement of water into the cell decreases cytoplasmic viscosity but causes an increase in cell volume without affecting surface area, thus adversely affecting deformability. Movement of water out of the cell increases cytoplasmic viscosity and consequently decreases deformability. Optimal deformability is noted at physiologic plasma osmolarity (290 mOsm). Membrane material properties are complex, as the membrane behaves as a solid, semi-solid or liquid depending upon the duration and strength of the deforming force exerted. The force required to increase surface area is primarily determined by the lipid bilayer, whereas most other behaviors such as elasticity, elastic recoil and yield shear stress are determined by the intrinsic and cytoskeletal protein network.[58] Many of the proteins of the red cell membrane are subject to post-translational modification by phosphorylation, glycosylation, myristylation, fatty acid acylation, sulfhydryl mediated oxidation, calmodulin, calpain-mediated proteolysis, and other processes. 1,2-diphosphoglycerate (1,2-DPG) disrupts spectrin-actin-protein 4.1 complexes. In experimental systems utilizing membrane ghosts, skeletons or purified membrane proteins, these modifications usually tend to weaken cytoskeletal protein interactions and adversely affect membrane mechanical properties, but whether similar effects are operative *in vivo* has not been fully established.[59]

MEMBRANE TRANSPORT

Water, urea, glucose, anions and many other molecules move across the red cell membrane. This discussion is limited to cations, as disorders of cation transport are those most frequently associated with various human red cell disorders. The normal red cell has an internal cation content quite different from that of the surrounding plasma.[60] The red cell K^+ concentration is high (about 140 mEq/l cell water) compared to plasma K^+ concentrations of 4–5 mEq/l, whereas the red cell Na^+ concentration is low (about 10 mEq/l cell water) compared to the plasma Na^+ concentration of about 140 mEq/l. These concentration gradients lead to a small passive movement across the lipid bilayer of Na^+ into and K^+ out of the cell.[61] Cation homeostasis is maintained by the active transport of Na^+ out of and K^+ into the cell with a 3:2 stoichiometry that exactly equals the normal passive movement of these cations. The Na^+/K^+-ATPase pump responsible for active transport couples the hydrolysis of ATP to the movement of Na^+ and K^+. The pump is a multimer composed of a catalytic α subunit and smaller β and γ subunits.[62] Two other cation transport pathways are of importance. The Gardos channel is activated by increased intracellular Ca^{2+}, usually the result of ATP depletion, and promotes loss of intracellular K^+ and ultimately cell dehydration.[61] The volume-activated K/Cl co-transport pathway, chiefly found in reticulocytes, also leads to cell dehydration secondary to the loss of K^+.[63] Finally, mechanical stretching of the membrane may lead to cation loss,[64] a process likely to be of importance in the cellular dehydration that follows sickling deformation of hemoglobin SS red cells.

FETAL AND NEONATAL RED CELL MEMBRANE

Because the life-span of neonatal red cells is only about half that of adult cells, considerable effort has been expended in cataloging the membrane differences between these two types of cells.[65] The blood group antigen systems of neonatal cells are not fully developed. The membrane protein pattern on SDS PAGE gels is normal,[66] but more detailed scrutiny has revealed an increase in red cell myosin[67] and a decrease in aquaporin (CHIP 28), the latter accounting for the reduced water transport that is characteristic of neonatal red cells.[68] Increased K^+ loss and reduced chloride/bicarbonate exchange are other transport features of neonatal red cells.[65] The membrane lipid profile is essentially normal,[70] except for a general increase in cholesterol and lipid phosphorus.[69] The latter probably reflects the presence of internalized normal membrane due to the increased amount of receptor-mediated endocytosis characteristic of neonatal red cells.[69] Perhaps due to this process of internalization, there is a striking loss of surface area as neonatal red cells age[69] and this, along with cation loss and dehydration, creates a sub-population of dense, poorly deformable older cells coated with immunoglobulin and thus presumably destined for early destruction.[66] Another contributor to the shortened life-span of neonatal red cells may be their oxidant susceptibility.[71] The deformability in vitro of unfractionated populations of neonatal red cells is normal,[72] but their ability to pass through filters with small pores is limited by their large size, which increases the minimal cylindrical diameter they can attain.[70,73] The contribution of these many structural and functional features of neonatal red cells to their shortened life-span has not been completely worked out.

HEREDITARY SPHEROCYTOSIS

As the name implies, the hallmark of this group of disorders is the presence of spherocytes on the peripheral blood smear. Hemolysis, sometimes fully compensated, but more commonly accompanied by anemia of variable severity is present. Family studies indicate autosomal dominant inheritance in about 75% of patients. In most of the remainder, inheritance is recessive. A small proportion prove to harbor new mutations that exhibit dominant inheritance in subsequent generations.[74–77] The incidence of hereditary spherocytosis is about 200–300/million in Northern European populations but this is likely to be an underestimate as mild cases are often not diagnosed.[78] In other parts of the world, the disease is thought to be less common, although comprehensive population survey data are unavailable.

CLINICAL FEATURES

Anemia in hereditary spherocytosis may be absent, mild, moderate or severe to the point of threatening life.[2,74]

- *Mildly affected individuals* exhibit no anemia, have modest reticulocytosis, and may not be detected until adolescence or adult life. They maintain normal hemoglobin levels in the face of accelerated erythrocyte destruction by virtue of an erythropoietin-driven increase in erythropoiesis. The stimulus for increased production of erythropoietin is not known but does not appear to be hypoxia.[79]
- *Moderately affected individuals* are more anemic, have higher reticulocyte counts and elevated serum bilirubin levels, may require occasional transfusions, and are usually detected in infancy or childhood.
- *Severely affected individuals* have marked hemolysis, anemia, hyperbilirubinemia, splenomegaly and a regular red cell transfusion requirement.[74] In the most severe cases, hydrops fetalis with death *in utero* may occur.[80]

When detected in the neonatal period, hereditary spherocytosis is commonly accompanied by jaundice, requiring treatment with phototherapy or exchange transfusion (see Chapter 9).[74] On the other hand, anemia, spherocytosis on the peripheral blood smear, and reticulocytosis are often minimal or absent.[81]

As in other chronic hemolytic anemias, exacerbations of anemia may be aplastic, hemolytic or megaloblastic in origin.

- An *aplastic crisis* may occur as a result of transient marrow suppression by parvovirus B19 or other viral infections.
- Increased *hemolysis* may accompany viral illnesses, probably as a consequence of concomitant splenomegaly associated with the illness (the crucial role of the spleen in spherocyte destruction is discussed below).
- In malnourished patients in particular, *megaloblastic anemia* may be superimposed on the chronic hemolytic anemia of

hereditary spherocytosis due to an unmet increased need for folate to support erythropoiesis.

An expected and common complication of hereditary spherocytosis is the formation of bilirubin gallstones, which may be present in at least half of all adult patients, particularly those with more severe hemolytic disease. Rare complications or associations include leg ulcers, extramedullary hematopoietic tumors,[82] spinocerebellar degenerative syndromes, hypertrophic cardiomyopathy and movement disorder with myopathy.[2]

LABORATORY DIAGNOSIS

Nearly all cases of hereditary spherocytosis are initially suspected because spherocytes are found on the peripheral blood smear (Fig. 13.1). In the newborn and in mild cases in later life, spherocytes may be few in number. Variant spherocytic morphologies include notched or pincered spherocytes in Band 3 deficiency,[83] acanthocytic spherocytes in β-spectrin deficiency[84] or dysfunction,[85] dense and irregularly shaped cells in combined spectrin-ankyrin deficiency,[86] and spherocytic elliptocytes in the disorder aptly named spherocytic elliptocytosis.[87] Analysis of the specific membrane protein molecular defects responsible for hereditary spherocytosis in individual families is beyond the capabilities of clinical laboratories and is limited to specialized research facilities. Therefore, the diagnosis is almost always made on clinical grounds, based on the presence of spherocytes in the setting of familial hemolytic anemia.

Spherocytes are a feature of many hemolytic anemias, so their identification on the peripheral blood smear alone is not sufficient to establish a diagnosis of hereditary spherocytosis. The mechanism of spherocyte production is usually loss of membrane surface area in excess of loss of cell volume. Loss of membrane may be secondary to oxidant injury as in G6PD deficiency or hemoglobin H disease. In immune hemolytic anemia, interaction of membrane-antibody complexes with the reticuloendothelial system leads to membrane loss through phagocytosis. Venoms may contain

phospholipases or other membrane active enzymes that induce spherocyte formation. Various types of mechanical hemolytic anemia may generate spherocytes in the process of erythrocyte fragmentation. With the exception of autoimmune hemolytic anemia, spherocytes are rarely the sole or dominant morphologic abnormality noted in these conditions. Macrospherocytes may be seen when red cell water content is increased and the cell swells, as is the case in hereditary hydrocytosis.

Acquired immune hemolytic disease is the condition that most closely resembles hereditary spherocytosis. It can be ruled out by the absence of a family history of hemolytic anemia, the presence of a positive direct antiglobulin test or other manifestations of autoimmune disease, and a relative lack of exacerbation of hemolysis in the incubated osmotic fragility test. In the newborn, ABO incompatibility is excluded by blood grouping of mother and infant and by a negative result upon antiglobulin testing of newborn red cells. Other diseases in which spherocytes may be seen, such as unstable hemoglobinopathies, G6PD deficiency, microangiopathic hemolytic anemia, or clostridial sepsis, are distinguished from hereditary spherocytosis by easily recognized differences in clinical course, red cell morphology and clinical laboratory tests specific for each disease.

Routine blood counts in hereditary spherocytosis reveal anemia and reticulocytosis to varying degrees, depending on the severity of the mutation. The mean corpuscular volume (MCV) is normal or slightly low and is of little diagnostic value. The most helpful red cell index is the MCHC which is routinely higher than normal, reflecting red cell dehydration.[88] An elevated red cell distribution width (RDW) also points to a diagnosis of hereditary spherocytosis. In unsplenectomized children, an elevated MCHC (>35 gm/dl) and RDW (>14) has a sensitivity of 63% and specificity of 100% for the diagnosis of hereditary spherocytosis, making these combined indices a powerful screening tool.[89]

The reduced surface area:volume ratio that is characteristic of spherocytes increases their susceptibility to osmotic lysis in hypotonic solutions. This is the basis of the well-known osmotic fragility test, in which red cells are suspended in buffered salt solutions of varying tonicities and the degree of hemolyis is determined. However, according to one recent report, the osmotic fragility test is normal in as many as one-third of hereditary spherocytosis samples.[88] The normal samples are those in which cell dehydration has reduced cell volume to a degree equivalent to the reduction in surface area characteristic of spherocytes. Incubation of blood specimens for 24 hours in the absence of metabolic substrate accentuates the osmotic fragility of spherocytes and makes easier the distinction of this disease from others. Surprisingly, even after incubation, 15% of the samples in the report cited above[88] had normal osmotic fragility. Osmotic gradient ektacytometry, although not widely available, is a more accurate way to distinguish hereditary spherocytes from normal red cells as it measures not only surface area:volume relationships but also cell hydration and intrinsic membrane

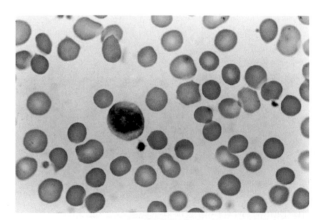

Fig. 13.1 Typical red cell morphology in hereditary spherocytosis.

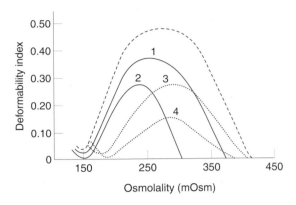

Fig. 13.2 Osmotic gradient ektacytometry in hereditary spherocytosis. Curves 1–4 display results for spherocytosis samples of increasing clinical severity. Results for normal red cells are indicated by the dashed line. Note that the minimum deformability on the hypotonic arm (left side of curve) of curves 1 and 2 is normal, indicating that the osmotic fragility of these red cell samples is normal, as is the case in as many as one-third of cases of hereditary spherocytosis. The maximum deformability of all spherocytosis samples is decreased, in rough proportion to clinical severity. The shift to the left in the hypertonic arm (right side of curve) reflects cell dehydration, which is present to varying degrees in each of the spherocytosis samples. Reproduced with permission from Ref. 88.

effects on deformability (Fig. 13.2).[88] A simple screening test, the acidified glycerol lysis test, in its most recently modified version appears to have the same sensitivity and selectivity as the osmotic fragility test,[78] as does a variant of the glycerol lysis test, the Pink test.[90] Another recently developed approach to screening is the cryohemolysis test, in which red cells are suspended in a hypertonic solution, briefly heated to 37°C, then cooled to 4°C for 10 min. Ease of performance and the wide separation in degree of hemolysis between spherocytes and normal cells are two attractive features of this test.[91]

PATHOPHYSIOLOGY

The vertical associations that ties the membrane skeleton to the lipid bilayer are impaired in hereditary spherocytosis by mutations in the proteins involved in these associations: spectrin, ankyrin, pallidin and Band 3. Spectrin deficiency is often present, even if the primary mutation is in a non-spectrin protein, because alterations in the non-spectrin proteins adversely affect assembly of spectrin onto the membrane skeleton. The clinical severity of the disorder correlates well with the degree of spectrin deficiency.[92] As in hereditary elliptocytosis, decreased membrane mechanical stability is noted in spectrin-deficient spherocytes and this probably contributes to red cell destruction in severe cases. However, the central abnormality that defines spherocytosis is progressive loss of elements of the lipid bilayer by micro-vesiculation, reflecting the weakened vertical association of the bilayer with the membrane skeleton. Loss of surface area without concomitant loss of volume imposes the spherocytic shape on affected red cells, reducing their ability to deform and pass through constricted regions of the microcirculation.

Two hypotheses have been advanced to explain how deficiencies or qualitative defects in the membrane proteins involved in the vertical association of the membrane skeleton with the lipid bilayer lead to vesiculation and membrane loss. In the first, spectrin deficiency acts directly on the bilayer to create areas of weakness that allow membrane loss. In the second, the integrity of the bilayer is maintained by Band 3 and deficiency of this protein or its dispersion as a result of abnormalities in the underlying membrane skeletal proteins is the proximate cause of vesiculation.[2]

Red cell ion transport abnormalities associated with hereditary spherocytosis are to some extent dependent upon the particular membrane protein abnormality present. For example, anion transport is decreased in Band 3 deficiency (an expected finding since Band 3 is the anion transporter), normal in spectrin-ankyrin deficiency, and increased in isolated pallidin deficiency.[93] On the other hand, increased passive permeability to monovalent cations (Na^+, K^+) is a general feature of human spherocytes with any of these 3 membrane protein defects[93] and is also found in spherocytic mice with deficiencies of ankyrin or spectrin.[94]

The spleen plays a crucial role in the generation and destruction of hereditary spherocytes. Reticulocytes are not spherocytic, indicating that the spherocytic change in shape appears after reticulocyte maturation in the circulation. Repeated passages through the splenic cords, a process termed splenic conditioning, promotes membrane lipid loss leading to a reduction in surface area and a progressively more spheroid red cell. Reflecting this process, red cells obtained from the splenic vein have greater osmotic fragility than those obtained from the splenic artery. The more spheroidal the red cell, the greater the likelihood that its lack of deformability will prevent its passage through the narrow fenestrations of the splenic cords. Detained in the spleen, the red cell is subjected to an acidotic, metabolically unfavorable enviroment where oxidants are prevalent and phagocytic reticulo-endothelial cells are ubiquitous. Secondary lesions such as 2,3-DPG depletion occur in this setting. Membrane protein methylation, a marker for damage, is greatly increased in spectrin-deficient spherocytes pre-splenectomy but drops to near normal levels after splenectomy. This abnormality may be a marker for splenic conditioning. When the molecular abnormality causing spherocytosis involves Band 3 instead of spectrin, little or no increase in membrane protein methylation occurs, suggesting that cytoskeletal damage is not a component of this type of spherocytosis.[95] The central importance of the spleen in the production and destruction of spherocytes is most clearly seen when the spleen is removed surgically, for this procedure virtually eliminates hemolysis and anemia in moderately severe cases and eliminates the need for transfusion and partially corrects the anemia in severe cases.

MOLECULAR PATHOLOGY AND GENETICS

Hereditary spherocytosis is the clinical consequence of mutations in the genes encoding ankyrin, Band 3, α and β spectrin or pallidin. One extensive survey of 166 hereditary sphero-cytosis kindreds found spectrin or spectrin-ankyrin defi-ciency in 60%, Band 3 deficiency in 23%, isolated pallidin deficiency in 2%, and no membrane protein abnormalities in the remaining 15%.[83] Similar findings have been reported by other laboratories.[96–99] The central role of mutations of these membrane proteins in the origin of spherocytosis has been underscored by study of transgenic mice which com-pletely lack Band 3[57,100] and by naturally occuring muta-tions that create severe ankyrin-spectrin or severe spectrin deficiency in mice[51] and complete Band 3 deficiency in cattle.[101]

Ankyrin

Ankyrin-spectrin deficiency is found in up to 60% of individuals with the dominant form of hereditary spherocy-tosis.[51] The responsible mutation is in the ankyrin gene; spectrin deficiency is secondary to the reduced amount of ankyrin present in the membrane. In one-third of such cases, 1 ankyrin mRNA allele is virtually missing, as a result of deletion, frameshift, or nonsense mutations that alter tran-scription, processing, or stability of ankyrin mRNA.[98,102] Oddly, the severity of hemolytic anemia varies widely from case to case, even though the molecular defect appears to be similar.[98] In 7 patients with hereditary spherocytosis who also had mental retardation and physical abnormalities, a chromosomal deletion [del (8)(p11–p21)] that included the ankyrin gene locus has been reported.[103] Obviously, these individuals also lack 1 ankyrin mRNA allele. Other ankyrin mutations in dominant hereditary spherocytosis include 1 truncated ankyrin (Prague) and 1 non-expressed isoform (Rakovnik).[104] Ankyrin mutations associated with recessive hereditary spherocytosis, in general, have been missense or promotor mutations.[98]

Band 3

In patients with hereditary spherocytosis with partial Band 3 deficiency, there is always an associated and roughly propor-tional deficiency of pallidin, but no spectrin deficiency.[83] Inheritance is dominant and the clinical picture is that of mild, usually compensated, hemolytic anemia A reduction in red cell anion transport proportional to the reduction in Band 3 is commonly found[105] and there may be abnormal-ities in renal bicarbonate handling.[106] A few cases of familial distal renal tubular acidosis are associated with mutations in erythrocyte band 3 and abnormalities in red cell ion trans-port. These cases, however, do not have hereditary spher-ocytosis.[107]

As is the case for ankyrin-spectrin deficiency, many Band 3-deficient individuals harbor frameshift or nonsense mutations that are associated with complete or near com-plete absence of mutant allele mRNA in reticulo-cytes.[83,99,106,108,109] Others have recombination or missense mutations involving highly conserved regions of the Band 3

molecule. In these, reticulocyte mRNA is normal in amount, but little or no mutant Band 3 is present in the membrane. The exact abnormality in Band 3 biosynthesis, transport or assembly in the membrane responsible for the absence of Band 3 is unknown.[83,99,105,109–112] The degree of Band 3 deficiency and the clinical severity of these dominantly inherited mutations is sometimes increased by the simulta-neous inheritance of a second Band 3 mutation in *trans*. These mutations produce very mild Band 3 deficiency when inherited alone, and are clinically silent.[112,113]

α-Spectrin

Severe hereditary spherocytosis with markedly low mem-brane spectrin levels is associated with recessive inheritance of 2 α-spectrin-deficiency mutations. Both homozygotes for a single α-spectrin mutation and compound heterozygotes for 2 different α-spectrin mutations have been described.[114] In one hereditary spherocytosis pedigree, the 2 α-spectrin mutations were found to be α-spectrin[PRAGUE], a truncated α-spectrin and α-spectrin[LEPRA], a splice-site mutation that causes a frameshift, premature termination of translation, and greatly reduced production of α-spectrin. Indirect evidence suggests that α-spectrin[LEPRA] may be found in as many as 50% of kindreds with recessive hereditary sphero-cytosis and marked spectrin deficiency.[115] Interestingly, α-spectrin[LELY], another mutation that is associated with α-spectrin deficiency (see below), does not reduce the output of α-spectrin polypeptides sufficiently to lead to sphero-cytosis, even when inherited in the homozygous state.[114] Although not yet described, if co-inherited with a severe α-spectrin deficiency in *trans*, α-spectrin[LELY] is theoretically capable of leading to recessive spectrin-deficiency hereditary spherocytosis.

β-Spectrin

Most mutations of β-spectrin are associated with mild-to-moderate autosomal dominant hereditary spherocytosis.[84] Numerous null mutations (missense or frameshift mutations that silence the affected allele)[84a] have been found in this setting. In addition, a β-spectrin missense mutation that generates a dysfunctional molecule, β-spectrin Kissammee, exhibits decreased binding affinity for protein 4.1 and is associated with mild spectrin deficiency has been reported.[118] Since synthesis of β-spectrin is rate limiting for the assembly of the spectrin tetramer, while α-spectrin is synthesized in excess, it is not surprising that deficiency or dysfunction of a single β-spectrin allele is sufficient to cause spherocytosis (dominant inheritance) while both α-spectrin alleles must be affected (recessive inheritance) for the same to occur. Missense mutations of β-spectrin associated with recessive inheritance have also been reported.[84] These are presumably milder mutations that either do not completely abolish transcription and translation or lead to production of normal or near normal amounts of a dysfunctional protein.

Pallidin (protein 4.2)

Hereditary spherocytosis associated with isolated pallidin deficiency is an autosomal recessive condition that is usually found in individuals of Japanese ancestry, in whom numerous missense mutations[119–121] and at least 1 splicing mutation[122] of the pallidin gene have been discovered. It should be distinguished from spherocytosis associated with Band 3 deficiency, in which the mutation and primary protein deficiency involve Band 3 but in which there is also a concomitant secondary deficiency of pallidin polypeptide, even though no pallidin mutation is present. In a third type of pallidin deficiency, mutations in Band 3 that adversely affect binding of pallidin to Band 3 produce pallidin deficiency and spherocytosis even though Band 3 levels remain normal.[123,124,124a] Of the 3 pedigrees exhibiting this type of defect, inheritance was autosomal recessive in 2 and not determined in the other.

TREATMENT

As with most hemolytic anemias, supportive care with daily oral folic acid (1 mg/day) and blood transfusions during periods of extreme anemia is warranted. An important element of treatment planning is consideration of splenectomy, which eliminates or minimizes anemia in patients with moderate spherocytosis.[74,88] In severely affected patients, life-threatening anemia and a need for regular transfusions is abolished by splenectomy, although an anemia of moderate degree usually persists.[125] Splenectomy prior to the formation of bilirubin gallstones can eliminate the need for a cholecystectomy later in life.

These benefits of splenectomy must be balanced against the immediate and long-term risks of the procedure. Immediate risks, which include hemorrhage at the operative site, post-operative infection, or injury to adjacent organs, are those associated with any surgical procedure and are relatively infrequent. Laparoscopic splenectomy is preferred in many centers as it shortens hospitalization, reduces post-operative pain, and may reduce operative bleeding. It is sometimes necessary to extend the incision, however, particularly when the spleen is enlarged.[126,127]

The most feared long-term complication of splenectomy is fatal overwhelming sepsis with encapsulated bacteria, most commonly *Streptococcus pneumonia*. A literature review in 1973 of 850 post-splenectomy hereditary spherocytosis cases, mostly infants and children, found that 30 (3.52%) developed sepsis and 19 (2.23%) died of infection.[128] A more recent retrospective review of 226 hereditary spherocytosis patients who underwent splenectomy up to 45 years earlier, estimated the mortality from overwhelming sepsis to be 0.73/1000 years. The 4 deaths from sepsis occurred 2, 18, 23 and 30 years post splenectomy. The mortality rates for the 35 children who underwent splenectomy prior to 6 years of age and for the 191 individuals who were older than 6 at the time of splenectomy were 1.12/1000 and 0.66/1000 years

of life after splenectomy, respectively.[129] As pointed out by the author, these rates are far higher than those seen in the general population. These rates and the 2.23% incidence of mortality from sepsis reported in 1973 by Singer[128] may overestimate the risk of sepsis for contemporary patients, since most of the participants underwent splenectomy prior to the introduction of the pneumococcal vaccine. The effectiveness of this vaccine in preventing overwhelming pneumococcal sepsis in splenectomized children was documented in a Danish study.[130]

Currently, the optimal strategy to prevent overwhelming sepsis post splenectomy includes administration of pneumococcal vaccine several weeks before the operation and daily oral penicillin prophylaxis (125 mg penicillin bid for children under 3 years and 250 mg bid for older individuals). Young children should also receive *Haemophilus influenzae* immunization before splenectomy. In view of reported deaths from sepsis up to 30 years or more post splenectomy, a case can be made for life-time penicillin prophylaxis. As an alternative, it is advisable to have antibiotics available at home for immediate treatment of any significant fever.[130] The emerging risk of penicillin-resistant pneumococcal infections[131] requires vigilance and prompt selection of alternative antibiotics in hospitalized individuals who have documented pneumococcal sepsis and remain febrile despite intravenous antibiotic therapy.[132] Splenectomy may pose special risks for individuals living in geographic regions where parasitic diseases such as malaria or babesiosis occur.[133,134]

The higher risk of overwhelming sepsis in young children who undergo splenectomy makes it important to defer the operation until at least age 6 years of age in all but the most severe patients. For young children who need an immediate splenectomy, Tchernia *et al*[135] tested the use of partial splenectomy, with a view to preserving the immunologic functions of the spleen while at the same time reducing the degree of splenic entrapment and destruction of spherocytic red cells. Removal of 80–90% of the spleen does reduce hemolysis, but not to the extent seen following complete removal. The phagocytic function of the spleen, assessed by red cell pit counts and/or splenic uptake of radiolabeled, heat-treated red cells, is normal and in more than 40 patients with hereditary spherocytosis followed for up to 11 years there have been no episodes of serious or fatal sepsis. The spleen does eventually regain its previous size and a second (complete) splenectomy will probably be required in most patients, but at a time when they are considerably older and the risk of sepsis is less.

Decisions regarding splenectomy must take into account the severity of hemolysis, age of the patient and the various risks described above. In mild hereditary spherocytosis, where the purpose of splenectomy is solely to prevent gallstone formation, the risks of operation may exceed those associated with expectant management.[136] When hemolysis and anemia are more severe and symptomatic, splenectomy is warranted. Long-term post-splenectomy thrombotic complications are reported to be uncommon in hereditary spherocytosis,[137] but there may be reason for concern since cases have been reported[138,139] and thromboembolic events are common in individuals splenectomized for other hereditary hemolytic anemias.[140,141] In addition, there appears to be an increased long-term risk of myocardial infarction after splenectomy for trauma.[142]

HEREDITARY ELLIPTOCYTOSIS

Elliptocytosis is a heterogeneous group of hereditary erythrocyte disorders that have in common the presence of elongated, oval or elliptically-shaped red cells on the peripheral blood smear. Inheritance is usually autosomal dominant. The incidence of elliptocytosis in the US is not greater than 1:2000–1:4000,[2] but in malarial regions of Africa it may reach 1.6% of the population[143] and in malarial areas of south-east Asia 30% or higher.[144]

CLINICAL SYNDROMES

Elliptocytic red cell morphology is the common denominator in all but the clinically silent forms of this group of patients (Figs 13.3 and 13.4). Hemolytic anemia ranges from absent to life-threatening. Severe hemolysis is usually a consequence of homozygosity or compound heterozygosity for one or more of the various membrane protein mutations associated with the disorder. The clinical features generally fall into one of the following categories defined by Palek.[2,87]

Silent carrier

These individuals are clinically and hematologically normal, but usually have subtle defects in membrane skeletal properties that can be detected in the laboratory. The responsible mutation is most commonly the low expression spectrin variant, α-spectrin[LELY], but occasionally one of the structural spectrin mutations usually associated with common hereditary elliptocytosis may be clinically silent. Silent carriers are usually only detected during analysis of pedigrees containing individuals with more clinically obvious forms of elliptocytosis.

Common hereditary elliptocytosis

This disorder is usually asymptomatic and comes to the attention of the clinician only because of the presence of elliptocytes on the peripheral blood smear (Fig. 13.3). Transient hemolytic anemia with more striking morphologic abnormalities (schistocytes, fragments, budding forms, and

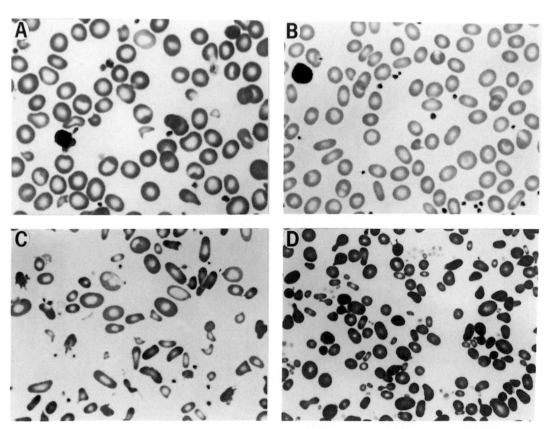

Fig. 13.3 Red cell morphology in elliptocytic disorders. (A) Transient neonatal poikilocytosis; (B) common hereditary elliptocytosis (asymptomatic); (C) common hereditary elliptocytosis with chronic hemolysis secondary to compound heterozygosity for 2 different α-spectrin mutations; (D) hereditary pyropoikilocytosis. Note the abundance of spherocytes. Reproduced with permission from Ref. 155.

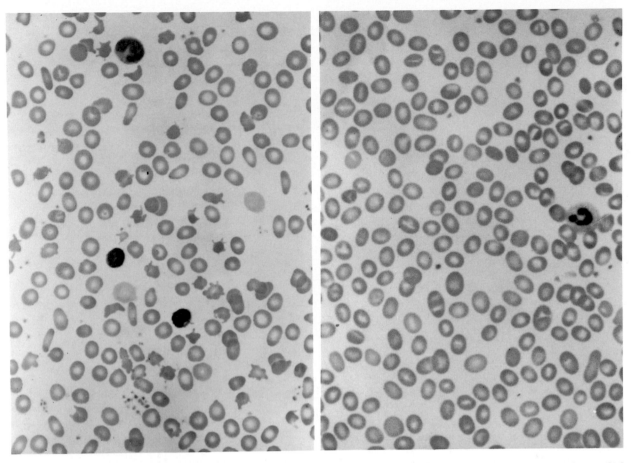

Fig. 13.4 Red cell morphology in elliptocytic disorders. (A) Transient neonatal poikilocytosis. Note the presence of numerous small, dense pyknocytes. (B) Southeast Asian ovalocytosis. Note the presence of frequent ovalocytes, occasional stomatocytes, and several ovalocytes with a transverse central band.

microcytes) (Fig. 13.4) may be encountered during the newborn period in infants with common hereditary elliptocytosis.[145,146] Episodic hemolysis and morphologic changes like those seen in transient neonatal poikilocytosis may also occur in CHE during acute or chronic illnesses characterized by reticuloendothelial hyperplasia,[147,148] B$_{12}$ deficiency[149] or altered microvasculature.[150] Sometimes, CHE may be associated with life-long hemolysis. This usually implies the inheritance of an unusually severe mutation or, in the case of α-spectrin, the co-inheritance of a low expression mutation that increases the relative amount of the mutant α spectrin polypeptide. Homozygous[151–154] or compound heterozygous CHE[154,155] is also often associated with chronic hemolysis, which ranges from moderate to life-threatening and may be accompanied by splenomegaly. Dramatic red cell poikilocytosis like that seen in CHE with episodic hemolysis is usually encountered.

Hereditary pyropoikilocytosis

Generally the severest type of hereditary elliptocytosis, this disorder acquired its name because the red cells resembled those seen in burn patients and, indeed, were susceptible to budding and fragmentation upon heating to 46°C, whereas

normal red cells were unaffected at temperatures below 50°.[156] Hereditary pyropoikilocytosis (HPP) is often an autosomal recessive disorder with both parents being clinically and hematologically normal. In other instances, CHE is found in 1 parent and the other is a silent carrier. Hemolytic anemia usually first appears in the neonatal period and resembles the transient neonatal hemolysis described above in CHE infants. However, in HPP the morphologic abnormalities of the red cells (poikilocytes, spherocytes, fragmentation, and extreme microcytosis) (Fig. 13.3) and the hemolytic anemia is life-long rather than transient. An abundance of spherocytes and, often, a paucity of elliptocytes on the peripheral blood smear are features that distinguish HPP from the hemolytic forms of CHE. HPP patients develop splenomegaly, may require transfusions for episodes of anemia, and often require splenectomy.

Spherocytic elliptocytosis

Seen only in caucasians, this is a dominantly inherited disorder producing mild-to-moderate hemolysis, splenomegaly and red cells that range from spherocytes to elliptocytes. The elliptocytes are often few in number and fragmentation, budding and extreme microcytosis are absent, distinguishing spherocytic elliptocytosis (SE) from HPP and the other hemolytic forms of CHE.

South-east Asian ovalocytosis

Common in New Guinea and other malaria-ridden regions of south-east Asia, south-east Asian ovalocytosis (SAO) is a dominant asymptomatic condition that is thought to confer protection against *Plasmodium falciparum* infection. The red cells are often described as stomatocytic elliptocytes and have a unique appearance on the peripheral blood smear (Fig. 13.4). Heterozygotes are not anemic. The homozygous state has never been seen and is thought to be lethal *in utero*.[157]

DIAGNOSIS

A careful inspection of the peripheral blood smear is the first step in identifying the various clinical forms of elliptocytosis (Figs 13.3 and 13.4). The red cell indices are normal in silent carriers and CHE, whereas profound microcytosis and an increased MCHC are features of HPP. Hematologic evaluation of the parents and siblings is usually helpful in defining the pattern of inheritance. Osmotic fragility is increased in HPP and homozygous CHE but normal in the less severe subtypes.[87] Osmotic gradient ektacytometry yields distinctive patterns that distinguish CHE from normal and from HPP (Fig. 13.5).[146,155]

Morphologic changes produced by heating red cells to 45–48°C suggest the presence of spectrin mutations such as are seen in HPP or CHE.[87] The test is easily done in any

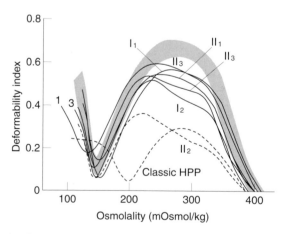

Fig. 13.5 Osmotic gradient ektacytometry in the elliptocytic disorders. The normal range is indicated by the shaded area. Results from a family in which various forms of elliptocytosis were present are shown. I_1 and II_1 = common hereditary elliptocytosis (CHE) (spectrin $\alpha^{I/50a}$ mutation). I_2 and II_3 = CHE (spectrin $\alpha^{I/65}$ mutation). II_3 curve 1 (top curve) = transient neonatal poikilocytosis at birth, II_3 curve 3 (lower curve) = same child at 7 months of age after conversion from transient neonatal poikilocytosis to CHE. II_2 = severe CHE (compound heterozygosity for spectrin $\alpha^{I/50a}$ and spectrin $\alpha^{I/65}$ mutations). A classic case of hereditary pyropoikilocytosis (HPP) is shown for comparison. Only the HPP red cells exhibit a shift to the right in the $Di_{minimum}$ indicating the presence of spherocytes (see Fig. 13.2). Reproduced with permission from Ref. 155.

laboratory, but is limited by the occurrence of occasional false positive and false negative results. Other tests require the facilities of specialized laboratories. SDS-denaturing polyacrylamide gel electrophoresis of red cell membrane proteins can detect spectrin deficiency and truncated α- or β-spectrins as well as protein 4.1 deficiency and abnormally large or small protein 4.1 mutant polypeptides. Non-denaturing acrylamide gel electrophoresis of spectrin extracted from membrane ghosts can detect and quantitate an abnormally high proportion of spectrin dimers relative to tetramers.

Tryptic peptide mapping by 2-dimensional gel electrophoresis of digested spectrin is a powerful way to define the presence and general location of a spectrin structural mutation.[87] Identification of specific mutations is best done by DNA analysis. Detection of frequently encountered mutations such as α-spectrin[LELY 158] or the Band III mutation responsible for SAO[159] by PCR-based DNA analysis is feasible, but these tests are not widely available. Prenatal diagnosis has been accomplished by direct examination of fetal red cells and membrane proteins.[160] If the specific mutation(s) present in the family are known, prenatal diagnosis by analysis of fetal DNA is also feasible.

PATHOPHYSIOLOGY

The elliptocytic shape is conferred by the red cell membrane skeleton as shown by persistence of the change in shape of red cell ghosts and skeletons prepared from ghosts by removal of the lipid bilayer.[161] Elliptocytes form as the red cell matures, since immature red cells in the hereditary elliptocytosis syndromes do not exhibit any morphologic abnormalities.[87] The elliptocytic change in shape is thought to be the result of the repeated episodes of elliptocytic deformation that all red cells experience during each circulatory cycle. Whereas normal red cells regain a discocytic configuration by a process of elastic recoil, hereditary elliptocytic red cells appear to be locked into the elliptocytic configuration by disruption of the normally abundant interconnections between the various cytoskeletal proteins.

The elliptocytic shape, *per se*, does not necessarily shorten the life-span of the red cell. For example, south-east Asian ovalocytes, despite being rigid cells with a membrane mechanical stability greater than normal, have a normal life-span.[87] It is the weakening of cytoskeletal protein interactions by mutations in protein structure or by deficiencies in the amount of a skeletal protein that leads to diminished membrane mechanical stability and ultimately to hemolysis. Mutations in α- or β-spectrin chains, protein 4.1, Band 3 or, rarely, glycophorin exert their effect by altering the horizontal stability of the membrane skeleton.[87] In the case of α- or β-spectrin mutations near the dimer-dimer association region, spectrin tetramer formation is impaired, while protein 4.1 or glycophorin deficiency affect the spectrin-actin-protein 4.1 complex and the vertical attachment to the membrane through glycophorin. In any event, membrane mechanical stability is reduced, which if severe may lead to red cell fragmentation, microcytosis and hemolysis. An elegant experimental confirmation of this proposed mechanism comes from the study of protein 4.1-deficient red cells. These cells exhibit striking membrane mechanical fragility on *in vitro* testing in the ektacytometer.[152] Reconstitution of normal protein 4.1 content in 4.1-deficient red cells by exchange hemolysis restores normal membrane mechanical fragility.[62] Even truncated fragments of the 4.1 peptide that contain the spectrin-actin binding domain are sufficient to correct the defect in mechanical stability.[63]

Although mechanical fragility is impaired, leading to fragmentation and microcytosis, intravascular hemolysis appears to play little role in red cell destruction since hemoglobinuria, hemoglobinemia or hemosiderinuria are not features of hemolytic elliptocytosis. In fact, considerable hemolysis must occur within the spleen, since splenectomy usually reduces the hemolytic rate.

In α- and β-spectrin mutations, the extent to which normal dimer-dimer self association is impaired is a major determinant of the degree of membrane mechanical instability and consequent hemolysis.[164,165] This is reflected by the degree of elevation in the concentration of spectrin dimers in the membrane. In HPP, where hemolysis is particularly severe, the spectrin content of the membrane is also reduced, leading to disruption in vertical associations of skeletal proteins with the lipid bilayer and loss of membrane surface area as is seen in spherocytosis.[87] The resulting spherocytes contribute to the shortened red cell life-span.

Alterations in the microcirculation or transient developmental factors present during fetal and early postnatal life[145] can generate poikilocytosis and hemolysis in individuals born with CHE. The microcirculatory changes include those associated with rejection of a renal transplant and those seen in thrombotic thrombocytopenic purpura.[150] Presumably, the added mechanical stress of passing through altered capillaries partly occluded by fibrin strands is responsible for fragmentation and hemolysis. Transient neonatal poikilocytosis and hemolysis is thought to occur as a consequence of the high concentrations of fetal hemoglobin in neonatal red cells. Because fetal hemoglobin does not bind 2,3-DPG, large amounts of free 2,3-DPG are available in the neonatal red cell to interact with and destabilize the membrane skeleton.[146] In normal neonatal red cells this does not appear to have a discernible effect on red cell shape or survival, but in red cells whose membrane skeleton is weakened by an inherited defect involving spectrin or other skeletal proteins, the sum of the effects of 2,3-DPG and the inherited defect is sufficient to decrease mechanical stability, producing poikilocytosis and hemolytic anemia. As fetal hemoglobin levels decline over the first few months of life, the contribution of 2,3-DPG to the hemolytic process wanes, hemolysis disappears and poikilocytes are replaced by the elliptocytes that are characteristic of common hereditary elliptocytosis.

MOLECULAR PATHOLOGY AND GENETICS

Two general types of mutation underlie the hereditary elliptocytic syndromes. The first alters the structure of a membrane protein, adversely affecting the normal interactions of the affected protein with its neighbors. The second reduces or abolishes the synthesis of a membrane protein, usually lowering its concentration in the membrane. The variable clinical severity of hereditary elliptocytosis is a consequence of the many possible combinations of these 2 types of mutations that may be inherited. Mutations in protein 4.1, α- and β-spectrin, Band 3, and glycophorin B have been described.[2,3,166]

Protein 4.1

Heterozygotes for 2 structural mutations and 5 mutations that lead to deficiency of protein 4.1 have been discovered (Table 13.2). All have elliptocytosis without hemolysis or anemia. Homozygotes for the deficiency mutations have no protein 4.1 in their red cells and exhibit a severe poikilocytic hemolytic anemia.

Table 13.2 Known mutations of red cell membrane protein 4.1.

Ref	Mutation site	Mutation	Result	Origin
201	Downstream initiation site	nt 161 (T→G) in exon 4	No RBC 4.1	Spain
202	Downstream initiation site	nt 161 (T→C) in exon 4	No RBC 4.1	France
53	Downstream initiation site	318 nt deletion of exons 4,5	No RBC 4.1	Algeria
203	Downstream initiation site and 5′ coding region	2 kb deletion	No RBC 4.1	France
204, 205	Spectrin/actin binding domain	Deletion of exons 16,17	Shortened RBC 4.1	Italy
204, 205	Spectrin/actin binding domain	Duplication of exons 16,17,18	Elongated RBC 4.1	Scotland, Ireland
205a	Upstream and downstream initiation sites	Deletion of exons 2–12	No RBC 4.1	France

α-Spectrin

Mutations in α-spectrin have usually been identified because they alter a tryptic cleavage site on spectrin, generating an abnormal peptide pattern following electrophoresis of spectrin tryptic digests. The majority of mutations are located near the N-terminal end of the spectrin polypeptide and alter the normal 80-kDa α1 tryptic fragment that arises from this region, creating fragments that are 78, 74, 65 or 46–50 kDa in size. An abnormal tryptic fragment may be the result of numerous mutations in the proximity of the tryptic cleavage site. Thus, 3 mutations are associated with the αI-78 fragment, 9 with the αI-74 fragment, 2 with the αI-65 fragment, and 7 (in 2 distinct regions of α spectrin) with the αI-46–50 fragment.[2,166–168] For the most part these are single nucleotide substitutions, nearly always occuring in helix C of one of the repeating polypeptide units of α spectrin. In the αII tryptic fragment, which is adjacent to the αI-80 fragment, 3 mutations have been discovered.[166,169,170] In addition, several truncated α-spectrin variants have been reported, one due to deletion of exon 18,[171] another to deletion of exon 39,[172] a third to deletion of exon 39,[173] a fourth to insertion of a novel mobile element into exon 5 which leads to deletion of this exon,[174] and a fifth whose molecular basis has yet to be established.[175]

The large number of α-spectrin mutations has allowed correlations to be established between clinical severity and the nature of the mutation. Mutations near the site of dimer-dimer self association at the N-terminus of the α-spectrin polypeptide, which are the commonest, are those most likely to interfere with tetramer formation and lead to clinical symptoms.[3,166] Another important determinant of clinical severity is the amount of mutant spectrin polypeptides present. In general, the greater the percentage of mutant spectrin, the more severe the clinical course.[164,165] Variation in the amount of mutant spectrin found in members of a given pedigree is sometimes due to homozygous or heterozygous inheritance of the structural mutation, but more often it is due to the presence or absence of a low-expression α-spectrin mutation inherited in *trans* to a single mutant α-spectrin allele.

The commonest example of such a low expression allele is α-spectrin[LELY] which is present in 20–30% of α-spectrin alleles in the normal population.[176] The primary mutation, which is in intron 45, leads to variable splicing and loss of exon 46 in about half of the mRNA synthesized.[158] α-Spectrin polypeptides lacking exon 46 sequences do not participate as avidly as do normal α-spectrin polypeptides in dimer and tetramer assembly and, therefore, are vulnerable to loss by proteolysis. The ultimate effect of such a mutation, then, is to reduce the quantity of α-spectrin available for assembly into the membrane. Since more α- than β-spectrin is normally synthesized, a moderate reduction in α-spectrin need not alter the number of α-β-spectrin dimers finally assembled into the membrane. It will however have the effect of increasing the fraction of α-spectrin from

the non-spectrin[LELY] allele in *trans* that participates in the final assembly. If this allele bears a mutation that is associated with elliptocytosis, the greater quantity of the mutant spectrin in the membrane will usually be associated with greater clinical severity.[167,168] In contrast, if the α-spectrin[LELY] mutation is inherited in *cis* with an elliptocytic mutation, there will be a reduced quantity of the mutant spectrin in the membrane and a milder clinical picture.[177]

There are several other interesting features of the spectrin[LELY] mutation. Homozygotes have normal amounts of spectrin in the red cell membrane and membrane function is normal, indicating that spectrin[LELY] polypeptides are capable of combining with β-spectrin to form a normal dimer. A tightly linked point mutation in exon 40 (Leu→Val) which alters the usual spectrin tryptic digestion pattern has been found in every spectrin[LELY] individual studied. This mutation does not alter α-spectrin synthesis or function but has served as a convenient marker for the presence of spectrin[LELY].[158,178]

Although spectrin[LELY] is the commonest low-expression α-spectrin mutation, at least 3 others have been found. Two pedigrees investigated by Hanspall *et al*[179] harbored an undefined mutation that greatly reduced the amount of α-spectrin mRNA synthesis, thus distinguishing it from the spectrin[LELY] mutation where mRNA synthesis is normal. Spectrin[Oran] is an αII splice site mutation which leads to the loss of exon 18.[171] Spectrin[St Claude], another αII mutation associated with a splicing defect, produces 2 mRNA species. One contains a terminator codon midway along the α-spectrin coding region, producing a small α-spectrin that is rapidly proteolyzed. The other is associated with skipping of exon 40 and a slightly truncated α-spectrin polypeptide.[173]

β-spectrin

Mutations of β-spectrin that lead to elliptocytosis are located at the C-end of the molecule and affect dimer-dimer association. Six single nucleotide substitutions in the β-17 repeat located at the C-terminus (4 within helix A and 2 within helix B) produce full length β-spectrin polypeptides with altered function. A surprising distant effect of each of these mutations is alteration of the tryptic digestion pattern of α-spectrin, a consequence of enhanced access of trypsin to the αI[74] cleavage site. The result is an increase in the quantity of the αI[74] fragment at the expense of the αI[80] fragment. Heterozygotes bearing these mutations are usually clinically silent or mildly affected, but homozygotes have severe or even lethal disease.[2,168,180–182] Another group of mutations at the C-terminus produce β-spectrin polypeptides that are truncated by 2,[183] 4,[184–187] or 10 kDa.[188,190] Like the previous group, these mutations lead to altered dimer-dimer associations. In some instances the truncated β-spectrin polypeptides may be produced in low abundance.[184,186,190] Since α-spectrin is normally produced in excess quantities, the amount of β-spectrin synthesized should determine the total quantity of spectrin that will ultimately be assembled on the red cell membrane. For this reason, low-abundance truncated β-spectrin mutants may be associated with spectrin deficiency as well as altered dimer-dimer associations,[184,186,190] sometimes,[190] but not always,[186] giving rise to a clinical picture of spherocytic elliptocytosis. An unstable extra long β-spectrin polypeptide has also been found in one kindred.[191] Heterozygotes have about 25% mutant β spectrin. Spectrin deficiency and reduced dimer–dimer association are both present, but the abnormalities are not sufficient to cause any clinical abnormalities.

Band 3

The mutation responsible for SAO is a deletion of 9 amino acids (codons 400–408) at the junction of the membrane-spanning domain and the cytoplasmic tail of Band 3.[159,192,193] The SAO mutation increases oligomerization and membrane skeletal association of Band 3, restricting lateral mobility and increasing membrane rigidity.[159,194] The SAO mutation is invariably linked to the Band 3 Memphis polymorphism, a separate point mutation at codon 56, near the N-terminus of the cytoplasmic tail.[195] The Band 3 Memphis mutation serves as a molecular marker for SAO but does not contribute to the membrane abnormalities characteristic of SAO.

Glycophorin

A complete deficiency of glycophorin C, known as the Leach phenotype, can be identified by absence of the Gerbich blood group antigen and by the presence of elliptocytosis (without hemolysis). A secondary partial deficiency of protein 4.1 and protein p55 is present in these cells and is thought to explain the elliptocytic morphology. In homozygous protein 4.1 deficiency, glycophorin C and the Gerbich blood group antigen are both reduced by about 70%.[196] The postulated binding of the normal cytoskeleton to the membrane through interactions between glycophorin C, 4.1 and p55 is consistent with these observations.[46]

RESISTANCE TO MALARIA

As is the case with mutations of hemoglobin and intra-erythrocytic enzymes, alterations in red cell membrane structure that lead to elliptocytosis may provide resistance against malaria and, due to positive evolutionary selection, be found in high prevalence in regions where malaria has been or is endemic. Resistance to malaria seems to be a reasonable hypothesis to explain the approximately 1% incidence of common hereditary elliptocytosis in inhabitants of Benin in West Africa,[143] although convincing evidence of a protective effect against malaria has yet to be obtained. More convincing data are available in the case of heterozygous south-east Asian ovalocytosis which was found to be present in about 15% of all inhabitants of the Madang area of Papua New Guinea, but in only 9% of those who had

uncomplicated *P. falciparum* malaria and in none of those with potentially life-threatening cerebral malaria.[197] The resistance of these ovalocytes to malaria may involve diminished invasion, poor intraerythrocytic growth or diminished cytoadherence of infected erythrocytes.[198]

Inherited red cell membrane protein defects have also been used to explore the details of the interaction between the malarial parasite and its intraerythrocytic environment. *P. falciparum* parasites that generate mature-parasite-infected erythrocyte surface antigen (MESA), a protein that is thought to play a role in regulating cytoadherence, do not grow well in protein 4.1-deficient red cells. MESA binds to protein 4.1 in normal red cells and the failure of this association probably explains the accumulation of large amounts of MESA in the cytoplasm of 4.1-deficient cells, an event that is presumably unfavorable for parasite development.[199] *P. falciparum* invasion into protein 4.1- or glycophorin C-deficient red cells is greatly reduced, but once inside parasites grow normally in the latter red cells but poorly in the former.[200] The importance of a normal 4.1-glycophorin C-protein 55 complex for parasite invasion and development is established by these studies.

TREATMENT

Most cases require no specific therapy. Supportive care measures such as supplemental folic acid or occasional red cell transfusions for episodes of anemia (usually related to infection) may be helpful. When hemolysis is severe, splenectomy may eliminate the need for regular red cell transfusions and improve the anemia. As in hereditary spherocytosis, the increased risk of bacterial infection following splenectomy in infancy or early childhood is a reason to wait until later childhood or adolescence before considering surgery.

SPICULATED RED CELLS (ECHINOCYTES AND ACANTHOCYTES)

Echinocytes and acanthocytes are types of spiculated red blood cells. *Echinocytes* have serrated edges over the entire surface of the cell and often appear crenated in a blood smear. *Acanthocytes* have only a few spicules of varying size that project from the cell surface at irregular intervals. They appear contracted and dense on stained peripheral blood smears. Wet preparations or scanning electron micrographs can be used to distinguish these 2 types of cells. Echinocytes can be produced *in vitro* by washing red cells in saline, by interactions between glass and red cells and by insertion of amphipathic compounds that localize to the exterior leaflet of the lipid bilayer.[4,206] High pH, ATP depletion and Ca^{2+} accumulation can also cause echinocytosis.[207] Echinocytes are seen in neonates and in patients with uremia,[208,209] those who have defects in glycolytic metabolism, after splenectomy and in some patients with microangiopathic hemolytic anemia. Acanthocytosis and echinocytes may be found in patients with liver damage,[210-216] abetalipoproteinemia, unusual neurologic symptoms, anorexia nervosa, McLeod and IN(Lu) blood groups, myelodysplasia and hypothyroidism.

ABETALIPOPROTEINEMIA

Progressive ataxia, retinitis pigmentosa, celiac syndrome and acanthocytosis are the primary manifestations of abetalipoproteinemia.[211,217] Absorption of lipids through the intestine is defective, serum cholesterol levels are extremely low, and serum β lipoprotein is absent in this hereditary disease. The disease is due to failure to synthesize or secrete lipoprotein containing products of the apolipoprotein B gene. A spectrum of clinical manifestations can be seen, depending upon the extent to which apolipoprotein B-mediated metabolic processes are affected. All patients have neurologic impairment and acanthocyes.[217] The red cell defect in shape is not present in young cells but accumulates with cell aging. In severe cases, 50–90% of the red cells are acanthocytes. Membrane lipids but not proteins are affected. Despite the profound morphologic abnormality, anemia and evidence for hemolysis are not found.

In the abetalipoproteinemic-acanthocytic red cell, the outer leaflet of the red cell membrane is enriched in sphingomyelin and cholesterol and the total red cell content of phosphatidyl choline is decreased by 20%.[218-220] These lipid abnormalities are thought to explain acanthocyte formation in this setting. As a consequence of fat malabsorption, patients may become deficient in vitamin E,[251] rendering their acanthocytic red cells susceptible to hemolysis following *in vitro* incubation in dilute solutions of hydrogen peroxide. Whether vitamin E deficiency influences the various clinical manifestations of this disease is not known. However, children who have chronic liver disease and develop vitamin E deficiency have been reported to develop acanthocytosis as well as neurologic dysfunction.[222-224] The neurologic abnormalities in these patients can be delayed or prevented by chronic parenteral administration of vitamin E.

ACANTHOCYTOSIS WITH NEUROLOGIC DISEASE AND NORMAL LIPOPROTEINS (AMYOTROPHIC CHOREA-ACANTHOCYTOSIS)

This syndrome is characterized by acanthocytes, normolipoproteinemia and progressive neurologic disease beginning in late childhood, adolescence or adult life. The neurologic manifestations are varied but always include chorea. Muscle wasting is prominent.[225,226] The relationship between the red cell changes and neurologic manifestations are unclear, although a defect in the red cell membrane is likely to exist. The basal ganglia and caudate nucleus show atrophic changes. A variety of conditions that are likely to be variants

of this disorder have been reported. These include syndromes with chorea-acanthocytosis and myopathy and with chorea-acanthocytosis, spherocytosis and hemolysis.[227-232] Other rare neurologic disorders have been reported to have acanthocytes; their cause is unknown but the presence of the acanthocytes suggests that a defect may exist in the red cell membrane. Studies of individual patients vary but suggest subtle changes in lipids and/or proteins. Further investigation of the precise defect in the red cell may provide insights into the pathophysiologic processes affecting the brain.

MISCELLANEOUS DISORDERS

A variety of additional disorders are associated with either acanthocytes or echinocytes.

Anorexia nervosa

Patients with anorexia nervosa may have acanthocytes.[212,233] The mechanisms responsible have not been defined and considerable variation in the number of acanthocytes exists between patients. Changes in plasma lipids or red cell membrane proteins may be involved. However, the anemia seen in patients with anorexia nervosa is more often hypoplastic and not hemolytic or related to the changes in red cell morphology.

Liver disease

Patients with liver disease may develop either target cells or spur cells.[234-236] Those with target cells have a reversible disorder primarily related to the increased unesterified cholesterol content of the plasma associated with lecithin-cholesterol acyl transferase inhibition (see below) and do not have hemolysis. In contrast, patients with advanced hepatocellular disease have 20–30% acanthocytes in their peripheral blood and moderate-to-severe hemolysis.[236,237] Echinocytes and target cells may also be present. In contrast to target cells, where there is a proportionate increase in red cell cholesterol and phospholipid, in spur cells or acanthocytes associated with hepatocellular liver disease, there is not only an increase in both cholesterol and phospholipid, but a dramatic increase in the ratio of cholesterol to phospholipid. The precise impact of this imbalance of lipids on membrane properties and the profound hemolysis associated with this condition have not been determined. In addition to these quantitative lipid abnormalities, a defect in the remodeling of membrane phospholipids is present.[238] To add additional complexity to the picture, some patients with advanced hepatocellular liver disease, particularly children, develop spur cells but do not have abnormalities in membrane lipids.

Vitamin E deficiency

Echinocytes and occasional acanthocytes are a feature of vitamin E deficiency.[234] Previously noted in premature infants due to inadequate dietary vitamin E content, this condition is now limited to patients who have fat malabsorption, often related to liver disease or cystic fibrosis. Parenteral administration of vitamin E will correct the deficiency in patients with impaired gastrointestinal absorption of this vitamin.[222,223]

Blood group abnormalities

Acanthocytes have been associated with certain abnormalities of the blood group systems. In McLeod's syndrome, an X-linked inherited anomaly of the Kell blood group system, red cells, leukocytes, or both cell types react poorly with Kell antisera but behave normally in other blood group reactions.[240] Affected cells lack the product of a membrane precursor related to the Kell antigens.[241] Males have variable acanthocytosis (8–85%) and mild compensated hemolysis. Females have only occasional acanthocytes and very mild hemolysis.[242,243] Some McLeod patients develop a neuropathy or myopathy. Psychiatric symptoms, seizures and peripheral neuropathy with muscle deneravation have also been reported.

The commonest cause of the null Lutheran phenotype Lu(a-b-) is the presence of an inhibitor called In(Lu) which partially suppresses expression of Lu_a and Lu_b so that these antigens are undetectable by standard agglutination tests.[214] About 1 person in 5000 inherits this dominantly acting inhibitor. Patients with this inhibitor have abnormally shaped red cells but no hemolysis. Red cell morphology may be normal, poikilocytic or acanthocytic.[244]

Uremia

Echinocytes are found in the blood smear of patients who develop uremia and hemolysis.[245] These are secondary to an extracorpuscular factor which appears to affect red cell metabolism and results in elevated levels of intracellular calcium, a factor known to induce echinocytosis.[242] Red cells from patients with uremia survive normally when infused into non-uremic recipients.

Other disorders

Woronet's trait is a benign, dominantly inherited condition associated with acanthocytosis (5–10%) and echinocytosis has been reported in a single family.[246] Red cell life-span is normal.

Approximately 50% of patients with *hypothyroidism* have a small number of acanthocytes (0.5–2%) on peripheral blood smears.[247] Therefore, thyroid testing may be indicated when acanthocytes are seen.[248]

TARGET CELLS

Target cells are red cells that have an increased surface area:volume ratio. The redundant membrane creates what appears to be a hyperchromic bullseye in the center of the red cell when viewed on a stained peripheral blood smear. Target cells are generated either by increasing the membrane lipid content and thus the surface area or by decreasing cell volume. The latter is the consequence of decreased hemoglobin synthesis (thalassemia or iron deficiency), the presence of certain structural mutations of hemoglobin (S, C, D, E), or as a result of primary disorders of cell hydration.[4] Generally, an increase in membrane surface area does not affect red cell survival, while reduced volume from cellular dehydration or reduced hemoglobin synthesis often may.

In the peripheral blood smear of patients who have obstructive liver disease, target cells are often seen, reflecting a balanced increase in phospholipids and cholesterol.[249–251] Unesterified cholesterol in the plasma increases in concentration as a result of the inhibition of lecithin-cholesterol acyl transferase (LCAT) by bile salts. The central role of abnormal plasma lipids in the formation of target cells can be shown *in vitro* by incubation of normal red cells in plasma from patients with obstructive liver disease or, conversely, by incubating target cells in normal plasma. In the former situation, target cells are formed and in the latter they disappear. This is the basis for the observation that in hereditary spherocytosis patients who develop temporary obstructive jaundice as a result of gallstones, the hemolytic process improves and osmotic fragility may become normal. In this setting, the increase in membrane surface area normalizes the previously abnormal surface area:volume ratio of spherocytes.[252]

Target cells are also seen in hereditary LCAT deficiency, a rare disease due to a mutation in the LCAT gene.[253,254] Plasma unesterified cholesterol and phospholipid concentrations are increased. The disorder, which exhibits an autosomal recessive mode of inheritance, is characterized by anemia, corneal opacities, hyperlipemia, proteinuria, chronic nephritis, and premature atherosclerosis.[255–257] A moderate normochromic, normocytic anemia accompanied by prominent target cell formation and decreased red cell osmotic fragility is noted. Serum and red cell lipids are improved *in vivo* when LCAT is provided by infusions of normal plasma.

In the first few weeks following splenectomy target cells appear, reaching levels of 2–10%. Like other target cells, membrane lipids are increased, osmotic fragility is decreased, and the mean surface area:volume ratio is increased.[258] The spleen normally removes excess membrane from red cells, a process called 'splenic conditioning'.[259,260] The exact mechanism responsible is not defined, although the reduction in red cell lipid content suggests that lipases may be involved. Post splenectomy, red cells may eventually lose their excess lipid by conditioning in non-splenic sites, gradually leading to the disappearance of target cells.

DISORDERS OF RED CELL HYDRATION AND CATION TRANSPORT

Either de- or over-hydration of red cells may be the consequence of inherited membrane disorders of cation transport. *Xerocytosis* and *hydrocytosis*, the names given to these 2 disorders, stand at the extremes of abnormalities of red cell hydration. Both are associated with chronic hemolytic anemia. There are also rare, poorly understood hemolytic disorders that involve cation transport but do not fit neatly into the xerocytosis-hydrocytosis dichotomy. Beyond this, primary disorders of metabolism or hemoglobinopathies may produce a secondary abnormality of cell hydration that contributes to the hemolytic process. This section focuses on the primary disorders of cell hydration; the secondary disorders are covered in Chapters 12 and 14.

XEROCYTOSIS

Clinical features

Little or no anemia is usually found in this disorder, although the red cell life-span may be considerably shortened.[2,261,262] Exercise-associated episodes of hemolysis were reported in a competitive swimmer who had xerocytosis.[263] Splenomegaly is uncommon. Inheritance has usually been autosomal dominant. In one family, linkage between Factor VII deficiency and xerocytosis was observed.[264]

Laboratory findings

The hallmark of xerocytosis is red cell dehydration, which is most easily detected by an examination of the red cell indices (high MCHC) or the osmotic fragility curve (increased osmotic resistance). Ektacytometry reveals a decreased deformability index (DI) minimum and a shift to the left in the hyperosmotic arm (Fig. 13.6). These tests serve to separate xerocytosis from spherocytosis, where the MCHC may be elevated but osmotic fragility is usually increased. A simple test may reveal resistance of xerocytes to heat-induced budding and fragmentation.[262] Target cells and occasional bizarre red cells where the hemoglobin is puddled at each pole are seen on the peripheral blood smear (Fig. 13.7).[265] The reticulocyte count is often increased to a level higher than that expected for the degree of anemia. Ultimately, the diagnosis of xerocytosis depends on recognizing the abnormalities listed above and eliminating from consideration other diseases such as hemoglobinopathies or pyruvate kinase deficiency that may produce similar abnormalities.

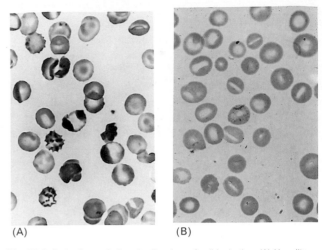

(A)   (B)

Fig. 13.6 Red cell morphology in disorders of cell hydration. (A) Hereditary xerocytosis; (B) hereditary hydrocytosis. Reproduced with permission from Ref. 261.

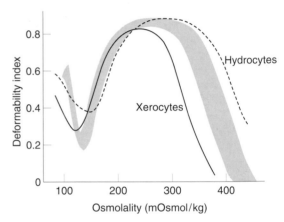

Fig. 13.7 Osmotic gradient ektacytometry of xerocytes and hydrocytes. The normal range is indicated by the shaded area. The deformability index (DI) minimum in hypotonic medium (normal about 140 mOsmol/kg) is shifted to the left in xerocytosis and to the right in hydrocytosis. Although the entire curves are shifted, both xerocytes and hydrocytes achieve a normal maximal DI (but not at the physiologic plasma osmolarity of 290 mOsmol). Reproduced with permission from Ref. 261.

Pathophysiology and nature of the primary defect

The basic red cell abnormality in xerocytosis is passive loss of intracellular K^+ in excess of accumulation of intracellular Na^+, leading to a gradual decline in total intracellular cations and an obligate loss of cell water to maintain osmotic balance. Active transport of cations via the Na^+/K^+-ATPase pump does not restore cation homeostasis but rather exaggerates the defect, since the fixed stoichiometry of the pump (3 Na^+ out:2 K^+ in) leads to a further net loss of cations from the cell.[266] A primary pathway for cellular dehydration in hemoglobinopathic red cells (HbS, HbC) is volume-dependent KCl co-transport. This pathway has not been characterized extensively in xerocytes, but in one family there was evidence that it was abnormal.[267] The dehydrated xerocyte is a rigid due both to its increased cytoplasmic viscosity[268] and perhaps also to intrinsic membrane rigidity induced by complexing of globin to spectrin.[269] The rigidity of the xerocyte may contribute to its shortened life-span by increasing its sensitivity to shear-induced hemolysis in the circulation.[263] *In vitro* following metabolic depletion, xerocytes resemble hereditary spherocytes in their proclivity to vesiculation and loss of membrane surface area.[270] Finally, xerocytes, like other dehydrated red cells, are susceptible to injury by exogenous oxidants, a susceptibility that can be prevented by prior rehydration of the cells.[271]

The primary molecular event responsible for xerocytosis is unknown. Red cell membrane protein composition has usually been normal but increased binding of globin[272] and glyceraldehyde-3-phosphate dehydrogenase[273] to membrane proteins has been noted. Increased hemoglobin-spectrin complexing has been observed, particularly in the densest xerocyte sub-population.[269] In one xerocytic family there was an excess of all the major red cell membrane proteins.[272] Consistent with this finding, the surface area of xerocytes is increased.[274] Red cell phosphatidylcholine content is often increased, but no linkage between this abnormality and the cation transport defects that lead to cellular dehydration has been established.[275] Red cell 2,3-DPG levels are low in xerocytes[265,270] for reasons that are unclear. The predicted leftward shift in the hemoglobin oxygen dissociation curve that accompanies low 2,3-DPG levels may lead to a functional deficit in oxygen transport despite normal or near normal hemoglobin levels, accounting for the often striking reticulocytosis that may be seen in xerocytosis patients.

Treatment

No specific treatment is available or usually required. Splenectomy is of little or no benefit.

HYDROCYTOSIS (STOMATOCYTOSIS)

Clinical features

Mild-to-moderate life-long hemolytic anemia, often accompanied by splenomegaly, jaundice, and the early development of pigment gallstones are seen in hydrocytosis.[261] Some affected individuals develop evidence of iron overload, even in the absence of blood transfusions.[140] Hydrocytosis is a rare disorder, but in informative pedigrees where >1 family member has been affected, the inheritance has been autosomal dominant.[140,261]

Laboratory findings

As implied by the name, cell water is increased in hydrocytes, causing them to swell and appear on the peripheral blood smear as stomatocytes (Fig. 13.7). The swollen, water-logged cells can also be recognized by the unusually high MCV (often >120 fl) and low MCHC that are seen in this condition. The osmotic fragility of hydrocytes is increased and osmotic gradient ektacytometry produces a characteristic profile (Fig. 13.6). Unlike normal red cells, hydrocytes are low in K^+ and high in Na^+. The total monovalent cation content (Na^+ and K^+) of hydrocytes is greater than that of normal red cells. Increased osmotic fragility is found in both hydrocytosis and hereditary spherocytosis, but the 2 disorders are easily distinguished on the basis of their morphology, red cell indices and red cell monovalent cation content.

Pathophysiology and nature of the primary defect

Like xerocytosis, hydrocytosis is caused by an abnormality in passive monovalent cation flux. The dominant abnormality is increased passive influx of Na^+, which is not matched by an equivalent outflow of K^+. Active cation transport by the Na^+/K^+-ATPase pump, although greatly increased, is unable to prevent the accumulation of intracellular Na^+ and the resulting increase in monovalent cation content causes an osmotic movement of water into the cell, cell swelling, and transformation from discocyte to stomatocyte morphology. Metabolic depletion, by preventing ATP generation for the Na^+/K^+-ATPase pump, inhibits active transport of Na^+ out of the cell and accelerates water accumulation and cell swelling.[276] As in spherocytosis, the favorable effect of splenectomy on the rate of hemolysis is most likely due to removal of the organ where metabolic depletion of red cells is most likely to occur. The importance of overhydration as the basis for shortening the life-span of hydrocytes was shown by experiments using the bifunctional cross-linking agent dimethyl adipimidate, an imidoester that reacts with lysine amino groups on proteins and phospholipids.[277] The passive influx of Na^+ into hydrocytes treated with dimethyl adipimidate became normal, allowing ATP-mediated active cation transport to restore to normal the content of intracellular cations and cell water. When the survival of treated cells was subsequently measured *in vivo* in a heterologous species experimental system, it was normal. The particular cross-linked groups responsible for the correction could not be identified, due to the ubiquity of lysine amino groups in red cell membrane proteins and phospholipids.[278]

The molecular basis for hydrocytosis is not known. Hydrocytic red cells from many patients lack stomatin, an integral red cell membrane protein, also termed protein 7.2b based on its migration pattern in SDS-PAGE gels.[279–283] Analysis of the sequence of normal erythrocyte stomatin cDNA indicates that the predicted polypeptide (MW 31 709 kDa) has a single transmembrane domain and a large C-terminal cytoplasmic tail.[282] These findings suggest that stomatin is not itself a transmembrane channel but that it may play a structural or regulatory role in cation transport.[284] Mutations that would alter the stomatin polypeptide sequence have not been found in stomatin cDNA from hydrocytosis patients and the stomatin mRNA content of

275

reticulocytes is normal.[282,285] A mutation affecting translation of stomatin mRNA may be responsible for the deficiency of this protein in hydrocytosis or, alternatively, an abnormality of an as yet unidentified neighboring protein, may affect stomatin binding and retention on the red cell membrane. Recent work in *C. elegans* indicates that a stomatin-like protein links the mechanosensory channel and the microtubule cytoskeleton of the touch receptor neurons, suggesting an interaction with ion channels consistent with the hypothesized role of stomatin in human red cells.[286]

Treatment

Splenectomy may diminish the rate of hemolysis,[276] but is to be avoided if at all possible because of an unusually high risk of serious thrombotic complications that persists for years after surgery.[140] An increased risk of thrombotic disease is seen in many hemolytic anemias if hemolysis persists after splenectomy.[287,141] Among the factors that may contribute to the thrombotic tendency are thrombocytosis, persistent reticulocytosis and interactions between the abnormal red cells and the vascular endothelium.[140,287,288] The basis for thromboembolic disease in hydrocytosis is unknown, but it is reasonable to suspect that the abnormal red cell membrane of these cells plays a role.

OTHER PRIMARY DISORDERS OF RED CELL HYDRATION

Cryohydrocytosis, another condition associated with abnormal cation transport and overhydrated red cells, is distinguished from hydrocytosis by the profound increase in cation permeability that occurs *in vitro* at low temperature (4°C).[289,290] A similar susceptibility to cold-induced cation permeability in which K^+ loss predominates and xerocytes instead of hydrocytes are present has also been described.[291] A third condition, the rH null syndrome, is peculiar in that stomatocytes are noted on the peripheral blood smear and osmotic fragility is increased, suggesting cellular overhydration, but cation content and cell water are actually decreased.[292]

REFERENCES

1. Palek J, Jarolim P. Clinical expression and laboratory detection of red blood cell membrane protein mutations. *Semin Hemat* 1993; **30**: 249–283

2. Lux SE, Palek J. Disorders of the red cell membrane. In: Handin RI, Lux SE, Stossel TP (eds) *Blood. Principles and Practice of Hematology*. Philadelphia: Lippencott, 1995, pp 1701–1818

3. Delaunay J. Genetic disorders of the red cell membrane. *Crit Rev Oncol Hematol* 1995; **19**: 79–110

4. Gallagher PG, Forget BG, Lux SE. Disorders of the erythrocyte membrane. In: Nathan DG, Orkin SH (eds) *Hematology of Infancy and Childhood*, 5th edn. Philadelphia: WB Saunders, 1997, pp 544–664

5. Sweeley CC, Dawson G. Lipids of the erythrocyte. In: Jamieson GA,

6. Greenwalt TJ (eds) *Red Cell Membrane Structure and Function*. Philadelphia: JB Lippincott, 1969, pp 172–227

6. Ways P, Hanahan DJ. Characterization and quantification of red cell lipids in normal man. *J Lipid Res* 1964; **5**: 318–328

7. Van Deenen LLM, DeGier J. Lipids of the red blood cell membrane. In: Surgenor DM (ed) *The Red Blood Cell*, 2nd edn. New York: Academic Press, 1974, p 148

8. Op den Kamp JAF. Lipid asymmetry in membranes. *Annu Rev Biochem* 1979; **48**: 47–71

9. Christiansson A, Kuypers FA, Roelofsen B, Op den Kamp JAF, van Deenen LLM. Lipid molecular shape effects erythrocyte morphology: A study involving replacement of native phosphatidylcholine with different species followed by treatment of cells with sphingomyelinase C or phospholipase A. *J Cell Biol* 1985; **101**: 1455–1462

10. Lubin BH, Kuypers FA. Phospholipid repair in human erythrocytes. In: Davies KJ (ed) *Oxidative Damage and Repair; Chemical, Biological, and Medical Aspects*. New York: Pergamon Press, 1991, pp 557–564

11. Ferrell JE Jr, Lee KJ, Huestis WH. Membrane bilayer balance and erythrocyte shape: A quantitative assessment. *Biochemistry* 1985; **24**: 2849–2857

12. Sheetz MP, Singer SJ. Biological membranes as bilayer couples: A molecular mechanism of drug-erythrocyte interactions. *Proc Natl Acad Sci USA* 1974; **71**: 4457–4461

13. Lange Y, Steck TL. Mechanism of red blood cell acanthocytosis and echinocytosis *in vivo*. *J Membr Biol* 1984; **77**: 153–159

14. Blau L, Bittman R. Cholesterol distribution between the two halves of the lipid bilayer of human erythrocyte ghost membranes. *J Biol Chem* 1978; **253**: 8366–8368

15. Lange Y, Dolde J, Steck TL. The rate of transmembrane movement of cholesterol in the human erythrocyte. *J Biol Chem* 1981; **256**: 5321–5323

16. Devaux PF. Lipid transmembrane asymmetry and flip-flip in biological membranes and in lipid bilayers. *Curr Opin Struct Biol* 1993; **3**: 489

17. Daleke DL, Huestis WH. Incorporation and translocation of aminophospholipids in human erythrocytes. *Biochemistry* 1985; **24**: 5406–5415

18. Devaux PF. Protein involvement in transmembrane lipid asymmetry. *Annu Rev Biophys Biomol Struct* 1992; **21**: 417–439

19. Devaux PF. Static and dynamic lipid asymmetry in cell membranes. *Biochemistry* 1991; **30**: 1163–1173

20. Zachowski A, Favre E, Cribiers S, Herve P, Devaux PF. Outside-inside translocation of aminophospholipids in the human erythrocyte membrane is mediated by a specific enzyme. *Biochemistry* 1986; **25**: 2585–2590

21. Williamson P, Kulick A, Zachowski A *et al*. Ca^{2+} induces transbilayer redistribution of all major phospholipids in human erythrocytes. *Biochemistry* 1992; **31**: 6355–6360

22. Seigneuret M, Devaux PF. ATP-dependent asymmetric distribution of spin-labeled phospholipids in the erythrocyte membrane: Relation to shape changes. *Proc Natl Acad Sci USA* 1984; **81**: 3751–3755

23. Tilley L, Cribier S, Roelofsen B, Op den Kamp JAF, van Deenan LLM. ATP-dependent translocation of amino phospholipids across the human erythrocyte membrane. *FEBS Lett* 1986; **194**: 21–27

24. Allen TM, Williamson P, Schlegel RA. Phosphatidylserine as a determinant of reticuloendothelial recognition of liposome models of the erythrocyte surface. *Proc Natl Acad Sci USA* 1988; **85**: 8067–8071

25. McEvoy L, Williamson P, Schlegel RA. Membrane phospholipid asymmetry as a determinant of erythrocyte recognition by macrophages. *Proc Natl Acad Sci USA* 1986; **83**: 3311–3315

26. Schwartz RS, Chiu DT, Lubin BH. Plasma membrane phospholipid organization in human erythrocytes. *Curr Topics Hematol* 1985; **5**: 63

27. Kuypers FA, Lubin BH, Yee M, Agre P, Devaux PF. The distribution of erythrocyte phospholipids in hereditary spherocytosis demonstrates a minimal role for erythrocyte spectrin on phospholipid diffusion and asymmetry. *Blood* 1993; **81**: 1051–1057

28. Haest CWM, Plasa G, Kamp D, Deuticke B. Spectrin as a stabilizer of

the phospholipid asymmetry in the human erythrocyte membrane. *Biochim Biophys Acta* 1978; **509**: 21–32

29. Lubin BH, Chiu D, Bastacky J, Roelofsen B, van Deenen LLM. Abnormalities in membrane phospholipid organization in sickled erythrocytes. *J Clin Invest* 1981; **67**: 1643–1649

30. Blumenfeld N, Zachowski A, Galacteros F, Beuzard E, Devaux PF. Transmembrane mobility of phospholipids in sickle erythrocytes: Effect of deoxygenation on diffusion and asymmetry. *Blood* 1991; **77**: 849–854

31. Franck PFH, Chiu D, Op den Kamp JA *et al*. Accerlerated transbilayer movement of phosphatidylcholine in sickled erythrocytes: A reversible process. *J Biol Chem* 1983; **258**: 8436.

32. Liu S-C, Derick LH, Zhai S, Palek J. Uncoupling of the spectrin-based skeleton from the lipid bilayer in sickled red cells. *Science* 1991; **252**: 574–576

33. Kuypers FA, Lewis RA, Ernst JD, Discher D, Lubin BH. Detection of altered membrane phospholipid asymmetry in subpopulations of human red cells using fluorescently labeled annexin V. *Blood* 1996; **87**: 1179–1187

34. Zwaal RFA, Comfurius P, Bevers EM. Mechanism and function of changes in membrane phospholipid asymmetry in platelets and erythrocytes. *Biochem Soc Trans* 1993; **21**: 248–253

35. Chiu D, Lubin BH, Roelofsen B, van Deenen LLM. Sickled erythrocytes accelerate clotting *in vitro*: An effect of abnormal membrane lipid asymmetry. *Blood* 1981; **58**: 398–401

36. Styles L, de Jong K, Vichinsky EV, Lubin BH, Adams R, Kuypers FA. Increased annexin binding in sickle cell disease patients at risk for stroke by transcranial doppler screening. *Proceedings 25th National Sickle Cell Disease Conference*, Washington DC, 1997, 98A

37. Wilson MJ, Richter-Loney K, Daleke DL. Hyperglycemia induces a loss of phospholipid asymmetry in human erythrocytes. *Biochemistry* 1993; **32**: 11302–11310

38. Berridge MJ. Inositol tripshosphate and calcium signaling. *Nature* 1993; **361**: 315–325

39. Rosse WF. Complement sensitivity of paroxysmal nocturnal hemoglobinuria cells. *Ser Haematol* 1972; **5**: 101–114

40. Test ST, Woolworth VS. Defective regulation of complement by the sickle erythrocyte: Evidence for a defect in control of membrane attack complex formation. *Blood* 1994; **83**: 842–852

41. Shohet SB, Nathan DG, Karnovsky ML. Stages in the incorporation of fatty acids into red blood cells. *J Clin Invest* 1968; **47**: 1096–1108

42. Farquhar JW, Ahrens EH Jr. Effects of dietary fats on human erythrocyte fatty acid patterns. *J Clin Invest* 1963; **42**: 675

43. Rosse W. The glycoprotein anchor of membrane surface proteins. *Semin Hematol* 1993; **30**: 219–231

44. Tanner, MJA. Molecular and cellular biology of the erythrocyte anion exchanger (AE1). *Semin Hematol* 1993; **30**: 34–57

45. Fukuda M. Molecular genetics of the glycophorin A gene cluster. *Semin Hematol* 1993; **30**: 138–151

46. Cartron JP, Kim CLV, Colin Y. Glycophorin C and related glycophorins: Structure, function, and regulation. *Semin Hematol* 1993; **30**: 152–168

47. Wang D, Mentzer WC, Cameron T, Johnson RM. Purification of band 7.2b, a 31-kDa integral phosphoprotein absent in hereditary stomatocytosis. *J Biol Chem* 1991; **266**: 17826–17831

48. Olives B, Mattei MG, Huet M *et al*. Kidd blood group and urea transport function of human erythrocytes are carried by the same protein. *J Biol Chem* 1995; **270**: 15607–15610.

49. Lee MD, King LS, Agre P. The aquaporin family of water channel proteins in clinical medicine. *Medicine* 1997; **76**: 141–156

50. Gallagher PG, Forget BG. Spectrin genes in health and disease. *Semin Hematol* 1993; **30**: 4–20

51. Peters LL, Lux SE. Ankyrins: Structure and function in normal cells and hereditary spherocytes. *Semin Hematol* 1993; **30**: 85–118

52. Cohen CM, Dotimas E, Korsgen C. Human erythrocyte membrane protein band 4.2 (pallidin). *Semin Hematol* 1993; **30**: 119–137

53. Conboy JG. Structure, function, and molecular genetics of erythroid membrane skeletal protein 4.1 in normal and abnormal red cells. *Semin Hematol* 1993; **30**: 58–74

54. Gilligan DM, Bennett V. The junctional complex of the membrane skeleton. *Semin Hematol* 1993; **30**: 74–83

55. Chasis, JA, Coulombel L, McGee S *et al*. Differential use of protein 4.1 translation initiation sites during erythropoiesis: Implications for a mutation-induced stage-specific deficiency of protein 4.1 during erythroid development. *Blood* 1996; **87**: 5324–5331

56. Hanspal M, Palek J. Biogenesis of normal and abnormal red blood cell membrane skeleton. *Semin Hematol* 1993; **30**: 305–319

57. Peters LL, Shivdasani RA, Liu SC *et al*. Anion exchanger 1 (Band 3) is required to prevent erythrocyte membrane surface loss but not to form the membrane skeleton. *Cell* 1996; **86**: 917–927

58. Mohandas N, Chasis JA. Red blood cell deformability, membrane material properties and shape: Regulation by transmembrane, skeletal, and cytosolic proteins and lipids. *Semin Hematol* 1993; **30**: 171–192

59. Cohen CM, Gascard P. Regulation and post-translational modification of erythrocyte membrane and membrane-skeletal proteins. *Semin Hematol* 1993; **30**: 244–292

60. Brugnara, C. Erythrocyte membrane transport physiology. *Curr Opin Hematol* 1997; **4**: 122–127

61. Mercer RW, Schneider JW, Benz EJ Jr. Na,K-ATPase structure. In: Agre P, Parker JC (eds) *Red Blood Cell Membranes*. New York: Marcel Dekker, 1989, pp 135–166

62. Parker JC, Dunham PB. Passive cation transport. In: Agre P, Parker JC (eds) *Red Blood Cell Membranes*. New York, Marcel Dekker, 1989, pp 507–562

63. Lauf PK, Bauer J, Adragna NC *et al*. Erythrocyte K-Cl cotransport: properties and regulation. *Am J Physiol* 1992; **263**: C917

64. Johnson RM. Membrane stress increases cation permeability in red cells. *Biophysic J* 1994; **67**: 1876–1881

65. Matovcik LM, Mentzer WC. The membrane of the human neonatal red cell. *Clin Haematol* 1985; **14**: 203–221

66. Lane PA, Galili U, Iarocci TA, Shew RL, Mentzer WC. Cellular dehydration and immunoglobulin binding in senescent neonatal erythrocytes. *Pediatr Res* 1988; **23**: 288–292

67. Matovcik LM, Groschel-Stewart U, Schrier SL. Myosin in adult and neonatal human erythrocyte membranes. *Blood* 1986; **67**: 1668–1674

68. Agre P, Smith BL, Baumgarten R *et al.*. Human red cell aquaporin CHIP. II. Expression during normal fetal development and in a novel form of congenital dyserythropoietic anemia. *J Clin Invest* 1994; **94**: 1050–1058

69. Matovcik LM, Chiu D, Lubin BH *et al*. The aging process of human neonatal erythrocytes. *Pediatr Res* 1986; **20**: 1091–1096.

70. Colin FC, Gallois Y, Rapin D *et al*. Impaired fetal erythrocytes' filterability: Relationship with cell size, membrane fluidity, and membrane lipid composition. *Blood* 1992; **79**: 2148–2153

71. Jain SK. The neonatal erythrocyte and its oxidative susceptibility. *Semin Hematol* 1989; **26**: 286–300

72. Linderkamp O, Nash GB, Wu PYK, Meiselman HJ. Deformability and intrinsic material properties of neonatal red blood cells. *Blood* 1986; **67**: 1244–1250

73. Linderkamp O, Hammer BJ, Miller R. Filterability of erythrocytes and whole blood in preterm and full-term neonates and adults. *Pediatr Res* 1986; **20**: 1269–1273

74. Eber SW, Armbrust R, Schroter W. Variable clinical severity of hereditary spherocytosis: Relation to erythrocytic spectrin concentration, osmotic fragility, and autohemolysis. *J Pediatr* 1990; **117**: 409–416

75. Randon J, Miraglia del Giudice E, Bozon *et al*. Frequent *de novo* mutations of the ANK1 gene mimic a recessive mode of transmission in hereditary spherocytosis: three new ANK1 variants: ankyrins Bari, Napoli II, and Anzio. *Br J Haematol* 1997; **96**: 500–506

76. Miraglia del Giudice E, Hayette S, Bozon M *et al*. Ankyrin Napoli: a de novo deletional frameshift mutation in exon 16 of ankyrin gene (ANK1) associated with spherocytosis. *Br J Haematol* 1996; **93**: 828–834

77. Morle L, Bozon M, Alloisio N *et al*. Ankyrin Bugey: A *de novo* deletional

frameshift variant in exon 6 of the ankyrin gene associated with spherocytosis. *Am J Hematol* 1997; **54**: 242–248

78. Eber SW, Pekrun A, Neufeldt A, Shroter W. Prevalence of increased osmotic fragility of erythrocytes in German blood donors: screening using a modified glycerol lysis test. *Ann Hematol* 1992; **64**: 88

79. Guarnone R, Centenara E, Zappa M, Zanella A, Barosi G. Erythropoietin production and erythropoiesis in compensated and anaemic states of hereditary spherocytosis. *Br J Haematol* 1996; **92**: 150–154

80. Whitfield CF, Follweiler JB, Lopresti-Morrow L, Miller BA. Deficiency of α-spectrin in burst-forming units-erythroid in lethal hereditary spherocytosis. *Blood* 1991; **78**: 3043–3051

81. Schroter W, Kahsnitz E. Diagnosis of hereditary spherocytosis in newborn infants. *J Pediatr* 1983; **103**: 460–463

82. Bastion Y, Coiffier B, Feiman P *et al.* Massive mediastinal extramedullary hematopoiesis in hereditary spherocytosis: A case report. *Am J Hematol* 1990; **35**: 263–265

83. Jarolim P, Murray JL, Rubin HL *et al.* Characterization of 13 novel Band 3 gene defects in hereditary spherocytosis with Band 3 deficiency. *Blood* 1996; **88**: 4366–4374

84. Hassoun H, Vassiliadis JN, Murray J *et al.* Characterization of the underlying molecular defect in hereditary spherocytosis associated with spectrin deficiency. *Blood* 1997; **90**: 398–406

84a. Garberz M, Galand C, Bibas D *et al.* A 5′ splice region G→C mutation in exon 3 of the human β-spectrum gene leads to decreased levels of β-spectrin MRNA and is responsible for dominant hereditary spherocytosis (spectrin Guemene–Penfao). *Br J Haematol* 1998; **100**: 90–98

85. Becker PS, Tse WT, Lux SE, Forget BG. β Spectrin Kissimmee: A spectrin variant associated with autosomal dominant hereditary spherocytosis and defective binding to protein 4.1. *J Clin Invest* 1993; **92**: 612–616

86. Coetzer T, Lawler J, Liu SC *et al.* Partial ankyrin and spectrin deficiency in severe, atypical hereditary spherocytosis. *N Engl J Med* 1988; **318**: 230–234

87. Palek J, Jarolim P. Clinical expression and laboratory detection of red blood cell membrane protein mutations. *Semin Hematol* 1993; **30**: 249–283

88. Cynober T, Mohandas N, Tchernia G. Red cell abnormalities in hereditary spherocytosis: Relevance to diagnosis and understanding of the variable expression of clinical severity. *J Lab Clin Med* 1996; **128**: 259–69

89. Michaels LA, Cohen AR, Zhao H, Raphael RI, Manno CS. Screening for hereditary spherocytosis by use of automated erythrocyte indexes. *J Pediatr* 1997; **130**: 957–960

90. Bucx MJL, Breed WPM, Hoffmann JJML. Comparison of acidified glycerol lysis test, Pink test and osmotic fragility test in hereditary spherocytosis. *Eur J Haematol* 1988; **40**: 227–231

91. Romero RR, Poo JL, Robles JA, Uriostegui A, Vargas F, Majluf-Cruz A. Usefulness of cryohemolysis test in the diagnosis of hereditary spherocytosis. *Arch Med Res* 1997; **28**: 247–251

92. Agre P, Orringer EP, Bennett V. Deficient red-cell spectrin in severe, recessively inherited spherocytosis. *N Engl J Med* 1982; **306**: 1155–1161

93. De Franceschi L, Olivieri O, Miraglia del Giudice E *et al.* Membrane cation and anion transport activities in erythrocytes of hereditary spherocytosis: Effects of different membrane protein defects. *Am J Hematol* 1997; **55**: 121–128

94. Joiner CH, Franco RS, Jiang M, Franco MS, Barker JE, Lux SE. Increased cation permeability in mutant mouse red blood cells with defective membrane skeletons. *Blood* 1995; **86**: 4307–4314

95. Ingrosso D, D'Angelo S, Perrotta S *et al.* Cytoskeletal behaviour in spectrin and in band 3 deficient spherocytic red cells: evidence for a differentiated splenic conditioning role. *Br J Haematol* 1996; **93**: 38–41

96. Peters L, Lux SE. Ankyrins: Structure and function in normal cells and hereditary spherocytes. *Semin Hematol* 1993; **30**: 85–118

97. Miraglia del Giudice E, Iolascon A, Pinto L, Nobili B, Perrotta S.

98. Eber SW, Gonzalez JM, Lux ML *et al.* Ankyrin-1 mutations are a major cause of dominant and recessive hereditary spherocytosis. *Nature Genet* 1996; **13**: 214–218

99. Dhermy D, Galand C, Bournier O *et al.* Heterogenous band 3 deficiency in hereditary spherocytosis related to different band 3 gene defects. *Br J Haematol* 1997; **98**: 32–40

100. Southgate CD, Chishti AH, Mitchell B, Yi SJ, Palek J. Targeted disruption of the murine erythroid band 3 gene results in spherocytosis and severe haemolytic anaemia despite a normal membrane skeleton. *Nature Genet* 1996; **14**: 227–230

101. Inaba M, Yawata A, Koshino I *et al.* Defective anion transport and marked spherocytosis with membrane instability caused by hereditary total deficiency of red cell band 3 in cattle due to a nonsense mutation. *J Clin Invest* 1996; **97**: 1804–1817

102. Jarolim P, Rubin HL, Brabec V, Palek J. Comparison of the ankyrin (AC)$_n$microsatellites in genomic DNA and mRNA reveals absence of one ankyrin mRNA allele in 20% of patients with hereditary spherocytosis. *Blood* 1995; **85**: 3278–3282

103. Okamoto N, Wada Y, Nakamura Y *et al.* Hereditary spherocytic anemia with deletion of the short arm of chromosome 8. *Am J Med Genet* 1995; **58**: 225–229

104. Jarolim P, Rubin HL, Brabec V, Palek J. Abnormal alternative splicing of erythroid ankyrin mRNA in two kindred with hereditary spherocytosis (ankyrin[PRAGUE] and ankyrin[RAKOVNIK]). *Blood* 1993; **82 (Suppl 1)**: 5A

105. Jarolim P, Rubin HL, Brabec V *et al.* Mutations of conserved arginines in the membrane domain of erythroid band 3 lead to a decrease in membrane-associated band 3 and to the phenotype of hereditary spherocytosis. *Blood* 1995; **85**: 634–640

106. Lima PRM, Gontijo JAR, Lopes de Faria JB, Costa FF, Saad STO. Band 3 Campinas: A novel splicing mutation the the Band 3 gene (AE1) associated with hereditary spherocytosis, hyperactivity of Na$^+$/Li$^+$ countertransport and an abnormal renal bicarbonate handling. *Blood* 1997; **90**: 2810–2818

107. Bruce LJ, Cope DL, Jones GK *et al.* Familial distal renal tubular acidosis is associated with mutations in the red cell anion exchanger (Band 3, AE1) gene. *J Clin Invest* 1997; **100**: 1693–1707

108. Jenkins PB, Abou-Alfa GK, Dhermy D *et al.* A nonsense mutation in the erythrocyte Band 3 gene associated with decreased mRNA accumulation in a kindred with dominant hereditary spherocytosis. *J Clin Invest* 1996; **97**: 373–380

109. Miraglia del Giudice E, Vallier A, Maillet P *et al.* Novel band 3 variants (bands 3 Foggia, Napoli I and Napoli II) associated with hereditary spherocytosis and band 3 deficiency: status of the D38A polymorphism within the EPB3 locus. *Br J Haematol* 1997; **96**: 70–76

110. Maillet P, Vallier A, Reinhart WH *et al.* Band 3 Chur: a variant associated with band 3-deficient hereditary spherocytosis and substitution in a highly conserved position of transmembrane segment 11. *Br J Haematol* 1995; **91**: 804–810

111. Bianchi P, Zanella A, Alloisio N *et al.* A variant of the EPB3 gene of the anti-Lepore type in hereditary spherocytosis. *Br J Haematol* 1997; **98**: 283–288.

112. Alloisio N, Texier P, Vallier A *et al.* Modulation of clinical expression and Band 3 deficiency in hereditary spherocytosis. *Blood* 1997; **90**: 414–420

113. Alloisio N, Maillet P, Carre G *et al.* Hereditary spherocytosis with Band 3 deficiency. Association with a nonsense mutation of the Band 3 gene (allele Lyon) and aggravation by a low-expression allele occurring in trans (allele Genas). *Blood* 1996; **88**: 1062–1069

114. Tse WT, Gallagher PG, Jenkins PB *et al.* Amino-acid substitution in α-spectrin commonly coinherited with nondominant hereditary spherocytosis. *Am J Hematol* 1997; **54**: 233–241

115. Wichterle H, Manspal M, Palek J, Jarolim P. Combination of two mutant alpha spectrin alleles underlies a severe spherocytic hemolytic anemia. *J Clin Invest* 1996; **98**: 2300–2307

116. Hassoun H, Vassiliadis JN, Murray J *et al*. Molecular basis of spectrin deficiency in β spectrin Durham. *J Clin Invest* 1995; **96**: 2623–2629

117. Hassoun H, Vassiliadis JN, Murray J *et al*. Hereditary spherocytosis with spectrin deficiency due to an unstable truncated β spectrin. *Blood* 1996; **87**: 2538–2545

118. Becker PS, Tse WT, Lux SE, Forget BG. β spectrin Kissammee: A spectrin variant associated with autosomal dominant hereditary spherocytosis and defective binding to protein 4.1. *J Clin Invest* 1993; **92**: 612–616

119. Bouhassira EE, Schwartz RS, Yawata Y *et al*. An alanine-to-threonine substitution in protein 4.2 cDNA is associated with a Japanese form of hereditary hemolytic anemia (protein 4.2 Nippon). *Blood* 1992; **79**: 1846–1854

120. Takaoka Y, Ideguchi H, Matsuda M, Sakamoto N, Takeuchi T, Fukamaki Y. A novel mutation in the erythrocyte protein 4.2 gene of Japanese patients with hereditary spherocytosis (protein 4.2 Fukuoka). *Br J Haematol* 1994; **88**: 527–533

121. Kanzaki A, Yasunaga M, Okamoto N *et al*. Band 4.2 Shiga: 317 CGC→TGC in compound heterozygotes with 142 GCT→ACT results in band 4.2 deficiency and microspherocytosis. *Br J Haematol* 1995; **91**: 333–340

122. Matsuda M, Hatano N, Ideguchi H, Takahira H, Fukumaki Y. A novel mutation causing an aberrant splicing in the protein 4.2 gene associated with hereditary spherocytosis (protein 4.2 Notame). *Hum Mol Genet* 1995; **4**: 1187–1191

123. Jarolim P, Palek J, Rubin HL, Prchal JT, Korsgren C, Cohen CM. Band 3 Tuscaloosa: Pro^{327}→Arg^{327} substitution in the cytoplasmic domain of erythrocyte band 3 protein associated with spherocytic hemolytic anemia and partial deficiency of protein 4.2. *Blood* 1992; **80**: 523–529

124. Rybicki AC, Qiu JJH, Musto S, Rosen NL, Nagel RL, Schwartz RS. Human erythrocyte protein 4.2 deficiency associated with hemolytic anemia and a homozygous ^{40}glutamic acid→lysine substitution in the cytoplasmic domain of band 3 (band 3^{Montefiore}). *Blood* 1993; **81**: 2155–2165

124a. Inoue T, Kanzaki A, Kaku M *et al*. Homozygous missense mutation (band 3 Fukuoka: G130R): a mild form of hereditary spherocytosis with near-normal band 3 content and minimal changes of membrane ultrastructure despite moderate protein 4.2 deficiency. *Br J Haematol* 1998; **102**: 932–939

125. Agre P, Asimos A, Cesella JF, McMillan C. Inheritance pattern and clinical response to splenectomy as a reflection of erythrocyte spectrin deficiency in hereditary spherocytosis. *N Engl J Med* 1986; **315**: 1579–1583

126. Gigot J-F, de Goyet J, Van Beers BE *et al*. Laparoscopic splenectomy in adults and children: Experience with 31 patients. *Surgery* 1996; **119**: 384–389

127. Patton ML, Moss BE, Haith LR Jr *et al*. Concomitant laparoscopic cholecystectomy and splenectomy for surgical management of hereditary spherocytosis. *Am Surg* 1997; **63**: 536–539

128. Singer DB. Postsplenectomy sepsis. *Perspect Pediatr Pathol* 1973; **1**: 285–311

129. Schilling RF. Estimating the risk for sepsis after splenectomy in hereditary spherocytosis. *Ann Int Med* 1995; **122**: 187–188

130. Konradsen HB, Henrichsen J. Pneumococcal infections in splenectomized children are preventable. *Acta Paediatr Scand* 1991; **80**: 423–427

131. Friedland IR, Med M, McCracken GH Jr. Management of infections caused by antibiotic-resistant *Streptococcus pneumoniae*. *N Engl J Med* 1994; **331**: 377–382

132. Wang WC, Wong W-Y, Rogers ZR, Wilimas JA, Buchanan GR, Powars DR. Antibiotic-resistant pneumococcal infection in children with sickle cell disease in the United States. *J Pediatr Hematol Oncol* 1996; **18**: 140–144

133. Persing DH, Herwaldt BL, Glaser C *et al*. Infection with a babesia-like organism in Northern California. *N Engl J Med* 1995; **332**: 298–303

134. Herwaldt BL, Persing DH, Precigout EA *et al*. A fatal case of babesiosis in Missouri: Identification of another piroplasm that infects humans. *Ann Intern Med* 1996; **124**: 643–650

135. Tchernia G, Bader-Meunier B, Berterottiere P, Eber S, Dommergues JP, Bauthier F. Effectiveness of partial splenectomy in hereditary spherocytosis. *Curr Opin Hematol* 1997; **4**: 136–141

136. Manno CS, Cohen AR. Splenectomy in mild hereditary spherocytosis: Is it worth the risk? *Am J Pediatr Hematol Oncol* 1989; **11**: 300–303

137. Dacie J. *The Haemolytic Anaemias*, vol I, 3rd edn. Edinburgh: Churchill Livingstone, 1985, p 179

138. Alani FSS, Dyer T, Hindle E, Newsome DA, Ormerod LP, Mahoney MP. Pseudohyperkalaemia associated with hereditary spherocytosis in four members of a family. *Postgrad Med J* 1994; **70**: 749–751

139. Verresen D, de Backer W, von Meerbeeck J *et al*. Spherocytosis and pulmonary hypertension. Coincidental occurrence or causal relationship? *Eur Respir J* 1991; **4**: 629–631

140. Stewart GW, Amess JAL, Eber SW *et al*. Thrombo-embolic disease after splenectomy for hereditary stomatocytosis. *Br J Haematol* 1996; **93**: 303–310

141. Tso S, Chan T, Todd D. Venous thrombosis in haemoglobin H disease after splenectomy. *Aust N Z J Med* 1982; **12**: 635–638

142. Robinette CD, Fraumeni JF Jr. Splenectomy and subsequent mortality in veterans of the 1939–45 war. *Lancet* 1977; **ii**: 127–129

143. Glele-Kakal C, Garbarz M, Lecomte M-C *et al*. Epidemiological studies of spectrin mutations related to hereditary elliptocytosis and spectrin polymorphisms in Benin. *Br J Haematol* 1996; **95**: 57–66

144. Nagel RL. Red-cell cytoskeletal abnormatities—implications for malaria. *N Engl J Med* 1990; **323**: 1558–1559

145. Austin RF, Desforges JF. Hereditary elliptocytosis: An unusual presentation of hemolysis in the newborn associated with transient morphological abnormalities. *Pediatrics* 1969; **44**: 196–200

146. Mentzer WC, Iarocci TA, Mohandas N *et al*. Modulation of erythrocyute membrane mechanical stability by 2,3-diphosphoglycerate in the neonatal poikilocytosis/elliptocytosis syndrome. *J Clin Invest* 1987; **79**: 943–949

147. Pui CH, Wang W, Wilimas J. Hereditary elliptocytosis. Morphologic abnormalities during acute hepatitis. *Clin Pediatr* 1982; **21**: 188–190

148. Nkrumah FK. Hereditary elliptocytosis associated with severe haemolytic anaemia and malaria. *Afr J Med Sci* 1972; **3**: 131–136

149. Schoomaker EB, Butler WM, Diehl LF. Increased heat sensitivity of red blood cells in hereditary elliptocytosis with acquired cobalamin (vitamin B12) deficiency. *Blood* 1982; **59**: 1213–1219

150. Jarolim P, Palek J, Coetzer TL *et al*. Severe hemolysis and red cell fragmentation caused by the combination of a spectrin mutation with a thrombotic microangiopathy. *Am J Hematol* 1989; **32**: 50–56

151. Garbarz M, Lecomte MC, Dhermy D *et al*. Double inheritance of an alpha I/65 spectrin variant in a child with homozygous elliptocytosis. *Blood* 1986; **67**: 1661–1667

152. Tchernia G, Mohandas N, Shohet SB. Deficiency of skeletal membrane protein band 4.1 in homozygous hereditary elliptocytosis. *J Clin Invest* 1981; **68**: 454–460

153. Alloisio N, Morle L, Pothier B *et al*. Spectrin Oran (α$^{II/21}$), a new spectrin variant concerning the αII domain and causing severe elliptocytosis in the homozygous state. *Blood* 1988; **71**: 1039–1047

154. Coetzer T, Palek J, Lawler J *et al*. Structural and functional heterogeneity of α spectrin mutations involving the spectrin heterodimer self-association site: Relationships to hematologic expression of homozygous hereditary elliptocytosis and hereditary pyropoikilocytosis. *Blood* 1990; **75**: 2235–2244

155. Iarocci TA, Wagner GM, Mohandas N, Lane PA, Mentzer WC. Hereditary poikilocytic anemia associated with the co-inheritance of two alpha spectrin abnormalities. *Blood* 1988; **71**: 1390–1396

156. Zarkowsky HS, Mohandas N, Speaker CB, Shohet SB. A congenital haemolytic anaemia with thermal sensitivity of the erythrocyte membrane. *Br J Haematol* 1975; **29**: 537–543

157. Liu SC, Jarolim P, Rubin HL *et al*. The homozygous state for the band

3 protein mutation in southeast asian ovalocytosis may be lethal. *Blood* 1994; **84**: 3590–3591

158. Wilmotte R, Marechal J, Morle L *et al.* Low expression allele α^{LELY} of red cell spectrin is associated with mutations in exon 40 ($\alpha^{V/41}$ polymorphism) and intron 45 and with partial skipping of exon 46. *J Clin Invest* 1993; **91**: 2091–2096

159. Mohandas N, Winardi R, Knowles D *et al.* Molecular basis for membrane rigidity of hereditary ovalocytosis. *J Clin Invest* 1992; **89**: 686–692

160. Dhermy D, Feo C, Garbarz M *et al.* Prenatal diagnosis of hereditary elliptocytosis with molecular defect of spectrin. *Prenat Diagn* 1987; **7**: 471–483

161. Tomaselli MB, John KM, Lux SE. Elliptical erythrocyte membrane skeletons and heat sensitive spectrin in hereditary elliptocytosis. *Proc Natl Acad Sci USA* 1981; **78**: 1911–1915

162. Takakuwa Y, Tchernia G, Rossi M, Benabadji M, Mohandas N. Restoration of normal membrane stability to unstable protein 4.1-deficient erythrocyte membranes by incorporation of purified protein 4.1. *J Clin Invest* 1986; **78**: 80–85

163. Discher DE, Winardi R, Schischmanoff PO, Parra M, Conboy JG, Mohandas N. Mechanochemistry of protein 4.1's spectrin-actin-binding domain: Ternary complex interactions, membrane binding, network integration, structural strengthening. *J Cell Biol* 1995; **130**: 897–907

164. Delaunay J, Dhermy D. Mutations involving the spectrin heterodimer contact site: Clinical expression and alterations in specific function. *Semin Hematol* 1993; **30**: 21–33

165. Lecomte MC, Garbarz M, Gautero H *et al.* Molecular basis of clinical and morphological heterogeneity in hereditary elliptocytosis (HE) with spectrin αI variants. *Br J Haematol* 1993; **85**: 584–595

166. Maillet P, Alloisio N, Morle L, Delaunay J. Spectrin mutations in hereditary elliptocytosis and hereditary spherocytosis. *Hum Mutat* 1996; **8**: 97–107

167. Perrotta S, Iolascon A, DeAngelis F *et al.* Spectrin Anastasia ($\alpha^{I/78}$): a new spectrin variant ($\alpha45$ Arg→Thr) with moderate elliptocytogenic potential. *Br J Haematol* 1995; **89**: 933–936

168. Parquet N, Devaux I, Boulanger L *et al.* Identification of three novel spectrin $\alpha I/74$ mutations in hereditary elliptocytosis: further support for a triple-stranded folding un it model of the spectrin heterodimer contact site. *Blood* 1994; **84**: 303–308

169. Lecomte MC, Feo C, Gautero H *et al.* Severe recessive poikilocytic anaemia with a new spectrin α chain variant. *Br J Haematol* 1990; **74**: 497–507

170. Alloisio N, Wilmotte R, Morle L *et al.* Spectrin Jendouba: An $\alpha^{II/31}$ spectrin variant that is associated with elliptocytosis and carries a mutation distant from the dimer self-association site. *Blood* 1992; **80**: 809–815

171. Alloisio N, Wilmotte R, Marechal J *et al.* A splice site mutation of α spectrin gene causing skipping of exon 18 in hereditary elliptocytosis. *Blood* 1993; **81**: 2991–2798

172. Ullmann S, Kugler W, Dornwell M *et al.* Spectrin α-Esche, a novel truncated spectrin α-chain variant due to skipping of exon 39, leading to severe infantile poikilocytosis. *Blood* 1996; **88 (Suppl 1)**: 4A

173. Fournier CM, Nicolas G, Gallagher PG, Dhermy D, Grandchamp B, Lecomte MC. Spectrin$^{St\ Claude}$, a splicing mutation of the human α-spectrin gene associated with severe poikilocytic anemia. *Blood* 1997; **89**: 4584–4590

174. Hassoun H, Coetzer TL, Vassiliadis JN *et al.* A novel mobile element inserted in the α spectrin gene: Spectrin Dayton. *J Clin Invest* 1994; **94**: 643–648

175. Lane PA, Shew RL, Iarocci TA, Mohandas N, Hays T, Mentzer WC. Unique alpha-spectrin mutant in a kindred with common hereditary elliptocytosis. *J Clin Invest* 1987; **79**: 989–996

176. Marechal J, Wilmotte R, Kanzaki A *et al.* Ethnic distribution of allele α^{LELY}, a low-expression allele of red-cell spectrin α-gene. *Br J Haematol* 1995; **90**: 553–556

177. Randon J, Boulanger L, Marechal J *et al.* A variant of spectrin low-expression allele α^{LELY} carrying a hereditary elliptocytosis mutation in codon 28. *Br J Haematol* 1994; **88**: 534–540

178. Alliosio N, Morle L, Marechal J *et al.* Sp$\alpha^{V/41}$41: a common spectrin polymorphism at the αIV-αV domain junction. *J Clin Invest* 1991; **87**: 2169–2177

179. Hanspal M, Hanspal JS, Sahr KE, Fibach E, Nachman J, Palek J. Molecular basis of spectrin deficiency in hereditary pyropoikilocytosis. *Blood* 1993; **82**: 1652–1660

180. Qualtieri A, Pasqua A, Bisconte MG, Le Pera M, Brancati C. Spectrin Cosenza: a novel β chain variant associated with Sp α^{I74} hereditary elliptocytosis. *Br J Haematol* 1997; **97**: 273–278

181. Gallagher PG, Weed SA, Tse WT *et al.* Recurrent fatal hydrops fetalis associated with a nucleotide substitution in the erythrocyte β-spectrin gene. *J Clin Invest* 1995; **95**: 1174–1182

182. Gallagher PG, Petruzzi MJ, Weed SA *et al.* Mutation of a highly conserved residue of βI spectrin associated with fatal and near-fatal neonatal hemolytic anemia. *J Clin Invest* 1997; **99**: 267–277

183. Lecomte MC, Gautero H, Bournier O *et al.* Elliptocytosis-associated spectrin Rouen ($\beta^{220/218}$) has a truncated but still phosphorylatable β chain. *Br J Haematol* 1992; **80**: 242–250

184. Kanzaki A, Rabodonirina M, Yawata Y *et al.* A deletional frameshift mutation of the β-spectrin gene associated with elliptocytosis in spectrin Tokyo ($\beta^{220/216}$). *Blood* 1992; **80**: 2115–2121

185. Garbarz M, Boulanger L, Pedroni S *et al.* Spectrin β^{TANDIL}, a novel shortened β-chain variant associated with hereditary elliptocytosis is due to a deletional frameshift mutation in the β-spectrin gene. *Blood* 1992; **80**: 1066–1073

186. Wilmotte R, Miraglia del Giudice E, Marechal J *et al.* A deletional frameshift mutation in spectrin β-gene associated with hereditary elliptocytosis in spectrin Napoli. *Br J Haematol* 1994; **88**: 437–439

187. Tse WT, Gallagher PG, Pothier B *et al.* An insertional frameshift mutation of the β-spectrin gene associated with elliptocytosis in spectrin Nice ($\beta^{220/216}$). *Blood* 1991; **78**: 517–523

188. Yoon SH, Yu H, Eber S, Prchal JT. Molecular defect of truncated β-spectrin associated with hereditary elliptocytosis: β-spectrin Gottingen. *J Biol Chem* 1991; **266**: 8490

189. Gallagher PG, Tse WT, Costa F *et al.* A splice site mutation of the β-spectrin gene causing exon skipping in hereditary elliptocytosis associated with a truncated β-spectrin chain. *J Biol Chem* 1991; **266**: 15154

190. Jarolim P, Wichterle H, Hanspal M, Murray J, Rubin HL, Palek J. β spectrin^{PRAGUE}: a truncated β spectrin producing spectrin deficiency, defective spectrin heterodimer self-association and a phenotype of spherocytic elliptocytosis. *Br J Haematol* 1995; **91**: 502–510

191. Johnson RM, Ravindranath Y, Brohn F, Mukarram H. A large erythroid spectrin β-chain variant. *Br J Haematol* 1992; **80**: 6–14

192. Schofield AE, Reardon DM, Tanner MJA. Defective anion transport activity of the abnormal band 3 in hereditary ovalocytic red blood cells. *Nature* 1992; **355**: 836–838

193. Sarabia VE, Casey JR, Reithmeier AF. Molecular characterization of the Band 3 protein from Southeast Asian ovalocytes. *J Biol Chem* 1993; **268**: 10676–10680

194. Liu SC, Palek J, Yi SJ *et al.* Molecular basis of altered red blood cell membrane properties in Southeastern Asian ovalocytosis: Role of the mutant Band 3 protein in Band 3 oligomerization and retention by the membrane skeleton. *Blood* 1995; **86**: 349–358

195. Jarolim P, Rubin HL, Zhai S *et al.* Band 3 Memphis: a widespread polymorphism with abnormal electrophoretic mobility of erythrocyte Band 3 protein caused by substitution AAG→GAG (Lys→Glu) in codon 56. *Blood* 1992; **80**: 1592–1598

196. Alloisio N, Venezia ND, Rana A. Evidence that red blood cell protein p55 may participate in the skeleton-membrane linkage that involves protein 4.1 and glycophorin C. *Blood* 1993; **82**: 1323–1327

197. Genton B, Al-Yaman F, Mgone CS *et al.* Ovalocytosis and cerebral malaria. *Nature* 1995; **378**: 564–565

198. Gratzer WB, Dluzewski AR. The red blood cell and malaria parasite invasion. *Semin Hematol* 1993; **30**: 232–247

199. Magowan C, Coppel RL, Lau AOT *et al*. Role of the *Plasmodium falciparum* mature-parasite-infected erythrocyte surface antigen (MESA/PfEMP-2) in malarial infection of erythrocytes. *Blood* 1995; **86**: 3196–3204

200. Chishti AH, Palek J, Fisher D *et al*. Reduced invasion and growth of Plasmodium falciparum into elliptocytic red blood cells with a combined deficiency of protein 4.1, glycophorin C, and p55. *Blood* 1996; **87**: 3462–3469

201. Dalla Venezia N, Gilsanz F, Alloisio N, Bucluzeau M-T, Benz EJ Jr, Delaunay J. Homozygous 4.1 (-) hereditary elliptocytosis associated with a point mutation in the downstream initiation codon of protein 4.1 gene. *J Clin Invest* 1992; **90**: 1713–1717

202. Garbarz M, Devaux I, Bournier B, Grandchamp B, Dhermy D. Protein 4.1 Lille, a novel mutation in the downstream initiation codon of protein 4.1 gene associated with heterozygous 4.1 (-) hereditary elliptocytosis. *Hum Mutat* 1995; **5**: 339–340

203. Feddal S, Brunet G, Roda S *et al*. Molecular analysis of hereditary elliptocytosis with reduced protein 4.1 in the French northern alps. *Blood* 1991; **78**: 2113–2119

204. Marchesi S, Conboy J, Agre P *et al*. Molecular analysis of insertion/deletion mutations in protein 4.1 in elliptocytosis. I. Biochemical identification of rearrangements in the spectrin/actin binding domain and functional characterizations. *J Clin Invest* 1990; **86**: 516–523

205. Conboy J, Marchesi S, Kim R, Agre P, Kan YW, Mohandas N. Molecular analysis of insertion/deletion mutations in protein 4.1 in elliptocytosis. II. Determination of molecular genetic origins of rearrangements. *J Clin Invest* 1990; **86**: 524–530

205a. Dalla Venezia N, Maillet P, Morle L, Roda L, Delaunay J, Baklouti F. A large deletion within the protein 4.1 gene associated with a stable truncated MRNA and an unaltered tissue-specific alternative splicing. *Blood* 1998; **91**: 4361–4367

206. Furchgott RF. Disk-sphere transformation in mammalian red cells. *J Exp Biol* 1940; **17**: 30

207. Palek J, Stewart G, Lionetti FJ. The dependence of shape of human erythrocyte ghosts on calcium, magnesium, and adenosine triphosphate. *Blood* 1974; **44**: 583–597

208. Aherne WA. The "burr" red cell and azotaemia. *J Clin Pathol* 1957; **10**: 252–257

209. Schwartz SO, Motto SA. The diagnostic significance of "burr" red blood cells. *Am J Med Sci* 1949; **218**: 563–566

210. Cooper RA. Anemia with spur cells: A red cell defect acquired in serum and modified in the circulation. *J Clin Invest* 1969; **48**: 1820–1831

211. Bassen FA, Kornzweig AL. Malformation of the erythrocytes in a case of atypical retinitis pigmentosa. *Blood* 1950; **5**: 381–387

212. Kay J, Stricker RB. Hematologic and immunologic abnormalities in anorexia nervosa. *South Med J* 1983; **76**: 1008–1010

213. Symmans WA, Shepard CS, Marsh WL *et al*. Hereditary acanthocytosis associated with the McLeod phenotype of the Kell blood group system. *Br J Haematol* 1979; **42**: 575–583

214. Udden MM, Umeda M, Hirano Y, Marcus DM. New abnormalities in the morphology, cell surface receptors, and electrolyte metabolism of In(Lu) erythrocytes. *Blood* 1987; **69**: 52–57

215. Wardrop C, Hutchison HE. Red-cell shape in hypothyroidism. *Lancet* 1969; **1**: 1243

216. Doll DC, List AF, Dayhoff DA, Loy TS, Ringenberg QS, Yarbro JW. Acanthocytosis associated with myelodysplasia. *J Clin Oncol* 1989; **7**: 1569–1572

217. Kane JP, Havel RJ. Disorders of the biogenesis and secretion of lipoproteins containing the B apolipoproteins. In: Scriver CS, Beaudet AL, Sly WS *et al* (eds) *The Metabolic and Molecular Bases of Inherited Disease*, 7th edn. New York: McGraw-Hill, 1995, pp 1853–1887

218. Barenholz Y, Yechiel E, Cohen R *et al*. Importance of cholesterol-phospholipid interaction in determining dynamics of normal and abetalipoproteinemia red blood cell membrane. *Cell Biophys* 1981; **3**: 115

219. Iida H, Takashima Y, Maeda S *et al*. Alterations in erythrocyte membrane lipids in abetalipoproteinemia: Phospholipid and fatty acyl composition. *Biochem Med* 1984; **32**: 79–87

220. Cooper RA, Gulbrandsen CL. The relationship between serum lipoproteins and red cell membranes in abetalipoproteinemia: Deficiency of lecithin:cholesterol acyltransferase. *J Lab Clin Med* 1971; **78**: 323–325

221. Dodge JT, Cohen G, Kayden HJ, Phillips GB. Peroxidative hemolysis of red blood cells from patients with abetalipoproteinemia (acanthocytosis). *J Clin Invest* 1967; **46**: 357–368

222. Elias E, Muller DP, Scott J. Association of spinocerebellar disorders with cystic fibrosis or chronic childhood cholestasis and very low serum vitamin E. *Lancet* 1981; **2**: 1319–1321

223. Sokol RJ, Guggenheim MA, Heubi JE *et al*. Frequency and clinical progression of the vitamin E deficiency neurologic disorder in children with prolonged neonatal cholestasis. *Am J Dis Child* 1985; **139**: 1211–1215

224. Muller DPR, Lloyd JK, Bird AC. Long-term management of abetalipoproteinaemia. *Arch Dis Child* 1977; **52**: 209–214

225. Hardie RJ. Acanthocytosis and neurological impairment—a review. *Q J Med* 1989; **71**: 291–306

226. Asano K, Osawa Y, Yanagisawa N *et al*. Erythrocyte membrane abnormalities in patients with amyotrophic chorea with acanthocytosis: II. Abnormal degradation of membrane proteins. *J Neurol Sci* 1985; **68**: 161

227. Clark MR, Aminoff MJ, Chiu DTY, Kuypers FA, Friend DS. Red cell deformability and lipid composition in two forms of acanthocytosis: Enrichment of acanthocytic populations by density gradient centrifugation. *J Lab Clin Med* 1989; **113**: 469–481

228. Critchley EM, Clark DB, Wikler A. Acanthocytosis and neurological disorder without abetalipoproteinemia. *Arch Neurol* 1968; **18**: 134–140

229. Hardie RJ, Pullon HW, Harding AE *et al*. Neuroacanthocytosis: A clinical, haematological and pathological study of 19 cases. *Brain* 1991; **114**: 13–49

230. Spitz MC, Jankovic J, Killian JM. Familial tic disorder, parkinsonism, motor neuron disease, and acanthodytosis: A new syndrome. *Neurology* 1985; **35**: 366–370

231. Higgins JJ, Patterson MC, Papadopoulos NM, Brady RO, Pentchev PG, Barton NW. Hypoprebetalipoproteinemia, acanthocytosis, retinitis pigmentosa, and pallidal degeneration (HARP syndrome). *Neurology* 1992; **42**: 194–198

232. Gracey M, Hilton HB. Acanthocytes and hypobetalipoproteinemia. *Lancet* 1973; **1**: 679

233. Mant MJ, Faragher BS. The haematology of anorexia nervosa. *Br J Haematol* 1972; **23**: 737–749

234. Cynamon HA, Isenberg JN, Gustavson LP, Gourley WK. Erythrocyte lipid alterations in pediatric cholestatic liver disease: Spur cell anemia of infancy. *J Pediatr Gastroenterol Nutr* 1985; **4**: 542–549

235. Grahn EP, Dietz AA, Stefani SS, Donnelly WJ. Burr cells, hemolytic anemia and cirrhosis. *Am J Med* 1968; **45**: 78–87

236. Smith JA, Lonergan ET, Sterling K *et al*. Spur cell anemia: Hemolytic anemia with red cells resembling acanthocytes in alcoholic cirrhosis. *N Engl J Med* 1964; **276**: 396

237. Salvioli G, Rioli G, Lugli R, Salati R. Membrane lipid composition of red blood cells in liver disease: Regression of spur cell anaemia after infusion of polyunsaturated phosphatidylcholine. *Gut* 1978; **19**: 844–850

238. Allen DW, Manning N. Abnormal phospholipid metabolism in spur cell anemia: decreased fatty acid incorporation into phosphatidylethanolamine and increased incorporation into acylcarnitine in spur cell anemia erythrocytes. *Blood* 1994; **84**: 1283–1287

239. Zipursky A. Vitamin E deficiency anemia in newborn infants. *Clin Perinatol* 1984; **11**: 393–402

240. Redman CM, Marsh WL. The Kell antigens and McLeod red cells. In: Agre PC, Cartron JP (eds) *Protein Blood Group Antigens of the Human Red Cell: Structure, Function and Clinical Significance*. Baltimore: Johns Hopkins University Press, 1992, pp 53–69

241. Ho MF, Chalmers RM, Davis MB, Harding AE, Monaco AP. A novel point mutation in the McLeod syndrome gene in neuroacanthocytosis. *Ann Neurol* 1996; **39**: 672–675

242. Taswell HF, Lewis JC, Marsh WL, Wimer BM, Pineda AA, Brzica SM. Erythrocyte morphology in genetic defects of the Rh and Kell blood group systems. *Mayo Clin Proc* 1977; **52**: 157–159

243. Takashima H, Sakai T, Iwashita H *et al*. A family of McLeod syndrome, masquerading as chorea-acanthocytosis. *J Neurol Sci* 1994; **124**: 56

244. Telen MJ. The Lutheran antigens and proteins affected by Lutheran regulatory genes. In: Agre PC, Cartron JP (eds) *Protein Blood Group Antigens of the Human Red Cell: Structure, Function and Clinical Significance.* Baltimore: Johns Hopkins University Press, 1992, pp 70–87

245. Loge JP, Lange RD, Moore CV. Characterization of the anemia associated with chronic renal insufficiency. *Am J Med* 1958; **24**: 4–18

246. Beutler E, West C, Tavassoli M, Grahn E. The Woronet's trait: A new familial erythrocyte anomaly. *Blood Cells* 1980; **6**: 281–287

247. Horton L, Coburn RJ, England JM, Himsworth RL. The haematology of hypothyroidism. *Q J Med* 1976; **45**: 101–124

248. Perillie PE, Tembrevilla C. Red-cell changes in hypothroidism. *Lancet* 1975; **2**: 1151–1152.

249. Cooper RA, Jandl JH. Bile salts and cholesterol in the pathogenesis of target cells in obstructive jaundice. *J Clin Invest* 1968; **47**: 809–822

250. Cooper RA, Diloy-Puray M, Lando P, Greenberg MS. An analysis of lipoproteins, bile acids, and red cell membranes associated with target cells and spur cells in patients with liver disease. *J Clin Invest* 1972; **31**: 3182–3192

251. Neerhout RC. Abnormalities of erythrocyte stromal lipids in hepatic disease: Erythrocyte stromal lipids in hyperlipemic states. *J Lab Clin Med* 1968; **71**: 438–447

252. Cooper RA, Jandl JH. The role of membrane lipids in the survival of red cells in hereditary spherocytosis. *J Clin Invest* 1969; **48**: 736–744

253. Norum KR, Gjone E. Familial serum-cholesterol esterification failure: A new inborn error of metabolism. *Biochim Biophys Acta* 1967; **144**: 698–700

254. Gjone E, Torsvik H, Norum KR. Familial plasma cholesterol ester deficiency: A study of the erythrocytes. *Scand J Clin Lab Invest* 1968; **21**: 327–332

255. Bujo H, Kusunoki J, Ogasawara T *et al*. Molecular defect in familial lecithin:cholesterol acyltransferase (LCAT) deficiency: A single nucleotide insertion in LCAT gene causes a complete deficient type of the disease. *Biochim Biophys Res Commun* 1991; **181**: 933–940

256. Funke H, von Eckardstein A, Pritchard PH *et al*. Genetic and phenotypic heterogeneity in familial lecithin:cholesterol acyltransferase (LCAT) deficiency: Six newly identified defective alleles further contribute to the structural heterogeneity in this disease. *J Clin Invest* 1993; **91**: 677–683

257. Norum KR, Gjone E. The influence of plasma from patients with familial lecithin:cholesterol acyltransferase deficiency on the lipid pattern of erythrocytes. *Scand J Clin Lab Invest* 1968; **22**: 94–98

258. Singer K, Miller EB, Dameshek W *et al*. Hematologic changes following splenectomy in man, with particular reference to target cells, hemolytic index, and lysolecithin. *Am J Med Sci* 1941; **202**: 171–187

259. Singer K, Weisz L. The life cycle of the erythrocyte after splenectomy and the problems of splenic hemolysis and target cell formation. *Am J Med Sci* 1945; **210**: 301–323

260. DeHaan LD, Werre JM, Ruben AMT, Huls HA, De Gier J, Staal GEJ. Alterations in size, shape and osmotic behavior of red cells after splenectomy: A study of their age dependence. *Br J Haematol* 1988; **69**: 71–80

261. Lande WM, Mentzer WC. Haemolytic anaemia associated with increased cation permeability. *Clin Haematol* 1985; **14**: 89–103

262. Vives Corrons JL, Besson I, Aymerich M *et al*. Hereditary xerocytosis: a report of six unrelated Spanish families with leaky red cell syndrome and increased heat stability of the erythrocyte membrane. *Br J Haematol* 1995; **90**: 817–822

263. Platt OS, Lux SE, Nathan DG. Exercise-induced hemolysis in xerocytosis. *J Clin Invest* 1981; **68**: 631–638

264. Vives Corrons, Besson I, Merino A *et al*. Occurrence of hereditary leaky red cell syndrome and partial coagulation factor VII deficiency in a Spanish family. *Acta Haematol* 1991; **86**: 194–199

265. Glader BE, Fortier N, Albala MM, Nathan DG. Congenital hemolytic anemia associated with dehydrated erythrocytes and increased potassium loss. *N Engl J Med* 1974; **291**: 491–496

266. Glader BE, Sullivan DW. Erythrocyte disorders leading to potassium loss and cellular dehydration. In: Lux SE, Marchesi VT, Fox CF (eds) *Normal and Abnormal Red Cell Membranes.* New York: Alan R Liss, 1979, pp 503–513

267. Fairbanks G, Dino JE, Snyder LM. Passive cation transport in hereditary xerocytosis. In: Kruckeberg WC, Eaton JW, Aster J, Brewer GJ (eds) *Erythrocyte Membranes 3: Recent Clinical and Experimental Advances.* New York: Alan R Liss, 1984, pp 205–217

268. Clark MR, Mohandas N, Caggiano V, Shohet SB. Effects of abnormal cation transport on deformability of desiccytes. *J Supramol Struct* 1978; **8**: 521–532

269. Fortier N, Snyder LM, Garver F, Kiefer C, McKenney J, Mohandas N. The relationship between in vivo generated hemoglobin skeletal protein complex and increased red cell membrane rigidity. *Blood* 1988; **71**: 1427–1431

270. Snyder LM, Lutz HU, Sauberman N, Jacobs J, Fortier NL. Fragmentation and myelin formation in hereditary xerocytosis and other hemolytic anemias. *Blood* 1978; **52**: 750–761

271. Snyder LM, Sauberman N, Condara H *et al*. Red cell membrane response to hydrogen peroxide-sensitivity in hereditary xerocytosis and in other abnormal red cells. *Br J Haematol* 1981; **48**: 435–444

272. Lane PA, Kuypers FA, Clark MR *et al*. Excess of red cell membrane proteins in hereditary high-phosphatidylcholine hemolytic anemia. *Am J Hematol* 1990; **34**: 186–192

273. Fairbanks G, Dino JE, Fortier NL, Snyder LM. Membrane alterations in hereditary xerocytosis: Elevated binding of glycrealdehyde-3 phosphate dehydrogenase. In: Kruckeberg WC, Eaton JW, Brewer GJ (eds) *Erythrocyte Membranes: Recent Clinical and Experimental Advances.* New York: Alan R Liss, 1977, pp 173–188

274. Sauberman N, Fairbanks G, Lutz HU, Fortier NL, Snyder LM. Altered red blood cell surface area in hereditary xerocytosis. *Clin Chim Med* 1981; **114**: 149

275. Clark MR, Shohet SB, Gottfried EL. Hereditary hemolytic disease with increased red blood cell phosphatidylcholine and dehydration: one, two, or many disorders? *Am J Hematol* 1993; **42**: 25–30

276. Mentzer WC, Smith WB, Goldstone J, Shohet SB. Hereditary stomatocytosis: membrane and metabolism studies. *Blood* 1975; **46**: 659–669

277. Mentzer WC, Lubin BH, Emmons S. Correction of the permeability defect in hereditary stomatocytosis by dimethyl adipimidate. *N Engl J Med* 1976; **294**: 1200–1204

278. Mentzer WC, Lam GKH, Lubin BH, Greenquist A. Schrier SL, Lande W. Membrane effects of imidoesters in hereditary stomatocytosis. *J Supramol Struct* 1978; **9**: 275–288

279. Lande WM, Thiemann PVW, Mentzer WC. Missing band 7 membrane protein in two patients with high Na, low K erythrocytes. *J Clin Invest* 1982; **70**: 1273–1280

280. Eber SW, Lande WM, Iarocci TA *et al*. Hereditary stomotocytosis: consistent association with an interral membrane protein deficiency. *Br J Haematol* 1989; **72**: 452–455

281. Morle L, Pothier B, Alloisio N *et al*. Reduction of membrane band 7 and activation of volume stimulated (K$^+$, Cl$^-$)-cotransport in a case of congenital stomatocytosis. *Br J Haematol* 1989; **71**: 141–146

282. Stewart GW, Hepworth-Jones BE, Keen BCJ, Dash BCJ, Argent AC, Casimir CM. Isolation of cDNA coding for an ubiquitous membrane protein deficient in high Na$^+$, low K$^+$ stomatocytic erythrocytes. *Blood* 1992; **79**: 1593–1601

283. Kanzaki A, Yawata Y. Hereditary stomatocytosis: phenotypical

expression of sodium transport and band 7 peptides in 44 cases. *Br J Haematol* 1992; **82**: 133–141

284. Stewart GW, Argent AC, Dash BCJ. Stomatin: a putative cation transport regulator in the red cell membrane. *Biochim Biophys Acta* 1993; **1225**: 15–25

285. Wang D, Turetsky T, Perrine S, Johnson RM, Mentzer WC. Further studies on RBC membrane protein 7.2b deficiency in hereditary stomatocytosis. *Blood* 1992; **80 (Suppl 1)**: 275A

286. Huang M, Gu G, Ferguson EL, Chalfie M. a stomatin-like protein necessary for mechanosensation in *C. elegans*. *Nature* 1995; **378**: 292–295

287. Hirsh J, Dacie JV. Persistent post-splenectomy thrombocytosis and thrombo-embolism: a consequence of continuing anemia. *Br J Haematol* 1966; **12**: 44–53

288. Smith BD, Segel GB. Abnormal erythrocyte endothelial adherence in hereditary stomatocytosis. *Blood* 1997; **89**: 3451–3456

289. Miller G, Townes PL, MacWhinney JB. A new congenital hemolytic anemia with deformed erythrocytes (? stomatocytes) and remarkable susceptibility of erythrocytes to cold hemolysis *in vitro*. I. Clinical and hematologic studies. *Pediatrics* 1965; **35**: 906–915

290. Mentzer WC, Clark MR. Disorders of erythrocyte cation permeability and water content associated with hemolytic anemia. In: Nowotny A (ed) *Biomembranes*, vol 11. New York: Plenum Publishing, 1983, pp 79–117

291. Stewart GW, Ellory JC. A family with mild hereditary xerocytosis showing high membrane cation permeability at low temperatures. *Clin Sci* 1985; **69**: 309–319

292. Ballas S, Clark MR, Mohandas N *et al*. Red cell membrane and cation deficiency in Rh null syndrome. *Blood* 1984; **63**: 1046–1055

Disorders of erythrocyte metabolism

D MARK LAYTON AND ALASTAIR J BELLINGHAM

RED CELL METABOLISM

To meet its energy requirements and ensure structural and functional integrity, the mature red cell has evolved a highly adapted metabolism.[1] Devoid of the capacity for protein synthesis and oxidative phosphorylation, the red cell depends solely on catabolism of glucose for the generation of adenosine triphosphate (ATP) required for cation homeostasis (Fig. 14.1). In the resting state, at least 90% of glucose is catabolized anaerobically via the Embden–Meyerhof pathway, the remaining 10% being metabolized through the hexose monophosphate shunt (pentose phosphate pathway). The deleterious effects of inborn errors of anaerobic glycolysis attest to the importance of the Embden–Meyerhof pathway in red cell metabolism. The same pathway generates nicotinamide adenine dinucleotide in its reduced form (NADH), a cofactor for cytochrome b_5 reductase which is the main enzyme responsible for restoration of methemoglobin to its functional state.

The principal role of the pentose phosphate pathway is production of the reduced form of nicotinamide adenine dinucleotide phosphate (NADPH) required for regeneration of reduced glutathione (GSH), which acts as a sacrificial reductant to protect the red cell membrane and hemoglobin against oxidative damage from oxygen radicals generated during methemoglobin formation and hydrogen peroxide (Fig. 14.2). Hydrogen peroxide may also be detoxified by catalase but the relative importance of this pathway in the red cell is disputed. The first and rate-limiting step in this pathway, the conversion of glucose-6-phosphate (G6P) to 6-phosphogluconate (6PG) is catalyzed by glucose-6-phosphate dehydrogenase (G6PD).

In addition to glycolysis, which provides high-energy phosphates—adenosine triphosphate (ATP) and 2,3-diphosphoglycerate (2,3-DPG)—and reducing power in the form of the pyridine nucleotides (NADH and NADPH) and GSH, nucleotide salvage pathways play a key role in red cell metabolism.[2] The mature red cell lacks the capacity for *de novo* synthesis of purines and pyrimidines. During maturation of the reticulocyte, ribosomal RNA is catabolized to its constituent nucleotides. Since adenine nucleotides in the form of ATP are essential to fulfill cellular energy needs, their reutilization is desirable. The existence of salvage pathways to maintain the adenine nucleotide pool was first suggested from studies directed towards blood storage by the observation that the nucleotides adenosine and inosine protect against depletion of the high-energy phosphates ATP and 2,3-DPG associated with loss of viability of stored red cells. The adenine nucleotide pool is composed predominantly of ATP (85–90%) with small amounts of adenosine di- and mono-phosphate (ADP and AMP). Their equilibrium is mediated by adenylate kinase (Fig. 14.3).

Pyrimidine ribonucleotides (uridine, cytidine and thymidine) are, at high concentrations, toxic to the red cell. To meet the need to catabolize pyrimidine nucleotides, red cells have evolved a nucleotidase, pyrimidine 5'-nucleotidase, which selectively dephosphorylates only pyrimidine nucleoside-5'-monophosphates (CMP, UMP), allowing their removal from the cell by passive diffusion. This substrate specificity ensures adenine nucleotides are conserved.

Elucidation of the key steps of intermediate metabolism

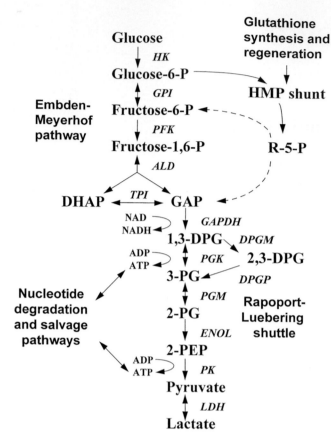

Fig. 14.1 Glycolytic pathways in the human red cell. HK = hexokinase; GPI = glucosephosphate kinase; PFK = phosphofructokinase; ALD = aldolase; TPI = triosephosphate isomerase; DPGM = diphosphoglycerate mutase; PGM = phosphoglycerate mutase; GAPDH = glyceraldehyde-3-phosphate dehydrogenase; PGK = phosphoglycerate kinase; 2,3-DPG = 2,3-diphosphoglycerate; DPGP = diphosphoglycerate phosphatase; ENOL = enolase; PK = pyruvate kinase; LDH = lactate dehydrogenase; HMP = hexose monophosphate pathway.

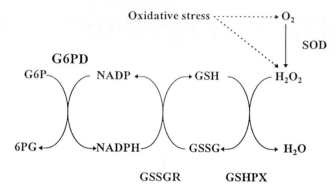

Fig. 14.2 Role of glucose-6-phosphate dehydrogenase (G6PD) in defense against oxidative damage. GSSGR = glutathione reductase; GSHPX = glutathione peroxidase; SOD = superoxide desmutase, H_2O_2 = hydrogen peroxide; GSH = glutathione; GSSG = oxidized glutathione.

during the first half of this century set the stage for the discovery of hereditary disorders of red cell metabolism. That an intrinsic defect could impair red cell survival was first shown by Alving in cross-transfusion studies among volunteers.[3] ^{51}Cr-labeled red cells from primaquine-sensitive subjects were selectively destroyed in normal recipients given primaquine. This culminated in recognition of G6PD deficiency as the mechanism underlying primaquine-induced hemolysis.[4] In 1953, Dacie *et al*[5] drew attention to a group of patients in whom the increased rate of autohemolysis was not reduced in the presence of excess glucose, a pattern (type II) which did not conform to that seen in hereditary spherocytosis, then the most commonly recognized form of congenital hemolytic anemia. This led to speculation that failure of glucose to correct autohemolysis reflected an underlying defect in energy generation via glycolysis, a notion that gained support from the observation that ATP levels were reduced in some patients with type II autohemolysis. This was confirmed in 1961 when Valentine *et al*[6] described the first cases of hemolytic anemia due to pyruvate kinase deficiency. Subsequently, between 1965 and 1974, deficien-

cies of triosephosphate isomerase,[7] phosphofructokinase,[8] hexokinase,[9] glucosephosphate isomerase,[10] phosphoglycerate kinase[11] and aldolase[12] were recognized to cause hemolysis.

GENETICS AND EPIDEMIOLOGY

G6PD deficiency, although a paradigm for X-linked disease, is not in the strict sense recessive. While hemizygous males and homozygous females generally suffer more severe effects, deficiency may also manifest in female heterozygotes. This is explained by the co-existence in heterozygotes of 2 distinct populations of normal (Gd^+) and deficient (Gd^-) red cells as a consequence of X chromosome inactivation. The mode of inheritance of other clinically significant erythroenzyme disorders is autosomal recessive with the exception of phosphoglycerate kinase (PGK deficiency (X-linked recessive), adenosine deaminase (ADA) overproduction (autosomal dominant)[13] and rare examples of pyruvate kinase (PK)[14] and hexokinase (HK)[15] deficiency (autosomal dominant).

With the exception of polymorphic G6PD variants, which affect an estimated 400 million people worldwide, most erythroenzymopathies are uncommon (Table 14.1). Deficiency of PK is the most frequently encountered inborn error of the Embden–Meyerhof pathway. Heterozygote frequencies in different populations vary between 0.14% (United States)[16] and 6% (Saudi Arabia).[17] The frequency in some populations may be influenced by consanguinity. While the majority of reported cases have been of European origin, PK deficiency has a wide geographic distribution. After deficiency of PK, the commonest glycolytic disorders are, in order of frequency, glucosephosphate isomerase (GPI), phosphofructokinase (PFK), triosephosphate isomerase (TPI), PGK and HK. Chronic hemolytic anemia due to G6PD deficiency appears at least as common as any of these disorders. Isolated families with deficiency of aldolase (ALD), glyceraldehyde-3-phosphate dehydrogenase (GAPDH), 2,3-diphosphoglycerate mutase (DPGM) or

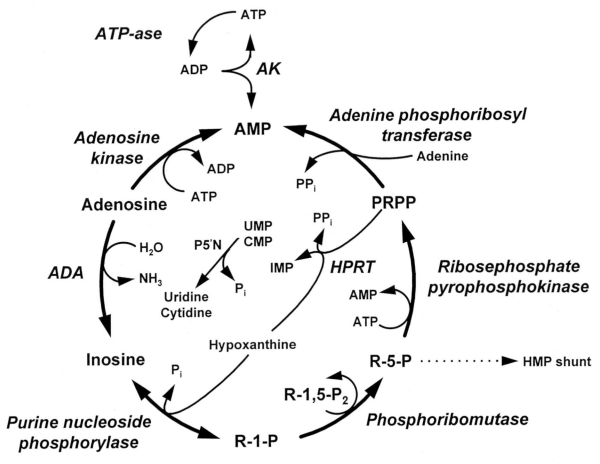

Fig. 14.3 Adenine nucleotide salvage pathways in the human red cell. P5′N = pyrimidine 5′-nucleotidase. HPRT = hypoxanthine-guanine phosphoribosyltransferase; PRPP = phosphoribosyl pyrophosphate.

enolase (ENOL), have been described. Only in the case of aldolase deficiency is a causal link with hemolysis convincingly established. Of enzymes outside the glycolytic pathway, deficiency of pyrimidine 5′-nucleotidase (P5′N)[18] occurs at appreciable frequency. Hereditary deficiency of P5′N is the commonest abnormality of erythrocyte nucleotide metabolism. The disorder has been described in northern European, Mediterranean, African, Middle Eastern,

Asian and Ashkenazi Jewish populations.[19] Other defects involving nucleotide salvage pathways which have been implicated in hemolytic anemia include overproduction of ADA[20] and deficiencies of adenylate kinase[20] or CDP-choline phosphotransferase.[21] All are rare.

Population studies have indicated heterozygosity rates which for most enzyme disorders parallel the number of reported cases of clinical deficiency. In the case of TPI

Table 14.1 Number of reported cases of erythroenzymopathies associated with hereditary hemolytic anemia.

Defect	Polymorphic	Common (>100)	Uncommon (10–100)	Rare (<10)
Emben–Meyerhof pathway	—	Pyruvate kinase	Glucosephosphate isomerase Phosphofructokinase Triosephosphate isomerase Phosphoglycerate kinase Hexokinase	Aldolase
Hexose monophosphate shunt/ glutathione synthesis	Glucose-6-phosphate dehydrogenase Class II and III	Glucose-6-phosphate dehydrogenase Class I	Glutathione synthetase	γ-Glutamylcysteine synthetase
Nucleotide metabolism	—	—	Pyrimidine 5′-nucleotidase	Adenosine deaminase Adenylate kinase CDP-choline phosphotransferase

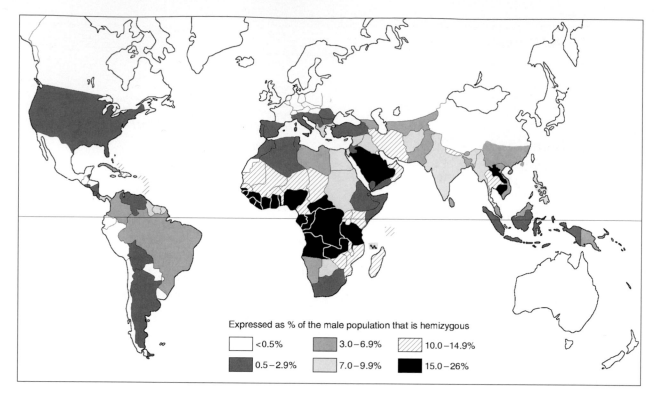

Fig. 14.4 World distribution of glucose-6-phosphate dehydrogenase (G6PD) deficiency.

deficiency, however, striking interethnic variation in hetero-zygote frequency has been observed.[22,23] In African-Americans the carrier frequency reaches 4.2%. This corresponds to a predicted birth prevalence for homozygous TPI deficiency of 1/2300 which is at odds with the extreme rarity of the disorder in this population. It has been proposed that this discrepancy may be attributed to one or several null alleles which in homozygotes are lethal.

The distribution of G6PD deficiency in different populations has been extensively studied.[24] Gene frequencies range from <0.5% in northern European populations to >25% in parts of Central and West Africa, the Middle East and South-East Asia (Fig. 14.4).[25] The highest prevalence of G6PD deficiency has been observed in Kurdish Jews. Of variants found at polymorphic frequency G6PD A⁻ and its non-deficient counterpart G6PD A are prevalent throughout Africa and among immigrant populations of African descent but also occur in southern Europe and the Middle East. G6PD Mediterranean is common throughout the Mediterranean basin and accounts for a significant proportion of G6PD deficient alleles in Middle Eastern and Asian Indian populations. A striking similarity between the world-wide distribution of G6PD deficiency and malaria endemi-city prompted the hypothesis that the high frequency of G6PD deficiency reflects positive selection. This is supported by evidence of lower levels of *Plasmodium falciparum* parasit-emia in female heterozygotes[26,27] compared with normal subjects and impaired growth of *P. falciparum* in G6PD deficient red cells *in vitro*.[28] The exact mechanism by which

G6PD deficiency confers resistance against malaria and why protection is confined to female heterozygotes is not fully understood.

A high prevalence of type I *(vide infra)* enzymopathic hereditary methemoglobinemia is found in indigenous Alaskan populations, native Americans, the Chuvash people of Siberia, Puerto Rica and parts of the Mediterranean.[29]

INVESTIGATION

From a clinical perspective, erythroenzyme defects associated with hemolytic anemia can be usefully divided into those in which hemolysis is the sole manifestation and those in which deficiency results in a multisystem disorder. Important distinguishing clinical features which aid diagnosis are summarized in Table 14.2. The mode of inheritance discerned from a family history and pattern of hemolysis may be informative. Disorders of the pentose phosphate and glutathione pathways characteristically exhibit episodic hemolysis under oxidative stress. By contrast, defects of the Embden–Meyerhof pathway, crucial for steady-state energy generation in the red cell, cause chronic hemolysis. This distinction is not, however, absolute and there may be overlap, examples being chronic non-spherocytic hemolytic anemia due to class I G6PD variants and exacerbation of hemolysis following oxidant exposure in GPI deficiency.

Table 14.2 Distinctive clinical features associated with erythroenzymopathies.

Enzyme	Inheritance	Hemolysis	Neurological	Myopathy	Other
Hexokinase	AR	+			
Glucosephosphate isomerase	AR	+	+ (Rare)	+ (Rare)	Fetal hydrops, recurrent infection
Phosphofructokinase	AR	±		+	Myoglobinuria, hyperuricemia
Aldolase	AR	+	(+)	±	
Triosephosphate isomerase	AR	+	+*	+*	Recurrent infection, sudden cardiac death
Phosphoglycerate kinase	XL	±	±	±	Myoglobinuria
Diphosphoglycerate mutase	AR				Erythrocytosis
Enolase	AD?	(+)			Spherocytosis
Pyruvate kinase L/R	AR (rarely AD)	+			Fetal hydrops
Lactate dehydrogenase M(B)	AR			+	
γ-Glutamylcysteine synthetase	AR	+	±		
Glutathione synthetase	AR	+	±		Acidosis, 5-oxoprolinuria, recurrent infection
Glutathione reductase	AR	+			Favism, cataract
Pyrimidine-5′-nucleotidase	AR	+	(+)		Basophilic stippling
					Acquired deficiency in plumbism and transient erythroblastopenia of childhood
CDP-choline phosphotransferase	AR	+			Basophilic stippling
Adenosine deaminase (↑)	AD	+			
Adenylate kinase	AR	+	±		

Parentheses indicate link to enzyme deficiency unproven.
AR = autosomal recessive; AD = autosomal dominant; XL = X-linked.
*Two cases of triosephosphate isomerase deficiency without neuromuscular manifestations have been reported.

Physical examination is frequently unhelpful. The presence of splenomegaly more commonly denotes chronic hemolysis. While both autohemolysis and osmotic fragility tests are abnormal in some red cell enzymopathies, their diagnostic value lies principally in the exclusion of membrane defects as a prelude to specific studies of erythrocyte metabolism in cases of unexplained hemolytic anemia.

Blood cell morphology

Examination of the blood film may reveal characteristic morphologic features, most prominent of which is the extensive basophilic stippling associated with pyrimidine 5′-nucleotidase deficiency. In general, however, red cell enzymopathies are not associated with characteristic abnormalities of red cell morphology. The presence of spheroechinocytes or 'sputnik-cells' dehydrated effete red cells, reflecting the consequences of severe ATP depletion, is most striking in PK deficiency particularly after splenectomy but also occurs in some cases of HK, GPI, TPI and PGK deficiency.[30]

Enzyme screening tests

For several erythroenzyme disorders screening methods have been devised of which that recommended by the International Committee for Standardization in Haematology for G6PD deficiency is the most useful.[31] The screening test for PK deficiency requires rigorous removal of leukocytes which have a PK activity 300-fold greater than red cells. The pattern of intracellular pyrimidine nucleotides that accumu-

late in P5′N deficiency forms the basis of a useful screening test based on spectral analysis (*vide infra*).

Analysis of intermediate metabolism

Quantitation of the major red cell metabolites 2,3-DPG, ATP and GSH which are present at millimolar concentration and can be assayed readily by spectrophotometric techniques provides valuable information on the identity of a suspected erythroenzyme disorder. While failure of ATP generation is regarded a *sine qua non* of glycolytic disorders and fundamental to their pathophysiologic consequences, reduced ATP concentration is an inconstant finding. This is largely explained by the relatively high ATP concentration in younger red cells which masks the overall deficit in production. An increase in red cell 2,3-DPG level occurs in most anemias as an adaptive response to facilitate oxygen delivery and is also seen irrespective of the presence of anemia in hypoxemia, alkalosis and hyperphosphatemia.[32,33] The 2,3-DPG level may, particularly in conjunction with ATP concentration, be helpful in localizing an enzyme defect to proximal or distal glycolysis (Table 14.3). Extremely low red cell 2,3-DPG concentration associated with secondary erythrocytosis has been reported in a kindred with complete 2,3-diphosphoglycerate mutase (DPGM) deficiency.[34]

In G6PD deficiency and disorders of anaerobic glycolysis associated with impaired hexose monophosphate shunt activity, e.g. GPI deficiency, GSH concentration is often moderately reduced. Red cell GSH levels are also diminished in patients with an unstable hemoglobin. A marked

Table 14.3 2,3-Diphosphoglycerate (2,3-DPG) and ATP patterns in some hereditary hemolytic anemias.

Defect	2,3-DPG	ATP	Comments
Proximal glycolysis, e.g. HK, GPI or PFK	N or ↓	N or ↓	Variable ↓ 2,3-DPG also seen in DPGM deficiency, stomatocytosis and some cases of hereditary spherocytosis before splenectomy
Distal glycolysis, e.g. PK or PGK	↑↑	N or ↓	2,3-DPG:ATP more useful in PK deficiency
Overproduction ADA	↓	N	

N = normal; HK = hexokinase; GPI = glucosephosphate isomerase; PGK = phosphoglycerate kinase; ADA = adenosine deaminase; DPGM = 2,3-diphosphoglycerate mutase; PK = pyruvate kinase.

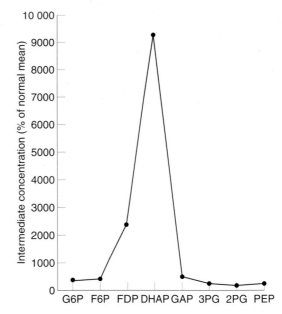

Fig. 14.5 Pattern of glycolytic intermediates in a patient with triosephosphate isomerase (TPI) deficiency demonstrating markedly elevated dihydroxyacetone phosphate (DHAP) concentration. Values are expressed as a percentage of the normal mean. G6P = glucose-6-phosphate; F6P = fructose-6-phosphate; FDP = fructose-1,6-diphosphate; GAP = glyceraldehyde-3-phosphate; 3PG = 3-phosphoglycerate; 2PG = 2-phosphoglycerate; PEP = phosphoenolpyruvate.

reduction in GSH suggests block in glutathione biosynthesis due to deficiency of glutathione synthetase[35] or γ-glutamyl-cysteine synthetase.[36] GSH concentration is increased in P5′N deficiency, the reason for which is unclear, and has been described as an isolated abnormality in a family with non-recessively inherited hemolytic anemia.[37]

Metabolic block in the glycolytic pathway is most accurately pinpointed by measurement of the *in vivo* concentration of glycolytic intermediates. This overcomes the limitation of assays of enzyme activity performed *in vitro* under conditions which may not accurately reflect enzyme function *in vivo*. Typically, a block in glycolysis will be evident from accumulation of metabolites proximal and depletion distal to the defective step. In some instances, e.g. TPI deficiency in which there is a dramatic increase in the concentration of dihydroxyacetone phosphate (DHAP) above other intermediates, the intermediate profile is pathognomonic (Fig. 14.5). A distinct metabolic 'crossover' is sometimes obscured by feedback regulation and the higher metabolic rate and intermediate concentrations in young red cells. Despite this, measurement of glycolytic intermediates extracted from fresh red cells constitutes the most valuable tool for demonstration of metabolic block in glycolysis and permits detailed studies of catalytic function to be targeted towards a specific enzyme.

Enzyme activity and other physicochemical properties

Definitive diagnosis of enzyme deficiency rests on quantitative assay of enzyme activity in red cells coupled with characterization of the biochemical properties of the mutant enzyme (Table 14.4). Particular attention must be paid to removal of leukocytes and correction for the increased activity of 'age-dependent' enzymes, particularly HK, PK, ALD, G6PD and P5′N in reticulocytes.[38] If control samples with a similar reticulocyte count are not available for comparison, assay of a second 'age-dependent' enzyme is

helpful. The physiologic changes in enzyme activity (and intermediate concentration) that accompany development must be taken into account when interpreting the results of assays in neonates.[39–41] In some cases the basis for defective enzyme function *in vivo* lies not in a reduction in activity demonstrable *in vitro* but in another abnormal property of the mutant enzyme, e.g. altered substrate kinetics, thermal stability or response to physiologic activators or inhibitors. Thus, it may be necessary to undertake detailed characterization of the mutant enzyme to establish a causal link with hemolysis. Family studies are frequently helpful in this respect as is illustrated in the case of PK deficiency shown in Table 14.5 and Figs 14.6 and 14.7. The proband exhibited normal activities of all glycolytic enzymes including PK but an increase in the ratio of 2,3-DPG:ATP indicative of metabolic block at the PK step. This was confirmed by abnormally low PK activity at reduced substrate (phosphoenolpyruvate) concentration. Futher investigation

Table 14.4 Properties used for characterization of mutant enzymes *in vitro*.

V_{Max}	Maximum enzyme velocity (activity) at saturating substrate concentration
K_M	Substrate concentration at which enzyme activity is 50% of V_{Max}
Thermolability	Resistance to heat denaturation
pH optimum	pH at which enzyme activity is maximal
Electrophoretic mobility	Altered charge relative to wild type enzyme

Table 14.5 Pyruvate kinase (PK) properties and concentrations of 2,3-diphosphoglycerate (2,3-DPG) and ATP in a family with PK deficiency.

PK properties	Normal range	Propositus	Father	Mother
Activity (IU/g Hb)	6.3–13.0	8.0	9.2	8.5
K_M PEP (mM)	0.75–1.20	3.50	1.80	0.75
Thermostability (% residual activity after 60 min at 55°C)	52–65	19	42	33
Electrophoretic mobility	Normal	Fast	Fast	Normal
2,3-DPG (μmol/g Hb)	12.6–17.2	24.5	NT	NT
ATP (μmol/g Hb)	3.9–5.4	2.3	NT	NT
2,3-DPG:ATP ratio	2.7–3.6	10.7	NT	NT

NT: not tested

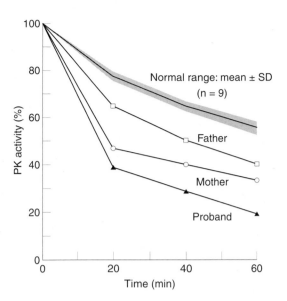

Fig. 14.7 Heat stability curves in pyruvate kinase (PK) deficiency. Residual PK activity after incubation at 55°C is abnormal in all 3 members of the family. The values at 60 min are shown in Table 14.5.

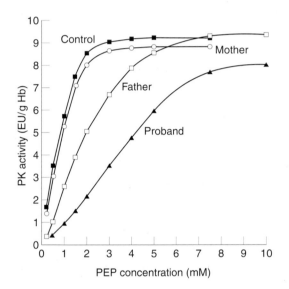

Fig. 14.6 Pyruvate kinase (PK) kinetics in the family shown in Table 14.5. Patient (proband, ▲), father (□), mother (○) and normal control (■). Although the maximum PK activity (V_{Max}) is normal, PK activity at 50% phosphoenolpyruvate (PEP) saturation ($K_{0.5s}$[PEP]) is reduced in the proband and father.

revealed the proband to be a compound heterozygote for 2 mutant enzymes which differ in their physicochemical properties.

Prenatal diagnosis

Prenatal diagnosis has been performed by biochemical analysis of umbilical venous blood or cultured amniocytes for several of the more severe enzymopathies, including deficiencies of TPI,[42] GPI,[43] PK[44] and cytochrome b_5 reductase.[45] To enable phenotypic diagnosis *in utero* normal ranges for red cell enzymes and intermediate metabolites in mid-gestation fetal blood have been established.[46–49] With expansion in knowledge of the genetic defects responsible for erythroenzyme disorders (*vide infra*), this approach has been superseded in some cases by molecular diagnosis,[50,51] which

allows prenatal testing by chorionic villus analysis in the first trimester of pregnancy.[52]

DISORDERS OF THE EMBDEN–MEYERHOF PATHWAY

HEXOKINASE DEFICIENCY

HK catalyzes the phosphorylation of glucose at the 6-carbon position providing a common substrate, G6P, for anaerobic and oxidative glycolysis. This reaction is rate limiting and thus crucial to the generation of energy via the glycolytic pathway. In most cases of HK deficiency, anemia is moderate but, in common with other disorders of glycolysis, there is a spectrum of clinical severity ranging from severe neonatal jaundice with subsequent transfusion dependence to compensated hemolysis. Poor effort tolerance relative to the degree of anemia is characteristic. This may be attributed to the low concentration of 2,3-DPG in HK-deficient red cells, the effect of which is to increase the oxygen affinity of hemoglobin and shift the oxygen dissociation curve to the left.[53,54] Red cell morphology is seldom remarkable.

The diagnosis of HK deficiency may be made on the basis of reduced cell enzyme activity in the presence of low concentrations of metabolic intermediates, particularly G6P and fructose-6-phosphate (F6P). Red cell ATP concentration is low or normal.[55,56] The reduction in enzyme activity in homozygotes may, because of the relatively high HK activity in young red cells, be no greater than in heterozygotes, making diagnosis difficult in some cases. Interpretation of HK activity is aided by comparison with the activity of another age-dependent enzyme.

GLUCOSEPHOSPHATE ISOMERASE DEFICIENCY

Deficiency of GPI, which catalyzes the interconversion of G6P and F6P, results in hemolytic anemia of variable severity. Onset is typically during infancy with neonatal jaundice in a third of cases. Hydrops fetalis due to GPI deficiency has been reported.[43,57] Hemolytic crises associated with intercurrent infection or exposure to oxidant drugs may occur. This may be reconciled with a greater susceptibility of GPI-deficient red cells to oxidative damage due to their inability to recycle F6P through the hexose monophosphate shunt.[10,58] The increased thermolability displayed by virtually all GPI-deficient variants in vitro may also contribute to red cell destruction in vivo during febrile episodes.

Isolated reports of non-hematologic manifestations of GPI deficiency of include impaired granulocyte function,[59,60] priapism,[61] myopathy and mental retardation.[62,63] Reduced deformability of GPI-deficient red cells has been invoked as a possible mechanism underlying priapism. In 2 well documented cases associated with multisystem disease, the basis for enzyme deficiency was shown to reside solely in abnormal kinetic properties of the mutant enzyme.[59,63] Such defects may cause a more global perturbance of glycolysis than structurally unstable variants, the effects of which will be mitigated partially in tissues that retain the ability to synthesize GPI.

In homozygous GPI deficiency, residual erythrocyte enzyme activity is typically 10–40% of normal and is accompanied by an increase in the ratio of G6P:F6P reflecting a block in glycolysis at the GPI step. In keeping with impaired hexose monophosphate pathway (HMP) activity, red cell glutathione concentration and glutathione stability may be diminished. Increased Heinz body (precipitates of denatured hemoglobin) formation and further reduction in glutathione stability is observed after incubation with acetylphenylhydrazine.[57]

PHOSPHOFRUCTOKINASE DEFICIENCY

PFK catalyzes the principal rate-limiting step in glycolysis—the phosphorylation of F6P to fructose-1,6-diphosphate (FDP). The heterogeneity of clinical syndromes associated with deficiency of PFK mirrors the complexity of its genetic control. The active form of PFK is a tetramer. Muscle (M), liver (L) and platelet (P) subunits are encoded by separate structural genes.[64] Muscle PFK is composed entirely of M subunits, whereas in red cells both M and L subunits combine to from different tetramers, the relative proportions of which vary during development. This may explain the lower activity of PFK in neonatal red cells, the composition of which includes the relatively unstable L_4 isoenzyme which is not found in normal adult red cells.

The association between PFK deficiency and shortened red cell survival in patients with myopathy and glycogen storage disease (type VII) was first noted by Tarui et al.[8] The presence of residual L subunits which combine to form an active tetramer explains why red cells are spared the full metabolic effects of M-subunit deficiency in classic PFK deficiency. Cases of PFK deficiency with isolated hemolysis and normal muscle enzyme activity have also been recognized.[65,66] Here the defect lies predominantly in instability of the active enzyme in red cells.[67]

In its most severe form, PFK deficiency may present at birth and follow an inexorable course with death from respiratory failure in infancy.[68] More usually, the onset of symptoms is delayed until later childhood or even adult life. The cardinal features of muscle weakness, fatigability aggravated by exertion or after a carbohydrate meal[69] and cramps raise suspicion of the diagnosis. Muscle weakness characteristically worsens during exercise because of the reliance of muscle cells on anaerobic glycolysis for energy generation. Exertional rhabdomyolysis with myoglobinuria may occur. Where present, anemia is usually mild or moderate. Hemolysis may be fully compensated and even mild erythrocytosis due to reduced 2,3-DPG concentration as a consequence of block at the PFK step has been reported. Red cell morphology is, with the exception of prominent basophilic stippling seen in a few cases, not helpful diagnostically. Increased purine generation in muscle and red cells may lead to hyperuricemia and arthropathy.

The diagnosis of PFK deficiency can be confirmed by assay of red cell enzyme activity and intermediates. Typically, red cell PFK activity is about 50% of normal. Reduced muscle PFK activity may be inferred from a failure of lactate production after anaerobic (ischemic) forearm exercise or magnetic resonance spectroscopy studies.[70] Direct confirmation may be obtained by assay of enzyme activity on biopsied muscle tissue. Since muscle contains exclusively M_4 tetramers, the reduction in enzyme activity is correspondingly greater than in red cells.[71]

ALDOLASE DEFICIENCY

Aldolase is responsible for conversion of FDP to glyceraldehyde-3-phosphate (GAP) and dihydroxyacetone phosphate (DHAP). Three tissue-specific isoenzymes, A, B and C, exist of which aldolase A is found in brain, muscle and red cells.[72] Only 3 cases of hemolytic anemia due to inherited aldolase deficiency have been described.[12,73,74] In the initial case, which occurred on a background of parental consanguinity, mental retardation, dysmorphism and glycogen storage disease were associated, but these features were not evident in the subsequent 2 cases. In one case myopathy characterized by exercise intolerance and rhabdomyolysis was a prominent manifestation.[74] Episodes of rhabdomyolysis were precipitated by fever. This was attributed to marked thermal instability of the mutant enzyme.

TRIOSEPHOSPHATE ISOMERASE DEFICIENCY

TPI catalyzes with high efficiency the interconversion of the triosephosphates DHAP and GAP, the equilibrium favoring DHAP formation by a factor of 22:1. The clinical phenotype first described by Schneider et al[7] that results from homozygous deficiency of TPI is the severest among disorders of the Embden–Meyerhof pathway. The active enzyme, a homodimer, is found in all tissues, a pattern of expression reflected in the multisystem nature of the clinical deficiency state.[75]

Around 40 cases of TPI deficiency have been reported. Typically, presentation is in the first year of life with neonatal jaundice or hemolytic anemia. Between 6 months and 2 years of age neuromuscular dysfunction becomes evident. The constellation of neurologic abnormalities observed in TPI deficiency includes motor delay or regression, spasticity, hypotonia, dystonic movements, opisthotonos, nystagmus and optic atrophy.[76–78] Neuromuscular impairment is usually progressive, although it may stabilize during childhood[79] and isolated cases in which there is no overt neurologic dysfunction have been described.[80,81] Cognitive function is usually spared. Most affected children fail to survive beyond 5 years of age. Death may be sudden and cardiac arrythmia has been invoked as a likely cause. Deficiency of leukocyte enzyme may account for the increased susceptibility to bacterial infection which has been noted among affected children. The degree of anemia in TPI deficiency is variable. Although severe anemia may be encountered, most patients require only occasional transfusion after the neonatal period. Morphologically, occasional spheroechinocytes may be visible on the blood film but there are no distinguishing features.

The mechanisms underlying the neuropathic effects of TPI deficiency are poorly delineated. Neuroimaging studies have failed to reveal extensive structural changes in the brain. Electrophysiologic studies show evidence of denervation myopathy in some cases. A kindred has been described in which only one of two affected siblings manifests neurologic dysfunction.[80] This informative case suggests factors other than the primary defect in glycolysis contribute to neurologic expression of the disease. DHAP is an essential precursor in biosynthesis of ether glycerolipids (plasmalogens). Plasmalogen biosynthesis is impaired in peroxisosmal disorders, e.g. Zellweger syndrome and neonatal adrenoleukodystrophy, in which neurologic manifestations are prominent.[82] It is more difficult to envisage how excess DHAP as a result of a block in glycolysis might cause such a defect but recent evidence suggests plasmalogen biosynthesis may be impaired in TPI deficiency.[83]

TPI deficiency is diagnosed by assay of red cell enzyme activity in conjunction with metabolic intermediates. The biochemical hallmark of homozygous TPI deficiency is intracellular accummulation of DHAP. This is most marked (20–100-fold) in red cells which, unlike other tissues, lack the capacity to metabolize DHAP in the glycerol phosphate shuttle via α-glycerophosphate dehydrogenase.

PHOSPHOGLYCERATE KINASE DEFICIENCY

PGK, a key enzyme in the glycolytic pathway, catalyses the conversion of 1,3-diphosphoglycerate (1,3-DPG) to 3-phosphoglycerate (3-PG) with the concomitant generation of ATP. Ironically for an X-linked disorder, deficiency of PGK was first recognized in a female with hemolytic anemia.[11] Soon thereafter a more severe phenotype accompanied by neurologic manifestations was recognized in hemizygous males.[84] The spectrum of neurologic abnormalities in affected males includes seizures, movement disorders, hemiplegia, aphasia, mental retardation and behavioral disturbance including emotional lability. While onset in the neonatal period with jaundice and seizures is reported,[85] there may be latency in the appearance of neurologic manifestations with normal development in infancy.[86] Isolated hemolytic anemia or myopathy and myopathy in combination with either hemolysis or neurologic abnormalities are described.[87–90] In patients with muscle disease, rhabdomyolysis with myoglobinuria may occur and are sometimes precipitated by exercise or convulsions. The basis for the differing patterns of clinical expression in PGK deficiency is not understood since the same isoenzyme is expressed in all somatic cells.[91] Heterozygote females may manifest mild hemolysis but have normal neurologic function.

In hemizygous males, red cell PGK activity is usually <20% of normal. Enzyme levels in female heterozygotes vary due not only to Lyonization, as in other X-linked disorders, but also the preferential survival of PGK-replete red cells that have the normal allele on their active X chromosome. The profile of red cell intermediates in affected males is consistent with a block in glycolysis at the PGK step. Reduction in the concentration of ATP is characteristic, whereas 2,3-DPG is usually elevated, reflecting increased flow through the Rapoport–Luebering shunt. Despite this attempt at metabolic compensation, accumulation of intermediates proximal to the PGK step attests to perturbance of glycolysis in vivo.

PYRUVATE KINASE DEFICIENCY

PK catalyzes the conversion of phosphoenolpyruvate (PEP) to pyruvate with the generation of ATP. PK deficiency is the commonest enzymopathic cause of chronic hemolytic anemia with 400 cases reported. Over 80% of cases present during childhood. The spectrum of clinical severity is wide.[92] Anemia may manifest in utero[93,94] or in the newborn period.[95] Neonatal jaundice is a common manifestation of PK deficiency and if pronounced may herald a severe course. Kernicterus, although rare, has been described. In severely affected cases, dependence on transfusion may be lifelong. A particularly severe form of PK deficiency has been described in the Dutch Amish population in Pennsylvania.[96] It should, however, be noted that owing to a high erythrocyte 2,3-DPG concentration in PK-deficient erythrocytes, which shifts the hemoglobin oxygen dissociation curve to the right,[97] favoring oxygen delivery to the tissues, haemoglobin levels as low as 6–7 g/dl may be remarkably well tolerated. At the opposite end of the spectrum are cases that evade diagnosis until later in life and in which anemia is mild or even absent. In the latter, unconjugated hyperbilirubinemia may be the sole clinical manifestation. Exacerbation of hemolysis in PK deficiency may occur during intercurrent infection and less consistently pregnancy[98] and oral contraceptive use.[99] Quite often pregnancy is uncomplicated with no adverse effects on maternal or fetal well-being.

Primary manifestations outside the erythropoietic system are rare, although in severely affected children there may be growth delay and skeletal changes due to expanded erythropoiesis. Spinal cord compression due to extramedullary hemopoiesis has been described.[100]

This restricted pattern of clinical expression may be reconciled with the genetic control of human PK. In its active form, PK is a tetramer composed of 4 identical subunits. Red cell (R) and liver (L) subunits are encoded by the PK-L/R gene[101] and produced by expression from different tissue-specific promoters.[102] This has prompted speculation as to whether deficiency of the liver enzyme may contribute to jaundice. Evidence of abnormal liver function in some cases of PK deficiency supports this possibility. All other tissues express the muscle (M) subunit which is encoded by a separate structural gene, PK-M.[103] Two forms of the M subunit, M_1 and M_2, probably reflect alternative splicing of the PK-M gene transcript. A switch takes place both during early human development and erythroid differentiation from the M_2 to R subunit.[104] In some cases of severe deficiency of the R subunit, reversion to synthesis of the M_2 form may partially rescue the deficient phenotype.[105] This has been likened to the persistence of fetal hemoglobin in β-thalassemia. Persistence of the M_2 isoenzyme in red cells may also account for the rare 'high ATP' syndrome in which supraphysiologic PK activity leads to metabolic depletion of 2,3-DPG with increased hemoglobin oxygen affinity and erythrocytosis.[106,107]

The presence of characteristic changes in red cell morphology, unusual among glycolytic disorders, may assist in the diagnosis of PK deficiency.[30] Typically, there is slight macrocytosis and poikilocytosis with ovalocytes and elliptocytes accompanied by polychromasia and occasional contracted crenated red cells (spheroechinocytes). The latter are accentuated after splenectomy. Removal of the spleen is accompanied by a rise in hemoglobin which typically stabilizes at 1–3 g/dl higher than the level pre-splenectomy. The paradoxic rise in reticulocyte count that accompanies splenectomy in PK deficiency may be dramatic, sometimes reaching 40–60%. This reflects preferential destruction of PK-deficient reticulocytes in the spleen which can be attrib-

uted to their dependence on mitochondrial oxidative phosphorylation to maintain ATP. In the acidic hypoxic environment of the spleen, oxidative generation of ATP is suppressed. This in turn leads to a cascade of events which includes loss of cation homeostasis with efflux of potassium and water that culminate in cellular dehydration and contraction. The rigid crenated cells which form are entrapped within the red pulp of the spleen. This sequence is supported by histologic evidence of splenic red cell sequestration in PK deficiency.[108]

Biochemically, PK deficiency is heterogeneous. Homozygotes typically exhibit <25% and heterozygotes 40–60% residual enzyme activity. There is, however, considerable overlap and some PK-deficient variants are associated with normal or minimally reduced activity in vitro. Quantitative assays should be performed at high and low substrate concentrations in the presence or absence of the allosteric effector FDP to detect PK variants with abnormal kinetic properties. Accumulation of glycolytic intermediates preceding the PK step in glycolysis, particularly PEP, 2-phosphoglycerate (2-PG), 3-PG and 2,3-DPG,[109] but sometimes extending proximally due to feedback inhibition of other glycolytic enzymes by 2,3-DPG provides evidence of defective function in vivo. ATP formation is reduced but in the presence of marked reticulocytosis absolute levels may be normal. An increase in the ratio of 2,3-DPG:ATP has been found to be a more reliable predictor of PK deficiency.[110] The majority of PK variants exhibit reduced stability and/or altered kinetic properties in vitro. The interpretation of kinetic studies in PK deficiency is complicated in compound heterozygotes by the varying proportion of tetramers formed by the 2 mutant subunits. Occasional reports of dominant inheritance[14,111,112] with clinical hemolysis in heterozygotes suggest in rare circumstances a single mutant subunit may disrupt catalytic function. Autohemolysis is variable but most frequently shows a type II pattern.

GLUCOSE-6-PHOSPHATE DEHYDROGENASE DEFICIENCY

Though ubiquitously expressed by all cells, the pathophysiologic consequences of G6PD deficiency are confined almost exclusively to red blood cells which lack the capacity to synthesize the enzyme and are inherently vulnerable to endogenous oxidative damage because of their role in oxygen transport. Since the landmark discovery that primaquine sensitivity was due to inherited deficiency of G6PD,[3,4] over 400 variants have been reported.[24] G6PD variants may be classified according to the level of residual enzyme activity and associated clinical manifestations (Table 14.6). Several well defined clinical syndromes due to G6PD deficiency are encountered during childhood. The commonest are neonatal jaundice and acute hemolysis triggered by exposure to oxidants or intercurrent infection. Much less commonly, G6PD deficiency causes chronic non-spherocytic hemolytic

Table 14.6 Classification of glucose-6-phosphate dehydrogenase (G6PD) variants.

Class	Enzyme activity (% of normal)	Example(s)	Clinical effects
I	Variable (typically <20)	San Diego	CNSHA
II	<10	Mediterranean, Canton	AHA, NNJ
III	10–60	A⁻	AHA, NNJ
IV	100	B,* A	None
V	>100	Verona	None

* Wild type.
NNJ = neonatal jaundice; AHA = acute hemolytic anemia; CNSHA = chronic non-spherocytic hemolytic anemia.

anemia (CNSHA). Rare class I G6PD variants have been described in which enzyme deficiency in leukocytes is associated with defective function *in vivo* and increased susceptibility to bacterial infection,[113] particularly with *Staphylococcus aureus*. This may be explained by reduced availability of NADPH, the substrate for the respiratory burst oxidase. The clinical picture in these cases resembles milder forms of chronic granulomatous disease. Other reported associations are an increase in the severity of viral hepatitis[114] and risk of cataract.[115] It should be emphasized that in the vast majority of individuals, G6PD deficiency is clinically silent.

ACUTE HEMOLYTIC ANEMIA

Under conditions of oxidative stress, acute hemolysis may occur abruptly in a child with G6PD deficiency who at other times is clinically well. Not all individuals even with the same G6PD variant are equally susceptible. The reasons for this are still poorly understood. The commonest trigger is infection followed by drugs or other exogenous oxidants (Table 14.7). The release of peroxides generated during phagocytosis of bacteria may be important in triggering hemolysis

Table 14.7 Drugs associated with hemolysis in glucose-6-phosphate dehydrogenase (G6PD) deficiency.

Class of drug	Examples
Antimalarials	Primaquine, pentaquine, pamaquine
Sulfonamides and sulfones	Sulfanilamide, sulfacetamide, sulfapyridine, sulfamethoxazole, dapsone
Other antibacterial agents	Nitrofurantoin, nalidixic acid, chloramphenicol, ciprofloxacin
Analgesic/antipyretic	Acetanilid, acetylsalicylic acid (Aspirin)
Miscellaneous	Probenecid Dimercaprol Vitamin K analogs Naphthalene (moth balls) Methylene blue Ascorbic acid

during bacterial infection. Pneumonia, viral hepatitis and typhoid are particularly likely to precipitate hemolysis in children with G6PD deficiency.[116] More tenuously, diabetic ketoacidosis[117] and hypoglycemia have been linked to acute hemolysis in G6PD-deficient subjects. The course and severity of acute hemolysis in G6PD deficiency is highly variable. Males are more frequently affected than females. The onset usually follows within 2–3 days of oxidative challenge but can be more rapid, notably in favism. Constitutional symptoms, including irritability and lethargy, may herald overt hemolysis. Typically, these are followed by the development of fever sometimes accompanied by gastrointestinal symptoms. Hemoglobinuria, the cardinal sign of intravascular hemolysis, ensues with dark red or brown urine often colloquially described as the color of Coca-Cola. This precedes or coincides with the onset of jaundice and is accompanied by signs of anemia with pallor, tachycardia and in severe cases hypovolemic shock. The degree of anemia is variable but may be extremely severe.

Characteristic poikilocytes, including 'hemighosts' and 'bite cells' are visible on examination of the blood film. There may be marked reticulocytosis. Heinz bodies may be visualized by supravital staining with methyl violet. Since Heinz bodies are removed by the spleen and red cells containing them are rapidly destroyed, their appearance is transient. Haptoglobin is absent. Oxidation of hemoglobin is occasionally sufficient to produce methemoglobinemia. Other causes of intravascular hemolysis, which include *P. falciparum* malaria ('blackwater fever'), hemolytic transfusion reaction, paroxysmal cold hemoglobinuria, paroxysmal nocturnal hemoglobinuria, *Clostridium welchii* septicemia and babesiosis, should, where appropriate, be considered in the differential diagnosis.

In the majority of cases, hemolysis is self limiting. Blood transfusion may be required and although no didactic rules apply, useful guidelines have been recommended by Luzzatto.[118] These advise immediate transfusion if the hemoglobin level is <7 g/dl or between 7 and 9 g/dl in the face of hemoglobinuria. At higher hemoglobin levels it may be justified to withhold transfusion, providing the child is kept under close observation and transfusion instigated if the hemoglobin falls below the threshold identified above. Avoidance of transfusion with G6PD-deficient red cells is theoretically desirable, although in practice difficult to achieve. Recovery of hemoglobin to steady-state levels may take 3–6 weeks. This is quicker in the case of G6PD variants, e.g. A⁻ in which enzyme activity is relatively well preserved in reticulocytes, making them less susceptible to destruction.

Hemolysis following ingestion of broad beans (*Vicia faba*), favism, although classically associated with more severe deficiencies, exemplified by G6PD Mediterranean, may occur in other variants including G6PD A⁻. Fresh beans are most often implicated. Variability in sensitivity to fava beans among individuals with G6PD deficiency and even in the same individual at different times suggests other

295

factors, including perhaps absorption and metabolism of the toxic constituents, probably the pyrimidine β-glycosides vicine and convicine, play a role. Maternal ingestion of fava beans[119] has been reported to cause hemolysis in breast-fed infants who are G6PD deficient and even hydrops fetalis.[120] Favism has been attributed to inhalation of bean pollen.[121]

NEONATAL JAUNDICE

Neonatal jaundice is potentially one of the most serious consequences of G6PD deficiency and, untreated, may have irreversible neurologic sequelae. In Africa and South East Asia, G6PD deficiency is the commonest cause of kernicterus.[24] Although early reports highlighted the prevalence of neonatal jaundice in Mediterranean and South East Asian infants, this complication affects all indigenous and immigrant populations in which G6PD deficiency occurs. Jaundice develops later than in Rhesus alloimmunization, typically on the second or third day of life. In the majority of cases, anemia is not conspicuous, suggesting the underlying mechanism of hyperbilirubinemia is primarily hepatic in origin.[122,123] A hemolytic component may predominate where neonatal exposure to oxidants,[124] e.g. drugs or naphthalene in the form of moth balls, occurs and after maternal consumption of fava beans.[125]

With respect to management, the degree of hyperbilirubinemia which triggers the need for phototherapy or exchange transfusion follows conventional criteria, adjusted for birth weight. A lower threshold may be applied in the face of rapid hemolysis. Prompt correction of hypoxia, acidosis, sepsis and other factors which exacerbate jaundice in the G6PD-deficient neonate is important.

The fact that not all G6PD-deficient neonates develop jaundice has been interpreted as suggesting additional genetic or environmental factors are involved. Recently, evidence has been provided that severe neonatal jaundice in some G6PD-deficient infants is due to synergism between G6PD deficiency and defective bilirubin conjugation linked to polymorphism of a TA repeat in the promoter of the gene for UDP-glucuronosyltransferase 1 associated with Gilbert syndrome.[126]

CHRONIC NON-SPHEROCYTIC HEMOLYTIC ANEMIA

In contrast to the episodic pattern of hemolysis associated with polymorphic G6PD variants, G6PD deficiency much less commonly results in a chronic hemolytic anemia.[24] Such cases are usually sporadic and show no geographic or ethnic predilection. All reported cases have been male. Neonatal jaundice, sometimes severe, is often the first manifestation. A spectrum of clinical expression varying from compensated hemolysis to transfusion dependence is seen. This reflects the heterogeneity of molecular defects among Class I G6PD variants. The spleen, although typically moderately increased in size, may be sufficiently enlarged to cause hypersplenism. In the steady state, hemolysis is primarily extravascular, as evidenced by the absence of hemoglobinuria. Oxidative stress, particularly during intercurrent infection, however exacerbates hemolysis and is occasionally accompanied by frank hemoglobinuria.

LABORATORY DIAGNOSIS

The diagnosis of G6PD deficiency may be readily confirmed by quantitative assay of red cell activity which measures by spectrophotometry the reduction of NADP to NADPH in the presence of G6P. Several simple semi-quantitative tests for G6PD deficiency are also available. These are of particular use in population screening and include dye-decolorization methods, the methemoglobin reduction test and fluorescent spot test.[31,121] A positive screening test should be confirmed by quantitative enzyme assay. Caution must be exercised in interpretation since false negative results may occur in heterozygous females and in the presence of reticulocytosis in males hemizygous for variants, e.g. G6PD A$^-$ in which enzyme activity is relatively well preserved in young red cells. This is most likely to be encountered if a child is investigated during or immediately following an acute hemolytic episode and is less common in class II variants, e.g. G6PD Mediterranean where enzyme activity is reduced in both young and old red cells. In practice, these limitations can usually be circumvented by assaying enzyme activity separately in old and young red cells fractionated by centrifugation, relating G6PD activity to that of another age-dependent enzyme, e.g. hexokinase, or performing a confirmatory test in the steady state. A specific problem arises in the diagnosis of chronic non-spherocytic hemolytic anemia in a G6PD-deficient child who originates from a population in which the prevalence of G6PD deficiency is high. In this situation biochemical characterization of the G6PD variant is necessary. If this proves to be a common variant, an alternative explanation for chronic hemolysis must be sought. Genotypic diagnosis, which is feasible by rapid techniques for several polymorphic G6PD variants, is also useful in this context.

The diagnosis of G6PD deficiency in heterozygous females warrants special mention. Unbalanced mosaicism in favor of cells in which the active chromosome carries the wild-type G6PD allele may render the enzyme activity of a red cell lysate normal. In this situation (and after red cell transfusion), cytochemical staining with tetrazolium which is capable of detecting minor populations of Gd^- red cells may be helpful.[127] Somatic selection in favor of Gd^+ red cells[128] may also mask the heterozygous phenotype, particularly in the case of severely deficient variants.

Increased GSH instability or Heinz body formation after exposure of red cells to acetylphenylhydrazine, although of considerable historic interest, are now seldom employed to diagnose G6PD deficiency.

DISORDERS OF ERYTHROCYTE NUCLEOTIDE METABOLISM

Several disorders of erythrocyte nucleotide metabolism associated with hemolytic anemia have been described. By comparison with disorders of glycolysis, the mechanism by which they mediate premature red cell destruction is poorly understood.

PYRIMIDINE 5′-NUCLEOTIDASE DEFICIENCY

P5′N exists as 2 isoenzymes, P5′N or uridine monophosphate hydrolase (UMPH) 1 and 2,[129] which have different substrate specificities and are encoded by separate structural loci. Hemolytic anemia is the result of deficiency in P5′N-1 (UMPH-1). Deficiency of P5′N is associated with hemolytic anemia of mild-to-moderate severity which may worsen during infection or pregnancy.[19] Over 40 cases have been reported.[18,130,131] As a consequence of failure to dephosphorylate pyrimidine products of RNA degradation during reticulocyte maturation, there is accumulation in the red cell of pyrimidine phosphates and their derivatives, particularly the phosphodiesters CDP–choline and CDP–ethanolamine. This forms the basis of a screening test to establish the diagnosis.[132] Normally, adenosine phosphates account for at least 97% of cellular nucleotides. In P5′N deficiency the presence in red cell perchloric acid extracts of significant concentrations of pyrimidine compounds shifts the ultraviolet absorption spectrum from the normal peak at 257 nm to 265–270 nm. The diagnosis may be confirmed by specific enzyme assay. A conspicuous feature of P5′N deficiency is basophilic stippling (ribonucleoprotein aggregates) due to impaired degradation of RNA and this may be visible in up to 5% of red cells. Blood collected in EDTA must be examined fresh since after 3 hours stippling is no longer discernible. Alternatively, a stained blood film may be prepared from heparinized blood.[133] The activity of P5′N is increased in young red cells.[134] When corrected for reticulocytosis, the enzyme activity in homozygous P5′N deficiency is generally about 5% of that in normal red cells. Typically, heterozygotes exhibit 50% P5′N activity, although overlap of values with those of normal subjects renders carier detection difficult in some cases.[135] P5′N is also expressed in brain, kidney and spleen tissue.[136] In this respect it is of interest to note that mental retardation has been described in some deficient individuals.[137]

How intracellular accumulation of pyrimidines causes hemolysis is not known. Selective accumulation of CDP–choline due to a putative defect in CDP–choline phosphotransferase has been reported in rare patients with a disorder that resembles P5′N deficiency characterized by hemolytic anemia and basophilic stippling.[21,138] This supports a direct role for pyrimidine nucleotides in erythrocyte destruction. Inhibition of glycolysis or adenine nucleotide salvage through competition of UTP and CTP with ATP has been postulated,[2] but the exact mechanism remains elusive.

Acquired P5′N deficiency is seen in lead poisoning[139] and underlies the mechanism of lead-induced hemolytic anemia.[140] P5′N is sensitive to inactivation by low concentrations of lead and exposed individuals show a dose-dependent depression of nucleotidase activity. Patients with severe acute lead toxicity have enzyme levels comparable to those found in homozygous deficiency states.

Recently, interaction of P5′N deficiency and hemoglobin E (HbE) has been shown to contribute to a marked increase in instability of HbE in a family in which the 2 defects cosegregated.[141] Although the underlying mechanism is unknown, this suggests the milieu of P5′N-deficient red cells may accentuate oxidative damage, a finding of potential importance to understanding the pathophysiology of HbE β-thalassemia.

OVERPRODUCTION OF ADENOSINE DEAMINASE

Three unrelated kindreds have been described in which hemolytic anemia is associated with an increase in red cell ADA activity[13,142,143] and depletion of ATP due to preferential deamination of adenosine to inosine at the expense of phosphorylation by adenylate kinase (AK). Clinically, overproduction of ADA is characterized by a well compensated hemolytic anemia showing dominant inheritance. Red cell ADA levels are increased up to 100-fold, reflecting upregulation of transcription of the ADA gene. This phenomenon appears specific to red cells, since ADA levels in other cells are normal. Linkage studies indicate the genetic defect responsible lies in *cis* rather than *trans* to the ADA gene[144] but its identity remains obscure.

ADENYLATE KINASE DEFICIENCY

AK plays an important role in regulation of adenosine phosphate equilibrium in the red cell through phosphorylation of AMP to ADP and interconversion of ADP and ATP. Three isoenzymes have been identified of which AK1 is found in red cells, muscle and brain. Only 6 families with AK deficiency and congenital hemolytic anemia have been reported.[20,145] Variable clinical expression among members of the same kindred with comparably reduced red cell AK activity has made it difficult to prove a clear relationship between AK deficiency and hemolysis.[146] Elevation of red cell ATP concentration has been observed in the majority of cases. Studies have failed to pinpoint any defect in red cells of energy generation or reducing potential and the mechanism of hemolysis remains obscure. In one family there was associated mental retardation.[147] It has been suggested that AK deficiency may be a marker for a hitherto unknown genetic defect responsible for hemolytic anemia.[148]

DISORDERS OF GLUTATHIONE METABOLISM

Glutathione, a tripeptide composed of glutamic acid, cysteine and glycine, is synthesized through sequential reactions catalyzed by γ-glutamylcysteine synthetase (GCS) and glutathione synthetase (GSHS). Glutathione is present in the red cell at millimolar concentrations and in its reduced form (GSH) provides the main defence against oxidative damage. The conversion of harmful peroxides to water is catalyzed by glutathione peroxidase (GSHPX). Intracellular levels of GSH are maintained by both regeneration from oxidized glutathione (GSSG), catalyzed by glutathione reductase (GSSGR) and de novo synthesis.

Three defects of glutathione metabolism associated with decreased red cell GSH have been implicated in hemolytic anemia; glutathione reductase, GCS and GSHS deficiencies. The first 2 of these are exceedingly rare. Many early cases of glutathione reductase deficiency were subsequently shown to be due to inadequate synthesis of its cofactor flavin-adenine dinucleotide secondary to nutritional riboflavin deficiency.[149] A single well documented case of glutathione reductase deficiency associated with favism and cataract showing apparent autosomal recessive inheritance has been described.[150] Reduced glutathione stability was demonstrated after incubation with acetylephenylhydrazine. Hemolytic anemia due to GCS deficiency has been reported in 4 families, in one of which the affected members developed progressive spinocerebellar ataxia.[36] In contrast, 3 other cases diagnosed during childhood or early adult life exhibited isolated hemolytic anemia.[151,152] This disparity might reflect the different ages of the probands as the onset of neurologic disease was delayed until the third decade of life.

GCS deficiency[35] is the commonest metabolic defect to cause GSH deficiency and over 20 families with the condition have been reported.[152] Two phenotypes are recognized: in the red cell type of GCS deficiency there is mild hemolytic anemia which may be exacerbated by oxidant stress; it may also result in a multisystem disorder characterized by hemolysis, metabolic acidosis, neurologic abnormalities, neutropenia and susceptibility to bacterial infection. Urinary excretion of 5-oxoproline is markedly elevated. Vitamin E has been used with clinical benefit in patients with recurrent infection.[153]

MANAGEMENT OF HEREDITARY HEMOLYTIC ANEMIAS

The management of children with hereditary hemolytic anemias may be conveniently viewed in terms of specific treatment aimed at avoidance or correction of anemia and supportive measures to prevent or treat secondary complications. Families should also receive appropriate genetic counselling. In common with other disorders associated with shortened red cell survival, parvovirus B19 infection may be associated with aplastic crises in patients with erythroenzymopathies.[154,155] The availability of an effective vaccine against parvovirus B19 should in future prevent this complication. Formation of pigment gallstones may lead to biliary colic, cholecystitis or pancreatitis requiring cholecystectomy. Cholelithiasis may be evident in early childhood in PK[95] and HK[156] deficiency.

Attempts to overcome the metabolic block by stimulation of alternative pathways have generally met with little success. A variety of pharmacologic approaches to treatment of hemolysis in G6PD deficiency, none of whose efficacy is indisputed, have been proposed. These include the use of deferoxamine (desferrioxamine), xylitol and the antioxidants vitamin E and selenium. The latter have been reported to be of benefit in some cases of chronic nonspherocytic hemolytic anemia due to G6PD deficiency.[24]

Prevention

Prevention plays an important role in reducing the risk of drug-induced hemolysis and favism in G6PD deficiency. In Sardinia prospective neonatal screening combined with health education has resulted in a decline in the incidence of favism among children with G6PD deficiency.[157] Once the diagnosis of G6PD deficiency has been made, parents should be advised regarding avoidance of oxidants and the risk of hemolysis during intercurrent infection, a list of culpable drugs provided and screening of siblings and other family members undertaken. If it is necessary, because no effective alternative exists, to consider administering a drug incriminated as a cause of hemolysis, e.g. primaquine for the treatment of P. vivax or P. malariae infection, to a child known to have G6PD deficiency, dosage reduction may reduce hemolysis to a tolerable level. Avoidance of oxidants is recommended in defects of glutathione synthesis. With few exceptions drug ingestion has not been implicated in hemolytic crises in other enzymopathies. Salicylates have been shown to pose a theoretic risk in PK deficiency[158] due to inhibition of mitochondrial oxidative phosphorylation which further depletes ATP, and are probably best avoided. Drug-induced hemolysis has been reported occasionally in GPI deficiency.[62]

Megaloblastic change due to folic acid deficiency is relatively uncommon in hemolytic anemia due to enzyme deficiency but should be suspected if the reticulocyte count is inappropriately low in relation to the degree of anemia, particularly if nutritional status is poor. Supplemental folic acid is warranted if there is severe chronic hemolysis and may be given following acute hemolytic episodes when the demand to meet the needs of regenerative erythropoiesis is greatest.

Transfusion

The role of blood transfusion has already been referred to in the context of G6PD deficiency. In this and other erythroenzymopathies, severe hemolytic disease of the newborn or neonatal jaundice necessitate exchange transfusion, as may subsequent hemolytic or aplastic crises. A minority of children remain transfusion dependent.

The threshold at which transfusion is indicated differs among enzyme disorders. As mentioned above, in PK deficiency a shift in the oxygen dissociation curve increases the efficiency of oxygen delivery to the tissues and consequently anemia is well tolerated. Conversely, poor effort tolerance is characteristic in HK deficiency due to the low erythrocyte 2,3-DPG concentration. Thus, the growth, developmental progress and well-being of a child rather than the hemoglobin level alone should guide the decision to transfuse.

The hemoglobin level can usually be maintained above 7–8 g/dl by a 6–8 weekly transfusion regimen. Maintenance of a higher hemoglobin level by hypertransfusion is unnecessary since there is no ineffective erythropoiesis. In children of non-northern European origin, it may be preferable to use phenotype-matched red cells to avoid alloimmunization.

Hepatitis A and B immunization is advised. Chelation therapy with deferoxamine may be needed to prevent transfusional siderosis in children who have received multiple transfusions. Iron overload may also develop in the absence of extensive transfusion due to enhanced absorption of dietary iron or inappropriate administration of medicinal iron.[159,160] It is possible that in some cases this reflects co-inheritance of the genetic defect for hereditary hemochromatosis.[161] Screening for the common C282Y mutant allele of the *HFE* gene is prudent in children with hemolytic anemia, particularly those of northern European descent, to detect predisposition to iron loading. As the pattern of iron loading is predominantly parenchymal, organ damage may develop relatively quickly. Plasma transferrin saturation and ferritin should be monitored and where indicated the presence and extent of organ damage assessed (see Chapter 5).

Splenectomy

Splenectomy results in substantial benefit in several erythro-enzyme disorders, most notably PK deficiency but also deficiencies of HK, GPI, PGK, AK, GSHS and some class I G6PD variants. It has not proved of value in PFK, TPI or P5′N deficiency.

Transfusion dependence is one of the few clearcut indications but unless a precedent exists on which to judge future clinical severity in the form of a previously affected family member or circumscribed phenotype, e.g. the Amish PK variant, splenectomy is best deferred until the child is at least 3 years of age. This minimizes the risk of post-splenectomy sepsis and allows time for spontaneous improvement that might obviate the need for splenectomy. ^{51}Cr-labeled red cell studies are not generally helpful in predicting the response to splenectomy.[162]

Splenectomy may also be considered if the spleen is sufficiently enlarged to cause mechanical discomfort or hypersplenism. Polyvalent pneumococcal, meningococcal and haemophilus vaccines should be given before splenectomy and penicillin prophylaxis thereafter. Persistent post-splenectomy thrombocytosis complicated by thromboembolism has been reported. The increased risk of malaria and certain other protozoal infections e.g. babesiosis, should be borne in mind when considering of splenectomy in a child returning to an area where these infections are endemic.

MOLECULAR BASIS OF ERYTHROENZYMOPATHIES ASSOCIATED WITH HEREDITARY HEMOLYTIC ANEMIA

During the past decade, the molecular alternations that underlie many of the hematologically important erythroenzyme disorders have been extensively studied.[163,164] The human genes encoding all known enzymes, other than P5′N, central to red cell metabolism have been cloned. Apart from a few examples due to mutations that result in premature termination of translation or aberrant mRNA splicing and ADA overproduction, in which the basic defect that upregulates transcription appears to lie outside the structural gene, the majority of erythroenzymopathies are caused by missense mutations (Table 14.8).[165–167] Most

Table 14.8 Mutations in enzymopathies associated with hereditary hemolytic anemia.

Enzyme	Acronym	Chromosomal locus	Missense	Nonsense	Deletion	Insertion	Splicing	Total
Hexokinase	HK1	10q 22	1	0	1	0	0	2
Glucosephosphate isomerase	GPI	19q13.1	16	1	0	0	0	17
Phosphofructokinase	PFK-M	1cen–q32	9	1	1	0	7	18
Aldolase	ALD-A	16q22–q24	2	0	0	0	0	2
Triosephosphate isomerase	TPI	12p13	6	2	1	0	0	9
Phosphoglycerate kinase	PGK1	Xq13	5	0	0	0	1	6
Pyruvate kinase	PK-L/R	1q21	57	3	7	2	6	75
Glucose-6-phosphate dehydrogenase	G6PD	Xq28	114	1	6	0	1	122
Adenylate kinase	AK1	9q34.1	2	0	0	0	0	2
Glutathione synthetase	GSHS	20q11.2	16	0	2	0	0	18
Total (%)			228 (84.1)	8 (2.9)	18 (6.6)	2 (0.7)	15 (5.5)	271

cases characterized have, in the absence of consanguinity, proved to be compound heterozygous for different mutations. Exceptions in this respect are PK[169] and TPI[78,81] deficiency, in which a single mutation predominates in certain populations due to a founder effect. The resulting change(s) in primary protein structure (amino acid sequence) may affect enzyme function quantitatively or qualitatively and not infrequently both effects are observed. Missense mutations that destabilize inter-subunit contact or alter the conformation of the active site are generally associated with markedly diminished enzyme activity and correspondingly more severe clinical expression.

Teleologically, the restricted pattern of mutation associated with erythroenzymopathies is not surprising since, in the case of a housekeeping gene, more deleterious alterations would be non-viable in the homozygous (and in X-linked disorders, hemizygous) state. This is supported by evidence from murine models that homozygosity for null alleles at GPI or TPI loci is lethal in early embryonic development.[169,170] Among human erythroenzymopathies, null mutations have been found only in the compound heterozygous state with a less severe mutation.

OTHER HEMATOLOGIC SYNDROMES ASSOCIATED WITH ERYTHROENZYMOPATHIES

CONGENITAL METHEMOGLOBINEMIA DUE TO DEFICIENCY OF CYTOCHROME b_5 REDUCTASE

The biologic role of hemoglobin in oxygen transport depends on maintenance of heme iron in the ferrous (Fe^{2+}) state. The formation of methemoglobin by oxidation of heme iron to the ferric (Fe^{3+}) state must therefore be counterbalanced by its reduction. This is reflected in the steady-state level of methemoglobin which normally comprises <1% of total hemoglobin. The principal pathway by which functional hemoglobin is restored involves the transfer of electrons from NADH to methemoglobin mediated by cytochrome b_5 reductase and cytochrome b_5.[29] As deduced with remarkable prescience by Gibson in 1948,[171] a defect in this pathway underlies hereditary methemoglobinemia. Homozygous deficiency of cytochrome b_5 reductase classically results in a benign clinical disorder characterized by congenital cyanosis. Most affected children are otherwise asymptomatic, even in the face of methemoglobin levels of up to 50%. Transient cyanosis may occur spontaneously in heterozygotes for cytochrome b_5 reductase deficiency in the neonatal period and after exposure to oxidizing compounds in later childhood. Cytochrome b_5 reductase deficiency must be distinguished from other causes of cyanosis at birth, including M hemoglobins due to α or rarely γ chain variants (see Chapter 12), cardiac or pulmonary disease and toxic methemoglobinemia, to which newborns and infants whose physiologic red cell cytochrome b_5 reductase activity is about 50% that of adult levels are particularly susceptible. Conjunctival cyanosis, a cardinal sign of hereditary methemoglobinemia, is usually absent in hypoxemia due to cyanotic cardiac or respiratory disease. The list of drugs and toxins that can induce methemoglobin formation includes nitrites, sulfonamides, dapsone, metoclopromide, doxorubicin, vitamin K analogs, antimalarials, benzocaine and aniline dyes. During attacks of gastroenteritis, endogenous nitrite production maybe enhanced sufficiently to cause toxic methemoglobinemia in infants. Congenital methemoglobinemia has been reported in a family with erythrocyte cytochrome b_5 deficiency.[172]

Deficiency of cytochrome b_5 reductase is limited to the red cells (type I) in the majority of cases. In contrast to this form in which affected individuals are 'more blue than sick', a severe lethal disorder (type II) results from deficiency of cytochrome b_5 reductase in all somatic cells. Generalized cytochrome b_5 reductase deficiency is characterized by failure to thrive, mental retardation and neurologic abnormalities, including microcephaly, opisthotonos, athetoid movements and hypertonia leading to early death. A third form of cytochrome b_5 reductase deficiency (type III) without neurologic involvement has been described in which there is enzyme deficiency in red cells, platelets and leukocytes but not other cells.[173]

The diagnosis of cytochrome b_5 reductase deficiency is based on the demonstration of methemoglobin in the absorption spectrum of hemolysate. This disappears upon the addition of cyanide, thus distinguishing enzymopathic methemoglobinemia from cases due to an M hemoglobin. The diagnosis is confirmed by evidence of reduced enzyme activity in red cells alone (type I) or in addition to leukocytes and platelets (types II or III). Reduction in the level of methemoglobin, although seldom indicated clinically, may if desired on cosmetic grounds be achieved by oral administration of methylene blue, ascorbic acid (vitamin C) or riboflavin (vitamin B_2). These measures reduce methemoglobin levels to around 5–10% but have no impact on the neurologic manifestations in generalized cytochrome b_5 reductase deficiency. Methylene blue should be avoided in children with G6PD deficiency since it is ineffective and may cause hemolysis. Renal stone formation may follow prolonged administration of ascorbic acid.

DIPHOSPHOGLYCERATE MUTASE DEFICIENCY

Diphosphoglycerate mutase (DPGM) acts in the Rapoport–Luebering shunt to regulate the metabolism of 2,3-DPG. Its main catalytic function is the conversion of 1,3-DPG to 2,3-DPG. In addition, DPGM possesses phosphatase activity that is responsible for the conversion of 2,3-DPG to 3-PG and functions, albeit at low efficiency, as a monophosphoglycerate mutase. Human DPGM activity is confined to red cells. 2,3-DPG is the most abundant glycolyic intermediate and serves to lower the affinity of hemoglobin for oxygen, thereby shifting the oxygen dissociation curve to the right. The phenotype of DPGM deficiency has been documented in most detail in a single kindred in which both homozygotes and heterozygotes exhibited erythrocytosis but no signs of hemolysis.[34,174]

HEREDITARY OROTIC ACIDURIA

Hereditary orotic aciduria is a rare inborn error of *de novo* pyrimidine synthesis characterized by megaloblastic anemia unresponsive to treatment with vitamin B_{12} or folic acid and increased urinary excretion of orotic acid accompanied by macroscopic crystalluria which may result in obstructive nephropathy.[19] Inheritance is autosomal recessive. Delayed development of motor and cognitive skills is apparent in the majority of cases. Other clinical features include sparse hair, poor nail growth, immune dysfunction, cardiac malformations, strabismus and malabsorption. Red cell hypochromia despite replete iron stores has been remarked upon in some cases. The underlying defect is a deficiency of uridine 5'-monophosphate synthetase, a bifunctional enzyme with orotatate phosphoribosyltransferase (OPRT) and orotodine 5'-monophosphate decarboxylate (ODC) activities which reside in separate functional domains of the protein. Hereditary orotic aciduria may be distinguished from other causes of megaloblastic anemia in infancy and childhood (see Chapter 8) by the presence of orotic aciduria and a specific enzyme assay. Long-term pyrimidine replacement therapy in the form of uridine given orally has led to clinical improvement in a significant proportion of cases with reversal of megaloblastosis and reduction in urinary orotic acid excretion.

ACQUIRED ERYTHROENZYME DISORDERS

Acquired alterations in erythroenzyme activity have been observed in a wide variety of hematologic and other disorders.[175] These may involve an increase or decrease in enzyme activity and affect one or several enzymes. In leukemia, myeloproliferative disorders, myelodysplastic syndrome and congenital dyserythropoietic anemia, reduced PK, PFK and P5'N activities are the most frequently observed abnormalities. Acquired deficiency of P5'N has also been described in thalassemia and transient erythroblastopenia of childhood. In some instances these epiphenomena may assist diagnosis. For example, the characteristic elevation in red cell ADA activity distinguishes Diamond–Blackfan anemia from other causes of pure red cell aplasia. Despite the presence in some cases of metabolic block as evidenced by intermediate studies, acquired erythroenzyme disorders are not generally associated with shortened red cell survival. In cases where doubt exists as to whether an erythroenzyme defect is primary or secondary in nature,

family studies are helpful. The mechanisms which underlie acquired alterations in erythroenzyme activity are heterogenous and ill defined. They may include reversion to a fetal pattern of erythropoiesis, modulation of gene expression, gene dosage effects—an example of which is seen in the increase in red cell PFK activity in trisomy 21, post-translational modification and somatic mutation.

REFERENCES

1. Beutler E. The red cell. In: *Hemolytic Anemia in Disorders of Red Cell Metabolism.* New York: Plenum, 1978, pp 1–21
2. Paglia DE, Valentine WN. Hemolytic anemia associated with disorders of the purine and pyrimidine salvage pathways. In: Mentzer WC (ed) Enzymopathies. *Clin Hematology* 1981; **10**: 81–98
3. Dern RJ, Weinstein IM, LeRoy GV *et al.* The hemolytic effect of primaquine. I. The localization of the drug-induced hemolytic defect in primaquine-sensitive individuals. *J Lab Clin Med* 1954; **43**: 303–309
4. Carson PE, Flanagan CL, Ickes CE, Alving AS. Enzymatic deficiency in primaquine-sensitive erythrocytes. *Science* 1956; **124**: 484–485
5. Dacie J, Mollison PL, Richardson N *et al.* Atypical congenital hemolytic anemia. *Q J Med* 1953; **22**: 79–98
6. Valentine WN, Tanaka KR, Miwa S *et al.* A specific erythrocyte glycolytic enzyme defect (pyruvate kinase) in three subjects with congenital non-spherocytic hemolytic anemia. *Trans Assoc Am Physicians* 1961; **74**: 100–110
7. Schneider AS, Valentine WN, Hattori M, Heins HL. Hereditary hemolytic anemia with triosephosphate isomerase deficiency. *N Engl J Med* 1965; **272**: 229–235
8. Tarui S, Okuno G, Ikura Y *et al.* Phosphofructokinase deficiency in skeletal muscle: a new type of glycogenosis. *Biochem Biophys Res Commun* 1965; **19**: 517–523
9. Valentine WN, Oski FA, Paglia DE *et al.* Hereditary hemolytic anemia with hexokinase deficiency. *N Engl J Med* 1967; **276**: 1–11
10. Baughan M, Valentine WN, Paglia DE *et al.* Hereditary hemolytic anemia associated with glucosephosphate isomerase (GPI) deficiency – a new enzyme defect of human erythrocytes. *Blood* 1968; **32**: 236–249
11. Kraus AP, Langston MF Jr, Lynch BL. Red cell phosphoglycerate kinase deficiency: a new cause of non-spherocytic hemolytic anemia. *Biochem Biophys Res Commun* 1968; **30**: 173–177
12. Beutler E, Scott S, Bishop A *et al.* Red cell aldolase deficiency and hemolytic anemia: A new syndrome. *Trans Assoc Am Physicians* 1973; **86**: 154–166
13. Valentine WN, Paglia DE, Tartaglia AP, Gilsanz F. Hereditary hemolytic anemia with incresed red cell adenosine deaminase (45 to 70 fold) and decreased adenosine triphosphate. *Science* 1977; **195**: 783–785
14. Etiemble J, Picat C, Dhermy D, Buc HA, Morin M, Boivin P. Erythrocytic pyruvate kinase deficiency and hemolytic anemia inherited as a dominant trait. *Am J Hematol* 1984; **17**: 251–260
15. Necheles TF, Rai US, Cameron D. Congenital non spherocytic hemolytic anemia sssociated with an unusual erythrocyte hexokinase abnormality. *J Lab Clin Med* 1970; **76**: 593–602
16. Mohrenweiser HW. Frequency of enzyme deficiency variants in erythrocytes of newborn infants. *Proc Natl Acad Sci USA* 1981; **78**: 5046–5050
17. El-Hazmi MAF, Al-Swailem AR, Al-Faleh FZ, Warsy AS. Frequency of glucose-6-phosphate dehydrogenase, pyruvate kinase and hexokinase deficiency in the Saudi population. *Hum Hered* 1986; **36**: 45–49
18. Valentine WN, Fink K, Paglia DE *et al.* Hereditary hemolytic anemia with human erythrocyte pyrimidine 5'-nucleotidase deficiency. *J Clin Invest* 1974; **54**: 866–879
19. Webster DR, Becroft DMO, Parker Suttle D. Hereditary orotic aciduria and other disorders of pyrimidine metabolism. In: Scriver

CH, Beaudet AL, Sly WS, Valle D (eds) *The Metabolic and Molecular Bases of Inherited Disease, Vol 2.* New York: McGraw Hill, 1995, pp 1799–1837

20. Boivin P, Galand C, Hakim J *et al.* Une nouvelle érythroenzymopathie. Anémie hémolytique congenitale non sphérocytaire et déficit héréditaire en adénylate-kinase érythrocytaire. *Presse Medicale* 1971; **79**: 215–218

21. Paglia DE, Valentine WN, Nakatani M *et al.* Selective accumulation of cytosol CDP-choline as an isolated erythrocyte defect in chronic hemolysis. *Proc Natl Acad Sci USA* 1983; **80**: 3081–3085

22. Mohrenweiser HW, Fielek S. Elevated frequency of carriers for triosephosphate isomerase deficiency in newborn infants. *Pediatr Res* 1982; **16**: 960–963

23. Mohrenweiser HW. Functional hemizygosity in the human genome: direct estimate from twelve erythrocyte enzyme loci. *Hum Genet* 1987; **77**: 241–245

24. Luzzatto L, Mehta A. Glucose 6-phosphate dehydrogenase deficiency. In: Scriver CH, Beaudet AL, Sly WS, Valle D (eds) *The Metabolic and Molecular Bases of Inherited Disease, Vol 3.* New York: McGraw Hill, 1995, pp 3367–3398

25. WHO Working Group. Glucose 6-phosphate dehydrogenase deficiency. *Bull WHO* 1989; **67**: 601

26. Bienzle U, Ayeni O, Lucas AO, Luzzatto L. Glucose-6-phosphate dehydrogenase deficiency and malaria. Greater resistance of females heterozygous for enzyme deficiency and of males with non-deficient variant. *Lancet* 1972; **1**: 107–110

27. Ruwende C, Khoo SC, Snow AW *et al.* Natural selection of hemi and heterozygotes for G6PD deficiency in Africa by resistance to severe malaria. *Nature* 1995; **376**: 246–249

28. Roth EF Jr, Raventos-Suarez C, Rinaldi A, Nagel RL. Glucose 6-phosphate dehydrogenase deficiency inhibits *in vitro* growth of *Plasmodium falciparum. Proc Natl Acad Sci USA* 1983; **80**: 298–299

29. Jaffé ER, Hultquist DE. Cytochrome b_5 reductase deficiency and enzymopenic hereditary methemoglobinemia. In: Scriver CH, Beaudet AL, Sly WS, Valle D (eds) *The Metabolic and Molecular Bases of Inherited Disease, Vol 3.* New York: McGraw Hill, 1995, pp 3399–3415

30. Dacie J. *The Haemolytic Anaemias, Vol 1. The Hereditary Haemolytic Anaemias Part I,* 3rd edn. Edinburgh: Churchill Livingstone, 1985

31. Beutler E, Blume KG, Kaplan JC *et al.* International Committee for Standardization in Haematology: Recommended screening test for glucose-6-phosphate dehydrogenase (G-6-PD) deficiency. *Br J Haematol* 1979; **43**: 469–477

32. Torrance J, Jacobs P. Restrepo A *et al.* Intraerythrocytic adaptation to anemia. *N Engl J Med* 1970; **283**: 165–169

33. Thomas HM III, Lefrak SS, Irwin RS *et al.* The oxyhemoglobin dissociation curve in health and disease. Role of 2,3-diphosphoglycerate. *Am J Med* 1974; **57**: 331–348

34. Rosa R, Prehu M-O, Beuzard Y, Rosa J. The first case of a complete deficiency of diphosphoglycerate mutase in human erythrocytes. *J Clin Invest* 1978; **62**: 907–915

35. Boivin P, Galand C, Andre R, Debray J. Anémies hémolytiques congenitales avec déficit isole en gluthathion reduit par déficit en glutathion synthetase. *Nouv Rev Fr Hématol* 1966; **6**: 859–866

36. Konrad PN, Richards II F, Valentine WN, Paglia DE. Gamma-glutamyl-cysteine synthetase deficiency. *N Engl J Med* 1972; **286**: 557–561

37. Valentine WN, Paglia DE. Nonrecessively transmitted nonspherocytic hereditary haemolytic anaemia associated with increased red cell gluthathion. *Br J Haematol* 1979; **42**: 231–237

38. Beutler E, Blume KG, Kaplan JC *et al.* International Committee for Standardisation in Hematology: Recommended methods for red cell enzyme analysis. *Br J Haematol* 1977; **35**: 331–340

39. Konrad PN, Valentine WN, Paglia DE. Enzymatic activities and glutathione content of erythrocytes in the newborn: comparison with red cells of older normal subjects and those with comparable reticulocytosis. *Acta Haematol* 1972; **48**: 193–201

40. Travis SF, Kumar SP, Delivoria-Papadopoulos M. Red cell metabolic alterations in postnatal life in term infants: glycolytic enzymes and glucose-6-phosphate dehydrogenase. *Pediatr Res* 1980; **14**: 1349–1352

41. Travis SF, Kumar SP, Delivoria-Papadopoulos M. Red cell metabolic alterations in postnatal life in term infants: glycolytic intermediates and adenosine triphosphate. *Pediatr Res* 1981; **15**: 34–37

42. Bellingham AJ, Lestas AN, Williams LHP, Nicolaides KH. Prenatal diagnosis of red cell enzymopathy: triose phosphate isomerase deficiency. *Lancet* 1989; **ii**: 419–421

43. Whitelaw AGL, Rogers PA, Hopkinson DA *et al.* Congenital haemolytic anaemia resulting from glucose phosphate isomerase deficiency: genetics, clinical picture, and prenatal diagnosis. *J Med Genet* 1979; **16**: 189–196

44. Lestas AN, Bellingham AJ, Nicolaides KH. Prenatal diagnosis of red cell pyruvate kinase deficiency. *Br J Haematol* 1989; **71 (Suppl 1)**: 29

45. Junien C, Leroux A, Lostanlen D *et al.* Prenatal diagnosis of congenital enzymopenic methaemeglobinaemia with mental retardation due to generalized cytochrome b5 reductase deficiency: first report of two cases. *Prenat Diagn* 1981; **1**: 17–24

46. Lestas AN, Rodeck CH, White JM. Normal activities of glycolytic enzymes in the fetal erythrocytes. *Br J Haematol* 1982; **50**: 439–444

47. Lestas AN, Rodeck CH. Normal gluthathione content and some related enzyme activities in the fetal erythrocytes. *Br J Haematol* 1984; **57**: 695–702

48. Lestas AN, Nicolaides KH, Rodeck CH, Bellingham AJ. Normal levels of ATP, total nucleotides and activities of three enzymes related to nucleotide metabolism in fetal erythrocytes. *Br J Haematol* 1986; **63**: 471–476

49. Lestas AN, Bellingham AJ, Nicolaides KH. Red cell glycolytic intermediates in normal, anaemic and transfused human fetuses. *Br J Haematol* 1989; **73**: 387–391

50. Beutler E, Kuhl W, Fox M *et al.* Prenatal diagnosis of glucose 6-phosphate dehydrogenase deficiency. *Acta Haematol* 1992; **87**: 103–104

51. Baronciani L, Beutler E. Prenatal diagnosis of pyruvate kinase deficiency. *Blood* 1994; **84**: 2354–2356

52. Arya R, Lalloz MRA, Nicolaides KH, Bellingham AJ, Layton DM. Prenatal diagnosis of triosephosphate isomerase deficiency. *Blood* 1996; **87**: 4507–4509

53. Delivoria-Papadopoulos M, Oski FA, Gottlieb AJ. Oxygen hemoglobin dissociation curves: effect of inherited enzyme defects of the red cell. *Science* 1969; **165**: 601–602

54. Oski FA, Marshall BE, Cohen PJ *et al.* Exercise with anemia: the role of the left-shifted or right-shifted oxygen hemoglobin equilibrium curve. *Ann Intern Med* 1971; **74**: 44–46

55. Newman P, Muir A, Parker AC. Non-spherocytic haemolytic anaemia in mother and son associated with hexokinase deficiency. *Br J Haematol* 1980; **46**: 537–547

56. Rijksen G, Akkerman JWN, Vandernwallbake AWL, Mofstede DP, Staal GEJ. Generalized hexokinase deficiency in the blood cells of a patient with nonspherocytic hemolytic anemia. *Blood* 1983; **61**: 12–18

57. Ravindranath Y, Paglia DE, Warrier I, Valentine W, Nakatani M, Brockway RA. Glucose phosphate isomerase deficiency as a cause of hydrops fetalis. *New Engl J Med* 1987; **316**: 258–261

58. Paglia DE, Holland P, Baughan MA, Valentine WN. Occurrence of defective hexosephosphate isomerization in human erythrocytes and leukocytes. *N Engl J Med* 1969; **280**: 66–71

59. Schroter W, Eber SW, Bardosi A *et al.* Generalised glucosephosphate isomerase (GPI) deficiency causing hemolytic anemia, neuromuscular symptoms and impairment of granulocytic function: a new syndrome due to a new stable GPI variant and diminished specific activity (GPI Homburg). *Eur J Pediatr* 1985; **144**: 301–305

60. Neubauer BA, Eber SW, Lakomek M, Gahr M, Schroter W. Combination of congenital non-spherocytic haemolytic anaemia and impairment of granulocyte function in severe glucose phosphate isomerase deficiency. *Acta Haematol* 1990; **83**: 206–210

61. Goulding FJ. Priapism caused by glucose phosphate isomerase deficiency. *J Urol* 1976; **116**: 819–820

62. Van Biervliet JPGM. Glucosephosphate isomerase deficiency in a Dutch family. *Acta Paediatr Scand* 1975; **64**: 868–872

63. Zanella A, Izzo C, Rebulla P *et al*. The first stable variant of erythrocyte glucose-phosphate isomerase associated with severe hemolytic anemia. *Am J Hematol* 1980; **9**: 1–11

64. Vora S. Isozymes of phosphofructokinase. In: Ratazzi MC, Scandalios JG, Whitt GS (eds) Isozymes. *Curr Topics Biol Med Res* 1982; **4**: 119

65. Miwa S, Sato T, Murao H *et al*. A new type of phosphofructokinase deficiency: hereditary nonspherocytic hemolytic anemia. *Acta Haematol Jpn* 1972; **35**: 113–118

66. Waterbury L, Frenkel EP. Hereditary nonspherocytic hemolysis with erythrocyte phosphofructokinase deficiency. *Blood* 1972; **39**: 415–425

67. Kahn A, Etiemble J, Merenhoffer MC. Erythrocyte phosphofructokinase deficiency associated with an unstable variant of muscle phosphofructokinase. *Clin Chim Acta* 1975; **61**: 415–419

68. Servidei S, Bonilla E, Diedrich RG *et al*. Fatal infantile form of phosphofructokinase deficiency. *Neurology* 1986; **36**: 1465–1470

69. Haller RG, Lewis SF. Glucose-induced exertional fatigue in muscle phosphofructokinase deficiency. *N Engl J Med* 1991; **324**: 364–369

70. Duboc D, Jehenson P, Dinh ST *et al*. Phosphorus NMR spectroscopy study of muscular enzyme deficiencies involving glycogenolysis and glycolysis. *Neurology* 1987; **37**: 663–671

71. Layzer RB, Rasmussen J. The molecular basis of muscle phosphofructokinase deficiency. *Arch Neurol* 1974; **31**: 411–417

72. Penhoet E, Rajkumar T, Rutter WJ. Multiple forms of fructose diphosphate aldolase in mammalian tissues. *Proc Natl Acad Sci USA* 1996; **56**: 1275–1282

73. Miwa S, Fujii H, Tani K *et al*. Two cases of red cell aldolase deficiency associated with hereditary hemolytic anemia in a Japanese family. *Am J Hematol* 1981; **11**: 425–437

74. Kreuder J, Borkhardt A, Repp R *et al*. Inherited metabolic myopathy and hemolysis due to a mutation in aldolase A. *N Engl J Med* 1996; **334**: 1100–1104

75. Schneider AS, Valentine WN, Baughan MA *et al*. A multisystem inherited enzyme disorder: clinical and genetic aspects. In: Beutler E (ed) *Hereditary Disorders of Erythrocyte Metabolism*. New York: Grune & Stratton, 1968, pp 265–272

76. Valentine WN, Schneider AS, Baughan MA *et al*. Hereditary hemolytic anemia with triosephosphate isomerase deficiency. *Am J Med* 1966; **41**: 27–41

77. Poll-The BW, Aicardi J, Girot R, Rosa R. Neurological findings in triosephosphate isomerase deficiency. *Ann Neurol* 1985; **17**: 439–443

78. Schneider A, Westwood B, Yim C *et al*. Triosephosphate isomerase deficiency: repetitive occurrence of point mutation in amino acid 104 in multiple apparently unrelated families. *Am J Hematol* 1995; **50**: 263–268

79. Harris SR, Paglia DE, Jaffe ER, Valentine WN, Klein RL. Triosephosphate isomerase deficiency in an adult. *Clin Res* 1970; **18**: 529 (abstract)

80. Hollan S, Fujii H, Hirono A *et al*. Hereditary triosephosphate isomerase (TPI) deficiency: two severely affected brothers, one with and one without neurological symptoms. *Hum Genet* 1993; **92**: 486–490

81. Arya R, Lalloz MRA, Bellingham AJ, Layton DM. Evidence for founder effect of the Glu104Asp substitution and identification of new mutations in triosephosphate isomerase deficiency. *Hum Mutat* 1997; **10**: 290–294

82. Lazarow PB, Moser HW. Disorders of peroxisome biogenesis. In: Scriver CH, Beaudet Al, Sly WS, Valle D (eds) *The Metabolic and Molecular Bases of Inherited Disease, Vol 2*. New York: McGraw Hill. 1995, pp 2287–2324

83. Hollan S, Magocsi M, Fodor E *et al*. Search for the pathogenesis of the differing phenotype in two compound heterozygote Hungarian brothers with the same genotype triosephosphate isomerase deficiency. *Proc Natl Acad Sci USA* 1997; **94**: 10362–10366

84. Valentine WN, Hsieh H-S, Paglia DE *et al*. Hereditary hemolytic anemia associated with phosphoglycerate kinase deficiency in erythrocytes and leukocytes: a probable X-chromosome-linked syndrome. *N Engl J Med* 1969; **280**: 528–534

85. Boivin P, Hakim J, Mandereau J *et al*. Erythrocyte and leucocyte 3-phosphoglycerate kinase deficiency. Studies of properties of the enzyme, phagocytic activity of the polymorphonuclear leucocytes and a review of the literature. *Nouv Rev Fr Hematol* 1974; **14**: 496–508

86. Konrad PNJ, McCarthy DJ, Mauer AM *et al*. Erythrocyte and leukocyte phosphoglycerate kinase deficiency with neurologic disease. *J Pediatr* 1973; **82**: 456–460

87. Guis MS, Karadsheh N, Mentzer WC. Phosphoglycerate kinase San Francisco: A new variant associated with hemolytic anemia but not with neuromuscular manifestations. *Am J Hematol* 1987; 25: 175–182

88. Tonin P, Shanske S, Miranda AF *et al* Phosphoglycerate kinase deficiency variant (PGK Alberta). *Neurology* 1993; **43**: 387–391

89. Sugie H, Sugie Y, Nishida M *et al*. Recurrent myoglobinuria in a child with mental retardation: phosphoglycerate kinase deficiency. *J Child Neurol* 1989; **4**: 95–99

90. Cohen-Solal M, Valentin C, Plassa F *et al*. Identification of new mutations in two phosphoglycerate kinase (PGK) variants expressing different clinical syndromes: PGK Creteil and PGK Amiens. *Blood* 1994; **84**: 898–903

91. Beutler E. Electrophoresis of phosphoglycerate kinase. *Biochem Genet* 1969; **3**: 189–195

92. Tanaka KR, Paglia DE. Pyruvate kinase deficiency. *Semin Hematol* 1971; **8**: 367–395

93. Gilsanz F, Vega MA, Gomez-Castillo E *et al*. Fetal anaemia due to pyruvate kinase deficiency. *Arch Dis Child* 1993; **69**: 523–524

94. Hennekam RCM, Beemer FA, Cats BP *et al*. Hydrops fetalis associated with red cell pyruvate kinase deficiency. *Genet Couns* 1990; **1**: 75–77

95. Gordon-Smith EC. Erythrocyte enzyme deficiencies. Pyruvate kinase deficiency. *J Clin Pathol* 1974; **27**: 128–133

96. Bowman HS, McKusick VA, Dronamraju KR. Pyruvate kinase deficient hemolytic anemia in an Amish isolate. *Am J Hum Genet* 1965; **17**: 1–8

97. Delivoria-Papadopoulos M, Oski FA, Gottlieb AJ. Oxygen-hemoglobin dissociation curves: Effect of inherited enzyme defects of the red cell. *Science* 1969; **165**: 601–602

98. Fanning J, Hinkle RS. Pyruvate kinase deficiency hemolytic anemia: Two successful pregnancy outcomes. *Am J Obstet Gynecol* 1985; **153**: 313–314.

99. Kendall AG, Charlow GF. Red cell pyruvate kinase deficiency: Adverse effect of oral contraceptives. *Acta Haematol* 1977; **57**: 116–120

100. Rutgers MJ, van der Lugt PJ, van Turnhout JM. Spinal cord compression by extramedullary hemopoietic tissue in pyruvate-kinase-deficiency-caused hemolytic anemia. *Neurology* 1979; **29**: 510–513

101. Tani K, Fujii H, Nagata S, Miwa S. Human liver type pyruvate kinase complete amino acid sequence and the expression in mammalian cells. *Proc Natl Acad Sci USA* 1988; **85**: 1792–1795

102. Takegawa S, Fujii H, Miwa S. Change of pyruvate kinase isozymes from M$_2$- to L-type during development of the red cell. *Br J Haematol* 1983; **54**: 467–474

103. Tani K, Yoshida MC, Satoh H *et al*. Human M$_2$-type pyruvate kinase: cDNA cloning, chromosomal assignment and expression in hepatoma. *Gene* 1988; **73**: 509–516

104. Marie J, Simon M-P, Dreyfus J-C, Kahn A. One gene, but two messenger RNAs encode liver L and red cell L' pyruvate kinase subunits. *Nature* 1981; **292**: 70–72.

105. Takegawa S, Miwa S. Change of pyruvate kinase (PK) isozymes in classical type PK deficiency and other PK deficiency cases during red cell maturation. *Am J Hematol* 1984; **16**: 53–58

106. Max-Audit I, Rosa R, Marie J. Pyruvate kinase hyperactivity genetically determined: Metabolic consequenes and molecular characterization. *Blood* 1980; **56**: 902–909

107. Staal GEJ, Vansen G, Roos D. Pyruvate kinase and the 'high ATP syndrome'. *J Clin Invest* 1984; **74**: 231–235

108. Bowman HS, Oski FA. Splenic macrophage interaction with red cells

in pyruvate kinase deficiency and hereditary spherocytosis. *Vox Sang* 1970; **19**: 168–175

109. Lestas AN, Kay LA, Bellingham AJ. Red cell 3-phosphoglycerate level as a diagnosic aid in pyruvate kinase deficiency. *Br J Haematol* 1987; **67**: 485–488

110. Buc HA, Leroux JP, Garreau H *et al.* Metabolic regulation in enzyme deficient red cells. *Enzyme* 1974; **18**: 19–36

111. Sachs JR, Wicker DJ, Gilcher RO *et al.* Familial hemolytic anemia resulting from an abnormal red blood cell pyruvate kinase. *J Lab Clin Med* 1968; **72**: 359–362

112. Paglia DE, Valentine WN, Williams KO, Konrad PN. An isozyme of erythrocyte pyruvate kinase (PK-Los Angeles) with impaired kinetics corrected by fructose 1,6-diphosphate. *Am J Clin Pathol* 1977; **68**: 229–234

113. Vives-Corrons JL, Feliu E, Pujades MA *et al.* Severe glucose-6-phosphate dehydrogenase (G6PD) deficiency associated with chronic hemolytic anemia, granulocyte dysfunction and increased susceptibility to infections. Description of a new molecular variant (G6PD_BARCELONA). *Blood* 1982; **59**: 428–434

114. Choremis C, Kattamis CA, Kyriazakou M, Gavrillidou E. Viral hepatitis in G6PD deficiency. *Lancet* 1966; **i**: 269–270

115. Moro F, Gorgone G, Li-Volti S *et al.* Glucose-6-phosphate dehydrogenase deficiency and incidence of cataract in Sicily. *Ophthal Paediatr Genet* 1985; **5**: 197–200

116. Gellady A, Greenwood RD. G-6-PD hemolytic anemia complicating diabetic ketoacidosis. *J Pediatr* 1972; **80**: 1037–1038

117. Glucose-6-phosphate dehydrogenase deficiency. In: Beutler E (ed) *Hemolytic Anemia in Disorders of Red Cell Metabolism*. New York: Plenum, 1978, pp 23–167

118. Luzzatto L. Glucose-6-phosphate dehydrogenase deficiency and hemolytic anemia. In: Nathan DG, Orkin SH (eds) *Nathan and Oski's Hematology of Infancy and Childhood*. Philadelphia: WB Saunders, 1998, pp 704–726

119. Kattamis CA, Kyriazakou M, Chaidas S. Favism. Clinical and biochemical data. *J Med Genet* 1969; **6**: 34–41

120. Mentzer WC Jr, Collier E. Hydrops fetalis associated with erythrocyte G-6-PD deficiency and maternal ingestion of fava beans and ascorbic acid. *J Pediatr* 1975; **86**: 565–567

121. Dacie J. Hereditary enzyme-deficiency haemolytic anaemias III: deficiency of glucose-6-phosphate dehydrogenase. In: *The Haemolytic Anaemias, vol 1. The Hereditary Haemolytic Anaemias*, 3rd edn. Edinburgh: Churchill Livingstone, 1985, pp 364–418

122. Meloni T, Costa S, Cutillo S. Haptoglobin, hemopexin, hemoglobin and hematocrit in newborns with erythrocyte glucose-6-phosphate dehydrogenase deficiency. *Acta Haematol* 1975; **54**: 284–288

123. Kaplan M, Vreman HJ, Hammerman C *et al.* Contribution of haemolysis to jaundice in Sephardic Jewish glucose-6-phosphate dehydrogenase deficient neonates. *Br J Haematol* 1996; **93**: 822–827

124. Owa JA. Relationship between exposure to icterogenic agents, glucose-6-phosphate dehydrogenase deficiency and neonatal jaundice in Nigeria. *Acta Paediatr Scand* 1989; **78**: 848–852

125. Corchia C, Balata A, Meloni GF *et al.* Favism in a female newborn infant whose mother ingested fava beans before delivery. *J Pediatr* 1995; **127**: 807–808

126. Kaplan M, Renbaum P, Levy Lahad E *et al.* Gilbert syndrome and glucose-6-phosphate dehydrogenase deficiency. A dose-dependent genetic interaction crucial to neonatal hyperbilirubinemia. *Proc Natl Acad Sci USA* 1997; **94**: 12128–12132

127. Van Noorden CJF, Vogels IMC. A sensitive cytochemical staining method for glucose-6-phosphate dehydrogenase activity in individual erythrocytes. II Further improvements of the staining procedure and some observations with glucose-6-phosphate dehydrogenase deficiency. *Br J Haematol* 1985; **60**: 57–63

128. Filosa S, Giacometti N, Cai WW *et al.* Somatic cell selection is a major determinant of the blood cell phenotype in heterozygotes for glucose 6-phosphate dehydrogenase mutations causing severe enzyme deficiency. *Am J Hum Genet* 1996; **59**: 887–895

129. Hirono A, Fujii H, Natori H *et al.* Chromatographic analysis of human erythrocyte pyrimidine 5′ nucleotidase from five patients with pyrimidine 5′ nucleotidase deficiency. *Br J Haematol* 1987; **65**: 35–41

130. Paglia DE, Fink K, Valentine WN. Additional data from two kindreds with genetically-induced deficiencies of erythrocyte pyrimidine nucleotidase. *Acta Haematol* 1980; **63**: 262–267

131. Hansen TWR, Siep M, De Verdier C-H, Ericson A. Erythrocyte pyrimidine 5′-nucleotidase deficiency. Report of 2 new cases, with a review of the literature. *Scand J Haematol* 1983; **31**: 122–128

132. International Committee for Standardization in Haematology. Recommended screening for pyrimidine 5′-nucleotidase deficiency. *Clin Lab Haematol* 1989; **11**: 55–56

133. Ben-Bassat I, Brok-Simoni F, Kende G *et al.* A family with red cell pyrimidine 5′-nucleotidase deficiency. *Blood* 1976; **47**: 919–922

134. Beutler E, Hartman G. Age-related red cell enzymes in children with transient erythroblastoma of childhood and with hemolytic anemia. *Pediatr Res* 1985; **19**: 44–47

135. Vives-Corrons JL, Montserrat-Costa E, Rozman C. Hereditary hemolytic anemia with erythrocyte pyrimidine 5′-nucleotidase deficiency in Spain. *Hum Genet* 1976; **34**: 285–292

136. Beutler E, West C. Tissue distribution of pyrimidine-5′-nucleotidase. *Biochem Med* 1982; **27**: 334–341

137. Beutler E, Baranko PV, Feagler J *et al.* Hemolytic anemia due to pyrimidine-5′-nucleotidase deficiency: report of eight cases in six families. *Blood* 1980; **56**: 251–255

138. Laurence A, Duley JA, Simmonds AH *et al.* Erythrocyte CDP-choline accumulation in hemolytic anemia and renal failure. *Advances in Experimental Medicine and Biology*. New York: Plenum, 1998, pp 155–159

139. Paglia DE, Valentine WN, Dahlgren JG. Effects of low-level lead exposure on pyrimidine 5′-nucleotidase and other erythrocyte enzymes. *J Clin Invest* 1975; **56**: 1164–1169

140. Valentine WN, Paglia DE, Fink K, Madokoro G. Lead poisoning. Association with hemolytic anemia, basophilic stippling, erythrocyte pyrimidine 5′-nucleotidase deficiency and intraerythrocyte accumulation of pyrimidines. *J Clin Invest* 1976; **58**: 926–932

141. Rees DC, Duley J, Simmonds HA *et al.* Interaction of hemoglobin E and pyrimidine 5′-nucleotidase deficiency. *Blood* 1996; **88**: 2761–2767

142. Miwa S, Fujii H, Matsumoto N *et al.* A case of red cell adenosine deaminase overproduction associated with hereditary hemolytic anaemia found in Japan. *Am J Hematol* 1978; **5**: 107–115

143. Perignon JL, Hamet M, Buc HA *et al.* Biochemical study of a case of hemolytic anemia with increased (85 fold) red cell adenosine deaminase. *Clin Chim Acta* 1982; **124**: 205–212

144. Chen FH, Tartaglia AP, Mitchell BS. Hereditary overexpression of adenosine deaminase in erythrocytes: evidence for a *cis*-acting mutation. *Am J Hum Genet* 1993; **53**: 889–893

145. Qualtieri A, Pedace V, Bisconte MG *et al.* Severe erythrocyte adenylate kinase deficiency due to homozygous A→G substitution at codon 164 of human AK1 gene associated with chronic haemolytic anaemia. *Br J Haematol* 1997; **99**: 770–776

146. Beutler E, Carson D, Dannawi H *et al.* Metabolic compensation for profound erythrocyte adenylate kinase deficiency: a hereditary enzyme defect without hemolytic anemia. *J Clin Invest* 1983; **72**: 648–655

147. Toren A, Brok-Simoni F, Ben-Bassat I *et al.* Congenital haemolytic anaemia associated with adenylate kinase deficiency. *Br J Haematol* 1994; **87**: 376–380

148. Lachant NA, Zerek CR, Barredo J *et al.* Hereditary erythrocyte adenylate kinase deficiency: a defect of multiple phosphotransferases? *Blood* 1991; **77**: 2774–2784

149. Beutler E. Effect of flavin compounds on glutathione reductase activity: *in vivo* and *in vitro* studies. *J Clin Invest* 1969; **48**: 1957–1966

150. Loos H, Roos D, Weening R, Houwerzijl J. Familial deficiency of glutathione reductase in human blood cells. *Blood* 1976; **48**: 53–62

151. Beutler E, Moroose R, Kramer L *et al.* Gamma-glutamylcysteine synthetase deficiency and hemolytic anemia. *Blood* 1990; **75**: 271–273

152. Hirono A, Iyori H, Sekine I *et al.* Three cases of hereditary non-

spherocytic hemolytic anemia associated with red blood cell glutathione deficiency. *Blood* 1996; **87**: 2071–2074

153. Boxer LA, Oliver JM, Spielberg SP. Protection of granulocytes by vitamin E in glutathione synthetase deficiency. *N Engl J Med* 1979; **301**: 901–905

154. Duncan JR, Potter CG, Cappellini MD *et al*. Aplastic crisis due to parvovirus infection in pyruvate kinase deficiency. *Lancet* 1983; **ii**: 14–16

155. Rechavi G, Vonsover A, Manor Y *et al*. Aplastic crisis due to human B-19 parvovirus infection in red cell pyrimidine-5′- nucleotidase deficiency. *Acta Haematol* 1989; **82**: 46

156. Board PG, Trueworthy R, Smith JE, Moore K. Congenital nonspherocytic hemolytic anemia with an unstable hexokinase variant. *Blood* 1978; **51**: 111–118

157. Meloni T, Forteleoni G, Meloni GF. Marked decline of favism after neonatal glucose-6-phosphate dehydrogenase screening and health education. The northern Sardinian experience. *Acta Haematol* 1992; **87**: 29–31

158. Glader BE. Salicylate-induced injury of pyruvate kinase deficient erythrocytes. *N Engl J Med* 1976; **294**: 916–918

159. Salem HH, van der Weyden MB, Firken BG. Iron overload in congenital erythrocyte pyruvate kinase deficiency. *Med J Aust* 1980; **1**: 531–532

160. Reeves G, Rigby PG, Rosen H *et al*. Hemochromatosis and congenital nonspherocytic hemolytic anemia in siblings. *J Am Med Assoc* 1963; **186**: 123–126

161. Feder JN, Gnirke A, Thomas W *et al*. A novel MHC class 1-like gene is mutated in patients with hereditary haemochromatosis. *Nature Genet* 1996; **13**: 399–408

162. Bowman HS, Oski FA. Laboratory studies of erythrocytic pyruvate kinase deficiency. Pathogenesis of the hemolysis. *Am J Clin Path* 1978; **70**: 259–270

163. Arya R, Layton DM, Bellingham AJ. Hereditary red cell enzymopathies. *Blood Rev* 1995; **9**: 165–175

164. Miwa S, Fujii H. Molecular basis of erythroenzympathies associated with hereditary hemolytic anemia: Tabulation of mutant enzymes. *Am J Hematol* 1996; **51**: 122–132

165. Krawczak M, Cooper DN. The human gene mutation database. *Trends Genet* 1977; **13**: 121–122

166. Schneider A, Cohen-Solal M. Hematologically important mutations: Triosephosphate isomerase. *Blood Cells Mol Dis* 1996; **22**: 82–84

167. Vulliamy T, Luzzatto L, Hirono A, Beutler E. Hematologically important mutations: Glucose-6-phosphate dehydrogenase. *Blood Cells Mol Dis* 1997; **23**: 302–313

168. Baronciani L, Beutler E. Molecular study of pyruvate kinase deficiency patients with hereditary nonspherocytic hemolytic anemia. *J Clin Invest* 1995; **95**: 1702–1709

169. Merkle S, Pretsch W. Characterisation of triosephosphate isomerase mutants with reduced enzyme activity in *Mus musculus*. *Genetics* 1989; **123**: 837–844

170. Merkle S, Pretsch W. Glucose-6-phosphate isomerase deficiency associated with non-spherocytic hemolytic anemia in the mouse: an animal model for the human disease. *Blood* 1993; **81**: 206–213

171. Gibson QH . The reduction of methaemoglobin in red blood cells and studies on the cause of idiopathic methaemoglobinaemia. *Biochem J* 1948; **42**: 13–23

172. Hegesh E, Hegesh J, Kaftory A. Congenital methemoglobinemia with a deficiency of cytochrome b_5. *N Engl J Med* 1986; **314**: 757–761

173. Tanishima K, Tanimoto K, Tomoda A *et al*. Hereditary methemoglobinemia due to cytochrome b_5 reductase deficiency in blood cells without associated neurologic and mental disorders. *Blood* 1985; **66**: 1288–1299

174. Lemarchandel V, Joulin V, Valentin C *et al* Compound heterozygosity in a complete erythrocyte bisphosphoglycerate mutase deficiency. *Blood* 1992; **80**: 2643–2649

175. Kahn A. Abnormalities of erythrocyte enzymes in dyserythropoiesis and malignancies. In: Mentzer WC (ed) Enzymopathies. *Clin Hematol* 1981; **10**: 123–138

Thalassemias

NANCY F OLIVIERI AND DJ WEATHERALL

The thalassemias, a heterogeneous family of inherited disorders of hemoglobin synthesis, were first recognized in their severe and milder forms quite independently in the US and Italy between 1925 and 1927.[1] The word 'thalassemia' owes its name to an attempt, mistaken as it turned out later, to relate the diseases to Mediterranean populations; thalassa is Greek for 'sea'.

It is now apparent that the thalassemias are the commonest monogenic diseases and they are widespread among races ranging from the Mediterranean region, through the Middle East and Indian sub-continent, to south-east Asia. Many countries in these regions have, over the last 30 years, gone through a remarkable demographic change in the pattern of their illnesses. With improvements in hygiene and public health measures, very high infant and childhood mortalities due to infection and malnutrition have fallen. In the past, babies born with serious genetic blood diseases would have been unlikely to survive the first years of life, but the scene has now changed dramatically; the majority of these children are now surviving long enough to come to diagnosis and to require management. As the symptomatic treatment of thalassemia is expensive, this change in the pattern of childhood illness will place an increasing drain on the resources of countries in which the disease occurs at a high frequency.[2]

The problems posed by the thalassemias for pediatric hematology are not confined to the high frequency countries of the world. Because of major population movements, these diseases are assuming an increasing importance in the clinical practice of pediatricians in the richer countries.

GENETICS AND CLASSIFICATION

Since the thalassemias are inherited disorders of hemoglobin, to appreciate their genetic transmission and how they are classified, it is necessary to understand the principles of the genetic control of hemoglobin synthesis and how it is regulated.

GENETIC CONTROL OF HEMOGLOBIN SYNTHESIS

A great deal is known about the structure, genetic regulation and synthesis of hemoglobin.[3-6] Only those aspects of particular importance for an understanding of the thalassemias are summarized here.

Different hemoglobins, each adapted to the particular oxygen requirements at each stage of development, are synthesized in the embryo, fetus and adult. They all have a similar tetrameric structure, consisting of 2 different pairs of globin chains, each attached to a heme moiety (see also Chapter 12). Adult and fetal hemoglobins have α chains combined with β chains (HbA, $\alpha_2\beta_2$), δ chains (HbA$_2$, $\alpha_2\delta_2$) and γ chains (HbF, $\alpha_2\gamma_2$). In embryonic life, α-like chains called ζ combine with γ chains to produce hemoglobin Portland ($\zeta_2\gamma_2$), or with ε chains to form hemoglobin Gower 1 ($\zeta_2\varepsilon_2$), and α and ε chains combine to form hemoglobin Gower 2 ($\alpha_2\varepsilon_2$). HbF is itself heterogeneous; there are two kinds of γ chains, which differ in their amino acid compositions only at position 136, where they have either glycine or alanine. Those γ chains with glycine are called $^G\gamma$ chains, and those with alanine, $^A\gamma$ chains. The $^G\gamma$ and $^A\gamma$ chains are the products of separate ($^G\gamma$ and $^A\gamma$) loci.

The different globin chains are controlled by 2 families of globin genes (Fig. 15.1). The β-like globin genes are arranged in a linked cluster on chromosome 11, which is distributed over approximately 60 kb. They are arranged in the order 5' to 3' (left to right) ε-$^G\gamma$-$^A\gamma$-$\psi\beta$-δ-β. (The symbol ψ is used to described a 'pseudo-gene', probably a burnt out evolutionary remnant of a once active gene.) The α-like globin genes also form a cluster, in this case on chromosome 16. They are distributed in the order 5'-ζ-$\psi\zeta$-$\psi\alpha1$-$\alpha2$-$\alpha1$-3'.

To appreciate the molecular basis for the thalassemias, it is important to understand, at least in outline, something of the structure of the globin genes, how they are regulated, and

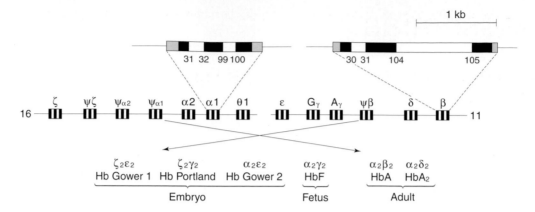

Fig. 15.1 Genetic control of human hemoglobin synthesis. The α- and β-globin gene clusters on chromosomes 16 and 11 are shown, together with the different hemoglobins produced in embryonic, fetal and adult life. In the extended representations of the α1- and β-globin genes the exons are shown in dark shading, the introns unshaded, and the 5′ and 3′ non-coding regions are shown in light shading.

how their products are synthesized and unite with heme to form hemoglobin molecules in the red cell precursors.[4,6]

Each globin gene consists of a string of nucleotide bases which are divided into coding sequences, called exons, and non-coding regions known as intervening sequences (IVS) or introns. In the 5′ non-coding or flanking regions of globin genes, there are blocks of nucleotide homology, which are found in similar positions in many species. There are 3 such regions, called promoter elements, which play a major role in the transcription of the structural genes. The globin gene clusters contain other elements that play an important part in promoting erythroid-specific gene expression, and in co-ordinating the changes in globin gene activity at different stages during development. These include enhancers, i.e. sequences that increase gene expression despite being located at a variable distance from a particular gene, and 'master' regulatory sequences, called the locus control region (LCR) in the case of the β-globin gene family and HS40 in the case of the α gene complex, which lie upstream from the globin gene clusters and are responsible for their activation in erythroid tissue. Each of these regulatory sequences has a modular structure made up of an array of short nucleotide motifs that represent binding sites for transcriptional activators or repressors, molecules involved in the activation or repression of globin gene production in different cell types and at different stages of development.

Each of these regulatory regions bind a number of erythroid-specific factors, including GATA-1 and NF-E2, thereby activating the LCR, which renders the entire β-globin gene cluster transcriptionally active. It seems likely that the LCR and HS40 regions come into apposition with the promoter regions of each of the globin genes in turn, and, together with a number of transcription factors and other proteins, form an initiation complex so that individual genes are transcribed.

When a globin gene is transcribed, mRNA is synthesized from one of its strands by the action of RNA polymerase. The primary transcription product is a large mRNA pre-cursor, which contains both intron and exon sequences. While in the nucleus this molecule undergoes a remarkable series of modifications; the introns are removed and the exons are spliced together. This is a multi-step process which requires certain structural features of the mRNA precursor, notably the nucleotides GT at the 5′ end, and AG at the 3′ end of intron-exon junctions. The importance of these sequences will be discussed when the mutations that cause thalassemia are considered. The mRNAs are now modified at both their 5′ and 3′ ends and move into the cytoplasm of the red cell precursor to act as a template for globin-chain production.

Amino acids are transported to the mRNA template on carrier molecules (tRNAs). There are specific tRNAs for each amino acid. The order of amino acids in a globin chain is determined by a triplet code, i.e. 3 bases (codons) code for a particular amino acid. The tRNAs also contain 3 bases, or anti-codons, which are complementary to the mRNA codons for particular amino acids. Hence, the tRNAs carry amino acids to the template, find the right position by codon-anti-codon base pairing, and initiate globin chain synthesis. When the first tRNA is in position, a complex is formed between several protein initiation factors and the subunits of the ribosome which is to hold the growing peptide chains together on the mRNA as it is translated. A second tRNA moves in alongside and the 2 amino acids are united by a peptide bond; the globin chain is now 2 amino acid residues long. This process is continued as the message is translated, from left to right, until a specific codon for termination is reached, whereupon the finished globin chain drops off the ribosome mRNA complex and the ribosomal subunits are recycled. The finished globin chain combines with heme and 3 of its fellows to form a definitive hemoglobin molecule.

The developmental switches from embryonic to fetal, and fetal to adult hemoglobin production are synchronized throughout the different organs of hemopoiesis that function at various times of development.[4,6] The way in which these switches are regulated is not understood. It is believed that the LCR becomes spatially related sequentially to the ε, γ and finally δ and β chains at different times during fetal development. Why this happens is not clear, although it is possible that specific DNA-binding proteins are involved in the activation or repression of these genes at different developmental stages.

CLASSIFICATION

The thalassemias are a heterogeneous group of genetic disorders of hemoglobin synthesis, all of which result from a reduced rate of production of one or more of the globin chains of hemoglobin. This causes imbalanced globin-chain synthesis, the hallmark of all forms of thalassemia.[1]

The thalassemias can be classified at different levels. Clinically, it is useful to divide them into 3 groups:

- severe transfusion-dependent (major) varieties;
- symptomless carrier states (minor) varieties;
- a group of conditions of intermediate severity which fall under the loose heading 'thalassemia intermedia'.

This classification is retained because it has implications for both diagnosis and management.

Thalassemias can also be classified at the genetic level into the α-, β-, $\delta\beta$- or $\varepsilon\gamma\delta\beta$-thalassemias, according to which globin chain is produced in reduced amounts (Table 15.1). In some thalassemias, no globin chain is synthesized, and hence these are called α^o- or β^o-thalassemias, whereas in others, some globin chain is produced but at a reduced rate; these are designated α^+- or β^+-thalassemias. The $\delta\beta$-thalassemias, in which there is defective δ- and β-chain synthesis,

Table 15.1 Classification of the common thalassemias and related disorders.

β-Thalassemia
    β^+ β^o

$\delta\beta$-Thalassemia
    $(\delta\beta)^+$ Hb Lepore thalassemia
    $(\delta\beta)^o$
    $(^A\gamma\delta\beta)^o$

$\varepsilon\gamma\delta\beta$-Thalassemia
    $(\varepsilon\gamma\delta\beta)^o$

δ-Thalassemia

β- or $\delta\beta$-thalassemia associated with β-chain variants
    Hb S β-thalassemia
    Hb E β-thalassemia
    Many others

α-Thalassemia
    α^+ (deletion)
    α^+ (non-deletion)
    α^o

Hereditary persistence of HbF
    Deletion $(\delta\beta)^o$
    Non-deletion $^A\gamma\beta^+$ $^G\gamma\beta^+$
    Unlinked to β-globin gene cluster

can be subdivided in the same way, i.e. into $(\delta\beta)^+$ and $(\delta\beta)^o$ varieties.

As the thalassemias occur in populations in which structural hemoglobin variants are also common, it is not unusual to inherit a thalassemia gene from one parent and a gene for a structural variant from the other. Furthermore, since both α- and β-thalassemia occur commonly in some countries, individuals may receive genes for both types. All these different interactions produce an extremely complex and clinically diverse family of genetic disorders, which range in severity from death *in utero* to extremely mild, symptomless hypochromic anemias.

Despite their genetic complexity, most thalassemias are inherited in a Mendelian recessive or co-dominant fashion. Heterozygotes are usually symptomless, while more severely affected patients are either homozygous for α- or β-thalassemia, or compound heterozygotes for different molecular forms of the diseases.

DISTRIBUTION

The world distributions of β- and α-thalassemias are shown in Figs 15.2 and 15.3, respectively. Several detailed accounts of their frequency and population genetics have been reported.[1,7]

The α^o-thalassemias are found predominantly in southeast Asia and in the Mediterranean islands. The α^+-thalassemias occur widely throughout Africa, the Mediterranean region, the Middle East, parts of the Indian subcontinent and throughout south-east Asia. They achieve carrier rates of 40–80% in some populations.

The β-thalassemias have a distribution similar to that of the α-thalassemias. With the exception of a few countries, the β-thalassemias are less common in Africa, extremely frequent in some of the Mediterranean island populations, and occur at variable frequencies throughout the Middle East, the Indian subcontinent and parts of south-east Asia. As discussed below, the structural hemoglobin variant, HbE, is associated with the phenotype of a mild form of β-thalassemia. This also reaches extremely high gene frequencies in eastern parts of India, Burma, and in many countries in south-east Asia. Thus the interaction of HbE and β-thalassemia, HbE-thalassemia, is the most important form of the disease in these regions.

There is increasing evidence that these high gene frequencies for the different forms of thalassemia have been maintained by heterozygote advantage against severe forms of malaria, predominantly *Plasmodium falciparum*. One of the most remarkable features of the world distribution of these diseases is that in each high-frequency population there are different sets of mutations (Figs 15.2 and 15.3). This indicates that these diseases have arisen by new mutations and have then been expanded very rapidly due to local selection by malaria. The fact that the mutations are so different

309

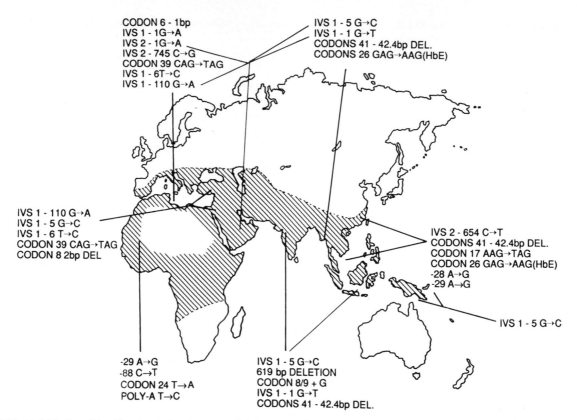

Fig. 15.2 World distribution of the different mutations that cause β-thalassemia. IVS = intervening sequence.

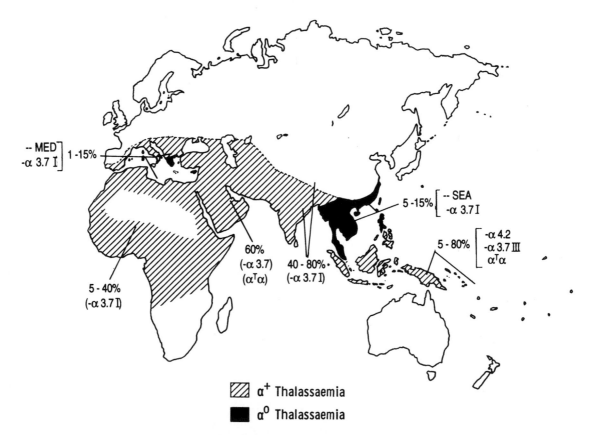

α⁺ Thalassaemia

α⁰ Thalassaemia

Fig. 15.3 World distribution of the different varieties of α-thalassemia. The 3 different forms of α⁺-thalassaemia due to deletions of a single α-globin gene involving the loss of 3.7 kb of the α gene cluster are represented as types I, II and III. The common deletional forms of α⁰-thalassaemia are designated MED (Mediterranean) and SEA (south-east Asian). The percentages indicate the approximate frequency of these different genes.

among populations indicates that this selective force is, in evolutionary terms, quite recent, probably not more than a few thousand years.

PATHOPHYSIOLOGY

To appreciate the pathophysiology of the thalassemias it is necessary to understand both their molecular pathology, and how globin chain imbalance causes the characteristic ineffective erythropoiesis and shortened red cell survival.

MOLECULAR PATHOLOGY

Although the basic principles are similar, the patterns of the mutations that cause α- and β-thalassemia are different. The β-thalassemias are considered first because of their greater clinical importance.

β-Thalassemias

Over 150 different mutations have been described in patients with β-thalassemia (Fig. 15.4).[8,9] Unlike the α-thalassemias, major deletions causing β-thalassemia are unusual. The bulk of β-thalassemia mutations are single base changes, small deletions or insertions of 1 or 2 bases at critical points along the genes. Remarkably, they occur in both introns and exons, and outside the coding regions of the genes.

Some substitutions, called nonsense mutations, result in a single base change in an exon that generates a stop codon in the coding region of the mRNA. This, of course, causes premature termination of globin chain synthesis and leads to the production of a shortened and non-viable β-globin chain. Other exon mutations cause 'frameshifts', i.e. one or more bases are lost or inserted so that the reading frame of the genetic code is thrown out of phase or a new stop codon is produced. Mutations within introns or exons, or at their junctions, may interfere with the mechanism of splicing the exons together after the introns have been removed during the processing of the mRNA precursor. For example, single substitutions at the invariant GT or AG sequences at the intron-exon junctions prevent splicing altogether and cause β^{o}-thalassemia. The sequences adjacent to the GT and AG sequences are highly conserved and are also involved in splicing; several β-thalassemia mutations involve this region and are associated with variable degrees of defective β-globin production. Mutations in exon sequences which resemble consensus sequences at the intron-exon junctions may activate 'cryptic' splice sites. For example, there is a sequence that resembles the IVS-1 consensus site and spans codons 24–27 of exon 1 of the β-globin gene; mutations at codons 19 (A→G), 26 (G→A) and 27 (G→T) result in both a reduced amount of mRNA due to abnormal splicing and to an amino acid substitution encoded by the mRNA which is spliced normally and is translated into protein. The abnormal hemoglobins produced are hemoglobins Malay, E and Knossos, each of which is associated with a mild β-thalassemia phenotype.

Single base substitutions are also found in the flanking regions of the β-globin genes. Those which involve the promoter elements down-regulate β-globin gene transcription, and are usually associated with a mild form of β-thalassemia. Other mutations, which involve the 3′ end of the β-globin mRNA interfere with its processing and produce severe β-thalassemia phenotypes.

Because there are so many different β-thalassemia mutations, it follows that many patients who are apparently homozygous for the disease are, in fact, compound heterozygotes for 2 different molecular lesions. Rarely, patients are encountered with forms of β-thalassemia in which the hemoglobin A_2 level, which is usually raised in carriers, is normal. Usually this results from the co-inheritance of β- and δ-thalassemia.

The $\delta\beta$ thalassemias are also divided into the $(\delta\beta)^{+}$ and $(\delta\beta)^{o}$ forms. The $(\delta\beta)^{+}$-thalassemias result from misalignment of the δ and β globin genes during meiosis with the

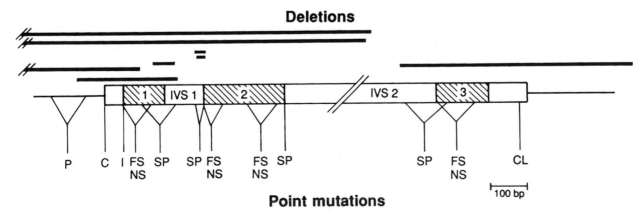

Fig. 15.4 Different classes of mutations of the β-globin gene involved in β-thalassemia. FS = Frameshift; NS = nonsense; SP = splicing; P = promoter; CL = polyA addition site mutations; IVS = intervening sequence.

production of $\delta\beta$ fusion genes. These give rise to structural hemoglobin variants called the Lepore hemoglobins, after the family name of the first patient to be identified with this condition. Because the genes that direct the $\delta\beta$ fusion chains have δ-globin gene promoter regions which contain mutations which result in their ineffective transcription, the $\delta\beta$ chains are synthesized at a reduced rate and hence are associated with the phenotype of $\delta\beta$-thalassemia. The different forms of $(\delta\beta)^o$ thalassemia all result from long deletions of the β-globin gene cluster which remove the δ and β genes, and leave either 1 or both the γ-globin genes intact. Longer deletions that remove the β-globin LCR and all or most of the cluster completely inactivate the gene complex and result in $(\varepsilon\gamma\delta\beta)^o$-thalassemia.[9,10]

α-Thalassemias

The molecular pathology and genetics of the α-thalassemias are more complicated than that of the β-thalassemias, largely because there are 2 functional α-globin genes on each pair of chromosomes 16.[9,11,12] The normal α-globin genotype can be written $\alpha\alpha/\alpha\alpha$. The α^o-thalassemias result from a family of different-sized deletions which remove both α-globin genes; the homozygous and heterozygous states are designated $-/-$ and $-/\alpha\alpha$, respectively. Rarely, α^o-thalassemia may result from deletions involving a region similar to the β-globin LCR, 40 kb upstream from the α-globin gene cluster, or from short truncations of the end of the short arm of chromosome 16.

The molecular basis for the α^+-thalassemias is more complicated. In some cases, they result from deletions that remove one of the linked pairs of α-globin genes, $-\alpha/\alpha\alpha$, leaving the other intact; in others both α-globin genes are intact but 1 of them has a mutation which either partially or completely inactivates it, $\alpha^T\alpha/\alpha\alpha$.

The deletion forms of α^+-thalassemia are further classified into the particular size of the underlying deletion. There are 2 common varieties involving loss of either 3.7 or 4.2 kb of DNA; they are designated $-\alpha^{3.7}$ and $-\alpha^{4.2}$ respectively. It turns out that the former is quite heterogeneous, depending on the site of the abnormal genetic crossing over event that underlies the deletion. These deletions are thought to be due to misalignment and reciprocal crossing over between the α-globin gene segments at meiosis; this mechanism results in 1 chromosome with a single $(-\alpha)$ α gene and the opposite of the pair with a triplicated $(\alpha\alpha\alpha)$ α-gene arrangement.

Non-deletional forms of α-thalassemia, in which the α globin genes are intact, are caused by mutations which are very similar to those that cause β-thalassemia. Some result from initiation or splice mutations, or the production of a highly unstable α globin which is incapable of producing a viable tetramer. Another particularly common form, found in south-east Asia, results from a single base change in the termination codon UAA, which changes to CAA. The latter is the code word for the amino acid glutamine. Hence, when the ribosomes reach this point, instead of the chain terminat-

ing, mRNA which is not normally transcribed is read through until another stop codon is reached. Thus, an elongated α-globin chain is produced which is synthesized at a reduced rate; the resulting variant is called hemoglobin Constant Spring after the name of the town in Jamaica in which it was first discovered. It occurs in 2–5% of the population of Thailand and other regions of south-east Asia. As the termination codon can change to yield several different codons, this variant is only one of a family of chain-termination mutants. Another common form of non-deletion α-thalassemia, which is found in the Middle East, results from a single base change in the highly conserved sequence of the 3' coding region of the α-globin gene, AATAAA, which is changed to AATAAG. This is the signal site for polyadenylation of globin mRNA, a process which appears to stabilize its passage into the cytoplasm. This mutation results in a marked reduction in α-globin chain production from the affected locus.

In addition to these common forms of α-thalassemia, there is a syndrome characterized by mild α-thalassemia and mental retardation (ATR), which is being recognized increasingly in many different populations. By combining clinical and molecular studies, it has been possible to subclassify this condition into two main syndromes, one encoded on chromosome 16 (ATR-16) and another on the X chromosome (ATR-X). ATR-16 is associated with relatively mild mental retardation and results from a variety of long deletions that remove the end of the short arm of chromosome 16. These may occur alone or as part of a chromosomal translocation. ATR-X, which is characterized by a more severe form of mental retardation and a characteristic dysmorphological picture, results from mutations at a locus on the X chromosome identified as *XH2*. The gene product is a DNA helicase which is thought to be a transcription factor involved in regulation of the α-globin genes, but which also must be involved in important phases in early fetal development, particularly of the renal tract and central nervous system.[12–14]

CELLULAR PATHOLOGY

Although the basic defect, imbalanced globin-chain synthesis, is similar in all types of thalassemia, the consequences of excess α- or β-chain production in the β- and α-thalassemias are quite different.[1] The excess α chains produced in β-thalassemia are unable to form a hemoglobin tetramer and precipitate in the red cell precursors. On the other hand, the excess of γ and β chains produced at different developmental stages in the α-thalassemias are able to form homotetramers which, although unstable, are viable and form soluble hemoglobin molecules called hemoglobins Bart's (γ_4) and H (β_4). It is these fundamental differences in the behavior of the excess chains in the 2 common classes of thalassemia that are responsible for the major differences in their cellular pathology.

312

β-Thalassemias

The excess of α chains produced in β-thalassemia is highly unstable, rapidly precipitates and becomes associated with the membrane of the red cell precursors and red cells. This leads to extensive intramedullary destruction of red cell precursors, probably through a variety of complex mechanisms, including interference with cell division and oxidative damage to the precursor membranes.[15-18] Such red cells as do reach the peripheral blood, because they contain large inclusion bodies, are damaged in their passage through the spleen and their membranes also suffer oxidative injury due to the action of heme liberated from denatured hemoglobin and the excess of iron that accumulates in the thalassemic red cell. Thus, the anemia of β-thalassemia reflects a combination of ineffective erythropoiesis combined with a reduced red cell survival.

Small populations of red cell precursors retain the capacity for producing the γ chains of HbF in extrauterine life. In β thalassemics these cells come under intense selection; the excess of α chains is smaller because some combine with γ chains to produce HbF. Thus, the baseline level of HbF is elevated in β-thalassemia. Cell selection occurs throughout the life-span of the HbF-rich population;[1] it is also apparent that there are a number of genetic factors which modify the ability to make HbF in response to severe anemia.[19] These factors combine to produce increased levels of hemoglobin F in all forms of severe β-thalassemia. Since δ-chain synthesis is unaffected in β-thalassemia, heterozygotes usually have an elevated level of hemoglobin A_2, which is another important diagnostic feature.

The profound anemia of β-thalassemia, together with the production of red cell populations rich in HbF and hence with a high oxygen affinity, combine to cause severe hypoxia and stimulate erythropoietin production. This, in turn, leads to extensive expansion of the ineffective erythroid mass with consequent bone changes, increased iron absorption, a high metabolic rate, and many of the other clinical features of severe β-thalassemia (see below). The bombardment of the spleen with abnormal red cells causes increasing splenomegaly; hence, the disease may be complicated by trapping of part of the circulating red cell mass in the spleen which, together with sequestration of white cells and platelets, may produce the classical picture of severe hypersplenism.

Many of these features can be reversed by suppressing ineffective erythropoiesis by transfusion, which leads in turn to increased iron overload. The resulting pathology can be best appreciated against the background of normal iron metabolism.[20] Iron *in vivo* is tightly bound to the transport protein transferrin. On delivery to tissues by transferrin, it is immediately available for chelation from a low-molecular-weight iron pool. This pool represents the major compartment through which all intracellular traffic of iron passes. When it is large, it may be toxic to cells. In patients with iron overload, excess iron is deposited in most tissues, but the bulk is found in reticulo-endothelial cells, where it is relatively

harmless, and in parenchymal tissue, primarily myocytes and hepatocytes, where it causes significant damage. The toxicity of iron is mediated, in part, by its catalysis of reactions which generate free hydroxyl radicals, propagators of oxygen-related damage.[21,22]

In normal individuals, tight binding of plasma iron to the transport protein transferrin prevents the catalytic activity of iron in free-radical production.[22] In very heavily iron-loaded patients, transferrin becomes fully saturated and a non-transferrin-bound fraction of iron becomes detectable in plasma. This may accelerate the formation of free hydroxyl radicals and also cause accelerated iron loading in the heart, liver and endocrine glands, with consequent organ damage and dysfunction.[22]

Clearly, therefore, it is possible to relate most of the clinical features of severe β-thalassemia to the consequences of defective β-globin production, the deleterious results of excess α-globin chain synthesis on erythroid maturation and survival, and the effects of iron loading resulting from increased absorption and blood transfusion (Fig. 15.5). If these principles are appreciated, it is easy to understand why some forms of β-thalassemia are associated with a much milder phenotype than others. Indeed, all the known factors which modify the phenotype of this disease act through reducing the amount of globin chain imbalance. They include the co-inheritance of α-thalassemia, the presence of a mild β-thalassemia allele, or the co-segregation of a gene that results in a higher than usual output of HbF.[19]

α-Thalassemias

The cellular pathology of α-thalassemia, because of the properties of HbH and Bart's, is different in many ways from that of β-thalassemia.[1,11,18] A result of the generation of these soluble tetramers is less ineffective erythropoiesis. Particularly in the case of HbH, the tetramer tends to precipitate as cells age, with the production of inclusion bodies, and hence a major hemolytic component is a feature of the disorder. The clinical effects of the anemia are exacerbated by the fact that both HbH and Hb Bart's are homotetramers, and therefore cannot undergo the allosteric changes required for normal oxygen delivery. They behave, in effect, like myoglobin and are unable to give up oxygen at physiologic tensions. Hence, high levels of hemoglobins Bart's or HbH are associated with severe hypoxia.

The pathophysiology of the α-thalassemias can be best understood in terms of simple gene-dosage effects.[11] In the homozygous state for α⁰-thalassemia (--/--), no α chains are produced. Affected infants have very high levels of hemoglobin Bart's with some embryonic hemoglobin. Although their hemoglobin concentration might be compatible with intrauterine life if the structure of their hemoglobin were normal, the fact that it is nearly all hemoglobin Bart's renders them seriously hypoxic. Most affected infants are stillborn with all the signs of gross intrauterine hypoxia. The

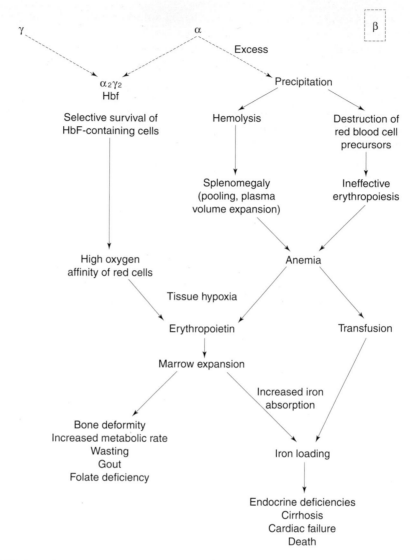

Fig. 15.5 Pathophysiology of β-thalassemia.

compound heterozygous state for α^{o}- and α^{+}-thalassemia ($--/\alpha-$) results in less chain imbalance and is compatible with survival, a condition called HbH disease. This disorder is characterized by a variable hemolytic anemia; adaptation to the level of anemia is often unsatisfactory because HbH, like hemoglobin Bart's, is unable to function as an oxygen carrier.

The heterozygous state for α^{o}-thalassemia ($--/\alpha\alpha$), and the homozygous state for the deletion form of α^{+}-thalassemia ($-\alpha/-\alpha$) are associated with a mild hypochromic anemia, very similar to β-thalassemia trait. Although a few red cells contain HbH inclusions in the α^{o}-thalassemia trait, they are not observed in the α^{+}-thalassemia trait, suggesting that there must be a critical level of excess β chains required to form viable β_4 tetramers. Interestingly, the homozygous states for the non-deletion forms of α-thalassemia ($\alpha^{T}\alpha/\alpha^{T}\alpha$) are associated with a more severe deficiency of α chains and the clinical phenotype of HbH disease.

CLINICAL FEATURES

β-THALASSEMIAS

Most children with the severe forms of homozygous or compound heterozygous β-thalassemia present within the first year of life, with failure to thrive, poor feeding, intermittent bouts of infection and general malaise. These infants are pale and, in many cases, splenomegaly is already present. At this stage there are no other specific clinical signs and the diagnosis rests on the hematologic changes (see below). If the infant receives regular red cell transfusions, subsequent development is usually normal and further symptoms do not occur until puberty, when, if they have not received adequate chelation therapy, the signs of iron loading start to appear. If, on the other hand, the infant is not adequately transfused, the typical clinical picture of thalassemia major develops. It follows, therefore, that clinical manifestations of the severe forms of β-thalassemia can be described in two contexts:

- the well-transfused child;
- the child with chronic anemia throughout early childhood.[1,23]

In the *adequately transfused child*, early growth and development are usually normal and splenomegaly is minimal or absent. If chelation therapy is effective, these children may enter normal puberty and continue to grow and develop normally into early adult life.[24,25] On the other hand, if chelation therapy is inadequate, there is a gradual accumulation of iron, the effects of which start to manifest by the end of the first decade. The normal adolescent growth spurt fails to occur and hepatic, endocrine and cardiac complications of iron overloading give rise to a variety of complications including diabetes, hyperthyroidism, hypoparathyroidism and progressive liver failure. Secondary sexual development is delayed or absent.

The commonest cause of death in iron-loaded children, which usually occurs towards the end of the second or early in the third decade, is iron-induced cardiac dysfunction; these patients die either in protracted cardiac failure or suddenly due to an acute arrythmia, often precipitated by infection.[26]

The clinical picture in *inadequately transfused patients* is quite different.[1] The rates of growth and development are retarded, and progressive splenomegaly may cause a worsening of the anemia, and is sometimes associated with thrombocytopenia. There may be extensive bone marrow expansion leading to deformities of the skull, with marked bossing and overgrowth of the zygomata giving rise to the classical 'mongoloid' appearance. These bone changes are associated with a characteristic radiologic picture, including a lacy, trabecular pattern of the long bones and phalanges (Fig. 15.6) and a characteristic 'hair on end' appearance of the skull. These children are prone to infection which may cause a catastrophic drop in the hemoglobin level. Because of the massive expansion of the ineffective erythroid mass, they are hypermetabolic, run intermittent fevers and fail to thrive. They have increased requirements for folic acid; deficiency is often associated with worsening of anemia. Because of the increased turnover of red cell precursors, hyperuricemia and secondary gout occur occasionally. There is also a bleeding tendency, which, although partly explained by the thrombocytopenia, may also be exacerbated by liver damage associated with iron loading, viral hepatitis or extramedullary hemopoiesis. If these children survive to puberty, they often develop the same complications of iron loading as well-transfused patients; in these cases, some of the iron accumulation results from an increased rate of gastrointestinal absorption.

The prognosis for the inadequately transfused thalassemic child is poor. If they receive no transfusions, they may die within the first 2 years; if maintained at a low hemoglobin

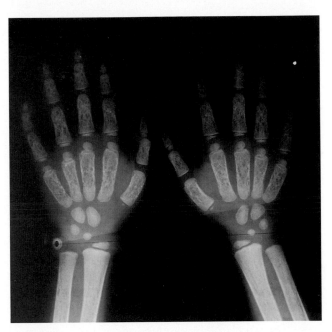

Fig. 15.6 Radiologic changes of the hands in severe β-thalassemia.

level throughout childhood, they usually die of infection or other intercurrent illness in early childhood. If they survive to reach puberty they succumb to the effects of iron accumulation in the same way as the adequately transfused but poorly chelated child.

It should be emphasized that poor growth in children with β-thalassemia is not restricted to those who are inadequately transfused or iron chelated. This problem is also observed in well-managed patients (Table 15.2).

The further complications, particularly those related to therapy, are considered in a later section.

Hematologic changes

On presentation, hemoglobin values range from 2 to 8 g/dl. The red cells show marked hypochromia and variation in shape and size; there are many hypochromic macrocytes and misshapen microcytes, some of which are mere fragments of cells. There is moderate basophilic stippling and nucleated red cells are always present in the peripheral blood; after

Table 15.2 Causes of poor growth in children with β-thalassemia.

Inadequate transfusions
Iron-induced selective central hypogonadism
Interference of iron with the production of insulin-like growth factor 1
Impaired growth hormone responses to growth hormone-releasing hormone
Abnormalities in growth hormone secretion
Abnormalities in the growth hormone-receptor itself
Hyposecretion of adrenal androgen
Delay in pubertal development
Zinc deficiency
Free hemoglobin-induced inhibition of cartilage growth
Intensive deferoxamine (desferrioxamine) administration

splenectomy these may appear in large numbers. The reticulocyte count is only moderately elevated. The white cell and platelet counts are normal unless hypersplenism is present. The bone marrow shows marked erythroid hyperplasia and many of the red cell precursors contain ragged inclusions, best demonstrated by staining with methyl violet, which represent α-globin precipitates.

The HbF level is always elevated and is heterogeneously distributed among the red cells. In β^o-thalassemia there is no HbA; the hemoglobin consists of HbF and HbA_2 only. In β^+-thalassemia the level of HbF ranges from 20 to >90%. The HbA_2 value is usually normal and of no diagnostic value. *In vitro* globin synthesis studies, involving the labeling of the globin chains with radioactive amino acids, reveals a marked degree of globin-chain imbalance with an excess of α over non-α chain production.

β-Thalassemia trait

This is almost invariably asymptomatic and is characterized by mild anemia; splenomegaly is unusual. There is a slightly reduced hemoglobin level and a marked reduction in the mean cell hemoglobin and volume. The blood film shows hypochromia, microcytosis and variable basophilic stippling. In the majority of cases, the HbA_2 level is elevated to about twice normal, i.e. in the 4–6% range, while there is a slight elevation of HbF in about 50% of cases. In some populations, notably those of the Mediterranean, β-thalassemia trait may be associated with a normal HbA_2 level. By far the commonest cause is the co-inheritance of a gene for δ-thalassemia. For genetic counseling (see below) it is vital to distinguish this condition from the different forms of α-thalassemia trait.

Intermediate forms of β-thalassemia

Not all forms of homozygous or compound heterozygous β-thalassemia are transfusion dependent from early life. The term 'β-thalassemia intermedia' is used to describe a wide spectrum of conditions ranging from those that are almost as severe as β-thalassemia, with marked anemia and growth retardation, to those which are almost as mild as β-thalassemia trait and which may only be discovered on routine hematologic examination.[19] In the more severe varieties, there is obvious growth retardation, bone deformity and failure to thrive from early life and, except for a later presentation, the condition differs little from the transfusion-dependent forms of the illness. For management, this type of thalassemia intermedia should be considered to be in the same category as the severe transfusion-dependent form. On the other hand, many varieties are associated with good early growth and development, a satisfactory steady-state hemoglobin level, and mild-to-moderate splenomegaly. Even in these patients, several important complications may develop as these patients grow older. They include increasing bone deformity, progressive osteoporosis with spontaneous fractures, leg ulcers, folate deficiency, hypersplenism, progressive anemia, and the effects of systemic iron overload due to increased intestinal absorption.

β-Thalassemia associated with β-globin structural variants

Although β-thalassemia has been found in association with many different β-globin chain variants the only common disorders of this type are due to the co-inheritance of hemoglobins S, C or E.[1,3]

HbS β-thalassemia

This varies considerably in its clinical manifestations, depending mainly on the nature of the associated β-thalassemia gene. HbS β^o-thalassemia, in which no HbA is produced, is often indistinguishable from sickle cell anemia. Similarly, HbS β^+-thalassemia, in which the thalassemia gene results in a very low output of normal β chains, and hence a level of HbA in the 5–10% range, often runs a severe course. On the other hand, HbS β^+-thalassemia in which the β-thalassemia allele is of the mild variety, particularly those forms seen in black populations, and in which levels of HbA are in the 30–40% range, may be extremely mild and are often asymptomatic. The clinical manifestations of the sickling disorders are described in Chapter 11.

HbC β-thalassemia

This occurs in West Africa and Mediterranean populations and is characterized by a mild-to-moderate form of thalassemia intermedia with the typical hematologic changes of thalassemia associated with the presence of nearly 100% of target cells (see Chapter 13) in the peripheral blood.

HbE β-thalassemia

This is a condition of major importance in eastern parts of India, Bangladesh, Burma and throughout south-east Asia. Since HbE behaves like a mild β-thalassemia allele, it is not surprising that this condition can behave like homozygous β-thalassemia. What is difficult to explain, however, is the remarkable clinical variability in its course. The clinical picture and complications may range from those of transfusion-dependent homozygous β-thalassemia (Fig. 15.7) through the milder forms of thalassemia intermedia, as described above. The pattern of complications of the more severe forms of HbE β-thalassemia are similar to those described earlier for β-thalassemia major; the milder forms behave like β-thalassemia intermedia. The hemoglobin pattern depends on the nature of the associated β-thalassemia gene; in HbE β^o-thalassemia the hemoglobin is made up of F and E, whereas in HbE β^+-thalassemia there are variable amounts of HbA.

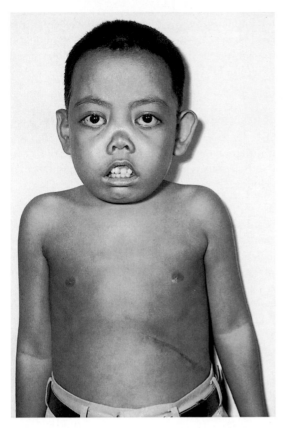

Fig. 15.7 Child with HbE β-thalassemia showing the typical facial appearance of the more severe forms of the disease. This child had undergone splenectomy for worsening anemia.

δβ-Thalassemia

The common forms of $(\delta\beta)^+$-thalassemia are the hemoglobin Lepore disorders.[1,19] The homozygous state is usually characterized by a clinical disorder which is indistinguishable from β-thalassemia major, although in some cases runs a milder course. The hemoglobin consists mainly of HbF, with up to 20% hemoglobin Lepore. Heterozygotes for the different hemoglobin Lepore disorders have the hematologic findings of thalassemia trait, with a hemoglobin pattern that consists of approximately 5–15% hemoglobin Lepore, and low or normal levels of HbA$_2$.

There are many different molecular varieties of $(\delta\beta)^\circ$-thalassemia. The homozygous states are characterized by a mild-to-moderate form of thalassemia intermedia with typical thalassemic red cell changes and a hemoglobin pattern characterized by 100% HbF. Heterozygotes have mild thalassemic red cell changes with levels of HbF in the 10–20% range and low-normal levels of HbA$_2$.

$(\epsilon\gamma\delta\beta)^\circ$-Thalassemia

This condition has not been observed in the homozygous state, presumably because it would be incompatible with fetal survival. Heterozygotes may be quite severely anemic at birth, with the clinical picture of hemolytic disease of the

newborn[27] associated with hypochromic red cells and globin chain imbalance typical of β-thalassemia trait. For reasons that are not understood, the anemia improves with age; in late childhood and in adult life, the blood picture is similar to β-thalassemia trait but with a normal HbA$_2$ level.

α-THALASSEMIAS

Homozygous α°-thalassemia

This condition, the hemoglobin Bart's hydrops syndrome, is usually characterized by death *in utero*.[1,12] These babies are either stillborn near term or, if liveborn and untreated, usually only survive for a short period. The clinical picture is typical of hydrops fetalis, with marked edema and hepatosplenomegaly. The blood picture shows a hemoglobin level in the 6–8 g/dl range and the red cells are hypochromic with numerous nucleated forms. The hemoglobin consists of approximately 80% hemoglobin Bart's, with the remainder the embryonic hemoglobin Portland. This disorder is associated with a high frequency of toxemia of pregnancy, with postpartum bleeding, and other problems due to massive hypertrophy of the placenta. Autopsy studies show an increased frequency of fetal abnormalities, although these are not always present; in a few babies that have been rescued by exchange transfusion and maintained on regular red cell transfusions, growth and development has been normal.

α°/α⁺-Thalassemia (HbH disease)

This condition is characterized by a moderate degree of anemia and splenomegaly. It has a remarkably variable clinical course; while some patients become transfusion dependent, the majority grow and develop normally without transfusion. The blood picture shows typical thalassemic red cell changes and the hemoglobin pattern is characterized by variable amounts of HbH, small amounts of hemoglobin Bart's, and a low-normal level of HbA$_2$. HbH may be demonstrated by incubating the red cells with a redox agent, e.g. brilliant cresyl blue, which causes it to precipitate with the formation of inclusion bodies. After splenectomy, large, pre-formed inclusion bodies are present in many of the red cells.

α-Thalassemia trait

The clinical picture of α thalassemia trait may result from the heterozygous state for α°-thalassemia (--/αα) or the homozygous state for α⁺-thalassemia (-α/-α) as described above. These conditions are asymptomatic and the hematologic findings are characterized by a mild hypochromic anemia with a marked reduction in the mean cell hemoglobin and volume. The hemoglobin pattern is normal and patients can only be diagnosed with certainty by DNA analyses. In the newborn period there are increased levels of hemoglobin Bart's, in the 5–10% range, but HbH is not demonstrable in adult life; occasional inclusions may be seen in the red cells in α^{0}-thalassemia carriers.

'Silent' α-thalassemia carriers

The heterozygous state for α^{+}-thalassemia (-$\alpha/\alpha\alpha$) is associated with no hematologic abnormalities and a normal hemoglobin pattern in adult life. At birth, approximately 50% of cases have slightly elevated levels of hemoglobin Bart's, in the 1–3% range, but its absence does not rule out the diagnosis.

α-Thalassemia mental retardation syndromes

The ATR-16 syndrome is characterized by moderate mental retardation and a very mild form of HbH disease or a blood picture resembling α-thalassemia trait. Patients with this disorder should undergo detailed cytogenetic analysis; in some cases chromosomal translocations may be found which are of importance for genetic counseling for future pregnancies. The ATR-X syndrome is characterized by severe mental retardation, seizures, an unusual facial appearance with flattening of the nose (Fig. 15.8), urogenital abnormalities and other dysmorphic features.[28] The blood picture

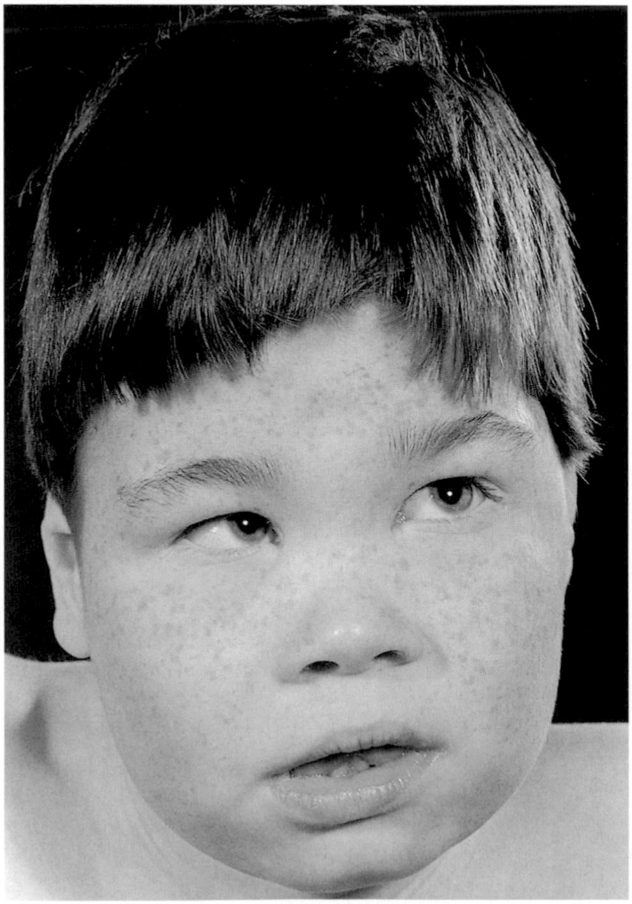

Fig. 15.8 Facial appearances in the α-thalassemia mental retardation syndrome encoded on the X chromosome (ATR-X).

shows a mild form of HbH disease or α-thalassemia trait and HbH inclusions can usually be demonstrated. The mothers of these children usually have small populations of red cells which contain HbH inclusions.

SCREENING AND PREVENTION

There are 2 major approaches to the avoidance of the thalassemias.

1. Since the carrier states for β-thalassemia can be easily recognized, it is possible to screen populations and provide genetic counseling about the choice of marriage partners. If 2 β-thalassemia heterozygotes have children, 1 in 4 of their children will have the severe compound heterozygous or homozygous disorder.
2. Alternatively, when a heterozygous mother is identified prenatally, the male partner may be tested; if he is also a carrier, the couple may be counseled and offered the possibility of prenatal diagnosis and termination of the pregnancy carrying a fetus with a severe form of β-thalassemia.

SCREENING

If populations wish to offer marital choice, it is essential to develop pre-marital screening programs, which are best carried out in schoolchildren. However, it is vital to have a very well organized genetic counseling program in place and to provide both verbal advice and written information about the results of screening.

The alternative approach is to screen every woman of an appropriate racial background in early pregnancy. Probably the most cost-effective way of screening for thalassemia is through the red cell indices.[29,30] If mean corpuscular volume (MCV) and MCH values are found to be in the range associated with the carrier states for thalassemia, an HbA_2 estimation should be carried out.[5] This will be elevated in the majority of cases of β-thalassemia. If the HbA_2 level is normal, it is essential to refer the patient to a center that can analyse the α-globin genes. It is important to distinguish between the homozygous state for α^{+}-thalassemia (-$\alpha/$-α) and the heterozygous state for α^{0}-thalassemia (- -$/\alpha\alpha$); in the former, the patient is not at risk for having a baby homozygous for α^{0}-thalassemia with its attendant obstetric risks. In those rare cases in which the blood picture resembles heterozygous β-thalassemia but the HbA_2 level is normal and the α globin genes are intact, the differential diagnosis lies between a non-deletion form of α-thalassemia and a normal HbA_2 form of β-thalassemia. These conditions have to be distinguished by globin-chain synthesis analysis and further DNA studies.[29] It is important, of course, to carry out a routine hemoglobin electrophoresis in all these cases to exclude a co-existing structural hemoglobin variant.

PRENATAL DIAGNOSIS

Prenatal diagnosis of different forms of thalassemia can be carried out in several ways.[29] It can be made by globin-chain synthesis studies of fetal blood samples obtained by fetoscopy at 18–20 weeks' gestation, although this approach has now been largely replaced by fetal DNA analysis. DNA is usually obtained by chorion villus sampling (CVS) between the 9th and 12th week of gestation. There is a small risk of fetal loss and fetal abnormalities following this approach.[30]

The diagnostic techniques used for DNA analysis after CVS have changed rapidly over recent years.[29] The first diagnoses were carried out by Southern blotting of fetal DNA, using either restriction fragment length polymorphisms (RFLPs) combined with linkage analysis, or direct detection of mutations. More recently, following the development of the polymerase chain reaction (PCR), the identification of thalassemia mutations in fetal DNA has been greatly facilitated. For example, PCR can be used for the rapid detection of mutations that alter restriction enzyme cutting sites. The particular fragment of the β-globin gene is amplified, after which the DNA fragments are digested with an appropriate enzyme and separated by electrophoresis; these fragments can be detected by either ethidium bromide or silver staining of DNA bands on gels, and radioactive probes are not required.

Now that the mutations have been identified in many forms of α- and β-thalassemia, it is possible to detect them directly as the first-line approach to fetal DNA analysis. The development of PCR, combined with the availability of oligonucleotide probes to detect individual mutations, has opened up a variety of new approaches for improving the speed and accuracy of carrier detection and prenatal diagnosis.[31,32] For example, a diagnosis can be made using hybridization of specific ^{32}P-end-labeled oligonucleotides to an amplified region of the β-globin genes dotted onto nylon membranes. Since the β-globin gene sequence of interest can be amplified $>10^6$-fold, hybridization times can be limited to 1 hour, and the entire procedure can be carried out in 2 hours.

There are many variations on the PCR approach to prenatal diagnosis. For example, a technique called ARMS (amplification refractory mutation system), based on the observation that, in many cases, oligonucleotides for the 3′ mismatched residue will, under appropriate conditions, not function as primers in the PCR, it is possible to construct two specific primers.[33] The normal primer is refractory to PCR on a mutant template DNA, while the mutant sequence is refractory to PCR on normal DNA. Other modifications of PCR involve the use of non-radioactively labeled probes.

The error rate using these different approaches in most laboratories is now well below 1%.[34] Potential sources of error include maternal contamination of fetal DNA, non-paternity, and, if RFLP linkage analysis is used, genetic recombination.

β-THALASSEMIAS

The development of better blood transfusion regimens combined with effective chelation therapy has completely transformed the outlook for children with severe forms of β-thalassemia, at least those for whom this treatment is available in richer countries.

Red cell transfusions

Regular red cell transfusions eliminate the complications of anemia and ineffective erythropoiesis, permit normal growth and development throughout childhood, and extend survival in thalassemia major.[20] The decision to initiate a transfusion program is usually based on the observation of a hemoglobin concentration of <6 g/dl at monthly intervals over 3 consecutive months, in association with poor growth, splenic enlargement and/or marrow expansion. Determination of the molecular basis for severe β-thalassemia is only occasionally of value in predicting a requirement for regular transfusions. Prior to the first transfusion, the iron and folate status should be assessed, hepatitis B vaccine series should be initiated, and a complete red cell phenotype should be obtained so that subsequent alloimmunization may be detected.

Adoption of a regimen to maintain pre-transfusion hemoglobin concentrations not exceeding 9.5 g/dl has been shown to result in a reduced transfusion requirement and improved control of body iron burden,[35] compared to previous regimens of transfusion in which baseline hemoglobins exceeded 11 g/dl. The individualization of a transfusion regimen for each patient is necessary. The pre-transfusion hemoglobin concentration, the volume of red cells administered, the weight of the patient, and the size of the spleen should be recorded at each visit to detect the development of hypersplenism.

Type of red cell concentrates

Studies of the use of neocytes, or young red blood cells, have confirmed that their prolonged survival reduces the red cell mass required to maintain appropriate baseline hemoglobin concentrations.[36] A recent analysis reported that an extension of approximately 15% in the interval between transfusions was observed during administration of neocyte concentrates. Although this would be expected minimally to reduce the requirement for iron chelation therapy, it was achieved only through increased exposure to donated units and a 5-fold increase in preparation costs over those of standard concentrates.[37] Hence, the use of neocytes would have a small impact on the long-term management of most chronically transfused patients.

Infective complications

Viral hepatitis. Liver disease is reported as a common cause of death in patients with thalassemia over the age of 15 years.[38] Iron-induced hepatic damage is influenced by a second complication of transfusions, infection with hepatitis C virus, which is the most frequent cause of hepatitis in thalassemic children.[38] The high incidence of liver failure and hepatocellular carcinoma in patients who acquire this virus through transfusions support the use of antiviral therapy for patients with thalassemia. Results of trials of α-interferon in hepatitis C-infected patients with thalassemia[39,40] suggest that the clinical and pathologic responses to this agent may be inversely related to body iron burden.

Yersinia infection. The growth of pathogenic strains of *Yersinia enterocolitica* is limited in the presence of normal hosts because this micro-organism does not synthesize iron scavenger molecules known as siderophores.[41] Both increased amounts of body iron, and the availability of siderophores from other microbes, can be exploited by *Yersinia enterocolitica* for its growth. Hence, the recognized risk factors for this infection include both increased body iron burden and treatment with the iron-chelating agent deferoxamine (desferrioxamine). Since the first description of invasive *Yersinia enterocolitica* in 2 children with β-thalassemia in 1970, reports of >80 patients with thalassemia who have developed this complication have been published.[42] Infection should be suspected in patients with iron overload who present with high fever and no obvious focus of infection; commonly, but not invariably, diarrhea is present. Even in the absence of a positive blood culture for *Yersinia enterocolitica* in this clinical setting, therapy with intravenous gentamicin and oral trimethoprim-sulfamethoxazole should be promptly instituted, and continued for at least 7 days.

Splenectomy

In the past, most patients with severe β-thalassemia developed significant hypersplenism and an increase in yearly red cell requirements during the first decade of life. While hypersplenism may sometimes be avoided by early and regular transfusion, many patients will nevertheless ultimately require splenectomy. Splenectomy should reduce red cell requirements by 30% in a patient whose transfusion index (calculated by addition of the total of packed cells administered over 1 year, divided by the mid-year weight in kg) exceeds 200 ml/kg/year.[23] Because of the risk of infection, splenectomy should usually be delayed until the age of 5 years.[43] At least 2–3 weeks prior to splenectomy, patients should be vaccinated with the pneumococcal and *Haemophilus influenzae* type B vaccines, and after surgery daily prophylactic penicillin should be administered at least during childhood and probably indefinitely. Erythromycin should be substituted for those who are allergic to penicillin.

Iron overload

Iron overload is the most important consequence of transfusions in thalassemia.[20] The mechanisms of iron toxicity were reviewed above.

Iron-chelating therapy with deferoxamine

Deferoxamine is poorly absorbed orally. Substantial iron excretion was first reported after short-term administration of intramuscular, intravenous and subcutaneous deferoxamine in the early 1960s.[20] Over the next two decades, long-term intramuscular administration was shown to slow iron accumulation and arrest hepatic fibrosis in transfused patients,[44] while the effectiveness of 24-hour infusions of deferoxamine, and subsequently of 12-hour infusions, were reported.[45–47] Together, these studies permitted the design of regimens of overnight infusions of subcutaneous deferoxamine, using portable ambulatory pumps, which are the standard method of deferoxamine administration today.[48,49]

Thalassemia major. The beneficial effects of deferoxamine therapy on survival in patients with thalassemia were first reported in the 1980s.[50] Studies from 4 North American centers in the 1990s have demonstrated unequivocally that effective long-term use of deferoxamine in thalassemia major is associated with long-term survival free of the complications of iron overload,[24,25] identifying the magnitude of the body iron burden as the principal determinant of clinical outcome. Over the period of follow-up, patients with adequate reduction of body iron burden enjoyed an estimated cardiac disease-free survival exceeding 90% after 15 years. By contrast, patients in whom iron was poorly controlled had a mean estimated cardiac disease-free survival of <20%. Effective chelation helped protect against impaired glucose tolerance and diabetes mellitus.

Reports of improvement in laboratory abnormalities of liver function and arrest of hepatic fibrosis support the benefits of subcutaneous deferoxamine with respect to the liver in thalassemia.[51]

The effectiveness of deferoxamine in the prevention of growth failure and gonadal dysfunction has been reported in a cross-sectional study of young adults with thalassemia major regularly treated since mid-childhood. Ninety percent of these patients reached normal puberty, in contrast to only 38% in a second group who had received relatively less deferoxamine beginning in the early teens.[52] In parallel, a striking increase in fertility in men and women with thalassemia major has been reported over the last decade.[53] Other studies have reported a high incidence of gonadal dysfunction and secondary amenorrhea in adolescents with thalassemia major.[54] Intensive deferoxamine administration in children may itself be associated with impaired linear growth.[55]

Reversal of established iron-induced cardiac, hepatic and thyroid dysfunction, and glucose intolerance, during intensive deferoxamine therapy in thalassemia major has been described. In patients with true 'end-stage' iron-related cardiac disease, both cardiac transplantation and combined cardiac and liver transplantation have been successful in extending survival in patients with thalassemia major.[56] By contrast, reversal of established pituitary failure has never been reported in thalassemia major; therefore, prevention of this complication with regular deferoxamine is an important goal in the management of thalassemic children.

Because the magnitude of the body iron burden is the principal determinant of clinical outcome,[24,25] the prime goal of iron-chelating therapy is *optimal control of body iron*. This should minimize both the risk of complications from iron overload and the adverse effects from deferoxamine, which are increased in the presence of a very reduced body iron burden.[57] Thus, therapy to maintain normal body iron stores (hepatic iron of 0.2–1.6 mg/ g dry weight liver tissue) increases the probability of deferoxamine toxicity and is not a goal of therapy in chelated patients. The minor degree of iron loading (corresponding to hepatic iron concentrations between 3.2 and 7 mg/g dry weight liver tissue) that develops in a proportion of individuals *heterozygous* for hereditary hemochromatosis, a disorder in which iron absorption is abnormally regulated,[58] is associated with a normal life expectancy and no evidence of iron-induced morbidity.[59] By contrast, *homozygotes* for this disorder who develop greater iron burdens (hepatic iron exceeding 7 mg/g dry weight liver tissue), have an increased risk of complications of iron overload.[60–62] Finally, in patients with much higher body iron burdens (hepatic iron exceeding 15 mg/g dry weight liver tissue), the risk of cardiac disease and early death is greatly increased.[24] These considerations suggest that a conservative goal for iron-chelating therapy in patients with thalassemia major is to maintain hepatic storage iron concentrations of approximately 3.2–7 mg/g dry weight liver tissue), in the range found in apparently healthy heterozygotes for hereditary hemochromatosis.[59] These ranges of hepatic iron concentration and the thresholds of risk are shown in Fig. 15.9.

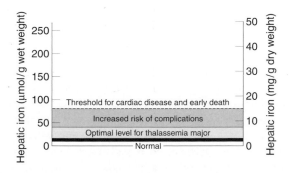

Fig. 15.9 Thresholds of hepatic iron concentration in thalassemia (see text).

As outlined above, in addition to the reduction of tissue iron stores, *reduction of the fraction of non-transferrin-bound plasma iron* is also a goal in iron-chelating therapy in thalassemia major. Reduction of non-transferrin-bound plasma iron has been demonstrated during subcutaneous and intravenous infusion of deferoxamine,[63] after which a *rebound* to pretreatment concentrations may be observed.

Management of chelation therapy

Several practical problems are posed by long-term chelation therapy:

- accurate assessment of body iron burden;
- appropriate time to initiate treatment;
- maintenance of a balance between effectiveness and toxicity.

Assessment of body iron burden (Table 15.3). Determination of plasma or serum ferritin concentration is the most commonly used indirect estimate of body iron stores in the management of chelated patients. A plasma ferritin concentration of about 4000 μg/l may represent the upper physiologic limit of the rate of ferritin synthesis; higher concentrations, due to the release of ferritin from damaged cells, do not reflect body iron stores directly.[64] The practical implication of this is that changes above a serum ferritin concentration of 4000 μg/l may have limited clinical relevance. Interpretation of ferritin values may be complicated by a variety of conditions that alter concentrations independently of changes in body iron burden, including ascorbate deficiency, fever, acute infection, chronic inflammation, acute and chronic hepatic damage, hemolysis and ineffective erythropoiesis, all of which are common in patients with thalassemia major. Hence, serum ferritin concentrations do not provide precise determination of body iron burden and reliance on these measurements may result in errors in management of chelated patients.[20]

Imaging techniques including computed tomography (CT) and magnetic resonance imaging (MRI) have been used to evalaute tissue iron stores *in vitro* and *in vivo*. MRI can identify the presence of tissue iron and is the method in clinical use with the potential to image iron within the heart. Neither method has been validated as one that provides measurements of tissue iron quantitatively equivalent to those determined at tissue biopsy.

Measurement of hepatic iron concentration is the most quantitative, specific and sensitive method of assessing body iron burden in patients with thalassemia major.[65,66] Liver biopsy represents the best means of evaluating the pattern of iron accumulation in hepatocytes and Kupffer cells, inflammatory activity and the histology of the liver. Under ultrasound guidance it is a safe procedure in children, with no complications in patients aged < 5 years in a series of > 1000 biopsies performed prior to marrow transplantation for

Table 15.3 Assessment of body iron burden in thalassemia.

Test	Comments
Indirect	Most tests widely available
Serum/plasma ferritin concentration	Non-invasive
	Lacks sensitivity and specificity
	Poorly correlated with hepatic iron concentration in individual patients
Serum transferrin saturation	Lacks sensitivity
Tests of 24-hour deferoxamine-induced urinary	Less than half of outpatient aliquots collected correctly
iron excretion	Ratio of stool:urine iron variable; poorly correlated with hepatic iron concentration
Imaging of tissue iron	
Computed tomography: Liver	Variable correlation with hepatic iron concentration reported
Magnetic resonance: Liver	Variable correlations with hepatic iron concentration reported
	Treatment-induced changes confirmed by liver biopsy
Heart	Only modality available to image cardiac iron stores; changes observed during chelating therapy consistent with reduction in cardiac iron
Anterior pituitary	Only modality available to image pituitary iron; signal moderately well correlated with pituitary reserve
Evaluation of organ function	Most tests lack sensitivity and specificity; may identify established organ dysfunction
Direct	Most tests not widely available
Cardiac iron quantitation: Biopsy	Imprecise due to inhomogeneous distribution of cardiac iron
Hepatic iron quantitation: Biopsy	Reference method; provides direct assessment of body iron burden, severity of fibrosis and inflammation
	Safe when performed under ultrasound guidance
Superconducting susceptometry (SQUID)	Non-invasive; excellent correlation with biopsy-determined hepatic iron

thalassemia.[67] Liver biopsy should be performed at important crossroads in the management of pediatric patients with thalassemia major (see below).

Initiation and management of chelating therapy. Few guidelines exist with respect to the appropriate time to start iron-chelating therapy. In practice, the usual approach is to determine the serum ferritin concentration after a period of regular transfusions and, based upon the value, to begin a regimen of nightly subcutaneous deferoxamine therapy. As emphasized above, reliance on serum ferritin measurements alone can lead to inaccurate assessment of body iron burden in individual patients. Given the safety of liver biospy under ultrasound guidance, the authors recommend that all children with thalassemia major undergo direct determination of liver iron concentration after 1 year of regular transfusions. The value of hepatic iron that should prompt therapy is in the range of the same concentrations which should be ideally maintained during chronic iron-chelating therapy, as discussed above. If a liver biopsy is not done at the start of therapy, treatment with subcutaneous deferoxamine not exceeding 25–35 mg deferoxamine/kg/24 hours in young children, should be initiated after approximately 1 year of regular transfusions. The basis for this recommendation is detailed below.

Balance between effectiveness and toxicity of deferoxamine. Most toxicities associated with deferoxamine have been observed in children during administration of doses exceeding 50 mg/kg, or during adminstration of smaller doses in the presence of very modest body iron burdens. The toxicities associated with deferoxamine and their management are summarized in Table 15.4. One important side-effect in children is reduction in both sitting and standing height, related in part to the effects of deferoxamine on spinal cartilage. As improvement in linear growth of patients with spinal abnormalities has not been observed, even following reduction of deferoxamine dose, it is important to prevent this toxicity.

Most of the well-described toxicities of intensive deferoxamine administration may be preventable with simple measures. These include regular, direct assessment of body iron burden, with the goal being the maintenance of hepatic iron between 3 and 7 mg/g dry weight liver tissue. If hepatic iron concentration is not regularly assessed, a 'toxicity' index, defined as the mean daily dose of deferoxamine (in mg/kg) divided by the serum ferritin concentration (in μg/l) should be calculated for each patient every 6 months, and should not exceed 0.025.[57] Deferoxamine doses should rarely exceed 50 mg/kg/day. Regular evaluation of deferoxamine toxicity is strongly recommended in all patients maintained on any dose of deferoxamine.

Alternatives to subcutaneous infusions of deferoxamine

The commonest difficulty associated with long-term therapy with subcutaneous deferoxamine is erratic compliance with therapy, especially in adolescents. One alternative which circumvents the problem of tissue irritation is the administration of the drug through implantable venous access ports.[68] These reduce the local pain and irritation of sub-

Table 15.4 Monitoring of deferoxamine (desferrioxamine)-related toxicity.

Toxicity	Investigations	Frequency	Alteration in therapy
High frequency sensorineural hearing loss	Audiogram	Yearly; if patient symptomatic, immediate reassessment	Interrupt DFO immediately Directly assess body iron burden Discontinue DFO × 6 months if HIC 3.2–7 mg/g dry weight liver tissue Repeat audiogram q3-months until normal or stable Adjust DFO to HIC as per Table 15.3
Retinal abnormalities	Retinal examination	Yearly; if patient symptomatic, immediate reassessment	Interrupt DFO immediately Directly assess body iron burden Discontinue DFO × 6 months if HIC 3.2–7 mg/g dry weight liver tissue Review q3-months until normal or stable Adjust DFO to HIC as per Table 15.3
Metaphyseal and spinal abnormalities	X-rays of wrists, knees, thoraco-lumbar-sacral spine Bone age of wrist	Yearly	Reduce DFO to 25 mg/kg/day × 4/week Directly assess body iron burden Discontinue DFO × 6 months if HIC ⩽3 mg/g dry weight liver tissue Reassess HIC after 6 months Adjust DFO to HIC as per Table 15.3
Decline in height velocity and/or sitting height	Determination of sitting and standing heights	Twice yearly	As for metaphyseal and spinal abnormalities Regular (6-monthly) assessment by pediatric endocrinologist

HIC = hepatic iron concentration; DFO = deferoxamine (desferrioxamine).

cutaneous infusions and are associated with rapid reduction of body iron burden. The need for nightly self-administration is removed with such regimens, and patients compliance has been shown to improve.

Orally-active iron-chelating agents. The expense and inconvenience of deferoxamine has led to a search for an orally-active iron chelator. The agent most extensively assessed is 1,2-dimethyl-3-hydroxypyridin-4-one (deferiprone; L1), patented in 1982 as an alternative to deferoxamine for the treatment of chronic iron overload.[69] The long-term effectiveness of this drug has been evaluated using serial quantitative determinations of hepatic iron in only 2 trials worldwide.[70] Both were terminated prematurely by their corporate sponsor, Apotex Pharamecuticals (Weston, Canada), in 1996. Follow-up of hepatic iron concentrations in both a long-term treatment cohort of deferiprone-treated patients, and patients in a randomized trial of deferiprone and deferoxamine, have provided information regarding the long-term effectiveness of deferiprone in thalassemia major. In the former, hepatic iron concentrations exceeded the threshold associated with increased risk of heart disease and early death in thalassemia major in one-third of patients.[71] In the latter, review of available hepatic iron concentrations in patients who had completed 2 years in the study by May 1997 showed a mean increase in hepatic iron concentration of nearly 50% over baseline in patients treated with deferiprone, but no significant change in those treated with deferoxamine.[72] These results, recently confirmed in other treatment cohorts of deferiprone in which single determinations of

hepatic iron were obtained after 2–6 years of therapy, raise concerns that long-term therapy with deferiprone may not provide adequate control of body iron in a substantial proportion of patients with thalassemia major. In parallel, concerns have been raised with respect to deferiprone-related complications of agranulocytosis and neutropenia, exceeding 8% in a large series. The inadequate effectiveness and toxicity of this agent mandates a careful evaluation of the balance between risk and benefit of deferiprone in patients with thalassemia, in most of whom deferoxamine is a safe and efficacious treatment.

Bone marrow transplantation

The cure of severe β-thalassemia with allogeneic bone marrow transplantation (BMT), first reported over a decade ago,[73] offers an alternative to standard clinical management and is now an accepted treatment for β-thalassemia; disease-free survival cannot be provided by any other therapy. Despite the cure of many patients with β-thalassemia with BMT, optimal procedures for the selection of patients, the timing of transplantation, and the preparative regimen have not yet been determined.

The most extensive experience has been reported by Lucarelli et al in Italy.[74,75] They have identified three characteristics as significantly associated the risk of complications after allogeneic BMT in thalassemia:

1. degree of hepatomegaly;
2. presence of portal fibrosis on liver biopsy;
3. effectiveness of chelation therapy prior to transplantation.

In patients with even 1 of these factors present before transplant, event-free survival was significantly poorer than in those who underwent transplantation in their absence. In patients in whom none of these factors was present prior to allogeneic BMT (identified as 'Class 1' patients), event-free survival exceeded 90%. By contrast, in those with all 3 ('Class 3' patients), it was only 56%. These factors may be related to the severity of iron overload at the time of transplantation.

Successful allogeneic BMT in thalassemia liberates patients from chronic transfusions, but does not eliminate the necessity for iron-chelating therapy in all cases. Timely reduction of hepatic iron concentration is observed only in younger patients with low pre-transplantation body iron burdens; parenchymal hepatic iron overload persists, up to 6 years after BMT, in most patients who do not receive post-transplant deferoxamine treatment. Both phlebotomy and short-term deferoxamine are safe and effective in the reduction of tissue iron in the 'ex-thalassemic' patient, and should be initiated 1 year following successful marrow transplantation if the hepatic iron concentration exceeds 7 mg/g dry weight liver tissue at that time.

Many parents of children with thalassemia major are inevitably confronted with the choice between standard therapy and BMT. The excellent results from Lucarelli et al[74,75] suggest that transplantation should be offered to any patient with a compatible donor. On the other hand, several factors need to be considered by families and their clinicians in deciding between these therapeutic options. The most important is the increased expectation of survival with standard therapy; the estimated 15-year cardiac disease-free survival of transfused patients regularly compliant with deferoxamine currently exceeds 90%, which is comparable to that achieved with BMT in 'Class I' patients. Secondly, event-free survival following BMT for thalassemia in North America is much lower than that reported from Italy. Lastly, the long-term outcomes of BMT for thalassemia, including the preservation of fertility, are not fully known. In support of BMT as a treatment option, this procedure renders patients not merely cardiac disease free, but also thalassemia free. Moreover, the long-term cost of transfusion and chelation therapy exceeds the cost of BMT. Finally, regular administration of deferoxamine is difficult and may be associated with toxicity; if compliance with this difficult regimen falters, the survival rate for 'medically-treated' patients would be expected to be considerably lower than 90%.

Experimental approaches

Augmentation of HbF in thalassemia major

The neonatal switch from fetal to adult hemoglobin was described above. In the majority of individuals with β-thalassemia, the γ-globin genes are intact and functional. Therefore, if their output could be augmented, HbF synth-

esis could be maintained at a higher level, ameliorating the severity of the disease. This notion is supported by observations of the mild phenotype of individuals with the co-inheritance of β-thalassemia and hereditary persistence of HbF, a condition in which γ-chain synthesis and HbF production continue throughout adult life and in which HbF synthesis appears to more than an adequate substitute for defective synthesis of adult hemoglobin.

Several cell cycle-specific agents, including 5-azacytidine, cytarabine, vinblastine, and hydroxyurea, as well as non-chemotherapeutic agents, including hematopoietic growth factors and short-chain fatty acids, stimulate γ-globin synthesis and HbF production in vitro and in animal models. Clinical trials aimed at augmentation of HbF synthesis in thalassemia have included short- and long-term administration of 5-azacytidine, hydroxyurea, recombinant human erythropoietin and butyric acid compounds, as well as combinations of these agents. The results in patients homozygous for β-thalassemia are summarized below.

5-azacytidine. In the first application of therapy to augment HbF in vivo, 5-azacytidine successfully increased hemoglobin and HbF levels in a patient homozygous for β-thalassemia.[77] Further studies have reported similar and consistent laboratory and clinical responses during intravenous administration. Predictably, 5-azacytidine caused bone marrow suppression, which limited drug administration in some patients, and was associated with serious infection in a few. Consideration of this and other potential adverse effects of 5-azacytidine has shifted interest to the use of alternative therapies.

Hydroxyurea. Although recent reports suggest some response to this agent adminstered alone, clinical responses associated with its administration in β-thalassemia have been detailed in a small number of patients only.

Recombinant human erythropoietin. The experience of recombinant human erythropoietin therapy in thalassemia suggests that clinical responses (increases in hemoglobin concentration) to pharmacologic doses of this agent may be observed in selected patients. In patients with thalassemia treated with erythropoietin as a single agent, the total hemoglobin concentration has increased in 10 patients, in general without observed effects on HbF synthesis but in parallel with increases in red blood cell counts. The effectiveness and safety of combination therapy with hydroxyurea or other agents, the effect of dose and dosing regimen, and the potential of adverse effects of recombinant human erythropoietin in thalassemia, all require further study.

Butyrate analogues. The observation that elevated plasma concentrations of α amino-n-butyric acid in infants of diabetic mothers delayed the switch from γ to β globin around the time of birth suggests that the butyric acid compounds, natural short-chain fatty acids, offer a potenital therapy for the β hemoglobinopathies.[78,79] Elevated levels of α amino-n-butyric acid did not delay other developmental processes in such infants, suggesting a relatively specific effect in maintaining expression of HbF.[80] Butyrate has been demonstrated to act on 5'-flanking sequences in the embryonic globin gene in the adult chicken, while in humans, evidence has been presented that it may act via sequences near the transcriptional start site of the γ-globin gene promotor. Hematologic responses to arginine butyrate[81] and sodium phenylbutyrate[82] have been reported in patients with specific genotypes of thalassemia major.

In summary, in the relatively few patients in whom clinically significant changes have been observed, as outlined above, the factors influencing the response are unknown. Encouraging changes in laboratory or clinical parameters observed during administration of new compounds in pilot studies should be followed by extended clinical trials to establish effectiveness in larger cohorts. As in chemotherapy for malignant disease, it is likely that combination therapies may prove useful in the augmentation of HbF in the β hemoglobinopathies, and studies to evaluate the effectiveness of combination therapies are proceeding.

OTHER FORMS OF THALASSEMIA

Thalassemia intermedia

Generally, patients in whom steady-state hemoglobin concentrations of 6–7 g/dl are maintained without transfusions benefit from conservative management. At the time of diagnosis, folate supplementation should be initiated and the hemoglobin concentration determined twice-monthly. A substantial decline should prompt investigations for secondary causes, including infection, folate deficiency or hypersplenism. If a precipitating cause can be identified and treated, steady-state hemoglobin concentrations may be maintained without further transfusions. In patients over 4 years of age, splenectomy may be indicated prior to initiation of a program of regular transfusions. Some patients may become less tolerant of anemia with advancing age, or may develop transfusion dependency in adolescence or early adulthood. Abnormal growth, delayed or absent pubertal development, severe symptomatic bone disease, including the occurrence of pathologic fractures, cardiac failure or other signs of intolerance of anemia should prompt consideration of a program of regular red cell transfusions. Spinal or nerve compression should be treated by local irradiation followed by a program of red cell transfusions.

Iron loading as a result of increased gastrointestinal absorption is slower than that resulting from transfusions in thalassemia major but the same clinical consequences of iron loading and the issues of iron-chelating therapy may apply. In particular, the time at which treatment for iron overload should be initiated is an important question. Only a few studies have attempted to define the extent of iron loading in patients with thalassemia intermedia.[83] The absorption of a standard dose of oral iron is greatly increased compared to that in normal iron-replete individuals. The percentage of iron absorbed in the presence of adequate iron stores suggests that the mechanisms regulating iron absorption may be abnormal in patients with thalassemia intermedia. One study reported a positive iron balance of 3–9 mg/day, which is 3–10-fold normal absorption of iron, and projected that iron loading in these patients may be of the order of 2–5 g/year. By contrast, in regularly transfused patients with thalassemia major, iron accumulation would be in the range of 6–7 g/year. Thus, the older patient with thalassemia intermedia might be expected to be at similar risk for iron-induced hepatic, cardiac and endocrine dysfunction to the patient with thalassemia major. Since reliance on serum ferritin measurements alone can lead to inaccurate assessment of body iron burden in individual patients, direct determination of body iron burden is thus indicated in patients with elevated serum ferritin concentrations, and iron-chelating therapy should be initiated if the hepatic iron concentration exceeds 6 mg/g dry weight liver tissue. Hepatic iron concentration and liver histology should be assessed at least every 2 years in patients receiving chelating therapy.

HbE β-thalassemia

As mentioned above, the natural history of HbE β-thalassemia is poorly characterized. Until more is known about this important disease, approaches to its management should follow the lines suggested above for thalassemia intermedia.

α-Thalassemias

Until recently the hemoglobin Bart's hydrope syndrome was always thought to be associated with fetal loss and no therapeutic options were considered. While some of these infants demonstrate congenital malformations or delayed postnatal neurologic development, the exact cause of which is uncertain but which may be related to intrauterine hypoxia, this is not always the case. There are now at least five reports of infants with this disorder who have been managed aggressively, including the use of prenatal transfusions and exchange transfusions in the first days of life, followed by a regular transfusion regimen similar to that employed in β-thalassemia.[84] Large numbers of south-east Asian α-thalassemia carriers are emigrating to developed countries and hence it is becoming increasingly important to learn more about the potential rescue of some of these babies. While there are considerable costs associated with the management of this disorder, any discussion of options with an at-risk family must acknowledge the fact that, in selected cases, intrauterine transfusion and careful postnatal management may offer a high probability of long-term survival.

Many patients with HbH disease can be managed conservatively with regular folate supplementation and avoidance of oxidant drugs, which tend to exacerbate their anemia. In some cases, the hemoglobin level is such that a regular transfusion regimen, similar to that employed for severe cases of β-thalassemia, may be required. Overall, the results of splenectomy are disappointing and in a few cases it has been followed by severe thrombotic complications.[1]

REFERENCES

1. Weatherall DJ, Clegg JB. *The Thalassaemia Syndromes*. 3rd edn. Oxford: Blackwell Scientific Publications, 1981

2. Weatherall DJ, Clegg JB. Thalassemia—a global public health problem. *Nature Med* 1996; **2**: 847–849

3. Bunn HF, Forget BG. *Hemoglobin: Molecular, Genetic and Clinical Aspects*. Philadelphia: WB Saunders, 1986

4. Grosveld F, Dillon N, Higgs D. The regulation of human globin gene expression. *Clin Haematol* 1993; **6**: 31–55

5. Huisman THJ. The structure and function of normal and abnormal haemoglobins. *Clin Haematol* 1993; **6**: 1–30

6. Weatherall DJ, Clegg JB, Higgs DR, Wood WG. The hemoglobinopathies. In: Scriver CR, Beaud AL, Sly WS, Valle D (eds) *The Metabolic Basis of Inherited Disease 7th Ed*. New York: McGraw-Hill, 1995, pp 3417–3484

7. Flint J, Harding RM, Boyce AJ, Clegg JB. The population genetics of the haemoglobinopathies. *Clin Haematol* 1993; **6**: 215–262

8. Thein SL. β-Thalassaemia. *Clin Haematol* 1993; **6**: 151–175

9. Huisman THJ, Carver MFH, Baysal E. *A Syllabus of Thalassemia Mutations*. Augusta: The Sickle Cell Anemia Foundation, 1997

10. Wood WG. Increased HbF in adult life. *Clin Haematol* 1993; **6**: 177–213

11. Higgs DR, Vickers MA, Wilkie AOM, Pretorius I-M, Jarman AP, Weatherall DJ. A review of the molecular genetics of the human α-globin gene cluster. *Blood* 1989; **73**: 1081–1104

12. Higgs DR. α-Thalassaemia. *Clin Haematol* 1993; **6**: 117–150

13. Weatherall DJ, Higgs DR, Bunch C *et al*. Hemoglobin H disease and mental retardation: a new syndrome or a remarkable coincidence? *N Engl J Med* 1981; **305**: 607–612

14. Gibbons RJ, Picketts DJ, Villard L, Higgs DR. Mutations in a putative global transcriptional regulator caused X-linked mental retardation with α thalassaemia (ATR-X syndrome). *Cell* 1995; **80**: 837–845

15. Shinar E, Rachmilewitz EA. Oxidative denaturation of red blood cells in thalassemia. *Semin Hematol* 1990; **27**: 70–82

16. Rund D, Rachmilewitz E. Advances in the pathophysiology and treatment of thalassemia. *Crit Rev Oncol Hematol* 1995; **20**: 237–254

17. Grinberg LN, Rachmilewitz EA. Oxidative stress in β-thalassemic red blood cells and potential use of antioxidants. In: Beuzard Y, Lubin B, Rosa, Colloque J (eds) Sickle Cell Disease and Thalassaemias: New Trends in Therapy. *INSERM/John Libbey Eurotext* 1995: **234**: 519–524

18. Schrier SL. Pathobiology of thalassemia erythrocytes. *Curr Opin Hematol* 1997; **4**: 75–78

19. Weatherall DJ. Thalassemia. In: Stamatoyannopoulos G, Nienhuis AW, Majerus PW, Varmus H (eds) *The Molecular Basis of Blood Diseases*. Philadelphia: WB Saunders, 1994, pp 157–206

20. Olivieri NF, Brittenham GM. Iron-chelating therapy and the treatment of thalassemia. *Blood* 1997; **89**: 739–761

21. Halliwell B, Gutteridge JMC: Oxygen toxicity, oxygen radicals, transition metals and disease. *Biochem J* 1984; **219**: 1–14

22. Hershko C, Weatherall DJ. Iron-chelating therapy. *Crit Rev Clin Lab Sci* 1988; **26**: 303–345

23. Modell B, Berdoukas V. *The Clinical Approach to Thalassaemia*. London: Grune and Stratton, 1984

24. Brittenham GM, Griffith PM, Nienhuis AW *et al*. Efficacy of deferox-

25. Olivieri NF, Nathan DG, MacMillan JH *et al*. Survival of medically treated patients with homozygous β thalassemia. *N Engl J Med* 1994; **331**: 574–578

26. Engle MA, Erlandson M, Smith CH: Late cardiac complications of chronic, severe, refractory anemia with hemochromatosis. *Circulation* 1964; **30**: 698–705

27. Kan YW, Forget BG, Nathan DG. Gamma-beta thalassemia: a cause of hemolytic disease of the newborn. *N Engl J Med* 1972; **286**: 129–134

28. Gibbons RJ, Brueton L, Buckle VJ *et al*. Clinical and hematologic aspects of the X-linked α-thalassemia/mental retardation syndrome (ATR-X). *Am J Med Genet* 1995; **55**: 288–299

29. Cao A, Rosatelli MC. Screening and prenatal diagnosis of the haemoglobinopathies. *Clin Haematol* 1993; **6**: 263–286

30. Weatherall DJ, Letsky EA. Screening and prenatal diagnosis of haematological disorders. In: Wald N (ed) *Antenatal and Neonatal Screening*. Oxford: Oxford University Press, 1997 (in Press)

31. Saiki RA, Gelfand DH, Stoffel S *et al*. Primer-directed enzymatic amplification of DNA with thermostable DNA polymerase. *Science* 1988; **239**: 487–491

32. Saiki RK, Chang C-A, Levenson CH *et al*. Diagnosis of sickle cell anemia and β-thalassemia with enzymatically amplified DNA and non-radioactive allele-specific oligonucleotide probes. *N Engl J Med* 1988; **319**: 537–541

33. Old JM, Varawalla NY, Weatherall DJ. The rapid detection and prenatal diagnosis of β-thalassaemia in the Asian Indian and Cypriot populations in the UK. *Lancet* 1990; **336**: 834–837

34. Modell B, Petrou M, Layton M *et al*. Audit of prenatal diagnosis for haemoglobin disorders in the United Kingdom: the first 20 years. *Br Med J* 1997; **315**: 779–784

35. Cazzola M, De Stefano P, Ponchio L *et al*. Relationship between transfusion regimen and suppression of erythropoiesis in beta thalassaemia major. *Br J Haematol* 1995; **89**: 473–478

36. Piomelli S, Seaman C, Reibman J, Tyrun A, Graziano J, Tabachnik N. Separation of younger red cells with improved survival in vivo: an approach to chronic transfusion therapy. *Proc Natl Acad Sci USA* 1978; **75**: 3474–3478

37. Collins AF, Dias GC, Haddad S *et al*. Evaluation of a new neocyte transfusion preparation vs. washed cell transfusion in patients with homozygous beta thalassemia. *Transfusion* 1994; **34**: 517–520

38. Lai ME, De Virgilis S, Argiolu F *et al*. Evaluation of antibodies to hepatitis C virus in a long-term prospective study of posttransfusion hepatitis among thalassemic children: comparison between first- and second-generation assay. *J Pediatr Gastroenterol Nutr* 1993; **16**: 458–464

39. Donohue SM, Wonke B, Hoffbrand AV *et al*. Alpha interferon in the treatment of chronic hepatitis C infection in thalassaemia major. *Br J Haematol* 1993; **83**: 491–497

40. Clemente MG, Congia M, Lai ME *et al*. Effect of iron overload on the response to recombinant interferon-alfa treatment in transfusion-dependent patients with thalassemia major and chronic hepatitis C. *J Pediatr* 1994; **125**: 123–128

41. Chambers CE, Sokol PA. Comparison of siderophore production and utilization in pathogenic and environmental isolates of *Yersinia enterocolitica*. *J Clin Microbiol* 1994; **32**: 32–39

42. Green NS. Yersinia infections in patients with homozygous beta-thalassemia associated with iron overload and its treatment. *Pediatr Hematol Oncol* 1992; **9**: 247–254

43. Fosburg M, Nathan DG. Treatment of Cooley's anemia: deferoxamine provocation test. *Blood* 1990; **76**: 1897

44. Barry M, Flynn D, Letsky E, Risdon RA. Long term chelation therapy in thalassemia major: effect on liver iron concentration, liver histology and clinical progress. *Br Med J* 1974; **2**: 16–20

45. Hussain MAM, Flynn DM, Green N, Hussein S, Hoffbrand AV. Subcutaneous infusion and intramuscular injection of desferrioxamine in patients with transfusional iron overload. *Lancet* 1976; **2**: 1278–1280

46. Propper RD, Cooper B, Rufo RR *et al*. Continuous subcutaneous

administration of deferoxamine in patients with iron overload. *N Engl J Med* 1977; **297**: 418–423

47. Propper RD, Shurin SB, Nathan DG. Reassessment of the use of desferrioxamine B in iron overload. *N Engl J Med* 1976; **294**: 1421–1423

48. Pippard MJ, Callender ST, Weatherall DJ. Intensive iron-chelation therapy with desferrioxamine in iron-loading anaemias. *Clin Sci Mol Med* 1978; **54**: 99–106

49. Pippard MJ, Callender ST, Letsky EA, Weatherall DJ. Prevention of iron loading in transfusion-dependent thalassaemia. *Lancet* 1978; **1**: 1178–1180

50. Zurlo MG, De Stefano P, Borgna-Pignatti C et al. Survival and causes of death in thalassaemia major. *Lancet* 1989; **2**: 27–30

51. Aldouri MA, Wonke B, Hoffbrand AV et al. Iron state and hepatic disease in patients with thalassaemia major treated with long term subcutaneous desferrioxamine. *J Clin Path* 1987; **40**: 1353–1359

52. Bronspeigel-Weintrob N, Olivieri NF, Tyler BJ, Andrews D, Freedman MH, Holland FJ. Effect of age at the start of iron chelation therapy on gonadal function in *β*-thalassaemia major. *N Engl J Med* 1990; **323**: 713–719

53. Jensen CE, Tuck SM, Wonke B. Fertility in thalassaemia major: a report of 16 pregnancies, preconceptual evaluation and a review of the literature. *Br J Obstet Gynaecol* 1995; **102**: 625–629

54. Chatterjee R, Katz M, Cox TF, Porter JB. Prospective study of the hypothalamic-pituitary axis in thalassaemic patients who developed secondary amenorrhea. *Clin Endocrinol* 1993; **39**: 287–296

55. DeVirgilis S, Congia M, Frau F et al. Deferoxamine-induced growth retardation in patients with thalassemia major. *J Pediatr* 1988; **113**: 661–669

56. Olivieri NF, Liu PP, Sher GD et al. Successful combined cardiac and liver transplantation in an adult with homozygous beta-thalassemia. *N Engl J Med* 1994; **330**: 1125–1127

57. Porter JB, Jaswon MS, Huehns ER, East CA, Hazell JWP. Desferrioxamine ototoxicity: evaluation of risk factors in thalassaemic patients and guidelines for safe dosage. *Br J Haematol* 1989; **73**: 403–409

58. Brittenham GM. Disorders of iron metabolism: deficiency and overload. In: Hoffman R, Benz E, Shattil S, Furie B, Cohen H (eds) *Hematology: Basic Principles and Practice.* New York: Churchill Livingstone, 1994, pp 492–523

59. Cartwright GE, Edwards CQ, Kravitz K et al. Hereditary hemochromatosis: phenotypic expression of the disease. *N Engl J Med* 1979; **301**: 175–179

60. Niederau C, Fischer R, Sonnenberg A, Stremmel W, Trampisch HJ, Strohmeyer G. Survival and causes of death in cirrhotic and in noncirrhotic patients with primary hemochromatosis. *N Engl J Med* 1985; **313**: 1256–1262

61. Loreal O, Deugnier Y, Moirand R et al. Liver fibrosis in genetic hemochromatosis. Repective roles of iron and non-iron related factors in 127 homozygous patients. *J Hepatol* 1992; **16**: 122–127

62. Niederau C, Fischer R, Purschel A, Stremmel W, Haussinger D, Strohmeyer G. Long-term survival in patients with hereditary hemochromatosis. *Gastroenterology* 1996; **110**: 1107–1179

63. Wang WC, Ahmed N, Hanna M. Non-transferrin-bound iron in long-term transfusion in children with congenital anemias. *J Pediatr* 1986; **108**: 552–557

64. Worwood M, Cragg SJ, McLaren C, Ricketts C, Economidou J.

Binding of serum ferritin to concanavalin A: patients with homozygous *β* thalassaemia and transfusional iron overload. *Br J Haematol* 1980; **46**: 409–416

65. Pippard MJ. Measurement of iron status. *Prog Clin Biol Res* 1989; **309**: 85–92

66. Pippard M. Desferrioxamine induced iron excretion in humans. *Baillière's Clin Hematol* 1989; **2**: 323–343

67. Angelucci E, Baronciani D, Lucarelli G et al. Needle liver biopsy in thalassaemia: analyses of diagnostic accuracy and safety in 1184 consecutive biopsies. *Br J Haematol* 1994; **89**: 757–761

68. Olivieri NF, Berriman AM, Davis SA, Tyler BJ, Ingram J, Francombe WH. Continuous intravenous administration of deferoxamine in adults with severe iron overload. *Am J Hematol* 1992; **41**: 61–63

69. Brittenham GM. Development of iron-chelating agents for clinical use. *Blood* 1992; **80**: 593–599

70. Olivieri NF, Brittenham GM, Matsui D et al. Iron-chelation therapy with oral deferiprone in patients with thalassemia major. *N Engl J Med* 1995; **332**: 918–922

71. Olivieri NF for the Toronto Iron Chelation Group. Long-term followup of body iron in patients with thalassemia major during therapy with the orally active iron chelator deferiprone (L1). *Blood* 1996; **88 (Suppl 1)**: 310A

72. Olivieri NF for the Toronto Iron Chelation Group. Randomized trial of deferiprone (L1) and deferoxamine in thalassemia major. Blood 1996; **88 (Suppl 1)**: 651A

73. Thomas ED, Buckner CD, Sanders JE et al. Marrow transplantation for thalassaemia. *Lancet* 1982; **2**: 227–229

74. Lucarelli G, Galimberti M, Polchi P et al. Bone marrow transplantation in patients with thalassemia. *N Engl J Med* 1990; **233**: 417–421

75. Lucarelli G, Galimberti M, Polchi P et al. Marrow transplantation in patients with thalassemia responsive to iron chelation therapy. *N Engl J Med* 1993; **329**: 840–844

76. Olivieri NF. Reactivation of fetal hemoglobin in patients with thalassemia. *Semin Hematol* 1996; **33**: 24–42

77. Ley TJ, DeSimone J, Anagnou NP et al. 5-Azacytidine selectively increases gamma-globin synthesis in a patient with β^+ thalassemia. *N Engl J Med* 1982; **307**: 1469–1475

78. Bard H, Prosmanne J. Relative rates of fetal hemoglobin and adult hemoglobin synthesis in cord blood of infants of insulin-dependent diabetic mothers. *Pediatrics* 1985; **75**: 1143–1147

79. Perrine SP, Greene MF, Faller DV. Delay in the fetal globin switch in infants of diabetic mothers. *N Engl J Med* 1985; **312**: 334–338

80. Burns LJ, Glauber J, Ginder GD. Butyrate induces selective transcriptional activation of a hypomethylated embryonic globin gene in adult erythroid cells: *Blood* 1988; **72**: 1536–1542

81. Perrine SP, Ginder GD, Faller DV. A short-term trial of butyrate to stimulate fetal-globin-gene expression in the b-globin disorders. *N Engl J Med* 1993; **328**: 81–86

82. Collins AF, Pearson HA, Giardina P, McDonagh KT, Brusilow SW, Dover GJ. Oral sodium phenylbutyrate therapy in homozygous beta thalassemia. *Blood* 1995; **85**: 43–49

83. Pippard MJ, Callender ST, Warner GT, Weatherall DJ. Iron absorption and loading in beta-thalassaemia intermedia. *Lancet* 1979; **ii**: 819–821

84. Carr S, Rubin L, Dixon D, Star J, Dailey J. Intrauterine therapy for homozygous α-thalassemia. *Obstet Gynecol* 1995; **85**: 876–879

Granulocyte and macrophage disorders

Disorders of granulopoiesis and granulocyte function

RICHARD F STEVENS

The healthy adult produces up to 60 billion neutrophils each day and yet their half-life in the blood is relatively short (in the order of 8 hours in the healthy individual). Neutrophils are the most important cellular constituents in the control of infection and the host defence system as can be inferred from the disease profile in patients who lack normal neutrophil numbers or function. When released from the bone marrow they circulate briefly, sometimes migrating along the vascular endothelium, before being attracted to foci of infection by chemotactic factors. There they ingest opsonized organisms and enclose the microbe within a vesicular phagosome into which they discharge their granule contents. Finally, they enzymatically reduce oxygen to reactive metabolites which aid in the killing of the micro-organisms.

The neutrophil is packed with granules which are essential for the killing and degradation of micro-organisms. Primary (azurophilic) granules contain proteases, hydrolytic enzymes, defensins and myeloperoxidase. Secondary granules contain enzymes such as collagenase, lysozyme, apolactoferrin and a C5-splitting enzyme.[1] Interaction with micro-organisms or other external stimuli triggers a cascade of events affecting neutrophil adhesion, migration and bacterial activity.

tive and cell cycle qualities leading to mixed marrow colonies that are heterogeneous in size.

Regulatory glycoproteins, known as colony-stimulating factors (CSFs), influence the growth of granulocytes and monocytes in culture. CSFs are produced by a variety of tissues including endothelial cells, T lymphocytes and mononuclear phagocytes. Several CSFs (e.g. GM-CSF, G-CSF, M-CSF) which are more selective in their stimulatory capacity have been isolated and cloned. G- and GM-CSF are now available in therapeutic quantities as a result of recombinant DNA technology.

Table 16.1 illustrates the kinetics of mature neutrophil production. In the peripheral blood a relatively small number of neutrophils make up the circulating and marginating pools. In the marrow there is an immense cellular reserve made up of dividing and maturing cells.

The release of neutrophils from the marrow into the circulation is multifactorial. Neutrophil deformability, cell-releasing factor, blood flow through the marrow and localization of cells in relation to the vascular channels can all affect release of granulocytes into the blood stream.

BONE MARROW GRANULOCYTE DEVELOPMENT

Granulocyte-macrophage progenitor cells can be demonstrated in bone marrow, blood, spleen and cord blood. Mature granulocyte and macrophage populations can develop from a common granulocyte-macrophage colony-forming unit (CFU-GM) that morphologically resembles a primitive blast cell or lymphocyte. The CFU-GM population represents a continuation of cells with varying prolifera-

Table 16.1 Neutrophil production and kinetics.

Compartment	Compartment size ($\times 10^9$ cells/kg)	Compartment transit time (h)
Myeloblast	0.15	18
Promyelocyte	0.5	24
Myelocyte	2.0	104
Meta-myelocyte	3.0	40
Segmented neutrophil	3.0	96
Peripheral neutrophil	0.7	10

NEUTROPENIA

Neutropenia is an absolute reduction in the number of circulating neutrophils. Normal values are age dependent (see Reference values at the front of this book). In general, these counts range from $1.8 \times 10^9/l$ to $4.0 \times 10^9/l$, with a mean of about $3.0 \times 10^9/l$. Infants between 2 weeks and 1 year of age tend to have lower neutrophil counts than older individuals, as do Africans compared with caucasians.[2] Classification of the neutropenias can be based on one of several approaches, including pathophysiology, kinetics, metabolism, function and the severity of the neutropenia. None of these is ideal, but in this chapter emphasis is given to the severity and variability of the neutropenia.

Symptoms are relatively uncommon with neutrophil counts $>1.0 \times 10^9/l$, but become increasingly severe as the count falls. A neutrophil count of $0.5-1.0 \times 10^9/l$ can be considered as moderate, and one $<0.5 \times 10^9/l$ as severe neutropenia. Within a particular neutrophil range there is considerable variation in infective symptoms both within a patient population and within a single individual.

Bacterial infections are the commonest problem associated with neutropenia. Fungal, viral and parasitic infections are relatively uncommon in isolated neutropenia as opposed to the severe pancytopenias associated with marrow hypoplasia (as seen after intensive chemotherapy, marrow transplantation and aplastic anemia). Cellulitis, superficial and deep abscess formation, pneumonia and septicemia are particularly associated with neutropenia. The typical inflammatory response may be much modified with a poor localization of infection and a tendency to rapid dissemination.

PROFOUND AND PROLONGED NEUTROPENIA

Reticular dysgenesis

This condition results from the failure of marrow progenitor cells which are committed to myeloid and lymphoid proliferation.[3] Affected infants are susceptible to fatal bacterial and viral infections because of severe neutropenia and lymphopenia. As well as a virtual absence of marrow myeloid precursors, there is a total lack of lymphoid cells, both marrow and thymic derived. Lymph nodes show absent germinal follicles. Lymphocytes are also lacking from the tonsils, spleen and Peyer's patches. Red cell and platelet maturation is normal. No specific treatment is available other than bone marrow transplantation (BMT).

Neutropenia and lymphocyte abnormalities

The association between X-linked hypogammaglobulinemia and neutropenia has been recognized for some time.[4] Approximately one-third of males with X-linked agammaglobulinemia have neutropenia at some stage during their illness. Absence of IgG and IgA with normal or raised IgM

has also been reported in association with severe neutropenia. Bone marrow examination usually reveals a maturation arrest, with early myeloid precursors but little maturation beyond the myelocyte stage. Children usually have severe recurrent bacterial infections, hepatosplenomegaly and failure to thrive. Patients may die in early childhood and no specific treatment is available other than immunoglobulin replacement therapy or BMT.

The syndrome of T-cell lymphocytosis and neutropenia, where an acquired excess of suppressor T cells is associated with a profound neutropenia, is occasionally seen in children, although it is more common in adults. The condition is not neoplastic, its cause is obscure and there is no effective therapy. Morbidity can be considerable.[5]

Severe congenital neutropenia (Kostmann's syndrome)

This autosomal recessive condition was first described by the Swedish physician Kostmann in 1956.[6] The neutropenia is severe, with absolute counts usually $<0.2 \times 10^9/l$, although the total white cell count may be normal because of the accompanying monocytosis and eosinophilia. Inheritance may be both autosomal dominant and recessive. Infective episodes usually begin shortly after birth and are frequently very severe. Bone marrow examination shows variable degrees of abnormality but there is usually normal myeloid maturation to the promyelocyte/myelocyte stage and a scarcity of more mature forms. Nevertheless, normal numbers of myeloid progenitor cells have been detected in many patients, and *in vitro* culture appears to progress beyond the myelocyte stage with the appearance of neutrophils.[7]

There is ultrastructural and cytochemical evidence of an intrinsic myeloid precursor cell defect, with defective primary granules, a reduced number of secondary granules and autologous ingestion of mature neutrophils. However, formation of monocytes and eosinophils usually remains normal. *In vitro* cultures demonstrate adequate numbers of CFU-GM, in which normal maturation of progenitor cells into mature neutrophils usually occurs.[8] With exposure to supraphysiologic doses of recombinant human growth factors, however, these CFU-GM often form mature neutrophils.[9] Biologic levels of G-CSF in these patients are either normal or high and therefore it is postulated that the G-CSF receptor somehow fails to transduce its signal properly.[10] G-CSF receptors appear to be normal in number and binding affinity in the majority of patients studied. However, some children with Kostmann's syndrome (usually those in transition to acute myeloid leukemia [AML]) have abnormalities of the receptor for G-CSF.[11] In these rare cases, somatic mutation in 1 of the 2 alleles prevents the receptor encoded by the remaining normal allele from functioning. This mutated receptor appears to disrupt the normal regulation of myeloid growth and might facilitate the evolution of leukemic sub-populations.

However, in the majority of patients with Kostmann's syndrome, no obvious defect has been identified, suggesting a post-receptor problem.

The majority of patients used to die of severe infection although leukemic transformation has also been reported.[12] Antibiotics may help prolong life, but androgens, steroids or splenectomy have been of no proven benefit. BMT has helped in some patients,[13] but may now have been super-seded by successful therapy with G-CSF.

VARIABLE NEUTROPENIA

Several syndromes have been described where neutropenia is associated with other phenotypic abnormalities. These include Shwachman's syndrome, cartilage hair hypoplasia, Fanconi's anemia and dyskeratosis congenita. Although of variable severity, these conditions are not usually as devas-tating as Kostmann's syndrome or reticular dysgenesis (see also Chapter 1).

Shwachman's syndrome

Shwachman's syndrome is a rare multiorgan disease of unknown cause which is probably transmitted as an auto-somal recessive trait.[14] Its features include exocrine pan-creatic insufficiency, growth retardation, metaphyseal dyschondroplasia, bone marrow hypoplasia, neutropenia, anemia, thrombocytopenia and a raised level of fetal hemo-globin (HbF). Diarrhea, weight loss, failure to thrive, eczema, otitis media and chest infections tend to occur in the neonatal period, whereas growth failure and dwarfism tend to become apparent in infancy and early childhood. Abnor-mal gait follows the metaphyseal chondroplasia. Other features include reduced thoracic gas volume and chest wall compliance, mild learning difficulties, hypotonia, deafness, retinitis pigmentosa, diabetes mellitus, dental abnormalities, delayed puberty and renal tubular acidosis.[15,16]

The degree of neutropenia is variable, usually averaging between 0.2 and 0.5 × 10^9/l. The bone marrow is usually hypoplastic or may show myeloid maturation arrest.[15]

If the neutropenia is not noted, then the diagnosis may be mistaken for cystic fibrosis in the young, although the sweat test is normal. The malabsorption tends to diminish with time, although the pancreatic insufficiency persists and is probably the result of pancreatic fatty infiltration and acinar degeneration.[15] Although the majority of patients are diag-nosed before the age of 2 years, occasional cases have been described as presenting during the second decade.[17]

Although the precise abnormality in Shwachman's syn-drome is unknown, it has been postulated that the condition is the result of a cytoskeletal defect in neutrophils as reflected by an abnormal distribution of concanavalin A receptors.[18] This does not, however, explain the non-neutrophil features of the condition. Aggett *et al*[15] have speculated that the syndrome may be the result of a defect in microtubular and microfilament cellular elements, but this hypothesis awaits

confirmation. The malabsorption of Shwachman's syn-drome responds to oral pancreatic enzymes. Associated infections can be treated with antibiotics.

The disorder is a pre-malignant condition and secondary leukemia is well described. Otherwise, the prognosis is probably better than that of cystic fibrosis, with most patients surviving to adulthood, given adequate supportive therapy.

Cartilage hair hypoplasia

This condition is characterized by short-limbed dwarfism, fine hair, frequent infections and a moderate neutropenia. Impaired cellular immunity together with more variable immunologic abnormalities are found.[19] Bone marrow transplantation has been used successfully to correct the condition.[20]

Dyskeratosis congenita

This X-linked recessive condition is associated with dys-trophic nails, leukoplakia and skin hyperpigmentation. Neutropenia is seen in approximately one-third of patients and is the result of marrow hypoplasia. The majority of patients reach adult life, and life-threatening infections are uncommon.

Fanconi's anemia

This condition is dealt with in Chapter 1. Patients often show some degree of leukopenia, which is usually of mild or moderate severity initially but eventually becomes profound with the development of marrow aplasia. Infections are relatively uncommon prior to the development of severe marrow hypoplasia or acute leukemia.

Chronic benign neutropenia

In the relatively common chronic benign neutropenia, the severity of illness and susceptibility to infection is closely related to the severity of the neutropenia. Except for the low neutrophil count, no other specific phenotypic features have been reported. The condition may be the result of a defect in committed myeloid progenitor cells[21] or a dimin-ished release of colony-stimulating activity by the marrow microenvironment.

The peripheral blood neutrophil count usually remains static over many years, but spontaneous remissions have been reported, usually in younger children.[22] The lack of associated dysmorphic or chromosomal features in chronic benign neutropenia may be connected with the lack of evidence for an increased incidence of secondary leukemia. In the majority of patients no genetic pattern has been identified.

Bone marrow appearances are variable. Most frequently, there are plentiful early myeloid forms but a marked reduction of mature segmented forms. This coincides with the presence of peripheral blood segmented ('band') forms but few mature neutrophils. Marrow myeloid progenitor cells are also very variable in number.[23]

Patients with chronic benign neutropenia have a relatively low risk of serious infections and hence should not be subjected to therapy with potential side-effects unless indicated. Therapy should be based on symptoms and not on the neutrophil count.

Myelokathexis

This is a form of neutropenia in which the granulocyte nuclei show marked morphologic abnormalities, with filaments connecting the nuclear lobes and cytoplasmic vacuolation. Bone marrow cellularity is usually increased and shows numerous degenerating neutrophils which may be hypersegmented. The peripheral blood neutropenia is probably the result of increased marrow granulocyte destruction.[24]

Metabolic neutropenia

Neutropenia has been associated with a variety of inherited metabolic disorders including propionic acidemia, isovaleric acidemia, methylmalonic acidemia and hyperglycinemia.[25] The neutropenia may be the result of a direct inhibition of progenitor cell maturation.

CYCLICAL NEUTROPENIA

Cyclical neutropenia is an unusual disorder characterized by regular recurring episodes of severe neutropenia ($<0.2 \times 10^9/l$), usually lasting 3–6 days and occurring approximately every 3 weeks. The condition was first reported by Leale in 1910.[26] Since then, over 100 cases have been described.

When the patient is neutropenic, symptoms such as oral ulceration, stomatitis and pharyngitis are common. More serious localized and disseminated infections can occur, the severity of which is usually related to the degree of neutropenia, although it is not unusual for patients to be asymptomatic throughout periods of neutropenia. Patients frequently know when they have a fall in neutrophils because they experience anorexia and malaise and develop oral ulcers and white exudates over the tongue. As the neutrophil count recovers, the patient's well-being also improves. There is no evidence that affected individuals are especially prone to viral, fungal or parasitic infections. Although usually considered benign, up to 10% of patients have died of infectious complications.[27]

In many patients, mild chronic neutropenia ($<2.0 \times 10^9/l$) is seen in addition to periods of severe neutropenia.[28] Monocytes, lymphocytes, eosinophils, platelets and reticulocytes are also seen to cycle. When a patient is at the neutrophil nadir, blood monocyte counts are elevated. Mild anemia is common, particularly when there is severe infec-

tion, and is probably a non-specific consequence of inflammation.

At the beginning of each period of neutropenia, the bone marrow shows a rapid increase in the number of promyelocytes and myelocytes followed by an increase in later forms (meta-myelocytes and segmented forms). About 10 days after the beginning of the neutropenic period, the marrow shows a high percentage of mature neutrophils and fewer early myeloid precursors. Because of the cyclical changes in marrow lymphoid, erythroid and platelet precursors, the name 'periodic or cyclic hematopoiesis' has also been used.[29]

Cyclic neutropenia should be suspected in patients with the typical pattern of regularly recurring symptoms. Total and differential white cell counts should be performed at least twice a week for 2 months to confirm the diagnosis. Greatest confusion occurs when differentiating cyclical neutropenia from chronic benign neutropenia, a more common diagnosis.[22] In both conditions, splenomegaly is usually absent, there is a monocytosis and the marrow shows a myeloid 'maturation arrest'. Although patients with chronic benign neutropenia may show fluctuating counts, they do not have the strict regularity of cyclical neutropenia, although it is probable that the conditions may in fact overlap to some extent. Families have been described with both cyclic and non-cyclical members.[30]

Family studies have demonstrated an inherited pattern to cyclical neutropenia and/or symptoms highly suggestive of the condition in almost one-third of reported cases. The pattern of occurrence suggests an autosomal dominant mode of inheritance. In nearly all the familial cases, symptoms start in infancy or early childhood.[30] In other cases the onset appears to be spontaneous and the condition is diagnosed in both children and adults.[27] The collie dog shows the veterinary equivalent of cyclical neutropenia, where inheritance is autosomal recessive.[31]

Two lines of evidence suggest that cyclical neutropenia may occur by heterogeneous mechanisms. First, it has been shown that some older patients with the disorder have a clonal proliferation of large granular lymphocytes,[32] whereas children usually do not. It appears that the cyclical neutropenia can be acquired late in life. Secondly, there are reports of cyclical neutropenia in adults responding to androgens and steroids.[33,34] There are reports of neutrophil cycling in association with leukemia,[35] but there are no reports of typical childhood-onset cyclical neutropenia evolving into malignancy. Based on these observations, Dale and Hammond[36] proposed the classification shown in Table 16.2.

Several lines of evidence suggest that the primary defect in cyclical neutropenia is in the regulation of hemopoietic stem cells or progenitors committed to the neutrophil cell line. For example, in dogs, it has been shown that the disease can be transmitted and cured by BMT.[37] In man, the marked swings in marrow cell populations seen in serial bone marrows support this idea. The condition has also been transferred between humans by allogeneic BMT.[38]

Table 16.2 Classification of cyclical neutropenia.[35]

Childhood onset
  Family history
  Without large granular lymphocytes
Adult onset
  With large granular lymphocytes
  Without large granular lymphocytes
Associated with hematologic malignancy
Associated with other cyclical phenomena
Possible cyclical neutropenia (inadequate data)

There are 3 suggested mechanisms for cyclical neutropenia:

1. a stem cell defect resulting in altered response to hemopoietic regulation;
2. a defect in humoral or cellular stem cell control;
3. a periodic accumulation of an inhibitor of stem cell proliferation.[36]

Cell culture studies of blood and bone marrow indicate that stem cells, or at least the committed stem cells of the neutrophil series, have little if any defect in their proliferative capacity.[39] It has not been substantiated whether specific CSFs or interleukins fluctuate cyclically and, if so, whether they are a cause or effect of the disease. Studies suggest that there may be a basic defect in endogenous generation of CSFs in some patients, which raises the possibility of treatment with recombinant growth factors.[36] Although cyclical variations in potentially toxic nucleotides have been demonstrated in cyclical neutropenia, these mitotic inhibitors may be secondary to recurrent inflammation and intense cyclical proliferation.[40]

The management of patients with cyclical neutropenia requires an understanding of symptoms associated with neutropenic episodes and appropriate treatment of infections during periods of neutropenia. Good oral hygiene and dental care are extremely important. Fortunately, symptoms are often milder as patients age. Prednisone, androgenic steroids and possibly plasmapheresis can affect the disease[41] but are not of practical value. Lithium therapy is of no benefit. Although BMT offers a definitive cure, the associated mortality and morbidity does not justify this treatment. Recombinant growth factors offer the possibility of disease modification and regulation and G-CSF looks particularly promising.

CHRONIC IDIOPATHIC NEUTROPENIA

This heterogeneous group of conditions is usually diagnosed by exclusion. Patients usually have a normal past medical history and often previously normal full blood counts. Other associated conditions such as malignant or pre-malignant hematologic conditions, recognized infections or autoimmune disease must be excluded. Often the neutropenia is seen on a routine blood count but skin, oral or perianal infections may arouse suspicion. The remainder of the blood count is usually normal although a moderate monocytosis is often seen. The disorder is often benign and may resolve spontaneously. Nevertheless, autoimmune and myelodysplastic syndromes must be excluded. Treatment is often not necessary except in children experiencing multiple infections in whom cytokine therapy may be beneficial.

TREATMENT OF SEVERE CHRONIC NEUTROPENIA

A major contribution to the treatment of patients with congenital, cyclical and idiopathic neutropenia was made by the publication of the results of a phase III randomized trial that showed a marked clinical efficacy of recombinant human G-CSF (rHuG-CSF).[42] Patients enrolled had confirmed severe congenital neutropenia and a history of infection. Approximately 90% showed a complete clinical response and were able to maintain neutrophil counts above 1.5×10^9/l, and a significant reduction in infections. As might be expected, patients with idiopathic and cyclical neutropenia required lower doses than those with Kostmann's syndrome. Many patients have now been treated with rHuG-CSF for a decade without significant variation in their clinical responses and children seem to tolerate the subcutaneous injections remarkably well. Bone pain and headache seem to be relatively uncommon side-effects.

It is well recognized that an occasional patient with severe neutropenia can eventually develop AML.[43] Unfortunately, the precise incidence or life-time risk is not known. Of the patients receiving rHuG-CSF, those that have developed AML have almost all had preceding monosomy 7 or some other chromosomal abnormality. It is of course possible that rHuG-CSF therapy only prolongs life expectancy by allowing latent marrow transformation to occur. Children with cyclical or idiopathic neutropenia have not generally developed such complications. It is strongly recommended that routine bone marrow examination and chromosomal analysis is performed.

DISORDERS OF NEUTROPHIL SURVIVIAL

Neonatal isoimmune neutropenia

This condition is analogous to isoimmune hemolytic disease and isoimmune thrombocytopenia in the neonate. It has been estimated to affect up to 3% of newborns.[44] Mothers are sensitized by the passage of fetal antigens across the placenta during gestation. IgG antineutrophil antibodies subsequently cross the placenta and destroy the infant's neutrophils. Despite the theoretically high incidence of this condition, less than 100 reported cases have been described.[45] Affected infants tend to suffer from fever, skin infections (particularly *Staphylococcus aureus*), and respiratory and urinary infections. Septicemia may also occur.

The bone marrow shows compensatory myeloid hyperplasia with a 'maturation arrest' and reduction in mature neutrophils. Erythroid precursors and megakaryocytes are normal. The peripheral blood shows severe neutropenia often with an associated monocytosis and eosinophilia.

Neutrophil antibodies may be found in the sera of the child and mother. The antibody reacts against the neutrophils of the patient, father and possibly some siblings, but does not react against the mother's neutrophils. Minchinton[46] has classified the neutrophil antigens as NA1, NA2, NB1 and NC1 and most commonly antibody is directed against paternal NA1 or NA2 which are inherited by the fetus. Neutrophil counts usually return to normal by 2 months of age, associated with the decay of the maternal antibody.

Isoimmune neonatal neutropenia is best treated with appropriate antibiotics. Occasionally, in severe cases, plasma or whole blood exchange may have to be considered to remove the antibody. Transfusion of maternal neutrophils (which will lack the antigen) may be helpful in exceptional circumstances.[47]

HLA antigens are also present on neutrophils and it might be expected that neonatal neutropenia could occur in the offspring of multiparous women with the transplacental transfer of maternal HLA antibodies.[48] This seldom happens, perhaps because HLA antigens are present on other tissues and the antibodies are rapidly absorbed so that insufficient remain to cause neutropenia.

Autoimmune neutropenia

Autoimmune neutropenia of infancy

This is an uncommon but well defined condition which has distinctive clinical features. After an initial asymptomatic period, infants develop recurrent mild infections. The majority of children present within the first year of life, and many patients have symptoms for several months before a blood count is performed. The neutrophil count is probably normal at birth. Neutropenia is usually severe ($<0.5 \times 10^9/l$) and is often associated with an eosinophilia and monocytosis. Bone marrow examination shows myeloid hyperplasia but reduced or absent mature neutrophils ('maturation arrest'). The condition does not appear to be familial and is more common in girls.

The autoimmune nature of this disease can be established in >98% of patients by demonstrating neutrophil-bound and circulating antibodies in the patient and the absence of antibodies in maternal blood.[49] Antibodies can be demonstrated by direct and indirect immunofluorescence in >80%, and by agglutination in approximately 75% of cases. Some antibodies can only be detected by one of these techniques. Neutrophil antibodies may be directed against neutrophil-specific antigens, whereas in other patients the antigen specificity remains undefined. Autoantibodies may be IgG, IgM, IgA or a mixture.[50] Late in the course of this self-limiting disease, antibodies may become undetectable even though the patient is still neutropenic. This may

present a diagnostic dilemma when a patient is seen for the first time late in the disease.

Approximately half the children show abnormal circulating immune complexes but these are probably not the cause of the neutropenia but, rather, a secondary phenomenon. The exact mechanism of neutrophil destruction remains unclear. The autoantibodies opsonize neutrophils *in vitro*.[51] Other suggested mechanisms for the neutropenia include intravascular lysis, antibody-dependent cell-mediated cytotoxicity and entrapment of agglutinated neutrophils in the microcapillaries.[52]

The disorder should be differentiated from other immunologically-induced neutropenias including:

- isoimmune neonatal neutropenia;
- transient neonatal neutropenia which occurs in infants born to mothers who have an immune neutropenia;
- the rare infant neutropenia associated with autoimmune hemolytic anemia and thrombocytopenia.

In general, patients with autoimmune neutropenia of infancy tolerate the disease well, and treatment should be based on antibiotics to control severe infective episodes. Systemic steroids may result in a temporary rise in the neutrophil count but carry the theoretical risk of disseminating infection. Temporary remission can be induced with high-dose intravenous immunoglobulin.[53]

Autoimmune neutropenia in older children

Acquired autoimmune neutropenias in older children are occasionally seen in patients with:

- no other obvious autoimmune phenomena;
- additional autoantibodies against platelets and/or red cells;
- associated multisystem disorders such as systemic lupus erythematosus, rheumatoid arthritis and chronic active hepatitis.

Morbidity can be considerable with bacterial and fungal infections (Fig. 16.1).

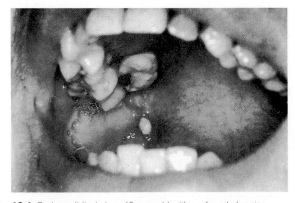

Fig. 16.1 Oral candidiasis in a 13-year-old with profound chronic autoimmune neutropenia. The condition has persisted for over 5 years with several life-threatening infections.

Felty's syndrome may also be associated with antineutrophil antibodies. It is characterized by rheumatoid arthritis, splenomegaly and leukopenia.[54] Its exact nature is not understood. Neutrophil survival appears to be shortened, with increased release of marrow neutrophils and impaired myelopoiesis. This may result from antineutrophil antibodies, immune complexes or circulating inhibitory factors.[55] It has also been suggested that the shortened neutrophil survival may be the result of impaired marrow release of neutrophils or increased neutrophil margination.[56]

Autoimmune neutropenia has also been reported following BMT, both autologous and allogeneic.[57] A variety of mechanisms for the formation of autoantibodies have been postulated and include:

1. neutrophil sensitization to alloantigens shared with engrafted progenitor cells as a result of sensitization by transfused blood products;
2. altered T-helper/suppressor cell ratios;
3. abnormal neutrophil antigen expression secondary to *in vitro* stem cell damage;
4. an altered immune state secondary to the underlying malignancy.

Infective neutropenia

In children, viral infections are a common cause of neutropenia. The commonest offending organisms include respiratory syncytial virus, influenza, hepatitis (A and B), measles, varicella and rubella.[58] The neutropenia usually corresponds to the period of viremia and may result from increased neutrophil utilization following viral-induced tissue damage.[59] Neutropenia in this setting usually develops over 1–2 days and can persist for up to a week without serious consequences. Transient neutropenia is also often seen in association with infectious mononucleosis and may be the result of neutrophil destruction by antineutrophil antibodies.[60] Neutropenia has also been described in association with tuberculosis, brucellosis, typhoid and paratyphoid fevers, malaria and rickettsial infections.[58] In most cases, the pathophysiology of the neutropenia remains obscure.

Septic neutropenia may be particularly profound and may be the result of severe marrow toxic changes affecting myelopoiesis.[61] Bacteremic neutropenia may also result from excessive destruction of neutrophils,[62] and the neutropenia may be the result of complement activation and aggregation of neutrophils in the pulmonary vasculature contributing to the adult respiratory distress syndrome. Other possible mechanisms include neutrophil destruction following microbial phagocytosis.

Drug-associated neutropenia

The commonest cause of drug-induced neutropenia is that associated with treatment for malignancy. Outside that context, drug-induced neutropenia can be defined as a severe and selective reduction in the numbers of circulating neutrophils ($<0.2 \times 10^9$/l) due to an idiosyncratic reaction to the offending drug. This also implies that drug-associated neutropenia is unpredictable in its frequency and distribution. The list of drugs which have been implicated in neutropenia is extensive[63] but is summarized in Table 16.3.

In most cases, the pathogenesis in children is unknown. Girls are more often affected than boys. Three basic mechanisms are suggested:

1. increased *sensitivity of myeloid progenitor cells* to drugs, e.g. phenothiazines.[63] Such compounds may act as haptens, stimulating the formation of antibodies which then complex with the drug and cause myeloid progenitor suppression. Penicillin, thiouracil and gold can also cause neutropenia by this mechanism.[64]
2. alterations in the *immune response* as a result of drug administration, e.g. quinidine, which can activate a cellular immune response, or phenytoin which produces a humoral response, both of which may suppress myelopoiesis.[63]
3. differences in *drug pharmacokinetics* leading to toxic drug (or metabolite) levels in the marrow microenvironment, e.g. sulfasalazine, where patients who are slow acetylators show greater toxicity than those who are fast acetylators.[65]

It is probable that genetic factors also contribute.

Bone marrow appearances in drug-induced neutropenia are very variable. Myeloid precursors may be normal, reduced or increased. Frequently there is a 'maturation arrest' with a reduction in mature forms. After withdrawal of the drug, there is an increase in early myeloid forms followed by a rapid expansion of all myeloid elements.

It is not usually practical or possible to predict the onset of neutropenia with serial blood counts. If neutropenia occurs, withdrawal of the offending drug is the most important therapeutic action. Antibiotics should be used to treat infective episodes. Corticosteroids and granulocyte transfusions are of little benefit. The duration of the neutropenia is very variable. Acute idiosyncratic reactions may last only a few days, whereas chronic episodes may persist for years. Immune-mediated neutropenia usually lasts for about 7 days.

EVALUATION OF NEUTROPENIA

Particular attention should focus on the frequency and duration of infective symptoms and any drugs or potentially

Table 16.3 Drugs causing neutropenia.

Antimicrobial agents—particularly penicillins and sulfonamides
Antirheumatics—particularly gold, phenylbutazone and penicillamine
Sedatives—including barbiturates and benzodiazepines
Antithyroid drugs
Phenothiazines
Antipyretics

Table 16.4 Investigation of the child with neutropenia.

Full blood counts at least weekly to check for cyclical neutropenia and to confirm persistent absolute neutropenia

Blood film examination for white cell morphology

Leukocyte alkaline phosphatase and peroxidase reactions, to detect abnormal neutrophil granulation

Quantitative immunoglobulins, to exclude hypogammaglobulinemia

Lymphocyte T and B subsets, to exclude reticular dysgenesis

Complement levels, to exclude dysgammaglobinemia

HLA antibodies, to exclude association with neutropenia*

Neutrophil antibodies, to exclude isoimmune and autoimmune neutropenia*

Bone marrow examination, to exclude agranulocytosis, maturation arrest, dyserythropoiesis or megaloblastic change

Bone marrow culture:
  Increased colonies with abnormal morphology suggests severe congenital neutropenia
  Increased colonies with normal morphology suggests Shwachman syndrome or chronic benign neutropenia
  Reduced colonies suggests immune neutropenia, chronic neutropenia or progenitor cell disorder

Autoantibodies to exclude systemic lupus erythematosus or Felty's syndrome

B$_{12}$ and folate assays to exclude megaloblastic neutropenia

Exocrine pancreatic function tests to exclude Shwachman's syndrome

Sucrose lysis and Ham's test to exclude paroxysmal nocturnal hemoglobinuria

Chromosomal analysis to exclude Fanconi's anemia

Skeletal survey to exclude cartilage hair syndrome, Fanconi's anemia, Shwachman's syndrome, dyskeratosis congenita

Rebuck skin window to exclude neutrophil chemotactic defect

Plasma and urine amino acids to exclude organic acidemia

Neutrophil stimulation tests (see Table 16.5)

*May be performed on the patient's mother in some cases.

toxic agents which may produce neutropenia. A family history may indicate other family members with repeated infections. Physical examination should concentrate on any evidence of superficial infection (e.g. skin and mucus membranes), hepatosplenomegaly, lymphadenopathy or any dysmorphic or phenotypic abnormality. Table 16.4 gives a basis for the investigation of a neutropenic child. This list should be considered only as a guide. In many cases, a large number of the tests may prove necessary. Table 16.5 indicates some neutrophil stimulation tests which may also occasionally be helpful.

Table 16.5 Neutrophil stimulation tests.

Hydrocortisone stress test
  5 mg/kg of hydrocortisone hemisuccinate intravenously and monitor neutrophil count hourly from 0 to 6 h
  A normal response is a rise in the absolute neutrophil count of >2.0 × 10^9/l
  Cells are released into the circulating pool from the bone marrow
  Abnormal results seen in chronic neutropenia, drug- or toxin-induced hypoplasia, infection-induced hypoplasia, ineffective myelopoiesis and increased peripheral neutrophil destruction

Epinephrine (adrenaline) stress test
  0.03 ml/kg of 1:10 000 epinephrine subcutaneously and monitor neutrophil count at 0, 5, 10, 15 and 30 min
  A normal response shows a doubling of the absolute neutrophil count within 20 min
  Cells are mobilized from the marginating pool

NEUTROPHILIA

In adults, neutrophilia can be applied to patients with an absolute neutrophil count $>7.5 \times 10^9$/l. This definition is too restrictive in children, as neutrophil counts are age-dependent (see Reference values at the front of this book).

An increase in the number of circulating neutrophils results from an alteration in the normal steady-state of neutrophil production, transit, migration and destruction. Neutrophilia is usually the result of one of the following mechanisms:

1. increased neutrophil mobilization from the marginating pools or bone marrow
2. prolonged neutrophil survival due to impaired transit into the tissues;
3. expansion of the neutrophil circulating pool due to (a) increased progenitor cell proliferation, and (b) increased frequency of cell division of committed neutrophil precursors.[66]

ACUTE NEUTROPHILIA

Neutrophils can be mobilized very rapidly, as indicated by the adrenaline stress test where they are released by the marginating cell pool in less than 20 min. It has been postulated that adrenaline stimulates receptors on endothelial cells, with the release of cyclic AMP, and reduces neutrophil adhesion. This mechanism is probably of particular importance when neutrophilia is associated with acute bacterial infection, stress, exercise and various toxic agents.

A slightly slower rise in neutrophil count occurs when cells are released from the bone marrow storage pool; this is demonstrated by the hydrocortisone stress test, where neutrophilia may not appear for a few hours. The response may also be mediated via endotoxins released by various microbial agents, or complement activation with the formation of C3e.[67] Corticosteroids may also reduce the passage of circulating neutrophils into the tissues, and congenital disorders of neutrophil motility, such as congenital neutrophil actin dysfunction syndrome, may have a similar effect. The phenomenon may be reflected by an abnormal Rebuck skin window test.[68]

CHRONIC NEUTROPHILIA

Chronic neutrophilia is usually the result of prolonged stimulation of neutrophil production resulting from increased marrow myeloid progenitor cell proliferation. The majority of reactions last a few days or weeks but some may persist for many months. Chronic neutrophilia may follow long-term corticosteroid therapy, long-standing inflammatory reactions, infections or chronic blood loss. Infections include less common organisms such as disseminated herpes and varicella, poliomyelitis and leptospira.

Chronic inflammatory conditions are frequently associated with neutrophilia, and include juvenile rheumatoid arthritis and Kawasaki's disease. Splenectomy or functional hyposplenism may result in neutrophilia due to reduced removal of neutrophils from the circulation. Other 'noninfectious' causes of neutrophilia include diabetic ketoacidosis, disseminated malignancy, hemolysis, severe burns, uremia and postoperative states.

LEUKEMOID REACTIONS

'Leukemoid reaction' is an overused term and is not pathognomonic of any disease process. It is usually applied to a chronic neutrophilia where there is a marked leukocytosis (usually $> 20 \times 10^9$/l). A usual feature is a 'shift to the left' of myeloid cells in the blood, including metamyelocytes, myelocytes, promyelocytes and occasional myeloblasts. The main causes are listed in Table 16.6. Leukemoid reactions may be confused with leukoerythroblastic anemias, where similar myeloid precursors may be seen, but the main differentiating feature is the co-existence of nucleated red cells in the peripheral blood, and the leukocyte count may not be raised.

Leukemoid reactions and myeloproliferative disease

A transient leukemoid reaction of the newborn may be seen in up to one-third of patients with Down's syndrome. The reaction usually regresses spontaneously within 12 months, but at its zenith may be indistinguishable from acute leukemia. Bone marrow chromosomal changes may also be found. The reaction appears to arise from an intrinsic intracellular defect in the regulation of neutrophil proliferation and maturation within the bone marrow.[69] A true leukemia may follow later in childhood in some cases.

A familial myeloproliferative disease resembling chronic myeloid leukemia (CML) has also been described.[70] As well as neutrophilia and immature precursors in the blood, such patients are anemic and have hepatosplenomegaly. Some of those described die in early life, whereas others improve with time.

Differentiation between a leukemoid reaction and chronic granulocytic leukemia is usually straightforward; the presence of massive splenomegaly, a low leukocyte alkaline phosphatase score and the Philadelphia chromosome indicate the latter condition. Juvenile CML (better known as chronic myelomonocytic leukemia [CMML]) is less likely to be confused with a leukemoid reaction, as thrombocytopenia is usually present and frequently there is a raised concentration of HbF.

NEONATAL NEUTROPHILIA

When compared to those of adults, neutrophil counts are relatively high in the first few days of life, being in the range $8-15 \times 10^9$/l, but by 3 days of age they usually fall to between 1.5 and 5×10^9/l. This early physiologic neutrophilia is often associated with a few myeloid precursors (promyelocytes and blast cells) in the peripheral blood, together with segmented forms. Persisting neutrophilia beyond the first few days of life requires explanation and may be associated with bacterial infection.

EOSINOPHILIA

Eosinophils are proportionately reduced in numbers during the neonatal period. They also exhibit a diurnal variation, being relatively higher during the evenings. Both of these features are of no clinical importance.

The causes of eosinophilia are legion but can be considered under the following headings: allergy, parasites, malignancy, drugs, skin disorders, gastrointestinal disorders, hypereosinophilic syndrome, and a group of miscellaneous disorders.

Allergy

This is the commonest cause of eosinophilia in the western world. Acute allergic reactions may cause 'leukemoid' eosinophilic responses with absolute eosinophil counts exceeding 20×10^9/l. Chronic allergic states are rarely associated with counts $> 2 \times 10^9$/l. Over 75% of asthmatic children have eosinophil counts of $> 0.6 \times 10^9$/l. Other allergic disorders such as hay fever and acute urticaria are also associated with modest eosinophilia.

Parasites

Outside the western world, invasive parasitic infections are the commonest cause of eosinophilia. The helminths usually produce a more marked response than do protozoan infections.[71] The eosinophilia associated with parasitic infections is probably not due to a specific factor in the parasites, but to a granulomatous response of the tissues requiring the participation of intact parasites. Some organisms, such as *Giardia lamblia*, do not induce eosinophilia, probably because they do not enter the circulation but remain localized in the gastrointestinal tract. *Toxicara canis* may result in a marked

---

Table 16.6 Causes of leukemoid reactions.

Infections
   Bacterial (especially *Staph. aureus* and *Strep. pneumoniae*)
   Tuberculosis
   Brucellosis
   Toxoplasmosis
Marrow infiltrative disease (often with leukoerythroblastosis)
Systemic disease
   Acute glomerulonephritis
   Acute liver failure

systemic involvement with respiratory, retinal and central nervous system signs. Marked leukocytosis and eosinophilia may persist for years.

Malignant disease

Mild eosinophilia may be associated with Hodgkin's disease in about one-quarter of patients, although occasionally a very marked eosinophilia may be seen. Eosinophilia is also seen occasionally in association with non-Hodgkin's lymphoma, CML (often with basophilia), acute leukemias (uncommon), malignant histiocytosis and brain tumors.

Drugs

Of the myriad of drugs causing raised eosinophil counts, many are preceded by the prefix 'anti', such as antibiotics (penicillin, ampicillin, cephalosporins, nitrofurantoin), antituberculins (para-aminosalicylic acid), antiepileptics (phenytoin) and antihypertensives (hydralazine).

Skin disorders

A variety of skin diseases have been associated with eosinophilia, including atopic dermatitis, eczema, acute urticaria, toxic epidermal necrolysis and dermatitis herpetiformis.

Gastrointestinal disorders

Crohn's disease is often associated with modest eosinophilia, whereas in ulcerative colitis there may be large numbers of eosinophils infiltrating the bowel and relatively few in the blood. Milk intolerance and gastrointestinal saccharide intolerance may be associated with a moderate eosinophilia. Chronic liver disease, in particular chronic hepatitis, may also produce a mild rise in circulating eosinophils.

Hypereosinophilic syndrome

In 1968, Hardy and Anderson[72] drew attention to the fact that persistent hypereosinophilia of any type could be associated with a range of similar complications, and they grouped these together as hypereosinophilic syndrome. Cushid et al[73] restricted the diagnosis to patients in whom no underlying cause for the hypereosinophilia could be shown.

To make the diagnosis, the following criteria have been suggested: a peripheral blood eosinophilia of $>1.5 \times 10^9/l$ persisting for >6 months, resulting in organ system dysfunction and the absence of any obvious cause for the eosinophilia.

The term encompasses various syndromes including disseminated eosinophilic collagen disease and Loeffler's fibroblastic endocarditis with eosinophilia.[74] Some patients have hypereosinophilia with only lung involvement and angioedema. Others present with, or develop, severe cardiac or edema.

central nervous system complications. A third group has eosinophilic cytogenetic abnormalities and features of an eosinophilic leukemic process (see below).

A cause for the condition remains to be identified, although it has been postulated that it may be autoimmune or neoplastic in nature.[75] Although it is commonest between the ages of 20 and 50 years, hypereosinophilic syndrome is well-recognized in children, although it is very rare below the age of 5.[74]

Involvement of the cardiovascular system is the main cause of morbidity and mortality. In the heart, both ventricles are usually involved but the cardiac outflow tracts are spared. Mitral and tricuspid regurgitation are common, and endocardial thrombi give rise to embolic disease. Disease of small blood vessels with intimal thickening also occurs. Cases previously described as Loeffler's syndrome are probably hypereosinophilia with cardiac involvement. Other organs may be involved, as indicated by hepatosplenomegaly, pulmonary fibrosis, central nervous system damage, fever, weight loss and anemia.

Eosinophilic leukemia

Rickles and Miller[76] suggest that the following criteria should be met for a diagnosis of eosinophilic leukemia: pronounced and persistent eosinophilia associated with immature forms, either in the peripheral blood or bone marrow, $>5\%$ of bone marrow blasts, tissue infiltration by immature eosinophilic cells, and an acute history with anemia, thrombocytopenia and increased infection.

Chromosomal abnormalities, abnormal leukocyte alkaline phosphatase activity, high serum B_{12} levels and an associated basophilia suggest leukemic change and a poor prognosis due to eventual bone marrow failure, but it is more common for patients to succumb to cardiac damage secondary to endocardial and myocardial fibrosis.

The mainstay of treatment for hypereosinophilic syndrome is corticosteroids. These have brought about a notable improvement in survival and prognosis. Hydroxyurea can be used in non-responders or to allow a reduction in steroid dosage. Vincristine has also been used in association with aggressive disease. Many patients are given anticoagulants. Treatment is given with the aim of reducing the leukocytosis and eosinophilia and alleviating organ dysfunction.

Miscellaneous causes

Most immune deficiency syndromes are associated with a mild eosinophilia. This is particularly noteworthy in Wiskott–Aldrich syndrome, but may be due in part to the severe eczema associated with that condition. In children with hypogammaglobulinemia, the presence of eosinophilia may be an indication of *Pneumocystis carinii* infection. Peritoneal dialysis and hemodialysis for chronic renal failure and congenital heart disease (with or without hyposplenism) have also been associated with a moderate eosinophilia,[77] as has thrombocytopenia/absent radius syndrome (see Chapter 24).

Two fungal conditions can produce a marked eosinophilia—coccidioidomycosis and allergic bronchopulmonary aspergillosis.

BASOPHILIA

As basophils are the least common of the granulocytes, they are the most subject to counting error. A true basophilia is most commonly associated with hypersensitivity reactions to drugs or food substances or in association with acute urticaria.

Inflammatory and infective conditions such as ulcerative colitis, juvenile rheumatoid arthritis, renal failure, influenza, chicken pox and tuberculosis are also associated with a mild-to-moderate basophilia.[78] Other conditions include Hodgkin's disease, cirrhosis, chronic hemolysis and post splenectomy.

Basophilia is particularly associated with adult-type (Philadelphia chromosome-positive) CML. The cells may appear abnormal both morphologically and ultrastructurally. Basophil counts may exceed 30% of the white cell population and may rise during the accelerated stage of the disease (see Chapter 20).

MONOCYTOSIS

The absolute monocyte count is age dependent, and during the first 2 weeks of life the level is $> 1.0 \times 10^9$/l. Thereafter, the monocyte count rarely exceeds this figure or 10% of the total leukocyte count.

Monocytes are derived from bone marrow progenitor cells, but as there is no substantial bone marrow reserve pool, mature monocytes are released into the peripheral circulation several days earlier than neutrophils following an

Table 16.7 Conditions associated with a reactive monocytosis.

Infections	Connective tissue disorder
Infective endocarditis	Ulcerative colitis
Tuberculosis	Sarcoidosis
Brucellosis	Crohn's disease
Typhoid fever	Miscellaneous
Congenital syphilis	Post splenectomy
Leishmaniasis	
Malignant disease	
Myelodysplastic syndromes	
Myeloid leukemias	
Hodgkin's disease	
Non-Hodgkin's lymphomas	

episode of myelosuppression. They are sometimes a useful harbinger of engraftment following allogeneic marrow transplantation.

Conditions associated with a monocytosis can be grouped into infections, malignant diseases, connective tissue disorders, granulomatous diseases and miscellaneous disease (Table 16.7).

DISORDERS OF GRANULOCYTE FUNCTION

Disorders of granulocyte function usually produce signs and symptoms similar to those associated with neutropenia or low levels of complement and immunoglobulins. The possibility of a granulocyte dysfunction should be considered after these disorders have been excluded.

Screening tests

Screening for abnormalities of neutrophil function may involve the following investigations:

- *Examination of the blood film.* This can identify large abnormal granules in Chédiak–Higashi disease, or bilobed nuclei with a distorted nuclear membrane in neutrophil-specific granule deficiency. The Pelger-Huet anomaly may be seen in various marrow stem cell disorders, Döhle-body-like inclusions in the May Hegglin anomaly, and hypersegmented neutrophils in megaloblastic anaemia.
- *Rebuck skin window.* This measures the migration of neutrophils on to a glass cover slip applied to a superficial skin abrasion. Another way of assessing neutrophil chemotaxis involves the Boyden chamber and neutrophil adhesion can be determined *in vitro* by the cells' adherence to nylon wool.
- *Respiratory burst.* This is evaluated using the nitrobluetetrazolium (NBT) reduction test. Neutrophils are activated in the presence of NBT which produces a dark precipitate in cells producing superoxide (O_2^-). Respiratory burst activity can be measured directly as oxygen consumption, O_2^- production (using cytochrome C reduction) or hydrogen peroxide production, and indirectly using neutrophil chemiluminescence.[79]
- *Special stains.* These can be used to detect deficiencies in the enzymes myeloperoxidase and alkaline phosphatase.
- *Additional tests.* These include measurement of neutrophil degranulation and can be used to differentiate between disorders of primary and secondary granules. Bacterial and fungal phagocytosis and killing can also be measured. These tests are more research tools than of value in screening.

It is convenient to consider the various granulocyte disorders under the same headings as neutrophil function, namely adherence and margination, chemotaxis, ingestion and recognition, degranulation, oxidative metabolism and oxidant scavenging.

DISORDERS OF ADHERENCE AND MARGINATION

Leukocyte adhesion deficiency

Leukocyte adhesion deficiency (LAD) is a rare disorder of neutrophil adhesion and chemotaxis that results in severe bacterial infections.[80] The molecular basis for LAD involves 3 integrins (adhesion molecules) all sharing an identical $\beta 2$ subunit (CD18) and distinct α subunit (CD11). Patients express either structurally abnormal or reduced amounts of β subunit, resulting in a deficiency of all 3 integrins. Different mutations leading to various degrees of clinical severity have been identified.[81]

Reduced or absent expression of all 3 $\beta 2$ integrins in LAD leukocytes results in 2 major functional defects. One is the failure of the phagocyte to adhere to or migrate through the endothelial lining. The other is the inability of the leukocyte to bind C3bi oposonized organisms. CD11/CD18 is the C3bi receptor for the neutrophil and all phagocytic functions (e.g. C3bi-mediated phagocytosis, enzyme release, and oxygen radical production) are severely affected. This combined dysfunction leads to a severe illness in most patients although children with a less severe propensity to infection have been described.

A second type of LAD has been described (LAD II).[82] In two unrelated children, the defect in leukocyte adhesion was due to the absence of the Sialyl-Lewis X ligand of the neutrophil E- and P-selectin receptors. There were normal levels of CD18 expression.

Children with LAD deficiency may present with delayed separation of the umbilical cord. Recurrent infections (particularly pseudomonal), poor pus formation and peripheral blood leukocytosis are frequently seen. The clinical presentation of LAD I is however very heterogeneous whereas children with LAD II may have associated mental retardation, short stature, abnormal facies and the Bombay (hh) red cell phenotype.

Diagnosis is usually made on the basis of decreased neutrophil chemotaxisis and adhesion. Deficient CD18 and CD11 on flow cytometry confirms LAD I whereas a deficiency of Sialyl-Lewis X is indicative of LAD II.

Long-term antibiotic therapy is usually necessary to control infections and acute exacerbations require intensive parenteral therapy. Severely affected patients (CD11 <0.3%) who have a matched sibling donor should be considered for transplantation.

Acquired neutrophil adherence disorders

Various drugs are known to affect the adhesion of neutrophils to surfaces and may result in a marked transient neutrophilia. Epinephrine (adrenaline) and corticosteroids are probably the best examples, and these responses form part of the basis of the epinepherine and corticosteroid stimulation tests. Epinephrine causes the stimulation of cyclic AMP in the vascular endothelium which appears to reduce neutrophil adherence, and hence marginating neutrophils are released into the circulating pool.[83] Steroids may change neutrophil adherence by affecting arachidonic acid metabolism, impairing neutrophil fatty acid metabolism, or interfering with the binding of chemotactic molecules to cells.[84,85]

Increased neutrophil aggregation has been reported with granulocyte transfusions that have been obtained by filtration rather than centrifugation, and with amphotericin B, particularly when these two therapies are combined. Neutrophil aggregation can result in the formation of pulmonary aggregates causing respiratory insufficiency.[86]

Complement activation, and the generation of C5a in particular, is an important trigger to the activation of neutrophils and increased adhesion. The reaction is probably mediated via membrane glycoproteins. Stimulating factors probably include bacterial sepsis, thermal injury, extensive tissue necrosis and possibly hemodialysis. Aggregated neutrophils may then result in the liberation of proteases, endothelial cell damage and, in the lungs, the development of adult respiratory distress syndrome.[87]

CHEMOTACTIC DISORDERS

Chemotaxis refers to the attractions of cells by chemical substances; it has been recognized since the turn of the century, when Metchnikoff[88] appreciated the importance of phagocytes and their ability to recognize bacterial products.

Normal chemotaxis is dependent upon an integrated chain of events. First, chemotactic factors must be produced in order to create a 'chemotactic gradient'. Monocytes and neutrophils must then process their appropriate receptors to identify these factors and be able to identify the direction of the gradient. Neutrophils must then be able to adhere to the endothelial wall and other connective tissues, and migrate to the point of inflammation (margination) with the aid of cytoplasmic contractile proteins. Finally, the stimulating chemotactic factors must be inactivated once an adequate neutrophil/monocyte response has taken place.

Phagocytes (i.e. neutrophils and monocytes) are known to contain plasma membrane receptors for leukokines, bacterial products, complement and CSFs. Receptors are more densely concentrated on the cell's leading edge, and intracellular receptors for the complement factor CR3 (C3bi) have also been identified.[89] Alcohols can increase phagocyte receptor affinity whereas amphotericin can produce the opposite effect.[90] Minute concentrations of GM-CSF can result in an initial rise and subsequent fall in receptor affinity.[91]

Neutrophils cannot swim; they crawl towards sites of inflammation. Chemotactic factors reduce the normal cellular negative charge and enhance endothelial adherence. Increased adhesion appears to involve the CD11/CD18 neutrophil glycoprotein complex as well as endotoxins and interleukins.[92] After surface attachment, neutrophils become more elongated, with the nucleus moving to the back of the cell with the granule-rich cytoplasm and the microtubular apparatus positioned between the nucleus and the front of the cell. Both the microtubule apparatus and actin polymerization changes play a critical role in cell orientation and locomotion.[93]

Lymphokines are also important in chemotaxis. γ-Interferon stimulates monocyte chemotaxis.[94] Tumor necrosis factor (TNF) causes increased adherence of neutrophils to endothelial cells and increased phagocytic capacity.[92]

Laboratory diagnosis

Most *in vitro* assays of chemotaxis measure the movement of neutrophils under agarose or through a cellulose nitrate filter (Boyden chamber). After a set period, the cells are fixed and stained and their patterns of movement analyzed. Migration under agarose is not as sensitive as through cellulose nitrate filters, and conditions such as Chédiak–Higashi syndrome may be missed as the agarose method does not detect defects in deformability. The agarose method, however, requires fewer neutrophils and identification of individual cell types is easier.

Radioisotope assays of chemotaxis using ^{51}Cr-labeled neutrophils are simple and, when used in the form of a multicell micro-assay, require small numbers of cells and minimal chemoattractant.[95]

In vivo assessment of neutrophil movement usually involves the Rebuck skin window or skin blister technique (see above). The Rebuck assay is rather non-specific as it measures not only chemotaxis but also the ability of leukocytes to adhere to glass. Nevertheless, the technique provides a simple screening test for the integrity of the inflammatory response. The suction blister apparatus yields information on neutrophil locomotion and is particularly useful for studying large numbers of functional neutrophils and quantitation of the number and types of cells arriving at inflammatory exudates.

Clinical features

Several chemotactic disorders have specific and distinct clinical features. These include Chédiak–Higashi syndrome, Job's syndrome, CR3-receptor deficiency and localized juvenile periodontitis. Other disorders may not be associated with such specific characteristics, but all are associated with increased susceptibility to a variety of infections, including sinusitis, gingivitis, pneumonia, bronchiectasis, otitis, dermatitis and other skin infections. Frequent and severe soft tissue abscesses are also commonly associated with chemotactic disorders, and recurrent or chronic fungal and bacterial infections can occur despite a peripheral blood leukocytosis.

Pneumonia and lung abscesses are the most frequent fatal complications.

Infections and dermatitis may present in the neonatal period but thereafter may be periodic and unpredictable. *Staphylococcus aureus* is the commonest infecting organism, but Gram-negative bacilli, fungi, *Haemophilus influenzae* and *Staph. epidermidis* may also be troublesome. Streptococci and particularly *Strep. pneumoniae* are not associated with chemotactic disorders, being more common in children with hypogammaglobulinemia.

It is important to remember that severe infections may be associated with minimal signs and symptoms, probably because of the delayed movement of leukocytes to the focus of infection. The infections tend to become indolent, with a high recurrence rate and poor antimicrobial response. Determined investigation and therapy is therefore required.

Cellular disorders

CR3 deficiency

CR3 (C3bi receptor) deficiency usually presents in infancy with delayed separation of the umbilicus. The children can exhibit poor wound healing, with recurrent bacterial and fungal infections and little or no pus formation. Mucositis and oral periodontal infections are particularly common, as are more serious osteomyelitis and pneumonia. *Pseudomonas* and *Staph. aureus* are the commonest infecting organisms.

As well as defective chemotaxis, a deficiency of neutrophil CR3 can be demonstrated using fluorescent, flow cytometry, or peroxidase-labeled anti-CR3 antibodies.

The mode of inheritance is autosomal recessive. CR3 is related to the CD11/CD18 neutrophil glycoprotein complex, and the severity of the glycoprotein deficiency correlates with the clinical severity of the condition. CR3 is also important in neutrophil adherence to endothelial cells, and its expression can be increased by endotoxin, interleukin-1 and TNF.

Chédiak–Higashi syndrome

This is a rare, recessively inherited abnormality characterized by partial oculocutaneous albinism, mental retardation, photophobia, peripheral neuropathy and recurrent infections, particularly oral and cutaneous. All cells containing lysosomal granules show giant forms which are the result of fusion of different granules (Fig. 16.2). The majority of patients enter a phase of accelerated morbidity, usually during their second decade, which is characterized by a stormy febrile course, pancytopenia and widespread lymphohistiocytic organ infiltrates. Those patients who do not suffer an accelerated phase fall prey to recurrent serious infections, progressive peripheral neuropathy and, sometimes, CNS disease with cerebellar ataxia, cranial nerve palsies and raised intracranial pressure.[93] The neurologic

343

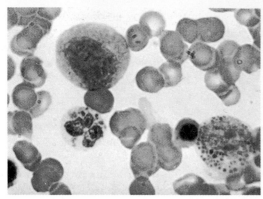

Fig. 16.2 Giant neutrophil inclusions seen in the Chédiak–Higashi syndrome. A myelocyte in the picture also shows abnormal giant granules.

Table 16.8 Laboratory features of the Chédiak–Higashi syndrome.[96]

Stable phase
Neutrophils
  Giant azurophilic and specific granules
  Neutropenia resulting from ineffective myelopoiesis
  Reduced bacterial activity:
  Impaired chemotaxis
  Delayed degranulation
  Reduced granule proteases

Monocytes/macrophages
  Giant inclusion bodies
  Impaired chemotaxis

Lymphocytes (NK cells) + platelets
  Giant cytoplasmic granules
  Absence of dense bodies
  Platelet storage pool defect

Accelerated phase
  Epstein–Barr infection
  Diffuse polyclonal non-neoplastic lymphohistiocytic infiltrate
  Histiocytic hemophagocytosis
  Massive hepatosplenomegaly resulting in pancytopenia

effects may be the result of giant granule infiltration of cells in the CNS, particularly Schwann cells.

The hematologic features of Chédiak–Higashi syndrome are summarized in Table 16.8. The abnormal cytoplasmic granules form during myelopoiesis, and the majority of marrow progenitor stem cells are defective as judged by in vitro colony assays.[97] This observation has led to the suggestion that the marrow stem cells are affected by the genetic defect, which is as yet unidentified.[98] The moderate neutropenia seen is the result of ineffective medullary myelopoiesis and recurrent infections are the result of neutropenia together with defective chemotaxis, degranulation and antibacterial activity.[99]

It has been suggested that natural killer (NK) cells in Chédiak–Higashi syndrome possess abnormal membrane and cytoplasmic structural components which are necessary for their function.[100] In addition, storage pool platelet defects have been described, resulting in prolonged bleeding times

and hemorrhagic manifestations associated with normal platelet counts.[101]

Both Gram-positive and -negative organisms are troublesome for children with Chédiak–Higashi syndrome. Infections are often repeated and debilitating, with the skin and mucous membranes most often affected. *Staph. aureus* is the commonest organism.

Although the basic nature of the underlying abnormality is unknown, it is likely that anomalous neutrophil membrane function is an important factor in the functional defect.[102] The neutrophils act as though unable to control membrane activation. They spontaneously aggregate molecules into caps, and show increased oxygen consumption, reduced surface adherence and impaired chemotactic responses.[103] They also form giant neutrophil granules, changing the primary granules into large secondary lysosomes which have a reduced enzyme content.[104] Despite normal ingestion, neutrophils kill micro-organisms slowly due to the reduced and erratic delivery of diluted hydrolytic enzymes from the giant granules.[105] An abnormal membrane fluidity has been demonstrated in neutrophils and red cells of patients,[106] and this concept may serve to link the abnormal motility, granule fusion, platelet abnormality and abnormal NK cell structure seen in the syndrome.

Management of Chédiak–Higashi syndrome is based predominantly on the treatment of infectious episodes. Prophylactic co-trimoxazole may be helpful, but acute infections should be treated aggressively. High doses of ascorbic acid have been found to be helpful in some, but not all, patients.[107] Treatment for the accelerated phase has included vincristine, corticosteroids and antithymocyte globulin, but without obvious benefit.[100] BMT has been successfully performed in a few patients.[108]

Kartagener's syndrome

Patients with this disorder experience recurrent infections of the respiratory tract, middle ear and sinuses, and have associated situs inversus. Neutrophils exhibit defective locomotion and chemotaxis.[109]

Specific granule deficiency

Specific (secondary) granules contain leukocyte adhesion molecules, enzymes important for the inflammatory cascade and components of the oxidase system.[110] Specific granule-deficient neutrophils lack the contents of secondary granules and are also devoid of defensins present in primary granules, suggesting defective regulation of the synthesis of various lysosomal proteins. This results in decreased chemotaxis, impaired superoxide production and low bactericidal activity.

This very rare disorder can be detected by blood film examination in patients who suffer from repeated infections.[96] Standard Romanowsky stains show agranular neutrophils, whereas peroxidase stain shows the primary granules to be intact. The absence of specific granules can be confirmed by immunochemical stains or demonstration of the absence of lactoferrin in either mature neutrophils or bone marrow precursors. There are also abnormalities of nuclear shape resembling the Pelger-Huet abnormality. Individuals with specific granule deficiency are prone to recurrent bacterial and fungal infections of the skin and deep tissues[111] and a variety of abnormalities of neutrophil function. These include poor chemotaxis, failure of neutrophil disaggregation following stimulation and reduced recruitment of monocytes to sites of inflammation by neutrophils.[112]

The precise molecular defect has not been identified but the fault appears to be confined to the myeloid series.

Treatment is based on the prompt use of appropriate antibiotics with surgical drainage of abscesses. Morbidity and mortality may be less than those associated with phagocytic defects.

Localized juvenile periodontitis

This familial condition usually affects older children and adolescents, and infection is usually localized to the mouth, with premature loss of teeth and periodontitis resulting in alveolar bone resorption.[113] There is a moderate defect of leukocyte chemotaxis due to the bacterium *Capnocytophaga* which infects the gums and secretes an inhibitor of neutrophil chemotaxis.[114]

Lazy leukocyte syndrome

Several miscellaneous disorders have been described in which there is abnormal neutrophil chemotaxis. The lazy leucocyte syndrome is characterized by recurrent dermatitis, otitis media, gingivitis, respiratory infections and congenital neutropenia.[115] Bone marrow examination shows normal myeloid precursors, but abnormal chemotaxis is demonstrable using the Rebuck skin window (see above). The condition is relatively mild.

Humoral disorders

Hyperimmunoglobulin-E syndrome (Job's syndrome)

Hyperimmunoglobuin-E (HIE) syndrome is characterized by recurrent skin and sinopulmonary infections beginning in infancy or early childhood. Typical infective problems include the development of subcutaneous abscesses and chronic mucocutaneous candidiasis, usually involving the esophagus, vagina and nails. Other problems include pneumonia, recurrent ear infections, dermatitis and chronic eczema. Chronic lung illnesses can be the most dangerous and debilitating, with bronchiectasis and fistula formation.[116] Patients frequently have characteristic facies with a broad nasal bridge and prominent jaw. The most com-

monly associated bacterial infections are *Staph. aureus* and *H. influenzae*.

HIE syndrome is extremely rare but should be considered in children and infants presenting with severe atopic dermatitis and recurrent staphylococcal skin infections. Most such patients will have other disorders, including primary skin complaints, hypogammaglobulinemia, Wiskott–Aldrich syndrome or Di George's syndrome (see Chapter 25). The diagnosis is based on the clinical history and the presence of an IgE level usually at least 10 times the age-related value.[117]

The associated neutrophil chemotactic defect[118] is present only intermittently. Although immune complexes have been shown to inhibit neutrophil chemotaxis, serum from patients with HIE syndrome does not affect normal phagocyte function; however, their mononuclear cells have been shown to produce an inhibitor of leukocyte chemotaxis. Thus, the suggestion is that the neutrophils themselves are not abnormal, but that some sporadically produced factor causes the reversible chemotactic defect, a factor which does not appear to be plasma derived, but may be of monocytic origin, or may be an IgE-mediated histamine release.[119] Increased IgE and abnormal neutrophil chemotaxis may be related to a decreased production of γ-interferon and TNF.

Treatment is much the same as for other leukocyte disorders and is based on the effective use of antibiotics. Surgery may be necessary for abscess drainage. Other therapies that have been tried include ascorbic acid, cimetidine and levamisole. None has been shown to be of proven benefit, and a double-blind placebo-controlled trial actually demonstrated an increased incidence of infection in patients receiving levamisole.[117] As patients with HIE syndrome have low levels of circulating antibody against bacterial antigens, a trial of intravenous immunoglobulin would appear logical, but no comparative study has been performed. There is anecdotal evidence that plasmapheresis may be beneficial for patients who fail to respond to antibiotics.[116] Administration of γ-interferon is under investigation as this cytokine has been shown to improve the chemotaxis of patients' neutrophils *in vitro*.[120]

Chemotactic inhibitors of the neutrophil response

Various clinical disorders have been described where the production of inhibitors interferes with the normal response of neutrophils to chemotactic factors. The mechanisms by which these inhibitors work are not known. Some immune complex diseases are associated with such chemotactic defects.[121] IgG-binding to neutrophils has been shown to inhibit locomotion. Similar effects have been seen in patients with IgA paraproteinemias and solid tumors (mainly melanoma and breast cancer in adults).

Viral and bacterial products can also interfere with chemotaxis. Herpes simplex and influenza viruses can inhibit monocyte chemotaxis but this has not been shown with vaccinia, polio or retroviruses. Mouse cytomegalovirus infection can reduce chemotaxis but this has not been demonstrated for human strains.[93] HIV infection may have a direct effect on neutrophil chemotaxis, or an indirect effect via raised, inhibitory levels of IgA.[122]

Neutrophils of donor origin in patients who have recently undergone BMT may show reduced chemotaxis particularly when associated with graft-versus-host disease.[123]

There are many other anecdotal reports of defective chemotaxis in association with systemic disease. These include α-mannosidase deficiency, myotonic dystrophy, α-1-antitrypsin deficiency, Pelger-Huet abnormality, cirrhosis and sarcoidosis.[93]

Chemotactic factor phagocyte deactivation

Abnormal phagocyte chemotaxis has been observed in Wiskott-Aldrich syndrome and appears to be the result of excessive production of lymphocyte-derived chemotactic factor.[124] This finding complements the other features of this X-linked disorder (eczema, thrombocytopenia, abnormal cell-mediated immune responses and a deficiency of IgM production to polysaccharide antigens). Plasma from Wiskott patients inhibits the chemotaxis of normal leukocytes. It has been suggested that the excessive production of this chemotactic lymphokine leads to deactivation of chemotactic receptors.

DISORDERS OF OXIDATIVE METABOLISM

Chronic granulomatous disease

Chronic granulomatous disease (CGD) refers to a group of inherited disorders in which phagocytes (neutrophils, eosinophils and monocytes) are unable to express the respiratory burst. There are both X-linked and autosomal recessive variants. Defects in the various components of the enzyme system nicotinamide-adenine dinucleotide phosphate (NADPH) oxidase result in CGD.[125] The enzyme responsible for the reduction of O_2 to O_2^- includes various cellular components present in the cytosol and cell membrane. This enzyme system contains a flavoprotein and a unique cytochrome b558 which consists of a large 91 kDa subunit (gp91-phox) and a small 22 kDa protein subunit (p22-phox). Two cytosolic components (p47-phox and p67-phox) form a complex with cytochrome b558 and interact with a cytosolic GTP-binding protein, rac2.[126] The commonest type of CGD is found in about two-thirds of patients and is due to an abnormality of the membrane-associated heavy chain of cytochrome b558 encoded on the X chromosome (Table 16.9). Deficiency of the cytosolic product, p47-phox encoded by a gene on chromosome 7 is present in about a quarter of patients. Deficiency of the light chain of cytochrome b558, p22-phox (which is linked to chromosome 16), and a lack of the larger protein, p67-phox, encoded by chromosome 1, each account for about 5% of patients suffering from CGD.

Table 16.9 Classification of chronic granulomatous disease.

Affected component	Gene locus	Inheritance	Location of defect	Frequency (% of cases)
gp91-phox	Xp21.1	X	Membrane	64
p22-phox	16p24	AR	Membrane	7
p47-phox	7q11.23	AR	Cytosol	23
p67-phox	1q25	AR	Cytosol	6

Table 16.10 Clinical features suggestive of chronic granulomatous disease.

Recurrent lymphadenitis
Multiple site osteomyelitis
Family history of recurrent infections
Hepatic bacterial abscesses
Unusual catalase-positive infections
Purulent, slowly healing skin lesions
Subcutaneous immunization related abscesses
Infantile rash of ears and nares
Ulcerative stomatitis
Persistent rhinitis
Conjunctivitis
Association of the above with chronic inflammatory bowel disease

Clinical manifestations

The main clinical manifestations of CGD are shown in Table 16.10. Children suffer from recurrent infections by catalase-positive micro-organisms of which Staphylococci, Enterococci and fungi are the most important (Figs. 16.3 and 16.4). Because the bacteria are ingested but not killed and digested, patients develop severe chronic tissue granulomas from which the condition gets its name. Chronic granuloma formation may lead to non-infectious complications such as hepatosplenomegaly, lymphadenopathy, hypergamma-globulinemia, chronic diarrhea and granulomatous obstruction of certain organs such as the gastric pylorus and colon. Patients become chronically ill and their ability to withstand the frequent infections gradually deteriorates. Death is often

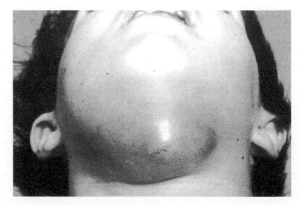

Fig. 16.3 Chronic granulomatous disease. Persisting submandibular soft tissue infection with incipient skin breakdown and chronic discharge.

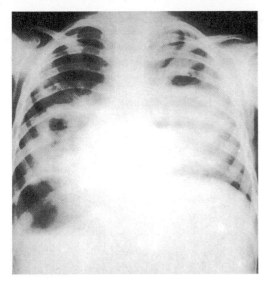

Fig. 16.4 Chronic granulomatous disease. Lung abscess and chronic inflammatory changes.

the result of fungal sepsis, mainly caused by *Aspergillus* species.[127]

Diagnosis

The diagnosis is made by the nitrobluetetrazolium (NBT) test or other tests demonstrating the lack of phagocyte O_2^- production. Characterization of the mutations in CGD now makes it possible to provide earlier and accurate prenatal diagnosis of CGD using fetal DNA from chorionic villi or amniocytes. However, this technology is only available in a limited number of laboratories. In the absence of molecular genetic facilities, prenatal diagnosis can be established using the NBT test on fetal blood obtained by percutaneous umbilical sampling.[128]

Treatment

Prophylactic antibiotic therapy, especially with trimethoprim-sulfamethoxazole reduces the incidence of life-threatening infections and should be given routinely to patients with CGD.[129] This has resulted in improved life expectancy and quality but at the cost of the emergence of severe fungal infections. Early vigorous antibiotic therapy is necessary particularly when resistant bacteria or fungal infections are present. Surgical drainage of granulomas may be necessary. In some life-threatening infections, white cell transfusions may be helpful. Granulomas causing obstruction to vital organs can respond to treatment with corticosteroids, presumably by affecting the production of cytokines such as interleukin-1, γ-interferon and TNF.[130] This form of treatment remains controversial, however, and should be used with caution.

γ-Interferon has been evaluated in the reduction of frequency and severity of infection in patients with CGD.[131]

The mechanism of action is thought to involve stimulation of the macrophage oxidative pathway, especially the heavy b cytochrome chain of NADPH oxidase.[132] However, in a phase III trial of γ-interferon, none of the patients showed an increase in neutrophil O_2^- production, despite clinical improvement.[133] This suggests that the cytokine does not augment the host system by reversing the respiratory burst defect, but by a mechanism that has still to be identified. γ-Interferon is indicated as a therapeutic agent in CGD patients along with antibiotics, with both on a continuous basis. Prophylactic antifungal therapy is currently under investigation. BMT is rarely performed because of improvement in the quality of life and survival of patients given prophylactic antibiotic therapy, and because the results of transplantation have usually proved disappointing.

Gene therapy. Theoretically, genes can be introduced into fetal cells, germ cells or specific somatic cells. Bone marrow provides a very suitable target tissue. Several methods are available for the introduction of genes into mammalian cells, and work has concentrated on the use of recombinant retrovirus vectors to effect gene transfer into bone marrow cells. Marrow cells are infected with a retrovirus gene vector and the gene transfer is quantitated by use of clonal assays, either *in vitro* agar culture or *in vivo* murine assays.

Several disorders of neutrophil function are potential candidates for gene transfer. These include CGD, myeloperoxidase deficiency, specific granule deficiency and leukocyte glycoprotein deficiency. The copy DNAs for both subunits of the CGD protein have been cloned.[134] The treatment of this and similar disorders, although rare, may provide useful models for gene therapy in the future.

Neutrophil glucose-6-phosphate dehydrogenase deficiency

NADPH is the basic substrate for the respiratory burst reaction necessary for the formation of superoxide (O_{2^-}). It is produced by glucose-6-phosphate dehydrogenase (G6PD) and 6-phosphogluconate dehydrogenase (6PGD), the first two enzymes of the hexose monophosphate shunt. Absence of G6PD results in reduced availability of NADPH, reduced respiratory burst activity and a clinical picture similar to chronic granulomatous disease. Similar micro-organisms are involved (i.e. predominantly catalase-positive bacteria).

The gene for leukocyte G6PD deficiency is identical to that for the red cell enzyme, and patients have the associated hemolytic anemia,[135] but unlike red cell G6PD deficiency, fewer than 10 patients with severe leukocyte G6PD deficiency have been described.[136] A possible explanation for this discrepancy in disease frequency is that neutrophils must have a severe (<5%) deficiency before neutrophil function is affected. Most cases of neutrophil dysfunction are found in Mediterranean G6PD deficiency, but even in this variant, clinically important leukocyte dysfunction is rare.

The treatment for neutrophil G6PD deficiency is the same as for CGD, except that the effect of γ-interferon is questionable and supportive therapy for chronic hemolysis is required.

Myeloperoxidase deficiency

Myeloperoxidase (MPO) is a heme-containing enzyme found in primary neutrophil granules. It is essential for the formation of hypochlorite ions which react with free amine groups to form potent microbicidal agents. MPO deficiency may affect up to 1 in 400 persons[137] and is the commonest inherited disorder of neutrophil function. However, the clinical disorder is usually mild and is mainly expressed by *Candida albicans* infections in individuals with co-existent diabetes. The gene encoding MPO is located on chromosome 17 at q22–p23, near the breakpoint for the t(15;17) translocation seen in M3 acute promyelocytic leukemia.[138]

MPO deficiency is inherited as an autosomal recessive trait. With blood counters which incorporate automated white cell differential counters based on a peroxidase stain, patients with MPO deficiency may be incorrectly indicated to have an absolute neutropenia.[139] The disorder is diagnosed by demonstrating the absence of cytochemically stainable enzyme. MPO-deficient neutrophils show normal chemotaxis, phagocytosis and degranulation. The respiratory burst is mildly prolonged and hydrogen peroxide production is mildly augmented.[140] Bacterial killing is delayed but does reach completion.

Cloning of cDNA for MPO has indicated that in some patients the deficiency may result from derangement of post-translocational processing of an abnormal precursor peptide.[141]

Since most patients do not experience life-threatening infections, antibiotic maintenance therapy is not recommended. Caution is necessary in diabetics who are more prone to pyogenic and fungal infections.

Disorders of oxidant scavenging

Superoxides produced by the respiratory burst are very efficient at destroying micro-organisms, but may diffuse into leukocyte cytoplasm resulting in serious cellular damage. Consequently, neutrophils are equipped with enzymes and antioxidants to remove these damaging oxygen derivatives from the cytoplasm,[142] whilst not interfering with the normal microbicidal reactions within the phagolysosomes.

Superoxide is destroyed by the reaction:

$$O_2^- + O_2^- + 2H^+ \rightarrow H_2O_2 + O_2$$

Hydrogen peroxide is then degraded into oxygen and water by cytoplasmic catalase or glutathione peroxidase and the glutathione reductase system.

Glutathione reductase maintains adequate amounts of reduced glutathione (GSH) by the reaction:

$$GSSG \text{ (glutathione)} + NADPH + H^+ \rightarrow$$
$$2\,GSH + NADP^+ \text{ (glutathione reductase)}$$

Reduced glutathione then destroys hydrogen peroxide with the aid of glutathione peroxide:

$$H_2O_2 + 2GSH \rightarrow 2H_2 + GSSG \text{ (glutathione peroxidase)}$$

Catalase deficiency

This very rare syndrome has not been associated with an increased incidence of infection. Roos *et al*[143] reported 2 patients with reduced levels of both erythrocyte ($<2\%$ activity) and neutrophil (10–20%) catalase activity. They proposed that whilst affected neutrophils may be able to cope with endogenously generated hydrogen peroxide, they may exhibit reduced activity against exogenous superoxides.

Glutathione reductase deficiency

One family has been reported in which 3 siblings of a consanguineous marriage showed marked neutrophil glutathione reductase deficiency.[144] The children had activity levels 10–15% of normal, whereas both parents showed neutrophil glutathione reductase levels of 50%, suggesting that the defect was inherited as an autosomal recessive trait. As with G6PD, both red cell and neutrophil glutathione reductase are under the control of the same gene, and affected patients hemolyze when subjected to oxidative stress.

None of the affected patients showed signs of excessive infections, but their neutrophils showed a reduced respiratory burst because of an inadequate production of GSH. This suggests that only a brief respiratory burst is necessary for complete destruction of bacteria.[145]

Glutathione peroxidase deficiency

Deficiency of glutathione peroxidase has been described in 3 unrelated patients where the neutrophil enzyme level was approximately 25% of normal and red cell levels were undetectable.[146,147] All 3 had a clinical syndrome resembling chronic granulomatous disease. It is not clear how the severity of the illness relates to the modest reduction in neutrophil enzyme levels and it is possible that these patients may not represent a distinct clinical entity[142] or may in fact have had CGD.[148]

Glutathione peroxidase deficiency has also been seen in cases of dietary selenium deficiency.[149]

Glutathione synthetase deficiency

GSH is a tripeptide synthesized from glutamyl-cysteine by the enzyme glutamyl synthetase. Deficiency results in reduced levels of glutathione and a mild phagocytic defect. Several types of enzyme deficiency have been described which show autosomal recessive inheritance. Phagocytic abnormalities are only seen in those cases in which the glutathione synthetase deficiency is severe.[150] Patients usually also have a hemolytic anemia (due to low erythrocyte enzyme levels) and a severe metabolic acidosis due to raised oxyproline levels (which cannot be metabolized to GSH because of the synthetase deficiency).

Boxer *et al*[151] suggested that increased sensitivity of neutrophils to oxidants resulting from glutathione synthetase deficiency could be corrected by administration of vitamin E, a powerful antioxidant.

SECONDARY NEUTROPHIL FUNCTION DEFECTS

Various neutrophil defects have been described in hematologic and non-hematologic disorders. These functional abnormalities are usually partial and therefore a tendency toward infection is uncommon and not severe.

HEMATOLOGIC DISORDERS

Acute myeloid leukaemia

AML patients sometimes suffer from infections despite a normal neutrophil count and therefore a neutrophil func-

tional defect has been postulated. In some cases a deficiency in one or more neutrophil enzymes has been described.[152]

Myeloproliferative disorders

Patients with CML do not usually suffer from severe infections during the chronic phase of their disease. However, functional abnormalities such as reduced alkaline phosphatase activity, abnormal adhesion and reduced migration are common.[153] On the other hand, children with myelodysplastic syndromes often have a predisposition to infection even in the presence of normal neutrophil counts. Monosomy 7 in particular is associated with abnormal migration. Other reports have shown qualitative abnormalities in neutrophil adhesion, migration, phagocytosis and bacterial killing.[154]

NON-HEMATOLOGIC DISORDERS

Diabetes mellitus is the most important non-hematologic disorder associated with a tendency towards infection and is particularly associated with uncontrolled hyperglycemia where chemotactic and adhesion defects have been described.[155] Depressed neutrophil activity, mainly chemotaxis, has been reported in liver disease, burns and premature neonates.[110] It is also known that during a septic episode or protracted infection neutrophil function may be altered.

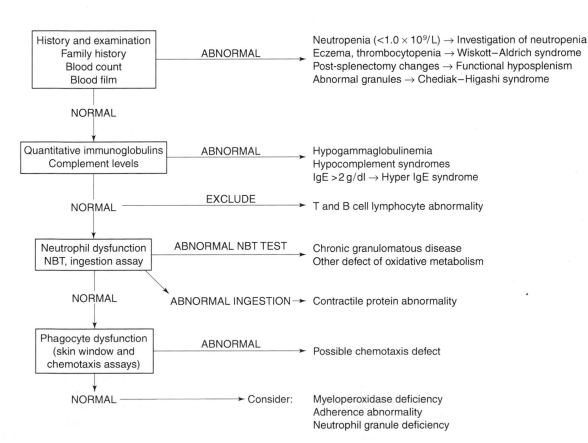

Fig. 16.5 Investigation of the child with recurrent infection.

Splenectomized patients are more susceptible to infection due to a defect in opsonization together with impairment of granulocyte chemotactic and phagocytic functions.[156] Cytotoxic agents, corticosteroids and ionizing irradiation can also modify neutrophil function.

INVESTIGATION OF THE CHILD WITH RECURRENT INFECTION

It is important to remember that neutrophils are only one component of the normal defence mechanisms against infection, and that many different phagocytic defects may present in a similar clinical fashion. The nature of the infecting organisms may be helpful, as in CGD, which is particularly associated with staphylococci and other catalase producers. Lymphopenia tends to result in fungal and pneumocystis infections. Fig. 16.5 attempts to lead the reader through the maze of clinical possibilities.

REFERENCES

1. Lehrer RI, Ganz T. Antimicrobial polypeptides of human neutrophils. *Blood* 1990; **76**: 2169–2181

2. Karayalcin G, Rosner F, Sawitsky A. Pseudo-neutropenia in African Negroes. *Lancet* 1972; **i**: 387

3. DeVaal OM, Seynhaeve V. Reticular dysgenesis. *Lancet* 1959; **2**: 1123–1125

4. Rosen FS, Craig J, Jones AP *et al*. The dysgammaglobulinaemias and X-linked thymic hypoplasia. In: Bergsma D (ed) *Immunologic Deficiency Diseases in Man*. New York: National Foundation—March of Dimes, 1968, p 67

5. Murray JA, Lilleyman JS. T cell lymphocytosis with neutropenia. *Arch Dis Child* 1983; **58**: 635–636

6. Kostmann R. Infantile genetic agranulocytosis. A review with presentation of ten new cases. *Acta Pediatr Scand* 1956; **64**: 362–366

7. Parmley RT, Crist WM, Ragab AH *et al*. Congenital dysgranulopoietic neutropenia: clinical, serologic, ultrastructural and *in vitro* proliferative characterisation. *Blood* 1980; **56**: 465–450

8. Parmley RT, Ogawa M, Darby CP *et al*. Congenital neutropenia: neutrophil proliferation with abnormal maturation. *Blood* 1975; **46**: 723–734

9. Bonilla MA, Gillio AP, Ruggeiro M *et al*. Effects of recombinant human granulocyte colony-stimulating factor on neutropenia in patients with congenital agranulocytosis. *N Engl J Med* 1989; **320**: 1574–1580

10. Mempel K, Pietsch T, Menzel T *et al*. Increased serum levels of granulocyte colony-stimulating factor in patients with severe congenital neutropenia. *Blood* 1991; **77**: 1919–1922

11. Dong F, Brynes RK, Tidow N *et al*. Mutations in the gene for the granulocyte colony-stimulating-factor receptor in patients with acute myeloid leukemia preceded by severe congenital neutropenia. *N Engl J Med* 1995; **333**: 487–493

12. Gilman PA, Jackson DP *et al*. Congenital agranulocytosis: prolonged survival and terminal acute leukaemia. *Blood* 1970; **36**: 576–579

13. Pahwa RN, O'Reilly RJ, Pahwa S *et al*. Partial correction of neutrophil deficiency in congenital neutropenia following bone marrow transplantation (BMT). *Exp Haematol* 1977; **5**: 45–50

14. Shwachman H, Diamond LK, Oski FA *et al*. The syndrome of pancreatic insufficiency and bone marrow dysfunction. *J Pediatr* 1964; **65**: 645–663

15. Aggett PJ, Cavanagh NP, Matthew DJ *et al*. Shwachman's syndrome: a review of 21 cases. *Arch Dis Child* 1980; **55**: 331–334

16. Marra G, Appiani AC, Romeo L *et al*. Renal tubular acidosis in a case of Shwachman's syndrome. *Acta Paediatr Scand* 1986; **75**: 682–684

17. Hislop WS, Hayes PC, Boyd EJS. Late presentation of Shwachman's syndrome. *Acta Paediatr Scand* 1982; **71**: 677–679

18. Rothbaum RJ, Williams DA, Daugherty CC. Unusual surface distribution of concanavolin A reflects a cytoskeletal defect in neutrophils in Shwachman's syndrome. *Lancet* 1982; **ii**: 800–801

19. McKusick VA, Eldridge R, Hostetler J *et al*. Dwarfism in the Amish. Cartilage hair hypoplasia. *Bull Johns Hopkins Hosp* 1965; **116**: 285–326

20. O'Reilly RJ, Bochstein J, Dinsmore R *et al*. Marrow transplantation for congenital disorders. *Semin Haemat* 1984; **21**: 188–221

21. Greenberg PL, Mara B, Steed S, Boxer LA. The chronic idiopathic neutropenic syndrome: Correlation of clinical features with *in vitro* parameters of granulopoiesis. *Blood* 1980; **55**: 915–921

22. Dale DC, Guerry D, Werweka JR *et al*. Chronic neutropenia. *Medicine* 1979; **58**: 128–144

23. Falk PM, Rich K, Feig S *et al*. Evaluation of congenital neutropenic disorders by *in vitro* bone marrow. *J Immunol Methods* 1980; **33**: 239–247

24. Zuelzer WW. Myelokathexis—new form of chronic granulocytopenia. *N Engl J Med* 1970; **282**: 231–236

25. Tanaka K, Rosenberg LE. Disorders of branched chain amino acid and organic acid metabolism. In: Stanbury JB, Wyngaarden JB (eds) *The Metabolic Basis of Inherited Disease*, 5th edn. New York: McGraw Hill, 1983, p 440

26. Leale M. Recurrent furniculosis in an infant showing an unusual blood picture. *JAMA* 1910; **54**: 1845

27. Lange RD. Cyclic hematopoiesis: human cyclic neutropenia. *Exp Hematol* 1983; **11**: 435–451

28. Wright DG, Dale DC, Fauci AS *et al*. Human cyclic neutropenia: clinical review and long-term follow-up of patients. *Medicine* 1981; **60**: 1–13

29. Guerry D, Dale DC, Omine M, Perry S, Wolf SM. Periodic hematopoiesis in human cyclic neutropenia. *J Clin Invest* 1973; **52**: 3220–3229

30. Morley AA, Carew JP, Baikie AG. Familial cyclical neutropenia. *Br J Haematol* 1967; **13**: 719–738

31. Lund JE, Pagett GA, Ott RL. Cyclic neutropenia in grey collie dogs. *Blood* 1967; **29**: 452–461

32. Loughran TP, Clark EA, Price TH, Hammond WP. Adult onset cyclic neutropenia is associated with increased large granular lymphocytes. *Blood* 1986; **68**: 1082–1087

33. Rodgers GM, Shuman MA. Acquired cyclic neutropenia: successful treatment with prednisone. *Am J Hematol* 1982; **13**: 83–89

34. Roozendaal KJ, Dicke KA, Boonzajer Flaes ML. Effect of oxymetholone on human cyclic haematopoiesis. *Br J Haematol* 1981; **47**: 185–193

35. Lensink DB, Barton A, Appelbaum FR, Hammond WP. Cyclic neutropenia as a premalignant manifestation of acute lymphoblastic leukemia. *Am J Hematol* 1986; **22**: 9–16

36. Dale DC, Hammond WP. Cyclic neutropenia: a clinical review. *Blood Rev* 1988; **2**: 178–185

37. Dale DC, Graw RG. Transplantation of allogeneic bone marrow in canine cyclic neutropenia. *Science* 1974; **183**: 83–84

38. Krance RA, Spruce WE, Forman SJ *et al*. Human cyclic neutropenia transferred in allogeneic bone marrow grafting. *Blood* 1982; **60**: 1263–1266

39. Engelhard D, Landreth KS, Kapoor N *et al*. Cycling of peripheral blood and marrow lymphocytes in cyclic neutropenia. *Proc Natl Acad Sci USA* 1983; **13**: 5734–5738

40. Osborne WRA, Hammond WP, Dale DC. Human cyclic haematopoiesis is associated with aberrant purine metabolism. *J Lab Clin Med* 1985; **105**: 403–409

41. von Schulthess GK, Fehr J, Dahinden C. Cyclic neutropenia: amplification of granulocyte oscillations by lithium and long term suppression of cycling by plasmapheresis. *Blood* 1983; **62**: 320–326

42. Dale DC, Bonilla MA, Zeidler C *et al*. A randomised controlled phase III trial of recombinant human granulocyte colony-stimulating factor

(filgrastim) in the treatment of severe chronic neutropenia. *Blood* 1993; **81**: 2496–2502

43. Rosen RB, Kang SJ. Congenital agranulocytosis terminating in acute myelomonocytic leukaemia. *J Pediatr* 1979; **94**: 406–408

44. Verheugt FWA, van Noord-Bokhurst J, von dem Borne AE *et al*. A family with allo-immune neutropenia: group specific pathogenicity of maternal antibodies. *Vox Sang* 1979; **36**: 1–8

45. Curnutte JT, Boxer LA. Disorders of granulopoiesis and granulocyte function. In: Nathan DG, Oski FA (eds) *Hematology of Infancy and Childhood*. Philadelphia: WB Saunders, 1987

46. Minchinton RM. The occurrence and significance of neutrophil antibodies. *Br J Haematol* 1984; **56**: 521–524

47. Boxer LA. Immune neutropenias. Clinical and biological implications. *Am J Pediatr Hematol Oncol* 1981; **3**: 89–96

48. Payne R. Neonatal neutropenia and leukoagglutinins. *Pediatrics* 1964; **33**: 194–197

49. Lalezari P, Khorshidi M, Petrosova M 1986 Autoimmune neutropenia of infancy. *J Pediatr* 109: 764–767

50. Verheugt FWA, von dem Borne AE, van Noord-Bokhorst JC *et al*. Autoimmune granulocytopenia: the detection of granulocyte auto-antibodies with the immunofluorescent test. *Br J Haematol* 1978; **39**: 339–350

51. Boxer LA, Greenberg MS, Boxer GJ, Stossel TP. Autoimmune neutropenia. *N Engl J Med* 1975; **293**: 748–753

52. Lalezari P. Autoimmune neutropenia. In: Rose MR, MacKay IR (eds) *The Autoimmune Diseases*. Blackwell, Oxford, 1985, p 523

53. Bussel J, Lalezari P, Hilgartner M *et al*. Reversal of neutropenia with intravenous gammaglobulin in autoimmune neutropenia of infancy. *Blood* 1983; **62**: 398–402

54. Logue GL, Shimm DS. Autoimmune granulocytopenia. *Annu Rev Med* 1980; **31**: 191–200

55. Joyce RA, Boggs DA, Chervenick PA, Lalezari P. Neutrophil kinetics in Felty's syndrome. *Am J Med* 1980; **69**: 695–702

56. Dancey JT, Brubaker LH. Neutrophil marrow profiles in patients with rheumatoid arthritis and neutropenia. *Br J Haematol* 1979; **43**: 607–617

57. Minchinton RM, Waters AH. Autoimmune thrombocytopenia and neutropenia after bone marrow transplantation. *Blood* 1985; **3**: 752–757

58. Murdoch RM, Smith CC. Hematological aspects of systemic disease: infection. *Clin Hematol* 1972; **1**: 619–625

59. MacGregor RR, Friedman HM, Macarak EJ *et al*. Virus infection of endothelial cells increases granulocyte adherence. *J Clin Invest* 1980; **65**: 1469–1477

60. Stevens DL, Everett ED, Boxer LA *et al*. Infectious mononucleosis with severe neutropenia and opsonic antineutrophil activity. *South Med J* 1979; **72**: 519–521

61. Christensen RD, Rothstein G. Exhaustion of mature marrow neutrophils in neonates with sepsis. *J Pediatr* 1980; **96**: 316–318

62. Craddock PR, Hammerschmidt DE, Moldow CF *et al*. Granulocyte aggregation as a manifestation of membrane interactions with complement: possible role in leukocyte margination, microvascular occlusion, and endothelial damage. *Semin Hematol* 1979; **16**: 140–147

63. Young GA, Vincent PC. Drug-induced agranulocytosis. *Clin Haematol* 1980; **9**: 438–504

64. Weitzman SA, Stossel TP. Drug-induced immunological neutropenia. *Lancet* 1978; **1**: 1068–1072

65. Schröder H, Evans DAP. Acetylator phenotype and adverse effects of sulphasalazine in healthy subjects. *Gut* 1972; **13**: 278–284

66. Cronkite EP. Kinetics of granulopoiesis. *Clin Haematol* 1976; **8**: 351–370

67. Ghebrehiwet B, Müller-Eberhart HJ. C3e: an acidic fragment of human C3 with leukocytosis-inducing activity. *J Immunol* 1979; **123**: 616–621

68. Crowley CA, Curnutte JT, Rosin RE *et al*. An inherited abnormality of neutrophil adhesion: its genetic transmission and its association with a missing protein. *N Engl J Med* 1980; **302**: 1163–1168

69. Engel RR, Hammond D, Eitzman DV *et al*. Transient congenital leukemia in seven children with mongolism. *J Pediatr* 1964; **65**: 303–305

70. Randall DL, Reiquam CN, Githens JH *et al*. Familial myeloprolifera-tive disease. A new syndrome closely simulating myelogenous leukae-mia in childhood. *Am J Dis Child* 1965; **110**: 479–500

71. Teo CG, Singh M, Ting WC *et al*. Evaluation of the common conditions associated with eosinophilia. *J Clin Pathol* 1985; **38**: 305–308

72. Hardy WR, Anderson RE. The hypereosinophilic syndrome. *Ann Intern Med* 1968; **68**: 1220–1229

73. Cushid MJ, Dale DC, West BC, Wolf SM. The hypereosinophilic syndrome: analysis of fourteen cases with review of the literature. *Medicine (Baltimore)* 1975; **54**: 1–5

74. Alfaham MA, Fergusson SD, Shira B, Davies J. The idiopathic hypereosinophilic syndrome. *Arch Dis Child* 1987; **62**: 601–613

75. Fauci AS, Harley JB, Roberts WC *et al*. The idiopathic hypereosino-philic syndrome: clinical, pathophysiologic and therapeutic considera-tions. *Ann Intern Med* 1982; **97**: 78–92

76. Rickles FR, Miller DR. Eosinophilic leukemoid reaction; report of a case, its relationship to eosinophilic leukemia and review of pediatric literature. *J Pediatr* 1972; **80**: 418–428

77. Beeson P B, Bass DA. *The Eosinophil*. Philadelphia: WB Saunders, 1977

78. May ME, Waddell CC. Basophils in peripheral blood and bone marrow. A retrospective review. *Am J Med* 1984; **76**: 509–511

79. Metcalfe JA, Gallin JI, Nauseef WM *et al*. *Laboratory Manual of Neutrophil Function*. New York: Raven Press, 1986

80. Anderson DC, Schmalsteig FC, Finegold MJ *et al*. The severe and moderate phenotype of heritable Mac-1, LFA-1 deficiency: their quantitative definition and relation to leukocyte dysfunction and clinical features. *J Infect Dis* 1985; **152**: 668–689

81. Harlan JM. Leukocyte adhesion deficiency syndrome: Insights into the molecular basis of leukocyte emigration. *Clin Immunol Immunopathol* 1993; **67**: S15-S24

82. Etzioni A, Frydman M, Pollack S *et al*. Recurrent infections caused by a novel leukocyte adhesion deficiency. *N Engl J Med* 1992; **327**: 1789–1792

83. Bryant RE, Sutcliff MC. The effect of 3'5'-adenosine monophosphate on granulocyte adhesion. *J Clin Invest* 1974; **54**: 1241–1244

84. Oseas RS, Allen J, Yang HH *et al*. Mechanism of dexamethasone inhibition of chemotactic factor-induced granulocyte aggregation. *Blood* 1982; **59**: 265–269

85. Hirata F, Schiffman E, Venkata Subramanian *et al*. A phospholipase A₂ inhibitory protein in rabbit neutrophils induced by glucocorticoids. *Proc Natl Acad Sci USA* 1980; **77**: 2533–2536

86. Boxer LA, Oseas RS, Oliver JM *et al*. Amphotericin B promotes leukocyte aggregation of nylon wool fibre treated polymorphonuclear leukocytes. *Blood* 1981; **58**: 518–521

87. Tate RM, Repine JE. Neutrophils and the adult respiratory distress syndrome. *Am Rev Resp Dis* 1983; **128**: 552–559

88. Metchnikoff E. *Immunity in Infective Disease*. Cambridge: Cambridge University Press, 1905

89. Fearon DT, Collins LA. Increased expression of C3b receptors on polymorphonuclear leukocytes induced by chemotactic factors and by purification procedures. *J Immunol* 1983; **130**: 370–375

90. Snyderman R, Pike MC. Transductional mechanisms of chemoattrac-tant receptors on leukocytes. In: Snyderman R (ed) *Regulation of Leukocyte Function*. New York: Plenum Press, 1984, p 1

91. Weisbart RH, Golde DW, Clark SC *et al*. Human granulocyte-macrophage colony stimulating factor is a neutrophil activator. *Nature* 1985; **314**: 361–362

92. Schleimer R, Rutledge B. Cultured human vascular endothelial cells acquire adhesiveness for neutrophils after stimulation with interleukin 1, endotoxin and tumour-promoting phorbol esters. *J Immunol* 1986; **136**: 649–654

93. Brown CC, Gallin JI. Chemotactic disorders. *Hematol Oncol Clin N Am* 1988; **2**: 61–79

94. Sechler J, Gallin JI. Recombinant gamma interferon is a chemo-attractant for human monocytes. *Fed Proc* 1987; **46**: 5523A

95. Falk W, Goodwin RH, Leonard EJ. A 48-well micro chemotaxis assembly for rapid and accurate measurements of leukocyte migration. *J Immunol Methods* 1980; **33**: 239–247

96. Boxer LA, Smolen JE. Neutrophil granule constituents and their release in health and disease. *Hematol Oncol Clin N Am* 1988; **2**: 101–134

97. Oliver C, Essner E. Formation of anomalous lysozomes in monocytes neutrophils and eosinophils from bone marrow of mice with Chédiak–Higashi syndrome. *Lab Invest* 1985; **32**: 17–21

98. Barak Y, Karov Y, Nir E *et al*. Chédiak–Higashi syndrome: Expression of the cytoplasmic defect by *in vitro* cultures on bone marrow progenitors. *Am J Pediatr Hematol Oncol* 1986; **8**: 128–133

99. Root RK, Rosenthal AS, Balestra DK. Abnormal bactericidal, metabolic and lysosomal functions of Chédiack–Higashi syndrome leukocytes. *J Invest* 1972; **51**: 649–665

100. Nair MP, Gray RH, Boxer LA, Schwartz S. Deficiency of inducible suppressor cell activity in the Chédiak–Higashi syndrome. *Am J Hematol* 1987; **26**: 55–66

101. Buchanan GB, Handin RI. Platelet function in the Chédiak–Higashi syndrome. *Blood* 1976; **47**: 941–945

102. White JG, Clawson CC. The Chédiak–Higashi syndrome. The nature of the giant neutrophil granules and their interaction with cytoplasm and foreign particles. *Am J Pathol* 1980; **98**: 151–196

103. Oliver JM. Cell biology of leukocyte abnormalities in membrane and cytoskeletal function in normal and defective cells. A review. *Am J Pathol* 1978; **93**: 221–270

104. Kimball HR, Ford GH, Wolff SM. Lysosomal enzymes in normal and Chédiak–Higashi blood leukocytes. *J Lab Clin Med* 1975; **86**: 616–630

105. Stossel TP, Root RK, Vaughan K. Phagocytosis in chronic granulomatous disease and the Chédiak–Higashi syndrome. *N Engl J Med* 1972; **286**: 120–123

106. Ingraham LM, Burns CP, Hack RA *et al*. Fluidity properties and lipid composition of erythrocyte membranes in Chédiak–Higashi syndrome. *J Cell Biol* 1981; **89**: 510–516

107. Gallin JI, Elin RJ, Hubert RT *et al*. Efficacy of ascorbic acid in Chédiak–Higashi syndrome. Studies in humans and mice. *Blood* 1979; **53**: 226–234

108. Fischer A, Griscelli C, Friedrich W *et al*. Bone marrow transplantation for immunodeficiencies and osteopetrosis: European survey, 1968–85. *Lancet* 1986; **ii**: 1080–1084

109. Malech HL, Englander L, Zakhinehb A. Abnormal polymorphonuclear neutrophil function in Kartagener's syndrome. *Clin Res* 1979; **27**: 590A

110. Bogomolski-Yahalom V, Matzner Y. Disorders of neutrophil function. *Blood Rev* 1995; **9**: 183–190

111. Gallin JI. Neutrophil-specific granule deficiency. *Annu Rev Med* 1985; **36**: 263–274

112. Lomax KJ, Malech HL, Gallin JI. The molecular biology of selected phagocyte defects. *Blood Rev* 1989; **3**: 94–104

113. van Dyke TE. Role of the neutrophil in oral disease: receptor deficiency in leukocytes from patients with juvenile periodontis. *Rev Infect Dis* 1985; **7**: 419–425

114. Wanatabe K. Prepubertal periodontitis: a review of diagnostic criteria, pathogenesis, and differential diagnosis. *J Periodon Res* 1990; **25**: 31–48

115. Miller ME, Oski FA, Harris MB. 'Lazy leukocyte' syndrome. A new disorder of neutrophil dysfunction. *Lancet* 1971; **i**: 665–669

116. Leung DY, Geha RS. Clinical and immunologic aspects of the hyperimmunoglobulin E syndrome. *Hematol Oncol Clin N Am* 1988; **2**: 81–100

117. Donabedian H, Alling DW, Gallin JI. Levamisole is inferior to placebo in the hyperimmunoglobulin E recurrent infection (Job's) syndrome. *N Engl J Med* 1982; **307**: 290–292

118. Clark RA, Root R, Kimball H *et al*. Defective neutrophil chemotaxis and cellular immunity in a child with recurrent infections. *Ann Intern Med* 1973; **78**: 515–519

119. Hill HR, Estensen RD, Hogan NA *et al*. Severe staphylococcal disease associated with allergic manifestations, hyperimmunoglobulin E and defective neutrophil chemotaxis. *J Lab Clin Med* 1976; **88**: 796–806

120. Jeppson JD, Jaffe HS, Hill HR. Use of recombinant human interferon gamma to enhance neutrophilic chemotactic responses in Job syndrome of hyperimmunoglobulinaemia E and recurrent infections. *J Pediatr* 1991; **118**: 383–387

121. Hanlon SM, Panayi GS, Laurent R. Defective polymorphonuclear leukocyte chemotaxis in rheumatoid arthritis associated with a serum inhibitor. *Ann Rheum Dis* 1980; **39**: 68–74

122. Estevez ME, Ballart IJ, Diez RA *et al*. Early defect of phagocytic cell function in subjects at risk for acquired immune deficiency syndrome. *Scand J Immunol* 1986; **24**: 215–221

123. Clark RA, Johnson FL, Klebanoff SJ *et al*. Defective neutrophil chemotaxis in bone marrow transplant patients. *J Clin Invest* 1976; **58**: 22–31

124. Ochs HD, Slichter SJ, Harker LA *et al*. The Wiskott–Aldrich syndrome: studies of lymphocytes, granulocytes and platelets. *Blood* 1980; **55**: 243–252

125. Curnutte JT. Chronic granulomatous disease: the solving of a clinical riddle at the molecular level. *Clin Immunol Immunopathol* 1993; **67**: S2-S15122.

126. Gallin JI, Leto TL, Rotrosen D *et al*. Delineation of the phagocyte NADPH oxidase through studues of chronic granulomatous disease of childhood. *Curr Opin Immunol* 1991; **4**: 53–56

127. Gallin JI (ed). *Disorders of Phagocytic Cells; Inflammation: Basic Principles and Clinical Correlates*, 2nd edn. New York: Raven Press, 1992

128. Levinsky RJ, Harvey BAM, Nikolaides K *et al*. Antenatal diagnosis of chronic granulomatous disease. *Lancet* 1986; **i**: 504

129. Gallin JI, Buesher ES, Seligmann BE *et al*. Recent advances in chronic granulomatous disease. *Ann Intern Med* 1983; **99**: 657–674

130. Chin TW, Stiehm ER, Falloon J *et al*. Corticosteroids in the treatment of obstructive lesions of chronic granulomatous disease. *J Pediatr* 1987; **111**: 349–352

131. Gallin JI, Malech HL, Melnick DA *et al*. A controlled trial of interferon gamma in chronic granulomatous disease. The International Chronic Granulomatous Disease Study Group. *N Engl J Med* 1991; **324**: 509–516

132. Ezekowitz RAB, Dinauer MC, Jaffe HS *et al*. Partial correction of the phagocyte defect in patients with X-linked chronic granulomatous disease by subcutaneous interferon gamma. *N Engl J Med* 1988; **319**: 146–151

133. Woodman RC, Erickson RW, Rae J *et al*. Prolonged recombinant interferon gamma therapy in chronic granulomatous disease: Evidence against enhanced neutrophil oxidase activity. *Blood* 1992; **79**: 1558–1562

134. Dinauer MC, Orkin SH, Brown R *et al*. The glycoprotein encoded by the X-linked chronic granulomatous disease locus is a component of the neutrophil cytochrome b locus. *Nature* 1987; 327: 717–720

135. Yoshida A, Stamatoyannopoulos G. Biochemical genetics of glucose-6-phosphate dehydrogenase variation. *Ann NY Acad Sci* 1968; **155**: 868–872

136. Gray GR, Stannatoyannopoulos G, Naiman SC *et al*. Neutrophil dysfunction, chronic granulomatous disease, and non-spherocytic haemolytic anaemia caused by complete deficiency of glucose-6-phosphate dehydrogenase. *Lancet* 1973; **ii**: 530–534

137. Parry MF, Root RK, Metcalf J A *et al*. Myeloperoxidase deficiency. Prevalence and clinical significance. *Ann Intern Med* 1981; **95**: 293–301

138. Chang KS, Schroeder W, Siciliano MJ *et al*. The localisation of the human myeloperoxidase gene is in close proximity to the translocation breakpoint in acute promyelocytic leukaemia. *Leukaemia* 1987; **1**: 458–462

139. Kitahara M, Simonian Y, Eyre HJ. Neutrophil myeloperioxidase: A simple reproducible technique to determine activity. *J Lab Clin Med* 1979; **93**: 232–237

140. Nauseef WM. Myeloperoxidase deficiency. *Hematol Pathol* 1990; **4**: 165–178

141. Nauseef WM. Aberrant restriction endonuclease digests of DNA from subjects with hereditary myeloperoxidase deficiency. *Blood* 1989; **73**: 290–295

142. Babior BM, Crowley CA. Chronic granulomatous disease and other disorders of oxidative killing by phagocytes. In: Stanbury JB, Wyngaarden JB, Frederickson DS *et al* (eds) *The Metabolic Basis of Inherited Disease*. New York: McGraw Hill, 1983, p 1956

143. Roos D, Weening RS, Wyss SR *et al*. Protection of human neutrophils by endogenous catalase. *J Clin Invest* 1980; **65**: 1515–1522

144. Loos H, Roos D, Weening R *et al*. Familial deficiency of glutathione reductase in human blood cells. *Blood* 1976; **48**: 53–62

145. Roos D, Weening RS, Wyss SR *et al*. Protection of phagocytic leukocytes by endogenous glutathione: studies in a family with glutathione reductase deficiency. *Blood* 1979; **53**: 851–866

146. Holmes B, Park BH, Malawista SE *et al*. Chronic granulomatous disease in females. A deficiency of leukocyte glutathione peroxidase. *N Engl J Med* 1970; **283**: 217–221

147. Matsuda I, Oka Y, Taniguchi N *et al* 1970 Leukocyte glutathione peroxidase deficiency in a male patient with chronic granulomatous disease. *J Pediatr* 88: 581–584

148. Whitin JC, Cohen HJ. Disorders of respiratory burst termination. *Hematol Oncol Clin N Am* 1988; **2**: 289–299

149. Baker SS, Cohen HJ. Altered oxidative metabolism in selenium-deficient rat granulocytes. *J Immunol* 1983; **130**: 2856–2860

150. Spielberg SP, Boxer LA, Oliver JM *et al*. Oxidative damage to neutrophils in glutathione synthetase deficiency. *Br J Haematol* 1979; **42**: 215–225

151. Boxer LA, Oliver JM, Spielberg SP *et al*. Protection of granulocytes by vitamin E in glutathione synthetase deficiency. *N Engl J Med* 1979; **301**: 901–905

152. Suda T, Onai T, Maekawa T. Studies of abnormal polymorphonuclear neutrophils in acute myelogenous leukemia: Clinical significance and changes after chemotherapy. *Am J Hematol* 1983; **15**: 45–56

153. Matzer Y. Granulocyte dysfunction in hematological disorders. *Cancer Invest* 1992; **10**: 155–161

154. Martin S, Baldock SC, Ghoneim ATM *et al*. Defective neutrophil function and microbicidal mechanism in the myelodysplastic disorders. *J Clin Pathol* 1983; **36**: 1120–1128

155. Andersen B, Goldsmith GH, Spagnuolo PJ. Neutrophil adhesive dysfunction in diabetes mellitus. *J Lab Clin Med* 1988; **111**: 275–285

156. Dahl M, Hakansson L, Kreuger A *et al*. Polymorphonuclear neutrophil function and infections following splenectomy in childhood. *Scand J Haematol* 1986; **37**: 137–143

Histiocytic syndromes

DAVID KH WEBB

Histiocyte disorders are a group of conditions characterized by infiltration of affected tissues with cells of monocyte/macrophage lineage, often mixed with other inflammatory cells. They may be divided into 2 broad categories:

1. reactive disorders believed to represent a disordered response to immune activation;
2. neoplastic conditions.

A number of other disorders with lymphohistiocytic infiltration of tissues are conventionally excluded, including immune disorders such as the X-linked lymphoproliferative syndrome, and Chédiak–Higashi syndrome (see Chapter 16). To aid study, the Histiocyte Society has proposed a classification subdividing the histiocyte disorders into 3 classes (Table 17.1),[1] namely abnormalities of dendritic cells, those affecting antigen-processing cells, and neoplastic disorders, although the boundaries between classes may be blurred, and more than one class of disorder may be present in the same child.[2] Abnormal responses to antigen stimulation mediated by inflammatory cytokines have been proposed as the mechanism for the 2 commonest disorders, Langerhans cell histiocytosis (LCH) and hemophagocytic lymphohistiocytosis (HLH), and it remains unclear whether the histiocytes themselves, or other immune active cells are the defective population.

HISTIOCYTES IN HEALTH

Most histiocytes are derived from the hemopoietic stem cell, via the granulocyte–macrophage colony-forming unit (GM-CFU),[3] although local proliferation in the tissues may occur following contact with antigen and in disease states. Growth and differentiation are controlled by hemopoietic growth factors, produced by stromal cells, macrophages, and lymphocytes.[4] These growth factors are glycoproteins that stimulate proliferation and differentiation of early precursors to monoblasts, promonocytes and monocytes, via specific, high-affinity surface membrane receptors. The bone marrow transit time has been estimated as 54 hours, and monocytes enter the blood, with a circulating half-life of 8 hours, prior to migration into the tissues.[5] Differentiation into tissue macrophages and dendritic cells occurs under the influence of growth factors and physical stimuli, including contact with antigen.

Histiocytes are widely spread throughout the tissues, and include Kupffer cells in the liver, microglia in the central nervous system, Langerhans cells in skin, and osteoclasts in bone, and these cells play a key role in host defence, acting as antigen-presenting cells, phagocytes and generators of inflammation through enzyme release and the production of inflammatory cytokines and cellular growth factors.[6] Macrophages possess a wide range of surface antigens or receptors, including those for HLA class I and II, the Fc fragment of IgG and IgE, complement and γ-interferon. Phagocytic macrophages internalize antigen by pinocytosis (ingestion of soluble antigen) or phagocytosis (ingestion of particulate antigen) within vesicles which then fuse with lysosomes, although some infective agents may survive in macrophages, providing a pool of infection. Products of these cells include lysozyme, proteases, hydrolases, complement,

Table 17.1 Classification of the histiocytosis syndromes.

Class I	Disorders of dendritic cells
	Langerhans cell histiocytosis
Class II	Disorders of macrophages
	Hemophagocytic lymphohistiocytosis
	Primary (genetic)
	Secondary
	Sinus histiocytosis with massive lymphadenopathy
	Juvenile xanthogranuloma
	Self-healing reticulo-histiocytosis
	Histiocytic necrotizing lymphadenitis
Class III	Malignant histiocyte disorders
	Acute monoblastic leukemia (FAB type M5)
	Malignant histiocytosis
	Reticulum cell and interdigitating reticulum cell sarcoma

coagulation factors, reactive oxygen species, prostaglandins, interleukin-1 (IL-1), colony stimulating factors (CSFs), interferons, tumor necrosis factor (TNF) and binding proteins. IL-1 is a key cytokine with wide inflammatory and immunomodulatory properties, including the stimulation of lymphocyte proliferation.

Normal histiocytes are divided into 2 subgroups: antigen-presenting or dendritic cells (Langerhans, dendritic reticulum and interdigitating reticulum cells); and antigen-processing cells (macrophages). Langerhans cells (LCs) are normally found in the epidermis, the mucosa of the bronchial tree and gut, and in lymph nodes and the thymus.[7,8] They are thought to undergo differentiation from bone marrow-derived precursor cells in the tissues under the influence of cytokines (IL-3, GM-CSF and TNF-α) and physical stimuli which, in the skin, include low temperature. Characteristic features of LCs include the expression of the CD1a surface antigen and the presence of specific cytoplasmic organelles termed Birbeck granules. Suggested origins for Birbeck granules are either the invagination of the surface membrane during endocytosis of antigen, or secretory organelles derived from the Golgi apparatus, and these organelles may be demonstrated on electron microscopy as rod-shaped structures, often with an expanded end (tennis-racket appearance). CD1a has considerable homology with HLA Class I molecules, and is generally specific for LCs, being otherwise expressed only by cortical thymocytes. The function of this antigen is unknown, but a role in the immune response, perhaps in antigen presentation to T cells is possible. LCs are fundamental to immune surveillance in skin where they are located in the supra-basal layer of the epidermis, aligned in a horizontal plane, with up to 9 dendrites which expand the area for interaction with antigen. Following stimulation by either soluble or particulate antigen, LCs migrate to lymph nodes, where they present antigen to T cells. Dendritic and interdigitating reticulum cells are localized to lymph nodes, where they present antigen to B and T cells, respectively. The location of these cells within the lymph nodes varies, with interdigitating reticulum cells primarily located in the paracortex, and dendritic cells in the lymph node follicle.

HISTIOCYTIC DISORDERS

CLASS I

This subgroup comprises reactive disorders of antigen-presenting (dendritic) histiocytes, predominantly Langerhans cell histiocytosis (LCH).

Langerhans cell histiocytosis

In 1959, Lichtenstein[9] identified the diagnostic entities of eosinophilic granuloma of bone, Hand–Schuller–Christian disease and Letterer-Siwe disease as part of a single disease spectrum which he termed histiocytosis X. Nezelhof et al[10] subsequently identified LCs as characteristic of lesions in the disease process, and the term Langerhans cell histiocytosis was proposed by the international Histiocyte Society in 1987.

LCH is rare, affecting 4/million children/year,[11] with a peak incidence between 1 and 3 years of age. The disorder is slightly more common in boys. Clinical presentation is variable and despite the restricted distribution of LCs in health, lesions which comprise LCs and other inflammatory cells, particularly eosinophils, lymphocytes, neutrophils and antigen-processing cells[12] may occur in a wide range of organs, including skin, bone, lymph nodes, liver, spleen, bone marrow, lungs, central nervous system and gut (Fig. 17.1). However, the proportion of LCs varies widely, and they may be few in number, or even absent, particularly in lesions of the gut and central nervous system. Morphologically, LCs in disease are indistinguishable from normal LCs, and studies of surface-antigen expression show a similar pattern to that of activated LCs in healthy individuals.[13] However, 3 histochemical markers which are negative in normal LCs are positive in LCH cells—peanut agglutinin, placental alkaline phosphatase and γ-interferon receptor.

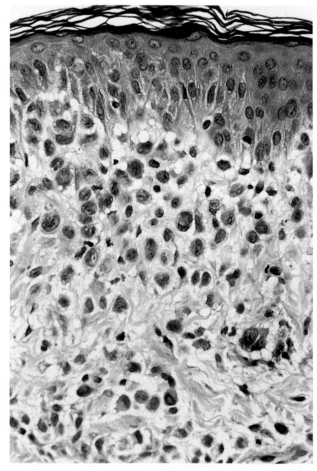

Fig. 17.1 Langerhans cell histiocytosis (LCH) in skin. H & E stain showing infiltrate of Langerhans cells, lymphocytes and eosinophils. Kindly provided by M Malone.

Later, lesions are characterized by reduced numbers of LCs and the accumulation of lipid-laden macrophages, and ultimate resolution is accompanied by residual fibrosis.

Etiology

The etiology is unknown, but LCH is generally considered to be a reactive disorder resulting from immune activation. Searches for potential triggers have been unsuccessful, and in general there is no evidence for a viral etiology,[14] although studies of the role of human herpes virus 6 are conflicting.[15,16] High levels of cytokines (GM-CSF, IL-1, -3, -4 and -8, TNF, and lymphocyte inhibitory factor [LIF]) have been demonstrated in lesions, with GM-CSF and LIF detected in the serum of children with multisystem disease.[17,18] As might be expected, studies using *in-situ* hybridization have revealed production of cytokines both by lesional lymphocytes and histiocytes. Although LCH is considered reactive rather than neoplastic, 2 studies of X-linked DNA polymorphisms have demonstrated clonality in lesional cells. Willman *et al*,[19] using a HUMARA (human androgen receptor gene) assay, demonstrated clonality in lesional tissues from 9 of 10 female cases with various forms of the disease—extreme constitutional lyonization precluded study of the tenth case. The percentage of clonal cells closely approximated the percentage of CD1a-positive cells in the lesions, and there was no evidence of lymphoid clonality by analysis of the immunoglobulin and T-cell receptor genes. Yu *et al*[20] studied 3 females with active multisystem disease, again by HUMARA assay, and demonstrated clonality in CD1a-positive but not other lesional cells. These data are unable to define whether LCH is a neoplastic or reactive disorder, however, as clonality has been demonstrated in a variety of non-neoplastic disorders.[21,22]

Investigation

In general, initial work-up for a suspected case requires confirmatory biopsy, and an accurate assessment of the extent of disease. An exception to this rule regarding the need for tissue biopsy may be made for asymptomatic children with typical lesions, e.g. isolated lytic lesions of bone, where no specific therapy is intended. Identification of LCs within the lesional inflammatory cell infiltrate is recommended for firm diagnosis, with demonstration of either the CD1a surface antigen on immunohistochemistry (Plate 5), or the presence of Birbeck granules on electron microscopy (Fig. 17.2).

In the assessment of each patient, the disease may be categorized as single- or multi-system, and children with single-system disease may have isolated or multiple sites of involvement. It is important carefully to assess the function of affected organs, as dysfunction carries prognostic significance (see below).[23] Thorough physical examination and investigations are required to determine the extent of disease, and these must include a full blood count, liver function tests,

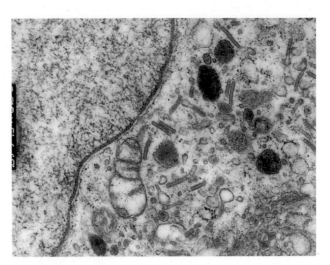

Fig. 17.2 Electron micrograph of a Langerhans cell demonstrating Birbeck granules.

serum proteins, a coagulation screen and skeletal survey by plain radiographs; technetium bone scans are generally less informative. The use of an indium-labeled murine monoclonal anti-CD1a antibody (NA1/34) in localization of active disease has been reported,[24] although this methodology currently remains a research tool. Further investigations should be guided by the need to explain specific symptoms and signs, and Lahey[23] described criteria for the diagnosis of organ/system disease and dysfunction, which remain valuable (Table 17.2).

Clinical features

The *skin rash* of LCH comprises red or yellow-brown papules on the trunk, erythema in skin folds and behind the ears, and scaling, particularly affecting the scalp (Plate 6). In mild cases, these changes are often mistaken for seborrhoeic dermatitis, eczema and cradle cap. Rarely, young infants develop a vesicular rash, similar to varicella (Plate 7), which may be present at birth, and which is generally self-limiting, although a minority of these children subsequently suffer recurrences or develop bone lesions.[25]

Ear discharge is a classic sign, and may be due either to skin involvement in the external auditory canal, or bone

Table 17.2 Criteria for the assessment of organ dysfunction in Langerhans cell histiocytosis (LCH).[23]

Liver	Total protein <55 g/l or albumin <25 g/l
	Edema, ascites
	Bilirubin' >25 μmol/l
Lungs	Tachypnea, cyanosis, cough, pneumothorax
	Pleural effusion not attributable to infection
Bone marrow	Hemoglobin <10 g/dl not due to hematinic deficiency
	White cells <4 × 10⁹/l
	Neutrophils <1.5 × 10⁹/l
	Platelets <100 × 10⁹/l

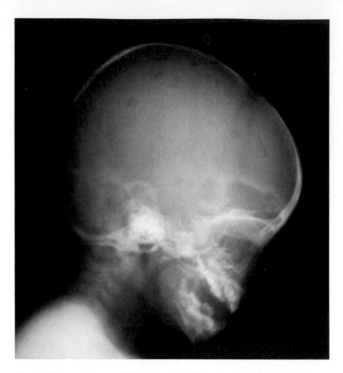

Fig. 17.3 Langerhans cell histiocytosis (LCH); radiograph showing lytic bone lesions of skull.

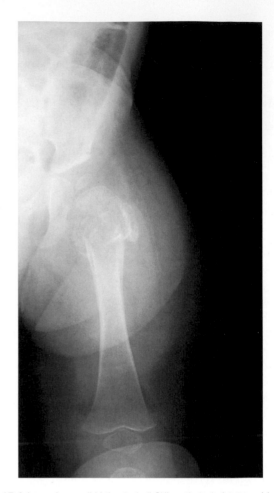

Fig. 17.4 Langerhans cell histiocytosis (LCH); pathologic fracture of femur.

destruction around and in the middle ear, with polyp formation. Such destructive lesions may result in hearing loss, and formal ENT assessment is essential.

Bone lesions may be occult, but present clinically with pain and soft tissue swelling, and are best seen on plain radiographs as irregular lytic areas sometimes with marked periosteal reaction, most commonly affecting the skull and long bones, although any bone may be involved, and there may be pathologic fractures (Figs 17.3 and 17.4).[26] Involvement of the axial skeleton may result in vertebral collapse and vertebral plana, although spinal cord compression is rare.

Orbital disease may cause proptosis, another 'classical' feature, but visual impairment is unusual.

Diabetes insipidus (DI) due to involvement of the hypothalamus and pituitary stalk may occur in both single- and multi-system disease, although this is far more common in the latter, reaching 40% in some series.[27] Besides multisystem disease, other risk factors for DI include skull lesions and proptosis. Because of this risk, study of paired early-morning plasma and urinary osmolalities is a standard part of initial assessment, and children with suggestive symptoms require a formal water deprivation test with measurement of urinary arginine vasopressin (AVP). In children with DI, magnetic resonance imaging (MRI) may demonstrate thickening of the pituitary stalk, with loss of the posterior pituitary bright signal on T2-weighted images due to the absence of AVP; the latter change occurs in DI from any cause and is not specific to LCH.[28] Some children demonstrate a transient phase of partial DI, but once true DI is established it appears to be irreversible.

Around 40% of children have multisystem disease, and although this group may include individuals with skin and bone disease, it is *visceral involvement* that carries particular significance with regard to prognosis. In particular, around 30% develop organ dysfunction and mortality in these children is 50%. Age is a significant risk factor and these more severely affected children are predominantly under 2 years of age at diagnosis.

Lung disease is characterized by cough and tachypnea, with diffuse micronodular shadowing on chest radiograph, which may progress to cyst formation and a honeycomb lung appearance and hypoxia; pleural effusions and pneumothorax may occur in advanced disease.[29] Amongst adults, tobacco smoking is a risk factor for pulmonary disease.[30] However, lung involvement *per se* has no effect on overall survival. Histology of affected lung shows peribronchiolar inflammatory infiltrates leading to fibrosis and cyst formation. On occasion, there may be doubt as to the cause of pulmonary signs, and the diagnosis can be confirmed, and infection excluded, by bronchoalveolar lavage or lung biopsy. As LCs are normally present in the bronchial tree, the presence of LCs in lavage fluid is not necessarily diagnostic of lung disease; one study indicated that >5% CD1a-positive cells should be present to support a diagnosis of lung disease.[31] High-resolution computed tomography (CT) scanning has been reported to offer good diagnostic discrimination.[32] In an international study of therapy, LCH 1 (see below) lung involvement occurred in 40 of 125 (32%) children with multi-system disease, but in only 1 of 283 with single-system disease.[33] Amongst the children with multi-system disease, 15 died. Concomitant involvement of the liver was identified as carrying a high risk of death, being present in 11 of these children.

Hepatomegaly is common, but documentation of liver dysfunction requires the demonstration of hypoalbuminemia (<30 g/dl), cholestatic jaundice, or prolonged coagulation tests, and hepatomegaly and elevated transaminases may occur without evidence of liver infiltration with lesional cells on biopsy.[34] Jaundice may also result from obstruction of the biliary tract by enlarged portal nodes, and therefore is not necessarily diagnostic of liver dysfunction. These provisos emphasize the need for careful assessment of mechanisms for clinical findings and investigation results in the initial evaluation. Severe liver disease may result in fibrosis, biliary cirrhosis and hepatic failure, and hepatic failure due to LCH has been successfully treated by orthoptic liver transplantation; 14 of 17 children reported in the literature were alive at a median follow-up of 3 years.[35]

A *low hemoglobin* is a common finding in active disease, which most often reflects anemia of chronic disease. However, pancytopenia with bone marrow infiltration by macrophages (usually not LCs), and marrow hypocellularity may occur. These changes often occur in infants with associated splenomegaly and these children have a poor prognosis. There are few studies of these changes, but McClain *et al*[36] found evidence of bone marrow disease in only 3 of 10 children with hemoglobin <10 g/dl, and in 3 of 5 with platelets <175 × 10^9/l. Several studies have identified that children with liver and bone marrow dysfunction combined fare extremely poorly.

Gut involvement with failure to thrive, vomiting, diarrhea, malabsorption, and protein-losing enteropathy occurs in under 5% of children, and requires full investigation, including adequate biopsy for confirmation.[37,38] Although infiltrates may be seen in the mucosa and submucosa, biopsy of the muscle wall may be required in some cases, and because of this previous estimates may represent underdiagnosis. Barium studies may reveal alternate dilated and stenotic segments throughout the intestine.

Mandibular and maxillary disease may result in floating teeth, and there may be gingivitis and buccal ulceration.

Disease in the central nervous system, excluding DI, occurs in around 4% of cases, and typically affects the cerebellar and cerebral white matter, with ataxia, dysarthria, nystagmus and cranial nerve palsies.[39] CNS disease usually develops at about 5 years from original presentation, and is rarely a feature at diagnosis. Most cases occur in children with multisystem disease, but also in the setting of single-system bone disease, especially of the skull, and in children with DI. On imaging, several patterns of changes are seen:

- poorly-defined changes in the white matter of the cerebellum, cerebrum and basal ganglia. Biopsy in these cases shows perivascular and parenchymal infiltrates of macrophages and lymphocytes with sparse LCs, associated with edema and demyelination;
- well-defined lesions in white and gray matter;
- extra-parenchymal masses, generally not in continuity with skull lesions, which on biopsy comprise xanthomatous histiocytes, diffusely infiltrating lymphocytes and Touton giant cells similar to those found in juvenile xanthogranuloma.

Lymphadenopathy occurs in both single- and multi-system disease, and cervical nodes in particular may be grossly enlarged. Local pressure effects may cause symptoms and signs due to obstruction of the airway, vasculature, or biliary tree, and discharging sinuses may form to the overlying skin. Involvement of the thymus may be detected on chest X-ray, and may be present on tissue examination, even without enlargement of the organ.[40]

Treatment

As the majority of cases of LCH eventually resolve spontaneously, and no therapy is uniformly effective, approaches to treatment have varied, with particular controversy regarding the role of intensive chemotherapy for children with multisystem disease. Deaths occur in 10–15% of cases, and are largely restricted to children with organ dysfunction. For most cases the primary objectives are control of symptoms and limitation of long-term disability which affects up to 50% of those with extensive disease.

Accordingly, observation alone may be appropriate, but for children with *skin disease* requiring therapy, topical application of corticosteroids may prove beneficial. For those with more severe skin involvement, topical mustine has proved highly effective—in one study rapid improvement within 10 days was seen in 16 children, with complete healing in 14.[41] The median duration of treatment was 3.5 months, and the only side-effect was contact sensitivity in one child. However, some children require systemic therapy, and oral corticosteroids result in improvement in over half of cases.

Bone lesions may resolve following diagnostic biopsy or pathologic fracture, but local therapies include curettage, injected steroids or radiotherapy, although the latter is now uncommon due to concerns over late effects—in particular, secondary malignancies have been described within the radiation field.[42] For children with multi-focal bone disease (30% of all children with bone disease), or single, symptomatic lesions unsuitable for local therapy, systemic therapy is indicated. However, further lesions and reactivations of initially responding lesions develop in up to a third of patients.

Even children with *multisystem disease* may be managed conservatively, with systemic therapy reserved for those who have organ dysfunction, pain, systemic upset or failure to thrive. The most commonly used agents for children who require systemic treatment are corticosteroids, vinblastine and etoposide, either alone or in combination, but a wide range of cytotoxic drugs have been used, including antimetabolites, alkylating agents and anthracyclines. Strategies which have failed to produce benefit include treatment with α-interferon, thymic extracts or thymic hormone. The paucity of randomized trials makes the determination of the relative efficacy of these approaches difficult, and the possibility of late effects from some of these agents argues against their use. In particular, secondary malignancy has been described in 1–5% of long-term survivors,[42–45] and treatments including etoposide, alkylating agents or radiotherapy carry particular risk.

Risk of malignancy

There is a recognized association between LCH and malignancy, which may precede or follow diagnosis. In one retrospective, registry-based study, 13 children developed acute leukemia (5 acute lymphoblastic [ALL] and 8 acute myeloid [AML]), 4 lymphomas and 10 other solid tumors. Four cases of ALL predated the LCH, whilst 7 cases of AML developed >2 years after diagnosis and treatment with chemotherapy and/or radiotherapy.[44] In another study, a literature review revealed details of 87 LCH-associated malignancies: 39 lymphomas, 62% of which occurred during the course of LCH; 22 acute leukemias, mostly AML diagnosed after the LCH; and the remainder solid tumors, including secondary tumors arising within fields of previous irradiation.[42] Amongst 341 children registered in 2 international treatment trials (LCH 1 and DAL-HX 83), however, the incidence of secondary malignancy was 1%. Accordingly, only a proportion of cases represent malignancy secondary to therapy for LCH, but this occurrence raises disquiet regarding the use of oncogenic drugs or radiotherapy in those children with little or no risk of a fatal outcome.

Evaluation of treatment approaches

Against this background, the outcome for children treated in the United Kingdom Children's Cancer Study Group (UKCCSG) centers and registered with the United Kingdom Children's Cancer Research Group are of interest (C Stiller, personal communication). Between 1977 and 1994, 370 children were registered, 191 of whom had single-system disease. When outcomes were compared between 3 time periods (1977–84, 1985–90, 1991–94), there was no change in prognosis for those with multisystem disease (Fig. 17.5). The great majority of deaths occurred in children with multisystem disease, with the poorest prognosis (60% survival) for children under 2 years of age at diagnosis (Fig. 17.6).

McLelland et al[46] reported 44 children with extensive disease managed conservatively: 36 required systemic therapy, 17 responded to prednisolone, and 19 required

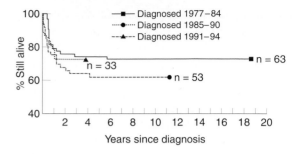

Fig. 17.5 Outcome subdivided by period of diagnosis for children treated for multisystem Langerhans cell histiocytosis (LCH) in UK Children's Cancer Study Group centers.

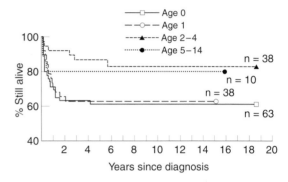

Fig. 17.6 Outcome for children treated at UK Children's Cancer Study Group centers: effect of age at diagnosis on outcome.

further treatment with vinblastine or etoposide. Overall survival was 82% (64% amongst those with organ dysfunction); 60% of survivors had late effects and 36% DI. In an Italian series, 84 children were stratified into good- and poor-risk groups depending on whether organ dysfunction was present.[47] Good-risk children received vinblastine, adriamycin and etoposide for a total of 9 months, whereas the poor-risk group was given 9 courses of cyclophosphamide, vincristine, adriamycin and prednisolone. The overall survival at 4 years was 92%, but there was a low complete response rate in the poor-risk group (2 of 11 cases) with 6 deaths, and the survivors had chronic disease. Overall, disease-related sequelae were noted in 45% and DI in 20%.

A Dutch study described the results of treatment with cytarabine, vincristine and prednisolone; 8 of 10 children without and 5 of 8 with organ dysfunction showed a complete response, with an incidence of DI of 20%.[48]

Gadner et al[49] treated children with multifocal bone or multisystem disease with 12 months combined therapy including prednisolone, vinblastine, etoposide and mercaptopurine, plus methotrexate in children with organ dysfunction. In this study (DAL-HX 83), 106 newly diagnosed children were stratified into 3 risk groups and treated with risk-directed therapy. Group A comprised 28 children with multifocal bone disease, Group B comprised 57 with soft tissue disease but no organ dysfunction, and Group C comprised 21 children with organ dysfunction. Complete resolution was achieved in 89%, 90% and 67%, respectively, with a median 4 months to complete resolution.

Recurrences occured in 12%, 23% and 42%, respectively, and overall 77% remained free of disease. Deaths were limited to Groups B and C, and mortality in group C was 38%.

Accordingly, there is little evidence that initial therapy with various combinations of cytotoxic drugs produces better survival than a more conservative, stepwise approach. However, this issue remains controversial, with claims of more rapid resolution, fewer reactivations and fewer late effects for the more intensively treated children. The uncertainty regarding the most effective and least toxic approach to treatment, together with the rarity of LCH, emphasizes the need for international collaborative randomized studies, and the Histiocyte Society has recently co-ordinated a trial (LCH 1) of vinblastine versus etoposide, both combined with initial prednisolone, in children with multisystem disease.[50]

By August 1995, 447 children had been registered (192 with multisystem disease), of whom 136 were randomized to receive 3 doses of high-dose methylprednisolone, and either weekly vinblastine or etoposide every 3 weeks. A further 134 patients were allocated to either therapy. After 6 weeks of treatment, 50% had responded and 19% had deteriorated. The remainder had stable disease. With a median follow-up of 2 years, 71% responded, 16% had progressive disease and 18% had died. Changing treatment arms provided no benefit to the majority of children with progressive disease. There was no difference in outcome for children treated with vinblastine or etoposide, and children with progressive disease after 6 weeks fared poorly, irrespective of therapy, with 90% of all study deaths occuring in this group. Joint analysis of individuals with multisystem disease treated in LCH 1 and DAL-HX 83 suggested improved disease control for children treated in the DAL series, and allowed identification of a group of 'low risk' children aged over 2 years at diagnosis, and without involvement of bone marrow, liver, lungs or spleen, who have 100% survival and a 90% probability of response to treatment.

The management of children with progressive disease despite therapy remains very difficult. Developments have included treatment with 2-chlorodeoxyadenosine,[51] anti-lymphocyte globulin, cyclosporin[52] or bone marrow transplantation,[53] and the availability of an anti-CD1a monoclonal antibody has raised the possibility of effective immunotherapy. The fundamental issue remains that assessment of all these strategies is impossible without adequate randomized trials, and there are currently insufficient data to evaluate the role of any of these treatments in either *de novo* or refractory disease.

Late effects

Although most children with LCH survive long term, there may be disability due to bone deformity, deafness, DI, lung fibrosis, cirrhosis and neurologic dysfunction. Other endocrinopathies may occur, but the commonest, growth hormone deficiency, is seen in <1% of patients.[54] However, suboptimal growth is common during active disease, although final height was normal in one Dutch study.[55] Assessment of late effects is an important aspect of comprehensive care because of the wide range of tissues at risk of involvement. Bernstrand and Henter[56] described a cross-sectional study of 75 children treated in Sweden, aged 0–15 years at diagnosis. Twenty-five children had multisystem disease (5 with organ dysfunction), 11 multifocal bone disease, 29 single-site bone involvement, 7 skin only, 1 lymph nodes only, and 2 DI. At a median follow-up of 15 years, 31 of 66 surviving patients had at least one late effect of disease or therapy: 10 had DI, 9 required other hormone replacement, 9 had short stature, 7 had orthopedic problems, 11 had facial asymetry, 6 had abnormal dentition, 6 had central nervous system abnormalities, and 3 developed a second malignancy. In the DAL series of clinical trials, permanent consequences (late effects) occurred in 20% and DI in 10%. Twelve children had orthopedic problems, 8 growth failure, 8 anterior pituitary dysfunction, 5 deafness, 3 liver fibrosis, 2 lung fibrosis, 2 dental problems and 1 psychomotor retardation. In another study assessing cognitive function, 22 children diagnosed before 5 years of age and 11–16 years of age at the time of study were compared to normal controls. Eighteen percent were below average for school work, especially reading and maths, and 23% had behavioral problems. The authors stressed the need for larger, prospective studies. These data emphasize the need for all trials of therapy to include long-term, prospective assessments of late effects.

CLASS II

This class comprises non-malignant disorders of macrophages.

Hemophagocytic lymphohistiocytosis

Hemophagocytic lymphohistiocytosis (HLH) is a rare disorder with typical histology showing tissue infiltration by morphologically benign histiocytes, some manifesting hemophagocytosis, and mature lymphocytes (Fig. 17.7).[57] The disorder occurs in primary and secondary forms with an incidence for primary HLH of 1–2 cases/million children/year in the UK and Sweden.[58,59] *Primary HLH* is a genetic disorder with autosomal recessive inheritance, but the nature of the gene defect is unknown. In a proportion of cases, there is a history of previously affected siblings indicating a familial predisposition (familial HLH), and parental consanguinity or onset in early infancy are further supportive features. It appears likely that there is an underlying disorder in T-lymphocyte function, with tissue infiltrates and hemophagocytosis generated by dysregulated secretion of cytokines, but studies of T-cell clonality have yielded conflicting results. The description of a lymphoproliferative syndrome with associated hemophagocytosis consequent on mutations

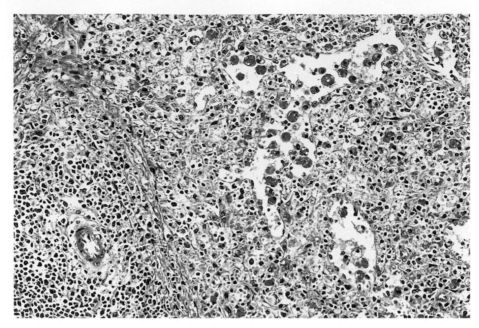

Fig. 17.7 H & E section of spleen showing lymphohistiocytic infiltrate with hemophagocytic histiocytes within the sinusoids. Kindly provided by M Malone.

affecting the Fas (CD 95) receptor raised speculation that this might be a mechanism for HLH, but this finding has not been substantiated in a large series of patients.[60]

Secondary HLH is considered to be at least as common as primary disease, and precipitants include viral, bacterial, fungal or protozoan infections, often in an immunocompromised host (infection-associated hemophagocytic syndrome [IAHS]).[61] Other precipitants include malignancy, particularly T-cell lymphoproliferative states,[62,63] and lipid infusions.[64]

Careful assessment is required to distinguish those children with true secondary disease whose disorder will resolve with reversal of any immune suppression, and treatment for or removal of the precipitant, from those with evidence of viral infection but underlying primary HLH. In one series of children and adults diagnosed with IAHS due to viral infection (virus-associated hemophagocytic syndrome [VAHS]), 14 of 19 patients were receiving immune suppression.[61] Supportive care with withdrawal of immunosuppression led to resolution in 13 cases. Amongst the 5 children with no prior immunosuppression, 2 died and 3 improved with steroids and/or azathioprine. However, not all reports show a favorable outcome, and Kikuta *et al*[65] described 6 children aged 112 years with fatal Epstein–Barr virus (EBV)-related VAHS. Furthermore, Henter *et al*[66] reported evidence of viral infection in 10 of 32 children with primary HLH, implicating EBV, cytomegalovirus and parvovirus, and amongst 93 children with HLH reported to the Histiocyte Society registry, there was no difference in outcome between 40 children with and 53 children without evidence of viral infection. These data emphasize the overlap between these disorders, and the need for circumspection in determining the best approach to therapy in each case.

Clinical features

Most children with primary HLH are young; in one series, 16 of 23 children presented before their first birthday.[67] Clinical manifestations include fever (84% of cases), splenomegaly (80%), hepatomegaly (88%), lymphadenopathy (50%), pancytopenia (88%), abnormal liver function (86%), coagulopathy (70%), and signs and symptoms referable to the central nervous system (40%). Occasionally, central nervous system involvement has been the only evidence of disease at presentation.[68] Splenomegaly is a reliable marker of disease and occurs early in the overwhelming majority of cases.[69] Initial blood changes may show anemia or thrombocytopenia, with the development of pancytopenia as the disease progresses. Other features include high fasting triglycerides, low fibrinogen, mononuclear pleocytosis and increased protein in the cerebrospinal fluid, high serum ferritin, and reduced or absent natural killer cell and cytotoxic T-cell function.[70–72] Many of these changes result from immune activation with cytokine production, and high levels of circulating IL-1 and -2, IL-2 receptor, GM-CSF and TNF have been reported.[73,74] In particular, disturbances in lipid metabolism with high triglycerides, low high density and raised very low density lipoproteins reflect reduced activity of lipoprotein lipase reductase consequent on cytokinemia.[70]

Involvement of the central nervous system varies from asymptomatic cerebrospinal fluid pleocytosis (usually to moderate levels and predominantly comprising lymphocytes with occasional macrophages [Plate 8]) to symptomatic disease with encephalitis, abnormal head movements, fits, cranial nerve palsies, ataxia, regression of developmental milestones and coma.[68,75] High levels of neopterins in cerebrospinal fluid are consistent with activation of

Table 17.3 Diagnostic guidelines for hemophagocytic lymphohistiocytosis (HLH).[67]

Clinical criteria
Fever
Splenomegaly

Laboratory criteria
Cytopenias (affecting >2 of 3 lineages in the peripheral blood)
 Hemoglobin (<9 g/dl)
 Platelets (<100 × 10^9/l)
 Neutrophils (<1.0 × 10^9/l)

Hypertriglyceridemia and/or hypofibrinogenemia
 Fasting triglycerides >2.00 mmol/l
 Fibrinogen <1.5 g/l

Histopathologic criteria
 Hemophagocytosis in bone marrow, spleen or lymph nodes
 No evidence of malignancy

All criteria required for the diagnosis of HLH. In addition, the diagnosis of familial HLH is justified by a positive family history and parental consanguinity is suggestive.

The following findings may provide strong supportive evidence for the diagnosis:
 Spinal fluid pleocytosis (mononuclear cells)
 Histologic picture in the liver resembling chronic persistent hepatitis
 Low natural killer cell activity
 High serum ferritin

macrophages, and may return to normal with adequate therapy resulting in resolution of disease.[76] In children with central nervous system disease, histology of the brain shows perivascular, parenchymal and leptomeningeal infiltrates, with necrosis and destruction, especially of white matter.

The Histiocyte Society has established criteria for the diagnosis of HLH (Table 17.3),[77] although not all features are present in every case, and repeated investigation or presumptive diagnosis may be necessary. The tissues which are most frequently sampled to substantiate the diagnosis are bone marrow, lymph node and liver, although fine needle aspiration of the spleen is reported to have a high diagnostic yield.[69,77] Diagnostic changes may be difficult to demonstrate, and the bone marrow in particular is hypercellular and reactive in the early stages of the disease, with hypocellularity and hemophagocytosis by histiocytes being later features (Plate 9).[80] Indeed, in epidemiologic surveys, diagnosis has been made post-mortem in many cases. Hemophagocytosis may not be a prominent feature of liver biopsies, and there may be prominent sinusoidal Kupffer cells and lymphoid portal infiltrates similar to those seen in chronic persistent hepatitis.

Treatment

There are two standard approaches to treatment, one using etoposide and corticosteroids,[79] and the other antithymocyte globulin (ATG), corticosteroids and cyclosporin,[79] suggesting that disordered T cells are central to pathogenesis. Around 80% of patients respond, but eventual disease recurrence is usual in primary HLH unless the child receives

an allogeneic bone marrow transplant (BMT). In one study, disease recurrence occurred in 8 of 10 children treated by etoposide, prednisolone and intrathecal methotrexate, at a median of 5 months from diagnosis. These children are at high risk of opportunistic infection due to reduced natural killer and cytotoxic T-cell function, as well as the immune suppressive effects of therapy. Age is an important determinant of prognosis; in a combined series of 23 cases treated in 2 London centers, survival was significantly higher in children aged over 2 years at presentation than in younger children (Fig. 17.8)[67] and was better for sporadic than familial cases. Inadequate disease control or reactivation may also occur in some secondary cases, and these children should then be treated in line with strategies for primary disease.

Adequate control of central nervous system involvement is very important, but the role of routine intrathecal methotrexate in this is controversial, and cranial radiation is no longer recommended. This treatment question is particularly important as some children manifest changes of leukoencephalopathy which may be related to intrathecal therapy, and the development or progression of central nervous system disease has been reported to be a feature in children receiving etoposide/corticosteroids or ATG unless they also receive a BMT.[81] Indeed, there is now evidence that changes on imaging and neurodevelopmental performance may improve following successful BMT.[75]

Experience with BMT is greatest using matched sibling donors, with around 70% of children remaining disease free, but increasing use of alternative donors, including matched and mismatched unrelated donors, and haploidentical grafts from a parent, has shown that similar results may be achieved with this approach.[82,83] Full engraftment following

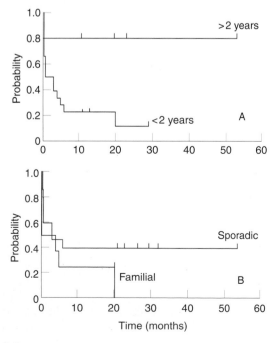

Fig. 17.8 Effects of (A) age and (B) positive family history on survival in children with primary hemophagocytic lymphohistiocytosis (HLH).[59]

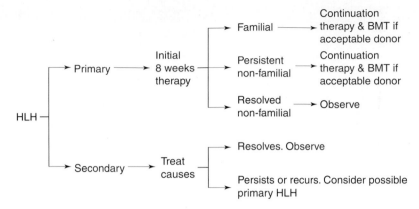

Fig. 17.9 HLH 94: a strategy for the treatment of hemophagocytic lymphohistiocytosis (HLH).[85]

transplantation is not a prerequisite for cure, as low levels of donor T cells may provide adequate disease control.[84] Clinical condition at the time of transplant affects outcome, and this emphasizes the importance of initial treatment to establish disease control. A particular worry regarding the use of a sibling donor is that in familial disease there is a 25% risk that the donor will also develop HLH, and continued improvement in the results of alternative donor procedures may make these the treatment of choice. It must also be remembered that some children, usually sporadic cases aged over 2 years at diagnosis, remain well following initial therapy and that BMT is not indicated for this group.

The Histiocyte Society has approved an international study for HLH (HLH 94) to provide a uniform approach to assessment, therapy and biologic study (Fig. 17.9).[85] Treatment is discontinued in children with a complete response to initial therapy with etoposide and dexamethasone and no evidence for familial disease, and only recom-

menced if there is reactivation. All children who require continued therapy receive cyclosporin, and intermittent etoposide and dexamethasone, and are eligible for BMT. One particular aspect under investigation is the approach to central nervous system involvement as it is possible that better systemic therapy, including dexamethasone which has good penetration to the cerebrospinal fluid, may obviate the need for methotrexate in some cases.

Other Class II disorders

Sinus histiocytosis with massive lymphadenopathy (SHML) was described in 1969 by Rosai and Dorfman as a syndrome of cervical lymphadenopathy with typical histology showing preserved lymph node structure and dilated lymph node sinuses containing mixed inflammatory cells, with vacuolated histiocytes manifesting hemophagocytosis and emperipolesis of lymphocytes (Fig. 17.10).[86–90] Fibrosis may be

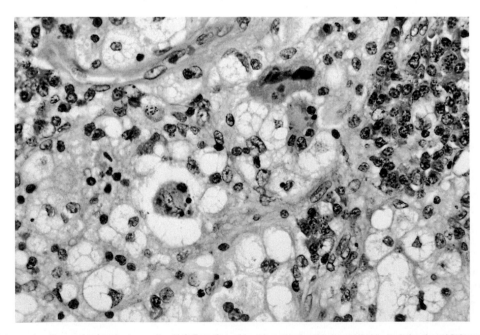

Fig. 17.10 Sinus histiocytosis with massive lymphadenopathy. H & E section of lymph node showing hemophagocytosis by sinus histiocytes. Kindly provided by M Malone.

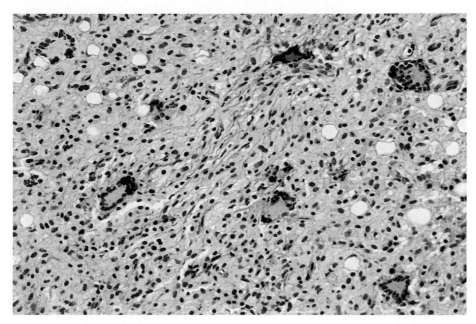

Fig. 17.11 *Juvenile xanthogranuloma.* H & E section of biopsy showing typical infiltrate and Touton giant cells. Kindly provided by M Malone.

marked. Histologic features in other tissues are similar, with increased fibrosis and less hemophagocytosis. Other features of SHML include systemic ill health with fever and weight loss, destructive infiltrates in skin, bone and other extranodal sites, hypergammaglobulinemia, elevated erythrocyte sedimentation rate, reactive leukocytosis, and immune dysfunction including autoimmune anemia and neutropenia. Although most cases are isolated, SHML has occurred in individuals with malignancy, autoimmune diseases or other histiocyte disorders, especially LCH. Involvement of cervical lymph nodes is present in most cases, but other groups are affected, either jointly or alone. The lymphadenopathy may be gross, and often painless, and may wax and wane with time. Extranodal disease of the head and neck, or a variety of other sites, is present in almost half of cases, either alone or in association with lymphoid masses. As with other histiocyte disorders, a possible role for EBV in pathogenesis has been postulated.

The natural history of the disorder is chronic with spontaneous resolution over months or years in many cases, although approximately 5% of patients die due to immune-mediated organ dysfunction, amyloidosis, or infection. Few individuals have died directly from lymphohistiocytic infiltrates. Therapy with steroids, cytotoxic drugs, particularly vincristine and alkylating agents, or radiotherapy has been variably effective, and is unnecessary in most cases.

Histiocytic necrotizing lymphadenopathy presents with nodal enlargement in the neck or axilla, which may be associated with fever and lethargy.[91] Histology reveals inflammatory infiltrates, prominent histiocytes and local necrosis. The etiology is unknown and spontaneous resolution can be expected.

Juvenile xanthogranuloma usually presents with single or multiple yellow-red skin lesions in newborns and infants; in one series, the median age at presentation in 36 children was 0.3 years (range birth–12 years).[92–94] Histology shows a cutaneous accumulation of lipid-filled macrophages, Touton giant cells and fibroblasts (Fig. 17.11). Extracutaneous disease may occur in around 10% of patients involving the central nervous system, liver, spleen, lung, eye, oropharynx and muscle. For lesions resulting in complications, excision may be indicated, but spontaneous resolution is usual and no treatment has been proven to be undoubtedly beneficial.

Self-healing reticulo-histiocytosis comprises cutaneous nodules composed of large histiocytes with cytologic atypia, multinucleated forms and mitotic figures, usually affecting young babies.[95] These lesions resolve spontaneously over several months, but there may be hematologic changes including neutropenia.

CLASS III

Acute monocytic leukemia (AML M5 by the FAB classification) accounts for 10% of AML in children (see Chapter 18). Considerable controversy exists regarding other malignancies of the monocyte/macrophage system due to difficulties in nosology. Malignant histiocytosis was described as a clinical picture of lymphadenopathy, hepatosplenomegaly, fever, wasting and pancytopenia, with histology showing tissue infiltration by large cells with copious cytoplasm and irregular nuclei.[96] However, recent studies of cell lineage in such cases with monoclonal antibodies, and of immunoglobulin or T-cell receptor gene rearrangements, indicate that the majority of these tumors are in fact of lymphoid origin, and reclassifiable as large cell (Ki 1-positive) anaplastic lymphomas (see Chapter 28).[97,98] In one overview of experience at the University of Minnesota combined with a literature review, only 19 of 164 cases originally diagnosed as malignant histiocytosis were confirmed as negative for B- and T-cell markers and positive for monocytic lineage surface antigens.[97]

Accordingly, true malignant histiocytosis is an extremely rare entity, requiring careful pathologic assessment to substantiate diagnosis. This uncertainty clouds issues regarding therapy, although a high response rate has been described for children receiving cyclophosphamide, prednisolone, vincristine and adriamycin.[99,100] Other agents employed in these cases have included methotrexate, cytarabine and etoposide, all drugs widely employed in lymphoma therapy. Due to these difficulties it is not possible to assess outcome for the few patients with true malignant histiocytosis, other than to report that occasional individuals appear to be long-term survivors following combination chemotherapy.

Finally, malignant tumors of both dendritic and interdigitating reticulum cells present as localized lymphadenopathy, although metastases have been described.[101,102] Both are very rare and neither tumor has been described in children.

REFERENCES

1. Chu T, D'Angio GJ, Favara B, Ladisch S, Nesbit M, Pritchard J. Histiocytosis syndromes in children. *Lancet* 1987; **i**: 208–209

2. Hesseling PB, Wessels G, Egeler RM, Rossouw DJ. Simultaneous occurrence of viral-associated hemophagocytic syndrome and Langerhans cell histiocytosis: a case report. *Pediatr Hematol Oncol* 1995; **12**; 135–141

3. Lasser A. The mononuclear phagocyte system: a review. *Hum Pathol* 1983; **14**: 108–126

4. Metcalf D. The granulocyte-macrophage colony-stimulating factors. *Science* 1985: **229**: 16–22

5. Meuret G, Hoffman G. Monocyte kinetics in normal and disease states. *Br J Haematol* 1973; **24**: 275–282

6. Weinberg JB, Athens JW. The mononuclear phagocyte system. In: Lee GR, Billell TC, Foerster J, Athens SW, Lukens JN (eds) *Wintrobe's Clinical Haematology*. Philadelphia: Lea and Febiger, 1993, pp 267–298

7. Austyn J. Lymphoid dendritic cells. *Immunology* 1987; **62**: 161–170

8. Chu T, Jaffe R. The normal Langerhans cell and the LCH cell. *Br J Cancer* 1994; **70 (Suppl xxiii)**: S4–S10

9. Lichtenstein L. Histiocytosis X. Integration of eosinophilic granuloma of bone, Letterer–Siwe disease, and Hand–Christian–Schuller disease as related manifestations of a single nosologic entity. *AMA Arch Pathol* 1953; **56**: 84–102

10. Nezelhof C, Basset F, Rousseau MF. Histiocytosis X; histogenetic arguments for a Langerhans cell origin. *Biomedecine* 1973; **18**: 365–371

11. Raney RB, D'Angio GJ. Langerhans cell histiocytosis (histiocytosis X): experience at the Children's Hospital of Philadelphia, 1970–1984. *Med Pediatr Oncol* 1989; **17**: 20–28

12. Favara BE, Jaffe R. The histopathology of Langerhans cell histiocytosis. *Br J Cancer* 1994; **70 (Suppl xxiii)**: S17–S23

13. Kapsenberg ML, Teuissen MBM, Boss JD. Langerhans cells; a unique subpopulation of antigen-presenting dendritic cells. In: Boss JD (ed) *Skin Immune System*. Boca Ratton: CRC Press, 1990, pp 125–157

14. McClain K, Jin H, Gresik V, Favara B. Langerhans cell histiocytosis: lack of a viral etiology. *Am J Hematol* 1994; **47**: 16–20

15. Leahy MA, Krejci SM, Friednash M *et al*. Human herpesvirus 6 is present in lesions of Langerhans cell histiocytosis. *J Invest Dermatol* 1993; **101**: 642–645

16. Mierau GW, Wills EJ, Steele PO. Ultrastructural studies in Langerhans cell histiocytosis: a search for evidence of viral etiology. *Pediatr Pathol* 1994; **14**: 895–904

17. Kannourakis G, Abbas A. The role of cytokines in the pathogenesis of Langerhans cell histiocytosis. *Br J Cancer* 1994; **70 (Suppl xxiii)**: S37–S40

18. Emile JF, Tartour E, Brugieres L *et al*. Detection of GM-CSF in the serum of children with Langerhans cell histiocytosis. *Pediatr Allergy Immunol* 1994; **5**: 162–163

19. Willman CL, Busque L, Griffith BB *et al*. Langerhans cell histiocytosis (histiocytosis X)—a clonal proliferative disease. *N Engl J Med* 1994; **331**: 154–160

20. Yu RC, Chu C, Buluwela L, Chu AC. Clonal proliferation of Langerhans cells in Langerhans cell histiocytosis. *Lancet* 1994; **343**: 767–768

21. Orphanos V, Anagnostou D, Papdaki T. Detection of gene rearrangements in reactive lymphoid processes. *Leukemia* 1993; **9**: 103–106

22. Van-Dongen JJ, Wolvers-Tettaro ILM. Analysis of immunoglobulin and T cell receptor genes. Possibilities and limitations in the diagnosis and management of lymphoproliferative diseases and related disorders. *Clin Chim Acta* 1991; **198**: 93–175

23. Lahey ME. Histiocytosis X: an analysis of prognostic factors. *J Pediatr* 1975; **87**: 184–189

24. Kelly KM, Beverley PC, Chu AC *et al*. Successful *in vivo* immunolocalisation of Langerhans cell histiocytosis with use of a monoclonal antibody, NA1/34. *J Pediatr* 1994; **125**: 717–722

25. Hashimoto K, Pritzker MS. Electron microscopic study of reticulohistiocytoma—an unusual case of self-healing reticulohistiocytosis. *Arch Dermatol* 1973; **107**: 283–289

26. Kilpatrick SE, Wenger DE, Gilchrist GS, Shives TC, Wollan PC, Unni KK. Langerhans cell histiocytosis of bone. *Cancer* 1995; **76**: 2471–2484

27. Dunger DB, Broadbent V, Yeomans E. The frequency and natural history of diabetes insipidus in children with Langerhans cell histiocytosis. *N Engl J Med* 1989; **321**: 1157–1162

28. Rosenfield NS, Abrahams J, Komp D. Brain MR in patients with Langerhans cell histiocytosis: findings and enhancement with Gd-DTPA. *Pediatr Radiol* 1990; **20**: 433–466

29. Ha SY, Helms P, Fletcher M, Broadbent V, Pritchard J. Lung involvement in Langerhans cell histiocytosis: prevalence, clinical features, and outcome. *Pediatrics* 1992; **89**: 466–469

30. Travis WD, Borok Z, Roum JH, Zhang J, Feuerstein I, Ferrans VJ, Crystal RG. Pulmonary Langerhans cell granulomatosis (histiocytosis X). A clinicopathological study. *Am J Surg Pathol* 1993; **17**: 971–986

31. Auerswald U, Barth J, Magnussen H. Value of CD1a positive cells in bronchoalveolar lavage fluid for the diagnosis of pulmonary histiocytosis X. *Lungs* 1991; **169**: 305–309

32. Kulweic EL, Lynch DA, Aguayo SM, Schwarz MI, King TE. Imaging of pulmonary histiocytosis X. *Radiographics* 1992; **12**: 515–526

33. Flucher-Wolfram B, Minkov M, Grois N *et al*. Pulmonary involvement in multisystem Langerhans cell histiocytosis. *Med Pediatr Oncol* 1997; 28: 155

34. Favara BE. The histiocytoses: clinical presentation and differential diagnosis. *Oncology* 1990; 4: 60–61

35. Melendez HV, Dhawan A, Mieli-Vergani G *et al*. Liver transplantation for Langerhans cell histiocytosis—a case report and literature review. *Transplantation* 1996; **62**: 1167–1171

36. McClain K, Ramsay NKC, Robinson L, Sundberg RD, Nesbit ME. Bone marrow involvement in histiocytosis X. *Med Pediatr Oncol* 1983; **11**: 167–171

37. Keeling JW, Harries JT. Intestinal malabsorption in infants with histiocytosis X. *Arch Dis Child* 1973; **48**: 350–354

38. Geissmann F, Thomas C, Emile J-F *et al*. Digestive tract involvement in Langerhans cell histiocytosis. *Med Pediatr Oncol* 1996; **28**: 161

39. Grois N, Barkovich AJ, Rosenau W, Ablin AR. Central nervous system disease associated with Langerhans cell histiocytosis. *Am J Pediatr Hematol Oncol* 1993; **15**: 245–254

40. Osband ME, Lipton JM, Lavin P *et al*. Histiocytosis X—demonstration of abnormal immunity, T-cell histamine H2-receptor deficiency, and successful treatment with thymic extract. *N Engl J Med* 1981; **304**: 146–153

41. Sheehan MP, Atherton DJ, Broadbent V, Pritchard J. Topical nitrogen mustard: an effective treatment for cutaneous Langerhans cell histiocytosis. *J Pediatr* 1991; **119**: 317–321

42. Egeler RM, Neglia JP, Puccetti DM, Brennan CA, Nesbit ME. Association of Langerhans cell histiocytosis with malignant neoplasms. *Cancer* 1993; **71**: 865–873

43. Selch MT, Parker RG. Radiation therapy in the management of Langerhans cell histiocytosis. *Med Pediatr Oncol* 1990; **18**: 97–102

44. Egeler RM, Neglia JP, Arico M, Favara BE, Heitger A, Nesbit ME. Acute leukemia in association with Langerhans cell histiocytosis. *Med Pediatr Oncol* 1994; **23**: 81–85

45. Haupt R, Fears TR, Rosso P *et al*. Increased risk of secondary leukemia after single-agent treatment with etoposide for Langerhan's cell histiocytosis. *Pediatr Hematol Oncol* 1994; **11**: 499–507

46. McLelland J, Broadbent V, Yeomans E, Malone M, Pritchard J. Langerhan's cell histiocytosis: the case for conservative treatment. *Arch Dis Child* 1990; **65**: 301–303

47. Ceci A, De Terlizzi M, Colella R *et al*. Langerhans cell histiocytosis in childhood: results from the Italian Cooperative AIEOP-CNR-HX'83 study. *Med Pediatr Oncol* 1993; **21**: 259–264

48. Egeler RM, De Kraker J, Voute PA. Cytosine arabinoside, vincristine, and prednisolone in the treatment of children with disseminated Langerhans cell histiocytosis with organ dysfunction. *Med Pediatr Oncol* 1993; **21**; 265–270

49. Gadner H, Heitger A, Grois N, Gatterer-Menz I, Ladisch S. Treatment strategy for disseminated Langerhan's cell histiocytosis. *Med Pediatr Oncol* 1994; **23**: 72–80

50. Ladisch S, Gadner H. Treatment of Langerhans cell histiocytosis—evolution and current approaches. *Br J Cancer* 1994; **70 (Suppl xxiii)**: S41–S46

51. Saven A, Foon KA, Piro LD. 2 chlorodeoxyadenosine induced complete remissions in Langerhans cell histiocytosis. *Ann Intern Med* 1994; **121**: 430–432

52. Arico M, Colella R, Conter V *et al*. Cyclosporine therapy for refractory Langerhans cell histiocytosis. *Med Pediatr Oncol* 1995; **25**: 12–16

53. Morgan G. Myeloablative therapy and bone marrow transplantation for Langerhans cell histiocytosis. *Br J Cancer* 1994; **70 (Suppl xxiii)**: S52–S53

54. Dean HJ, Bishop A, Winter JSD. Growth hormone deficiency in patients with histiocytosis X. *J Pediatr* 1986; **109**: 615–618

55. Van den Hoek ACJ, Karstens A, Egeler RM, Hahlen K. Growth of children with Langerhans cell histiocytosis. *Eur J Pediatr* 1995; **154**: 822–825

56. Bernstrand C, Henter J-I. Long term follow up of 83 patients with Langerhans cell histiocytosis (LCH)—a single centre study. *Med Pediatr Oncol* 1997; **28**: 158

57. Perry MC, Harrison EG, Burgert EO *et al*. Familial erythrophagocytic lymphohistiocytosis: report of 2 cases and clinicopathological review. *Cancer* 1976; **38**: 209–218

58. Henter J-I, Soder O, Ost A, Elinder G. Incidence and clinical features of familial hemophagocytic lymphohistiocytosis. *Acta Pediatr Scand* 1991; **80**: 428–435

59. Layton DM, Pritchard J, Mieli-Vergani G, Strobel S. A prospective study of haemophagocytic lymphohistiocytosis in the UK. *Br J Haematol* 1995; **89 (suppl 1)**: 2

60. Lalloz MRA, Layton DM. FAS receptor and FAS ligand defects are excluded as major determinants of haemophagocytic lymphohistiocytosis. *Br J Haematol* 1997; **97 (Suppl 1)**: 12

61. Risdall RJ, McKenna RW, Nesbit ME *et al*. Virus-associated hemophagocytic syndrome. *Cancer* 1979; **44**: 993–1002

62. Su I-H, Wang C-H, Cheng A-L, Chen R-L. Hemophagocytic syndrome in Epstein–Barr virus T-lymphocyte disorders: disease spectrum, pathogenesis, and management. *Leukemia Lymphoma* 1995; **19**: 401–406

63. Wong KF, Chan JK. Reactive hemophagocytic syndrome—a clinico-pathological study of 40 patients in an Oriental population. *Am J Med* 1992; **93**: 177–180

64. Goulet O, Girot R, Maier-Redelsperger M *et al*. Hematologic disorders following prolonged use of intravenous fat emulsions in children. *J Parenter Enter Nutr* 1986; **10**: 284–288

65. Kikuta H, Sakiyama Y, Matsumoto S *et al*. Fatal Epstein–Barr virus-associated hemophagocytic syndrome. *Blood* 1993; **82**: 3259–3264

66. Henter J-I, Ehrnst A, Andersson J, Elinder G. Familial hemophagocytic lymphohistiocytosis and viral infections. *Acta Paediatr* 1993; **82**: 369–372

67. Hirst WJR, Layton DM, Singh S *et al*. Haemophagocytic lymphohistiocytosis: experience at two UK centres. *Br J Haematol* 1994; **88**: 731–739

68. Henter J-I, Elinder G. Cerebromeningeal haemophagocytic lymphohistiocytosis. *Lancet* 1992; **339**: 104–107

69. Henter J-I, Elinder G. Familial hemophagocytic lymphohistiocytosis: clinical review based on the findings in seven children. *Acta Pediatr Scand* 1991; **80**: 269–277

70. Henter J-I, Carlson LA, Soder O, Nilsson-Ehle P, Elinder G. Lipoprotein alterations and plasma lipoprotein lipase reductase reduction in familial hemophagocytic lymphohistiocytosis. *Acta Pediatr Scand* 1991; **80**: 675–681

71. Esumi N, Ikushima S, Todo S, Imashuku S. Hyperferritinemia in malignant histiocytosis, virus-associated hemophagocytic syndrome and familial erythrophagocytic lymphohistiocytosis. *Acta Pediatr Scand* 1989; **78**: 268–270

72. Perez N, Virelizier J-L, Arenzana-Seisedos F, Fischer A, Griscelli C. Impaired natural killer activity in lymphohistiocytosis syndrome. *J Pediatr* 1984; **104**: 569–573

73. Henter JI, Elinder G, Soder O, Hansson M, Andersson B, Andersson U. Hypercytokinemia in familial hemophagocytic lymphohistiocytosis. *Blood* 1991; **78**: 2918–2922

74. Fujiwara F, Hibi S, Imashuku S. Hypercytokinemia in hemophagocytic syndrome. *Am J Pediatr Hematol Oncol* 1993; **15**: 92–98

75. Filipovich AH, Madison M. Central nervous system (CNS) complications of infantile hemophagocytic lymphohistiocytosis (HLH): neuroradiologic findings pre and post bone marrow transplant (BMT). *Med Pediatr Oncol* 1997; **28**: 161

76. Howells DW, Strobel S, Smith RI, Levinsky RJ, Hyland K. Central nervous system involvement in erythrophagocytic disorders of infancy: the role of cerebrospinal neopterins in their differential diagnosis and clinical management. *Pediatr Res* 1990; **28**: 116–119

77. Henter J-I., Elinder G, Ost A. Diagnostic guidelines for haemophagocytic lymphohistiocytosis. *Semin Oncol* 1991; **18**: 29–33

78. Janka G.E. Familial hemophagocytic lymphohistiocytosis. *Eur J Pediatr* 1983; **140**: 221–230

79. Blanche S, Caniglia M, Girault D, Landman J, Griscelli C, Fischer A. Treatment of hemophagocytic lymphohistiocytosis with chemotherapy and bone marrow transplantation: a single-centre study of 22 cases. *Blood* 1991; **78**: 51–54

80. Stephan JL, Donadieu J, Ledeist F, Blanche S, Griscelli C, Fischer A. Treatment of familial hemophagocytic lymphohistiocytosis with antithymocyte globulins, steroids, and cyclosporin A. *Blood* 1993; **82**: 2319–2323

81. Haddad E, Sulis ML, Jabado N, Blanche S, Fischer A, Tardieu M. Frequency and severity of CNS lesions in haemophagocytic lymphohistiocytosis. *Blood* 1997; 89: 794–800

82. Bolme P, Henter J-I, Winiarski J *et al*. Allogeneic bone marrow transplantaion for haemophagocytic lymphohistiocytosis in Sweden. *Bone Marrow Transplant* 1995; **15**: 331–335

83. Filipovich AH, Porta F, Kollman C. Unrelated donor (URD) bone marrow transplantation (BMT) for primary immunodeficiencies: an international review. *Blood* 1994; **84 (Suppl 1)**: 394A

84. Landman-Parker J, Le Diest F, Blaise A, Brison O, Fischer A. Partial engraftment of donor bone marrow cells associated with long term remission of haemophagocytic lymphohistiocytosis. *Br J Haematol* 1993; **85**: 37–41

85. Henter J-I, Arico M, Egeler RM *et al*. HLH 94: a treatment protocol for hemophagocytic lymphohistiocytosis. *Med Pediatr Oncol* 1997; **28**: 342–347

86. Sacchi S, Artusi T, Torelli U, Emilia G. Sinus histiocytosis with massive lymphadenopathy. *Leukemia Lymphoma* 1992; **7**: 189–194

87. Horneff G, Jurgens H, Hort W, Karitzky D, Gobel U. Sinus histiocytosis with massive lymphadenopathy (Rosai–Dorfman disease): response to methotrexate and mercaptopurine. *Med Pediatr Oncol* 1996; **27**: 187–192

88. Foucar E, Rosai J, Dorfman F. Sinus histiocytosis with massive lympadenopathy: an analysis of 15 deaths occuring in a registry. *Cancer* 1984; **54**: 1834–1840

89. Suarez CR, Zeller WP, Silberman S, Rust G, Messmore H. Sinus histiocytosis with massive lymphadenopathy: remission with chemotherapy. *Am J Pediatr Hematol Oncol* 1983; **5**: 235–241

90. Lampert F, Lennert K. Sinus histiocytosis with massive lymphadenopathy. *Cancer* 1976; **37**: 783–789

91. Turner RR, Martin J, Dorfman RF. Necrotizing lympadenitis: a study of 30 cases. *Am J Surg Pathol* 1983; **7**: 115–123

92. Freyer DR, Kennedy R, Bostrom BC, Kohut G, Dehner LP. Juvenile xanthogranuloma: forms of systemic disease and their clinical implications. *J Pediatr* 1996; **129**: 227–236

93. Helwig EB, Hackney VC. Juvenile xanthogranuloma. *Am J Pathol* 1954; **30**: 625–630

94. Seo S, Min KW, Mirkin LD. Juvenile xanthogranuloma: ultrastructural and immunocytochemical studies. *Arch Pathol Lab Med* 1986; **110**: 911–915

95. Hashimoto K, Griffin D, Kohsbaki M. Self-healing reticulohistiocytosis: a clinical, histologic, and ultrastructural study. *Cancer* 1982; **49**: 331–337

96. Schmidt D. Monocyte/macrophage system and malignancies. *Med Pediatr Oncol* 1994; **23**: 444–451

97. Egeler RM, Schmitz L, Sonneveld P, Mannival C, Nesbit ME. Malignant histiocytosis: a reassessment of cases formerly classified as histiocytic neoplasms and review of the literature. *Med Pediatr Oncol* 1995; **25**: 1–7

98. Bucksky P, Favara B, Feller AC *et al*. Malignant histiocytosis and large cell anaplastic lymphoma in childhood: guidelines for differential diagnosis—report of the Histiocyte Society. *Med Pediatr Oncol* 1994; **22**: 200–203

99. Tseng A, Coleman CN, Cox RS *et al*. The treatment of malignant histiocytosis. *Blood* 1984; **64**: 48–53

100. Brugieres L, Caillaud JM, Patte C *et al*. Malignant histiocytosis: therapeutic results in 27 children treated with a single polychemotherapy regimen. *Med Pediatr Oncol* 1989; **17**: 193–196

101. Chan JK, Ng CS, Law CK *et al*. Lymph node interdigitating reticulum cell sarcoma. *Am J Clin Pathol* 1986; **85**: 739–744

102. Manda L, Warnke R, Rosai J. A primary lymph node malignancy with features suggestive of dendritic reticulum cell differentiation. *Am J Pathol* 1986; **122**: 562–572

Pathology of acute myeloid leukemia

CHING-HON PUI AND FREDERICK G BEHM

Leukemia, the commonest form of childhood cancer, affects approximately 3000 children under the age of 15 years in the US/year, accounting for almost one-third of all childhood malignancies.[1] Acute myeloid (non-lymphoblastic) leukemia (AML) accounts for 17% of all childhood leukemias.[2] The annual incidence rate of AML is 5.6/million children/year.[1] Except for a slightly higher rate in infants <1 year of age, the incidence of AML is relatively stable throughout childhood until the age of 20, after which it begins to rise.[3] In adults, the annual incidence rate increases progressively with age, exceeding 150 cases/million persons older than 65 years of age, an approximate 30-fold increase over that in children.[4] In contrast to findings in acute lymphoid leukemia (ALL) (see Chapters 26 and 27), the biology and treatment of AML are very similar in children and younger adults (<60 years of age) and studies of adult cases have contributed importantly to current knowledge of childhood AML. This chapter summarizes the clinical and biologic characteristics of childhood AML, while Chapter 19 provides a detailed account of modern leukemia therapy.

EPIDEMIOLOGY

The incidence of AML shows considerable geographic and ethnic variation. Incidence rates are highest in Asia, similar in North America, Europe and Australia, and somewhat lower in South America and India.[5] In the US, the incidence is higher in white (5.8 cases/million) than black children (4.8 cases/million),[1] with the highest rate occurring among Latin Americans in Los Angeles.[5] Unlike the clear pattern of male dominance in childhood ALL, AML lacks any consistent variation in incidence by gender.[3] Limited data suggest an increased incidence of childhood AML in the US from 1974 to 1991,[6,7] but it is still uncertain whether this finding reflects a true increase or merely random statistical variability.

Although certain genetic diseases and environmental factors have been implicated in the development of AML (Table 18.1), predisposing factors are not identified in the majority of patients. Down's syndrome increases the risk of leukemia development by 10–20-fold.[8–10] In several large studies of newly diagnosed childhood AML, 4.2–13% of patients had this syndrome.[11–16] Although the ratio of AML:ALL cases in patients with Down's syndrome is the same overall as that in the general population, the megakaryoblastic subtype of AML predominates in younger children with this congenital disorder (4 years or younger), while ALL is commoner in older patients.[17–19]

Compared to other children with AML, Down's patients are younger, have a lower leukocyte count, are more likely to have myelodysplasia, megakaryoblastic leukemia or undifferentiated AML, and have a more favorable treatment outcome.[19] Neonates with Down's frequently develop a transient myeloproliferative syndrome, characterized as a monoclonal disorder involving a multipotent stem cell with a

Table 18.1 Conditions associated with an increased risk of acute myeloid leukemia.

Genetic and constitutional factors
Down's syndrome
Fanconi's anemia
Bloom's syndrome
Kostmann's syndrome
Diamond–Blackfan anemia
Neurofibromatosis
Shwachman's syndrome*
Klinefelter's syndrome*
Identical twin of child with leukemia

Prenatal factors
Parental exposure to pesticides, solvents or petroleum products
Maternal alcohol consumption and marijuana use

Postnatal factors
Exposure to pesticides and petroleum products
Cytotoxic chemotherapy (alkylating agents, epipodophyllotoxins)
Aplastic anemia

*Insufficient data to establish the association.

preference for megakaryoblastic differentiation, that resolves spontaneously within the first 3 months of life.[20–23] Up to 30% of cases with transient myeloproliferative syndrome develop AML in the first 3 years of life.[10] Thus, the seemingly benign leukocyte proliferation in some Down's neonates represents a pre-leukemic disorder.

Syndromes with increased chromosomal breakage are also associated with an increased risk of AML, including Fanconi's anemia, Bloom's syndrome, congenital disorders of hematopoiesis such as Kostmann's syndrome, idiopathic congenital neutropenia and Diamond–Blackfan anemia, and neurofibromatosis (Table 18.1).[3,24–28] Several patients with severe congenital neutropenia who developed AML all had a truncated C-terminal region of the granulocyte colony-stimulating factor (G-CSF) receptor, suggesting that interruptions in the signals required for the maturation of myeloid cells are involved in the pathogenesis of both processes.[29,30] Although frequently listed as a risk factor for AML, ataxia-telangiectasia is actually associated with lymphoid neoplasia.[31] The identical twin of a young child (<6 years old) with leukemia is at high risk (approx 25%) for developing concordant leukemia, especially during the first year of life.[32] There is unequivocal evidence that intraplacental metastasis is the cause of concordant leukemia.[33]

Exposures to ionizing radiation, petroleum products, benzene and other solvents have been associated with an increased risk of AML in adults. Similar epidemiologic findings are limited in children who rarely come into contact with carcinogens capable of causing leukemia. In one study, occupational exposures of either parent to pesticides, paternal exposures to solvents and petroleum products, and postnatal exposures to pesticides and petroleum products were associated with an increased risk of childhood AML.[34] A higher risk of childhood AML after maternal occupational exposure to benzene and gasoline during pregnancy was also demonstrated in a study from Shanghai.[35] In addition, maternal use of marijuana and alcohol consumption during pregnancy have been related to the development of AML in offspring, especially during infancy.[36,37] Studies of the leukemogenic potential of parental smoking, radon exposure and residential exposure to electromagnetic fields have yielded inconsistent results.[3,38] It is well recognized that treatment with alkylating agents and topoisomerase II inhibitors (the epipodophyllotoxins especially) can induce AML.[39–41] Cases induced by alkylators are characterized by a latency period of 4–6 years, a myelodysplastic phase, and a loss or deletions of part of chromosomes 5, 7 or both, while those related to topoisomerase II inhibitors have a relatively short latency, 1–3 years, lack a myelodysplastic phase, and have 11q23 chromosomal translocations involving the *MLL* (myeloid/lymphoid leukemia) gene.[39–41]

Finally, approximately 10% of children with severe aplastic anemia will develop AML or myelodysplastic syndrome.[42,43]

LEUKEMIC PROGENITOR CELLS

Acute leukemia arises in a single transformed hematopoietic progenitor cell that spawns a clone of leukemic blast cells. The clonal nature of leukemia has been confirmed by numerous lines of research, including glucose-6-phosphate dehydrogenase (G6PD) enzyme studies and recombinant DNA analysis based on X-linked restriction fragment length polymorphisms (RFLPs) in heterozygous females whose normal tissues are mosaics with respect to X-chromosome expression but whose leukemic cells show a single active parental allele.[44] Morphologic, cytogenetic, fluorescence *in situ* hybridization (FISH), and G6PD isoenzyme studies indicate differences in the leukemic cell of origin depending on the age of the patient and the mechanism of transformation. In the elderly and in patients with secondary AML, the target cell appears to be capable of trilineage development, indicative of transformation at the level of a pluripotent stem cell.[45–47] By contrast, the disease in children generally arises in lineage-restricted, committed granulocytic progenitor cells.[47] The increased capacity for self-renewal of leukemic cells and their growth advantage over normal marrow progenitors is ultimately responsible for the failure of normal hematopoiesis, the hallmark of leukemia.

MORPHOLOGY

CYTOCHEMICAL ANALYSES

Examination of the bone marrow is crucial to establishing the diagnosis of AML and properly classifying the blast cells, as some patients lack circulating leukemic blasts and the morphology of the cells in peripheral blood may differ from that of bone marrow cells. Marrow aspiration generally yields an interpretable specimen, although in cases with myelofibrosis or a tightly packed marrow cavity, a biopsy may be the only method that will ensure a high-quality sample. Touch preparations should be made from all biopsy specimens, as they provide cytologic details not appreciable in histologic preparations.

The initial morphologic assessment begins with Romanowsky-stained (Wright, Wright-Giemsa or May-Grünwald-Giemsa) smears. Myeloblasts are usually larger than lymphoblasts and contain more cytoplasm. The nucleus varies from round to indented and usually contains fine chromatin and 1–4 distinct nucleoli. The cytoplasm is pale to moderately basophilic, often displaying a variable number of primary granules (Plate 10). Auer rods or elongated red crystalline bodies consisting of coalescence of primary granules are pathognomonic of malignant myeloblasts (Plate 11).[48] Monoblasts are large, with a folded or indented nucleus, lacy chromatin, 1–3 large nucleoli, and generally abundant cytoplasm that is intensely basophilic, occasion-

SECTION 1 MARROW FAILURE SYNDROMES

Chapter 3 Failure of red cell production

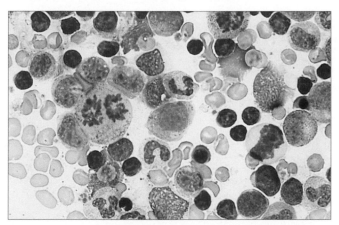

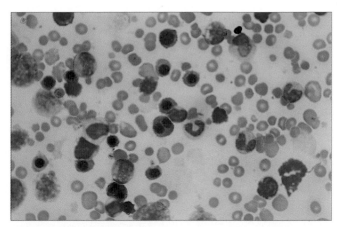

Plate 1 Bone marrow aspirate from a 6-week-old baby with familial Diamond–Blackfan anemia, showing a cellular marrow with active myelopoiesis but virtually absent erythroid maturation.

Plate 2 Abnormal erythroblasts seen in human parvovirus B19 infection. Kindly supplied by IM Hann.

Chapter 4 Myelodysplastic syndromes

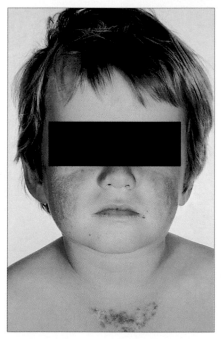

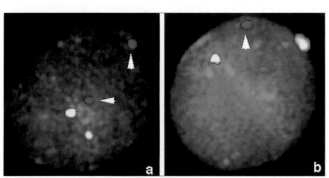

Plate 4 Fluorescent *in situ* hybridization using α-satellite centrometric probes to demonstrate monosomy for chromosome 7. (a) Normal cell showing two signals for both the normal control probe (yellow signal) and chromosome 7 (red signal). (b) Cell monosomic for chromosome 7 showing 2 copies for the control of probe (yellow signal) and only 1 copy for chromosome 7 (red signal).

Plate 3 Skin rash in a 5-year-old boy who presented with CMML: Hb 8.7 g/dl, platelet count 15 × 10⁹/l and WBC 4.7 × 10⁹/l. Bone marrow cytogenetics were normal and the fetal Hb was 39%.

Colour plates

SECTION 3 GRANULOCYTE AND MACROPHAGE DISORDERS

Chapter 17 Histiocytic syndromes

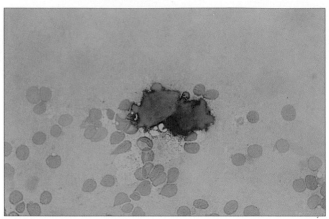

Plate 5 Langerhans cells demonstrating positivity for the monoclonal anti-CD1a antibody NA1/34.

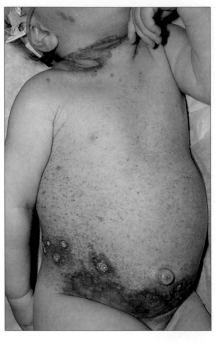

Plate 6 Severe skin involvement in Langerhans cell histiocytosis (LCH).

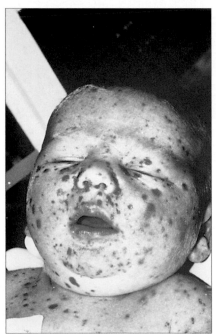

Plate 7 Congenital Langerhans cell histiocytosis (LCH) of skin; varicelliform rash.

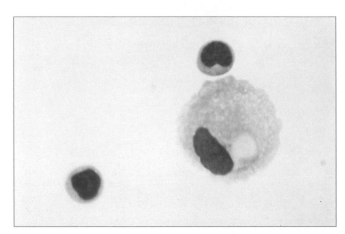

Plate 8 Cerebrospinal fluid cytospin in hemophagocytic lymphohistiocytosis (HLH), showing 2 lymphocytes and a histiocyte (CSF white cell count 40/mm³, protein 0.8 g/l).

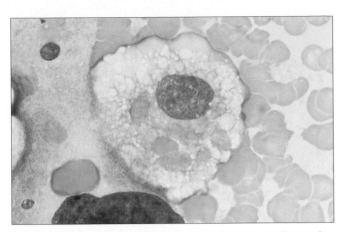

Plate 9 Hemophagocytic lymphohistiocytosis (HLH); hemophagocytic histiocyte in bone marrow.

Chapter 18 Pathology of acute myeloid leukemia

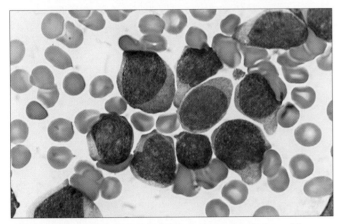

Plate 10 Myeloblasts of M1. Myeloblasts show abundant, weakly basophilic cytoplasm, fine nuclear chromatin, and indistinct nucleoli. A few blasts contain fine azurophilic granules in their cytoplasm. Wright stain, ×100.

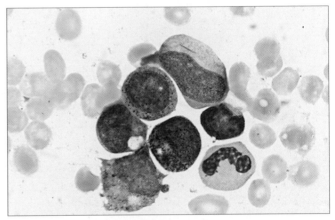

Plate 11 Leukemic cells of M2. In addition to myeloblasts, more mature myeloid elements are also present. A myeloblast containing an Auer rod is shown. Auer rods consist of crystalline coalescence of primary granules. Wright stain, ×100.

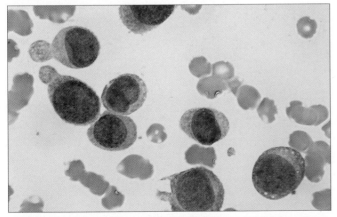

Plate 12 Monoblasts of M5a. Blasts are large with copious amounts of basophilic cytoplasm, round to reniform nucleus, and prominent nucleoli. Wright stain, ×63.

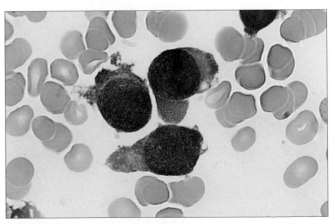

Plate 13 Megakaryoblasts of M7. The leukemic cells of this leukemic subtype may range from small lymphoblast-like to large undifferentiated blasts. The blasts shown here display moderate amounts of basophilic cytoplasm with foot-like protrusions and blebs. Nuclear chromatin is dense and nucleoli are not visible. Wright stain, ×100.

Colour plates

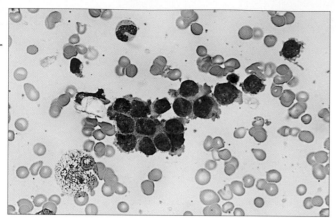

Plate 14 Clustered megakaryoblasts of M7. Aggregates or clusters of adherent blasts are common to M7 and may be confused with metastatic small cell tumors. Wright stain, ×50.

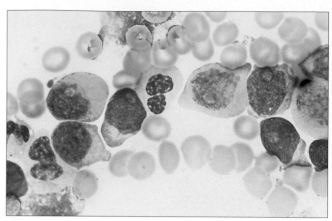

Plate 15 Myeloperoxidase stain. Leukemic cells of M2 show yellow reaction product of myeloperoxidase reaction. Myeloperoxidase stain with O-toludine and Giemsa counterstain, ×100.

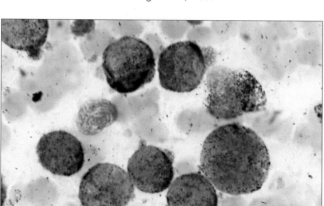

Plate 16 Sudan black B stain. Leukemic cells of M2 demonstrate a black staining of lipid material of primary granules. The Sudan black B may be a more sensitive stain than myeloperoxidase for myeloblasts but may also stain lipid material in non-myeloid leukemic blasts. Crystal violet counterstain, ×100.

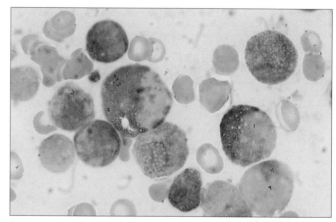

Plate 17 Naphthol ASD chloroacetate esterase stain of M2 (also termed the specific esterase or Leder stain). The enzymes identified by this stain may also be present in monoblasts. Hematoxylin counter stain, ×100.

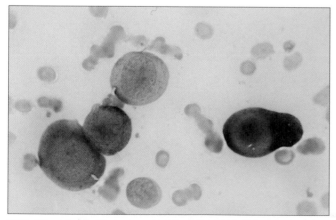

Plate 18 α-Naphthyl butyrate esterase stain of AML-M5a. Positive staining for this esterase is largely limited to the monocytic (M4 and M5) types of AML and produces an intense diffuse, finely granular reaction pattern that is totally inhibited by treatment with sodium fluoride. Hematoxylin counter stain, ×100.

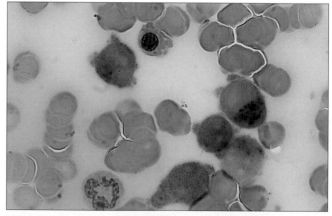

Plate 19 α-Naphthyl acetate esterase stain of M7. A positive reaction with this stain may be observed with all FAB subtypes of AML. The reaction is inhibited by sodium fluoride in the monocytic leukemias but not in the myeloid and megakaryoblastic types. The typical reaction in M7 blasts produces a punctate or large granular pattern that is not inhibited by sodium fluoride. Hematoxylin counterstain, ×100.

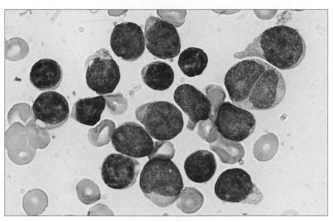

Plate 20 Leukemia blasts of M0. The leukemic cells of M0 may resemble the blasts of M1, M7 or ALL. To qualify for an M0 diagnosis, <3% of the leukemic blasts should demonstrate a positive cytochemical reaction for myeloperoxidase. Wright stain, ×100.

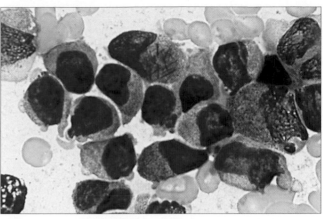

Plate 21 Leukemic cells of M3. Leukemic cells of M3 have folded, lobated and sometimes monocytoid nuclei. Intense primary granulation may sometimes obscure the nuclear detail. A leukemic cell with multiple Auer rods (faggot cell) is shown and is a common feature of this subtype of AML. Wright stain, ×100.

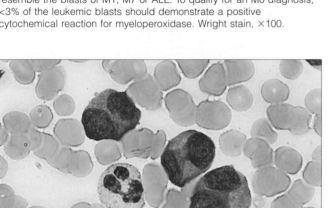

Plate 22 Hypogranular variant of M3 (M3v). The leukemic cells show the nuclear features of hypergranular M3 but lack the intense cytoplasmic granulation. Auer rods may be difficult to find. Wright stain, ×100.

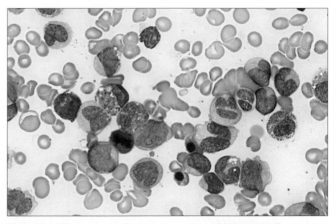

Plate 23 M4Eo leukemia. The bone marrows of M4 and M4Eo contain a mixture of myeloid and monocytic cells. A combined chloroacetate esterase and α-naphthyl butyrate esterase stain may be necessary to identify both leukemic elements. As shown here, the marrows of M4Eo contain increased numbers of immature and mature eosinophils. The basophilic granules of the promyelocytic stage of eosinophilic development are retained in the later stages of maturation. Wright stain, ×50.

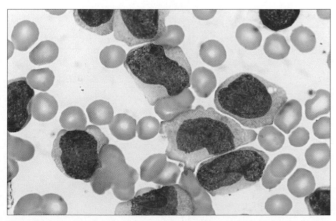

Plate 24 M5b leukemia. Leukemic cells of this subtype of monocytic leukemia show more mature cytologic features, including monocytoid nuclei, cytoplasmic granules and large amounts of pale blue cytoplasm. Wright stain, ×100.

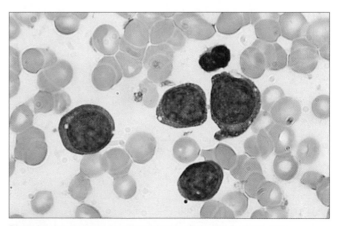

Plate 25 Acute erythroblastic leukemia. The blasts of this rare leukemia may resemble lymphoblasts or megakaryoblasts to which they are closely related. Unlike M6, myeloblasts are absent. The diagnosis is established by immunophenotyping and ultrastructural studies. Wright stain, ×100.

5

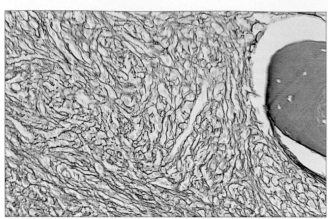

Plate 26 Bone marrow needle biopsy of M7. An intense reticulin fibrosis entraps the leukemic blasts. The increase of reticulin is thought to be the result of release of factors, including PDGF, TGFβ, and PF4, by the leukemic megakaryoblasts that stimulate collagen formation and angiogenesis. Silver stain, ×60.

Chapter 20 Adult type chronic myeloid leukemia

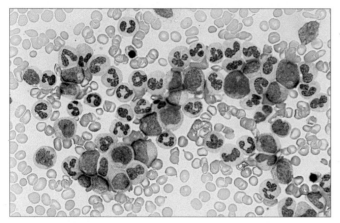

Plate 27 Peripheral blood smear showing increased numbers of immature granulocytes in chronic phase ATCML, ×400. Kindly provided by David Swirsky.

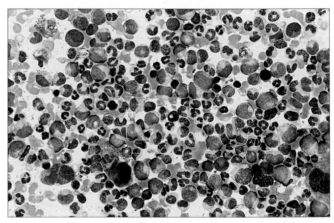

Plate 28 Bone marrow smear of chronic-phase ATCML showing increased cellularity and increased numbers of granulocytes at all stages, ×400. Kindly provided by David Swirsky.

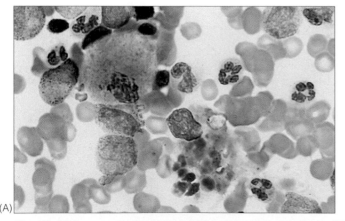

(A)

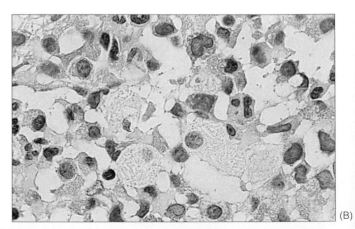

(B)

Plate 29 (A) Bone marrow aspirate and (B) trephine of chronic-phase ATCML showing 'sea-blue histiocytes', ×1000. Kindly provided by David Swirsky.

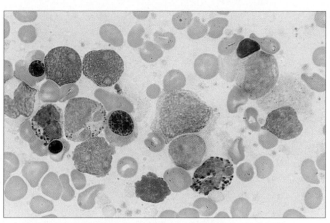

Plate 30 Bone marrow smear of myeloid blast crisis showing myeloblasts and basophils, ×1000. Kindly provided by David Swirsky.

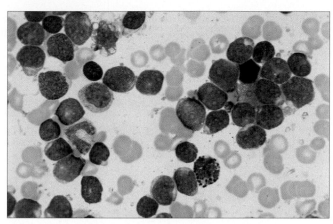

Plate 31 Bone marrow smear showing lymphoid blast crisis, ×630. Kindly provided by David Swirsky.

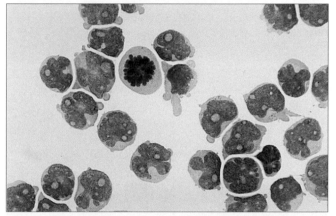

Plate 32 Cytospin of CSF showing lymphoid blasts, ×1000. Kindly provided by David Swirsky.

SECTION 4 PLATELET DISORDERS

Chapter 24 Platelet functional disorders

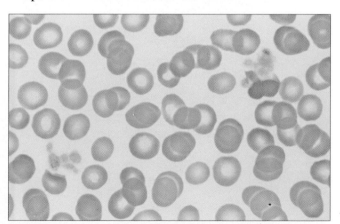

Plate 33 Romanowsky-stained blood film from a patient with gray platelet syndrome. Kindly supplied by James G White.

Colour plates

SECTION 5 LYMPHOCYTE DISORDERS

Chapter 26 Pathology of acute lymphoblastic leukemias

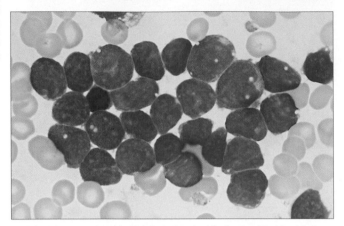

Plate 34 L1 acute lymphoblastic leukemia. Kindly provided by Marie-Thérèse Daniel.

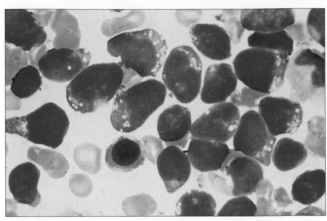

Plate 35 L2 acute lymphoblastic leukemia. Kindly provided by Marie-Thérèse Daniel.

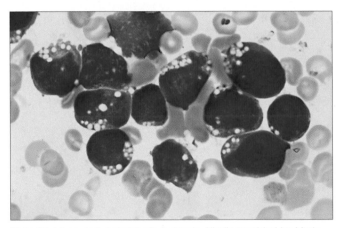

Plate 36 L3 acute lymphoblastic leukemia. Kindly provided by Marie-Thérèse Daniel.

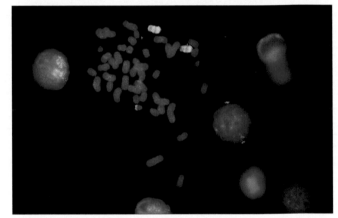

Plate 37 Flourescent *in situ* hybridization (FISH) (chromosome painting) for t(12;21) (yellow probe for chromosome 12). Kindly provided by Roland Berger.

Table 18.2 Cytochemical characteristics of major cell types in acute leukemia.

Stain	Lymphoblast	Myeloblast	Monoblast	Erythroblast	Megakaryoblast
Myeloperoxidase	Negative	Positive	Positive or negative	Negative	Negative
Sudan black B	Negative, occasionally weakly positive	Positive	Positive or negative	Negative	Negative
Esterases					
Naphthol ASD-chloroacetate	Negative, rarely weakly positive	Positive	Negative or weakly positive	Negative	Negative
α-Naphthyl acetate	Negative, occasionally weakly positive	Positive (not inhibited by sodium fluoride)	Diffusely positive (inhibited by sodium fluoride)	Positive (not inhibited by sodium fluoride)	Granular positive (resistant to sodium fluoride)
α-Naphthyl butyrate	Negative or weakly positive	Negative	Positive (inhibited by sodium fluoride)	Negative	Negative (occasionally positive)
Periodic acid-Schiff	Fine to coarse granules or blocks	Negative or diffusely positive	Negative or fine granulation	Strongly granular positive	Negative or granular positive

ally with fine azurophilic granules (Plate 12). Erythroblasts and other erythroid precursors often show bizarre morphologic features, including multiple, often multilobulated nuclei, the presence of one or more nuclear fragments, and megaloblastic changes.[49,50] Megakaryoblasts are highly polymorphic, ranging from small round cells with scanty cytoplasm and dense chromatin to large cells with abundant cytoplasm, fine nuclear chromatin and 1–3 nucleoli (Plate 13).[51] Blast cells may be bi- or multi-nucleated,[52–54] may have cytoplasmic blebs,[51] or may form clumps (Plate 14), mimicking metastatic tumor cells.[55,56]

Because Romanowsky stains cannot be relied upon to assign the lineage of leukemic cells, cytochemical staining with myeloperoxidase, Sudan black B and esterases (naphthol ASD chloroacetate esterase, α-naphthyl butyrate esterase or α-naphthyl acetate esterase) should be performed (Table 18.2). Myeloperoxidase stain detects the enzyme in peroxisomes of neutrophilic, eosinophilic and monocytic cells; myeloperoxidase may be expressed in myeloblasts and monoblasts (Plate 15) but not in lymphoblasts. It also identifies Auer rods more reliably than Romanowsky staining.[57] The French-American-British (FAB) Co-operative Group recommends a 3% positivity threshold for a definitive classification of myeloid leukemia.[49] However, minimally differentiated AML, megakaryoblastic leukemia, and many cases of acute monoblastic leukemia lack myeloperoxidase reactivity,[58–60] and a low percentage of positive cells may indicate residual normal myeloid precursors. Sudan black B stain non-enzymatically identifies phospholipid in the membranes of primary and secondary granules with reactivity generally parallel to but more intense than that of myeloperoxidase (Plate 16). In some cases of ALL, Sudan black B stains the phospholipid membrane of lysosomal granules of lymphoblasts, producing a gray and granular pattern instead of the black and often Golgi-localized reaction of myeloblasts.[61,62]

Reactivity to naphthol ASD chloroacetate esterase stain probably reflects the presence of several different enzymes in

secondary granules and for the most part is confined to cells of the myeloid lineage (Plate 17).[49] Such reactions tend to be positive in the differentiated myeloid leukemias but not as frequently as with myeloperoxidase stains. As many as half of all monoblastic leukemia cases are weakly positive when stained for this esterase, with rare cases showing strong positivity.[63,64] The enzymes identified by this stain are preserved in paraffin-embedded tissue and provide a useful laboratory test for granulocytic sarcoma or chloroma (tumorous growth of granulocytic or monocytic precursor cells) in tissue sections.[65]

Non-specific esterases are enzymes found in many different cell types that can be identified by using α-naphthyl butyrate or α-naphthyl acetate as substrates; sodium fluoride inhibits these reactions.[66] Enzymatic activity is detected in monocytic and myeloid cells with α-naphthyl acetate esterase stain at neutral pH. At an acidic pH, α-naphthyl butyrate esterase staining produces reactions in monocytes and T lymphocytes, but not myeloid cells (Plate 18). Myeloblasts may produce a diffuse granular reaction that is not inhibited by sodium fluoride. Megakaryoblasts are usually negative for α-naphthyl butyrate esterase but positive for α-naphthyl acetate esterase; their granular or punctate cytoplasmic reaction pattern can be partially inhibited with sodium fluoride (Plate 19).[67,68]

MORPHOLOGIC CLASSIFICATION

Although several attempts have been made to subclassify AML on the basis of cell morphology, most have been unsuccessful because of lack of reproducibility and lack of meaningful clinical correlations. In 1976, a group of French, American and British (FAB) investigators proposed a classification scheme for AML that relied on the morphologic features and cytochemical staining properties of bone marrow blast cells.[49] The FAB classification system, which has been modified several times over the years,[50,51,59] distinguishes AML from myelodysplastic syndrome by virtue of

Table 18.3 Classification of childhood acute myeloid leukemias by French–American–British (FAB) criteria.

FAB designation	Common name	Prominent features
M0	Acute myeloblastic leukemia with minimal differentiation	Large blasts with minimal myeloid differentiation; negative by myeloperoxidase and Sudan black B staining; myeloperoxidase demonstrable by ultrastructural or immunophenotype studies or the expression of at least 1 myeloid antigen (e.g. CD13, CD33)
M1	Acute myeloblastic leukemia with poor differentiation	Poorly differentiated myeloblasts with occasional Auer rods
M2	Acute myeloblastic leukemia with differentiation	Myeloblastic with differentiation (<20% monoblasts); Auer rods sometimes prominent
M3	Acute promyelocytic leukemia	Hypergranular, abnormal pro-myelocytes with bundles of Auer rods and often reniform or bilobed nuclei; M3v variant characterized by deeply notched or folded nucleus, a few fine granules and infrequent Auer rods
M4	Acute myelomonoblastic leukemia	Myeloblastic and monoblastic differentiation (20–80% of non-erythroid cells are monoblastic); M4Eo variant associated with >5% esoinophil precursors in marrow
M5	Acute monoblastic leukemia	Monoblastic differentiation (≥80% monocytic cells); M5a subtype has ≥25% monoblasts; M5b subtype shows differentiation with <25% monoblasts
M6	Erythroleukemia	Bizarre dyserythropoiesis and megaloblastic features
M7	Acute megakaryoblastic leukemia	Small to large undifferentiated blasts; tendency for blasts to aggregate; frequent bone marrow reticulin fibrosis

the percentages of myeloblasts and erythroblasts in the bone marrow.[50] AML is diagnosed when:

- 30% or more of the nucleated cells are blasts in a sample containing <50% erythroblasts; or
- 30% or more of non-erythroid cells are blasts in a sample containing 50% or more erythroblasts.

Cases with lower percentages of blast cells are classified as myelodysplastic syndrome.

The FAB classification recognizes 8 major morphologic subtypes of AML (M0–M7; Table 18.3).

M0 subtype

The M0 subtype is minimally differentiated and lacks cytochemical markers for AML (Plate 20); however, myeloperoxidase may be detected with antimyeloperoxidase antibodies or by ultrastructural studies (Table 18.3).[59,60,69,70] In the absence of myeloperoxidase reactivity, detection of the expression of 1 or more myeloid-associated antigens by immunologic techniques facilitates the diagnosis of M0.[59,60]

M1, M2 and M3 subtypes

AML cases in the granulocytic differentiation pathway are subdivided by increasing level of maturation as M1, M2 or M3.[50] M1 is separated from M2 by the finding of <10% non-erythroid cells at the promyelocytic stage and beyond (Plates 10, 11, 15 to 17). In the M3 subtype, blasts and promyelocytes together must comprise >30% of all nucleated cells. The predominant population consists of hypergranular promyelocytes with a grooved or bilobed nucleus (Plate 21) and Auer rods. Numerous Auer rods can be observed in some cells (faggot cells) (Plate 21). A micro-

granular variant (M3V) is characterized by a distinct folding and lobulation of the nucleus which resembles monoblasts but displays strong myeloperoxidase and no or weak non-specific esterase reactivity (Plate 22).[71,72] However, circulating blasts of this variant, unlike those in the bone marrow, may have prominent cytoplasmic granules characteristic of classic M3 blasts.[72,73] The prevalence of the M3, as well as M3v, subtype varies between certain geographic regions or ethnic groups. In the US, Germany and France, 5–10% of AML cases are classified as M3, compared with as many as 30% in Italy and Latin America.[73–75] In Italy, M3v AML accounts for up to one-third of all M3 cases, whereas in the US this proportion is only 15%.[71,72] Whether this difference reflects genetic or environmental influences is uncertain.

M4 and M5 subtypes

AML with monoblastic differentiation is classified as either M4 and M5, depending on the size of the myeloid component. M4 cases have a mixture of myelocytic and monocytic cells, with the latter comprising 20–80% of the non-erythroid population. In the M4Eo variant, eosinophilic precursors account for 5% or more of non-erythroid cells in the bone marrow (Plate 23). The eosinophilic population often contains immature forms with a monocytoid nucleus and basophilic granules. Unlike normal eosinophils, the granules of these cells produce positive reactions with chloroacetate esterase and periodic acid-Schiff stains.[76] FISH analysis has shown that the eosinophils are part of the leukemic cell clone.[77] Diagnosis of the M5 subtype requires only a single criterion: 80% or more of the non-erythroid cells in the bone marrow must be monoblasts, promonocytes or monocytes. Depending on the degree of differentiation,

M5 leukemia is further classified as M5a (Plate 12) with little or no monocytic differentiation or M5b with monocytic maturation (Plate 24).

M6 subtype

M6 leukemia is diagnosed when >50% of all marrow nucleated cells are erythroblasts in various stages of maturation, and >30% of the non-erythroid cells are myeloblasts.[50] In some M6 cases, the main leukemic component consists of myeloblasts, and the erythroid component shows a variety of dysplastic changes; both cell populations have been shown to derive from the same malignant clone.[78] The M6 subtype is exceedingly rare in childhood, most often evolving from a myelodysplastic syndrome and affecting a disproportionally large number of patients with Down's syndrome.[78,79] A rare type of acute erythroblastic leukemia has been described in children (primarily those with Down's syndrome) and some adults.[80,81] Unlike M6 leukemia, this subtype has an insignificant myeloblastic component and small undifferentiated blasts (Plate 25), and it can be identified only by ultrastructural and immunophenotyping studies. The erythroblasts may demonstrate platelet peroxidase and the platelet-associated antigens CD41 and CD61, as found in megakaryoblasts, but also show membrane-bound collections of ferritin molecules or theta granules.[78]

M7 subtype

In M7 leukemia, megakaryoblasts comprise 30% or more of the bone marrow cellularity (Plates 13 and 14),[51] requiring that the diagnosis is confirmed by platelet peroxidase (Fig. 18.1) or immunophenotyping. In cases with extensive myelofibrosis (Plate 26) precluding bone marrow aspiration, the diagnosis of M7 depends on a bone marrow biopsy showing an excess of blasts and, at times, an increased number of immature and mature megakaryocytes.

Table 18.4 shows the frequency of FAB-AML subtypes in several major co-operative groups or institutional

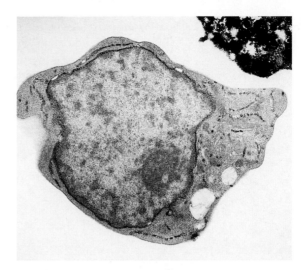

Fig. 18.1 Platelet peroxidase study of M7. Peroxidase enzymes are demonstrable in megakaryoblasts with fixation in special buffers and subsequent ultrastructural examination. Megakaryoblasts show dense reaction product deposits in the endoplasmic reticulum and perinuclear space.

studies.[14,16,82–85] It should be noted that the concordance of FAB classifications of individual cases assigned by different observers is relatively low (65–80%) with discordance found mainly between the M1 and M2, M2 and M4, and M4 and M5 subtypes.[86,87] Moreover, the FAB system fails to accommodate several distinct, albeit rare, subgroups of AML: hypocellular AML (>30% blasts in a bone marrow with <30% cellularity on biopsy),[88] so-called mixed-lineage leukemia,[89] and AML with basophilic differentiation.[90,91]

IMMUNOPHENOTYPIC ANALYSIS

Large panels of monoclonal antibodies have been developed to detect antigenic determinants expressed on normal and leukemic myeloid cells. Monoclonal antibodies commonly used in the immunophenotyping of AML cases include those detecting myeloperoxidase; a cluster of differentiation antigens CD11b, CD11c, CD13, CD14, CD15, CD33, CD36, CD41, CD42, CD61, CD65, CD66, and CD117 (c-kit); and

Table 18.4 Frequency (%) of acute myeloid leukemia subtypes according to French–American–British (FAB) classification in recent studies.

	AIEOP[82] (n = 161)	BFM[83] (n = 307)	CCG[16] (n = 559)	NOPHO[18] (n = 223)	POG[14] (n = 510)	SJCRH[84] (n = 328)
M0	?	6	–	–	–	2
M1	12	10	15	21	37 (includes M2)	18
M2	27	27	28	30		29
M3	17	5	10	7	6	8
M4	16	21	25	18	16	16
M5	19	22	15	15	13	17
M6	?	3	3	5	1	2
M7	?	6	4	4	6	8

AIEOP = Associazione Italiana Ematologia Oncologia Pediatrics; BFM = Berlin–Frankfurt–Münster; CCG = Children's Cancer Group; NOPHO = Nordic Society of Paediatric Haematology and Oncology; POG = Pediatric Oncology Group; SJCRH = St Jude Children's Research Hospital.

glycophorin A.[92,93] Except for antimyeloperoxidase,[94,95] these antibodies are not specific for AML and many do not distinguish the different myeloid lineages. Thus, the assessment of cell lineage is based on the reactivity pattern obtained with a panel of myeloid-associated antibodies (Table 18.5, Fig. 18.2). Some investigators advocate the use of 2 or more selected myeloid-associated markers to diagnose AML.[92] However, it is equally important that lack of

Table 18.5 Typical immunophenotype patterns of acute myeloid leukemia.*

FAB subtype	CD34	DR	CD13	CD14	CD15	CD33	CD36	CD41/61	CD65	CD2	CD4	CD7	CD19	CD56
M0	+ +	+ +	+ +	±	+	+ +	±	0	+ +	+	±	+	+	±
M1	+ +	+ +	+ +	0	+ +	+ + +	±	0	+ + +	+	±	+	+	±
M2	+ + +	+ + +	+ + +	0	+ +	+ + +	±	0	+ + +	+	±	+	+	+
M3	±	±	+ + +	0	+ +	+ + +	±	0	+ + +	+	±	±	0	±
M4	+ +	+ + +	+ +	+ +	+ +	+ + +	+ +	0	+ + +	+	+ + +	+	±	+
M5	±	+ + +	+ +	+ +	+ +	+ + +	+ +	+ **	+ + +	±	+ + +	+	±	+
M7	+	+	+	0	±	+ +	+ +	+ + +	+	+ +	+ +	+ +	0	+

FAB = French–American–British classification.
*Percent of cases expressing CD antigen: 0 = none; ± = <10%; + = 10–49%; + + = 50–80%; + + + = >80%.
**CD41/CD61 positivity in the M5 subtype of AML is usually due to non-specific adhesion of platelets or gpIIb/IIIa to blast cells.

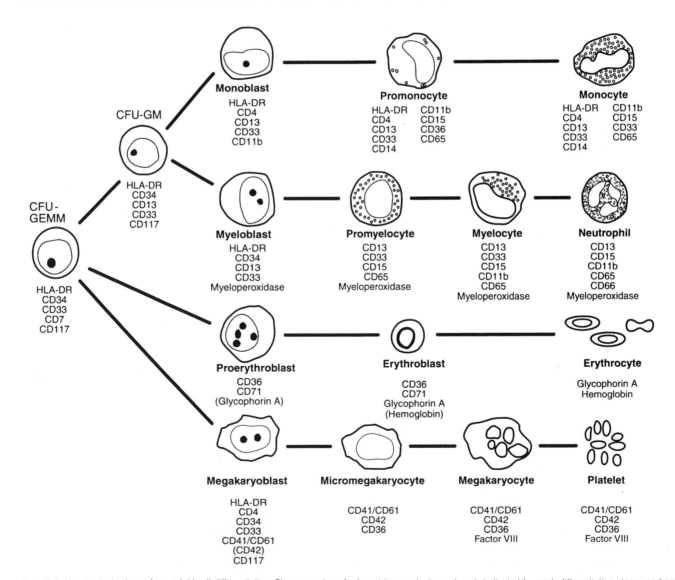

Fig. 18.2 Hypothetical scheme for myeloid cell differentiation. The expression of relevant immunologic markers is indicated for each differentiation stage; markers in parentheses are not always expressed.

Table 18.6 Diagnostic criteria for acute myeloid leukemia with minimal differentiation (AML-M0).

SJCRH criteria	FAB Co-operative Group criteria[59]
<3% of blasts positive with MPO or SBB	<3% of blasts positive for MPO or SBB
<3% of blasts positive with ANB esterase	Blasts negative for all lymphoid antigens except CD2, CD4, or CD7
<3% of blasts express platelet antigens CD36, CD41, CD42, or CD61	plus
<3% of blasts express cytoplasmic CD3 and CD79	Ultrastructural evidence of MPO
plus	or
Ultrastructural evidence of MPO	Blasts react with anti-MPO antibody
or	or
>10% of blasts react with anti-MPO antibody	Blasts express one or more of the following antigens: CD11b, CD13, CD14, CD15, or CD33
or	
>10% of blasts express 2 or more of the following antigens: CD13, CD14, CD15, CD33, CD65, CD117	

FAB = French–American–British classification; SJCRH = St Jude Children's Research Hospital; MPO = myeloperoxidase; SBB = Sudan black B; ANB = α-naphthyl butyrate.

expression of 'lymphoid lineage-restricted' markers is also included as a criterion because, as discussed below, the so-called myeloid antigen-positive ALL cases can also express 2 or more myeloid-associated antigens.[89]

Although the FAB-AML subtypes show considerable heterogeneity in cell-surface antigen expression, several dominant patterns have emerged (Table 18.5).[83,92,93,96,97] The chief value of immunophenotyping in AML is diagnosis of morphologically and cytochemically undifferentiated cases (e.g. M0 leukemia; Table 18.6) and confirmation of the M6 and M7 subtypes.[95] By comparison with other subtypes of AML, M0 cases are less likely to express late panmyeloid antigens, especially CD13, CD14 and CD15, and are more likely to express T-associated antigens (CD7 or CD2) as well as terminal deoxynucleotidyl transferase.[83] The blast cells of the M6 subtype express glycophorin,[78,93] while those of the M7 subtype express platelet-associated surface antigens (glycoproteins Ib [CD42], IIb [CD41] and IIIa [CD61]) and occasionally Factor VIII-related antigens.[51] It should be noted that platelet adherence to or adsorption of CD41 by monoblasts, and sometimes myeloblasts, can yield false-positive results.[98]

Since the early 1980s, it has been recognized that leukemic blast cells frequently co-express antigens associated with more than one lineage.[99–101] With the use of more comprehensive panels of monoclonal antibodies and more sensitive flow cytometric methods in immunophenotyping, increasing numbers of cases are being classified as 'mixed-lineage' or 'biphenotypic' leukemia.[84,89,102–109] Excluding a few markers (e.g. cytoplasmic CD22, CD79a and immunoglobulin in B-lineage ALL, cytoplasmic CD3 and T-cell receptor in T-lineage ALL, myeloperoxidase for myeloid differentiation, and cytoplasmic CD41 for megakaryoblasts), most antigens studied are not lineage-specific.[92,95] For example, CD2 (E-rosette receptor) is expressed in almost one-half of all M3 cases,[110] especially in the microgranular variant and in cases with M4Eo and inv(16).[111] CD4, a T-cell and monocytic antigen, is expressed in many cases of granulocytic and megakaryocytic as well as almost all monocytic subtypes of AML.[112] CD7, another T-associated

marker, is expressed by a quarter of AML cases, usually M0, M1, M2, M5 and M7 subtypes (FG Behm and C-H Pui, unpublished observation). B-lineage-associated antigens, such as CD19, can be found on blasts cells of most M2 cases with t(8;21).[113–115] An unconfirmed report has described CD79a on most M3 cases with the t(15;17).[116] Conversely, CD15, a myeloid-associated antigen, is expressed in two-thirds of ALL cases with t(4;11).[117] There is a conspicious lack of agreement on criteria for the diagnosis of mixed-lineage leukemia. The authors recommend a rigorous definition—expression of 2 or more antigens associated with the opposite lineage—and believe it important to distinguish AML with lymphoid-associated antigen expression (Ly$^+$ AML) from ALL with myeloid-associated antigen expression (My$^+$ ALL), as each variant requires treatment directed at the dominant phenotype.[89,118] The immunophenotypic criteria used at the authors' center are presented in Table 18.7.

Several studies have attempted to correlate immunophenotyping results with response to therapy in childhood AML. Unlike findings in some adult studies, the lymphoid- or myeloid-associated antigens as well as CD34 antigen, CD56 (NK cell-associated) antigen, CD117 and p-glycoprotein have not shown prognostic significance in this disease.[106–109,119,120] In one study, a monoclonal antibody, 7.1, was found to correlate with M5 morphology, 11q23 chromosomal abnormalities and a poorer clinical outcome.[121] Ly$^+$ AML cases often co-express CD2 and CD7, have dual populations of large myeloperoxidase-positive blasts and small myeloperoxidase-negative blasts with hand mirror morphology, low overall myeloperoxidase reactivity, and benefit from the addition of lymphoid-targeted therapy.[89,122] These observations require confirmation.

Finally, there are rare cases of so-called bilineal leukemia, characterized by mixed populations of blast cells displaying either lymphoid or myeloid features, but not both, and arising from a single progenitor cell.[123] In other rare cases, lineage switch from ALL to AML or vice versa, with retention of the original karyotype, has been observed at

Table 18.7 St Jude Children's Research Hospital criteria for My⁺ALL, Ly⁺AML and true mixed-lineage leukemia.

B-lineage My⁺ ALL*	Ly⁺ AML*
≥90% of blasts are CD19⁺ plus CD79a⁺ or CD22⁺	≥3% blasts are MPO⁺***
Leukemic blasts are cytoplasmic CD3⁻	Leukemic blasts are cytoplasmic CD3⁻
Leukemic blasts are MPO⁻**	Leukemic blasts are CD79a⁻ and CD22⁻
Leukemic blasts express ≥1 myeloid-associated antigen: CD13, CD15, CD33, CD36, or CD65	Leukemic blasts express ≥1 lymphoid-associated antigens: CD2, CD5, CD7, CD19, CD56
T-lineage My⁺ ALL*	True mixed-lineage leukemia
≥90% of blasts are CD7⁺ plus cytoplasmic CD3⁺	Blasts co-express MPO*** plus CD79a or μ immunoglobulin
Leukemic blasts are CD79a⁻ and CD22⁻	or
Leukemic blasts are MPO⁻**	Blasts co-express MPO*** plus cytoplasmic CD3
Leukemic blasts express ≥1 myeloid-associated antigens: CD13, CD15, CD33, CD36, or CD65	or
	Blasts co-express CD3 plus CD79a

My⁺ ALL = acute lymphoblastic leukemia expressing myeloid-associated antigens; Ly⁺ AML = acute myeloid leukemia expressing lymphoid-associated antigens; MPO = myeloperoxidase.
*All four criteria must be met.
**MPO-negative by cytochemical, anti-MPO antibody testing or ultrastructural analysis.
***MPO-positive by cytochemistry, anti-MPO antibody testing or ultrastructural analysis.

the time of relapse. Such cases often have 11q23 chromosomal abnormalities involving the *MLL* gene,[124,125] but these should not be confused with therapy-induced AML with *MLL* rearrangement.[39–41]

GENETIC FEATURES

Clonal chromosomal abnormalities are found in the leukemic cells of 80–90% of children with AML,[83,126–134] and are non-random in two-thirds (Table 18.8). The commonest recurring abnormalities are t(8;21),[113,114,129,132,135] t(15;17),[110,136–139] inv(16),[111,132] t(9;11),[129,132,140,141] t(11q23),[132,141] monosomy 7,[132,142] t(1;22),[143,144] inv(3)/t(3;3),[145] and t(6;9),[146] each of which is associated with characteristic clinical and biologic features (Table 18.9). Because of the paucity of large series of consecutively

registered patients, the exact frequency of these chromosomal aberrations is uncertain. Also, their prevalence may differ according to ethnic group or geographic region, as illustrated by the very high frequency of t(15;17) in Italian and Latin American patients.[73–75] Among infants, the commonest structural rearrangements (40–45% of cases) affect the q23 region of chromosome 11; chromosomes 9 and 19 are the most frequently involved reciprocal partners.[140,147–150] t(1;22) is also common (approx 10% of infant cases).[143,144]

Many of these genetic lesions are associated with particular morphologic features, but only t(15;17) and t(1;22) show an absolute correlation with acute promyelocytic leukemia (FAB M3) and acute megakaryoblastic leukemia (FAB M7), respectively. As mentioned earlier, most of the antigens on leukemic cells are not lineage specific and, in fact, a large proportion of cases can be expected to express some lymphoid-associated antigens in conjunction with recurring

Table 18.8 Cytogenetic abnormalities in childhood acute myeloid leukemia and myelodysplastic syndrome.

Chromosomal abnormality	Involved genes	FAB Group	Frequency
Normal			<10%
t(8;21)(q22;q22)	ETO;AML1	M1; M2	8–15% (45% of M2)
t(15;17)(q22;q12)	PML;RARA	M3	7–20%
t(11;17)(q23;q12)	LZF;RARA	M3-like	Rare
inv(16)(p13q22)	MYH11;CBFβ	M4; M2	7–12%
t(16;16)(p13;q22)	MYH11;CBFβ	M4	Rare
t(8;16)(p11;p13)	MOZ;CBP	M5	Rare
t(9;11)(p22;q23)	AF9;MLL	M4; M5	7–10% (25–35% of M5)
t(10;11)(p12;q23)	MLL;AF10	M5	Rare
t(11;19)(q23;p13.3)	MLL;ENL	M4; M5	<2%
t(11;19)(q23;p13.1)	MLL;ELL	M4; M5	<2%
t(11;17)(q23;q21)	MLL;AF17	M5	Rare
t(1;22)(p13;q13)	?	M7	2–3%
t(6;9)(p23;q34)	DEK;CAN	MDS; M4; M2	<1%
−7/del(7q)	?	MDS; M1; M2; M4; M6	2–5%
inv(3)(q21q26)/t(3;3)(q21;q26)	EVI1	MDS; M2; M4	<1%
i(17)(q10)		MDS; AML	Rare

FAB = French–American–British classification; MDS = myelodysplastic syndrome.

Table 18.9 Clinical and biologic characteristics of common non-random chromosomal abnormalities in childhood acute myeloid leukemia.

Abnormality	Molecular genetic alteration	Associated features	Estimated 3-year event-free survival (%)
t(8;21)(q22;q22)	AML1-ETO fusion	M2 morphology; Auer rods, increased expression of CD19, CD34 and CD56; granulocytic sarcoma	30–50
t(15;17)(q22;q12)	PML-RARA fusion	M3 morphology; Auer rods; increased expression of CD2, CD9, CD33, and CD65; CD34$^-$, HLA-DR$^-$; older age group; female predominance; lower leukocyte count; absence of extramedullary leukemia; coagulopathy; differentiates in response to all-trans-retinoic acid	50–75
inv(16)(p13q22)	CBFβ-MYH11 fusion	Predominant M4Eo morphology; increased expression of CD2, CD13, CD14, CD34 and c-kit; CNS leukemia; hepatomegaly and lymphadenopathy; hyperleukocytosis; favorable response to high-dose cytarabine	40–60
t(9;11)(p22;q23)	MLL-AF9 fusion	M4/M5 morphology; infant age group predominance; male predominance; CD14$^+$, CD34$^-$, DR$^-$; coagulopathy	50–70
11q23 translocation other than t(9;11)	MLL rearrangement	M4/M5 morphology; male predominance; hyperleukocytosis; CNS leukemia; skin involvement; coagulopathy	10–20
Monosomy 7/7q-	Unknown	Myelodysplastic syndrome; constitutional disorders; organomegaly; increased expression of CD7; unfavorable prognosis with chemotherapy	<10
t(1;22)(p13;q13)	Unknown	M7 morphology; infant <12 months old; hepatosplenomegaly; lytic bone lesion; myelofibrosis; low initial leukocyte count	20–30
inv(3)(q21q26)/ t(3;3)(q21;q26)	EVI1 actication	Preceding myelodysplastic syndrome; thrombocytosis; abnormal platelets	Unknown
t(6;9)(p23;q34)	DEK-CAN fusion	M2, M4 or myelodysplastic syndrome; unfavorable prognosis	10–20

translocations: CD2 (E-rosette receptor) in AML with t(15;17)[110,137] or inv(16)[111] cases and CD19 in cases with t(8;21).[113–115]

The chromosomal abnormalities identified in leukemic myeloid cells not only have diagnostic value but therapeutic implications as well. For example, cases with t(15;17) respond well to treatment that includes retinoic acid and high-dose anthracyclines;[139,151,152] those with t(8;21) or inv(16) have a better outcome when treated with high-dose cytarabine in combination with other agents,[152] and those with monosomy 7 or t(1;22), t(6;9) or 11q23 translocations other than t(9;11) have a particularly poor prognosis with the use of chemotherapy.[132,142,146,152]

Molecular genetic studies offer advantages over cytogenetic analysis for cell classification and treatment assignment. They are not limited by the technical difficulties and sampling problems that have led to failure to recognize critical genetic rearrangements in specimens prepared for cytogenetic examination,[149] and can be relied upon to detect submicroscopic lesions.[153] By molecular analysis, there are 2 general mechanisms of leukemogenesis: one involves the activation of dominant cellular proto-oncogenes and the other the inactivation of tumor suppressor genes.[131,154] The genes involved in leukemic transformation have a variety of normal functions, including signal transduction, transcriptional activation, cell differentiation, programed cell death and tumor suppression (Table 18.10).[153–166] While some genetic abnormalities are not tissue specific and appear in a wide range of cancers (e.g. RAS mutations and RB1, P53 or WT1 mutations or deletions), others are restricted to particular types of leukemia, including AML.[154] Fusion genes resulting from chromosomal rearrangements are good examples of this class of genetic anomalies.[167–170] In general, the activation of proto-oncogenes is thought to initiate leukemogenesis, whereas the loss of tumor-suppressor gene function promotes more aggressive proliferation of leukemic cells.

Table 18.10 Molecular genetic abnormalities in acute myeloid leukemia.[154]

Type of gene	Function	Molecular alteration	Common chromosomal abnormality	Frequency (%)
RAS	Signal transduction	N-RAS mutations	None	15–50
Homeodomain	Differentiation and gene transcription	MLL rearrangement	t(11q23)	12–18
Runt homology	Gene transcription	AML1-ETO	t(8;21)	8–15
Receptor	Differentiation	PML-RARA fusion	t(15;17)	7–20
Tumor suppressor gene	Tumor suppression, transcription, cell cycle control, apoptosis	Mutation, loss, or rearrangement of P53	del(17)	5–15
		Disruption of RB1	13q	3–10
		Loss of WT1	11p	?20

CLINICAL PRESENTATION

The presenting signs and symptoms of AML are the consequences of bone marrow failure and organ infiltration and include fever, pallor, cutaneous or mucosal bleeding, bone or joint pain, fatigue and anorexia. The leukemias may present insidiously or with acute manifestations. Prodromal symptoms last 2 days to 12 months (median 6 weeks).[84] Unexplained menorrhagia is a common presenting feature in teenage girls.

Table 18.11 summarizes the commonly recognized presenting clinical and laboratory features of children with newly diagnosed AML.[15–17,82–84,171–177] Half have some degree of hepatomegaly and splenomegaly. Other extramedullary manifestations include granulocytic sarcoma (affecting 2–13% of children), leukemia cutis (4–9%), gingival hypertrophy (9–15%), and lymphadenopathy (13–20%), which are commoner in infant cases.[178] While chloroma can involve virtually all organs, the commonest site of involvement is the orbit,[178] especially in Turkish children.[179] Some children present with ptosis from periorbital chloroma, cauda equina syndrome or paraparesis

Table 18.11 Presenting features of children with acute myeloid leukemia (based on a literature review of 3751 patients).[15–18,82–84,171–177]

Feature	Frequency (% of total)
Age (years)	
<1	10–12
1-2	9–19
2-9	35–41
≥10	30–46
Male	52–54
Symptoms	
Fever	30
Bleeding	33
Bone or joint pain	18
Liver ≥5 cm below costal margin	19–21
Spleen ≥5 cm below costal margin	16–18
Chloroma	2–16
Central nevous system leukemia*	6–25
Leukocyte count (x10^9/l)	
<25	54–60
25–49	14–15
50–100	12–14
>100	13–18
Median (range)	24 (0.46–750)
Hemoglobin (g/d)	
<9	56
Median (range)	8.2 (2–15)
Platelet count (x10^9/l)	
<100	70–72
Median (range)	51 (1–520)
Auer rods	42–46
Coagulopathy	13–17

*Variable frequency according to definition of CNS disease.

from epidural tumor.[84] Occasionally, detection of chloroma precedes the development of AML by a few weeks to as long as 2 years (median 7 months).[178] The frequency of central nervous system (CNS) involvement varies from 4% to 25%, depending on the definition used.[15–18,82–84,171–177] Infants and patients with M4 or M5 leukemia have a particularly high rate of CNS leukemia.[180–182] In most cases, CNS leukemia is asymptomatic, revealed only by detection of leukemic cells in cerebrospinal fluid; occasionally, it presents as cranial nerve palsy or intracerebral chloroma. Testicular leukemia is very rare in AML.[183]

The median leukocyte count in patients with AML is 24 × 10^9/l. In 13–18% of cases, the presenting leukocyte count exceeds 100 × 10^9/l. The risk of early death from intracerebral hemorrhage and respiratory failure, presumably due to leukostasis, correlates positively with hyperleukocytosis, especially when the cell count exceeds 300 × 10^9/l.[184,185] Disseminated intravascular coagulation or increased fibrinolytic activity associated with hemorrhagic complications may occur in any subtype of AML, but is more common in the M3, M4 and M5 subtypes.[186–189]

A chest X-ray may demonstrate infiltrates caused by pulmonary edema, leukemic infiltration or pneumonia. Patients with M4 or M5 leukemia have increased serum and urine levels of muramidase (lysozyme), a hydrolytic enzyme in the primary granules of myeloblasts or monoblasts, leading to renal tubular dysfunction with secondary hypokalemia.[190]

PROGNOSTIC FACTORS

The ability to relate prognosis to clinical and biologic markers, and to devise appropriate therapy for the risk groups defined in this manner, has been central to treatment successes in ALL. Unfortunately, the generally poor clinical outcome in patients with AML has thwarted similar efforts in this childhood disease. Although numerous prognostic factors have been identified in recent major studies of AML,[14,15,18,82,83,171–173,176,191] the results have not been consistent. Some variables have had apparent clinical significance that disappeared as therapy improved, while others have shown predictive strength in only a single trial. Among clinical features, only an increased leukemic cell burden (as reflected by a high leukocyte count) appears to provide uniformly reliable prognostic information (Table 18.12). The Berlin-Frankfurt-Münster (BFM) group found that age <2 years conferred a poor prognosis in their patients,[83,173,176] but this marker lacked prognostic significance in trials conducted at St. Jude Children's Research Hospital[182] and was even associated with a favorable outcome in a Pediatric Oncology Group study.[175]

Genetic abnormalities have begun to emerge as the most relevant predictors of treatment outcome in childhood AML. Several specific translocations—t(8;21), t(15;17),

Table 18.12 Adverse prognostic factors in acute myeloid leukemia.

Study group	Adverse prognostic factors
AIEOP[82]	WBC $>100 \times 10^9$/l
BFM[83,173,176]	WBC $>100 \times 10^9$/l; age <2 years; FAB subtypes other than M1/M2 with Auer rods, M3 or M4Eo; >5 % blasts in day 15 bone marrow
CCG[12]	WBC $>20 \times 10^9$/l; CNS leukemia
Dana-Farber[171]	WBC $\geqslant 100 \times 10^9$/l; M5 subtype
NOPHO[15]	Male gender
POG[175]	WBC $\geqslant 100 \times 10^9$/l; WBC $>10 \times 10^9$/l; age $\geqslant 2$ years
SJCRH[191]	WBC $\geqslant 10 \times 10^9$/l; age >14 years; splenomegaly; presence of coagulopathy

AIEOP = Associazione Italiana Ematologia Oncologica Pediatrica; BFM = Berlin–Frankfurt–Münster; CCG = Children's Cancer Group; Dana-Farber = Dana-Farber Cancer Institute; NOPHO = Nordic Society of Paediatric Haematology and Oncology; POG = Pediatric Oncology Group; SJCRH = St Jude Children's Research Hospital; WBC = white blood cells.

Table 18.13 Genetic abnormalities and immunophenotypes that can be used as targets for minimal residual disease detection in acute myeloid leukemia.

	Frequency (%)
Fusion gene	
AML1-ETO (RNA)	8–15
PML-RARA (RNA)	7–20
CBFβ-MYH11 (RNA)	7–12
MLL-AF9 (RNA)	7–10
BCR-ABL (RNA)	<1
Immunophenotype	
CD34/CD56	20
CD13/CD33/TdT	20
CD7/CD13/CD33	10
p53	10
7.1	10

t(9;11) and inv(16)—are associated with a favorable prognosis, while monosomy 7, t(1;22) and 11q23 translocations other than t(9;11) confer a particularly poor outcome.[118,132,142,146,152] Among patients with constitutional genetic abnormalities, those with trisomy 21 have a favorable response to cytarabine-containing regimens.[14,16,19,192] To avoid life-threatening toxicities in children with Down's syndrome, it is important to reduce the intensity of chemotherapy to a level commensurate with the patient's unique tolerance. Recent studies showed that myeloblasts from Down's patients were approximately 10-fold more sensitive to cytarabine and accumulated more 1-β-D-arabinofuranosylcytosine 5'-triphosphate than did otherwise comparable blast cells from patients without this disorder, providing an explanation for the generally favorable prognosis of AML in this genetically-defined subgroup.[193]

Studies on the multidrug resistance gene product (MDR1, also known as P-glycoprotein) in childhood AML are limited. In one study, it was found in 30% of infants with AML and 5% of older patients, but its presence did not correlate with poor prognosis.[194] There have also been reports of increased P-glycoprotein function in patients in relapse[195] and a higher frequency of expression in cases with t(8;21).[196] Standard assays to determine P-glycoprotein expression and function are needed to stimulate progress in this potentially important research area. Finally, autonomous growth of blast cells *in vitro* correlated with a poor outcome in a study of pediatric and adult patients,[197] an observation which warrants further testing in children with AML.

MINIMAL RESIDUAL DISEASE DETECTION

Children with AML in remission may harbor as many as 10^{10} leukemic cells, yet they are likely to receive essentially

the same type and intensity of treatment as patients with a much smaller leukemia burden or no leukemia at all. In theory, a reliable estimate of minimal residual disease (MRD), defined as leukemic cells not detectable by morphologic examination, would allow more rationale clinical management decisions (e.g. intensification of therapy for patients with residual leukemia or perhaps elective cessation of treatment in those without residual disease).

There are no universally reliable genetic changes in AML (such as immunoglobulin heavy-chain rearrangements or T-cell receptor V-D-J recombination in lymphoid leukemias) that facilitate detection of MRD. Rather, the emphasis in MRD detection is molecular detection of specific translocations and immunologic identification of phenotypes that are expressed aberrantly on leukemic cells.[198] The commonly recognized targets are shown in Table 18.13.

Leukemia-specific chromosomal translocations provide disease markers that can be detected by polymerase chain reaction (PCR) analysis at a high level of sensitivity (10^{-4}–10^{-6}).[198] Up to 45% of AML cases in children have identifiable chromosomal translocations that are candidates for PCR analysis (Table 18.13). A number of studies have established the predictive value of PCR reactivity in acute promyelocytic leukemia with the *PML-RARA* fusion gene.[199–203] The clinical value of PCR monitoring in acute myeloblastic leukemia with the *AML1* (also termed *CBFA2*)-*ETO* fusion gene is less certain, as the fusion transcripts may be detected in bone marrow or even peripheral blood from patients who have completed chemotherapy and remained in remission for as long as 12 years.[204–207] While allogeneic hematopoietic stem cell transplantation may eradicate cells expressing *AML1-ETO* in some patients,[207,208] a recent study suggested that this outcome does not extend to the majority of patients and that a positive PCR result is compatible with long-term continuous remission.[209] Whether expression of the fusion gene does not itself constitute a transformed phenotype or whether the 'quiescent cells' in patients with only PCR reactivity were suppressed by host immunity is unclear. PCR studies of MRD in patients with the *CBFβ-MYH11* fusion gene are limited to only a few patients.[210–212] However, future results will probably be similar to those obtained with *AML1-ETO* because the *AML1* and *CBFβ* gene products normally form a transcriptionally active dimer complex. In this regard, the persistence of PCR positivity for *CBFβ-MYH11* has been noted in some patients in long-term remission.[212] That the Wilms' tumor zinc-finger tumor suppressor gene (*WT1*) is expressed in virtually all human leukemias, at levels exceeding 10^3 times normal, renders this marker potentially useful for MRD detection.[213] Preliminary results suggest that monitoring of *WT1* expression in bone marrow and even peripheral blood is predictive of relapse.[214]

Since aberrant expression of certain combinations of antigens is a characteristic feature of some AML cases, multiparameter flow cytometric analysis measuring 2 or more cell-surface antigens simultaneously is being used to detect MRD.[215–219] Other immunologic methods rely on the use of leukemia-specific monoclonal antibodies (e.g. the 7.1 antibody in cases defined by 11q23 abnormalities)[121] or the overexpression of certain antigens (e.g. CD34 in cases with t(8;21)[115] and *WT1* gene product in the majority of AML cells).[220] In general, flow cytometry allows the detection of at least 1 target cell in 10^3–10^4 normal cells,[198] and in most instances the detection of phenotypically abnormal cells has correlated with outcome.[198,215–217,219] Although false-negative results due to phenotypic switches may occur, they have not been a limiting factor in the reported studies.[198,221]

Carefully controlled prospective studies are needed to evaluate the predictive utility of serial MRD determinations in childhood AML patients. The expectation is that accurate measurement of the leukemic cell burden remaining after initial chemotherapy will have a profound impact on the clinical management of patients with this disease.

Acknowledgement

Supported in part by grants PO1 CA 20180 and P30 CA 21765 from the National Cancer Institute, and by the American Lebanese Syrian Associated Charities (ALSAC).

REFERENCES

1. Gurney JG, Severson RK, Davis S, Robison LL. Incidence of cancer in children in the United States. Sex-, race-, and 1-year age-specific rates by histologic type. *Cancer* 1995; **75**: 2186–2195
2. Miller RW, Young JL Jr, Novakovic B. Childhood cancer. *Cancer* 1994; **75**: 395–405
3. Bhatia S, Neglia JP. Epidemiology of childhood acute myelogenous leukemia. *J Pediatr Hematol Oncol* 1995; **17**: 94–100
4. *Cancer Statistics Review, May 1989*. NIH publication no. 89–2789. Bethesda, MD: US Department of Health and Human Services, 1989
5. Parkin DM, Stiller CA, Draper GJ *et al. International Incidence of Childhood Cancer.* IARC scientific publication no. 87. Lyon: IARC, 1988
6. Gordis L, Szklo M, Thompson B, Kaplan E, Tonascia JA. An apparent increase in the incidence of acute nonlymphocytic leukemia in Black children. *Cancer* 1981; **47**: 2763–2768
7. Ries LAG, Hankey BF, Miller BA, Hartman AM, Edwards BK (eds). *Cancer Statistics Review 1973–1988*. NIH publication no. 91–2789. Bethesda, MD: National Cancer Institute, 1991
8. Fong C-T, Brodeur GM. Down's syndrome and leukemia: eipdemiology, genetics, cytogenetics and mechanisms of leukemogenesis. *Cancer Genet Cytogenet* 1987; **28**: 55–76
9. Robison LL. Down syndrome and leukemia. *Leukemia* 1992; **6 (Suppl 1)**: 5–7
10. Zipursky A, Poon A, Doyle J. Leukemia in Down syndrome: a review. *Pediatr Hematol Oncol* 1992; **9**: 139–149
11. Ravindranath Y, Abella E, Kirscher JP *et al.* Acute myeloid leukemia (AML) in Down's syndrome is highly responsive to chemotherapy: experience on Pediatric Oncology Group AML Study 8498. *Blood* 1992; **80**: 2210–2214
12. Woods WG, Kobrinsky N, Buckley J *et al.* Intensively timed induction therapy followed by autologous or allogeneic bone marrow transplantation for children with acute myeloid leukemia or myelodysplastic syndrome: a Children's Cancer Group Pilot Study. *J Clin Oncol* 1993; **11**: 1448–1457
13. Woods WG, Kobrinsky N, Buckley JD *et al.* Timed-sequential induction therapy improves postremission outcome in acute myeloid leukemia: a report from the Children's Cancer Group. *Blood* 1996; **87**: 4979–4989
14. Ravindranath Y, Yeager AM, Chang MN *et al.* Autologous bone marrow transplantation versus intensive consolidation chemotherapy for acute myeloid leukemia in childhood. *N Engl J Med* 1996; **334**: 1428–1434
15. Lie SO, Jonmundsson G, Mellander L, Siimes MA, Yssing M, Gustafsson G on behalf of the Nordic Society of Paediatric Haematology and Oncology (NOPHO). A population-based study of 272 children with acute myeloid leukaemia treated on two consecutive protocols with different intensity: best outcome in girls, infants, and children with Down's syndrome. *Br J Haematol* 1996; **94**: 82–88
16. Lange BJ, Kobrinsky N, Barnard DR *et al.* Distinctive demography, biology, and outcome of acute myeloid leukemia and myelodysplastic syndrome in children with Down syndrome: Children's Cancer Center Group studies 2861 and 2891. *Blood* 1998; **91**: 608–615
17. Kojima S, Matsuyama T, Sato T *et al.* Down's syndrome and acute leukemia in children: an analysis of phenotype by use of monoclonal antibodies and electron microscopic platelet peroxidase reaction. *Blood* 1990; **76**: 2348–2353
18. Pui C-H, Raimondi SC, Borowitz MJ *et al.* Immunophenotypes and karyotypes of leukemic cells in children with Down syndrome and acute lymphoblastic leukemia. *J Clin Oncol* 1993; **11**: 1361–1367
19. Creutzig U, Ritter J, Vormoor J *et al.* Myelodysplasia and acute myelogenous leukemia in Down's syndrome. A report of 40 children of the AML-BFM Study Group. *Leukemia* 1996; **10**: 1677–1686
20. Suda J, Eguchi M, Ozawa T *et al.* Platelet peroxidase-positive blasts cells in transient myeloproliferative disorder with Down's syndrome. *Br J Haematol* 1988; **68**: 181–187
21. Hayashi Y, Eguchi M, Sugita K *et al.* Cytogenetic findings and clinical features in acute leukemia and transient myeloproliferative disorder in Down's syndrome. *Blood* 1988; **72**: 15–23
22. Kurahashi H, Hara J, Yumura-Yagi K, *et al.* Monoclonal nature of transient abnormal myelopoiesis in Down's syndrome. *Blood* 1991; **77**: 1161–1163
23. Kurahashi H, Hara J, Yumura-Yagi K, Tawa A, Kawa-Ha K. Transient abnormal myelopoiesis in Down's syndrome. *Leuk Lymphoma* 1992; **8**: 465–475
24. Shannon KM, Watterson J, Johnson P, *et al.* Monosomy 7 myeloproliferative disease in children with neurofibromatosis, Type 1: epidemiology and molecular analysis. *Blood* 1992; **79**: 1311–1318
25. Gillio AP, Gabrilove JL. Cytokine treatment of inherited bone marrow failure syndromes. *Blood* 1993; **81**: 1669–1674
26. Kalra R, Dale D, Freedman M *et al.* Monosomy 7 and activating *RAS*

mutations accompany malignant transformation in patients with congenital neutropenia. *Blood* 1995; **86**: 4579–4586

27. Maarek O, Jonveaux P, Le Coniat M, Berger R. Fanconi anemia and bone marrow clonal chromosome abnormalities. *Leukemia* 1996; **10**: 1700–1704

28. Miles DK, Freedman MH, Stephens K *et al*. Patterns of hematopoietic lineage involvement in children with neurofibromatosis type 1 and malignant myeloid disorders. *Blood* 1996; **88**: 4314–4320

29. Dong F, Brynes RK, Tidow N, Welte K, Löwenberg B, Touw IP. Mutations in the gene for the granulocyte colony-stimulating-factor receptor in patients with acute myeloid leukemia preceded by severe congenital neutropenia. *N Engl J Med* 1995; **333**: 487–493

30. Naparstek E. Granulocyte colony-stimulating factor, congenital neutropenia, and acute myeloid leukemia. *N Engl J Med* 1995; **333**: 516–518

31. Taylor AMR, Metcalfe JA, Mak Y-F. Leukemia and lymphoma in ataxia telangiectasia. *Blood* 1996; **87**: 423–438

32. Miller RW. Deaths from childhood leukemia and solid tumors among twins and other sibs in the United States, 1960–67. *J Natl Cancer Inst* 1971; **46**: 203–209

33. Ford AM, Ridge SA, Cabrera ME *et al*. In utero rearrangements in the trithorax-related oncogene in infant leukaemias. *Nature* 1993; **363**: 358–360

34. Buckley JD, Robinson LL, Swotinsky R *et al*. Occupational exposures of parents of children with acute nonlymphocytic leukemia: a report from the Children's Cancer Study Group. *Cancer Res* 1989; **49**: 4030–4037

35. Shu XO, Gao YT, Brinton LA *et al*. A population-based case-control study of childhood leukemia in Shanghai. *Cancer* 1988; **62**: 635–644

36. Robison LL, Buckley JD, Daigle AE *et al*. Maternal drug use and risk of childhood nonlymphoblastic leukemia among offspring. *Cancer* 1989; **63**: 1904–1911

37. Shu X-O, Ross JA, Pendergrass TW, Reaman GH, Lampkin B, Robison LL. Parental alcohol consumption, cigarette smoking and risk of infant leukemia: a Children's Cancer Group Study. *J Natl Cancer Inst* 1996; **88**: 24–31

38. Sandler DP. Recent studies in leukemia epidemiology. *Curr Opin Oncol* 1995; **7**: 12–18

39. Smith MA, McCaffrey RP, Karp JE. The secondary leukemias: challenges and research directions. *J Natl Cancer Inst* 1996; **88**: 407–418

40. Pui C-H, Behm FG, Raimondi SC *et al*. Secondary acute myeloid leukemia in children treated for acute lymphoid leukemia. *N Engl J Med* 1989; **321**: 136–142.

41. Pui C-H, Ribeiro RC, Hancock ML *et al*. Acute myeloid leukemia in children treated with epipodophyllotoxins for acute lymphoblastic leukemia. *N Engl J Med* 1991; **325**: 1682–1687

42. Imashuku S, Hibi S, Nakajima F *et al*. A review of 125 cases to determine the risk of myelodysplasia and leukemia in pediatric neutropenic patients after treatment with recombinant human granulocyte colony-stimulating factor. *Blood* 1994; **84**: 2380–2381

43. Socié G, Henry-Amar M, Bacigalupo A *et al*. Malignant tumors occurring after treatment of aplastic anemia. *N Engl J Med* 1993; **329**: 1152–1157

44. Russell NH. Biology of acute leukaemia. *Lancet* 1997; **349**: 118–122

45. Van Lom K, Hagemeijer A, Vanderkerckhove F, Smit B, Lowenberg B. Cytogenetic clonality analysis: typical patterns in myelodysplastic syndrome and acute myeloid leukemia. *Br J Haematol* 1996; **93**: 594–600

46. Keinanen M, Griffin JD, Bloomfield CD, Mackniki J, de la Chapelle A. Clonal chromosome abnormalities showing mutliple lineage involvement in acute myeloid leukaemia. *N Engl J Med* 1988; **318**: 1153–1158

47. Fialkow PJ, Singer J, Raskind W *et al*. Clonal development, stem cell differentiation, and clinical remissions in acute nonlymphocytic leukaemia. *N Engl J Med* 1987; **317**: 468–473

48. Hayhoe FG, Quaglino D, Flemans RJ. Consecutive use of Rama-

nowsky and periodic-acid-Schiff techniques in the study of blood and bone-marrow cells. *Br J Haematol* 1960; **6**: 23–25

49. Bennett JM, Catovsky D, Daniel M-T *et al*. Proposals for the classification of the acute leukaemias. *Br J Haematol* 1976; **33**: 451–458

50. Bennett JM, Catovsky D, Daniel MT *et al*. Proposed revised criteria for the classification of acute myeloid leukemia. A report of the French-American-British Co-operative Group. *Ann Intern Med* 1985; **103**: 626–629

51. Bennett JM, Catovsky D, Daniel M-T *et al*. Criteria for the diagnosis of acute leukemia of megakaryocyte lineage (M7). A report of the French-American-British Cooperative Group. *Ann Intern Med* 1985; **103**: 460–462

52. Huang M-J, Li C-Y, Nichols WL, Young J-H, Katzman JA. Acute leukemia with megakaryocytic differentiation: a study of 12 cases identified immunocytochemically. *Blood* 1984; **64**: 427–439

53. Bevan D, Rose M, Greaves M. Leukaemia of platelet precursors: diverse features in four cases. *Br J Haematol* 1982; **51**: 147–164

54. Mirchandani I, Palutke M. Acute megakaryoblastic leukaemia. *Cancer* 1983; **50**: 2866–2872

55. Pui C-H, Rivera G, Mirro J, Stass S, Peiper S, Murphy SB. Acute megakaryoblastic leukaemia. *Arch Pathol Lab Med* 1985; **109**: 1033–1035

56. Penchansky L, Taylor SR, Krause JR. Three infants with acute megakaryoblastic leukemia simulating metastatic tumor. *Cancer* 1989; **64**: 1366–1371

57. Hanker JS, Ambrose WW, James CJ. Facilitated light microscopic cytochemical diagnosis of acute myelogenous leukemia. *Cancer Res* 1979; **39**: 1635–1639

58. van der Schoot CE, Daams GM, Pinkster J, Vet R, von dem Brone AEGK. Monoclonal antibodies against myeloperoxidase are valuable immunological reagents for the diagnosis of acute myeloid leukaemia. *Br J Haematol* 1990; **74**: 173–178

59. Bennett JM, Catovsky D, Daniel M-T *et al*. Proposal for the recognition of minimally differentiated acute myeloid leukaemia (AML-M0). *Br J Haematol* 1991; **78**: 325–329

60. Venditti A, Del Poeta G, Stasi R *et al*. Minimally differentiated acute myeloid leukaemia (AML-M0): cytochemical, immunophenotypic and cytogenetic analysis of 19 cases. *Br J Haematol* 1994; **88**: 784–793

61. Stass SA, Pui C-H, Melvin S *et al*. Sudan black B positive acute lymphoblastic leukaemia. *Br J Haematol* 1984; **57**: 413–421

62. Charak BS, Advani SH, Karandikar SM *et al*. Sudan black B positivity in acute lymphoblastic leukaemia. *Acta Haematol* 1988; **80**: 199–202

63. Hayhoe FGJ, Quaglino D. *Haematological Cytochemistry*, 3rd edn. Edinburgh: Churchill Livingstone, 1994

64. Rosenthal NS, Farhi DC. Acute monocytic leukemia with chloroacetate esterase positivity. FAB M4 or M5? *Am J Clin Pathol* 1992; **98**: 41–45

65. Neiman RS, Barcos M, Berard C *et al*. Granulocytic sarcoma: a clinicopathologic study of 61 biopsied cases. *Cancer* 1981; **48**: 1426–1437

66. Li CY, Lam KW, Yam LT. Esterases in human leukocytes. *J Histochem Cytochem* 1973; **21**: 1–12

67. Pui C-H, Williams DL, Scarborough V, Jackson CW, Price R, Murphy S. Acute megakaryoblastic leukaemia associated with intrinsic platelet dysfunction and constitutional ring 21 chromosome in a young boy. *Br J Haematol* 1982; **50**: 191–200

68. Peterson BA, Levine EG. Uncommon subtypes of acute nonlymphocytic leukemia: clinical features and management of FAB M5, M6 and M7. *Semin Oncol* 1987; **14**: 425–434

69. van der Schoot CE, Daams GM, Pinkster J, Vet R, von dem Borne AEGK. Monoclonal antibodies against myeloperoxidase are valuable immunological reagents for the diagnosis of acute myeloid leukaemia. *Br J Haematol* 1990; **74**: 173–178

70. Stoor J, Dolan G, Coustan-Smith E, Barnett D, Reilly JT. Value of monoclonal anti-myeloperoxidase (MPO7) for diagnosing acute leukaemia. *J Clin Pathol* 1990; **43**: 847–849

71. Rovelli A, Biondi A, Cantu-Rajnoldi A *et al*. Microgranular variant of

acute promyelocytic leukemia in children. *J Clin Oncol* 1992; **10**: 1413–1418

72. Cantú-Rajnoldi A, Biondi A, Jankovic M *et al*. Diagnosis and incidence of acute promyelocytic leukemia (FAB M3 and M3 variant) in childhood. *Blood* 1993; **81**: 2209–2210

73. Biondi A, Rovelli A, Cantu-Rajnoldi A *et al*. Acute promyelocytic leukemia in children: experience of the Italian Pediatric Hematology and Oncology Group (AIEOP). *Leukemia* 1994; **8**: 1264–1268

74. Douer D, Preston-Martin S, Chang E, Nichols PW, Watkins KJ, Levine AM. High frequency of acute promyelocytic leukemia among Latinos with acute myeloid leukemia. *Blood* 1996; **87**: 308–313

75. Otero JC, Santillana S, Fereyros G. High frequency of acute promyelocytic leukemia among Latinos with acute myeloid leukemia. *Blood* 1996; **88**: 377–379

76. Le Beau MM, Larson RA, Bitter MA, Vardiman JW, Golomb HM, Rowley JD. Association of an inversion of chromosome 16 with abnormal marrow eosinophils in acute myelomonocytic leukemia. A unique cytogenetic-clinicopathological association. *N Engl J Med* 1983; **309**: 630–636

77. Haferlach T, Winkemann M, Löffler H *et al*. The abnormal eosinophils are part of the leukemic cell population in acute myelomonocytic leukemia with abnormal eosinophils (AML M4Eo) and carry the pericentric inversion 16: a combination of May-Grünwald-Giemsa staining and fluroescence *in situ* hybridization. *Blood* 1996; **87**: 2459–2463

78. Malkin D, Freedman MH. Childhood erythroleukemia: review of clinical and biological features. *Am J Pediatr Hematol Oncol* 1989; **11**: 348–359

79. Villeval JL, Cramer P, Lemoine F *et al*. Phenotype of early erythroblastic leukemias. *Blood* 1986; **68**: 1167–1174

80. Breton-Gorius J, Villeval JL, Mitjavila MT *et al*. Ultrastructural and cytochemical characterization of blasts from early erythroblastic leukemias. *Leukemia* 1987; **1**: 173–181

81. Garland R, Duchayne E, Blanchard D *et al*. Minimally differentiated erythroleukaemia (AML M6 'variant'): a rare subset of AML distinct from AML M6. *Br J Haematol* 1995; **90**: 868–875

82. Amadori S, Testi AM, Aricò M *et al*. Prospective comparative study of bone marrow transplantation and postremission chemotherapy for childhood acute myelogenous leukemia. *J Clin Oncol* 1993; **11**: 1046–1054

83. Creutzig U, Harbott J, Sperling C *et al*. Clinical significance of surface antigen expression in children with acute myeloid leukemia: results of study AML-BFM-87. *Blood* 1995; **86**: 3097–3108

84. Pui C-H. Childhood leukemia. In: Murphy GP, Lawrence W Jr, Lenhard RE Jr (eds) *American Cancer Society Textbook of Clinical Oncology*, 2nd edn. Atlanta, GA: American Cancer Society, Inc, 1995, pp 501–523

85. Hann IM, Stevens RF, Goldstone AH *et al*. Randomized comparison of DAT versus ADE as induction chemotherapy in children and younger adults with acute myeloid leukemia. Results of the medical research council's 10th AML trial (MRC AML 10). *Blood* 1997; **89**: 2311–2318

86. Argyle JC, Benjamin DR, Lampkin B, Hammond D. Acute non-lymphocytic leukemias of childhood. Inter-observer variability and problems in the use of the FAB classification. *Cancer* 1989; **63**: 295–301

87. Barnard DR, Kalousek DK, Wiersma SR, *et al*. Morphologic, immunologic and cytogenetic classification of acute myeloid leukemia and myelodysplastic syndrome in childhood: a report from the Children's Cancer Group. *Leukemia* 1996; **10**: 5–12

88. Cheson BD, Cassileth PA, Head DR *et al*. Report of the National Cancer Institute-sponsored workshop on definitions of diagnosis and response in acute myeloid leukemia. *J Clin Oncol* 1990; **8**: 813–819

89. Pui C-H, Raimondi SC, Head DR *et al*. Characterization of childhood acute leukemia with multiple myeloid and lymphoid markers at diagnosis and at relapse. *Blood* 1991; **78**: 1327–1337

90. Peterson LC, Parkin IL, Arthur DC, Brunning RD. Acute basophilic leukemia: a clinical, morphologic, and cytogenetic study of eight cases. *Am J Clin Pathol* 1991; **96**: 160–170

91. Bernini JC, Timmons CF, Sandler ES. Acute basophilic leukemia in a child. Anaphylactoid reaction and coagulopathy secondary to vincristine-mediated degranulation. *Cancer* 1995; **75**: 110–114

92. Bene MC, Castoldi G, Knapp W. Proposals for the immunological classification of acute leukemias. *Leukemia* 1995; **9**: 1783–1786

93. Smith FO, Raskind WH, Fialkow PJ, Bernstein ID. Cellular biology of acute myelogenous leukemia. *J Pediatr Hematol Oncol* 1995; **17**: 113–122

94. Buccheri V, Shetty V, Yoshida N, Morilla R, Matutes E, Catovsky D. The role of an anti-myeloperoxidase antibody in the diagnosis and classification of acute leukaemia: a comparison with light and electron microscopy cytochemistry. *Br J Haematol* 1992; **80**: 62–68

95. Pui C-H, Campana D, Crist WM. Toward a clinically useful classification of the acute leukemias. *Leukemia* 1995; **9**: 2154–2157

96. Drexler HG. Classification of acute myeloid leukemias—a comparison of FAB and immunophenotyping. *Leukemia* 1987; **1**: 697–705

97. Second MIC Co-operative Study Group. Morphologic, immunologic and cytogenetic (MIC) working classification of the acute myeloid leukaemias. *Br J Haematol* 1988; **68**: 487–494

98. Betz SA, Foucar K, Head DR, Chen I-M, Willman CL. False-positive flow cytometric platelet glycoprotein IIb/IIIa expression in myeloid leukemias secondary to platelet adherence to blasts. *Blood* 1992; **79**: 2399–2403

99. Smith LJ, Curtis JE, Messner HA, Senn JS, Furthmayr H, McCulloch EA. Lineage infidelity in acute leukemia. *Blood* 1983; **61**: 1138–1145

100. Pui C-H, Dahl GV, Melvin S *et al*. Acute leukaemia with mixed lymphoid and myeloid phenotype. *Br J Haematol* 1984; **56**: 121–130

101. Greaves MF, Chan LC, Furley AJW, Watt SM, Molgaard HV. Lineage promiscuity in hemopoietic differentiation and leukemia. *Blood* 1986; **67**: 1–11

102. Mirro J, Zipf TF, Pui C-H *et al*. Acute mixed lineage leukemia: clinicopathologic correlations and prognostic significance. *Blood* 1985; **66**: 1115–1123

103. Pui C-H, Behm FG, Singh B *et al*. Myeloid-associated antigen expression lacks prognostic value in childhood acute lymphoblastic leukemia treated with intensive multiagent chemotherapy. *Blood* 1990; **75**: 198–202

104. Wiersma SR, Ortega J, Sobel E, Weinberg KI. Clinical importance of myeloid-antigen expression in acute lymphoblastic leukemia of childhood. *N Engl J Med* 1991; **324**: 800–808

105. Drexler HG, Thiel E, Ludwig W-D. Review of the incidence and clinical relevance of myeloid antigen-positive acute lymphoblastic leukemia. *Leukemia* 1991; **5**: 637–645

106. Smith FO, Lampkin BC, Versteeg C *et al*. Expression of lymphoid-associated cell surface antigens by childhood acute myeloid leukemia cells lacks prognostic significance. *Blood* 1992; **79**: 2415–2422

107. Kuerbitz SJ, Civin CI, Krischer JP *et al*. Expression of myeloid-associated and lymphoid-associated cell-surface antigens in acute myeloid leukemia of childhood: a Pediatric Oncology Group Study. *J Clin Oncol* 1992; **10**: 1419–1429

108. Drexler HG, Thiel E, Ludwig W-D. Acute myeloid leukemias expressing lymphoid-associated antigens: diagnostic incidence and prognostic significance. *Leukemia* 1993; **7**: 489–498

109. Kawai S, Zha Z, Yamamoto Y, Shimizu H, Fujimoto T. Clinical significance of childhood acute myeloid leukemias expressing lymphoid-associated antigens. *Pediatr Hematol Oncol* 1995; **12**: 463–469

110. Claxton DF, Reading CL, Nagarajan L *et al*. Correlation of CD2 expression with PML gene breakpoints in patients with acute promyelocytic leukemia. *Blood* 1992; **80**: 582–586

111. Adriaansen HJ, te Boekhorst PAW, Hagemeijer AM, van der Schoot CE, Delwel HR, van Dongen JJM. Acute myeloid leukemia M4 with bone marrow eosinophilia (M4Eo) and inv(16)(p13q22) exhibits a specific immunophenotype with CD2 expression. *Blood* 1993; **81**: 3043–3051

112. Pui C-H, Schell MJ, Vodian MA *et al*. Serum CD4, CD8, and

interleukin-2 receptor levels in childhood acute myeloid leukemia. *Leukemia* 1991; **5**: 249–254

113. Kita K, Nakase K, Miwa H *et al*. Phenotypical characteristics of acute myelocytic leukemia associated with the t(8;21)(q22;q22) chromosomal abnormality: frequent expression of immature B-cell antigen CD19 together with stem cell antigen CD34. *Blood* 1992; **80**: 470–477

114. Hurwitz CA, Raimondi SC, Head D *et al*. Distinctive immunophenotypic features of t(8;21)(q22;q22) acute myeloblastic leukemia in children. *Blood* 1992; **80**: 3182–3188

115. Porwit-MacDonald A, Janossy G, Ivory K *et al*. Leukemia-associated changes identified by quantitative flow cytometry. IV. CD34 overexpression in acute myelogenous leukemia M2 with t(8;21). *Blood* 1996; **87**: 1162–1169

116. Arber DA, Jenkins KA, Slovak ML. CD79α expression in acute myeloid leukemia. High frequency of expression in acute promyelocytic leukemia. *Am J Pathol* 1996; **149**: 1105–1110

117. Pui C-H, Frankel LS, Carroll AJ *et al*. Clinical characteristics and treatment outcome of childhood acute lymphoblastic leukemia with the t(4;11)(q21;q23): a collaborative study of 40 cases. *Blood* 1991; **77**: 440–447

118. Pui C-H. Childhood leukemias. *N Engl J Med* 1995; **332**: 1618–1630

119. Smith FO, Broudy VC, Zsebo KM *et al*. Cell surface expression of c-kit receptors by childhood acute myeloid leukemia blasts is not of prognostic value: a report from the Children's Cancer Group. *Blood* 1994; **84**: 847–852

120. Sievers EL, Smith FO, Woods WG *et al*. Cell surface expression of the multidrug resistance P-glycoprotein (P-170) as detected by monoclonal antibody MRK-16 in pediatric acute myeloid leukemia fails to define a poor prognostic group: a report from the Children's Cancer Group. *Leukemia* 1995; **9**: 2042–2048

121. Smith FO, Rauch C, Williams DE *et al*. The human homologue of rat NG2, a chondroitin sulfate proteoglycan, is not expressed on the cell surface of normal hematopoietic cells but is expressed by acute myeloid leukemia blasts from poor-prognosis patients with abnormalities of chromosome band 11q23. *Blood* 1996; **87**: 1123–1133

122. Pui C-H, Behm FG, Kalwinsky DK *et al*. Clinical significance of low levels of myeloperoxidase positivity in childhood acute nonlymphoblastic leukemia. *Blood* 1987; **70**: 51–54

123. Gale RP, Bassat IB. Annotation: Hybrid acute leukaemia. *Br J Haematol* 1987; **65**: 261–26

124. Pui C-H, Relling MV, Behm FG *et al*. L-asparaginase may potentiate the leukomogenic effect of the epipodophyllotoxins. *Leukemia* 1995; **9**: 1680–1684

125. Pui C-H, Relling MV, Rivera GK *et al*. Epipodophyllotoxin-related acute myeloid leukemia: a study of 35 cases. *Leukemia* 1995; **9**: 1990–1996

126. Woods WG, Nesbit ME, Buckley J *et al*. Correlation of chromosome abnormalities with patient characteristics, histologic subtype, and induction success in children with acute nonlymphocytic leukemia. *J Clin Oncol* 1985; **3**: 3–11

127. Keverger G, Bernheim A, Daniel M-T *et al*. Cytogenetic study of 130 childhood acute nonlymphocytic leukemias. *Med Pediatr Oncol* 1988; **16**: 227–232

128. Raimondi SC, Kalwinsky DK, Hayashi Y, Behm FG, Mirro J Jr, Williams DL. Cytogenetics of childhood acute nonlymphocytic leukemia. *Cancer Genet Cytogenet* 1989; **40**: 13–27

129. Kalwinsky DK, Raimondi SC, Schell MJ *et al*. Prognostic importance of cytogenetic subgroups in de novo pediatric acute nonlymphocytic leukemia. *J Clin Oncol* 1990; **8**: 75–83

130. Haas OA, Kornberger M, Mayerhofer L. Cytogenetic abnormalities associated with childhood acute myeloblastic leukemia. Recent results. *Cancer Res* 1993; **131**: 103–112

131. Rabbitts TH. Chromosomal translocations in human cancer. *Nature* 1994; **372**: 143–149

132. Martinez-Climent JA, Lane NJ, Rubin CM *et al*. Clinical and prognostic significance of chromosomal abnormalities in childhood acute myeloid leukemia de novo. *Leukemia* 1995; **9**: 95–101

133. Borrow J, Stanton VP, Andersen M *et al*. The transloction t(8;16)(p11;p13) of acute myeloid leukaemia fuses a putative acetyltransferase to the CREB-binding protein. *Nature Genet* 1996; **14**: 33–41

134. Mrózek K, Heinonen K, de la Chapelle A, Bloomfield C. Clinical significance of cytogenetics in acute myeloid leukemia. *Semin Oncol* 1997; **24**: 17–31

135. Tallman MS, Hakimian D, Shaw JM, Lissner GS, Russell EJ, Variakojis D. Granulocytic sarcoma is associated with the 8:21 translocation in acute myeloid leukemia. *J Clin Oncol* 1993; **11**: 690–697

136. Carter M, Kalwinsky DK, Dahl GV, Santana VM, Mason CA, Schell MJ. Childhood acute promyelocytic leukemia: a rare variant of nonlymphoid leukemia with distinctive clinical and biologic features. *Leukemia* 1989; **3**: 298–302

137. Biondi A, Luciano A, Bassan R *et al*. CD2 expression in acute promyelocytic leukemia is associated with microgranular morphology (FAB M3v) but not with any PML gene breakpoint. *Leukemia* 1995; **9**: 1461–1466

138. Erber WN, Asbahr H, Rule SA, Scott CS. Unique immunophenotype of acute promyelocytic leukaemia as defined by CD9 and CD68 antibodies. *Br J Haematol* 1994; **88**: 101–104

139. Lemons RS, Keller S, Gietzen D *et al*. Acute promyelocytic leukemia. *J Pediatr Hematol Oncol* 1995; **17**: 198–210

140. Pui C-H, Raimondi SC, Murphy SB *et al*. An analysis of leukemic cell chromosomal features in infants. *Blood* 1987; **69**: 1289–1293

141. Martinez-Climent JA, Espinosa R III, Thirman MJ, Le Beau MM, Rowley JD. Abnormalities of chromosome band 11q23 and the *MLL* gene in pediatric myelomonocytic and monoblastic leukemias. Identification of the t(9;11) as an indicator of long survival. *J Pediatr Hematol Oncol* 1995; **17**: 277–283

142. Luna-Fineman S, Shannon KM, Lange BJ. Childhood monosomy 7: epidemiology, biology, and mechanistic implications. *Blood* 1995; **85**: 1985–1999

143. Lion T, Haas OA. Acute megakaryocytic leukemia with the t(1;22)(p13;q13). *Leukemia Lymphoma* 1993; **11**: 15–20

144. Carroll A, Civin C, Schneider N *et al*. The t(1;22)(p13;q13) is nonrandom and restricted to infants with acute megakaryoblastic leukemia: a Pediatric Oncology Group study. *Blood* 1991; **78**: 748–752

145. Fonatsch C, Gudat H, Lengfelder E *et al*. Correlation of cytogenetic findings with clinical features in 18 patients with inv(3)(q21q26) or t(3;3)(q21;q26). *Leukemia* 1994; **8**: 1318–1326

146. Soekarman D, von Lindern M, Daenen S *et al*. The translocation (6;9)(p23;q34) shows consistent rearrangement of two genes and defines a myeloproliferative disorder with specific clinical features. *Blood* 1992; **79**: 2990–2997

147. Köller U, Haas OA, Ludwig W-D *et al*. Phenotypic and genotypic heterogeneity in infant acute leukemia. II. Acute nonlymphoblastic leukemia. *Leukemia* 1989; **3**: 708–714

148. Lampert F, Harbott J, Ritterbach J. Cytogenetic findings in acute leukaemias of infants. *Br J Cancer* 1992; **66**: S20-S22

149. Sorensen PHB, Chen C-S, Smith FO *et al*. Molecular rearrangements of the *MLL* gene are present in most cases of infant acute myeloid leukemia and are strongly correlated with monocytic or myelomonocytic phenotypes. *J Clin Invest* 1994; **93**: 429–437

150. Pui C-H, Kane JR, Crist WM. Biology and treatment of infant leukemias. *Leukemia* 1995; **9**: 762–769

151. Warrell RP Jr, de Thé H, Wang Z-Y, Degos L. Acute promyelocytic leukemia. *N Engl J Med* 1993; **329**: 177–189

152. Pui C-H. Acute leukemia in children. *Curr Opin Hematol* 1996; **3**: 249–258

153. Ahuja HG, Foti A, Bar-Eli M, Cline MJ. The pattern of mutational involvement of *RAS* genes in human hematologic malignancies determined by DNA amplification and direct sequencing. *Blood* 1990; **75**: 1684–1690

154. Cline MJ. The molecular basis of leukemia. *N Engl J Med* 1994; **330**: 328–336

155. Imamura J, Miyoshi I, Koeffler HP. p53 in hematologic malignancies. *Blood* 1994; **84**: 2412–2421

156. Wattel E, Preudhomme C, Hecquet B *et al.* p53 mutations are associated with resistance to chemotherapy and short survival in hematologic malignances. *Blood* 1994; **84**: 3148–3157

157. Yamagami T, Sugiyama H, Inoue K *et al.* Growth inhibition of human leukemic cells by WT1 (Wilms' tumor gene) antisense oligodeoxynucleotides: implications for the involvement of WT1 in leukemogenesis. *Blood* 1996; **87**: 2878–2884

158. King-Underwood L, Renshaw J, Pritchard-Jones K. Mutations in the Wilms' tumor gene WT1 in leukemias. *Blood* 1996; **87**: 2171–2179

159. Paggi MG, de Fabritiis P, Bonetto F *et al.* The retinoblastoma gene product in acute myeloid leukemia: a possible involvement in promyelocytic leukemia. *Cancer Res* 1995; **55**: 4552–4556

160. Lotem J, Sachs L. Control of apoptosis in hematopoiesis and leukemia by cytokines, tumor suppressor and oncogenes. *Leukemia* 1996; **10**: 925–931

161. Liu P, Tarlé SA, Hajra A *et al.* Fusion between transcription factor CBFβ/PEBP2β and a myosin heavy chain in acute myeloid leukemia. *Science* 1993; **261**: 1041–1044

162. Dyck JA, Maul GG, Miller WH Jr, Chen JD, Kakizuka A, Evans RM. A novel macromolecular structure in a target of the promyelocyte-retinoic acid receptor oncoprotein. *Cell* 1994; **76**: 333–343

163. Okuda T, van Deursen J, Heibert SW, Grosveld G, Downing JR. AML1, the target of multiple chromosomal translocations in human leukemia, is essential for normal fetal liver hematopoiesis. *Cell* 1996; **84**: 321–330

164. Castilla LH, Wijmenga C, Wang Q *et al.* Failure of embryonic hematopoiesis and lethal hemorrhages in mouse embryos heterozygous for a knocked-in leukemia gene *CBFβ-MYH11*. *Cell* 1996; **87**: 687–696

165. Caligiuri MA, Strout MP, Gilliland DG. Molecular biology of acute myeloid leukemia. *Semin Oncol* 1997; **24**: 32–44

166. Sawyers CL. Molecular genetics of acute leukaemia. *Lancet* 1997; **349**: 196–200

167. Grignani F, Ferrucci PF, Testa U, *et al.* The acute promyelocytic leukemia-specific PML-RARα fusion protein inhibits differentiation and promotes survival of myeloid precursor cells. *Cell* 1993; **74**: 423–431

168. Nucifora G, Rowley JD. *AML1* and the 8;21 and 3;21 translocations in acute and chronic myeloid leukemia. *Blood* 1995; **86**: 1–14

169. Corral J, Lavenir I, Impey H *et al.* An *Mll-AF9* fusion gene made by homologos recombination causes acute leukemia in chimeric mice: a method to crease fusion oncogenes. *Cell* 1996; **85**: 853–861

170. Liu PP, Hajra A, Wijmenga C, Collins FS. Molecular pathogenesis of the chromosome 16 inversion in the M4Eo subtype of acute myeloid leukemia. *Blood* 1995; **85**: 2289–2302

171. Grier HE, Gelber RD, Camitta BM *et al.* Prognostic factors in childhood acute myelogenous leukemia. *J Clin Oncol* 1987; **5**: 1026–1032

172. Krischer JP, Steuber CP, Vietti TJ *et al.* Long-term results in the treatment of acute nonlymphocytic leukemia: a Pediatric Oncology Group Study. *Med Pediatr Oncol* 1989; **17**: 401–408

173. Creutzig U, Ritter J, Schellong G for the AML-BFM Study Group. Identification of two risk groups in childhood acute myelogenous leukemia after therapy intensification in study AML-BFM-83 as compared with Study AML-BFM-78. *Blood* 1990; **75**: 1932–1940

174. Steuber CP, Civin C, Krischer J *et al.* A comparison of induction and maintenance therapy for acute nonlymphocytic leukemia in childhood: results of a Pediatic Oncology Group Study. *J Clin Oncol* 1991; **9**: 247–258

175. Ravindranath Y, Steuber CP, Krischer J *et al.* High-dose cytarabine for intensification of early therapy of childhood acute myeloid leukemia: a Pediatric Oncology Group Study. *J Clin Oncol* 1991; **9**: 572–580

176. Creutzig U, Ritter J, Zimmermann M, Schellong G. Does cranial irradiation reduce the risk for bone marrow relapse in acute myelogenous leukemia? Unexpected results of the childhood acute myelogenous leukemia study BFM-87. *J Clin Oncol* 1993; **11**: 279–286

177. Nesbit ME Jr, Buckley JD, Feig SA *et al.* Chemotherapy for induction of remission of childhood acute myeloid leukemia followed by marrow transplantation or multiagent chemotherapy: a report from the Children's Cancer Group. *J Clin Oncol* 1994; **12**: 127–135

178. Byrd JC, Edenfield WJ, Shields DJ, Dawson NA. Extramedullary myeloid cell tumors in acute nonlymphocytic leukemia: a clinical review. *J Clin Oncol* 1995; **13**: 1800–1816

179. Cavdar AO, Babacan E, Gözdasoglu S *et al.* High risk subgroup of acute myelomonocytic leukemia (AMML) with orbito-ocular granulocytic sarcoma (OOGS) in Turkish children. Retrospetive analysis of clinical, hematological, ultrastructural and therapeutical findings of thirty-three OOGS. *Acta Haemaol* 1989; **81**: 80–85

180. Pui C-H, Dahl GV, Kalwinsky DK *et al.* Central nervous system leukemia in children with acute nonlymphoblastic leukemia. *Blood* 1985; **66**: 1062–1067

181. Pui C-H, Kalwinsky DK, Schell MJ, Mason CA, Mirro J Jr, Dahl GV. Acute nonlymphoblastic leukemia in infants: clinical presentation and outcome. *J Clin Oncol* 1988; **6**: 1008–1013

182. Pui C-H, Ribeiro RC, Campana D *et al.* Prognostic factors in the acute lymphoid and myeloid leukemias of infants. *Leukemia* 1996; **10**: 952–956

183. Odom LF, Gordon EM. Acute monoblastic leukemia in infancy and early childhood: successful treatment with an epipodophyllotoxin. *Blood* 1984; **64**: 875–882

184. Bunin NJ, Pui C-H. Differing complications of hyperleukocytosis in children with acute lymphoblastic or acute nonlymphoblastic leukemia. *J Clin Oncol* 1985; **3**: 1590–1595

185. Creutzig U, Ritter J, Budde M, Sutor A, Schellong G, and the German BFM Study Group. Early deaths due to hemorrhage and leukostasis in childhood acute myelogenous leukemia. *Cancer* 1987; **60**: 3071–3079

186. Ribeiro RC, Pui C-H. The clinical and biological correlates of coagulopathy in children with acute leukemia. *J Clin Oncol* 1986; **4**: 1212–1218

187. Sakata Y, Murakami T, Noro A, Mori K, Matsuda M. The specific activity of plasminogen activator inhibitor-1 in disseminated intravascular coagulation with acute promyelocytic leukemia. *Blood* 1991; **77**: 1949–1957

188. Tallman MS, Hakimian D, Kwaan HC, Rickles FR. New insights into the pathogenesis of coagulation dysfunction in acute promyelocytic leukemia. *Leukemia Lymphoma* 1993; **11**: 27–36

189. Nur S, Anwar M, Saleen M, Ahmad PA. Disseminated intravascular coagulation in acute leukaemias at first diagnosis. *Eur J Haematol* 1995; **55**: 78–82

190. Tobelem G, Jacquillat C, Chastang C *et al.* Acute monoblastic leukemia: a clinical and biologic study of 74 cases. *Blood* 1980; **55**: 71–76

191. Hurwitz CA, Schell MJ, Pui C-H, Crist WM, Behm F, Mirro J Jr. Adverse prognostic features in 251 children treated for acute myeloid leukemia. *Med Pediatr Oncol* 1993; **21**: 1–7

192. Boulad F, Kernan NA. Treatment of childhood acute nonlymphoblastic leukemia: A review. *Cancer Invest* 1993; **11**: 534–553

193. Taub JW, Matherly LH, Stout ML, Buck SA, Gurney JG, Ravindranath Y. Enhanced metabolism of 1-β-D-arabinofuranosylcytosine in Down syndrome cells: a contributing factor to the superior event free survival of Down syndrome children with acute myeloid leukemia. *Blood* 1996; **87**: 3395–3403

194. Sievers EL, Smith FO, Woods WG *et al.* Cell surface expression of the multidrug resistance P-glycoprotein (P-170) as detected by monoclonal antibody MRK-16 in pediatric acute myeloid leukemia fails to define a poor prognostic group: a report from the Children's Cancer Group. *Leukemia* 1995; **9**: 2042–2048

195. Ivy SP, Olshefski RS, Taylor BJ, Patel KM, Reaman GH. Correlation of P-glycoprotein expression and function in childhood acute leukemia: a Children's Cancer Group study. *Blood* 1996; **88**: 309–318

196. Pearson L, Leith CP, Chen I-M *et al.* Multidrug resistance-1 (MDR1) expression and functional dye/drug efflux is highly correlated with the

t(8;21) chromosomal translocation in pediatric acute myeloid leukemia (AML). *Blood* 1994; **84 (Suppl 1)**: 46A

197. Hunter AE, Rogers SY, Roberts IAG, Barrett JA, Russell N. Autonomous growth of blast cells is associated with reduced survival in acute myeloblastic leukemia. *Blood* 1993; **82**: 899–903

198. Campana D, Pui C-H. Detection of minimal residual disease in acute leukemia: methodologic advances and clinical significance. *Blood* 1995; **85**: 1416–1434

199. Lo Coco F, Diverio D, Pandolfi PP *et al*. Molecular evaluation of residual disease as a predictor of relapse in acute promyelocytic leukaemia. *Lancet* 1992; **340**: 1437–1438

200. Huang W, Sun G-L, Li X-S *et al*. Acute promyelocytic leukemia: clinical relevance of two major PML-RARα isoforms and detection of minimal residual disease by retrotranscriptase/polymerase chain reaction to predict relapse. *Blood* 1993; **82**: 1264–1269

201. Miller WH Jr, Levine K, DeBlasio A, Frankel SR, Dmitrovsky E, Warrell RP Jr. Detection of minimal residual disease in acute promyelocytic leukemia by a reverse transcription polymerase chain reaction assay for the PML/RAR-α fusion mRNA. *Blood* 1993; **82**: 1689–1694

202. Diverio D, Pandolfi PP, Biondi A *et al*. Absence of reverse transcription-polymerase chain reaction detectable residual disease in patients with acute promyelocytic leukemia in long-term remission. *Blood* 1993; **82**: 3556–3559

203. Workshop Report. RT-PCR in acute promyelocytic leukemia: second workshop of the European Retinoic Group. *Leukemia* 1996; **10**: 368–371

204. Nucifora G, Larson RA, Rowley JD. Persistence of the 8;21 translocation in patients with acute myeloid leukemia type M2 in long-term remission. *Blood* 1993; **82**: 712–715

205. Kusec R, Laczika K, Knöbl P *et al*. *AML1/ETO* fusion mRNA can be detected in remission blood samples of all patients with t(8;21) acute myeloid leukemia after chemotherapy or autologous bone marrow transplantation. *Leukemia* 1994; **8**: 735–739

206. Guerrasio A, Rosso C, Martinelli G *et al*. Polyclonal haemopoiesis associated with long-term persistence of the AML1-ETO transcript in patients with FAB M2 acute myeloid leukaemia in continuous clinical remission. *Br J Haematol* 1995; **90**: 364–368

207. Miyamoto T, Nagafuji K, Akashi K *et al*. Persistence of multipotent progenitors expressing *AML1/ETO* transcripts in long-term remission patients with t(8;21) acute myelogenous leukemia. *Blood* 1996; **87**: 4789–4796

208. Satake N, Maseki N, Kozu T *et al*. Disappearance of *AML1-MTG8 (ETO)* fusion transcript in acute myeloid leukaemia patients with t(8;21) in long-term remission. *Br J Haematol* 1995; **91**: 892–898

209. Jurlander J, Caligiuri MA, Ruutu T *et al*. Persistence of the *AML1/ETO* fusion transcript in patients treated with allogeneic bone marrow transplantation for t(8;21) leukemia. *Blood* 1996; **88**: 2183–2191

210. Claxton DF, Liu P, Hsu HB *et al*. Detection of fusion transcripts generated by the inversion 16 chromosome in acute myelogenous leukemia. *Blood* 1994; **83**: 1750–1756

211. Hébert J, Cayuela J-M, Daniel M-T, Berger R, Sigaux F. Detection of minimal residual disease in acute myelomonocytic leukemia with abnormal marrow eosinophils by nested polymerase chain reaction with allele specific amplification. *Blood* 1994; **84**: 2291–2296

212. Tobal K, Johnson PRE, Saunders MJ, Harrison CJ, Liu Yin JA. Detection of CBFB/MYH11 transcripts in patients with inversion and other abnormalities of chromosome 16 at presentation and remission. *Br J Haematol* 1995; **91**: 104–108

213. Inoue K, Sugiyama H, Ogawa H *et al*. *WT1* as a new prognostic factor and a new marker for the detection of minimal residual disease in acute leukemia. *Blood* 1994; **84**: 3071–3079

214. Inoue K, Ogawa H, Yamagami T *et al*. Long-term follow-up of minimal residual disease in leukemia patients by monitoring WT1 (Wilms' tumor gene) expression levels. *Blood* 1996; **88**: 2267–2278

215. Campana D, Coustan-Smith E, Janossy G. The immunologic detection of minimal residual disease in acute leukemia. *Blood* 1990; **76**: 163–171

216. Adriaansen HJ, Jacobs BC, Kappers-Klunne MC, Hählen K, Hooijkaas H, van Dongen JJM. Detection of residual disease in AML patients by use of double immunological marker analysis for terminal deoxynucleotidyl transferase and myeloid markers. *Leukemia* 1993; **7**: 472–481

217. Coustan-Smith E, Behm FG, Hurwitz CA, Rivera GK, Campana D. N-CAM (CD56) expression by CD34⁺ malignant myeloblasts has implications for minimal residual disease detection in acute myeloid leukemia. *Leukemia* 1993; **7**: 853–858

218. Campana D, Freitas RO, Coustan-Smith E. Detection of residual leukemia with immunologic methods: technical developments and clinical implications. *Leukemia Lymphoma* 1994; **13**: 31–34

219. Sievers EL, Lange BJ, Buckley JD *et al*. Prediction of relapse of pediatric acute myeloid leukemia by use of multidimensional flow cytometry. *J Natl Cancer Inst* 1996; **88**: 1483–1488

220. Menssen HD, Renkl H-J, Rodeck U *et al*. Presence of Wilms' tumor gene (*wt1*) transcripts and the WT1 nuclear protein in the majority of human acute leukemias. *Leukemia* 1995; **9**: 1060–1067

221. Macedo A, San Miguel JF, Vidriales MB *et al*. Phenotypic changes in acute myeloid leukaemia: implications in the detection of minimal residual disease. *J Clin Pathol* 1996; **49**: 15–18

Therapy of acute myeloid leukemia

BEVERLY J LANGE AND NANCY J BUNIN

Most clinical trials of the 1980s achieved long-term survival in one-third of children and adolescents with acute myeloid leukemia (AML).[1–5] The National Cancer Institutes SEER survival statistics suggest that this fraction has not changed in a decade (Table 19.1).[6] However, many trials of the 1990s anticipate 5-year event-free survivals (EFSs) of >40%,[7–12] and a few recent studies project 5-year survival rates approaching 50%.[9,13–16] Cure eludes most AML patients for several reasons: the vast heterogeneity of the disease, heterogeneity of the host, a limited repertoire of treatment strategies and a high treatment-associated mortality.

This chapter reviews the principles of AML therapy and its associated supportive care. Because AML in children and adults have many similarities, relevant studies in adults are cited.

TREATMENT STRATEGY

Treatment of AML involves antineoplastic agents and anticipatory supportive care. The former consists of remission induction therapy, central nervous system prophylaxis and post-remission therapy, which includes consolidation therapy, intensification therapy[17] and, in some trials, maintenance therapy and central nervous system prophylaxis (Fig. 19.1). Initially, all post-remission therapy was modeled after that of acute lymphoblastic leukemia (ALL) with cranial irradition and years of maintenance therapy. Today, most protocols have increased the intensity of therapy, shortened its duration and eliminated prophylactic cranial irradiation.

Table 19.1 Trends in survival for children under 5 years of age with acute myeloid leukemia in the United States, 1960–1991 (NCI SEER Program Statistics).[6]

Interval	5-Year survival (%)
1960–63	3
1970–73	5
1974–76	14
1977–79	26 ± 5–10
1980–82	21 ± 5–10
1983–85	33 ± 5–10
1986–91	28 ± 5–10

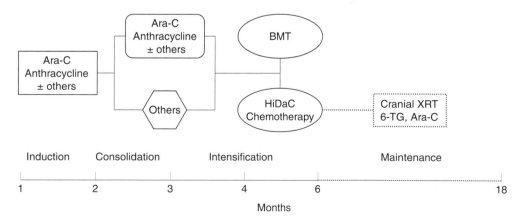

Fig. 19.1 Current general treatment strategy for acute myeloid leukemia in children. Ara-C = cytosine arabinoside; BMT = bone marrow transplantation; HiDaC = high-dose ara-C; cranial XRT = prophylactic cranial radiation; 6-TG = 6-thioguanine.

Steuber[18] has summarized the evolution of pediatric AML therapy from ALL-derived strategies to the present arabinosylcytosine (ara-C) and anthracycline-based strategies. Hurwitz et al[19] have reviewed the clinical trials of the 1980s. Pivotal studies are the VAPA-10 protocol with rotating intensive chemotherapy,[20] Children's Cancer Group (CCG)-251, which biologically randomized allogeneic BMT in first remission,[2,21,22] and the Berlin–Frankfurt–Münster (BFM) '83 study.[16]

INDUCTION THERAPY

There are 3 purposes to induction therapy:

1. to reduce the proportion of leukemic cells in the marrow to <5% and/or eradicate extramedullary disease;
2. to restore normal trilineage hematopoiesis;
3. to establish the foundation for a durable remission.

With the exception of therapy for acute promyelocytic leukemia (APL), AML induction therapy entails highly myelosuppressive chemotherapy followed by finite periods of marrow aplasia. In practice, the combined effects of leukemia replacing normal marrow and therapy inducing aplasia give rise to pancytopenia of 3–6 weeks' duration or longer. Mortality during induction ranges from 6–20% depending on intensity of therapy and the age of the patient.[1,3,7–16] Infants and the elderly suffer higher mortality unless adjustments are made. In infants, this is accomplished by calculating doses by weight or reducing doses by 33–50%. These adjustments reduce toxicity but also may reduce efficacy, as found in the studies CCG-251 and LAME 89/91.[2,14]

Ara-C and anthracyclines are the most effective single agents for inducing and sustaining remission in AML.[22] Results of clinical trials suggest that ara-C and anthracyclines are additive *in vivo*.[23] Ara-C is an S-phase agent.[24] Only a minority of leukemic myeloblasts are in S phase.[25,26] As cells die or are killed by ara-C, new ones are recruited. Continuous infusions of ara-C, frequent subcutaneous injections, or b.i.d. infusions of very high doses expose the maximal number of cells to the drug. Kinetic studies *in vitro* and randomized trials of the Cancer and Acute Leukemia Group B (CALGB) established the superior efficacy of continuous exposure.[27,28]

The recognized standard AML induction regimen is called '7 and 3', i.e. 7 days of ara-C at 100 mg/m²/day continuous infusion and 3 days of daunorubicin at 45–60 mg/m²/day. One or 2 courses of '7 and 3' induce remission in about 75–80% of children (Table 19.2).[2,19,22,23,29–30]

Many trials have attempted to improve on '7 and 3' by increasing the dose of ara-C or adding other agents.[30–37] In adults, randomized comparisons of 100–200 mg/m² of ara-C have not shown any advantage to the higher dose.[31,32] Randomized comparisons of '7 and 3' to logarithmic

increases in ara-C with 3-hour pulses of 1000–3000 mg/m² every 12 hours for 8–12 doses have either shown modest improvements in remission duration or no benefit.[33,34] Addition of etoposide to '7 and 3' (ADE) extended the duration of remission.[35] CALGB found no increase in complete remission with 6-thioguanine (6-TG).[36] Stasi et al[37] conclude that dose intensification in AML in adults results in minimal improvement in outcome.[37]

In pediatric AML, there are a few randomized comparisons of '7 and 3' to other regimens. CCG-213 compared '7 and 3' to a 5-drug combination called 'Denver'.[5,38] There was no difference in remission induction rate or long-term outcome.[5] Despite the lack of formal evidence for benefits of embellishment of '7 and 3', no current clinical trial in pediatric AML uses standard '7 and 3' (Table 19.2). BFM '83 and '87 protocols and BFM-derived protocols add etoposide and increase the cumulative dose of ara-C (Table 19.2). Their remission induction rates are comparable to '7 and 3'.[7–9,12,16]

Several trials in Table 19.2 achieve induction rates higher than the historical 75–80% of '7 and 3'. The Pediatric Oncology Group (POG) trial 8821 used TD '7 and 3' plus 6-TG (TAD); the remission induction rate was 85% (Table 19.2),[3] the same as in the previous trial POG 8498, which used TAD with ara-C 200 mg/m².[39] UK AML 10 extended ara-C to 10 days plus either 6-TG (TAD) or etoposide (ADE). Remission induction rate was 85% after 1 or 2 courses and 92% with additional agents.[15] LAME 89/91 increased the dose of ara-C to 1000 mg/m² continuous infusion for only 5 days and replaced daunorubicin for 3 days with mitoxantrone for 5 days, approximately a 40% increase in anthracycline dose.[14]

Idarubicin may effect both a higher remission induction rate and more durable remissions than daunorubicin, especially in patients aged under 50 years.[40–42] The MRC/ICRF Cancer Studies Unit evaluated randomized comparisons of idarubicin (IDA) or mitoxantrone versus daunomycin.[43] The remission induction was higher with IDA (68% versus 59%, p <0.001) with a trend toward better results with younger age.[43] Five-year disease-free survival (DFS) with IDA was not superior, but this analysis did not separate out the younger patients.[43] Although there was a trend for mitoxantrone to be superior to daunomycin, evidence of benefit was less substantial than that supporting IDA.[43] In one of the first pediatric trials to use idarubicin in a BFM '87-derived induction regimen, the Garrahan Institute achieved a 78% remission rate, i.e. the same as with daunorubicin (Table 19.2).[12]

CCG-2891 has tested a kinetically-based timed-sequencing approach to induction therapy. *In vitro* AML blasts show maximal recruitment and synchronization 6–8 days after cessation of ara-C.[25,26,44–46] To exploit this putative recruitment *in vivo*, CCG-2891 compared standard timing of a 5-drug induction regimen called DCTER to intensive timing of DCTER (Table 19.2).[47,48] With standard timing the second course of DCTER is given only if the day 14

Table 19.2 Complete response rates after 1 or 2 courses of induction therapy for recent co-operative group studies of pediatric acute myeloid leukemia.

| Study | Regimen[a] | N | Cumulative dose in first 14 days | | | | Complete response (%)[e] |
			Ara-C (mg/m²)[b]	Dnm (mg/m²)[c]	Dnm equiv (mg/m²)[d]	Other agents	
CCG-213[5]	Standard '7 and 3'	597	700	135			79
POG-8821[3]	TAD	649	700	135		6-TG	85
UK AML 10[15]	TA$_{10}$D	318	1000	150		6-TG	85–92
	A$_{10}$DE		1000	150		Etoposide	
BFM '87[9]	A$_8$DE	210	1400	180		Etoposide	78
EORTC[7]	A$_8$ME	106	1400		Mitox 36 Dnm 144	Etoposide	78
Garrahan[12]	A$_8$IE	68	1400		IDA 36 Dnm 144	Etoposide	78
LAME '89/91[14]	A$_5$M	171	5000		Mitox 60 Dnm 225	Etoposide	87
CCG-2891[13]	DCTER standard timing	294	800	80		Etoposide 6-TG Dexamethasone	74
CCG-2891[13]	DCTER intensive timing	295	1600	60		Etoposide 6-TG Dexamethasone	78

[a]The standard AML induction regimen is '7 and 3', i.e. 7 days of continuous infusion cytosine arabinoside (ara-C) at 100 mg/m²/day and 3 days of daunorubicin at 45–60 mg/m²/day. TAD = '7 and 3' + 6-thioguanine (6-TG). Subscripts after 'A' indicate the number of days of ara-C. Thus, TA$_{10}$ refers to standard daily doses of ara-C and daunomycin + 6-TG but 10 days of ara-C rather than 7. ADE = ara-C, daunorubicin and etoposide; A$_{10}$DE = 10 days of ara-C rather than the standard 7. DCTER = dexamethasone, ara-C, 6-TG, etoposide and rubidomycin. AM = ara-C mitxantrone. AIE = ara-C, idarubicin and etoposide.
[b]Cumulative dose of ara-C during the first 14 days of therapy.
[c]Cumulative dose of anthracycline during the first 14 days of therapy. Several recent studies have replaced daunomycin (Dnm) with newer anthracyclines mitxantrone (Mitox) or idarubicin (IDA).
[d]Estimated equivalent of daunorubicin is listed below the anthracycline.
[e]Complete response rates are for 1 or 2 courses of induction therapy with the exception of UK-AML 10 where the 92% figure includes 8% of patients who had 3 or 4 courses.

marrow shows residual leukemia. Intensive DCTER was given on days 0–3 and repeated on days 10–13 regardless of marrow status. Remission induction rate was 78% with intensively-timed therapy and 74% with conventionally-timed therapy (p = ns). Induction mortality was significantly higher with the former; refractory leukemia was less; 3-year EFS was significantly higher with intensive timing (41% versus 30%, p = 0.008; Fig. 19.2).[48] These results illustrate 2 points about AML induction therapy:

1. intensification of therapy will not improve the remission induction rate if the increase in mortality equals the reduction in failure rate;
2. not all remissions are equal: the more toxic regimen achieves a higher quality, more durable remission.

POST-REMISSION THERAPY

The Eastern Co-operative Oncology Group (ECOG) demonstrated that it is necessary to continue AML therapy beyond morphologic remission.[49,50] Currently, in pediatric AML there are 2 valid, disparate approaches to AML post-remission therapy. BFM '83 and BFM '87 (Fig. 19.3) protocols and many BFM-derivative protocols epitomize a modified ALL strategy.[8,9,51–53] CCG-2891, LAME-89/91, UK AML 10, POG and 8821 exemplify the short duration, maximal dose intensity strategy. Matched related allogeneic BMT in first remission represents the extreme example of dose intensification.

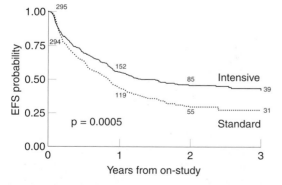

Fig. 19.2 Event-free survival (EFS) from time of study for patients with acute myeloid leukemia, comparing patients randomized to intensive induction timing (n = 295) versus standard induction timing (n = 294). Reproduced with permission from Ref. 48.

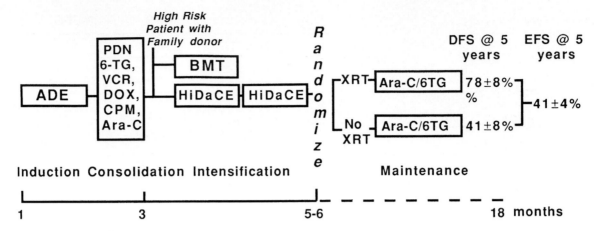

Fig. 19.3 Treatment scheme for the BFM '97 protocol. ADE = cytosine arabinoside, daunorubicin and etoposide; PDN = prednisone; 6-TG = 6-thioguanine; VCR = vincristine; DOX = doxorubicin; Ara-C = cytosine arabinoside; CPM = cyclophosphamide; BMT = bone marrow transplantation; HiDaCE = high-dose ara-C and etoposide intensification; XRT = prophylactic cranial radiation.[53]

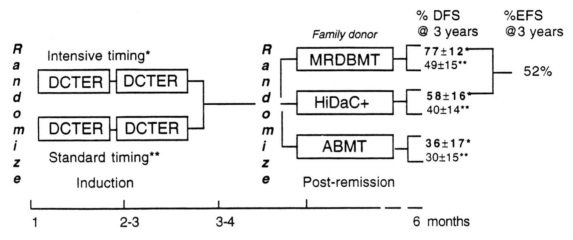

Fig. 19.4 CCG-2891 treatment scheme. Patients are randomly assigned to an intensively-timed 5-drug regimen DCTER (dexamethasone, cytosine arabinoside, 6-thioguanine, etoposide and rubidomycin). At the end of the induction (patients with a matched family donor) biologically randomized to matched related marrow transplant (MRDBMT); the others are randomly assigned to high-dose ara-C/L-asparaginase chemotherapy (HiDaC+) and 3 months of less intensive post-remission therapy for autologous bone marrow transplantation (ABMT). DFS = disease-free survival; EFS = event-free survival.[13,47,48]

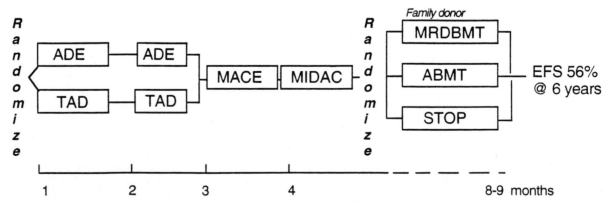

Fig. 19.5 UK MRC AML 10 treatment scheme.

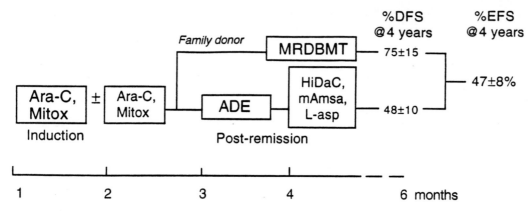

Fig. 19.6 French LAME 89/91 protocol. Induction consists of cytosine arabinoside (ara-C) and mitxantrone (mitox) (see Table 19.2). Patients with a family donor undergo a matched related bone marrow transplant (MRDBMT) or post-remission chemotherapy with ara-C, daunorubicin and etoposide (ADE) followed by high-dose ara-C (HiDaC) and amasarcine mAmsa; and L-asparaginase (L-asp). DFS = disease-free survival; EFS = event-free survival.[14]

Figs 19.3–19.6 depict treatment schemes from 4 recent Co-operative Group studies which had encouraging results. In these figures, post-remission outcomes are expressed in terms of EFS from the time of diagnosis and disease-free survival (DFS) from the end of induction. Separation of induction and post-remission analyses arose because the availability of a matched related donor (MRD) is not usually known at diagnosis. In trials comparing bone marrow transplantation (BMT) to post-remission chemotherapy, patients with a suitable donor are 'biologically randomized' to BMT. Not all patients with donors can undergo BMT. To avoid selection bias, DFS is evaluated according to an intention-to-treat analysis, i.e. patients are considered as having received a BMT or chemotherapy based on existence of a donor whether or not they received the randomized therapy.

CHEMOTHERAPY

In the mid 1980s, it became apparent that very high dose ara-C (HiDaC, 1–3 g/m^2/dose repeated 8–12 times) could eradicate leukemia resistant to standard dose ara-C.[24,54,55] This dose of ara-C exceeds by about 5-fold the extracellular concentration needed to transport sufficient ara-C into myeloblasts to phosphorylate maximally ara-C to ara-CTP.[24] CNS penetration of HiDaC is excellent and HiDaC can eradicate established CNS disease.[56] HiDaC is toxic. Most patients have grade III or IV febrile neutropenia and half may have documented infections; mortality in children related to myelosuppression ranges from <1 to 10%.[39,57,58] Cerebellar toxicity, which is frequently irreversible, occurs in elderly patients or those with renal impairment.[59]

A seminal randomized CALGB study illustrates the benefits of HiDaC post-remission therapy: DFS at 4 years in patients <60 years of age was 24% with consolidation ara-C 100 mg/m^2, 29% with 400 mg/m^2 and 44% with 3 g/m^2 (p = 0.003).[60] In pediatric AML, sequentially or historically controlled investigations of HiDaC infer the benefits of post-remission HiDaC.[4,39,58] For example, addi-

tion of post-remission Capizzi II HiDaC/L-asparaginase raised 5-year survival from 29% in CCG-251 to 36% in CCG-213 (p < 0.02).[4,54,61]

Various combinations of HiDaC effective in recurrent AML have entered pediatric Phase III trials as post-remission therapy (Table 19.3).[62–69] There is no clear superiority of one regimen over another. Two highly successful studies in pediatric AML, UK AML 10 and LAME 89/91, use at least 2 post-remission courses of HiDaC (Figs 19.5 and 19.6).[14,15]

Randomized pediatric studies have failed to show differences among various maintenance strategies and 2 have documented harm. CCG-251 compared high-dose pulses of combinations of 10 different agents and a 5-drug ALL-style maintenance consisting of monthly vincristine and 4 days of 5-azacytidine, cyclophosphamide and ara-C and daily 6-TG.[2] There was no difference in outcome between the two. CCG-213 compared 16 months of the 5-drug daily 6-TG regimen to none. EPS was the same with and without maintenance, but no maintenance conferred a significantly better survival.[4] In a non-randomized comparison of

Table 19.3 High-dose cytosine arabinoside (ara-C) regimens in recurrent or refractory pediatric acute myeloid leukemia.

Regimen	N	Complete response (%)
Ara-C/L-asparaginase 'Capizzi II'[57]	19	42
Ara-C/mitoxantrone[66]	37	73
Ara-C/VP-16[67]	5	80
Ara-C/6-meracaptopurine[63]	13	46
Ara-C/fludarabine[62]	85	53
Ara-C/fludarabine/IDA[68]		
Phase I	7	28
Phase II	10	80
Ara-C/fludarabine/IDA[69]		
Phase I/II	15	67

IDA = idarubicin.

maintenance versus none, Michel et al[14] found that both survival and EFS were compromised by maintenance therapy. It is difficult to reconcile these results with BFM therapy where maintenance is though to be an essential component (Fig. 19.3).[9,51]

BONE MARROW TRANSPLANTATION

Thomas et al[70] first used BMT to salvage patients with multiply relapsed or refractory AML: 6 of 54 end-stage patients with AML survived 6–10 years. Success led to the use of BMT in first remission AML.[71,72] In the first Seattle series, 10 of 19 patients survived over 10 years. Subsequently, the majority of biologically randomized trials have shown that younger patients transplanted in first remission with matched related donors have significantly better DFS and survival than those receiving chemotherapy (Table 19.4).[1,5,14,48,73]

The randomization of post-remission therapy in CCG-2891 shows that allogeneic transplant is superior to autologous transplant or chemotherapy (Fig. 19.4).[13] Outcomes of the respective transplant regimens are consistently better in the intensively timed induction regimen (IB). The implications are that the success of the transplant depends on the quality of the remission. Hence, it is possible that differences in the outcomes of apparently similar BMT studies in AML are due to different pre-transplant experiences.

There is no standard BMT therapy for AML. Preparative regimens, source of stem cells and graft-versus-host disease (GVHD) prophylaxis vary from study to study.

Preparative therapy

Preparative or conditioning therapy has 3 purposes:

1. to eradicate residual leukemia;
2. to immunosuppress sufficiently to prevent graft rejection;
3. to make space for new marrow.

Preparative regimens include high-dose chemotherapy $\pm$ total body irradiation (TBI). In the initial transplants in Seattle, cyclophosphamide (60 mg/kg × 2 doses) was followed by TBI,[74] the preparative regimen to which others are compared. Other drugs, such as etoposide, ara-C and melphalan, have been used alone and with TBI and/or cyclophosphamide.[75–78] These agents may increase mucositis and hepatic injury and are of unproven benefit (Fig. 19.7).[79]

Initially, TBI was delivered as 1 fraction of 1000 cGy. Currently, TBI usually involves fractionation of the total dose with lower daily doses given over several days. Fractionation favors normal tissue repair whilst maintaining leukemic kill.[80] Fractionation may also decrease the incidence of interstitial pneumonitis and cataracts. Hyperfractionation, i.e. giving smaller fractions of radiation 2–3 times daily, is used in some centers to decrease morbidity further. Most protocols prescribe doses of 1000–1340 cGy in 5–11 fractions. A fractionated dose of 1575 cGy increases

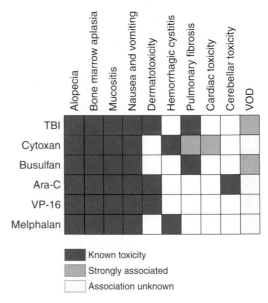

Fig. 19.7 Comparison of toxicities that have been associated with total body irradiation (TBI) and chemotherapeutic agents used in preparative regimens for BMT. VOD = veno-occlusive disease. Reproduced with permission from Ref. 79.

Table 19.4 Outcomes of matched related donor marrow transplants in children.

Center/study	Number of patients	Conditioning	GVH prophylaxis	Disease-free survival (3 years) (%)
Seattle[72]	38	Cy TBI	MTX or CSA	64
Minnesota[71]	41	Cy TBI	MTX = ATG	61
CCG-251[2]	85	Cy TBI	MTX or CSA	52
AIEOP[1]	22	Cy TBI	CSA	56
LAME 89/91[14]	33	Cy TBI (10) Bu Cy (23)	CSA + MTX	72
CCG 2891[13]	95	Bu/Cy	MTX	77 (Intensive) 49 (Standard)

Cy = cyclophosphamide; Bu = busulfan; TBI = total body irradiation; MTX = methrotrexate; CSA = cyclosporin; ATG = antithymocyte globulin.

mortality from organ toxicity with no improvement in survival.[81] Two small studies suggest greater leukemic cell kill with TBI prior to chemotherapy.[82,83]

Limited access to radiation therapy facilities and the morbidity of radiation led to investigations of chemotherapy-based preparative regimens.[84] Busulfan has gained wide acceptance in many centers as a radiation alternative.[85,86] In adults, 2 randomized trials show that TBI/cyclophosphamide is superior to busulfan/cyclophosphamide.[87,88] However, in children, regimens utilizing busulfan/cyclophosphamide appear to be of comparable and possibly greater efficacy than TBI/cyclophosphamide regimens, provided the cumulative dose of cyclophosphamide is 200 mg/kg.[89–92]

Children have widely variable absorption of busulfan.[93–96] Systemic exposure is 4-fold lower in children <3 years old and 2-fold lower in children <15 years old compared with adults.[94] Relapse rate appears to correlate with adequate systemic exposure.[97] Higher levels are associated with a greater risk of veno-occlusive disease.[98] Dosage of busulfan based upon body surface area rather than weight may improve systemic exposure in children. Currently, busulfan is given orally; a new intravenous preparation may reduce variability in absorption and exposure. Alternatively, individualized dosing based on the area under the curve may optimize exposure.

TBI has potential short- and long-term toxicity which may impact upon survival and quality of survival. Acutely, TBI contributes to idiopathic interstitial pneumonitis and nephritis. Pneumonitis is usually fatal. Growth retardation, cataracts, hypothyroidism, infertility and other endocrine function disturbances have been well documented; long-term cardiac and pulmonary effects are less well established.[99–101] The effects of TBI upon neuropsychologic function in children are unknown and under investigation. Busulfan has fewer deleterious effects on growth (Fig. 19.8), and is rarely associated with cataracts or hypothyroidism;

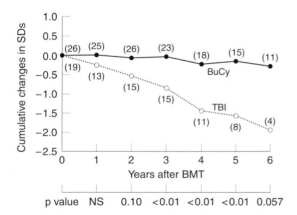

Fig. 19.8 Growth according to preparative regimen. Comparisons are made using the Wilcoxon sum-rank test. Numbers in parentheses indicate number of patients who had height determination each time. BuCy = busulfan; TBI = total body irradiation; BMT = bone marrow transplantation. Reproduced with permission from Ref. 92.

both forms of therapy cause infertility and pubertal delay.[92] Busulfan may increase the risk of pulmonary fibrosis. As busulfan administration results in high levels in the CSF, there may be potential for untoward effects on neurophysiologic functioning.

Allogeneic bone marrow transplantation

Allogeneic marrow may be obtained either from an HLA-identical sibling, partially matched relation or unrelated donor. A 1-antigen mismatched related donor appears to be as good as a fully matched related donor.[120] Most pediatric studies prospectively comparing MRD BMT to chemotherapy, favor BMT (Table 19.4). They show 40->70% DFS with a MRD BMT in first remission. Among pre-transplant prognostic factors, induction regimen,[13,48] initial leukocyte count $>20 \times 10^9$ and FAB M4 or M5 predict a poorer outcome in some studies,[103–105] but not in others.[106–108] Comparisons of the late effects of BMT and chemotherapy show that BMT with TBI causes growth failure, infertility, cataracts and thyroid dysfunction; cardiac and renal complications are similar.[109] With the exception of high rate of infertility in BMT recipients, late effects are similar when TBI is not a part of cytoreduction.[110]

Only 25–30% of patients have a matched or 1-antigen mismatched sibling or parent. The success of MRD BMT in first remission AML has led to investigations of alternative donors and development of other potential sources of stem cells to extend the benefits of MRD BMT to all patients. Other types of allogeneic BMT using stem cells from mismatched relatives, matched or partially mismatched unrelated donors, and cord blood are generally not used in first remission AML.

Autologous bone marrow transplantation

Autologous marrow is obtained from a patient in morphologic remission. It may be chemically, immunologically or physically 'purged' of occult residual leukemia. Studies of 4-hydroxyperoxycyclophosphamide (4-HC) autologous BMT in first relapse or second remission report a DFS of 30–40%.[111–113] CCG, POG, MRC and AIEOP have compared unpurged or purged autologous BMT to allogeneic BMT or chemotherapy in first remission (Table 14.5).[1,3,13,15] In none of these is autologous BMT superior to chemotherapy.[1,3,13,15] IEOP has recently re-examined its accumulated experience with 110 autologous BMTs in first remission and found that TBI-containing regimens achieved a DFS of 79%, which is comparable to the best of allogeneic BMT, while those prepared with chemotherapy alone had a DFS of 27% (p = 0.0001).[114]

Failure of unpurged autologous BMT is attributed to contamination with residual leukemia cells[115] and absence of the putative allogeneic graft-versus-leukemia (GVL) effect. Attempts to generate GVL cells include the use of IL-2 with or without lymphokine-activated killer cells.[116]

Table 19.5 Intention-to-treat disease-free survival at 3 years of biologically randomized comparisons of chemotherapy to matched related donor bone marrow transplant (BMT) or autologous transplant in first remission pediatric acute myeloid leukemia.

Group/center	Number of patients	Chemotherapy disease-free survival (%)	Allogeneic BMT disease-free survival (%)	Autologous BMT disease-free survival (%)
AIEOP[1]	161	27	51	21
CCG-251[2]	508	43	52	ND
CCG-213[5]	591	38	46	ND
CCG-2891[13]	589	58 (Intensive)	77 (Intensive)	36 (Intensive)
		40 (Standard)	49 (Standard)	30 (Standard)
LAME 89/91[14]	171	48	72	ND
POG[3]	649	36	52	38
SJCRH[73]	87	31	43	ND

Transplantation-specific complications

Tranplant-related mortality of MRD BMT in children has decreased over from over 30% 20 years ago to 3–10% today.[2,14,21] Mortality from alternative forms of allogeneic BMT remains high.[117] Infection and GVHD are the major causes of transplant-related morbidity and mortality.

Up to 40% of children receiving a matched sibling donor BMT will develop acute GVHD. This number may be doubled following a matched unrelated BMT. Some studies suggest that acute GVHD confers a GVL effect but that chronic GVHD has no therapeutic benefit.[118] In studies from France, the absence of both acute and chronic GVHD were associated with a better outcome in children transplanted for AML.[91]

While the benefits of GVHD are controversial, its risk are formidable, drugs used to prevent GVHD include cyclosporine, FK506, methotrexate and steroids. With methotrexate alone, 46% of patients developed acute GVHD.[119] A subsequent study using both cyclosporine and methotrexate decreased transplant-related mortality from 31 to 11%, but there was a trend toward increase in relapse risk.[119] A retrospective review has confirmed that GVHD prophylaxis combined with cyclosporine and methotrexate was associated with a higher relapse rate; acute GVHD was associated with a higher non-relapse mortality.[120] Standard practice includes methotrexate and cyclosporine. Recent CCG studies have shown both a lower relapse rate and a lower mortality with methotrexate alone.[13,48]

The success of allogeneic BMT in myeloid leukemia apparently derives from the intensity of the cytoreduction therapy and a GVL effect, although evidence for a GVL effect in AML is less compelling than in chronic myeloid leukemia (CML).[118,121] Experiments with donor-derived T lymphocytes transduced with the Herpes simplex thymidine kinase gene (HSV-TK) generated a GVL response with transfusion of donor T lymphocytes at the time of relapse.[122] The GVL response was accompanied by GVHD. When GVHD became life-threatening, administration of gan-cyclovir killed the cells with the HSV-TK gene and attenuated GVHD.[122]

Perspective on bone marrow transplantation

Perhaps the most controversial questions in pediatric AML concern marrow transplants: which patients should receive transplants; what type of transplant should be given; and when should the transplant be performed.[123,124] MRD BMT has been the standard post-remission therapy for children with AML who have a matched sibling or parent. Some argue that outcome for certain subsets of patients with chemotherapy is so good that BMT should be reserved for second remission or possibly first relapse with low tumor burden. BMT offers no advantage for Down's syndrome patients with AML in first remission,[125] or in patients with APL. Studies of pediatric and adult AML show inversion 16 karyotype to be a favorable subtype, often curable with chemotherapy alone.[53,126] In contrast, in most studies, AML with monosomy 7 has a <10% EFS with chemotherapy.[127] Alternative allogeneic BMT strategies for AML in first remission are a consideration for this group.

PREVENTION AND TREATMENT OF EXTRAMEDULLARY DISEASE

Without CNS prophylaxis, incidence of CNS relapse is about 50%.[20] CNS relapse is usually a harbinger of marrow relapse.[20] Most co-operative groups have accomplished CNS prophylaxis with intrathecal methotrexate/ara-C or both plus hydrocortisone.[19,128] With intrathecal CNS prophylaxis, the incidence of CNS relapse is about 5%.[48,128] BFM '83 used prophylactic cranial irradiation and intrathecal chemotherapy; BFM '87 attempted to replace the prophylactic CNS irradiation used in BFM '83 with HiDaC: surprisingly, marrow relapses were more common in those randomized to HiDaC (Fig. 19.3), suggesting that cranial irradiation had systemic effects superior to those of HiDaC.[9]

In pediatric AML, intrathecal and systemic chemotherapy may suffice to sterilize the CNS of patients with CNS disease at diagnosis.[48,128] CNS disease rarely recurs as the site of first relapse.[128] Craniospinal irradiation compromises the ability to administer highly immunosuppressive or myelosuppressive systemic therapy.

Chloromas occur in about 10% of pediatric patients with AML. Patients who present with isolated chloromas and no marrow disease invariably experience a marrow relapse if they are not given systemic therapy.[129] In CCG-2891, a significant increase was not seen in recurrence in the site of the chloroma in patients who did not receive radiation compared to those who did, nor did lack of irradiation compromise the EFS.[130] The CCG data raise questions about the value of radiation to chloromas, but the size and location of the chloromas were not considered. Chloromas are more common in Turkish children with AML, and Turkish investigators recommend irradiation.[131]

ACUTE PROMYELOCYTIC LEUKEMIA

APL stands apart from the rest of AML.[132] Many studies have confirmed the observation of Huang et al[133] that all-*trans*-retinoic acid (ATRA) induces remission in most patients with APL by differentiating the leukemic promyelocytes.[133] The NCI/CTG randomized study of 401 patients with APL showed that exposure to ATRA during induction, consolidation or maintenance achieved an EFS of approximately 70% at 2 years compared to 28% with chemotherapy alone, and reduced the relapse rate (17/116 versus 29/40; $p < 0.0001$).[134] No major differences in disease or response to ATRA between children and adults were apparent. Children are more likely to experience *pseudotumor cerebri*.[135] Children and adults are equally at risk of rapid onset pulmonary failure, the 'retinoic acid syndrome'.[136] This syndrome responds to dexamethasone.[136] ATRA has not eliminated the early hemorrhagic death that occurs in 10% of patients. Benefits of ATRA are limited to those with the 15;17 translocation: FAB M3 NK cell leukemia or the FAB M3 with the 11;17 translocation do not respond.[137,138]

Optimal therapy for APL is ATRA plus cytotoxic chemotherapy which includes anthracyclines. Several studies in adults suggest that anthracyclines may be more important than ara-C in APL.[139]

Chinese investigators have presented *in vitro* and *in vivo* evidence that arsenic trioxide is also an effective agent in APL and does not appear to be cross-resistant with ATRA.[140]

AML IN CHILDREN WITH DOWN'S SYNDROME

Infants under 2 months of age with Down's syndrome or trisomy 21 mosaicism may develop a transient myeloproliferative syndrome (TMS).[141–143] TMS is most often a megakaryoblastic proliferation and may have acquired cytogenetic abnormalities.[1] Neonates with Down's syndrome and TMS need good supportive care. They require little or no cytotoxic therapy as their leukemia spontaneously regresses.

Older infants and children with Down's syndrome with AML require cytotoxic therapy. Their disease is uniquely responsive to therapy with EFS ranging from 68 to 100%.[125,141,144] There is no apparent benefit from BMT in first remission in these children and their induction mortality is higher than that of other children with more intensive induction regimens.[125]

CONGENITAL LEUKEMIA

Congenital AML in constitutionally normal neonates occasionally regresses spontaneously, but most ultimately require cytotoxic therapy.[145,146] Any neonate who has experienced a regression of leukemia needs to be monitored for the development of AML months or years later.

SUPPORTIVE CARE

Patients with AML experience prolonged myelosuppression and severe mucositis. In the transplant setting, immunosuppression and defects in neutrophil function also occur. As therapy for AML has become more aggressive, supportive care has had to be equally aggressive. It is impossible to separate the contributions of supportive care from those of antineoplastic therapy.

Because AML patients spend much time in hospital, staff and environmental contributions to the prevention of infection are important (see Chapter 37). Hand-washing remains the prime prophylactic measure. Staff familiarity with the complications of AML and its treatment facilitates prompt and appropriate therapy. This is best accomplished through the development of policies, procedures and algorithms for the management of complications based on the prevailing institutional flora.

Many of the principles of supportive care were developed through a series of randomized trials at the National Cancer Institute (NCI) in the 1980s. Three recent reviews of infectious complications summarize the results of these studies, discuss the evolution of new patterns of disease and are the basis for the guidelines presented below.[147–149] The commonest complication is febrile neutropenia and the commonest cause of death is bacterial infection, followed in frequency by fungal infection. Pseudomonas sepsis was the major cause of death in the early 1980s, but Gram-positive sepsis has increased because of central venous catheter associated staphylococcal infections and *Streptococcus viridans* sepsis.[150] It is standard practice to culture blood and any potential infectious sites and to start empiric broad-spectrum parenteral antibiotics immediately in any AML patient with a fever of $>38°C \times 3$ in 24 hours or $>39.4°C$ once. These antibiotics are continued until the phagocyte count begins to rise or for a minimum of 14 days. It is standard practice to start amphotericin B in any AML patient with recurrent fever or fever persistent for 7 days or less if the patient is unwell. History, physical examinations, and radiological studies, particularly chest radiographs, and CT scans of the chest, brain and retroperitoneum are helpful in the search for fungi.

It is not clear if any form of antibacterial prophylactic prevents febrile neutropenia or infection in AML patients. Trimethoprim sulfamethoxazole, often used as antibacterial prophylaxis a decade ago, has fallen into disuse in many places for this purpose because of plasmid-mediated resistance and possible association with a sepsis syndrome caused by *Strep. viridans*. Attempts to prevent *Strep. viridans* with vancomycin oral paste have been thwarted by the emergence of vancomycin-resistant enterococcus. Oral penicillin may offer an alternative where *Strep. viridans* is a common pathogen. Gut sterilization is not of benefit in AML patients receiving chemotherapy, but is commonly used in allogeneic BMT. Antifungal prophylaxis with imidazole antibiotics is controversial because of the emergence of *Candida kruzei* and aspergillus species. In the BMT setting, antiviral prophylaxis with acyclovir is given to patients seropositive for Herpes simplex and gancyclovir to patients at risk of cytomegalovirus. HEPA-filtered air is a *sine qua non* where aspergillus infections have been documented and in hospitals undergoing construction and renovation. Laminar air flow is used mostly for patients undergoing allogeneic BMT, but has not been documented to be more beneficial than HEPA filtration. Reverse isolation is no longer used for AML patients.

Patients with AML rarely experience tumor lysis syndrome except with high-dose ara-C therapy.[151] Nonetheless, allopurinol and hydration are administered prior to starting chemotherapy and continued for several days. Patients with white blood cell counts $>200\,000/ml^3$ are at risk of cerebrovascular accidents (CVAs) and pulmonary leukostasis.[151] Many oncologists use leukopheresis to reduce the white blood cell count. Ten percent of patients with APL die of hemorrhage early in treatment.[132,152] Aggressive use of platelets and plasma has replaced heparin for the treatment of the coagulopathy of APL.[132,152]

The hematopoietic growth factors G-CSF, GM-CSF and IL-3 have been introduced into clinical trials in AML to reduce infection and mortality by shortening the duration of neutropenia and, based on studies *in vitro*, to enhance the cytotoxicity of ara-C by recruiting and synchronizing leukemic cells in S phase.[153,154] In both randomized and histori-

cally controlled trials, G-CSF and GM-CSF reduce the duration of neutropenia by an average of 4 days.[154] Their impact on documented infection, days in hospital, mortality and the leukemia itself is modest or none at all. G-CSF and GM-CSF are probably safe when used in the setting of low tumor burden.[154] There is no imperative to use growth factors.

The leukemic blasts of about half the pediatric patients with AML proliferate in response to G-CSF, GM-CSF or IL-3.[155] There are no randomized trials of these growth factors in children with AML. In consecutive series of patients in CCG-2891, the addition of G-CSF on day 6 of intensively timed therapy and continued to a neutrophil count of $500/ml^3$ reduced the induction mortality from 13 to 9% (p = 0.09).[156]

TREATMENT OF REFRACTORY OR RECURRENT AML

Half of patients with AML have disease which is either refractory to induction therapy or which recurs. The most successful salvage regimens include HiDaC (Table 19.3). The combinations in Table 19.3 can effect a marrow remission in half or more of young patients, even in those who have previously been given HiDaC.[57,63,64,67–69] Two reports document salvage chemotherapy alone.[64,157] The POG has reviewed its results with single agent or combination Phase II therapies in patients with refractory or recurrent cancer in the past decade.[158] AML is one of the more responsive diseases. Among 140 pediatric AML patients treated with combination therapy, 36% had a complete/partial remission and 9% survived 2 years and 3% 5 years, which is the best outcome of any pediatric neoplasms. Among 81 patients treated with single agents, 15% had complete/partial remissions but none was alive at 2 years.[158] Single agents with activity include carboplatinum, the purine analogs fludarabine or 2-chlorodeoxyadenosine, and IL-2.[159] Table 19.6 lists active single agents that have not as yet been incorporated into most Phase III studies.

Although chemotherapy can effect cure in recurrent AML, BMT following second remission induction with chemotherapy is generally considered the treatment of choice. Most patients with a well-matched related donor will already have undergone an allogeneic BMT. For those without a matched first-degree relative, an extended family search will locate a more distant relative who is a 1-antigen mismatch in 5–10% of cases.[117] Expansion of an international donor registry has made locating a suitable unrelated donor feasible for many patients.[160–165] DFS for alternative donor transplants ranges from 20 to 50%. Transplant-related mortality may exceed 50% when all age groups are considered; risk of relapse is higher with each degree of mismatch.[117] Children have a lower mortality as they appear to tolerate HLA disparity better than adults can.[162–164,166] Improvements in tissue typing technology

Table 19.6 New single agents active in recurrent or refractory pediatric acute myeloid leukemia.[158]

Agent	N Adult (A) Pediatric (P)	(N trials)	Dose (mg/m²)	Complete remission (%)
Amsacrine	90–120 A/P	(3)	90–120 × 5	20–31
Carboplatinum	55 A	(2)	175–420 × 5	30
2-Chlorodeoxyadenosine	17 P	(1)	8.9 × 5	47
Homoharringtonine	120 A/P	(4)	6–12 × 5–10	0–29
Interleukin-2	22 A/P	(2)	0.1–0.5 × 5	25
			8 × 10⁶ units × 5	20

may improve matching and outcome.[167] Outcomes are better the less advanced the disease.[117]

Studies using peripheral blood stem cells and cord blood are in their infancy.[168–171] Many questions remain regarding engraftment kinetics, control of leukemia and the risk of complications. Review of the European data shows good engraftment and minimal risk of GVHD with matched related cord blood transplants in patients under the age of 6 years.[171]

Curative therapy is usually limited following a post-transplant marrow relapse. Either a second BMT from the same or alternative donors are used. Failure of second BMT is almost universal when recurrence occurs within 6 months of the first transplant, but long-term survival has occurred in patients with relapses after 1 year.[172,173] An approach used in CML is infusion of donor leukocytes to provoke a GVL effect.[174] However, this approach is less successful in patients with AML, although there are small numbers of patients who benefit.[175]

CONCLUSIONS

AML in children is rare. The question of what constitutes cure in AML is debated. Most events occur in the first 2 years from diagnosis. In CCG-251, deaths occurred in 2–3% of patients between 5 and 8 years from diagnosis.[2] It is probably reasonable to say that a patient who is 10 years from diagnosis who has not experienced a recurrence and who has no life-threatening complications of treatment is cured of AML.

Treatment has cured a minority of patients. Only with a substantial number of long-term survivors will it be possible to dissect out prognostic factors. As in pediatric ALL, future therapies most probably will be stratified by risk of relapse. It is possible that therapy directed at cytogenetic translocation breakpoints or their gene products will provide more subset-specific therapy for this heterogeneous group of diseases. In contrast to generic therapy is disease-specific targeted therapy, of which there is currently only one example: all-*trans* retinoic acid (ATRA) therapy in APL. ATRA corrects

the abnormalities of proliferation and differentiation resulting from the characteristic 15;17 translocation in APL. Disease-specific targeted therapy for other forms of AML is a distant goal.

REFERENCES

1. Amadori S, Testi AM, Arico M *et al*. Prospective comparative study of bone marrow transplantation and post-remission chemotherapy for childhood acute myelogenous leukemia. *J Clin Oncol* 1993; **11**: 1046–1054

2. Nesbit M, Buckley J, Feig S *et al*. Chemotherapy for induction of remission of childhood acute myeloid leukemia followed by marrow transplantation or multi-agent chemotherapy. *J Clin Oncol* 1994; **12**: 127–135

3. Ravindranath Y, Yeager AM, Chang MN *et al*. Autologous bone marrow transplantation versus intensive consolidation chemotherapy for acute myeloid leukemia in childhood. *N Engl J Med* 1996; **334**: 1428–1434

4. Wells R, Woods W, Lampkin B *et al*. Impact of high-dose cytarabine and aparaginase intensification on childhood acute myeloid leukemia: A report from the Children's Cancer Group. *J Clin Oncol* 1993; **11**: 538–545

5. Wells R, Woods W, Buckley J *et al*. Treatment of newly diagnosed children and adolescents with acute myeloid leukemia: a Children's Cancer Group Study. *J Clin Oncol* 1994; **12**: 2367–2377

6. Parker S, Tong T, Bolden S, Wingo P. Cancer statistics, 1996. *CA Cancer J Clin* 1996; **46**: 5–25

7. Behar C, Suciu S, Benoit Y *et al*. Mitoxantrone-containing regimen for treatment of childhood acute leukemia (AML) and analysis of prognostic factors: results of the EORTC Children Leukemia Cooperative Study 58872. *Med Pediatr Oncol* 1996; **26**: 173–179

8. Sartori PCE, Taylor MH, Stevens MCG, Darbyshire PJ, Mann JR. Treatment of childhood acute myeloid leukemia using the BFM-83 protocol. *Med Pediatr Oncol* 1993; **21**: 8–13

9. Creutzig U, Ritter J, Zimmerman M, Schellong G. Does cranial irradiation reduce the risk for bone marrow relapse in acute myelogenous leukemia? Unexpected results of the childhood acute myelogenous leukemia study BFM-87. *J Clin Oncol* 1993; **11**: 279–286

10. Amadori S, Testi AM, Moleti ML, Giuliano M, Pession A, Mandelli F. Intensive consolidation therapy in children with acute myeloid leukemia (AML) with high-dose cytarabine and an anthracycline: preliminary results of AIEOP LAM/87M-92P. *Proc ASCO* 1994; **13**: 319

11. Lie SO, Jonmundsson G, Mellander L, Simes MA, Yssing M, Gustafsson G. A population-based study of 272 children with acute myeloid leukaemia treated on two consecutive protocols with different intensity: best outcome in girls, infants and children with Down's

syndrome. Nordic Society of Paediatric Haematology and Oncology (NOPHO). *Br J Haematol* 1996; **94**: 82–88

12. Sackmann-Muriel F, Zubizarreta P, Felice MS *et al*. Results of treatment with an intensive induction regimen using idarubicin in combination with cytarabine and etoposide in children with acute myeloblastic leukemia. *Leukemia Res* 1996; **20**: 973–981

13. Woods WG, Neudorf S, Gold S *et al*. Aggressive post-remission (REM) chemotherapy is better than autologous bone marrow transplantation (BMT) and allogeneic BMT is superior to both in children with acute myeloid leukemia (AML). *Proc Am Soc Clin Oncol* 1996; **14**: 271A

14. Michel G, Leverger G, Leblanc T *et al*. Allogeneic bone marrow transplantation vs aggressive post-remission chemotherapy for children with acute myeloid leukemia in first complete remission. A prospective study from the French Society of Pediatric Hematology and Immunology. *Bone Marrow Transplant* 1996; **17**: 191–196

15. Hann IM, Stevens RF, Goldstone AH *et al*. Randomized comparison of DAT versus ADE as induction chemotherapy in children and younger adults with acute myeloid leukemia. Results of the Medical Research Council's 10th AML trial (MRC AML10). Adult and Childhood Leukaemia Working Parties of the Medical Research Council. *Blood* 1997; **89**: 2311–2318

16. Creutzig U, Ritter J, Schellong G, for the AML-BFM Study Group. Identification of two risk groups in childhood acute myelogenous leukemia after therapy intensification in study AML-BFM-83 as compared with AML-BFM-78. *Blood* 1990; **75**: 1932–1941

17. Bloomfield C. Post-remission therapy in acute myeloid leukemia. *J Clin Oncol* 1985; **3**: 1570–1572

18. Steuber C. Therapy in childhood acute non-lymphocytic leukemia (ANLL): evolution of current concepts of chemotherapy. *Am J Pediatr Hematol Oncol* 1981; **3**: 379

19. Hurwitz CA, Mounce KG, Grier HE. Treatment of patients with acute myelogenous leukemia: review of clinical trials of the past decade. *J Pediatr Hematol Oncol* 1995; **17**: 185–197

20. Weinstein H, Mayer R, Rosenthal D *et al*. Treatment of acute myelogenous leukemia in children and adults. *N Engl J Med* 1980; **303**: 473–478

21. Feig SA, Lampkin B, Nesbit ME, Woods WG. Outcome of BMT during complete remission of AML: a comparison of two sequential studies by the Children's Cancer Group. *Bone Marrow Transplant* 1993; **12**: 65–71

22. Yates J, Glidewell O, Wiernick P *et al*. Cytosine arabinoside with daunorubicin or adriamycin for therapy of acute myelocytic leukemia: a CALBG study. *Blood* 1982; **60**: 454–461

23. Buckley JD, Lampkin B, Nesbit M *et al*. Remission induction in children with acute non-lymphocytic leukemia using cytosine arabinoside and doxorubicin or daunorubicin: A report from the Children's Cancer Study Group. *Med Pediatr Oncol* 1989; **17**: 382–390

24. Capizzi R, White J, Powell B, Perrino F. Effect of dose on the pharmacokinetic and pharmacodynamic effects of cytarabine. *Semin Hematol* 1991; **28**: 54–69

25. Karp J, Burke P. Enhancement of drug cytotoxicity by recruitment of malignant myeloblasts with humeral stimulation. *Cancer Res* 1976; **36**: 3600–3603

26. Karp J, Donehower R, Burke P. An *in vitro* model to predict clinical response in adult acute myelogenous leukemia. *Semin Oncol* 1987; **14**: 172–181

27. Skipper H, Schabel FM, Wilcox WM *et al*. Experimental evaluation of potential anticancer agents XXI. Scheduling of arabinosyl-cytosine to take advantage of its S-phase specificity against leukemic cells. *Cancer Chemother Rep* 1967; **51**: 125

28. Wiernik P, Jones B, Weinberg V *et al*. Present day results in young patients with acute nonlymphocytic leukemia (ANLL): the Cancer and Leukemia Group B experience. In: Madelli F (ed) *Therapy of Acute Leukemias*. Milan: Loambarado Editore, 1979, pp 430–443

29. Rowe JM, Tallman MS. Intensifying induction therapy in acute myeloid leukemia: has a new standard of care emerged? *Blood* 1997; **90**: 2121–2126

30. Lampkin BC, Lange B, Bernstein ID *et al*. Biologic characteristics and treatment of nonlymphocytic leukemia in children: report of the ANLL Strategy Group of the Children's Cancer Study Group. *Pediatr Clin North Am* 1988; **35**: 743–764

31. Steuber CP, Civin C, Krischer J *et al*. A comparison of induction and maintenance therapy for acute non lymphocytic leukemia in childhood: results of a Pediatric Oncology Group Study. *J Clin Oncol* 1991; **9**: 247–258

32. Dillman R, David R, Green M *et al*. Comparative study of two remission induction regimens in acute myelocytic leukemia (AML). *Blood* 1991; **78**: 2520–2526

33. Bishop JF, Matthews JP, Young GA *et al*. A randomized study of high-dose cytarabine in induction in acute myeloid leukemia [see comments]. *Blood* 1996; **87**: 1710–1717

34. Weick JK, Kopecky KJ, Appelbaum FR *et al*. A randomized investigation of high-dose versus standard-dose cytosine arabinoside with daunorubicin in patients with previously untreated acute myeloid leukemia: a Southwest Oncology Group study. *Blood* 1996; **88**: 2841–2851

35. Bishop JF, Lowenthal R, Joshua D *et al*. Etoposide in leukemia. *Cancer* 1991; **67**: 285–291

36. Preisler H, Anderson K, Rai K *et al*. Comparison of three remission induction regimens and two post-induction strategies for treatment of acute non-lymphocytic leukemia: a Cancer and Acute Leukemia Group B study. *Br J Haematol* 1987; **5**: 75

37. Stasi R, Venditti A, Del Poeta G *et al*. High-dose chemotherapy in adult acute myeloid leukemia: rationale and results. *Leukemia Res* 1996; 20: 535–549

38. Odom L, Morse H, Tubergen D, Blake M. Long-term survival in acute non-lymphoblastic leukemia. *Med Pediatr Oncol* 1988; **16**: 248–254

39. Ravindranath Y, Steuber C, Krisher J *et al*. High dose cytarabine for intensification of early therapy of childhood myeloid leukemia: a Pediatric Oncology Group study. *J Clin Oncol* 1991; **9**: 572–580

40. Wiernik PH, Banks PLC, Case DC *et al*. Cytarabine plus idarubicin or daunorubicin as induction and consolidation therapy for previously untreated adult patients with acute myeloid leukemia. *Blood* 1992; **79**: 313–320

41. Vogler WR, Velex-Garcia E, Weiner RS *et al*. A Phase III trial comparing idarubicin and daunorubicin in combination with cytarabine in acute myelogenous leukemia. A Southeastern Cancer Study Group study. *J Clin Oncol* 1992; **10**: 1103–1111

42. Berman E, Heller G, Santorsa J *et al*. Results of a randomized trial comparing idarubicin and cytosine arabinoside with daunorubicin and cytosine arabinoside in adult patients with newly diagnosed acute myeloid leukemia. *Blood* 1991; **77**: 1666–1674

43. Wheatley K. Meta-analysis of randomized trials of idarubicin (IDAR) or metozantrone (Mito) versus daunorubicin (DNR) as induction therapy for acute myeloid leukaemia (AML). *Blood* 1995; **86**: 434A

44. Karp JE, Burch PA, Merz WG. An approach to intensive antileukemia therapy in patients with previous invasive Aspergillosis. *Am J Med* 1988; **85**: 203–206

45. Karp J, Donehower R, Enterline J, Dole G, Fox M, Burke P. In vivo cell growth and pharmacologic determinants of clinical response in acute myelogenous leukemia. *Blood* 1989; **73**: 24–30

46. Burke P, Karp J, Vaughan WP. Chemotherapy of leukemia in mice, rats and humans relating time of humoral stimulation, tumor growth and clinical response. *J Natl Cancer Inst* 1981; **64**: 529–538

47. Woods W, Kobrinsky N, Buckley J *et al*. Intensively timed induction therapy followed by autologous or allogeneic bone marrow transplantation for children with acute myeloid leukemia or myelodysplastic syndrome: A Children's Cancer Study Group Pilot Study. *J Clin Oncol* 1993; **11**: 1448–1457

48. Woods WG, Kobrinsky N, Buckley J *et al*. Timed sequential induction therapy improves post-remission outcome in acute myeloid leukemia (AML). *Blood* 1996; **87**: 4979–4989

49. Cassileth P, Begg CB, Silber R *et al*. Prolonged unmaintained remission

after intensive consolidation therapy in adult acute nonlymphocytic leukemia. *Cancer Treat Rep* 1987; **71**: 137

50. Cassileth PA, Lynch E, Hines J *et al*. Varying intensity or postremission therapy in acute myeloid leukemia. *Blood* 1992; **79**: 1924–1930

51. Creutzig U, Ritter J, Riehm H *et al*. Improved treatment results in childhood acute myelogenous leukemia. A report of the German Cooperative Study AML-BFM-78. *Blood* 1985; **65**: 298–304

52. Behar C, Bertrand Y, Rubie H *et al*. Mitoxantrone and high dose ara-C for the treatment of AML in childhood: a pilot study of the CLCG (EORTG 58 872). *Leukemia* 1992; **6 (Suppl)**: 63

53. Creutzig U, Harbott J, Sperling C *et al*. Clinical significance of surface antigen expression in children with acute myeloid leukemia: Results of study AML-BFM-87. *Blood* 1995; **86**: 3097–3108

54. Capizzi R, Poole M, Cooper M *et al*. Treatment of poor risk acute leukemia with sequential high dose Ara-C and Asparaginase. *Blood* 1984; **63**: 694–700

55. Preisler H, Raza A, Barcos M *et al*. High-dose cytosine arabinoside as the initial treatment of poor-risk patients with acute nonlymphocytic leukemia. A leukemia intergroup study. *J Clin Oncol* 1987; **5**: 75–82

56. Amadori S, Papa G, Avvisati GEA. Sequential combination of systemic high-dose cytarabine in the treatment of central nervous system leukemia. *Cancer* 1984; **72**: 439

57. Wells R, Feusner J, Devney R *et al*. Sequential high-dose cytosine arabinoside-asparaginase treatment in advanced childhood leukemia. *J Clin Oncol* 1985; **3**: 998–1004

58. Woods W, Ruymann F, Lampkin B *et al*. The role of timing of high-dose cytosine arabinoside intensification and of maintenance therapy in the treatment of children with acute nonlymphocytic leukemia. *Cancer* 1990; **66**: 1106–1113

59. Rubin E, Anderson J, Berg DEA. Risk factors for high dose cytarabine neurotoxicity: an analysis of a Cancer and Leukemia Group B trial in patients with acute myeloid leukemia. *J Clin Oncol* 1992; **10**: 948

60. Mayer RJ, Davis RB, Schiffer CA *et al*. Intensive postremission chemotherapy in adults with acute myeloid leukemia. Cancer and Leukemia Group B [see comments]. *N Engl J Med* 1994; **331**: 896–903

61. Capizzi R, Davis R, Powell B *et al*. Synergy between high-dose cytarabine and asparaginase in the treatment of adults with refractory and relapsed acute myelogenous leukemia – A cancer and leukemia group B study. *J Clin Oncol* 1988; **6**: 499–508

62. Sato JK, Weirsma S, Krailo M *et al*. Phase I clinical and pharmacodynamic study of continuous infusion fludarabine followed by continuous infusion cytosine arabinoside in relapsed leukemia. *Proc Am Assoc Cancer Res* 1990; **33**: 211A

63. Lockhart S, Plunkett W, Jeha S *et al*. High-dose mercaptopurine followed by intermediate-dose cytarabine in relapsed acute leukemia. *J Clin Oncol* 1994; **12**: 587–595

64. Wells R, Odom L, Gold S *et al*. Mitoxantrone (Mx) and Ara-C (AC) treatment of relapsed or refractory childhood leukemia: induction results and significance of multidrug resistance gene (MDR1). *Proc Am Soc Clin Oncol* 1992; **11**: 277

65. Wells RJ, Feusner J, Devney R *et al*. Sequential high-dose cytosine arabinoside-asparaginase treatment in advanced childhood leukemia. *J Clin Oncol* 1985; **3**: 998–1004

66. Wells RJ, Gold SH, Krill CE *et al*. Cytosine arabinoside and mitoxantrone induction chemotherapy followed by bone marrow transplantation or chemotherapy for relapsed or refractory pediatric acute myeloid leukemia. *Leukemia* 1994; **8**: 1626–1630

67. Whitlock JA, Wells RJ, Hord JD *et al*. High-dose cytosine arabinoside and etoposide: an effective regimen without anthracyclines for refractory childhood acute non-lymphocytic leukemia. *Leukemia* 1997; **11**: 185–189

68. Dinndorf PA, Avramis VI, Wiersma S *et al*. A Phase I/II study of idarubicin given with continuous infusion cytosine arabinoside in children with acute leukemia: a report from the Children's Cancer Group. *J Clin Oncol* 1997; **15**: 2780–2785

69. Leahey A, Kelly K, Rorke L, Lange B. A phase I study of idarubicin (Ida) with continuous infusion fludarabine and cytarabine (Fara-A/

Ara-C) for refractory or relapsed pediatric acute myeloid leukemia (AML). *J Pediatr Hematol Oncol* 1997; **19**: 304–308

70. Thomas E, Buckner C, Banaji M *et al*. One hundred patients with acute leukemia treated by chemotherapy total body irradiation; and allogeneic marrow transplantation. *Blood* 1997; **49**: 511–533

71. Kersey J, Ramsay N, Kim T *et al*. Allogeneic bone marrow transplantation in acute nonlymphocytic leukemia: A pilot study. *Blood* 1982; **60**: 400–404

72. Sanders JE, Thomas ED, Buckner CD *et al*. Marrow transplantation for children in first remission of acute nonlymphoblastic leukemia: an update. *Bone Marrow Transplant* 1985; **66**: 460

73. Dahl G, Kalwinsky D, Schell M *et al*. Allogeneic bone marrow transplantation in a program of intensive sequential chemotherapy for children and young adults with acute nonlymphocytic leukemia in first remission. *J Clin Oncol* 1990; **8**: 295–303

74. Thomas E, Storb R, Clift R *et al*. Bone marrow transplantation. *N Engl J Med* 1975; **29**: 832–843, 896–903

75. Riddell S, Appelbaum F, Buckner C *et al*. High dose cytarabine and total body irradiation with or without cyclophosphamide as a preparative regimen for marrow transplantation for acute leukemia. *J Clin Oncol* 1988; **6**: 576–582

76. Spitzer T, Cottler-Fox M, Torrisi J *et al*. Escalating doses of etoposide with cyclophosphamide and fractionated total body irradiation or busulfan as conditioning for bone marrow transplantation. *Bone Marrow Transplant* 1989; **4**: 559–565

77. Herzig R, Coccia P, Strandford S *et al*. Bone marrow transplantation for acute leukemia and lymphoma with high dose cytosine arabinoside and total body irradiation. *Semin Oncol* 1987; **14 (Suppl 1)**: 139–140

78. Helenglass G, Powles R, McElwain T *et al*. Melphalan and total body irradiation (TBI) versus cyclophosphamide and TBI as conditioning for allogeneic matched sibling bone marrow transplants for acute myeloblastic leukaemia in first remission. *Bone Marrow Transplant* 1988; **3**: 21–29

79. Dinndorf P, Bunin N. Bone marrow transplantation for children with acute myelogenous leukemia. *J Pediatr Hematol Oncol* 1995; **17**: 211–224

80. Peters L, Withers H, Cundiff J *et al*. Radiological considerations in the use of total body irradiation for bone marrow transplantation. *Radiology* 1979; **131**: 243–247

81. Clift R, Buckner C, Appelbaum F *et al*. Allogeneic marrow transplantation in patients with acute myeloid leukemia in first remission: A randomized trial of two irradiation regimens. *Blood* 1990; **76**: 1867–1871

82. Brochstein J, Kernan N, Groshen S *et al*. Allogeneic bone marrow transplantation after hyperfractionated total body irradiation and cyclophosphamide in children with acute leukemia. *N Engl J Med* 1987; **317**: 1618–1624

83. Snyder D, Findley D, Forman SJ *et al*. Fractionated total body irradiation and high dose cyclophosphamide: A preparative regimen for bone marrow transplantation for patients with hematologic malignancies in first complete remission. *Blut* 1988; **57**: 7–13

84. Copelan EA, Deeg HH. Conditioning for allogeneic transplantation in patients with lymphohematopoietic malignancies without the use of total body irradiation. *Blood* 1992; **80**: 1648–1658

85. Tutschka P, Copelan E, Kapoor N. Replacing total body irradiation with busulfan as conditioning of patients with leukemia for allogeneic marrow transplantation. *Transpl Proc* 1989; **21**: 2952–2954

86. Santos G, Tutschka P, Brookmeyer R *et al*. Marrow transplantation for acute nonlymphocytic leukemia after treatment with busulfan and cyclophosphamide. *N Engl J Med* 1983; **309**: 1347–1353

87. Blaise D, Stoppa A, Viens P *et al*. Intensive immunotherapy with recombinant IL2 after autologous bone marrow transplantation is associated with a high incidence of bacterial infections. *Bone Marrow Transplant* 1992; **10**: 193–195

88. Ringden O, Ruutu T, Remberger M *et al*. A randomized trial comparing busulfan with total body irradiation as conditioning in allogeneic marrow transplant recipients with leukemia: A report from

the Nordic Bone Marrow Transplantation Group. *Blood* 1994; **83**: 2723–2730

89. Geller R, Saral R, Piantadosi S *et al*. Allogeneic bone marrow transplantation after high-dose busulfan and cyclophosphamide in patients with acute nonlymphocytic leukemia. *Blood* 1989; **73**: 2209–2218

90. Nevill T, Barne M, Klinemann H *et al*. Regimen related toxicity of a busulfan-cyclophosphamide conditioning regimen in 70 patients undergoing allogeneic bone marrow transplantation. *J Clin Oncol* 1991; **9**: 1224–1232

91. Michel G, Gluckman E, Blaise D *et al*. Improvement in outcome for children receiving allogeneic bone marrow transplantation in first remission of acute myeloid leukemia: A report from the Groupe d'Etude des Greffes de Moelle Osseuse. *J Clin Oncol* 1992; **10**: 1865–1869

92. Michel G, Socié G, Gebhard F, Bernaudin F, Thuret I, Vannier J. Late effects of allogeneic bone marrow transplantation for children with acute myeloblastic leukemia in first complete remission: the impact of conditioning regimen without total body irradiation – a report from the Société Française de Greffe de Moelle. *J Clin Oncol* 1997; **15**: 2238–2246

93. Shaw P, Hugh-Jones K, Hobbs J *et al*. Busulphan and cyclophosphamide cause little early toxicity during displacement bone marrow transplantation in fifty children. *Bone Marrow Transplant* 1986; **1**: 193–198

94. Grochow L, Krivit W, Blazar B. Busulfan disposition in children. *Blood* 1990; **75**: 1723–1727

95. Hartmann O, Benhamou E, Beaujean F *et al*. High-dose busulfan and cyclophosphamide with autologous bone marrow transplantation support in advanced malignancies in children: A phase II study. *J Clin Oncol* 1986; **4**: 1804–1811

96. Yeager AM, Wagner JE, Graham ML, Jones RJ, Santos GW, Grochow LB. Optimization of busulfan dosage in children undergoing bone marrow transplantation: a pharmacokinetic study of dose escalation. *Blood* 1992; **80**: 2425–2428

97. Stattery JT, Clift RA, Buckner CD *et al*. Marrow transplantation for chronic myeloid leukemia: the influence of plasma busulfan levels of outcome of transplantation. *Blood* 1997; **89**: 3055–3060

98. Vassal G, Deroussent A, Challine D *et al*. Is 600 mg/m^2 the appropriate dosage of busulfan in children undergoing bone marrow transplantation? *Blood* 1992; **79**: 2475–2479

99. Sanders JE, Team SMT. The impact of marrow transplant preparative regimens on subsequent growth and development. *Semin Hematol* 1991; **28**: 244–249

100. Wingard JR, Curbow B, Baker F, Piantadosi S. Health, functional status and employment of adult survivors of bone marrow transplantation. *Ann Intern Med* 1991; **114**: 113–118

101. Wingard JR, Plotnick LP, Freeman CS *et al*. Growth in children after bone marrow transplantation: busulfan plus cyclophosphamide versus cyclophosphamide total body irradiation. *Blood* 1992; **79**: 1068–1073

102. Beatty P, Clift R, Mickleson E *et al*. Marrow transplantation from related donors other than HLA-identical siblings. *N Engl J Med* 1985; **313**: 765–771

103. McGlave P, Haake R, Bostrom B *et al*. Allogeneic bone marrow transplantation for acute nonlymphoblastic leukemia in first remission. *Blood* 1988; **72**: 1512–1517

104. Dini G, Boni L, Abla O *et al*. Allogeneic bone marrow transplantation in children with acute myelogenous leukemia in first remission. *Bone Marrow Transplant* 1994; **13**: 771–776

105. Zwaan F, Hermans J, Barrett A, Speck B. Bone marrow transplantation for acute nonlymphoblastic leukaemia: a survey of the European Group for Bone Marrow Transplantation. *Br J Haematol* 1984; **56**: 645–653

106. Weisdorf D, McGlave P, Ramsay N *et al*. Allogeneic bone marrow transplantation for acute leukaemia: comparative outcomes for adults and children. *Br J Haematol* 1988; **69**: 351–358

107. Forman S, Krance R, O'Donnell M *et al*. Bone marrow transplantation for acute leukemia: comparative outcomes for adults and children. *Br J Haematol* 1988; **69**: 351–358

108. Clift R, Buckner C, Thomas E *et al*. The treatment of acute non-lymphoblastic leukemia by allogeneic marrow transplantation. *Bone Marrow Transplant* 1987; **2**: 243–258

109. Liesner RJ, Leiper AD, Hann IM, Chessells JM. Late effects of intensive treatment for acute myeloid leukemia and myelodysplasia in childhood. *J Clin Oncol* 1994; **12**: 916–924

110. Teunissen E, Leahey A, Bunin G, Meadows A. Late effects of chemotherapy vs bone marrow transplantation in the treatment of acute myeloid leukemia and myelodysplasia. *Med Pediatr Oncol* 1997; **22**: 242A

111. Yeager AM, Kaizer H, Santos GW. Autologous bone marrow transplantation in patients with acute non-lymphocytic leukemia, using ex-vivo marrow treatment with 4-hydroperoxycyclophosphamide. *N Engl J Med* 1986; **315**: 141

112. Phillips G, Shepherd J, Barnett M *et al*. Busulfan, cyclophosphamide, and melphalan conditioning for autologous bone marrow transplantation in hematologic malignancy. *J Clin Oncol* 1991; **9**: 1880–1888

113. Petersen FB, Lynch MHE, Clift RA *et al*. Autologous marrow transplantation for patients with acute myeloid leukemia in untreated first relapse or second complete remission. *J Clin Oncol* 1993; **11**: 1353–1360

114. Vignetti M, Rondelli R, Locatelli F *et al*. Autologous bone marrow transplantation in children with acute myeloblastic leukemia: a report from the Italian National Pediatric Registry (AIEOP-BMT). *Bone Marrow Transplant* 1996; **18 (Suppl 2)**: 59–62

115. Brenner M, Rill D, Moen R *et al*. Gene-marking to trace origin of relapse after autologous bone-marrow transplantation. *Lancet* 1993; **341**: 85–86

116. Benyunes MC, Massumoto C, Higuchi CM *et al*. Interleukin-2 with or without lymphokine-activated killer cells as consolidative immunotherapy after autologous bone marrow transplantation for acute myelogenous leukemia. *Bone Marrow Transplant* 1993; **12**: 159–163

117. Szydlo R, Goldman JM, Klein JP *et al*. Results of allogeneic bone marrow transplants for leukemia using donors other than HLA-identical siblings. *J Clin Oncol* 1997; **15**: 1767–1777

118. Weiden P, Flourney N, Thomas E *et al*. Antileukemic effects of graft vs host disease in human recipients of allogeneic marrow grafts. *N Engl J Med* 1979; **300**: 1068–1079

119. Feig S, Nesbit M, Lampkin B *et al* (eds). What is the optimal strategy to prevent relapse in children with acute myeloid leukemia. *Cancer Chemotherapy: Challenges for the Future*, vol 8. Tokyo: Excerpta Medica Ltd, 1993

120. Weaver C, Clift R, Deeg H *et al*. Effect of graft-versus-host disease prophylaxis on relapse in patients transplanted for acute myeloid leukemia. *Bone Marrow Transplant* 1994; **14**: 885–893

121. Horowitz M, Gale R, Sondel P *et al*. Graft-vs-leukemia reactions after bone marrow transplantation. *Blood* 1990; **75**: 555–562

122. Bonini C, Ferrari G, Verzeletti S *et al*. HSV-TK gene transfer into donor T lymphocytes for contol of allogeneic graft-versus-leukemia. *Science* 1997; **276**: 1719–1724

123. Pinkel D. Bone marrow transplantation in children. *J Pediatr* 1993; **122**: 331–340

124. Mayer RJ. Allogeneic transplantation versus chemotherapy in first-remission acute leukemia: is there a 'best choice'? *J Clin Oncol* 1988; **6**: 1532–1536

125. Lange B, Kobrinsky N, Barnard D *et al*. Distinctive demography, biology and outcome of acute myeloid leukemia and myelodysplastic syndrome in children with Down syndrome in Children's Cancer Group Studies 2861 and 2961. *Blood* 1998; **91**: 608–615

126. LeBlanc T, Auvirigon A, Michel G *et al*. Prognosis value of cytogenetics in 250 children with acute myeloblastic leukemia treated in Lame 89/91. *Blood* 1996; **88 (Suppl 1)**: 634A

127. Woods WG, Nesbit ME, Buckley J *et al*. Correlation of chromosome abnormalities with patient characteristics, histologic subtype and

induction success in children with acute nonlymphoblastic leukemia. *J Clin Oncol* 1985; **3**: 3–11

128. Pui CH, Dahl GV, Kalwinsky DK *et al*. Central nervous system leukemia in children with acute nonlymphoblastic leukemia. *Blood* 1985; **66**: 1062–1067

129. Eshghabadi M, Shojania M, Carr I. Isolated granulocytic sarcoma: report of a case and review of the literature. *J Clin Oncol* 1986; **4**: 912–917

130. Dusenbery KE, Arthur DC, Howells W *et al*. Granulocytic sarcomas (chloromas) in pediatric patients with newly diagnosed acute myeloid leukemia. *Proc Am Soc Clin Oncol* 1996; **15**: 369 (abstract)

131. Truker A, Cadver AO, Yavuz G *et al*. Cytogenetic heterogeneity in Turkish children with acute myeloid leukemia (AML) and orbito-ocular granulocytic sarcoma (chloroma). *Blood* 1993; **82**: 550A

132. Lemons R, Keller S, Gietzen D *et al*. Acute promyelocytic leukemia. *J Pediatr Hematol Oncol* 1995; **17**: 198–210

133. Huang M, Ye Y, Chai J *et al*. Use of all-*trans* retinoic acid in the treatment of acute promyelocytic leukemia. *Blood* 1988; **72**: 567–572

134. Tallman MS, Anderson J, Schiffer CA *et al*. All-*trans* retinoic acid in acute promyelocytic leukemia. *N Engl J Med* 1997; **337**: 1021–1028

135. Mahmoud HH, Jurwitz CA, Roberts WM, Santana VM, Ribeiro RC, Krance RA. Tretinoin toxicity in children with acute promyelocytic leukemia. *Lancet* 1993; **342**: 1394–1396

136. Frankel SR, Eardley A, Lauwers G, Weiss M, Warrell R. The 'retinoic acid syndrome' in acute promyelocytic leukemia. *Ann Intern Med* 1992; **117**: 292–298

137. Scott AA, Head DR, Kopecky KJ *et al*. HLA-DR-, CD33+, CD56+, CD16- Myeloid/natural killer cell acute leukemia: a previously unrecognized form of acute leukemia potentially misdiagnosed a French-British-American acute myeloid leukemia-M3. *Blood* 1994; **84**: 244–255

138. Warrell R, de The H, Wang Z-Y, Degos L. Acute promyelocytic leukemia. *N Engl J Med* 1993; **329**: 177–189

139. Estey E, Thall PF, Pierce S, Kantarjian H, Keating M. Treatment of newly diagnosed acute promyelocytic leukemia without cytarabine. *J Clin Oncol* 1997; **15**: 483–490

140. Shen X-Z, Chen G-Q, Ni J-H *et al*. Use of arsenic trioxide in the treatment of acute promyelocytic leukemia. II: clinical efficacy and pharmacokinetics in relapsed patients. *Blood* 1997; **89**: 3354–3360

141. Zipursky A. The treatment of children with acute megakaryoblastic leukemia who have Down syndrome. *J Pediatr Hematol Oncol* 1996; **8**: 10–12

142. Zipursky A, Peeters M, Poon A. Megakaryoblastic leukemia and Down syndrome: a review. *Pediatr Hematol Oncol* 1987; **4**: 211–230

143. Zipursky A, Thorner P, De Harven E, Christensen H, Doyle J. Myelodysplasia and acute megakaryoblastic leukemia in Down's syndrome. *Leukemia Res* 1994; **18**: 163–171

144. Ravindranath Y, Abella E, Krischer JP *et al*. Acute myeloid leukemia (AML) in Down's syndrome is highly responsive to chemotherapy: experience on Pediatric Oncology Group AML Study 8498 [see comments]. *Blood* 1992; **80**: 2210–2214

145. Lampkin BC, Peipon JJ, Price JK, Bove KE, Srivastava AK, Jones MM. Spontaneous remission of presumed congenital acute nonlymphoblastic leukemia (ANLL) in a karyotypically normal neonate. *Am J Pediatr Hematol Oncol* 1985; **7**: 346–351

146. Dinulos JG, Hawkins DS, Clark BS, Francis JS. Spontaneous remission of congenital leukemia. *J Pediatr* 1997; **131**: 300–303

147. Feusner J, Hastings C. Infections in children with acute myeloid leukemia: concepts of management and prevention. *J Pediatr Hematol Oncol* 1995; **17**: 234–247

148. Chanock S, Pizzo P. Fever in the neutropenic host. *Infect Dis Clin North Am* 1996; **10**: 77–96

149. Chanock S, Pizzo P. Infectious complications in patients undergoing therapy for acute leukemia: current status and future prospects. *Semin Oncol* 1997; **24**: 132–140

150. Weisman S, Scoopo F, Johnson G, Altman A, Quinn J. Septicemia in pediatric oncology patients: The significance of viridans streptococcal infections. *J Clin Oncol* 1990; **8**: 453–459

151. Bunin NJ, Pui CH. Differing complications of hyperleukocytosis in children with acute lymphoblastic or acute nonlymphoblastic leukemia. *J Clin Oncol* 1985; **3**: 1590–1595

152. Goldberg M, Ginsberg D, Mayer RA. Is heparin necessary during induction chemotherapy for patients with acute promyelocytic leukemia? *Blood* 1987; **69**: 187–191

153. Geller RB. Use of cytokines in the treatment of acute myelocytic leukemia: a critical review. *J Clin Oncol* 1996; 14: 1371–1382

154. Schiffer CA. Hematopoietic growth factors as adjuncts to the treatment of acute myeloid leukemia. *Blood* 1996; **88**: 3675–3685

155. Mirro J, Hurwitz CA, Behm FG *et al*. Effects of recombinant human hematopoietic growth factors on leukemic blasts from children with acute myeloblastic or lymphoblastic leukemia. *Leukemia* 1993; **7**: 1026–1033

156. Woods WG, Kobrinsky N, Buckley J *et al*. Timed sequential induction therapy improves post-remission outcome in acute myeloid leukemia (AML). *Med Pediatr Oncol* 1995; **25**: 271A

157. Archimbaud E, Thomas X, Leblond V *et al*. Timed sequential chemotherapy for previously treated patients with acute myeloid leukemia: Longterm follow-up of the etoposide, mitoxantrone and cytarabine – 86 trial. *J Clin Oncol* 1995; **13**: 11–18

158. Weitman S, Ochoa S, Sullivan J *et al*. Pediatric phase II cancer chemotherapy trials: a Pediatric Oncology Group Study. *J Pediatr Hematol Oncol* 1997; **19**: 187–191

159. Wells RJ, Arndt CAS. New agents for treatment of children with acute myelogenous leukemia. *J Pediatr Hematol Oncol* 1995; **17**: 225–23

160. Bunin NJ, Casper JT, Chitambar C *et al*. Partially matched bone marrow transplantation in patients with myelodysplastic syndromes. *J Clin Oncol* 1988; **6**: 1851–1855

161. Bunin NJ, Casper JT, Lawton C *et al*. Allogeneic marrow transplantation using T cell depletion for patients with juvenile chronic myelogenous leukemia without HLA-identical siblings. *Bone Marrow Transplant* 1992; **9**: 119–122

162. Casper J, Camitta B, Truitt R *et al*. Unrelated bone marrow transplants for children with leukemia or myelodysplasia. *Blood* 1995; **85**: 2354–2363

163. Balduzzi A, Gooley T, Anasetti C *et al*. Unrelated marrow donor transplantation in children. *Blood* 1995; **86**: 3247–3256

164. Davies SM, Wagner JE, Shu XO *et al*. Unrelated donor bone marrow transplantation for children with acute leukemia. *J Clin Oncol* 1997; **15**: 557–565

165. Davies SM, Wagner JE, Weisdorf DJ *et al*. Unrelated donor bone marrow transplantation for hematological malignancies – current status. *Leukemia Lymphoma* 1996; **23**: 221–226

166. Beatty PG, Anasetti C, Hansen JA *et al*. Marrow transplantation from unrelated donors for treatment of hematologic malignancies: effect of mismatching for one HLA locus. *Blood* 1993; **81**: 249–253

167. Nademanee A, Schmidt GM, Parker P *et al*. The outcome of matched unrelated donor bone marrow transplantation in patients with hematologic malignancies using molecular typing for donor selection and graft-versus-host disease prophylaxis regimen of cyclosporine, methotrexate and prednisone. *Blood* 1995; **86**: 1228–1234

168. Kurtzberg J, Laughlin M, Graham ML *et al*. Placental blood as a source of hematopoietic stem cells for transplantation into unrelated recipients. *N Engl J Med* 1996; **335**: 157–166

169. Wagner J, Kernan N, Steinbuch M, Broxmeyer H, Gluckman E. Allogeneic sibling umbilical cord blood transplantation in children with malignant and non malignant disease. *Lancet* 1995; **i**: 214–219

170. Wagner JE, Rosenthal J, Sweetman R *et al*. Successful transplantation of HLA-matched and HLA-mismatched umbilical cord blood from unrelated donors: analysis of engraftment and acute graft-vs-host disease. *N Engl J Med* 1996; **88**: 795–802

171. Gluckman E, Rocha V, Boyer-Chammard *et al*. Outcome of cord blood transplantation from related and unrelated donors. *N Engl J Med* 1997; **337**: 373–381

172. Wagner J, Santos G, Burns W, Saral R. Second bone marrow transplantation after leukemia relapse in 11 patients. *Bone Marrow Transplant* 1989; **4**: 115–118

173. Sanders JE, Buckner CD, Martin PJ *et al.* Second allogeneic marrow transplantation for patients with recurrent leukemia after intial transplant with total body irradiation-containing regimens. *J Clin Oncol* 1993; **11**: 304–313

174. Kolb H, Mittermuller J, Clemm C *et al.* Donor leukocyte infusions for treatment of recurrent chronic myelogenous leukemia in marrow transplant patients. *Blood* 1990; **76**: 2462–2465

175. Kolb HJ, Schattenberg A, Goldman JM *et al.* Graft-versus-leukemia effect of donor lymphocyte transfusions in marrow grafted patients. European Group for Blood and Marrow Transplantation Working Party Chronic Leukemia (see comments). *Blood* 1995; **86**: 2041–2050

Adult-type chronic myeloid leukemia

IRENE AG ROBERTS AND INDERJEET S DOKAL

EPIDEMIOLOGY

Chronic myeloid leukemia (CML) in childhood presents as one of two clinically and biologically distinct syndromes: adult-type CML (ATCML), which appears to be identical to CML in adults, and juvenile CML (JCML), which is a form of myelodysplasia (see Chapter 4). Together these diseases constitute around 2–5% of all childhood leukemias, ATCML being rather more common than JCML.[1] The incidence of ATCML in childhood is <1/100 000; just under 20 and 100 new cases are diagnosed each year in the UK and US, respectively.[2,3] In all age groups ATCML is slightly more common in males than females, with a male:female ratio varying from just over 1.0 to 2.8.[3,4] ATCML tends to affect older children. It is exceptionally rare in infancy, although it has been reported in a 3-month old baby, and 60% of children are >6 years old at diagnosis.[4]

ETIOLOGY

Although the molecular basis of ATCML has been well characterized for some time, its etiology is unknown in the vast majority of children. There is no clear evidence of a hereditary predisposition; with 1 exception,[5] identical twins appear to be discordant for the disease and ATCML is no more common in siblings of affected children. There is also no increased risk of ATCML in pre-leukemic chromosomal disorders such as Fanconi's anemia and Down's syndrome.

In occasional cases, an association with ionizing radiation has been described;[6] a 7-fold increase in ATCML, particularly in children under 5 years of age, was reported in Japan following the nuclear explosions in the 1940s.

MOLECULAR BIOLOGY

As in CML in adults, ATCML in children is characterized by the presence of the Philadelphia (Ph) chromosome in all, or most, hemopoietic stem cells.[7,8] The Ph chromosome (22q-) results from the reciprocal translocation of the distal parts of the long arms of chromosomes 9 and 22 (Fig. 20.1). The translocation breakpoints disrupt genes on both chromosomes; the *ABL* (Abelson) proto-oncogene on chromosome 9 (9q34) and breakpoint cluster region (*BCR*) gene on chromosome 22 (22q11).[9–12] The consequence of this molecular rearrangement is the formation of an abnormal *BCR-ABL* fusion gene which encodes a 210-kDa *bcr-abl* fusion protein (Fig. 20.2). Breakpoints in *ABL* almost invariably occur upstream of exon 1b, between Ib and Ia, or between Ia and a2. The breakpoints in *BCR* usually occur within M-*bcr* (major breakpoint cluster region) (Fig. 20.2).

In around 90% of cases of ATCML, the Ph chromosome is readily detectable by standard cytogenetic preparations of bone marrow cells; in most of the remaining 10%, chromosomes 9 and 22 appear normal but identical patterns of *BCR-ABL* rearrangement to those found in cases of ATCML with the Ph chromosome can be clearly demonstrated by molecular techniques. A small proportion of children with ATCML (probably <5%) either have variant translocations (see below) or no evidence of *BCR-ABL* rearrangement even after extensive investigation at the molecular level.

Despite the fact that the Ph chromosome was first described in 1960 and its molecular basis in the 1980s, the exact role played by the novel *BCR-ABL* fusion gene in the pathogenesis of CML and ATCML remains unclear. Most evidence points to *BCR-ABL* being the major factor determining the leukemic phenotype;[13–15] however, *BCR-ABL* rearrangement may not always be the initiating step in the development of CML or ATCML. The identification of families in which several members have developed CML or another malignancy suggests an inherited predisposing factor;[5] the *BCR-ABL* rearrangement in these cases is likely

(a)

der(9)

9

22

der(22)
"Ph"

(b)

t (9;22) (q34;q11)

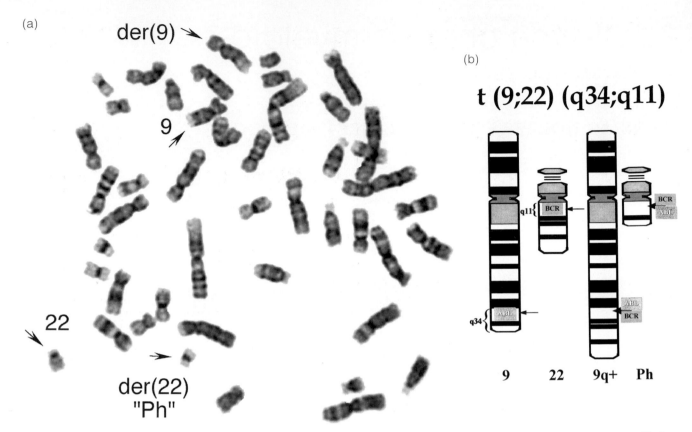

q11 BCR

q34 ABL

BCR
ABL

ABL
BCR

9   22   9q+   Ph

Fig. 20.1 (A) Metaphase showing the normal chromosomes 9 and 22, and the 9q+ and 22q- (Ph) derivatives from the t(9;22)(q34;q11) rearrangement. Kindly provided by Andy Chase. (B) Schematic diagram of the normal chromosomes 9 and 22, and of the 9q+ and 22q- (Ph) derivatives from the t(9;22)(q34;q11). The arrows indicate the breakpoints on 9 and 22 which disrupt the *ABL* and *BCRy* genes, respectively. Kindly provided by Junia Melo.

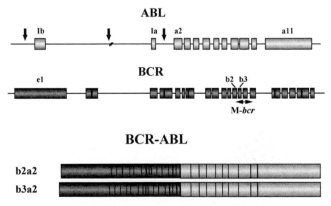

ABL

Ib   Ia a2   a11

BCR

e1   b2 b3

M-bcr

BCR-ABL

b2a2

b3a2

Fig. 20.2 Schematic representation of the *ABL* and the *BCR* genes disrupted in the t(9;22)(q34;q11). Exons are represented by boxes and introns by connecting horizontal lines. Breakpoints in *ABL*, illustrated as vertical arrows, almost invariably occur either upstream of exon 1b, between Ib and Ia, or between Ia and a2. The *BCR* gene contains 25 exons, including two putative alternative first (e1′) and second (e2′) exons. The breakpoints in *BCR* usually occur within M-*bcr* (major breakpoint cluster region), the location of which is shown by the double-headed horizontal arrows. The lower half of the figure shows the structure of the *BCR-ABL* mRNA transcripts The breaks in M-*bcr* occur either between exons b2(e13) and b3 (e14) or between b3 and b4 (e15), generating fusion transcripts with a b2a2 or a b3a2 junction, respectively. Kindly provided by Junia Melo.

to represent the second step in the neoplastic process. In addition, both epidemiologic data[16] and animal models of CML suggest that a minimum of 2 mutations is necessary for the development of chronic-phase CML.[14,15]

It is clear that the *bcr-abl* fusion protein is a potent, constitutively active tyrosine kinase and, like other tyrosine kinases in hemopoietic cells, it is likely to play a direct role in stimulating cell proliferation, perhaps in an unregulated or dysregulated fashion. The functional significance of the reciprocal fusion gene, *ABL-BCR*, remains unknown.[17] The p210 *bcr-abl* fusion protein characteristic of CML and ATCML is distinct from that seen in Ph-positive acute lymphoid leukemia (ALL), in which rearrangement of ABL and BCR results in a 185-kDa fusion (p185*bcr-abl*) protein (see Chapter 26).[18]

The oncogenic potential of the *bcr-abl* protein has been demonstrated in a number of *in vitro* and *in vivo* model systems. *Bcr-abl* binds and/or phosphorylates >20 proteins, many of which can be directly linked to signal transduction pathways.[19] For example, *bcr-abl* activates *ras*, and an intact *ras* protein is required for *bcr-abl* transformation and anti-apoptotic activities.[20–22]

BIOLOGY

ATCML, like other hematologic malignancies, is a clonal disorder originating in a multipotent stem cell. This is clear from well-defined subpopulations of stem and progenitor cells studied by immunophenotyping and colony growth *in vitro* and *in vivo*.[23] Thus, the Ph chromosome and/or *BCR-ABL* rearrangement can be demonstrated and expression of *BCR-ABL* found in progenitor and mature cells of the granulocytic, erythroid and megakaryocytic lineages. In some, but not all, cases B lymphocytes and, less often, T lymphocytes have also been shown to be part of the malignant clone.[24] This suggests that leukemic transformation in these cases has occurred in a pluripotent lymphohemopoietic stem cell. In other cases, where the lymphocytes do not contain the Ph chromosome, ATCML may have arisen in a more mature multipotent stem cell, 'sparing' the lymphoid lineage. However, the interpretation of such data is difficult and it remains uncertain whether the clonal origin of CML/ATCML is truly heterogeneous or whether all cases arise in the pluripotent lymphohemopoietic stem cell, lymphocytes without the Ph chromosome representing long-lived cells arising prior to leukemic transformation. An alternative explanation, for which there is some evidence, is that in a proportion of patients with CML/ATCML defective hemopoiesis precedes the acquisition of the Ph chromosome, i.e. the Ph translocation may not be the initiating leukemogenic event.[25]

The clinical hallmark of ATCML is the hyperproliferation of the *BCR-ABL*-containing clone leading to expansion of the granulocytic compartment at all stages of maturation and variable suppression of normal hemopoiesis. Expansion of the abnormal clone presumably occurs because of failure of the normal control mechanisms which regulate hemopoiesis. Interestingly, despite predominantly granulocytic hyperplasia, all lineages and classes of committed progenitor cell appear to be similarly dysregulated. Thus, in addition to granulocyte/monocyte progenitors, erythroid and megakaryocyte progenitors are also increased.

The exact mechanism(s) mediating the expansion of the *BCR-ABL*-positive clone are complex and controversial. Some studies indicate that there is increased proliferative activity of CML stem cells; others that there is increased self-renewal of more mature, committed progenitors and this does seem more likely than myeloid expansion secondary to enhanced differentiation of progenitor cells.[23,26] There is also some evidence for reduced susceptibility of CML cells to apoptosis,[27] although whether this property is relevant to the myeloid expansion in CML is unclear. In addition, CML progenitors have been shown to have diminished adhesive properties which result in reduced contact with stromal cells, possibly releasing them from physiologic inhibitory regulatory mechanisms.[28] Although the exact mechanisms remain unclear, the abnormal growth characteristics of CML cells and their progenitors are thought to be the result of the *BCR-ABL* rearrangement. Direct evidence in support of this is provided by studies in cell lines and animal models of CML. The *BCR-ABL* gene can confer growth factor-independence on previously factor-dependent cell lines.[29,30] Complementary evidence for a pathogenetic role of the *BCR-ABL* rearrangement is provided by the demonstration that it is possible to induce a CML-like disorder in a mouse model by insertion of the *BCR-ABL* gene into hemopoietic cells.[14,15]

CLINICAL FEATURES

ATCML, like CML in adults, most commonly presents with non-specific symptoms, such as fatigue and malaise (Table 20.1). Abdominal discomfort, due to an enlarging spleen, and bone and joint pain due to marrow hyperplasia are also fairly common.[31] If there is a marked leukocytosis ($>100 \times 10^9$/l), affected children may present with symptoms of an hypermetabolic state, including weight loss, fever and, occasionally, night sweats. While mild anemia is frequently seen and may contribute to the presenting symptoms, hemorrhagic problems are rarely seen at presentation unless there is advanced disease or marked hypersplenism.[31]

Examination

The majority of children have mild or moderate splenomegaly; otherwise findings on examination are usually unremarkable.[1,31] Palpable hepatomegaly (1–2 cm) is sometimes found but gross hepatomegaly and lymphadenopathy are very uncommon unless the disease has progressed to accelerated phase or blast crisis. Signs of leukostasis (e.g. retinal hemorrhages, papilloedema, priapism) are usually only seen if the leukocyte count at presentation is very high ($>300 \times 10^9$/l). Some reports have suggested that such signs are more common in association with ATCML than in CML in adults.[32] Skin nodules due to leukemic deposits (chloromas) are occasionally seen, usually in association with advanced-phase disease.

Table 20.1 Clinical features at diagnosis of ATCML.

Common
Fatigue
Weight loss
Fever
Sweating
Abdominal discomfort/splenomegaly
Bone pains
Anemia
Rare
Hemorrhagic complications (e.g. retinal hemorrhages)
Leukostasis (e.g. priapism)
Gout
Splenic infarction

DIAGNOSIS

Peripheral blood

The most consistent finding at presentation is the characteristic leukocytosis made up predominantly of mature granulocytic cells (neutrophils, bands and metamyelocytes) and their precursors (myelocytes and promyelocytes) (Plate 27). In chronic-phase ATCML, blasts constitute <5% of peripheral blood leukocytes. As in CML in adults, eosinophilia and basophilia are commonly present at diagnosis. The total white count at presentation is usually $>100 \times 10^9/l$. Most children have a normal or slightly increased platelet count at presentation; the presence either of thrombocytopenia or of marked thrombocytosis ($>1000 \times 10^9/l$) suggests more advanced-phase disease. By contrast, mild or moderate anemia is a presenting finding in the majority of children.

Bone marrow

The marrow in ATCML is markedly hypercellular due mainly to hyperplasia of granulocytic cells (Plate 28). A characteristic 'myelocyte' peak is commonly seen at presentation and blast cells constitute <5% of nucleated cells in chronic-phase ATCML. Eosinophils, basophils and their precursors are frequently increased and are sometimes dysplastic. In addition, pseudo-Gaucher cells similar to sea-blue histiocytes are seen in a small proportion of cases (Plate 29A and 29B). Megakaryocytes are usually present in increased numbers but they are usually morphologically normal.

The trephine biopsy is often useful in ATCML and should be performed at presentation if a bone marrow harvest is planned and if accelerated-phase disease is suspected. At presentation, the main features seen on biopsy in chronic phase are hypercellularity, granulocytic hyperplasia and increased megakaryocyte numbers. However, the biopsy is useful for assessing the extent of accompanying myelofibrosis and may show increases in blast cells in advanced-phase disease. Myelofibrosis is not usually prominent at presentation but it is a common feature of advanced-phase disease and may make marrow harvesting extremely difficult.

Cytogenetics

Cytogenetic studies on bone marrow at presentation show the classic Ph chromosome in around 90% of patients with chronic-phase ATCML. In almost all such patients, the Ph chromosome is seen in 100% of the metaphases but occasionally small numbers of cytogenetically normal cells are still detectable at presentation. Variant translocations are seen in <5% of children in chronic phase. These are of 2 types: rearrangements involving 2 chromosomes, 1 of which is chromosome 22; and rearrangements involving chromosomes 22 and 9 together with at least 1 other chromosome. Variant translocations, and some cases which are cytogen-

etically normal, virtually always show *BCR* rearrangement by Southern blotting despite the absence of the Ph chromosome using classical cytogenetics.[33] Recent work shows that fluorescent *in situ* hybridization (FISH) is almost as accurate in detecting the Ph chromosome *BCR-ABL* fusion gene in bone marrow from adults with CML.[34] More widespread introduction of FISH may make the diagnosis of ATCML easier, quicker and cheaper and may also render the miscellaneous rapid confirmatory tests described below redundant in ATCML.

There remains a very small number of children with ATCML who are Ph-negative and who have no evidence of *BCR-ABL* rearrangement even after extensive molecular investigation. Most, if not all, such children meet the diagnostic criteria for JCML or other types of myelodysplasia or myeloproliferative disorders (see Chapter 4). Thus, the existence of true Ph-negative ATCML is extremely unlikely and in adults, although of scientific interest, the distinction does not appear to be of practical clinical importance since the clinical features, laboratory findings and natural history of Ph-positive and -negative, *BCR-ABL*-negative CML/ATCML are so similar that their treatment is the same.[35]

A number of cytogenetic abnormalities, such as isochromosome 17q, in addition to the Ph chromosome may be seen in bone marrow cells in ATCML.[33] However, these changes are associated with accelerated disease or blast crisis (see below) and therefore cast doubt on the diagnosis of ATCML still in chronic phase.

Miscellaneous tests

A number of other laboratory tests are abnormal in ATCML and may be used to substantiate the diagnosis where cytogenetic or molecular studies are unavailable. These include reduced leukocyte alkaline phosphatase (LAP) activity (measured cytochemically as a low LAP 'score') and increased vitamin B_{12}-binding protein (usually measured as a reduced serum B_{12} level). In addition, the serum uric acid is often elevated although clinical gout appears to be unusual.

ACCELERATED-PHASE ATCML

Although there are no specific laboratory findings diagnostic of accelerated phase ATCML, there are a number of features which suggest that the disease has entered a more advanced stage and predict the onset of blast crisis within the ensuing 6–12 months. One of the commonest is a change in the platelet count; this may manifest either as thrombocytopenia or thrombocytosis increasingly resistant to chemotherapy. Similarly, the leukocyte count may become refractory to treatment and there may be increased numbers of basophils and/or eosinophils in comparison with earlier in the disease course. Blast cells in the marrow may also increase. Many patients become anemic. In part this may be due to increasing myelofibrosis, a common feature of accelerated-phase ATCML, and in part due to hypersplenism in association with a larger spleen.

The progression of ATCML to accelerated phase is often associated with the acquisition of new cytogenetic abnormalities. The commonest are a second Ph chromosome, isochromosome 17, trisomy 8 and trisomy 19.[33,36,37] The genes involved in the evolution of CML in adults and children have not yet been fully characterized (see below).

BLAST CRISIS

Blast crisis usually evolves relatively gradually from accelerated phase, but not infrequently the switch from chronic phase is dramatic, blast cells appearing in the peripheral blood without a distinct period of 'acceleration'. Occasionally, children with ATCML present in blast crisis or relapse straight into blast crisis following allogeneic BMT. The majority of patients with blast crisis have a rapidly rising leukocyte count together with anemia and are frequently thrombocytopenic. In >60% of cases, the blast cells have the morphologic and immunophenotypic characteristics of myeloblasts (Plate 30).[37,38] However, 20–30% of patients undergo lymphoid blast transformation, most commonly with a pre-B phenotype (Plates 31 and 32);[37–39] among adults, their median age is younger than patients developing myeloblastic crisis but there are no large series to confirm whether or not children are more likely to undergo lymphoid rather than myeloid transformation. Classification into lymphoid versus myeloid blast crisis on morphologic grounds is often very difficult; immunophenotyping to confirm the myeloid or lymphoid characteristics of the blasts is therefore very important since this has a major impact on treatment and prognosis.

As in accelerated phase, cytogenetic changes in addition to the Ph chromosome are common. As well as those affecting chromosomes 8, 17 and 19, the translocations associated with acute myeloid leukemia (AML) and ALL are sometimes seen in blastic crisis (see Chapters 18 and 26). At the molecular level, blast crisis has been variably associated with abnormalities of tumor suppressor genes, in particular *p53*, p16 and *rb*, or proto-oncogenes, such as *ras* and *myc*, or with the generation of chimeric transcription factors, as in the *AML-EVI1* gene fusion.[40–44] It is likely, therefore, that multiple and alternative molecular defects underlie the acute transformation of the disease.

DIFFERENTIAL DIAGNOSIS

The most important differential diagnosis in young children is *juvenile chronic myeloid leukemia* (JCML) (see Chapter 4). JCML is seen more commonly in children <2 years of age in contrast to ATCML which occurs predominantly in children >6 years. The profile of clinical signs is also rather different: skin rashes and lymphadenopathy are very common in JCML but rare in chronic-phase ATCML, while prominent splenomegaly is suggestive of ATCML

since it is usually less marked in JCML. The laboratory features are also usually distinct: in JCML the white cell count tends to be <100 × 10^9/l and there is a monocytosis, thrombocytopenia and a raised fetal hemoglobin (HbF), none of which is common in ATCML. The diagnosis is generally not in doubt once the bone marrow karyotype is available but the absence of the Ph chromosome in up to 10% of cases of ATCML may lead to diagnostic uncertainty in occasional cases.

A transient CML-like blood picture is also occasionally seen in association with severe bacterial infections, chronic Epstein–Barr virus (EBV) infection and non-hematologic cancers. Similar granulocytic hyperplasia may also be found during the first year of life in 60–70% of cases of thrombocytopenia with absent radii (TAR) syndrome. Finally, the blood film and marrow of children who present in lymphoid blast crisis may be difficult to distinguish from *de novo* Ph-positive ALL on morphologic grounds: molecular analysis for the p210 and p185 *bcr-abl* proteins in ATCML and ALL, respectively, may clarify the underlying diagnosis.

MANAGEMENT

CHRONIC PHASE

Initial management

For children presenting in chronic phase it is rarely necessary to start treatment immediately. It is important to spend time with the family explaining the natural history of the disease, particularly since it differs in so many ways from most childhood malignancies. Unlike acute leukemia, ATCML can only be cured by bone marrow transplantation (BMT). It is therefore appropriate to raise this with families and to proceed to HLA typing of family members at an early stage since the availability of an HLA-identical sibling donor has a major impact on the choice of treatment.

In addition, prior to initiating treatment, hemopoietic stem cells should be collected from all children in chronic phase and cryopreserved for possible later autologous transplantation. In the majority of children, sufficient stem cells can be collected by leukapheresis (aim for 10 × 10^8 cells/kg), but where this is not possible (e.g. poor vascular access) autologous bone marrow harvesting is a satisfactory alternative (aim to cryopreserve 2 × 10^8 cells/ kg). In the rare cases presenting with symptoms of hyperviscosity, leukapheresis should be carried out as soon as possible.

Once stem cell cryopreservation has been completed, treatment should be instituted to bring the disease under control pending a decision about allogeneic BMT. This is usually best achieved using oral chemotherapy. In symptomatic children and/or those with white cell counts >100 ×

10^9/l, chemotherapy should be started promptly and most will feel considerably better after only a few days. For asymptomatic children the aim of chemotherapy is to 'normalize' the blood count and thereby delay onset of symptoms.

Several well known oral agents are active in ATCML, including hydroxyurea, busulfan, 6-mercaptopurine (6-MP) and 6-thioguanine (6-TG). Hydroxyurea has a number of advantages and is usually the best drug for initial disease control. It causes a rapid fall in both white cell and platelet counts, usually within 1–2 weeks; myelo-suppressive hydroxyurea-associated pancytopenia is usually rapidly reversible, particularly in comparison with busulfan; and it has fewer serious side-effects. In contrast to busulfan, there is no evidence that hydroxyurea is leukemogenic or tumorigenic in humans; it does not appear to cause pulmonary fibrosis even with long-term use and, in the doses used, it does not cause infertility. Furthermore, a history of busulfan use in adults prior to BMT has been identified as one of the factors predicting a poorer outcome compared to the use of no chemotherapy or hydroxyurea for disease control before BMT.[45] The usual starting dose of hydroxyurea is 20 mg/kg, increasing up to 30 mg/kg depending on response, with the aim of bringing the white cell count down below 10×10^9/l.

Soon after diagnosis a decision must be made about long-term treatment since there are several treatment options with the potential to cure or significantly to prolong survival compared to oral chemotherapy.[46–49] A suggested treatment algorithm is shown in Fig. 20.3. For children with an HLA-identical sibling, the treatment of choice is allogeneic BMT. For those without a sibling marrow donor, an alternative donor should be sought, although the decision to transplant may be difficult if a well matched donor is not available and in this situation α-interferon may be a useful option.

α-Interferon

α-Interferon (IFN-α) was first introduced as treatment for CML in adults in the early 1980s.[50] There have been 7 large randomized trials of interferon in CML involving >2000 patients.[51] Some of these trials and other published studies have included children but the results for children have not been separately analyzed. Nevertheless, it seems unlikely that there is any significant difference between the response of children to IFN-α compared to the response of young adults (<30 years).

In adults the overall response rate is 70%, with around 20% of patients achieving a major or complete cytogenetic response.[51] While the majority of those destined to respond cytogenetically do so within 6 months of starting IFN-α, in a small proportion it takes up to 2 years for a response to become apparent. There is now overwhelming evidence that patients who achieve a complete cytogenetic response to IFN-α live longer than those treated with hydroxyurea.[52] It is not clear, however, whether those with a minor response or

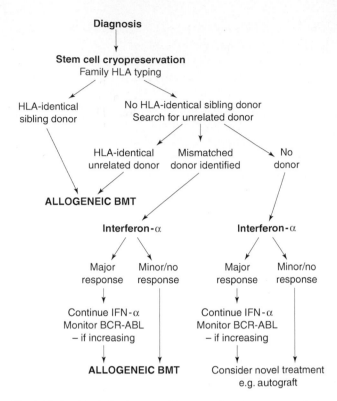

Fig. 20.3 Algorithm indicating a possible approach to the management of a newly diagnosed child with ATCML. A major response to interferon-α is one in which there is complete cytogenetic remission. BMT = bone marrow transplantation.

non-responders have any survival advantage with IFN-α compared to conventional cytotoxic drugs. The role of IFN-α in the management of children with ATCML is also not clear since allogeneic BMT is the treatment of choice for all those with an HLA-identical donor (Fig. 20.3). However, IFN-α may well be the best option for the small group of children with no suitable donor or for whom BMT is delayed >6–12 months after diagnosis.

Mode of action

The mechanism of action of IFN-α in ATCML is not fully understood. It is clear that IFN-α reduces cellular proliferation and in CML and ATCML it may exert its beneficial effects by directly inhibiting the proliferation of progenitor cells or by facilitating their programed cell death. IFN-α also seems to play a role, at least *in vitro*, in modulating the abnormal progenitor cell-stromal cell interactions characteristic of CML cells, leading to their growth arrest and selective repopulation of the marrow with normal progenitors.[27,28] Finally, IFN may have immunomodulatory effects which enhance cellular antigen presentation, leading to increased recognition of CML cells in affected patients. In addition to these direct effects of IFN-α on CML cells, it seems likely that a response to IFN-α identifies a group of patients with an inherently better prognosis.

Dose

IFN-α is generally started once the white cell count has been brought under control (5–10 × 10^9/l) using hydroxyurea. The standard starting dose in adults is 3 mega units (MU) daily by subcutaneous injection; this is also the dose used in most published series including children. The dose of IFN-α should be adjusted after the first few weeks of treatment to maintain the white cell count between 2 and 5 × 10^9/l. In fact, the optimal dose of IFN-α has yet to be established; since at least one study has suggested that higher doses may be associated with a higher response rate, this question is currently being investigated in the UK in adults with CML in the CML V MRC trial.

Duration of treatment

This is controversial. Response to IFN-α is usually assessed both by hematologic parameters and by assessing marrow cytogenetics at 3–6-month intervals. It normally takes at least 6 months to determine whether patients are going to show a major cytogenetic response to IFN-α. It therefore seems appropriate to continue IFN-α in all patients with an hematologic response for at least 6 months. For children who have only had a minor cytogenetic response (<30% Ph negative), or no response by 6 months, it is unlikely that continuing IFN-α will confer a survival advantage. In these children, allogeneic BMT or cord blood transplantation with the best donor available is the treatment of choice. Finally, there is a small group of patients who initially have a good partial cytogenetic response and for whom it may take 2 years or more to assess whether they will achieve a complete cytogenetic response. There is a case for continuing IFN-α in such children for 2 years and proceeding to BMT if a complete cytogenetic remission has not been achieved after 2 years.

Monitoring the level of *BCR-ABL* transcripts[53,54] may in future prove to be helpful in guiding the duration of therapy since there are preliminary data to suggest that rising numbers of transcripts in IFN-α responders who are 100% Ph-negative may herald relapse to chronic-phase disease or acceleration. For those patients for whom BMT was not the first choice, this may allow time to proceed to BMT (allogeneic or autologous) without the vastly reduced chance of success normally associated with BMT carried out where there is conventional laboratory evidence of disease acceleration or transformation.

Side-effects

The commonest complaints are of flu-like symptoms (including fever, chills, rigors, headache, muscle aches and malaise), which usually occur during the first 2 weeks of treatment. In the majority of patients, the symptoms resolve completely on continuing therapy; however, it may be helpful to administer the IFN-α just before bed-time and to give a dose of paracetamol half an hour beforehand, particularly if fever is a prominent feature. Convulsions in association with fever have also occasionally been reported in children treated with IFN-α. If symptoms persist, and are intolerable despite ameliorative measures, dosage reduction may be considered. Other side-effects include lethargy, depression, alopecia, myelosuppression, anorexia, weight loss, abnormal liver function and autoimmune phenomena (idiopathic thrombocytopenic purpura, hypothyroidism and hemolytic anemia).

Combination treatment

The significant improvement in survival of patients who achieve a complete cytogenetic response to IFN-α has led to the suggestion that combination treatment of IFN-α with chemotherapy might further improve the response rate and/ or prolong survival. Recent data from a French multicenter study[55] in which adult patients were randomized to IFN-α with or without cytosine arabinoside suggested that this combination can prolong survival; the 3-year survival in the IFN-cytarabine group was 86% compared to 79% for the IFN group. This difference appeared to be due to an increased proportion of patients achieving a major or complete cytogenetic response in the combination group at 12 months: 41% in the IFN-cytarabine group versus 24% in the IFN group. If these results are confirmed, this approach, perhaps combined with autologous BMT, may provide a reasonable alternative for those children unable to undergo allogeneic BMT.

Allogeneic bone marrow transplantation

Allogeneic BMT remains the only curative treatment for ATCML. For those children with an HLA-identical sibling donor, BMT is the treatment of choice and if carried out within a year of diagnosis should be associated with a long-term leukemia-free survival of 80–90%.[56,57] For children without an HLA-identical sibling, BMT from an alternative donor should also be considered at an early stage since alternative strategies, such as IFN-α, are associated with a 5-year survival of 60% at best.[50] Data from the largest series of children transplanted for ACTML supports this view.[58] This recent analysis of transplants on >500 children with ACTML reported to the European Group for Blood and Marrow Transplantation (EBMT) found that for the 78 children transplanted in first chronic phase overall survival and leukemia-free survival after BMT from volunteer unrelated donors were 64% and 60%, respectively.[58] Recent advances in fertility treatment mean that it is important to consider the feasibility of cryopreservation of sperm or ovarian/testicular tissue in all children prior to myeloablative therapy since the vast majority of such children would otherwise become infertile.

Timing

In recommending the optimum timing for BMT a number of factors need to be considered. For children with an HLA-identical sibling, the data from 2 large adult series suggest that there is likely to be a survival advantage in undergoing BMT within a year of diagnosis.[45,57,59] This also reduces the time interval in which transformation to accelerated phase or blast crisis may occur since around 10% of children progress to more advanced disease within a year of diagnosis. The principal disadvantage of early BMT is that it remains a hazardous procedure with an average transplant-related mortality of around 10–20% in patients <20 years old.[56] Nevertheless, since the risks of BMT are directly related to age,[45,59] and since the biology of ATCML is still impossible to predict accurately, the evidence favors offering BMT to all children with sibling donors within the first year.

The timing of BMT in children without an HLA-identical sibling is much more difficult since transplant-related mortality is likely to be higher with an alternative donor, even in children (25–40%).[58,60,61] For those with an HLA-compatible donor matched at the molecular level, BMT remains the treatment of choice since leukemia-free survival is currently 50–75% for young patients transplanted early.[58,60,62,63] However, for those without an HLA-identical alternative donor, one approach is to be guided by the IFN-α response as outlined in Fig. 20.3. For children who show a complete cytogenetic response, although BMT is the only curative option, the survival rate 5 years after diagnosis is likely to be higher with IFN-α (60%) than BMT from a mismatched donor (~40%).[50,64] Therefore, for these children, delaying BMT would be reasonable, particularly if there was some way of predicting acceleration/transformation from chronic phase disease. Preliminary evidence suggests that serial quantitative RT-PCR for *BCR-ABL* may allow acceleration to be detected and this would help to guide the timing of BMT.[54,65]

Finally, for the unfortunate group of children who are non-responders or poor responders to IFN-α and who have no HLA-identical donors, BMT with a mismatched donor needs to be considered since overall long-term survival following BMT would be be predicted to be superior to IFN-α (5-year survival in non-responders is 30–40%).[66]

Conditioning

Early experience showed that the combination of high-dose cyclophosphamide and total body irradiation (TBI) is an effective conditioning regimen for cure of CML in adults and children.[45,59,67,68] This regimen is still used by many centers. However, more recent results indicate an equivalent anti-leukemic efficacy for cyclophosphamide in combination with busulfan,[56,69] thus eliminating the need for radiotherapy. Experience suggests that this regimen is more convenient and better tolerated. Long-term toxicity may also be less than with TBI regimens, although this has not yet been established.

The issue of the need for splenic radiation has now been addressed. There appears to be no benefit of additional splenic irradiation where the spleen is small or impalpable.[70] In accelerated phase or blast crisis where there is significant splenomegaly (>5 cm), splenectomy prior to BMT may enable the disease to be controlled better and will facilitate engraftment, although there is no effect on overall survival.[71]

Donors

Since only around 25% of children will have a compatible sibling donor, a number of alternative approaches has been explored for those without such donors, including HLA-identical unrelated marrow donors, cord blood donors and mismatched family donors.[60–62,64,72–76] In chronic phase, 2 major factors which determine the outcome of BMT from these alternative donors are the cytomegalovirus (CMV) status and the degree of HLA disparity, survival being better in CMV-negative patients and those with no detectable mismatches of the HLA class I or II genes using molecular subtyping.[62,64] Thus, the donor characteristics may well influence the timing of BMT; BMT using a CMV-positive donor with disparity at 1 or 2 major HLA loci is likely to be an unattractive option for most patients while a good cytogenetic response to IFN-α is sustained.

Graft-versus-host disease

Graft-versus-host disease (GVHD) remains an important cause of transplant-related mortality and morbidity and there are several approaches to its prevention and treatment. However, it appears that in CML more than any other hematologic malignancy the occurence and clinical behavior of GVHD mediated by allogeneic donor cells is intimately linked with the 'graft-versus- leukemia' (GVL) effect of the donor cells.[77–79] While it is not yet known whether these two processes are mediated by the same or distinct cell types or subtypes, it is clear that the need to maintain an effective GVL effect of allogeneic donor cells has a major impact on the choice of regimen employed to prevent GVHD after BMT for CML and ATCML. Broadly, the two approaches to GVHD prevention are T-cell depletion and pharmacologic immunosuppression.

T-cell depletion. A number of methods of T-cell depletion have been employed in CML. These include *ex vivo* T-cell depletion of donor marrow using monoclonal antibodies (e.g. anti-CD6, anti-CD8, anti-CD2 or CD52 [Campath-1M]), counterflow elutriation or soybean lectin agglutination and *in vivo* T-cell depletion by intravenous infusion of antibodies such as Campath-1H.[62,63,80–82] There is a large amount of data on the impact of T-cell depletion on the outcome of BMT for CML in adults; many of these trials have included children and it is likely that the conclusions from the adult studies apply also to pediatric practice. The principal benefit of T-cell depletion is that it is highly effective in reducing the incidence and severity of GVHD both from HLA-matched siblings and alternative donors.[63] However, the benefits of T-cell depletion are achieved at the expense of a significantly increased rate of early graft rejection and relapse of CML.[83,84] The rate of relapse after sibling transplants may be as high as 60%[82,85] and this has led several groups to abandon T-cell depletion in favor of immunosuppression, particularly in patients under 20 years of age who have a lower incidence of severe GVHD. The clear association between a low rate of GVHD and a high rate of relapse after BMT for CML (and *vice versa*) provides strong clinical evidence for the GVL effect of allogeneic T cells[33,34,82] and has led to the development of a number of possible strategies to prevent GVHD without sacrificing important elements of GVL (see below).

Immunosuppression. There is clear evidence that combination treatment with cyclosporin A and methotrexate is, apart from T-cell depletion, the most effective way of preventing GVHD.[47,86] Most regimens combine short-course methotrexate during the first 2 weeks after BMT with 6–12 months' maintenance treatment with oral cyclosporin. Acute GVHD still develops in around 30% of children treated with these regimens but in the majority of cases this is mild and responds to topical or low-dose steroids. In children who develop GVHD of >grade II severity the treatment of choice is high-dose steroids usually by the intravenous route.

Graft-versus-leukemia effect

As mentioned above, GVL and GVHD are closely linked and it seems likely that similar mechanisms control both processes.[77] In GVHD, donor T cells recognize antigens presented by major histocompatiblity complex molecules on recipient cells (in skin, gut, biliary tree, etc.) leading to the clinical features of acute and chronic GVHD. In GVL, donor T cells instead suppress or eradicate residual leukemia. The target antigens for the GVL effect have not been identified but they are likely to include not only leukemia-specific antigens (e.g. *BCR-ABL*), but also minor histocompatability antigens expressed either ubiquitously or in a tissue-restricted fashion (e.g. those on normal lymphoid or myeloid cells).[77,78] The effector T cells which mediate GVL are now known from clinical studies and *in vitro* experiments to be mainly CD4$^+$ T cells, rather than CD8$^+$ T cells.[87,88] It seems likely that dendritic cells also play an important role in presenting target antigens to enhance the alloreactive T-cell response and so increase the GVL effect.[89] Despite the uncertainities about the exact mechanisms involved in the GVL effect, clinical protocols which utilize the GVL activity of donor T cells are already in widespread

use in the treatment of children and adults with leukemia relapsing after BMT, particularly for CML.[79,88,90–93]

Outcome

Both the International Bone Marrow Transplant Registry (IBMTR) and the European Group for Blood and Marrow Transplant (EBMT) have collected outcome data on several 1000 patients with CML, around 10% of whom were <20 years old at the time of BMT.[45,58,64,83,94] The largest analysis of outcome for children transplanted for ATCML was recently reported by the EBMT Chronic Leukaemia Working Party. A total of 559 transplants had been carried out in patients <18 years over the period 1982–1998. Overall survival and leukemia-free survival for patients transplanted in first chronic phase from an HLA-identical sibling are 74% and 66%, respectively, 3 years after BMT.[58] The outcome for patients transplanted with marrow from volunteer unrelated donors is very similar: in first chronic phase the 3-year survival and leukemia-free survival are around 64% and 60%, respectively, for patients <18 years.[58]

In advanced-phase disease, leukemia-free survival from sibling or unrelated donors is considerably less. The poorest outcome is for those transplanted in blast crisis for whom the chance of long-term survival is 10–20%.[58,94,95] For accelerated-phase disease, the Seattle group have reported 4-year leukemia-free survival of 43% in 58 patients with a wide age range (6–59 years) transplanted using marrow from HLA-identical siblings.[96] Similar results using sibling donors, also in a wide age group (1–57 years), were recently reported by the IBMTR[95] and the EBMT study in children which found a 3-year overall survival of 36% and leukemia-free survival of 26% for children transplanted in accelerated phase from HLA-identical siblings.[58] Unrelated donor marrow transplantation for accelerated phase remains a worthwhile therapeutic option since leukemia-free survival of around 30% is consistently reported by a number of groups, including the 2 series in children.[58,59,61,62,94]

Prognostic factors

The principal factors determining outcome after transplant from an HLA-identical sibling are:

- phase of ATCML at the time of transplant with the best results in chronic phase and the worst in accelerated phase and blast crisis;[58,96]
- interval between diagnosis and BMT with the best results in those transplanted within 1 year of diagnosis;[45,57]
- age at the time of BMT with young patients faring better than those >30 years of age.[97,98]

Other factors contributing to outcome include: *ex vivo* T-cell depletion (increased relapse)[82,85] and the presence/severity of GVHD (best outcome in those with Grade I rather than those with either higher grades of GVHD or no GVHD).[98,99]

For patients transplanted using marrow from alternative donors, the principal factors determining outcome are:

- phase of ATCML at the time of transplant;
- age at the time of BMT with young patients again faring better;
- CMV serologic status of the patient, the survival of CMV-negative patients being significantly higher;
- degree of HLA disparity, survival being better in those with no detectable mismatches of the HLA class I or II genes using molecular subtyping.[62,64]

Management of relapse

Although the majority of patients who relapse after BMT do so into chronic-phase ATCML, a small proportion relapse straight into blast crisis. The options for managing relapse into chronic phase are: donor lymphocyte infusion (DLI), second BMT and IFN-α.

For those children with a sibling donor, the best option is DLI followed, if unsuccessful, by a second transplant unless there has been substantial transplant-related morbidity following the first (e.g. significant pulmonary, liver or renal impairment).[100–102] The available literature suggests that the second procedure should be delayed for at least 12 months after the first to reduce transplant-related mortality.[100] For children conditioned with busulfan/cyclophosphamide for the first transplant, a TBI regimen may be preferable for the second, although there is no definite evidence of greater antileukemic efficacy; for those who received TBI for the first transplant, second transplants with busulfan alone have been successful.[101] However, there is little information in the literature to guide the clinician.

Where there is relapse into chronic phase after an unrelated donor transplant for ATCML, DLI is also the treatment of choice using lymphocytes from the original bone marrow donor. Where this is not possible, or where DLI is unsuccessful, the choice lies with a second transplant from an alternative donor or IFN-α. Since the morbidity and mortality of a second transplant are likely to be high, the decision must be made on an individual patient basis; it is clearly difficult and will be influenced by many factors including previous BMT course, current health and IFN-responsiveness.

For children who relapse into blast crisis, particularly myeloid blast crisis, following BMT the outlook is often, but not always, bleak. The management is that for blast crisis (see below). If chronic-phase disease is re-established, consideration should be given to DLI if donor cells remain detectable, or a second BMT where there is no evidence of residual donor cells.

Donor lymphocyte infusion. Since the first successful reports of DLI to treat leukemia relapsing after BMT in 1990, this approach has become part of the routine management of this difficult problem.[79,88,90–93] DLI

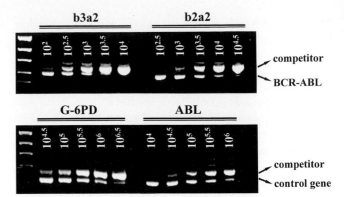

Fig. 20.4 Examples of competitive RT-PCR in peripheral blood leukocytes from CML patients: ethidium bromide-stained agarose gels for quantification of *BCR-ABL* (b3a2 and b2a2 junctions) and of G6PD and ABL transcripts as internal controls. Serial dilutions of a linearized competitor were added to fixed amounts of patient cDNA. The number of competitor molecules added is shown above each track. The equivalence point, at which competitor and sample bands have the same intensity, can be estimated by visual inspection or, more accurately, by densitometry. This point permits calculation of the number of target-transcript molecules in the sample per unit-volume of cDNA. Kindly provided by Junia Melo.

appears to be particularly successful in CML. There is a variety of protocols but all involve infusion of donor lymphocytes at intervals following BMT where there is evidence of recurrence of CML either manifest as overt hematologic relapse or occult relapse at the cytogenetic or molecular level (persistent and rising numbers of BCR-ABL mRNA transcripts detectable on serial blood samples by RT-PCR; Fig. 20.4).

There is good evidence that the success rate of DLI is higher where there is molecular or cytogenetic relapse rather than hematologic relapse and therefore DLI should be considered as soon as any measure of recurrent disease is detected and recommended where there is evidence of disease progression.[91,93] Overall the response rate is around 90% and 70% for patients treated in molecular/cytogenetic and hematologic relapse, respectively.[79,91–93] For those patients who respond, the response is usually apparent by 3–6 months after DLI. Unfortunately for patients relapsing into blast crisis, the outlook has been poor since with no successful responses to this approach, although a current EBMT study is investigating the effect of adding IFN-α and/or chemotherapy.

While DLI has an established role in re-inducing complete remission and long-term cure, it also has significant side-effects. GVHD of > grade II severity occurs in around 10% of patients treated in molecular/cytogenetic relapse and in ~40% of patients treated in hematologic relapse. It may be fatal, although in most cases it responds to re-institution of cyclosporin A ± steroids. Prolonged or irreversible aplasia also occurs in around 25% of patients treated in hematologic relapse but has not been seen in patients treated in molecular/cytogenetic relapse. The preliminary data suggest that not only is DLI less successful if patients are treated in hematologic relapse, but it is also associated with greater risks of GVHD and marrow hypoplasia which may need to be followed by a further donor stem cell 'top up'.

Autologous bone marrow transplantation

Whilst the exact role of autologous BMT for CML is still unclear, in adults there is considerable experience in the use of autologous stem cells.[104–106] The role of autologous stem cells in the treatment of CML is being actively investigated, including a MRC trial and EBMT studies. However, there are no data on this approach in children. Of the 559 transplants for ATCML in children reported to the EMBT since 1982, only 30 were autologous transplants and no data on the outcome of this small group of children have been published.[58]

ACCELERATED-PHASE ATCML AND BLAST CRISIS

Accelerated-phase ATCML

The management of accelerated-phase depends both upon the nature of any previous treatment and the specific problems experienced by the child. Any child who develops evidence of acceleration while awaiting BMT should be transplanted at the earliest opportunity; hydroxyurea, 6-TG or 6-MP are usually the most useful drugs for disease control until the transplant is carried out. For children who have been transplanted and relapse into advanced phase, DLI is usually ineffective[79,91,92] and a second BMT is likely to offer the best prospect of long-term survival.

The commonest manifestations of accelerated-phase disease are splenomegaly and thrombocytosis. Splenectomy is indicated for massive splenomegaly and, if BMT is planned, should preferably be carried out at least 6 weeks beforehand. Routine splenectomy and splenic irradiation prior to BMT are no longer recommended as they have not been shown to improve survival. On the other hand, if moderate splenomegaly is present prior to BMT, then splenic irradiation should be included in the conditioning protocol. Thrombocytosis may be difficult to control since it is often resistant to hydroxyurea and busulfan or the doses required lead to unacceptable leukopenia. Fortunately, even platelet counts in excess of 1000×10^9/l are usually well tolerated and are rarely associated with thrombosis or hemorrhage in children.[107] Where thrombocytosis is resistant to oral chemotherapy, particularly if there are associated clinical problems, interferon is often effective. A possible alternative might be anagrelide which has been used in adults and children for the treatment of primary proliferative thrombocytosis.[108]

Lymphoid blast crisis

The approach to treatment of lymphoid blast crisis of CML in children is very similar to that of ALL. Remission induction with vincristine and steroids is successful in the majority of children.[39,109] For those with a bone marrow donor (either related or unrelated), allogeneic BMT is the treatment of choice following remission induction. For children in whom it is possible to proceed straight to BMT, further chemotherapy prior to BMT should not be necessary. In most cases, however, BMT is likely to be delayed for a few months and in this situation some form of intensification chemotherapy should be given as in childhood ALL protocols, followed by maintenance if there is a prolonged delay. The most appropriate CNS-directed treatment for such children is not clear. It seems wise to give regular intrathecal methotrexate as is standard in most ALL protocols, but for children proceeding to BMT cranial irradiation and high dose methotrexate should be avoided to reduce toxicity.

Where no HLA-identical marrow donors can be identified, there are 3 main options: BMT from a mismatched donor, cord-blood transplantation and maintenance chemotherapy as for ALL. The last option is never curative since those children achieving complete remission of lymphoid blast crisis return to chronic-phase ATCML and will inevitably relapse. This must be balanced against the potentially severe morbidity and relatively high mortality[60,62,64] of BMT where there is a disparity of >1 HLA antigen. Nevertheless, survival after mismatched BMT in second chronic-phase CML for patients <20 years is likely to be 25–40%.[61,62,72]

An alternative option is cord-blood transplantation where preliminary data suggested that it was possible to achieve a reasonable rate of engraftment without severe GVHD in a substantial proportion of children with leukemia even with a disparity of 2 or 3 antigens.[73] Recent analysis suggests that the outcome of such transplants for CML may be less good (P Rubinstein, personal communication). However, the number of patients is small and the size of the cord-blood bank registries is growing rapidly which should enhance the chances of identifying a well-matched donor and improve the outcome for children without HLA-identical sibling donors.

Myeloid blast crisis

The remission rate for myeloid blast crisis remains poor, even with the most recent AML-type chemotherapy regimens and, in contrast to lymphoid blast crisis, vincristine and steroids are of little benefit. Most centers, including the Hammersmith Hospital, use combination chemotherapy similar to that for AML and including daunorubicin or mitoxantrone, cytosine arabinoside and etoposide or thioguanine. Children who show a complete or good partial remission should proceed to BMT (or cord blood transplantation) as soon as possible since the median survival is only 6 months even in those who respond to chemotherapy. Where allogeneic BMT is not possible, autologous BMT may have a role in prolonging survival; 'mini' autografts

413

using intermediate-dose busulfan have been carried out in adults with advanced-phase CML and appear to prolong survival with acceptable morbidity and most of the procedure can be carried out on an outpatient basis.[110]

FUTURE DIRECTIONS

Since ATCML is a stem cell disorder, successful therapy will continue to require elimination of all of the CML clone or at least reduction in the CML clone to levels barely detectable by current techniques (around 1 in 10^5 cells). It is likely that low levels of disease can persist for long peroids, and possibly indefinitely, clonal expansion being prevented by the patient's own immune response. For these reasons, stem cell transplantation will remain the principal therapeutic approach to ATCML and improvement in the outcome of the disease in children will most likely derive from progress in stem cell transplantation, particularly advances in donor matching, GVHD prevention and treatment, management of CMV infection and increased understanding of the GVL response. In adults with CML, where a significant proportion of patients is >50 years old and the risks of allogeneic transplantation may be too great, most attention is currently focused on autografting using novel strategies to remove Ph-positive cells.

Acknowledgements

We are grateful to Andy Chase for providing Figure 1a, Junio Melo for Figures 1b, 2, 9 and David Swirsky for many of the morphology slides.

REFERENCES

1. Grier HE, Civin CI. Acute and chronic myeloproliferative disorders and myelodysplasia. In: Nathan DG, Oski FA (eds) *Hematology of Infancy and Childhood*. Philadelphia: WB Saunders, 1992, p 1289
2. Cartwright RA, Alexander FE, McKinney PA *et al*. *Leukaemia and Lymphoma. An Atlas of Distribution within Areas of England and Wales. 1984–88*. London: Leukaemia Research Fund, 1990
3. Altman AJ. Chronic leukemias of childhood. *Pediatr Clin N Am* 1988; **35**: 765–787
4. Finch SC, Linet MS. Chronic leukaemias. *Clin Haematol* 1982; **5**: 27–56.
5. Tokuhata GK, Neely CL, Williams DL. Chronic myelocytic leukemia in identical twins and a sibling. *Blood* 1968; **31**: 216–225
6. Preston DL, Kusumi S, Tomonaga M *et al*. Cancer incidence in atomic bomb survivors. Part III: leukaemia, lymphoma and multiple myeloma, 1950–1987. *Radiation Res* 1994; **137**: 68–97
7. Nowell PC, Hungerford DA. A minute chromosome in human granulocytic leukemia. *Science* 1960; **132**: 1497–1501
8. Rowley JD. A new consistent abnormality in chronic myelogenous leukaemia. *Nature* 1982; **243**: 290–291
9. DeKlein A, Van Kessel AG, Grosveld G *et al*. A cellular oncogene is translocated to the Philadelphia chromosome in chronic myelocytic leukaemia. *Nature* 1982; **300**: 765–767
10. Kurzrock R, Gutterman JU, Talpaz M. The molecular genetics of Philadelphia chromosome-positive leukemias. *N Engl J Med* 1988; **319**: 990–998
11. Chissoe SL, Bodenteich A, Wang YF *et al*. Sequence and analysis of the human ABL gene, the BCR gene, and regions involved in the Philadelphia chromosomal translocation. *Genomics* 1995; **27**: 67–82
12. Melo JV. The molecular biology of chronic myeloid leukemia. *Leukemia* 1996; **10**: 751–756
13. Lugo TG, Pendergast AM, Muller AJ, Witte ON. Tyrosine kinase activity and transformation potency of bcr-abl oncogene products. *Science* 1990; **247**: 1079–1082
14. Daley GQ, Van Etten RA, Baltimore D. Induction of chronic myelogenous leukemia in mice by the P210bcr/abl gene of the Philadelphia chromosome. *Science* 1990; **247**: 824–830
15. Kelliher MA, McLaughlin J, Witte ON, Rosenberg N. Induction of chronic myelogenous leukemia-like syndrome in mice with v-abl and BCR-ABL. *Proc Natl Acad Sci USA* 1990; **87**: 6649–6653
16. Vickers M. Estimation of the number of mutations necessary to cause chronic myeloid leukaemia from epidemiological data. *Br J Haematol* 1996; **94**: 1–4
17. Melo JV, Gordon DE, Cross NC, Goldman JM. The ABL-BCR fusion gene is expressed in chronic myeloid leukemia. *Blood* 1993; **81**: 158–165
18. Melo JV. The diversity of BCR-ABL fusion proteins and their relationship to leukemia phenotype. *Blood* 1996; **88**: 2375–2384
19. Sawyers C. Signal transduction pathways involved in BCR-ABL transformation. *Baillière's Clin Haematol* 1997; **10**: 223–231
20. Sawyers CL, McLaughlin J, Witte O. Genetic requirement for Ras in the transformation of fibroblasts and hematopoietic cells by the Bcr-Abl oncogene. *J Exp Med* 1995; **181**: 307–313
21. Cortez D, Stoica G, Pierce JH, Pendergast AM. The BCR-ABL tyrosine kinase inhibits apoptosis by activating a Ras-dependent signalling pathway. *Oncogene* 1996; **13**: 2589–2594
22. Mandanas RA, Leibowitz DS, Gharehbaghi K *et al*. Role of p21 RAS in bcr/abl transformation of murine myeloid cells. *Blood* 1993; **82**: 1838–1847
23. Jonas D, Lubbert M, Kawasaki ES *et al*. Clonal analysis of bcr-abl rearrangement in T lymphocytes from patients with chronic myelogenous leukemia. *Blood* 1992; **79**: 1017–1023
24. Raskind W, Ferraris AM, Najfeld V, Jacobson RH, Moohr JW, Fialkow PJ. Further evidence for the existence of a clonal Ph-negative stage in some cases of Ph-positive chronic myelocytic leukemia. *Leukemia* 1993; **7**: 1163–1167
25. Eaves CJ, Eaves AC. Stem cell kinetics. *Baillière's Clin Haematol* 1997; **10**: 233–257
26. Gordon MY, Goldman JM. Cellular and molecular mechanisms in chronic myeloid leukaemia: biology and treatment. *Br J Haematol* 1996; **95**: 10–20
27. Bedi A, Zehnbauer BA, Barber J *et al*. Inhibition of apoptosis by BCR-ABL in chronic myeloid leukemia. *Blood* 1994; **83**: 2038–2044.
28. Gordon MY, Dowding CR, Riley GP, Goldman JM, Greaves MF. Altered adhesive interactions with marrow stroma of haematopoietic progenitor cells in chronic myeloid leukaemia. *Nature* 1987; **328**: 342–344
29. Harihan IK, Adams JM, Cory S. BCR-ABL oncogene renders myeloid cell line factor-independent: potential autocrine mechanism in chronic myeloid leukemia. *Oncogene Res* 1988; **3**: 387–399
30. Sirard C, Laneuville P, Dick J. Expression of bcr-abl abrogates factor-dependent growth of human hematopoietic MO7E cells by an autocrine mechanism. *Blood* 1994; **83**: 1575–1585
31. Castro-Malaspina H, Schaison G, Briere J *et al*. Philadelphia chromosome positive chronic myelocytic leukemia in children. Survival and prognostic factors. *Cancer* 1983; **52**: 721–727
32. Rowe JM, Lichtman MA. Hyperleukocytosis and leukostasis: common features of childhood chronic myelogenous leukemia. *Blood* 1984; **63**: 1230–1234
33. Mitelman F. The cytogenetic scenario of chronic myeloid leukemia. *Leukemia Lymphoma* 1993; **11**: 11–15
34. Seong DC, Kantarjian HM, Ro JY *et al*. 'Hypermetaphase FISH' for quantitative monitoring of Philadelphia chromosome positive cells in

chronic myelogenous leukemia patients during treatment. *Blood* 1995; **86**: 2343–2349

35. van de Plas DC, Grosveld G, Hagermeijer A. Review of clinical, cytogenetic and molecular aspects of Ph-negative CML. *Cancer Genet Cytogenet* 1991; **52**: 143–156

36. Majlis A, Smith TL, Talpaz M *et al*. Significance of cytogenetic clonal evolution in chronic myelogenous leukemia. *J Clin Oncol* 1996; **14**: 196–203

37. Kantarjian HM, Keating MJ, Talpaz M *et al*. Chronic myelogenous leukemia in blast crisis. *Am J Med* 1987; **83**: 445–454

38. Ruff P, Saragas E, Poulos M, Weaving A. Patterns of clonal evolution in transformed chronic myelogenous leukemia. *Cancer Genet Cytogenet* 1995; **81**: 182–184

39. Janossy G, Woodruff RK, Pippard AJ *et al*. Relation of "lymphoid" phenotype and response to chemotherapy incorporating vincristine-prednisolone in the acute phase of Ph′-positive leukemia. *Cancer* 1979; **43**: 426–434.

40. Sawyers C. The role of MYC in transformation by BCR-ABL. *Leukemia Lymphoma* 1993; **11**: 45–46

41. Feinstein E, Cimino G, Gale RP *et al*. p53 in chronic myelogenous leukemia in acute phase. *Proc Natl Acad Sci USA* 1991; **88**: 6293–6297

42. Ahuja HG, Jat PS, Foti A, Bar-Eli M, Cline MJ. Abnormalities of the retinoblastoma gene in the pathogenesis of acute leukemia. *Blood* 1991; **78**: 3259–3268

43. Sill H, Goldman JM, Cross NCP. Homozygous deletions of the p16 tumor suppressor gene are associated with lymphoid transformation of chronic myeloid leukemia. *Blood* 1995; **85**: 2013–2016

44. Mitani K, Ogawa S, Tanaka T *et al*. Generation of the AML-EVI1 fusion gene in the t(3;21)(q26;q22) causes blastic crisis in chronic myelocytic leukaemia. *EMBO J* 1994; **13**: 504–510

45. Goldman JM, Szydlo R, Horowitz MM *et al*. Choice of pre-transplant treatment and timing of transplants for chronic myelogenous leukemia in chronic phase. *Blood* 1993; **82**: 2235–2238

46. Goldman JM. Management of chronic myeloid leukaemia. *Blood Rev* 1994; **8**: 21–29

47. Spencer A, O'Brien SG, Goldman JM. Chronic myeloid leukemia—options for therapy. *Br J Haematol* 1995; **91**: 2–7

48. Kantarjian HM, O'Brien S, Anderlini P, Talpaz M. Treatment of chronic myelogenous leukemia: current status and investigational options. *Blood* 1996; **87**: 3069–3081

49. Goldman JM. Optimizing treatment for chronic myeloid leukemia. *N Engl J Med* 1997; **337**: 270–271

50. Kantarjian HM, Smith TI, O'Brien S, Beran M, Pierce S, Talpaz M. Prolonged survival in chronic myelogenous leukemia after cyto-genetic response to interferon-α therapy. *Ann Intern Med* 1995; **122**: 254–261

51. Richards SM. Interferon-α: results from randomized trials. *Baillière's Clin Haematol* 1997; **10**: 307–318

52. The Italian Cooperative Study Group on Chronic Myeloid Leukemia. Interferon alfa 2a as compared with conventional chemotherapy for the treatment of chronic myeloid leukemia. *N Engl J Med* 1994; **330**: 820–825

53. Cross NCP, Lin F, Chase A *et al*. Competitive polymerase chain reaction to estimate the number of BCR-ABL transcripts in chronic myeloid leukemia patients after bone marrow transplantation. *Blood* 1993; **6**: 1929–1936

54. Hochhaus A, Lin F, Reiter A *et al*. Quantification of residual disease in chronic myelogenous leukemia on interferon-α therapy by competitive polymerase chain reaction. *Blood* 1996; **87**: 1549–1555

55. Guilhot F, Chastang C, Michallet M *et al*. Interferon alfa-2b combined with cytarabine versus interferon alone in chronic myelogenous leukemia. *N Engl J Med* 1997; **337**: 223–229

56. Clift RA, Buckner CD, Thomas ED *et al*. Marrow transplantation for chronic myeloid leukemia: a randomized study comparing cyclophos-phamide and total body irradiation with busulfan and cyclophos-phamide. *Blood* 1994; **84**: 2036–2043

57. Thomas ED, Clift RA, Fefer A *et al*. Marrow transplantation for the treatment of chronic myelogenous leukemia. *Ann Intern Med* 1986; **104**: 155–163

58. Roberts IAG, Niethammer D, van Biezen A *et al*. Outcome of transplant for children with adult type CML (ATCML). *Bone Marrow Transplant* 1988; **21 (Suppl 1)**: S85

59. Enright H, Daniels K, Arthur DC *et al*. Related donor marrow transplant for chronic myeloid leukemia: patient characteristics predictive of outcome. *Bone Marrow Transplant* 17: 537–542

60. Balduzzi A, Gooley T, Anasetti C *et al*. Unrelated donor marrow transplantation in children. *Blood* 1995; **86**: 3247–3256

61. Dini G, Rondelli R, Miano M *et al*. Unrelated-donor bone marrow transplantation for Philadelphia chromosome-positive chronic myelo-genous leukemia in children: experience in eight European countries. *Bone Marrow Transplant* 1996; **18 (Suppl 2)**: 80–85

62. Spencer A, Szydlo R, Brookes PA *et al*. Bone marrow transplantation for chronic myeloid leukemia with volunteer unrelated donors using *ex vivo* or *in vivo* T-cell depletion: major prognostic impact of HLA Class I identity between donor and recipient. *Blood* 1995; **86**: 3590–3597

63. Drobyski WR, Ash RC, Casper JT *et al*. Effect of T-cell depletion as graft-versus-host disease prophylaxis on engraftment, relapse, and disease-free survival in unrelated marrow transplantation for chronic myelogenous leukemia. *Blood* 1994; **83**: 1980–1987

64. Devergie A, Madrigal A, Apperley JF *et al*. European results of matched unrelated donor bone marrow transplantation for chronic myeloid leukemia. Impact of HLA Class II matching. *Bone Marrow Transplant* 1997; **20**: 11–20

65. Gaiger A, Henn T, Horth E *et al*. Increase of BCR-ABL chimeric mRNA expression in tumor cells of patients with chronic myeloid leukemia precedes disease progression. *Blood* 1995; **86**: 2371–2378

66. Talpaz M, Kantarjian HM, O'Brien S, Kurzrock R. The MD Anderson Cancer Center experience with interferon-α therapy in chronic myelogenous leukemia. *Baillière's Clin Haematol* 1997; **10**: 291–305

67. Goldman JM, Apperley JF, Jones L *et al*. Bone marrow transplant-tion for patients with chronic myeloid leukemia. *N Engl J Med* 1986; **314**: 202–207

68. Clift RA, Buckner CD, Appelbaum FR *et al*. Allogeneic marrow transplantation in patients with chronic myeloid leukemia in chronic phase. A randomized trial of two irradiation regimens. *Blood* 1991; **77**: 1660–65

69. Devergie A, Blaise D, Attal M *et al*. Allogeneic bone marrow transplantation for chronic myeloid leukemia in first chronic phase: a randomized trial of busulfan-cytoxan versus cytoxan-total body irra-diation as a preparative regimen: a report from the French Society of Bone Marrow Graft (SFGM). *Blood* 1995; **85**: 2263–2268

70. Gratwohl A, Hermans J, Biezen AV *et al*. No advantage for patients who receive splenic irradiation before bone marrow transplantation for chronic myeloid leukemia: results of a prospective randomized study. *Bone Marrow Transplant* 1992; **10**: 147–152

71. Kalhs P, Schwarzinger I, Anderson G *et al*. A retrospective analysis of the long-term effect of splenectomy on late infections, graft-versus-host disease, relapse and survival after allogeneic marrow transplantation for chronic myelogenous leukemia. *Blood* 1995; **86**: 2028–2032.

72. Gamis AS, Haake R, McGlave P *et al*. Unrelated donor bone marrow transplantation for Philadelphia chromosome-positive chronic myelo-genous leukemia in children. *J Clin Oncol* 1993; **11**: 834–838

73. Gluckman E, Rocha V, Boyer-Chammard A *et al*. Outcome of cord-blood transplantation from related and unrelated donors. *N Engl J Med* 1997; **337**: 373–381

74. Bogdanic V, Nemet D, Kastelan A *et al*. Umbilical cord blood transplantation in a patient with Philadelphia chromosome positive chronic myeloid leukemia. *Transplantation* 1993; **56**: 477–479

75. Szydlo R, Goldman JM, Klein JP *et al*. Results of allogeneic bone marrow transplants using donors other than HLA-identical siblings. *J Clin Oncol* 1997; **15**: 1767–1777

76. Speiser DE, Hermans J, van Biezen A *et al*. Haploidentical family member transplants for patients with chronic myeloid leukaemia: a

415

report of the Chronic Leukaemia Working Party of the European Group for Blood and Marrow Transplantation. *Bone Marrow Transplant* 1997; **19**: 1197–1203

77. Barrett AJ, Malkovska V. Graft-versus-leukaemia: understanding and using the alloimmune response to treat haematological malignancies. *Br J Haematol* 1996; **93**: 754–761

78. Lim S, Coleman S. Chronic myeloid leukemia as an immunological target. *Am J Hematol* 1997; **54**: 61–67

79. Kolb HJ, Schattenberg A, Goldman JM *et al*. Graft-versus-leukemia effect of donor lymphocyte transfusion in marrow grafted patients. *Blood* 1995; **86**: 2041–2050

80. Prentice HG, Blacklock HA, Janossy G *et al*. Depletion of T-lymphocytes in donor marrow prevents significant graft-versus-host-disease in matched allogeneic leukaemic marrow transplant recipients. *Lancet* 1984; **1**: 472–475

81. Hale G, Waldmann H. Recent results using CAMPATH-1 antibodies to control GVHD and graft rejection. *Bone Marrow Transplant* 1996; **17**: 305–308

82. Apperley JF, Jones L, Hale G *et al*. Bone marrow transplantation for chronic myeloid leukaemia: T cell depletion with Campath-1 reduces the incidence of acute graft-versus-host disease but may increase the risk of leukaemic relapse. *Bone Marrow Transplant* 1986; **1**: 53–66

83. McGlave P, Bartsch G, Anasetti C *et al*. Unrelated donor marrow transplantation therapy for chronic myelogenous leukemia: initial experience of the National Marrow Donor Program. *Blood* 1993; **81**: 543–550

84. Champlin R, Pasweg J, Horowitz M *et al*. T-cell depleted (TCD) BMT for leukemic patients with donors other than HLA-identical siblings. *Blood* 1995; **86 (Suppl 1)**: 94A

85. Goldman JM, Gale RP, Horowitz M *et al*. Bone marrow transplantation for chronic myelogenous leukemia in chronic phase. Increased risk of relapse associated with T-cell depletion. *Ann Intern Med* 1988; **108**: 806–814

86. Storb R, Deeg HJ, Whitehead J. Methotrexate and cyclosporine compared with cyclosporine alone for prophylaxis of acute graft versus host disease after marrow transplantation for leukemia. *N Engl J Med* 1986; **314**: 729–735

87. Yiang YZ, Mavroudis DA, Dermine S *et al*. Alloreactive CD4$^+$ T lymphocytes can exert cytotoxicity to CML cells processing and presenting exogenous antigen. *Br J Haematol* 1996; **93**: 606–614

88. Giralt S, Hester J, Huh Y *et al*. CD8-depleted donor lymphocyte infusion as treatment for relapsed chronic myelogenous leukemia after allogeneic bone marrow transplantation. *Blood* 1995; **86**: 4337–4343

89. Reid CDL. The dendritic cell lineage in haemopoiesis. *Br J Haematol* 1997; **96**: 217–223

90. Kolb HJ, Mittermuller J, Clemm C *et al*. Donor leukocyte transfusions for the treatment of recurrent chronic myelogenous leukemia in marrow transplant patients. *Blood* 1990; **76**: 2462–2465

91. Van Rhee F, Feng L, Cullis JO *et al*. Relapse of chronic myeloid leukemia after allogeneic bone marrow transplant: the case of giving donor leukocyte transfusions before the onset of hematologic relapse. *Blood* 1994; **83**: 3377–3383

92. MacKinnon S, Papadopoulos EP, Carabasi MH *et al*. Adoptive immunotherapy evaluating escalating doses of donor leukocytes for relapse of chronic myeloid leukemia following bone marrow trans-

plantation: separation of graft-versus-leukemia responses from graft-versus-host disease. *Blood* 1995; **86**: 1261–1268

93. Dazzi F, Raanani P, van Rhee F *et al*. Donor lymphocyte infusion (DLI) for relapse of CML after allo-BMT: comparison of two regimens. *Bone Marrow Transplant* 1992; **10**: 113–114

94. Bortin M, Horowitz M, Rimm AA. Progress report from the International Bone Marrow Transplant Registry. *Bone Marrow Transplant* 1992; **10**: 113–122

95. Clift RA, Anasetti C. Allografting for chronic myeloid leukaemia. *Baillière's Clin Haematol* 1997; **10**: 319–336

96. Clift RA, Buckner CD, Thomas ED *et al*. Bone marrow transplantation for patients in accelerated phase of chronic myeloid leukemia. *Blood* 1994; **84**: 4368–4373

97. Kernan NA, Bartsch G, Ash RC *et al*. Analysis of 462 transplantations from unrelated donors facilitated by the National Marrow Donor Program. *N Engl J Med* 1993; **328**: 593–602

98. Gratwohl A, Hermans J, Apperley JF *et al*. Acute graft-versus-host disease grade and outcome in patients with chronic myelogenous leukemia. *Blood* 1995; **86**: 813–818

99. Ringden O, Hermans J, Labopin M *et al*. The highest leukaemia-free survival after allogeneic bone marrow transplantation is seen in patients with Grade I acute graft-versus-host disease. *Leukemia Lymphoma* 1996; **24**: 71–79

100. Barrett AJ, Locatelli F, Treleaven JG *et al*. Second transplant for leukaemic relapse after bone marrow transplantation: high early mortality but favourable effect of chronic GVHD on continuing remission. *Br J Haematol* 1991; **79**: 567–574

101. Mrsic M, Horowitz M, Atkinson K *et al*. Second HLA-identical sibling transplants for leukemic recurrence. *Bone Marrow Transplant* 1992; **9**: 269–275

102. Arcese W, Goldman JM, D'Arcangelo E *et al*. Outcome for patients who relapse after allogeneic bone marrow transplantation for chronic myeloid leukemia. *Blood* 1993; **82**: 3211–3219

103. Cullis JO, Schwarer AP, Hughes TP *et al*. Second transplants for patients with chronic myeloid leukaemia in relapse after original transplant with T-depleted marrow: feasibility of using busulphan alone for re-conditioning. *Br J Haematol* 1992; **80**: 33–39

104. Hoyle C, Gray R, Goldman J. Autografting for patients with CML in chronic phase: An update. *Br J Haematol* 1994; **86**: 76

105. Carella AM, Cunningham I, Benvenuto F *et al*. Mobilization and transplantation of Philadelphia-negative peripheral blood progenitor cells early in chronic myelogenous leukemia. *J Clin Oncol* 1997; **15**: 1575–1582

106. Bhatia R, Verfaille CM, Miller JS, McGlave PB. Autologous transplantation therapy for chronic myelogenous leukemia. *Blood* 1997; **89**: 2623–2634

107. Mitus AJ, Schafer A. Thrombocytosis and thrombocythemia. *Hematol Oncol Clin N Am* 1990; **4**: 157–178

108. Chintagumpala MM, Kennedy LL, Steubler CP. Treatment of essential thrombocythemia with anagrelide. *J Pediatr* 1995; **127**: 495–498

109. Rosenthal S, Canellos GP, Whang-Peng J, Gralnick HR. Blast crisis of chronic granulocytic leukemia: morphologic variants and therapeutic implications. *Am J Med* 1977; **63**: 542–547

110. Rule SA, Savage DG, O'Brien SG *et al*. Intermediate dose busulphan before autografting for advanced phase disease. *Br J Haematol* 1996; **94**: 694–698

Platelet disorders

Inherited and congenital thrombocytopenia

OWEN P SMITH

The normal range of the platelet count in fetal life is similar to that seen in adulthood, being in the range 150–400 $\times$ 10^9/l. Neonatal thrombocytopenia, defined as a platelet count of <150 $\times$ 10^9/l is common, with a reported frequency of approximately 0.9% in unselected newborns, and 40% in infants in intensive care units.[1] The differential diagnosis of thrombocytopenia in the neonatal period is similar to thrombocytopenia in older children with a number of exceptions that include the inherited thrombocytopenias and those that arise due to pathophysiologic events unique to the ante- and peri-natal periods. It is important to remember to confirm that the low platelet count is genuine by careful inspection of the blood sample and smear before initiating further investigations. Once established, the approach to the diagnosis of the thrombocytopenia should be tailored to the individual infant and his mother. For example, assessment of the child's general well-being is very important as healthy neonates usually have an immune or an inherited etiology, whereas the presence of lymphadenopathy, hepatosplenomegaly, mass lesions, hemangiomas, bruits and congenital anomalies point towards a totally different spectrum of causes. It should also be emphasized that obtaining a detailed maternal history, including bleeding problems, pre-eclampsia and drug ingestion in the present and past pregnancies and any history of viral infections (cytomegalovirus, rubella, herpes simplex and HIV) or connective tissue disease (systemic lupus erythematosus [SLE]), will save time and unnecessary investigation.

In this chapter the causes of thrombocytopenia are divided into 2 broad categories:

- those arising on a background of an established genetic defect (inherited thrombocytopenia);
- those associated with birth (congenital thrombocytopenia).

HISTORIC PERSPECTIVE

Although Donne,[2] Geber,[3] Addison[4] and Simon[5] are said independently to have first described the platelet in 1842, the first true description is generally credited to Max Schultze of Freiburg, who in 1865 described them as:

> "gray, colorless spherical bodies in the blood from which, when clumped, rays of finely granular protoplasm often spread, in conjunction with fibrin coagulation."[6]

In 1882, Julius Bizzozero, who coined the term 'Blut Plattchen', wrote his classic paper describing "viscous metamorphosis" of platelets in which he stated:

> "Platelets become granular within the lumen of an injured vessel: and this change produces a substance which activates the coagulation system to form fibrin."[7]

By 1906, Wright[8] confirmed Bizzozero's theory of the origin of the platelet from bone marrow megakaryocytes by observing that the cytoplamsic pseudopodia from megakaryocytes have the same staining characteristics as platelets and concluded that the pseudopodia produced new platelets. These findings were subsequently confirmed in the late 1940s and early 1950s with the arrival of electron microscopy. Over the following 3 decades, steady, albeit limited, progress was made in characterizing platelet pathophysiologic states.

The 1970s witnessed the birth of the modern era of platelet and megakaryocyte research as newer methods of analysis (molecular biologic tools and *in vitro* systems) became available to study megakaryocytopoiesis and platelet structure and function. The fruits of this endeavor have been the recognition of different stages of normal megakaryoctyopoiesis and a greater understanding of the molecular events responsible for dysmegakaryocytopoiesis. During this period, the cloning of cytokines that act on the megakaryocytic lineage and their clinical application was realized. In 1993, Wendling *et al*[9] identified the *c-mpl* proto-oncogene as the receptor of a major regulator of thrombocytopoiesis and this greatly facilitated the subsequent isolation and cloning of *c-mpl* ligand or thrombopoietin by several groups.[10] These two discoveries represent the most important recent advance in platelet/megakaryocyte research.

INHERITED THROMBOCYTOPENIA

The inherited thrombocytopenias comprise a group of platelet formation abnormalities in which platelet numbers are reduced. In the vast majority of patients the platelet count is only mild-to-moderately reduced ($50–100 \times 10^9$/l) and therefore significant spontaneous hemorrhage tends not be problematic. There are, however, a number of notable exceptions where spontaneous bleeding is a prominent clinical feature of the syndrome:

- Wiskott–Aldrich syndrome, amegakaryocytic thrombocytopenia and thrombocytopenia with absent radii (TAR) where the platelet count is usually very low;
- Bernard–Soulier and Chédiak–Higashi syndromes where there is a marked platelet dysfunction.

Immune-mediated thrombocytopenia is a major differential diagnosis in children with low platelet counts and therefore making the correct diagnosis of these conditions is important, as it usually prevents the useless and potentially dangerous prescribing of immunosuppressants such as corticosteroids. Although the inherited nature of these conditions has been known for the past 30 years, the molecular basis for the thrombocytopenia has only been fully elucidated in a very small number of these conditions, in particular those arising from defects in von Willebrand factor (VWF) and its platelet receptor, GpIb-V-IX complex.

It is convenient to divide this etiologically heterogeneous group of disorders into 2 broad categories based on the association of a significant concomitant platelet function abnormality (Table 21.1).

DISORDERS WITH DYSFUNCTIONAL PLATELETS

GpIb-V-IX complex

The GpIb-V-IX complex is one of the major adhesion receptors on the platelet surface and plays a pivitol role in primary hemostasis by mediating VWF attachment following collagen exposure on the damaged vessel wall. Its structure is well known with each gene product possessing one or more characteristic leucine-rich domains.[11,12] Binding of VWF occurs to one or more sites within or close to a double disulfide-bonded and sulfated loop region close to the amino terminal of the receptor during high shear conditions involving the platelet cytoskeleton. Three inherited bleeding

Table 21.1 Inherited thrombocytopenias.

Disorder	Inheritance	Platelet feature	Platelet size	Other findings
With dysfunctional platelets				
Bernard–Soulier syndrome	AR	↓ Aggregation to ristocetin	Large	Qualitative and or quantitative in platelet GpIb–V–IX
Pseudo-von Willebrand disease	AD	↑ Aggregation to ristocetin	Normal	Spontaneous ↑ platelet binding of VWF due to GpIb defect
Type 2b-von Willebrand disease	AD	↑ Aggregation to ristocetin	Large	Spontaneous ↑ VWF binding to platelets due to VWF defect
Montreal syndrome	AD	Spontaneous aggregation	Large	Calpain defect, pale-staining platelets, agranular megakaryocytes
Gray platelet syndrome	AR	α-Granule defect	Normal	Bone marrow fibrosis
Paris–Trousseau syndrome	AD	Giant α-granules	Normal	Chromosome 11 (del(11)(q23.3;qter))
Wiskott–Aldrich syndrome	X-linked	↓ Dense granules in some	Small	*WASP* mutations at Xp11.22–11.23, infections, eczema
X-linked thrombocytopenia	X-linked	↓ Dense granules in some	Small	*WASP* mutations at Xp11.22–11.23
Chédiak–Higashi syndrome	AD	↓ Aggregation to Ep and Co	Normal	Oculocutaneous albinism, recurrent infections, large white cell inclusions
Factor V Quebec	AD	↓ Aggregation to Ep	Normal	↓ Platelet Fg', VWF, FV, Ts, osteonectin, normal platelet plasma factor 4 and β-TG
Without dysfunctional platelets				
May–Hegglin anomaly	AD	Function studies vary	Large	Döhle bodies in neutrophils
Alport's syndrome variants				
Epstein's syndrome	AD	↓ Aggregation to Ep and Co	Large	Nephritis, deafness, congenital cataract, white cell inclusions
Eckstein's syndrome	AD	Normal platelet function	Large	White cell inclusions with features of Alport's syndrome
Fechtner's syndrome	AD	Function studies vary	Large	Nephritis, deafness, congenital cataract, white cell inclusions
Sebastian's syndrome	AD	Normal platelet function	Large	White cell inclusions but *no* nephritis or deafness
Thrombocytopenia with absent radii	AR	↓ Aggregation to Ep and Co	Normal	↓ Marrow megakaryocytes
Pure genetic thrombocytopenia	AD	Not known	Large	Normal morphologically and platelet survival
Mediterranean thrombocytopenia	AD	Not known	Large	

AR = autosomal recessive; AD = autosomal dominant; Ep = epinephrine (adrenaline); Co = collagen; Fg' = fibrinogen; VWF = von Willebrand factor protein; FV = factor V; Ts = thrombospondin; β-TG = β-thromboglobulin.

disorders associated with gene defects within this complex are Bernard–Soulier syndrome (BSS), pseudo-von Willebrand disease (VWD) and type 2B VWD.

Bernard–Soulier syndrome (see also Chapter 24)

This is the best characterized inherited thrombocytopenia which has in association an abnormal platelet function.[13] Typically, there is moderate-to-severe thrombocytopenia, a prolonged bleeding time and platelet morphology usually reveals 'giant' forms. The platelets in this condition are incapable of interacting with VWF and hence the bleeding seen is typical of a primary hemostatic defect. Whilst BSS platelets show normal shape change, secretion, signal transduction and aggregation in the presence of ADP, epinephrine (adrenaline), collagen and arachidonic acid, they do not aggregate with ristocetin in the presence of VWF.

BSS is inherited in an autosomal recessive manner with the underlying molecular defects due to quantitative or qualitative defects in the GpIb-V-IX complex. Numerous variants of BSS have been described at the molecular level ranging from 'classic' BSS, where the entire glycoprotein complex is missing from the membrane, to full platelet expression of the GpIb-V-IX complex but with a point mutation in codon 156, the crucial leucine-repeat region $(Ala^{156} \rightarrow Val^{156})$ of the subunit GpIbα, which in turn prevents VWF binding, the so-called 'Bolzano' variant.[13–15]

Pseudo-von Willebrand disease (see also Chapter 24)

This is an autosomal dominant disorder characterized by mild intermittent thrombocytopenia, mild bleeding, absence of high molecular weight VWF multimers, and increased ristocetin-induced platelet aggregation.[13] It is caused by a mutation(s) in the major double-loop structure of GpIbα causing a conformational change in the receptor which in turn leads to enhanced VWF binding and hence spontaneous platelet aggregation and thrombocytopenia.[14–16] It can be differentiated from type 2B VWD, where the mutation resides in the VWF protein by spontaneous aggregation of the patient's platelets with normal plasma (see below).

Bolin–Jamieson syndrome is a mild bleeding disorder, characterized by 1 allele of the GpIbα gene producing a molecule of about 10 kDa larger than the normal range.[17] How this defect leads to an increased bleeding susceptibility is not known.

Type 2B von Willebrand's disease

This subtype of VWD is clinically and biochemically very similar to pseudo-VWD. It is usually diagnosed by the increased platelet agglutination induced by low concentrations of ristocetin. However, it should be remembered that in some cases defects can be delineated in the absence of ristocetin. Like type 2A VWD, the mutations causing type 2B are clustered within exon 28 of the VWF gene.[18] These

mutations result in 'gain-of-function', i.e. there is spontaneous binding of the mutant VWF to GpIb, with consequent loss of high molecular weight multimers from the plasma and a tendency to thrombocytopenia.

Montreal platelet syndrome

This syndrome is characterized by thrombocytopenia, large platelets, spontaneous platelet aggregation, and a reduced response to thrombin-induced aggregation.[19] It can be distinguished from BSS by its autosomal dominant inheritance and normal platelet agglutinability response to ristocetin. The platelets have a quantitative and qualitative reduction of the calcium-dependent proteinase calpain which prevents them from returning to a normal volume after agonist stimulation.[20,21]

Gray platelet syndrome (see also Chapter 24)

This is an extremely rare autosomally inherited syndrome characterized by a markedly reduced platelet α-granule content but normal dense-bodies and lysosomes.[22] The name gray platelet comes from the bland gray agranular appearance of platelets on Wright-Giemsa-stained blood smears which reflects the reduced numbers of platelet α-granules (see Fig. 24.5). Other features include a prolonged skin bleeding time, morphologically large platelets and highly variable platelet aggregation profiles. The platelet α-granules which are present, albeit in reduced numbers, are deficient in the storage proteins, coagulation Factor V, VWF, platelet Factor 4, β-thromboglobulin, fibrinogen, platelet-derived growth factor (PDGF) and thrombospondin.[23] Concomitant elevation in plasma levels of platelet Factor 4 and β-thromboglobulin are seen, implying that there is an abnormality in α-granule protein packaging within the megakaryocyte; this would appear to be lineage restricted to megakaryocytes as VWF biosynthesis within endothelial cells is normal.[24] Myelofibrosis is not an uncommon finding in these patients and the continuous premature release of α-granule proteins such as PDGF into the bone marrow microenvironment may be key to its development.[25] The accompanying thrombocytopenia and bleeding symptoms are usually mild. The mechanism responsible for the bleeding propensity is not fully understood but is likely to be multifactorial, involving mild impairment of platelet aggregation and adhesion together with impaired thrombin and fibrin generation as there is probably a paucity of coagulation Factor V within the α-granules.[26]

Appropriate on demand or prophylactic treatment needs to be individualized. For example, those patients with moderate thrombocytopenia and evidence of abnormal platelet aggregation are most likely to benefit from a combination of platelet transfusion and desmopressin (DDAVP), whilst for those with very mild thrombocytopenia and a prolonged bleeding time, desmopressin alone is all that is needed.

Paris–Trousseau syndrome

This is a recently described autosomal dominant syndrome comprised of mild thrombocytopenia, a moderate hemorrhagic tendency, giant α-granules in a subpopulation of platelets, bone marrow micromegakaryocytes with enhanced megakaryocyte apoptosis and a deletion of the distal part of chromosome 11 at position 11q23 (del (11)(q23.3;qter)).[27] The giant α-granules fail to release their content following thrombin exposure and this may explain the moderate bleeding events seen in this disorder. The cytogenetic abnormality seen in this syndrome is probably responsible for the abnormal megakaryocytopoiesis as the 2 proto-oncogenes *ETS1* and *FL1* map to 11q23–24 and are involved in normal expression of megakaryocyte-specific genes.[27]

Wiskott–Aldrich syndrome

Wiskott–Aldrich syndrome (WAS) is inhertied as an X-linked recessive trait and is characterized by eczema, microthrombocytopenia and combined immunodeficiency.[28,29] It is often fatal by the early teens due to infection, lymphoreticular malignancy or bleeding. Hemorrhagic events are common during the first 2 years of life and the reason for this is multifactorial. For example, platelet survival is modestly reduced to half normal,[30] ineffective megakaryocytopoiesis is prominent as reflected by a platelet turnover of 25% that of normal with a normal megakaryocyte mass[30] and there is evidence of platelet functional abnormalities related to abnormal storage of adenine nucleotides and impaired platelet energy metabolism.[31,32]

Allogeneic bone marrow transplantation (BMT) is the treatment of choice when there is a fully matched donor available as this corrects the abnormal stem cell compartment.[33] When there is no suitable donor, splenectomy is the therapeutic first choice as this usually raises the platelet count into the normal range, improves platelet survival and normalizes platelet size.[34] It should be remembered that splenectomy is *not* advocated for the other hereditary thrombocytopenic disorders as it usually gives little benefit.

Wiskott–Aldrich syndrome variants (X-linked thrombocytopenia)

This is a heterogeneous group of thrombocytopenic disorders with X-linked inheritance. Some families have microthrombocytopenia and no associated abnormalities, while others have mild eczema and impaired immune responses.[35] The thrombocytopenia is usually less severe in WAS variants and requires no treatment but in the rare case with severe thrombocytopenia splenectomy has been shown to be effective.[36]

Both WAS and WAS variants appear to be caused by different mutations of the same gene on the short arm of the X chromosome (Xp11.2).[37,38]

Oculocutaneous albinism (Hermanksy–Pudlak and Chédiak–Higashi syndromes)

Oculocutaneous albinism denotes a group of inherited disorders characterized by reduced or absent pigmentation of skin, hair and eyes. Whilst the majority of these patients have an isolated platelet storage pool defect, in some an accompanying low platelet count can occur.

Hermansky–Pudlak syndrome is an autosomal recessive disorder with the classic triad of oculocutaneous albinism (tyrosinase positive), platelet dense-body or combined dense-body and α-granule storage pool deficiency, and deposits of ceroid-like material in the monocyte-macrophage system (see Chapter 24). The bleeding tendency is usually mild (related to the storage pool defect and not thrombocytopenia, as the latter is not a feature of the syndrome); however, excessive bleeding following tooth extractions and tonsillectomy is the rule. The ceroid-like deposits in the lungs, gastrointestinal tract and renal tubule cells may lead to restrictive lung disease, colitis or renal failure, respectively.

The features of *Chédiak–Higashi syndrome* include partial oculocutaneous albinism, the presence of giant granules in all granule-containing cells, neutropenia, peripheral neuropathy and platelet storage pool deficiency which usually involves the dense bodies. Thrombocytopenia usually occurs during the accelerated phase of the disease, which involves the development of pancytopenia, hepatosplenomegaly, lymphadenopathy and extensive tissue infiltration with lymphoid cells (see Chapter 24). The accelerated phase, which is clinically similar to virus-associated hemophagocytic lymphohistiocytosis, unfortunately occurs in most patients and the majority die. The precise molecular basis of Chédiak–Higashi syndrome has not been fully elucidated and the only curable therapeutic modality is allogeneic BMT which in one report was successful in 6 of 7 patients grafted.[39]

Factor V Quebec

This condition is characterized by an autosomal dominant inheritance pattern, mild thrombocytopenia, quantitative and qualitative defects in platelet Factor V, an epinephrine platelet aggregation defect, and a severe post-traumatic bleeding tendency.[40] Defects in multimerin, a large complex multimeric protein expressed in platelet α-granules and endothelial cell Weibel-Palade bodies, is most likely to be responsible for the lower platelet Factor V but its deficiency also plays a role in the reduced levels of the other α-granule proteins, fibrinogen, VWF, thrombospondin and osteonectin.[41] As platelet Factor 4 and β-thromboglobulin levels are normal in platelets from these patients and there is failure to aggregate with epinephrine,[42] it is most likely that α-granule assembly and protein packaging interact. Whilst the precise mechanism responsible for the coagulopathy is not known, deficiency in multimerin probably leads to a defect either in stabilizing or enhancing the proteolytic degradation of α-granule hemostatic proteins.

DISORDERS WITHOUT DYSFUNCTIONAL PLATELETS

May-Hegglin anomaly

This is an autosomal dominant disorder, characterized by giant platelets, variable thrombocytopenia and Döhle-like inclusions within granulocytic cells, including monocytes.[43–45] These structures are blue on Wright-Giemsa staining (denoting RNA), spindle-shaped and occur 1/cell and have a distinctive ultrastructure of 7–10 nm filaments of remnant rough endoplasmic reticulum oriented in parallel in the long axis.[46] A small percentage of patients have persistent leukopenia which has been associated with occasional infections and in 1 case neutrophil chemotaxis and chemokinetic responses were impaired.[46] Platelet function has been reported to be normal in some and impaired in others.[45,47–51] Troublesome primary hemostatic bleeding,[45,47] which is seen in approximately 40% of these patients, is felt to be most likely secondary to the degree of thrombocytopenia at the time of hemorrhage.

Alport's syndome

This is associated with sensorineural deafness (usually high tone), hematuria, cataracts and progressive renal failure.[52] The disorder is a heterogeneous group with the majority having autosomal dominant inheritance. Many variants of Alport's syndrome have been described, the commonest being associated with hyperprolinemia. The genetic basis of this syndrome is believed to involve deletions or rearrangements in the $\alpha 5(IV)$ collagen gene located on Xq22.[53] Three variants have been described with associated thrombocytopenia. It is not known whether the gene defect seen in 'classic' Alport's syndrome is linked to the thrombocytopenia seen in the variants described below.

Epstein's and Eckstein's syndromes

Epstein's syndrome was first described in 1972 in a family with features of Alport's syndrome, macrothrombocytopenia and defective platelet aggregation and secretion in response to ADP and collagen.[54] Three years later, *Eckstein's syndrome* was reported and described to have all the features that characterized Epstein's syndrome but in contrast had normal platelet function.[55]

Fechtner's syndrome

This is characterized by the same morphologic features as those seen in the Sebastian platelet syndrome (see below) but in addition is associated with deafness, cataracts and renal failure.[56] The white cell inclusion bodies (Fechtner's inclusions) are characteristic of the syndrome and resemble toxic Döhle bodies (seen with infection and malignancies) and May-Hegglin granulocyte inclusions. They can be differen-tiated by light and electron microscopy as Fechtner's inclusion bodies are smaller and lighter-staining than those seen in May-Hegglin granulocytes and are composed of dispersed filament, ribosome and endoplasmic reticulum. Fechtner's inclusion bodies lack the parallel bundles of fine filaments seen in May-Hegglin inclusions.[57]

Whilst these syndromes are associated with a mild-to-moderate bleeding tendency, significant hemorrhagic morbidity is usually encountered following trauma, dental extraction and other forms of surgery and platelet concentrates are the main therapeutic intervention. It should be remembered that the progressive renal failure seen in these patients usually adds to the hemorrhagic tendency and is also the main etiological factor contributing to overall morbidity and indeed mortality.

Sebastian platelet syndrome

Sebastian platelet syndrome resembles May-Hegglin anomaly but the Döhle-body-like inclusions seen in granulocytes are different in that they are smaller and ultrastructural analysis shows them to consist of ribosomes and dispersed filaments without an enclosing membrane. They are detected by light microscopy only if the blood smears are stained within 4 hours after venepuncture,[58] which implies that this syndrome is probably an under-reported cause of hereditary thrombocytopenia.[59] This syndrome is felt to be a variant of Fechtner's syndrome without the associated Alport's syndrome features.[58] It is inherited in an autosomal dominant manner and whilst the bleeding tendency is considered to be mild-to-moderate, hemorrhagic deaths have been reported.[60]

Inherited bone marrow failure syndromes

Thrombocytopenia with absent radii (see also Chapter 1)

This is a rare, autosomal recessive disorder that is usually diagnosed at birth as the vast majority of these patients are thrombocytopenic and have the pathognomic physical signs of bilateral absent radii.[61] Other skeletal abnormalities involving the ulnae, fingers and lower limbs are also seen but are much rarer.[62] Thrombocytopenia with absent radii (TAR) differs from Fanconi's anemia in several ways: the absent radii are accompanied by the presence of thumbs (see Fig. 1.4), the thrombocytopenia is the only cytopenia, there is absence of spontaneous or clastogenic stress-induced chromosomal breakage and evolution of aplastic anemia and leukemia has not been reported.[62] It is not uncommon for these children to be anemic and have transient white cell counts at presentation (the former is felt to be secondary to bleeding as it is always accompanied by a reticulocytosis and the latter usually subsides by 6 months of age). The striking morphologic feature within the bone marrow is the absent or greatly reduced numbers of megakaryocytes with normal

423

granulopoietic and erythroid compartments.[63,64] The precise pathophysiologic defect responsible for TAR is not known; however, the restoration of platelet count seen following sibling allogeneic BMT supports the idea that the thrombopoietic defect lies within the hematopoietic stem cell compartment rather than a deficiency of thrombopoietin or another platelet humoral factor.[65]

The majority of children with TAR have recurrent significant bleeding episodes in the first 6 months of life. Intracerebral and gastrointestinal hemorrhage are the usual cause of mortality with previously 1 in 4 of these children dying by 4 years of age.[62] The majority of these deaths, however, occurred in the first year of life. The severity of the bleeding problem is related to the degree of thrombocytopenia which in the majority of children is usually $<20 \times 10^9/l$ and in some there is evidence of qualitative platelet defects (storage pool and abnormal aggregation profiles).[62,66] The mainstay of treatment is the judicious use of single donor platelet concentrates, aiming to keep the platelet count above $20 \times 10^9/l$, especially in the first year of life as this is the time of maximum morbidity and mortality. This more aggressive platelet transfusion approach should reduce dramatically the unacceptable hemorrhagic mortality and morbidity rate. If the patient survives the first year of life, survival appears to be normal.[62] All elective reconstructive orthopedic surgery should be postponed during the first few years of life.

Prenatal diagnosis of TAR is possible with absent radii easily visualized with radiography and/or ultrasound and thrombocytopenia diagnosed following fetal blood sampling obtained by fetoscopy or cordocentesis.[67,68] This relatively recent advance in obstetric care allows for the possibility of prophylactic antenatal management.

Amegakaryocytic thrombocytopenia (see also Chapter 1)

This is an extremely rare disorder of infancy and early childhood. The thrombocytopenia is non-immune and usually severe and early bone marrow examination shows a normal karyotype, absent or greatly reduced numbers of megakaryocytes with normal granulopoietic and erythroid elements.[69] Some patients have macrocytic red cells with increased expression of i antigen and elevated hemoglobin F levels,[70] implying that the pathophysiologic trigger occurs at the stem cell level. The inheritance pattern in the majority of cases is X-linked, the remainder being autosomal recessive. Amegarkaryocytic thrombocytopenia (AMEGA) patients can be broadly divided into 2 groups, those with physical anomalies and those without. The pattern of somatic anomalies is not unlike that seen with Fanconi's anemia; however, in those children tested, there was no evidence of DNA repair abnormality. The presence of anomalies influences outcome; projected median survivals are 6 years for those with no anomalies and 2 years when anomalies are present.[70] Those with isolated thrombocytopenia usually die from hemorrhagic complications whilst those with aplasia, which usually occurs after a relatively long period of thrombocytopenia, succumb to infection and bleeding.[62] AMEGA is considered to be a leukemia predisposition syndrome.[62,71]

Platelet transfusions are the main therapeutic intervention following diagnosis. Treatment with corticosteroids alone or in combination with androgens has been disappointing and splenectomy has no role. Encouraging platelet responses following the administration of interleukin 3 have been reported[69] and clinical trial results with thrombopoietin are eagerly awaited. Allogeneic BMT offers the only probable chance of cure.

Fanconi's anemia (see also Chapter 1)

This is a premalignant disorder, inherited as an autosomal recessive trait, with genetic heterogeneity and a gene frequency of about 1 in 600.[72] Thrombocytopenia is usually the first cytopenia to appear, followed by granulocytopenia and ultimately severe aplasia which occurs in the majority of patients.[73] The average age of onset of the hematologic abnormalties varies, with boys developing pancytopenia earlier than girls at 6.6 years and 8.8 years, respectively, with ranges from 18 months to 22 years.[74] The diagnosis of Fanconi's anemia should always be considered in a child with an isolated cytopenia even when somatic anomalies are absent as a significant number of these cases are physically normal.

Trisomy syndromes

Moderately severe thrombocytopenia is seen in some cases of trisomy-18,[75] -13[76] and to a lesser extent -21 syndromes.[76] Both trisomy-13 and -18 are usually diagnosed at birth as the associated abnormalities are usually quite striking. The majority of these cases die in the neonatal period from non-hemorrhagic sequelae.[77]

Pure genetic thrombocytopenia

This is an autosomal dominant macrothrombocytopenic disorder characterized by a chronic low platelet count, a normal platelet half-life, normal platelet function (aggregation and adhesion), normal skin bleeding time, absent platelet-associated immunoglobulins and a morphologically normal bone marrow megakaryoctye compartment.[78] Although the molecular lesion causing the thrombocytopenia has not been elucidated, platelet isotope studies using homologous and autologous platelets are highly suggestive that there is a pure production defect within the bone marrow.[78,79] The majority of cases are picked up following routine blood tests carried out for non-hematologic indications. The diagnosis is usually considered when there is a negative surrogate marker profile for inherited thrombocytopenia and is confirmed with isotope studies using the tracer [111]Indium-oxinate and autologous platelets showing a normal platelet life-span.[79] The dose of radioactivity administered and necessary to perform the study is approximately 1.5 μC (50 kBq)/kg of [111]Indium, which is negligible and perfectly acceptable in children, although not all pediatricians are comfortable with this view. Failure in differentiating this pure genetic thrombocytopenia from the commoner immune thrombocytopenias may expose the child to potentially toxic and unnecessary expensive therapeutics such as corticosteroids, chemotherapy and immunoglobulin. As the majority of these patients have platelet counts in the region of 50–100 $\times$ 10^9/l with normal skin bleeding times, the hemorrhagic potential for spontaneous bleeding is low and only rises at menses, following trauma or surgery.[79]

Mediterranean macrothrombocytopenia

This type of macrothrombocytopenia was initially reported from Australia in blood donors with Greek and Italian ancestry and has subsequently been shown to be present in the North African immigrant population in France.[80,81] The thrombocytopenia is mild with platelet counts ranging between 100 and 150 $\times$ 10^9/l and platelet morphology showing only a mild increase in platelet size. Inheritance is autosomal dominant and the low platelet count is very rarely if ever associated with troublesome bleeding.[82]

CONGENITAL THROMBOCYTOPENIA

Congenital thrombocytopenia is defined as a low platelet count at birth and not resulting from the association of a specific gene defect; it accounts for the majority of cases of neonatal thrombocytopenia. Thrombocytopenia is a common finding in sick neonates, however, and since the introduction of automated cell counters it is now considered a relatively common (approximately 1%) finding in apparently normal infants. In the vast majority of cases the thrombocytopenia results from increased platelet destruction which can arise by several mechanisms, the majority of which are not known. It is helpful to consider etiological factors contributing to neonatal thrombocytopenia in terms of whether the insult is maternal, infant or placentally based (Table 21.2).

MATERNAL FACTORS

Immune thrombocytopenia

Immune-mediated thrombocytopenia is usually seen in term babies who are clinically well and may be responsible for one-third of cases of thrombocytopenia seen in the general neonatal population.[1] There are 2 broad categories of conditions:

- those mediated by an alloimmune mechanism;
- those with associated autoimmune phenomena.

Table 21.2 Congenital thrombocytopenias.

Maternal factors
Immune thrombocytopenia
   Neonatal alloimmune thrombocytopenia
   Maternal autoimmune thrombocytopenia
Intrauterine infections (TORCH syndromes)
   Toxoplasmosis
   Rubella
   Cytomegalovirus
   Herpes simplex
   Other (including HIV and parvovirus B19)
Pre-eclampsia/hypertension
Drugs

Infant factors
Disseminated intravascular coagulation
Primary microangiopathic hemolytic anemias
   Hemolytic uremic syndrome
   Thrombotic thrombocytopenic purpura
Giant hemangioma syndrome (Kasabach–Merritt syndrome)
Hypercoagulable states
   Birth asphyxia
   Cyanotic congenital heart disease
   Respiratory distress syndrome
   Necrotizing enterocolitis
   Bacterial infection
   Rhesus hemolytic disease
   Anticoagulant deficiency (homozygous antithrombin, protein C and S deficiency)
   Heparin-induced thrombocytopenia
Rare bone marrow diseases
   Transient abnormal myelopoiesis
   Hemophagocytic lymphohistiocytosis
   Osteopetrosis
   Congenital leukemia
   Metastatic neuroblastoma

Placental factors
Infarction
Angiomas (chorioangiomas)
Lupus anticoagulants/anticardiolipin antibodies

Neonatal alloimmune thrombocytopenia (see also Chapter 33)

This arises following maternal sensitization to paternal antigens present on fetal platelets.[83] It occurs in approximately 1 in 1500–2000 births, with the mother having a normal platelet count and a negative history of bleeding.[84,85] The maternal alloantibody produced does not react with the mother's platelets but crosses the placenta and destroys fetal platelets. The paternal-derived fetal platelet antigen target against which the maternal alloantibody is directed is usually HPA-1a (also called P1^{A1} or Zw^a), which is present on the platelets of 98% of the population and is responsible for neonatal immune thrombocytopenia (NAIT) in approximately 80% of cases.[84] The second commonest platelet antigen involved in NAIT is HPA-5b (also called Br^a, Zav^a or Hc^a).[86] Whilst NAIT is in other ways analogous to hemolytic disease of the newborn due to Rhesus or ABO incompatibility (see Chapter 10), in NAIT the first child is usually affected with thrombocytopenia.[83] Given that 2% of the population is HPA-1a negative it is somewhat surprising that the frequency of NAIT is lower than would be predicted from the prevalence of the alloantigen.[85,87] The most likely reason for this discrepancy is that certain HLA-types are more likely to be associated with alloantibody formation, e.g. women who have the HLA-DR3 alloantigen account for the majority of affected cases of HPA-1a-induced NAIT.[85,88–90] A similar finding is seen with the Br[a] alloantigen and HLA-DRw6.[91]

NAIT typically presents as an isolated severe thrombocytopenia in an otherwise healthy child at birth. Severe thrombocytopenia may be present early in gestation and at least 20% of cases suffer intracranial hemorrhage (ICH),[92] some sustaining it *in utero* which usually results in long-term severe neurologic sequelae such as porencephalic cysts and optic hypoplasia.[93,94] Widespread petechial hemorrhage is present in >90% of cases, while cephalohematomata, hematuria and gastrointestinal bleeding occur in a significantly smaller number of children. Typically, the platelet count spontaneously returns into the normal range within 3 weeks after birth.

Neonates with alloimmune thrombocytopenia usually have platelet counts $< 20 \times 10^9/l$. Making the distinction from autoimmune causes is usually facilitated by the maternal platelet count, in that the mother has no thrombocytopenia nor is there any history of immune thrombocytopenic purpura (ITP). The diagnosis of NAIT is usually confirmed by platelet antigen typing of the parents, showing the antigen to be absent on the mother's platelets, present on the father's platelets or by demonstrating in the mother's serum antibody activity to the antigen using indirect immunofluorescence assay,[94,95] or enzyme-linked immunoassay.[97] It should be remembered that failure to detect a platelet-specific alloantibody in the maternal serum does not exclude the diagnosis,[97,98] and testing for NAIT does not require testing of the baby.

The mainstay of treatment for affected infant is washed, irradiated, maternal platelet concentrates.[99–101] The reason for washing the platelets is to remove antibody-laden plasma,[97,98] and irradiation to destroy maternal lymphocytes that are capable of stimulating transfusion-associated graft-versus-host disease (GVHD).[102] Both unrelated matched and maternal platelets can be administered; however, the latter are preferred because of their certain compatibility, availability and perhaps most importantly, safety. With *de novo* cases of NAIT, platelets can be rapidly procured from the mother and following washing and γ-irradiation given to the infant in a matter of a few hours. Random donor platelets should be given to infants who are actively bleeding while awaiting maternal platelets. In less severe cases, high-dose (1 g/kg) immunoglobulin therapy on 2 consecutive days will usually increase the platelet count within 2 days of administration.[102–105] In those cases of known NAIT where elective caesarian section is the preferred route of delivery, platelets are usually collected from the mother a few days before surgery and if this is deemed

logistically problematic, then platelets can be collected early in the pregnancy or indeed when the mother is not pregnant and frozen for use at a later stage.[106] Alternatively, non-maternal HPA-1a-negative platelets can be ordered in advance from a blood bank.

All children born to a father homozygous for the implicated antigen will harbor the antigen and half of the offspring will have it if there is paternal heterozygosity. This has important implications for future pregnancies as imaging with ultrasound early in the pregancy will indicate if intervention is required. Sampling fetal blood at 20 weeks' gestation allows an accurate assessment of the platelet count and fetal alloantigen genotyping can also be carried out on the sample.[107,108] Knowing the fetal platelet count and whether there is intracranial bleeding present usually dictates the most appropriate therapeutic intervention. For example, a fetus with severe thrombocytopenia and high risk of ICH will probably benefit from antigen-negative platelets transfused weekly.[97] At the other end of the clinical spectrum, a fetus who is at risk of NAIT, who has mild thrombocytopenia and a normal cranial ultrasound may equally benefit from maternal high dose immunoglobulin therapy alone.[109,110] It should be noted, however, that there is no published randomized trial comparing the more aggressive approach of intrauterine platelet transfusion with the least aggressive therapeutic modality of maternal immunoglobulin infusion. Elective caesarian section is recommended for all affected mature fetuses as this optimizes postnatal management.[111]

Maternal autoimmune thrombocytopenia (see also Chapter 33)

Autoimmune thrombocytopenia (AIT) is due to the passive transfer of autoantibodies from mothers with isolated ITP or it may be seen in association with conditions that have immune dysregulatory features such as maternal SLE, hypothryroidism and lymphoproliferative states.[112,113] Unlike NAIT, the specificity of the platelet antibody seen in AIT is towards antigen(s) common to maternal and fetal platelets.[114] Approximately 1 in 10 000 pregnancies are complicated by maternal ITP.[115] The risk of significant infant morbidity and mortality is minimal as the infant platelet count is rarely $< 50 \times 10^9/l$ and ICH rarely if ever occurs and when it does, it is not related to birth trauma.[115,116] It is also clear that there is no correlation between the platelet count and the level of autoantibody seen in the mother to the severity of thrombocytopenia observed in the infant; in fact, it has been well documented that women with normal platelet counts following splenectomy for ITP still deliver babies who are thrombocytopenic.[117] AIT needs to be distinguished from incidental or 'gestational' thrombocytopenia where the thrombocytopenia is usually mild ($70–100 \times 10^9/l$) with no history of bleeding of thrombocytopenia outside pregnancy, and the platelet count swiftly returns to normal following delivery.[118,119] Infants born to mothers with 'gestational' thrombocytopenia never or extremely rarely have a low platelet count.

The bleeding manifestations, including the risk of ICH, in children of mothers with AIT is significantly less than in children with NAIT.[115, 116,120] These infants are usually very well and born at term. The neonatal platelet count often falls after birth to a nadir on days 1–3 and it is during this time frame that bleeding occurs.[121] Spontaneous recovery of the infant platelet count is usually observed within 3 weeks after birth. However, if the platelet count is $<20 \times 10^9/l$ or if there is significant bleeding, then intravenous immunoglobulin (1 g/kg) should be given on 2 consecutive days and if this fails to raise the platelet count, then a short course of prednisolone (2–4 mg/kg/day per os) for 7–14 days should be added.[122] The mother's immune thrombocytopenia should be treated in accordance with the severity of the platelet count and not for a theoretical risk estimate of bleeding in the baby. As there are no reliable maternal predictors of severe thrombocytopenia in the infant, prenatal treatment of the mother with immunoglobulin and/or steroids does not make therapeutic sense.[123] Birth is usually by spontaneous vaginal delivery and caesarian section should only be contemplated in those pregnancies where problems are anticipated or if there is an history of a previous complicated delivery.

Intrauterine infections (**TORCH syndromes,** see also Chapter 38)

Intrauterine viral infections rarely produce thrombocytopenia ($<20 \times 10^9/l$) and therefore therapeutic intervention in the form of platelet concentrate and/or antiviral therapy is only indicated when there is active bleeding or surgical intervention is being considered. The mechanism(s) responsible for thrombocytopenia secondary to intrauterine infection is not fully understood but is probably multifactorial, including megakaryocyte injury with decreased platelet production, splenic removal, liver dysfunction and platelet-endothelial cell injury. In the vast majority of cases, the platelet count returns into the normal range within 2–4 weeks after birth but may persist to 4 months of age.[124] The well established intrauterine infections that cause congenital thrombocytopenia are outlined below.

Toxoplasmosis

Contracted during pregnancy, toxoplasmosis can result in serious damage to the fetus, including hydrocephaly, intracranial calcification, chorioretinitis and neurologic manifestations. Fortunately, as maternal screeening for toxoplasmosis in pregrancy and good antenatal treatment is now available, the severe form is less frequently seen. Subclinical forms are now more frequently encountered with chorioretinitis occurring in approximately one-third of cases. Thrombocytopenia is seen in a quarter of cases of congenital toxoplasmosis and in approximately 20% of these cases the platelet count is $<50 \times 10^9/l$.[125] Blood eosinophilia is also a common hematologic manifestation of this disease.

Congenital rubella

This is always due to a primary infection occurring in the first 3 months of pregnancy. The risk of serious malformation is highest if the infection is contracted in the first trimester. Mild-to-moderate thrombocytopenia is seen in approximately 20% of affected cases.[125] Hemolytic anemia and dermal extramedullary hematopoiesis, which resembles the skin manifestation seen in congenital leukemia (so-called 'blueberry muffin'), and other hematologic abnormalities are seen.

Cytomegalovirus

Like the other herpes viruses, and especially herpes simplex (types I and II), cytomegalovirus (CMV) can cause thrombocytopenia in the fetus and newborn. Approximately 1 in 5000 births have evidence of CMV inclusion disease, characterized by hypotrophy, jaundice, hepatosplenomegaly, thrombocytopenia, anemia, microcephaly, intracerebral calcification and/or chorioretinitis. While most newborns congenitally infected with CMV are asymptomatic, symptoms and sequelae are much more likely to occur in infants congenitally infected as a result of the mother's primary infection during pregnancy than those infected from reactivation of latent virus.[125,126] In 2 studies, thrombocytopenia was observed in 36% and 77% of infants infected with CMV, respectively,[125,126] and in the former study, the platelet count was $<50 \times 10^9/l$ in more than one-third of infants.[126]

Herpes simplex

Herpes simplex infection only causes problems to the fetus when the mother has a primary infection prior to 20 weeks' gestation. The risk of congenital malformation is very low; however, the frequency of fetal loss may be as high as 25% if the mother is infected during this time period. Thrombocytopenia is a well established hematologic abnormality associated with congenital herpes simplex infection.[127]

Other causes

Other causes of intrauterine viral-induced neonatal thrombocytopenia include human immunodeficiency virus (HIV)[128,129] and parvovirus B19.[130] Estimates of the rates of HIV transmission from mother to newborn range from 20 to 60% depending on the study.[131] The risk is reduced significantly when the mother is asymptomatic but increases with the length of time that she is seropositive.[131] Thrombocytopenia is rarely if ever the first clinical manifestation of congenital HIV and like parvovirus B19 infection, thrombocytopenia seems to be less frequently seen than with the other well established causes of intrauterine viral-induced thrombocytopenia.[128–130]

Maternal pre-eclampsia

The association of neonatal thrombocytopenia and maternal pre-eclampsia and maternal hypertension is a controversial one. As there are more premature infants born to mothers with hypertensive disorders of pregnancy, it is most likely that the increased rate of thrombocytopenia seen in these infants is more a reflection of how sick and premature the child is at birth, rather than a direct result of the maternal hypertension. Very few of these infants have severe thrombocytopenia and ICH is exceedingly rare.[132]

Maternal use of drugs

Drug-induced thrombocytopenia in the mother may also affect the neonate and when it occurs it is usually mediated by immune destruction of platelets.[132] It should be stressed that maternal usage of drugs is an extremely rare cause of low platelets in the newborn and the drugs that have been implicated include anticonvulsants (valproic acid, phenytoin, carbamazapine), quinidine and possibly thiazides and hydralazine.[132]

INFANT FACTORS

Disseminated intravascular coagulation (see also Chapter 32)

Disseminated intravascular coagulation (DIC) is an acquired hemostatic syndrome usually seen in association with well-defined clinical disorders. It is characterized by consumption of procoagulant and natural anticoagulant proteins which contribute to a state of mixed hemorrhage and thrombosis. The classic laboratory markers are thrombocytopenia, prolonged thrombin, prothrombin (PT) and activated partial thromboplastin (APTT) times, elevated D-dimers, and reductions in the plasma levels of fibrinogen, Factors II, V and VIII, protein C and antithrombin. The causes of DIC in infants and children are legion (see Chapter 32).

As a general axiom in medicine, when a pathologic syndrome is secondary to another primary disease state, the appropriate therapy should be directed when at all possible towards the underlying disease in order to correct the associated problem. For example, the appropriate treatment of the thrombotic DIC seen in children shortly after birth with homozygous protein C deficiency is replacement with protein C concentrate. As the plasma protein C level comes into the normal range following protein C concentrate infusion, the laboratory markers of DIC are corrected and resolution of skin purpura then becomes apparent.[133] The same clinical and laboratory response is seen following administration of protein C in children with severe acquired protein C deficiency secondary to meningococcemia.[134] Supportive treatment in the form of clotting factor replacement (fresh frozen plasma [FFP] 15 ml/kg to maintain the PT below 17 s), cryoprecipitate (1 bag/5 kg to maintain the fibrinogen above 1 g/l) and platelets (5 bags/m^2 to keep the count above 50×10^9/l) is usually administered as initial therapy, especially when there is evidence of active surface bleeding.[135] Usage of heparin and natural anticoagulant concentrates (antithrombin and protein C) should also be considered.

Primary microangiopathic hemolytic anemias

Microangiopathic hemolytic anemia (MAHA) is a term that describes intravascular destruction of red cells in the presence of an abnormal microcirculation. In a significant number of clinical syndromes associated with MAHA there is also thrombocytopenia. The thrombocytopenia results from platelet activation and thus platelet thrombi formation and the red cell fragmentation as a consequence of the shearing force produced by the abnormal flow within the abnormal microvasculature in concert with the microthrombi. The hallmark of MAHA is red cell fragmentation, polychromasia and thrombocytopenia on the blood smear with absent haptoglobulins, hemoglobinuria and elevated serum lactate dehydrogenase and bilirubin levels. The PT and APTT are usually within the normal range as are the plasma levels of clotting Factors V and VIII.

Hemolytic uremic syndrome (see also Chapters 32 and 37)

Hemolytic uremic syndrome (HUS) with its classic triad of MAHA, low platelets and renal failure, is usually seen in infants and children following seasonal epidemics of gastroenteritis caused by *Escherichia coli* (0157:H7 strain) producing verotoxin. It is one of the commonest causes of renal failure in childhood and while the precise pathogenic mechanism responsible for it is not fully understood, renovascular endothelial damage is probably a key event in promoting platelet activation and fibrin deposition that ultimately leads to microthrombi formation.[136] The other important contributing factor may be elevated levels of abnormal VWF multimer released from the damaged endothelium which enhance platelet aggregation and adhesion.[137,138] Treatment is essentially supportive with early renal dialysis allowing for better control of fluid and electrolyte balance. Unlike the situation in thrombotic thrombocytopenia purpura (TTP; see below), the role of plasma infusions and plasma exchange remains to be proven and therefore they are not used in the treatment of classic HUS.[139]

Thrombotic thrombocytopenic purpura

Whilst Moschcowitz initially described thrombotic thrombocytopenic purpura (TTP) in a 16-year-old girl,[140] it is more commonly seen in young adults with <20% of all patients reported to be <21 years of age.[139] It is characterized by MAHA, low platelets, fluctuating neurologic symptoms, fever and renal failure. However, severe thrombocytopenia, intravascular hemolysis with many red cell fragments on the blood smear and neurologic symptoms and signs constitute the characteristic TTP clinical triad. Like HUS, the pathophysiologic events involved in TTP are not fully understood but again they probably involve abnormalities in endothelial and VWF multimer composition, in particular the presence of unusually large VWF factor multimers in the circulation causing platelet activation with resultant platelet thrombi formation.[141,142] TTP should not be considered as a single disorder but as a heterogeneous group with at least 4 subtypes:[141]

- single-episode TTP (occurs *de novo* and seldom if ever recurs);
- intermittent TTP (characterized by occasional relapses at infrequent intervals);
- secondary TTP (usually seen in association with recognized clinical entities such as BMT, chemotherapy, pregnancy and infection, e.g. HIV);
- chronic relapsing TTP (frequent episodes occurring at regular intervals).

The commonest form seen in infancy and childhood is the chronic relapsing variety which may be different from its adult counterpart as there is usually no end-organ damage and only very small quantities of FFP (without plasma exchange) are needed to reverse the anemia and thrombocytopenia.[143] However, the VWF multimer profiles characterized by the presence of unusually large VWF multimers seen in both chronic relapsing types are similar, making it most likely that they are indeed the same disease state.[144,145]

The mainstay of treatment is plasma exchange with FFP or plasma devoid of the large VWF multimers (cryosupernatant or solvent detergent treated). Plasma infusions have also been shown to be efficacious, but plasma exchange is now considered the therapeutic modality of choice as controlled clinical trials have shown it to have superior efficacy.[146] Plasma exchange is continued until the platelet count and lactate dehydrogenase level return into the normal range. For those patients who do not respond to first-line treatment, a variety of other therapeutic approaches can be considered. These include corticosteroids, immunosuppression (vincristine, azathioprine, immunoglobulins), antiplatelet-aggregating agents (aspirin, dipyridamole) and splenectomy. It should be stated that all of these approaches have been reported to be successful anecdotally and not in a controlled clinical setting.

Giant hemangioma syndrome (Kasabach–Merritt syndrome)

Kasabach–Merritt syndrome (KMS) is the association of giant cavernous hemantiomata and DIC.[147] The consumptive coagulopathy seen in approximately 25% of cases of KMS is usually low grade and compensated. However, acceleration into the fulminant form, which is characterized by hypofibrinogenemia, raised D-dimers, red cell microangiopathy and severe thrombocytopenia, is not uncommon. This transformation can arise without an identifiable precipitating cause but it is usually accompanied by an expansion of the vascular tumor. The tumors are usually present at birth, grow in size over the first few months of life and then gradually recede. Therefore, the thrombocytopenia and indeed hemostatic failure that can be seen with these tumors may not be manifest until well into infancy. The majority of the hemangiomata is cutaneous; however 'hidden' visceral tumors, especially splenic, should always be included in the differential diagnosis of a child with unexplained thrombocytopenia with or without evidence of compensated intravascular coagulopathy as these forms of KMS have a high mortality rate if appropriate therapeutic measures are not undertaken.[148,149] Imaging with CT/MRI is useful, but the use of [111]Indium oxine-labeled platelets is probably a more sensitive modality in delineating the size and number of hemagniomata present.

Fortunately, spontaneous regression of these tumors occurs in the majority of patients.[148] A number of therapeutic approaches can be instituted in those who fail to undergo spontaneous regression and depend on the severity of the hemostatic failure, anatomic location and size of the hemangiomata. Treatment modalities that have been used with varying success include corticosteroids,[149,150] surgical resection,[149,150] α-interferon,[151] embolization,[152,153] and radiotherapy.[154] Replacement therapy with platelets, fibrinogen concentrate, FFP, cryoprecipitate and antifibrinolytic drugs and antiplatelet agents have a role in the fulminant phase of severe forms.

Hypercoagulable states

Consumptive thrombocytopenia, mainly secondary to DIC following thrombin generation, can be the first manifestation of an acquired or inherited hypercoagulable state. The clinical hallmark in a significant number of these disorders is an inappropriate thrombotic event(s) (see Chapter 34). It should be remembered, however, that venous and arterial thrombotic events in young children and neonates are rare, but when they do occur they can be associated with morbidity and significant mortality such as limb loss and organ impairment. Most events occur in the neonatal period and while the majority are usually associated with indwelling vascular catheters,[155] other etiological factors, both inherited and acquired, characteristic of the neonatal period may predispose to hypercoagulability and these are discussed below.

Birth asphyxia

Birth asphyxia as reflected by low Apgar scores is strongly associated with neonatal thrombocytopenia.[156,157] The mechanism responsible for the low platelet count has not been fully elucidated but consumption secondary to thrombin generation/DIC is probably the key event as hypoxia is known to upregulate tissue factor expression, reduce thrombomodulin activity and enhance plasminogen activator inhibitor-1 production by endothelial cells.[158]

Cyanotic congenital heart disease

The same mechanism probably plays a role in the thrombocytopenia seen in association with polycythemia in some cases of cyanotic congenital heart disease; however, other factors such as increased platelet destruction on abnormal anatomic vascular beds[159] and an artifactual low platelet count secondary to a high hematocrit may also be operating.

Respiratory distress syndrome

A significant number of infants with respiratory distress syndrome (RDS) also develop thrombocytopenia,[160] which is usually accompanied by evidence of DIC. Postmortem findings in some infants who die from RDS show pulmonary microvascular thrombosis[161] and again, like most of the other perinatal conditions seen in association with thrombocytopenia, the precise mechanism(s) responsible for the low platelet count in RDS is not known. The degree of thrombocytopenia may be exacerbated with treatment as it is known that mechanical ventilation can induce mild thrombocytopenia in newborn infants.[162]

Necrotizing enterocolitis

The majority of infants with necrotizing enterocolitis (NEC) have evidence of thrombocytopenia. In one study, 90% of infants studied had a platelet count of $<150 \times 10^9/l$ and over half a platelet count $<50 \times 10^9/l$. Over 50% of the severe thrombocytopenic group had bleeding complications, with one-third having serious sequelae which were felt to be a contributing factor to infant mortality. A significant number of the severe cases had evidence of DIC.[163] Increased platelet destruction is thought to be the principle mechanism contributing to NEC-associated thrombocytopenia.

Bacterial infections

Thrombocytopenia is frequently seen in septic infants and probably results from consumptive coagulopathy, especially in those with bacterial infections.[164–166] Immune-mediated platelet destruction as well as impaired platelet production secondary to bone marrow infection have also been shown to contribute to the thrombocytopenia.[167] A low platelet count is usually seen after the onset of infectious symptoms and resolution of the platelet count occurs promptly when infection control is achieved.[168–171]

Rhesus hemolytic disease

Severe Rhesus hemolytic disease of the newborn may be associated with thrombocytopenia, especially in the setting of liver dysfunction and DIC.[172–174] The mechanism of the thrombocytopenia has not been fully elucidated but is probably multifactorial, involving hyperbilirubinemia, phototherapy, consumptive coagulopathy and the immune process. The thrombocytopenia usually improves during the first week of life and following exchange transfusion.[175] It should be remembered that exchange transfusion itself may cause thrombocytopenia, a process felt to be due to a dilutional effect, which can be prevented in some infants by using whole blood.[174,175]

Protein C and S deficiency

Hereditary protein C (PC) and S (PS) deficiency (homozygosity or compound heterozygosity) are associated with a high venous thromboembolic risk at birth or in the first few months of life.[176,177] The first clinical manifestation is usually necrotic purpura mainly affecting the extremities and in some cases massive large vessel thrombosis (renal, vena caval and iliac veins) can also be a presenting feature. Laboratory markers of DIC are usually present within the first week of life. Low levels of PC and PS are also usually seen in DIC associated with other etiologies, especially infection, and therefore it is important to make the correct diagnosis of hereditary PC or PS deficiency as optimum therapy involves factor replacement (protein C concentrate in PC deficiency or FFP in PS deficiency) and heparin in the acute phase and oral anticoagulation in the long term. Within hours of factor replacement restoration of plasma coagulation proteins and platelets levels is apparent.[176,177] Homozygotes of antithrombin deficiency producing functional defects are also associated with a high risk of venous thromboembolic disease; however, at the time of writing, only 1 case of thrombosis presenting in childhood has been reported.[178] Like PC deficiency, emergency or elective therapy involves antithrombin concentrate and heparin infusions.[179] Heterozygotes of PC, PS and antithrombin generally do not experience thrombosis until adolescence or early adulthood.

Heparin-induced thrombocytopenia

Heparin-induced thrombocytopenia (HIT) constitutes the severest adverse effect of heparin therapy. It is of highly variable incidence, depending on the type of heparin used and whether the patient was infected/inflamed at the time of administration, but generally varies between $>1\%$ and $<15\%$ of patients receiving unfractionated heparin.[180] There are 2 types of HIT:

- type I occurs within 1–2 days, is non-immune and is usually totally benign;
- type II usually occurs after a latent period of 7–14 days, is

immune mediated and is associated with paradoxical thrombosis/thromboembolism.[181]

Fortunately, the latter is an extremely rare event in neonates; nevertheless, when an infant is receiving heparin, no matter how small the dose, whether to keep a catheter patent or in total parenteral nutrition, a watchful eye should always be kept on the daily platelet count.

Rare bone marrow diseases

Transient abnormal myelopoiesis (see also Chapter 4)

Transient abnormal myelopoiesis (TAM) associated with Down's syndrome (trisomy 21) or trisomy 21 mosaicism is a clonal disorder usually affecting children under 3 months of age. It is classically manifest as a myeloproliferative syndrome with hepatosplenomegaly, elevated white cell count, normal hemoglobin and commonly thrombocytopenia. Blood smear examination usually reveals increased numbers of eosinophils and basophils but also blast cells that in the majority resemble megakaryoblasts.[182] Essentially, TAM looks like congenital leukemia; however, spontaneous remission is usually seen. Approximately 1 in 4 of these children develop megakaryoblastic leukemia by their third birthday.[183]

Hemophagocytic lymphohistiocytosis (see also Chapter 17)

Hemophagocytic lymphohistiocytosis (HLH) is a rare, probably autosomal recessive disorder of the monocyte-macrophage lineage. It usually occurs within the first 6 months of life and is characterized by fever, maculopapular rash, jaundice, hepatosplenomegaly, lymphadenopathy, pancytopenia, hypofibrionogenemia, hypertriglyceridemia and abnormal liver chemistry. Bone marrow examination shows numerous macrophages actively engulfing bone marrow elements including platelets. This disorder is usually rapidly fatal and allogeneic BMT offers the only real chance of cure.[184] Infection-associated hemophagocytic syndrome, especially in the immunocompromised host, can also present with thrombocytopenia as can the systemic variety of Langerhans' cell histiocytosis; however, older children are those usually affected.[184]

Osteopetrosis

Variable cytopenias and a leukoerythroblastic blood smear are not an uncommon feature of autosomal recessive osteopetrosis (severe form). This usually presents during the first few months of life as failure to thrive, hypocalcemia, thrombocytopenia and anemia with or without infection. Generalized hyperostosis leads to bone marrow cavity obliteration and thus induces extramedullary hematopoiesis which results in hepatosplenomegaly. Allogeneic BMT is the optimal therapeutic option for the severe disease as a significant number of these children die early in childhood.

Congenital leukemia

Congenital leukemia is a rare disease, usually of the myelomonoblastic, monoblastic or megakaryoblastic phenotype.[185] Nodular skin infiltration, the so-called 'blueberry muffin' appearance, and hepatosplenomegaly are not uncommon associations. Thrombocytopenia alone or in association with other cytopenias is usually present at diagnosis.

Metastatic neuroblastoma

Metastatic neuroblastoma may also cause cytopenias secondary to marrow infiltration. Neuroblastoma cells are usually easily identifiable on marrow smears as they usually appear in tight groups and/or rosettes. Whilst thrombocytopenia occurs in metastatic neuroblastoma, thrombocytosis is more common as a presenting hematologic abnormality.[186]

PLACENTAL FACTORS

Placental infarction, which is not uncommon in women with circulating lupus anticoagulants and anticardiolipin antibodies, together with circulating lupus (chorioangiomas) can lead to thrombocytopenia which is usually present early in neonatal life. The mechanism(s) responsible for the thrombocytopenia has not been fully elucidated but is probably the end result of a localized DIC within the abnormal vascular bed.

CONCLUSIONS

The inherited and congenital thrombocytopenias represent a very diverse group of disorders ranging from those with little or no hemorrhagic problems to those where significant mortality occurs within the neonatal period if appropriate therapy is not initiated. The inherited thrombocytopenias are very rare disorders when compared to the congenital or acquired thrombocytopenia group and making the correct diagnosis at the outset is very important as it usually avoids the prescribing of unnecessary and potentially toxic therapies. The differential diagnosis of neonatal thrombocytopenia differs enormously depending on the general well being of the infant and therefore, a detailed maternal history and neonatal examination are essential in making a speedy diagnosis. Platelet concentrate transfusions are the mainstay of therapy in the inherited group and treating the underlying cause in the congenital group usually raises the platelet count into the normal range.

The past 25 years have witnessed remarkable progress in

the understanding, at the molecular level, of the mechanism by which platelet production and survival is controlled. Despite these impressive breakthroughs, much remains to be learned about the molecular defects responsible for the majority of inherited thrombocytopenias. No doubt, the next 25 years will see not only the isolation of the rogue genes responsible for these conditions but also gene therapies for these disorders will become a reality.

REFERENCES

1. Clemetson KH, Clemetson JM. Platelet GpIb-V-IX complex: structure, function, physiology and pathology. *Semin Thromb Hemostas* 1995; **21**: 130–136

2. Donne AD. L'origine des globules der san, de leur mode de formation et de leur fin. *CK Acad Sci* 1842; **14**: 366–371

3. Geber F. *Elements of General and Minute Anatomy of Man and Mammals*. London: G Gulliver, 1942

4. Addison W. On the colorless corpuscles and on the molecules and cytoblasts in the blood. *London Med Gas (NS)* 1842; **30**: 144–148

5. Simon F. Physiologische und pathologische antropochemic mit Berucksichtigung der eigentlichen Zoochemie. *Handbuch derangewandten medizinischen chemie nach dem neusten Standpunkte der wissengraft und nach zahlreichen eigenen untersuchungen. Theil II*. Berlin: Forstner, 1842

6. Wintrobe MM. Early beginnings. In: *Hematology, the Blossoming of a New Science: A Story of Inspiration and Effort*. Philadelphia: Lea & Febiger, 1985, pp 28–29

7. Bizzozero J. Uber einen neuen Formbestandtheil des Blutes und die rolle bei der Thrombose und der Blutgrinning. *Virchows Arch [A]* 1882; **90**: 264

8. Wright JH. The origin and nature of blood plates. *Boston Med Surg J* 1906; **154**: 643–645

9. Wendling F, Maraskovsky E, Debili N *et al*. The Mpl ligand is a humoral regulator of megakaryocytopoiesis. *Nature* 1994; **369**: 571–574

10. Eaton D. The purification and cloning of human thrombopoietin. In: Kuter DJ, Hunt P, Sheridan, Zucker-Franklin D (eds) *Thrombopoiesis and Thrombopoietins: Molecular, Cellular, Preclinical and Clinical Biology*. Totowa, NJ: Humana Press, 1997, pp 135–142

11. Dreyfus M, Kaplan C, Verdy E *et al*. Frequency of immune thrombocytopenia in newborns. A prospective study. *Blood* 1997; **89**: 4402–4406

12. Tuddenham EGD, Cooper DN. The von Willebrand factor and von Willebrand disease. In: Tuddenham EGD, Cooper DN (eds) *The Molecular Genetics of Haemostasis and its Inherited Disorders*. Oxford: Oxford University Press, 1994, pp 374–401

13. Clemetson KH, Clemetson JM. Molecular abnormalities in Glanzman's thrombasthenia, Bernard–Soulier syndrome and platelet type von Willebrand's disease. *Curr Opin Hematol* 1994; **1**: 388–393

14. Lopez JA. The platelet glycoprotein Ib-IX. *Blood Coag Fibrinol* 1994; **5**: 97–118

15. Roth GJ. Developing relationships: arterial platelet adhesion, glycoprotein Ib, and leucine-rich glycoproteins. *Blood* 1991; **77**: 5–19

16. Miller JL, Cunningham D, Lyle VA, Finch CN. Mutation in the gene encoding the α chain of platelet glycoprotein Ib in platelet-type von-Willebrand disease. *Proc Natl Acad Sci USA* 1991; **88**: 4761–1765

17. Bolin RB, Okumura T, Jamieson GA. New polymorphism of platelet membrane glycoproteins. *Nature* 1977; **269**: 69–70

18. Bowen DF, Hampton KK. von Willebrand disease and its diagnosis. In: Poller L, Ludlam CA (eds) *Recent Advances in Blood Coagulation*. Edinburgh: Churchill Livingstone, 1997, pp 201–219

19. Milton JG, Frojmovic MM, Tacry SS, White JG. Spontaneous platelet aggregation in an hereditary giant platelet syndrome (MPS). *Am J Pathol* 1984; **74**: 715–721

20. Okita JR, Frojmovic MM, Kristopeit S, Wong T, Kunicki TJ. Montreal platelet syndrome: A defect in calcium-activated neutral proteins (Calpain). *Blood* 1989; **74**: 715–721

21. Milton JG, Frojmovic MM. Shape-changing agents produce abnormally large platelets in a hereditary "giant platelet syndrome (MPS)". *J Lab Clin Med* 1979; **93**: 154–159

22. Bennett JS, Shattil SJ. Congenital qualitative platelet disorders. In: Williams WJ (ed) *Hematology*. New York: McGraw Hill, 1990, pp 1407–1419

23. Jantunen E. Inherited giant platelet disorders. *Eur J Haematol* 1994; **53**: 191–196

24. Gebrane-Younes J, Martin Cramer E, Orcel L, Caen JP. Gray platelet syndrome. Dissociation between abnormal sorting in megakaryocyte alpha-granules and normal sorting in Weibel-Palade bodies of endothelial cells. *J Clin Invest* 1993; **92**: 3023–3028

25. Jantunen E, Hanninen A, Naukkarinen A, Vornanen M, Lahtinen R. Gray platelet syndrome with splenomegaly and signs of extramedullary hematopoiesis. *Am J Hematol* 1994; **46**: 218–224

26. George JN, Nurden AT, Phillips DR. Molecular defects in interactions of platelets with the vessel wall. *N Engl J Med* 1984; **311**: 1084–1089

27. Breton-Gorius J, Favier R, Guichard J *et al*. A new congenital dysmegakaryopoietic thrombocytopenia (Paris–Trousseau) associated with giant α-granules and chromosome 11 deletion at 11q23. *Blood* 1995; **85**: 1805–1814

28. Aldrich RA, Steinberg AG, Campbell DC. Pedigree demonstrating a sex-linked recessive condition characterised by draining ears, eczematoid dermatitis and bloody diarrhea. *Blood* 1995; **85**: 1805–1814

29. Cooper MD, Chase HP, Lowman JT *et al*. Wiskott–Aldrich syndrome: an immunologic deficiency disease involving the afferent limb of the immunity. *Am J Med* 1968; **44**: 499–513

30. Ochs HD, Slichter SJ, Harker LA *et al*. The Wiskott–Aldrich syndrome: studies of lymphocytes, granulocytes and platelets. *Blood* 1980; **55**: 243–252

31. Grottum KA, Hovig T, Holmsen H *et al*. Wiskott–Aldrich syndrome: qualitative platelet defects and short survival. *Br J Haematol* 1969; **17**: 373–377

32. Verhoeven AJM, Oostrum IEA, van Haarlem H. Impaired energy metabolism in platelets from patients with Wiskott–Aldrich syndrome. *Thromb Haemostas* 1989; **61**: 10–15

33. Mullen CA, Anderson KD, Blaese M. Splenectomy and/or bone marrow transplantation in the management of Wiskott–Aldrich syndrome: long term follow-up of 62 cases. *Blood* 1993; **82**: 2961–2965

34. Lum LG, Tubergen DG, Corash L, Blaese M. Splenectomy in the management of the thrombocytopenia of the Wiskott–Aldrich syndrome. *N Engl J Med* 1980; **302**: 892–895

35. Stomorken H, Hellum B, Egeland T *et al*. X-linked thrombocytopenia and thrombocytopathia: attenuated Wiskott–Aldrich syndrome. Functional and morphological studies of platelets and lymphoctyes. *Thromb Haemostas* 1991; **65**: 300–305

36. Ata M, Fisher OD, Holman CA. Inherited thrombocytopenia. *Lancet* 1965; **i**: 119–121

37. Donner M, Schwarte M, Carlsson KM *et al*. Hereditary X-linked thrombocytopenia maps to the same chromosomal region as the Wiskott–Aldrich syndrome. *Blood* 1988; **72**: 1849–1852

38. Zhu Q, Zhang M, Bles RM *et al*. The Wiskott–Aldrich syndrome and X-linked congenital thrombocytopenia are caused by mutations of the same gene. *Blood* 1995; **86**: 3797–3802

39. Haddad WM *et al*. Treatment of Chediak-Highasi syndrome by allogeneic bone marrow transplantation: report of 10 cases. *Blood* 1995; **85**: 3328–3342

40. Tracy PB, Giles AE, Mann KG *et al*. Factor V (Quebec): A bleeding diathesis associated with a qualitative platelet factor V deficiency. *J Clin Invest* 1984; **74**: 1221–1228

41. Janeway CM, Rivard GE, Tracy PB, Mann KG. Factor V Quebec revisited. *Blood* 1996; **87**: 3571–3578

42. Haward CPM, Rivard GE, Kane WH *et al*. An autosomal dominant, qualitative platelet disorder associated with multimerin deficiency, abnormality of platelet factor V, thrombospondin, von Willebrand

factor, and fibrinogen and an epinephrine aggregation defect. *Blood* 1996; **87**: 4967–4978

43. Hegglin R. Gleichzeitige knostitutionelle Veranderungen an Neutrophylen und Thrombozyten. *Helv Med Acta* 1945; **12**: 439–444

44. Greinacher A, Muller-Eckhart C. Hereditary types of thrombocytopenia with giant platelets and inclusion bodies in the leukocytes. *Blut* 1990; **60**: 53–59

45. Godwin HA, Ginsburg AD. May-Hegglin anomaly: a defect in megakaryocyte fragmentation? *Br J Haematol* 1974; **26**: 117–124

46. Cabrera JR, Fonton G, Lorente F *et al.* Defective neutrophil mobility in the May-Hegglin anomaly. *Br J Haematol* 1981; **47**: 337–341

47. Buchanan JG *et al.* The May-Hegglin anomaly. A family report and chromosome study. *Br J Haematol* 1964; **10**: 508–514

48. Hamilton RW, Shaikh BS, Ottie JN *et al.* Platelet function, ultrastructure and survival in the May-Hegglin anomaly. *Am J Clin Pathol* 1980; **74**: 663–671

49. Davis JW, Wilson SJ. Platelet survival in the May-Hegglin anomaly. *Br J Haematol* 1966; **12**: 61–64

50. Greinacher A, Bux J, Kiefel V *et al.* May-Hegglin anomaly: a rare cause of thrombocytopenia. *Eur J Pediatr* 1994; **53**: 191–196

51. Jantunen E. Inherited giant platelet disorders. *Eur J Haematol* 1994; **53**: 191–196

53. Alport CA. Hereditary familial congenital haemorrhagic nephritis. *Br Med J* 1927; **1**: 504–505

54. Epstein CJ, Sahud MA, Piel CF *et al.* Hereditary macrothrombocytopenia, nephritis and deafness. *Am J Med* 1972; **52**: 299–310

55. Eckstein JD, Filip DJ, Watts JC. Hereditary thrombocytopenia, deafness and renal disease. *Ann Intern Med* 1975; **82**: 639–645

56. Peterson LC, Rao KV, Crosson JT, White JG. Fechtner syndrome – A variant of Alport's syndrome with leucocyte inclusion and macrothrombocytopenia. *Blood* 1985; **65**: 397–406

57. Gershoni-Baruch R, Viener A, Lichtig C. Fechtner syndrome: clinical and genetic aspects. *Am J Med Genet* 1988; **31**: 357–367

58. Greinacher A, Niewenhuis HK, White JG. Sebastian platelet syndrome: A new variant of hereditary macrothrombocytopenia with leukocyte inclusions. *Blut* 1990; **61**: 282–288

59. Pujol-Moix N, Muniz-Diaz E, Moreno-Torres MLB, Hernandez A, Madox P, Domingo A. Sebastian platelet syndrome. *Ann Hematol* 1991; **62**: 235–237

60. Greinacher A, Muller-Eckhart C. Hereditary types of thrombocytopenia with giant platelets and inclusion bodies in the leukocytes. *Blut* 1990; **60**: 53–59

61. Hall JG. Thrombocytopenia and absent radius (TAR) syndrome. *J Med Genet* 1987; **24**: 79–83

62. Alter BP. Inherited bone marrow failure syndrome. In: Handin RI, Stossel TP, Lux SE (eds) *Blood: Principles and Practice of Hematology.* Philadelphia: JB Lippincott Co, 1995, pp 227–291

63. Bessman JD, Harrison RL, Howard LC, Peterson D. The megakaryocyte abnormality in thrombocytopenia-absent radius syndrome. *Blood* 1983; **62**: 143–148

64. Homans AC, Cohen JL, Mazur EM. Defective megakaryocytopoiesis in the sydrome of thrombocytopenia with absent radii. *Br J Haematol* 1988; **70**: 205–210

65. Brochstein JA, Shank B, Kernan NA, Terwillinger JW, O'Reilly RJ. Marrow transplantation for thrombocytopenia-absent radii syndrome. *J Pediatr* 1992; **121**: 587–589

66. Day HJ, Holmsen H. Platelet adenine nucleotide 'storage pool deficiency' in thrombocytopenia absent radii syndrome. *JAMA* 1972; **221**: 1053–1056

67. Filkins K, Russo J, Bilinki I, Diamond N, Searle B. Prenatal diagnosis of thrombocytopenia absent radius syndrome using ultrasound and fetoscopy. *Prenat Diagn* 1984; **4**: 139–144

68. Daffos F, Forestier F, Kaplan C, Cox W. Prenatal diagnosis and management of bleeding disorders with fetal blood sampling. *Am J Obstet Gynecol* 1988; **158**: 939–942

69. Guinan EC, Lee Y, Lopez KD *et al.* Effects of interleukin-3 and granulocyte-macrophage colony-stimulating factor on thrombopoiesis

in congenital amegakaryocytic thrombocytopenia. *Blood* 1993; **81**: 1691–1698

70. Van Oostrom CG, Wilms RHH. Congential thrombocytopenia, associated with raised concentrations of haemoglobin F. *Helv Paediatr Acta* 1978; **33**: 59–64

71. O'Gorman Hughes DW. Aplastic anemia in childhood III. Constitutional aplastic anaemia and related cytopenias. *Med J Aust* 1974; **1**: 519–526

72. Schroeder-Kurt TM, Auerbach AD, Obe G. *Fanconi Anemia. Clinical, Cytogenetic and Experimental Aspects.* Berlin: Springer-Verlag, 1989, p 264

73. Minagi HJ, Steinbach H. Roentgen appearance of anomalies associated with hypoplastic anemia of childhood: Fanconi's anemia and congential hypoplastic anemia (erythrogenesis imperfecta). *Am J Roentgenol* 1966; **97**: 100–105

74. McIntosh S, Breg WR, Lubiniecki AS. Fanconi's anemia: the pre-anemic phase. *Am J Pediatri Hematol Oncol* 1979; **1**: 107–110

75. Rabinowitz JG, Mosely JE, Mitty HA, Hirshorn K. Trisomy-18, esophageal atresia, anomalies of the radius and congenital hypoplastic thrombocytopenia. *Radiology* 1967; **89**: 488–491

76. De Alarcon PA. Thrombopoiesis in the fetus and newborn. In: Stockman JA, Pochedly C (eds) *Developmental and Neonatal Hematology.* New York: Raven Press, 1988, pp 103–130

77. Oski FA, De Angelis CD, Feigin RD, Warshaw JB (eds). *Principles and Practice of Pediatrics.* 6th edn. Philadelphia: JB Lippincott Co, 1990

78. Najean Y, Lecompte T. Genetic thrombocytopenia with autosomal dominant transmission. *Br J Haematol* 1990; **74**: 203–208

79. Najean Y, Lecompte T. Hereditary thrombocytopenia in childhood. *Semin Thromb Hemostas* 1995; **21**: 294–304

80. Von Behrens WC. Mediterranean thrombocytopenia. *Blood* 1975; **46**: 199–208

81. Najean Y. The congenital thrombocytopenias due to a production defect. In: Sutor AH, Thomas KB (eds) *Thrombocytopenia in Childhood.* Basel: Roche Schattauer, 1994, pp 199–208

82. Guerois G, Gruel Y, Petit A *et al.* Familial macrothrombocytopenia. *Curr Studies Hematol Blood Transfusion* 1988; **55**: 153–161

83. Pearson HA, Shulman NR, Marder VJ, Cone TE. Isoimmune neonatal thrombocytopenic purpura: Clinical and therapeutic considerations. *Blood* 1964; **23**: 154–177

84. Blanchette VS, Peters MA, Pegg-Feige K. Alloimmune thrombocytopenia. Review from a neonatal intensive care unit. *Curr Studies Hematol Blood Transfusion* 1986; **52**: 87–96

85. Mueller-Eckhardt C, Kiefel V, Grubert A *et al.* 348 cases of suspected neonatal alloimmune thrombocytopenia. *Lancet* 1989; **i**: 363–366

86. Kaplan C, Morel-Kopp MC, Kroll H *et al.* HPA-5b (Brᵃ) neonatal alloimmune thrombocytopenia. Clinical and immunological analysis of 39 cases. *Br J Haematol* 1991; **78**: 425–429

87. Blanchette VS, Chen L, Salomon de Friedberg Z, Hogan VA, Trudel E, Decary F. Alloimmunization to the Plᴬ¹ platelet antigen: Results of a prospective study. *Br J Haematol* 1990; **74**: 209–215

88. Reznikoff-Etievant MF, Kaplan C, Durieux I, Huchet J, Salmon C, Neter A. Alloimmune thrombocytopenia, definition of a group at risk: A prospective study. *Curr Studies Blood Transfusion* 1988; **55**: 119–125

89. De Wall LP, Van Dalen CM, Englefriet CP, von dem Borne AEG. Alloimmunisation against the platelet-specific Zwa antigen, resulting in neonatal thrombocytopenia or post-transfusion purpura, is associated with the supertypic Drw52 antigen including DR3 and Drw6. *Hum Immunol* 1986; **17**: 45–53

90. Reznikoff-Etievant MR, Dangu C. ALA-B8 antigens and anti-Pl^A1 and alloimmunisation. *Tissue Antigens* 1981; **18**: 66–72

91. Mueller-Eckhardt C, Kiefel V. HLA-DRw6, a new immune response marker for immunisation against the platelet alloantigen Brᵃ. *Vox Sang* 1986; **50**: 94–99

92. Bussel J, Berkowitz R, McFarland J. *In-utero* platelet transfusion for alloimmune thrombocytopenia. *Lancet* 1988; **ii**: 506

93. Herman JH, Jumbelic MI, Ancona RJ, Kickler TS. *In utero* cerebral hemorrhage in alloimmune thrombocytopenia. *Am J Pediatr Hematol Oncol* 1986; **8**: 312–317

94. Davidson JE, McWilliam RC, Evans TJ, Stephenson JB. Porencephaly and optic hypoplasia in neonatal isoimmune thrombocytopenia. *Arch Dis Child* 1989; **64**: 858–860

95. Mueller-Eckhardt C, Kayser W, Forster C, Muller-Eckhardt G, Ringenberg C. Improved assay for detection of platelet-specific PlA1 antibodies in neonatal immune thrombocytopenia. *Vox Sang* 1982; **43**: 76–81

96. Kiefel V, Santoso S, Katzmann B, Mueller-Eckhardt C. A new platelet-specific alloantigen Bra. Report of 4 cases with neonatal alloimmune thrombocytopenia. *Vox Sang* 1988; **54**: 101–106

97. Kaplan C, Daffos F, Forestier F. Management of alloimmune thrombocytopenia: antenatal diagnosis and in-utero transfusion of maternal platelets. *Blood* 1988; **72**: 340–343

98. McFarland JG, Frenzke M, Aster RH. Testing of maternal sera in pregnancies at risk for neonatal alloimmune thrombocytopenia. *Transfusion* 1989; **29**: 128–133

99. Adner MM, Fisch GR, Starobin SG, Aster RH. Use of "compatible" platelet transfusions in the treatment of congenital isoimmune thrombocytopenic purpura. *N Engl J Med* 1969; **280**: 244–247

100. Katz J, Hodder FS, Aster RS, Bennetts GA, Cairo MS. Neonatal isoimmune thrombocytopenia. The natural course and management and the detection of maternal antibody. *Clin Pediatr* 1984; **23**: 159–162

101. Sanders MR, Graeber JE. Posttransfusion graft-versus-host-disease in infancy. *J Pediatr* 1990; **117**: 159–163

102. Sidiropoulos D, Straume B. The treatment of neonatal thrombocytopenia with intravenous immunoglobulin (IgG i.v.). *Blut* 1984; **48**: 383–386

103. Derycke M, Dreyfus M, Ropert JC, Tchernia G. Intravenous immunoglobulin for neonatal isoimmune thrombocytopenia. *Arch Dis Child* 1985; **60**: 667–669

104. Suarez CR, Anderson C. High-dose intravenous gammaglobulin (IVIG) in neonatal immune thrombocytopenia. *Am J Hematol* 1987; **26**: 247–253

105. Massey GV, McWilliams NB, Mueller DG, Napolitano A, Mauer HM. Intravenous immunoglobulin in the treatment of neonatal isoimmune thrombocytopenia. *J Pediatr* 1987; **111**: 133–135

106. McGill M, Mayhaus C, Hoff R, Carey P. Frozen maternal platelets for neonatal thrombocytopenia. *Transfusion* 1982; **27**: 341–347

107. McFarland JG, Aster RH, Bussel JB, Gianopoulos JG, Derbes RS, Newman PJ. Prenatal diagnosis of neonatal alloimmune thrombocytopenia using allele specific oligonucleotide probes. *Blood* 1991; **78**: 2276–2282

108. Kuijpers RW, Faber NM, Kanhai HH, von dem Borne AE. Typing of fetal platelet alloantigens when platelets are not available. *Lancet* 1990; **336**: 1391

109. Bussel JB, Berkowitz RL, McFarland JG, Lynch L, Chitkara U. Antenatal treatment of neonatal alloimmune thrombocytopenia. *N Engl J Med* 1988; **319**: 1374–1378

110. Lynch L, Bussel JB, McFarland JG, Chitkara U, Berkowitz RL. Antenatal treatment of alloimmune thrombocytopenia. *Obstet Gynecol* 1992; **80**: 67–71

111. Anon. Management of alloimmune neonatal thrombocytopenia. *Lancet* 1989; **i**: 137–139

112. Kapatkin S, Stick N, Kapatkin MB, Siskind GW. Cumulative experience in the detection of antiplatelet antibody in 234 patients with idiopathic thrombocytopenic purpura, systemic lupus erythematosus and other clinical disorders. *Am J Med* 1972; **52**: 776–785

113. de Swiet M. Maternal alloimmune disease and the fetus. *Arch Dis Child* 1985; **60**: 749–797

114. Dixon RH, Rosse WF. Platelet antibody in autoimmune thrombocytopenia. *Br J Haematol* 1975; **31**: 129–137

115. George D, Bussel JB. Neonatal thrombocytopenia. *Semin Thromb Hemostas* 1995; **21**: 276–293

116. Burrows RF, Kelton JG. Low fetal risks in pregnancies associated with idiopathic thrombocytopenic purpura. *Am J Obstet Gynecol* 1990; **163**: 1147–1150

117. Barbui T, Cortelazzo S, Viero P, Buelli M, Casarotto C. Idiopathic thrombocytopenic purpura and pregnancy. Maternal platelet count and antiplatelet antibodies do not predict the risk of neonatal thrombocytopenia. *La Ric Clin Lab* 1985; **15**: 139–145

118. Burrows RF, Kelton JG. Incidentally detected thrombocytopenia in healthy mothers and their infants. *N Engl J Med* 1988; **319**: 142–145

119. Aster RH. "Gestational" thrombocytopenia. A plea for conservative management. *N Engl J Med* 1990; **323**: 264–266

120. Sauels P, Bussel JB, Braitman LE *et al*. Estimation of the risk of thrombocytopenia in the offspring of pregnant women with presumed immune thrombocytopenia purpura. *N Engl J Med* 1990; **323**: 229–235

121. Kapatkin M, Porges RF, Karpatkin S. Platelet counts in infants of women with autoimmune thrombocytopenia: effects of steroid administration to the mother. *N Engl J Med* 1981; **52**: 776–785

122. Bussel JB, Kaplan C, McFarland J. Recommendations for the evaluation and treatment of neonatal autoimmune and alloimmune thrombocytopenia. *Thromb Haemostas* 1991; **65**: 631–635

123. Blanchette VS, Sacher RA, Ballem PJ, Bussel JB, Imbash P. Commentary on the management of autoimmune thrombocytopenia during pregnancy and the neonatal period. *Blut* 1989; **59**: 121–126

124. Cooper LZ, Green RH, Krugman S. Neonatal thrombocytopenic purpura and other manifestations of rubella contracted in utero. *Am J Dis Child* 1965; **110**: 416–419

125. Hohlfield P, Forestier F, Kaplan C *et al*. Fetal thrombocytopenia: A retrospective survey of 5,914 fetal blood samplings. *Blood* 1994; **84**: 1851–1856

126. Boppana SB, Pass RF, Britt WJ, Stagno S, Alford CA. Symptomatic congenital cytomegalovirus infection: neonatal morbidity and mortality. *Pediatr Infect Dis J* 1992; **11**: 93–99

127. Malbrunot C, Boue A. Herpes. In: Boue A (ed) *Fetal Medicine, Prenatal Diagnosis and Management*. Oxford: Oxford University Press, 1995, pp 233–240

128. Rigaud M, Leibovitz E, Quee CS *et al*. Thrombocytopenia in children infected with human immunodeficiency virus: Long-term follow-up and therapeutic considerations. *J Acquir Immune Deficiency Syndrome* 1992; **5**: 450–455

129. Mandlebrot L, Schlienger I, Bongain A *et al*. Thrombocytopenia in pregnant women infected with human immunodeficiency virus. Maternal and neonatal outcome. *Am J Obstet Gynecol* 1994; **171**: 252–257

130. Srivastava A, Bruno E, Briddell R *et al*. Parvovirus B19-induced perturbation of human megakaryocytopoiesis in vitro. *Blood* 1990; **76**: 1997–2004

131. Malbrunot C, Boue A. AIDS. In: Boue A (ed) *Fetal Medicine, Prenatal Diagnosis and Management*. Oxford: Oxford University Press, 1995, pp 242–246

132. George D, Bussel JB. Neonatal thromboctyopenia. *Semin Thromb Hemostas* 1995; **21**: 276–293

133. Dreyfus M, Magny JF, Bridey F. Treatment of homozygous protein C deficiency and neonatal purpura fulminans with a purified protein C concentrate. *N Engl J Med* 1991; **325**: 1565–1568

134. Smith OP, White B, Vaughan D *et al*. Use of protein C concentrate, heparin and haemodiafiltration in meningococcus-induced purpura fulminans. *Lancet* 1997; **350**: 1590–1593

135. Hilgartner NW, Corrigan JJ Jr. Coagulation disorders. In: Miller DR, Baehnwer RL (eds) *Blood Diseases of Infancy and Childhood*. St Louis: CV Mosby, 1995, pp 924–986

136. Kaplan BS, Cleary TG, Obrig TG. Recent advances in understanding the pathogenesis of hemolytic uremic syndrome. *Pediatr Nephrol* 1990; **4**: 276–283

137. Beningi A, Boccardo P, Noris M *et al*. Urinary excretion of platelet-activating factor in haemolytic-uraemic syndrome. *Lancet* 1992; **339**: 835–836

138. Moake JL, McPherson PD. Abnormalities of von Willebrand factor multimers in TTP and HUS. *Am J Med* 1989; **87 (Suppl 3N)**: 9N–15N

139. McSherry KJ, Sills RH. Acquired microangiopathic haemolytic anaemias. *Int J Paediatr Haematol Oncol* 1994; **1**: 25–42

140. Moschcowitz E. Hyaline thrombosis of the terminal arterioles and capillaries: A hitherto undescribed disease. *Proc N York Pathol Soc* 1924; **24**: 21–24

141. Byrnes JJ, Moake JL. Thrombotic thrombocytopenic purpura and the haemolytic-uraemic syndrome. Evolving concepts of pathogenesis and therapy. *Clin Haematol* 1986; **15**: 413–442

142. Moake JL. Thrombotic thrombocytopenic purpura. Pathophysiologic and therapeutic studies. In: Brubaker DB, Simpson MB Jr (eds) *Dynamics of Hemostasis and Thrombosis*. Bethesda, MD: American Association of Blood Banks, 1995, pp 123–132

143. Upshaw JD Jr. Congenital deficiency of a factor in normal plasma that reverses microangiopathic hemolysis and thrombocytopenia. *N Engl J Med* 1978; **298**: 1350–1352

144. Miura M, Koizumi S, Nakamura K *et al*. Efficacy of several plasma components in a young boy with chronic thrombocytopenia and hemolytic anemia who responds repeatedly to normal plasma infusions. *Am J Hematol* 1984; **17**: 307–319

145. Chintagumpala M, Hurwitz R, Moake J *et al*. Chronic relapsing thrombotic thrombocytopenic purpura in infants with large von Willebrand factor multimers during remission. *J Pediatr* 1992; **120**: 49–53

146. Rock GA, Shumak KH, Buskard NA *et al*. Comparison of plasma exchange with plasma infusion in the treatment of thrombotic thrombocytopenic purpura. *N Engl J Med* 1991; **325**: 393–397

147. Kasabach HH, Merritt KK. Capillary hemagioma with extensive purpura: report of a case. *Am J Dis Child* 1940; **59**: 1063–1070

148. Berman B, Lim HW-P. Concurrent cutaneous and hepatic haemagiomata in infancy. Report of a case and review of the literature. *J Dermatol Surg Oncol* 1978; **4**: 869–873

149. Enjolras O, Riche MC, Merland JJ, Escande JP. Management of alarming hemangiomas in infancy. A review of 25 cases. *Pediatrics* 1990; **85**: 491–498

150. Kushner BJ. The treatment of periorbital infantile hemangiomas with intralesional steroids. *Plast Reconst Surg* 1985; **76**: 517–526

151. Ezekowitz RAB, Mulliken JB, Folkman J. Interferon alpha-2a therapy for life-threatening hemagiomas in infancy. *N Engl J Med* 1992; **326**: 1456–1463

152. Argenta LC, Bishop E, Cho KL, Andrews AF, Coran AG. Complete resolution of life-threatening haemangioma by embolisation and corticosteroids. *Plast Reconst Surg* 1982; **70**: 739–744

153. Stanley P, Gomperts E, Woolley MM. Kasabach–Merritt syndrome treated by therapeutic embolisation with polyvinyl alcohol. *Am J Pediatr Hematol Oncol* 1986; **8**: 308–311

154. Schild SE, Buskrit SJ, Frick LM, Cupps RE. Radiotherapy for large symptomatic hemangiomas. *Int J Radiat Oncol Biol Phys* 1991; **21**: 729–735

155. David M, Andrew M. Venous thromboembolism complications in children: a critical review of the literature. *J Pediatr* 1993; **123**: 337–342

156. Chessells JM, Wigglesworth JS. Coagulation studies in severe birth asphyxia. *Arch Dis Child* 1971; **46**: 253–256

157. Chadd MA, Elwood PC, Grey OP, Muxworthy SM. Coagulation studies in hypoxia fullterm newborn infants. *Br Med J* 1971; **4**: 516–518

158. van Hinsbergh VWM. The vessel wall and hemostasis. In: van Hinsbergh VWM (ed) *Vascular Control of Hemostasis*. Australia: Harwood Academic Publishers, 1996, pp 1–9

159. Henriksson P, Varendh G, Lundstrom NR. Haemostatic defects in cyanotic congenital heart disease. *Br Heart J* 1979; **41**: 23–27

160. Segal ML, Goetzman BW, Schick JB. Thrombocytopenia and pulmonary hypertension in perinatal aspiration syndromes. *J Pediatr* 1980; **96**: 727–730

161. George D, Bussel JB. Neonatal thrombocytopenia. *Semin Thromb Hemostas* 1995; **21**: 276–293

162. Ballin A, Koren G, Kohelet D *et al*. Reduction of platelet counts induced by mechanical ventilation in newborn infants. *J Pediatr* 1987; **111**: 445–449

163. Hutter JJ, Hathaway WE, Wayne ER. Hematologic abnormalities in severe neonatal necrotising enterocolitis. *J Pediatr* 1976; **88**: 1026–1031

164. Castle V, Andrew M, Kelton J, Giron D, Johnston M, Carter C. Frequency and mechanism of neonatal thrombocytopenia. *J Pediatr* 1986; **108**: 749–755

165. De Alarcon PA. Thrombopoiesis in the fetus and newborn. In: Syockman JA, Pochedly C (eds) *Developmental and Neonatal Hematology*. New York: Raven Press, 1988, pp 103–130

166. Naiman JL. Disorders of platelets. In: Oski FA, Naiman J (eds) *Hematologic Problems of the Newborn*. Philadelphia: WB Saunders , 1982, pp 175–222

167. Desforges JF, O'Connell LG. Hematologic observations of the course of erythroblastosis fetalis. *Blood* 1955; **10**: 802–810

168. Tate DY, Carlton GT, Johnson D *et al*. Immune thrombocytopenia in severe neonatal infections. *J Pediatr* 1981; **98**: 449–453

169. Mehta P, Vasa R, Neumann L, Karpartkin M. Thrombocytopenia in the high risk infant. *J Pediatr* 1980; **97**: 791–794

170. Zipursky A, Jaber HM. The haematology of bacterial infection in newborn infants. *Clin Haematol* 1978; **7**: 175–193

171. Mondanlou HD, Ortiz OB. Thrombocytopenia in neonatal infection. *Clin Pediatr* 1981; **20**: 402–407

172. Chessells JM, Wigglesworth JS. Haemostatic failure in babies with rhesus isoimmuisation. *Arch Dis Child* 1971; **46**: 38–45

173. Andrew M. The hemostatic system in the infant. In: Nathan DG, Oski FA (eds) *Hematology of Infancy and Childhood*, 4th edn. Philadelphia: WB Saunders, 1993, 115–153

174. Andrew M, Castle V, Saigal S, Carter C, Kelton JG. Clinical impact of neonatal thrombocytopenia. *J Pediatr* 1987; **110**: 457–464

175. Andrew M, Vegh P, Caco C *et al*. A randomised, controlled trial of platelet transfusions in thrombocytopenic premature infants. *J Pediatr* 1993; **123**: 285–291

176. Dreyfus M, Magny JF, Bridey F. Treatment of homozygous protein C deficiency and neonatal purpura fulminans with a purified protein C concentrate. *N Engl J Med* 1991; **325**: 1565–1569

177. Mahasandana C, Suvatte V, Marlar RA. Neonatal purpura fulminans associated with homozygous protein S deficiency. *Lancet* 1990; **22**: 61–62

178. Boyer C, Wolf M, Vendrenne J. Homozygous variant of antithrombin III: AT III Fontaineblue. *Thromb Haemostas* 1986; **56**: 18–21

179. Schwartz RS, Bauer KA, Rosenberg RD, Kavanaugh EJ, Davies DC, Bogdanoff DA. Clinical experience with antithrombin III concentrate in treatment of congenital and acquired deficiency of antithrombin. *Am J Med* 1989; **87**: 53S

180. Bick RL. Heparin-induced thrombocytopenia and paradoxical thromboembolism: Diagnostic and therapeutic dilemmas. *Clin Appl Thromb Hemostas* 1997; **3**: 63–65

181. Spadone D, Clark F, James E, Laster J, Hoch J, Silver D. Heparin-induced thrombocytopenia in the newborn. *J Vasc Surg* 1992; **15**: 306–311

182. Iselius L, Jacobs P, Morton, N. Leukaemia and transient leukaemia in Down syndrome. *Hum Genet* 1990; **85**: 477–481

183. Zipursky A, Poon A, Doyle J. Hematologic and oncologic disorders in Down's syndrome. In: Lott I, McCoy E (eds) *Down Syndrome: Today's Health Care Issues*. New York: John Wiley & Sons, 1991; pp 42–56

184. Pritchard J, Malone M. Histiocyte disorders. In: Peckham M, Pinedo HM, Veronesi U (eds) *Oxford Textbook of Oncology*. Oxford: Oxford University Press, 1995, pp 1878–1894

185. Koller U, Haas HA, Ludwig W-D. Phenotypic and genotypic heterogeneity in infant acute leukaemia. II. Acute nonlymphoblastic leukaemia. *Leukaemia* 1989; **3**: 708–712

186. Roald B, Ninane J. Neuroblastoma. In: Peckham M, Pinedo HM, Veronesi U (eds) *Oxford Textbook of Oncology*. Oxford: Oxford University Press, 1995, pp 1992–2000

Immune thrombocytopenic purpura

PAUL IMBACH

Immune thrombocytopenic purpura (ITP) is a bleeding disorder which occurs either as an acute, self-limiting condition, or as a recurrent or chronic autoimmune disorder. Synonyms are autoimmune thrombocytopenic purpura (AITP; often used for chronic ITP in adults), Morbus Werlhof and purpura hemorrhagica. Pathophysiologically, it is characterized by early platelet destruction due to antibody binding and subsequent removal of platelets by the mononuclear phagocytic system. ITP also presents in association with other disorders such as infections, connective tissue diseases, or as thrombocytopenia after bone marrow transplantation. Moreover, ITP may also occur with alloimmune platelet destruction as observed in neonatal purpura and post-transfusion purpura. Finally, drug-induced ITP is seen more frequently in adults than in children.

HISTORY

In 1735, Werlhof described a bleeding disorder which he called Morbus maculosus hemorrhagicus.[1] In 1883, Krauss observed decreased platelets and in 1890, Hayem performed the first platelet count and found a low number of platelets in the disease. The first splenectomy in ITP was successfully performed in Prague in 1916.[2] Subsequently, splenectomy became the main treatment for chronic ITP despite a lack of knowledge concerning the pathophysiologic role of the spleen in this disorder.

Since 1950 there has been increasing clinical evidence for an immuno-pathogenetic mechanism of ITP. In 1951, Harrington et al[3,4] observed that newborns of mothers with chronic ITP often had a transient decrease in their platelet counts, suggesting the transfer of an humoral antiplatelet factor from the mother to her baby. Harrington developed classical transient ITP after self-administration of plasma from a patient with ITP, as did other volunteers (Fig. 22.1A). Later, Shulman et al[5] showed that the thrombocytopenic factor was associated with the 7S IgG fraction of ITP plasma and, importantly, that this factor binds to autologous as well as homologous platelets. Since 1975, laboratory techniques have demonstrated elevated platelet-associated IgG (PAIgG) in the majority of patients with thrombocytopenia.[6] In 1980, Imbach et al[7] observed that the intravenous administration of intact 7S IgG, fractionated and pooled from single blood donors, raises the platelet counts in patients with acute and chronic ITP (Fig. 22.1B).

In 1982, Van Leeuwen et al[8] provided the first evidence for autoantibodies in chronic ITP. They reported that 32 of 42 eluates from ITP platelets would bind to normal but not to thrombasthenic platelets. Since these latter platelets are deficient in glycoproteins (Gp) IIb and IIIa, they postulated that ITP patients have autoantibodies to one of these glycoproteins. In 1987, 2 assays were developed that can detect both platelet-associated and free plasmic autoantibodies: the immunobead assay[9] and the monoclonal antibody-specific immobilization of platelet antigens (MAIPA) assay.[10]

INCIDENCE

ITP is diagnosed more frequently than any other form of destructive thrombocytopenia. In its acute form, it affects mostly children, while the chronic form is frequently seen in young adults. ITP is more common in white than black children and its severity and duration may display geographic variations.

Eighty to 90% of children with ITP have an acute transient bleeding episode, resolving within a few days or weeks and, by definition, ending within 6 months. In acute ITP, both sexes are equally affected[11,12] with a peak occurrence between 2 and 5 years of age. There is frequently a history of viral or bacterial infection or vaccination 1–6 weeks prior to the onset of acute ITP. The onset of bleeding is often abrupt and is associated with a platelet count $<20 \times 10^9/l$.

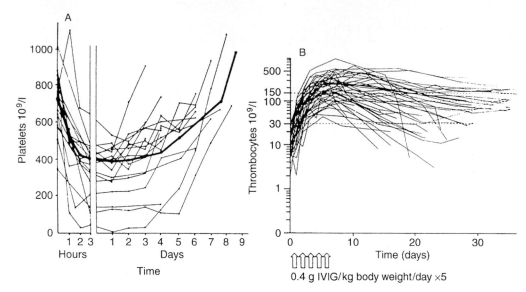

Fig. 22.1 (A) Platelet counts of volunteers after infusion of immune thrombocytopenic purpura (ITP) plasma. (B) Platelet counts of 42 children with ITP during and after intravenous immunoglobulin (IVIG) treatment. Reproduced with permission from Ref. 246.

Chronic ITP in children manifests with similar clinical features to those seen in adults, i.e. the onset is usually insidious and there is a predominance among females.[13,14] Most children with chronic ITP are >7 years of age.

The recurrent form of ITP is defined as episodes of thrombocytopenia at intervals of >3 months and occurs in 1–4% of children with ITP.[15,16]

Familial ITP is a rare disorder[17–22] and the precise nature of inheritance remains unclear.

PATHOGENESIS

The clinical signs and symptoms of ITP are caused by an increased rate of premature platelet destruction which occurs preferentially in the spleen, liver, bone marrow and lung. The severity of thrombocytopenia thus reflects the balance between platelet production by megakaryocytes and the accelerated clearance of sensitized platelets. Thrombocytopenic bleeding occurs when the platelet counts fall below $10–50 \times 10^9/l$.

The pathogenesis of acute ITP is often regarded as a consequence of inappropriate immune recovery after an infection. Circulating antigens or antibodies may alter the platelet membrane. Alternatively, immune complexes derived from primary or underlying disease processes may non-specifically adsorb to platelet surfaces resulting in opsonization and destruction of young platelets (Fig. 22.2).[23–26] Chronic ITP can be attributed to autoantibodies directed against platelet constituents such as glycoproteins. Corroborating these findings, labeling studies[27,28] of autologous or homologous platelets using ^{51}Cr or ^{111}Indium-oxine have shown that platelet survival is decreased in patients with ITP.[29–34]

PLATELET ANTIGEN AND AUTOANTIBODY

The main epitope for ITP-associated antibody binding lies on either the platelet GpIIb-IIIa or the GpIb-IX complex.[9,10,35,36] There is also evidence that some antibodies implicated in ITP bind to glycolipids.[37] In a controlled laboratory study,[38] platelet and plasma samples from 67 children and 23 adults with chronic ITP were evaluated for glycoprotein autoantibodies. At the time of sampling, 36 children had thrombocytopenia (mean duration 2–9 years, range 0.5–9). Of the adult patients with chronic ITP, 18 had thrombocytopenia and 5 had normal platelet counts. As shown in Table 22.1, platelet-associated autoantibodies were detected in 26 of 36 (72.2%) children with thrombocytopenia of the chronic form while 15 of 31 (48.4%) with an history of ITP but normal platelet counts at the time of sampling had these findings. Of 23 adults with chronic ITP, 12 of 18 (66.7%) with thrombocytopenia displayed platelet-associated antibodies. A significant correlation was noted between the platelet-associated autoantibody level and the patient's age at the time of diagnosis. Children with high platelet-associated autoantibody levels were older, with a mean age of 12.4 years (range 8–17 years), compared with an average age of 7.1 years (1–16) for children with moderate or negative autoantibody levels.

These data suggest that there may be different forms of childhood ITP. Younger children with moderate autoantibody levels appear to have an increased likelihood for spontaneous remission or compensated disease with a platelet count $>20–150 \times 10^9/l$. The course of adolescents with high autoantibody levels seems similar to that of adults, in whom spontaneous remission or compensation of ITP is unusual. In the above study,[38] children with an history of chronic ITP but normal platelet counts at the time of blood sampling had elevated autoantibody levels. This suggests a

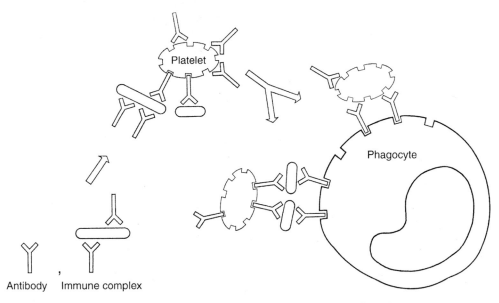

Fig. 22.2 Pathogenic aspects of platelet opsonization and phagocytosis. Reproduced with permisson from Ref. 247.

Table 22.1 Antiglycoprotein antiplatelet autoantibody in chronic thrombocytopenic purpura.[38]

	Ongoing ITP*	Prior ITP†
Children (n = 67)		
AAb level‡ elevated	26/36	15/31
AAb level‡ negative	10/36	16/31
Adults (n = 23)		
AAb level‡ elevated	12/18	4/5
AAb level‡ negative	6/18	1/5

*Ongoing immune thrombocytopenic purpura (ITP, platelet count at the time of sampling <150 × 10⁹/l).
†Prior ITP, history of platelet count <50 × 10⁹/l for at least 6 months but with normal counts, without therapy, at the end of sampling.
‡Autoantibody (AAb) level, ratio of patient AAb value to that of the mean control value plus 3 standard deviations.

compensated form of ITP. However, recurrence of disease is likely to occur if this balance is altered by factors that decrease platelet production (i.e. viral infection) or that increase autoantibody production and/or platelet consumption. Furthermore, the offspring of a mother with the compensated stage of ITP and platelet autoantibodies may be at risk of neonatal thrombocytopenia.

The mechanisms of platelet destruction are outlined in Fig. 22.2. The rapid destruction of platelets is due either to autoantibodies that bind via the antigenic site or immune complexes that bind via Fc receptors on platelets. These opsonized cells are rapidly removed by cells of the mononuclear phagocytic system. The quantity of antibodies correlates with the degree of thrombocytopenia.[39] Phagocytosis of platelets has been demonstrated by *in vivo* studies using reticuloendothelial blockade with monoclonal anti-Fc receptor antibodies.[40] The role of complement is documented by increased platelet-associated C4 and C3. *In vitro* studies show binding of C4 and C3 followed by platelet lysis after incubation of platelets with patients' plasma and fresh serum.[41]

For effective platelet destruction, there must be sufficient antigens and autoantibodies on platelets. The specific anatomic configuration of the spleen is optimal for engulfment and subsequent phagocytosis.[42] In some patients with ITP, the reticuloendothelial system of the liver may also be efficient in removing platelets. In the bone marrow, thrombopoiesis and intramedullary platelet destruction could be concomitantly inhibited as there is antibody production[43] and antibody binding to platelets and megakaryocytes.[44] In addition, platelet kinetic studies showing decreased platelet delivery into the bloodstream suggest that intramedullary events may also be critical for clinical disease in many patients with ITP.[34,45,46]

IMMUNE REGULATION

Normally, the immune response to an antigenic challenge is well regulated. Initiated by antigen-presenting cells, the pathways of humoral and cell-mediated immunity are activated via cell-cell interactions and lymphokine production resulting among other events in the generation of cytotoxic T-effector cells and the secretion of specific antibodies. Regulatory mechanisms, possibly involving suppressor T cells and anti-idiotypic antibodies, down-modulate the degree and duration of the immune response to a specific stimulus.

In ITP, the maintenance of self-tolerance and the effective immune response may be altered in the presence of an inflammatory process directed at another target cell than platelets. As shown in Table 22.2 and Fig. 22.3, multiple defects related to cellular immunity have been described in patients with ITP.[47–63] Enhanced serum levels of HLA-DR

Table 22.2 Defects related to cellular immunity in chronic immune thrombocytopenic purpura.[47]

Antigen-specific autoantibodies[48,49]	↑
Lymphocyte defects	
Phenotype	
CD19+ or CD20+ CD5+ B cells[50,51]	↑
CD3+ DR+ T cells[51–53]	↑
CD3+ CD57+ T cells[54]	↑
CD3– CD57+ NK cells[54]	↑
Functional PHA	
Stimulation of PBMC[51–53,55]	normal
[56]	or ↑
Platelet induced IL-2 secretion[51,57]	↑
T-cell-mediated autoantibody production[58]	↑
T suppressor cells[59]	↓
NK-mediated cytolysis[60,61]	↓

PHA = phytohemagglutine; PBMC = peripheral blood mononuclear cell; NK = natural killer.

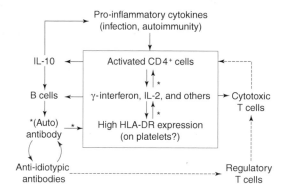

Fig. 22.3 Model of the immunopathogenesis of acute and chronic immune thrombocytopenic purpura (ITP). Dotted line represents hypothetical feedback. *Only in chronic ITP. Reproduced with permission from Ref. 248.

molecules have been detected.[64–66] In acute ITP, the transient increase in surface expression of HLA-DR molecules may be induced by proinflammatory cytokines such as interferon gamma (IFN-γ). As a consequence of immune activation, increased serum levels of interleukin (IL)-2 have been observed in various autoimmune disorders, including ITP.[60,67–72] In parallel, high levels of IL-10 have also been detected. IL-10 is a potent stimulator of human B cells[73] and down-modulates the production of inflammatory cytokines by T cells (Th 1) and monocytes/macrophages.[74] Increased serum concentrations of IL-2, interferon and/or IL-10 reflecting *in vivo* T-cell activation have been observed in patients with chronic ITP, but not in those with the acute form.[60,75] Moreover, an increased serum concentration of IL-2 in chronic ITP correlates significantly with *in vitro* IL-2 secretion by platelet-stimulated T-helper cells.[60]

The difference in the serum detection of IFN-γ, IL-2 and IL-10 expression suggests that different mechanisms operate in the pathogenesis of chronic versus acute ITP. It has been proposed that acute ITP may be due to a cross-reactive immune response directed against an infectious agent.[76] In

contrast, chronic ITP may be perpetuated by a constant HLA-DR-stimulated immune response with enhanced cytokine production, increased activation of T-cells and increased production of specific autoantibodies (Fig. 22.3). Therefore, both forms of ITP appear to result from an altered feedback mechanism critical for the termination of an immune response.

CLINICAL FEATURES AND DIAGNOSIS

In most children, thrombocytopenia occurs within 1–3 weeks after an infectious disease. Commonly, the infection is a bacterial or non-specific viral (upper respiratory or gastrointestinal) infection. ITP may also occur after rubella, rubeola, chickenpox or live virus vaccination. As mentioned above, the hemorrhagic manifestations depend on the degree of thrombocytopenia (Table 22.3). Common first bleeding signs are easy bruising and skin petechiae. These signs occur with platelet counts below 20×10^9/l. Severe mucosal bleeding, hematuria and genital bleeding usually occur with platelet counts below 10×10^9/l. Adolescent girls may have prolonged menorrhagia. Intracranial hemorrhage (ICH) occurs in 0.5–1% of hospitalized children with ITP and is fatal in one-third.[77] The risk is greater during the initial days of thrombocytopenia but can occur at any time in ongoing ITP. Salicylate-containing medications or antihistamines may increase the risk of bleeding.[77]

The characteristic features of history, physical examination and laboratory analysis are summarized in Table 22.4. Apart from bleeding and thrombocytopenia there should be no other abnormal physical findings. Bone marrow examination is not necessary in patients displaying the typical signs and symptoms of ITP. In one study, 127 children with ITP diagnosed clinically were subjected to bone marrow examination but only 5 (4%) had abnormal cytologic findings not compatible with the diagnosis of ITP and upon closer examination, all 5 had additional atypical features on presentation.[79] Importantly, bone marrow examination is indicated to establish the diagnosis in patients who fail to respond to treatment after 3–6 months.

Table 22.3 Staging due to platelet count and clinical manifestation and intervention guidelines in children with immune thrombocytopenic purpura.

Stage	Platelet count ($\times 10^9$/l)	Symptoms, physical findings	Recommendation
1	>50–150	None	None
2	>20	None	Individual treatment (therapeutic/preventive)
3	>20 and/or <10	Mucosal bleeding } Minor bleeding }	Hospitalization and IVIG or corticosteroids

Table 22.4 Elements of the history, physical examination and peripheral blood analysis in a child with suspected immune thrombocytopenic purpura.[78]

History
Bleeding symptoms
  Type of bleeding
  Severity of bleeding
  Duration of bleeding
  History of prior bleedings
Systemic symptoms
  Especially of recent (within 6 weeks) infectious illness; exposure or vaccination or recurrent infections suggesting immunodeficiency; symptoms of an autoimmune disorder
Medications
  Heparin, sulfonamides and quinidine/quinine, which may cause thrombocytopenia, and aspirin, which may exacerbate bleeding
Risk of HIV infection, including maternal HIV status
Family history of thrombocytopenia or hematologic disorder
In an infant <6 months old, include perinatal and maternal history
Co-morbid conditions, which may increase the risk of bleeding
Lifestyle, including vigorous and potentially traumatic activities

Physical examination
Bleeding signs
  Type of bleeding (including retinal hemorrhages)
  Severity of bleeding
Liver, spleen and lymph nodes
Evidence for infection
Presence of dysmorphic features suggestive of congenital disorder, including skeletal anomalies, auditory acuity
Exclude specific congenital syndomes
  Fanconi's syndrome
  Thrombocytopenia with absent radii
  Wiskott–Aldrich syndrome
  Alport syndrome (and its variants)
  Bernard–Soulier syndrome
  May–Hegglin anomaly
  Gray platelet syndrome

Peripheral blood analysis
Thrombocytopenia: platelet are normal in size or may appear larger than normal, but consistently giant platelets (approaching the size of red blood cells) should be absent
Normal red blood cell morphology
Normal white blood morphology, normal reticulocyte count

DIFFERENTIAL DIAGNOSIS

Initially, ITP has to be differentiated from other forms of thrombocytopenic bleeding disorders (Table 22.5). The bleeding manifestations in ITP are similar in presentation to the findings in patients with thrombocytopenia associated, for example, with bone marrow hypoproliferation. A decreased mean platelet volume suggests marrow hypoproduction of platelets or indicates findings characteristic of the Wiskott–Aldrich syndrome. If there is anemia and leukocyte abnormalities, a bone marrow examination is required to rule out marrow diseases such as acute leukemia, aplastic anemia, myelodysplasia, lymphoma or metastatic disease. Autoimmune hemolysis, if suspected, can be confirmed by a Coombs' test. If risk factors are present for human immunodeficiency virus (HIV) infection, serologic testing must be performed. Thrombotic thrombocytopenic purpura and hemolytic uremic syndrome can be distinguished by the presence of hemolysis, a negative Coombs' test, and microangiopathic red cell changes. Disseminated intravascular coagulation (DIC) is associated with characteristic coagulation abnormalities. Splenomegaly may indicate hypersplenism.

CLINICAL COURSE

Independent of treatment, complete remission of ITP occurs in 80–90% of children after 6 months and in >90% after 3–37 years (Fig. 22.4).[12–14,80,81] The 3–5% of children who do not display remission have chronic ITP (Table 22.6). Children who develop chronic ITP are mostly over 7 years of age and are rarely those with postinfectious ITP. Recurrent ITP, defined as periodic episodes of thombocytopenia at intervals of >3 months, occurs in 14% of children with acute ITP.[15,16] In children with persistent ITP of 3–6 months' duration, additional laboratory testing is indicated (Table 22.7).

Table 22.5 Differential diagnosis in childhood thrombocytopenia.*

	Onset	MPV	PAlgG	Coagulation	Marrow	Other
Destructive thrombocytopenia						
ITP	Sudden	Increased	Increased	ND	ND	—
Wiskott–Aldrich	Insidious	Decreased*	Increased	ND	ND	—
HIV–ITP	Variable	Increased	Increased	ND	ND	HIV-positive*
DIC, TTP, HUS	Sudden	Increased	Increased	Diagnostic*	ND	—
Hypersplenism	Insidious	Increased	ND	ND	ND	Splenomegaly*
Decreased production						
Amegakaryocytic	Insidious	Decreased	ND	ND	Diagnostic*	±Radius*
Aplastic anemia	Insidious	Decreased	ND	ND	Diagnostic*	—
Myelodysplasia	Insidious	Decreased	ND	ND	Diagnostic*	—
Acute leukemia	Insidious	Decreased	ND	ND	Diagnostic*	—
Lymphoma	Insidious	Decreased	ND	ND	Diagnostic*	—
Metastatic disease	Insidious	Decreased	Variable	ND	Diagnostic	—

MPV = mean platelet volume; PAlgG = plasma-associated IgG; ITP = immune thrombocytopenic purpura; HIV = human immunodeficiency virus; DIC = disseminated intravascular coagulation; TTP = thrombotic thrombocytopenic purpura; HUS = hemolytic uremic syndrome; ND = non-diagnostic.
*Characteristic.

Table 22.6 Summary of the clinical course of immune thrombocytopenic purpura from a series of 12 reports.[78]

Number of children	Remission at 6 months without treatment*	Remission at 6 months**	ICH (fatal)	Other deaths	Persistent ITP after 6 resp. 12 months	Spontaneous remission	Deaths
1693[80,82–92]	389/467 (83%)	1207/1597 (76%)	16 (13) 0.9% (0.7%)	4 0.2%	179 10.6%	66/179 37%	3 2%

ICH = intracranial hemorrhage.
*Number of patients managed without specific initial therapy. The response rate for untreated patients is greater than the overall response at 6 months because of selection of patients with good prognostic features for no treatment.
**A different denominator from the original number of patients indicates that some patients were not followed long enough to be included in the estimate.

Table 22.7 Routine testing in addition to initial laboratory analysis in children with persistent immune thrombocytopenic purpura of 3–6 months' duration.

Bone marrow analysis, thyroid function, urine analysis, abdominal ultrasound

Antinuclear antibody, direct antiglobin, lupus anticoagulant, platelet antigen-specific antibodies, serum immunoglobulins with IgG subclasses, platelet function test, coagulation studies

Viral serology (HIV, CMV, EBV, VZV, rubeola, parvovirus B19 and others)

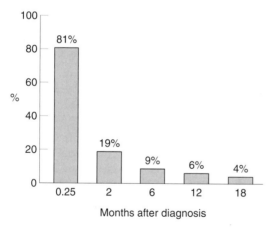

Fig. 22.4 Clinical course of immune thrombocytopenic purpura (ITP) in children. Percentage of children with ITP and platelet counts <20 × 10⁹/l 2, 6, 12 and 18 months after diagnosis. Swiss Canadian retrospective analysis (n = 554). Reproduced with permission from Ref. 127.

As mentioned above, ICH occurs in 0.5–1% of hospitalized children with ITP and is fatal in one-third despite treatment with corticosteroids[77] or intravenous immunoglobulin (IVIG).[93] Postsplenectomy sepsis constitutes the other major cause of death in children with ITP (Table 22.6). Only limited observational data are available regarding the complications of ICH. In a review of 14 children with ICH, Woerner et al[77] reported that 4 children died and 2 others may have had neurologic long-term effects. Of 30 children with ICH described in a retrospective study by the American Society of Hematology,[78] this complication occurred in 12 patients (40%) within 12 days after diagnosis, including in 2 with a history of head trauma. The ICHs in the other 18 patients occurred after 1 month to 5 years of diagnosis, and

were typically associated with the administration of glucocorticoids and/or splenectomy subsequent to a lack of remission. At least 24 of these 30 patients were reported prior to 1981 when the benefits of IVIG therapy in ITP were initially described.[7] This finding argues against immunosuppression and/or splenectomy in the long-term treatment of ITP.

Unlike ITP in adults, persistent thrombocytopenia is uncommon in children. In the 12 series summarized in Table 22.6, ITP resolved in 1207 (76%) of the 1597 children. Clinical features of the presenting illness and parameters associated with an increased risk of chronic persistent thrombocytopenia included a history of purpura for >2–4 weeks before diagnosis,[80–84,93] female sex,[80,85–87] age over 10 years[85–87] and a platelet count at presentation >20 × 10⁹/l.[85] The fate of children with chronic ITP is uncertain, although about one-third appear to have spontaneous remission several months to many years after diagnosis (Fig. 22.4).[80,94,95]

MANAGEMENT

Treatment is indicated in children either at risk of or with overt signs of bleeding. Table 22.3 summarizes the recommendations for the treatment of ITP in children according to a staging system. Hospitalization is required for severe bleeding regardless of the platelet count. Treatment is necessary for a child with mucosal bleeding and platelet counts below 20 × 10⁹/l and one with mild bleeding and platelet counts below 10 × 10⁹/l. Therapeutic measures in the acute management of ITP should be maintained until bleeding has ceased and the platelet counts have reached hemostatic levels (i.e. >20 × 10⁹/l). Continued treatment beyond this defined point is, however, not indicated. Moreover, it also seems unnecessary to treat patients without signs of bleeding and with platelet counts >20 × 10⁹/l.

Recent insight into the immunopathogenesis of ITP (see above) has formed the clinical base for novel therapeutic strategies. The therapy of ITP focuses on measures modulating the immune response and includes IVIG,[7,96] anti-Rh(D) immunoglobulin[97] and α-interferon.[98] Immunosuppressive treatment with corticosteroids[99–101] is used as an alternative therapeutic strategy and cytostatic agents,[102–110] splenectomy [80–87,93–95,111–114] and other treatment possibilities are only indicated in special situations.

The following recommendations focus on children with bleeding symptoms (stage 2 or 3, see Table 22.3) and are generally in accordance with the recently published practical guidelines of the American Society of Hematology (ASH) for diagnosis and treatment of ITP.[78]

ACUTE BLEEDING

Acute bleeding in children with ITP (stage 3, see Table 22.3) may warrant a rapid increase in platelets. As a follow-up of earlier studies,[115] 2 Canadian multicenter studies have analyzed prospectively children diagnosed with acute ITP and platelet counts $<20 \times 10^9$/l.[116,117] The first study compared treatment of IVIG or corticosteroids with no intervention, supportive care and observation.[116] The second trial randomized treatment with IVIG, oral corticosteroids or intravenous anti-Rh(D).[117] The results are summarized in Table 22.8, detailing specifically the effect of each therapeutic regimen within 72 hours after initiation. Both studies demonstrated that IVIG produced the fastest recovery to safe, hemostatic platelet counts. Treatment with 4 mg corticosteroids/kg body weight given daily for 7 days was recommended as the second choice. However, long-term corticosteroid treatment in children should be avoided due to unacceptable side-effects. In addition, the second study found that a single dose of 0.8 g IVIG/kg body weight was sufficient and comparable to the more traditional larger dose of 2 g/kg body weight given over 48 hours. Treatment with the lower IVIG dose decreases the duration and cost of hospitalization. Based on these findings, the ASH panel recommends the use of IVIG in preference to corticosteroids for the treatment of children with ITP.[78]

Table 22.9 summarizes studies of the effectiveness of corticosteroids, IVIG and anti-Rh(D), and Table 22.10 shows treatment possibilities and dosages.

Emergency treatment

The morbidity and mortality associated with severe hemorrhage from thrombocytopenia is extensive.[80,88,166] Severe, life-threatening bleeding justifies intervention, including IVIG (0.8–1 g/kg body weight/dose), high-dose intravenous methylprednisolone 30 mg/kg or dexamethasone 1–2 mg/kg and platelet transfusions. The latter should be given as a third line of treatment because transfused platelets may survive longer *in vivo* after IVIG and/or corticosteroid administration. Emergency splenectomy in case of urgent life-threatening bleeding is not recommended.[78]

MILD BLEEDING AND MANAGEMENT OF LONG-TERM BLEEDING PROBLEMS

Children with a history of mild bleeding or recurrent bleeding should receive treatment aimed at maintaining their platelet counts at a level that renders them free of symptoms (stage 2, see Tables 22.3 and 22.10). This level is individual and patients at increased risk of hemorrhage (i.e. those playing contact sports, undergoing surgery, etc.) may benefit from additional therapy. Recommended treatment modalities are IVIG (0.4–0.8 kg body weight at 2–8-week intervals) or corticosteroids (2–4 mg/kg body weight for 4 days). Children and adolescents who fail to respond to IVIG or to corticosteroids, i.e. do not maintain safe platelet counts, may benefit from one of the following treatment regimens (see below): anti-Rh(D); α-interferon; or - in special circumstances - plasma exchange, protein A immunoadsorption of antibodies, or the administration of cytostatic agents. The role of ascorbic acid in the treatment of ITP remains uncertain.

Prolonged response to long-term cyclic treatment versus natural course of ITP

The long-term effects of treatment in ITP must be interpreted with caution, since the natural history of ITP in children and in some young adults is one of gradual spontaneous resolution.[127–130] Several uncontrolled studies have reported that patients with chronic ITP display long-lasting recovery (sustained platelet counts $>20 \times 10^9$/l) when treated with repeated courses of IVIG (Table 22.10)[131–133] or with a high-dose, cyclic dexamethasone regimen.[101] In the latter,[101] 10 adults with persistent symptomatic ITP were treated with 6 cycles of oral dexamethasone: 40 mg/day for 4 days every 4 weeks. All patients demonstrated a therapeutic response with platelet counts $>100 \times 10^9$/l for at least 6 months after completion of treatment. Adult patients tolerated this treatment well. In contrast, children with chronic ITP given a comparable dexamethasone regimen demonstrated not only a less impressive response to treatment but also suffered from significant side-effects (fatigue, weight gain, difficulty in sleeping, significant behavioral changes, hyperadrenocorticism, transient increase of blood glucose levels).[134] Based on these observations, there is a need for adequately controlled studies to determine whether long-term or cyclic treatments can alter the natural course of chronic ITP in children.

Table 22.8 Immediate response rate (platelet rate $>20 \times 10^9$/l) to different treatment regimens.[116,117]

Randomized group	Rapid responders (⩾72 hours) (%)
No treatment	9/16 (56)
Intravenous anti-R(D), 25 μg/kg for 2 days	31/38 (82)
Corticosteroids, 4 mg/kg/day for 7 days	45/57 (79)
IVIG, 1 g/kg/day for 2 days	50/53 (94)
IVIG, 0.8 g/kg once	34/35 (97)

IVIG = intravenous immunoglobulin.

Table 22.9 Effectiveness of corticosteroids, intravenous immunoglobulin (IVIG) and anti-R(D).[78]

Reference	Study population			Randomized treatment arms	Outcome		
	Number	Age	Follow-up		Outcome measure		Adverse effects
118	27	6 years (mean)	NR	Prednisone (2mg/kg/day × 21 days) No treatment	Median time to platelet count of 150 × 10⁹/l	21 days 60 days (p ≤ 0.3)	NR NR
119	93	6 months– 16 years	>6 months	Prednisone (60 mg/m²/day × 21 days, then tapered Placebo	Proportion with platelet count >30 K and >100 K, and with negative Rumpel–Leede test	Prednisone > placebo (p < 0.01)	NR
120	27	<11 years	28 days	Prednisone (2 mg/kg/day × 14 days, then tapered to day 21) Placebo	Platelet count, bleeding time, clinical bleeding score at day 0–28	Prednisone > placebo (p < 0.05) only at day 7	Increased appetite, weight gain
115	94	<16 years	1 year	Prednisone (60 mg/m²/day × 21 days, follow-up protocol for poor response/ remissions) IVIG (0.4 g/kg/day × 5 days, follow-up protocol for poor response/remissions)	Proportion with platelet count >100 K	77% 83% (no difference)	77% with weight gain or acne 22% with headache, fever, vomiting, vertigo
121	61	2–12 years	>6 months	Prednisone (0.5 mg/kd/day × 1 month or until platelet normalization) Prednisone (1.5 mg/kg/day × 1 month or until platelet normalization)	Proportion with platelet count >150 K	62% 81% (p < 0.05)	NR NR
122	160	<15 years	>12 months	Prednisone (0.25 mg/kg/day × 3 weeks) Prednisone (1 mg/kg/day × 3 weeks)	Proportion with platelet count >100 K for >3 months	71% 77% (no difference)	NR NR
123	30	2 months– 15 years	>6 months	Methylprednisolone (IV, 10 mg/kg/day × 5 days) Prednisone (2 mg/kg/d × 4 weeks) IVIG (0.4 g/kg/day × 5 days)	Mean platelet count on days 1–14	Methylprednisolone = IVIG > prednisone (p < 0.001)	NR NR NR
124	20	2 months– 11 years	>6 months	Methylprednisolone (po 30 mg/kg/day × 3 days, then 20 mg/kg/day × 4 days) IVIG (0.4 g/kg/day × 5 days)	Proportion with platelet count >150 K at 3 days, 6 months	60%, 90% (no difference) 60%, 75%	NR NR
116	53	7 months– 14 years	180 days	Prednisone (4 mg/kg/day × 7 days, then tapered to day 21) IVIG (1g/kg/day × 2 days) No therapy	Median time to platelet count >20 K, >50 K	2 days, 4 days 1 day, 2 days (p < 0.01 v prednisone) 4 days, 16 days (p < 0.1 v either treatment)	Weight gain, behavioral change 75% with nausea, vomiting, headache, fever
117	146	6 months– 18 years	6–32 months	Prednisone (4 mg/kg/day × 7 days then tapered to day 21) IVIG (1 g/kg/day × 2 days) IVIG (0.8 g/kg once) Anti-R(D) (25 μg/kg/day × 2 days)	Median time to platelet count >20 K, >50 K	2 days, 3 days 2 days, 2 days 1 day, 2 days (p < 0.05 v prednisone) 2 days, 2.5 days (p < 0.05 v both IVIG regimens)	None 16–18% with fever, nausea, vomiting, headache 24% with hemoglobin <10 g/dl
125	57	2 months– 17 years	6 months	Methylprednisolone (po, 30 mg/kg/d × 7 days) Methylprednisolone (po, 50 mg/kg/d × 7 days) IVIG (0.5 g/kg/day × 5 days)	Mean platelet count on days 0–30	Mean >100 K by day 4. No difference among groups	Increased appetite and Cushingoid appearance Increased appetite and Cushingoid appearance 1 patient with aseptic meningitis; 2 with headache, vomiting

*NR = Not reported.

Table 22.10 Treatment possibilities for children with immune thrombocytopenic purpura.

Intravenous immunoglobulin (IVIG)	Initial treatment 0.8 g/kg body weight once. Repeat the same dose if platelet count is $<30 \times 10^9$/l on day 3 (72 hours after first infusion) In emergency bleeding: 1–2 times 0.8 g/kg body weight, eventually together with corticosteroids and platelet transfusion Treatment in chronic ITP: 0.4 g/kg body weight once every 2–8 weeks
Corticosteroids	4 mg/kg prednisone/day orally or intravenously for 7 days, then tapering over a 7-day period In emergency bleeding: 8–12 mg methylprednisone/kg body weight intravenously or 0.5–1.0 mg dexamethasone/kg body weight intravenously or orally, together with IVIG or platelet transfusion
Anti-R(D) antibody	10–25 μg/kg/day for 2–5 days intravenously in 50 cc of normal saline over 30 min
α-Interferon	3×10^6 units subcutaneously 3 times per week for 4 weeks
Cyclosporine	3–8 mg/kg/day orally divided in 2 or 3 doses
Azathioprine	50–300 mg/m^2 per os daily during 4 months or longer

IMMUNOGLOBULIN

Initial IVIG treatment of children with ITP due to platelets $<20 \times 10^9$/l resulted in a quicker and more extensive increase in platelet counts[7,115–117,132,133] in comparison to patients receiving corticosteroid therapy. Importantly, a single daily dose of 0.8 g IVIG/kg body weight appears to have the identical initial effect as 5×0.4 g or 2×1.0 g/kg body weight of IVIG given each day.[117]

Adverse effects noted with IVIG include flu-like symptoms such as headache, backache, nausea and fever.[116,117,135,136] Aseptic, transient meningitis is a rare complication.[131] It is important to use quality controlled, commercially available (not experimental) intact 7S IgG preparations from which there is no risk of hepatitis C infection.[137–140]

Mechanism of action

There are immediate and long-term effects. The immediate effect of IVIG on the immune system is reflected in an alteration in activity of membrane- bound Fc receptors. Following the observation that IVIG is clinically effective, it was hypothesized that the inhibition of platelet destruction by phagocytosis may have resulted from blockade of Fc receptors (FcRs). FcRs are expressed on a range of cells and are functionally important for scavenging immunoglobulin-sensitized cells such as platelets. The plausibility of this explanation is underscored by the finding that anti-Rh (D)-coated erythrocytes also show prolonged survival with IVIG treatment.[141] A decrease in leukocyte counts or the size of the various lymphocyte subpopulations is inversely proportional to the platelet counts during IVIG treatment.[142,143] These observations suggest that not only FcRs on mononuclear phagocytes but also those on other cells are affected by IVIG infusion. Since the humoral immune response *in vivo* works in concert with the cellular immune response and *vice versa*, IVIG could modulate the synthesis and release of cytokines from FcR-bearing lymphocytes and monocytes.[47,144,145] In this context, different speculations and experimental observations appear to exist but no unifying explanation for the

immunologic findings associated with IVIG treatment. *In vitro*, IgG administration induces down-regulation of IL-6, IL-2, IL-10, IFN-γ and tumor necrosis factor (TNF)-β in lipopolysaccharide-stimulated monocytes, and reduces IL-2 receptor expression in activated lymphocytes.[146,147] In ITP, overproduction of IL-4 has been reported in one study,[148] while high levels of IL-2, IL-10, INF-γ and TNF-α have been described in other studies.[65,149] Availablility of FcRs may be altered by IgG dimers or larger complexes in the IVIG preparations, or by erythrocyte alloantibodies.[150] Inhibition of complement activation by IVIG may be another possible mechanism of action.[151]

Long-term effects following IVIG administration (Table 22.11) may be induced by anti-idiotypic antibodies. As mentioned above, antibodies against glycoprotein GpIIb-IIIa and Ib-IX can be identified in 70–80% of children and adults with chronic ITP.[9,38] It has been demonstrated that IVIG contains anti-idiotypic antibodies against anti-GpIIb-IIIa autoantibodies and these inhibit the binding of auto-antibodies to platelet GpIIb-IIIa.[152] Thus, restoration of the balance within the anti-idiotype network or, alternatively, suppression of secretion of anti-idiotypic antibodies, may lead to long-term improvement of ITP.[153–155] In this context, it is of note that the size of the donor pool from which IVIG is prepared may be relevant as the chance that a given antibody idiotype is recognized and bound by a complementary anti-idiotypic antibody is obviously dependent on the donor-pool size.[156]

Table 22.11 Studies showing long-term improvement for therapy with intravenous immunoglobulin (IVIG).

Study	Total in study	Number	Long-term improvement %
Children			
Imholz et al[132]	42	22	52
Bussel et al[238]	12	5	42
Adults			
Bussel et al[244]	40	16	40
Godeau et al[245]	18	7	39

CORTICOSTEROIDS

The mechanism of action of corticosteroids in ITP remains uncertain. Corticosteroids may inhibit the phagocytosis of antibody-bearing platelets[157] and may suppress antibody production by B lymphocytes.[158,159] Other indirect mechanisms may account for the beneficial therapeutic effect of corticosteroids: maintenance of capillary integrity[160–167] or inhibition of vascular prostacyclin synthesis leading to a normalization of the possible prolonged bleeding time in ITP.[168,169]

In randomized clinical trials[116,117] the median time to achieve a platelet count $>50 \times 10^9/l$ was 4 days if the patients received 4 mg/kg/day prednisone for 7 days. In contrast, children receiving no treatment displayed comparable platelet counts only 16 days after onset of disease. The higher dosage of steroids (4 mg/kg/day) is preferable to the classical dose of 2 mg/kg/day of oral prednisone for 21 days[119–122] because the side-effects are fewer and less extensive. Methylprednisolone in very high doses for several days (10–30 mg oral or intravenous methylprednisolone/kg/day) has been administered in uncontrolled studies and resulted in a dramatic increase in platelet counts with long-term improvement in some but not all patients.[124,125,170–174] Adverse effects include signs and symptoms of hypercortisolism, such as facial swelling, weight gain, hyperglycemia, hypertension and behavioral abnormalities. Long-term application of high corticosteroid dosages has the risk of growth retardation and cataracts,[175] and should thus be avoided. Sustained corticosteroid doses of 0.5–0.7 mg/kg body weight/day may suppress platelet formation as well.[176,177]

ANTI-RH(D)

The rationale for using anti-Rh(D) as a therapeutic measure in ITP is based on the hypothesis that an increase in platelet counts following IVIG therapy may be due to competitive inhibition of the monocyte/phagocyte system as effected by the preferential sequestration of autologous erythrocytes sensitized by alloantibodies present in the IgG preparations. Indeed, a clinical trial by Salama *et al*[178] demonstrated a clinical effect. Administration of anti-Rh(D) globulin to Rh-positive patients with ITP resulted in a significant increase in platelet counts ($>20 \times 10^9/l$) in 6 of 10 patients. Other uncontrolled studies have demonstrated that anti-Rh(D) treatment may increase the platelet count in approximately 80% of Rh-positive children.[179–182] A controlled clinical study showed, however, that anti-Rh(D) therapy was less effective in comparison to IVIG or corticosteroids, demonstrating a prolonged delay to achieve platelet counts of $20 \times 10^9/l$ as well as $50 \times 10^9/l$.[117] The therapeutic effect of anti-Rh(D) usually lasts for 1–5 weeks and appears to depend on the presence of an intact spleen.

The recommended dosage is intravenous 50 μg/kg body weight in a short infusion. Adverse effects include alloimmune hemolysis. With this treatment, children develop a positive direct Coombs' test which is accompanied by a transient decrease in hemoglobin concentrations for 1–2 weeks.[117,181]

OTHER TREATMENTS

α-Interferon

Although the precise mechanism of action awaits elucidation, 25% of adult patients treated with IFN-α displayed a significant increase in platelet counts lasting 1 week to 7 months.[183–188] Despite this possibly beneficial effect, there are reports suggesting an aggravation of the thrombocytopenia after administration of IFN-α.[189,190]

The recommended dosage is 3×10^6 units subcutaneously 3 times per week. Adverse effects include fever, fatigue and myalgia.

Plasma exchange and protein A-immunoadsorption

Plasma exchange[191–193] and protein-A-immunoadsorption[194–197] are *ex vivo* physical measures to remove antiplatelet antibodies. In 20–30% of patients with chronic ITP, plasma exchange may transiently result in a response. In one report[194] using protein A-immunoadsorption to remove antiplatelet antibodies, 16 of 72 patients demonstrated a sustained platelet increase. This extracorporal treatment is required daily for 3–5 days.

Vinca alkaloids

The use of vinca alkaloids in ITP is based on the observation that the administration of vincristine and vinblastine can cause lymphocytopenia and suppression of antibody production. The increase in platelets after treatment with vincristine or vinblastine lasts 1–3 weeks in two-thirds of patients.[103,104,198–206]

The recommended dosage of vincristine is 1–1.5 mg/m² intravenously (maximal single dose 2 mg) every 1–2 weeks. A combination with 1–2 mg corticosteroid/kg body weight/day × 3 per os may enhance the effect. For vinblastine the recommended dosage is 6 mg/m² intravenously every 1–2 weeks. Adverse effects include neuropathy, constipation, leukopenia and fever. The infusion of vinblastine-loaded platelets has not shown convincing results.[200]

Danazol

The use of danazol, an androgenic steroid with minimal virilizing effects, was suggested for the treatment of ITP because one of the documented side-effects is thrombocytosis. There is a broad range of response to danazol in patients with ITP (10–80%).[104,207–224]

The recommend dosage is 100–150 mg/m² per os 3 × daily. Adverse effects include weight gain, headache, hair loss, liver dysfunction, myalgia, amenorrhea, some virilization and even thrombocytopenia.

Ascorbic acid (vitamin C)

Although a response rate of 15% has been reported, the role of ascorbic acid in the treatment of ITP remains to be determined.[105,225–237] The recommended dosage is 1–1.5 g/m² per os daily.

Azathioprine

Azathioprine, an immunosuppressive drug, was the first compound reported to be effective in chronic ITP patients refractory to glucocorticoid treatment and splenectomy; 50–70% of patients may achieve an improvement.[105,233–237] Continuous treatment for 4 months appears to be necessary before a patient is considered unresponsive. The recommended dosage is 50–300 mg/m² per os daily. Adverse effects are mainly leukopenia and the risk of developing malformations during pregnancy.

Cyclophosphamide

Sixty to 80% of patients treated with cyclophosphamide will respond with an increase in platelet counts.[105–110] Although of similar therapeutic potency, cyclophosphamide has more severe side-effects in comparison to azathioprine. The recommended dosage is 3–8 mg/kg body weight per os daily. Adverse effects are leukopenia, alopecia, infertility, teratogenecity and urinary bladder hemorrhage.

Splenectomy

Splenectomy as a therapeutic intervention in children with ITP should be restricted to those with uncontrollable bleeding. Recent studies document the decline in rates of splenectomy.[95,173,238] Splenectomy is indicated in children in whom thrombocytopenia has persisted for >1 year in association with substantial bleeding episodes. In 16 reports (277 children in total), 72% of patients with ITP achieved a remission following surgical splenectomy.[80–87,93–95,111–114]

Elective splenectomy in children with chronic ITP is only recommended if platelet counts remain below 10×10^9/l in the absence of treatment (IVIG, corticosteroids, anti-Rh [D]) for >14 days or in instances of severe and repetitive hemorrhage. It is paramount that children are immunized against *Haemophilus influenzae*, pneumococci and meningococci prior to splenectomy.[239]

Adverse effects

The important late effect of splenectomy is the increased risk of fatal bacterial infections, particularly in children below 5 years of age; a fatality of 1/300–1000 patient years has been calculated.[239–241] The difficulty is therefore to decide whether the adverse effects of splenectomy outweigh its potential benefits since spontaneous recovery from ITP has been observed many years after diagnosis.[242,243]

REFERENCES

1. Jones HW, Tocantins LM. The history of purpura hemorrhagica. *Ann Med Hist* 1933; **5**: 349
2. Kasnelson P. Verschwinden der hämorrhagischen Diathese bei einem Falle von essentieller Thrombopenie (Frank) nach Milzexstirpation. *Wein Klin Wochenschr* 1916; **29**: 1451
3. Harrington WJ, Minnich V. Demonstration of a thrombocytopenic factor in the *Blood* of patients with thrombocytopenic purpura. *J Lab Clin Med* 1951; **38**: 1–10
4. Harrington WJ, Sprague CC, Minnich V, Moore CV, Aulvin RC, Dubach R. Immunologic mechanisms in idiopathic and neonatal thrombocytopenic purpura. *Ann Intern Med* 1953; **38**: 433–469
5. Shulman NR, Marder VJ, Weinrach RS. Similarities between known antiplatelet antibodies and the factor responsible for thrombocytopenia in idiopathic purpura: physiologic, serologic and isotopic studies. *Ann NY Acad Sci* 1965; **124**: 499–542
6. Dixon RH, Rosse WF. Platelet antibody in immune thrombocytopenia. *Br J Haematol* 1975; **31**: 129–134
7. Imbach P, d'Appuzzo V, Hirt A, Rossi E, Vest M, Barandun S, Baumgartner C, Morell A, Schoni M, Wagner HP. High-dose intravenous gammaglobulin for idiopathic thrombocytopenic purpura in childdhood. *Lancet* 1981; **i**: 1228–1231
8. van Leeuwen EF, van der Ven JTH, Engelfriet CP, von dem Borne AEG. Specificity of autoantibodies in autoimmune thrombocytopenia. *Blood* 1982; **59**: 23–26
9. McMillan R, Tani P, Millard F, Berchtold L, Renshaw L, Woods VL. Platelet-associated and plasma anti-glycoprotein autoantibodies in chronic ITP. *Blood* 1987; **70**: 1040–1045
10. Kiefel V, Santoso S, Weisheit M, Mueller-Eckhardt C. Monolocal antibody-specific immobilization of platelet antigens (MAIPA): a new tool for the identification of platelet-reactive antibodies. *Blood* 1987; **70**: 1722–1726
11. Lammi AT, Lovric VA. Idiopathic thrombocytopenic purpura: an epidemiologic study. *J Pediatr* 1973; **83**: 31
12. Lusher JM, Zuelzer WW. Idiopathic thrombocytopenic purpura in childhood. *J Pediatr* 1966; **68**: 971
13. Hirsch EO, Dameshek W. Idiopathic thrombocytopenia. *Arch Intern Med* 1951; **88**: 701
14. Simons SM, Main CA, Yaish HM *et al*. Idiopathic thrombocytopenic purpura in children. *J Pediatr* 1975; **87**: 16
15. Dameshek W, Ebbe S. Recurrent acute idiopathic thrombocytopenic purpura. *N Engl J Med* 1963; **269**: 647
16. Figueroa M, Gehlsen J, Hammond D *et al*. Combination chemotherapy in refractory immune thrombocytopenic purpura. *N Engl J Med* 1993; **328**: 1226–1229
17. Ata M, Fisher OD, Holman CA. Inherited thrombocytopenia. *Lancet* 1965; **i**: 119
18. Chiaro JJ, Ayut D, Bloom GE. X-linked thrombocytopenic purpura. I. Clinical and genetic studies of a kindred. *Am J Dis Child* 1972; **123**: 565
19. Roberts MH, Smith MH. Thrombocytopenic purpura: a report of four cases in one family. *Am J Dis Child* 1950; **79**: 820
20. Schaar FE. Familial idiopathic thrombocytopenic purpura. *J Pediatr* 1963; **62**: 546
21. Bithell TC, Didisheim GE, Wintrobe MM. Thrombocytopenia inherited as an autosomal dominant trait. *Blood* 1965; **25**: 231
22. Stuart MJ, Tomar RH, Miller ML *et al*. Chronic idiopathic thrombocytopenic purpura: a familial immunodeficiency syndrome? *JAMA* 1978; **239**: 939
23. Lightsey AL, Koenig HM, McMilan R, Stone JR. Platelet-

associated immunglobulin G in childhood idiopathic thrombocytopenic purpura. *J Pediatr* 1979; **94**: 201–204

24. Lightsey AL, McMilan R. The role of spleen in 'autoimmune' blood disorders. *Am J Pediatr Hematol Oncol* 1979; **1**: 331

25. McIntosh S, Johnson C, Hartigan P *et al*. Immunoregulatory abnormalities in children with thrombocytopenic purpura. *J Pediatr* 1981; **99**: 525

26. Myllylä G, Vaheri A, Vesikari T *et al*. Interaction between human *Blood* platelets, viruses and antibodies. IV. Post-rubella thrombocytopenic purpura and platelet aggregation by rubella antigen-antibody interaction. *Clin Exp Immunol* 1969; **4**: 323

27. Panel on Diagnostic Application of Radioisotopes in Hematology. International Committee for Standardization in Hematology. Recommanded methods for radioisotope platelet survival studies. *Blood* 1977; **50**: 1137–1144

28. Panel on Diagnostic Applications of Radionuclides in Hematology. Recommended method for indium-111 platelet survival studies. *J Nucl Med* 1988; **29**: 564–566

29. Branehog I, Kutti J, Weinfeld A. Platelet survival and production in idiopathic thrombocytopenic purpura (ITP). *Br J Haematol* 1974; **27**: 127–143

30. Harker LA, Finch CA. Thrombokinetics in man. *J Clin Invest* 1969; **48**: 963–974

31. Aster RH, Keene WR. Sites of platelet destruction in idiopathic thrombocytopenic purpura. *Br J Haematol* 1969; **16**: 61–73

32. Heyns AP, Lotter MG, Badenhorst PN *et al*. Kinetics and sites of destruction of 111-indium-oxine-labeled platelets in idiopathic thrombocytopenic purpura: a quantitative study. *Am J Hematol* 1982; **12**: 167–177

33. Schmidt KG, Rasmussen JW. Kinetics and distribution in vivo of 111-In-labeled autologus platelets in idiopathic thrombocytopenic purpura. *Scand J Haematol* 1985; **34**: 47–56

34. Ballem PJ, Segal GM, Stratton JR, Gernsheimer T, Adamson JW, Slichter S. Mechanisms of thrombocytopenia in chronic autoimmune thrombocytopenic purpura. Evidence for both impaired platelet production and increased platelet clearance. *J Clin Invest* 1987; **80**: 33–40

35. Kiefel V, Santoso S, Kaufmann E *et al*. Autoantibodies against platelet glycoprotein Ib/IX: a frequent finding in autoimmune thrombocytopenic purpura. *Br J Haematol* 1991; **79**: 256–262

36. McMillan R. Antigen-specific assays in immune thrombocytopenic. *Trans Med Rev* 1990; **4**: 136–143

37. Koerner TAW, Weinfeld HM, Bullard LSB, Williams LCJ. Antibodies against platelet glycosphingolipids: detection in serum by quantitative HPTLC-autoradiography and association with autoimmune and alloimmune processes. *Blood* 1989; **74**: 274–284

38. Imbach P, Tani P, Berchtold W *et al*. Different forms of chronic ITP in children defined by antiplatelet autoantibodies. *J Pediatr* 1991; **118**: 535–539

39. Kurata Y, Curd JG, Tamerius JD, McMillan R. Platelet-associated complement in chronic ITP. *Br J Haematol* 1985; **60**: 723–733

40. Clarkson SB, Bussel HB, Kimberly RP, Valinsky JE, Nachman RL, Unkeless JC. Treatment of refractory immune thrombocytopenic purpura with anti-Fcg-receptor antibody. *N Engl J Med* 1986; **314**: 1236–1239

41. Tsubakio T, Tani P, Curd JG, McMillan R. Complement activation in vitro by antiplatelet antibodies in chronic immune thrombocytopenic purpura. *Br J Haematol* 1985; **63**: 293–300.

42. McMillan R, Longmire RL, Yelenosky R, Donnell RL, Armstrong S. Quantitation of platelet-binding IgG produced *in vitro* by spleens from patients with idiopathic thrombocytopenic purpura. *N Engl J Med* 1974; **291**: 812–817

43. McMillan R, Yelenosky RJ, Longmire RL. Antiplatelet antibody production by the spleen and bone marrow in immune thrombocytopenic purpura. In: Battisto JR, Streinlein JW (eds) *Immunoaspects of the Spleen*. Amsterdam: North Holland Biomedical Press, 1976, pp 227–237

44. McMillan R, Luiken GA, Levy R, Yelenosky R, Longmire RL. Antibody against megakaryocytes in idiopathic thrombocytopenic purpura. *JAMA* 1978; **239**: 2460–2462

45. Heyns AP, Bdenhorst PN, Lotter MG, Pieters H, Wessels P, Kotze HF. Platelet turnover and kinetics in immune thrombocytopenic purpura: Results with autologus 111-In-labeled and homologous 51-Cr-labeled platelets differ. *Blood* 1986; **67**: 86–92

46. Stoll D, Cines DB, Aster RH, Murphy S. Platelet kinetics in patients with idiopathic thrombocytopenic purpura and moderate thrombocytopenia. *Blood* 1985; **65**: 584–588

47. Semple JW, Freedman J. Abnormal cellular immune mechanisms associated with autoimmune thrombocytopenia. *Trans Med Rev* 1995; **4**: 327–338

48. Fujisawa K, O'Toole TE, Tani P *et al*. Autoantibodies to the presumptive cytoplasmic domain of platelet glycoprotein IIIa in patients with chronic immune thrombocytopenic purpura. *Blood* 1991; **77**: 2207–2213

49. Kekomaki R, Dawson B, McFarland J *et al*. Localization of human platelet autoantigen to the cysteine-rich region of glycoprotein IIIa. *J Clin Invest* 1991; **88**: 847–854

50. Mizutani H, Furubayashi T, Kashiwagi H *et al*. B cells expressing CD5 antigen are markedly increased in peripheral blood and spleen lymphocytes from patients with immune thrombocytopenic purpura. *Br J Haematol* 1991; **78**: 474–479

51. Semple JW, Freedman J. Increased anti-platelet T helper lymphocyte reactivity in patients with autoimmune thrombocytopenic purpura. *Blood* 1991; **78**: 2619–2625

52. Ware R, Howard TA. Elevated numbers of gamma–delta ($\gamma\delta+$) lymphocytes in children with immune thrombocytopenic purpura. *J Clin Immunol* 1994; **11**: 237–247

53. Garcia-Suarez J, Prieto A, Manzano L *et al*. T lymphocytes from autoimmune thrombocytopenic purpura show a defective activation and proliferation after cytoplasmic membrane and intracytoplasmic mitogenic signals. *Am J Hematol* 1993; **44**: 1–8

54. Garcia-Suarez J, Prieto A, Ryes E. Severe chronic autoimmune thrombocytopenic purpura is associated with an expansion of CD56 + CD3-natural killer cell subset. *Blood* 1993; **82**: 1538–1545

55. Quagliata F, Karpatkin S. Impaired lymphocyte transformation and capping in autoimmune thrombocytopenic purpura. *Blood* 1979; **53**: 341–349

56. Garcia-Suarez J, Prieto A, Reyes E *et al*. The clinical outcome of autoimmune thrombocytopenic purpura patients is related to their T cell immunodeficiency. *Br J Haematol* 1993; **84**: 464–470

57. Ware RE, Howard TA. Phenotypic and clonal analysis of T lymphocytes in childhood immune thrombocytopenic purpura. *Blood* 1993; **82**: 2137–2142

58. Semple JW, Allen DA, Gross P *et al*. CD19 + B lymphocytes from patients with chronic ATP require stimulation of CD40 and CD4 + T cell contact for antiplatet autoantibody production. *Platelets* 1998 (in press)

59. Hymes KB, Karpatkin S. *In vitro* suppressor T lymphocyte dysfunction in autoimmune thrombocytopenic purpura associated with complement fixing antibody. *Br J Haematol* 1990; **74**: 330–335

60. Semple JW, Bruce S, Freedman J. Supressed natural killer cell activity in patients with chronic autoimmune thromboxytopenic purpura. *Am J Hematol* 1991; **37**: 258–262

61. Gardiner RA, Smith JG. A study of natural killer cells and interferon-gamma in patients with immune thrombocytopenic purpura. *Blood* 1990; **76**: 206A

62. Mizutani H, Tsubakio T, Tomiyama Y *et al*. Increased circulating Ia-positive T cells in patients with idiopathic thrombocytopenic purpura. *Clin Exp Immunol* 1987; **67**: 191–197

63. Semple JW, Freedam J. Increased anti platelet T helper lymphocyte reactivity in patients with autoimmune thrombocytopenic purpura. *Blood* 1991; **78**: 474

64. Boshkov LK, Kelton JG, Halloran PF. HLA-DR expression by

platelets in acute idiopathic thromocytopenic purpura. *Br J Haematol* 1992; **81**: 552–557

65. Semple JW, Milev Y, Cosgrave D *et al*. Differences in serum cytokine levels in acute and chronic autoimmune thrombocytopenic purpura: Relationship to platelet phenotype and antiplatelet T-Cell reactivity. *Blood* 1996; **87**: 4245–4254

66. Santoso S, Kalb R, Kiefel V, Mueller-Eckhardt C. The presence of messenger RNA for HLA class I in human platelets and its capability for protein biosynthesis. *Br J Haematol* 1993: **84**: 451

67. Nepom G. Erlich H. MHC class-II molecules and autoimmunity. *Annu Rev Immunol* 1991; **9**: 493

68. Bottazzo GF, Dean BM, McNally JM, McKay EH, Swift PGF, Gamble DR. *In situ* characterization of autoimmune phenomena and expression of HLA molecules in the pancreas in diabetes mellitus. *N Engl J Med* 1985; **313**: 353

69. Traugott U, Scheinberg LC, Raine CS. On the presence of Ia-positive endothelial cells and astrocytes in multiple sclerosis lesions and its relevance to antigen presentation. *J Neuroimmuol* 1985; **8**: 1

70. Trotter JL. Serial studies of serum interleukin-2 in chronic progressive multiple sclerosis patients: occurrence of bursts and effects of cyclosporine. *J Neuroimmunol* 1990; **28**: 1

71. Tebib JG, Boughaba H, Letroublon MC. Serum IL-2 level in rheumatoid arthritis: Correlation with joint destruciton and disease progression. *Eur Cytokine Network* 1991; **2**: 239

72. Huang Y-P, Perrin LH, Miescher PA, Zubler RH. Correlation of T and B cell activites *in vitro* and serum IL-2 levels in systemic lupus erythmatosus. *J Immunol* 1991; **141**: 827

73. DeFrance T, Vandeviliet B, Briere F, Durand I, Rousset F, Banchereau J. Interleukin 10 and transforming growth factor β co-operate to induce anti-CD40-activated naive human B cells to secrete immunoglobulin A. *J Exp Med* 1992; **175**: 671

74. Howard M, Muchamuel T, Audrade S, Mennon S. Anti-inflammatory effect of IL-10. *J Exp Med* 1993; **177**: 1205

75. Garcia-Suarez J, Prieto A, Reyes E, Manzano L, Arribalzago K, Alverez Mon M. Abnormal γ-IFN and αTNF secretion in purified CD2 + cells from autoimmune thrombocytopenic purpura (ATP) patients: Their implication in the clinical course of the disease. *Am J Hematol* 1995; **49**: 271

76. Kaplan C, Morinet F, Carton J. Virus-induced autoimmune thrombocytopenia and neutropenia. *Semin Hematol* 1992; **1**: 34

77. Woerner SJ, Abildgaard CF, French BN. Intracranial hemorrhage in children with idiopathic thromboxytopenic purpura. *Pediatrics* 1981; **67**: 453

78. George JN, Woolf SH, Raskob GE *et al*. Idiopathic thrombocytopenic purpura; A practice guideline developed by explicit methods for the American Society of Hematology. *Blood* 1996; **88**: 3–40

79. Halperin DS, Doyle JJ. Is bone marrow examination justified in idiopathic thrombocytopenic purpura? *Am J Dis Child* 1988; **142**: 509

80. Ramos MEG, Newman AJ, Gross S. Chronic thrombocytopenia in childhood. *J Pediatr* 1978; **92**: 584

81. Venetz U, Willi P, Hirt A, Imbach P, Wagner HP. Chronische idiopathische thrombozytopenische Purpura im Kindesalter. *Helv Paediatr Acta* 1982; **37**: 27

82. Benham ES, Taft LI. Idiopathic thrombocytopenic purpura in children: Results of steroid therapy and splenectomy. *Aust Paediatr J* 1972; **8**: 311

83. Hoyle C, Darbyshire P, Eden OB. Idiopathic thrombocytopenia in childhood. *Scott Med J* 1986; **31**: 174

84. Robb LG, Tiedeman K. Idiopathic thrombocytopenic purpura: Predictors of chronic disease. *Arch Dis Child* 1990; **65**: 502

85. Lusher JM, Zuelzer WW. Idiopathic thrombocytopenic purpura in childhood. *J Pediatr* 1966; **68**: 971

86. Simons SM, Main CA, Yaish HM, Rutzky J. Idiopathic thrombocytopenic purpura in children. *Pediatrics* 1975; **87**: 16

87. Zaki M, Hassanein AA, Khalil AF. Childhood idiopathic thrombocytopenic purpura: Report of 60 cases from Kuwait. *J Trop Pediatr* 1990; **36**: 10

88. Komrower GM, Watson GH. Prognosis in idiopathic thrombocytopenic purpura of childhood. *Arch Dis Child* 1954; **29**: 502

89. Choi SI, McClure PD. Idiopathic thrombocytopenic purpura in childhood. *Can Med Assoc J* 1967; **97**: 562

90. Walker RW, Walker W. Idiopathic thrombocytopenia, initial illness and long term follow up. *Arch Dis Child* 1984; **59**: 316

91. Lammi AT, Lovric VA. Idiopathic thrombocytopenic purpura: An epidemiologic study. *Pediatrics* 1973; **83**: 31

92. den Ottolander GJ, Gratama JW, deKoning J, Brand A. Longterm follow-up study of 168 patients with immune thrombocytopenia. *Scand Haematol* 1984; **32**: 101

93. Imbach P, Berchtold W, Hirt A *et al*. Intravenous immunoglobulin versus oral corticosteroids in acute immune thrombocytopenic purpura in childhood. *Lancet* 1985; **ii**: 464–468

94. Tamary H, Kaplinsky C, Levy I *et al*. Chronic childhood idiopathic thrombocytopenia purpura: Long-term follow-up. *Acta Paediatr* 1994; **83**: 931

95. Reid MM. Chronic idiopathic thrombocytopenic purpura: incidence, treatment and outcome. *Arch Dis Child* 1995; **72**: 125

96. Imbach P, Blanchette V, Nugent D, Kühne T. *Immune Thrombocytopenic Purpura: Immediate and Long-term Effects of Intravenous Immunoglobulin. Advances in IVIG Research and Therapy*. London: Parthenon Publishing Group, 1996

97. Andrew M, Blanchette VS, Adams M *et al*. A multicenter study of the treatment of childhood chronic idiopathic thrombocytopenic purpura with anti-D. *J Pediatr* 1991; **120**: 522–527

98. Proctor SJ, Jackson G, Carey P *et al*. Improvement of platelet counts in steroid-unresponsive idiopathic immune thrombocytopenic purpura after short-course therapy with recombinant alpha 2b interferon. *Blood* 1989; **74**: 1894–1897

99. Sartorius JA. Steroid treatment of idiopathic thrombocytopenic purpura in children. Preliminary results of a randomized cooperative study. *Am J Pediatr Hematol Oncol* 1984; **6**: 165

100. Ozsoylu S, Irken G, Karabent A. High-dose intravenous methyl-prednisolone for acute childhood idiopathic thrombocytopenic purpura. *Eur J Haematol* 1989; **42**: 431

101. Andersen JC. Response of resistant idiopathic thrombocytopenic purpura to pulsed high-dose dexamethasone therapy. *N Engl J Med* 1994; **330**: 1560–1564

102. Facon T, Caulier MT, Wattel E, Jouet JP, Bauters F, Fenaux P. A randomized trial comparing vinblastine in slow infusion and by bolus i.v. injection in idiopathic thrombocytopenic purpura: A report on 42 patients. *Br J Haematol* 1994; **86**: 678

103. Ahn YS, Harrington WJ, Seelman RC, Eytel CS. Vincristine therapy of idiopathic and secondary thrombocytopenias. *N Engl J Med* 1974; **291**: 376

104. Facon T, Caulier MT, Wattel E, Jouet JP, Bauters F, Fenaux P. A randomized trial comparing vinblastine in slow infusion and by bolus i.v. injection in idiopathic thrombocytopenic purpura: A report on 42 patients. *Br J Haematol* 1994; **86**: 678

105. Pizzuto J, Ambriz R. Therapeutic experience on 934 adults with idiopathic thrombocytopenic purpura: multicentric trial of the cooperative Latin American group on hemostasis and thrombosis. *Blood* 1984; **64**: 1179

106. Laros RK, Penner JA. Refractory thrombocytopenic purpura treated successfully with cyclophosphamide. *JAMA* 1971; **215**: 445

107. Verlin M, Laros RK, Penner JA. Treatment of refractory thrombocytopenic purpura with cyclophosphamide. *Am J Hematol* 1976; **1**: 97

108. Weinerman B, Maxwell I, Hryniuk W. Intermittent cyclophosphamide treatment of autoimmune thrombocytopenia. *Can Med Assoc J* 1974; **111**: 1100

109. Srichaikul T, Boonpucknavig S, Archararit N, Chaisiri-pumkeeree W. Chronic immunologic thrombocytopenic purpura. Results of

cyclophosphamide therapy before splenectomy. *Arch Intern Med* 1980; **140**: 636

110. Reiner A, Gernsheimer T, Slichter SJ. Pulse cyclophosphamide therapy for refractory autoimmune thrombocytopenic purpura. *Blood* 1995; **85**: 351

111. Brooks PL, O'Shea MJ, Pryor JP. Splenectomy in the treatment of idiopathic thrombocytopenic purpura. *Br J Surg* 1969; **56**: 861

112. Grosfeld JL, Naffis D, Boles ET Jr, Newton WA Jr. The role of splenectomy in neonatal idiopathic thrombocytopenic purpura. *J Pediatr Surg* 1970; **5**: 166

113. Zarella JT, Martin LW, Lampkin BC. Emergency splenectomy for idiopathic thrombocytopenic purpura in children. *J Pediatr Surg* 1978; **13**: 243

114. Davis PW, Williams DA, Shamberger RC. Immune thrombocytopenia: Surgical therapy and predictors of response. *J Pediatr Surg* 1991; **26**: 407

115. Imbach P, Wagner HP, Berchtold W *et al*. Intravenous immunoglobulin versus oral corticosteroids in acute immune thrombocytopenic purpura in childhood. *Lancet* 1985; **2**: 464

116. Blanchette VS, Luke B, Anrew M *et al*. A prospective, randomized trial of high-dose intravenous immune globulin G therapy, oral prednisone therapy, and no therapy in childhood acute immune thrombocytopenic purpura. *J Pediatr* 1993; **123**: 989

117. Blanchette V, Imbach P, Andrew M *et al*. Randomized trial of intravenous immunoglobulin G, intravenous anti-D, and oral prednisone in childhood acute immune thrombocytopenic purpura. *Lancet* 1994; **344**: 703

118. McWilliams NB, Maurer HM. Acute idiopathic thrombocytopenic purpura in children. *Am J Hematol* 1979; **7**: 87

119. Sartorius JA. Steroid treatment of idiopathic thrombocytopenic purpura in children. Preliminary results of a randomized cooperative study. *Am J Pediatr Hematol Oncol* 1984; **6**: 165

120. Buchanan GR, Holtkamp CA. Prednisone therapy for children with newly diagnosed idiopathic thrombocytopenic purpura. A randomized clinical trial. *Am J Pediatr Hematol Oncol* 1984; **6**: 355

121. Mazzucconi MG, Francesconi M, Fidani P *et al*. Treatment of idiopathic thrombocytopenic purpura: results of a multicentric protocol. *Haematologia* 1985; **70**: 329

122. Bellucci S, Charpak Y, Chastang C, Tobelem G. Low doses v conventional doses of corticoids in immune thrombocytopenic purpura (ITP). Results of a randomized clinical trial in 160 children, 223 adults. *Blood* 1988; **71**: 1165

123. Khalifa AS, Tolba KA, El-Alfy MS, Gadallah M, Ibrahim FH. Idiopathic thrombocytopenic purpura in Egyptian children. *Acta Haematol* 1993; **90**: 125

124. Ozsoylu S, Sayli TR, Ozturk G. Oral megadose methylprednisolone versus intravenous immunoglobulin for acute childhood idiopathic thrombocytopenic purpura. *Pediatr Hematol Oncol* 1993; **10**: 317

125. Albayrak D, Islek I, Kalayci AG, Gürses N. Acute immune thrombocytopenic purpura: A comparative study of very high oral doses of methylprednisolone and intravenously administered immune globulin. *J Pediatr* 1994; **125**: 1004

126. Schattner E, Bussel J. Mortality in immune thrombocytopenic purpura: Report of seven cases and consideration of prognostic indicators. *Am J Hematol* 1994; **46**: 120

127. Imbach P, Akatsuka J, Blanchette V *et al*. Immunthrombocytopenic purpura as a model for pathogenesis and treatment of autoimmunity. *Eur J Pediatr* 1995; **154**: 60–64

128. Oezsoylu S. Treatment of chronic ITP. *Pediatr Hematol Oncol* 1995; **12**: 407–408

129. Aronis S, Platokouki H, Mitsika A, Haidas S, Constantopoulos A. Seventeen years of experience with chronic idiopathic thrombocytopenic purpura in childhood. Is therapy always better? *Pediatr Hematol Oncol* 1994; **11**: 487–498

130. Aronis S, Platokouki H, Mitsika A, Haidas S, Constantopoulos A. Treatment of chronic idopathic thrombocytopenic purpura. *Pediatr Hematol Oncol* 1995; **12**: 409–410

131. Kattamis AC, Shankar S, Cohen AR. Neurologic complications of treatment of childhood acute immune thrombocytopenic purpura with intravenously administered immunoglobulin G. *J Pediatr* 1997; **130**: 281–283

132. Imholz B, Imbach P, Baumgartner C *et al*. Intravenous immunoglobulin (i.v. IgG) for previously treated acute or for chronic idiopathic thrombocytopenic purpura (ITP) in childhood: A prospective multicenter study. *Blut* 1988; **56**: 63

133. Warrier IA, Lusher JM. Intravenous gammaglobulin (gamimune) for treatment of chronic idiopathic thrombocytopenic purpura (ITP): A two-year follow-up. *Am J Hematol* 1990; **33**: 184

134. Nugent D, English M, Hawkins D, Pendergrass T, Tarantino M. High dose dexamethasone therapy for pediatric patients with refractory immune-mediated thrombocytopenic purpura (ITP). *Blood* 1994; **94**: 731A

135. Duhem C, Dicato MA, Ries F. Side-effects of intravenous immune globulins. *Clin Exp Immunol* 1994; **97 (Suppl 1)**: 79

136. Thomas MJ, Misbah SA, Chapel HM, Jones M, Elrington G, Newsom-Davis J. Hemolysis after high-dose intravenous Ig. *Blood* 1993; **82**: 3789

137. Centers for Disease Control and Prevention. Outbreak of hepatitis C associated with intravenous immunoglobulin administration – United States, October 1993–June 1994. *Morb Mortal Wkly Rep* 1994; **43**: 505

138. Bjoro K, Froland SS, Yun Z, Samdal H, Haaland T. Hepatitis C infection in patients with primary hypogammaglobulinemia after treatment with contaminated immune globulin. *N Engl J Med* 1994; **331**: 1607

139. Yu MW, Mason BL, Guo ZP *et al*. Hepatitis C transmission associated with intravenous immunoglobulins. *Lancet* 1995; **345**: 1173

140. Schiano TD, Bellary SV, Black M. Possible transmission of hepatitis C virus infection with intravenous immunoglobulin. *Ann Intern Med* 1995; **122**: 802

141. Fehr J, Hofmann V, Kappeler U. Transient reversal of thrombocytopenia in idiopathic thrombocytopenic purpura by high-dose intravenous gamma globulin. *N Engl J Med* 1982; **306**: 1254–1258

142. Dammacco F, Jodice G, Campobasso N. Treatment of adult patients with ITP with intravenous immunoglobulin effect on T cell subsets and PWM induced antibody synthesis *in vitro*. *Br J Haematol* 1986; **62**: 125–135

143. Macey MG, Newland AG. CD4 and CD8 subpopulation changes during high dose intravenous immunoglobulin treatment. *Br J Haematol* 1990; **76**: 513–520

144. Leung DYM, Cotran RS, Kurf-Jones E, Burns JC, Newburger JW, Pober JS. Endothelial cell activation and high interleukin-secretion in the pathogenesis of acute Kawasaki disease. *Lancet* 1989: **ii**: 1298–1302

145. Ross C, Hansen MB, Schyberg T, Berk K. Autoantibodies to crude human leukocyte interferon (IFN), native human IFN, recombinant human IFN alpha 2b and human IFN gamma in healthy blood donors. *Clin Exp Immunol* 1990; **32**: 695–701

146. Andersson JP, Andersson UG. Human intravenous immunoglobulin modulates monokine production *in vitro*. *Immunology* 1990; **71**: 372–376

147. Andersson UG, Björk L, Skansen-Saphir U, Andersson JP. Downregulation of cytokine production and interleukin-2 receptor expression by pooled human IgG. *Immunology* 1993; **79**: 211–216

148. Nugent D, Wang Z, Sandborg C, Berman M. Reduced levels of JL-4 in immune mediated thrombocytopenia (ITP): role of cytokine imbalances in autoimmune disease. *Immunohematology* 1988; **2**: 65A

149. Garcia-Suarez J, Prieto A, Reyes E *et al*. Abnormal γIFN and αTNF secretion in purified CD2 + cells from autoimmune thrombocytopenic purpura (ATP) patients. Their implication in the clinical course of the disease. *Am J Hematol* 1995; **49**: 271–276

150. Templeton JG, Cocker JE, Crawford RJ *et al*. Fcγ-receptor blocking antibodies in hyperimmune and normal pooled gammaglobulin. *Lancet* 1985; **i**: 1337

151. Basta M, Langlois PF, Marques M *et al*. High dose intravenous immunoglobulin modifies complement-mediated *in vivo* clearance. *Blood* 1989; **74**: 326–333

152. Berchtold P, Dale GL, Tani P, McMillan R. Inhibition of autoantibody binding to platelet glycoprotein IIb/IIa by anti-idiotypic antibodies in intravenous gammaglobulin. *Blood* 1989; **74**: 2414–2417

153. Rossi F, Kazatchkine MD. Antiidiotypes against autoantibodies in pooled normal human polyspecific Ig. *J Immunol* 1989; **143**: 4104–4109

154. Dietrich G, Kazatchkine MD. Normal immunoglobulin G (IgG) for therapeutic use (intravenous Ig) contain anti-idiotypic specificities against an immunodominant, disease-associated, cross-reactive idiotype of human anti-thyroglobulin autoantibodies. *J Clin Invest* 1990; **85**: 620–625

155. Dietrich S, Kaverl SV, Kazatchkine MD. Modulation of autoimmunity by intravenous globulin through interaction with the functions of the immune/idiotypic network. *Clin Immunol Immunopathol* 1992; **62**: 873–881

156. Roux KH, Tankersley DL. A view of the human idiotypic repertoire. Electron microscopic and immunologic analyses of spontaneous idiotype-anti-idiotype dimers in pooled human IgG. *J Immunol* 1990; **84**: 2136–2143

157. McMillan R, Longmire RL *et al*. *In vitro* platelet phagocytosis by splenic leucocytes in idiopathic thrombocytopenic purpura. *N Engl J Med* 1974; **290**: 249

158. Dixon R, Rosse W. Platelet antibody in autoimmune thrombocytopenia. *Br J Haematol* 1975; **31**: 129

159. McMillan R, Longmire R *et al*. The effect of corticosteroids on human IgG synthesis. *J Immunol* 1976; **116**: 1592

160. Robson HN, Duthie JJR. Capillary resistance and adrenocortical activity. *Br Med J* 1950; **2**: 971

161. Labran C. Etude de l'action vaso-constrictrice de la prednisone. *Rev Francaise Etude Clin Biol* 1963; **8**: 765

162. Hutter JJ, Hathaway WE. Prednisone-induced hemostasis in a platelet function abnormality. *Am J Dis Child* 1975; **129**: 641

163. Alexander M, van den Bogart N *et al*. Le pronostic et le traitement du purpura thrombopénique idiopathique de l'enfant. *Arch Française Pediatr* 1976; **33**: 329

164. Johnson SA. Endothelial supporting function of platelets. In: Johnson SA (ed) *The Circulating Platelet*. New York: Academic Press, 1971, p 283

165. Kitchens CS, Weiss L. Ultrastructural changes of endothelium associated with thrombocytopenia. *Blood* 1975; **46**: 567

166. Kitchens CS, Weiss L. Amelioration of endothelial abnormalities by prednisone in experimental thrombocytopenia in the rabbit. *J Clin Invest* 1977; **60**: 1129

167. Kitchens CS, Pendergast JF. Human thrombocytopenia is associated with structural abnormalities of the endothelium that are ameliorated by glucocorticoid administration. *Blood* 1986; **67**: 203

168. Senyi A, Blajchman MA *et al*. The experimental corrective effect of hydrocortisone on the bleeding time in thrombocytopenic rabbits. *American Society of Hematology, 18th Annual Meeting*, 1975, p 80A

169. Blajchman MA, Senyi AF *et al*. Shortening of the bleeding time in rabbits by hydrocortisone caused by inhibition of prostacyclin generation by the vessel wall. *J Clin Invest* 1979; **63**: 1026

170. Ozsoylu S, Irken G, Karabent A. High-dose intravenous methylprednisolone for acute childhood idiopathic thrombocytopenic purpura. *Eur J Haematol* 1989; **42**: 431

171. Gaulier MT, Rose C, Roussel MT, Huart C, Bauters F, Fenaux P. Pulsed high-dose dexamethasone in refractory chronic idiopathic thrombocytopenic purpura: a report on 10 cases. *Br J Haematol* 1995; **91**: 477–479

172. del Principe D, Menichelli A, Mori PG *et al*. Phase II trial of methylprednisolone pulse therapy in childhood chronic thrombocytopenia. *Acta Haematol* 1987; **77**: 226

173. van Hoff J, Ritchey AK. Pulse methylprednisolone therapy for acute childhood idiopathic thrombocytopenic purpura. *J Pediatr* 1988; **113**: 563

174. Adams DM, Kinney TR, Obranksirupp E, Ware RE. High-dose oral dexamethasone therapy for chronic childhood idiopathic thrombocytopenic purpura. *J Pediatr* 1996; **2**: 281–283

175. Saag KG, Koehnke R, Caldwell JR *et al*. Low dose long-term corticosteroid therapy in rheumatoid arthritis: an analysis of serious adverse effects. *Am J Med* 1994; **96**: 115

176. Cohen P, Gardner FH. The thrombocytopenic effect of sustained high-dosage prednisone therapy in thrombocytopenic purpura. *N Engl J Med* 1961; **265**: 611

177. Giles AHB, Shellshear ID. Unwanted corticosteroid effects in childhood bone marrow failure, renal failure and brain damage: Case report. *NZ Med J* 1975; **539**: 424

178. Salama A, Kiefel V, Mueller-Eckhardt C. Effect of IgG anti Rho(D) in adult patients with chronic autoimmune thrombocytopenia. *Am J Hematol* 1986; **22**: 241–250

179. Becker T, Kuenzlen E, Salama A *et al*. Treatment of childhood idiopathic thrombocytopenic purpura with Rhesus antibodies (anti-D). *Eur J Pediatr* 1986; **145**: 166

180. Bussel JB, Graziano JN, Kimberly RP, Pahwa S, Aledort LM. Intravenous anti-D treatment of immune thrombocytopenic purpura: Analysis of efficacy, toxicity, and mechanism of effect. *Blood* 1991; **77**: 1884

181. Andrew M, Blanchette VS, Adams M *et al*. A multicenter study of the treatment of childhood chronic idiopathic thrombocytopenic purpura with anti-D. *J Pediatr* 1992; **120**: 522

182. Borgna-Pignatti C, Battisti L, Zecca M, Locatelli F. Treatment of chronic childhood immune thrombocytopenic purpura with intramuscular anti-D immunoglobulins. *Br J Haematol* 1994; **88**: 618

183. Proctor SJ, Jackson G, Carey P *et al*. Improvement of platelet counts in steroid-unresponsive idiopathic immune thrombocytopenic purpura after short-course therapy with recombinant α 2b interferon. *Blood* 1989; **74**: 1894–1897

184. Proctor SJ. Alpha interferon therapy in the treatment of idiopathic thrombocytopenic purpura. *Eur J Cancer* 1991; **27 (Suppl 4)**: S63

185. Bellucci S, Bordessoule D, Coiffier B, Tabah I. Interferon alpha-2b therapy in adult chronic thrombocytopenic purpura (ITP). *Br J Haematol* 1989; **73**: 578

186. Iannaccaro P, Molica S, Santoro R. Recombinant alpha-2b interferon in refractory idiopathic immune thrombocytopenia. *Eur J Haematol* 1992; **48**: 271

187. Dubbeld P, Hillen HFP, Schouten HC. Interferon treatment of refractory idiopathic thrombocytopenic purpura (ITP). *Eur J Haematol* 1994; **52**: 233

188. Cohn RJ, Schwyzer R, Hesseling PB, Poole JE, Naidoo J, Van Heerden C. α-Interferon therapy for severe chronic idiopathic thrombocytopenic purpura in children. *Am J Hematol* 1993; **43**: 246

189. Matthey F, Ardeman S, Jones L, Newland AC. Bleeding in immune thrombocytopenic purpura after alpha-interferon. *Lancet* 1990; **335**: 471

190. Hudson JG, Yates P, Scott GL. Further concern over use of alpha-interferon in immune thrombocytopenic purpura. *Br J Haematol* 1992; **82**: 630

191. Marder VJ, Nusbacher J, Anderson FW. One-year follow-up of plasma exchange therapy in 14 patients with idiopathic thrombocytopenic purpura. *Transfusion* 1981; **21**: 291

192. Blanchette VS, Hogan VA, McCombie NE *et al*. Intensive plasma exchange therapy in ten patients with idiopathic thrombocytopenic purpura. *Transfusion* 1984; **24**: 388

193. Bussel JB, Saal S, Gordon B. Combined plasma exchange and intravenous gammaglobulin in the treatment of patients with refractory immune thrombocytopenic purpura. *Transfusion* 1988; **28**: 38

194. Snyder HW, Cochran SK, Balint JP *et al*. Experience with protein

A-immunoadsorption in treatment-resistant adult immune thrombocytopenic purpura. *Blood* 1992; **79**: 2237

195. Balint JP Jr, Snyder HW Jr, Cochran SK, Jones FR. Longterm response of immune thrombocytopenia to extracorporeal immunoadsorption. *Lancet* 1991; **337**: 1106

196. Guthrie TH, Oral A. Immunethrombocytopenic purpura: A pilot study of staphylococcal protein A immunomodulation in refractory patients. *Semin Hematol* 1989; **26**: 3

197. Balint J, Quagliata F, Cochran SK, Jones FR. Association of antiplatelet IgG antibody levels with response to extracorporeal protein A/silica Immunoadsorption in ITP patients. *Am J Hematol* 1995; **50**: 74–75

198. Ahn YS, Byrnes JJ, Harrington WJ *et al*. The treatment of idiopathic thrombocytopenia with vinblastine-loaded platelets. *N Engl J Med* 1978; **298**: 1101

199. Cervantes F, Rozman C, Feliu E, Montserrat E, Diumenjo C, Granena A. Low-dose vincristine in the treatment of corticosteroid-refractory idiopathic thrombocytopenic purpura (ITP) in non-splenectomized patients. *Postgrad Med J* 1980; **56**: 711

200. Kelton JG, McDonald JWD, Barr RM *et al*. The reversible binding of vinblastine to platelets: implications for therapy. *Blood* 1981; **57**: 431

201. Ahn YS, Harrington WJ, Mylvaganam R, Allen LM, Pall LM. Slow infusion of vinca alkaloids in the treatment of idiopathic thrombocytopenic purpura. *Ann Intern Med* 1984; **100**: 192

202. Manoharan A. Slow infusion of vincristine in the treatment of idiopathic thrombocytopenic purpura. *Am J Hematol* 1986; **21**: 135

203. Simon M, Jouet J, Fenaux P, Pollet J, Walter M, Bauters F. The treatment of adult idiopathic thrombocytopenic purpura. Infusion of vinblastine in ITP. *Eur J Haematol* 1987; **39**: 193

204. Linares M, Cervero A, Sanchez M *et al*. Slow infusion of vincristine in the treatment of refractory thrombocytopenic purpura. *Acta Haematol* 1988; **80**: 173

205. Fenaux P, Quiquandon I, Caulier MT, Simon M, Walter MP, Bauters F. Slow infusions of vinblastine in the treatment of adult idiopathic thrombocytopenic purpura: a report on 43 cases. *Blut* 1990; **60**: 238

206. Manoharan A. Targeted-immunosuppression with vincristine infusion in the treatment of immune thrombocytopenia. *Aus NZ J Med* 1991; **21**: 405

207. Ahn YS, Harrington WJ, Simon SR, Mylvaganam R, Pall LM, So AG. Danazol for the treatment of idiopathic thrombocytopenic purpura. *N Engl J Med* 1983; **308**: 1396

208. Buelli M, Cortelazzo S, Viero P *et al*. Danazol for the treatment of idiopathic thrombocytopenic purpura. *Acta Haematol* 1985; **74**: 97

209. McVerry BA, Auger M, Bellingham AJ. The use of danazol in the management of chronic immune thrombocytopenic purpura. *Br J Haematol* 1985; **61**: 145

210. Almargo D. Danazol in idiopathic thrombocytopenic purpura. *Acta Haematol* 1985; **74**: 120

211. Ambriz R, Pizzuto J, Morales M, Chavez G, Guillen C, Aviles A. Therapeutic effect of danazol on metrorrhagia in patients with idiopathic thrombocytopenic purpura (ITP). *Nouv Rev Francaise Hematol* 1986; **28**: 275

212. Mazzucconi MG, Francesconi M, Falcione E *et al*. Danazol therapy in refractory chronic immune thrombocytopenic purpura. *Acta Haematol* 1987; **77**: 45

213. Manoharan A. Danazol therapy in patients with immune cytopenias. *Aust NZ J Med* 1987; **17**: 613

214. Schreiber AD, Chien P, Tomaski A, Cines DB. Effect of danazol in immune thrombocytopenic purpura. *N Engl J Med* 1987; **316**: 503.

215. Kotlarek-Haus S, Podolak-Dawidziak M. Danazol in chronic idiopathic thrombocytopenic purpura resistant to corticosteroids. *Folia Haematol* 1987; **114**: 768

216. Ahn YS, Mylvaganam R, Garcia RO, Kim CI, Palow D, Harrington WJ. Low-dose danazol therapy in idiopathic thrombocytopenic purpura. *Ann Intern Med* 1987; **107**: 177

217. Nalli G, Sajeva MR, Maffe GC, Ascari E. Danazol therapy for idiopathic thrombocytopenic purpura (ITP). *Haematologia* 1988; **73**: 55

218. Ahn YS, Rocha R, Mylvaganam R, Garcia R, Duncan R, Harrington WJ. Long-term danazol therapy in autoimmune thrombocytopenia: unmaintained remission and age-dependent response in women. *Ann Intern Med* 1989; **111**: 723

219. Edelmann DZ, Knobel B, Virag I, Meytes D. Danazol in non-splenectomized patients with refractory idiopathic thrombocytopenic purpura. *Postgrad Med J* 1990; **66**: 827

220. Flores A, Carles J, Junca J, Abella E. Danazol therapy in chronic immune thrombocytopenic purpura. *Eur J Haematol* 1990; **45**: 109

221. Arrowsmith JB, Dreis M. Thrombocytopenia after treatment with Danazol. *N Engl J Med* 1986; **314**: 585

222. Rabinowe SN, Miller KB. Danazol-induced thrombocytopenia. *Br J Haematol* 1987; **65**: 383

223. Laveder F, Marcolongo R, Zamboni S. Thrombocytopenic purpura following treatment with danazol. *Br J Haematol* 1995; **90**: 970

224. Weinblatt ME, Kochen J, Ortega J. Danazol for children with immune thrombocytopenic purpura. *Am J Dis Child* 1988; **142**: 1317

225. Brox AG, Howson-Jan K, Fauser AA. Treatment of idiopathic thrombocytopenic purpura with ascorbate. *Br J Haematol* 1988; **70**: 341

226. Toyama K, Ohyashiki K, Nehashi Y, Ohyashiki JH. Ascorbate for the treatment of idiopathic thrombocytopenic purpura. *Br J Haematol* 1990; **75**: 623

227. Win N, Matthey F, Davies SC. Ascorbate for the treatment of idiopathic thrombocytopenic purpura. *Br J Haematol* 1990; **75**: 626

228. Verhoef GEG, Boonen S, Boogaerts MA. Ascorbate for the treatment of refractory idiopathic thrombocytopenic purpura. *Br J Haematol* 1990; **74**: 234

229. Godeau B, Bierling P. Treatment of chronic autoimmune thrombocytopenic purpura with ascorbate. *Br J Haematol* 1990; 75: 289

230. Novitzky N, Wood L, Jacobs P. Treatment of refractory immune thrombocytopenic purpura with ascorbate. *South Afr Med J* 1992; **81**: 44

231. Van der Beek-Boter JW, Van Oers MHJ, Von dem Borne AEKG, Klaassen RJL. Ascorbate for the treatment of ITP. *Eur J Haematol* 1992; **48**: 61

232. Jubelirer SJ. Pilot study of ascorbic acid for the treatment of refractory immune thrombocytopenic purpura. *Am J Hematol* 1993; **43**: 44

233. Bouroncle BA, Doan CA. Refractory idiopathic thrombocytopenic purpura treated with azathioprine. *N Engl J Med* 1966; **275**: 630

234. Bouroncle BA, Doan CA. Treatment of refractory idiopathic thrombocytopenic purpura. *JAMA* 1969; **207**: 2049

235. Sussman LN. Azathioprine in refractory idiopathic thrombocytopenic purpura. *JAMA* 1967; **202**: 259

236. Quiquandon I, Fenaux P, Caulier MT, Pagniez D, Huart JJ, Bauters F. Re-evaluation of the role of azathioprine in the treatment of adult chronic idiopathic thrombocytopenic purpura: A report on 53 cases. *Br J Haematol* 1990; **74**: 223

237. Hilgartner MW, Lanzkowsky P, Smith CH. The use of azathioprine in refractory idiopathic thrombocytopenic purpura in children. *Acta Paediatr Scand* 1970; **59**: 409

238. Bussel JB, Schulman I, Hilgartner MW, Barandun S. Intravenous use of gammaglobulin in the treatment of chronic immune thrombocytopenic purpura as a means to defer splenectomy. *J Pediatr* 1983; **103**: 651

239. Lortan JE. Clinical annotation. Management of asplenic patients. *Br J Haematol* 1993; **84**: 566

240. Styrt B. Infection associated with asplenia: Risks, mechanisms, and prevention. *Am J Med* 1990; **88**: 5–33N

241. Schilling RF. Estimating the risk for sepsis after splenectomy in hereditary spherocytosis. *Ann Intern Med* 1995; **122**: 187

242. Dickermann JD. Splenectomy and sepsis: a warning. *Pediatrics* 1979; **63**: 938–941

243. Tamary H, Kaplinsky C, Levy I *et al.* Chronic childhood idiopathic thrombocytopenic purpura; Longterm follow-up. *Acta Paediatr* 1994; **83**: 931

244. Bussel JB, Pham LC, Aledort L, Nachman R. Maintenance treatment of adults with chronic refractory immune thrombocytopenic purpura using repeated intravenous infusions of gammaglobulin. *Blood* 1988; **72**: 121–127

245. Godeau B, Bierling P, Oksenhendler E, Castaigne S, Dexoninck E,

Wechsler B. High-dose dexamethasone therapy for resistant auto-immune thrombocytopenic purpura. *Am J Hematol* 1996; **51**: 334

246. Imbach P. Harmful and beneficial antibodies in immune thrombo-cytopenic purpura. *Clin Exp Immunol* 1994; **97 (Suppl 1)**: 25–30

247. Imbach P, Morell A. Idiopathic thrombocytopenic purpura (ITP): Immunomodulation by intravenous immunoglobulin. *Int Rev Immunol* 1989; **5**: 181–188

248. Imbach P, Kühne T, Holländer G. Immunologic aspects in the pathogenesis and treatment of immune thrombocytopenic purpura in children. *Curr Opin Pediatr* 1997; **9**: 35–40

Thrombocytosis

AH SUTOR

Thrombocytosis is defined as a thrombocyte count above the normal value for age. It requires a knowledge of normal values and information about the method of platelet counting.

Normal upper thrombocyte levels in childhood

There are no gold standards for the method of sampling (venous or capillary blood) or method of counting (in an electronic particle counter or under the microscope, in whole blood or platelet-rich plasma [PRP]). Upper normal limits for the pediatric age group, and particularly for infants, vary widely from 290 to 666 $\times$ 10^9/l.[1] Thrombocytosis, as defined in the pediatric literature, varies between platelet counts of $>400->1000$ $\times$ 10^9/l (Table 23.1).[2] To compare the incidence, pathophysiology and clinical picture of thrombocytosis, the degree of platelet elevation has to be taken into consideration. The following arbitrary classification, which refers to the platelet count and not the clinical state, is chosen to allow comparison of recent studies on childhood thrombocytosis:

- mild: $>500-<700$ $\times$ 10^9/l;
- moderate: $700-900$ $\times$ 10^9/l;
- severe: >900 $\times$ 10^9/l;
- extreme: >1000 $\times$ 10^9/l.

PHYSIOLOGY OF PLATELET PRODUCTION

Platelet production is complex and depends on a balance between stimulating and inhibiting factors. For the last 30 years a factor promoting platelet production has been postulated and tentatively called thrombopoietin (TPO), but since TPO could not be isolated, its existence was quenstioned and other cytokines, such as interleukin (IL)-1, -3, -6 or -11, were suggested to be the putative lineage-

Table 23.1 Definition of thrombocytosis in childhood. Updated from Ref. 1.

Study	Number of patients	Platelets ($\times 10^9$/l)	Predominant age group
Sutor and Hank (1992)[2]	227	>500	25% <2 months, 72% <2 years
	41	>800	
Addiego et al (1974)[37]	10	>800	90% <3 years
Heyne et al (1988)[8]	10	>500	80% <2 years*
Chan et al (1989)[38]	94	>900	65% <2 years
Vora and Lilleyman (1993)[36]	458	>500	40% <6 months, median 13 months
	38	>800	
Heath and Pearson (1989)[39]	119	>500	Median age 22 months
	15	>700	
Yohannan et al (1994)[41]	663	>500	
Buss et al (1994)[15]	82	>1000	75% <10 years, 50% of those <1 year

*Only patients with hemophilus infections are included.

specific regulator of megakaryopoiesis.[3,4] Recently, however, several groups published almost simultaneously their work on the identification, purification, cloning and characterization of the myeloproliferative leukemia virus-ligand (mpl-ligand), which is the long sought TPO.[5] It has considerable structural and functional similarities to erythropoietin. TPO promotes the proliferation of combined megakaryocyte progenitors,[3] the maturation of megakaryocytes and blood platelets by an interaction with the Mpl-receptor.[6] Although the boundaries are fluid, 3 stages of the stem-cell-megakaryocyte-platelet system can be distinguished.[3]

- the first extends from stem-cells to promegakaryocytes;
- the second is that of endomitotic reduplication or polyploidization;
- the third is that of cytoplasmic maturation of megakaryocytes.

At the end of their maturation process, megakaryocytes divide their cytoplasm into several 1000 fairly uniform platelets. Platelets are not only produced in the bone marrow but also in the lung, most probably in the pulmonary microvasculature, by physical fragmentation of megakaryocyte plasma. According to some investigators, whole megakaryocytes or large cytoplasmic fragments leave the bone marrow and travel through the large veins into the right heart ventricle where they are propelled into the pulmonary circulation.[7]

TERMINOLOGY AND CLASSIFICATION

Some authors[8,9] define thrombocythemia as a long-lasting and very pronounced thrombocytosis ($>1000 \times 10^9$/l). In internal medicine, the term thrombocythemia—corresponding to leukemia—is used for thrombocytosis due to an autonomous stem cell defect (e.g. in myeloproliferative disorders [MPDs]), where the term 'esssential thrombocythemia' is applied.[10–12]

More practical is the classification of thrombocytoses according to their origin into primary and secondary forms. An increase in platelet count generally has 1 of 3 causes:

- a primary disorder, such as a myelo-proliferative or -dysplastic syndrome;
- increased production due to stimuli (a prolonged platelet survival time as cause for thrombocytosis has not been described);
- a shift in platelets from the splenic pool into the peripheral circulation.

The first cause is classified as essential (or primary) thrombocytosis (ET), and causes 2 and 3 as reactive (or secondary) thrombocytosis (RT) (Table 23.2). In this chapter, the terms essential and reactive thrombocytosis are used.

With the advent of automated platelet counting, ET is diagnosed with increasing frequency in asymptomatic

Table 23.2 Differences between essential and reactive thrombocytosis. Updated from Ref. 1, includes data from Refs 12–14, 25.

	Essential (primary)	Reactive (secondary)
Age (years)	Mostly >20, often >40	Mostly <20 years
Duration	Over 2 years	Days or weeks, sometimes months
Origin	Stem-cell defect	Reaction to hypoxemia, infection, platelet loss; shift of platelet pool
Microvascular symptoms	Often	Extremely rare
Thrombosis	Often	Extremely rare
Bleeding	Often	Extremely rare
Splenomegaly	Often	Rare
Platelet count ($\times 10^9$/l)	Mostly >1000	Mostly <1000
Platelet morphology	Large, dysmorphic	Large, normal appearance
Platelet function	Disturbed	Normal
Platelet distribution	Elevated	Normal width
Iron stores	Normal	Low
Acute phase reagents such as IL-6, CRP, fibrinogen	Normal	High, if thrombocytosis caused by infection

CRP = C-reactive protein.

patients, in young adults and even in childhood. However, it is still extremely rare in children. A recent large series of >1500 children with thrombocytosis did not encounter 1 case of ET.[1] For this reason this chapter concentrates on RT.

ESSENTIAL THROMBOCYTOSIS

AGE DISTRIBUTION

ET is extremely rare in children and rare in young or middle-aged adults, and most commonly presents in the fifth or sixth decade of life.[12–14] Over a period of 13 years, Randi et al[11] found ET in 57 patients under the age of 40 years and only 8 of these fell in the pediatric age group. Michiels and van Genderen[12] reviewed 11 patients with ET who were between 6 and 11 years of age. Buss et al[15] observed 280 patients with extreme thrombocytosis, 82 of whom were under the age of 20 years, but only 2 of these had ET.

DISTINCTION FROM REACTIVE THROMBOCYTOSIS

Table 23.2 lists the criteria for the differential diagnosis of ET and RT.[1,12,16,17] ET results from a stem-cell defect and is associated with MPDs such as idiopathic thrombocythemia, polycythemia vera (PCV), chronic myeloid leukemia and idiopathic myelofibrosis.[18] In RT, a reason for the increased platelet level can usually be found. Predisposing conditions are, for example, acute and chronic infections, hypoxemia, surgery, other kinds of trauma, malignant disease, hemorrhage, iron deficiency, stress, injection of epinephrine (adrenaline) and splenectomy.[3]

In ET the platelet count usually persists at $> 1000 \times 10^9/l$, while in RT platelet counts are usually lower and as a rule decline within weeks of recovery from the underlying disease.[19,20] In ET platelet function is usually disturbed and spontaneous aggregation as well as hypofunction can be observed.[21] This may explain why the bleeding time in these patients is frequently prolonged despite thrombocytosis.

In ET as well as RT the number of megakaryocytes in the bone marrow is elevated. In ET, dysmorphic megakaryocytes are found, not infrequently in clusters, but this does not help greatly in differentiating between ET and RT.[20] In RT, peripheral platelets are large and round, whereas the large platelets of ET are dysmorphic.

There are practically no thromboses in RT. Patients with ET, however, may suffer from thrombohemorrhagic events, more often from microvascular circulation disturbances or thrombosis of major vessels than from hemorrhage; when they do arise from hemorrhage, this is mainly from mucous membranes.[12,22,23] In children, bleeding seems to be more frequent than microcirculatory disturbances. An enlarged spleen is more frequent in ET than RT.

Several attempts have been made to formulate positive criteria for distinguishing patients with ET from those with RT.[1,12–14,24] Suggested positive criteria for the diagnosis of ET are increased values for platelet count, platelet nucleotide ratio (ATP:ADP), mean platelet volume (MPV), platelet distribution width (PDW), unstimulated erythroid burst-forming unit (BFU-E) derived from erythroid colony formation from peripheral blood and bone marrow, splenic enlargement on radionuclide scan or ultrasound examination and clinical evidence of specific platelet-dependent and aspirin-responsive microvascular circulation disturbances.

Knowledge of bone marrow findings in ET of childhood is limited. According to Michiels and van Genderen,[12] the bone marrow criteria for adult ET, i.e. megakaryocyte hyperplasia and abundant platelet clumps in bone marrow smears in the absence of PCV, Philadelphia chromosome, significant myelofibrosis and myelodysplasia, may also apply to childhood ET.

Since RT is often associated with infections, patients have—in addition to elevated platelet counts—increased values for erythrocyte sedimentation rate, plasma fibrinogen, von Willebrand factor antigen, C-reactive protein (CRP) and IL-6 in the presence of an underlying disorder.[16,25]

A simple scoring system was introduced by Dudley et al[26] to differentiate ET from RT based on the presence of splenomegaly (scores 2), spontaneous BFU-E (2) and an elevated ATP:ADP ratio (1). When a total score of $\geqslant 3$ was taken as a predictor of ET and a score of < 3 as a predictor of RT, there were no false predictions of ET, but some false predictions of RT in the patients studied. However, this proposed scoring system is currently not used as the gold standard for diagnosing ET since its predictive value needs to be established in appropriate clinical trials. There are currently no trials in the pediatric age group.

CLINICAL MANIFESTATIONS

Michiels and van Genderen[12] reviewed 11 pediatric patients with ET (aged 6–12 years) and persistent elevated platelet counts in excess of $1000 \times 10^9/l$; 9 of the 11 patients had splenomegaly and 2 were asymptomatic. Four cases presented with recurrent mucocutaneous bleeding and/or bleeding after minor surgery and 1 developed bleeding symptoms during long-term treatment with aspirin 500 mg/day for recurrent attacks of headache. Two cases had no bleeding symptoms, but presented with microcirculatory disturbances including acrocyanosis, myocardial infarction, focal transient cerebral ischemic attacks (TIA), atypical TIAs such as dysarthria and hemianopia and headache. In one of these, TIAs recurred during relapse of ET after treatment with ^{32}P at platelet counts between 650 and 850 $\times 10^9/l$.

In the absence of a bone marrow biopsy at presentation in 6 cases, the diagnosis of ET remains unresolved. Four of these remained asymptomatic with no treatment or responded well to platelet reductive therapy with remissions lasting for 5–14 years without progression, which is consistent with the benign course of ET. One case transformed into overt idiopathic myelofibrosis (IMF) or chronic megakaryocytic granulocyte metaplasia (CMGM) with severe anemia, leukoerythroblastosis and massive splenomegaly after 11 years. The findings of increased mature megakaryocytes and platelet clumps on bone marrow smears with normal erythroid and myeloid series and no fibrosis in bone marrow biopsy material from 2 cases are compatible with the diagnosis of ET. In contrast, excess of megakaryocytes with a predominance of early forms and/or hypercellularity of the initial bone marrow with no fibrosis in biopsy material in 2 cases may have been indicative of atypical variants of ET. As the follow-up in the latter cases was very short (<2 years), the question of whether a correct diagnosis has been made remains unanswered.

TREATMENT OPTIONS

Procedures to prevent obstruction of large vessels or disturbances of microvascular circulation include:

- platelet-lowering therapy (e.g. hydroxyurea, busulfan, anagrelide, interferon, radioactive phosphorus, platelet apheresis);
- platelet aggregation inhibitors (e.g. aspirin and dipyridamole).

No general recommendations can be made as information is restricted to case reports.[12] The case described above with atypical ET and transformation into acute myeloblastic leukemia (AML) did not respond to recurrent treatment with ^{32}P. Two symptomatic children and 1 asymptomatic child with ET remained asymptomatic with no treatment during follow-up for 2, 8 and 11 years, respectively. Long-term or maintained remission of ET with correction of platelet counts to normal levels was obtained by treatment with 2 subsequent courses of ^{32}P in 1 case, with 3 courses of busulfan in 2 cases, and with continuous treatment with hydroxyurea in 1 and anagrelide in another case. No side-effects were reported.

Tefferi et al[16] recommend specific platelet lowering therapy for young patients with symptoms of thrombosis and bleeding. The platelet count should always be maintained at $<400 \times 10^9/l$. The author found no preference for anagrelide or hydroxyurea in a review of 56 young adults aged 12–40 years.

Chintagumpala et al[27] treated 3 ET patients (16, 15 and 10 years old) with anagrelide. Symptoms were recurrent headaches and abdominal pain in 1 case, severe headaches and epistaxis in another, and swelling of one knee and splenomegaly in the third. There were no episodes of bleeding or thromboses during therapy and all 3 patients have been relatively free of symptoms for 5, 4 and 2 years, respectively.

Plateletpheresis may be used in emergency situations, such as major bleeding at platelets counts $>1000 \times 10^9/l$.[28]

REACTIVE THROMBOCYTOSIS

PATHOPHYSIOLOGY

Stimulation of thrombocyte production has been observed after peripheral loss of platelets, e.g. after immunologic, septic, oncogenic or traumatic events, blood loss or hypoxemia of respiratory or cardiac origin. Elevated numbers of megakaryocytes were found in the bone marrow of affected patients.[29] Kanz[30] observed increased ploidy (>16 N) in patients with RT. In adults with immune thrombocytopenia (ITP), megakaryocytes in the bone marrow were markedly increased. The portion of megakaryocyte colony-forming units (CFU-Meg) in the S-phase was elevated, while the total CFU-Meg was normal with regard to number and size. This observation leads to the assumption that the cyclic activity of the quantitatively unchanged CFU-Meg pool is increased and adds to the elevated number of megakaryocytes in the bone marrow.[31] Morphologic peculiarities have not been described; inert ingestion of other bone marrow cells by megakaryocytes (emperipoiesis) is physiologic and is increased in patients with ET and RT.[32] Elevated levels of TPO have been found in patients with malignant liver tumors, hepatoblastoma and hepatocellular carcinoma,[33] active lung tuberculosis and acute megakaryocytic leukemia.[34,35] Data suggest that the CFU-

Meg pool of patients with RT is quantitatively and qualitatively normal. They also imply that the local marrow environment may contain a factor that increases megakaryocyte production at the post-CFU-Meg level. Such a putative growth factor might be elevated by activated T cells or natural killer (NK) cells.[7]

Another reactive cause of thombocytosis is a shift of the splenic pool into the peripheral blood. This can be provoked by exercise or stress situations or by injection of epinephrine and isoprenaline,[29] and can be found with functional or anatomical asplenia.

INCIDENCE

Thombocytosis in childhood is not as rare as was assumed until recently. Newer studies estimate an incidence between 6 and 13% in hospitalized children[2,36–40] and 15% in pediatric outpatients.[39] The variation is due to different definitions of the degree of thrombocytosis. In general, there is no difference in frequency between boys and girls,[36,41] but in children with thrombocytosis due to infections, Yohannan et al[41] observed significantly more boys. A review of the medical records of in- and out-patients with at least 1 platelet count $>1000 \times 10^9$ was performed during a $5\frac{1}{2}$-year period by Buss et al.[15] There were 280 patients with thrombocytosis, ranging in age from 12 days to 100 years, with a mean age of 37 years (82 under 20 years, 22 between 10 and 19 and 60 under 10 of whom 33 were under 1 year of age). Most of these patients had RT (82% versus 18% with ET), with only 2 patients under 20 years having ET. Infection was the commonest cause of RT in the first decade (39 of 60 patients) and trauma in the second decade (9 of 20).

DEGREE OF THROMBOCYTOSIS

In most cases, thrombocyte numbers are only slightly elevated. Between 78 and 86% of children with thrombocytosis had a platelet count between 500 and 700 $\times 10^9/l$ (Table 23.1).[2,36–39] Over 6 months, Sutor and Hank[2] saw 227 children with thrombocytosis, 78% of whom had the mild form, 15% the moderate form and only 7% the severe form with a platelet count exceeding $900 \times 10^9/l$; 3% had platelet counts $>1000 \times 10^9/l$ ('platelet millionaires'). A similar distribution was found by Vora and Lilleyman,[36] who saw 458 children with thrombocytosis over a 1-year period; 35 (8%) had at least 1 platelet count of $>800 \times 10^9/l$ and 7 (1.5%) were 'platelet millionaires'. Addiego et al[37] saw 10 children with counts $>800 \times 10^9/l$ at a university children's hospital in less than 1 year. Chan et al[38] found in 1 year 94 children with platelet counts $>900 \times 10^9/l$. The absolute number is comparable to the above mentioned studies when it is considered that the authors operate a referral center serving a population of 3 million.

Table 23.3 Predominant diseases in children with thrombocytosis. Updated from Ref. 2.

Disease	Sutor and Hank[2]	Yohannan et al[41]	Vora and Lilleyman[36]**	Buss et al[15]
Number of patients (platelets $\times 10^9$/l)	227 (>500)	663 (>500)	139 (>800)	82 (>1000)
Infection, total (%)	37	31	38	50
Respiratory tract	41	38		
Gastrointestinal	16	18		
Trauma/surgery (%)	15	15	21	11
Hypoxemia (%)	12	33*	14	
Anemia	8	33*	6	
Respiratory distress	4		8	
Gastroesophageal reflux (%)	6.5			
Renal disease (%)	6	4		
Autoimmune disease (Kawasaki, juvenile rheumatoid arthritis, vasculitis, Henoch–Schönlein) (%)	4	2	9	

*Data from a country with a high incidence of hemolytic disease.
**Includes data from Refs 37 and 38.

AGE DISTRIBUTION

Sutor and Hank[2] found the frequency of thrombocytosis to be exceptionally high in neonates, infants and young children; 72% occurred in patients under 2 years of age, 56% in infants and 25% during the first 2 months of life,[2] which is in agreement with the results of other studies (Table 23.1), including those that reported only moderate and severe thrombocytosis.[36,38] Buss et al,[15] who reported only on patients with extreme thrombocytosis of >1000 × 10^9/l, found that approximately 55% of their patients under 10 years with thrombocytosis were infants under 1 year. It is conceivable that thrombocytic precursor cells in the bone marrow of young children have an intensified ability to react to stress. Another reason might be that infants normally have higher platelet values,[42] and therefore develop mild thrombocytosis with the slightest platelet-producing stimulus. This is particularly true for low-birth-weight infants.[2,43]

CAUSES

Possible causes for thrombocytosis are summarized in Table 23.4.

Infection

Infection is by far the commonest cause of thrombocytosis (Table 23.3).[2,37,38,41] An incidence of 51% was found by Felici et al[40] and Buss et al[15] found that 65% of their children under 10 years of age with a platelet count >1 × 10^6 suffered from an infectious process. In the study of Heath and Pearson,[39] all 15 children with platelet counts >700 × 10^9/l had infections. The 2 children with the highest platelet counts (>1000 × 10^9/l) were recovering

Table 23.4 Conditions associated with reactive thrombocytosis (predominantly in infants and young children).

Infection (bacterial, viral)
  Respiratory
  Meningitis
  Gastrointestinal

Tissue damage (surgery, trauma)

Splenectomy

Hypoxemia
  Anemia
    Iron-deficiency anemia
    Hemolytic anemia
    Anemia due to blood loss, chemotherapy
    Anemia caused by nephrotic disease
  Respiratory disease
  Cardiac hypoxemia

Autoimmune disease
  Juvenile rheumatoid arthritis
  Kawasaki syndrome
  Henoch-Schönlein disease

Renal disease

Malignancy
  Hepatoblastoma
  Hodgkin's disease
  Histiocytosis
  Sarcoma
  Acute lymphoblastic leukemia and non-Hodgkin lymphoma

Prematurity

Stress situation

Medication
  Epinephrine (adrenaline)
  Corticosteroids
  Vinca alkaloids
  Miconazole
  Penicillamine
  Methadone (during pregnancy)
  Hydantoin (during pregnancy)

Miscellaneous
  Gastroesophageal reflux
  Caffey's disease

from pyogenic abscesses, one involving the brain and the other the soft tissue of the arm. Heyne and Tegtmeyer[8] found thrombocytosis in all 10 children treated for *Haemophilus influenzae* meningitis. Usually, a drop in platelet count was noted during the first 2 days of treatment, followed by a rise in platelet number after day 5, resulting in thrombocytosis in all observed cases. The plasma level of CRP was inversely related to the thrombocyte concentration. *In vitro*, aggregated CRP (H-CRP) induces thrombocyte aggregation. The rise in platelets in the course of an infection could be considered a compensatory, exaggerated platelet production following initial thrombocyte consumption by septic processes with intravascular coagulation, CRP induction and loss of platelets due to defense mechanisms.[44] Kilpi *et al*[45] found thrombocytosis in 49% of 311 children with bacterial meningitis after the first week of treatment. There was no relation between thrombocytosis and neurologic complications. A patient who died, however, developed thrombocytopenia instead of thrombocytosis. The authors speculate that the difference between the thrombocyte curves of the surviving and dying patients might be useful in predicting the outcome in the severest cases of bacterial meningitis.

Weissbach *et al*[46] found elevated thrombocyte counts in sepsis after the neonatal period. They reported what appear to be different stages of consumption and compensation at the beginning of the clinical symptoms, and these might be influenced by the type of pathogen and mode of invasion. Heath and Pearson,[39] on the other hand, conclude that the amount of thrombocytosis is not influenced by the infectious agent, the duration or localization of the infection, or the degree of fever. In agreement with this finding and with Yohannan *et al*,[41] the author's studies showed that respiratory tract infections are the commonest cause of thrombocytosis due to infection. Wolach *et al*[47] observed thrombocytosis in 92.5% of patients with pneumonia and empyema. No correlation between thrombocytosis and prognosis was found.[47] Inflammatory pulmonary disorders such as bronchitis and bronchopneumonia also induced elevation of pulmonary megakaryocytes. Whether the enhanced number of trapped pulmonary megakaryocytes in these disorders is due to changes in microvasculature or simply reflects enhanced platelet production in these conditions is not clear.[48] Bone marrow aspiration of 3 children with pneumonia and empyema showed megakaryocytic hyperplasia.[47]

Gastrointestinal infections accounted for 16% of the thrombocytopenias due to infection (Table 23.3). It cannot be concluded from the author's studies or the pediatric literature that thrombocytosis due to infection results in thrombosis. However, in adults with thrombocytosis, rare cases of severe, but often lethal, thromboembolic complications, predominantly in patients with ulcerative colitis and Crohn's disease, have been reported.[49]

Tissue damage

Thrombocytosis after traumatic or surgical tissue damage occurred in 15% of patients with thrombocytosis.[2] Similar figures are reported in the review by Vora and Lilleyman[36] and Yohannan *et al*.[41] Buss *et al*[15] found that 9 of 20 patients between 10 and 19 years of age had RT due to trauma. The highest elevation of platelet count is observed between the first and second postoperative weeks.[2,19] The increased platelet numbers can be looked upon as a reaction to blood loss or platelet consumption to restore hemostasis, which is especially pronounced after splenectomy.[19,29] In the author's studies there was a single case of thrombosis due to postoperative thrombocytosis. Postsurgical thromboembolic complications in patients with thombocytosis have been reported when additional risk factors, such as cyanotic heart disease and cardiac arrhythmia,[50] are present or when splenectomy has been performed because of myeloproliferative syndrome.[11,29]

Whether thrombocytosis, which develops after splenectomy, indicates a risk for thromboembolic complications is controversial. Thromboembolic complications are very rare in children; however, they have been observed after splenectomy for hematologic abnormalities such as autoimmune hemolytic anemia and portal hypertension.[51]

Hypoxemia

In the author's study, 28 children (12.3%) with thrombocytosis had hypoxemia due to anemia or respiratory distress syndrome. The 10 premature infants with respiratory distress accounted for 4.4% of all children with thrombocytosis. Eighteen children (7.9%) had anemia of different origin: iron deficiency and hemolytic anemia were found in 11 patients (4.8%) and 7 patients (3.1%) had developed anemic conditions following chronic blood loss, renal disease with anemia and transient erythroblastosis.[2] Iron deficiency as a cause of thrombocytosis was described as early as 1904.[52] Chan *et al*[38] found that 6% of their patients with thrombocytosis had anemia, mostly irondeficiency anemia. According to Dickerhoff and von Rücker,[10] 35% of children with iron-deficiency anemia have thrombocytosis. Yohannan *et al*[41] classified thrombocytosis in children with iron deficiency as rebound thrombocytosis, which is the same as thrombocytosis after hemorrhage and recovery from chemotherapy. They sorted 15% of their patients into this rebound group; about 10% had iron deficiency and 5% had chronic blood loss or had received chemotherapy. Of their children, 19.3% with thrombocytosis had hemolytic anemia which reflects the higher incidence of hereditary hemolytic disease in the population of Saudi Arabia. Thrombocytosis has also been observed in infants with blood loss due to vitamin K deficiency bleeding[53] and after extreme hemodilution in open heart surgery.[54]

Autoimmune disease

Autoimmune disease accounted for the increased platelet count in 4–10% of the patients reported by Sutor[1] and Vora and Lilleyman.[36] Chan et al[38] observed an underlying autoimmune disease in 11% of their patients with thrombocytosis; 3% of these cases had juvenile rheumatoid arthritis (JRA) and 2% had Kawasaki's syndrome. Thrombocytosis as a common feature of Kawasaki's syndrome was described by Limbach and Lindinger.[55] The author found JRA in 2% of patients with thrombocytosis, some of whom were treated with corticosteroids.[2] In adults, Robbins and Barnard[19] observed autoimmune disease in 7.8% of patients with thrombocytosis; except for 2, all had rheumatoid arthritis. Gonzenbach et al[56] reported on rheumatoid arthritis, lupus erythematosus and other collagen disease and subsumed under chronic infections, these were the reason for 11% of cases of thrombocytosis. De Benedetti et al[57] measured elevated serum IL-6 in patients with JRA and this correlated with the extent and severity of joint involvement and with platelet counts. Patients with Henoch-Schönlein purpura have only mild thrombocytosis.[2,58,59] The coincidence of abdominal pain due to hemorrhage and thrombocytosis is remarkable.

Gastrointestinal disease without infection

Of the author's patients, 6.5% suffered from gastroesophageal reflux.[2] The increased platelet production could reflect a reaction of the esophageal mucosa to constant irritation by acid gastric contents. Regurgitation and aspiration frequently result in recurrent bronchitis. Vomiting of hematin may in some cases lead to iron-deficiency anemia.

Thrombocytosis has been reported in children with allergy to cows' milk, which in some cases leads to colitis.[60] Of patients with Crohn's disease, 75% presented with thrombocytosis.[61]

Renal disease

Of the author's children with thrombocytosis, 14 (6%) had some kind of renal disease and in 11 of these, this was in connection with anemia due to macrohematuria or renal failure. Thrombocytosis in children with nephrotic syndrome is not rare: among the author's patients, 3 had nephrotic syndrome.[2] There is a predisposition to bacterial infections in this condition, which is possibly explained by decreased splenic function.[62] In 1 nephrotic patient, excessive thrombocytosis was observed after therapy with cyclosporin.[63]

Oncologic disease

When patients undergoing chemotherapy are excluded, children with malignancies constitute approximately 1–3% of all patients with thrombocytosis.[2,5,38] In the author's study, 2 children with a tumor of the CNS were seen. Blatt et al[64] reported 7 children with acute lymphoid leukemia (ALL) (3.2% of all newly diagnosed cases) with a platelet count of $>400 \times 10^9/l$ before diagnosis. Two of these had major complications during the induction phase of therapy; 1 developed thrombosis of the cavernous sinus during therapy for ALL and the other had bleeding from the gastrointestinal tract following perforation of a duodenal ulcer. These complications are rare but not unknown during ALL treatment and it is conceivable that they are caused by medications, such as glucocorticoids or asparaginase.[65]

Elevated levels of thrombopoietin have been shown in patients with malignant liver disease, such as hepatoblastoma and hepatocellular carcinoma.[35] Since excessive thrombocytosis is usually present before chemotherapy, the platelet count may be a strong diagnostic pointer in a child with a newly diagnosed abdominal mass.[33] Vora and Lilleyman[36] found malignant disease in 16 of 139 patients with very high platelet counts. However, since most of them were tested during or after surgery or chemotherapy, anemia[41] or drugs could also be the reason for thrombocytosis.

Medications

The following medications are claimed to cause thrombocytosis in children: epinephrine (adrenaline), corticosteroids, cyclosporin, vinca alkaloids, miconazole, penicillamine and citroforum.[61,66,67] Epinephrine increases the platelet count by shifting the splenic pool into the peripheral blood. Thrombocytosis in patients treated with penicillamine for Wilson's disease has been explained as a rebound effect to the low pre-treatment values.[61] Ten of 11 patients with oncologic disease (solid tumors, ALL) developed thrombocytopenia during therapy with corticosteroids and/or vinca alkaloids.[1] Both of these medications can cause thrombocytosis.[20,61,67]

In immune thrombocytopenias, advantage is taken of the fact that corticosteroids suppress platelet phagocytosis by macrophages.[68] It is possible that the rise in platelets in patients who have been treated with corticosteroids is due to the same mechanim. Therefore, the inclusion of corticosteroid therapy in the differential diagnosis of thrombocytosis is recommended.

Transient thrombocytosis has been described in infants born to mothers taking methadone during pregnancy.[69] Thrombocytosis as part of the fetal hydantoin syndrome was observed by Alvarez et al.[70]

Other causes

Prematurity

Elevated thrombocyte counts have been observed in otherwise healthy premature babies (2.6% of the author's pediatric patients with thrombocytosis). These values may be physiologic as they are within the limits which Lundström[43] set for premature infants. The 95% range was between 160 and 675 × 10^9/l with a median value of 375 × 10^9/l. The author and Lundström[43] have not observed a single thrombosis in preterm infants.

Exercise

The human spleen normally retains about one-third of the total platelets in an exchangeable pool which can be released into the circulation on α-adrenergic stimulation.[71,72] Redistribution of this pool into the peripheral blood stream immediately leads to marked thrombocytosis. It has not been possible to explain the association between thrombocytosis and various diseases, such as allergies, metabolic disease, myopathies, convulsive disorders (without steroid treatment), preoperative stages and deformities of the skeletal system, in pediatric[40] and adult[56] patients.

Discounting the cohort of premature infants, the reason for one-fifth of all thrombocytosis is not clear. If the patients with gastroesophageal reflux are added to the proportion of unexplained thrombocytosis, a quarter of all thrombocytoses could not be explained in our study.[2] Felici *et al*[40] and Gonzenbach *et al*[56] found no explanation for 29% and 32% of their cases with thrombocytosis, respectively.

COMPLICATIONS

A review of the literature over the past 18 years revealed 2 pediatric patients who had developed thrombosis in the course of iron-deficiency anemia with RT. One was a 22-month-old boy with iron-deficiency anemia who on admission had a hemoglobin of 4 g/dl and a thrombocyte count of 1000 × 10^9/l. On day 2 of his hospital stay he developed headache, confusion and convulsions. The CT showed infarction of the basal ganglia and thalamus and MRI indicated hemorrhagic infarction. Control of the blood count revealed a hemoglobin of 6 g/dl, a mean corpuscular volume (MCV) of 57 fl and a thrombocyte count of 540 × 10^9/l.[73]

The second case was an 8-month-old Japanese girl who had developed left hemiparesis after a slight head injury. Her CT and MRI demonstrated a cerebral infarction. Laboratory findings revealed iron-deficiency anemia and thrombocytosis with a platelet count of 1075 × 10^9/l. Serum iron was only 18 μg/dl.[74]

Interestingly, thrombotic complications in connection with thrombocytosis due to iron-deficiency anemia have been reported in rare adult cases. In the absence of other risk factors, thrombocytosis secondary to iron-deficiency anemia due to polymenorrhea was considered to be the reason for multiple cerebral infarctions in a 30-year-old woman. Platelet count was normalized after iron therapy.[75] A 45-year-old woman with mild thrombocytosis secondary to iron-deficiency anemia suffered from hemispheric infarc-

tion in the absence of vascular, cardiac or coagulation pathologies.[76]

The question remains whether thrombocytosis was the only reason for infarction in these patients. In neither of the case reports was the method of platelet counting mentioned; small erythrocytes resulting from iron deficiency can be counted as platelets in electronic particle counters and falsely indicate a platelet count of >1 million/μl (author's own observation). The rigidity of the iron-deficiency erythrocytes may play a role as well.[77] Iron deficiency in patients with polycythemia because of cyanotic heart disease with constant hypoxemia may act as continuous stimulation for erythro- and thrombo-cytogenesis. Thus, in polycythemia, increased rigidity of iron-deficient erythrocytes and thrombocytosis combine to give a high-risk for thrombosis. The vicious circle is better interrupted by therapy with iron than with anticoagulants.

The stimulant effect of erythropoietin on thrombocytogenesis is controversial: animal experiments favor it but experience of erythropoietin administration in patients with renal insufficiency does not.[78]

Turba *et al*[79] reported 3 newborns with subcutaneous fat necrosis that appeared between the 4th and 21st day of life. All patients showed a marked increase in platelets before the onset of clinical manifestations. The question is raised whether thrombocytosis might lower blood perfusion with relative hypoxia and hypothermia and thus lead to necrosis of adipose tissue.[79]

Thrombosis is the severest complication of thrombocytosis after splenectomy; however, it is not yet proven that the elevated number of platelets is a causative or concomitant factor.[51]

INDICATIONS FOR PROPHYLAXIS

RT in children does not justify general prophylaxis with anticoagulants or platelet aggregation inhibitors. Even an RT of 1000 × 10^9/l or more has no clinical importance in terms of morbidity. No prophylaxis with platelet aggregation inhibitors should be recommended.[10] Individually tailored thrombosis prophylaxis should be considered if additional risk factors exist, such as immobilization in a cast, some cases of leukemia,[63] alterations of other plasmatic thrombophilic factors,[29,80] iron-deficiency anemia,[38,52] cyanotic heart disease and cardiac arrhythmias after Fontan surgery,[50] splenectomy for a myeloproliferative syndrome or hematologic disease such as autoimmune hemolytic anemia,[29,51,81] or increased incidence of thrombosis in connection with postoperative thrombocytosis after pancreas transplantation.[82]

REFERENCES

1. Sutor AH. Thrombocytosis in childhood. *Semin Thromb Hemostas* 1995; **21**: 330–339
2. Sutor AH, Hank D. Thrombosen bei Thrombozytosen im Kindesalter.

In: Sutor AH (ed) *Thombosen im Kindesalter. Risikofaktoren–Diagnose–Prophylaxe–Therapie*. Basel: Roche, 1992, pp 113–136

3. Schneider W, Gattermann N. Evolution of cellular haemostasis. *Haemostaseologie* 1996; **16**: 88–96
4. Williams N. Is thrombopoietin interleukin 6? *Exp Hematol* 1991; **19**: 714–718
5. Metcalf D. Thrombopoietin—at last. *Nature* 1994; **369**: 519–520
6. Baatout S. Thrombopoietin. A review. *Haemostasis* 1997; **27**: 1–8
7. Gewirtz AM, Schick B. Platelet production and function. In: Colman RW, Hirst J, Marder VJ, Salzman EW (eds) *Hemostasis and Thrombosis*. Philadelphia: JB Lippincott, 1994, pp 353–396
8. Heyne K, Tegtmeyer FK. Postinfektiöse Thrombozytose als Akute Phase-Reaktion: das Beispiel *Haemophilus influenzae*-Meningitis. *Monatsschr Kinderheilk* 1988; **136**: 622–625
9. Göbel U. Thrombozytäre Erkrankungen. In: Reinhardt D, Harnack von GA (eds) *Therapie der Krankheiten des Kindesalters*. Berlin: Springer Verlag, 1990, p 377
10. Dickerhoff R, von Rücker A. Thrombozytose im Kindesalter. Differentialdiagnose und klinische Bedeutung. *Pädiatrische Praxis* 1991; **41**: 25–28
11. Randi ML, Fabris F, Girolani A. Thrombocytosis in young people: Evaluation of 57 cases diagnosed before the age of 40. *Blut* 1990; **60**: 233–237
12. Michiels JJ, van Genderen PJJ. Essential thrombocythemia in childhood. *Semin Thromb Hemostas* 1997; **23**: 295–301
13. Schafer AI. Essential thrombocythemia. *Prog Hemostas Thromb* 1991; **10**: 69–96
14. Van Genderen PJJ, Michiels JJ. Primary thrombocythemia: Diagnosis, clinical manifestations and management. *Ann Hematol* 1993; **67**: 57–62
15. Buss DH, Cashell AW, O'Connor ML, Richards FII, Case LD. Occurrence, etiology and clinical significance of extreme thrombocytosis: A study of 280 cases. *Am J Med* 1994; **96**: 247–253
16. Tefferi A, Silverstein MN, Hoagland HC. Primary thrombocythemia. Review. *Semin Oncol* 1995; **22**: 334–340
17. Murphy S, Iland H, Rosenthal D, Laszlo J. Essential thrombocythemia: an interim report from the Polycythemia Vera Study Group. *Semin Hematol* 1986; **23**: 177–182
18. Schafer AI. Bleeding and thrombosis in the myeloproliferative disorders. *Blood* 1984; **64**: 1–12
19. Robbins G, Barnard DL. Thrombocytosis and microthrombocytosis: A clinical evaluation of 372 cases. *Acta Haematol* 1983; **70**: 175–182
20. Mitus AJ, Schafer AI. Thrombocytosis and thrombocythemia. *Hematol Oncol Clin North Am* 1990; **4**: 157–178
21. Hochhaus A, Mindner K, Ostermann G, Hoche D. Aggregationsverhalten und Calciumgehalt der Plättchen bei Thrombozythämien und Thrombozytosen. *Folia Haematol* 1990; **117**: 765–770
22. Schwartz CL, Cohen HJ. Myeloproliferative and myelodysplastic syndromes. In: Pizzo PA, Poplack DG (eds) *Principles and Practice of Pediatric Oncology*. Philadelphia: JB Lippincott, 1997, pp 505–521
23. Frezzato M, Ruggeri M, Castaman G, Rodeghiero F. Polycythemia vera and essential thrombocythemia in young patients. *Haematologica* 1993; **78**: 11–17
24. Laszlo J. Myeloproliferative disorders (MPD): myelofibrosis, myelosclerosis, extramedullary hematopoiesis, undifferentiated MPD and hemorrhagic thrombocythemia. *Semin Hematol* 1975; **12**: 409–432
25. Kutti J, Wadenik H. Diagnostic and differential criteria of essential thrombocythemia and reactive thrombocytosis. *Leukemia Lymphoma* 1996; **22 (Suppl 1)**: 41–45
26. Dudley JM, Messinezy M, Eridani S *et al*. Primary thrombocythemia: diagnostic criteria and a simple scoring system for positive diagnosis. *Br J Haematol* 1992; **39**: 131–136
27. Chintagumpala MM, Kennedy LL, Steuber CP. Treatment of essential thrombocythemia with anagrelide. *J Pediatr* 1995; **127**: 495–498
28. Griesshammer M, Heimpel H, Pearson TC. Essential thrombocythemia and pregnancy. *Semin Thromb Hemostas* 1996; **22 (Suppl 1)**: 57–63
29. Kutti J. The managment of thrombocytosis. *Eur J Haematol* 1990; **44**: 81–88
30. Kanz L. Human megakaryocytopoiesis: Stimulation of platelet production. In: Sutor AH, Thomas KB (eds) *Thrombocytopenia in childhood*. Stuttgart: Schattauer, 1994, pp 3–11
31. Dan K, Gomi S, Nomura T. Kinetics of megakaryocyte progenitor cells in idiopathic thrombocytopenic purpura. *Blut* 1990; **61**: 303–306
32. Cashell AW, Buss DH. The frequency and significance of megakaryocytic emperipolesis in myeloproliferative and reactive states. *Ann Hematol* 1992; **64**: 273–276
33. Shafford EA, Pritchard J. Extreme thrombocytosis as a diagnostic clue to hepatoblastoma. *Arch Dis Child* 1993; **69**: 171
34. Nickerson HJ, Silberman TL, McDonald TP. Hepatoblastoma, thrombocytosis and increased thrombopoietin. *Cancer* 1980; **45**: 315–317
35. McDonald TP. Thrombopoietin. Its biology, clinical aspects and possibilities. *Am J Pediatr Hematol Oncol* 1992; **14**: 8–21
36. Vora AJ, Lilleyman JS. Secondary thrombosis. *Arch Dis Child* 1993; **68**: 88–90
37. Addiego JE, Mentzer WC, Dallmann PR. Thrombocytosis in infants and children. *J Pediatr* 1974; **85**: 805–807
38. Chan KW, Kaikow Y, Wadsworth LD. Thrombocytosis in childhood: A survey of 94 patients. *Pediatrics* 1989; **84**: 1064–1067
39. Heath HW, Pearson HA. Thrombocytosis in pediatric outpatients. *J Pediatr* 1989; **114**: 805–807
40. Felici L, Freddara R, Pierani P, Coppa GV, Girogi PL. Thrombocytosis in hospitalized children. *J Pediatr* 1990; **116**: 835
41. Yohannan MD, Higgy KE, Al-Mashhadani SA, Santhosh-Kumar CR. Thrombocytosis. Etiologic analysis of 663 patients. *Clin Pediatr* 1994; **33**: 340–343
42. Artmann C, Mayr K. Spezifische Einflüsse des Lebensalters und des Geschlechts auf Thrombozytenzahl, Grösse und Grössenverteilung. Referenzbereiche für ein mechanisiertes Analysengerät. *Lab Med* 1983; **7**: 379–383
43. Lundström U. Thrombocytosis in low birthweight infants. A physiological phenomenon in infancy. *Arch Dis Child* 1979; **54**: 715–717
44. Sutor AH. Blutgerinnungsstörung und Infektion in der Pädiatrie. In: Tilsner V, Matthias FR (eds) *Infektion, Entzündung und Blutgerinnung. XXXII. Hamburger Symposion über Blutgerinnung*. Basel: Roche 1990, pp 135–150
45. Kilpi T, Anttila M, Kallio MJ, Peltola H. Thrombocytosis and thrombocytopenia in childhood bacterial meningitis. *Pediatr Infect Dis J* 1992; **11**: 456–460
46. Weissbach G, Domula M, Handrick W. Beeinflussung von Hämostase und Thrombogenese durch septische Prozesse speziell im Kindesalter. *Z Ges Inn Med* 1984; **39**: 214–218
47. Wolach B, Morag H, Drucker M, Sadan N. Thrombocytosis after pneumonia with empyema and other bacterial infections in children. *Pediatr Infect Dis J* 1990; **9**: 718–721
48. Eldor A, Vlodavsky I, Deutsch V, Levine RF. Megakaryocyte function and dysfunction. *Baillière's Clin Haematol* 1989; **3**: 543–568
49. Talbot RW, Heppell J, Dozois RR, Beart RW Jr. Vascular complications of inflammatory bowel disease. *Mayo Clin Proc* 1986; **61**: 140–145
50. Mathews K, Bale JF, Clark EB, Marvin WJ, Doty DB. Cerebral infarction complicating Fontan surgery for cyanotic heart disease. *Pediatr Cardiol* 1986; **7**: 161–166
51. Eber SW, Grosche M, Ditzig M, Pekrun A, Lakomek M, Schröter W. Komplikationen nach Splenektomie bei gutartigen hämatologischen Erkrankungen im Kindesalter. *Monatsschr Kinderheilkd* 1996; **114**: 275–280
52. Richardson FL. Effect of severe hemorrhage on the number of blood platelets in blood from the peripheral circulation of rabbits. *J Med Res* 1904; **13**: 99
53. Sutor AH. Vitamin-K-deficiency bleeding in infancy. *Semin Thromb Hemostas* 1995; **21**: 317–329
54. Dale J, Lilleaasen P, Erikssen J. Hemostasis after open heart surgery with extreme or moderate hemodilution. *Eur Surg Res* 1987; **19**: 339–347
55. Limbach HG, Lindinger A. Kawasaki syndrome in infants in the first 6 months of life. *Klin Pädiatr* 1991; **203**: 133–136
56. Gonzenbach R, Grimm J, Trachsler M, Rhyner K. Häufigkeit und

klinische Relvanz von Thrombozytosen. *Schweiz Med Wschr* 1982; **112**: 38–41

57. De Benedetti F, Massa M, Robbioni P, Ravelli A, Burgio GR, Martini A. Correlation of serum interleukin-6 levels with joint involvement in systemic juvenile rheumatoid arthritis. *Arthritis Rheumat* 1991; **34**: 1158–1163

58. Sauslbury FT, Kesler RW. Thrombocytosis in Henoch–Schönlein purpura. *Clin Pediatr* 1983; **22**: 185–187

59. Bost M, Kolodie L, Pouzol P, Dechelette E, Joannard A, Andreani P. L'hyperplaquettose et la baisse du factor XIII dans le purpura rheumatoide de l'enfant. *Pediatrie* 1986; **41**: 401–411

60. Harms HK. Die Kuhmilcheiweiss-abhängige Darmerkrankung des jungen Säuglings. *Klin Pädiatr* 1982; **194**: 375–380

61. Lascari AD. *Hematologic Manifestations of Childhood Diseases*. New York: Georg Thieme Verlag 1984, pp 250–251, 283, 341

62. McVicar MJ, Chandra M, Margouleff D, Zanzi J. Splenic hypofunction in the nephrotic syndrome of childhood. *Am J Kidney Dis* 1986; **7**: 395–401

63. Itami N, Akutsu Y, Yasoshima K. Thrombocytosis after cyclosporin therapy in a child with nephrotic syndrome. *Lancet* 1988; **ii**: 1018

64. Blatt J, Penchansky L, Horn M. Thrombocytosis as a presenting feature of acute lymphoblastic leukemia in childhood. *Am J Hematol* 1989; **31**: 46–49

65. Sutor AH, Niemeyer C, Sauter S *et al.* Gerinnungsveränderungen bei Behandlung mit den Protokollen ALL-BFM 90 und NHL-BFM 90. *Klin Pädiatr* 1993; **204**: 264–273

66. Stevens DA. Miconazole in the treatment of coccidioidomycosis. *Drugs* 1983; **26**: 347–354

67. Frye JL, Thompson DF. Drug-induced thrombocytosis. *J Clin Pharmacy Therapeut* 1993; **18**: 45–48

68. Belluci S. Autoimmune thrombocytopenias. *Baillière's Clin Haematol* 1989; **3**: 695–718

69. Burstein Y, Giardina PJV, Rausen AR. Thrombocytosis and increased circulating platelet aggregates in newborn infants of polydrug users. *J Pediatr* 1979; **94**: 895–899

70. Alvarez O, Miller JH, Coates TD. Thrombocytosis and hyposplenism in an infant with fetal hydantoin syndrome. *Am J Pediatr Hematol Oncol* 1992; **14**: 62–65

71. Chamberlain KG, Tong M, Penington DG. Properties of the exchangeable splenic platelets released into the circulation during exercise-induced thrombocytosis. *Am J Hematol* 1990; **34**: 161–168

72. Ricci G, Masotti M, Mazzoni G, Grazzi I, Casoni I. Platelet count, mean platelet volume and platelet dimensional width in professional cyclists during races. *Thromb Res* 1991; **62**: 791–792

73. Belman AL, Roque CT, Ancona R, Anand AK, Davis RP. Cerebral venous thrombosis in a child with iron deficiency anemia and thrombocytosis. *Stroke* 1990; **21**: 488–493

74. Tamura T, Konno K, Matsumoto S, Gotou T. An infantile case of cerebral infarction associated with thrombocytosis [Japanese]. *No to Hattatsu* 1992; **24**: 257–261

75. Saxena VK, Brands C, Crosl R, Moens E, Marien P, de Deyn PP. Multiple cerebral infarctions in a young patient with secondary thrombocythemia due to iron deficiency anemia. *Acta Neurol* 1993; **15**: 297–302 [see erratum in *Acta Neurol* 1993; **15**: 321]

76. Scoditti U, Colonna F, Ludovico L, Trabattoni G. Mild thrombocytosis secondary to iron deficiency anemia and stroke. *Rivista Neurologia* 1990; **60**: 146–147

77. Schrieber R. Thrombosen bei angeborenen Herz–Gefäss-Fehlern. In: Sutor AH (ed) *Thrombosen im Kindesalter*. Basel: Roche, 1992, pp 29–46

78. Gewirtz AM, Hoffman R. Human megakaryocyte production: Cell biology and clinical considerations. *Hematol Oncol Clin North Am* 1990; **4**: 43–64

79. Turba F, Bianchi C, Cella D, Rondanini GF. Thrombocytosis and neonatal subcutaneous adiponecrosis. *Minerva Pediatr* 1994; **46**: 343–346

80. Nowak-Göttl U, Kreuz WD, Hach-Wunderle V *et al.* Untersuchungen bei "idiopathischen" venösen Thrombosen im Kindes- und Jugendalter. In: Sutor AH (ed) *Thrombosen im Kindesalter. Risikofaktoren–Diagnose–Prophylaxe–Therapie*. Basel: Roche, 1992: 11–25

81. Randi ML, Fabris F, Dona S, Girolami A. Evaluation of platelet function in postsplenectomy thrombocytosis. *Folia Haematol (Leipzig)* 1987; **114**: 252–256

82. Hunziker D, Schlumpf R, Decrutins M, Keusch G, Largiader F. Thrombozytose nach Pankreastransplantation. *Helv Chir Acta* 1989; **56**: 543–547

Platelet functional disorders

ROGER M HARDISTY*

Bleeding disorders may result from defects of many different aspects of platelet function, even when the platelet count is normal. Functional defects may also accompany thrombocytopenia and aggravate the severity of the bleeding tendency which results. The most clearly characterized are the inherited disorders, which usually present clinically in infancy or childhood. Despite their comparative rarity, these conditions are important for the extensive information which their study has provided concerning the physiology of the hemostatic mechanism and the relative clinical significance of its component parts. Platelet function may also be disturbed in a wide range of acquired diseases involving patients of all ages, or by a variety of drugs, but in most of these instances the pathogenetic mechanisms involved are much less clearly defined.

HEMOSTATIC FUNCTIONS OF PLATELETS

The characteristic clinical diagnostic features of a platelet disorder, whether quantitative or functional, are a long bleeding time and spontaneous purpuric lesions; these show that the platelets are essential not only for the arrest of hemorrhage after injury to small vessels, but also for the maintenance of integrity of apparently uninjured vessels. The platelets do indeed play a central role in both these aspects of the hemostatic process. Originating as anucleate fragments of megakaryocyte cytoplasm, enveloped by a highly organized unit membrane, they circulate in the form of smooth discs. When the endothelial lining of the vessel wall is breached, bringing platelets into contact with subendothelium or deeper layers of the vessel wall, they rapidly adhere to these tissues, spread over their surface, undergo morphologic changes with the formation of pseudopodia, and aggregate together to form a hemostatic plug.

*Deceased.

These processes, which begin within seconds of injury, involve:

- interaction of platelet membrane components with adhesive proteins in the vessel wall and the plasma;
- secretion from the platelet of many active principles which themselves contribute to aggregation, vasoconstriction and vessel wall repair;
- activation of blood coagulation on the platelet surface.

Defects of any of these steps in platelet plug formation can lead to hemostatic failure, while, in certain circumstances, increased platelet reactivity may contribute to a thrombotic tendency.

PLATELET ULTRASTRUCTURE

The ultrastructural features of the unstimulated discoid platelet are shown in Fig. 24.1. The *plasma membrane* consists of a lipid bilayer, partially or completely penetrated by many glycoprotein (Gp) molecules. These carry receptors for many different agonists and for adhesive proteins as well as specific alloantigenic sites, and are linked to elements of the platelet cytoskeleton. Several have been extensively characterized and shown to play key roles in the hemostatic process (Table 24.1), particularly as receptors for collagen, for adhesive proteins in the vessel wall, and for fibrinogen and von Willebrand factor (VWF), which are essential for the processes of aggregation and adhesion.

The most abundant glycoproteins are GpIIb and IIIa, which form a calcium-dependent heterodimer complex which carries receptors for fibrinogen, VWF, fibronectin and vitronectin, and is of crucial importance in hemostasis and thrombosis (see below). The GpIIb–IIIa complex[1] is a member of the super-family of adhesion receptors known as *integrins*:[2] these are heterodimers, present on many cell types, and consist of an α subunit non-covalently linked to one of a restricted number of β subunits. GpIIb–IIIa is thus designated as the integrin $\alpha_{IIb}\beta_3$. The integrins are transmembrane proteins, providing binding sites for adhesive proteins

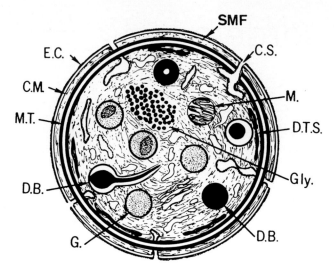

Fig. 24.1 Platelet in equatorial section. EC = external coat; CM = cell surface membrane; SMF = submembranous microfilaments; MT = microtubules; DTS = dense tubular system; CS = surface-connected canalicular system; G = α-granule; DB = dense body; M = mitochondrion; Gly = glycogen granules. Kindly provided by James G White.

and its cytoplasmic domain is linked through actin-binding protein to actin.

Closely subjacent to the plasma membrane, in the equatorial plane, runs the circumferential band of *microtubules* which maintains the discoid shape of the resting platelet and disassembles on stimulation with aggregating agents. The *surface-connected canalicular system (SCCS)* consists of invaginations of the plasma membrane, through which granule contents are chiefly discharged during the secretory process, and the *dense tubular system* or smooth endoplasmic reticulum is the chief site of thromboxane synthesis and of the sequestration and release of calcium ions for the control of intracellular calcium-dependent processes.

Other organelles within the platelet include mitochondria, glycogen granules, lysosomes, peroxisomes and 2 other specific types of storage organelle: the *dense osmiophilic granules* and *α-granules* (Table 24.2). The dense bodies contain the storage pool of adenine nucleotides and 5-hydroxytryptamine (5-HT, serotonin), and the α-granules contain many different proteins. Many of the α-granule proteins are synthesized in the megakaryocyte and include those specific to the platelet (platelet factor 4, β-thromboglobulin, platelet-derived growth factor), as well as VWF, Factor V and other proteins which are also found in other cell types and/or in the plasma; others, including fibrinogen and immunoglobulins, are taken up into the α-granules by endocytosis from the plasma. The contents of these granules are secreted by exocytosis in response to many stimuli, following the fusion of their membranes with the plasma membrane or SCCS. This process can be recognized by the appearance of specific granule contents in the plasma or by the identification of glycoproteins specific to the granule membranes (e.g.

on their extracellular domains and attachment to cytoskeletal elements on their cytoplasmic domains. The platelet GpIa–IIa and Ic–IIa complexes are also integrins, providing binding sites for collagen and fibronectin, respectively, and having identical structures ($\alpha_2\beta_1$ and $\alpha_5\beta_1$) to the VLA-2 and VLA-5 proteins of lymphocytes.[3] The leucine-rich glycoprotein Ib[4] carries receptors for VWF and thrombin on its α subunit and plays an essential part in platelet-vessel wall interaction (see below). It is closely associated in the membrane with 2 other leucine-rich glycoproteins, GpIX and V,

Table 24.1 Platelet membrane glycoproteins.

Glycoprotein		Copies per platelet (10^3)	Receptors	Alloantigens state	Deficiency
Ia (α_2)	VLA-2	2–4	Collagen	Br(HPA-5)	*
IIa (β_1)		5–10	Fibronectin, laminin		
Ic (α_5)	VLA-5				
Ib		25–30	VWF, (thrombin)	Ko(HPA-2)	Bernard–Soulier syndrome
IX					
IIb (α_{IIb})		40–50	Fibrinogen, VWF, fibronectin, vitronectin	Bak[a] (HPA-3)	Glanzmann's thrombasthenia
IIIa (β_3)				Pen(HPA-4) PI[A](HPA-1)	
IV (CD36)			Collagen type V thrombospondin	Nak[a]	**
V			Thrombin, Cl$_q$		
VI (p62)			Collagen		*

*Collagen-dependent defect.
**Asymptomatic.

Table 24.2 Platelet storage organelles and their contents.

Dense granules
  ATP, ADP
  5-HT
  Ca^{2+}

α-Granules
  Platelet factor 4
  β-thromboglobulin
  Platelet-derived growth factor
  von Willebrand factor
  Multimerin
  Factor V
  Thrombospondin
  High molecular weight kininogen
  Plasminogen
  Plasminogen activator inhibitor I
  $α_2$-Antiplasmin
  $α_2$-Macroglobulin
  $α_1$-Antitrypsin
  Histidine-rich glycoprotein
  Fibrinogen
  Fibronectin
  Albumin
  Immunoglobulins

P-selectin for α-granules; granulophysin for dense bodies) on the outer surface of the platelet.

HEMOSTATIC PROCESSES

Adhesion

The adhesion of platelets to subendothelium involves inter-actions between platelet membrane glycoproteins, elements of the vessel wall including collagen, and adhesive proteins including VWF and fibronectin. The relative importance of the various interactions varies with the conditions of flow.[5] Thus, at high shear rates, such as those that obtain in the microvasculature, the initial attachment of platelets to sub-endothelium is mediated chiefly through the binding of VWF (conformationally modified by its prior binding to the subendothelium)[6] to GpIb.[7,8] Under these conditions, however, VWF will also bind to GpIIb–IIIa, as does the VWF secreted from the α-granules, and this interaction probably contributes to the subsequent spreading of the platelets on the subendothelial surface as well as to thrombus formation.[9,10] At low shear rates similar to those on the venous side of the circulation, GpIb and IIb–IIIa are still involved, but the role of VWF is less important and other adhesive proteins, including fibronectin, also play a role in the adhesion reaction.

Aggregation

Adhesion to collagen, and many other stimuli, lead to a further series of reactions in the platelets, including a change of shape from discoid to spherical with the formation of many small pseudopodia, secretion of the contents of dense bodies and α-granules and the formation of aggregates. Aggregation in response to collagen is chiefly dependent on the secretion of active principles, including ADP and throm-boxane A_2 from the platelets themselves, but aggregation in the absence of significant secretion can be studied *in vitro* in response to ADP and various other agonists. However induced, platelet aggregation is dependent on the binding of fibrinogen to specific receptors on the GpIIb–IIIa complex. These receptors are not available for fibrinogen binding on the surface of unstimulated platelets, but become expressed when the platelets are stimulated by an aggregat-ing agent.[11,12] The nature of the signal transmitted from the receptor for the aggregating agent to GpIIb–IIIa is not known, but the binding of fibrinogen, unlike that of VWF to GpIb, is calcium-dependent, and involves at least 2 Arg-Gly-Asp sequences on the Aα chain and a C-terminal peptide on the γ chain of fibrinogen. GpIIb–IIIa also binds Arg-Gly-Asp sequences in VWF and fibronectin, but these adhesive proteins play no important physiologic role in platelet aggregation, since fibrinogen is present at much higher molar concentration in plasma.

Secretion

Binding of many agonists to their receptors on the platelet membrane not only leads to expression of fibrinogen recep-tors and so to aggregation, but sets in train a series of signal transduction mechanisms (Fig. 24.2). Agonist-receptor interaction leads, via the activation of guanine nucleotide-binding proteins (G proteins), to the hydrolysis of phospha-tidyl inositides in the platelet membrane by phospholipase C. The inositol trisphosphate thus produced promotes the mobilization of Ca^{2+} from its intracellular storage sites (chiefly the dense tubular system) and the influx of Ca^{2+} from the extracellular environment, while diacylglycerol activates protein kinase C (PKC). Amongst the intracellular reactions for which raised cytosolic Ca^{2+} is required are the phosphorylation of myosin light chain (P20) and the 47 kDa contractile protein (pleckstrin, P47) by PKC, and the liberation of arachidonic acid for thromboxane synthesis from membrane phospholipids by phospholipase A2 (Fig. 24.3).

Phosphorylation of the contractile proteins is an essential step in the structural rearrangement leading to secretion of granule contents by exocytosis, and pleckstrin phosphoryla-tion is also involved in the expression of fibrinogen-binding sites on GpIIb–IIIa. These processes are also regulated by cyclic AMP, the production of which by adenylate cyclase is also under the control of G proteins. Raised cAMP concen-trations lower cytosolic free Ca^{2+} levels and inhibit aggrega-tion and secretion. Meanwhile, cyclic endoperoxides and thromboxane A_2 themselves bind to specific receptors on secretion, and stimulate further activation of these pathways, as do ADP and 5-HT secreted from the dense bodies.

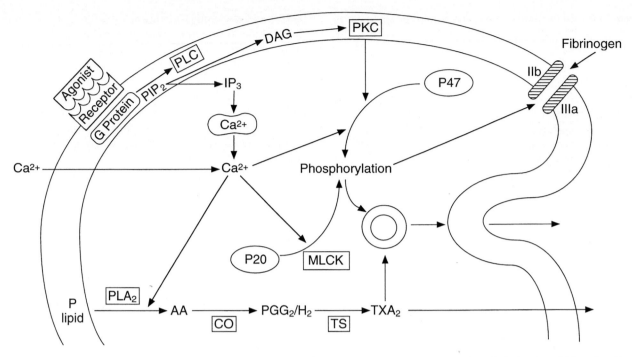

Fig. 24.2 Signal transduction mechanisms in the platelet. PIP_2 = phosphatidylinositol 4,5-bisphosphate; IP_3 = inositol 1, 4, 5-trisphosphate; DAG = diacylglycerol; PLC = phospholipase C; PKC = protein kinase C; P47 = pleckstrin; MLCK = myosin light chain kinase; P20 = myosin light chain; PLA_2 = phospholipase A_2; AA = arachidonic acid; CO = cyclo-oxygenase; TS = thromboxane synthetase.

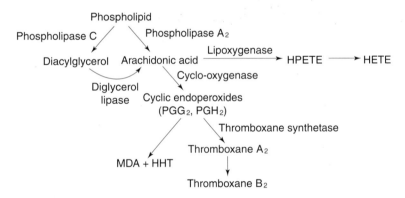

Fig. 24.3 Arachidonic acid metabolism in platelets. HPETE = 12-hydroperoxy-eicosatetraenoic acid; HETE = 12-hydroxy-eicosatetraenoic acid; MDA = malonyldialdehyde; HHT = 12-hydroxy-heptadecatrienoic acid.

Platelet procoagulant activity

Amongst the contents of platelet α-granules are several coagulation proteins—fibrinogen, factor V and high-molecular-weight kininogen (HMWK)—as well as a number of proteinase inhibitors; all of these may therefore reach high local concentrations when secreted from the platelets at sites of vascular injury. Probably the most important contribution of the platelets to blood coagulation, however, is in providing an active surface for the interaction of clotting factors. Much the most active phospholipid in this regard is phosphatidylserine. In the unstimulated platelet, most of this is situated in the inner leaflet of the membrane, but on stimulation by collagen and thrombin, a redistribution of the phospholipids in the bilayer occurs, resulting in

translocation of phosphatidylserine to the outer leaflet.[13] This change, which is associated with the formation of plasma membrane vesicles,[14] greatly increases the ability of the platelets to enhance the activation of Factor X and the conversion of prothrombin to thrombin, by providing binding sites for Factors VIIIa–IXa and Va-Xa complexes, respectively.[15] It is these activities of the platelets which were formerly loosely described as platelet factor 3.

PLATELET FUNCTION IN THE FETUS AND NEWBORN INFANT

Prolonged bleeding from puncture wounds has been noted in fetuses at about 20 weeks' gestation,[16] and studies of the platelets of a small number of fetuses at about this stage of development have shown profoundly defective aggregation, relative to adult platelets, in response to epinephrine (adrenaline) and collagen, and a lesser defect in response to ADP.[17] Although healthy newborn infants have normal bleeding times[18] and do not suffer from a bleeding tendency, their platelets have been shown to be functionally defective compared with adult platelets in a number of respects. They have usually been found to aggregate less completely in response to various agonists, including ADP, collagen and thrombin, but the aggregation defect is most marked in response to epinephrine,[19] apparently because newborn platelets lack α-adrenergic receptors.[20,21] The response to ristocetin, in contrast, appears to be enhanced relative to that of maternal platelets, perhaps because of a higher plasma concentration of VWF.[22] Neonatal platelets are also more sensitive than maternal platelets to the inhibitory effects of prostacyclin and nitric oxide on ADP-induced aggregation.[23]

Flow cytometry on small samples of cord and peripheral whole blood, using monoclonal antibodies to P-selectin and GpIIb–IIIa, showed no evidence of circulating degranulated platelets in neonates, but confirmed the diminished reactivity of neonatal platelets to thrombin, a combination of ADP and epinephrine, and a thromboxane analog.[24] Previous evidence of platelet degranulation[25,26] probably reflected *in vitro* artefacts due to the difficulty in obtaining clean platelet and plasma samples from cord blood.

Neonatal platelets appear to generate thromboxane A_2 and other arachidonic acid metabolites at least as effectively as do adult platelets,[27,28] and show enhanced release of arachidonate from membrane phospholipids on stimulation by thrombin.[29] No significant differences from adult platelets have been observed in respect of the platelet membrane glycoproteins IIb–IIIa or Ib, or the alloantigens Pl[A1] or Lek[a], in fetuses at 18–26 weeks' gestation,[30] and indeed the expression of both GpIb and GpIIIa has been shown to be within the adult range from as early as 8 weeks onwards.[31]

Such functional differences as have been observed between newborn and adult platelets are evidently of little clinical significance, since they do not of themselves cause an enhanced tendency to bleed. They may, however, lead to an increased susceptibility to additional hemostatic stresses, such as the maternal ingestion of aspirin prior to delivery.[32,33]

INHERITED DISORDERS OF PLATELET FUNCTION

These disorders are most conveniently classified according to the site and nature of the genetically determined defect (Table 24.3):

1. abnormalities affecting plasma membrane glycoproteins or phospholipids, and resulting in impairment of

Table 24.3 Inherited disorders of platelet function.

Defects of the plasma membrane
Glanzmann's thrombasthenia
Bernard–Soulier syndrome
Platelet-type von Willebrand disease
Glycoprotein Ia deficiency
Glycoprotein IV deficiency
Glycoprotein VI deficiency
Scott syndrome

Deficiency of storage organelles (storage pool deficiency)
δ-SPD (dense-body deficiency)
  Idiopathic (non-albino)
  Hermansky–Pudlak syndrome
  Chédiak–Higashi syndrome
  Wiskott–Aldrich syndrome
  Thrombocytopenia with absent radii
α-SPD (α-granule deficiency)
  Gray platelet syndrome
  Quebec platelet disorder
$\alpha\delta$-spdD (dense-body and α-granule deficiency)

Defects of thromboxane generation
Impaired liberation of arachidonic acid
Cyclo-oxygenase deficiency
Thromboxane synthetase deficiency

Defects in signal transduction
Defects of response to weak agonists
Defective response to thromboxane A_2
Defective response to epinephrine (adrenaline)

Miscellaneous disorders of uncertain pathogenesis
Giant platelet syndromes
  Montreal platelet syndrome
  May–Hegglin anomaly
  Epstein's syndrome, Fechtner's syndrome
  Sebastian platelet syndrome
Other disorders with normal platelet size

adhesion, aggregation or procoagulant activity of the platelets;
2. deficiency of specific intracellular organelles;
3. defects of thromboxane generation;
4. defects of the signal transduction mechanisms involved in secretion of granule contents.

A miscellaneous group of hereditary defects remains less well characterized with respect to their pathogenesis.

PLASMA MEMBRANE DISORDERS

Glycoprotein abnormalities

Glanzmann's thrombasthenia

Glanzmann[34] gave the first description of an hereditary disorder of platelet function, characterized by a long bleeding time and impaired clot retraction in the presence of a normal platelet count; he named it 'hereditary hemorrhagic thrombasthenia'. Nearly half a century later, the development of methods for measuring platelet aggregation led to the redefinition of Glanzmann's thrombasthenia (GT) as an autosomal recessive disorder of which the salient feature is a complete failure of the platelets to aggregate in response to ADP, collagen, thrombin or other agonists, although platelet adhesion to connective tissue occurs normally.[35–37] Subsequent investigations have shown that this functional abnormality is due to a deficiency or molecular defect of the GpIIb–IIIa complex in the plasma membrane of the platelet,[38–40] resulting in a failure of the platelets to bind fibrinogen—an essential step in the aggregation process.[11,41,42]

Clinical features. GT is an autosomal recessive disorder, rare in a global context but relatively more common in those communities where consanguineous marriages are frequent. It cannot be distinguished on clinical grounds alone from other congenital platelet disorders or severe von Willebrand disease (VWD). It commonly presents in infancy or early childhood with multiple bruises following minimal or unrecognized trauma, or with crops of petechiae or ecchymoses. George et al[43] reported the incidence and severity of bleeding symptoms in a series of 177 patients. Epistaxes are very common, and may be difficult to control with local measures, and may even be life-threatening; gingival hemorrhage is a frequent result of the shedding of deciduous teeth, or even tooth brushing, and is likely to lead to iron deficiency. Large muscle hematomata and hemarthroses seldom occur, but menorrhagia is virtually inevitable and may present a serious hazard in pubertal girls. Serious accidental and surgical trauma will be life-threatening and will certainly call for intensive replacement therapy with platelet concentrates. In the absence of major trauma, the overall severity may appear to diminish as years of discretion are attained. Although the failure of platelet aggregation *in vitro* is always virtually complete, the clinical severity correlates poorly with the nature and degree of the molecular abnormality, with even siblings sometimes being very differently affected.[43]

Laboratory diagnosis. The essential diagnostic features are a normal platelet count and morphology and a greatly prolonged bleeding time, associated with a complete failure of platelet aggregation in response to ADP at any concentration. The aggregation defect is also seen in response to epinephrine, collagen, thrombin and, indeed, to all other aggregating agents which ultimately depend on fibrinogen binding to the platelet for their effect. These include arachidonic acid, thromboxane A_2 and its synthetic analogs, calcium ionophores and platelet-activating factor (PAF-acether). Agglutination occurs normally, however, in response to ristocetin or bovine VWF, which act through the binding of VWF to platelet GpIb.

Having demonstrated the aggregation defect, the diagnosis can be confirmed—and in the case of unusual variants, extended—by measuring the amounts of GpIIb and IIIa in the platelet surface membrane. The methods available for this include 1- and 2-dimensional polyacrylamide gel electrophoresis, crossed immunoelectrophoresis using specific antibodies, and binding assays or flow cytometry with monoclonal antibodies to the constituent glycoproteins. The last of these has the advantage of being simply performed on very small volumes of whole blood,[44,45] making it particularly appropriate for prenatal diagnosis (see below) or the investigation of small children. Fibrinogen binding can also be measured by flow cytometry on microliter volumes of whole blood,[46] and this method can be useful for primary diagnosis of GT if sufficient blood cannot be obtained for platelet aggregation studies.

Clot retraction, platelet fibrinogen and platelet factor 3 availability are all defective in GT, but contribute no more to the diagnosis when the defective aggregation or fibrinogen binding has been demonstrated. Thrombasthenic platelets secrete their granule contents normally in response to strong agonists such as thrombin or high concentrations of collagen, but not in response to ADP or epinephrine, which depend on aggregation for their secretory effect.

Molecular heterogeneity. Although, by definition, all patients with GT have a virtually complete failure of platelet aggregation, the underlying biochemical abnormality varies between kindreds. Caen[47] was the first to draw attention to a functional heterogeneity between cases, and proposed classifying GT into types I and II: type I patients, who were clinically more severely affected, had absent clot retraction and greatly reduced platelet fibrinogen, while in the rarer type II, clot retraction and platelet fibrinogen were only slightly diminished, although aggregation was equally defective. Since the recognition of the GpIIb–IIIa deficiency, it has been shown that type I results from a severe deficiency of the complex ($<5\%$) and type II from a relatively mild deficiency (5–20%). In addition to these deficiency states, a number of variant forms of GT have been described (sometimes designated type III), in which the glycoproteins are present in normal or near-normal amount (50–100% of normal), but are functionally defective.

The genes for both glycoproteins IIb and IIIa are contained within a single 260 kb segment in the q21–23 band on chromosome 17.[48] Although human umbilical vein endothelial cells also synthesize GpIIb–IIIa,[49,50] this is evidently under separate genetic control from that synthesized in the megakaryocyte, since endothelial cells from the umbilical cord of an infant with GT were found to express the complex normally.[51] That deficiencies of the GpIIb–IIIa complex may result from genetically determined defects of either of the constituent glycoproteins was first clearly shown by Coller et al[52] in GT patients in Israel: they found that patients of Iraqi–Jewish origin had no demonstrable major GpIIIa band on immunoblots of their solubilized platelets, while Arab patients' platelets had clearly detectable amounts of this protein. Subsequent work[53] has shown that the abnormality in Arab patients results from a 13 base-pair deletion in the GpIIb α-chain gene, and that in Iraqi-

Jewish patients from an 11 base-pair deletion in the GpIIIa gene. The genetic basis for the disease has subsequently been established in many other families, and it is clear that various defects in either the GpIIb or the GpIIIa gene can give rise to the thrombasthenia phenotype. Of 14 mutant alleles resulting in type I GT reported in the literature up to 1994, 6 involved the GpIIIa gene and 8 the gene for GpIIb: most had point mutations, but 2 were due to larger gene rearrangements.[54]

Of the variant (type III) forms of GT, all those so far investigated have point mutations in the GpIIIa gene, resulting in amino acid substitutions. The first such variant, designated the Cam variant, was described in a family from Guam, of which the platelets of 2 members had near-normal amounts of GpIIb–IIIa but greatly defective binding of fibrinogen or other RGD-containing ligands.[55,56] This defect was shown to involve the substitution of Asp[119] by Tyr in GpIIIa. Further variants are frequently being described and most appear to involve amino acid substitutions either in the fibrinogen binding region of GpIIIa or in the region concerned with GpIIb–IIIa assembly or expression on the cell surface. It has been suggested that missense mutations in the GpIIb gene may prove to cause type I GT, while missense mutations in the GpIIIa gene cause type III GT.[54]

Detection of heterozygotes. Heterozygotes for GT usually have no significant bleeding symptoms, and no demonstrable defect of platelet aggregation. Characteristically, however, their platelets express about half the normal number of GpIIb–IIIa complexes in the plasma membrane, and have a corresponding partial defect of fibrinogen binding. This provides a means of carrier detection, using a variety of methods for quantitative GpIIb–IIIa determination[45,57–59] or fibrinogen binding.[46] Coller et al[59] found good agreement betwen the results of monoclonal antibody binding, polyacrylamide gel electrophoresis and electroimmunoassay methods in a large series of obligatory carriers, who had about 60% of normal GpIIb–IIIa by all 3 methods. None of these methods is completely reliable, but in kindreds in which the precise genetic defect has been identified, unequivocal carrier detection can be provided using DNA probes specific for the abnormal DNA sequence, or the detection of deletions by polymerase chain reaction analysis.[53,60] The latter method can be carried out on DNA recovered from cells in routine urine samples.

Prenatal diagnosis. Since platelet GpIIb–IIIa has reached adult levels by 18 weeks of gestation, its expression and functional integrity can be determined on fetal blood samples. Seligsohn et al[61] measured GpIIb–IIIa in such samples by a monoclonal antibody binding assay, and Kaplan et al[62] by the somewhat less direct method of Pl[A1] typing. These methods are applicable to families with the classical form of the disease, characterized by GpIIb–

IIIa deficiency, and can even detect the heterozygous state in utero,[63] but are less appropriate for the prenatal diagnosis of GT variants with molecular defects of the glycoprotein complex. In such cases, prenatal blood testing depends on the demonstration of a defect of aggregation[64] or fibrinogen binding; micromethods for the latter[46] are particularly appropriate. When the molecular genetic abnormality is known, diagnosis can be performed at 8–10 weeks' gestation by chorionic villus sampling and the use of appropriate DNA probes.

The experience of Champeix et al[64] and Seligsohn et al[65] shows that fetal sampling for the prenatal diagnosis of GT carries a high risk to the affected fetus of death from continuing hemorrhage. This underlines the importance of detailed counselling of the parents before the procedure is undertaken: it is clearly contraindicated if the parents wish the pregnancy to continue even if the fetus is affected.

Treatment. The only available curative treatment for GT is bone marrow transplantation (BMT), which has been successfully performed in a number of patients.[66,67] The risks of this procedure, however, are such as to confine its use to cases in which severe bleeding cannot be adequately controlled by more conservative measures. Gene therapy remains a more distant prospect in this, as in other, serious genetic disorders. Meanwhile, the management of GT consists of the avoidance of trauma and drugs, such as aspirin, which may further interfere with platelet function, and the treatment of major bleeding episodes by platelet transfusion. Minor bleeding from accessible sites, such as deciduous tooth sockets, can usually be controlled by local measures, although epistaxis may continue despite packing and require platelet transfusion in addition. The use of antifibrinolytic agents, such as tranexamic acid, may help to control bleeding after dental extractions, but has no other place in treatment. Nor has desmopressin (DDAVP), despite its occasional slight shortening of the bleeding time. Good dental care is obviously essential if gum bleeding is to be minimized and tooth extraction avoided, as also is the management of iron deficiency. Menorrhagia is likely to be a problem from the time of the first period, and may require hormonal therapy for its control.[43] Prepubertal counseling is important in this regard.

The chief limiting factor in the replacement therapy of GT is the risk of development of platelet antibodies. These may be directed against one or more of the platelet-specific alloantigens expressed on the GpIIb–IIIa complex (Pl[A1], Bak[a], Pen[a]) but probably arise more commonly against HLA determinants. For this reason, HLA-matched platelets, preferably from a single donor, should be used whenever possible. There is evidence that leukocyte depletion of platelet and red cell concentrates by filtration may reduce the likelihood of alloimmunization as well as of febrile transfusion reactions, and this procedure is therefore also to be recommended.[68]

471

Bernard–Soulier syndrome

Bernard and Soulier[69] described a severe hereditary bleeding disorder characterized by a long bleeding time, moderate thrombocytopenia with giant and morphologically abnormal platelets, normal clot retraction but defective prothrombin consumption. Subsequent investigation of similar cases showed that their platelets aggregated normally with ADP, epinephrine and collagen,[70,71] but were not agglutinated by bovine VWF,[72] or ristocetin.[70] In contrast to VWD, in which the defective response to ristocetin is due to deficiency of the plasma VWF, in Bernard–Soulier syndrome (BSS) it is the platelet membrane which is defective, lacking receptors for VWF.

Gröttum and Solum[73] had previously postulated a membrane abnormality in BSS platelets, which they found to have a reduced sialic acid content, and this was confirmed by Nurden and Caen,[74] who demonstrated a specific deficiency of the sialic acid-rich glycoprotein I complex in the platelet membrane. This deficiency is now known to involve components of the GpIb–IX complex, of which the individual subunits (GpIb α and β chains and GpIX) are members of the 'leucine-rich family' of glycoproteins.[75,76] The complex, which is non-covalently linked to another leucine-rich glycoprotein, GpV,[77] carries a binding site for VWF on the outermost extracellular portion of the GpIbα subunit. This is induced *in vitro* by ristocetin, and binds *in vivo* to VWF which has undergone a conformational change as a result of its prior binding to the vascular subendothelium.[78] This platelet-VWF-subendothelium interaction is an essential step in the initial adhesion of platelets to damaged blood vessels, particularly at the shear rates which obtain in small arteries and capillaries, and it is the failure of this initial step in platelet plug formation which accounts for the bleeding tendency of BSS.[7,79]

The thrombocytopenia of BSS is chiefly due to a shortened platelet life-span, which may be an end result of the deficiency of the sialic acid-rich glycoprotein. Other abnormalities which have been described include disordered phospholipid organization in the platelet membrane,[80] a failure of the platelets to bind and activate Factor XI on stimulation by collagen,[81] and a high basal prothrombinase activity in unstimulated platelets.[82] The partial defect of thrombin binding and aggregation reported by Jamieson and Okumura[83] suggested that the GpIb–IX complex carries a thrombin receptor, and this has subsequently been confirmed, and shown to be distinct from the VWF receptor.[84] The binding site for quinine/quinidine drug-dependent antibodies has also been shown to be lacking on BSS platelets;[85] it has been localized within the membrane-associated region of the GpIb–IX complex,[86] and more specifically to GpV.[87] The Pl[E1] alloantigen is also lacking in BSS platelets, and has been localized to the α subunit of GpIb.[88] The abnormally deformable membrane of BSS platelets[89] is evidently also related to the GpIb–IX deficiency, since this complex plays

an important part in linking the plasma membrane to the cytoskeleton of the platelet.[90]

Clinical features. BSS is an extremely rare autosomal recessive disorder; fewer than 100 published cases, many of them consanguineous, meet the full diagnostic criteria. It is clinically indistinguishable from Glanzmann's thrombasthenia (see above) and, like it, usually presents early in life with multiple bruises and ecchymoses, and bleeding from mucous membranes and superficial grazes and cuts. Epistaxes and menorrhagia are amongst the commonest symptoms, and can present difficult problems in management. Several children have died from uncontrollable bleeding, and the original patient of Bernard and Soulier, who presented with epistaxis and anal hemorrhage at the age of 15 days, had numerous bleeding episodes during his first 7 years, after which hemorrhage occurred less frequently and usually after injury; he died at the age of 28 from a cerebral hemorrhage following a bar-room brawl.[91] As in Glanzmann's thrombasthenia, clinical severity may vary widely between affected family members.

Laboratory diagnosis. The platelet count in BSS is usually only moderately reduced (commonly 50–100 $\times 10^9/l$), but the bleeding time is very prolonged. The giant platelets may not be recognized as such by electronic cell counters, leading to spuriously low counts, but their presence in the blood film will suggest the diagnosis. It is difficult to prepare platelet-rich plasma for aggregation and other tests, since the large dense platelets tend to sediment with the red and white cells. The failure to agglutinate in response to ristocetin (even in the presence of normal plasma or VWF), together with the normal or even increased aggregation response to ADP, epinephrine and collagen, and the demonstration of normal VWF in the patient's plasma, further establishes the diagnosis, which can be confirmed by demonstrating the deficiency of GpIb–IX complex in the platelet membrane. As for GpIIb–IIIa in thrombasthenia, this can be achieved by biochemical methods such as polyacrylamide gel electrophoresis, or by the use of specific monoclonal antibodies for flow cytometric or immunochemical tests.

Molecular genetics. Assembly of all 3 subunits of the GpIb–IX complex is required for optimum expression in the plasma membrane,[92] and point mutations in both the GpIbα and GpIX genes have been found to give rise to the BSS phenotype.[93-95] The first of these variants[93] is characterized by the heterozygous substitution of Leu[57] with Phe in the leucine-rich repeat area of GpIbα, and an unusual dominant inheritance; the second,[94] termed the Bolzano variant, is homozygous for an Ala[156]→Val substitution, resulting in a failure to bind VWF in the presence of ristocetin, but a normal thrombin-binding capacity.

Detection of heterozygotes and prenatal diagnosis. George et al[96] studied 2 families with BSS and found that the heterozygous parents, who were asymptomatic, had normal bleeding times, platelet counts and ristocetin-induced agglutination; 3 of them, however, had abnormally large platelets, with reduced GpIb and decreased sensitivity to a quinidine-dependent antibody. Quantitation of the GpIb–IX complex in small volumes of whole blood by means of monoclonal antibodies and flow cytometry provides the most suitable method for detecting heterozygotes and for prenatal diagnosis, but insufficient families have been studied to establish quantitative criteria. It is to be expected that prenatal blood sampling will carry a high risk to the affected fetus, as in the case of Glanzmann's thrombasthenia (see above). In those few cases in which the genetic defect has been identified, early prenatal diagnosis by chorionic villus sampling may be feasible.

Treatment. The general principles of treatment are the same as for Glanzmann's thrombasthenia: avoidance of injury and potentially harmful drugs, careful local hemostatic measures, platelet transfusions (preferably HLA-matched) for major bleeding episodes and hormonal control of menorrhagia if necessary. Treatment as for other thrombocytopenic conditions, such as steroids, intravenous immunoglobulin (IVIG) and splenectomy, is in general contraindicated, underlining the need for accurate diagnosis. IVIG and plasmapheresis have both been used, however, in patients who have become refractory to platelet transfusions.

Platelet-type von Willebrand disease

This is an autosomal dominant bleeding disorder characterized by mild thrombocytopenia, a deficiency of the higher molecular weight multimers of VWF in the plasma, and increased ristocetin-induced platelet agglutination, first described under this name by Miller and Castella[97] and as 'pseudo-von Willebrand's disease' by Weiss et al.[98] The platelet VWF has a normal multimeric structure, and the essential abnormality appears to be an enhanced affinity of the platelet membrane GpIb–IX for high-molecular-weight VWF multimers, which are selectively bound to the platelets from the plasma. This is therefore the functional opposite of Bernard–Soulier syndrome. Two distinct point mutations have been identified in such patients, both resulting in amino acid substitutions ($Gly^{233} \rightarrow Val$ and $Met^{239} \rightarrow Val$) in the VWF binding domain of GPIbα.[99,100]

Reported cases have varied from clinically mild to severe. Most have had moderately prolonged bleeding times and a degree of thrombocytopenia, perhaps due to platelet aggregation *in vivo*, and some have had an increased platelet volume. Platelet agglutination by low-dose ristocetin is increased, and indeed the patient's platelets are usually agglutinated by the addition of normal plasma or VWF in the absence of ristocetin. The distinction from type 2B VWD depends on the demonstration of binding of normal VWF to isolated platelets: lower concentrations of ristocetin are required for binding to platelets from patients with platelet-type VWD than to either normal platelets or those from patients with type 2B VWD. Treatment with desmopressin is contraindicated in both these conditions, since the large VWF multimers released into the plasma are quickly bound to the platelets and induce further thrombocytopenia by aggravating their *in vivo* aggregation. Careful use of low-dose cryoprecipitate has sometimes supported hemostasis adequately,[101] but platelet concentrates would seem to be the replacement therapy of choice in platelet-type VWD.

Glycoprotein Ia deficiency

Nieuwenhuis et al[102] reported the case of a young woman who had suffered from easy bruising and menorrhagia since her teens, with a constantly prolonged bleeding time, whose platelets failed to respond by aggregation, secretion or thromboxane synthesis to collagen (although they responded normally to other agonists), or to adhere to purified type I or type III collagen or subendothelial microfibrils. They found that her platelet membranes were deficient in glycoprotein Ia, which together with GpIIa forms the integrin $\alpha_2\beta_1$ (VLA-2),[3] an important collagen receptor. Although no corresponding abnormality could be found in the platelets of this patient's parents, sister or son, the defect seems likely to have been genetically determined. A similar patient has subsequently been described with a lifelong bleeding tendency and a decreased reaction with collagen, in whom GpIa deficiency was associated with a lack of platelet thrombospondin.[103] The symptoms and platelet defect disappeared at the time of the menopause, perhaps suggesting that they were related to hormonal influences.

Abnormalities of glycoproteins IV and VI

Both of these glycoproteins have been implicated as collagen receptors, and deficiency of each has been recorded. GpIV (CD36) carries the Nak[a] alloantigen, and is undetectable in Nak[a-] individuals,[104] who make up 3–11% of the Japanese donor population, but only about 0.3% of the population of the US. The deficiency does not result in a bleeding tendency, however; Nak[a-] donors are asymptomatic. Deficiency of GpVI (p62), on the other hand, has been found in association with defective collagen-induced adhesion and aggregation in 2 Japanese patients with mild bleeding tendencies.[105,106] In the first of these, whose symptoms were life-long, both parents' platelets reacted normally with collagen, but expressed about half the normal amount of GpVI, suggesting autosomal recessive heredity.

Abnormalities of platelet coagulant activity

Scott syndrome

Weiss et al[107] reported the case of a woman (Mrs Scott) who had suffered from a moderately severe bleeding disorder since her teens, and whose only demonstrable abnormality was a defect of platelet procoagulant activity. The bleeding time was consistently normal, as were platelet aggregation and secretion. The abnormality appeared to consist of a failure to express binding sites for Factors Va and Xa on the platelet membrane,[108] as a result of a defect in the mechanism by which phosphatidyl serine becomes exposed on the outer leaflet of the membrane on activation of the platelets.[109] This was associated with a failure to generate platelet microparticles on activation with various agonists,[110] and a similar defect of microparticle formation from red cells on stimulation with the Ca^{2+} ionophore A23187.[111] There was no family history, nor any detectable defect in the patient's parents' platelets, so that the hereditary nature of the defect remained in doubt. A second family has recently been described,[112] however, in which the proposita had a severe defect of phospholipid externalization, and 2 of her children a partial defect, suggesting heterozygosity for an autosomal recessive gene. The bleeding symptoms resemble those of a plasma coagulation disorder rather than a platelet defect, but surgical hemostasis has been achieved by means of platelet transfusion.

Quebec platelet disorder

Tracy et al[113] described an autosomal dominant bleeding disorder in 5 generations of a French-Canadian family, characterized by moderate to severe post-traumatic hemorrhage from birth, and by mild thrombocytopenia and a severe deficiency of platelet Factor V in the presence of only mild deficiency of plasma Factor V. Subsequent investigations on members of the same family[114] showed that their platelets were deficient in multimerin, a large multimeric protein to which platelet Factor V is normally complexed within the α-granules.[115] Although the multimerin deficiency was evidently not due to proteolysis, there was evidence of proteolytic degradation of 3 other α-granule proteins—thrombospondin, VWF and fibrinogen—as well as defective aggregation in response to epinephrine, despite normal α_2-adrenergic receptors. The pathogenic relationship between these multiple abnormalities, and their relative contribution to the bleeding tendency, remain unclear. This disorder is considered here as an abnormality of platelet coagulant activity, but should probably be more appropriately classed, together with the gray platelet syndrome, as one primarily involving α-granule proteins. None of platelets, fresh frozen plasma and cryoprecipitate has proven effective as replacement therapy.

INTRACELLULAR DISORDERS

All the conditions considered under this heading (Table 24.3) result in a failure of secretion of granule contents on stimulation of the platelets. They may be divided into those in which the dense bodies and/or α-granules themselves are deficient or defective (storage pool deficiency) and those in which these storage organelles are normally present but the secretory mechanisms are at fault. The latter group comprises defects of thromboxane generation and of the other signal transduction mechanisms leading to secretion and aggregation. Disorders of platelet secretion most commonly result from the ingestion of aspirin and other non-steroidal anti-inflammatory drugs, and are also seen in various acquired diseases (see below), but here refers only to hereditable disorders. Most of these usually result in relatively mild bleeding states, less severe than the membrane disorders described above, and clinical presentation and diagnosis are therefore often delayed until later in childhood or even until adult life. Common presenting symptoms include easy bruising and somewhat prolonged bleeding from superficial cuts, epistaxes and menorrhagia. Apart from the risks of excessive hemorrhage following major surgical or accidental trauma, most patients are not seriously incommoded by their disorder.

Storage pool deficiency

This term was first applied to deficiency of the osmiophilic dense bodies of the platelet, the site of the storage pool of adenine nucleotides and of 5-HT (serotonin). Following the suggestion of Weiss et al,[116] its use has been extended to include deficiency of the α-granules: pure dense-body deficiency is designated δ-storage pool deficiency (SPD), pure deficiency of α-granules (gray platelet syndrome) α-SPD, and the combined deficiency of both types of organelle, αδ-SPD.

Dense-body deficiency

Laboratory diagnosis. The definitive diagnosis of δ-SPD depends on direct demonstration of the dense-body deficiency, whether biochemically, morphologically or both. The bleeding time is usually moderately prolonged, and the aggregation pattern commonly reflects the defect of secretion, although it will not clearly distinguish dense-body deficiency from other secretory disorders. The typical features are normal primary aggregation in response to ADP and epinephrine, but without a second wave, a marked defect of aggregation and ATP secretion in response to collagen, and a normal response to arachidonic acid, which serves to exclude a defect of thromboxane generation.[117,118] This typical pattern, however, may not be seen in milder cases: Nieuwenhuis et al[119] studied over 100 patients with long bleeding times and a deficiency of total platelet ADP and 5-HT, of which about

(A)

(B)

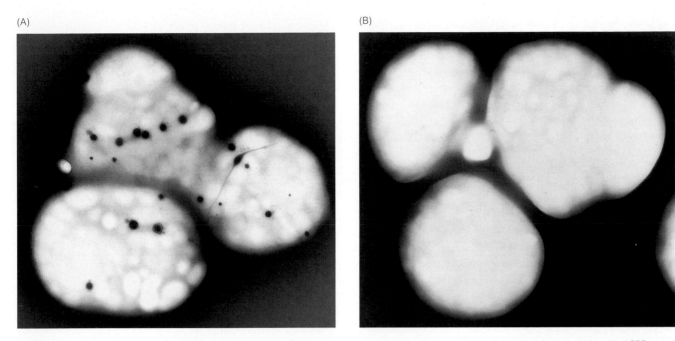

Fig. 24.4 Unstained whole mount preparations of (A) normal platelets, showing several dense bodies per cell; and (B) platelets from a patient with d-SPD (Hermansky–Pudlak syndrome), showing no dense bodies. Kindly supplied by James G White.

half were congenital in origin, and found that about a quarter had a normal aggregation pattern with ADP, epinephine and collagen, while only one-third showed a pattern completely typical of a secretory defect. The hallmarks of δ-SPD, therefore, are the actual deficiency of the dense bodies and their contents.

Dense bodies can be enumerated in platelets either by electron microscopy (Fig. 24.4) or by fluorescence microscopy after incubation with the fluorescent dye mepacrine, which is taken up and localized in the dense bodies.[120] A simple flow cytometric method for studying mepacrine uptake has also been described.[121] Biochemical evidence of dense-body deficiency depends on measurement of the platelet content of adenine nucleotides and 5-HT and their uptake and secretion. The storage pool of nucleotides in the dense bodies (which is largely deficient in δ-SPD) has an ATP:ADP ratio of about 2:3, while that of the metabolic pool in the cytosol is about 8:1.[122] In δ-SPD, therefore, the ATP:ADP ratio of whole platelets (normally 1.5–2.5:1) is much increased, approximating to that of the metabolic pool alone of normal platelets.[123] The defective secretion of adenine nucleotides is best demonstrated by lumiaggregometry after thrombin activation.

Gerrard et al[124] raised a monoclonal antibody to a dense-body membrane constituent, which they called *granulophysin*, and used it to show that the platelets of a patient with the Hermansky–Pudlak syndrome (see below) were profoundly deficient in this protein. Although it has subsequently been shown that granulophysin is not specific to the dense-body membrane, being identical with the protein CD63, a constituent of the membranes of lysosomes and melanocytes,[125]

it provides a useful further diagnostic and investigational approach in δ-SPD. Various immunologic methods are available for its measurement, including immunofluorescence, an ELISA method on whole platelets, and flow cytometry after activation of the platelets to translocate the protein to the plasma membrane.

Clinical associations. Dense-body deficiency has been observed in a number of families as an isolated platelet defect, and also occurs as an integral part of two well defined syndromes in association with albinism and lysosomal abnormalities: Hermansky–Pudlak and Chédiak–Higashi syndromes. The *non-albino group* (idiopathic δ-SPD) shows considerable heterogeneity with respect to both heredity and the degree of dense-body deficiency, and is usually more mildly affected than the albino patients. While in several families the isolated defect appears to be transmitted as an autosomal dominant trait,[117,125,126] others exhibit recessive heredity.[128] In contrast to the albino patients, whose platelets are profoundly deficient in both dense-body membranes and contents, the idiopathic non-albino group shows various degrees of dissociation between these 2 features. An extreme degree of such dissociation has been described in 2 sisters as the *empty sack syndrome*, in which deficiency of 5-HT and adenine nucleotides was associated with essentially normal amounts of dense-body membranes, as measured by their granulophysin content.[128] In at least some of these non-albino cases, therefore, the defect appears to be one of targeting of granule contents rather than of dense body formation.

Hermansky–Pudlak syndrome is an autosomal recessive disorder characterized by the triad of tyrosinase-positive oculocutaneous albinism, a life-long moderate bleeding tendency and the presence of ceroid-like pigment in cells of the reticuloendothelial system.[129] The pigment was first observed in bone marrow macrophages, but may also be deposited in the lungs and intestine—when it leads to pulmonary fibrosis and inflammatory bowel disease[130,131]—as well as in the buccal mucosa and urinary bladder. The bleeding tendency is primarily attributable to the deficiency of platelet dense bodies,[123,132] although defects of phospholipase activation have also been observed.[139,140] The dense-body deficiency is more severe than in the non-albino patients, and affects both membranes and contents,[135,136] suggesting that the defect is a structural one, involving dense-body formation in the megakaryocyte. Heterozygotes are clinically unaffected, and their platelets have been found to contain normal amounts of adenine nucleotides and to aggregate normally. Gerritsen *et al*,[137] however, found that heterozygotes in a large Dutch family had platelet 5-HT contents intermediate between homozygotes and normal controls.

Chédiak–Higashi syndrome, an autosomal recessive disorder of lysosome formation in neutrophils and other cells, is more fully described in Chapter 16. Thrombocytopenia is common and is the chief cause of the bleeding tendency, but dense-body deficiency is also characteristic.[138–141] As in the Hermansky–Pudlak syndrome, granulophysin is deficient, indicating a defect of dense-body membrane formation. Like the neutrophils, the platelets also contain large abnormal granules.[142,143]

Wiskott–Aldrich syndrome is an X-borne recessive disorder and is fully described in Chapter 25; the thrombocytopenia, which is the chief cause of the bleeding tendency, is discussed in Chapter 21. It is mentioned here only because the various structural and functional platelet defects which have also been described include dense-body deficiency.[144,145] The platelets are smaller than normal[146,147] and have also been found to have defects of mitochondrial ATP synthesis,[148] and sometimes of membrane glycoproteins,[149] although this is evidently not a constant feature.[150]

While the hemorrhagic tendency of the congenital disorder *thrombocytopenia with absent radii* (TAR syndrome) (see Chapter 21) is fully explained by the thrombocytopenia, storage pool deficiency has also been observed.[151]

Combined deficiency

Weiss and his colleagues[116,152] have shown that a proportion of patients with the non-albino variety of hereditary dense-body deficiency also have various degrees of α-granule deficiency: they use the term αδ-SPD to denote the combined defect. One such patient had severe α-granule deficiency, with deficiency of the α-granule membrane protein P-selectin, while another kindred had only a slight reduction in α-granules and normal amounts of P-selectin.[152] The clinical severity does not appear to be significantly greater in patients with the combined deficiency than in those with pure δ-SPD.

An apparent association with acute myeloid leukemia (AML) has been reported in 2 families with SPD: 2 affected members of the family with mild αδ-SPD had leukemia,[152] while a large family with apparent δ-SPD (in whom α-granules were not studied) included 7 patients with myeloid leukemias, of whom at least 4 had a pre-existing platelet disorder.[153] It seems possible that both these families were expressing defects in a proto-oncogene that regulates the maturation of both granulocytes and megakaryocytes.

α-Granule deficiency (gray platelet syndrome) (see also Chapter 21)

Unlike dense-body deficiency, a pure deficiency of α-granules occurs in only a single hereditary disorder, described by Raccuglia[154] as the gray platelet syndrome, from the appearance of the agranular platelets on a stained blood film. This extremely rare hereditary platelet disorder, which shows autosomal dominant heredity in some reported families,[155,156] is sometimes surprisingly mild clinically, considering the profound nature of the structural and biochemical platelet defect. Epistaxes, menorrhagia and prolonged bleeding after serious injury are the commonest symptoms.

Laboratory findings. The bleeding time is usually moderately prolonged, and unlike most other defects of platelet function, the first diagnostic clue comes from examination of the blood film, which reveals the characteristic gray agranular platelets. The platelet count is usually slightly below normal and the mean platelet volume increased. The profound α-granule deficiency can be confirmed by electron microscopy (Fig. 24.5),

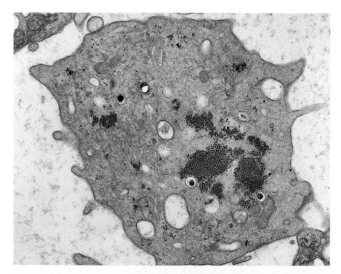

Fig. 24.5 Thin section of a platelet from a patient with gray platelet syndrome, showing dense bodies, mitochondria, glycogen granules and dilated vacuoles, but no α-granules. Kindly supplied by James G White.

which also shows normal numbers of dense bodies and mitochondria[157,158] and numerous large vesicles (Plate 33); the latter probably represent both abortive α-granules and elements of the open canalicular system. Small abnormal granules may also be seen, recognizable as α-granule precursors by their content of fibrinogen and VWF,[159] and also by the specific proteins, including P-selectin, in their membranes.

Gray platelets have been shown to be profoundly deficient in many of the proteins normally contained in α-granules, including β-thromboglobulin (β-TG), platelet Factor 4 (PF4), thrombospondin, platelet-derived growth factor (PDGF), VWF and Factor V,[158,160,161] all of which are synthesized within the megakaryocyte. The defect is one of packaging of these endogenous proteins within the organelles rather than of protein synthesis, as shown by normal or even slightly raised levels of β-TG and PF4 in the plasma. It has been suggested that this failure of packaging may lead to the premature release of PDGF and PF4 from the megakaryocyte, and so account for the myelofibrosis which is seen in some of these patients,[162,163] and perhaps for the pulmonary fibrosis which has also been described.[164] The failure of packaging does not extend, however, to the plasma proteins, including fibrinogen, fibronectin, immunoglobulins and albumin, which are taken up essentially normally into the α-granule precursors.

Gray platelets typically show a partial defect of aggregation and dense-body secretion, particularly in response to thrombin and collagen. This appears to be due to a defect of phosphoinositide hydrolysis and cytosolic calcium transport,[165,166] associated with an increased rate of transport of calcium into membrane vesicles;[167] this in turn may be related to an abnormality of the monomeric GTP-binding protein Rap-1, which is normally expressed in intracellular membranes from gray platelets, but abnormally phosphorylated by cAMP.[168]

Gray platelet syndrome has not yet been diagnosed prenatally, but Wautier and Gruel[63] were able to exclude the condition in the 19-week fetus of a woman with gray platelet syndrome by demonstrating normal platelet β-TG content and ultrastructure.

Defects of thromboxane generation

Aspirin ingestion is the commonest cause of defective thromboxane generation, and other drugs and even foods may have a similar effect. In a few cases, however, such abnormalities appear to have been congenital in origin, and some have shown a familial incidence. The characteristic laboratory features are an absence of the second wave of aggregation in response to ADP or epinephrine, and severe impairment of aggregation and dense body secretion in response to collagen, despite evidence of normal platelet nucleotides and 5-HT.

Impaired liberation of arachidonic acid

Rao et al[169] studied 3 patients with a life-long bleeding history, and the asymptomatic father of 1 of them; all had defective platelet aggregation in response to ADP, epinephrine and collagen, but a normal response to arachidonic acid and normal platelet ATP and ADP content. Liberation of ^{3}H-arachidonic acid from labeled platelet membrane phospholipids in response to thrombin was severely impaired. Subsequent investigation showed a defect of Ca^{2+} mobilization in 1 of the patients, suggesting that the impaired arachidonate liberation was secondary to reduced activation of the calcium-dependent phospholipase A_2.[170]

Impaired liberation of arachidonic acid has also been reported in several patients with storage pool deficiency,[117,133,134] and in a patient with inherited thrombocytopenia and giant platelets.[171]

Cyclo-oxygenase deficiency

It is to naturally-occurring deficiency of platelet cyclo-oxygenase that the term 'aspirin-like defect' ought properly to be confined. The distinction from the drug-induced defect may be somewhat easier to achieve in children than in adults, depending as it does on exclusion of drug ingestion and a life-long history of bleeding symptoms. The best evidence that the defect is genetically determined will be its demonstration in other family members; most reported cases have had negative family histories, but Horellou et al[172] observed the defect in a mother and 2 of her children, suggesting autosomal dominant inheritance. This family was unusual in the severity of the bleeding symptoms, which included hemarthroses.

The characteristic laboratory findings, in addition to those described above, are defective aggregation and secretion in response to arachidonic acid, but a normal response to exogenous prostaglandin G_2, thromboxane A_2 or their synthetic analogs.[173–175] In some patients,[176] normal levels of cyclo-oxygenase have been found by radioimmunoassay, suggesting a functional defect of the enzyme rather than an absolute deficiency.

Most patients with congenital cyclo-oxygenase deficiency suffer no more severe bleeding symptoms than subjects on regular aspirin therapy. This may be because PGI_2 generation in vascular endothelial cells is also impaired, as shown by Pareti et al[175] in their patient.

Thromboxane synthetase deficiency

Mestel et al[177] and Defreyn et al[178] have both described families in which a moderately severe life-long bleeding tendency was shown to be due to a defect of thromboxane formation from arachidonic acid or from cyclic endoperoxides. The condition can be distinguished from cyclo-oxygenase deficiency by the failure of the platelets to aggregate in response to the cyclic endoperoxides PGG_2 and PGH_2, or their synthetic analogs, as well as to arachidonic acid. The patient of Mestel et al[177] was a 3-year-old girl whose father and 2 siblings were similarly but less severely affected, suggesting an autosomal recessive mode of inheritance. In the family reported by Defreyn et al,[178] the degree of the defect appeared to be similar in a young woman and her father and daughter, making dominant inheritance more likely.

Defects in signal transduction

A miscellaneous group of life-long bleeding tendencies has been found to be associated with primary defects of platelet secretion, due neither to deficiency of organelles nor to defects of thromboxane synthesis, but purely to abnormalities of the secretory mechanisms themselves. These defects, which probably make up the majority of platelet secretion disorders, are usually associated with fairly mild bleeding symptoms, with or without a long bleeding time. The defect is often observed only in response to 'weak' agonists, including ADP, epinephrine and low concentrations of collagen, which induce secretion only as a result of aggregation, responses to strong agonists, such as thrombin and higher concentrations of collagen, being normal. Lages and Weiss[179] found that the initial rate of aggregation, as well as secretion, was impaired in 8 such patients, and coined the designation *'weak agonist response defects' (WARD)* for this heterogeneous group of disorders. It is likely that abnormalities of this type reflect various defects in signal transduction mechanisms within the platelet, and indeed several such defects have been identified. These are of course not mutually exclusive, including as they do defects of phosphatidyl inositide metabolism,[180] calcium mobilization[181] and phosphorylation of pleckstrin (P47),[182] all detected in separate studies on the same patient. Similarly, a mother and son in whom an abnormality of calcium influx and mobilization had been identified[183,184] were subsequently shown to have impaired activation of phospholipase C.[185] The precise identification of the primary defect in this heterogeneous group of patients will probably have to await the application of molecular genetic techniques, e.g. a dominantly inherited bleeding disorder characterized by defective responses to thromboxane A_2 has recently been shown to be due to a single amino acid substitution ($Arg^{60} \rightarrow Leu$) in the thromboxane A_2 receptor.[186]

Defective response to epinephrine

The aggregatory response of normal platelets to epinephrine is notably variable,[187] and Scrutton et al[188] and Gaxiola et al[189] have shown that decreased responsiveness may be inherited without conferring any hemostatic failure. It can therefore be argued that tests of epinephrine-induced aggregation are best avoided in the investigation of bleeding disorders, or at least discounted in the absence of other demonstrable abnormalities. Stormorken et al,[190] however,

reported a 16-year-old boy who had had frequent bleeding episodes since early childhood and whose platelets completely failed to aggregate in response to epinephrine. Like the hemostatically normal subjects studied by Scrutton et al,[188] his platelets had normal α_2-adrenergic receptors. The exact nature of the defect was not explained.

Management of intracellular platelet disorders

These disorders are usually of only mild or moderate clinical severity, and interfere little with everyday life. Excessive bleeding is likely to result from serious trauma, however, and may require replacement therapy as well as local hemostatic measures, although Mielke et al[191] were able to reduce the bleeding time and surgical blood loss in a miscellaneous series of patients with platelet disorders by a short pre- and post-operative course of prednisone. Platelet transfusions have been used successfully in many such cases, but cryoprecipitate[192] and desmopressin[193,194] have, somewhat surprisingly, also been found to shorten the bleeding time and control surgical bleeding in patients with various defects of platelet secretion. Nieuwenhuis and Sixma[195] found that desmopressin at 0.4 μg/kg shortened the bleeding time in 18 of 23 patients with δ-SPD, while Rao et al[196] found that the lower dose of 0.3 μg/kg had no effect in such patients, although it shortened the bleeding time for 50 min or more in most of those with other defects of secretion. In practice, a preoperative trial of desmopressin will permit responders to be identified and treated with the drug, while non-responders are more likely to require platelet transfusion to control surgical bleeding.

The mode of action of desmopressin in these platelet disorders remains to be fully explained: no direct effect on platelet adhesion or secretion has been observed,[196] but platelet aggregation at high shear rate is potentiated,[197] presumably owing to the raised plasma VWF concentration, and perhaps also to increased membrane expression of GpIb.[198] Pfueller et al[199] showed that desmopressin also shortened the bleeding time of a patient with gray platelet syndrome, despite undetectable platelet VWF, suggesting that desmopressin does not exert its hemostatic effect in this group of disorders through stimulation of the secretion of platelet VWF.

MISCELLANEOUS HEREDITARY DISORDERS

A number of other hereditary defects of platelet function have been described, whether as part of well-defined clinical syndromes or as isolated platelet abnormalities, which do not fall into any of the categories discussed above. Several of these are characterized by the presence of giant platelets, and therefore need to be distinguished from Bernard–Soulier syndrome in particular.

Giant platelet syndromes

Montreal platelet syndrome

First described by Lacombe and d'Angelo,[200] and subsequently studied in detail by Milton *et al*,[201–203] this is an autosomal dominant form of thrombocytopenia in which the platelets increase abnormally in size during the shape change which follows activation. Ristocetin-induced agglutination is normal, as are platelet aggregation responses to ADP and other agonists, but there is reduced sensitivity to thrombin and an increased tendency to spontaneous aggregation. The surface glycoprotein composition is normal, but a defect in calcium-activated neutral protease (calpain) has been observed, which may account for the other defects.[204]

May–Hegglin anomaly (see Chapter 21)

This is an autosomal dominant trait comprising the presence of giant platelets and pseudo-Döhle bodies in the neutrophils. About one-third of patients have had some degree of thrombocytopenia, and an increase in giant platelet granules has been seen, but there is no significant disorder of platelet function.[205] The bleeding tendency, which is usually mild, if present, reflects the degree of thrombocytopenia. The condition is mentioned here only to distinguish it from other giant platelet syndromes.

Epstein's syndrome (see also Chapter 21)

This is an autosomal dominant trait in which mild thrombocytopenia with giant platelets is associated with Alport's syndrome of nephritis and nerve deafness. Minor defects of platelet function have been reported in most cases,[206–208] but the bleeding tendency is probably chiefly attributable to the thrombocytopenia. A variant of this condition has been described under the name of *Fechtner syndrome;*[209] 8 of 17 members of 4 generations of a family had various combinations of nephritis, deafness, congenital cataracts, giant platelets and leukocyte inclusions. The inclusions resembled those of the May–Hegglin anomaly on stained blood films, but could be distinguished from them by electron microscopy. Apart from a partial defect of thromboxane synthesis from arachidonic acid, no significant abnormality of platelet function was observed.

Sebastian platelet syndrome (see Chapter 21)

This is an autosomal dominant trait characterized by giant platelets and neutrophil inclusions in the absence of other congenital abnormalities.[210]

Other disorders

Other examples of familial thrombocytopenia with giant platelets, with or without demonstrable defects of platelet function, have been described by various authors (see also Chapter 21). Greaves *et al*[171] studied a family in which congenital thrombocytopenia was dominantly inherited and associated with gross abnormalities of platelet ultrastructure, impaired arachidonic acid mobilization from membrane phospholipids and defective aggregation in response to ADP, epinephrine and collagen. Several affected members of this family had required transfusion for serious bleeding episodes during childhood. Stewart *et al*[211] reported the case of a 13-year-old girl in whom thrombocytopenia and giant platelets were associated with stomatocytosis and pseudo-homozygous type II hypercholesterolemia; platelet adhesion was reported to be slightly reduced, but aggregation was normal.

Disorders with normal platelet size

Dowton *et al*[212] described a large family of which 22 members suffered from an autosomal dominant bleeding disorder of moderate severity, usually presenting during their first decade, with mild-to-moderate thrombocytopenia, a long bleeding time and normal platelet survival. Several of the affected members had defective aggregation in response to ADP, epinephrine and collagen. One patient also had congenital neuroblastoma, successfully treated but followed at the age of 7 years by acute monocytic leukemia, and 5 other family members, 4 of whom had the bleeding tendency, developed hematologic neoplasms between the ages of 10 and 62 years.

Biochemical and/or functional abnormalities of the platelets have been described in Down's syndrome,[213,214] adenosine deaminase deficiency (see Chapter 25) and idiopathic scoliosis,[215] but none of these conditions is associated with abnormal bleeding. Various platelet abnormalities have been reported in hereditary disorders of connective tissue, including Ehlers–Danlos and Marfan's syndromes and osteogenesis imperfecta, but the bleeding tendency in these is more likely to result from the abnormality of the connective tissue itself. In Ehlers–Danlos syndrome, for example, skin collagen has been shown to be defective in aggregating normal platelets,[216] and the aggregation defect in 1 family could be corrected by purified fibronectin.[217] It is notable that the bleeding tendency is most severe in type IV Ehlers–Danlos syndrome, in which type III collagen, the most potent in activating the platelets, is deficient.[218]

Defective platelet aggregation has also been described in Bartter's syndrome, but is due to a plasma factor, the probable consequence of the metabolic disturbance.[219]

DIAGNOSTIC APPROACH TO INHERITED PLATELET DISORDERS

A life-long history of 'easy bruising', prolonged bleeding after superficial injuries, or even apparently spontaneous bleeding from mucosal surfaces or into the skin, suggests the diagnosis

Table 24.4 Diagnosis of inherited disorders of platelet function.

Disorder	Inheritance	Platelet count	Platelet size	Platelet aggregation				Confirmatory findings	Associated abnormalities
				ADP	Collagen	Arachidonate	Ristocetin		
Glanzmann's thrombasthenia	Autosomal recessive	N	N	O	O	O	(1)*	GpIIb-IIIa deficiency	
Bernard–Soulier syndrome	Autosomal recessive	↓	↑	N	N	N	O	GpIb-IX deficiency	
Glycoprotein Ia deficiency		N	N	N	O	N		GpIa deficiency	
Idiopathic storage-pool deficiency	Autosomal dominant	N	N or ↓	(1)*	↓	N	(1)*	Dense-body deficiency	
Hermansky–Pudlak syndrome	Autosomal recessive	N	N	(1)*	↓	N		Deficiency and failure of secretion of ATP, ADP, 5-HT	Tyrosinase-positive albinism Pigmented macrophages in marrow
Wiskott–Aldrich syndrome	X-borne recessive	↓	↓	(1)*	↓				Eczema Recurrent infections
Chédiak–Higashi syndrome	Autosomal recessive	N or ↓	N	(1)*	↓				Partial albinism Recurrent bacterial infections Abnormal neutrophil granules
Gray platelet syndrome	Autosomal dominant	↓	↑	N	N or ↓	N	N	α-Granule deficiency	Myelofibrosis
Cyclo-oxygenase deficiency Thromboxane synthetase deficiency	?	N	N	(1)*	O	O	N	Defective TXB₂ synthesis	

*First-phase aggregation only. N = normal. O = absent. TXB$_2$ = Thromboxane B$_2$.

either of a hereditary platelet disorder or VWD. In the investigation of such a patient, the first clues to a more specific diagnosis may come from the family history or the association of the bleeding symptoms with other clinical features typical of particular conditions (Table 24.4); Bernard–Soulier and gray platelet syndromes may first reveal themselves by the abnormal platelet morphology on the stained blood film, but a long bleeding time is the characteristic hallmark of this whole group of disorders. The combination of a long bleeding time with a normal (or perhaps moderately reduced) platelet count indicate the need for platelet function tests, as may a strongly suggestive clinical history even in the presence of a normal bleeding time. VWD can be excluded by appropriate investigations (see Chapter 30), and most of the recognized platelet abnormalities can be provisionally identified in the first instance by means of tests of aggregation and secretion in response to ADP, collagen, arachidonic acid and ristocetin, supplemented where necessary by determination of platelet size (Table 24.4). These tests of aggregation should, however, be regarded as screening rather than final diagnostic procedures; normal aggregation patterns are seen, for

example, in a proportion of cases of storage pool deficiency (see above).

Confirmation of the diagnosis of thrombasthenia, Bernard–Soulier syndrome or other membrane glycoprotein disorders requires biochemical tests for the glycoproteins or binding assays with specific monoclonal antibodies. Defects of aggregation in response to collagen and/or arachidonate call for a distinction to be made between deficiency of storage organelles, defective thromboxane synthesis and defects in signal transduction. The relevant tests for dense-body deficiency are uptake and secretion of 5-HT, content and secretion of adenine nucleotides and enumeration of dense bodies by fluorescence microscopy of mepacrine-treated platelets or by electron microscopy; α-granule deficiency is identified by electron microscopy and by assay of β-thromboglobulin, PF4 or other α-granule constituents (Table 24.2). The final analysis of other secretory defects may require measurement of thromboxane B$_2$ production in response to collagen, arachidonate and endoperoxide analogs, and of phosphatidyl inositol hydrolysis and Ca^{2+} mobilization in response to various stimuli.

ACQUIRED DISORDERS OF PLATELET FUNCTION

Abnormalities of platelet function occur in a wide range of conditions, often in association with other hemostatic defects including both thrombocytopenia and disorders of blood coagulation, so that it may be difficult to assess the relative importance of several observed abnormalities in the pathogenesis of the bleeding tendency. In most of these disorders, the nature of the platelet abnormality is much less clear cut than in the genetic disorders of platelet function, and a predominantly clinical rather than a pathogenetic classification is appropriate (Table 24.5). Many drugs may also interfere with platelet function (Table 24.6).

Enhanced platelet activity has been recorded in a number of conditions characterized by a thrombotic tendency. Although it is by no means always clear whether the observed changes in platelet behavior are of primary pathogenetic significance, or merely secondary to other prothrombotic influences, a list of such conditions which may occur in

Table 24.5 Causes of acquired platelet dysfunction in childhood.

Renal failure

Myeloproliferative disorders and myelodysplasia

Acute leukemias and pre-leukemic states

Liver disease

Chronic hypoglycemia
  Glycogen storage disease type I
  Fructose-1,6-diphosphatase deficiency
Cardiopulmonary bypass, extracorporeal circulations

Acquired storage-pool deficiency
  Autoimmune disease
  Disseminated intravascular coagulation
  Hemolytic uremic syndrome, thrombotic thrombocytopenic purpura
  Severe burns
  Valvular heart disease

Antibodies against platelet membrane glycoproteins

Drugs (Table 24.6)

Table 24.6 Drugs that may cause bleeding through interference with platelet function.

Non-steroidal anti-inflammatory drugs
  Aspirin
  Indomethacin
  Phenylbutazone
  Sulfinpyrazone

β-Lactam antibiotics
  Penicillins
  Cephalosporins

Dextrans

Heparin

Sodium valproate

Intravascular radiographic contrast agents

Table 24.7 Conditions associated with increased platelet activity.

Diabetes mellitus
Nephrotic syndrome
Kawasaki disease
Hyperlipoproteinemia
Homocystinuria
Renal allograft rejection

childhood is given in Table 24.7, and some of these are briefly discussed.

CONDITIONS ASSOCIATED WITH DEFECTIVE PLATELET FUNCTION

Renal failure

Coagulation defects and thrombocytopenia may both occur in patients in renal failure, but defective platelet function and anemia are evidently the chief causes of abnormal bleeding. This commonly presents as purpura, epistaxis or bleeding from the gums, although serious internal hemorrhage may also occur, and renal biopsy or surgical procedures present a special hazard. The pathogenesis of bleeding in renal failure, and its clinical management, have been reviewed by Remuzzi.[220] The bleeding time is typically prolonged, and abnormalities have been reported in a variety of aspects of platelet function, including aggregation,[221,222] adhesion to subendothelium[223] (perhaps related to a reduction in membrane GpIb[224]), elevation of cytoplasmic free calcium[225] and thromboxane formation.[226] The aggregation defect correlates poorly with the severity of the renal failure, but can be at least partially corrected by hemodialysis or peritoneal dialysis.[227,228] No general agreement has been reached on the identity of the dialysable component responsible for the effect on the platelets: urea,[229] guanidinosuccinic acid,[230] phenolic acids[231] and uremic middle molecules[232] have all been incriminated. Various defects of arachidonate metabolism have been described in uremic patients, leading to both impaired generation of thromboxane A_2[226] and increased prostacyclin production.[233,234] Remuzzi et al[235] have also shown that parathyroid hormone inhibits platelet aggregation and secretion in vitro, and suggested that the raised concentrations found in uremic plasma might contribute towards the bleeding tendency in this way. Docci et al,[236] however, found no correlation between secondary hyperparathyroidism and bleeding in uremic patients.

Apart from dialysis, uremic bleeding has been treated successfully, and the bleeding time corrected with desmopressin.[237] The most effective therapeutic measure, however, is correction of the hematocrit, whether by red cell transfusions[238,239] or by administration of human recombinant erythropoietin.[240,241] The beneficial effect on hemostasis of correcting the anemia in uremic patients remains to be fully explained: the mechanical effect of red cells in influencing flow conditions so as to promote interaction of platelets with the vessel wall[242] is probably part of the explanation, but erythropoietin treatment also appears to diminish the inhibitory effect of uremic plasma on platelet adhesion and aggregation.[243,244] Conjugated estrogens have also been shown to correct the bleeding time of uremic patients;[245,246] the effect lasts for several days, and appears to depend on reduction of endothelial synthesis of nitric oxide.[247]

Myeloproliferative disorders and myelodysplasia

Both hemorrhagic symptoms and arterial thromboses are common in adults with this group of disorders, and both may occur in the same patient. The commonest bleeding symptoms are large superficial ecchymoses, epistaxes and hemorrhage from the gastrointestinal tract; thrombosis usually involves either the cerebral arteries or the peripheral arteries of the limbs. The platelet defects which have been described are not specifically associated with any one of the adult myeloproliferative disorders; similar defects have been observed in essential thrombocythemia, polycythemia vera, chronic granulocytic leukemia and myelofibrosis. All these conditions are very rare in childhood, particularly the first two, but when they do occur may also be associated with functional platelet disorders. Bleeding in the juvenile form of chronic myeloid leukemia (JCML) typically results from thrombocytopenia, however, which is a usual presenting feature. Structural platelet abnormalities are commonly seen in the myeloproliferative disorders, and amongst the disturbances of platelet function which have been described are: defects of aggregation, particularly in response to epinephrine;[248] storage pool deficiency;[249–252] defects of arachidonate metabolism[253–255] and of platelet coagulant activities;[256,257] resistance to the action of the antiaggregatory prostaglandin D$_2$;[258] and various abnormalities of the membrane glycoproteins.[259] Many of these are probably due to the presence of activated platelets in the circulation.[260]

Michelson[261] studied 4 children with juvenile (Ph-negative) CML and with Ph-positive adult CML, all of whom (in contrast to age-matched controls and adults with Ph-positive CML) showed 2 subpopulations of platelets, positive and negative respectively for both glycoproteins Ib and IIb–IIIa. Berndt et al[262] described the case of a 9-year-old girl with a myelodysplastic syndrome characterized by monosomy 7, thrombocytopenia and giant platelets, who had had a bleeding tendency from the age of 5. She was also found to have 2 populations of platelets, the majority being large and deficient in GpIb–IX complex, as in Bernard–Soulier syndrome, and the minority normal.

Some of the platelet abnormalities which have been observed would be expected to lead to abnormal bleeding and others to predispose to thrombotic episodes, but in practice the laboratory findings have usually been found to correlate poorly with the clinical course of the disease. When thrombocythemia occurs in childhood, there is seldom any need for specific management of bleeding or thrombosis as

such, and the treatment is that of the underlying disorder. Restoration of the platelet count to normal will usually correct any hemostatic abnormality.

Acute leukemias and pre-leukemic states

Bleeding in the acute leukemias is usually the result of thrombocytopenia, but platelet dysfunction may also contribute, particularly in the myeloid leukemias. Defects of aggregation and secretion have been described and attributed variously to storage pool deficiency and defects of secretory mechanisms,[263] impaired thromboxane production,[264] and a deficiency of thrombin-binding sites on the platelet membrane.[265] Fäldt et al[266] showed that myeloid leukemia cells of various FAB types, like HL60 cells, but not normal polymorphs, secreted a low molecular weight inhibitor of platelet aggregation on incubation in vitro.

Bleeding in patients with pre-leukemic states, including those with normal platelet counts, has also been attributed to defective platelet aggregation.[267,268]

Liver disease

The hemostatic failure of liver disease results chiefly from defective synthesis of clotting factors, but low-grade intravascular coagulation and increased fibrinolysis may also occur. Defective platelet aggregation may be another contributory factor: acquired storage pool deficiency (see below) is a likely mechanism, and defects of thromboxane synthesis[269] and membrane glycoproteins[270] have also been reported. Although patients with liver disease usually have normal or raised levels of VWF, desmopressin has been found to shorten the prolonged bleeding time,[271] as well as improving the results of coagulation tests.

Chronic hypoglycemia

Patients with glycogen storage disease type I (glucose-6-phosphatase deficiency) and fructose-1,6-diphosphatase deficiency typically suffer from a mild bleeding tendency and have long bleeding times. The defect of platelet aggregation and adenine nucleotide secretion, to which the hemostatic failure appears to be due,[272,273] can be corrected by intravenous glucose administration; it appears that the chronic hypoglycemia of these conditions leads to a failure of nucleotide synthesis within the platelets, affecting both the storage and metabolic pool.[274]

Cardiopulmonary bypass

Bleeding during and after cardiopulmonary bypass may have many contributory causes, including defective surgical hemostasis, but transient thrombocytopenia and platelet dysfunction are near constant features.[275] The platelet dysfunction results in progressive prolongation of the bleeding time throughout the procedure, with normalization during the subsequent 2–4 hours. It is evidently attributable to platelet activation and membrane damage from contact with the bypass apparatus, and perhaps also from activation of clotting factors and complement components,[276–278] leading to a transient refractory state. It can be largely prevented by infusion of prostacyclin,[279,280] with correction of the bleeding time. Desmopressin has also been found to reduce excessive perioperative bleeding,[281] although its prophylactic use in uncomplicated cardiac surgery does not appear to be justified by the results.[282,283]

Acquired storage-pool deficiency

Many different stimuli can induce the secretion from platelets of their dense-body and α-granule contents, and if this occurs on a large scale in the circulation it may result in hemostatic failure due to the functional inadequacy of the depleted platelets, possibly combined with local thrombus formation at the site of platelet damage. A variety of conditions in which the platelets are subjected to either immune-mediated or mechanical damage (Table 24.5) may lead to abnormal bleeding and/or thrombosis in this way, and many of the platelet defects observed in clonal myeloproliferative disorders (see above) are probably attributable to a similar mechanism. The term 'acquired storage-pool deficiency' derives from the original observations of depleted granule contents[284–286] or raised concentrations of platelet-specific proteins in the plasma,[276] but these methods have now been largely superseded by the detection of activated platelets by flow cytometry, using specific monoclonal antibodies.[277,278] Many of these disorders are likely also to result in thrombocytopenia, but the functional may precede the quantitative platelet defect.

Antibodies against membrane glycoproteins

Many patients with immune thrombocytopenic purpura (ITP) have autoantibodies directed against determinants on GpIIb–IIIa or GpIb (see Chapter 22). Such antibodies have been detected in patients with acquired bleeding disorders and long bleeding times, but normal platelet counts, resulting in functional defects resembling those of Glanzmann's thrombasthenia[287,288] and Bernard–Soulier syndrome,[289] respectively. Deckmyn et al[290] reported a similar case in which the autoantibody was directed against GpIa and resulted in a specific failure of the platelets to aggregate in response to collagen. Of these 5 patients, 1 had Hodgkin's disease, 1 an unspecified lymphoproliferative disease and 1 myasthenia gravis and a thymoma; the others had had chronic ITP, but the antibody-induced functional defect persisted after recovery of the platelet count. The patients of Stricker et al[289] and Deckmyn et al[290] responded to repeated plasma exchange, and steroid therapy had a more lasting beneficial effect in 2 of the cases, but no effect in a third.

Platelet dysfunction due to drugs

Apart from the deliberate use of platelet inhibitory drugs as antithrombotic agents, interference with platelet function may occur as a side-effect of drugs used for other purposes. The defects induced are usually of minor degree, and observed only on laboratory testing, and the following account is largely confined to those drugs (Table 24.6) which have been recognized as potential causes of clinical bleeding.

Non-steroidal anti-inflammatory drugs

Aspirin ingestion is the commonest cause of platelet dysfunction, and may occasionally precipitate gastrointestinal or other hemorrhage, particularly in susceptible individuals. It is of proven value as an antithrombotic drug, but should be forbidden in patients with known bleeding disorders. Aspirin inhibits the formation of cyclic endoperoxides and thromboxane A_2 by irreversible acetylation of cyclo-oxygenase (Fig. 24.5); this results in a moderate prolongation of the bleeding time, which may last up to 2–4 days, absence of the second wave of aggregation with ADP and a failure of aggregation and secretion in response to collagen and arachidonic acid. These latter effects, which may follow the ingestion of as little as 75 mg, last throughout the life-span of the platelet—hence the importance of ensuring abstention from aspirin for at least 10 days before platelet function testing for diagnostic purposes. Since aspirin crosses the placenta, and can contribute to neonatal bleeding,[33] it should be withheld during the week before delivery.

Other non-steroidal anti-inflammatory drugs, including indomethacin, phenylbutazone and sulfinpyrazone, have a similar but reversible, and therefore less prolonged, effect on platelet function. They have not been reported to cause clinically important bleeding.

Antibiotics

Many of the β-lactam antibiotics, particularly the penicillins, can cause a bleeding tendency by interfering with platelet function. This side-effect, which may persist for up to 12 days after withdrawal of the drug,[291] is seen only with high dosage regimes; patients in renal failure are at particular risk, since high drug concentrations resulting from impaired clearance may co-exist with other hemostatic defects, and thrombocytopenic bleeding in patients on chemotherapy for malignant disease may be exacerbated by antibiotic-induced platelet dysfunction. Both penicillins and cephalosporins have been shown to inhibit platelet adhesion, aggregation and secretion in vitro: the underlying mechanisms appear to involve the inhibition of agonist binding to membrane receptors and impairment of thromboxane synthesis and calcium mobilization.[292,293]

483

Dextrans

Dextrans, particularly those of high molecular weight, have complex effects on the hemostatic mechanism. These include prolongation of the bleeding time and defects of platelet aggregation and secretion.[294] The effects, which are dose related, reach a maximum 4–8 hours after the end of the infusion, and may be due to refractoriness of the platelets following transient aggregation by the dextran itself.[295]

Heparin

The chief platelet-related complication of heparin therapy is heparin-induced thrombocytopenia, due to the activation of platelets by heparin-dependent IgG, and leading to the generation of procoagulant platelet microparticles and arterial and venous thrombotic complications (see Chapter 22).[296] Apart from this, unfractionated heparins have been found to bind to the platelet membrane and to inhibit platelet function in certain experimental systems, possibly by inducing a refractory state following partial activation,[297] and these effects might also theoretically contribute towards the bleeding tendency of heparin overdosage. Heparin fractions of low molecular weight and high antithrombin affinity are the least likely to bind to platelets[298] and interfere with platelet function,[299] and this may partly account for the lower incidence of bleeding complications seen with low molecular weight than with unfractionated heparin.[300]

Other drugs

Amongst drugs used in pediatric practice which have occasionally been found to cause bleeding symptoms through an effect on platelet function are the anticonvulsant sodium valproate[301] and intravascular radiographic contrast media.[302,303] Sodium valproate may also cause thrombocytopenia and minor coagulation abnormalities. Various other classes of drugs, including antihistamines, phenothiazines, tricyclic antidepressants, frusemide, daunorubicin, and both local and general anesthetics, have been shown to inhibit platelet function in vitro, but do not significantly impair hemostasis at pharmacologic doses. It is possible, however, that they may aggravate the bleeding tendency of patients with pre-existing hemostatic defects. Corby and Schulman[304] found that the platelets of newborn infants were more susceptible than those of their mothers to the effects of promethazine and aspirin taken before delivery.

Blue fluorescent light, as used in the phototherapy of neonatal hyperbilirubinemia, has been shown to damage platelets in vitro, depleting them of adenine nucleotides and glycogen,[305] and a fall in platelet count has sometimes been observed during such treatment.

While foodstuffs do not inhibit platelet function to the extent of causing a bleeding tendency, they may do so sufficiently to interfere with the results of laboratory tests. Onions, garlic, ginger and the chinese black tree fungus,

Mo-er, have all been incriminated, and should probably be avoided before diagnostic platelet function tests are performed.

CONDITIONS ASSOCIATED WITH INCREASED PLATELET ACTIVITY (Table 24.7)

Diabetes mellitus

Diabetes mellitus is well known to be associated with vascular disease and thrombotic events at all ages, manifested by retinopathy, peripheral neuropathy, renal vascular disease, and an increased risk of cerebral and myocardial infarction. While raised levels of coagulation factors have been observed, as well as decreased fibrinolysis, the chief pathogenetic mechanism appears to involve platelet-vessel wall reactivity. The presence of functionally hyperactive platelets in the circulation is shown by their increased volume, increased expression of glycoproteins Ib and IIb–IIIa, and increased thromboxane formation, while evidence of in vivo activation comes from the surface expression of the activation-dependent antigens CD62 (P-selectin) and CD63,[306] confirming the earlier observation of increased in vivo secretion of α-granule proteins.[307] Reduced synthesis of prostacyclin by endothelial cells[308] and an increased sensitivity of the platelet thromboxane receptor[309] have also been reported.

The platelet abnormalities appear early in the course of the disease, even in childhood diabetes,[310] sometimes predating symptoms, and are not fully corrected by glycemic control.[311,312] Increased platelet activity has also been seen in infants born to mothers with inadequately controlled diabetes;[313,314] such infants are known to have an increased incidence of thrombosis.[315] Low-dose aspirin therapy has proved of value in the primary and secondary prevention of vascular complications in adult diabetics.[316]

Nephrotic syndrome

Thrombosis is a common and serious complication of the nephrotic syndrome in childhood, as in later life, and platelet hyperaggregability and hypercoagulability both appear to be important factors in its pathogenesis.[317] The platelets are hyper-responsive to arachidonic acid, in terms of both aggregation and thromboxane production, and this effect is proportional to the degree of depletion of serum albumin and can be reversed by the addition of albumin in vitro or in vivo. This suggests that the hypoalbuminemia is largely responsible for the functional platelet abnormality, probably as a result of decreased binding of arachidonic acid, which thus becomes available in excess for thromboxane synthesis.[318] The platelet hyperaggregability seen in response to collagen and ristocetin, however, is not related to hypoalbuminemia,[319,320] but to the raised plasma concentrations of fibrinogen and VWF which are also found in these patients. Indeed, recent perfusion studies under carefully controlled flow conditions suggest that hyperfibrinogenemia itself, rather than platelet hyperaggregability, is responsible for the increased risk of thrombosis.[321] While the correction of the thrombotic tendency must rely chiefly on the management of the renal disorder and the consequent correction of the plasma protein changes, the use of low-dose aspirin as an inhibitor of the excessive thromboxane production would also seem appropriate.

Kawasaki disease

In this acute febrile vasculitis of infants and young children,[322] involvement of the coronary arteries occurs in >20% of untreated cases, and coronary aneurysm formation and thrombosis are important causes of sudden death. The inflammatory process results from the activation of an immunological cascade, perhaps triggered by endotoxins acting as superantigens.[323] Evidence of intravascular coagulation includes raised factor VIII and fibrinogen concentrations and raised platelet counts during the first 3 weeks of the illness, together with depletion of fibrinolytic activity;[324] increased platelet consumption, denoted by raised plasma β-thromboglobulin levels[324] and early thrombocytopenia,[325] was observed only in children who developed aneurysms and myocardial infarction, suggesting increased in vivo platelet activation specifically in this group. Yamada et al[326] found heightened in vitro aggregability of the platelets for as long as 9 months after the onset of disease, which could be suppressed by aspirin treatment.

Aspirin has an important place in the treatment of Kawasaki disease, both for its antiplatelet and anti-inflammatory effects, but the early infusion of a single large dose (2 g/kg) of intravenous gamma globulin in addition to aspirin greatly reduces the incidence of coronary arterial disease.[327]

Hyperlipoproteinemia

Hyperlipidemia is well known to predispose to atherosclerosis and thrombotic disease, but the relationship between plasma lipids and platelet function remains a matter for debate. Tremoli et al[328] studied a large group of patients with type II hyperlipoproteinemia aged from 11 years upwards, and found enhanced sensitivity of their platelets to aggregation by ADP, epinephrine and collagen, and increased production of thromboxane B_2 from endogenous arachidonic acid on stimulation with collagen. These abnormalities did not correlate with plasma cholesterol levels, but may have resulted from an increased cholesterol:phospholipid ratio in the platelet membrane. Platelet adhesion to collagen, but not thrombus formation, was significantly raised in flowing blood from patients with types IIa and IIb hyperlipoproteinemia examined in a perfusion system at high shear rate, equivalent to that obtaining in the arterial circulation.[329]

Homocystinuria

The commonest cause of homocystinuria, cystathionine-β-synthase deficiency, is associated with a high incidence of thromboembolic disease, which is a major cause of death, sometimes even in the first decade of life. The most likely explanation for this is endothelial cell injury induced by the homocystine in plasma, leading to platelet-mediated intimal proliferation, as in the genesis of other atherosclerotic lesions.[330] Patients with homocystinuria, although they show no evidence of increased platelet aggregability or ATP secretion in response to thrombin, exhibit abnormally high thromboxane biosynthesis, reflecting in vivo platelet activation; this is largely corrected by low-dose aspirin, and also by the cholesterol-lowering drug probucol.[331] Whether the primary injury is inflicted on the platelets themselves or the vascular endothelium, low-dose aspirin is the most appropriate antithrombotic treatment.

REFERENCES

1. Phillips DR, Charo IF, Parise LV, Fitzgerald LA. The platelet membrane glycoprotein IIb-IIIa complex. *Blood* 1988; **71**: 831–843
2. Hynes RO. Integrins: a family of cell surface receptors. *Cell* 1987; **48**: 549–554
3. Pischel KD, Bluestein HG, Woods VL. Platelet glycoproteins Ia, Ic and IIa are physicochemically indistinguishable from the very late activation antigens adhesion-related proteins of lymphocytes and other cell types. *J Clin Invest* 1988; **81**: 505–513
4. Wicki AN, Clemetson KJ. Structure and function of platelet membrane glycoproteins Ib and V. Effects of leukocyte elastase and other proteases on platelet response to von Willebrand factor and thrombin. *Eur J Biochem* 1985; **153**: 1–11
5. Turitto VT, Baumgartner HR. Platelet interaction with subendothelium in flowing rabbit blood—effect of blood sheer rate. *Microvasc Res* 1979; **17**: 38–54
6. Bolhuis PA, Sakariassen KS, Sander HJ, Bouma BN, Sixma JJ. Binding of factor VIII-von Willebrand factor to human arterial subendothelium precedes increased platelet adherence and enhances platelet spreading. *Journal Lab Clin Med* 1981; **97**: 568–576
7. Weiss HJ, Tschopp TB, Baumgartner HR, Sussman II, Johnson MM, Egan JJ. Decreased adhesion of giant (Bernard–Soulier) platelets to subendothelium. Further implications on the role of the von Willebrand factor in hemostasis. *Am J Med* 1974; **57**: 920–925
8. Coller BS, Peerschke EI, Scudder LE, Sullivan CA. Studies with a murine monoclonal antibody that abolishes ristocetin-induced binding of von Willebrand factor to platelets: additional evidence in support of GPIb as a platelet receptor for von Willebrand factor. *Blood* 1983; **61**: 99–110
9. Weiss HJ, Turitto VT, Baumgartner HR. Platelet adhesion and thrombus formation on subendothelium in platelets deficient in glycoproteins IIb-IIIa, Ib and storage granules. *Blood* 1986; **67**: 322–330
10. Sakariassen KS, Nievelstein PFEM, Coller BS, Sixma JJ. The role of platelet membrane glycoproteins Ib and IIb-IIIa in platelet adherence in human artery subendothelium. *Br J Haematol* 1986; **63**: 681–691
11. Bennett S, Vilaire G. Exposure of platelet fibrinogen receptors by ADP and epinephrine. *J Clin Invest* 1979; **64**: 1393–1401
12. Marguerie GA, Plow EF, Edgington TS. Human platelets possess an inducible and saturable receptor specific for fibrinogen. *J Biol Chem* 1979; **254**: 5357–5363
13. Bevers EM, Comfurius P, Zwaal RFA. Changes in membrane

phospholipid distribution during platelet activation. *Biochim Biophys Acta* 1983; **736**: 57–66

14. Sims PJ, Faioni EM, Wiedmer T *et al.* Complement proteins C5b-9 cause release of membrane vesicles from the platelet surface that are enriched in the membrane receptor for coagulation factor Va and express prothrombinase activity. *J Biol Chem* 1988; **263**: 18205–18212

15. Rosing J, van Rijn JLML, Bevers EM, van Dieijen G, Comfurius P, Zwaal RFA. The role of activated human platelets in prothrombin and factor X activation. *Blood* 1985; **65**: 319–332

16. Bleyer WA, Hakami N, Shepard TH. The development of hemostasis in the human fetus and newborn infant. *J Pediatr* 1971; **79**: 838–853

17. Pandolfi M, Åstedt B, Cronberg L, Nilsson IM. Failure of fetal platelets to aggregate in reponse to adrenaline and collagen. *Proc Soc Exp Biol Med* 1972; **141**: 1081–1083

18. Feusner JH. Normal and abnormal bleeding times in neonates and young children utilizing a fully standardized template technique. *Am J Pathol* 1980; **74**: 73–77

19. Mull MM, Hathaway WE. Altered platelet function in newborns. *Pediatr Res* 1970; **4**: 229–237

20. Corby DG, O'Barr TP. Decreased α-adrenergic receptors in newborn platelets: cause of abnormal response to epinephrine. *Dev Pharmacol Therap* 1981; **2**: 215–225

21. Jones CR, McCabe R, Hamilton CA, Reid JL. Maternal and fetal platelet responses and adrenoceptor binding characteristics. *Thromb Haemostasis* 1985; **53**: 95–98

22. Ts'ao C, Green D, Schultz K. Function and ultrastructure of platelets of neonates: enhanced ristocetin aggregation of neonatal platelets. *Br J Haematol* 1976; **32**: 225–233

23. Varela AF, Runge A, Ignarro LJ, Chaudhuri G. Nitric oxide and prostacyclin inhibit fetal platelet aggregation: a response similar to that observed in adults. *Am J Obstet Gynecol* 1992; **167**: 1599–1604

24. Rajasekhar D, Kestin AS, Bednarek FJ, Ellis PA, Barnard MR, Michelson AD. Neonatal platelets are less reactive than adult platelets to physiological agonists in whole blood. *Thromb Haemostasis* 1994; **72**: 957–963

25. Whaun JM. The platelet of the newborn infant—adenine nucleotide metabolism and release. *Thromb Haemostasis* 1980; **43**: 99–103

26. Suarez CR, Gonzalez J, Menendez C, Fareed J, Fresco R, Walenga J. Neonatal and maternal platelets: activation at time of birth. *Am J Hematol* 1988; **29**: 18–21

27. Stuart MJ, Duss EJ, Clark DA, Walenga RW. Differences in thromboxane production between neonatal and adult platelets in response to arachidonic acid and epinephrine. *Pediatr Res* 1984; **18**: 823–826

28. Kääpä P, Viinikka L, Ylikorkala O. Thromboxane B$_2$ production by fetal and neonatal platelets: effects of idiopathic respiratory distress syndrome and birth asphyxia. *Pediatr Res* 1984; **18**: 756–758

29. Stuart MJ, Allen JB. Arachidonic acid metabolism in the neonatal platelet. *Pediatrics* 1982; **69**: 714–718

30. Gruel Y, Boizard B, Daffos F, Forestier F, Caen J, Wautier JL. Determination of platelet antigens and glycoproteins in the human fetus. *Blood* 1986; **68**: 488–492

31. Meher-Homji NJ, Montemagno R, Thilaganathan B, Nicolaides KH. Platelet size and glycoprotein Ib and IIIa expression in normal fetal and maternal blood. *Am J Obstet Gynecol* 1994; **171**: 791–796

32. Bleyer WA, Breckenridge RT. Studies on the detection of adverse drug reactions in the newborn. II The effects of prenatal aspirin on newborn hemostasis. *JAMA* 1970; **213**: 2049–2053

33. Stuart MJ, Gross SJ, Elrad H, Graeber JE. Effects of acetysalicylic-acid ingestion on maternal and neonatal hemostasis. *N Engl J Med* 1982; **307**: 909–912

34. Glanzmann E. Hereditäre hämorrhagische Thrombasthenie. Ein Beitrag zur Pathologie der Blutplättchen. *Jahrbuch Kinderheilkunde* 1918; **88**: 1–42

35. Hardisty RM, Dormandy KM, Hutton RA. Thrombasthenia: studies on three cases. *Br J Haematol* 1964; **10**: 371–387

36. Caen JP, Castaldi PA, Leclerc JC *et al.* Congenital bleeding disorders with long bleeding time and normal platelet count. I. Glanzmann's thrombasthenia (report of 15 patients). *Am J Med* 1966; **41**: 4–26

37. Zucker MB, Pert JH, Hilgartner MW. Platelet function in a patient with thrombasthenia. *Blood* 1966; **28**: 524–534

38. Nurden AT, Caen JP. An abnormal platelet glycoprotein pattern in three cases of Glanzmann's thrombasthenia. *Br J Haematol* 1974; **28**: 253–260

39. Phillips DR, Agin PP. Platelet membrane defects in Glanzmann's thrombasthenia. Evidence for decreased amounts of two major glycoproteins. *J Clin Invest* 1977; **60**: 535–545

40. George JN, Nurden AT, Phillips DR. Molecular defects in interactions of platelets with the vessel wall. *N Engl J Med* 1984; **311**: 1084–1098

41. Mustard JF, Kinlough-Rathbone RL, Packham MA, Perry D, Harfenist EJ, Pai KRM. Comparison of fibrinogen association with normal and thrombasthenic platelets on exposure to ADP or chymotrypsin. *Blood* 1979; **54**: 987–993

42. Peerschke EI, Zucker MB, Grant RA, Egan JJ, Johnson MM. Correlation between fibrinogen binding to human platelets and platelet aggregability. *Blood* 1980; **55**: 841–847

43. George JN, Caen JP, Nurden AT. Glanzmann's thrombasthenia: the spectrum of clinical disease. *Blood* 1990; **75**: 1383–1395

44. Montgomery RR, Kunicki TJ, Taves C, Pidard D, Corcoran M. Diagnosis of Bernard–Soulier syndrome and Glanzmann's thrombasthenia with a monoclonal assay on whole blood. *J Clin Invest* 1983; **71**: 385–389

45. Jennings LK, Ashmun RA, Wang WC, Dockter ME. Analysis of human platelet glycoproteins IIb-IIIa in Glanzmann's thrombasthenia whole blood by flow cytometry. *Blood* 1986; **68**: 173–179

46. Warkentin TE, Powling MJ, Hardisty RM. Measurement of fibrinogen binding to platelets in whole blood by flow cytometry: a micromethod for the detection of platelet activation. *Br J Haematol* 1990; **76**: 387–394

47. Caen J. Glanzmann thrombasthenia. *Clin Hematol* 1972; **1**: 383–392

48. Sosnoski DM, Emanuel BS, Hawkins AL *et al.* Chromosomal localization of the genes for the vitronectin and fibronectin receptors alpha-subunits and for platelet glycoproteins IIb and IIIa. *J Clin Invest* 1988; **81**: 1993–1998

49. Newman PJ, Kawai Y, Montgomery RR, Kunicki TJ. Synthesis by cultured human umbilical vein endothelial cells of two proteins structurally and immunologically related to platelet membrane glycoproteins IIb and IIIa. *J Cell Biol* 1986; **103**: 81–86

50. Leeksma OC, Zandbergen-Spaargaren J, Giltay JC, Van Mourik JA. Cultured human endothelial cells synthesise a plasma membrane protein complex immunologically related to the platelet glycoprotein IIb/IIIa complex. *Blood* 1986; **67**: 1176–1180

51. Giltay JC, Leeksma OC, Breederveld C, Van Mourik JA. Normal synthesis and expression of endothelial IIb/IIIa in Glanzmann's thrombasthenia. *Blood* 1987; **69**: 809–812

52. Coller BS, Seligsohn U, Little PA. Type I Glanzmann thrombasthenia patients from the Iraqi–Jewish and Arab populations in Israel can be differentiated by platelet glycoprotein IIIa immunoblot analysis. *Blood* 1987; **69**: 1696–1703

53. Newman PJ, Seligsohn U, Lyman S, Coller BS. The molecular genetic basis of Glanzmann thrombasthenia in the Iraqi–Jewish and Arab populations in Israel. *Proc Natl Acad Sci USA* 1991; **88**: 3160–3164

54. Bray PF. Inherited diseases of platelet glycoproteins: considerations for rapid molecular characterizati. *Thromb Haemostasis* 1994; **72**: 492–502

55. Ginsberg MH, Lightsey A, Kunicki TJ, Kaufmann A, Marguerie G, Plow EF. Divalent cation regulation of the surface orientation of platelet membrane glycoprotein IIb. Correlation with fibrinogen binding function and definition of a novel variant of Glanzmann's thrombasthenia. *J Clin Invest* 1986; **78**: 1103–1111

56. Ginsberg MH, Frelinger AL, Lam SCT *et al.* Analysis of platelet aggregation disorders based on flow cytometric analysis of membrane glycoprotein IIb-IIIa with conformation-specific monoclonal antibodies. *Blood* 1990; **76**: 2017–2023

57. Kunicki TJ, Pidard D, Cazenave JP, Nurden AT, Caen J. Inheritance

of the human alloantigen Pl^{A1} in type I Glanzmann's thrombasthenia. *J Clin Invest* 1981; **62**: 717–724

58. Stormorken H, Gogstad G, Solum NO, Pande H. Diagnosis of heterozygotes in Glanzmann's thrombasthenia. *Thromb Haemostasis* 1982; **48**: 217–221

59. Coller BS, Seligsohn U, Zivelin A, Zwang E, Lusky A, Modan M. Immunologic and biochemical characterization of homozygous and heterozygous Glanzmann thrombasthenia in the Iraqi–Jewish and Arab populations of Israel: comparison of techniques for carrier detection. *Br J Haematol* 1986; **62**: 723–735

60. Peretz H, Seligsohn U, Zwang E, Coller BS, Newman PJ. Detection of the Glanzmann's thrombasthenia mutations in Arab and Iraqi–Jewish patients by polymerase chain reaction and restriction analysis of blood or urine samples. *Thromb Haemostasis* 1991; **66**: 500–504

61. Seligsohn U, Mibashan RS, Rodeck CH, Nicolaides KH, Millar DS, Coller BS. Prenatal diagnosis of Glanzmann's thrombasthenia. *Lancet* 1985; **ii**: 1419 (letter)

62. Kaplan C, Patereau C, Reznikoff-Etievant MF, Muller JY, Dumez Y, Kesseler A. Antenatal Pl^{A1} typing and detection of GPIIb-IIIa complex. *Br J Haematol* 1985; **60**: 586–588

63. Wautier JL, Gruel Y. Prenatal diagnosis of platelet disorders. *Baillière's Clin Haematol* 1989; **2**: 569–583

64. Champeix P, Forestier F, Daffos F, Kaplan C. Prenatal diagnosis of a molecular variant of Glanzmann's thrombasthenia. *Curr Studies Hematol Blood Transfusion* 1988; **55**: 180–183

65. Seligsohn U, Mibashan RS, Rodeck CH et al. Prevention program of type I Glanzmann's thrombasthenia in Israel: prenatal diagnosis. *Curr Studies Hematol Blood Transfusion* 1988; **55**: 174–179

66. Bellucci S, Devergie A, Gluckman E et al. Complete correction of Glanzmann's thrombasthenia by allogeneic bone-marrow transplantation. *Br J Haematol* 1985; **59**: 635–641

67. Johnson A, Goodall AH, Downie CJ, Vellodi A, Michael DP. Bone marrow transplantation for Glanzmann's thrombasthenia. *Bone Marrow Transplant* 1994; **14**: 147–150

68. Slichter SJ. Platelet transfusions a constantly evolving therapy. *Thromb Haemostasis* 1991; **66**: 178–188

69. Bernard J, Soulier JP. Sur une nouvelle variété de dystrophie thrombocytaire hémorrhagipare congenitale. *Semaine Hôpitaux Paris* 1948; **24**: 3217–3223

70. Howard MA, Hutton RA, Hardisty RM. Hereditary giant platelet syndrome: a disorder of a new aspect of platelet function. *Br Med J* 1973; **2**: 586–588

71. Caen JP, Nurden AT, Jeanneau C et al. Bernard–Soulier syndrome—a new platelet glycoprotein abnormality. Its relationship with platelet adhesion to subendothelium and with the factor VIII von Willebrand protein. *J Lab Clin Med* 1976; **87**: 586–596

72. Bithell TC, Parekh SJ, Strong RR. Platelet function in the Bernard–Soulier syndrome. *Ann NY Acad Sci* 1972; **201**: 145–160

73. Gröttum KA, Solum NO. Congenital thrombocytopenia with giant platelets: a defect in the platelet membrane. *Br J Haematol* 1969; **16**: 277–290

74. Nurden AT, Caen JP. Specific roles for platelet surface glycoproteins in platelet function. *Nature* 1975; **253**: 720–722

75. Roth GJ. Developing relationships: arterial platelet adhesion, glycoprotein Ib, and leucine-rich glycoproteins. *Blood* 1991; **77**: 5–19

76. Lopez JA. The platelet glycoprotein Ib-IX complex. *Blood Coag Fibrinol* 1994; **5**: 97–119

77. Modderman PW, Admiraal LG, Sonnenberg A, von dem Borne AEGK. Glycoproteins V and Ib-IX form a non-covalent complex in the platelet membrane. *J Biol Chem* 1992; **267**: 364–369

78. Sakariassen KS, Bolhuis PA, Sixma JJ. Human blood platelet adhesion to artery subendothelium is mediated by factor VIII-von Willebrand factor bound to the subendothelium. *Nature* 1979; **279**: 636–638

79. Weiss HJ, Turitto VT, Baumgartner HR. Effect of shear rate on platelet interaction with subendothelium in citrated and native blood. I. Shear rate-dependent decrease of adhesion in von Willebrand's disease and the Bernard–Soulier syndrome. *J Lab Clin Med* 1978; **92**: 750–764

80. Perret B, Levy-Toledano S, Plantavid M et al. Abnormal phospholipid organization in Bernard–Soulier platelets. *Thromb Res* 1983; **31**: 529–537

81. Walsh PN, Mills DCB, Pareti F et al. Hereditary giant platelet syndrome: absence of collagen activity and deficiency of factor XI binding to platelets. *Br J Haematol* 1975; **29**: 639–655

82. Bevers EM, Comfurius P, Nieuwenhuis HK et al. Platelet prothrombin converting activity in hereditary disorders of platelet function. *Br J Haematol* 1986; **63**: 335–345

83. Jamieson GA, Okumura T. Reduced thrombin binding and aggregation in Bernard–Soulier platelets. *J Clin Invest* 1978; **61**: 861–864

84. Gralnick HR, Williams S, McKeown LP, Hansmann K, Fenton JW II, Krutsch H. High-affinity α-thrombin binding to platelet glycoprotein Ibα: identification of two binding domains. *Proc Natl Acad Sci USA* 1994; **91**: 6334–6338

85. Kunicki TJ, Johnson MM, Aster RH. Absence of the platelet receptor for drug-dependent antibodies in the Bernard–Soulier syndrome. *J Clin Invest* 1978; **62**: 716–719

86. Berndt MC, Chong BH, Bull HA, Zola H, Castaldi PA. Molecular characterization of quinine/quinidine drug-dependent antibody platelet interaction using monoclonal antibodies. *Blood* 1985; **66**: 1292–1301

87. Stricker RB, Shuman MA. Quinidine purpura: evidence that glycoprotein V is a target platelet antigen. *Blood* 1986; **67**: 1377–1381

88. Furihata K, Hunter J, Aster RH, Koewing GR, Shulman NR, Kunicki TJ. Human anti-PlE1 antibody recognises epitopes associated with the alpha subunit of platelet glycoprotein Ib. *Br J Haematol* 1988; **68**: 103–110

89. White JG, Burris SM, Hasegawa D, Johnson M. Micropipette aspiration of human blood platelets: a defect in Bernard–Soulier's syndrome. *Blood* 1984; **63**: 1249–1252

90. Fox JEB. Linkage of a membrane skeleton to integral membrane glycoproteins in human platelets. Identification of one of the glycoproteins as GPIb. *J Clin Invest* 1985; **76**: 1673–1683

91. Bernard J. History of congenital hemorrhagic thrombocytopathic dystrophy. *Blood Cells* 1983; **9**: 179–193

92. Lopez J, Leung B, Reynolds CC, Li CQ, Fox JB. Efficient plasma membrane expression of a functional platelet glycoprotein Ib-IX complex requires the presence of its three subunits. *J Biol Chem* 1992; **267**: 12851–12859

93. Miller JL, Lyle VA, Cunningham D. Mutation of leucine-57 to phenylalanine in a platelet glycoprotein Ibα leucine tandem repeat occurring in patients with an autosomal dominant variant of Bernard–Soulier disease. *Blood* 1992; **79**: 439–446

94. Ware J, Russell SR, Marchese P et al. Point mutation in a leucine-rich repeat of platelet glycoprotein Ibα resulting in the Bernard–Soulier syndrome. *J Clin Invest* 1993; **92**: 1213–1220

95. Wright SD, Michaelides K, Johnson DJ, West NC, Tuddenham EG. Double heterozygosity for mutations in the platelet glycoprotein IX gene in three siblings with Bernard–Soulier syndrome. *Blood* 1993; **81**: 2339–2347

96. George JN, Reimann TA, Moake JL, Morgan RK, Cimo PL, Sears DA. Bernard–Soulier disease: a study of four patients and their parents. *Br J Haematol* 1981; **48**: 459–467

97. Miller JL, Castella A. Platelet-type von Willebrand's disease: characterization of a new bleeding disorder. *Blood* 1982; **60**: 790–794

98. Weiss HJ, Meyer D, Rabinowitz R et al. Pseudo-von Willebrand's disease. An intrinsic platelet defect with aggregation by unmodified human factor VIII/von Willebrand factor and enhanced absorption of its high-molecular-weight multimers. *N Engl J Med* 1982; **306**: 326–333

99. Miller JL, Cunningham D, Lyle VA, Finch CA. Mutation in the gene encoding the α chain of platelet glycoprotein Ib in platelet-type von Willebrand disease. *Proc Natl Acad Sci USA* 1991; **88**: 4761–4765

100. Russell SD, Roth GJ. Pseudo-von Willebrand disease: a mutation in

the platelet glycoprotein Ibα gene associated with a hyperactive surface receptor. *Blood* 1993; **81**: 1787–1791

101. Takahashi H. Replacement therapy in platelet-type von Willebrand disease. *Am J Hematol* 1985; **18**: 351–362

102. Nieuwenhuis HK, Akkerman JWN, Houdijk WPM, Sixma JJ. Human blood platelets showing no reponse to collagen fail to express surface glycoprotein Ia. *Nature* 1985; **318**: 470–472

103. Kehrel B, Balleisen L, Kokott R *et al.* Deficiency of intact thrombospondin and membrane glycoprotein Ia in platelets with defective collagen-induced aggregation and spontaneous loss of disorder. *Blood* 1988; **71**: 1074–1078

104. Yamamoto N, Ikeda H, Tandon NN *et al.* A platelet membrane glycoprotein (GP) deficiency in healthy blood donors: Nak^a-platelets lack detectable GP IV (CD 36). *Blood* 1990; **76**: 1698–1703

105. Moroi M, Jung SM, Okuma M, Shinmyoza K. A patient with platelets deficient in glycoprotein VI that lack both collagen-induced aggregation and adhesion. *J Clin Invest* 1989; **84**: 1440–1445

106. Ryo R, Yoshida A, Sugano W *et al.* Deficiency of P62, a putative collagen receptor, in platelets from a patient with defective collagen-induced platelet aggregation. *Am J Hematol* 1992; **39**: 25–31

107. Weiss HJ, Vicic WJ, Lages BA, Rogers J. Isolated deficiency of platelet procoagulant activity. *Am J Med* 1979; **67**: 206–213

108. Miletich JP, Kane WH, Hofmann SL, Stanford N, Majerus PW. Deficiency of factor Xa-factor Va binding sites on the platelets of a patient with a bleeding disorder. *Blood* 1979; **54**: 1015–1022

109. Rosing J, Bevers EM, Comfurius P *et al.* Impaired factor X- and prothrombin activation associated with decreased phospholipid exposure in platelets from a patient with a bleeding disorder. *Blood* 1985; **65**: 1557–1561

110. Sims PJ, Wiedmer T, Esmon CT, Weiss HJ, Shattil SJ. Assembly of the platelet prothrombinase complex is linked to vesiculation of the platelet plasma membrane. Studies in Scott syndrome: an isolated defect in platelet procoagulant activity. *J Biol Chem* 1989; **264**: 17049–17057

111. Bevers EM, Wiedmer T, Comfurius P *et al.* Defective Ca^{2+}-induced microvesiculation and deficient expression of procoagulant activity in erythrocytes from a patient with a bleeding disorder: a study of the red blood cells of Scott syndrome. *Blood* 1992; **79**: 380–388

112. Toti F, Satta N, Fressinaud E, Meyer D, Freyssinet JM. Scott syndrome, characterized by impaired transmembrane migration of procoagulant phosphatidylserine and hemorrhagic complications, is an inherited disorder. *Blood* 1996; **87**: 1409–1415

113. Tracy PB, Giles AR, Mann KG, Eide LL, Hoogendoorn H, Rivard GE. Factor V (Quebec): a bleeding diathesis associated with a qualitative platelet factor V deficiency. *J Clin Invest* 1984; **74**: 1221–1228

114. Hayward CPM, Rivard GE, Kane WH *et al.* An autosomal dominant, qualitative platelet disorder associated with multimerin deficiency, abnormalities in platelet factor V, thrombospondin, von Willebrand factor and fibrinogen and an epinephrine aggregation defect. *Blood* 1996; **87**: 4967–4978

115. Hayward CP, Furmaniak-Kazmierczak E, Cieutat AM *et al.* Factor V is complexed with multimerin in resting platelet lysates and colocalizes with multimerin in platelet alpha-granules. *J Biol Chem* 1995; **270**: 19217–19224

116. Weiss HJ, Witte LD, Kaplan KL *et al.* Heterogeneity in storage pool deficiency: studies on granule-bound substances in 18 patients including variants deficient in α-granules, platelet factor 4, β-thromboglobulin and platelet-derived growth factor. *Blood* 1979; **54**: 1296–1319

117. Ingerman CM, Smith JB, Shapiro S, Sedar A, Silver MJ. Hereditary abnormality of platelet aggregation attributable to nucleotide storage pool deficiency. *Blood* 1978; **52**: 332–344

118. Minkes MS, Joist JH, Needleman P. Arachidonic acid-induced platelet aggregation independent of ADP-release in a patient with a bleeding disorder due to platelet storage pool disease. *Thromb Res* 1979; **15**: 169–179

119. Nieuwenhuis HK, Akkerman JWN, Sixma JJ. Patients with a pro-

longed bleeding time and normal aggregation tests may have storage pool deficiency: studies on one hundred and six patients. *Blood* 1987; **70**: 620–623

120. Rendu F, Nurden AT, Lebret M, Caen JP. Relationship between mepacrine-labelled dense body number, platelet capacity to accumulate ^{14}C-5HT and platelet density in the Bernard–Soulier and Hermansky–Pudlak syndromes. *Thromb Haemostasis* 1979; **42**: 694–704

121. Gordon N, Thom J, Cole C, Baker R. Rapid detection of hereditary and acquired platelet storage pool deficiency by flow cytometry. *Br J Haematol* 1995; **89**: 117–123

122. Holmsen H, Weiss HJ. Secretable storage pools in platelets. *Annu Rev Med* 1979; **30**: 119–134

123. Hardisty RM, Mills DCB, Ketsa-Ard K. The platelet defect associated with albinism. *Br J Haematol* 1972; **23**: 679–692

124. Gerrard JM, Lint D, Sims PJ *et al.* Identification of a platelet dense granule membrane protein that is deficient in a patient with Hermansky–Pudlak syndrome. *Blood* 1991; **77**: 101–112

125. Nishibori M, Cham B, McNicol A, Shalev A, Jain N, Gerrard JM. The protein CD 63 is in platelet dense granules, is deficient in a patient with Hermansky–Pudlak syndrome, and appears identical to granulophysin. *J Clin Invest* 1993; **91**: 1775–1782

126. Weiss HJ, Chervenick PA, Zalusky R, Factor A. A familial defect in platelet function associated with impaired release of adenosine diphosphate. *N Engl J Med* 1969; **281**: 1264–1270

127. Maurer HM, Still WJS, Caul J. Familial bleeding tendency associated with microcytic platelets and impaired release of platelet adenosine diphosphate. *J Pediatr* 1971; **78**: 86–94

128. McNicol A, Israels SJ, Robertson C, Gerrard JM. The empty sack syndrome: a platelet storage pool deficiency associated with empty dense granules. *Br J Haematol* 1994; **86**: 574–582

129. Hermansky F, Pudlak P. Albinism associated with hemorrhagic diathesis and unusual pigmented reticular cells in the bone marrow: report of two cases with histochemical studies. *Blood* 1959; **14**: 162–169

130. Davies B, Tuddenham EGD. Familial pulmonary fibrosis associated with oculocutaneous albinism and platelet function defect. *Q J Med* 1976; **45**: 219–232

131. Garay SM, Gardella JE, Fazzini EP, Goldring RM. Hermansky–Pudlak syndrome: pulmonary manifestations of a ceroid storage disorder. *Am J Med* 1979; **66**: 737–747

132. White JG, Edson JR, Desnick SJ, Witkop CJ. Studies of platelets in a variant of the Hermansky–Pudlak syndrome. *Am J Pathol* 1971; **63**: 319–332

133. Rendu F, Breton-Gorius J, Trugnan G *et al.* Studies on a new variant of the Hermansky–Pudlak syndrome: qualitative, ultrastuctural and functional abnormalities of the platelet-dense bodies associated with a phospholipase A defect. *Am J Haematol* 1978; **4**: 387–399

134. Weiss HJ, Lages B. Platelet malondialdehyde production and aggregation responses induced by arachidonate, prostaglandin-G$_2$, collagen and epinephrine in 12 patients with storage pool deficiency. *Blood* 1981; **58**: 27–33

135. Weiss HJ, Lages B, Vicic W, Tsung LY, White JG. Heterogeneous abnormalities of platelet dense granule ultrastructure in 20 patients with congenital storage pool deficiency. *Br J Haematol* 1993; **83**: 282–295

136. Shalev A, Michaud G, Israels SJ *et al.* Quantification of a novel dense granule protein (granulophysin) in platelets of patients with dense granule storage pool deficiency. *Blood* 1992; **80**: 1231–1237

137. Gerritsen SM, Akkerman JWN, Nijmeijer B, Sixma JJ, Witkop CJ, White J. The Hermansky–Pudlak syndrome: evidence for a lowered 5-hydroxytryptamine content in platelets of heterozygotes. *Scand J Haematol* 1977; **18**: 249–256

138. Buchanan GR, Handin RI. Platelet function in the Chédiak–Higashi syndrome. *Blood* 1976; **47**: 941–948

139. Boxer GJ, Holmsen H, Robkin L, Bang NU, Boxer LA, Baehner RL. Abnormal platelet function in Chédiak–Higashi syndrome. *Br J Haematol* 1977; **35**: 521–533

140. Rendu F, Breton-Gorius J, Lebret M *et al.* Evidence that abnormal

platelet functions in human Chédiak–Higashi syndrome are the result of a lack of dense bodies. *Am J Pathol* 1983; **111**: 307–314

141. Apitz-Castro R, Cruz MR, Ledezma E *et al*. The storage pool deficiency in platelets from humans with the Chédiak–Higashi syndrome: study of six patients. *Br J Haematol* 1985; **59**: 471–483

142. Parmley RT, Poon MS, Crist WM, Malluh A. Giant platelet granules in a child with the Chédiak–Higashi syndrome. *Am J Hematol* 1979; **6**: 51–60

143. White JG. Platelet microtubules and giant granules in the Chédiak–Higashi syndrome. *Am J Med Technol* 1978; **44**: 273–278

144. Gröttum KA, Hovig T, Holmsen H, Abrahamsen AF, Jeremic M, Seip M. Wiskott–Aldrich syndrome: quantitative platelet defects and short platelet survival. *Br J Haematol* 1969; **17**: 373–388

145. Stormorken H, Hellum B, Egeland T, Abrahamsen TG, Hovig T. X-linked thrombocytopenia and thrombocytopathia: attenuated Wiskott–Aldrich syndrome. Functional and morphological studies of platelets and lymphocytes. *Thromb Haemostasis* 1991; **65**: 300–305

146. Murphy S, Oski FA, Naiman L, Lusch CJ, Goldberg S, Gardner FH. Platelet size and kinetics in hereditary and acquired thrombocytopenia. *N Engl J Med* 1972; **286**: 499–504

147. Ochs HD, Slichter SJ, Harker LA, von Behrens WE, Clark RA, Wedgwood RJ. The Wiskott–Aldrich syndrome: studies of lymphocytes, granulocytes, and platelets. *Blood* 1980; **55**: 243–252

148. Akkerman JWN, Van Brederode W, Gorter G, Zegers BJM, Kuis W. The Wiskott–Aldrich syndrome: studies on a possible defect in mitochondrial ATP resynthesis in platelets. *Br J Haematol* 1982; **51**: 561–568

149. Parkman R, Remold-O'Donnell E, Kenney DM, Perrine S, Rosen FS. Surface protein abnormalities in lymphocytes and platelets from patients with Wiskott–Aldrich syndrome. *Lancet* 1981; **ii**: 1387–1389

150. Pidard D, Didry D, Le Deist F *et al*. Analysis of the membrane glycoproteins of platelets in the Wiskott–Aldrich syndrome. *Br J Haematol* 1988; **69**: 529–535

151. Day HJ, Holmsen H. Platelet adenine nucleotide 'storage pool deficiency' in thrombocytopenic absent radii syndrome. *JAMA* 1972; **221**: 1053–1054

152. Lages B, Shattil SJ, Bainton DF, Weiss HJ. Decreased content and surface expression of alpha-granule membrane protein GMP-140 in one of two types of platelet *al*pha delta storage pool deficiency. *J Clin Invest* 1991; **87**: 919–929

153. Gerrard JM, Israels ED, Bishop AJ *et al*. Inherited platelet storage pool deficiency associated with a high incidence of acute myeloid leukaemia. *Br J Haematol* 1991; **79**: 246–255

154. Raccuglia G. Gray platelet syndrome. A variety of qualitative platelet disorder. *Am J Med* 1971; **51**: 818–828

155. Kurstjens R, Bolt C, Vossen M, Haanen C. Familial thrombopathic thrombocytopenia. *Br J Haematol* 1968; **15**: 305–317

156. Libanska J, Falcão L, Gautier A *et al*. Thrombocytopénie thrombocytopathique hypogranulaire héréditaire. *Nouv Rev Française Hématol* 1975; **15**: 165–182

157. White JG. Ultrastructural studies of the gray platelet syndrome. *Am J Pathol* 1979; **95**: 445–462

158. Gerrard JM, Phillips DR, Rao GHR *et al*. Biochemical studies of two patients with the gray platelet syndrome. Selective deficiency of platelet alpha granules. *J Clin Invest* 1980; **66**: 102–109

159. Cramer EM, Vainchenker W, Vinci G, Guichard J, Breton-Gorius J. Gray platelet syndrome: immunoelectron microscopic localization of fibrinogen and von Willebrand factor in platelets and megakaryocytes. *Blood* 1985; **66**: 1309–1316

160. Levy-Toledano S, Caen JP, Breton-Gorius J *et al*. Gray platelet syndrome: α-granule deficiency. Its influence on platelet function. *J Lab Clin Med* 1981; **98**: 831–848

161. Nurden AT, Kunicki TJ, Dupuis D, Soria C, Caen JP. Specific protein and glycoprotein deficiencies in platelets isolated from two patients with the gray platelet syndrome. *Blood* 1982; **59**: 709–718

162. Breton-Gorius J, Vainchenker W, Nurden A, Levy-Toledano S, Caen J. Defective α-granule production in megakaryocytes from gray plate-let syndrome. Ultrastructural studies of bone marrow cells and megakaryocytes growing in culture from blood precursors. *Am J Pathol* 1981; **102**: 10–19

163. Drouet L, Praloran V, Cywiner-Golenzer C *et al*. Déficit congénital en α-granules plaquettaires et fibrose reticulinique médullaire. Hypothèse physiopathogenique. *Nouv Rev Française Hématol* 1981; **23**: 95–100

164. Facon T, Goudemand J, Caron C *et al*. Simultaneous occurrence of grey platelet syndrome and idiopathic pulmonary fibrosis: a role for abnormal megakaryocytes in the pathogenesis of pulmonary fibrosis? *Br J Haematol* 1990; **74**: 542–543

165. Rendu F, Marche P, Hovig T *et al* Abnormal phosphoinositide metabolism and protein phosphorylation in platelets from a patient with the gray platelet syndrome. *Br J Haematol* 1987; **67**: 199–206

166. Srivastava PC, Powling MJ, Nokes TJC, Patrick AD, Dawes J, Hardisty RM. Grey platelet syndrome: studies on platelet alpha-granules, lysosomes and defective response to thrombin. *Br J Haematol* 1987; **65**: 441–446

167. Enouf J, Lebret M, Bredoux R, Levy-Toledano S, Caen JP. Abnormal calcium transport into microsomes of grey platelet syndrome. *Br J Haematol* 1987; **65**: 437–440

168. Enouf J, Corvazier E, Papp B *et al*. Abnormal cAMP-induced phosphorylation of rap 1 protein in grey platelet syndrome platelets. *Br J Haematol* 1994; **86**: 338–346

169. Rao AK, Koike K, Willis J *et al*. Platelet secretion defect associated with impaired liberation of arachidonic acid and normal myosin light chain phosphorylation. *Blood* 1984; **64**: 914–921

170. Rao AK. Congenital disorders of platelet function. *Hematol Oncol Clin N Am* 1990; **4**: 65–86

171. Greaves M, Pickering C, Martin J, Cartwright I, Preston FE. A new familial 'giant platelet syndrome' with structural, metabolic and functional abnormalities of platelets due to a primary megakaryocyte defect. *Br J Haematol* 1987; **65**: 429–435

172. Horellou MH, Lecompte T, Lecrubier C *et al*. Familial and constitutional bleeding disorder due to platelet cyclooxygenase deficiency. *Am J Hematol* 1983; **14**: 1–9

173. Malmsten C, Hamberg M, Svensson J, Samuelsson B. Physiological role of an endoperoxide in human platelets: hemostatic defect due to platelet cyclo-oxygenase deficiency. *Proc Natl Acad Sci USA* 1975; **72**: 1446–1450

174. Lagarde M, Bryon PA, Vargaftig BB, Dechavanne M. Impairment of platelet thromboxane A_2 generation and of the platelet release reaction in two patients with congenital deficiency of platelet cyclo-oxygenase. *Br J Haematol* 1978; **38**: 251–266

175. Pareti FI, Mannucci PM, D'Angelo A, Smith JB, Sautebin L, Galli G. Congenital deficiency of thromboxane and prostacyclin. *Lancet* 1980; **i**: 898–901

176. Roth GJ, Machuga R. Radioimmune assay of human platelet prostaglandin synthetase. *J Lab Clin Med* 1982; **99**: 187–196

177. Mestel F, Oetliker O, Beck E, Felix R, Imbach P, Wagner HP. Severe bleeding associated with defective thromboxane synthetase. *Lancet* 1980; **i**: 157 (letter)

178. Defreyn G, Machin SJ, Carreras LO, Dauden MV, Chamone DAF, Vermylen J. Familial bleeding tendency with partial platelet thromboxane synthetase deficiency: variation of cyclic endoperoxide metabolism. *Br J Haematol* 1981; **49**: 29–41

179. Lages B, Weiss HJ. Heterogeneous defects of platelet secretion and responses to weak agonists in patients with bleeding disorders. *Br J Haematol* 1988; **68**: 53–62

180. Lages B, Weiss HJ. Impairment of phosphatidylinositol metabolism in a patient with a bleeding disorder associated with defects of initial platelet responses. *Thromb Haemostasis* 1988; **59**: 175–179

181. Lages B, Malmsten C, Weiss HJ, Samuelsson B. Impaired platelet response to thromboxane A_2 and defective calcium mobilization in a patient with a bleeding disorder. *Blood* 1981; **57**: 545–552

182. Speiser-Ellerton S, Weiss HJ. Studies on platelet protein phosphorylation in patients with impaired responses to platelet agonists. *J Lab Clin Med* 1990; **115**: 104–111

183. Rao AK, Kowalska MA, Disa J. Impaired cytoplasmic ionized calcium mobilization in inherited platelet secretion defects. *Blood* 1989; **74**: 664–672

184. Rao AK, Disa J, Yang X. Concomitant defect in internal release and influx of calcium in patients with congenital platelet function and impaired agonist-induced calcium mobilization. Thromboxane production is not required for internal release of calcium. *J Lab Clin Med* 1993; **121**: 52–63

185. Yang X, Lee SB, Lee KH *et al.* Human platelet signaling defect Characterized by diminished inositol phosphate production, pleckstrin phosphorylation and expression of phospholipase C-β_2 isozyme. *Blood* 1995; **86**: 547A

186. Hirata T, Kakizuka A, Ushikubi F, Fuse I, Okuma M, Narumiya S. Arg^{60} to Leu mutation of the human thromboxane A_2 receptor in a dominantly inherited bleeding disorder. *J Clin Invest* 1994; **94**: 1662–1667

187. O'Brien JR. Variability in the aggregation of human platelets by adrenaline. *Nature* 1964; **202**: 1188–1190

188. Scrutton MC, Clare KA, Hutton RA, Bruckdorfer KR. Depressed responsiveness to adrenaline in platelets from apparently normal human donors: a familial trait. *Br J Haematol* 1981; **49**: 303–314

189. Gaxiola B, Friedl W, Propping P. Epinephrine-induced platelet aggregation. A twin study. *Clin Genet* 1984; **26**: 543–548

190. Stormorken H, Gogstad G, Solum NO. A new bleeding disorder: lack of platelet aggregatory response to adrenalin and lack of secondary aggregation to ADP and platelet activating factor (PAF). *Thromb Res* 1983; **29**: 391–402

191. Mielke CH Jr, Levine PH, Zucker S. Preoperative prednisone therapy in platelet function disorders. *Thromb Res* 1981; **21**: 655–662

192. Gerritsen SW, Akkerman JWN, Sixma JJ. Correction of the bleeding time in patients with storage pool deficiency by infusion of cryoprecipitate. *Br J Haematol* 1978; **40**: 153–160

193. Kobrinsky NL, Israels ED, Gerrard JM *et al.* Shortening of bleeding time by 1-deamino-8-D-arginine vasopressin in various bleeding disorders. *Lancet* 1984; **i**: 1145–1148

194. Schulman S, Johnsson H, Egberg N, Blombäck M. DDAVP-induced correction of prolonged bleeding time in patients with congenital platelet function defects. *Thromb Res* 1987; **45**: 165–174

195. Nieuwenhuis HK, Sixma JJ. 1-desamino-8-D-arginine vasopressin (desmopressin) shortens the bleeding time in storage pool deficiency. *Ann Intern Med* 1988; **108**: 65–67

196. Rao AK, Ghosh S, Sun L *et al.* Mechanisms of platelet dysfunction and response to DDAVP in patients with congenital platelet function defects. A double-blind placebo-controlled trial. *Thromb Haemostasis* 1995; **74**: 1071–1078

197. Cattaneo M, Pareti F, Zighetti ML, Lecchi A, Lombardi R, Mannucci PM. Platelet aggregation at high shear is impaired in patients with congenital defects of platelet secretion and is corrected by DDAVP: correlation with the bleeding time. *J Lab Clin Med* 1995; **125**: 540–547

198. Sloand EM, Alyono D, Klein HG *et al.* 1-deamino-8-D-arginine vasopressin (DDAVP) increases platelet membrane expression of glycoprotein Ib in patients with disorders of platelet function and after cardiopulmonary bypass. *Am J Hematol* 1994; **46**: 199–207

199. Pfueller SL, Howard MA, White JG, Menon C, Berry EW. Shortening of bleeding time by 1-deamino-8-arginine vasopressin (DDAVP) in the absence of platelet von Willebrand factor in gray platelet syndrome. *Thromb Haemostasis* 1987; **58**: 1060–1063

200. Lacombe M, D'Angelo G. Etudes sur une thrombopathie familiale. *Nouv Rev Française Hématol* 1963; **3**: 611–614

201. Milton JG, Frojmovic MM. Shape-changing agents produce abnormally large platelets in a hereditary 'giant platelets syndrome' (MPS). *J Lab Clin Med* 1979; **93**: 154161

202. Milton JG, Frojmovic MM, Tang SS, White JG. Spontaneous platelet aggregation in a hereditary giant platelet syndrome (MPS). *Am J Pathol* 1984; **114**: 336–345

203. Milton JG, Hutton RA, Tuddenham EGD, Frojmovic MM. Platelet

204. Okita JR, Frojmovic MM, Kristopeit S, Wong T, Kunicki TJ. Montreal platelet syndrome: a defect in calcium-activated neutral protease (calpain). *Blood* 1989; **74**: 715–721

205. Hamilton RW, Shaikh BS, Ottie JN, Storch AE, Saleem A, White JG. Platelet function, ultrastucture and survival in the May–Hegglin anomaly. *Am J Clin Pathol* 1980; **74**: 663–668

206. Epstein CJ, Sahud MA, Piel CF *et al.* Hereditary macrothrombocytopathia, nephritis and deafness. *Am J Med* 1972; **52**: 299–310

207. Bernheim J, Dechavanne M, Bryon PA *et al.* Thrombocytopenia, macrothrombocytopathia, nephritis and deafness. *Am J Med* 1976; **61**: 145–150

208. Clare NM, Montiel MM, Lifshitz MD, Bannayan GA. Alport's syndrome associated with macrothrombopathic thrombocytopenia. *Am J Clin Pathol* 1979; **72**: 111–117

209. Peterson LA, Rao KV, Crosson JT, White JG. Fechtner syndrome—a variant of Alport's syndrome with leukocyte inclusions and macrothrombocytopenia. *Blood* 1985; **65**: 397–406

210. Greinacher A, Nieuwenhuis HK, White JG. Sebastian platelet syndrome: a new variant of hereditary macrothrombocytopenia with leukocyte inclusions. *Blut* 1990; **61**: 282–288

211. Stewart GW, O'Brien H, Morris SA, Owen JS, Lloyd JK, Ames JAL. Stomatocytosis, abnormal platelets and pseudo-homozygous hypercholesterolaemia. *Eur J Haematol* 1987; **38**: 376–380

212. Dowton SB, Beardsley D, Jamison D, Blattner S, Li FP. Studies of a familial platelet disorder. *Blood* 1985; **65**: 557–563

213. Lott IT, Chase TN, Murphy DL. Down's syndrome: transport, storage and metabolism of serotonin in blood platelets. *Pediatr Res* 1972; **6**: 730–735

214. McCoy EE, Snedden JM. Decreased calcium content and $^{45}\text{Ca}^{2+}$ uptake in Down's syndrome blood platelets. *Pediatr Res* 1984; **18**: 914–916

215. Yarom R, Muhlrad A, Hodges A, Robin GC. Platelet pathology in patients with idiopathic scoliosis: ultrastructural morphometry, aggregation, x-ray spectrometry and biochemical analysis. *Lab Invest* 1980; **43**: 208–216

216. Karaca M, Cronberg L, Nilsson IM. Abnormal platelet-collagen reaction in Ehlers–Danlos syndrome. *Scand J Haematol* 1972; **9**: 465–469

217. Furcht LT, Wendelschafer-Crabb G, Mosher DF, Arneson M, Hammerschmidt D, Woodbridge P. The role of fibronectin in normal platelet aggregation and demonstration of an inherited disease with defective platelet aggregation correctable with normal fibronectin. *J Cell Biol* 1979; **83**: 61A

218. Pope FM, Martin GR, Lichtenstein JR *et al.* Patients with Ehlers–Danlos syndrome type IV lack type III collagen. *Proc Natl Acad Sci USA* 1975; **72**: 1314–1316

219. Solomon LR, Bobinski H, Astley P, Goldby FS, Mallick NP. Bartter's syndrome—observation on the pathophysiology. *Q J Med* 1982; **51**: 251–270

220. Remuzzi G. Bleeding in renal failure. *Lancet* 1988; **i**: 1205–1208

221. Castaldi PA, Rozenberg MC, Stewart JH. The bleeding disorder of uraemia. *Lancet* 1966; **ii**: 66–69

222. Di Minno G, Martinez J, McKean MR *et al.* Platelet dysfunction in uremia. Multifaceted defect partially corrected by dialysis. *Am J Med* 1985; **79**: 552–559

223. Castillo R, Lozano T, Escolar G, Revert L, Lopez J, Ordinas A. Defective platelet adhesion on vessel subendothelium in uremic patients. *Blood* 1986; **68**: 337–342

224. Sloand EM, Sloand JA, Prodouz K *et al.* Reduction of platelet glycoprotein Ib in uraemia. *Br J Haematol* 1991; **77**: 375–381

225. Ware JA, Clark BA, Smith M, Salzman EW. Abnormalities of cytoplasmic Ca^{2+} in platelets from patients with uremia. *Blood* 1989; **73**: 172–176

226. Remuzzi G, Benigni A, Dodesini P *et al.* Reduced platelet thromboxane formation in uremia. Evidence for a functional cyclooxygenase defect. *J Clin Invest* 1983; **71**: 762–768

size and shape in hereditary giant platelet syndromes on blood smear and in suspension. *J Lab Clin Med* 1985; **106**: 326–335

227. Stewart JH, Castaldi PA. Uraemic bleeding: a reversible platelet defect corrected by dialysis. *Q J Med* 1967; **36**: 409–423

228. Remuzzi G, Livio M, Marchiaro G, Mecca G, De Gaetano G. Bleeding in renal failure: altered platelet function in chronic uraemia only partially corrected by haemodialysis. *Nephron* 1978; **22**: 347–353

229. Eknoyan G, Wacksman SJ, Glueck HI, Will JJ. Platelet function in renal failure. *N Engl J Med* 1969; **280**: 677–681

230. Horowitz HI, Stein IM, Cohen BD, White JG. Further studies on the platelet inhibitory effect of guanidinosuccinic acid: its role in uremic bleeding. *Am J Med* 1970; **49**: 336–345

231. Rabiner SF, Molinas F. The role of phenol and phenolic acids on the thrombocytopathy and defective platelet aggregation of patients with renal failure. *Am J Med* 1970; **49**: 346–351

232. Bazilinski N, Shaykh M, Dunea G et al. Inhibition of platelet function by uremic middle molecules. *Nephron* 1985; **40**: 423–428

233. Deckmyn H, Proesmans W, Vermylen J. Prostacyclin production by whole *Blood* from children: impairment in the hemolytic uremic syndrome and excessive formation in chronic renal failure. *Thromb Res* 1983; **30**: 13–18

234. Kyrle PA, Stockenhuber F, Brenner B et al. Evidence for an increased generation of prostacyclin in the microvasculature and an impairment of the platelet α-granule release in chronic renal failure. *Thromb Haemostasis* 1988; **60**: 205–208

235. Remuzzi G, Benigni A, Dodesini P et al. Parathyroid hormone inhibits human platelet function. *Lancet* 1981; **ii**: 1321–1323

236. Docci D, Turci F, Delvecchio C et al. Lack of evidence for the role of secondary hyperparathyroidism in the pathogenesis of uremic thrombocytopathy. *Nephron* 1986; **43**: 28–32

237. Mannucci PM, Remuzzi G, Pusineri F et al. Deamino-8-D-arginine vasopressin shortens the bleeding time in uremia. *N Engl J Med* 1983; **308**: 8–12

238. Livio M, Gotti E, Marchesi D, Mecca G, Remuzzi G, De Gaetano G. Uraemic bleeding: role of anaemia and beneficial effect of red cell transfusions. *Lancet* 1982; **ii**: 1013–1015

239. Fernandez F, Goudable C, Sie P et al. Low haematocrit and prolonged bleeding time in uraemic patients: effect of red cell transfusions. *Br J Haematol* 1985; **59**: 139–148

240. Moia M, Vizzotto L, Cattanes M et al. Improvement of the haemostatic defect in uraemia after treatment with recombinant human erythropoietin. *Lancet* 1987; **ii**: 1227–1229

241. Van Geet C, Hauglustaine D, Verresen L, Vanrusselt M, Vermylen J. Haemostatic effects of recombinant human erythropoietin in chronic haemodialysis patients. *Thromb Haemostasis* 1989; **61**: 117–121

242. Turitto VT, Baumgartner HR. Platelet interaction with subendothelium in a perfusion system. Physical role of red blood cells. *Microvasc Res* 1975; **9**: 335–344

243. Zwaginga JJ, Ijsseldijk MJW, de Groot PG et al. Treatment of uremic anemia with recombinant erythropoietin also reduces the defects in platelet adhesion and aggregation caused by uremic plasma. *Thromb Haemostasis* 1991; **66**: 638–647

244. Zwaginga JJ, Ijsseldijk MJW, de Groot PG, Vos J, de Boskuil R, Sixma JJ. Platelet adhesion and aggregate formation are defective in the uremic blood disorder and are caused by a toxin in plasma. *Arterioscler Thromb* 1991; **11**: 733–744

245. Liu Y, Kosfeld RE, Marcum SG. Treatment of uraemic bleeding with conjugated oestrogen. *Lancet* 1984; **ii**: 887–890

246. Livio M, Mannucci PM, Vigano G et al. Conjugated estrogens for the management of bleeding associated with renal failure. *N Engl J Med* 1986; **315**: 731–735

247. Remuzzi G, Perico N, Zoja C, Corna D, Macconi D, Viganò G. Role of endothelium-derived nitric oxide in the bleeding tendency of uremia. *J Clin Invest* 1990; **86**: 1768–1771

248. Schafer AI. Bleeding and thrombosis in the myeloproliferative disorders. *Blood* 1984; **64**: 1–12

249. Gerrard JM, Stoddard SF, Shapiro RS et al. Platelet storage pool deficiency and prostaglandin synthesis in chronic granulocytic leukaemia. *Br J Haematol* 1978; **40**: 597–607

250. Rendu F, Lebret M, Nurden A, Caen JP. Detection of an acquired platelet storage pool disease in three patients with a myeloproliferative disorder. *Thromb Haemostasis* 1979; **42**: 794–796

251. Russell NH, Salmon J, Keenan JP, Bellingham AJ. Platelet adenine nucleotides and arachidonic acid metabolism in the myeloprolifetative disorders. *Thromb Res* 1981; **22**: 389–307

252. Malpass TW, Savage B, Hanson SR, Slichter SJ, Harker LA. Correlation between prolonged bleeding time and depletion of platelet dense granule ADP in patients with myelodysplastic and myeloproliferative disorders. *J Lab Clin Med* 1984; **103**: 894–904

253. Okuma M, Uchino H. Altered arachidonate metabolism by platelets in patients with myeloproliferative disorders. *Blood* 1979; **54**: 1258–1271

254. Jubelirer SJ, Russell F, Vaillancourt R, Deykin D. Platelet arachidonic acid metabolism and platelet function in ten patients with chronic myelogenous leukemia. *Blood* 1980; **56**: 728–731

255. Schafer AI. Deficiency of platelet lipoxygenase activity in myeloproliferative disorders. *N Engl J Med* 1982; **306**: 381–386

256. Walsh PN, Murphy S, Barry WE. The role of platelets in the pathogenesis of thrombosis and hemorrhage in patients with thrombocytosis. *Thromb Haemostasis* 1977; **38**: 1085–1096

257. Semeraro N, Cortellazzo S, Colucci M, Barbui T. A hitherto undescribed defect of platelet coagulant activity in polycythaemia vera and essential thrombocythaemia. *Thromb Res* 1979; **16**: 795–802

258. Cooper B, Schafer AI, Puchalsky D, Handin RI. Platelet resistance to prostaglandin D2 in patients with myeloproliferative disorders. *Blood* 1978; **52**: 618–626

259. Clezardin P, McGregor JL, Dechavanne M, Clemetson KJ. Platelet membrane glycoprotein abnormalities in patients with myeloproliferative disorders and secondary thrombocytosis. *Br J Haematol* 1985; **60**: 331–344

260. Wehmeier A, Tschöpe D, Esser J, Menzel C, Nieuwenhuis HK, Schneider W. Circulating activated platelets in myeloproliferative disorders. *Thromb Res* 1991; **61**: 271–278

261. Michelson AD. Flow cytometric analysis of platelet surface glycoproteins: phenotypically distinct subpopulations of platelets in children with chronic myeloid leukemia. *J Lab Clin Med* 1987; **110**: 346–354

262. Berndt MC, Kabral A, Grimsley P, Watson N, Robertson TI, Bradstock KF. An acquired Bernard–Soulier-like platelet defect associated with juvenile myelodysplastic syndrome. *Br J Haematol* 1988; **68**: 97–101

263. Cowan DH, Graham RC, Baunach D. The platelet defect in leukemia, platelet ultrastructure, adhesive nucleotide metabolism and the release reaction. *J Clin Invest* 1975; **56**: 188–200

264. Woodcock BE, Cooper PC, Brown PR, Pickering C, Winfield DA, Preston FE. The platelet defect in acute myeloid leukaemia. *J Clin Pathol* 1984; **37**: 1339–1342

265. Ganguly P, Sutherland SB, Bradford HR. Defective binding of thrombin to platelets in myeloid leukaemia. *Br J Haematol* 1978; **39**: 599–605

266. Fäldt R, Ankerst J, Zoukas E. Inhibition of platelet aggregation by myeloid leukaemic cells demonstrated *in vitro*. *Br J Haematol* 1987; **66**: 529–534

267. Russell NH, Keenan JP, Bellingham AJ. Thrombocytopathy in preleukaemia; association with a defect of thromboxane A2 activity. *Br J Haematol* 1979; **41**: 417–425

268. Stuart JJ, Lewis JC. Platelet aggregation and electron microscopic studies of platelets in preleukemia. *Arch Pathol Lab Med* 1982; **106**: 458–461

269. Laffi G, La Villa G, Pinzani M et al. Altered renal and platelet arachidonic acid metabolism in cirrhosis. *Gastroenterology* 1986; **90**: 274–282

270. Ordinas A, Maragall S, Castillo R, Nurden AT. A glycoprotein I defect in platelets in three patients with severe cirrhosis of the liver. *Thromb Res* 1978; **13**: 297–302

271. Mannucci P M, Vicente V, Vianello L et al. Controlled trial of

491

desmopressin in liver cirrhosis and other conditions associated with a prolonged bleeding time. *Blood* 1986; **67**: 1148–1153

272. Czapek EE, Deykin D, Salzman EW. Platelet dysfunction in glycogen storage disease type I. *Blood* 1973; **41**: 235–247

273. Corby DG, Putnam CW, Greene HL. Impaired platelet function in glucose-6-phoshatase deficiency. *J Pediatr* 1974; **85**: 71–76

274. Hutton RA, Macnab AJ, Rivers RPA. Defect of platelet function associated with chronic hypoglycaemia. *Arch Dis Child* 1976; **51**: 49–55

275. Woodman RC, Harker LA. Bleeding complications associated with cardiopulmonary bypass. *Blood* 1990; **76**: 1680–1697

276. Harker LA, Malpass TW, Branson HE, Hessel EA II, Slichter SJ. Mechanism of abnormal bleeding in patients undergoing cardiopulmonary bypass: acquired transient platelet dysfunction associated with selective α-granule release. *Blood* 1980; **56**: 824–834

277. George JN, Pickett EB, Saucerman S et al. Platelet surface glycoproteins. Studies on resting and activated platelets and platelet membrane microparticles in normal subjects and observations in patients during adult respiratory distress syndrome and cardiac surgery. *J Clin Invest* 1986; **78**: 340–348

278. Abrams CS, Ellison N, Budzynsi AZ, Shattil SJ. Direct detection of activated platelets and platelet-derived microparticles in humans. *Blood* 1990; **75**: 128–138

279. Longmore DS, Bennett G, Gueirra D et al. Prostacyclin: a solution to some problems of extracorporeal circulation. *Lancet* 1979; **i**: 1002–1005

280. Walker ID, Davidson JF, Faichney A, Wheatley DJ, Davidson KG. A double blind study of prostacyclin in cardiopulmonary bypass surgery. *Br J Haematol* 1981; **49**: 415–423

281. Salzman EW, Weinstein MJ, Weintraub RM et al. Treatment with desmopressin acetate to reduce blood loss after cardiac surgery. A double-blind randomized trial. *N Engl J Med* 1986; **314**: 1402–1406

282. Rocha E, Llorens R, Paramo JA, Arcas R, Cuesta B, Trenor AM. Does desmopressin acetate reduce blood loss after surgery in patients on cardiopulmonary bypass? *Circulation* 1988; **77**: 1319–1323

283. Hackmann T, Gascoyne RD, Naiman SC et al. A trial of desmopressin (1-desamino-8-D-arginine vasopressin) to reduce blood loss in uncomplicated cardiac surgery. *N Engl J Med* 1989; **321**: 1437–1443

284. Zahavi J, Marder VJ. Acquired 'storage pool disease' of platelets associated with circulating anti-platelet antibodies. *Am J Med* 1974; **56**: 883–890

285. Khurana MS, Lian ECY, Harkness DR. 'Storage pool disease' of platelets: association with multiple congenital cavernous hemangiomas. *JAMA* 1980; **244**: 169–171

286. Hourdillé P, Bernard P, Belloc F, Pradet A, Sanchez R, Boisseau MR. Platelet abnormalities in thermal injury. Study of platelet-dense bodies stained with mepacrine. *Haemostasis* 1981; **10**: 141–152

287. Niessner H, Clemetson KJ, Panzer S, Mueller-Eckhardt C, Santoso S, Bettelheim P. Acquired thrombasthenia due to GPIIb/IIIa-specific platelet autoantibodies. *Blood* 1986; **68**: 571–576

288. Balduini CL, Grignani G, Sinigaglia F et al. Severe platelet dysfunction in a patient with autoantibodies against membrane glycoproteins IIb-IIIa. *Haemostasis* 1987; **17**: 98–104

289. Stricker RB, Wong D, Saks SR, Corash L, Shuman MA. Acquired Bernard–Soulier syndrome. Evidence for the role of a 210 000 molecular weight protein in the interaction of platelets with von Willebrand factor. *J Clin Invest* 1985; **76**: 1274–1278

290. Deckmyn H, Chew SL, Vermylen J. Lack of platelet response to collagen associated with an autoantibody against glycoprotein Ia: a novel cause of acquired platelet dysfunction. *Thromb Haemostasis* 1990; **64**: 74–79

291. Brown CH, Natelson EA, Bradshaw MW, Williams TW, Alfrey CP. The hemostatic defect produced by carbenicillin. *N Engl J Med* 1974; **291**: 265–270

292. Shattil SJ, Bennett JS, McDonough M, Turnbull J. Carbenicillin and penicillin G inhibit platelet function in vitro by impairing the interaction of agonists with the platelet surface. *J Clin Invest* 1980; **65**: 329–337

293. Burroughs SF, Johnson GJ. β-lactam antibiotic-induced platelet dysfunction: evidence for irreversible inhibition of platelet activation *in vitro* and *in vivo* after prolonged exposure to penicillin. *Blood* 1990; **75**: 1473–1480

294. Weiss HJ. The effect of clinical dextran on platelet aggregation, adhesion, and ADP release in man: *in vivo* and *in vitro* studies. *J Lab Clin Med* 1967; **69**: 37–46

295. Evans RJ, Gordon JL. Mechanisms of the antithrombotic action of dextran. *N Engl J Med* 1974; **290**: 748 (letter)

296. Warkentin TE. Heparin-induced thrombocytopenia: IgG-mediated platelet activation, platelet microparticle generation, and altered procoagulant/anticoagulant balance in the pathogenesis of thrombosis and venous limb gangrene complicating heparin-induced thrombocytopenia. *Transfusion Med Rev* 1996; **10**: 249–258

297. Zucker MB. Heparin and platelet function. *Fed Proc* 1977; **36**: 47–49

298. Horne MK III, Chao ES. The effect of molecular weight on heparin binding to platelets. *Br J Haematol* 1990; **74**: 306–312

299. Salzman EW, Rosenberg RD, Smith MH, Lindon JN, Favreau L. Effect of heparin and heparin fractions on platelet aggregation. *J Clin Invest* 1980; **65**: 64–73

300. Levine MN, Hirsh J, Gent M et al. Prevention of deep vein thrombosis after elective hip surgery. A randomized trial comparing low molecular weight heparin with standard unfractionated heparin. *Ann Intern Med* 1991; **114**: 545–551

301. Richardson SGN, Fletcher DJ, Jeavons PM, Stuart J. Sodium valproate and platelet function. *Br Med J* 1976; **1**: 221–222

302. Parvez Z, Moncada R, Fareed J, Messmore HL. Antiplatelet action of intravascular contrast media. Implications in diagnostic procedures. *Invest Radiol* 1984; **19**: 208–211

303. Verdirame JD, Davis JW, Phillips PE. The effects of radiographic contrast agents on bleeding time and platelet aggregation. *Clin Cardiol* 1984; **7**: 31–34

304. Corby DG, Schulman I. The effects of antenatal drug administration on aggregation of platelets of newborn infants. *J Pediatr* 1971; **79**: 307–313

305. Maurer HM, Haggins JC, Still WJS. Platelet injury during phototherapy. *Am J Hematol* 1976; **1**: 89–96

306. Tschoepe D, Roesen P, Schwippert B, Gries FA. Platelets in diabetes: the role of the hemostatic regulation in atherosclerosis. *Semin Thromb Hemostasis* 1993; **19**: 122–128

307. Preston FE, Ward JD, Marcola BH, Porter NR, Timperley WR, O'Malley BC. Elevated beta-thromboglobulin levels and circulating platelet aggregates in diabetic microangiopathy. *Lancet* 1978; **i**: 238–240

308. Gerrard JM, Stuart MJ, Rao GHR et al. Alterations in the balance of prostaglandin and thromboxane synthesis in diabetes. *J Lab Clin Med* 1980; **95**: 950–958

309. Collier A, Tymkewycz P, Armstrong R, Young RJ, Jones RL, Clarke BF. Increased platelet thromboxane receptor sensitivity in diabetic patients with proliferative retinopathy. *Diabetologia* 1986; **29**: 471–474

310. Kobbah M, Ewald U, Tuvemo T. Platelet aggregation during the first year of diabetes in childhood. *Acta Paediatr Scand* 1985; **320 (Suppl)**: 50–55

311. Jackson CA, Greaves M, Boulton AJM, Ward JD, Preston FE. Near-normal glycaemic control does not correct abnormal platelet reactivity in diabetes mellitus. *Clin Sci* 1984; **67**: 551–555

312. Collier A, Tymkewycz PM, Matthews DM, Jones RL, Clarke BF. Changes in some aspects of platelet function with improvement of glycaemic control over 6 months. *Diabetes Res* 1987; **5**: 79–82

313. Stuart MJ, Elrad H, Graeber JE, Hakanson DO, Sunderji SG, Barvinchak MK. Increased synthesis of platelet malonyldialdehyde and platelet hyperfunction in infants of mothers with diabetes mellitus. *J Lab Clin Med* 1979; **94**: 12–26

314. Stuart MJ, Sunderji SG, Walenga RW, Setty BNY. Abnormalities in vascular arachidonic acid metabolism in the infant of the diabetic mother. *Br Med J* 1985; **290**: 1700–1702

315. Oppenheimer EH, Esterly JR. Thrombosis in the newborn: comparison between infants of diabetic and nondiabetic mothers. *J Pediatr* 1965; **67**: 549–556

316. Colwell JA. Clinical trials of antiplatelet agents in diabetes mellitus: rationale and results. *Semin Thromb Hemostat* 1991; **17**: 439–444

317. Cameron JS. Coagulation and thromboembolic complications in the nephrotic syndrome. *Adv Nephrol* 1984; **3**: 75–114

318. Jackson CA, Greaves M, Patterson AD, Brown CB, Preston FE. Relationship between platelet aggregation, thromboxane synthesis and albumin concentration in nephrotic syndrome. *Br J Haematol* 1982; **52**: 69–77

319. Bennett A, Cameron JS. Platelet hyperaggregability in the nephrotic syndrome which is not dependent on arachidonic acid metabolism or on plasma albumin concentration. *Clin Nephrol* 1987; **27**: 182–188

320. Machleidt C, Mettang T, Stärz E, Weber J, Risler T, Kuhlmann U. Multifactorial genesis of enhanced platelet aggregability in patients with nephrotic syndrome. *Kidney Int* 1989; **36**: 1119–1124

321. Zwaginga JJ, Koomans HA, Sixma JJ, Rabelink TJ. Thrombus formation and platelet-vessel wall interaction in the nephrotic syndrome under flow conditions. *J Clin Invest* 1994; **93**: 204–211

322. Kawasaki T, Kosaki F, Okawa S, Shigematsu I, Yanagawa H. A new infantile acute febrile mucocutaneous lymph node syndrome (MLNS) prevailing in Japan. *Pediatrics* 1974; **54**: 271–276

323. Leung DYM, Meissner HC, Fulton DR, Murray DL, Kotzin BL, Schlievert PM. Toxic shock syndrome toxin-secreting staphylococcus aureus in Kawasaki syndrome. *Lancet* 1993; **342**: 1385–1388

324. Burns JC, Glode MP, Clarke SH, Wiggins J, Hathaway WE. Coagulopathy and platelet activation in Kawasaki syndrome: identification of patients at high risk for development of coronary artery aneurysms. *J Pediatr* 1984; **105**: 206–211

325. Niwa K, Aotsuka H, Hamada H, Uchishiba M, Terai M, Niimi H. Thrombocytopenia: a risk factor for acute myocardial infarction during the acute phase of Kawasaki disease. *Coronary Artery Dis* 1995; **6**: 857–864

326. Yamada K, Fukumoto T, Shinkai A, Shirahata A, Meguro T. The platelet functions in acute febrile mucocutaneous lymph node syndrome and a trial of prevention for thrombosis by antiplatelet agents. *Acta Haematol Jpn* 1978; **41**: 113–124

327. Newburger JW, Takahashi M, Beiser AS *et al*. A single intravenous infusion of gamma globulin as compared with four infusions in the treatment of acute Kawasaki syndrome. *N Engl J Med* 1991; **324**: 1633–1639

328. Tremoli E, Maderna P, Colli S, Morazzoni G, Sirtori M, Sirtori CR. Increased platelet sensitivity and thromboxane B2 formation in type-II hyperlipoproteinaemic patients. *Eur J Clin Invest* 1984; **14**: 329–333

329. Cadroy Y, Lemozy S, Diquelou A *et al*. Human type II hyperlipoproteinemia enhances platelet-collagen adhesion in flowing nonanticoagulated blood. *Arterioscler Thromb* 1993; **13**: 1650–1653

330. Harker LA, Ross R, Slichter SJ, Scott CR. Homocystine-induced arteriosclerosis. The role of endothelial cell injury and platelet response in its genesis. *J Clin Invest* 1976; **58**: 731–741

331. Di Minno G, Davi G, Margaglione M *et al*. Abnormally high thromboxane biosynthesis in homozygous homocystinuria. Evidence for platelet involvement and probucol-sensitive mechanism. *J Clin Invest* 1993; **92**: 1440–1406

Lymphocyte disorders

Primary and acquired specific immunodeficiency diseases and disorders of opsonization

25

ADAM FINN AND ANDREW CANT

OVERVIEW OF SPECIFIC IMMUNITY

Eukaryotic organisms evolved a fundamental survival principle—manifest as the immune response—very early, namely: 'if it's inside me but isn't me, kill it before it kills me'. This process remains the unifying dogma of specific immunity because, despite important exceptions such as the mitochondria in all cells (thought to derive from exogenous microbes), individuals with immune systems which give invading microbes the benefit of the doubt do not survive well. Immune responses set clear boundaries to the hoards of microbes both outside and inside the individual. Secreted protein and phagocyte defences endeavor to inflict instant death on the invader, sometimes causing significant host tissue injury in the process, and specific immunity acts as a slower but highly organized search and destroy machinery for viruses or larger microbes which succeed in penetrating the initial defences. Individuals with inherited or acquired deficiencies in their specific immunity are rendered susceptible to unusual or abnormally frequent or severe infectious diseases.

RECOGNITION OF ANTIGEN AND HETEROGENEITY

The evolution of specific immunity in higher animals depends upon the development of a genomic machinery that can produce $> 10^8$ different clones of cells each bearing a single distinct specific receptor, so that there are lymphocytes available to recognize virtually every imaginable antigen. This is achieved using a series of genes designed (unusually) to produce somatic hypermutation by combining a single copy from a large number of alternatives lined up along the gene for each of a series of 2 or 3 segments (V, D and J) in each progenitor lymphocyte of each clone (Fig. 25.1). The large number of arithmetic possibilities allowed by this mechanism is further amplified by the combination of 2 distinct proteins at each binding site (Fig. 25.2). Finally, for immunoglobulin genes, further modification and 'improvement' of the receptor-binding site occurs by variable splicing between the gene segments and selection from the varied progeny—a process dubbed 'affinity maturation'.

Antigen recognition by the cells of the specific immune system depends therefore upon random events of gene splicing giving rise to such a large number of distinct binding receptors that, effectively, almost any distinct stereotypic epitope will be recognized. Under these circumstances it is essential that there is a mechanism to eliminate lymphocytes whose receptors recognize self antigens and this is thought to occur by a process of negative selection as lymphocytes develop in the thymus. Since 'recognition' is based on the chemical 'shape' of the epitope, there will inevitably be examples of cross-reaction between self epitopes and foreign antigens leading either to autoimmune phenomena or gaps in protection. It is thought that this results, for example, in post-infectious phenomena following Group A streptococcal infection (rheumatic fever, glomerulonephritis) and the immunologic 'invisibility' of antigens such as *Neisseria meningitidis* Group B capsular polysaccharide.

B AND T CELLS AND THE MAJOR HISTOCOMPATIBILITY COMPLEX

The gene loci for generating these diverse receptors are reduplicated. One set provides diversity for antibody production in B lymphocytes (humoral specific immunity) and the other does the same in T lymphocytes whose receptors mediate cell-mediated specific immunity. While antibodies

497

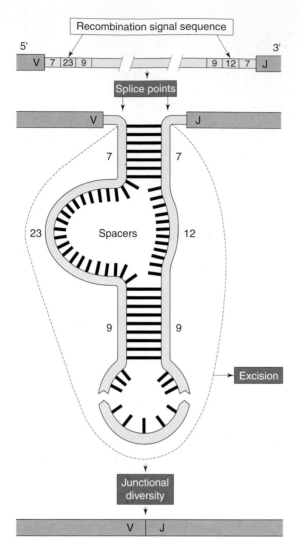

Fig. 25.1 Genetic mechanism for generating diversity in antibodies/T-cell receptors. Recombinase enzymes control recombination of a single VJ sequence at random from the many possible combinations of 70 V and 4 J sequences on the immunoglobulin light chain gene. The heavy chain gene has 100 V, 4 D and 6 J sequences. Reproduced with permission from Ref. 117.

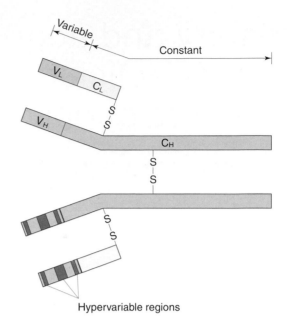

Fig. 25. 2 Structure of the immunoglobulin molecule. –S–S– = disulfide links; V = variable region; C = constant region; H = heavy chain; L = light chain. Reproduced with permission from Ref. 117.

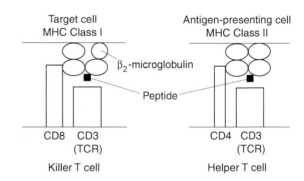

Fig 25.3 Interactions of CD3 (T-cell receptor complex) and CD8 or CD4 with Class I and Class II major histocompatibility complex (MHC), respectively.

recognize 'native' or unmodified antigens in solution, T-cell receptors are adapted to recognize and respond only to peptide antigens which are presented by host cells on surface major histocompatibility complex (MHC) antigens (Fig. 25.3). In this way T cells recognize, respond to, interact with and, under certain circumstances, kill infected host cells and host cells which have phagocytosed and internalized antigen. A process of positive selection of lymphocytes which recognize self MHC also occurs as they develop in the thymus.

While heterogeneity in T- and B-cell receptor expression occurs within individuals, heterogeneity in MHC expression occurs between individuals. The importance of this diversity to individual species, such as man, is often overlooked and this phenomenon dismissed as an annoying obstacle to organ transplantation. However, since the structure of MHC antigens determines the manner of antigen presentation to

T cells, different individuals vary in the manner and effectiveness with which they handle infection due to a particular micro-organism, thus greatly reducing the likelihood of a single epidemic eliminating a whole community or even the entire species.

B cells express antibody (immunoglobulin) on their surface during development and in this way the cells recognize the presence of antigen. Subsequently, antibodies are secreted in large quantities by the mature B cell (plasma cell). T-cell receptors by contrast are only surface expressed and exist in a complex of co-receptors and signaling molecules. Individual lymphocytes and their progeny do not change the antigen specificity of the receptor they express. However, B cells can change the isotype of the antibody they produce (e.g. from IgM to IgG). This switching process is controlled by interactions between B and T cells both through direct cell-cell receptor ligand

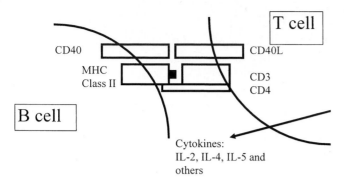

Fig. 25.4 Interactions between T and B cells: T cell help. L = ligand; MHC = major histocompatibility complex; CD = differentiation cluster, IL = interleukin.

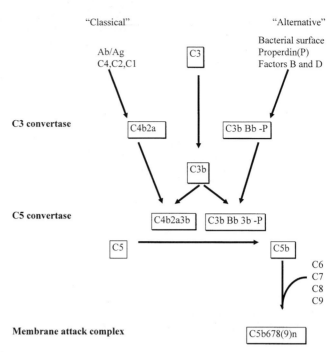

Fig. 25.5 Complement cascade.

contact and through release of soluble factors (cytokines) (Fig. 25.4). Thus, T cells are vital not only in specific cell-mediated but also most specific humoral (antibody-mediated) immune responses.

ANTIBODIES

Antibodies bind to antigen with high affinity and act as effectors of several responses which have evolved to neutralize and eliminate infectious pathogens. Thereby, they opsonize (literally to 'make more tasty') pathogens to facilitate phagocytosis mediated by Fc (the constant tail region of the antibody; Fig. 25.2) receptors on granulocytes and macrophages. Such responses appear to be vital in immunity to infections due to encapsulated bacteria (such as *Streptococcus pneumoniae*, *Neisseria meningitidis* and *Haemophilus influenzae* type b). These infections are common in early childhood principally because of immunologic immaturity and consequent poor responses to capsular polysaccharide antigens. Antibodies of IgE isotype are important in eosinophil-mediated defences against parasitic infection, responses which appear to become dysregulated in individuals with atopy and which involve antibody-dependent cell-mediated cytotoxicity.

Natural killer (NK) cells of lymphocyte lineage as well as myeloid leukocytes are also able to kill target cells which have been coated with antibody by binding the immunoglobulin through low-affinity Fc receptors such as FcγRIII (CD16). This binding to antibody acts both as a recognition and an activating signal to the attacking leukocyte and the process is thus termed antibody-dependent cell-mediated cytotoxicity.

COMPLEMENT

The cascade of serum proteins designated complement (Fig. 25.5) is phylogenetically older than the elements of specific immunity discussed above. This complex network mediates immune responses in several ways. The pathway originally evolved, like granulocytes, to be activated in a non-specific

way by foreign material (via the so-called 'alternative' activation pathway, because it was described second). As with granulocytes, evolution has since found a way to link this potent arm of the non-specific immune response to specific responses. Antibody-antigen (immune) complexes can activate the classical activation pathway (Fig. 25.5). Complement activation results in release of a series of vasoactive and pro-inflammatory peptides (anaphylotoxins: C_3a, C_4a and C_5a) as well as opsonic proteins (e.g. C_3b and C_3bi), and culminates in the assembly of a large complex of proteins ($C_5b \rightarrow C9$) (Fig. 25.5) which can punch holes in cell (or microbial cell) membranes and modulates other inflammatory effects.

Many other non-specific opsonic proteins exist (see below) and some certainly remain undescribed.

PRIMARY IMMUNODEFICIENCY DISEASES

As knowledge of immunology has advanced, the scene has been set for the recognition of an ever-growing list of specific inherited defects. Often, a particular clinical syndrome has been recognized first and then the underlying defect has been elucidated at the protein level and then the genetic level or, more recently, the obverse. In this way, clinical immunology has contributed richly to advances in basic immunology and *vice versa*. However, developments in the understanding and measurement of immune responses has also revealed apparent defects not only in patients but also in seemingly healthy individuals. What is certain is that everybody is, to some extent, 'immunodeficient'. In infancy humoral responses are universally poor and later many individuals have relatively poor opsonic, IgA or IgG subclass responses; as a species man is heterogeneous in MHC (HLA) haplotypes and thus the ability to mount cell-mediated responses to any single pathogen is variable; furthermore, with age, the potency of immunity fades.

The following section describes specific defects in immunity. The list of defects is continuously growing as is the wealth of detail about each individual syndrome and its underlying mutations. Inevitably, the severest conditions, which are also the rarest, have been the swiftest to yield their secrets. A golden era in pediatric immunology is beginning as the milder commoner disorders which affect many children who get 'more than their fair share' of infections are uncovered.

T-CELL AND 'COMBINED' IMMUNODEFICIENCY

Severe combined immunodeficiency

Severe combined immunodeficiency (SCID) describes the severest form of primary immunodeficiency where failure of T- and B-lymphocyte function leads inevitably to death from infection within the first year of life. The different forms of SCID represent experiments of nature with naturally-occurring blocks in T cell and, in some conditions, B and NK cell differentiation. The main types of SCID can be broadly classified into 5 groups according to their immunologic and clinical characteristics. Table 25.1 shows the numbers of each type reported to the European Bone Marrow Transplant Group Working Party.[1]

Recently, several SCID-associated gene mutations have been identified which provide a fascinating insight into the role of key molecules involved in lymphocyte precursor differentiation and enabling the broad groups of SCID to be further subclassified. Reticular dysgenesis with absence of lymphoid and myeloid cells is rare, red cell and platelet production are usually preserved; it may be due to a failure of stem cell differentiation but may also represent a form of SCID where maternal lymphocytes cross the placenta and prevent the development of cells of the fetal lymphoid and myeloid series.

$T^- B^-$ SCID

$T^- B^-$ SCID (absent T and B cells) is usually inherited as an autosomal recessive condition. It appears to be due to the same defect as that seen in the SCID mouse model,[2] where there is defective repair of DNA double-strand breaks and thus of the (VDJ) gene rearrangement in the generation of T- and B-cell receptors.[3] Recently, a similar defect has indeed been described in $T^- B^-$ SCID patients.[4] SCID presenting with the $T^- B^-$ phenotype may also be due to deficiency of enzymes of the purine pyrimidine salvage pathways (see below).

$T^- B^+$ SCID

$T^- B^+$ (T cells absent, B cells present) is the commonest form of SCID seen in Europe and North America. It is usually an X-linked disorder, but can be inherited in an autosomal recessive manner. A major advance in understanding this defect came with the finding that 3 unrelated infants with the X-linked form of $T^- B^+$ SCID had abnormalities of the gene coding for the γ chain of the interleukin (IL)-2 receptor.[5] It is now known that this γ chain is shared by the IL-2, -4, -7, -9 and -15 receptors. If these receptors are non-functional, there is failure of signaling to the JAK-3 + STAT sets of signaling proteins which stimulate activation and cell division of lymphocytes. Perhaps it was not surprising, therefore, when it emerged that the autosomal recessive form of $T^- B^+$ SCID is due to defects in the gene coding for the JAK-3 protein.[6]

T^+ SCID

SCID with T lymphocytes is significantly less common than the other forms of SCID, and represents a very heterogeneous group of rare defects (Table 25.2).

SCID with materno-fetal engraftment

In immunocompetent individuals, lymphocytes probably pass from mother to fetus and are quickly rejected by the fetal immune system. However, sensitive molecular techniques show that circulating T lymphocytes of maternal origin may be found in up to 50% of infants with SCID.[7] Maternally-engrafted lymphocytes show a profoundly restricted Vβ gene usage, suggesting they have a very

Table 25.1 Broad classification of severe combined immunodeficiency (SCID) with number of each type reported to the European Bone Marrow Transplant Group. Reproduced with permission from Ref. 1.

Type of SCID	Number (%)
Reticular dysgenesis	6 (3)
Adenosine deaminase deficiency	30 (16)
$T^- B^-$	50 (27)
$T^- B^+$	81 (44)
T^+	16 (9)

Table 25.2 Unusual forms of severe combined immunodeficiency (SCID) (mostly SCID with T lymphocytes).

SCID with materno-fetal engraftment
Omenn's syndrome
MHC Class II deficiency (bare lymphocyte syndrome)
T-lymphocyte stimulation and activation defects
SCID with short limbed dwarfism
Purine nucleoside phosphorylase deficiency

reduced T-cell receptor diversity and come from a small number of lymphocyte clones. They usually bear the phenotype of activated mature T lymphocytes but give markedly diminished or absent proliferative responses to PHA, allogeneic cells or specific antigens.[8] Such cells may be clinically silent but can cause severe congenital graft-versus-host disease (GVHD).

Omenn's syndrome

Omenn[9,10] first described 12 infants in 6 sibships from an inbred Irish–American kindred who all developed an infiltrating skin rash, hepatosplenomegaly and lymphadenopathy, together with diarrhea, failure to thrive and recurrent persistent infections leading to death. Most of the parents were first or second cousins, suggesting an autosomal recessive inheritance. T cells in these patients are not of maternal origin but in many cases the features are similar to those seen in SCID with materno-fetal GVHD. Proliferating T cells exhibit a T-helper (Th)-2 phenotype secreting high levels of IL-4 and -5.[11] In many cases, the T-receptor repertoire is very restricted with a small number of clones, suggesting that Omenn's syndrome represents an oligoclonal proliferation of T cells which localize and react on epithelia but do not traffic to peripheral lymphoid organs and the thymus. It may be that a small number of T-cell clones escape a block in differentiation and exert an autoimmune-like reactivity for reasons that are unclear. It is probably best described as a 'leaky form of SCID' where most T-cell lymphocyte clones do not differentiate but a few highly restricted ones are able to do so.

MHC Class II deficiency (bare lymphocyte syndrome)

This is an autosomal recessive condition in which MHC Class II molecules are absent. In most cases there is also a variable reduction in HLA Class I expression. The underlying defects described to date have all been due to mutations in genes coding for the regulatory proteins controlling the expression of Class II molecules rather than in the genes coding for the Class II molecules themselves.[12,13] Most affected children are Mediterranean in origin and present with recurrent infections similar to those seen in the more classical forms of SCID; neutropenia occurs in about a third of cases, together with autoimmune hemolytic anemia.[14]

T-lymphocyte stimulation and activation defects

Following antigen presentation by an appropriate MHC molecule and binding to a T-cell receptor specific to that antigen, a powerful clonal proliferation is induced which is dependent on proper signaling by the T-cell receptor and the associated CD3 molecular complex (see above). Following antigen binding to the T-cell receptor, appropriate secondary binding events between other T-cell lymphocyte surface receptors and their complementary molecules (ligands) on

the antigen-presenting cell must occur if T-cell lymphocyte activation and proliferation is to proceed. Both sets of events then cause a series of proteins within the T lymphocyte to be activated by phosphorylation of their tyrosine residues. Once phosphorylated, these proteins phosphorylate further proteins, thus setting up a signal transduction pathway. A number of defects in T-cell receptor molecules and other proteins in this pathway have been described in infants with SCID-like clinical features. The best described of these is associated with an anomaly of one of the activation proteins: Zap 70 kinase. T lymphocytes and immunoglobulin are present, but there is a marked lack of mature $CD8^+$ T cells reflecting a defect in positive selection within the thymus, and although $CD4^+$ cells are present, they are unresponsive to mitogens.[15]

Short-limbed dwarfism

Although McKusick-type metaphyseal chondrodysplasia (cartilage hair hypoplasia) is often associated with a T-lymphocyte disorder,[16] the range of severity varies wildly and only a very small proportion of cases has markedly reduced T-cell activity and the features of SCID. Phenotypically, patients have disproportionate short stature with height exceeding span and lower segments shorter than upper segments. Hands are short with stubby fingers and there is usually joint laxity. Hair is often fine and sparse and there is an association both with anorectal anomalies such as Hirschsprung's disease and with neutropenia. One child with this form of SCID developed features characteristic of Omenn's syndrome (see above).[17]

Purine/pyrimidine salvage pathway enzyme deficiency

Adenosine deaminase deficiency. This autosomal recessively inherited condition accounts for nearly one-sixth of the cases of typical SCID. Adenosine deaminase (ADA) is an enzyme of the purine salvage pathway that catalyzes the irreversible deamination of adenosine and deoxyadenosine to inosine and deoxyinosine. These metabolites can then be converted into other purines for re-utilization or removal by eventual degradation to uric acid, the end-product of purine metabolism in man. This pathway is particularly important for cells such as lymphocytes and erythrocytes which either lack or have very low activity of *de novo* purine synthesis. Failure of enzyme activity allows the accumulation of toxic metabolites such as deoxyadenosine which inhibits DNA synthesis by more than one mechanism. The gene for ADA has been located on chromosome 20q13.4 and many different mutations have been defined. Gene deletion leads to very little ADA activity and a profound T and B lymphopenia with an early onset of clinical symptoms. Partial gene deletions and some point mutations can also cause severe deficiency, but other point mutations are associated with low but not absent levels of ADA activity, and in these cases there is a less severe lymphopenia and a milder immunodeficiency. Bony defects are found in about 50% of patients with flared costochondral junctions, mild metaphyseal dysplasia and, occasionally, there are neurologic disturbances.[18] Eighty to 90% of patients present with the clinical features of SCID in the first few months of life. It is now becoming clear, however, that the clinical spectrum is much broader than classical SCID and an increasing number of patients are being diagnosed in childhood with features that include sinopulmonary bacterial infections, markedly elevated IgE and/or eosinophilia, variable elevation of IgM and IgG and autoimmune features including autoimmune hemolytic anemia and thrombocytopenia. In 2 cases, the diagnosis was not made until early adult life, although clinical features were present during adolescence.[18]

Where an infant with ADA-deficient SCID has an HLA identical sibling, bone marrow transplantation (BMT) is the best treatment (see below). Where no such donor is available, it has proved possible to restore a considerable degree of immune function by enzyme replacement therapy. This is achieved by infusing polyethylene glycol-modified ADA (PEG-ADA), a treatment which has been available for a decade. Some patients develop antibodies against the PEG-ADA complex and about 20% do not respond at all. Nevertheless, other patients have improved considerably, even though immune function has not been fully restored to normal. Gene replacement therapy by transfecting the ADA gene into bone marrow stem cells has been attempted, and although some initial results showed promise, it is not yet possible to evaluate this treatment fully.[19]

Purine nucleoside phosphorylase deficiency. Like ADA deficiency, this extremely rare form of SCID is caused by an inherited defect in the purine pyrimidine salvage pathway. Toxic metabolites poison the lymphoid system rather more slowly than in ADA deficiency so that there is a progressive T lymphopenia whilst B cells seem less affected. Recurrent infections usually begin during the first year of life, although some patients have been asymptomatic until as late as 6 years of age. Infections are similar to those found in typical SCID patients, but in addition, patients with purine nucleotide phosphorylase (PNP) deficiency show striking neurologic abnormalities, particularly spastic diplegia, ataxia and dysarthria as well as autoimmune problems, most notably autoimmune hemolytic anemia.[20]

Clinical features and diagnosis

With the exception of infants with reticular dysgenesis, most patients are asymptomatic for the first few weeks of life. Intractable diarrhea, often due to persistent rotavirus infection, which then leads to failure to thrive, is probably the commonest presenting feature, occurring in 80% of patients, and is usually seen by 3–4 months of age.

Respiratory infections occur in 60–90% of cases, although they take a variety of different forms. Some infants present with a steadily progressive interstitial pneumonitis due to *Pneumocystis carinii*, cytomegalovirus (CMV) or, occasionally, Aspergillus spp: Others suffer from a bronchiolitic illness characterized by coryza, a harsh brassy cough, a rapid respiratory rate and hyperinflation of the chest, accompanied by wheeze and crepitation. Respiratory syncytial and/or parainfluenza viruses are often isolated, and whereas in normal infants virus excretion ceases and symptoms resolve within 2–3 weeks, babies with SCID persistently excrete the virus and their respiratory state slowly worsens over weeks or even months. They are often misdiagnosed as having 'infantile asthma'.

Recurrent persistent superficial candidal infection involving the mouth and diaper area affects 30–50% of babies, although invasive candidiasis is unusual. Bacterial skin sepsis is a feature often overlooked, and in one series was seen in nearly a third of affected infants.[7]

By the time a diagnosis is made, most infants will have > 1 of the above features and over half will have 3 of them. Unfortunately, only interstitial pneumonitis is pathognomonic of immunodeficiency, and so unless there is a high index of suspicion, infants with respiratory infection may well be severely ill and needing assisted ventilation before immunodeficiency is considered. Children with SCID can also present with a wide range of rare infective problems. Bacillus Calmette-Guérin (BCG) vaccination, for example, can lead to disseminated infection causing hepatosplenomegaly and anemia; other children present with disseminated adenoviral or enteroviral infection, causing encephalitis, pneumonitis or even pericarditis, whilst in others Epstein–Barr virus infection can cause a lymphoproliferative state which leads to frank lymphomatous change.

None of the clinical features is in itself pathognomonic, and so many children are diagnosed late with significant organ damage from infection, which seriously reduces the chance of a successful BMT. This is particularly true for children with respiratory infection. In a UK series, symptoms developed at a median age of 5 weeks, but diagnosis of SCID was not made until a median age of 7 months (range 4 weeks to 16 months).[21] In a single-center French series, first clinical signs appeared by 2½ months and the diagnosis was made, on average, at 4½ months.

Lymphopenia is the most useful clue to the diagnosis of SCID but is often overlooked, partly because there is confusion concerning the normal range of lymphocyte counts in infancy, and partly because the absolute lymphocyte count is rarely observed or noted when a full blood count is performed on hospital admission. Age-related normal lymphocyte counts in infancy have a higher lower limit of normal than in adults and range from $2 \times 10^9/l$ at birth to $4 \times 10^9/l$ at 1 year (see Reference values at the front of this book). In the UK series of 45 infants with SCID, 44 had a lymphocyte count >2 standard deviations below the mean for age, whereas of a control group of sex- and age-matched infants with normal immunity and similar presenting illnesses, only 8 had low lymphocyte counts which were all normal on repeat testing after a few days.[21]

Once SCID is suspected, diagnosis should not be difficult. Lymphocyte subset analysis will show low numbers of lymphocytes bearing mature T-lymphocyte markers, and B lymphocytes may or may not be reduced. Whilst lymphocyte subset analysis gives a clear-cut result, interpretation of immunoglobulin levels is more difficult as IgG levels may be normal due to the presence of transplacentally transferred maternal IgG and many laboratories cannot distinguish between absent levels of IgA and IgM and the low levels normally seen between 3 and 6 months of age. Furthermore, many infants with SCID make low levels of IgM which may not appear abnormal. Measuring immunoglobulins may thus give a falsely reassuring result, and if SCID is suspected, lymphocyte subset analysis should always be performed. Failure of lymphocyte proliferation to stimuli such as phytohemagglutinin helps confirm the diagnosis, as does the absence of a response on mixed lymphocyte culture with allogeneic cells. ADA deficiency (see above) should be looked for by studying red cell enzyme activity and urinary metabolite levels.

Once an immunologic diagnosis has been made, careful studies should be carried out to determine the nature and extent of infection. Serology is not useful because of the inability of infants with SCID to produce antibody, so that screening must include viral culture and immunofluorescence studies of nasopharyngeal suction specimens, as well as electron microscopy of stool, and stool and urine viral culture, together with bacterial stool, urine and surface swab cultures. CMV must be looked for assiduously, and in children with a respiratory disease, bronchoalveolar lavage should be performed to look for pathogens such as *Pneumocystis carinii*, bacteria and viruses. Finding a respiratory virus in a nasopharyngeal suction specimen should not preclude carrying out a bronchoalveolar lavage as many infants may have dual infections, and *Pneumocystis carinii* is usually found only in deep and not in upper respiratory secretions. As *Pneumocystis carinii* pneumonia is treatable, it is vital to identify this. Infants should be nursed in strict style isolation, particularly to prevent opportunistic viral and fungal infections, and most babies with SCID need total parental nutrition to ensure that they are in optimum condition to survive the rigours of BMT.

Other X-linked combined immunodeficiency

Wiskott–Aldrich syndrome

This rare condition is characterized by the triad of infection, eczema and thrombocytopenia with bleeding. It is X-linked but its cause was a mystery until affected individuals were all found to have mutations in the gene encoding for the Wiskott–Aldrich syndrome (WAS) protein (WASP).[22] This protein is implicated in the regulation of the actin skeleton of hemopoietic cells.[23] Lack of a proper actin skeleton may lead to failure of polarization of T cells towards antigen-presenting cells and B cells, leading to a failure of cognate immune responses.

Molecular analysis has shown that patients with X-linked hereditary thrombocytopenia (XLT) and WAS both have mutations in the WASP gene, confirming that XLT is a mild variant of WAS. Clinical features vary from thrombocytopenia with small sized platelets (XLT) through eczema of increasing severity with recurrent infections, and in more severe cases, the development of autoimmunity and in due course B-lymphoid malignancy. On this basis, a severity scoring system grading patients from 1 to 5 has been devised, and it has been suggested that clinical severity is related to the severity of the genetic defects.[24] This has not been fully proven, but the scoring system does help assess disease severity.

The initial manifestation of WAS is the presence of petechial bleeding, particularly in the first 6 months of life. An eczematous rash of increasing severity then appears, and bacterial and viral infections including otitis media and pneumonia are also seen. During infections, the thrombocytopenia worsens and frank bleeding may occur. *Herpes simplex* infection can be particularly severe, as can infection with Epstein–Barr, varicella zoster and CMV. Hemolytic anemia is the commonest autoimmune manifestation and is associated with an increased risk of early malignancy. Boys who survive infection and bleeding seem to have a very great risk of developing lymphoid malignancy which may even approach 100% by early-to-middle adult life.

Treatment consists of prophylactic antibiotics, as well as aggressive treatment of viral and bacterial infections when they occur. Intravenous immunoglobulin is increasingly being used and splenectomy is indicated when there is severe autoimmune hemolytic anemia. However, splenectomy greatly increases the risk of fatal infection, and splenectomized boys with WAS should all be on prophylactic penicillin and/or cotrimoxazole and intravenous immunoglobulin (see below).[25] If there is an HLA-identical sibling or a good matched unrelated donor, BMT should be considered, particularly in boys under 5 years of age who seem to have a particularly good prognosis with 80% disease-free survival.

X-Linked lymphoproliferative disease (Duncan's syndrome)

X-Linked lymphoproliferative syndrome (XLP) is an inherited immunodeficiency to Epstein–Barr virus (EBV) infections that has been mapped to chromosome Xq25. Immunity develops normally until a primary EBV infection occurs and then there is an abnormal proliferation of transformed B cells that cannot be controlled by T lymphocytes, leading to the development of deranged immune function.[26] Severe infectious mononucleosis occurs in approximately 75% of cases and is fatal in about half. Somewhat less than half have other manifestations, including acquired hypogammaglobulinemia, aplastic anemia and malignant lymphomas (mostly affecting the gut or central nervous system).[27] After exposure to EBV, patients develop antibodies to EBV capsid antigen and nuclear antigens in the normal way, but do not maintain antibodies to EBV nuclear antigens in the way that normal individuals do. Natural killer function steadily falls and there may be high levels of IgM.

Conservative treatment is unsatisfactory; acyclovir seems to be of little benefit in EBV infection and although the hypogammaglobulinemia can be treated with intravenous immunoglobulin replacement, infection, aplastic anemia and malignant lymphoma mean that the prognosis is very poor. In younger boys, BMT seems to be increasingly successful and all children with this condition should be considered for transplant.[28]

DiGeorge anomaly (3rd and 4th branchial arch syndrome, thymic hypoplasia, cell-mediated immunodeficiency with hypoparathyroidism, CATCH-22)

The syndromal absence or hypoplasia of the thymus and parathyroid glands with congenital heart disease (particularly but not exclusively aortic arch defects) and abnormal facies is associated with microdeletion in chromosome 22q11, which is detected by fluorescence *in situ* hybridisation. Only 25% of cases have a demonstrable immunodeficiency as in most the thymus is present but small and maldescended.[29]

It is important to consider this diagnosis in infants with this kind of heart lesion or hypocalcemic fits. These infants often need to undergo urgent cardiac surgery. All blood products should be irradiated before transfusion to avoid potentially fatal GVHD in the minority of cases where there is total thymic aplasia. An absent thymus on chest radiograph is an interesting but unreliable finding. Immunologic investigations should include a lymphocyte and CD3[+], CD4[+] and CD8[+] T-cell counts, and a test of mitogen-induced proliferative responses (PHA). Whilst some cases show normal results, many show modestly reduced numbers of CD4[+] and CD8[+] T cells with normal mitogen-induced proliferation. These individuals often show no increased predisposition to infection and respond well to vaccination, including MMR. Some have an increased susceptibility to sinopulmonary bacterial infection due to a sluggish development of antipolysaccharide humoral immunity; occasionally, such children need immunoglobulin replacement (see below). Rarely, T-cell and mitogen responses are absent. In such cases of severe immunodeficiency, cotrimoxazole prophylaxis against pneumocystis and immunoglobulin replacement therapy should be given. Such children should be treated like those with SCID. Surprisingly, BMT has been a successful treatment.[30]

Ataxia telangiectasia and chromosome breakage syndromes

Ataxia telangiectasia is a rare autosomal recessive disorder and illustrates how a single gene defect can affect many different body systems. It has long been known that cells from these patients show chromosome instability with a high rate of chromosomal breaks and profound radiosensitivity. In all cases studied, a mutation has been found in the ataxia telangiectasia mutation (ATM) gene identified by positional cloning on chromosome 11q22–23. A portion of the ATM gene's protein sequence is very similar to that found in the PI-3 kinases, suggesting that the gene is involved in cellular growth control, a known function of PI-3 kinase.[31] The ATM protein is also similar to a group of proteins that arrest the cell cycle in cells whose DNA has been damaged by ultraviolet radiation; thus, the ATM protein may help cells recognize damaged DNA so that it can be repaired before cell division.[31]

Cerebellar ataxia is the earliest manifestation, usually first noticed when the child begins to walk. The ataxia is progressive, later developing into generalized neuromotor dysfunction with an increasing dysarthria, associated with degeneration of Purkinje cells. Telangiectases appear between 2 and 8 years of age, first in the eyes and then affecting the face and ears. Elevated levels of α-fetoprotein and carcinoembryonic antigen are also seen.

Sinopulmonary infections are the commonest manifestation of the immunodeficiency which affects both humoral and cellular components of the immune system. There is a progressive failure of antibody production, often beginning with poor responses to polysaccharide antigens and progressing to hypogammaglobulinemia. There is usually a fall in the number of CD4[+] T lymphocytes with a relative increase in T lymphocytes bearing the γδ receptor, as opposed to the αβ receptor.

The thymus is rather small. Patients also suffer from an increased risk of diabetes and delayed sexual maturation and a profound predisposition to malignancy which develops during childhood in about 10% of patients, lymphomas and acute lymphoblastic leukemia (ALL) accounting for 85% of these. Because of the chromosome fragility, treatment with radiotherapy is extremely damaging. Heterozygous carriers are also at increased risk of malignancy,[32] so that although ataxia telangiectasia is itself rare, approximately 0.5–1.4% of the population carry a single defective ATM gene, and this could account for up to 8% of all breast cancers.

There is no curative treatment for ataxia telangiectasia, but patients with symptomatic infections often benefit considerably from intravenous immunoglobulin therapy with or without prophylactic antibiotics.

It is now becoming clear that other immunodeficiency disorders are associated with defects in the enzymes responsible for repairing damaged DNA. The best characterized is the *Nijmegen breakage syndrome*, which is an autosomal recessive chromosomal instability syndrome associated with microcephaly, mild developmental delay, bird-like faces, growth retardation, humoral and cellular immuno-deficiency, and a marked susceptibility to malignancy. Details of the molecular pathogenesis have recently been elucidated.[32a,32b] Although patients share many of the characteristics of ataxia telangiectasia, they do not exhibit telangiectasia nor a raised α-fetoprotein.[33] In the SCID mouse model there is defective double-strand DNA break repair and VDJ coding joint formation which results in arrested lymphocyte development. It appears that a similar mechanism may account for some cases of T⁻B⁻ SCID.

Natural killer cell deficiency

NK cells are lymphocytes that do not bear B or T lymphocyte markers and can kill target cells without being previously sensitized. They are not limited by MHC restriction and look like large granular lymphocytes bearing CD56 as a distinguishing surface marker. Isolated complete absence of NK cells is extremely rare, and whilst some patients have suffered severe infection with viruses of the herpes family, including varicella zoster virus and CMV, other siblings also found to have no NK cells were essentially asymptomatic. NK-cell dysfunction is seen in other primary immunodeficiencies such as the Chédiak–Higashi syndrome (see Chapter 21) and leukocyte adhesion deficiency (see below), but in these cases the other defects of the primary disorder seem to account for the clinical picture, and the NK deficiency appears to be a secondary phenomenon.

Other combined immunodeficiencies

A number different diseases have been described which do not fit well into the classification of known primary immunodeficiencies. Mostly, there have only been single case reports or very small series of patients. In idiopathic CD4 lymphocytopenia, there is a profound lack of T-helper cells but no evidence of HIV infection.[34] Nevertheless, the clinical symptoms are often reminiscent of acquired immunodeficiency (AIDS). Patients have also been described whose T cells fail to express important surface molecules such as CD45 and CD7. In general, patients have low T-cell numbers and poor but not absent responses to T-cell mitogens. There is also variable production of immunoglobulin, but usually even if immunoglobulin is made, specific antibody responses are poor. In some cases, molecular studies reveal a minor defect (e.g. a 1-nucleotide substitution in the common γ chain of the interleukin receptors causing X-linked B⁺ SCID; see above). Such cases thus appear to represent an attenuated phenotype. In other cases, however, no molecular basis has been characterized.

In exceptional cases, there appears to be completely normal humoral immunity, despite profound T-cell immunodeficiency, a condition sometimes referred to as *Nezelof's syndrome*.[35] Infants with combined immunodeficiency usually present with opportunistic infections such as *Pneumocystis*

carinii pneumonia, CMV infection or cryptosporidiosis, as well as suffering from recurrent bacterial infections and recurrent candidiasis. Very often there is failure to thrive. In some, there are features of autoimmunity, particularly autoimmune hemolytic anemia and thrombocytopenia and there may be hepatosplenomegaly. This is perhaps due to a failure of T-cell orchestrated immune regulation.

Recently, a condition named *autoimmune lymphoproliferative syndrome* has been described which appears to be due to a failure of programmed T-cell death. This appears to occur when there is a defect in one of the genes coding for the surface receptors on T cells (Fasth and Fasth ligand) which trigger a programed cell death or apoptosis. Such children, who are often are born into consanguinous marriages, exhibit marked lymphoproliferation, thrombocytopenia, anemia, hepatosplenomegaly and hypoimmunoglobulin G and A. In some patients there is evidence of vasculitis and glomerulonephritis.[36]

Chronic mucocutaneous candidiasis

Chronic mucocutaneous candidiasis (CMC) is a complex disorder characterized by chronic and recurrent candidal infection of the skin and mucous membranes. Invasive candidal infection rarely occurs. There is a strong association with both organ-specific and -non-specific autoimmune disease, and, in a minority of patients, with either a humoral or a combined immunodeficiency. For these reasons, it is usually considered to be due to a defect in T-cell regulation, although there has been little direct evidence to support this view. Recent work, however, suggests an imbalance of T-cell cytokines, so that in patients with CMC, candida triggers a predominantly Th-2 response with increased IL-4 and IL-6 production, rather than a Th-1 response with mainly IL-2 and γ-interferon production, as is seen in normal controls.[37] A candidate gene for CMC has been reported.[38,39]

Most patients present in the first few months of life with persistent candida of the mouth, diaper area and, sometimes, esophagus. When present, the esophagitis is often severe and associated with esophageal reflux and failure to thrive. The candida is often very difficult to eradicate, but is ameliorated by long-term treatment with fluconazole or itraconazole. Autoimmune endocrinopathy is common, occurring in about one-third of patients. Symptomatic endocrine disease is not normally apparent in childhood, but becomes increasingly common from the second and third decades of life onwards. In one large series, hypoparathyroidism was found in 79%, adrenocortical failure in 72%, and gonadal failure in 60% of female patients over 30 years of age, and 4% of the males over 16 years of age.[40] Other less common autoimmune findings have included hemolytic anemia, thrombocytopenia and neutropenia, chronic active hepatitis and uveitis. Patients may also have evidence of dental enamel hypoplasia and keratopathy. A smaller proportion of patients show degrees of humoral immunodeficiency, particularly IgG2 and IgG4 deficiency and failure to make good quality specific antibodies,[41] and these patients are at risk of chronic recurrent pulmonary infection leading to bronchiectasis. Significant non-candidal infections occurred in a surprising number of patients in one series.[42] In this series as in others, CMC has been found to occur in several family members inherited as an autosomal dominant trait with variable penetrance. Given the spectrum and variability of clinical signs and symptoms, it may well be that CMC does not represent a single entity, but a group of similar disorders, only some of which are inherited in a familial fashion.

Most patients do not show delayed-type cutaneous hypersensitivity but do show proliferation of peripheral blood lymphocytes to candida. Some patients are also lymphopenic with decreased proliferation studies. Most patients do not respond well to oral nystatin and/or amphotericin treatment, but systemic fluconazole and itraconazole are more effective agents, and often need to be given on a long-term basis. Liver enzymes must be monitored when using these agents, particularly if there is evidence of autoimmune hepatitis. Immunotherapy with various agents including thymic peptides has not been very helpful. In a few severe cases the condition has been cured by BMT.[43]

Common variable immunodeficiency

Common variable immuodeficiency (CVID) is a heterogeneous group of disorders of antibody production usually, but not always, associated with some degree of abnormality of T-cell function.[44] Essentially it represents what is left over when all the more well-defined specific immunodeficiencies are ruled out and it can be supposed the term will be used less as the underlying basis for more disorders of immunity are elucidated.

Most patients with CVID present in adult life and it is rare in the pediatric clinic. Patients appear to have dysregulated B-cell maturation but the underlying cause for this is not clear. Low levels of several immunoglobulin isotypes are usually seen and these abnormalities may be progressive. Clinical manifestations are usually sinopulmonary infections due to common bacterial pathogens and occasionally opportunistic organisms, gastrointestinal problems, recurrent herpes virus infections autoimmune problems and a higher than average incidence of lymphoid and gastrointestinal malignancy.

Treatment is with IgG replacement and antibiotic prophylaxis (see below).

Leukocyte adhesion deficiency

The importance to immunology of the family of cell adhesion molecules called β_2 integrins (CD11/CD18) was first recognized in homotypic interactions between lymphocytes expressing LFA-1 (CD11a/CD18) and its counter-receptor ICAM1 (CD54). Patients with mutations in the common β_2 integrin β chain CD18, leading to low or absent expression of this family of proteins, suffer from leukocyte adhesion deficiency (LAD) type 1 which is manifest as delayed umbilical separation and then recurrent bacterial infection without pus formation but very high peripheral leukocyte counts.[45] This is because neutrophils also depend on β_2 integrins for adhesion to endothelium and migration out of the circulation. Umbilical separation is also a neutrophil-dependent event. Some patients have been successfully treated by BMT.[46]

A second type of LAD (type 2) has been described in patients lacking the ability to make fucosylated carbohydrates including sialyl Lewis-X, an important ligand for the selectins, the family of adhesion molecules which mediate the initial rolling phase of leukocyte-endothelial adhesion. As in LAD type 1, patients have high leukocyte counts and severe recurrent infections but in addition they suffer neurodevelopmental problems.[47]

DISORDERS OF B-CELL FUNCTION

X-Linked agammaglobulinemia (Bruton tyrosine kinase deficiency)

Boys with this condition have mutations in the gene for Bruton tyrosine kinase (BTK) (locus: Xq22),[48,49] which results in failure of B-cell development,[50] and consequently greatly reduced or absent antibody production. As a result, these children contract abnormally severe and frequent infections—most usually upper and lower bacterial respiratory infections but also gastrointestinal infections, pyoderma, septic arthritis, septicemia and meningitis.[51] These are usually manifest by the second year of life as maternal antibody wanes and are associated with growth failure. Unfortunately, diagnosis is often delayed resulting in severe chronic lung injury or other complications of invasive infection. Antibody plays an important role in protection against disseminated enteroviral infection and these children are prone to severe infection due to coxsackie and echoviruses,[52] which can cause chronic meningitis, dermatomyositis and hepatitis. Polio viruses, including the attenuated virus strains in oral polio vaccine, can cause paralytic poliomyelitis, so the injectable inactivated vaccine should be always be used in affected individuals.

Where there is a family history, diagnosis can be confirmed at birth by the absence or very low numbers of B cells (expressing CD19 or CD20) in peripheral venous blood on immunofluorescence analysis. A similar approach can be used for late prenatal diagnosis using a sample of cord blood, but early in pregnancy linkage analysis on amniotic fluid cells or chorionic villus is needed. Analysis of immunoglobulin levels only becomes meaningful at around 6 months of age as all infants have high levels of IgG acquired transplacentally from the mother and low levels of other isotypes (IgA, IgM, IgE) prior to this. After this age, boys with X-linked agammaglobulinemia (XLA) have consistently low or absent levels of all isotypes, although it should be noted that BTK mutations often appear to result in incomplete antibody production failure. Molecular genetic analysis of the BTK gene is also possible in patients and mothers for the purpose of carrier diagnosis and genetic counseling. Non-random X-chromosome inactivation in B cells of carrier mothers can also be demonstrated.

Treatment consists of IgG replacement therapy (see below).[53] Some immunologists give children antibiotic prophylaxis as well (see below) and this may be essential where lung damage has already occurred by the time of diagnosis, together with physiotherapy and normal programs of care for children with chronic lung disease. However, with timely diagnosis, current therapy permits these boys to lead entirely normal lives but for the inconvenience of treatments.

Rare associations of X-linked agammaglobulinemia are growth hormone deficiency, neutropenia, malabsorption and protein-losing enteropathy, although the basis for these problems is unknown and it is not known if they are causally linked to BTK mutations.

Hyper-IgM syndrome (CD40 ligand deficiency)

Most cases of this condition are X-linked and have mutations in the gene for the CD40 ligand (CD40L, gp39) (locus: Xq26), a T-cell surface signaling protein whose counter-receptor CD40 is expressed on B cells and other antigen presenting cells (Fig 25.4).[54–57] The interaction of these proteins is central to the regulation of isotype switching by B cells and the formation of memory B cells so that, in this disorder, they remain 'stuck' producing IgM and are unable to switch to producing IgA, M or E even though, unlike boys with XLA, the B cells are normal. CD40L may also be crucial for other aspects of T-cell function, including regulation of myelopoiesis and activation of monocyte-derived cells such as pulmonary alveolar macrophages and Kuppfer cells in the liver.

Thus, while these children may present with recurrent or severe bacterial infection and growth failure like those with XLA, *Pneumocystis carinii* pneumonia is the presenting complaint in 40% of cases, usually between 6 months and 1 year of age; 67% have neutropenia with its associated problems (see Chapter 37).[58,59] Patients may have chronic lymphoid hyperplasia, cytopenias and arthritis, and other autoimmune phenomena have been reported, although it is not clear whether these are secondary to chronic immune activation by infections. Gastrointestinal problems are emerging as a major problem for patients who survive into the second and third decades of life. In a recent survey, 12 of 16 patients reaching 20 years of age had significant liver disease.[60] It appears that chronic gastrointestinal infection with cryptosporidium provokes sclerosing cholangitis, followed by cirrhosis and ultimately hepatocellular carcinoma.[61] CD40 is expressed on Kuppfer cells and it may be that these cells cannot clear the cryptosporidia without T-cell stimulation via CD40L; thus, boys with hyper IgM suffer chronic cholangitis and its fatal sequelae.

Diagnosis is usually made during the pre-school years on the basis of a characteristic picture of normal or high serum levels of polyclonal IgM with low or absent IgG, IgA and IgE. B-cell numbers in blood are normal. Absence of CD40L on T cells by immunofluorescence confirms the diagnosis. Molecular genetic analysis of the CD40L gene is also possible in patients and mothers for the purpose of carrier diagnosis and genetic counseling.

Treatment consists of IgG replacement therapy (see below) and cotrimoxazole prophylaxis against *Pneumocystis carinii* pneumonia which may also serve to inhibit bacterial infections (see below). Granulocyte colony-stimulating factor (G-CSF) therapy is sometimes used when neutropenia is present.[62] BMT has been advocated since it became clear that this is a T-cell immunodeficiency with an appalling long-term outlook. This has been successful in a few cases, but needs to be performed before there is serious liver damage.[63]

Isotype (IgA, IgM and IgG subclass) deficiency

With the widespread availability of serum analysis for imunoglobulin isotypes has come the recognition that many children presenting with abnormally frequent or severe infections, as well as many with atopy and asthma, have total levels of one or more of these isotypes 2 standard deviations below the mean for age. This group of disorders is much less well defined than XLA. There is often a poor correlation between the deficiencies measured in the laboratory and the severity of the clinical problems which vary from none to those seen in XLA. The degree of functional impairment in antibody production must vary widely between cases and other unelucidated factors are likely to be involved.[64] Case definition is made more difficult by several factors: different methods are used to measure antibody concentrations; laboratories often do not have serum from healthy children to prepare age-matched normal ranges using their own assays in their own populations; and isotype levels change with time in response to infections and with age so that abnormalities are often transient.

In practice, assays for IgG, IgA, IgM, IgE and IgG subclasses are usually performed on serum from any child under investigation because of abnormally frequent or severe infections. If an abnormality is found, and is still present when the assay is repeated, the child is considered to be deficient. It should be noted that standard procedures for the definition of normal ranges dictate that an abnormality in at least 1 subclass will occur by chance alone in 1 in every 5 tests of IgG subclasses. Selective IgA deficiency is thought to occur in around 1 in 500 individuals. Deficiency of IgM and IgE are also reported and IgG-subclass deficiency (with normal total IgG) is rather common in pediatric clinics. Levels of IgG2 are low and responsiveness to unconjugated pneumococcal vaccine is often absent in children under 2 years of age. Some children develop this facet of the humoral immune system rather late and so up to the age of 5–6 years such findings may simply represent slow maturation that will resolve with time. Certain combinations of isotype deficiency are well recognized (e.g. low IgA with IgG2).

It will be clear that these disorders form a spectrum with CVID and a small proportion of these children appear to develop CVID in adolescence. However, while such findings add weight to concerns about immunodeficiency, management of such children is not standardized but tailored to the individual case. Sometimes, advice to seek early medical attention and, if necessary, antibiotics is sufficient. Many children appear to benefit from antibiotic prophylaxis (see below). Very occasional cases require IgG replacement therapy (see below), although this is never logical in cases of selective IgA deficiency. What is certain is that such children require immunologic review and revision of their management at regular intervals so that reassurance is given as matters improve (as is usually the case) or early appropriate treatment instituted in the rare cases that progress to CVID.

Specific antibody production defects

Following reports of children with severe or recurrent infection and an apparent inability to make antibodies to specific antigens (in particular polysaccharides), but with normal total circulating levels of all immunoglobulin isotypes and other tests of immune function,[65,66] it has become common to check children's specific antibody responses to vaccine antigens as part of the investigation for immunodeficiency. To delineate these cases effectively, sensitive and specific serologic assays are needed and, again, heterogeneity between centers hampers interpretation of results. Furthermore, there are several possible explanations for such abnormalities, including heterogeneity between individuals, immunologic immaturity and environmental factors such as large tolerizing doses of antigen. There has been no report of clustering of this group of conditions within families.

However, it is clear that certain individuals who experience severe or recurrent infection and have normal total isotype levels, fail to mount detectable responses to particular antigens, often despite repeated immunization. It is also clear that some individuals with persistently abnormally low isotypes respond well to protein and polysaccharide vaccines. Patients in both groups are managed according to the severity of their clinical picture, with IgG replacement therapy only indicated in rare severe cases.

Transient hypogammaglobulinemia of infancy

Normally, serum IgG levels at birth are higher than adult levels due to active transport of IgG across the placenta during the third trimester of pregnancy. Levels fall progressively at first, reaching a nadir at around 4–5 months and then rising progressively throughout the first decade of life towards adult levels. In a small proportion of infants, immunoglobulin levels of one or more isotypes are low during the second half of the first year of life, later catching up and approaching normal levels.[67] This is usually uncovered during investigations following one or a series of infections in a baby who is well by the time the result comes to light. Once again, it is unclear which if any of these infants form a distinct group as opposed to one extreme of normal. In practice, all that is usually required is reassurance and a repeat test at 18 months of age.

Other B-cell disorders

A number of other rare B-cell disorders have been described in children. Hyper IgD syndrome is an autosomal familial disorder characterized by high serum IgD levels and attacks of fever, rash, abdominal pain and arthritis.[68] Patients with transcobalamin II deficiency, among other problems, develop hypogammaglobulinemia which responds to high-dose vitamin B_{12} treatment.[69] Children with Down's syndrome often have demonstrable abnormalities of immunoglobulin production, although these are heterogeneous and occur alongside other immunologic defects. Patients with deficiencies in early complement components may have associated reduced antibody production (see below) as may patients with reduced splenic function (see below) or HIV infection (see below).

DEFICIENCY OF PLASMA PROTEINS

Specific complement component deficiencies (C1–C9)

Complement component deficiency is rare, although it has been described for virtually all the proteins in the pathways.[70] It may manifest as increased susceptibility to infection, collagen vascular disease or both. Many factors show 'autosomal co-dominant' inheritance so that heterozygote individuals (with 1 'null' or mutated gene) have half normal levels of the component.[71,72] The commonest deficiency is of C2, with a mutation in the C2 gene in around 1 in 100 of the population (homozygote frequency around 1 in 10 000). It exemplifies this group of disorders in that affected individuals may be asymptomatic, may suffer from a variety of autoimmune and vasculitic disorders or may develop recurrent bacteremia, particularly with encapsulated organisms such as *Strep. pneumoniae* and *Neisseria meningitidis*. Terminal pathway component deficiency is particularly associated with neisserial infection and in some populations as many as 14% of children with invasive meningococcal infection may have a such a deficiency,[72] although it is thought to be rarer than this in the UK.

Mannose-binding lectin deficiency

Yeasts such as candida species, mycobacteria and Gram-negative bacteria express high quantities of mannose-rich sugars on their surfaces, whereas eukaryotic cells do not. Mannose-binding lectin (MBL) is an opsonic protein synthesized in the liver, which recognizes foreign microbes by binding to such sugars—a non-specific immune response. As well as facilitating phagocytosis of micro-rganisms to which it binds, it can also promote C3 cleavage and complement activation.[73] Individuals with abnormally low levels of MBL are common (approximately 1 in 100)[74] and most appear well. However, there is evidence suggesting that mutations in the MBL gene are found more frequently in individuals with severe or recurrent infections of different types.[75] It may therefore be appropriate to measure serum levels of this protein with other investigations in these patients. Where the clinical picture suggests it is necessary, it may be appropriate to compensate for the defect with regular prophylactic antibiotics (see below).

Control protein deficiencies

Deficiency of C1esterase inhibitor (C1 INH) is an autosomal dominant disorder which causes hereditary angioedema, demonstrating the importance of this serum protein in negative feedback control on the release of vasoactive peptides. Affected patients have low levels of functional C1 INH or normal or high levels of a non-functional form. They are prone to episodes of spontaneous severe localized edema, usually lasting 2–3 days and without the redness and itching seen in urticaria. Laryngeal edema may be fatal. In childhood, abdominal cramps without obvious swelling are the commonest feature, angioedema becoming more prominent after puberty. Although there may be no obvious precipitating cause, trauma including surgery, menses and stress may trigger attacks. Diagnosis, often obvious when there is a family history, can be confirmed by assaying C1 INH, including a functional test as immunoassays for the protein can give misleadingly high results. Preventive treatment with the androgenic steroid danazol is not generally used in children. There is limited data to support the use of epsilon-aminocaproic acid or tranexemic acid on a regular basis. Recombinant C1 INH is available and is often used to treat acute attacks as well as prophylactically to cover surgery.

Described deficiencies of other complement regulatory proteins (e.g. Factors I and H, Properdin) result in phenotypes similar to complement factor deficiencies. Familial Mediterranean fever manifests as recurrent fever with joint and serosal inflammation. It appears to be due to deficiency in a serum protease which inactivates the chemoattractants C_5a and IL-8.[76]

TREATMENT OF PRIMARY IMMUNODEFICIENCY DISORDERS

Cure became possible for certain severe primary immunodeficiency disorders in the 1980s through BMT. Theoretically, this ideal could be extended through gene therapy to a wider group but this remains an experimental approach at present. For the rest, treatment consists of various approaches designed to prevent complications by compensating for deficiency and treating infection when prophylaxis fails.

BONE MARROW TRANSPLANTATION

Following early unsuccessful attempts at immune reconstitution by fetal liver and thymic transplantation, BMT has emerged as the most successful form of treatment for SCID and the more severe forms of combined immunodeficiency, as well as certain T-cell immunodeficiencies such as Wiskott–Aldrich syndrome and CD40-ligand deficiency. There is a 1 in 4 chance that any 2 siblings will have inherited exactly the same tissue types from their parents. In such cases, their lymphocytes will not proliferate in a mixed lymphocyte culture, and there is little capacity for graft rejection or GVHD. In 1968, an infant with SCID was successfully given a new immune system by transplanting bone marrow from an HLA-identical sibling. The results of such transplants have steadily improved and in a European survey of 183 patients transplanted for severe combined immunodeficiency, the survival rate of 60% for patients transplanted between 1968 and 1982 had risen to >90% for those transplanted between 1982 and 1989.[77] Usually, cytoreductive conditioning is not required and whole marrow can be infused without GVHD prophylaxis. Immune reconstitution is rapid with evidence of T-cell function within 2 weeks and full immune activity by 6–8 weeks. The improvement in outcome is probably mainly due to sterile isolation to prevent Aspergillus infection, early treatment with cotrimoxazole as prophylaxis against *Pneumocystis carinii* pneumonia, together with intravenous immunoglobulin replacement therapy and broad-spectrum antibiotic cover at the first sign of bacterial infection.

For the majority of children who lack an HLA-matched sibling, treatment by BMT is much more difficult and was not possible until 1981 when 3 patients with SCID were successfully transplanted using HLA non-identical marrow from a parent. Previous attempts to correct SCID using non-identical marrow had always ended in failure with fulminating fatal GVHD, but were successful after the bone marrow graft had been depleted of mature T lymphocytes by rosetting with sheep red blood cells. This technique has become well established, but is usually only successful in the small number of national centers with extensive experience in the difficult supportive care that is necessary. The data from a European network of such centers currently shows a survival rate of between 50% and 60% (unpublished observations). Some workers use E-rosetting as the method of T-cell depletion while other groups use the rat monoclonal antibody Campath-1M.[77] It has been difficult to compare the success of these different methods of T-cell depletion as there has also been variation in the way different centers treat their patients, particularly with regard to pre-transplant cytoreductive conditioning therapy.

Although there is general agreement that such conditioning is not needed when unmodified HLA-identical sibling grafts are given, there is wide variation in practice before T-cell depleted parental mismatched BMT. Although it is possible to achieve engraftment without conditioning therapy, there is often incomplete engraftment with only T-cell function and therefore greater long-term morbidity. Following conditioning therapy (usually with busulfan 60 mg/kg over 4 days and cyclophosphamide 200 mg/kg over 4 days), there is a higher engraftment rate and better long-term immune function with relatively little increase in infection-related mortality during the transplant period.

At presentation, infants with SCID often have multiple infections complicated by severe failure to thrive; their infections must be treated promptly and aggressively after appropriate swabs, cultures and biopsies have been taken. Total parental nutrition is almost always needed and has to be given by central venous catheter which adds to the risks of sepsis. Children need to be nursed in a sterile environment, particularly to prevent infection with fungi such as Aspergillus and great care must be taken to avoid contact with people excreting viruses, particularly respiratory viruses such as respiratory syncytial virus, parainfluenza virus and adenovirus. Children must always be given CMV-negative irradiated blood products. At the first sign of infection or temperature, cultures must be taken and broad-spectrum antibiotics started empirically.

Following transplantation with a T-cell depleted graft, neutrophil engraftment and platelet independence may be achieved quite quickly, but T-lymphocyte function often takes 120 days or more to develop and B-lymphocyte function 200–250 days. During this time infants need continuing support with antiviral and antimicrobial therapy, together with parental nutrition and intravenous immunoglobulin. GVHD is characterized by dermatitis and diarrhea, and liver dysfunction develops in a proportion of cases and is treated with steroid and cyclosporin therapy. Both the GVHD and its treatment are immunosuppressive, increasing the risk of further morbidity and mortality from infection. B-lymphoproliferative disease seems to be less common than in solid-organ transplant recipients, perhaps because EBV infection is less common in small infants.

Although treatment for SCID by mismatched BMT can be a very long and arduous process, most survivors (especially those given conditioning therapy) have full donor lymphoid chimerism and normal immune function. Furthermore, most appear to lead full and active lives, although it is still too early to say whether there are any very late complications.

Babies with SCID and respiratory viral infections pose a particularly difficult problem. European data showed that of the 49% of patients with such infections, only 31% survived, compared to 78% of those not infected.[77] Cytoreductive conditioning is often associated with a worsening of such infections, and so minimal conditioning should be given prior to transplantation. In an American series of 75 T-cell-depleted grafts without cytoreductive conditioning, 30% failed to achieve sustained engraftment.[78] However,

without conditioning, there is probably a poorer quality of immune function, and long-term survival may not be as good. Even without conditioning, an immune-mediated pneumonitis may still occur at the time of engraftment, probably due to cytokines released by newly matured lymphocytes reacting with virus and virally-damaged lung tissues. Only when this problem has been successfully overcome will survival rates be likely to rise to those seen for HLA-identical sibling transplants.

With the development of bone marrow donor programs, it is often possible to find HLA phenotypically-matched donors for patients lacking an HLA-identical sibling donor. Transplantation using these donors has been increasingly successful for patients with leukemia.[79] Severe GVHD and graft rejection were both more common than following HLA identical-sibling BMT, but for leukemic patients the results were much better than using an HLA mismatched graft. Despite increasingly sensitive methods of tissue typing, it is still not possible to detect all the 'minor' mismatches between 2 unrelated individuals who appear to share the same major tissue types, whereas HLA-identical siblings who have inherited the same major tissue types, also appear to inherit the same minor ones. Relatively few matched unrelated-donor transplants have been performed in SCID, mainly because of the protracted time (4–6 months) which it has usually taken to identify and recruit donors. This is simply too long for infants who are often already very ill with infection and need treatment urgently. European data also suggest that in SCID the results of matched unrelated-donor transplantation may not be much better than mismatched T-cell-depleted parental BMT, probably because parental donors can be worked up and harvested very quickly (<2 weeks), and also because an infant without an immune system is much less able to reject mismatched T-cell depleted marrow (A Fischer, unpublished communication). Most European centers would consider using a matched unrelated donor to transplant a child with SCID if the donor still appeared matched when tissue typing had been done at molecular level, and if the donor could be harvested and the transplant performed within 6 weeks of diagnosis. As neither of these criteria is easy to fulfil, most SCID babies in Europe without an HLA-identical sibling donor are still being transplanted using parental mismatched marrow.

Matched unrelated-donor transplantation may well have a role in treating children with T-cell immunodeficiencies such as Wiskott–Aldrich syndrome and hyper-IgM syndrome (CD40-ligand deficiency). In these cases, transplantation is not needed as urgently, so the donor work-up and harvest can be carried through in the usual way. It is also possible to use whole matched unrelated-donor marrow, particularly if prophylaxis against GVHD has been given by including antithymocyte globulin (ATG) immediately prior to transplant or by using cyclosporin with or without methotrexate after transplant. In transplants for leukemia, a degree of GVHD can be beneficial because the associated graft versus leukemia affect helps prevent relapse. This is, of course, of no benefit to children being transplanted for immunodeficiencies, and GVHD and its associated immune suppression may be more dangerous because of the risk of infection by reactivation of latent pathogens such as adenovirus. Nevertheless, early results for matched unrelated-donor transplants in immunodeficiency show promise.[80]

Umbilical cord blood has proved to be a useful source of allogeneic hemopoietic stem cells and banks of such stored material have now been set up. This offers potential for treating children with immunodeficiencies, not least because transplantation can proceed very quickly, and because there are sufficient hemopoietic stem cells present in a cord blood sample for a baby with SCID but not for an older patient.[81] Stem cells may also be obtained from peripheral blood, and using this as a source, larger numbers of stem cells can be given, which may improve engraftment rates, particularly following T-cell depletion.[82]

Correcting congenital immunodeficiencies by replacing defective genes with molecularly-engineered functional genes has been attempted in adenosine deaminase deficiency, and pre-clinical work is underway for other congenital primary immunodeficiencies. To date this does not seem to offer a robust and reliable form of treatment, but there is much ongoing work in this area and it remains to be seen whether this will prove a more useful technique than enhanced methods of BMT such as that using peripheral blood stem cells.

Another interesting new development is the treatment of severe combined immunodeficiency by *in utero* infusion of T-cell-depleted parental marrow. This can only be done when an earlier sibling has been shown to be affected and a diagnosis has been made early in pregnancy. This technique has the potential advantage of treating the child before he is exposed to infection, and giving the immune system time to develop *in utero* before birth, so that the child does not need to stay in hospital following delivery. There is however the potential disadvantage that GVHD will also occur *in utero* and will not be detected. There is a case report of successful treatment for SCID by this technique.[83]

IMMUNOGLOBULIN

Preparations of purified immunoglobulin first became available in the early 1950s. Administered intramuscularly, they were effective in reducing problems with infection in hypogammaglobulinemic patients.[84] However, this route of administration was associated with unpredictable absorption, frequent reactions and much discomfort and only limited volumes could be administered so serum levels were not adequate to prevent chronic infective lung damage. During the 1980s, intravenous immunoglobulin (IVIG) became widely available and has now superseded the intramuscular preparations. Current preparations are pooled from large numbers of donors (usually circa 10 000) who are screened for antibodies to HIV and hepatitis B and C, purified by Cohn cold ethanol fractionation and modified

to remove aggregates by low pH treatment (which fortuitously also inactivates hepatitis B virus) or by ion exchange chromatography. Many manufacturers also include a specific viral inactivation step such as detergent inactivation, which is effective against enveloped viruses such as hepatitis C and HIV, or heat treatment, which is effective against both enveloped and non-enveloped viruses such as hepatitis B. The immunoglobulin in standard preparations is almost entirely IgG, sometimes with IgG subclasses in physiologic proportions. However, there are certainly other undefined plasma proteins also present which may vary between preparations and batches and which may account for some of the observed clinical effects.

Administration of pooled immunoglobulin can only, at best, partially compensate for an inability to mount a specific humoral immune response to an invading pathogen, since the quantity of specific antibody present will always be limited to that present in the donor population and by the time of the most recent infusion. However, this therapy, when correctly managed, allows individuals who cannot make antibodies themselves, such as boys with XLA, to lead a normal healthy life. It is much more effective if started before there is lung damage from repeated infection, highlighting the importance of early diagnosis. Patients with humoral immunodeficiency, including XLA, common variable immunodeficiency, Wiskott–Aldrich syndrome, hyper-IgE syndrome, ataxia telangiectasia and occasionally combined isotype deficiencies and specific antibody production defects, may receive immunoglobulin prophylactic treatment if their clinical course, or predicted clinical course, suggests it to be appropriate. This therapy is also commonly used before BMT in patients with SCID and after transplantation while immune function remains suppressed and may need to be prolonged if GVHD is present.

The optimal dose interval for prophylactic replacement IVIG therapy is around 2–3 weeks and a dose of 0.3–0.4 g/kg is usually used.[85] However, higher doses may be used to overcome persistent problems in severely affected acutely or chronically infected patients and the dose is often adjusted according to serum IgG levels measured pre-infusion, which should remain in the upper part of the normal range for age. Where total IgG levels are normal, as for example in IgG subclass deficiency, trough subclass levels may be monitored. It is important that children on this treatment are monitored regularly to ensure good clinical progress and normal growth and that the practical aspects of regular infusions are trouble-free. It is a good idea to obtain blood to check for anemia and liver enzyme elevation on a regular basis. The dose and batch numbers of each infusion must always be carefully documented.

Immunoglobulin therapy is generally very safe and large doses can usually be given without adverse effects. However, hypersensitivity reactions do occur in a minority of patients causing one or a combination of fevers, rigors, headaches, nausea, myalgia and rashes. Rarely, severe anaphylactic reactions have been reported with associated collapse, shock or acute respiratory distress requiring urgent resuscitation.[86] Aseptic meningitis has also been reported as a complication of high-dose treatment.[87] In general, milder reactions can be managed by slowing or temporarily suspending the infusion and then proceeding at a slower rate with or without administration of non-steroidal anti-inflammatory medication. Antihistamine or steroid premedication is occasionally necessary. Occasionally, patients react specifically to a certain preparation and improve when an alternative is used. Some reactions are due to the presence of IgA autoantibodies in the patient so that preparations with little or no IgA present are better tolerated. Anaphylaxis in patients with selective IgA deficiency is likely to be due to this mechanism and provides another reason to avoid this therapeutic approach in such patients. There is a small but real risk of transmission of blood-borne viral infection in immunoglobulin, as with all blood products. Outbreaks of hepatitis C have occurred, reflecting the fact that screening for antibodies does not exclude donors who are newly infected and have not made a detectable antibody response.[88–90] It is highly inadvisable to change patients established on immunoglobulin therapy between different preparations, except for good clinical reasons, both because this will make it difficult to ascertain the source in the event of such an infection and because it will jeopardize the patient's chances of finding a well tolerated preparation in the event that adverse reactions become a problem in the future.

A major problem with immunoglobulin therapy is the inconvenience of infusions lasting several hours every 2–3 weeks. Children can miss significant amounts of school and parents' time is also taken up. This can be overcome to a great extent by establishing patients on treatment at home and such programs are now widespread. Suitable patients include those established on treatment and free of all but the most minor adverse effects. Appropriate liaison with primary care services is needed. Usually, a parent or carer learns to site intravenous access and to monitor infusions, although older patients can do this themselves provided another adult is present to seek or provide help if necessary. Patients or their parents need a well-formulated treatment plan with space to document problems with venepuncture, the immunoglobulin batches used and dose given and details of the progress of the infusion on each occasion. In some children, venous access is a problem. One solution is to use an indwelling central line with percutaneous access, although such lines are not without problems including infections which may be of great concern in the immunodeficient child. Another approach has been to use weekly rapid subcutaneous infusions of immunoglobulin.[91] Experience with this method of administration has been very encouraging to date and it may permit trouble-free home therapy in many more children. However, at the time of writing there is no licensed preparation available and an immunoglobulin preparation for intramuscular use is being used which has no viral inactivation step in its manufacture.

IVIG is also used in the treatment of a number of other infections and immunologic disorders. Where modulation of the immune response is the aim, higher doses (around 1–2 g/kg) are generally used on an empirical basis. In some cases (such as Kawasaki disease, chronic lymphocytic leukemia and idiopathic thrombocytopenic purpura), this is supported by good evidence; in others (such as pediatric HIV infection, Guillain–Barré syndrome, toxic shock syndrome and treatment of neonatal infection) indications for its use are not well defined.

ANTIMICROBIAL TREATMENT

Antimicrobial drugs are generally used for defined limited periods therapeutically in response to the clinical or microbiologic diagnosis of a specific infection or occasionally, prophylactically, to cover a short period of perceived high risk of infection (such as dental manipulation in children with congenital heart lesions thought to carry a significant risk of infectious endocarditis or surgical procedures associated with either a high risk of or high morbidity with postoperative infection). In children with specific immunodeficiency, the likelihood of developing common treatable infectious diseases of childhood, such as bacterial otitis media, sinusitis and pneumonia or complications thereof is elevated so that the threshold at which to intervene with standard treatment or to augment treatment to parenteral or high-dose administration is lowered. In addition, certain immunodeficiencies carry a risk of treatable infections not normally seen in children, such as *Pneumocystis carinii* pneumonia in those with combined immunodeficiencies, hyper-IgM syndrome and HIV infection, and require high-dose specific intravenous therapy (usually trimethoprim-sulfamethoxazole (cotrimoxazole)) if they present with the appropriate clinical picture.

There are several sound reasons why antimicrobial drugs should not, in principle, be administered for prolonged periods. Currently, the most pressing of these is the widespread emergence of highly and multiply antibiotic-resistant pathogens, particularly in countries where antibiotics are widely available and excessively used. This is, of course, not only a risk to the individual patient taking the drug but to all members of society as well. In addition, there may be concerns that long-term use of drugs may lead to unforeseen toxic effects—a particular worry in children whose growth and development are incomplete.

Despite this, antibiotics are used extensively for prolonged periods to reduce recurrence rates of urinary tract infections. There are also certain immunodeficient individuals in whom the likelihood of acute serious infection or an accumulation of repeated infections with chronic debilitating consequences such as chronic lung injury or significant school absence is sufficiently high to merit long-term regular prophylactic intervention with certain antimicrobial drugs. Low daily or alternate-day doses of trimethoprim-sulfamethoxazole (cotrimoxazole) prevents *Pneumocystis carinii* pneumonia in adults with AIDS[92] and is also used in children with severe primary or secondary cellular immunodeficiency. There is also a clear case for using both topical (e.g. nystatin) and systemic (e.g. fluconazole, itraconazole) long-term antifungal agents in some patients with chronic mucocutaneous candidiasis, as otherwise they remain chronically symptomatic. Antibiotic prophylaxis is also widely recommended for patients with reduced splenic function or asplenia.[115]

However, the commonest clinical situation in pediatric immunology is the need to prevent chronic or recurrent bacterial upper respiratory infections, including otitis media and lower respiratory tract infections, in children with demonstrable humoral or other opsonic immunodeficiency or a clear predisposition to recurrent infection without a defined underlying cause. A meta-analysis published in 1993 indicates that antibiotic prophylaxis does have an impact on occurrence of recurrent acute otitis media, although not on chronic otitis media with effusion or 'glue ear'.[93] Several small placebo-controlled studies have shown that a single daily dose of sulfonamide antibiotic reduces the incidence of recurrence of otitis media over a period of a few months in otitis-prone children[94,95] and that such drugs are as efficacious as amoxycillin[96,97] which costs more, causes more side-effects and for which resistance is more widespread. However, larger studies over longer periods have not been done nor have trials in children with diagnosed immunodeficiency, probably because placebo controls among such cases would be considered unethical. Nor are there good controlled data on the efficacy of antibiotic prophylaxis in preventing bacterial lower respiratory tract infection in such children, although it is widely assumed that it is effective.

None of the mainstream antibiotics is specifically licensed for prevention of respiratory infection anywhere in the world, and the majority of pediatric immunologists use trimethoprim-sulfamethoxazole (cotrimoxazole) given once daily at approximately a third to quarter the therapeutic dose (60–120 mg in infants and toddlers, 240 mg in children up to approximately 40 kg, then 480 mg). This drug combination has a relatively long half-life, is well absorbed orally and has extremely good penetration into all body fluids, cells and mucosal surfaces. It is not now widely used as a first-line routine pediatric antibiotic so there are fewer concerns regarding emergence of bacterial resistance in the individual patient and more generally. It seems to be remarkably well tolerated by almost all children who usually seem to like the taste of at least one of the currently available preparations and their parents who can usually remember to give it once a day at bedtime. The drug, once used widely in the prophylaxis of urinary tract infection in both adults and children, has fallen into disfavor in that setting as trimethoprim alone is equally effective and is less likely to cause the very rare cases of severe Stevens–Johnson syndrome (most or all in adults) associated with the combination. However, there is good microbiologic evidence to support the preferred use of the combination against the main bacterial respiratory pathogens (Table 25.3).

Table 25.3 Percentages of laboratory isolates of common respiratory pathogens sensitive to trimethoprim alone and trimethoprim-sulfamethoxazole (co-trimoxazole). Data were collected from UK clinical laboratories between 1986 and 1997. (Dr T Winstanley, Dept Microbiology, Royal Hallamshire Hospital, Sheffield, UK—'Microbe Base', sponsored by GlaxoWellcome UK.) Reproduced with permission from Ref. 116.

Organism	% Trimethoprim sensitive (n)	% Trimethoprim-sulfamethoxazole sensitive (n)
Haemophilus spp	90 (32 892)	92.4 (15 558)
Strep. pneumoniae	46.4 (7921)	88.1 (5385)
Moraxella	5.3 (3929)	78.6 (2002)
Group A streptococcus	73 (8515)	80.7 (3276)

It is unusual for children to develop a rash early after starting the drug and necessitating discontinuation of treatment[98] and the drug does not seem to cause the gastrointestinal symptoms commonly associated with β-lactams and some macrolides. The latter are the alternatives and amoxycillin with or without clavulanic acid, an oral cephalosporin or erythromycin given once or twice daily are all occasionally used in this setting. Children with immunodeficiency treated with immunoglobulin replacement therapy are usually also given regular antibiotic prophylaxis as an extra insurance against invasive or persistent bacterial infection.

ACQUIRED (SECONDARY) IMMUNODEFICIENCY DISEASES

The bulk of human disease is the direct or indirect result of infection. New roles for infectious agents are constantly emerging, e.g. Helicobacter pylori in duodenal ulceration and gastric cancer. Infectious agents can cause disease by direct or toxin-mediated tissue injury (e.g. in gas gangrene and tetanus) but the inflammatory and immune responses to infection often cause much of disease pathophysiology (e.g. in bacterial meningitis and post-infectious arthritis). Many infections can also induce an immunodeficient state in which the child is at enhanced risk of other infectious diseases. This is most commonly exemplified in the widely studied, although poorly understood, vicious spiral that occurs in children affected by infections and malnutrition (Fig. 25.6). Infections lead to much morbidity and mortality in children who have borderline nutrition, not only directly but also by induction of secondary immunodeficiency and thus other infections.

In settings where nutrition is adequate, many childhood infections are recognized to cause secondary immunodeficiency directly or at least to predispose to further infection. Measles was widely recognized as doing this before it became uncommon as a result of immunization. However, other examples are regularly encountered in clinical practice such as the occurrence of secondary perioral Herpes simplex infection in association with pneumococcal pneumonia and of

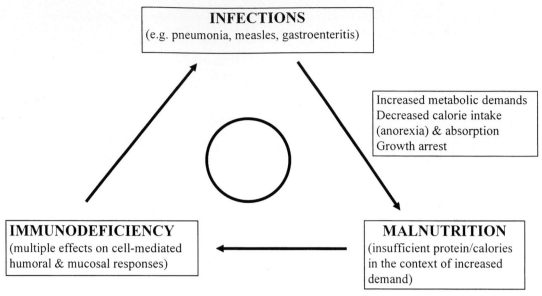

Fig. 25.6 Malnutrition cycle.

bacterial pneumonia following an apparent viral upper respiratory prodrome. Epidemiologic observations can also offer intriguing insights into phenomena of this kind; e.g. the apparent temporal association of outbreaks of meningococcal disease shortly after epidemics of influenza.[99] The precise immunologic mechanism of these effects remain obscure. A large number of hypotheses, including local mucosal injury, consumption of available immune resources, and cytokine-mediated suppressive effects, can be postulated and related observational studies are also sometimes feasible. However, it remains difficult to ascertain the precise role and significance of such effects in predisposing to infection and disease.

HUMAN IMMUNODEFICIENCY VIRUS 1 AND 2

The recognition of the epidemic of infection due to HIV in the early 1980s was remarkable not so much for the emergence of secondary immunodeficiency on a large scale, as this was already common as indicated above, but for the severity and unrelenting progression of the immunodeficiency it caused. The RNA lentivirus HIV has now been extensively characterized and is known to have high replication rates even in the early asymptomatic stages of infection as well as high rates of spontaneous mutation permitting rapid adaptation and acquisition of resistance to antiviral agents.

Transmission and its prevention

The main mode of acquisition in children is by vertical transmission from the infected mother either transplacentally *in utero*, perinatally in the birth canal or postnatally by breast feeding. Horizontal transmission sexually and in inoculated infected blood and blood products may also occur. Breast feeding by HIV-positive mothers should be avoided in developed countries but the balance of risk and benefit may be reversed in other settings. Intervention with antiretroviral therapy in the mother pre- and post-natally and the baby postnatally has also been shown to reduce substantially the rate of transmission from mother to infant.[100] Different drug regimens in this setting are certain to be introduced as further trials are completed. The role of elective caesarean delivery is controversial. Low cost measures such as vaginal viricides are also urgently needed in the countries where perinatal infection is common and systemic antiviral agents unavailable. Use of barrier contraception not only prevents the spread of HIV but also other sexually transmitted diseases which may act as cofactors in HIV-related illness. Since these forms of intervention have the potential to prevent many cases of pediatric HIV infection there is an urgent need to institute effective programs of antenatal testing, particularly in areas of relatively high prevalence. Such programs have been hampered by the prejudicial attitudes towards HIV infection and fears about its consequences which are held by health professionals and many of the public and which act to prevent tests being offered and from being accepted.[101]

Manifestations

Clinical definitions of progression of HIV-related infectious and malignant diseases in children have evolved over the years and are currently as shown in Table 25.4. The features, although overlapping, are distinct from those seen in adults. In some children there is rapid and often fatal progression during the first year of life—possibly as a consequence of prenatal infection—whereas the remainder progress heterogeneously towards severe immunosuppression usually between 5 and 10 years of age. Infections with encapsulated bacteria, in particular *Strep. pneumoniae*, including septicemia,

Table 25.4 Clinical staging of HIV-related disease in children. Reproduced with permission from Ref. 101.

Category	Features
N	Asymptomatic
A	Mildly symptomatic At least 2 of: Lymphadenopathy Hepatomegaly Splenomegaly Parotitis Rash Ear, nose and throat infections
B	Moderately symptomatic Single episode of a severe bacterial infection Lymphocytic interstitial pneumonitis Anemia, neutropenia, thrombocytopenia Cardiomyopathy, nephropathy, hepatitis, diarrhea Candidiasis, severe varicella/zoster or herpes simplex virus
C	Severely symptomatic Two serious bacterial infections Encephalopathy (acquired microcephaly, cognitive delay, abnormal neurology) Wasting syndrome (severe failure to thrive or downward crossing 2 weight centiles) Opportunistic infections (*Pneumocystis carinii* pneumonia, cytomegalovirus, toxoplasmosis, disseminated fungal infections) Disseminated mycobacterial disease Cancer (Kaposi's sarcoma, lymphomas)

pneumonia and otitis are a particular problem. As immunosuppression advances, opportunistic infections including *Pneumocystis carinii* pneumonia, mycobacterial infection both typical and atypical and cryptosporidial diarrhea can occur, although some which are commonly problematic in adults with AIDS such as CMV and toxoplasma infection are seen more rarely in children.

An insidious progressive lymphocytic intestinal pneumonitis is seen in some cases. Although really a histologic diagnosis, it is usually made in practice on clinical and radiologic evidence alone. Its etiology is obscure but may be due to chronic viral infection. It is associated with significant respiratory morbidity.[102] Neurologic disease is also well described in children with HIV manifesting variously as developmental delay and regression, paresis and encephalopathy. Malignancies are also a feature, in particular lymphoma,[103] and growth failure can be a major problem.

The progression of the immunodeficiency can be followed by monitoring the fall in the peripheral blood count of CD4$^+$ T lymphocytes which are selectively infected and destroyed by HIV. The normal range for CD4 counts varies with age and so must be monitored appropriately.[104] Quantitative measurement of HIV genomic RNA by polymerase chain reaction in plasma is now the standard for monitoring disease progression and response to therapy. Other less specific abnormalities, such as hypergammaglobulinemia and poor antibody responses to vaccine antigens, which reflect dysregulation of B-cell function, are commonly present.

Specific and adjunctive treatment

Until the mid 1990s medical management of pediatric HIV infection consisted mainly of prophylaxis and treatment of secondary infections with antimicrobial agents combined with the use of one widely available antiretroviral drug, azidothymidine (AZT). Cotrimoxazole is widely used as prophylaxis against *Pneumocystis carinii* pneumonia as well as bacterial respiratory infection and, where it is poorly tolerated, since pentamidine is not generally used in children, dapsone can be used as an alternative. In such cases, it is advisable to add a macrolide or β-lactam antibiotic as prophylaxis against bacterial infection. The importance of appropriate neurodevelopmental, dietetic, social and psychologic support for the children and their families has been clearly established.[105] 1996–97 saw the arrival of a large number of new antiretroviral agents for assessment in pediatric use. Agents can now be classified into 3 main groups:

- nucleoside analog reverse transcriptase inhibitors (RTIs), such as azidothymidine or zidovudine (AZT, ZVD), didanosine (ddI), lamivudine (3TC), zalcitabine (ddC) and stavusdine (d4T);
- non-nucleoside RTIs such as nevirapine and delavirdine;
- protease inhibitors such as ritonavir, indinavir, saquinavir and nelfinavir.

Current trials in children focus on the use of combinations of these agents to reduce viral load and to delay or reverse disease progression. Studies will need to address the optimal timing of institution of such treatments as well as the best combinations. Short- and long-term toxicities are also major issues as are convenience of use and palatability, all of which may affect compliance. The other major issue is cost.

In developed countries, children with HIV should be followed in a center with sufficient experience to ensure adequate and up-to-date management and to offer participation in multicenter therapeutic trials which are essential to evaluate how best to treat these patients. HIV in children is usually accompanied by HIV in the mother or both parents often together with degrees of social deprivation and isolation. Combining medical and health services with psychologic and social support services in a single clinic for both adults and children is an attractive model for provision of care for these families.[105] It should also be remembered that the number of children affected indirectly by HIV, e.g. through illness or death in their parents or other family members, greatly exceeds those actually infected with the virus. From the global perspective, the main hope for effective control of the infection must be through development of a vaccine.

HYPOSPLENISM

Post-traumatic splenectomy is unusual in childhood. However, children may have primary asplenia or hyposplenia, may undergo operative splenectomy for a number of malignant, hematologic or immunologic indications or may have reduced splenic function secondary to conditons such as hemoglobinopathies, lymphoproliferative diseases, inflammatory bowel disease or following BMT. Hyposplenism for whatever reason is associated with an enhanced the risk of fulminant infection,[106] particularly in early childhood. This is because the spleen acts as a filter for bacteria and parasitized erythrocytes.[107] Furthermore, many of the primary disorders associated with hyposplenism or indicating splenectomy themselves cause immunodeficiency either directly (e.g. Wiskott–Aldrich syndrome and hematologic malignancy) or through their treatment (e.g. chemotherapy or steroids). An ultrasound scan of the spleen is now a routine part of many immunologists' work-up of a child with recurrent bacteremia or invasive bacterial infection.

The main organisms which are prominent in hyposplenic patients are *Strep. pneumoniae* (the commonest, with a mortality of up to 60%) *Neisseria meningitidis* and *Haemophilus influenzae* type b (although the latter is now seen rarely since the introduction of universal immunization).[108,109] These are the main invasive encapsulated bacterial pathogens of early life after the end of the neonatal period. Patients are also at enhanced risk of *Escherichia coli* infection,[110] malaria,[111] babesiosis[112] and DF-2 bacillus (*Capnocytophaga canimorsus*) infection following dog bites.[113]

All children with hyposplenism should receive continous daily oral antibiotic prophylaxis[114] with phenoxymethyl penicillin, amoxycillin or, in allergic patients, erythromycin.[115] Some experts use cotrimoxazole prophylaxis in children up to the age of 5 years. However, these treatments do not guarantee protection against invasive infection, so patients and their parents need to understand the need to seek urgent medical advice when feverish or unwell so that appropriate intravenous antimicrobial therapy can be instituted if necessary.

Children with hyposplenism should receive all routine immunizations, including live vaccines. The polysaccharide 23 valent pneumococcal and 2 and 4 valent meningococcal vaccines are poorly immunogenic in children under 2 years old but can be given to hyposplenic children at age 2. New protein-conjugated vaccines with enhanced immunogenicity are expected to be available shortly and may join *Haemophilus influenzae* type b ('Hib') vaccine in the routine infant schedule in many countries. Influenza vaccine can sensibily be given to these patients each autumn as it may reduce the risk of secondary bacterial infection.

REFERENCES

1. Fischer A, Landais P, Friedrich W *et al*. European experience of bone-marrow transplantation for severe combined immunodeficiency. *Lancet* 1990; **336**: 850–854

2. Bosma GC, Custer RP, Bosma MJ. A severe combined immunodeficiency mutation in the mouse. *Nature* 1983; **301**: 527–530

3. Bosma MJ, Carroll AM. The SCID mouse mutant: definition, characterization, and potential uses. *Annu Rev Immunol* 1991; **9**: 323–350.

4. Schwarz K, Gauss GH, Ludwig L *et al*. RAG mutations in human B cell-negative SCID. *Science* 1996; **274**: 97–99

5. Noguchi M, Yi H, Rosenblatt HM *et al*. Interleukin-2 receptor gamma chain mutation results in X-linked severe combined immunodeficiency in humans. *Cell* 1993; **73**: 147–157

6. Russell SM, Johnston JA, Noguchi M *et al*. Interaction of IL-2R beta and gamma c chains with Jak1 and Jak3: implications for XSCID and XCID. *Science* 1994; **266**: 1042–1045

7. Stephan JL, Vlekova V, Le Deist F *et al*. Severe combined immunodeficiency: a retrospective single-center study of clinical presentation and outcome in 117 patients. *J Pediatr* 1993; **123**: 564–572

8. Knobloch C, Goldmann SF, Friedrich W. Limited T cell receptor diversity of transplacentally acquired maternal T cells in severe combined immunodeficiency. *J Immunol* 1991; **146**: 4157–4164

9. Omenn GS. Familial reticuloendotheliosis with eosinophilia. *N Engl J Med* 1965; **273**: 427–432

10. Omenn GS. Familial reticuloendotheliosis with eosinophilia: a follow-up. *Birth Defects* 1971; **7**: 196

11. Chilosi M, Facchetti F, Notarangelo LD *et al*. CD30 cell expression and abnormal soluble CD30 serum accumulation in Omenn's syndrome: evidence for a T helper 2-mediated condition. *Eur J Immunol* 1996; **26**: 329–334

12. Villard J, Lisowska Grospierre B, van den Elsen P *et al*. Mutation of RFXAP, a regulator of MHC class II genes, in primary MHC class II deficiency [see comments]. *N Engl J Med* 1997; **337**: 748–753

13. Elhasid R, Etzioni A. Major histocompatibility complex class II deficiency: a clinical review. *Blood* 1996; **10**: 242–248

14. Klein C, Lisowska Grospierre B, LeDeist F *et al*. Major histocompatibility complex class II deficiency: clinical manifestations, immunologic features, and outcome. *J Pediatr* 1993; **123**: 921–928

15. Negishi I, Motoyama N, Nakayama K *et al*. Essential role for ZAP-70 in both positive and negative selection of thymocytes. *Nature* 1995; **376**: 435–438

16. Makitie O, Kaitila I. Cartilage-hair hypoplasia—clinical manifestations in 108 Finnish patients. *Eur J Pediatr* 1993; **152**: 211–217

17. Schofer O, Blaha I, Mannhardt W *et al*. Omenn phenotype with short-limbed dwarfism. *J Pediatr* 1991; **118**: 86–89

18. Hirschhorn R. Adenosine deaminase deficiency: molecular basis and recent developments. *Clin Immunol Immunopathol* 1995; **76**: S219–227

19. Hershfield MS. PEG-ADA replacement therapy for adenosine deaminase deficiency: an update after 8.5 years. *Clin Immunol Immunopathol* 1995; **76**: S228–232.

20. Markert ML. Purine nucleoside phosphorylase deficiency. *Immunodeficiency Rev* 1991; **3**: 45–81

21. Hague RA, Rassam S, Morgan G *et al*. Early diagnosis of severe combined immunodeficiency syndrome. *Arch Dis Child* 1994; **70**: 260–263

22. Derry JM, Ochs HD, Francke U. Isolation of a novel gene mutated in Wiskott–Aldrich syndrome. *Cell* 1994; **78**: 635–644 (published erratum appears in *Cell* 1994; **79**: 922)

23. Aspenstrom P, Lindberg U, Hall A. Two GTPases, CDC 42 and Rac, bind directly to approach an implicated immunodeficiency disorder Wiskott Aldrich Syndrome. *Curr Biol* 1996; **6**: 70–75

24. Ox HD, Zhu QT, Watanabe C, Kanner SB, Hollenbauch D, Aruffo A. Wiskott Aldrich syndrome: The WASP protein phenotype and genotype. In: Fasth A, Bjork E, Kander J (eds) *Progress in Immunodeficiency*. Amsterdam: Elsevier; 1996, pp 85–96

25. Teare EL, Fairley CK, White J *et al*. Efficacy of Hib vaccine. *Lancet* 1994; **344**: 828–829

26. Sullivan JL, Byron KS, Brewster FE *et al*. X-linked lymphoproliferative syndrome. Natural history of the immunodeficiency. *J Clin Invest* 1983; **71**: 1765–1778

27. Seemayer TA, Gross TG, Egeler RM *et al*. X-linked lymphoproliferative disease: twenty-five years after the discovery. *Pediatr Res* 1995; **38**: 471–478

28. Gross TG, Filipovich AH, Conley ME *et al*. Cure of X-linked lymphoproliferative disease (XLP) with allogeneic hematopoietic

stem cell transplantation (HSCT): report from the XLP registry. *Bone Marrow Transplant* 1996; **17**: 741–744

29. Bastian J, Law S, Vogler L et al. Prediction of persistent immunodeficiency in the DiGeorge anomaly. *J Pediatr* 1989; **115**: 391–396

30. Goldsobel AB, Haas A, Stiehm ER. Bone marrow transplantation in DiGeorge syndrome. *J Pediatr* 1987; **111**: 40–44

31. Savitsky K, Bar Shira A, Gilad S et al. A single ataxia telangiectasia gene with a product similar to PI-3 kinase [see comments]. *Science* 1995; **268**: 1749–1753

32. Lavin MF, Shiloh Y. The genetic defect in ataxia telangiectasia. *Annu Rev Immunol* 1997; **15**: 177–202

32a. Carney JP, Maser RS, Olivares H et al. The hMre11/hRad50 protein complex and Nijmegen breakage syndrome: linkage of double-strand break repair to the cellular DNA damage response. *Cell* 1998; **93**: 477–486

32b. Varon R, Vissinga C, Platzer M et al. Nibrin, a novel DNA double-strand break repair protein, is mutated in Nijmegen breakage syndrome. *Cell* 1998; **93**: 467–476

33. Weemaes CM, Smeets DF, van der Burgt CJ. Nijmegen breakage syndrome: a progress report. *Int J Radiat Biol* 1994; **66**: S185–188

34. Freier S, Kerem E, Dranitzki Z et al. Hereditary CD4$^+$ T lymphocytopenia. *Arch Dis Child* 1998; **78**: 371–372

35. Nezelof C, Jammet ML, Lortholary P et al. L'hypoplasie hereditaire du thymus. Sa place et sa responsabilite dans une observation d'aplasie lymphocytaire, normoplasmocytaire et normolglobulinemique du nourrisson. *Arch Françaises Pediatr* 1998; **21**: 897–920

36. Le Deist F, Emile JF, Rieux Laucat F et al. Clinical, immunological, and pathological consequences of Fas-deficient conditions. *Lancet* 1996; **348**: 719–723

37. Lillic D, Cant AJ, Abinun M et al. Chronic mucocutaneous candidiasis 1. altered antigen stimulated IL-2, IL-4, IL-6 and Interferon gamma production. *Clin Exp Immunol* 1996; **105**: 205–212

38. Nagamine K, Peterson P, Scott H et al. Positional cloning of the APECED gene. *Nature Genet* 1997; **17**: 393–398

39. Aaltonen J, Bjorses P, Perheentupa J et al. An autoimmune disease, APECED, caused by mutations in a novel gene featuring two PHD-type zinc-finger domains. *Nature Genet* 1997; **17**: 399–403

40. Ahonen P, Myllarniemi S, Sipila I et al. Clinical variation of autoimmune polyendocrinopathy-candidiasis-ectodermal dystrophy (APECED) in a series of 68 patients. *N Engl J Med* 1990; **322**: 1829–1836

41. Bentur L, Nisbet Brown E, Levison H et al. Lung disease associated with IgG subclass deficiency in chronic mucocutaneous candidiasis. *J Pediatr* 1991; **118**: 82–86.

42. Herrod HG. Chronic mucocutaneous candidiasis in childhood and complications of non-Candida infection: a report of the Pediatric Immunodeficiency Collaborative Study Group. *J Pediatr* 1990; **116**: 377–382

43. Hoh MC, Lynn HP, Chan LL et al. Successful allogeneic bone marrow transplantation in severe chronic mucocutaneous candidiasis syndrome. *Bone Marrow Transplant* 1986; **18**: 797–800

44. Sneller MC, Strober W, Eisenstein E et al. NIH conference. New insights into common variable immunodeficiency. *Ann Intern Med* 1993; **118**: 720–730

45. Anderson DC, Springer TA. Leukocyte adhesion deficiency: an inherited defect in the Mac-1, LFA-1, and p150,95 glycoproteins. *Annu Rev Med* 1987; **38**: 175–194

46. Thomas C, Le Deist F, Cavazzana Calvo M et al. Results of allogeneic bone marrow transplantation in patients with leukocyte adhesion deficiency. *Blood* 1995; **86**: 1629–1635

47. Etzioni A, Frydman M, Pollack S et al. Recurrent severe infections caused by a novel leukocyte adhesion deficiency. *N Engl J Med* 1992; **327**: 1789–1792

48. Tsukada S, Saffran DC, Rawlings DJ et al. Deficient expression of a B cell cytoplasmic tyrosine kinase in human X-linked agammaglobulinemia. *Cell* 1993; **72**: 279–290

49. Vetrie D, Vorechovsky I, Sideras P et al. The gene involved in X-linked agammaglobulinaemia is a member of the src family of protein-tyrosine kinases. *Nature* 1993; **361**: 226–233 (published erratum appears in *Nature* 1993; **364**: 362)

50. Conley ME. B cells in patients with X-linked agammaglobulinemia. *J Immunol* 1985; **134**: 3070–3074

51. Lederman HM, Winkelstein JA. X-linked agammaglobulinemia: an analysis of 96 patients. *Medicine Baltimore* 1985; **64**: 145–156

52. McKinney RE Jr, Katz SL, Wilfert CM. Chronic enteroviral meningoencephalitis in agammaglobulinemic patients. *Rev Infect Dis* 1987; **9**: 334–356

53. Liese JG, Wintergerst U, Tympner KD et al. High- vs low-dose immunoglobulin therapy in the long-term treatment of X-linked agammaglobulinemia. *Am J Dis Child* 1992; **146**: 335–339

54. Allen RC, Armitage RJ, Conley ME et al. CD40 ligand gene defects responsible for X-linked hyper-IgM syndrome. *Science* 1993; **259**: 990–993

55. DiSanto JP, Bonnefoy JY, Gauchat JF et al. CD40 ligand mutations in X-linked immunodeficiency with hyper-IgM [see comments]. *Nature* 1993; **361**: 541–543

56. Fuleihan R, Ramesh N, Loh R et al. Defective expression of the CD40 ligand in X chromosome-linked immunoglobulin deficiency with normal or elevated IgM. *Proc Natl Acad Sci USA* 1993; **90**: 2170–2173

57. Korthauer U, Graf D, Mages HW et al. Defective expression of T-cell CD40 ligand causes X-linked immunodeficiency with hyper-IgM. *Nature* 1993; **361**: 539–541

58. Notarangelo LD, Duse M, Ugazio AG. Immunodeficiency with hyper-IgM (HIM). *Immunodeficiency Rev* 1992; **3**: 101–121

59. Levy J, Espanol Boren T, Thomas C et al. Clinical spectrum of X-linked hyper-IgM syndrome [see comments]. *J Pediatr* 1997; **131**: 47–54

60. Hayward AR, Levy J, Facchetti F et al. Cholangiopathy and tumors of the pancreas, liver and biliary tree in boys with X-linked immunodeficiency and hyper-IgM. *J Immunol* 1997; **158**: 977–983

61. Hayward AR, Levy J, Facchetti F et al. Cholangiopathy and tumors of the pancreas, liver, and biliary tree in boys with X-linked immunodeficiency with hyper-IgM. *J Immunol* 1997; **158**: 977–983

62. Banatvala N, Davies J, Kanariou M et al. Hypogammaglobulinaemia associated with normal or increased IgM (the hyper IgM syndrome): a case series review. *Arch Dis Child* 1994; **71**: 150–152

63. Thomas C, de Saint Basile G, Le Deist F et al. Brief report: correction of X-linked hyper-IgM syndrome by allogeneic bone marrow transplantation. *N Engl J Med* 1995; **333**: 426–429

64. Hanson LA, Soderstrom R, Avanzini A et al. Immunoglobulin subclass deficiency. *Pediatr Infect Dis J* 1988; **7**: S17–21

65. Ambrosino DM, Siber GR, Chilmonczyk BA et al. An immunodeficiency characterized by impaired antibody responses to polysaccharides. *N Engl J Med* 1987; **316**: 790–793

66. Gigliotti F, Herrod HG, Kalwinsky DK et al. Immunodeficiency associated with recurrent infections and an isolated *in vivo* inability to respond to bacterial polysaccharides. *Pediatr Infect Dis J* 1988; **7**: 417–420

67. Dressler F, Peter HH, Muller W et al. Transient hypogammaglobulinemia of infancy: Five new cases, review of the literature and redefinition. *Acta Paediatr Scand* 1989; **78**: 767–774

68. Drenth JP, Haagsma CJ, van der Meer JW. Hyperimmunoglobulinemia D and periodic fever syndrome. The clinical spectrum in a series of 50 patients. International Hyper-IgD Study Group. *Medicine Baltimore* 1994; **73**: 133–144

69. Zeitlin HC, Sheppard K, Baum JD et al. Homozygous transcobalamin II deficiency maintained on oral hydroxocobalamin. *Blood* 1985; **66**: 1022–1027

70. Johnston RB. The complement system in host defense and inflammation: the cutting edges of a double edged sword. *Pediatr Infect Dis J* 1993; **12**: 933–941

71. Kolble K, Reid KB. Genetic deficiencies of the complement system and association with disease—early components. *Int Rev Immunol* 1993; **10**: 17–36

72. Tedesco F, Nurnberger W, Perissutti S. Inherited deficiencies of the terminal complement components. *Int Rev Immunol* 1993; **10**: 51–64

73. Kuhlman M, Joiner K, Ezekowitz RA. The human mannose-binding protein functions as an opsonin. *J Exp Med* 1989; **169**: 1733–1745

74. Super M, Thiel S, Lu J *et al.* Association of low levels of mannan-binding protein with a common defect of opsonisation. *Lancet* 1989; **2**: 1236–1239

75. Summerfield JA, Sumiya M, Levin M *et al.* Association of mutations in mannose binding protein gene with childhood infection in consecutive hospital series. *Br Med J* 1997; **314**: 1229–1232

76. Matzner Y, Ayesh SK, Hochner Celniker D *et al.* Proposed mechanism of the inflammatory attacks in familial Mediterranean fever. *Arch Intern Med* 1990; **150**: 1289–1291

77. Fischer A, Landais P, Friedrich W *et al.* European experience of bone-marrow transplantation for severe combined immunodeficiency. *Lancet* 1990; **336**: 850–854

78. O'Reilly RJ, Keever CA, Small TN *et al.* The use of HLA-non-identical T-cell-depleted marrow transplants for correction of severe combined immunodeficiency disease. *Immunodeficiency Rev* 1989; **1**: 273–309

79. Kernan NA, Bartsch G, Ash RC *et al.* An analysis of 462 transplantations from unrelated donors facilitated by the National Marrow Donor Program. *N Engl J Med* 1993; **328**: 593–602

80. Filipovich AH, Shapiro RS, Ramsay NK *et al.* Unrelated donor bone marrow transplantation for correction of lethal congenital immunodeficiencies. *Blood* 1992; **80**: 270–276

81. Wagner JE, Kernan NA, Steinbuch M *et al.* Allogeneic sibling umbilical-cord-blood transplantation in children with malignant and non-malignant disease [see comments]. *Lancet* 1995; **346**: 214–219

82. Russel N, Gratwohl A, Schmitz N. The place of blood stem cells in allogeneic transplantation. *Br J Haematol* 1996; **93**: 747–753

83. Flake AW, Ron Carolo MG, Puck JM *et al.* Treatment of X-linked severe combined immunodeficiency by *in utero* transplantation of paternal marrow. *N Engl J Med* 1996; **335**: 1806–1810

84. Good RA, Lorenz E. Historic aspects of intravenous immunoglobulin therapy. *Cancer* 1991; **68**: 1415–1421

85. Chapel HM. Consensus on diagnosis and management of primary antibody deficiencies. Consensus Panel for the Diagnosis and Management of Primary Antibody Deficiencies. *Br Med J* 1994; **308**: 581–585

86. Wahn V, Good RA, Gupta S, Pahwa S, Day NK. Evidence of persistent IgA/IgG circulating immune complexes associated with activation of the complement system in serum of a patient with common variable immune deficiency: anaphylactic reactions to intravenous gammaglobulin. *Acta Pathol Microbiol Immunol Scand* 1984; **284** (**Suppl**): 49–58

87. Sekul EA, Cupler EJ, Dalakas MC. Aseptic meningitis associated with high-dose intravenous immunoglobulin therapy: frequency and risk factors. *Ann Intern Med* 1994; **121**: 259–262

88. Widell A, Zhang YY, Andersson Gare B *et al.* At least three hepatitis C virus strains implicated in Swedish and Danish patients with intravenous immunoglobulin-associated hepatitis C. *Transfusion* 1997; **37**: 313–320

89. Echevarria JM, Leon P, Domingo CJ *et al.* Laboratory diagnosis and molecular epidemiology of an outbreak of hepatitis C virus infection among recipients of human intravenous immunoglobulin in Spain. *Transfusion* 1996; **36**: 725–730

90. Healey CJ, Sabharwal NK, Daub J *et al.* Outbreak of acute hepatitis C following the use of anti-hepatitis C virus—screened intravenous immunoglobulin therapy. *Gastroenterology* 1996; **110**: 1120–1126

91. Abrahamsen TG, Sandersen H, Bustnes A. Home therapy with subcutaneous immunoglobulin infusions in children with congenital immunodeficiencies. *Pediatrics* 1996; **98**: 1127–1131

92. Fischl MA, Dickinson GM, La Voie L. Safety and efficacy of sulfamethoxazole and trimethoprim chemoprophylaxis for *Pneumocystis carinii* pneumonia in AIDS. *JAMA* 1988; **259**: 1185–1189

93. Williams RL, Chalmers TC, Stange KC *et al.* Use of antibiotics in preventing recurrent acute otitis media and in treating otitis media with effusion. A meta-analytic attempt to resolve the brouhaha. *JAMA* 1993; **270**: 1344–1351

94. Liston TE, Foshee WS, Pierson WD. Sulfisoxazole chemoprophylaxis for frequent otitis media. *Pediatrics* 1983; **71**: 524–530

95. Varsano I, Volovitz B, Mimouni F. Sulfisoxazole prophylaxis of middle ear effusion and recurrent acute otitis media. *Am J Dis Child* 1985; **139**: 632–635

96. Principi N, Marchisio P, Massironi E *et al.* Prophylaxis of recurrent acute otitis media and middle-ear effusion. Comparison of amoxicillin with sulfamethoxazole and trimethoprim. *Am J Dis Child* 1989; **143**: 1414–1418

97. Sih T, Moura R, Caldas S *et al.* Prophylaxis for recurrent acute otitis media: a Brazilian study. *Int J Pediatr Otorhinolaryngol* 1993; **25**: 19–24

98. Gutman LT. The use of trimethoprim-sulfamethoxazole in children: a review of adverse reactions and indications. *Pediatr Infect Dis J* 1984; **3**: 349–357

99. Hubert B, Watier L, Garnerin P *et al.* Meningococcal disease and influenza-like syndrome: a new approach to an old question. *J Infect Dis* 1992; **166**: 542–545

100. Connor EM, Sperling RS, Gelber R *et al.* Reduction of maternal-infant transmission of human immunodeficiency virus type 1 with zidovudine treatment. Pediatric AIDS Clinical Trials Group Protocol 076 Study Group. *N Engl J Med* 1994; **331**: 1173–1180

101. Sharland M, Gibb D, Tudor Williams G *et al.* Paediatric HIV infection. *Arch Dis Child* 1997; **76**: 293–296

102. Sharland M, Gibb DM, Holland F. Respiratory morbidity from lymphocytic interstitial pneumonitis (LIP) in vertically acquired HIV infection. *Arch Dis Child* 1997; **76**: 334–336

103. Evans JA, Gibb DM, Holland FJ *et al.* Malignancies in UK children with HIV infection acquired from mother to child transmission. *Arch Dis Child* 1997; **76**: 330–333

104. Gibb D, Walters S (eds) *Guidelines for Managment of Children with HIV Infection*, 3rd edn. Horsham: AVERT, 1998

105. Gibb DM, Masters J, Shingadia D *et al.* A family clinic – optimising care for HIV infected children and their families. *Arch Dis Child* 1997; **77**: 478–482

106. Cullingford GL, Watkins DN, Watts AD *et al.* Severe late post-splenectomy infection. *Br J Surg* 1991; **78**: 716–721

107. Rosse WF. The spleen as a filter. *N Engl J Med* 1987; **317**: 704–706

108. Traub A, Giebink GS, Smith C *et al.* Splenic reticuloendothelial function after splenectomy, spleen repair, and spleen autotransplantation. *N Engl J Med* 1987; **317**: 1559–1564

109. Holdsworth RJ, Irving AD, Cuschieri A. Postsplenectomy sepsis and its mortality rate: actual versus perceived risks. *Br J Surg* 1991; **78**: 1031–1038

110. Edwards LD, Digioia R. Infections in splenectomized patients. A study of 131 patients. *Scand J Infect Dis* 1976; **8**: 255–261

111. Oster CN, Koontz LC, Wyler DJ. Malaria in asplenic mice: effects of splenectomy, congenital asplenia, and splenic reconstitution on the course of infection. *Am J Trop Med Hyg* 1980; **29**: 1138–1142

112. Rosner F, Zarrabi MH, Benach JL *et al.* Babesiosis in splenectomized adults. Review of 22 reported cases. *Am J Med* 1984; **76**: 696–701

113. McCarthy M, Zumla A. DF-2 infection. *Br Med J* 1988; **297**: 1355–1356

114. Scopes JW. Continued need for pneumococcal prophylaxis after splenectomy. *Arch Dis Child* 1991; **66**: 750

115. Working Party of the British Committee for Standards in Haematology Clinical Haematology Task Force. Guidelines for the Prevention and Treatment of Infection in Patients with an Absent or Dysfunctional Spleen. *Br Med J* 1996; **312**: 430–434

116. Finn A, Smith J. The use of antimicrobial prophylaxis to prevent infections in childhood. *Arch Dis Child* 1998 (in press)

117. Roitt I. *Essential Immunology*, 8th edn. Oxford, Blackwell Scientific Publications, 1994

Pathology of acute lymphoblastic leukemias

26

ANDRÉ BARUCHEL, THIERRY LEBLANC AND GÉRARD SCHAISON

Leukemia comprises a group of diverse diseases that result from the neoplastic transformation of hematopoietic progenitors. Studies of morphology, immunology, cytogenetics and molecular genetics of leukemic lymphoblasts have confirmed that acute lymphoblastic leukemia (ALL) is a biologically heterogeneous disorder. This heterogeneity is linked to the fact that leukemogenesis may develop at any point during the multiple stages of lymphoid differentiation. Progress in stratification, design of therapies and supportive care have led to a 70% cure rate in developed countries. This chapter reviews the epidemiology of ALL, the classifications derived from morphology, immunology, cytogenetics and molecular biology, including considerations linked to leukemogenesis, and diagnostic issues.

EPIDEMIOLOGY

The childhood leukemias represent about 35% of all childhood malignancies. ALL is the commonest form of childhood cancer in the western world and is much more frequent in children than acute myeloid leukemia (AML), representing 80–85% of all leukemias. The incidence in western countries is approximately 4/100 000 children younger than 15 years, representing around 2000 new cases/year in the US, 380 in the UK and 400 in France. Worldwide variation can be explained by genetic or environmental etiologic factors, by early deaths from other causes, and by underreporting. The lowest incidence is observed in Africa (1.18–1.61/100 000) and the highest among Hispanic children (Costa Rica and Los Angeles, 5.94 and 5.02/100 000, respectively).[1,2] The low incidence in Africa could be attributed to the diminished incidence of common ALL of the B lineage.

There is a peak incidence of ALL between 2 and 5 years of age and this is especially marked in developed countries (Fig. 26.1) and weaker in Asia and Africa. A peak incidence has been seen at different times in different countries—in the UK in the 1920s, in the US in the 1940s and in Japan in the 1960s.[3] The appearance of these peaks corresponds to phases of industrialization in these countries, suggesting exposure to new environmental leukemogens.

Sex and immunophenotype are other factors of variation in the distribution of ALL. The gender ratio is 1.2 male:female in developed countries, but 4.0 for children with T-lineage ALL.[4] ALL is commoner among white than black American children.

In the past 2 decades, attention has focused on reported clusters of patients who have developed leukemia or solid tumors. The majority of these 'clusters' have not been confirmed by prolonged periods of analysis.[5]

ALL resulting from a known cause accounts for <1% of all cases and more comprehensive epidemiologic research is needed, taking into account the clinical and biologic heterogeneity of ALL.

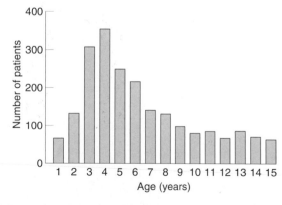

Fig. 26.1 Age distribution of 2157 patients with acute lymphoblastic leukemia in two consecutive French protocols (FRALLE).

GENETIC FACTORS

Genetic factors probably play a role given the:

- occurrence of familial cases;
- high incidence in twins;
- frequent association of ALL with some constitutional karyotypic aberrations, genetic instability syndromes or genetic diseases.

The deregulation of genes involved in cellular proliferation by acquired chromosomal translocations in leukemic cells is also an indirect argument for such genetic factors.

FAMILIAL CASES

Siblings of an affected child have an approximately 2–4-fold greater risk of developing an acute leukemia than the general population.[6,7] True familial aggregations of leukemia where a genetic origin is likely are very rare. Some fit with Li–Fraumeni syndrome in which mutations of the tumor suppressor gene p53 are generally found.[8] ALLs represented 7% of the cancers observed in a series of 24 kindreds.[9] Of course, nearly all these elements could represent shared environmental factors as well as genetic factors.

TWINS AND IN UTERO ORIGIN

The concordance rate (onset of leukemia in the second twin) is considered to be around 25%. This probability is even higher in monozygotic monochorial twins if the first child is affected in infancy, and then diminishes to around the normal rate after 10 years of age.[10] There is molecular evidence to support the fact that a leukemogenic event occurs in utero in one twin which is followed by the migration of the malignant cells to the second through a shared placental circulation, as suggested in 1971 by Clarkson and Boyse.[11] In 1986, Pombo de Oliveira et al[12] identified the same gene rearrangement (immunoglobulin heavy chain) in the ALL cells of siamese twins. In 1993, the MLL gene rearrangement involved in the translocation t(11;19)(q23;p13) was identified in 3 pairs of twins.[13] Comparable evidence has been shown in 2 identical twins affected with a CD2+, CD3+, CD7+ T-ALL at 9 and 11 years of age, respectively. The T-cell receptor β-gene rearrangement has been shown to occur particularly in the highly variable junctional region (Dβ1-(N)-Jβ2).[14] Another example of 'molecular concordance' in twins is the description of identical clonotypic TEL-AML1 fusion sequences in 2 monozygotic twins who were diagnosed with BCP-ALL at the age of 3 years 6 months and 4 years 10 months, respectively.[15] The TEL-AML1 fusion gene is the result of the most frequent (but cryptic) translocation observed in childhood ALL—the t(12;21) translocation.

An elegant confirmation of the intrauterine initiation of the leukemogenic events has been demonstrated using the stored Guthrie cards of 3 non-twin children who developed leukemia with the t(4;11) translocation at 5, 6 and 24 months, respectively. After the cloning of the translocation breakpoint, a DNA-based PCR technique was applied to the DNA extracted from the Guthrie card-eluted blood.[16] The demonstration of the amplification of the fusion gene at diagnosis and on day 1 of life is proof of the intrauterine initiation of the first leukemogenic event.

CONSTITUTIONAL CHROMOSOMAL ABNORMALITIES

Children with trisomy 21 carry a 14–38-fold increased risk of developing leukemia compared to normal children.[2,17] There is an overrepresentation of AML, particularly acute megakaryoblastic leukemia under the age of 4 years. Nevertheless, the global distribution of ALL/AML is identical to that in the general population (82% versus 18% in a series of 115 leukemia patients with Down's syndrome).[18] The cell involved in the leukemic transformation is the trisomic cell as shown in patients with mosaicism. However, the increased risk of leukemia in patients with Down's syndrome is poorly understood. There is no definite proof of an increased risk of leukemia and particularly ALL in children or adults with Klinefelter's or Turner's syndrome or other constitutional chromosomal aberrations.

CHROMOSOMAL BREAKAGE SYNDROMES

The incidence of acute leukemia in Bloom's syndrome and Fanconi's anemia is well documented.[19,20] In both, and particularly the latter, acute non-lymphoblastic leukemia (ANLL) predominates.[20] The increased incidence of non-Hodgkin lymphomas (NHL) and leukemias in patients with ataxia telangiectasia (AT) has been reviewed recently.[21] In the UK registry, 13% of the patients with AT were affected with ALL or NHL. Fourteen children (mean age 6 years) were studied between 1974 and 1994 and there was a higher incidence of T-lymphoid proliferation (ALL = 4, NHL = 5) but no myeloid proliferation. The role of the recently cloned AT gene in T-ALL/NHL is currently being studied.

OTHER GENETIC CONDITIONS

An increased risk of leukemia is reported for children with Shwachman's syndrome,[22] neurofibromatosis[23] and Diamond–Blackfan anemia.[24] ANLL predominates in all of these cases.

PATHOGENESIS

Environmental factors, viral infections and immunodeficiency are thought to play a role in leukemogenesis in addition to genetic factors.

ENVIRONMENTAL FACTORS

Ionizing radiation

Exposure to high doses of radiation is associated with an increased risk of leukemia. The survivors of the atomic bomb explosions in Japan during World War II had a 1 in 60 risk of developing a leukemia within the 12 years following exposure. ALL was commoner in the irradiated children with a peak incidence around 8 years after exposure.[25] Risk correlated with proximity to the explosion.

In utero exposure to low-dose irradiation for diagnostic procedures during the first trimester has been reported to be associated with an increased risk of leukemia. This contrasts with the absence of increased risk in survivors of the atomic bomb exposed to radiation *in utero*.[26] Prenatal X-ray exposure is now thought to account for a very small proportion of childhood ALL cases.

A European group (ECLIS) has been formed to study the epidemiology of leukemias after the 1986 Chernobyl accident.[27] Among a total of 23 756 cases observed in the 1980–1991 interval, a slight increase in the annual incidence of ALL was seen, but this increase started before the accident: 0.6% between 1980 and 1986, 0.4% between 1987 and 1991. Currently, there is thus no obvious link between leukemia and the Chernobyl accident. A longer follow-up and a detailed study with knowledge of ALL subentities are nevertheless necessary, especially in the light of a controversial report suggesting a link between the Chernobyl accident and a small increase in infant leukemia in Greece.[28]

Controversy exists about the risks from exposure to ionizing radiation from routine emissions from nuclear power plants[29] as so-called clusters are also encountered in areas without nuclear plants.[30] Complex studies (sufficient numbers, valid registries, studies of incidence and not only mortality, subclassifications of leukemias according to clinical, morphologic, immunophenotypic, cytogenetic and molecular criteria, quality of the control groups) are needed definitely to exclude such a risk.

Electromagnetic fields

The possibility of a potential increased risk for ALL linked to the electromagnetic fields (EMFs) generated by high-voltage cabling and home appliances was raised in 1979. Linet *et al*[31] have recently provided compelling evidence against this possibility with a large prospective study comparing the EMF exposure of 638 children with ALL included in the Children's Cancer Group protocols and 620 control subjects. There was no correlation between the exposure and risk of ALL.[31,32]

Chemicals and drugs

Parental exposure

Most drugs implicated as causative of leukemia (e.g. benzene) result mainly in ANLL in adults. An increasing list of occupations in adults is associated with an increased incidence of leukemia and NHL. No direct demonstration of a risk for their offspring is available although an increased relative risk has been observed in some studies concerning the children of parents exposed to hydrocarbons, solvents and pesticides.[33]

Tobacco

Cigarette smoke contains potential leukemogens: benzene, urethane, styrene, naphthalene and nitrosamines. A recent epidemiologic study has shown a correlation between cigarette smoking and ANLL in adults.[34] A Scandinavian study suggested a dose–response correlation between maternal smoking during pregnancy and an increased risk of ALL in children, but this has not been confirmed.[35]

Chemotherapy

The vast majority of secondary leukemias are ANLL. Alkylating agents, podophyllotoxins and anthracyclines are the most leukemognic agents.[36] Secondary ALLs are very rare and can be associated with 11q23 abnormalities.[37]

Immunosuppressive treatments

The course of acquired aplastic anemias treated with immunosuppressive agents (antithymocyte globulin, cyclosporin) can be complicated by acute leukemia, most of which are of the ANLL type. Nevertheless, these diseases must be considered as preleukemic states.

Growth hormone

Since the first descriptions in 1988, 46 cases of leukemia after growth hormone therapy have been reported,[38] and among these a high incidence of ANLL is observed (around 50%). The incidence for treated children not at risk for leukemia does not seem to differ from that of the general population.[39] Moreover, there is no suggestion of an increased risk of relapse for children with ALL treated for growth hormone deficiency.

INFECTION

Some epidemiologic studies favor the hypothesis of an infectious etiology for ALL,[40–42] but no known virus, including retroviruses, has been convincingly shown to be involved in the pathogenesis of common ALL. However, the Epstein–Barr virus (EBV) is associated with the development of

521

Burkitt's lymphoma (see Chapter 28) and the L3 subtype of ALL.[43] The EBV genome is found in 95% of the African Burkitt's tumor but only 20% of the tumors observed in Europe and North America. Early EBV infection is observed in Africa (>90% seropositivity before the age of 3 years). It has been demonstrated that the late membrane protein (LMP) 1 of the EBV can induce the expression of bcl-2, which inhibits the apoptosis of B-lymphoid cells. Complex interactions between EBV and plasmodium have been demonstrated. Plasmodium diminishes the function of the cytotoxic T cells responsible for the lysis of EBV-infected T cells and augments EBV replication. The BCRF1 peptide secreted by EBV is an interleukin (IL)-10-like peptide with immunosuppressive properties on immune cells involved in antimalaria immunity. Thus, it is thought that the interaction between EBV and plasmodium is of paramount importance in the genesis of the African type of Burkitt's lymphoma.

Rare cases of acute leukemia-lymphoma associated with HTLV-1 infection have been described in children.[43]

IMMUNE DEFICIENCY

Children with various congenital immune deficiencies, including Wiskott–Aldrich syndrome, hypogammaglobulinemia and ataxia telangiectasia may develop lymphoid malignancies, generally NHL, as do patients under treatment with immunosuppressive drugs. ALL is very uncommon in this setting.[44]

Abnormally low serum immunoglobulin levels have been observed in as many as 30% of patients with ALL,[45] which raises the possibility that some of these children could have an underlying immunodeficiency predisposing to ALL.

GREAVES' HYPOTHESIS

Normal lymphoid development is a period at high risk for mutation, particularly for the lymphoid precursors, due to a high rate of proliferation and important genomic constraints (gene rearrangements, with junctional additions and deletions of nucleotides). Greaves[46] suggested a 2-step pathogenesis for B-cell precursor ALL: the first event happens during fetal life and drives a clonal expansion; the second happens during childhood, due to viral stimuli of cellular proliferation. Intrauterine initiation of the leukemic events is now well documented in twins and a few non-twin cases (see above). ALL could arise as a rare response to common infection after relative immunologic isolation.

MORPHOLOGIC CLASSIFICATION

The French–American–British (FAB) system of classification defines 3 categories of lymphoblasts, depending on the size of the cells and nuclear and cytoplasmic features (Table 26.1; Plates 34–36).[47] Staining for peroxidase must be systematically performed for differentiation from AML. Refinements of the FAB classification have been proposed by the Children's Cancer Group to take into account the heterogeneity of the cell population.[48] Nevertheless, the FAB classification has gained wide acceptance and the concordance among investigators is relatively high.[49] The proportions of patients in each group are roughly 80–85% L1, 15–20% L2 and 2–3% L3. Patients with L2 morphology have been considered to be those with the worst prognosis, but this criterium does not have independent prognostic value in multivariate analyses of 'modern protocols'. There is no correlation between immunophenotype and L1 and L2 morphology (Plates 34 and 35). The L3 type (Plate 36) corresponds to B-cell ALL (expression of surface immunoglobulin) and translocations involving the c-myc gene on chromosome 8q14.

Some morphologic variants have been described from considering the degree of vacuolation or some cellular aspects (hand-mirror cells), but their value in clinical practice appears to be limited. Bone marrow eosinophilia is rare and is often associated with a t(5;14) translocation.[50]

Table 26.1 FAB classification of acute lymphoblastic leukemia.

Cytologic features	L1	L2	L3
Cell size	Small cells predominate	Large, heterogeneous in size	Large and homogeneous
Nuclear chromatin	Homogeneous in any one case	Variable, heterogeneous in any one case	Finely stippled and homogeneous
Nuclear shape	Regular, occasional clefting or indentation	Irregular, clefting or indentation common	Regular oval or round
Nucleoli	Not visible or small and inconspicuous, more vesicular	One or more present, often large	Prominent, one or more
Amount of cytoplasm	Scanty	Variable, often moderately abundant	Moderately abundant
Basophilia of cytoplasm	Slight or moderate, rarely intense	Variable, deep in some	Very deep
Cytoplasmic vacuolation	Variable	Variable	Often prominent

IMMUNOPHENOTYPIC STUDIES

The variable expression by leukemic cells of membrane or cytoplasmic antigens that can be detected by monoclonal antibodies allows determination of the B or T lineage of the lymphoid proliferation, generally by flow cytometry. The immunophenotype is defined by the pattern of CDs (clusters of differentiation) expressed by the leukemic cells. The list of leukocyte differentiation antigens has grown rapidly (166 CDs were defined at the 6th International Workshop on Leukocyte Differentiation Antigens).[51] However, few markers have lineage specificity. The simplified approach of testing the association of sensitive and specific markers is used in numerous laboratories.[52] Sensitive markers include CD19 for B lineage, CD7 for T lineage and CD13 and CD33 for myeloid lineage. Specific markers include CD79a for B lineage, cytoplasmic CD3 for T lineage and α-myeloperoxidase for myeloid lineage. With this approach, a lineage assignment can be made in >98% of cases.[52] The most helpful antibodies for immunologic classification of ALL are shown in Table 26.2.

The immunophenotype has some prognostic value but this is erased by the protocol intensity. However, this investigation is nevertheless of importance in defining the subgroup of ALL, which allows some stratification of treatment and comparison of the results of different protocols on a more homogeneous basis. Moreover, its usefulness in evaluating minimal residual disease in morphologic complete remission has been demonstrated (see below).[53]

B-Lineage ALL

The main clinically relevant distinction is between B-cell precursor (BCP) ALL and B-cell ALL. Classifications according to the expression of some important CDs have been proposed (Table 26.3).[54–56] Their main value is in allowing definition of subentities of childhood ALL frequently associated with different cytogenetic and molecular findings. Correlations between morphology, immunophenotype and cytogenetics in B-lineage ALL are summarized in Table 26.4.

Table 26.2 Monoclonal antibodies useful in immunologic classification of acute lymphoblastic leukemia.

	B-lineage	T-lineage
Constant lineage markers	CD19, CD79a	Cytoplasmic CD3
Non-constant lineage markers	CD20, CD22 Cytoplasmic μ heavy chain Surface Ig	Membrane CD3, CD2, CD5, CD7
Non-lineage specific markers (sometimes present)	CD10 (CALLA), CD34	CD10 (CALLA), CD34
Myeloid markers (sometimes present)	CD13, CD33, CD15, CDw65	CD13, CD33
Megakaryocytic markers (always absent)	CD41, CD42, CD61	CD41, CD42, CD61

Table 26.3 Immunologic classification of acute lymphoblastic leukemia (ALL). Adapted from Ref. 52.

Subtype	Profile of antigen expression	Frequency (%)
Pro-B ALL	CD19$^\pm$, CD22$^-$, CD79a$^+$, CD10$^-$, CD7$^-$, cCD3$^-$,* clgμ$^-$, slg$^-$	5–10
Early pre-B	CD19$^+$, CD22$^+$, CD79a$^+$, CD10$^+$, CD7$^-$, cCD3$^-$,* clgμ$^-$, slg$^-$	55–65
Pre-B	CD19$^+$, CD22$^+$, CD79a$^+$, CD10$^\pm$, CD7$^-$, cCD3$^-$,* clgμ$^+$, slg$^-$	20–25
Transitional	CD19$^+$, CD22$^+$, CD79a$^+$, CD10$^-$, CD7$^-$, cCD3$^-$,* clgμ$^+$, slgμ$^+$, slgκ$^-$, slgλ$^-$	2–3
B cell	CD19$^+$, CD22$^+$, CD79a$^+$, CD10$^\pm$, CD7$^-$, cCD3$^-$,* clgμ$^+$, slgμ$^+$, slgκ$^+$ or slgλ$^+$	2–3
T cell	CD19$^-$,** CD22$^-$, CD79a$^-$, CD10$^\pm$, CD7$^+$, cCD3$^+$,* clgμ$^-$, slg$^-$	13–15

clg = Cytoplasmic immunoglobulin; slg = surface immunoglobulin.; μ = immunoglobulin heavy chain; κ and λ = immunoglobulin light chains.
*Cytoplasmic CD3.
**Positive in approximately 5% of cases.

Table 26.4 Correlations between morphology, immunophenotype and cytogenetics in childhood B-lineage acute lymphoblastic leukemia.

	Pro-B CD19$^+$/CD10$^-$ (My$^\pm$)	Early pre-B CD19$^+$/CD10$^+$ (My$^\pm$)	Pre-B CD19$^+$/CD10$^+$ Cμ$^+$	Transitional pre-B CD19$^+$/CD10$^+$ Cμ$^+$/Sμ$^+$	B CD19$^+$/CD10$^\pm$ slg$^+$
L1 or L2	t(4;11) t(11;19)	t(12;21) t(9;22) Hyperdiploidy	t(1;19)	? Hyperdiploidy	
L3					t(8;14) t(2;8) t(8;22)

My = expression of at least 1 myeloid marker (CD13, CD15, CDw65, CD33); Cμ = presence of an intracytoplasmic immunoglobulin heavy chain; Sμ = presence of surface immunoglobulin heavy chain; slg$^+$ = presence of surface immunoglobulin.

BCP-ALL

This represents 85% of childhood ALL.[57] The most frequent form (55–65%) is early pre-B ALL expressing CD19 and CD10. Pre-B ALL (20–25%), is characterized by the presence of cytoplasmic immunoglobulin heavy chain. Features associated with pre-B ALL are: black race, CD10 positivity (>90%) and the translocation t(1;19) in 25% of cases. Pro-B ALL cells generally express CD19 but lack CD10. This is the commonest phenotype of infant ALL and is frequently associated with translocation t(4;11) or other translocations involving 11q23.

A rare subgroup has been recently identified, transitional pre-B ALL, where the leukemic cells express surface immunoglobulin heavy chain.[58]

B-Cell ALL

Expression of complete surface immunoglobulins with κ or λ chain defines this rare subgroup (<3% of childhood ALL) with L3 morphology.

T-Cell ALL

T-ALL represents 15% of childhood ALL in most developed countries and is defined by positivity for cytoplasmic CD3. Features associated with T-ALL include: male gender, greater age, high tumor burden, enlargement of the mediastinum, central nervous system (CNS) involvement, high white blood cell count (EBC) and normal hemoglobin level.[52]

Myeloid markers

CD13, CD14, CD15 and CD33 are myeloid antigens normally not expressed on lymphoid cells. Their expression on lymphoblasts can be considered as a marker of an early bipotent progenitor (lymphomyeloid) or of lineage infidelity due to the aberrant gene deregulation driven by the leukemic process. Their positivity is encountered in 5–20% of cases of childhood ALL, depending on the number of myeloid antigen markers studied, the chosen threshold of positivity (10, 20 and 30%), and the use of direct or indirect fluorescent methods. Features associated with myeloid antigen positivity include: L2 morphology, T-ALL and BCP-ALL, particularly when associated with some cytogenetic abnormalities, i.e. t(12;21), t(9;22) or 11q23 abnormalities.[59] Initial suggestions of their prognostic value[60] have not been fulfilled.[61] However, it seems probable that the prognostic value of myeloid antigen expression is actually related to the associated translocations, and should be re-evaluated in the light of molecular cytogenetics.

Other useful markers

CD34 is thought to be a marker of the hematopoietic stem cell. It is associated with childhood ALL in roughly two-thirds of cases. Its positivity has been claimed to be associated with a good prognosis in BCP-ALL.[62]

Megakaryocytic antigens are systematically looked for to discriminate ALL and megakaryoblastic leukemia which sometimes exhibits a typical lymphoid morphology without the classic features of M7 (cytoplasmic blebs) (see Plate 37).

CYTOGENETICS

Cytogenetic analysis of leukemic cells has become a major tool in studies of leukemia. Important advances have resulted from:

- improvements in high-resolution banding techniques, characterization of chromosomes or regions of chromosomes by fluorescent *in situ* hybridization (FISH) and cell culture techniques;
- identification of cytogenetic abnormalities specific for a given leukemia subtype, which allows a better diagnostic or prognostic approach.

Major advances in molecular biology have resulted in the cloning of genes involved in the leukemogenic process. A better definition of minimal residual disease is now possible with these techniques (see below).

METHODS AND NOMENCLATURE

The study of the malignant cell population is based on a bone marrow aspirate or, alternatively, a blood specimen if there are circulating blasts. The specimen is either processed immediately (direct preparation) or cultured for 24, 48 or 72 hours. G (trypsinization followed by Giemsa staining) and R (reverse) banding are the commonest techniques. About 350 bands are routinely obtained, each band corresponding to $0.5–1.0 \times 10^7$ DNA base pairs. Synchronization techniques, using methotrexate, may allow the definition of 1000–2000 bands. By comparison, the scale in molecular biology is the nucleotide. Nevertheless, cytogenetic analyses have allowed the idenfication of translocation breakpoints, which have been extremely useful in facilitating their molecular cloning.

Chromosomal abnormalities are described according to a universally accepted International System for Human Cytogenetic Nomenclature.[63] Long arm (p) and short arm (q) are divided into regions and these in turn are divided into bands in a centromere to telomere orientation, e.g. the second band on the third region on the short arm of chromosome 14 is denoted 14q32.

The chromosomal abnormalities of leukemic cells are acquired, limited to the tumor cells, clonal (deriving from the same cell) and non-random. The observation of at least 2 cells with identical structural abnormalities or chromosome gain, or at least 3 cells with identical chromosome losses is evidence of an abnormal clone.

CYTOGENETIC ABNORMALITIES

An abnormal karyotype is detected in 70–95% of ALL depending on the technique used.[64] Some of the abnormalities correlate with a distinct immunophenotype. Their prognostic value is recognized and may be taken into account in treatment stratification. The most frequent abnormalities in childhood ALL are numerical abnormalities (gain or loss of 1 or more chromosome) and structural abnormalities—translocations (exchange of material between 2 or more chromosomes) and deletions. A wider use of new karyotyping techniques, including multicolor spectral karyotyping, is likely to uncover subtle translocations not detected by conventional techniques.[65]

Numerical abnormalities

ALL can be divided into 5 subtypes based on modal number of chromosomes:

- high hyperdiploid with >50 chromosomes;
- hyperdiploid with 47–50 chromosomes;
- pseudodiploid (46 chromosomes with structural or numerical abnormalities);
- diploid (normal 46 chromosomes);
- hypodiploid (<46 chromosomes).

The frequency of each ploidy group in B- and T-lineage ALL is shown in Table 26.5.

Hyperdiploidy

Hyperdiploidy, whose mechanism is still unclear, is a well known prognostic factor. It is generally linked to a trisomy of chromosomes 4, 6, 10, 14, 17, 18, 20, 21 and X. A tetrasomy of chromosome 21 is also frequent. The frequency of high hyperdiploidy is about 25–30%, the major group having 53–56 chromosomes. High hyperdiploidy is associated with a DNA index $\geqslant 1.16$,[66] an early pre-B phenotype and a good prognosis.[67] This good prognosis of high hyperdiploidy has been attributed to low leukemic burden, a tendency to accumulate an increased amount of polyglutamates,[68] an increased sensitivity to antimetabolites[69] and a marked

tendency to spontaneous apoptosis.[70] Nevertheless, there is heterogeneity, depending on the modal chromosome number; hyperdiploidy with 51–55 chromosomes is associated with a worse prognosis than hyperdiploidy with 56–67 chromosomes (event-free survival [EFS] was 72% versus 86%, p = 0.04, in a recent series from the St Jude Research Children's Hospital).[71] This inferior prognosis seems to be linked to the greater frequency in the first subgroup of hyperleukocytosis $>50 \times 10^9/l$ and isochromosome 17q and to the diminished frequency of trisomy 4 and trisomy 10. Indeed, in one study, the association of trisomy 4 and 10 has been associated with a subgroup with a very good prognosis even with antimetabolite-based therapy (EFS = 96.6% at 4 years).[72] Hyperploidy (>50 chromosomes) was rare in T-ALL (1.2%) in a recent series (Table 26.5).[73]

Near tetraploidy (82–94 chromosomes) is rare (1%) and seems to be most frequently associated with T-ALL and an inferior prognosis.[74]

Hypodiploidy

Hypodiploidy (<46 chromosomes) is observed in 5–8% of cases of ALL, most of whom have a modal chromosome number of 45. Chromosome 20 is the one most frequently lost. Additional structural abnormalities have been observed in the majority of hypodiploid cases. Hypodiploidy, particularly when near-haploid karyotypes are found (0.7%), is reported to be associated with a poor prognosis.[76,77] The prognostic value in current protocols is not known.

Structural abnormalities

Gene abnormalities involved in translocations are reviewed below.

B-lineage associated translocations

t(8;14) and its variants in B-cell ALL. Expression of complete surface immunoglobulin with κ and λ chains defines this rare subgroup (<3% of childhood ALL) with L3 morphology. A reciprocal t(8;14)(q24;q23) has been

Table 26.5 Comparison of modal chromosome number in B and T lineage in 983 children with acute lymphoblastic leukemia included in the Children's Cancer Group protocols. Reproduced with permission from Ref. 73.

	T lineage (n = 169)		B lineage (n = 814)		
	Number	%	Number	%	p*
Normal	66	39.1	218	26.8	<0.0001
Hypodiploid (<46)	4	2.4	51	6.3	
Pseudodiploid	80	47.3	211	25.9	
Hyperdiploid (47–50)	17	10.1	95	11.7	
Hyperdiploid (>50)	2	1.2	239	29.4	

*Log rank of ploidy group, B versus T lineage.

detected in Burkitt's lymphoma of both African and non-African origin, independent of whether they are EBV positive or negative. Fewer than 10% of patients have 1 or 2 variant translocations, t(2;8)(p12;q24) and t(8;22)(p24;q11). CNS involvement as well as abdominal tumors are frequently associated with Burkitt's leukemia. The dismal prognosis associated with B-cell ALL has been completely transformed by current protocols based on short but very intensive chemotherapy resulting in a cure rate of > 70%.[78]

t(12;21)(p13;q22) translocation in BCP-ALL. This translocation was first identified in 1994 as a recurring abnormality by the use of FISH (Plate 37).[79] Indeed, it cannot be identified by the standard banding techniques. It was subsequently cloned. Through the use of a variety of techniques (FISH, Southern blot, RT-PCR), this rearrangement has been shown to be the commonest event in childhood BCP-ALL, occurring in 20–25% of cases.[80–83] Features associated with t(12;21) include age between 1 and 10 years and BCP immunophenotype (sometimes cIg-positive) with a high incidence of myleoid markers (CD13 and/or CD33),[59,84] pseudo-diploid karyotype, and suggested good prognosis in retrospective studies.[81,84–87]

t(1;19)(q23;p13) translocation and pre-B ALL. This translocation has an overall incidence of 5% (Fig. 26.2). Two cytogenetic forms have been described. A balanced translocation is found in 25% of cases and an unbalanced form, with a partial trisomy of the long arm of chromosome 1, accounts for the remaining 75%. This is written as der(19)t(1;19)(q23;p13). There is a close association between this translocation and pre-B (cIg$^+$) immunophenotype. At(1;19) is found in 25% of pre-B ALL cases. However, it may occasionally be found in early pre-B ALL. A pseudo-Burkitt morphology has been described in cases with t(1;19)(q23;p13), +8 (trisomy 8).[88] The poor prognosis initially suggested to be associated with the presence of t(1;19) is not found in current intensive protocols,[89] and a negative prognostic impact of the unbalanced form is controversial. A very rare variant, t(17;19)(q22;q13), has been described in association with the early pre-B immunophenotype and disseminated intravascular coagulopathy (DIC).

t(4;11)(q21;q23) translocation and pro-B ALL. There is a clustering of ALL with the t(4;11) in infants (< 1 year of age) (Fig. 26.2). This form represents about 2–3% of all childhood ALL. Abnormalities of the gene located at 11q23 (*MLL/ALL1*) can be detected by molecular techniques in 70% of infants with ALL. Features associated with t(4;11) are summarized in Table 26.6. The prognosis of this form remains very poor.[90,91] Rearrangements involving 11q23 with other chromosomes can also be encountered in children with ALL. The t(11;19)(q23;p13.3) is

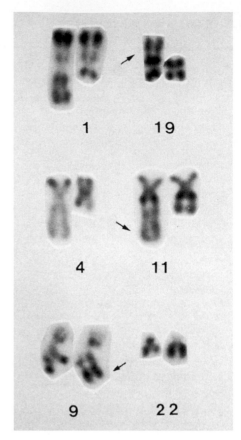

Fig. 26.2 Conventional cytogenetics (R bonding) for t(9;22), t(4;11) and t(1;19). Arrows indicate breakpoints. Reproduced with permission of Flammarion Ed, France.

Table 26.6 Features associated with t(4;11)(q21;q23) acute lymphoblastic leukemia.

Age <1 year
Female sex predominance
High hyperleukocytosis
Initial CNS involvement
CD19$^+$, CD10$^-$ immunophenotype
Positivity of myeloid markers: CD15$^+$, CDw65$^+$
No hyperdiploidy
Potential to differentiate in both lymphoid and myeloid pathways *in vitro*
Dismal prognosis

the second most frequent translocation. The t(9;11)(p22;q23) and t(11;19)(q23;p13.1) are rarely found in ALL.

t(9;22)(q34;q11) translocation in B-cell precursor ALL (Philadelphia [Ph] chromosome-positive ALL). Ph-positive ALL is the most frequently encountered translocation in adult ALL (about 30% of cases) but represents only 2–3% of childhood ALL (Fig. 26.2). At the cytogenetic level, t(9;22)(q34;q11) translocation is identical to that of chronic myelogenous leukemia (CML). Other cytogenetic abnormalities are also found in >50% of cases.[64] The most consistent secondary abnormality is loss or partial deletion of the long arm of chromosome 7 (-7/7q-) which seems to identify a subgroup with a particularly poor prognosis.[92] It is important but sometimes difficult to distinguish Ph-positive ALL and CML in lymphoid blast crisis. Distinguishing features are:

- In CML, the Ph chromosome is nearly always found in 100% of the metaphase cells; in contrast, in ALL a mixture of Ph-positive and normal metaphases is found.
- In the acute phase of CML, 70% of cases have a second Ph chromosome, an isochromosome 17q or a trisomy 8, which is very rarely the case in ALL (<10%).
- At complete remission after induction chemotherapy, an absence of Ph-positive metaphases is generally observed in ALL but this is extremely rare in CML.
- At the molecular level, the size and types of the chimeric mRNAs generated by the translocations are different, even if the correlations are not absolute.

Initial features include median age 8–9 years, hyperleukocytosis, CNS involvement, L2 morphology, early pre-B phenotype (sometimes with myeloid marker expression), whereas T-ALL phenotype is exceptional. A low remission rate and occurrence of very early relapses result in a dismal prognosis.[93] Nevertheless, some recent studies have suggested a standard prognosis in some subgroups ($<25 \times 10^9$ white blood cells/l and good response to prednisone).[94,95]

t(5;14)(q31–q32;q32) and BCP-ALL. This is a rare form of ALL (<1%) associated with eosinophilia and BCP phenotype.[50]

Rearrangements in T-ALL

About 45–50% of the karyotypes show pseudodiploidy in T-ALL. Forty percent of the abnormalities involve the 14q11, 7q35 and 7p35 bands which correspond at the molecular level to the T-cell receptor genes *TCRA/D*, *TCRB* and *TCRG* (Table 26.7).

As prognosis of T-ALL has evolved, no single karyotype abnormality is consistently associated with prognostic features.

Table 26.7 Chromosomal translocations, T-ALL and transcription factors.

Overexpressed gene	Translocation	Enhancer
TAL1 (1p32)	t(1;14)(p32;q11)	*TCRA* (14q11)
TAL2 (9q34)	t(7;9)(q35;q34)	*TCRB* (7q35)
RBTN1 (11p15)	t(11;14)(p15;q11)	*TCRD* (14q11)
RBTN2 (11p13)	t(11;14)(p13;q11)	*TCRD* (14q11)
LYL1 (19p13)	t(7;19)(q35;p13)	*TCRB* (7q35)
c-MYC (8q24)	t(8;14)(q24;q11)	*TCRA* (14q11)
HOX11 (10q14)	t(10;14)(q24;q11)	*TCRA* (14q11)

Non-lineage-specific rearrangements

Abnormalities of the short arm of chromosome 9. These are observed in 7–12% of childhood ALL,[64] consisting largely of interstitial deletions encompassing the 9q21–22 region. Translocations and other rare abnormalities have been described, particularly a dicentric chromosome 9 and 12—dic(9;12)(p11–13)(p11–12). The critical region involved in 9p abnormalities is 9p21–22. It encompasses the IFNα cluster and IFNβ1. ALL with the dic(9;12)(p11–13)(p11–12) has been associated with a good prognosis.[96] Poor prognostic features appear to be associated with the other 9p abnormalities: hyperleukocytosis, splenomegaly and T-ALL, and an increased rate of CNS relapses has been reported.[97]

Abnormalities of the short arm of chromosome 12. These are found in approximately 10% of cases of ALL, mostly associated with a B-lineage immunophenotype. A good prognosis has been reported in recent studies.[89] A cryptic t(12;21) is revealed by its fusion transcript in two-thirds of cases with 12p abnormality.[98]

Abnormalites of the long arm of chromosome 6. Deletion of the long arm of chromosome 6 is a relatively common abnormality in ALL with an incidence of 4–13%. Breakpoints are localized to 6q15 and 6q21. No specific immunophenotype or clinical features of the 6q- have been reported.

FLUORESCENT *IN SITU* HYBRIDIZATION (FISH)

A satisfying cellular growth and obtention of numerous metaphases are mandatory for a successful cytogenetic analysis. The FISH probes specific for a given chromosome allow the recognition of the corresponding sequences on metaphasic or even interphasic nuclei if an appropriately sized probe is used. The use of interphase cytogenetics is increasing as it has some advantages:

- screening of a large number of nuclei;
- easy detection of numerical abnormalities;[99]
- easy detection of some structural abnormalities, sometimes using 2 or more probes with different fluorochromes.[100]

The discovery and now routine detection of the cryptic t(12;21) is one of the great successes of this method in childhood ALL (Plate 37).[79]

MOLECULAR BIOLOGY

It is apparent that leukemia can arise as a result of many genetic abnormalities, ranging from defects in cell-surface receptors to transcription factors to cell cycle regulators, disrupting the usual controls of cell proliferation and differentiation. Cytogenetic analyses have allowed the regions of chromosomal rearrangement to be identified. However, molecular biology has been the revolution of the last 2 decades, permitting the cloning of the genes involved in the leukemogenic process. Moreover, the study of the biology of leukemic cells has been a key step in the understanding of lymphoid ontogeny and in the definition of the genes and mechanisms involved in antigen recognition by the lymphoid cells (T-cell receptor and immunoglobulin). Finally, the new molecular techniques allow a sensitive diagnostic approach to minimal residual disease (see below).

ACQUIRED GENETIC ABNORMALITIES AND LEUKEMOGENESIS (Tables 26.8 and 26.9)

Five families of genes involved in leukemogenesis can be described:[101]

- genes involved in the transmission of growth-stimulating signals from the cell membrane to the nucleus;
- factors activating the transcription of specific sequences;
- genes involved in tissue differentiation. Some of these contain homeobox domains. Many if not all of the products of these differentiation-associated genes alter the transcription of other genes;
- genes involved in programed cell death (apoptosis);

Table 26.8 Genetic abnormalities not involving transcription factors observed in childhood acute lymphoblastic leukemia.

Type of gene	Function	Molecular alteration	Structural abnormality or localization	Lineage (approximate frequency %)
Tyrosine kinase	Signal transduction	bcr-abl	t(9;22)(q34;q11)	Ph$^+$ BCP-ALL (2–4)
ras	Signal transduction	Mutations of N-ras	—	ALL (10–15)
Antioncogenes	Tumor suppression, transcription, cell cycle control, apoptosis	Mutation, deletion or rearrangement of p53	± del17	Early pre-B ALL (<2) B-ALL/B-NHL (30) T-ALL (<2)
		Rearrangement of RB1	13q	Ph$^+$ ALL (<30) BCP-ALL (?) T-ALL (?)
		Deletion of WT-1	11p	ALL (?)
		Deletion of MTS1 (p16/p19)	9p	BCP-ALL (10–40) T-ALL (75)
Other	Cellular proliferation	Gene fusion (IL-3–IgH)	t(5;14)(q31;q32)	BCP-ALL (<1)

Table 26.9 Chromosomal translocations involving transcription factors observed in childhood acute lymphoblastic leukemia.

Family of transcription (DNA binding domain)	Involved genes		Translocation	Lineage (approximate frequency, %)
Helix-loop-helix proteins	**MYC**	**IGH**	**t(8;14)(q24;q32)**	B-ALL/B-NHL (2–3)
	MYC	IGL	t(8;22)(q24;q11)	
	MYC	IGK	t(2;8)(p11;q24)	
	MYC	TCRA	t(8;14)(q24;q11)	T-ALL (<10)
	TAL1	TCRD[a]	t(1;14)(p32;q11)	T-ALL (20)[b]
	TCRB	TAL2	t(7;9)(q35;q34)	T-ALL (<10)
	TCRB	LYL1	t(7;19)(q35;p13)	T-ALL (<5)
	PBX[c]	**E2A**[a]	**t(1;19)(q23;p13)**	Pre-B ALL (25)
	HLF[c]	E2A[a]	t(17;19)(q22;p13)	
Cysteine-rich proteins (LIM)	RBTN1	TCRD	t(11;14)(p15;q11)	T-ALL (<10)
	RBTN2	TCRD	t(11;14)(p13;q11)	
Homeotic proteins	HOX11	TCRD	t(10;14)(q24;q11)	T-ALL (7)
AT-hook proteins	**FEL/AF4**	**MLL**[a]	**t(4;11)(q21;q23)**	Pro-B ALL
	AF9	MLL[a]	t(9;11)(p21;q23)	(60–70 if age <1 year)
	ENL, ELL	MLL[a]	t(11;19)(q23;p13)	
Other	**TEL**	**AML1**[a]	**t(12;21)(p12;q22)**	LAL B (25)
	TCRB	TAN1	t(7;9)(q34;q34.3)	T-ALL (?)

[a]Fusion mRNA generating translocation.
[b]Percentage considering all TAL gene abnormalities.
[c]PBX and HLF are homeotic proteins.

- anti-oncogenes which may normally function to suppress tumor development.

This distinction is to some extent arbitrary, since the product of a given gene may have more than one function, e.g. the product of the p53 gene has a role in tumor suppression, apoptosis and the control of transcription of other genes.

Abnormality of membrane signal transduction and leukemogenesis: the Philadelphia chromosome positive ALL example

The translocation t(9;22)(q34;q11) generates a chimeric mRNA, *BCR-ABL*, which in ALL cells encodes a hybrid protein of 190 kDa with an increased tyrosine kinase activity compared to the normal ABL protein.[102] The proto-oncogene *c-ABL* is the gene for a transmission molecule that is apparently linked to the *RAS* signalling pathway controlling cell proliferation. The accidental fusion with *BCR* (breakpoint cluster region) results in a deregulated proliferation signal. The p190 protein has a transforming activity superior to that of the p210 protein found in CML. It should be noted that a CML-type transcript can be found in ALL. The fusion transcripts are easily detected by the RT-PCR technique.[103–105]

Transcription factors

The transcription factors (TFs) are proteins with the ability to bind specific sequences of DNA, resulting in the inhibition of the activation of transcription. The abnormal activity of a TF results in the deregulation of the expression of target gene(s). The frequent involvement of these TF abnormalities in childhood ALL exemplifies their fundamental role in the normal process of proliferation, differentiation and cellular death. Two domains of a TF can be distinguished—the DNA-binding site and the transcriptional activation domain, which interacts with other proteins of the transcription complex. TFs frequently dimerize to make homodimers and heterodimers. Several classes of TF are described: helix–loop–helix, leucine zipper, zinc finger protein and homeotic proteins.[106]

Several mechanisms involve TFs in leukemogenesis: generation of fusion proteins with altered properties or inappropriate expression of TFs, both resulting from the chromosomal translocations (Table 26.9).

Transcription factors and B-lineage ALL

TEL–AML1 fusion in BCP-ALL with t(12;21)(p13;q22).
As mentioned above, this translocation can be identified by FISH or molecular techniques (Southern blot and RT-PCR). The consequences of the translocation is fusion of the 5′ end of the *TEL* gene, which encodes a highly conserved oligomerization motif, to essentially the full length of the *AML1* gene, including

the DNA binding and transcriptional activation domains.[80,107] Loss of the other *TEL* allele is usually associated with the *TEL–AML1* fusion.[82] This is unusual for genes involved in chromosomal translocations in which the wild-type alleles are retained and suggests that both *AML1* abnormality and loss of *TEL* function are important in the leukemogenic process. It should be noted that *TEL–AML1* can act as a repressor of the *TCRB* enhancer and can exert a dominant negative inhibition of *AML1* at this locus. However, the mechanism of transformation is unclear. The *TEL–AML1* fusion represents a new example of alteration of the core-binding factor (CBF). CBF is an heterodimeric TF normally involved in the transcriptional activation of important target genes: IL-3, myeloperoxidase, GM-CSF, M-CSF and T-cell receptor genes. Both heterodimeric components of CBF (*CBFα/AML1* and *CBFβ*) are involved in myeloid and lymphoid leukemias (Fig. 26.3).

E2A–PBX1 fusion and pre-B ALL with t(1;19)(q23;p13).
The t(1;19)(q23;p13) creates a fusion of the *E2A* and *PBX1* genes on chromosome 19p13 and 1q23, respectively.[108] The *E2A* gene encodes for a TF that binds to an enhancer sequence of the immunoglobulin κ light chain gene. *PBX1* encodes for an homeodomain protein. The *E2A–PBX1* fusion can cause leukemia in transgenic mice. RT-PCR allows detection and monitoring of the fusion transcript.[109]

MLL–AF4 fusion, t(4;11)(q21;q23) and other 11q23 rearrangements.
The *MLL* gene (also known as *ALL1*, *HRX*, *Htrx*)[110,111] has been localized to chromosome 11q23. The molecular sequence of the t(4;11) is the fusion of the *MLL* gene to a gene of unknown function on chromosome 4, *AF4*. The t(11;19)(q23;p13) is the second commonest fusion in infant ALL, generating a *MLL–ENL* fusion.

MLL is a very large gene composed of 34 exons and spanning 100 kb of genomic DNA. It has 3 domains of homology with the Drosophila *trithorax* gene, a complex gene

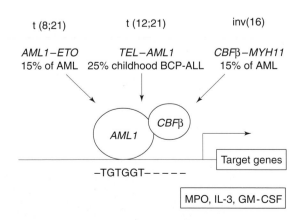

Fig. 26.3 The CBF transcription complex and its alterations in acute leukemias.

regulating a set of genes that is essential for normal Drosophila development. The targeted disruption of *MLL* in the mouse is lethal to the embryo. *MLL*-/- embryonic stem cells give immature or biphenotypic hematopoietic progenitors in colony forming assays, mimicking the aberrant hematopoiesis seen in leukemic patients. Finally, *MLL–AF9* transgenic mice have been created by the knock-out technology. These mice develop leukemia that is analogous to the t(9;11)(p22;q23) AML seen in humans. Thus, all experiments suggest a role for homeotic proteins in both normal and malignant hematopoiesis but the mechanism of transformation of the *MLL* fusions is not known. *MLL* rearrangements can be detected by Southern blotting or RT-PCR if the fusion partner is known or suspected.[112]

8q24 abnormalities, overexpression of c-MYC and B-cell ALL. *c-MYC* is a member of the basic helix–loop–helix (bHLH) family of TF and contains a leucine zipper dimerization motif. In both B-cell ALL and Burkitt's tumors, the t(8;14)(q24;q32) juxtaposes *c-MYC* to the immunoglobulin heavy chain enhancer, leading to an overexpression of *c-MYC*.[113] In the variant translocations—t(2;8)(p12;q24) and t(8;22)(q24;q11)—*c-MYC* is translocated to the κ light chain (2p12) or λ chain (22q11) loci, respectively. The overexpression of *c-MYC* seems to be critical in the malignant process. *c-MYC* is a paradigm of the 'master gene' controlling the expression of several responding genes due to its ability to dimerize with different TFs.[114]

The distribution of translocation breakpoints differs in sporadic and epidemic cases.[115] *c-MYC* is rearranged in sporadic Burkitt's lymphoma (breakpoint within the gene, with alteration of the promoting regions). *c-MYC* is not rearranged in epidemic Burkitt's lymphoma (breakpoint outside the gene), although point mutations or insertions can be present. The transfection of *c-MYC* in embryonic cells is under the control of an immunoglobulin gene promoter and produces transgenic mice which initially develop a polyclonal lymphoid proliferation followed by a monoclonal lymphoma.

Other genetic events are likely to be involved in the malignant transformation. Acquired mutations of the p53 tumor suppressor gene are frequently found in Burkitt's lymphoma and L3 ALL.[116] It is thus possible that 2 or more events co-operate in deregulating the cell cycle leading to the maintenance of the proliferative state.

Transcription factors and T-ALL

T-cell receptor genes α, β, γ and δ are normally rearranged in T cells. Forty percent of the abnormalities observed in T-ALL involve the α-δ locus at 14q11, the β locus at 7q35 and the γ locus at 7p15.[64] Errors in the V-D-J recombination, involving the recombinase complex encoded by the *RAG1* and *RAG2* genes, lead to translocations. These errors occur in the early stages of T-cell ontogeny, leading to the juxta-

position of T-cell receptor genes with TF genes normally not transcribed in T cells. This aberrant expression is thought to be the key process in T leukemogenesis.

The genes involved in the T-ALL-associated translocations are described in Table 26.7. An important example of aberrant expression leading to T-cell leukemogenesis is the *TAL1* gene. *TAL1* is a TF with a fundamental role in hematopoiesis as demonstrated by knock-out experiments: murine embryos die during mid-embryonic development with an absence of fetal liver-derived hematopoiesis. *TAL1* is normally expressed in immature hematopoietic tissues but not in normal T cells. The *TAL1* gene is involved in the very rare t(1;14)(p23;q11) translocation. Moreover, a 90-kb submicroscopic deletion of chromosome 1p23 is observed in 10–25% of children with T-ALL.[117,118] This deletion is driven by recombination signals (heptamere-nonamere sequences) and leads to the fusion of *TAL1* to the 5′ region of *SIL*, a gene ubiquitously expressed in hematopoietic cells. The expression of *TAL1* is then under the control of the *SIL* promoter, resulting in the ectopic expression of *TAL1* which is involved in leukemogenesis. It should be noted that *SIL–TAL1* regions are clone-specific and can be used for minimal residual disease detection.[118]

Proto-oncogenes and tumor suppressor genes

The mutations of these genes are not specific for acute leukemias, but are frequently found in numerous cancers. With some exceptions, these mutations occur during the course of the disease and seem to be more involved in progression than initiation of leukemogenesis. Two classes can be distinguished:

- proto-oncogenes, which become oncogenic after a mutation ('dominant genes');
- tumor suppressor genes (mutation or deletion of both alleles is necessary, 'recessive genes').

RAS family of oncogenes

The *RAS* family members are involved in the transduction of proliferative and differentiation signals from activated transmembrane receptors to downstream protein kinases and other effectors. The biochemical consequence of the mutation is that the mutant RAS protein remains in the GTP-bound activated state, mimicking constitutive signalling from the transmembrane receptors. The upregulated proliferation of cells is thus the consequence of codon 12, 13, 61 mutations in *RAS* oncogenes. Mutations of *N-RAS* have been described in 10–15% of childhood ALL.[101]

Genes that regulate the cell cycle

Retinoblastoma gene (RB). This is localized at 13q14 and encodes for a nuclear phosphoprotein which has a major role in the control of the cell cycle (transition from

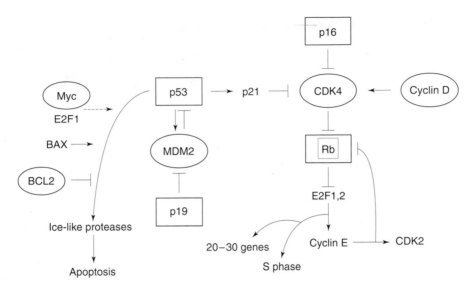

Fig. 26.4 Schematic regulation of the cell cycle with emphasis on p53–Rb interactions.

G1 to S phase) (Fig. 26.4). Alteration of the 2 copies of the RB gene have been reported in 10–30% of acute leukemias but rarely in childhood ALL.[101]

p16/MTS1 and p19/ARF. p16[INKa] (also called *MTS1*—multiple tumor suppressor—*CDK4I* or *CDKN2*) is a cyclin-dependent kinase inhibitor (CKI), a new class of regulatory protein involved in cell cycle progression. It is now thought to be a major tumor suppressor gene located at 9p21. The cell cycle is controlled by the sequential activation and inactivation of the serine-threonine kinases known as cyclin-dependent kinases (CDKs). Two families of CKI have been identified:

- p16[INKa] family which also includes p15[INK4B] (homologous to p16[INK4a] and located at the same locus), p18[INK4c] and p16[INK4D]. p16[INK4a] and its relative inhibit CDK4 and CDK6, 2 closely related G1 cyclins.
- p21[Waf1/CIPI] family which includes p27[Kip1] and p57[Kip2]. These CKIs inhibit a wide spectrum of CDK.

During G1 phase, CDK4 and CDK6 are activated by cyclins D and phosphorylate the retinoblastoma protein (pRB). When non-phosphorylated, pRB negatively controls passage from G1 to S phase by sequestering *E2F* TFs which are required for the transcription of S-phase genes. Phosphorylation *abolishes* its ability to bind *E2F* TFs and allows transition from G1 to S phase (Fig. 26.4).

The main identified function of p16[INK4a] is the inhibition of pRB phosphorylation and it has been demonstrated that overexpression of p16[INK4a] results in G1 arrest in cells with functional pRB. Deletions of the *MTS1* locus have been observed in 75% of T-ALL and 15–40% of BCP-ALL.[119–121] Its prognostic value is controversial due to the small size of the published series, but it seems to be limited.[122–124]

A complication stems from the fact that the *MTS1* locus

encodes a second alternative reading frame (ARF) protein (p19), sharing no homology with p16. Mice selectively nullizygous for p19 develop tumors. It has been demonstrated that in the majority of T-ALL, the complete locus is deleted (i.e. p16 and p19). Synergy between these 2 events can be deduced from Fig. 26.4: deletion of p16 allows the cell to enter S phase and deletion of p19 drives an overexpression of mdmd-2 which functionally inactivates p53, closing the way to apoptosis.

p53 gene. This tumor suppressor gene, located at 17p, is involved in Li–Fraumeni syndrome (familial susceptibility to cancer) and is mutated in about 50% of cancers. Loss of p53 function impairs arrest of the DNA synthesis at the G/S checkpoint in response to DNA damage and confers resistance to chemotherapeutic agents and γ-irradiation.

Mutations of the p53 gene are very rare at diagnosis of BCP-ALL in childhood (<2%).[125] Refractory or relapsed T-ALL forms exhibit more frequently mutations which seem to be associated with a poor prognosis.[126] Other mechanisms of p53 inactivation can be envisaged, i.e. overexpression of MDM2 which can bind inactive p53.[127]

WT1 gene. The Wilms' tumor gene is a tumor suppressor gene located at 11q13 which encodes for a nuclear transcription factor. Acquired mutations have been reported in leukemia, mainly AML.[128]

***NF1* gene.** This gene, located at 17q11.2, encodes for the neurofibromin, a member of the GTP-ase activating proteins. Inactivating mutations of *NF1* increase signaling through the *ras* pathway, potentially leading to the abnormal proliferation of cells. *NF1* mutations have been described in leukemia, mostly AML and juvenile myelomonocytic leukemia.[129]

CLINICAL VALUE OF MOLECULAR BIOLOGY

Two main applications are currently being explored.

Determination of the exact frequency of chromosomal translocations at diagnosis

A substantial underestimation of genetic lesions by conventional cytogenetics has been demonstrated due to technical failures and cryptic translocations. A fusion transcript, detectable by RT-PCR, is found in around 35% of children with BCP-ALL, corresponding to the 4 major translocations identified. Currently, those associated with a dismal prognosis (i.e. t(9;22) and t(4;11)) are used to direct treatment stratification and their molecular equivalents, i.e. fusion transcripts, must be systematically looked for. Multicenter prospective studies are underway and will help to define precisely the value of these methods.

Study of minimal residual disease

It has been estimated that the number of leukemic cells at diagnosis of acute leukemia is about 10^{12}. After induction therapy, when a complete morphologic remission is obtained (blast cells $<5\%$), this number can in fact be as high as 10^9–10^{10}. Minimal residual disease (MRD) is defined as the pool of malignant cells present in the organism but non detectable by standard morphologic methods. From a theoretical point of view, the better detection of MRD must allow a more rational basis for therapy intensification for a subset of 'poor responder' patients. A decrease in therapy for very good responders can also be envisaged.

The ideal marker for MRD is specific for the tumoral clone present on all tumoral cells and stable throughout the disease course. The ideal technique is sensitive, specific, reproducible, quantitative and allows the representative compartments of the tumor pool to be studied. Two orders of technique are being developed.[130]

Immunophenotypic studies

Flow cytometry screening after double or triple labeling allows the so-called 'leukemia-associated phenotypes' to be defined.[130] The sensitivity threshold for detecting ALL cells is around 1/10 000. Its applicability is around 50% for BCP-ALL and 90% for T-ALL. Its predictive value has been demonstrated in a single center study,[53] and further studies on a multicenter basis will be necessary to define its applicability.

Molecular tools

Two types of markers can be used.

T-cell receptor/Ig receptor genes. The genes encoding for the immunoglobulin heavy chain are rearranged

Table 26.10 Frequency of T-cell receptor (TCR)/Ig gene rearrangements in childhood acute lymphoblastic leukemia.

	B lineage (%)	T lineage (%)
IgH	90–98	10–15
γ	50–60	>90
δ	$V\delta_2$-$D\delta_3$ 20–40	$V\delta_1$-$J\delta_1$ 55–65

in the vast majority of BCP-ALL (Table 26.10). Moreover, as a mark of lineage infidelity, rearrangements of the γ and δ genes also occur. A rearrangement of the gene encoding for the γ chain of the T-cell receptor is observed in 90% of T-ALL cases and a preferential rearrangement $V\delta 1$-$J\delta 1$ is observed in 60%.[131,132]

These rearrangements can be easily amplified by the PCR technique using tumoral DNA. They are highly clone specific, due to the junctional diversity generated by the rearrangement. After cloning and sequencing, a clone-specific oligo-probe can be constructed, allowing detection of leukemic cells with a sensitivity of 10^{-4} to 10^{-6}.[133]

The problems associated with these methods include:

- clonal evolution, i.e. the possible disappearance of a rearrangement without disappearance of the tumor cell.[134] In fact, these rearrangements are only markers of events not linked to the oncogenic ones.
- time consuming, difficult and expensive.

Less sensitive but simplified strategies that do not require sequencing have been proposed.[135]

Fusion transcripts. Problems associated with the detection of fusion transcripts for MRD study include:

- limited applicability (30–35% of BCP-ALL);
- use of RNA which is fragile;
- difficult quantitation and thus requiring competitive PCR or more recently 'real time' PCR;
- risk of false positives due to contamination.

Advantages include a high sensitivity $(10^{-5}$–$10^{-6})$ and stability (the marker here is related to the oncogenic event).

Retrospective studies and two prospective studies suggest the predictive value of MRD study at the end of induction therapy for childhood ALL.[53,136,137,138] Nevertheless, the value of basing clinical decisions on these results in multicenter trials of children with ALL remains to be demonstrated.

CONCLUSION

The modern investigation of ALL requires complex studies, including molecular biology. This implies that children affected with ALL have to be referred to specialized units where all of these investigations can be done, allowing a proper diagnostic and prognostic classification. This is of major importance for therapy stratification and comparison of treatment outcomes (see Chapter 27).

REFERENCES

1. Parkin DM, Stiller CA, Draper GJ, Bieber CA. The international incidence of childhood cancer. *Int J Cancer* 1988; **42**: 511–520

2. Pendergrass TW. Epidemiology of acute lymphoblastic leukemia. *Semin Oncol* 1985; **12**: 80–91

3. Miller RW. Ethnic differences in cancer occurrence: genetic and environmental influences with particular reference to neuroblastoma. In: Mulvihill JJ, Miller RW *et al* (eds) *Genetics in Human Cancer*. New York: Raven Press, 1977, pp 1–39

4. Neglia J, Robison L. Epidemiology of childhood leukemias. *Pediatr Clin North Am* 1988; **35**: 675–692

5. Caldwell GG. Twenty-two years of cancer cluster investigations at the Centers for Disease Control. *Am J Epidemiol* 1990; **132 (Suppl 1)**: S43–S47

6. Draper GJ, Heaf MM, Kennier-Wilson LM. Occurrence of childhood cancers among sibs and estimation of familial risk. *J Med Genet* 1977; **14**: 81–90

7. Miller RW. Deaths from childhood leukemia and solid tumors among twins and other sibs in the United States. *J Natl Cancer Inst* 1971; **46**: 203–209

8. Malkin D, Li FP, Strong LC *et al*. Germline p53 mutations in a familial syndrome of breast cancer, sarcomas and other neoplasms. *Science* 1990; **250**: 1233–1238

9. Li FP, Fraumeni JF, Mulvihill JJ *et al*. A cancer family syndrome in twenty four kindreds. *Cancer Res* 1988; **48**: 5358–5362

10. Zuelzer W, Cox D. Genetic aspects of leukemia. *Semin Hematol* 1969; **6**: 228–249

11. Clarkson BD, Boyse EA. Possible explanation of the high concordance for acute leukemia in monozygotic twins. *Lancet* 1971; **1**: 699–701

12. Pombo de Oliveira MS, Awad el Seed FE, Foroni L *et al*. Lymphoblastic leukaemia in Siamese twins: evidence for identity. *Lancet* 1986; **ii**: 969–970

13. Ford AM, Ridge SA, Cabrera ME *et al*. *In utero* rearrangements in the trithorax-related oncogene in infant leukaemias. *Nature* 1993; **363**: 358–360

14. Ford AM, Pombo de Oliviera MS, McCarthy KP *et al*. Monoclonal origin of concordant T-cell malignancy in identical twins. *Blood* 1997; **89**: 281–285

15. Ford AM, Bennett CS, Price CM, Bruin MCA, Van Wering ER, Greaves M. Fetal origins of the TEL-AML1 fusion gene in identical twins with leukemia. *Proc Natl Acad Sci USA* 1998; **95**: 4584–4588

16. Gale KB, Ford AM, Repp R *et al*. Backtracking leukemia to birth: identification of clonotypic gene fusion sequences in neonatal blood spots. *Proc Natl Acad Sci USA* 1997; **94**: 13950–13954

17. Zipursky A, Poon A, Doyle J. Leukemia in Down syndrome: a review. *Pediatr Hematol Oncol* 1992; **9**: 139–149

18. Robison LL, Nesbit ME, Harland N *et al*. Down syndrome and acute leukemia in children: a 10 year retrospective survey from the Children's Cancer Study Group. *J Pediatr* 1984; **105**: 235–242

19. Passarge E. Bloom's syndrome. In: German J (ed) *Chromosome Mutation and Neoplasia*. New York: Alan R Liss, 1983, pp 11–22

20. Auerbach AD, Allen RG. Leukemia and preleukemia in Fanconi anemia patients. *Cancer Genet Cytogenet* 1991; **51**: 1–12

21. Taylor AMR, Metcalfe JA, Thick J, Mak YF. Leukemia and lymphoma in ataxia-telangiectasia. *Blood* 1996; **87**: 423–438

22. Woods W, Roloff J, Lukens J *et al*. The occurrence of leukemia in patients with Shwachman syndrome. *J Pediatr* 1981; **99**: 425–428

23. Bader JL, Miller RW. Neurofibromatosis and childhood leukemia. *J Pediatr* 1978; **92**: 925–929

24. Krijanovski OI, Sieff CA. Diamond–Blackfan anemia. *Hematol Oncol Clin North Am* 1997; **11**: 1061–1077

25. Moloney W. Leukemia in survivors of atomic bombing. *N Engl J Med* 1955; **253**: 88–90

26. Jablon S, Tachikawa K, Belsky JL, Steer A. Cancer in Japanese exposed as children to atomic bombs. *Lancet* 1971; **i**: 927–932

27. Parkin DM, Clayton D, Black RJ *et al*. Childhood leukemia in Europe after Chernobyl. *Br J Cancer* 1996; **73**: 1006–1012

28. Petridou E, Trichopoulos D, Dessypris N *et al*. Infant leukaemia after *in utero* exposure to radiation from Chernobyl. *Nature* 1996; **382**: 352–356

29. Gardner MJ, Snee MP, Hall AJ, Poxell CA, Downes S, Terrel JD. Results of case-control study of leukaemia and lymphoma among young people near Sellafield nuclear plant in West Cumbria. *Br Med J* 1990; **300**: 423–429

30. Openshaw S, Charlton M, Craft AW, Birch JM. Investigation of leukemia clusters by use of a geographical analysis machine. *Lancet* 1988; **1 (8590)**: 272–273

31. Linet MS, Hatch EE, Kleinerman RA *et al*. Residential exposure to magnetic fields and acute lymphoblastic leukemia in children. *N Engl J Med* 1997; **337**: 1–7

32. Campion EW. Power lines, cancer and fear. *N Engl J Med* 1997; **337**: 44–46

33. Miller DR, Miller LP. Acute lymphoblastic leukemia in children: an update of clinical, biological and therapeutic aspects. *Crit Rev Oncol Hematol* 1990; **10**: 132–164

34. Sandler DP, Shore DL, Anderson JR *et al*. Cigarette smoking and risk of acute leukemia: associations with morphology and cytogenetic abnormalities in bone marrow. *J Natl Cancer Inst* 1993; **85**: 1994–2003

35. Stjernfeldt M, Berglund K, Lindsten J, Ludwigson J. Maternal smoking during pregnancy and risk of childhood cancer. *Lancet* 1986; **i**: 1350

36. Pui C-H, Ribiero RC, Hancocks MI *et al*. Acute myeloid leukemia in children treated with epidophyllotoxins in acute lymphoblastic leukemia. *N Engl J Med* 1991; **325**: 1682–1687

37. Hunger SP, Sklar J, Link MP *et al*. Acute lymphoblastic leukemia occurring as a second malignant neoplasm in childhood: report of three cases and review of the literature. *J Clin Oncol* 1992; **10**: 156–163

38. Allen DB. Safety of human growth hormone therapy: current topics. *J Pediatr* 1996; **128 (Part 2)**: S8–S13

39. Allen DB, Rundle AC, Graves DA, Blethen SL. Risk of leukemia in children treated with human growth hormone: review and reanalysis. *J Pediatr* 1997; **131 (Part 2)**: S32–S36

40. Kinlen L. Evidence for an infective cause of childhood leukaemia: comparison of a Scottish new town with nuclear reprocessing sites in Britain. *Lancet* 1988; **ii**: 1323–1327

41. Alexander FE, Ricketts TJ, McKinney PA *et al*. Community lifestyle characteristics and risk of acute lymphoblastic leukemia in children. *Lancet* 1990; **336**: 1461–1465

42. Greaves MF, Alexander FE. An infectious etiology for common acute lymphoblastic leukemia in childhood? *Leukemia* 1993; **7**: 349–360

43. Ambinder RF. Human lymphotrophic viruses associated with lymphoid malignancy: Epstein–Barr and HTLV-1. *Hematol Oncol Clin North Am* 1990; **4**: 821–833

44. Filipovich AH, Zerbe D, Spector DB, Kersey JH. Lymphomas in persons with naturally occurring immunodeficiencies. In: Magrath IT (ed) *Pathogenesis of Leukemias and Lymphomas: Environmental Influences*. New York: Raven Press, 1984, pp 225–234

45. Leiken S, Miller DR, Sather H *et al*. Immunologic evaluation in the prognosis of acute lymphoblastic leukemia: a report from the Children's Cancer Group Study. *Blood* 1981; **58**: 5601

46. Greaves MF. Speculations on the cause of childhood acute lymphoblastic leukemia. *Leukemia* 1988; **2**: 120–125

47. Bennet JM, Catovsky D, Daniel MT *et al*. Proposals for the classification of the acute leukaemias. *Br J Haematol* 1976; **33**: 451–460

48. Miller DR, Leikin S, Albo V *et al*. Prognostic importance of morphology (FAB classification) in childhood acute lymphoblastic leukaemia. *Br J Haematol* 1981; **48**: 199–206

49. Bennet JM, Catovsky D, Daniel MT *et al*. The morphological classification of acute lymphoblastic leukaemia: concordance among observers and clinical correlations. *Br J Haematol* 1981; **47**: 553–561

50. Meeker TC, Hardy D, Willman C, Hogan T, Abrams J. Activation of the interleukin-3 gene by chromosome translocation in acute lymphocytic leukemia with eosinophilia. *Blood* 1990; **76**: 285–289

51. Kishimoto T, Goyert S, Kikutani H *et al* (eds). *Leucocyte Typing VI: White Cell Differentiation Antigens*. New York: Garland (in press)

52. Pui C-H, Behm FG, Crist WM. Clinical and biologic relevance of immunologic marker studies in childhood acute lymphoblastic leukemia. *Blood* 1993; **82**: 343–362

53. Coustan-Smith E, Behm FG *et al*. Immunological detection of minimal residual disease in children with acute lymphoblastic leukaemia. *Lancet* 1997; **351**: 550–554

54. Nadler LM, Korsmeyer SJ, Anderson KC *et al*. B-cell origin of non-T cell acute lymphoblastic leukemia. A model for discrete stages of neoplastic and normal pre-B cell differentiation. *J Clin Invest* 1984; **74**: 332

55. Foon KA, Todd RF. Immunologic classification of leukemia and lymphoma. *Blood* 1986; **68**: 1–31

56. Bene MC, Castoldi G, Knapp W *et al*. Proposals for the immunological classification of acute leukemias. European Group for the Immunological Characterization of Leukemias (EGIL). *Leukemia* 1995; **9**: 1783–1786

57. Pui C-H. Childhood leukemias. *N Engl J Med* 1995; **332**: 1618–1630

58. Koehler M, Behm FG, Shuster J *et al*. Transitional pre-B-cell acute lymphoblastic leukemia of childhood is associated with favorable prognostic clinical features and an excellent outcome: a Pediatric Oncology Group study. *Leukemia* 1993; **7**: 2064–2068

59. Baruchel A, Cayuela JM, Ballerini P *et al*. The majority of myeloid-antigen positive (My$^+$) childhood B-cell precursor acute lymphoblastic leukaemias express TEL-AML1 fusion transcripts. *Br J Haematol* 1997; **99**: 101–106

60. Wiersma SR, Ortega J, Sobel E, Weinberg KI. Clinical importance of myeloid-antigen expression in acute lymphoblastic leukemia of childhood. *N Engl J Med* 1991; **324**: 800–808

61. Uckun FM, Sather HN, Gaynon PS *et al*. Clinical features and treatment outcome of children with myeloid antigen positive acute lymphoblastic leukemia: a report from the Children's Cancer Group. *Blood* 1997; **90**: 28–35

62. Pui C-H, Hancock ML, Head DR *et al*. Clinical significance of CD34 expression in childhood acute lymphoblastic leukemia. *Blood* 1993; **82**: 889–894

63. Mitelman F (ed). *ISCN (1995). An International System for Human Cytogenetic Nomenclature*. Basel: S Karger AG, 1995

64. Berger R. The cytogenetics of haematological malignancies. *Baillière's Clin Haematol* 1992; **5**: 791–814

65. Veldman T, Vignon C, Schrock E, Rowley JD, Ried T. Hidden chromosome abnormalities in haematological malignancies detected by multicolour spectral karyotyping. *Nature Genet* 1997; **15**: 406–410

66. Look AT, Roberson PK, Murphy SB. Prognostic value of cellular DNA content in acute lymphoblastic leukemia in childhood. *N Engl J Med* 1987; **317**: 1666

67. Trueworthy R, Shuster J, Look TA *et al*. Ploidy of lymphoblasts is the strongest predictor of treatment outcome in B-progenitor cell acute lymphoblastic leukemia of childhood: a Pediatric Oncology Group study. *J Clin Oncol* 1992; **10**: 606–613

68. Synold TW, Relling MV, Boyett JM *et al*. Blast cell methotrexate-polyglutamate accumulation *in vivo* differs by lineage, ploidy and methotrexate dose in acute lymphoblastic leukemia. *J Clin Invest* 1994; **94**: 1996–2001

69. Kaspers GJ, Smets LA, Pieters R, Van Zantwijk CH, Van Wering ER, Veerman AJP. Favorable prognosis of hyperdiploid common acute lymphoblastic leukemia may be explained by sensitivity to antimetabolites and other drugs: results of an *in vitro* study. *Blood* 1995; **85**: 751–756

70. Kumagai M, Manabe A, Pui C-H *et al*. Stroma-supported culture in childhood B-lineage acute lymphoblastic leukemia cells predicts treatment outcome. *J Clin Invest* 1996; **97**: 755–760

71. Raimondi SC, Pui C-H, Hancock ML, Behm FG, Filatov L, Rivera GK. Heterogeneity of hyperdiploid (51–67) childhood acute lymphoblastic leukemia. *Leukemia* 1996; **10**: 213–224

72. Harris MB, Shuster JJ, Carroll A *et al*. Trisomy of leukemic cell chromosomes 4 and 10 identifies children with B-progenitor cell acute lymphoblastic leukemia with a very low risk of treatment failure: a Pediatric Oncology Group study. *Blood* 1992; **79**: 3316–3324

73. Heerema N, Sather HN, Sensel MG *et al*. Frequency and clinical significance of cytogenetic abnormalities in Pediatric T-lineage acute lymphoblastic leukemia: a report from the Children's Cancer Group. *J Clin Oncol* 1998; **16**: 1270–1278

74. Pui CH, Carroll AJ, Head D *et al*. Near-triploid and near-tetraploid acute lymphoblastic leukemia of childhood. *Blood* 1990; **76**: 590–596

75. Pui C-H, Williams DL, Raimondi SC *et al*. Hypodiploidy is associated with a poor prognosis in childhood acute lymphoblastic leukemia. *Blood* 1987; **70**: 247–253

76. Pui CH, Carroll AJ, Raimondi SC *et al*. Clinical presentation, karyotypic characterization and treatment outcome of childhood acute lymphoblastic leukemia with a near-haploid or hypodiploid less than 45 line. *Blood* 1990; **75**: 1170–1177

77. Pui C-H, Crist WM, Look T. Biology and clinical significance of cytogenetic abnormalities in childhood acute lymphoblastic leukemia. *Blood* 1990; **76**: 1449–1463

78. Patte C, Michon J, Frappaz D *et al*. Therapy of Burkitt and other B cell acute lymphoblastic leukemia and lymphoma. Experience with the LMB protocol of the SFOP in children and adults. *Baillière's Clin Haematol* 1994; **7**: 339–348

79. Romana SP, Mauchauffe M, Le Coniat M *et al*. The t(12;21) of acute lymphoblastic leukemia results in a TEL-AML1 gene fusion. *Blood* 1994; **85**: 3662–3670

80. Romana SP, Poirel H, Leconiat M *et al*. High frequency of t(12;21) in childhood B-lineage acute lymphoblastic leukemia. *Blood* 1995; **86**: 4263–4269

81. Shurtleff SA, Buijs A, Behm FG *et al*. TEL/AML1 fusion resulting from a cryptic t(12;21) is the most common genetic lesion in pediatric ALL and defines a subgroup with an excellent prognosis. *Leukemia* 1995; **9**: 1985–1989

82. Raynaud S, Cave H, Baens M *et al*. The t(12;21) translocation involving TEL and deletion of the other allele: two frequently associated alterations found in childhood acute lymphoblastic leukemia. *Blood* 1996; **87**: 2891–2899

83. Cayuela JM, Baruchel A, Orange C *et al*. *TEL-AML1* fusion mRNA as a new target to detect minimal residual disease in childhood B-cell precursor acute lymphoblastic leukemia. *Blood* 1996; **88**: 302–308

84. Borkhardt A, Cazzaniga G, Viehmann S *et al*. Incidence and clinical relevance of TEL/AML1 fusion genes in children with acute lymphoblastic leukemia enrolled in the German and Italian multicenter therapy trials. Associazione Italiana Ematologia Oncologia Pediatrica and the Berlin–Frankfurt–Munster Study Group. *Blood* 1997; **90**: 571–577

85. McLean TW, Ringold S, Neuberg D *et al*. TEL/AML1 dimerizes and is associated with a favorable outcome in childhood acute lymphoblastic leukemia. *Blood* 1996; **88**: 4252–4258

86. Rubnitz JE, Shuster JJ, Land VJ *et al*. Case-control study suggests a favorable impact of TEL rearrangements in patients with B-lineage acute lymphoblastic leukemia treated with antimetabolite-based therapy: a Pediatric Oncology study. *Blood* 1997; **89**: 1143–1146

87. Rubnitz JE, Downing JR, Pui Ch *et al*. TEL gene rearrangement in acute lymphoblastic leukemia: a new genetic marker with prognostic significance. *J Clin Oncol* 1997; **15**: 1150–1157

88. Troussard X, Rimokh R, Valensi F *et al*. Heterogeneity of t(1;19)(q23;p13) acute leukaemias. French Haematological Cytology Group. *Br J Haematol* 1995; **89**: 516–526

89. Rivera GK, Raimondi SC, Hancock ML *et al*. Improved outcome in childhood acute lymphoblastic leukaemia with reinforced early

treatment and rotational combination chemotherapy. *Lancet* 1991; **337**: 61–66

90. Pui C-H, Frankel LS, Carroll AJ *et al.* Clinical characteristics and treatment outcome of childhood acute lymphoblastic leukemia with t(4;11)(q21;q23): a collaborative study of 40 cases. *Blood* 1991; **77**: 440–447

91. Pui CH, Behm FG, Downing JR *et al.* 11q23/*MLL* rearrangement confers a poor prognosis in infants with acute lymphoblastic leukemia. *J Clin Invest* 1994; **12**: 909–915

92. Russo C, Carroll AJ, Kohler S *et al.* Philadelphia chromosome and monosomy 7 in childhood acute lymphoblastic leukemia: a Pediatric Oncology Group study. *Blood* 1991; **77**: 1050–1056

93. Fletcher JA, Lynch EA, Kimball VM *et al.* Translocation t(9;22) is associated with extremely poor prognosis in intensively treated children with acute lymphoblastic leukemia. *Blood* 1991; **77**: 435–439

94. Ribeiro RC, Broniscer A, Rivera GK *et al.* Philadelphia chromosome-positive acute lymphoblastic leukemia in children: durable responses to chemotherapy assoicated with low initial white blood cell counts. *Leukemia* 1997; **11**: 1493–1496

95. Arico M, Schrappe M, Harbott J *et al.* Prednisone good response identifies a subset of t(9;22) childhood acute lymphoblastic leukemia at lower risk for early relapse. *Blood* 1998; **Suppl 1**: 2494 (abstract)

96. Mahmoud H, Carroll AJ, Behm F *et al.* The non-random dic(9;12) translocation in acute lymphoblastic leukemia is associated with B-progenitor phenotype and an excellent prognosis. *Leukemia* 1992; **6**: 703–707

97. Murphy SB, Raimondi SC, Riveria GK *et al.* Non random abnormalities on chromosome 9p in childhood acute lymphoblastic leukemia: association with high-risk features. *Blood* 1989; **74**: 409–412

98. Raimondi SC, Shurtleff SA, Downing JR *et al.* 12 p abnormalities and the TEL gene (ETV6) in childhood acute lymphoblastic leukemia. *Blood* 1997; **90**: 4559–4566

99. Bauman H, Cherif D, Berger R. Interphase cytogenetics by fluorescent *in situ* hybridization (FISH) for characterization of monosomy 7-associated myeloid disorders. *Leukemia* 1993; **7**: 384–391

100. Seong DC, Song MY, Henske EP *et al.* Analysis of interphase cells for the Philadelphia translocation using painting probe made by inter-Alu-polymerase chain reaction from a radiation hybrid. *Blood* 1994; **83**: 2268–2273

101. Cline MJ. The molecular basis of leukemia. *N Engl J Med* 1994; **330**: 328–336

102. Allen PB, Morgan GJ, Wiederman LM. Philadelphia chromosome-positive leukemia: the translocated genes and their gene products. *Baillière's Clin Haematol* 1992; **5**: 897–930

103. Kawasaki ES, Clark SS, Coyne MY *et al.* Diagnosis of chronic myelogenous and acute lymphocytic leukemias by detection of leukemia-specific mRNA sequences amplified *in vitro*. *Proc Natl Acad Sci USA* 1988; **85**: 5698–5702

104. Maurer J, Janssen JW, Thiel E *et al.* Detection of chimeric BCR-ABL genes in acute lymphoblastic leukaemia by the polymerase chain reaction. *Lancet* 1991; **337**: 1055–1058

105. Melo JV, Gordon DE, Tuszynski A, Dhut S, Young BD, Goldman JM. Expression of the ABL–BCR fusion gene in Philadelphia-positive acute lymphoblastic leukemia. *Blood* 1993; **81**: 2488–2491

106. Nichols J, Nimer SD. Transcription factors, translocations and leukemia. *Blood* 1992; **80**: 2953–2963

107. Golub TR, Barker GF, Bohlander SK *et al.* Fusion of the TEL gene on 12p13 to the AML1 gene on 21q22 in acute lymphoblastic leukemia. *Proc Natl Acad Sci USA* 1995; **92**: 4917–4921

108. Cleary ML. Oncogenic conversion of transcription factors by chromosomal translocations. *Cell* 1991; **66**: 619–622

109. Hunger SP, Galili N, Carroll AJ, Crist WM, Link MP, Cleary ML. The t(1;19)(q23;p13) results in consistent fusion of E2A and PBX1 coding sequences in acute lymphoblastic leukemias. *Blood* 1991; **77**: 687–693

110. Cimino G, Lo Coco F, Biondi A *et al.* ALL-1 gene at chromosome

11q23 is consistently altered in acute leukemia of early infancy. *Blood* 1993; **82**: 544–546

111. Gu Y, Cimino G, Alder H. The t(4;11)(q21;q23) chromosome translocations in acute leukemias involve the VDJ recombinase. *Proc Natl Acad Sci USA* 1992; **89**: 10464–10468

112. Biondi A, Rambaldi A, Rossi V *et al.* Detection of ALL-1/AF4 fusion transcript by polymerase chain reaction for diagnosis and monitoring of acute lymphoblastic leukemias with the t(4;11) translocation. *Blood* 1993; **82**: 2943–2947

113. Taub R, Kirsch I, Morton C *et al.* Translocation of the c-myc gene into the immunoglobulin heavy chain locus in human Burkitt lymphoma and murine plasmocytoma cells. *Proc Natl Acad Sci USA* 1982; **79**: 7837–7841

114. Rabbitts TH. Translocations, master genes and differences between the origins of acute and chronic leukemias. *Cell* 1991; **67**: 641–644

115. Shiramizu B, Barriga F, Neequaye J *et al.* Pattern of chromosomal breakpoint locations in Burkitt's lymphoma: relevance of geography and Epstein–Barr virus association. *Blood* 1991; **77**: 1516–1526

116. Gaidano G, Ballerini P, Gong JZ *et al.* p53 mutations in human lymphoid malignancies: Association with Burkitt lymphoma and chronic lymphocytic leukemia. *Proc Natl Acad Sci USA* 1991; **88**: 5413–5417

117. Borkhardt A, Repp R, Harbott J *et al.* Frequency and DNA sequence of tal-1 rearrangement in children with T-cell acute lymphoblastic leukemia. *Ann Hematol* 1992; **64**: 305–308

118. Jonsson OG, Kitchens RL, Baer RJ, Buchanan GR, Smith RG. Rearrangements of the tal-1 locus as clonal markers for T-cell acute lymphoblastic leukemia. *J Clin Invest* 1991; **87**: 2029–2035

119. Cayuela JM, Madani A, Sanhes L, Stern MH, Sigaux F. Multiple tumor suppressor gene 1 inactivation is the most frequent genetic alteration in T-cell acute lymphoblastic leukemia. *Blood* 1996; **87**: 2180

120. Takeuchi S, Bartram CR, Seriu T *et al.* Analysis of a family of cyclin-dependent kinase inhibitors: p15/MTS2/INK4B, p16/MTS1/INK4A, and p18 genes in acute lymphoblastic leukemia of childhood. *Blood* 1995; **86**: 755–760

121. Nakao M, Yokota S, Kanako H *et al.* Alterations of the CDKN2 gene structure in childhood acute lymphoblastic leukemia: mutations of CDKN2 are observed preferentially in the T-lineage. *Leukemia* 1996; **10**: 249

122. Heyman M, Rasool O, Borgonovo Brandter L *et al.* Prognostic importance of p15INK4B and p16INK4 gene inactivation in childhood acute lymphocytic leukemia. *J Clin Oncol* 1996; **14**: 1512–1520

123. Kees UR, Burton PR, Lu C, Baker DL. Homozygous deletion of the p16/MTS1 gene in pediatric acute lymphoblastic leukemia is associated with unfavorable clinical outcome. *Blood* 1997; **89**: 4161–4166

124. Rubnitz JE, Behm FG, Pui CH *et al.* Genetic studies of childhood acute lymphoblastic leukemia with emphasis on p16, MLL and ETV6 abnormalities: results of St Jude total therapy study XII. *Leukemia* 1997; **11**: 1201–1206

125. Felix CA, Nau MM, Takahashi T *et al.* Hereditary and acquired p53 gene mutations in childhood acute lymphoblastic leukemia. *J Clin Invest* 1992; **89**: 640–647

126. Hsiao MH, Yu AL, Yeargin J, Ku D, Haas M. Non hereditary p53 mutations in T-cell acute lymphoblastic leukemia are associated with the relapse phase. *Blood* 1994; **83**: 2922–2930

127. Marks DI, Kurz BW, Link MP *et al.* Altered expression of p53 and mdm-2 proteins at diagnosis is associated with early treatment failure in childhood acute lymphoblastic leukemia. *J Clin Oncol* 1997; **15**: 1158–1162

128. Miwa H, Beran M, Saunders GF. Expression of the Wilms' tumor gene (WT1) in human leukemias. *Leukemia* 1992; **6**: 405–409

129. Shannon KM, O'Connell P, Martin GA *et al.* Loss of the normal NF1 allele from the bone marrow of children with type 1 neurofibromatosis and malignant myeloid disorders. *N Engl J Med* 1994; **330**: 597–601

130. Campana D, Pui CH. Detection of minimal residual disease in acute

leukemia: Methodologic advances and clinical significance. *Blood* 1995; **85**: 1416

131. Breit TM, Wolvers-Tettero IL, Beishuizen A, Verhoeven MA, van Wering ER, van Dongen JJ. Southern blot patterns, frequencies and junctional diversity of T-cell receptor-delta gene rearrangements in acute lymphoblastic leukemia. *Blood* 1993; **82**: 3063–3074

132. van Dongen JJM, Breit TM, Adraansen HJ *et al*. Detection of minimal residual disease in acute leukemia by immunological markers analysis and polymerase chain reaction. *Leukemia* 1992; **6**: 47–59

133. Macintyre E, D'Auriol L, Duparc N *et al*. Use of oligonucleotide probes directed against T cell antigen receptor gamma-delta genes variable-(diversity)-joining junctional sequences as a general method for detecting minimal residual disease in acute lymphoblastic leukemias. *J Clin Invest* 1990; **86**: 2125–2135

134. Baruchel A, Cayuela JM, Berger R, McIntyre E, Sigaux F. Assessment of clonal evolution of Ig/TCR loci in acute lymphoblastic leukemia by single-strand conformation polymorphism studies and highly resolutive PCR derived methods: Implication for a general strategy of minimal residual disease detection. *Br J Haematol* 1995; **90**: 85–93

135. Landman-Parker J, Aubin J, Delabesse E *et al*. Simplified strategies for minimal residual disease detection in B-cell precursor acute lymphoblastic leukaemia. *Br J Haematol* 1996; **95**: 281–290

136. Brisco MJ, Condon J, Hughes E *et al*. Outcome prediction in childhood acute lymphoblastic leukemia by molecular quantification of residual disease at the end of induction. *Lancet* 1994; **343**: 196–199

137. Wasserman R, Galili N, Ito Y *et al*. Residual disease at the end of induction therapy as a predictor of relapse during therapy in childhood B-lineage acute lymphoblastic leukemia. *J Clin Oncol* 1992; **10**: 1879–1888

138. Cavé H, Van der Werff Ten Bosch J, Suciu S *et al*. Clinical significance of minimal residual disease in childhood acute lymphoblastic leukemia. *N Engl J Med* 1998; **339**: 591–598

Clinical features and therapy of lymphoblastic leukemia

JÖRG RITTER AND MARTIN SCHRAPPE

Acute lymphoblastic leukemia (ALL) is the single commonest malignancy in children, comprising about 30–35% of all childhood neoplasias. Only 30 years ago this disease was fatal within 6 months in the vast majority of children.[1] In 1965, <1% of children with ALL were expected to be long-term survivors.[2] Today, owing to multimodal concepts of therapy, including appropriate supportive care, approximately 70–75% of children with ALL have an unmaintained remission, and the vast majority are eventually cured of their leukemia.[3–5] Furthermore, 20–30% of relapsed children have a long-lasting second remission with the chance of cure with second-line treatment.[6,7] This 'success story' was made possible by a series of carefully designed clinical trials both in the US and Europe, pioneered by Pinkel at St Jude Children's Research Hospital in Memphis, and Riehm in Berlin. The development of childhood ALL therapy during the last 4 decades is shown in Table 27.1.

Despite this progress in treatment outcome, the absolute number of children with ALL who relapse and eventually die of their leukemia still exceeds the absolute number of children with newly diagnosed acute myeloid leukemia (AML). Thus, childhood ALL continues to contribute significantly to the overall mortality of childhood cancer.

CLINICAL CHARACTERISTICS

The genetics of childhood ALL are covered in Chapter 26. Further evidence for a hereditary basis of childhood leukemia stems from the ever increasing list of genetic diseases associated with a high risk of developing ALL (Table 27.2). The absolute number of children with ALL and a defined genetic disorder is quite low. Sixty-one of 4110 (1.5%) children treated according to the Berlin–Frankfurt–Münster (BFM) protocols between 1981 and 1994 were known to have Down's syndrome,[8] which is in accordance with the range of 1.6–2.1% reported by other large multicenter trials.[9–11]

The clinical presentation of ALL is determined by the degree of marrow failure, caused by the infiltration of lymphoblasts and extramedullary organ infiltration. About two-thirds of children with ALL will have had signs and symptoms of disease for <4 weeks at the time of diagnosis; however, a history of some months is also compatible with the diagnosis ALL. The first symptoms are usually nonspecific and include lethargy, rapid exhaustion or lack of appetite. More specific symptoms such as anemia, hemorrhage and infections are a consequence of lymphoblasts occupying the bone marrow and disturbing the residual normal hematopoiesis. Signs and symptoms of childhood ALL are listed in Table 27.3.

Once leukemia is suspected from the history and clinical symptoms, the evaluation of a whole blood picture including

Table 27.1 Development of childhood acute lymphoblastic leukemia therapy.

1950–1960	Single agent chemotherapy (e.g. steroids, methotrexate), single centers
1960–1970	Combination chemotherapy, CNS-directed therapy (cranial/craniospinal irradiation), intrathecal chemotherapy, single centers
1970–1980	Intensification of polychemotherapy, definition of risk factors, single and multicenter trials
1980–today	Risk-adapted therapy, definition of biological subgroups, specific therapy for B-ALL/non-Hodgkin's lymphoma, definition of late effects of therapy, multicenter trials
The future	Individually adapted therapy approaches, specific therapy for biologically defined subgroups, inclusion of bone marrow transplantation into treatment schedules

Table 27.2 Genetic susceptibility to leukemia.

Disorder	Comment
Chromosomal syndromes	
Trisomy 21	Risk is 15 times normal
Trisomy 8	
Monosomy 5 or 7	Recurrent infections may precede neoplasia
DNA fragility	
Xeroderma pigmentosum	Autosomal recessive; failure to repair solar-damaged DNA
Fanconi's anemia	Autosomal recessive; 10% risk for acute myelogenous leukemia; chromosome fragility; positive diepoxybutane test
Bloom's syndrome	Autosomal recessive; chromosome fragility; high risk for malignancy
Ataxia–telangiectasia	Autosomal recessive; sensitive to X-radiation, radiomimetic drugs; chromosome fragility
Immunodeficiency syndromes	
Wiskott–Aldrich syndrome	Immunodeficiency; X-linked recessive
X-linked immunodeficiency (Duncan's syndrome)	Epstein–Barr virus is inciting agent
X-linked agammaglobulinemia	Immunodeficiency
Severe combined immunodeficiency	X-linked recessive immunodeficiency
Other	
Neurofibromatosis (NF1)	Autosomal dominant
Kostmann's syndrome	Mutation of G-CSF receptor

Table 27.3 Signs and symptoms in children with acute leukemias.

Signs of anemia	Weariness, fatigue, rapid exhaustion, lack of appetite Laboratory: normochromic, normocytic, hyporegenerative anemia (exception: condition following severe blood loss due to bleeding tendency)
Signs of susceptibility to infections	Feverish infections (e.g. nasopharynx, anal region) Laboratory: reduced absolute number of granulocytes
Signs of bleeding tendency	Purpura, mucosal bleeding, tendency to develop hematomas Laboratory: hyporegenerative thrombocytopenia, plasmatic coagulopathy (AML, especially promyelocytic leukemia)
Signs of organ infiltration	Bone and joint discomfort, hepatomegaly and splenomegaly, generalized lymph node swelling, infiltration of thymus
Signs of systemic disease	Fever of unknown origin, weight loss, night sweats

platelet and reticulocyte counts and especially microscopic evaluation of a blood smear allows an immediate diagnosis in many cases. However, a normal blood picture and normal blood smear do not rule out ALL. Thus, bone marrow aspiration must be performed immediately if there is still suspicion of ALL.

The differential diagnosis of ALL includes infections, other pediatric malignancies that involve the bone marrow, collagen vascular diseases and other hematologic diseases such as idiopathic thrombocytopenic purpura (ITP) and aplastic anemia (Table 27.4).

ALL may present as an incidental finding on a routine blood count of an asymptomatic child or as a life-threatening hemorrhagic infection or episode of respiratory distress, especially in children with hyperleukocytosis, e.g. in T-ALL. Lymphadenopathy is especially present in children with T-ALL and mostly correlates with a high white blood count (WBC) (lymphoma type of ALL). In about 30–60% of children with ALL, marked hepato- and/or spleno-

Table 27.4 Differential diagnosis of acute leukemia in children and adolescents.

Aplastic anemia	Less common than leukemia, trephine biopsy
Rheumatic disease (e.g. Still's disease, rheumatic fever)	Rare, bone marrow aspiration
Osteomyelitis	X-ray, skeletal scintigraphy, bone marrow aspiration
Bone marrow dissemination of different malignancies (e.g. neuroblastoma, rhabdomyosarcoma)	Tumor markers, immunophenotyping, immunohistochemistry, bone marrow aspiration, trephine biopsy
Myeloproliferative/myelodysplastic syndrome	Bone marrow aspiration, trephine biopsy, close monitoring
Viral infection (e.g. infectious mononucleosis, CMV infection)	Specific serology, bone marrow aspiration
Leukemoid reaction (e.g. in whooping cough, sepsis)	Bone marrow aspiration, close monitoring
Acute erythroblastopenia with normochromic anemia	Normal platelet and granulocyte count, bone marrow aspiration
Idiopathic thrombocytopenia	Normal granulocyte and red blood count, bone marrow aspiration

megaly is found at diagnosis. Hepatosplenomegaly also correlates with a high WBC at diagnosis.

Although ALL is primarily a disease of the bone marrow and peripheral blood, any other organ may be infiltrated by leukemic blasts. Such infiltration may easily be clinically apparent, such as lymphadenopathy or hepatosplenomegaly. However, leukemic infiltration of other organs may be occult and detectable only by histologic or cytologic examination or diagnostic imaging.

MEDIASTINAL MANIFESTATIONS

Anterior mediastinal masses, mostly within the thymus, are present in about two-thirds of children with T-ALL but are extremely rare in other immunologic subtypes (Table 27.5). Leukemic pleural effusion may be associated with mediastinal masses in some children with T-ALL.[12] Superior vena cava syndrome and severe respiratory distress may occur in these children and may lead to medical emergencies. During induction chemotherapy these children may develop pronounced tumor lysis syndrome.

CENTRAL NERVOUS SYSTEM MANIFESTATIONS

Overt central nervous system (CNS) leukemia as defined by the presence of lymphoblasts in the cerebrospinal fluid

(CSF) is found in 1.5–10% of children with newly diagnosed ALL, depending on their immunologic subtype (Table 27.5). CNS leukemia is more common in children with B-ALL and T-ALL and children with high WBCs. Children with CNS leukemia may present with diffuse or focal neurologic signs such as increased intracranial pressure—headache, vomiting, papilledema and lethargy, mostly without nuchal rigidity. Cranial nerve involvement, mostly of the 3rd, 4th, 6th and 7th nerves, may be found on careful neurologic evaluation. CNS leukemia rarely presents with hypothalamic involvement, resulting in excessive weight gain and behavior disturbances.[13]

Leukemic blasts may enter the CNS by hematogenous spread or by direct extension of involved skull bone marrow through bridging veins to the superficial arachnoidea. With progressive CNS leukemia, the blasts eventually infiltrate the deep arachnoidea and then the pia/glial membrane and eventually invade brain parenchyma. In a severe combined immunodeficiency (SCID) mouse model, histologically detectable engraftment of leukemic cells in the skull, vertebral bone marrow and meninges preceded engraftment at other sites.[14]

Most children with CNS leukemia at presentation have CNS pleocytoses as a result of the presence of leukemic blasts. These blasts can be identified with the use of cytocentrifugation and May–Grünewald–Giemsa staining. Careful morphologic evaluation is necessary to distinguish leukemic

Table 27.5 Correlation of immunophenotype with clinical characteristics in study ALL-BFM '86 according to Ref. 3.

	Pro-B	Early pre-B	Pre-B	B	Pre-T/T
Patients (%, n = 1037)*	52 (5)	635 (63)	156 (16)	39 (4)	124 (12)
Sex (% male)	38.5	52.8	50.0	84.6	75.0
Age (years)					
< 1 (%)	32.7	0.8	5.8	2.6	0.8
1–<10 (%)	50.0	82.4	80.1	64.1	62.1
⩾10 (%)	17.3	16.9	14.1	33.3	37.1
White blood count					
median × 10^9/l	37.9	7.5	16.2	13.5	59.8
⩽20 × 10^9/l (%)	37.7	75.1	52.6	69.2	22.6
>50 × 10^9/l (%)	44.2	10.7	20.5	5.1	56.5
Platelets					
⩽100 × 10^9/l (%)	76.9	74.5	80.8	56.4	55.6
Hemoglobin					
⩽8 g/dl (%)	57.7	61.9	59.6	20.5	15.3
Splenomegaly					
>4 cm below costal margin (%)	50.0	33.7	45.5	28.2	57.2
Hepatomegaly					
⩾4 cm below costal margin (%)	55.8	45.7	48.1	35.9	61.3
Mediastinal mass (%)	–	–	0.6	–	71.8
Lymphadenopathy					
>2 cm (%)	34.6	35.6	41.0	53.8	78.2
CNS disease (%)	9.6	1.4	1.3	–**	10.5

*27 patients were enrolled without identification of immunophenotype based on morphologic and cytochemical criteria; 1 patient was diagnosed as acute hybrid leukemia, 3 patients were diagnosed as acute undifferentiated leukemia.
**In the previous 2 studies ALL-BFM '81 and '83 the incidence of CNS disease was 36% and 29%, respectively.

blasts from reactive blood cells, which may be seen after intrathecal chemotherapy or during CNS infection. Contamination of the CNS with peripheral blood as indicated by the presence of red blood cells often makes the interpretation of morphologic examination difficult or even impossible. The incidence of CNS leukemia at presentation varies considerably depending on the diagnostic criteria used.[15] In 1986, the Rome International Workshop recommended an absolute cell count of ⩾5 leukocytes/μl with unequivocal blasts in a cytocentrifuge preparation as the definition of cerebromenigeal leukemia.[16]

With contemporary trials to reduce the intensity of CNS-directed treatment and its associated toxicity, attention has been drawn to the prognostic influence of leukemic blasts within the CSF without pleocytosis. While some investigators reported that a low number of blasts in the CSF at presentation did not predict later development of overt CNS leukemia or CNS relapse,[17] one retrospective single-center study showed an increased risk of subsequent CNS relapse in children with no leukocytes/μl but detectable blasts in the cytocentrifuged preparation at diagnosis, using a special technique.[18] To study the significance of a low number of CNS blasts in the context of the different treatment strategies, CNS disease status at presentation should be reported using the following definitions:

- CNS-1 (no blast cells);
- CNS-2 (<5 leukocytes/μl with morphologically detectable blasts);
- CNS-3 (⩾5 leukocytes/μl with morphologically detectable blasts and/or cranial nerve involvement).[19]

In addition to this morphologic definition of CNS leukemia, other methods of classification of WBCs within the CSF, such as terminaldeoxynucleotidyltransferase (TdT), immunophenotype, cytogenetics and molecular genetics, should be used to differentiate between leukemic blasts and reactive blood cells within the CSF.

Leukemic blasts may persist within the CNS throughout induction chemotherapy because most drugs used in the treatment of ALL inadequately penetrate the CNS, thus allowing progressive growth of lymphoblasts or the emergence of resistant clones. Cytogenetic studies and patterns of systemic relapse following the appearance of CNS disease strongly suggest that the hematologic recurrence may be due to reseeding of leukemic blasts from the CNS to the marrow.[20,21]

Spinal cord involvement due to a localized epidural leukemic infiltrate may lead to spinal cord compression with back pain, weakness of the extremities, paralysis and bladder or bowel incontinence.[22] Gadolinium-enhanced magnetic resonance tomography is helpful in localizing the leukemic infiltrate and in differentiating epidural hematoma and vertebral body collapse due to leukemic osteopathy.

GENITOURINARY MANIFESTATIONS

Overt testicular disease, found by careful palpation or sonography, is rare at presentation of a boy with ALL. However, leukemic blasts were found by testicular biopsy in as many 25% of boys at presentation.[23] Occult testicular involvement occurred only in boys with a WBC > 25 000/μl. The leukemic infiltration of testis is found mainly in the interstitium.

Clinically overt testicular relapse is usually painless and unilateral. Some boys have in addition the involvement of intra-abdominal lymph nodes. Bilateral testicular biopsy often shows an occult leukemic infiltration of the contralateral testis at the time of unilateral testicular relapse. The relatively high incidence of testicular relapse compared to, for example, ovarian relapse may be due to a blood-testes barrier analogous to the blood-brain barrier. However, the wider use of intensified multidrug regimens, including high-dose chemotherapy with methotrexate, in recent years has significantly reduced the overt relapse of the testes.[3] Thus, the use of bilateral testicular biopsies which was recommended for many years in some trials,[24] is no longer recommended.[25]

Renal infiltrates may lead to oliguria or may be asymptomatic and discovered by their presentation in large kidneys shown by sonography or computed tomography (CT). The incidence of pretherapeutic renal infiltration was 18% in one BFM study.[26] Priapism is rarely found in boys with T-ALL and the hyperleukocytosis/leukostasis syndrome.[27]

SKELETAL MANIFESTATIONS

About 20–30% of children with ALL present with severe pain, mainly in the lower extremities, leading to a limp or refusal to walk. These children suffer nearly exclusively from common ALL (c-ALL) and often present with a normal blood count and low number or even absence of peripheral lymphoblasts (aleukemic leukemia), which often results in a delayed diagnosis.[28] Up to 20% of children with ALL present with characteristic bony radiographic changes, including transverse radiolucent lines in metaphyses, subperiostal new bone formation or osteolytic lesions mimicking primary bone tumors, diffuse demineralization (osteopenia) or vertrebral collapse, mimicking Langerhans cell histiocytosis.[29,30] Pathologic fractures and vertrebral collapses may occur secondary to severe osteopenia (leukemic osteopathy). Osteonecrosis, especially of the hip and knee, may also produce severe bone pain and is a rare complication of antileukemic therapy, especially with steroids.[31]

GASTROINTESTINAL MANIFESTATIONS

Specific problems of the oral cavity are common in children with acute leukemia. Infection with Candida albicans (oral thrush) is common at diagnosis and during polychemotherapy, and regular mouth care with antifungal agents is an essential part of supportive care. Petechiae, hemorrhage and gum bleeding occur frequently, especially in children with severe thrombocytopenia. Gum infiltration by leukemic blasts has a characteristic appearance and is particularly associated with AML-M5 and -M4. Mucosal ulceration is also common, particularly in the presence of profound neutropenia in addition to fungal or bacterial infections, particularly with anaerobic organisms and *Streptococcus viridans* (*Strep. mitis, sanguis, hominis*). Viral infections, mainly due to herpes simplex virus (HSV), can be a problem in neutropenic children. Candida- or HSV-esophagitis characterized by retrosternal pain often occurs in neutropenic children with leukemia.

Bleeding as reflected by gross or occult blood in the stool is the commonest gastrointestinal manifestation of leukemia and may be due to thrombocytopenia, disseminated intravascular coagulation (DIC) or infiltration with leukemic cells.

Massive infiltration of intra-abdominal lymph nodes, especially in the right lower quadrant, is frequently found in children with B-ALL, which may be the result of rapid leukemic transformation of an abdominal B-non-Hodgkin's lymphoma (B-NHL).

A characteristic syndrome of right lower quadrant pain with tenderness, abdominal tension, vomiting and sepsis is often seen during profound neutropenia due to intensive polychemotherapy (neutropenic perityphlitis or neutropenic necrotizing enterocolitis).[32] Sonography may show a characteristic thickening of the gut wall in the right lower quadrant.[33] Peptic ulcers of the stomach and duodenum may be seen in children with ALL, especially during steroid treatment.

Severe hemorrhage or necrotizing pancreatitis can be found in children with ALL during asparaginase treatment.[34] Management of these conditions includes bowel rest, intravenous fluids and broad-spectrum antibiotics. Surgery is rarely indicated except in rare cases of perforation.[35] The differential diagnosis must include common childhood surgical problems, including appendicitis, cholangitis and intussusception.

Malabsorption is rarely seen in children with ALL and is mainly due to leukemic infiltration of the gut or anti-leukemia therapy. Perirectal inflammation or abscess formation is a characteristic sign of infection due to pseudomonas *spp* or anaerobic organisms.[36]

Impairment of liver function with or without elevated bilirubin levels may be due to liver infiltration by leukemic blasts, chemotherapy-induced hepatotoxity, especially during treatment with asparaginase, methotrexate and purine analogs, or viral hepatitis, especially with the hepatitis B or C virus (HBV and HCV).[37]

OCULAR MANIFESTATIONS

Occult ocular involvement seen on careful ophthalmologic investigation may be found in up to one-third of newly diagnosed children with ALL.[38] Virtually all ocular structures have been found to be involved.[39] Retinal hemorrhages are presumably due to thrombocytopenia and may precede intracranial hemorrhage, especially in children with the hyperleukocytosis/leukostasis syndrome.[40] Overt leukemic infiltration of the eye is uncommon at presentation and is usually associated with leukemic relapse.[41] About half of children with leukemic eye infiltration present with overt CNS relapse.[42] Oculomotor palsies and papilloedema are frequent signs of meningeal leukemia at presentation or at the time of relapse. Thus, it has been suggested that the eye could be a sanctuary site in ALL, like the CNS and testes.[43]

Under the conditions of today's intensive polychemotherapy protocols, which include high-dose chemotherapy and CNS-directed treatment, the incidence of ocular manifestations of ALL is lower than in the past, as are the incidences of CNS and testicular manifestations.[3,44]

CARDIOPULMONARY MANIFESTATIONS

Leukemic involvement of the lungs and heart is rare. However, these manifestations may cause life-threatening problems in a child with ALL. Pericardial leukemic effusions are found by echocardiographic examination in about one-third of children with T-ALL and are often associated with leukemic pleural effusion and a mediastinal mass. In children with a very high initial WBC, a life-threatening hyperleukocytosis/leukostasis syndrome may cause massive respiratory distress due to infiltration and leukostasis within the lung. Emergency leukapheresis or exchange transfusion can be a life-saving emergency measure in this situation.[45,46]

During polychemotherapy, pulmonary complications in children with leukemia almost always have an infectious origin. Differentiation between bacterial and fungal infections, leukemic infiltrations and hemorrhage is often possible with the help of diagnostic imaging, including high-resolution CT of the lungs (HR-CT).[47]

Severe cardiomyopathy in children with leukemia is seen during severe septicemia or metabolic disturbance in children with high blood counts and a rapid lysis of lymphoblasts (tumor lysis syndrome). Late cardiomyopathy is found after extensive treatment with anthracyclines.[48,49]

The rare ALL subtype with hypereosinophilia[50] may present with life-threatening involvement of the heart with mural thrombi of the myocardium or Löfflers' endocardial fibrosis.[51]

SKIN MANIFESTATIONS

Skin infiltration is rarely seen in children with ALL in contrast to children with AML M4 and M5. However, lymphoblasts may proliferate within the skin due to intradermal bleeding due to thrombocytopenia. In the rare case of congenital leukemia, skin infiltration has been reported in about 50% of neonates.[52]

LABORATORY FINDINGS

Laboratory data may show a broad spectrum of abnormal findings at presentation of ALL. Normochromic (mean cellular hemoglobin [MCH] normal), normocytic (mean corpuscular volume [MCV] normal) and hyporegeneratory (low reticulocytes) anemia is present in about two-thirds of children with ALL and reflects progressive bone marrow failure. The WBC is raised $> 10\,000/\mu l$ in about half of children with newly diagnosed ALL, reflecting the proliferative capacity of their lymphoblasts. However, in about 5% of children with ALL, the WBC is $< 2000/\mu l$, often without detectable lymphoblasts in the peripheral blood (aleukemic leukemia). Rarely, ALL presents with an aplastic blood profile. Hypereosinophilia in the peripheral blood is rarely found and is associated with the t(5;14) translocation.[50] This hypereosinophilia has to be differentiated from AML M4 eosinophilia, where atypical eosinophils are found in the bone marrow.

Peripheral blasts may not always reflect the bone marrow status. In some patients a pathologic shift to the left with increased numbers of pro-myelocytes or even myeloblasts can be found as a result of the leukoerythroblastic response to bone marrow infiltration which can be found in ALL, NHL, granulomatous infections and metastatic tumors (e.g. neuroblastoma, Ewing's sarcoma, rhabdomyosarcoma). Thus, the definitive diagnosis of leukemia should not be made from peripheral blood smears alone.

Thrombocytopenia $< 100\,000/\mu l$ is present in about 80% of children with ALL at diagnosis. The platelets in leukemia are morphologically normal. Thrombocytopenia is accompanied by other hematologic or physical manifestations of leukemia in the vast majority of children.[53]

BONE MARROW

Inspection of bone marrow smears is essential to establish the diagnosis of leukemia. Whereas a normal bone marrow contains $< 5\%$ of blast cells (M1 marrow), leukemic marrows generally contain $> 40\%$ and in most cases $> 80\%$ of blasts. By arbitrary convention, $> 25\%$ blasts (M3 marrow) is required to confirm the diagnosis of acute leukemia and to distinguish leukemia from NHL with bone marrow infiltration (Stage IV NHL). For cytomorphologic purposes, anterior or posterior iliac crest aspirates smeared in the same way as blood smears are required. The sternum is not used for bone marrow aspiration in children because this procedure may be hazardous, especially to young children. In very young infants, some physicians prefer the tibia. A 'dry tap' may be caused by bone infarction, myelofibrosis or bone necrosis,[54,55] and in such cases a bone marrow trephine biopsy should be performed. Imprint or rolled preparations of these specimens can be used for further classification.

ALL is subclassified according to morphologic, immunologic and genetic features of the leukemic blasts cells. The definite diagnosis is generally based on the examination of the bone marrow aspirate. The cytologic appearance of the blast cells in ALL can be highly variable, even in a single specimen, and no completely satisfactory morphologic classification has been devised. The French–American–British (FAB) classification distinguishes 3 morphologic subtypes (L1, L2 and L3).[56] L1 lymphoblasts are predominantly small with little cytoplasm; L2 cells are larger and pleomorphic with increased cytoplasm and sometimes an irregular nuclear shape and prominent nucleoli; L3 blasts have a deep blue cytoplasm with a prominent vacuolization and homogenous nuclear chromatin with prominent nucleoli. L3 lymphoblasts represent an immunophenotypically distinct population (B-ALL).

Granular ALL has been described as a rare variant in about 3% of cases.[28] In contrast to myeloblasts, the myeloperoxidase stain is always negative in granular ALL. Immunophenotyping reveals CD10 positivity in nearly all cases with this strange morphologic subtype.[57]

In approximately 80% of cases of ALL, lymphoblasts are reactive with periodic acid-Schiff (PAS) which stains cytoplasmatic glycogen. Cytoplasmic stains for myeloid enzymes (myeloperoxidase) and cytoplasmic lipids (Sudan black) are negative in lymphoblasts (with a few exceptions for the latter stain).[58] The presence of myeloperoxidase-positive Auer rods is specific for myeloid differentiation and excludes the diagnosis ALL. Diffuse positivity with non-specific esterases (e.g. alfanaphytlacetatesterase) is specific for monoblasts and also excludes the diagnosis of ALL. A strong positivity with acid phosphatase within the Golgi region correlates with a T-cell differentiation (T-ALL).[59,60]

In about 10% of children with ALL, morphologic and cytochemical classification does not allow an appropriate diagnosis, thus opening the field for immunophenotyping and genetic classification (see Chapter 26).

The introduction of immunophenotyping and genetic classification of acute leukemias revealed that some blasts show an ambigous phenotype and genotype which do not allow clear differentiation between ALL and AML.[61] These leukemias have been referred to as mixed lineage,[62] biphenotypic[63] or acute hybrid leukemias.[64] They may arise from malignant transformation of a progenitor cell capable of differentiation into more than one lineage (lineage promiscuity).[65] Alternatively, they may result from aberrant gene regulation not representative of normal hematopoiesis (lineage infidelity).[66] In B-precursor ALL, co-expression of one or more myeloid markers (e.g. CD13, CD33, CDw65) ranges from 4 to $> 20\%$ depending on the criteria applied.[67–69] The prognostic significance of co-expression of myeloid markers is unclear. In some trials My$^+$ ALL has been an independent predictor of poor outcome,[70] but not in others.[68,71] Thus, ALL defined by morphologic and cytochemical criteria in which blasts cells co-express myeloid antigens, most probably represents phenotypic deviations and should be classified as ALL.[72] True biphenotypic leukemias with 2 separate blast cell populations are rare (<1% of children with newly diagnosed acute leukemia).

Most cases of morphologically and cytochemically undifferentiated acute leukemias can be immunophenotypically classified as either B-precursor ALL or AML M0. However, in about 2% of childhood ALL,[3] the cellular origin of blasts remains obscure.[73,74] These leukemias are probably derived from a very immature hematopoietic progenitor cell.

Table 27.6 gives an overview of the diagnostic work-up in a newly diagnosed child with ALL. Levels of lactate dehydrogenase (LDH), liver enzymes and serum uric acid are often abnormal at presentation, due to leukemic cell turnover or kidney infiltration. In children with hyperleukocytosis and a high leukemic cell burden, metabolic abnormalities such as hypercalcemia, hyperphosphatemia or hyperkalemia may not preclude the immediate start of antileukemic treatment. In these cases, leukapheresis or exchange transfusion may be useful. Renal dialysis may be required in the occasional patient with B-ALL and a high leukemic cell turnover as demonstrated by very high levels of LDH (mostly >1000/ μl).[75] Most ALL children with hyperleukocytosis can, however, be managed by careful steroid-based cytoreductive treatment and preventive measures for hyperuricemia such as allopurinol or urate oxidase.

Table 27.6 Basic investigations required at diagnosis of childhood acute lymphoblastic leukemia.

Blood tests
Whole blood count, including platelets and reticulocytes
Differential blood count
Lactate dehydrogenase (LDH)
Electrolytes (Ca, K, Na, Cl, Phosphate, Mg)
Renal function (creatinine, urea, uric acid)
Liver function tests (GOT, GPT, CHE, AP, γ-GT, bilirubin)
Coagulation tests (Quick, PT, partial thromboplastin time, fibrinogen, antithrombin III, protein C, protein S, resistance to activated protein C [APC resistance], D dimer)
Immunoglobulin levels (IgG, A, M, E)
Viral serology (HBV, EBV, VZV, CMV, measles, hepatitis A, B, C)

Urinalysis

Bone marrow diagnostics
Bone marrow aspiration; if unsuccessful: trephine biopsy
Morphology and cytochemistry (periodic acid-Schiff [PAS], POX, acidic phosphatase, non-specific esterase)
Immunophenotyping
Cytogenetics, DNA content
Molecular genetics

CNS diagnostics
CSF cell count, cytospin preparation, protein, glucose
Cranial CT or MRT
EEG
Neurologic examination

Cardiology
ECG, echocardiography

Diagnostic imaging
Chest X-ray/sonography
Abdominal sonography for liver, spleen, kidney size

CHE = choline esterase; AP = alkaline phosphatase; γ-GT = γ-glutamate transferase; POX = myeloperoxidase.

Coagulation tests, including fibrinogen, antithrombin III and resistance to the activated form of protein C (APC resistance), are recommended during treatment with asparaginase.

In addition to a careful history recording previous infections, recent contact with infections and immunizations, baseline viral serologies are recommended, especially for measles, varicella zoster virus, cytomegalovirus, herpes simplex virus and hepatitis A, B and C. A diagnostic lumbar puncture—in most modern treatment protocols combined with intrathecal injection of methotrexate—for CSF examination (cell count including the number of red cells because of possible contamination with peripheral blood) and a cytospin is required at the beginning of treatment. This initial lumbar puncture should be delayed for a couple of days in children in a poor clinical condition or with a very high WBC.

Chest X-ray or sonography of the mediastinum may reveal a mediastinal mass, which may lead to severe obstruction of the airways and/or the vena cava superior. Sonography of the abdomen is recommended for the determination of liver, spleen and kidney size. Before the start of treatment with potential cardiotoxic and neurotoxic drugs, most protocols recommend echocardiography and an EEG.

Because of the high incidence of severe infections during remission induction treatment (see below), most protocols recommend a pre-therapeutic infection screen, including urinalysis and cultures of nose, throat and rectum. Blood cultures are recommended in children with fever and in those with central catheters.

PROGNOSTIC FACTORS

A retrospective analysis of clinical trials established many important prognostic factors which were subsequently applied prospectively to stratify children into different treatment groups according to their relative risk of treatment failure. Children at higher risk of relapse are treated more intensively,[3,76,77] whereas in those with a lower risk of relapse the more toxic components of treatment, such as cranial irradiation, anthracyclines, oxazaphorines and epipodophyllotoxins, are reduced or even eliminated.[76–79] Thus, treatment tailored to the individual risk of relapse is an essential prerequisite for current clinical trials. This approach greatly complicates any comparative analysis of treatment results.[80] Recently, an uniform approach to risk classification and the classification of special prognostic factors has been agreed by clinicians in the US.[19]

Since ALL is a heterogeneous disease, there may be multiple populations of patients with different prognosis on identical treatments. Various clinical and laboratory findings at the time of diagnosis have been correlated with prognosis (Table 27.7). The relative importance of a given prognostic factor varies between different treatment

Table 27.7 Prognostic factors in the therapy of *de novo* acute lymphoblastic leukemia.

Factor	Favorable	Unfavorable
Age	>1–<6 years	<1 year
White blood count (× 10⁹/l)	<20	>100
Response to initial 7-day prednisone monotherapy plus one IT methotrexate on day 1 (peripheral blood) (blasts × 10⁹/l blood)	<1	≥1
Response to initial induction therapy (bone marrow on day 14)	M1 marrow*	M2, M3 marrow*
Chromosome count	>50	<45
DNA index	≥1.16	<1.16
Chromosomal translocations	t(12;21)	t(9;22); t(4;11)
Probability of 5-year event-free survival	>80%	10–60%, depending on specific constellation

*M1 marrow, <5% blasts *and* complete regeneration of hematopoiesis; M2 marrow, >5%–<25% blasts and/or incomplete regeneration of hematopoiesis; M3 marrow, >25% blasts in the bone marrow.

protocols.[3,77,81] Intensification of treatment can eliminate the prognostic significance of some of the unfavorable features, illustrating that treatment *per se* is probably the most important risk factor in childhood ALL. Although all prognostic factors should be considered treatment specific, certain features appear to be consistently valuable (Table 27.7).

Prognostic factors according to clinical parameters

The initial WBC shows independent significance in most studies, with a linear relationship between the number of leukemic cells and the risk of relapse.[76,82,83] Organ infiltration is strongly correlated with WBC but has no additional prognostic significance in most trials.[3]

Age at presentation is an important prognostic factor: whereas infants younger than 1 year of age have the worst prognosis of any age group,[3,84] children aged 2–6 years do best of all.[3,4,78] Adolescents have faired poorly in many trials and adults with ALL have a poorer outcome as compared to children.[3,4,85] The prognostic importance of age may be due to the fact, for unknown reasons, that specific biologic subtypes of ALL occur more or less frequently in different age groups.

In the past, girls have had a better prognosis than boys, which is not completely explained by testicular relapse or the higher incidence of T-ALL in males. However, some recent trials do not find male sex to be an adverse prognostic factor.[5,86]

Black children, who account for about 10% of all newly diagnosed children with ALL in the US, have been reported to have a worse prognosis than white children. This has been attributed to the higher frequency of specific biologic subtypes of ALL with a poorer prognosis in black children.[87] However, a recent trial found race to lack prognostic importance.[5]

Prognostic factors according to cell biology

The immunophenotype of lymphoblasts was thought to be the most important factor in childhood ALL. This is still true for B-ALL which is now treated completely differently from B-precursor ALL and T-ALL. However, T-ALL is no longer an unfavorable entity using contemporary risk-adapted polychemotherapy.[3,77,81]

A pre-B cell phenotype has been reported to confer a worse prognosis compared to the early pre-B phenotype.[88,89] However, results of a recent trial using intensive polychemotherapy revealed no difference in outcome between these 2 immunologic subgroups.[3] ALL derived from an even earlier B-cell precursor (CD10-, CD19+) (pro-B ALL) has also been associated with a poor response to therapy.[90,91] However, in one recent study the adverse impact of this immune phenotype was abolished when infants were excluded from the analysis.[3] The prognostic significance of co-expression of myeloid antigens is still controversial.[68,70,71]

Children with hyperdiploid leukemia (DNA index ≥1.16) were reported to have a better prognosis as compared to children without this feature.[92,93] The translocation t(12;21), (p13; q22) with the TEL-AML 1 fusion transcript found in about 20% of children with ALL confers a favorable outcome with long-term survival exceeding 90%.[94,95] Children with t(9;22)[96–100] and the translocation (4;11)[101,102] have a particularly poor prognosis irrespective of other presenting features or treatment regimens. However, a recent study identified a subset of t(9;22) childhood ALL with a lower risk for relapse.[103]

Prognostic factors according to early response to treatment

Response to induction polychemotherapy[104,105] or monotherapy with steroids,[3,106,107] as measured by the absolute number of leukemic blasts in the peripheral blood on day 7 or the percentage of bone marrow blasts on days 14 and 33, has been defined as a new important predictor of outcome in many recent trials, again illustrating the importance of treatment response as a prognostic factor.

New technologies for the detection of minimal residual leukemic cells permit the identification of up to one leukemic blast within 10⁶ nucleated cells (Table 27.8), which could be important for the evaluation of post-induction response. The detection of clone-specific immunoglobulin and T-cell receptor (TCR) gene rearrangements by the polymerase chain reaction (PCR) is used in some multicenter trials. In a recent study of the international BFM study group using this

Table 27.8 Methods for the detection of minimal residual leukemic cells in childhood acute lymphoblastic leukemia (ALL).

Technique	Detection limit	Applicability
Morphology and cytochemistry	10^{-1}–10^{-2}	All leukemias
Cytogenetics	10^{-1}–10^{-2}	Leukemias with microscopically detectable numeric or structural aberrations (only cells in mitosis)
Fluorescence *in situ* hybridization (FISH)	10^{-1}–10^{-2}	Leukemias with known numeric or structural aberrations (interphase cells)
Flow cytometry for DNA content	10^{-1}–10^{-2}	About 30% of B-precursor ALL; <5% of T-ALL
Flow cytometry for leukemia-associated immunophenotype (LAIP)	10^{-3}–10^{-4}	50–90% of ALL
PCR techniques		
DNA level:		
Rearranged immunoglobulin and T-cell receptor genes	10^{-3}–10^{-6}	90% of ALL
Chromosomal aberrations with known breakpoints	10^{-4}–10^{-6}	10–20% of T-ALL, >5% of B-ALL
RNA level:		
Chromosomal aberrations resulting in leukemia-specific fusion genes and fusion mRNA	10^{-3}–10^{-5}	10–15% of B-precursor ALL

technology, minimal residual disease (MRD) analyses gave insight into the efficacy of the different treatment blocks. A negative PCR result at the end of remission induction treatment identifies children with a very good prognosis ($\geq$90% complete continuous remission [CCR]). A positive PCR signal during consolidation or at the beginning of maintenance therapy identifies children with an increased risk of relapse. Thus, the evaluation of residual tumor burden and monitoring of early response to treatment using PCR technology may provide a better risk stratification of ALL patients for future controlled clinical trials.[108]

TREATMENT OF NEWLY DIAGNOSED ACUTE LYMPHOBLASTIC LEUKEMIA

The ability of a cytotoxic drug to induce complete remission of ALL was first reported in 1948,[109] and since then a multitude of effective agents has been discovered. Despite the fact that single-agent therapy has no place in the curative treatment of ALL, knowledge of the administration and action of each of the available cytotoxic drugs is necessary so that optimal combinations and a sequential strategy can be determined.

ANTILEUKEMIC DRUGS

Steroids

Of all agents currently used in ALL treatment, the adrenocorticosteroids are of upmost importance in remission induction treatment. Steroids are lympholytic through a mechanism that is as yet poorly understood but which probably involves the activation of nucleases leading to DNA fragmentation (apoptosis). The particular susceptibility of lymphoblasts to steroids permits rapid reduction of leukemic cell number with minimal myelosuppression. The steroid most often used in polychemotherapy protocols is prednisone in oral doses of 40–80 mg/m^2 or its soluble analog, prednisolone, which is given intravenously. Other steroids have essentially identical remission induction capability, although dexamethasone may provide greater control of leukemia in the CNS and other extramedullary sites.[110]

Vinca alkaloids

Vinca alkaloids together with steroids are the most important agents for remission induction in ALL. Vincristine (VCR) in a weekly dose of 1.5 mg/m^2 (maximal dose 2.0 mg/m^2) is by far the most frequently used vinca alkaloid in ALL. Using this schedule, only mild myelosuppression is to be expected; however, neurotoxicity with paresthesia or paralytic ileus may occur, especially in older children. More frequent injections and continuous infusion increase the efficacy of VCR but also increase the neurotoxicity considerably. Other vinca alkaloids such as vinblastine (VBL) and vindesine (VDS) appear to be less effective than VCR in ALL.

L-asparaginase

L-asparaginase, an enzyme that splits asparagine into aspartic acid and ammonia, has a restricted activity against lymphoblasts. Asparaginases of two different origins are in current use, namely from *Escherichia coli* and *Erwinia carotovora*, later renamed *Erwinia chrysanthemis*, and have different pharmacokinetics.[111] Side-effects result from the inhibition of protein synthesis, especially of clotting and fibrinolytic factors,[112] and anaphylactoid reactions. With polyethylene glycol (PEG)-bound asparaginase, the risk of the latter may be reduced; however, PEG-binding alters the

545

pharmacokinetics.[111] L-asparaginase is given at various doses and schedules in modern polychemotherapy protocols.

Anthracyclines

Daunorubicin (DNR) was the first anthracycline antibiotic to show significant antileukemic activity. It is a highly myelosuppressive drug and its cardiotoxicity is cumulative. Cumulative doses should not exceed 300–400 mg/m^2 in children. Doxorubicine (adriamycin, ADR) has been less extensively tested in childhood ALL but may have a similar activity and at least the same toxicity compared to DNR. Of the newer anthracyclines, idarubicin (IDR) has substantial antileukemic efficacy; however, its relative value in comparison to DNR has not been established in childhood ALL.

Folic acid antimetabolites

Folic acid antagonists initiated the revolution in treatment of childhood ALL.[109] Methotrexate (MTX), the only compound in current use, together with 6-mercaptopurine (6-MP) is the basis of maintenance chemotherapy in ALL. Given intrathecally, MTX is the key component in CNS-directed chemotherapy. High-dose MTX introduced in the 1960s may provide effective antileukemic MTX concentrations in extramedullary sites, especially the CNS and testes.[113]

Purine antagonists

6-Mercaptopurine (6-MP) is the traditional purine antagonist in childhood ALL, whereas 6-thioguanine (6-TG) is preferred in AML. There is no convincing rationale for this choice, because these 2 drugs have not been directly compared in ALL. In many protocols, 6-MP and 6-TG are now used sequentially in remission induction and consolidation polychemotherapy. 6-MP remains the drug most often combined with MTX in virtually all maintenance chemotherapy protocols in childhood ALL. Drug dosage, patient compliance and route of administration determine the antileukemic efficacy during maintenance treatment. Several pharmacologic studies show that the bioavailability following oral administration of 6-MP is highly variable.[114–116] Information on the new purine analogs, such as 2-deoxycoformicin, 2-chlorodeoxyadenosine and fludarabine, in childhood ALL are scarce.

Pyrimidine antagonists

Cytosine-arabinoside (ara-C) is the only pyrimidine antagonist used in childhood ALL. *In vitro* studies suggest that T lymphoblasts may be especially sensitive to ara-C. High-dose ara-C (HD-ara-C) is a potent inducer of remissions in refractory and relapsed ALL, both in children and adults, and is now included in most protocols for high-risk patients.

Alkylating agents

Cyclophosphamide (Cyc) is the most commonly used alkylating drug for the treatment of childhood ALL. It is effective in both T- and B-ALL.[44,117,118] Ifosfamide (IFO) is at least as effective as Cyc and is included in most modern intensive polychemotherapy protocols for B-ALL.[44,118]

Epipodophyllotoxines

The 2 most important epipodophyllotoxins are teniposide (VM-26) and etoposide (VP-16). These compounds interact with topoisomerase-II to prevent the reannealing of DNA after it has been disrupted by the enzyme. This in turn leads to apoptosis. VP-16 particularly is included in some polychemotherapy protocols for high-risk patients. However, there is some concern about the development of secondary AML.[119]

The major toxic effects of drugs used in the therapy of childhood ALL are listed in Table 27.10.

The major advances achieved during the past 3 decades in the treatment of ALL in children and adolescents have dramatically changed the prognosis for this disease which was always fatal in the past. While treatment was purely palliative until the 1960s, the aim of current treatment protocols is cure; 70–75% of all children and adolescents with ALL can be expected to be cured of their leukemia. This altered prognosis of ALL is mainly the result of very intensive chemotherapy associated with severe suppression of both the normal hematopoietic stem cells and the immune system. Thus, the improvement of supportive measures such as packed red blood cells, effective platelet support and highly effective antimicrobial agents, including broad-spectrum antibiotics, antifungal agents and antiviral drugs, has been a prerequisite for the use of increasingly intensive polychemotherapy protocols (see below).

The aim of treatment is the elimination of the neoplastic cell clone and the restoration of normal hematopoiesis. The different phases of antileukemic treatment are shown in Table 27.9. As an example, the outline of 3 consecutive BMM studies ALL-BFM '81, '83 and '86 are shown in Fig. 27.1.

Table 27.9 Phases of treatment in acute lymphoblastic leukemia.

Remission induction therapy

Postremission therapy
   Consolidation therapy
   Intensification therapy
   CNS-directed treatment
   High-dose radiochemotherapy with subsequent support by autologous or allogeneic hematopoietic stem cell infusion (autologous or allogeneic bone marrow/peripheral stem cell transplantation)
   Maintenance therapy

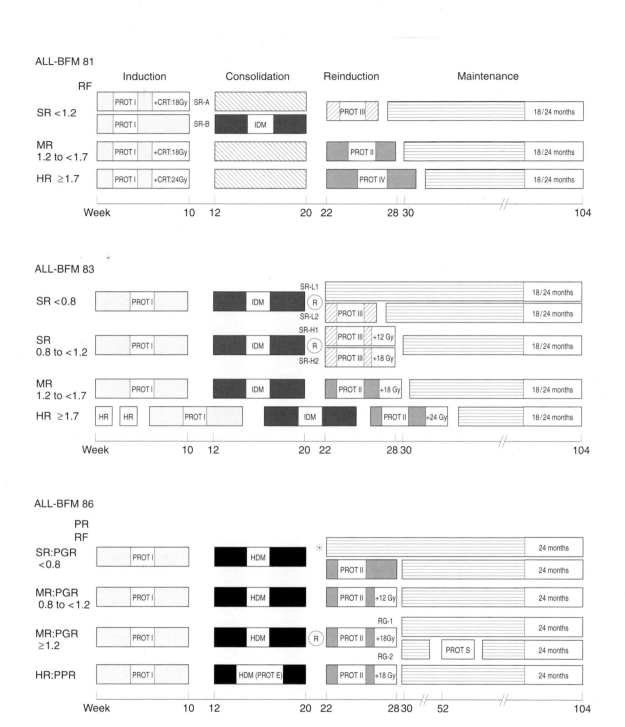

Fig. 27.1 Outline of studies ALL BFM '81, '83, and '86.

Table 27.10 Toxic effects of drugs used in the therapy of childhood acute lymphoblastic lymphoma.

Drug	Myelo-suppression	Immuno-suppression	Tissue irritant	Nausea and vomiting	Mucositis	Nephrotoxicity	Cardiotoxicity	Neuropathy	Hepato-toxicity	Hyper-sensitivity
STEROIDS	-	+++	High-dose IV painful	-				-		-
VINCRISTINE	±	++	+++	-	-	-	-	+++ (+SIADH)	-	±
ASPARAGINASE	+	++	-	±	-	-	-	Encephalopathy	++ Pancreatitis	+++
ANTHRACYCLINES										
Adriamycin	++	+	+++	+++	+++	-	+++		Radiation recall effect	±
Daunomycin	+	+	+++	++	++	-	+++	-		
ANTIMETABOLITES										
Methotrexate (oral, IV, IM, IT)	++	++	-	±	++	++ (esp. high dose)	-	++ (high dose + chronic IM + IT)	++	±
6-Mercaptopurine (+thioguanine)	+	+	-	rare	+	-	-	-	+	-
Cytosine arabinoside (IV, IM, IT)	++	++	- HD-ARA-C eye irritation	++	++	-	-	Cerebellar in high dose	-	±
ALKYLATING AGENTS										
Cyclophosphamide	++	++	++	+++	++	+ (cystitis ++)	+ (high dose)	+ (SIADH)	-	±
EPIPODOPHYLLOTOXINS (e.g. etoposide)	++	+	+	±	++	-	± (hypotension)	+ (mild peripheral)	+ (enzymes)	++

SIADH = syndrome of inadequate antidiuretic hormone.

REMISSION INDUCTION

After stabilization of the clinical status in a child with ALL (treatment of metabolic changes, infections, bleeding complications), remission induction polychemotherapy should be started without delay. The initial phase of treatment is designed to reduce the leukemic cell burden to a clinically and hematologically undetectable level. Complete remission is achieved when the marrow cellularity has returned to normal with <5% of blasts, the peripheral blood values are within the normal range and all clinical signs and symptoms of the disease have disappeared.

Clinical trials in the 1960s demonstrated that the combination of 2 antileukemic agents gives superior remission rates compared to single agents. The combination of vincristine and prednisone led to complete remission in about 90% of children with ALL.[120] The addition of a third drug, namely an anthracycline or asparaginase, increased the complete remission rate to >95%. This increased remission rate was later shown to translate into an increased long-term relapse-free survival,[76,121] thus demonstrating the importance of maximal early cell kill for the overall effectiveness of treatment. Current induction regimens therefore consist of 3 or more drugs. A large Children's Cancer Study Group (CCSG) study has demonstrated similar event-free survival (EFS) in intermediate risk (IR)-ALL treated with a 4- and 3-drug induction if intensive reintensification was given.[85]

CNS-directed treatment is integrated in most current remission induction regimens, most often in the form of intrathecally given methotrexate or triple drug (methotrexate, ara-C and hydrocortisone) intrathecal therapy.

Current polychemotherapy treatment protocols give a remission rate of >95%.[3–5] Induction failures are divided equally between children with refractory leukemia and those dying from complications of leukemia or toxicity of treatment. Thus, intensive induction polychemotherapy can increase long-term survival but may result in increased short-term morbidity and mortality, especially if supportive care is suboptimal, which illustrates the delicate balance required between intensive polychemotherapy and sometimes life-threatening toxicity.

INTENSIFICATION TREATMENT

Remission induction treatment is followed by intensification (reinduction treatment) early in remission in most current polychemotherapy regimens to maximize early leukemic cell kill. Intensification therapy is less standardized compared to remission induction treatment. While some regimens use single agents in high dosages, such as asparaginase, methotrexate or ara-C, other trials rely on reinduction with the same drug combinations or related drugs to those administered during remission induction. In most trials, children with presumed higher risk for relapse are treated with more intensive polychemotherapy compared to those with presumed standard risk. However, reintensification therapy is an important phase of therapy for all children with B-precursor ALL, as first demonstrated by the BFM group[76] and later confirmed by the CCSG.[85]

In *standard risk patients* the improvement in treatment outcome by addition of reinduction treatment early in remission was first demonstrated in study ALL BFM '83. In this randomized trial, children receiving reinduction did significantly better compared to those who were not (probability of complete continuous remission [pCCR] after 5 years 84%; SD 5%, versus 62%; SD 7%).[76] These results were confirmed by ALL BFM '86, which had to be amended after 2 years so that all children with standard risk features received intensive reinduction treatment (protocol II).[3] The importance of reinduction treatment was also confirmed by the CCSG demonstration of a 7-year EFS of 63% for standard risk children receiving BFM-type intensification compared to 42% for children not given such treatment.[85]

The importance of intensification therapy in *children with high-risk features* was first demonstrated by the BFM Group,[76,122] and confirmed by other trials.[4,5,123–125] In children with very high-risk features as defined by slow early response, prednisone non-response or unique biologic features such as t(9;22); t(4;11), the BFM Group could not demonstrate an improved outcome with further treatment intensification.[3,126] However, a recent CCSG trial did demonstrate that further prolongation and intensification of therapy (augmented BFM protocol) improved the outcome of children with high-risk features and slow response to early treatment as defined by an M3 marrow on day 7.[127]

CNS-DIRECTED TREATMENT

The use of CNS-directed treatment—CNS irradiation, intrathecal chemotherapy and high-dose chemotherapy—has been considered a prerequisite for long-term leukemia-free survival. Before its introduction >50% of children with ALL developed overt CNS disease whilst in systemic remission. The concept of CNS preventive therapy is based on the premise that the CNS is a sanctuary site in which leukemic cells are protected by the blood-brain barrier from therapeutic concentrations of systemically administered anti-leukemic drugs.

The use of CNS irradiation as preventive therapy was first demonstrated in a series of studies at St Jude Children's Hospital.[128] Relatively low doses of craniospinal irradiation (5 or 12 Gy) demonstrated no preventive effect, whereas 24 Gy cranial irradiation together with 5 doses of intrathecal methotrexate or 24 Gy of craniospinal irradiation reduced the incidence of CNS relapse from >50% to approximately 10%.[128] Because craniospinal irradiation was associated with excessive myelosuppression due to irra-

diation of large parts of the bone marrow and retardation of spinal growth, cranial irradiation (24 Gy) together with intrathecal methotrexate became the standard form of CNS preventive therapy during the 1970s. The identification of brain abnormalities on CT scans,[129] altered intellectual and psychometric functions and neuroendocrine dysfunction in children treated with 24 Gy of cranial irradiation and intrathecal chemotherapy prompted a reappraisal of CNS-preventive treatment strategies and stimulated the search for alternative less toxic treatments.[130]

Alternatives include intrathecal chemotherapy with 1 or more cytotoxic drugs such as methotrexate, ara-C with or without prednisolone as well as high doses of intravenous methotrexate to overcome the blood-brain barrier. With intermediate $(500 \, mg/m^2)$ or high $(\geqslant 1 \, g/m^2)$ doses of methotrexate some trials reported a higher CNS relapse rate than that observed with inclusion of cranial irradiation. The CNS relapse rate was found to depend on pre-therapy risk factors, the response to treatment and the intensity of systemic chemotherapy. Thus, in the context of more intensive systemic therapy, patients at lower risk of CNS relapse may require less intensive CNS-directed therapy with lower doses of cranial irradiation or even no cranial irradiation. The BFM Group demonstrated that the use of 12 Gy administered in a protocol with high-dose methotrexate and intensive reinduction/consolidation therapy was as effective in the prevention of CNS disease as 18 Gy in a selected group of standard risk patients.[3,76]

The optimal choice of CNS-directed therapy in childhood ALL is controversial, mostly because of the potential for adverse effects. Therefore, it should be emphasized that the results of such treatment have to be interpreted in the context of the overall treatment results. Furthermore, the late effects of high-dose systemic chemotherapy without cranial irradiation and prolonged intrathecal cytotoxic therapy are largely unknown and may be similar to those of cranial irradiation with minimal effective doses.[131]

CNS preventive treatment may be associated with acute neurotoxic sequelae such as headache, nausea and vomiting and other signs of increased intracranial pressure. In addition, 5–7 weeks after cranial irradiation some children develop a characteristic subacute neurotoxic reaction with somnolence, lethargy, anorexia, fever and irritability. This somnolence syndrome, which may be accompanied by EEG abnormalities and CSF pleocytosis, usually resolves within 1–3 weeks.[132]

MAINTENANCE TREATMENT

Unlike most other childhood malignancies, childhood ALL requires the continuation of therapy for a long time. Early studies in which no maintenance therapy was given after remission induction were associated with the rapid relapse of almost all children.[133] Furthermore, early studies demonstrated that interrupted treatment resulted in inferior results as compared to continued maintenance therapy in childhood ALL.[134] In early clinical studies a variety of single agents were evaluated as maintenance agents. Drugs particularly effective as induction agents were surprisingly not useful for maintenance therapy. The combination of methotrexate and 6-mercaptopurine administered continuously together is now used most widely and is a principal constituant of nearly all maintenance regimens.

Pharmacologic studies have demonstrated that the bioavailability of oral 6-mercaptopurine and oral methotrexate is highly variable. However, a randomized trial demonstrated that for maintenance therapy oral methotrexate is as effective as intramuscular.[135] In most trials, the interindividual variation in bioavailability of 6-mercaptopurine and methotrexate is compensated for by adjusting the dose of both drugs according to the actual WBC. The addition of vincristine and prednisone or dexamethasone to 6-mercaptopurine and methotrexate during maintenance therapy was found to be effective in some trials[79,136] but not in others.[76]

DURATION OF TREATMENT

The use of intensive induction polychemotherapy has significantly decreased the proportion of children suffering relapse after the cessation of treatment.[137] The BFM trials using very intensive induction polychemotherapy clearly demonstrated that the frequency of relapse after cessation of treatment could be reduced by further intensifying induction and reinduction polychemotherapy.[76] The relapse frequency after cessation of therapy is in the range of 15% for all children at risk in most trials.[5,138] Most of those children eventually relapsing did so within the first year off therapy.[138] In the second, third and fourth years after cessation of treatment, the risk of relapse was only about 2–3%/year. Relapses after the fourth year off therapy are extremely rare. However, very late relapses can occur; in a recent MRC study, 11 of 1000 long-term survivors (older than 10 years in their first remission) relapsed very late (10–24 years after diagnosis).[139] Molecular studies showed that in 5 patients the second presentation of ALL revealed an identical clonal IgH or T-cell receptor gene rearrangement, thus confirming that these second presentations were true relapses rather than a second or secondary ALL. The current practice of treating children for 2–3 years with maintenance chemotherapy derives from older studies in which patients were treated with less intensive polychemotherapy than in current use. For this reason, conclusions drawn from these studies on the duration of maintenance may not be applicable to current treatment protocols. In an attempt to address this question, the BFM Group randomized patients to receive 18 or 24 months of treatment. A significant advantage was observed for children receiving longer treatment.[76] The MRC UKALL-8 trial using less intensive induction polychemotherapy reported similar results between patients randomized to receive 2 or 3 years of maintenance therapy.[140]

The optimal duration of therapy may be different for boys and girls. Boys with standard risk features of ALL demonstrated a significant relapse cascade after cessation of therapy in both studies ALL BFM '86 and '90 (unpublished results). This confirms treatment results from CCSG 141[141] and MRC UKALL-10,[86] both demonstrating a higher incidence of relapses after cessation of therapy in males, even after excluding boys with occult testicular disease. Thus, in the ongoing ALL-BFM '95 study, as in most other trials, boys with standard risk features are treated for a total of 36 months, whereas girls receive treatment for 24 months.

Closer monitoring of early response parameters, including the assessment of minimal residual disease at regular intervals, may provide new guidelines for the optimal duration of therapy in the individual child with ALL which can be used for further stratification of therapy intensity and duration.[142,143] However, differences in rearrangement patterns at the time of diagnosis and relapse, most probably due to clonal evalution, have been described.[144–146] Thus, 2 or more junctional regions of different genes need to be monitored for detection of minimal residual disease.[144,147–149]

B-ACUTE LYMPHOBLASTIC LEUKEMIA

The lymphoblasts of about 4% of all children with ALL demonstrate features of more mature lymphocytes, an unique immunophenotype with the expression of surface immunoglobulin with light chain restriction (either κ or λ chains) and specific chromosomal translocations—t(8;14), t(2;8) and t(8;22).

Clinically, B-ALL is characterized by a high tumor burden, especially within the abdomen, a high LDH and a high propensity to invade the CNS.[44] Differentiation between B-ALL (>25% B lymphoblasts in the bone marrow) and B-NHL (stage IV) (<25% lymphoblasts in the bone marrow) is arbitrary in some patients. Thus, most protocols recommend identical treatment for B-ALL and B-NHL stage IV.[44,118] Children with B-ALL had a poor outcome when treated with the regimen used for B-precursor ALL. Using a very intensive therapy approach including high-dose methotrexate, ara-C and cyclophosphamide or ifosfamide, as well as intensive intrathecal chemotherapy, the EFS of children with B-ALL has increased up to 70%.[44,118] The duration of treatment for B-ALL is short, usually no more than 4–6 months. Nearly all relapses, often with involvement of the CNS, occur within the first year after initial presentation.[44, 118]

INFANT LEUKEMIA

About 3–5% of children with ALL are infants (<12 months of age). ALL in infancy differs from that in older children with respect to clinical and biologic features and outcome of therapy. At presentation, infants demonstrate a high tumor burden, including a high WBC, hepatosplenomegaly, a high LDH and a higher incidence of CNS leukemia, compared to older children. The lymphoblasts appear to arise from a very early stage of comittment to B-cell differentiation with an immunophenotype of $CD19^+$, $CD10^-$ and $HLA-DR^+$ and frequent co-expression of myeloid markers such as CD13, CD33 or CD65.

Infants with ALL have an increased incidence of chromosomal abnormalities associated with a poor prognosis. Structural abnormalities of chromosome 11, especially rearrangement of band 11q23 within the MLL gene, are frequently observed. The t(4;11) abnormality is particularly common in infants with hyperleukocytosis. Hyperdiploidy, a common finding in ALL of older age groups, is extremly rare in infant ALL.[150,151]

Although the complete response rate of infants appears to be no different from that for older children, the eventual outcome is much poorer. Five-year EFS in infant ALL ranges from 25 to 50% in most trials.[3] This is especially true for infants under 6 months of age.[152]

Because the pharmacokinetics of cytotoxic drugs may differ between infants and older children, the optimal dosage of polychemotherapy in infants with ALL is unclear. Most protocols recommend a reduced dosage or calculation according to body weight instead of body surface area.[3] Although polychemotherapy is generally well tolerated by infants and cranial irradiation is deferred until the second year of life, late effects of therapy are more often seen in this age group compared to older children.[153,154]

Congenital ALL, i.e. ALL diagnosed within the first 4 weeks of life, is especially rare and has to be differentiated from transient myeloproliferative disorders, which are mostly seen in children with Down's syndrome.[155]

TREATMENT OF RELAPSED ACUTE LYMPHOBLASTIC LEUKEMIA

Despite progress in treatment outcome of childhood ALL, 15–20% of children with ALL do suffer from relapse. Most relapses occur within the bone marrow, followed by the CNS, testes and other rare sites such as the eye, ovary or skin. Combined relapses may occur within bone marrow and CNS, followed by bone marrow and testes in boys. However, a leukemic relapse at any site should always be considered as a localized manifestation of a systemic disease, thus leading to careful staging procedures for other occult disease manifestations and to reinduction of systemic polychemotherapy in addition to local treatment including CNS-directed therapy.[7,156,157]

Since most, if not all, effective antileukemic drugs have already been delivered during primary polychemotherapy, treatment of relapse has to rely on combinations of the same drugs. Such an approach has been used by the BFM Group in a number of consecutive studies beginning in 1983,

which used cytotoxic drugs in intermittent blocks of polychemotherapy followed by maintenance treatment for 24 months.[7]

Careful documentation of relapse sites is of great importance in the individual child, including examination of extramedullary sites such as the CNS (lumbar puncture and diagnostic imaging of the neuroaxis), testes, including diagnostic imaging, and eye. Bone marrow relapse is diagnosed if > 25% unequivocal lymphoblasts are found. In some patients, the immunophenotype may be different from that found at presentation (phenotypic shift).[158] Similarly, there can be differences in chromosomal aberration and in gene rearrangement patterns at the time of diagnosis and relapse due to clonal evolution.[144,145,158] In most children with CNS relapse, more than 5 lymphoblasts/μl are found in the CSF. In rare cases, the differentiation between reactive cerebrospinal fluid (CSF) pleocytosis and true CNS relapse may be difficult and further immunologic and cytogentic/molecular genetic studies are warranted. In doubtful cases, another lumbar puncture is indicated after a couple of days. Testicular relapse is documented by biopsy or fine needle aspiration. However, the latter technique may give false positive results if lymphoblasts are present in the peripheral blood. A combined relapse is diagnosed if in addition to extramedullary relapse >5% unequivocal lymphoblasts are present in the bone marrow.[7]

Different mechanisms may be responsible for the occurrence of relapse of childhood ALL. One reason for treatment failure may be the existence of an anatomic barrier which prevents antileukemic drugs from reaching their target at therapeutically effective concentrations. This may be the reason for most CNS and testicular relapses (sanctuary sites). Another reason for relapse is drug resistance, either primary or secondary, resulting in non-response to treatment for early systemic relapse. Clinical resistance to antileukemic drugs is multifactorial and the cellular mechanisms are still poorly understood. Multiple drug resistance (MDR) is due to the overexpression of p-glycoprotein, which acts as a drug transport protein.[159] The third reason for relapse might be that cells are hidden in metabolic sancturaries, thus being prevented from recruitment into the cell cycle (G_o-phase) and therefore not accessible to the cytotoxic drug. This may be due either to intrinsic properties of the leukemic cell or altered metabolic environmental conditions which may exist in the CNS or the testes, resulting in much lower proliferative activity. In the individual child with relapsing ALL, one or more of these possible reasons may be responsible and have different treatment implications.[7]

As in the primary treatment of childhood ALL, a number of prognostic factors has emerged from long-term observation of multicenter ALL relapse trials (Table 27.11) implicating that different relapse situations should be treated differently.[7,160–162]

Table 27.11 Prognostic factors in the therapy of relapsed acute lymphoblastic leukemia.

Factor	Favorable	Unfavorable
Duration of first complete remission	Late (>6–12 months after cessation of treatment)	Early
Site of relapse	Extramedullary relapse	Bone marrow relapse
Peripheral blasts at relapse ($\times 10^9$/l)	<10	>10
Immunophenotype	B-precursor ALL	T-ALL; B-ALL
Cytogenetics/molecular genetics	t(12;21)	t(4;11), t(9;22)
Response to relapse treatment	Complete remission within 6 weeks	Complete remission after 6 weeks

Very early relapse

Children relapsing at any site within the first 18 months after presentation (very early relapse) and children with any relapse of T-ALL have a dismal prognosis with chemotherapy alone.[7,163,164] Thus, if the relapsing leukemia again responds to intensive polychemotherapy, allogeneic bone marrow transplantation (BMT) in second complete remission from a related or an unrelated donor is the treatment of choice in such patients.[165–168]

Early isolated bone marrow relapse

Most children with isolated bone marrow relapse within the first 6 months after cessation of therapy (early relapse) initially respond to second-line polychemotherapy. However, since prognosis is also dismal in this group,[7,169] allogeneic BMT from a related or unrelated donor is indicated in this subgroup of relapsing patients as well.

CNS relapse

After bone marrow the CNS is the second commonest site for relapse in childhood ALL. The incidence of CNS relapses depends largely on the CNS-directed treatment applied in first-line treatment.[80] With adaequate CNS-directed treatment, isolated and combined CNS relapses occur in <5% of children in first remission.[3–5,81,170] As in other presumed isolated extramedullary relapses of ALL, CNS relapses should be considered as a localized manifestation of systemic leukemia and thus treatment should always include intensive systemic polychemotherapy as well as local therapy. Most successful treatment regimens use intensive polychemotherapy together with extended intrathecal therapy and cranial or cranio-spinal irradiation at a dose dependent on the dose given during first-line treatment.[7,171,172]

A study from St Jude Children's Hospital reported a 5-year disease-free survival in second remission of >70% in children with isolated CNS relapse. About one-half of all children with CNS relapse with or without concomitant bone marrow involvement have achieved long-term (>5 years) second remission and possible cure in the ongoing ALL-BFM relapse trials.[173]

Testicular relapse

The testes are the third most frequent site of extramedullary relapse of childhood ALL. Testicular relapse probably arises in a sanctuary area. In early ALL trials with less intensive polychemotherapy and without intermediate or high-dose methotroxate, up to 50% of males exhibited testicular relapse, either with or without concomitant bone marrow involvement.[174–177] The incidence of testicular relapse has been dramatically decreased after intensification of front-line regimens, mainly by the introduction of intermediate- or high-dose MTX. In recent trials, <5% of boys with ALL developed an overt testicular relapse with or without bone marrow involvement.[3–5,170]

Treatment of testicular relapse with or without bone marrow involvement must include intensive polychemotherapy including CNS-directed therapy together with local therapy. In case of unilateral disease, most trials recommend orchidectomy of the enlarged testes, and after achievement of second remission radiotherapy to the contralateral testes with a dose dependent on the detection of occult disease. This approach minimizes the impairment of endocrine function of the contralateral testicle. Using this approach, the ALL Rez-BFM study reported a similar outcome in boys with isolated and combined testicular relapse with more than half achieving a long-lasting second remission. Boys with late isolated testicular relapse occurring later than 6 months after cessation of therapy may have a 70% or greater probability of cure.[7,178,179] Because of the similar treatment outcome in boys with isolated and combined testicular relapse, the practice of elective testicular biopsies during clinical remission is no longer advocated.[180]

Late bone marrow relapse

Children with B-precursor ALL relapsing >6 months after cessation of therapy may experience extended second remission or even cure with a second course of intensive polychemotherapy.[7,163,181,182] A second remission can be induced by intensive polychemotherapy in >90% of children with late bone marrow relapse[7,181] with a second EFS of >5 years in about 35%.[183,184] Duration of first remission[6,7,185] is the most important predictive factor for the length of a second remission. In addition, a peripheral lymphoblast count of <10 000/μl[183] and a low WBC[185] at the time of relapse have been associated with a high second EFS rate. Furthermore, the presence of t(12;21) at relapse predicts a favorable outcome.[186] Most relapse trials demonstrate a superior outcome in children with combined compared to isolated bone marrow relapse.[7,182]

Relapse at other sites

Leukemia may very rarely reoccur at other sites (e.g. eye, ovary, tonsils and skin). As in other extramedullary relapses, intensive polychemotherapy including CNS-directed treatment together with appropriate local therapy is recommended in these rare situations.

BONE MARROW TRANSPLANTATION

Over the past 2 decades, BMT has evolved as an effective treatment modality for hematologic malignancies.[187,188] Several sources of hematopoietic stem cells are available for BMT (Table 27.12).

In the past, much progress has been made in reducing treatment-related problems, which occur especially in older patients. However, BMT is still burdened by distinct toxic side-effects and infectious complications, resulting in a treatment-related mortality (TRM) of up to 30%, depending on the source of hematopoietic stem cells.[165,187]

Graft-versus-host disease (GVHD), which is mediated by cytotoxic T lymphocytes, may cause severe morbidity and even mortality, but may also provide additional anti-leukemic efficacy (graft-versus-leukemia [GVL] reaction). Attempts to seperate GVHD and GVL reaction have been unsuccessful. T-cell depletion of donor marrow results in a significant reduction in GVHD, but also an increased graft failure rate and an increased leukemic relapse rate.[165]

Matched related sibling or family donor transplantation is limited by the availability of a matched HLA identical family member (available in ≤30% of children with leukemia).[165,187] This limitation may be overcome with increasing numbers of volunteer bone marrow donors on worldwide registries for matched unrelated donor transplantation. However, transplantation-related mortality after matched unrelated donor transplantation is significantly higher compared to matched sibling transplantation in the majority of published trials.[167,168] Another alternative source of hematopoietic stem cells may be cord blood; long-term results are not yet available after cord blood stem cell transplantation.[189]

Predictive factors for the outcome after allogeneic BMT may at least in part be similar to those seen in polychemo-therapy, such as high-risk features at diagnosis and the duration of first remission.[166,190]

The most commonly used preparatory regimen consists of total body irradiation (TBI) and cyclophosphamide, the original Seattle regimen,[191] or TBI and etoposide.[192–194] Myeloablative chemotherapy with high-dose ara-C followed by TBI[155] or a preparative regimen without TBI such as busulfan/cyclophosphamide[196] did not decrease relapse rates or improve overall survival.

The high cure rate of ALL in children and adolescents implies that BMT is generally reserved for children who relapse. However, under the conditions of recent risk-adapted polychemotherapy, some patients with very poor risk factors may benefit from allogeneic transplantation in first remission.

Although BMT is widely accepted as an appropriate form of therapy in second remission, the exact impact of BMT for the different subsets of children in second remission, the possible use of matched unrelated donors and the possible impact of autologous transplantation are matters of intensive debate. The role of BMT has to be measured against the efficacy of polychemotherapy within controlled trials. In the absence of randomized trials, matched-pair analyses were used to try to answer some of the most important questions.[165,197]

In early bone marrow relapse (≤6 months after cessation of treatment) BMT increases the probability of EFS in second complete remission compared to chemotherapy.[184,193] This is especially true for T-ALL relapses and for relapses of Philadelphia-positive ALL. In these situations, the prognosis after conventional chemotherapy is dismal. Therefore, allogeneic BMT from a matched unrelated donor should be considered if no matched related donor is available.

In late bone marrow relapse (>6 months after cessation of therapy) about 35% of children with non-T-ALL may be cured by intensive polychemotherapy alone;[7] thus allogeneic BMT is not recommended by most investigators in this situation. However, a recent retrospective analysis of the ALL-BFM relapse study demonstrated that a peripheral blast count of >10 000/μl at relapse confers a dismal prognosis in late isolated bone marrow relapse. Thus, BMT should be considered in this subgroup of patients.[184]

It is expected that new technologies such as monitoring response to polychemotherapy for relapse, including monitoring of minimal residual disease, will help with the difficult decision of which child should receive an allogeneic BMT in second complete remission.

Possible indications for bone marrow transplantation using hematopoietic stem cells are summarized in Table 27.13.

Autologous stem cell transplantation has the advantage of applicability to all patients in the absence of GVHD. However, there exists a risk of reinfusing residual leukemic blasts.[198,199] In a recent matched-pair analysis, the outcome after autotransplantation was no different from intensive

---

Table 27.12 Types of bone marrow transplantation (BMT).

Autologous BMT

Allogeneic BMT
  Syngeneic (identical twin)
  Matched sibling donor
  Matched family donor
  Mismatched related donor (e.g. haploidentical BMT)
  Matched unrelated donor
  Mismatched unrelated donor

Table 27.13
Possible indications for bone marrow transplantation (BMT) in childhood acute lymphoblastic leukemia (ALL).

BMT in first complete remission
  Philadelphia chromosome⁺ (*BCR/ABL*⁺) ALL
  t (4;11)
  Poor response to treatment (e.g. no complete remission after 4 weeks of induction therapy)

BMT in second complete remission
  Early (<6 months after cessation of therapy) bone marrow relapse
  Late bone marrow relapse with unfavorable features (*BCR/ABL*⁺ ALL; *TEL/AML*⁻ ALL; poor response to relapse therapy after 6 weeks)
  All relapses of T-ALL

BMT in >second complete remission
  All patients

chemotherapy.[197] Thus, the role of autologous transplantation for the treatment of relapsed ALL still needs to be defined. The value of autologous transplantation of hematopoietic stem cells followed by intensive maintenance polychemotherapy with additional immunotherapy is being evaluated in ongoing studies.

COMPLICATIONS OF TREATMENT

EARLY COMPLICATIONS

At presentation major complications can be expected in children with a high leukemic cell burden and a high proliferation capacity, such as T-ALL, B-ALL and c-ALL with hyperleukocytosis (WBC $> 100\,000/\mu l$). Life-threatening metabolic complications can result from spontaneous leukemic cell turnover and chemotherapeutically-induced leukemic cell death (tumor lysis syndrome), presenting with hyperuricemia, hyperkalemia and hyperphosphatemia.[200,201] Massive release of cellular nucleic acids and their conversion to uric acid may result in the precipitation of uric acid in the renal collecting system and urethers.[202,203] Careful hydration and alkalinization with bicarbonate, together with the administration of allopurinol prior to chemotherapy[204-206] or the application of urate oxidase, help avert these metabolic complications.

Potassium is released from lysed lymphoblasts and requires dialysis in some children with decreased renal function due to leukemic infiltration.[205]

In children with hyperleukocytosis (WBC $> 100\,000/\mu l$) the microcirculation may be impaired by intravascular clumping of leukemic blasts, resulting in local hypoxemia, endothelial damage, hemorrhage and infarction, especially within the CNS and lungs (hyperleukocytosis/leukostasis syndrome).[45] This syndrome is seen more often in children with AML but has been reported in children with ALL.[75] Treatment consists of vigorous intravenous hydration, alka-

linization and urate oxidase before chemotherapy. Alternatively, allopurinol may be given. Occasionally, emergency leukapheresis or exchange transfusion have been used.[46] Packed red blood cell transfusion should not be given in this situation to avoid further increasing blood viscosity and thus worsening the symptoms of hyperleukocytosis/leukostasis syndrome.[45,46]

In children with T-ALL and an enlarged mediastinal mass, life-threatening bronchial and/or cardiovascular (vena cava superior syndrome) compression may occur. Immediate application of systemic chemotherapy (steroids, cyclophosphamide) is necessary in this oncologic emergency.

Signs and symptoms of meningeal or intracranial involvement, such as headache, vomiting, meningism and cranial nerve palsies, are rare at presentation. Differentiation between intracranial bleeding and leukemic infiltration of the CNS is sometimes impossible even with the help of diagnostic imaging (cranial CT, MRT), especially in children with the hyperleukocytosis/leukostasis syndrome. Immediate lumbar puncture may be dangerous in this situation. Prompt administration of systemic chemotherapy should be considered.

Leukemic infiltration of the optic nerve and/or the retina is extremely rare.[207,208] Immediate systemic chemotherapy including high doses of steroids together with local radiotherapy and intrathecal therapy should be given to prevent blindness.

SUPPORTIVE CARE

Optimal treatment of children with ALL requires appropriate supportive care, including the rational use of blood products, an aggressive approach to detection and treatment of bleeding and infectious complications, and continuous psychosocial support for the patient and his family. Some of these topics are addressed elsewhere (see Chapters 32, 36 and 37), and only the most important issues, namely the diagnosis, treatment and prophylaxis of bleeding and infectious complications are discussed here.

Bleeding

Bleeding in children with leukemia is usually due to thrombocytopenia, the differential diagnosis including decreased production due to marrow infiltration and/or chemotherapy-induced marrow aplasia, DIC and septicemia. In rare cases, heparin-induced thrombocytopenia (HIT) has also to be considered.[209]

Venous thrombosis (e.g. intracranial sinus vein thrombosis) may occur during treatment of childhood ALL, especially when asparaginase is given.[210,211] A recent study described 15 thromboembolic episodes in 243 consecutive children with ALL. Most of these children had central venous catheters and at least one of the following thrombophilic defects were found in all children: Factor V Leiden mutation (resistance against the activated form of protein C,

APCR), protein C deficiency, protein S deficiency, anti-thrombin (AT) III deficiency and increased level of lipoprotein (a).[212] Prophylaxis with AT III and avoidance of central venous catheters during asparaginase therapy may be useful in children with defined thrombophilic disorders.[112]

Infections

Infections during granulocytopenia are an important complication of intensive polychemotherapy. Most are presumably bacterial, but a significant micro-organism can often not be found by standard methods. Therefore, any febrile child with leukemia and an absolute neutrophil count (ANC) of $<500/\mu l$ should be considered bacteremic and treated with broad-spectrum antibiotics covering Gram-positive and -negative organisms.

A variety of non-bacterial opportunistic micro-organisms can invade the immunocompromised host. Fungal infections, especially candida and aspergillus species, are increasingly observed during prolonged periods of neutropenia and immunosuppression.[47]

The administration of the hematopoietic growth factor granulocyte colony-stimulating factor (G-CSF) to intensively treated children with high-risk ALL can reduce febrile neutropenia and culture-confirmed infections.[213]

Viral infections, especially due to varicella zoster virus (VZV), complicated by pneumonia, hepatitis and cerebral infection had a high morbidity and mortality in earlier studies.[214,215] Prophylaxis with VZV hyperimmunoglobulin[216] and treatment with acyclovir in overt VZV infection[217,218] have significantly reduced the frequency of disease. Rare cases of measles in severely compromised children with leukemia still have a high mortality.[219–221]

Pneumocystis carinii, now believed to be a fungus, in early trials was the cause of severe, often fatal interstitial pneumonia in children with leukemia receiving polychemotherapy, especially with steroids.[222] Prophylaxis with trimetoprim-sulfamethoxazol almost completely abolished the incidence of severe infection with this organism.[223]

LATE COMPLICATIONS

The improved survival of childhood ALL has focused attention on the late effects of antileukemic therapy (Table 27.14).

Gonadal sequelae

Normal sexual development can be expected in most girls regardless of the form of CNS-directed treatment.[224,225] Sexual maturation is also normal in most boys,[226,227] although gonadal dysfunction is common following testicular irradiation.[228] Testosterone replacement is recommended in this situation. Currently, there is no evidence

Table 27.14
Late sequelae of leukemia treatment.

Organ	Etiology
Gonads	
Infertility	Alkylating agents, radiotherapy
Liver	
Fibrosis/cirrhosis	Methotrexate, 6-mercaptopurine, hepatitis B, C virus
Hepatocellular carcinoma	Hepatitis B virus
Veno-occlusive disease	Busulfan, bone marrow transplantation
Lung	
Fibrosis/pneumonitis	Busulfan, radiotherapy
Kidney	
Tubulopathy (Fanconi's syndrome)	Ifosfamide
Thyroid	
Tumors; hypothyroidism	Radiotherapy
Spleen	
Overwhelming sepsis	Splenectomy/radiotherapy
Bone	
Osteonecrosis	Steroids
Heart	
Cardiomyopathy	Anthracyclines, radiotherapy
Central nervous system	
Leukoencephalopathy	Radiotherapy; intrathecal chemotherapy
IQ ↓, cognition ↓	Radiotherapy, intrathecal chemotherapy
Psychomotor skills ↓	Radiotherapy, intrathecal chemotherapy
Growth ↓	Radiotherapy, intrathecal chemotherapy
Second malignancies	Genetic predisposition; radiotherapy; alkylating agents, epipodophyllotoxins

that the progeny of survivors of childhood ALL are at increased risk of congenital abnormalities.[229]

Liver sequelae

Children receiving maintenance treatment with methotrexate frequently have elevated liver function tests. After cessation of therapy these tests return to normal. Chronic liver diseases may occur in children with a history of hepatitis B or C infection.[37,230]

Cardiac sequelae

Antracyclines are known to exhibit a cumulative dose-related cardiotoxicity. Children receiving a cumulative anthracycline dose of $200–260 \, mg/m^2$ are usually asymptomatic, although in some a reduced contractility has been measured after cessation of therapy.[48] Younger age, female sex and a greater cumulative dose of anthracyclines were found to be risk factors for late cardiotoxicity.[49] Additional cardiotoxicity may be caused by other cytotoxic drugs, such as high-dose cyclophosphamide and spinal or mediastinal irradiation.[231]

555

Central nervous system sequelae

A number of CNS sequelae have been described after different modalities of CNS-directed treatment.[154] The incidence of neuroradiologically-observed structural abnormalities varies greatly between different trials and may be as high as 75%.[232-235] Four radiologically distinct forms have been identified in children with ALL: subacute leukoencephalopathy, mineralizing angiopathy, subacute necrotizing leukomyelopathy and cortical atrophy.[236] Although a higher incidence of structural pathology was observed after more intensive CNS-directed treatment, the role of the different components of this treatment (namely high-dose systemic chemotherapy, intrathecal drug application and cranial irradiation) remains to be determined. Several trials revealed no difference in the CT abnormalities between patients receiving cranial irradiation and those who did not.[237,238]

Often a discrepancy between neurologic findings and clinical measurements of neurologic or neurocognitive function is found.[239,240] Children who receive cranial irradiation at a younger age tend to show greater neurologic decrements.[241,242] While most children in these studies had received cranial irradiation, the potential adverse sequelae with intensive intrathecal and systemic high-dose chemotherapy must also be appreciated.[243,244]

Children with CNS relapse who receive a second course of CNS-directed treatment are at particular risk of significant cerebral dysfunction in addition to neuropsychologic deficits, seizures and leukoencephalopathy.[245,246]

Growth

Cranial irradiation with doses of 18–24 Gy may have a negative impact on final growth, depending on age at radiation, fraction schedule, type of systemic chemotherapy and pubertal status at radiation. In general, the slowing of growth during treatment of ALL is followed by catch-up growth.[247,248] The effects of cranial irradiation on final growth are more marked in children treated at a young age,[249,250] and in female patients.[251] Endocrine studies revealed growth hormone deficiencies in some of these children and treatment with growth hormone has been evaluated in some of the most severely affected children.[252]

Other sequelae

Hypothyroidism is relatively common after radiation treatment.[253] Avascular osteonecrosis[254,255] has been reported during and after treatment with high doses of corticosteroids. Subcapsular cataracts have been described after treatment with corticosteroids and after cranial radiation.[256,257]

Second malignancies

The risk of developing second malignancy after successful treatment of ALL is low. Two large cohort studies from the Nordic countries and US estimated a cumulative risk of 2.9% by 20 years[258] and 2.5% by 15 years,[259] respectively. The majority of second malignancies were brain tumors, mostly gliomas, developing in the radiation field. Exposure to radiotherapy appears to be associated with a continuous risk of second neoplasm, especially within the thyroid gland.[260,261]

The use of epipodophyllotoxins has been described to be associated with substantial risk of secondary AML,[119] a complication which is not observed in treatment protocols without these drugs.[262]

REFERENCES

1. Zuelzer WW, Inoue S et al. Long-term cytogenetic studies in acute leukemia of children: the nature of relapse. Am J Hematol 1976; **1**: 143

2. Burchenal JH, Murphy ML. Long term survivors in acute leukemia. Cancer Res 1965; **25**: 1491–1494

3. Reiter A, Schrappe M, Ludwig W-D et al. Chemotherapy in 998 unselected childhood ALL patients. Results and conclusions of the multicenter trial ALL-BFM'86. Blood 1994; **84**: 3122–3133

4. Gaynon PS, Steinherz PG, Bleyer WA et al. Improved therapy for children with acute lymphoblastic leukemia and unfavorable presenting features: a follow-up report of the Children's Cancer Group Study CCG-106. J Clin Oncol 1993; **11**: 2234–2242

5. Rivera GK, Raimondi SC et al. Improved outcome in childhood acute lymphoblastic leukemia with reinforced early treatment and rotational combination chemotherapy. Lancet 1991; **337**: 61

6. Buchanan GR, Rivera GK et al. Reinduction therapy in 297 children with acute lymphoblastic leukemia in first bone marrow relapse: A Pediatric Oncology Group study. Blood 1988; **72**: 1286

7. Henze G, Fengler R, Hartmann R et al. Six-year experience with a comprehensive approach to the treatment of recurrent childhood acute lymphoblastic leukemia (ALL-REZ BFM 85). A relapse study of the BFM group. Blood 1991; **78**: 1166–1172

8. Dordelmann M, Schrappe M, Reiter A et al. Down's syndrome in childhood acute lymphoblastic leukemia: clinical characteristics and treatment outcome in four consecutive BFM trials. Berlin–Frankfurt–Munster Group. Leukemia 1998; **12**: 645–651

9. Pui CH, Raimondi SC, Borowitz MJ et al. Immunophenotypes and karyotypes of leukemic cells in children with Down syndrome and acute lymphoblastic leukemia. J Clin Oncol 1993; **11**: 1361–1367

10. Ragab AH, Abdel Mageed A, Shuster JJ et al. Clinical characteristics and treatment outcome of children with acute lymphocytic leukemia and Down's syndrome. A Pediatric Oncology Group study. Cancer 1991; **67**: 1057–1063

11. Robison LL, Nesbit ME Jr, Sather HN et al. Down syndrome and acute leukemia in children: a 10-year retrospective survey from Children's Cancer Study Group. J Pediatr 1984; **105**: 235–242

12. Mainzer R, Taybi H. Thymic enlargement and pleural effusion: an unusual roentgenographic complex in childhood leukemia. Am J Roentgenol 1971; **112**: 35

13. Greydanus DE, Burgert O et al. Hypothalamic syndrome in children with acute lymphocytic leukemia. Mayo Clin Proc 1978; **53**: 217

14. Gunther R, Chelstrom LM, Tuel-Ahlgren L, Simon J, Myers DE, Uckun FM. Biotherapy for xenografted human central nervous system leukemia in mice with severe combined immunodeficiency

using B43 (anti-CD19)-pokeweed antiviral protein immunotoxin. *Blood* 1995; **85**: 2537

15. Lauer SJ, Kirchner PAE. Identification of leukemic cells in the cerebrospinal fluid from children with acute lymphoblastic leukemia: advances and dilemmas. *Am J Pediatr Hematol Oncol* 1989; **11**: 64

16. Mastrangelo R, Poplack D *et al*. Report and recommendations of the Rome workshop concerning poor-prognosis acute lymphoblastic leukemia in children: biologic bases for staging, stratification, and treatment. *Med Pediatr Oncol* 1986; **14**: 191

17. Gilchrist GS, Tubergen DG, Sather HN *et al*. Low numbers of CSF blasts at diagnosis do not predict for the development of CNS leukemia in children with intermediate-risk acute lymphoblastic leukemia: a Children's Cancer Group report. *J Clin Oncol* 1994; **12**: 2594–2600

18. Mahmoud HH, Rivera GK, Hancock ML *et al*. Low leukocyte counts with blast cells in cerebrospinal fluid of children with newly diagnosed acute lymphoblastic leukemia. *N Engl J Med* 1993; **329**: 314–319

19. Smith M, Arthur D, Camitta B *et al*. Uniform approach to risk classification and treatment assignment for children with acute lymphoblastic leukemia. *J Clin Oncol* 1996; **14**: 18–24

20. Hustu HO, Aur RJA. Extramedullary leukemia. *Clin Haematol* 1978; **7**: 313

21. Mastrangelo R, Zuelzer WW *et al*. Chromosomes in the spinal fluid: evidence for metastatic origin of meningeal leukemia. *Blood* 1970; **35**: 227

22. Kataoka A, Shimizu K, Matsumoto T *et al*. Epidural spinal cord compression as an initial symptom in childhood acute lymphoblastic leukemia: rapid decompression by local irradiation and systemic chemotherapy. *Pediatr Hematol Oncol* 1995; **12**: 179–184

23. Kim TH, Hargreaves HK *et al*. Sequential testicular biopsies in childhood acute lymphocytic leukemia. *Cancer* 1986; **57**: 1038

24. Hudson MM, Frankel LS *et al*. Diagnostic value of surgical testicular biopsy after therapy for acute lymhocytic leukemia. *Pediatrics* 1985; **107**: 50

25. Pui C-H, Dahl GV *et al*. Elective testicular biopsy during chemotherapy for childhood leukaemia is of no clincial value. *Lancet* 1985; **ii**: 410

26. Schrappe M, Beck J *et al*. Treatment of acute lymphoblastic leukemia in young age: Results of multicenter study ALL-BFM 81. *Klin Pädiatr* 1987; **199**: 133

27. Steinhardt GF, Steinhardt E. Priapism in children with leukemia. *Urology* 1981; **18**: 604–606

28. Ritter J, Hiddemann W. *Akute Leukämie bei Kindern*. Munich: Urban & Schwarzenberger, 1985

29. Hughes RG, Kay HEM. Major bone lesions in acute lymphoblastic leukemia. *Med Pediatr Oncol* 1982; **10**: 67–70

30. Kushner DC, Weinstein HJ *et al*. The radiologic diagnosis of leukemia and lymphoma in children. *Semin Oncol* 1980; **15**: 316

31. Murphy RG, Greenberg ML. Osteonecrosis in pediatric patients with acute lymphoblastic leukemia. *Cancer* 1990; **65**: 1717

32. Katz JA, Milton L *et al*. Typhlitis: an 18-year experience and postmortem review. *Cancer* 1990; **65**: 1041

33. Gootenberg JE, Abbondanzo SL. Rapid diagnosis of neutropenic enterocolitis by ultrasonsography. *Am J Pediatr Hematol Oncol* 1987; **9**: 222

34. Weetman RM, Baehner RL. Latent onset of clinical pancreatitis in children receiving L-asparaginase therapy. *Cancer* 1974; **34**: 780

35. Shamberger RC, Weinstein HJ *et al*. The medical and surgical management of typhlitis in children with acute nonlymphocytic (myelogenous) leukemia. *Cancer* 1986; **57**: 603

36. Boddie AWJ, Bines SD. Management of acute rectal problems in leukemic patients. *J Surg Oncol* 1986; **33**: 53–56

37. Aricò M, Maggiore G, Sillni E *et al*. Hepatitis C virus infection in children treated for acute lymphoblastic leukemia. *Blood* 1994; **84**: 2919–2922.

38. Schachat A, Markowitz JA. Ophthalmic manifestations of leukemia. *Arch Ophthalmol* 1989; **107**: 697

39. Leonardy NJ, Rupani M, Dent G, Klintworth GK. Analysis of 135 autopsy eyes for ocular involvement in leukemia. *Am J Ophthalmol* 1990; **109**: 436–444

40. Creutzig U, Ritter J, Budde M, Sutor A, Schellong G. Early deaths due to hemorrhage and leukostasis in childhood acute myelogenous leukemia. Associations with hyperleukocytosis and acute monocytic leukemia. *Cancer* 1987; **60**: 3071–3079

41. Robb RM, Ervin LD *et al*. A pathological study of eye involvement in acute leukemia childhood. *Med Pediatr Oncol* 1979; **6**: 171

42. Lo Curto M, D'Angelo P, Lumia F *et al*. Leukemic ophthalmopathy: a report of 21 pediatric cases. *Med Pediatr Oncol* 1994; **23**: 8–13

43. Ninane J, Taylor D *et al*. The eye as a sanctuary in acute lymphoblastic leukaemia. *Lancet* 1980; **i**: 452

44. Reiter A, Schrappe M, Ludwig WD *et al*. Favorable outcome of B-cell acute lymphoblastic leukemia in childhood: a report of three consecutive studies of the BFM group. *Blood* 1992; **80**: 2471–2478

45. Lichtman M, Rowe J. Hyperleukocytic leukemias: rheological, clinical and therapeutic considerations. *Blood* 1982; **60**: 279

46. Strauss RA, Gloster ES *et al*. Acute cytoreduction techniques in the treatment of hyperleukocytosis associated with childhood hematologic malignancies. *Med Pediatr Oncol* 1985; **13**: 346

47. Ritter J, Roos N. Special aspects related to invasive fungal infections in children with cancer. *Baillière's Clin Infect Dis* 1995; **2**: 179–204

48. Lipshultz SE, Colan SD *et al*. Late cardiac effects of doxorubicin therapy for acute lymphoblastic leukemia in childhood. *N Engl J Med* 1991; **324**: 808

49. Lipshultz SE, Lipsitz SR, Mone SM *et al*. Female sex and higher drug dose as risk factors for late cardiotoxic effects of doxorubicin therapy for childhood cancer. *N Engl J Med* 1995; **332**: 1738–1743

50. Meeker TC, Hardy D *et al*. Activation of the interleukin-3 gene by chromosome translocation in acute lymphocytic leukemia with eosinophilia. *Blood* 1990; **76**: 285

51. Pereira F, Moreno H *et al*. Loffler's endomyocardial fibrosis, eosinophilia, and acute lymphoblastic leukemia. *Pediatrics* 1977; **59**: 950

52. Spier CM, Kjeldsberg CR *et al*. Pre-B-cell acute lymphoblastic leukemia in the newborn. *Blood* 1984; **64**: 1064

53. Dubansky AS, Boyett JM *et al*. Isolated thrombocytopenia in children with acute lymphoblastic leukemia: a rare event in a Pediatric Oncology Group study. *Pediatrics* 1989; **84**: 1068

54. Eguiguren JM, Pui C-H. Bone marrow necrosis and thrombotic complications in childhood acute lymphoblastic leukemia. *Med Pediatr Oncol* 1992; **20**: 58–60

55. Hann IM, Evans DIK *et al*. Bone marrow fibrosis in acute lymphoblastic leukaemia of childhood. *J Clin Pathol* 1978; **31**: 313

56. Bennett JM, Catovsky D *et al*. Proposals for the classification of the acute leukemias. French–American–British (FAB) co-operative group. *Br J Haematol* 1976; **33**: 451

57. Cerezo L, Shuster JJ, Pullen DJ *et al*. Laboratory correlates and prognostic significance of granular acute lymphoblastic leukemia in children. A Pediatric Oncology Group study. *Am J Clin Pathol* 1991; **95**: 526–531

58. Stass SA, Pui C-H *et al*. Sudan black B positive acute lymphoblastic leukaemia. *Br J Haematol* 1984; **57**: 413

59. Catovsky D, Greaves MF *et al*. Acid-phosphatase reaction in acute lymphoblastic leukaemia. *Lancet* 1978; **i**: 749

60. Ritter J, Gaedicke G, Winkler K, Beckmann H, Landbeck G. Possible T-cell origin of lymphoblasts in acid-phosphatase-positive leukemia. *Lancet* 1975; **ii**: 75

61. Ludwig WD, Bartram CR *et al*. Ambigous phenotypes and genotypes in 16 children with acute leukemia as characterized by multiparameter analysis. *Blood* 1988; **71**: 1515–1528

62. Mirro J, Zipf TF *et al*. Acute mixed lineage leukemia: clinicopathologic correlations and prognostic significance. *Blood* 1985; **66**: 1115

63. Perentesis J, Ramsay N *et al*. Biphenotypic leukemia: Immunologic and morphologic evidence for a common lymphoid-myeloid progenitor in humans. *J Pediatr* 1983; **102**: 63

64. Ben-Bassat I, Gale RP. Hybrid acute leukemia. *Leukemia Res* 1984; **8**: 929

65. Greaves MF, Chan LC *et al*. Lineage promiscuity in hemopoietic differentiation and leukemia. *Blood* 1986; **67**: 1

66. Smith LJ, Curtis JE *et al*. Lineage infidelity in acute leukemia. *Blood* 1983; **61**: 1138

67. Fink FM, Köller U, Mayer H *et al*. Prognostic significance of myeloid-associated antigen expression on blast cells in children with acute lymphoblastic leukemia. *Med Pediatr Oncol* 1993; **21**: 340–346

68. Ludwig WD, Harbott J, Bartram CR *et al*. Incidence and prognostic significance of immunophenotypic subgroups in childhood acute lymphoblastic leukemia: Experience of the BFM study 86. In: Ludwig WD, Thiel E (eds) *Recent Results in Cancer Research*. Berlin/Heidelberg: Springer-Verlag, 1993, pp 269–282

69. Pui C-H, Behm F *et al*. Myeloid-associated antigen expression lacks prognostic value in childhood acute lymphoblastic leukemia treated with intensive multiagent chemotherapy. *Blood* 1990; **75**: 198

70. Wiersma SR, Ortega J *et al*. Clinical importance of myeloid-antigen expression in acute lymphoblastic leukemia of childhood. *N Engl J Med* 1991; **324**: 800

71. Pui C-H, Raimondi SC, Head DR *et al*. Characterization of childhood acute leukemia with multiple myeloid and lymphoid markers at diagnosis and at relapse. *Blood* 1991; **78**: 1327–1337

72. Catovsky D, Matutes E, Buccheri V *et al*. A classification of acute leukaemia for the 1990s. *Ann Hematol* 1991; **62**: 16–21

73. Campana D, Hansen-Hagge TE, Matutes E *et al*. Phenotypic, genotypic, cytochemical and ultrastructural characterization of acute undifferentiated leukemia. *Leukemia* 1990; **4**: 620–624

74. Matutes E, Buccheri V, Morilla R, Shetty V, Dyer M. Immunological, ultrastructural and molecular features of unclassifiable acute leukaemia. In: Ludwig WD, Thiel E (eds) *Recent Results in Cancer Research*. Berlin/Heidelberg: Springer-Verlag, 1993, pp 41–52

75. Bunin NJ, Pui C-H. Differing complications of hyperleukocytosis in children with acute lymphoblastic or acute nonlymphoblastic leukemia. *J Clin Oncol* 1985; **12**: 1590

76. Riehm H, Gadner H, Henze G *et al*. Results and significance of six randomized trials in four consecutive ALL-BFM studies. In: Büchner T, Schellong G, Hiddemann W, Ritter J (eds) *Haematology and Blood Transfusion*. Berlin/Heidelberg: Springer-Verlag, 1990, pp 439–450

77. Rivera GK, Pinkel D, Simone JV, Hancock ML, Crist WM. Treatment of acute lymphoblastic leukemia: 30 years' experience at St. Jude Children's Research Hospital. *N Engl J Med* 1993; **329**: 1289–1295

78. Pullen J, Boyett J, Shuster J *et al*. Extended triple intrathecal chemotherapy trial for prevention of CNS relapse in good risk and poor-risk patients with B-progenitor acute lymphoblastic leukemia: a Pediatric Oncology Group Study. *J Clin Oncol* 1993; **11**: 839–849

79. Veerman AJP, Hählen K, Kamps WA *et al*. High cure rate with a moderately intensive treatment regimen in non-high-risk childhood acute lymphoblastic leukemia: Results of protocol ALL VI from the Dutch Childhood Leukemia Study Group. *J Clin Oncol* 1996; **14**: 911–918

80. Niemeyer CM, Hitchcock-Bryan S *et al*. Comparative analysis of treatment programs for childhood acute lymphoblastic leukemia. *Semin Oncol* 1985; **12**: 122

81. Schorin MA, Blattner S, Gelber RD *et al*. Treatment of childhood acute lymphoblastic leukemia: results of Dana-Farber Cancer Institute Children's Hospital Acute Lymphoblastic Leukemia Consortium Protocol 85–01. *J Clin Oncol* 1994; **12**: 740–747

82. Lilleyman JS, Hann IM, Stevens RF *et al*. Cytomorphology of childhood lymphoblastic leukaemia: a prospective study of 2000 patients. *Br J Haematol* 1992; **81**: 52–57

83. Steinherz PG, Siegel SE, Bleyer WA *et al*. Lymphomatous presentation of childhood acute lymphoblastic leukemia: a subgroup at high risk of early treatment failure. *Cancer* 1991; **68**: 751–758

84. Crist W, Pullen J *et al*. Clinical and biologic features predict a poor prognosis in acute lymphoid leukemias in infants: A Pediatric Oncology Group Study. *Blood* 1986; **67**: 135

85. Tubergen DG, Gilchrist GS, O'Brien RT *et al*. Improved outcome with delayed intensification for children with acute lymphoblastic leukemia and intermediate presenting features: a Children's Cancer Group phase III trial. *J Clin Oncol* 1993; **11**: 527–537

86. Chessells JM, Richards SM, Bailey CC, Lilleyman JS, Eden OB. Gender and treatment outcome in childhood lymphoblastic leukaemia: report from the MRC UKALL trials. *Br J Haematol* 1995; **89**: 364–372

87. Pui C-H, Boyett JM, Hancock ML, Pratt CB, Meyer WH, Crist WM. Outcome of treatment for childhood cancer in black as compared with white children. The St. Jude Children's Research Hospital experience, 1962 through 1992. *JAMA* 1995; **273**: 633–637

88. Crist WM, Boyett J. Pre B-cell leukemia responds poorly to treatment: A Pediatric Oncology Group Study. *Blood* 1984; **63**: 407

89. Crist WM, Caroll AJ *et al*. Poor prognosis of children with pre-B acute lymphoblastic leukemia is associated with the t(1;19)(q23;q13): A Pediatric Oncology Group study. *Blood* 1990; **76**: 117

90. Pui C-H, Williams DL *et al*. Unfavorable presenting clinical and laboratory features are associated with CALLA-negative non-T, non-B lymphoblastic leukemia in children. *Leukemia Res* 1986; **11**: 1287

91. Vannier JP, Bene MC *et al*. Investigation of the CD 10 (cALLA) negative acute lymphoblastic leukaemia: further description of a group with a poor prognosis. *Br J Haematol* 1989; **72**: 156

92. Kaspers GJ, Smets LA, Pieters R, van Zantwijk CH, van Wering ER, Veerman AJ. Favorable prognosis of hyperdiploid common acute lymphoblastic leukemia may be explained by sensitivity to antimetabolites and other drugs: results of an *in vitro* study. *Blood* 1995; **85**: 751–756

93. Raimondi SC, Pui C-H, Hancock ML, Behm FG, Filatov L, Rivera GK. Heterogeneity of hyperdiploid (51–67) childhood acute lymphoblastic leukemia. *Leukemia* 1996; **10**: 213–224

94. McLean TW, Ringold S, Neuberg D *et al*. TEL/AML-1 dimerizes and is associated with a favorable outcome in childhood acute lymphoblastic leukemia. *Blood* 1996; **88**: 4252–4258

95. Borkhardt A, Cazzaniga G, Viehmann S *et al*. Incidence and clinical relevance of TEL/AML1 fusion genes in children with acute lymphoblastic leukemia enrolled in the German and Italian multicenter therapy trials. Associazione Italiana Ematologia Oncologia Pediatrica and the Berlin–Frankfurt–Munster Study Group. *Blood* 1997; **90**: 571–577

96. Crist W, Carroll A *et al*. Philadelphia chromosome positive childhood acute lymphoblastic leukemia: clinical and cytogenetic characteristics and treatment outcome. A Pediatric Oncology Group study. *Blood* 1990; **76**: 489

97. Beyermann B, Agthe AG, Adams H-P *et al*. Clinical features and outcome of children with first marrow relapse of acute lymphoblastic leukemia expressing BCR-ABL fusion transcripts. *Blood* 1996; **87**: 1532–1538

98. Fletscher JA, Lynch EA *et al*. Translocation (9;22) is associated with extremely poor prognosis in intensively treated children with acute lymphoblastic leukemia. *Blood* 1991; **77**: 435

99. Ribeiro RC, Abromowitch M *et al*. Clinical and biologic hallmarks of the Philadelphia chromosome in childhood acute lymphoblastic leukemia. *Blood* 1987; **70**: 948

100. Roberts WM, Rivera GK, Raimondi SC *et al*. Intensive chemotherapy for Philadelphia-chromosome-positive acute lymphoblastic leukaemia. *Lancet* 1994; **343**: 331–332

101. Lampert F, Harbott J, Ludwig W-D *et al*. Acute leukemia with chromosome translocation (4;11): 7 new patients and analysis of 71 cases. *Blut* 1987; **54**: 325

102. Pui C-H, Frankel LS *et al*. Clinical characteristics and treatment outcome of childhood acute lymphoblastic leukemia with the t(4;11) (q21;q23): a collaborative study of 40 cases. *Blood* 1991; **77**: 440

103. Aricó M, Schrappe M, Harbott J *et al*. Prednisone good response (PGR) identifies a subset of t(9;22) childhood acute lymphoblastic leukemia (ALL) at lower risk for early leukemia relapse. *Blood* 1997; **90 (Suppl)**: 2494

104. Gaynon PS, Bleyer WA *et al*. Day 7 marrow response and outcome for children with acute lymphoblastic leukemia and unfavorable presenting features. *Med Pediatr Oncol* 1990; **18**: 273

105. Miller DR, Coccia PF. Early response to induction therapy as a predictor of disease-free survival and late recurrence of childhood acute lymphoblastic leukemia: A report from the Children's Cancer Study Group. *J Clin Oncol* 1989; **7**: 1807

106. Riehm H, Reiter A, Schrappe M *et al*. Die Corticosteroid-abhängige Dezimierung der Leukämiezellzahl im Blut als Prognosefaktor bei der akuten lymphoblastischen Leukämie im Kindesalter (Theraiestudie ALL-BFM 83). *Klin Pädiatr* 1987; **199**: 151–160

107. Schrappe M, Reiter A, Sauter S *et al*. Concept and interim result of the ALL-BFM 90 therapy study in treatment of acute lymphoblastic leukemia in children and adolescents: the significance of initial therapy response in blood and bone marrow. *Klin Padiatr* 1994; **206**: 208–221

108. Biondi A, van Dongen JJM, Seriu T *et al*. Predictive value of minimal residual disease measurement during remission in childhood acute lymphoblastic leukemia: The results of the International-BFM Study Group (I-BFM-SG). *Blood* 1997; **10 (Suppl)**: 1878

109. Farber S, Diamond LK *et al*. Temporary remissions in acute leukemia in children produced by folic acid antagonist, 4-amionopteroyl-glutamic acid (aminopterin). *N Engl J Med* 1948; **238**: 787

110. Jones B, Freeman AI, Shuster JJ *et al*. Lower incidence of meningeal leukemia when prednisone is replaced by dexamethasone in the treatment of acute lymphocytic leukemia. *Med Pediatr Oncol* 1991; **19**: 269–275

111. Boos J, Werber G, Ahlke E *et al*. Monitoring of asparaginase activity and asparagine levels in children on different asparaginase preparations. *Eur J Cancer* 1996; **32A**: 1544–1550

112. Nowak-Göttl U, Kuhn N, Wolff JE *et al*. Inhibition of hypercoagulation by antithrombin substitution in *E. coli* L-asparaginase-treated children. *Eur J Haematol* 1996; **56**: 35–38

113. Freeman AI, Weinberg V *et al*. Comparison of intermediate-dose methotrexate with cranial irradiation for the post-induction treatment of acute lymphocytic leukemia in children. *N Engl J Med* 1983; **308**: 477

114. Lennard L, Lilleyman JS. Variable mercaptopurine metabolism and treatment outcome in childhood lymphoblastic leukemia. *J Clin Oncol* 1989; **7**: 1816

115. Riccardi R, Balis FM *et al*. Influence of food intake on bioavailability of oral 6-mercaptopurine in children with acute lymphoblastic leukemia. *Pediatr Hematol Oncol* 1986; **3**: 319

116. Schmiegelow K, Schroder H, Gustafsson G *et al*. Risk of relapse in childhood acute lymphoblastic leukemia is related to RBC methotrexate and mercaptopurine metabolites during maintenance chemotherapy. *J Clin Oncol* 1995; **13**: 345–351

117. Lauer SJ, Camitta BM, Leventhal BG *et al*. Intensive alternating drug pairs for treatment of high-risk childhood acute lymphoblastic leukemia. A Pediatric Oncology Group pilot study. *Cancer* 1993; **71**: 2854–2861

118. Patte C, Philip T, Rodary C *et al*. High survival rate in advanced-stage B-cell lymphomas and leukemias without CNS involvement with a short intensive polychemotherapy: Results from the French Pediatric Oncology Society of a randomized trial of 216 children. *J Clin Oncol* 1991; **9**: 123

119. Pui CH, Behn FG *et al*. Secondary acute myeloid leukemia in children treated for acute lymphoid leukemia. *N Engl J Med* 1989; **321**: 136

120. Selawry OS, Hananian J *et al*. New treatment schedule with improved survival in childhood leukemia. *JAMA* 1965; **194**: 75

121. Clavell LA, Gelber RD *et al*. Four-agent induction and intensive asparaginase therapy for treatment of childhood acute lymphoblastic leukemia. *N Engl J Med* 1986; **315**: 657

122. Henze G, Langermann HJ *et al*. Treatment strategy for different risk groups in childhood acute lymphoblastic leukemia: A report form the BFM Study Group. *Haematol Bluttransfus* 1981; **26**: 87

123. Camitta B, Mahoney D, Leventhal B *et al*. Intensive intravenous methotrexate and mercaptopurine treatment of higher-risk non-T, non-B acute lymphocytic leukemia. *J Clin Oncol* 1994; **12**: 1383–1389

124. Raimondi SC, Behm FG, Roberson PK *et al*. Cytogenetics of childhood T-cell leukemia. *Blood* 1988; **72**: 1560

125. Sallan SE, Gelber RD *et al*. More is better! Update of Dana-Farber Cancer Institute/Children's Hospital childhood acute lymphoblastic leukemia trials. In: Büchner T, Schellong G *et al* (eds) *Haematology and Blood Transfusion 33. Acute Leukemias II*. Heidelberg: Springer, 1990, p 459

126. Schrappe M, Reiter A, Sauter S *et al*. Risk-oriented treatment of childhood ALL: Favorable outcome despite reduced intensity of treatment in trial ALL-BFM 90. *Blood* 1997; **90 (Suppl)**: 2488

127. Nachman J, Sather H, Lukens J *et al*. Acute lymphocytic leukemia—clinical investigation and pathophysiology. Augmented Berlin–Frankfurt–Münster (A-BFM) chemotherapy improves event free survival (EFS) for children with acute lymphoblastic leukemia (ALL) and unfavorable presenting features who show a slow early response (SER) to induction chemotherapy. *Blood* 1997; **90 (Suppl)**: 2487

128. Aur RJA, Simone JV *et al*. A comparative study of central nervous system irradiation and intensive chemotherapy early in remission of childhood acute lymphocytic leukemia. *Cancer* 1972; **29**: 381

129. Peylan-Ramu N, Poplack DG *et al*. Abnormal CT scans of the brain in asymptomatic children with acute lymphocytic leukemia after prophylactic treatment of the central nervous system with radiation and intrathecal chemotherapy. *N Engl J Med* 1978; **298**: 815

130. Ochs J, Rivera G *et al*. Central nervous system morbidity following an inital isolated central nervous system relapse and its subsequent therapy in childhood acute lymphoblastic leukemia. *J Clin Oncol* 1985; **3**: 622

131. Mulhern RK, Wasserman AL. Memory function in disease-free survivors of childhood acute lymphocytic leukemia given CNS prophylaxis with or without 1800 cGy cranial irradiation. *J Clin Oncol* 1988; **6**: 315

132. Freeman JE, Johnston PGB *et al*. Somnolence after prophylactic cranial irradiation in children with acute lymphoblastic leukaemia. *Br Med J* 1973; **1**: 523

133. Frei E, III, Karon M *et al*. The effectiveness of combinations of antileukemia agents in inducing and maintaining remission in children with acute leukemia. *Blood* 1965; **26**: 642

134. Lonsdale D, Gehan EA *et al*. Interrupted vs. continued maintenance therapy in childhood acute leukemia. *Cancer* 1975; **36**: 341

135. Chessells JM, Leiper AD *et al*. Oral methotrexate is as effective as intramuscular in maintenance therapy of acute lymphoblastic leukaemia. *Arch Dis Child* 1987; **62**: 172

136. Bleyer WA, Sather HN, Nickerson HJ *et al*. Monthly pulses of vincristine and prednisone prevent bone marrow and testicular relapse in low-risk childhood acute lymphoblastic leukemia: a report from the CCSG-161 Study by the Children's Cancer Study Group. *J Clin Oncol* 1991; **9**: 1012–1021

137. Childhood ALL Collaborative Group. Duration and intensity of maintenance chemotherapy in acute lymphoblastic leukaemia:

overview of 42 trials involving 12 000 randomised children. *Lancet* 1996; **347**: 1783–1788

138. George SL, Aur RJA *et al*. A reappraisal of the results of stopping therapy in childhood leukemia. *N Engl J Med* 1979; **330**: 269

139. Frost L, Richards DS, Goodeve A *et al*. Late relapsing childhood lymphoblastic leukemia. *Blood* 1997; **90**: 560A

140. Eden OB, Lilleyman JS, Richards S, Shaw MP, Peto J. Results of medical research council childhood leukaemia trial UKALL VIII (report to the Medical Research Council on behalf of the Working Party on Leukaemia in Childhood). *Br J Haematol* 1991; **78**: 196

141. Miller DR, Leikin S *et al*. Prognostic factors and therapy in acute lymphoblastic leukemia of childhood: CCG-141. *Cancer* 1983; **51**: 1041

142. Steenbergen EJ, Verhagen OJ, van Leeuwen EF *et al*. Prolonged persistence of PCR-detectable minimal residual disease after diagnosis or first relapse predicts poor outcome in childhood B-precursor acute lymphoblastic leukemia. *Leukemia* 1995; **9**: 1726–1734

143. Wasserman R, Galili N, Ito Y *et al*. Residual disease at the end of induction therapy as a predictor of relapse during therapy in childhood B-lineage acute lymphoblastic leukemia. *J Clin Oncol* 1992; **10**: 1879–1888

144. Beishuizen A, Verhoeven MA, van Wering ER, Hählen K, Hooijkaas H, van Dongen JJ. Analysis of Ig and T-cell receptor genes in 40 childhood acute lymphoblastic leukemias at diagnosis and subsequent relapse: Implications for the detection of minimal residual disease by polymerase chain reaction analysis. *Blood* 1994; **83**: 2238–2247

145. Raghavachar A, Ludwig W-D *et al*. Clonal variation in childhood acute lymphoblastic leukaemia at early and late relapse detected by analyses of phenotype and genotype. *Eur J Pediatr* 1988; **147**: 503

146. Wright JJ, Poplack DG *et al*. Gene rearrangements as markers of clonal variation and minimal residual disease in acute lymphoblastic leukemia. *J Clin Oncol* 1987; **5**: 735

147. Baruchel A, Cayuela JM, Macintyre E, Berger R, Sigaux F. Assessment of clonal evolution at Ig/TCR loci in acute lymphoblastic leukemia by single-strand conformation polymorphism studies and highly resolutive PCR derived methods: Implication for a general strategy of minimal residual disease detection. *Br J Haematol* 1995; **90**: 85–93

148. Steenbergen EJ, Verhagen OJ, van Leeuwen EF, van den Berg H, von dem Borne AE, van der Schoot CE. Frequent ongoing T-cell receptor rearrangements in childhood B-precursor acute lymphoblastic leukemia: Implications for monitoring minimal residual disease. *Blood* 1995; **86**: 692–702

149. Steward CG, Goulden NJ, Katz F *et al*. A polymerase chain reaction study of the stability of Ig heavy-chain and T-cell receptor delta gene rearrangements between presentation and relapse of childhood B-lineage acute lymphoblastic leukemia. *Blood* 1994; **83**: 1355–1362

150. Lampert R, Harbott J, Ritterbach J. Cytogenetic findings in acute leukaemias of infants. *Br J Cancer* 1992; **66**: 20–22

151. Pui C-H, Kane JR, Crist WM. Biology and treatment of infant leukemias. *Leukemia* 1995; **9**: 762–769

152. Bucsky P, Reiter A *et al*. Die akute lymphoblastische Leukämie im Säuglingsalter: Ergebnisse aus fünf multizentrischen Therapiestudien ALL-BFM 1970–1986. *Klin Pädiatr* 1988; **200**: 177

153. Ochs J, Mulhern RK. Late effects of antileukemic treatment. *Pediatr Clinic North Am* 1988; **35**: 815

154. Ochs JJ. Neurotoxicity due to central nervous system therapy for childhood leukemia. *Am J Pediatr Hematol Oncol* 1989; **11**: 93–105

155. Creutzig U, Ritter J, Vormoor J *et al*. Myelodysplasia and acute myelogenous leukemia in Down's syndrome. A report of 40 children of the AML-BFM Study Group. *Leukemia* 1996; **10**: 1677–1686

156. Neale GA, Pui CH, Mahmoud HH *et al*. Molecular evidence for minimal residual bone marrow disease in children with "isolated" extra-medullary relapse of T-cell acute lymphoblastic leukemia. *Leukemia* 1994; **8**: 768–775

157. Rivera G, Aur RJA *et al*. Second central nervous system prophylaxis in children with acute lymphoblastic leukemia who relapse after elective cessation of therapy. *J Clin Oncol* 1983; **1**: 471

158. Pui C-H, Raimondi SC *et al*. Shifts in blast cell phenotype and karyotype at relapse of childhood lymphoblastic leukemia. *Blood* 1986; **68**: 1306

159. Nooter K, Sonneveld P. Multidrug resistance (MDR) genes in haematological malignancies. *Cytotechnology* 1993; **12**: 213–230

160. Buchanan GR, Boyett JM, Pollock BH *et al*. Improved treatment results in boys with overt testicular relapse during or shortly following initial therapy for acute lymphoblastic leukemia: a Pediatric Oncology Group study. *Cancer* 1991; **68**: 48–55

161. Bührer C, Hartmann R, Fengler R *et al*. Superior prognosis in combined compared to isolated bone marrow relapses in salvage therapy of childhood acute lymphoblastic leukemia. *Med Pediatr Oncol* 1993; **21**: 470–476

162. Bührer C, Hartmann R, Fengler R *et al*. Importance of effective central nervous system therapy in isolated bone marrow relapse of childhood acute lymphoblastic leukemia. *Blood* 1994; **83**: 3468–3472

163. Bleyer WA, Sather H *et al*. Prognosis and treatment after relapse of acute lymphoblastic leukemia and non-Hodgkin's lymphoma: 1985. A report from the Children's Cancer Study Group. *Cancer* 1986; **58**: 590

164. Rivera GK, Buchanan G *et al*. Intensive retreatment of childhood acute lymphoblastic leukemia in first bone marrow relapse. A Pediatric Oncology Group study. *N Engl J Med* 1986; **315**: 274

165. Barrett AJ, Horowitz MM, Pollock BH *et al*. Bone marrow transplants from HLA-identical siblings as compared with chemotherapy for children with acute lymphoblastic leukemia in a second remission. *N Engl J Med* 1994; **331**: 1253–1258

166. Butturini A, Rivera GK *et al*. Which treatment for childhood acute lymphoblastic leukemia in second remission? *Lancet* 1987; **i**: 429

167. Casper J, Camitta B, Truitt R *et al*. Unrelated bone marrow donor transplants for children with leukemia or myelodysplasia. *Blood* 1995; **85**: 2345–2363

168. Oakhill A, Pamphilon DH, Potter MN *et al*. Unrelated donor bone marrow transplantation for children with relapsed acute lymphoblastic leukaemia in second complete remission. *Br J Haematol* 1996; **94**: 574–578

169. Pinkerton CR, Mills S *et al*. Modified Capizzi maintenance regimen in children with relapsed acute lymphoblastic leukaemia. *Med Pediatr Oncol* 1989; **14**: 69

170. Chessells JM, Bailey CC, Richards SM. Intensification of treatment and survival in all children with lymphoblastic leukemia. *Lancet* 1995; **345**: 143–148

171. Ribeiro RC, Rivera GK, Hudson M *et al*. An intensive re-treatment protocol for children with an isolated CNS relapse of acute lymphoblastic leukemia. *J Clin Oncol* 1995; **13**: 333–338

172. Winick NJ, Smith SD, Shuster J *et al*. Treatment of CNS relapse in children with acute lymphoblastic leukemia: a Pediatric Oncology Group study. *J Clin Oncol* 1993; **11**: 27

173. Henze G, Fengler R, Hartmann R, for the BFM Relapse Study Group. Chemotherapy for relapsed childhood acute lymphoblastic leukemia: Results of the BFM Study Group. *Haematol Blood Transfusion* 1993; **36**: 374–379

174. Bowman WP, Rhodes JA *et al*. Isolated testicular relapse in acute lymphocytic leukemia of childhood: categories and influence on survial. *J Clin Oncol* 1984; **2**: 924

175. Eden OB, Hardisty RM *et al*. Testicular disease in acute lymphoblastic leukaemia in childhood. Report on behalf of the Medical Research Council's Working Party on Leukaemia in Childhood. *Br Med J* 1978; **1**: 334

176. Tiedemann K, Chessells JM. Isolated testicular relapse in boys with acute lymphoblastic leukaemia: treatment and outcome. *Br Med J* 1982; **285**: 1614

177. Wong KY, Ballard ET *et al*. Clinical and occult testicular leukemia

in long-term survivors of acute lymphoblastic leukemia. *J Pediatr* 1980; **96**: 569

178. Chessells JM, Eden OB, Bailey C, Lilleyman JS, Richards SM. Acute lymphoblastic leukaemia in infancy: experience in MRC UKALL trials: report from the Medical Research Council Working Party on Childhood Leukaemia. *Leukemia* 1994; **8**: 1275–1279

179. Uderzo C, Zurlo G *et al*. Treatment of isolated testicular relapse in childhood acute lymphoblastic leukemia: an Italian multicenter study. *J Clin Oncol* 1990; **8**: 672

180. Nachman J, Palmer NF *et al*. Open-wedge testicular biopsy in childhood acute lymphoblastic leukaemia after two years of maintenance therapy: Diagnostic accuracy and influence on outcome—a report from Children's Cancer Study Group. *Blood* 1990; **75**: 1051

181. Chessells J, Leiper A, Rogers D. Ouctome following late marrow relapse in childhood acute lymphoblastic leukemia. *J Clin Oncol* 1984; **2**: 1099

182. Pui C-H, Behm F *et al*. Cyclic combination chemotherapy for acute lymphoblastic leukemia recurring after elective cessation of therapy. *Med Pediatr Oncol* 1988; **16**: 21

183. Bührer C, Hartmann R, Fengler R *et al*. Peripheral blast counts at diagnosis of late isolated bone marrow relapse of childhood acute lymphoblastic leukemia predict response to salvage chemotherapy and outcome. *J Clin Oncol* 1996; **14**: 2812–2817

184. Schmid H, von Schenck U, Hartmann R, Borgmann A, Henze G. Allogeneic BMT vs. chemotherapy in late bone marrow relapsed childhood non-T/non-B ALL: results of BFM ALL relapse studies. BFM Relapse Study Group. *Bone Marrow Transplant* 1996; **18** (**Suppl 2**): 28–30

185. Sadowitz PD, Smith SD, Shuster J, Wharam MD, Buchanan GR, Rivera GK. Treatment of late bone marrow relapse in children with acute lymphoblastic leukemia: a Pediatric Oncology Group study. *Blood* 1993; **81**: 602

186. Harbott J, Viehmann S, Borkhardt A, Henze G, Lampert F. Incidence of *TEL/AML1* fusion gene analyzed consecutively in children with acute lymphoblastic leukemia in relapse. *Blood* 1997; **90**: 4933–4937

187. Ramsay NKC, Kersey JH. Indications for marrow transplantation in acute lymphoblastic leukemia. *Blood* 1990; **75**: 815

188. Thomas ED. Marrow transplantation for malignant diseases. *J Clin Oncol* 1983; **1**: 517–531

189. Kurtzberg J, Laughlin M, Graham ML *et al*. Placental blood as a source of hematopoietic stem cells for transplantation into unrelated recipients. *N Engl J Med* 1996; **335**: 157–166

190. Kersey JH, Weisdorf D *et al*. Comparison of autologous and allogeneic bone marrow transplantation for treatment of high risk refractory acute lymphoblastic leukemia. *N Engl J Med* 1987; **317**: 461

191. Sanders JE, Thomas ED, Buckner CD, Doney K. Marrow transplantation for children with acute lymphoblastic leukemia in second remission. *Blood* 1987; **70**: 324

192. Blume KG, Forman SJ *et al*. Total body irradiation and high dose etoposide: a new preparatory regimen for bone marrow transplantation of patients with advanced hematologic malignancy. *Blood* 1987; **69**: 1015

193. Dopfer R, Henze G, Bender-Götze C *et al*. Allogeneic bone marrow transplantation for childhood acute lymphoblastic leukaemia in second remission after intensive primary and relapse therapy according to the BFM- and CoALL-protocols: results of the German Cooperative Study. *Blood* 1991; **78**: 2780–2784

194. Suttorp M, Schmitz N *et al*. Fractionated total body irradiation plus high-dose VP-16 prior to allogeneic bone marrow transplantation in children with poor risk acute leukaemias. *Bone Marrow Transplant* 1989; **4**: 144

195. Woods WG, Ramsay NKC *et al*. Bone marrow transplantation for acute lymphocytic leukemia utilizing total body irradiation fol-

lowed by high doses of cytosine arabinoside: lack of superiority over cyclophosphamide-containing regimens. *Bone Marrow Transplant* 1990; **6**: 9

196. Ringdén O, Ruutu T, Remberger M *et al*. A randomized trial comparing busulfan with total body irradiation as conditioning in allogeneic marrow transplant receipts with leukemia: a report from the Nordic Bone Marrow Transplantation Group. *Blood* 1994; **83**: 2723–2730

197. Borgmann A, Schmid H, Hartmann R *et al*. Autologous bone-marrow transplants compared with chemotherapy for children with acute lymphoblastic leukaemia in a second remission: a matched-pair analysis. *Lancet* 1995; **346**: 873–876

198. Brenner MK, Rill DR, Moen RC *et al*. Gene-marking to trace origin of relapse after autologous bone-marrow transplantation. *Lancet* 1993; **341**: 85

199. Brenner MK. Autologous bone marrow transplantation in childhood acute lymphoblastic leukaemia. *Lancet* 1995; **346**: 856–857

200. Maidment CG, Greaves MF *et al*. T-cell leukaemia presenting with hyperuricaemia, acute renal failure and gout. *Clin Lab Haematol* 1983; **5**: 423

201. Zusman J, Brown DM *et al*. Hyperphosphatemia, hyperphosphaturia and hypocalcemia in acute lymphoblastic leukemia. *N Engl J Med* 1973; **289**: 1335

202. Andreoli SP, Cark JH *et al*. Purine excretion during tumor lysis in children with acute lymphocytic leukemia receiving allopurinol: relationship to acute renal failure. *J Pediatr* 1986; **109**: 292

203. Jones DP, Stapleton FB *et al*. Renal dysfunction and hyperuricemia at presentation and relapse of acute lymphoblastic leukemia. *Med Pediatr Oncol* 1990; **18**: 283

204. Basade M, Dhar AK, Kulkarni SS *et al*. Rapid cytoreduction in childhood leukemic hyperleukocytosis by conservative therapy. *Med Pediatr Oncol* 1995; **25**: 204–207

205. Maurer HS, Steinherz PG, Gaynon PS *et al*. The effect of initial mangement of hyperleukocytosis on early complications and outcome of children with acute lymphoblastic leukemia. *J Clin Oncol* 1988; **6**: 1425

206. Nelson SC, Bruggers CS, Kurtzberg J, Friedman HS. Management of leukemic hyperleukocytosis with hydration, urinary alkalinization, and allopurinol. Are cranial irradiation and invasive cytoreduction necessary? *Am J Pediatr Hematol Oncol* 1993; **15**: 351–355

207. Lo Curto ML, Zingone A *et al*. Leukemic infiltration of the eye: Results of therapy in a retrospective multicentric study. *Med Pediatr Oncol* 1989; **17**: 134

208. Murray KM, Goldman JM *et al*. Ocular involvement in leukaemia. Report of three cases. *Lancet* 1977; **i**: 829

209. Warkentin TE, Kelton JG. Heparin-induced thrombocytopenia. *Prog Hemostas Thromb* 1991; **10**: 1–34

210. Ott N, Ramsay NKC *et al*. Sequelae of thrombotic or hemorrhagic complications following L-asparaginase therapy for childhood lymphoblastic leukemia. *Am J Pediatr Hematol Oncol* 1988; **10**: 191

211. Priest JR, Ramsey NKC *et al*. A syndrome of thrombosis and hemorrhage complicating L-asparaginase therapy for childhood acute lymphoblastic leukemia. *J Pediatr* 1982; **100**: 984

212. Nowak Göttl U, Auberger K, Göbel U *et al*. Inherited defects of the protein C anticoagulant system in childhood thrombo-embolism. *Eur J Pediatr* 1996; **155**: 921–927

213. Welte K, Reiter A, Mempel K *et al*. A randomized phase-III study of the efficacy of granulocyte colony-stimulating factor in children with high-risk acute lymphoblastic leukemia. *Blood* 1996; **87**: 3143–3150

214. Feldman S, Hughes WT *et al*. Varicella in children with cancer: seventy-seven cases. *Pediatrics* 1975; **56**: 388

215. Rowland P, Wald ER, Mirro JR *et al*. Progressive varicella presenting with pain and minimal skin involvement in children with acute lymphoblastic leukemia. *J Clin Oncol*. 1995; **13**: 1697–1703

216. Zaia JA, Levin MJ *et al*. Evaluation of varicella-zoster immune globulin: protection of immunosuppressed children after household exposure to varicella. *J Infect Dis* 1983; **147**: 171

217. Balfour HH Jr, Bean B *et al*. Acyclovir halts progression of herpes zoster in immunocompromised patients. *N Engl J Med* 1983; **308**: 1448

218. Prober CG, Kirk LE *et al*. Acyclovir therapy of chickenpox in immunosuppressed children-a collaborative study. *J Pediatr* 1982; **101**: 622

219. Gray MM, Hann IM, Glass S, Eden OB, Jones PM, Stevens RF. Mortality and morbidity caused by measles in children with malignant disease attending four major treatment centres: a retrospective study review. *Br Med J* 1987; **295**: 19–21

220. Gururangan S, Stevens RF, Morris DJ. Ribavirin response in measles pneumonia. *J Infection* 1990; **20**: 219–221

221. Hughes I, Jenney MEM, Newton RW, Morris DJ, Klapper PE. Measles encephalitis during immunosuppressive treatment for acute lymphoblastic leukaemia. *Arch Dis Child* 1993; **68**: 775–778

222. Pifer LL, Hughes WT *et al*. Pneumocystis carinii infection: evidence for high prevalence in normal and immunosuppressed children. *Pediatrics* 1978; **61**: 35

223. Hughes WT, Rivera GK *et al*. Successful intermittent chemoprophylaxis for *Pneumocystis carinii* pneumonitis. *N Engl J Med* 1987; **316**: 1627

224. Pasqualini T, Escobar ME *et al*. Evaluation of gonadal function following long-term treatment for acute lymphoblastic leukemia in girls. *Am J Pediatr Hematol Oncol* 1987; **9**: 15

225. Siris ES, Leventhal BG *et al*. Effects of childhood leukemia and chemotherapy on puberty and reproductive function in girls. *N Engl J Med* 1976; **294**: 1143

226. Lentz RD, Bergstein J *et al*. Postpubertal evaluation of gonadal function following cyclophosphamide therapy before and during puberty. *J Pediatr* 1977; 91: 385

227. Wallace WH, Shalet SM, Lendon M, Morris-Jones PH. Male fertility in long-term survivors of childhood acute lymphoblastic leukaemia. *Int J Androl* 1991; **14**: 312–319

228. Sklar CA, Robison LL *et al*. Effects of radiation on testicular function in long-term survivors of childhood acute lymphoblastic leukemia: A report from the Children's Cancer Study Group. *J Clin Oncol* 1990; **8**: 1981

229. Kenney LB, Nicholson HS, Brasseux C *et al*. Birth defects in offspring of adult survivors of childhood acute lymphoblastic leukemia. *Cancer* 1996; **78**: 169–176

230. Bessho F, Kinumaki H, Yokota S, Hayashi Y, Kobayashi M, Kamoshita S. Liver function studies in children with acute lymphocytic leukemia after cessation of therapy. *Med Pediatr Oncol* 1994; **23**: 111–115

231. Goldberg MA, Antin JH *et al*. Cyclophosphamide cardiotoxicity: An analysis of dosing as a risk factor. *Blood* 1986; **68**: 1114

232. Habermalz E, Habermalz H *et al*. Cranial computed tomography of 64 children in continuous complete remission of leukemia: I. Relations to therapy modalities. *Neuropediatrics* 1983; **14**: 144

233. Hara T, Kishikawa T *et al*. Central nervous system complications in childhood leukemia. *Am J Pediatr Hematol Oncol* 1984; **6**: 129

234. Ochs JJ, Parvey LS *et al*. Serial cranial computed tomography scans in children with leukemia given two different forms of central nervous system therapy. *J Clin Oncol* 1983; **1**: 793

235. Riccardi R, Brouwers P *et al*. Abnormal computed tomography brain scans in children with acute lymphoblastic leukemia: serial long-term follow-up. *J Clin Oncol* 1985; **3**: 12

236. Poplack DG, Brouwers P. Adverse sequelae of central nervous system therapy. *Clin Oncol* 1985; **4**: 263

237. Esseltine DW, Freeman CR *et al*. Computerized tomography brain scans in long-term survivors of childhood acute lymphoblastic leukemia. *Med Pediatr Oncol* 1981; **9**: 429

238. Jankovic M, Scotti G *et al*. Correlation between cranial computed tomographic scans at diagnosis in children with acute lymphoblastic leukaemia and central nervous system relapse. *Lancet* 1988; **ii**: 1212

239. Kramer JH, Crittenden MR, Halberg FE, Wara WM, Cowan MJ. A prospective study of cognitive functioning following low-dose cranial radiation for bone marrow transplantation. *Pediatrics* 1992; **90**: 447–450

240. Obetz WW, Smithson WA *et al*. Neuropsychologic follow-up study of children with acute lymphocytic leukemia. *Am J Pediatr Hematol Oncol* 1979; **3**: 207

241. Christie D, Leiper AD, Chessells JM, Vargha-Khadem F. Intellectual performance after presymptomatic cranial radiotherapy for leukaemia: effects of age and sex. *Arch Dis Child* 1995; **73**: 136–140

242. Jannoun L. Are cognitive and educational development affected by age at which therapy is given in acute lymphoblastic leukaemia? *Arch Dis Child* 1983; **58**: 953

243. Chessells JM, Cox TCS, Kendall B, Cavanagh NPC, Jannoun L, Richards S. Neurotoxicity in lymphoblastic leukaemia: Comparison of oral and intramuscular methotrexate and two doses of radiation. *Arch Dis Child* 1990; **65**: 416–422

244. Meadows AT, Evans AE. Effects of chemotherapy on the central nervous system: a study of parenteral methotrexate in longterm survivors of leukemia and lymphoma in childhood. *Cancer* 1976; **37**: 1079–1085

245. Kumar P, Mulhern RK, Regine WF, Rivera GK, Kun LE. A prospective neurocognitive evaluation of children treated with additional chemotherapy and craniospinal irradiation following isolated central nervous system relapse in acute lymphoblastic leukemia. *Int J Radiat Oncol Biol Phys* 1995; **31**: 561–566

246. Longeway K, Mulhern R *et al*. Treatment of meningeal relapse in childhood acute lymphoblastic leukemia: II. A prospective study of intellectual loss specific to CNS relapse and therapy. *Am J Pediatr Hematol Oncol* 1990; **12**: 45

247. Berglund G, Karlberg J *et al*. A longitudinal study of growth in children with acute lymphoblastic leukaemia. *Acta Paediatr Scand* 1985; **74**: 5300

248. Voorhess ML, Brecher ML *et al*. Growth in children treated for acute lymphoblastic leukaemia. *Lancet* 1988; **i**: 460

249. Kirk JA, Raghupathy P *et al*. Growth failure and growth-hormone deficiency after treatment for acute lymphoblastic leukaemia. *Pediatr Hematol Oncol* 1988; **5**: 187

250. Robison LL, Nesbit ME Jr. Height of children successfully treated for acute lymphoblastic leukemia: A report from the Late Effects Committee of the Children's Cancer Study Group. *Med Pediatr Oncol* 1985; **13**: 114–121

251. Moell C, Marky I, Hovi L *et al*. Cerebral irradiation causes blunted pubertal growth in girls treated for acute leukemia. *Med Pediatr Oncol* 1994; **22**: 375–379

252. Rappaport R, Brauner R. Growth and endocrine disorders secondary to cranial irridation. *Pediatr Res* 1989; **25**: 561

253. Pasqualini T, McCalla J, Berg S *et al*. Subtle primary hypothyroidism in patients treated for acute lymphoblastic leukemia. *Acta Endocrinol* 1991; **124**: 375–380

254. Hanif I, Mahmoud H, Pui C-H. Avascular femoral head necrosis in pediatric cancer patients. *Med Pediatr Oncol* 1993; **21**: 655–660

255. Pieters R, van der Schans-Dop AM *et al*. Osteonecrosis following chemotherpy for leukemia. *Eur J Haematol* 1989; **43**: 262

256. Hoover DL, Smith LE *et al*. Ophthalmic evaluation of survivors of acute lymphoblastic leukemia. *Ophthalmology* 1988; **95**: 151

257. Weaver G Jr, Chauvenet AR *et al*. Ophthalmic evaluation of long-term survivors of childhood acute lymphoblastic leukemia. *Cancer* 1986; **58**: 963

258. Nygaard R, Garwicz S, Haldorsen T *et al*. Second malignant neoplasms in patients treated for childhood leukemia. A population-based cohort study from the Nordic countries. *Acta Paediatr Scand* 1991; **80**: 1220–1228

259. Neglia JP, Meadows AT, Robison LL *et al.* Second neoplasms after acute lymphoblastic leukemia in childhood. *N Engl J Med* 1991; **325**: 1330–1336241.

260. Tang TT, Holcenberg JS *et al.* Thyroid carcinoma following treatment for acute lymphoblastic leukemia. *Cancer* 1980; **46**: 1572

261. Bessho F, Ohta K, Akanuma A. Dosimetry of radiation scattered to thyroid gland from prophylactic cranial irradiation for childhood leukemia. *Pediatr Hematol Oncol* 1994; **11**: 47–53

262. Kreissmann SG, Gelber RD, Cohen HJ, Clavell LA, Leavitt P, Sallan SE. Incidence of secondary acute myelogenous leukemia after treatment of childhood acute lymphoblastic leukemia. *Cancer* 1992; **70**: 2208–2213

Lymphomas

OB EDEN

NON-HODGKIN'S LYMPHOMA

Childhood non-Hodgkin's lymphomas (NHL) represent a heterogeneous group of disorders that are quite different from adult NHL in that they are almost invariably disseminated, diffuse not nodular, high-grade malignancies of immature T- or B-cell lineage, with frequent extra-nodal disease, marrow and central nervous system involvement. Over the last 3 decades, empirical chemotherapeutic management has transformed survival figures, and more recently greater understanding of the biology is offering hope for improved management of resistant disease.

EPIDEMIOLOGY

Age-standardized incidence rates for NHL vary from 6.1/million children (0–15 years) in the UK and Japan, to 90.1/million reported from Ibadan, Nigeria.[1] Hidden within these statistics are very different patterns of disease, particularly the incidence of B-cell lymphomas. Of all childhood cancers reported from Ibadan between 1960 and 1984, 47% were Burkitt's lymphoma (BL) with an age-standardized incidence rate of 80/million. Even higher rates have been reported from Uganda.

In endemic malarial areas of Africa, especially where BL is common, the peak age incidence is between 5 and 9 years with a ratio of 1.5–3 boys to each girl affected. The primary tumor is most frequently in the jaw. Other areas with an NHL incidence intermediate between the African and UK experience also report high BL rates (e.g. the Middle East, Latin America, Mediterranean area and North Africa), but in these regions the tumors occur more commonly in the abdomen and over a wider age range (0–9 years). The age-standardized incidence for BL in the UK is 0.2/million for girls and 0.3 for boys, whilst in the US it is 3.6 in white males, 0.4 in white females, 0.7 in black males and of a very low incidence in black girls.[1]

In western Europe, the male:female ratio for all NHL is approximately 2:1 and NHL constitutes 5–6% of all childhood cancers, although the relative and absolute incidence rises southwards towards the Mediterranean. In the UK the peak age incidence is between 7 and 10 years, but all ages can be affected. Over the last 30 years there appears to have been a steady increase in the overall incidence of NHL.

ETIOLOGY AND CELL BIOLOGY

The childhood immune system consists of many different end-stage functional cells as well as a wide array of precursor and stem cells. Malignancy can occur at any stage in lymphocyte ontogeny, and monoclonal antibodies have helped to define the differentiation process of both normal and malignant lymphocytes. Like adults, young children are constantly exposed to antigens, but unlike adults they do not have a large immune memory bank to help them to recognize and repel such antigens. As a result, a large proportion of lymphoid cells during childhood are in a very active state, undergoing molecular rearrangements to produce specific immunoglobulins and other factors required for the normal immune response. For B cells to function, the genes which regulate the different components of immunoglobulin production have to be brought together or rearranged. In T cells, the genes which control T-cell antigen receptor molecules similarly need to be organized. The immunoglobulin heavy chain genes are on chromosome 14 (q32), the λ light chain genes on chromosome 22 (q11), and the κ light chain genes on chromosome 2 (p12). For B cells to function properly the rearrangements must occur in an ordered sequence.

The human T-cell receptor α-chain gene maps to the long arm of chromosome 14 (14q11–12) and harbors the T-cell receptor δ genes between its V and J region gene sequences. The T-cell receptor β-chain locus is on chromosome 7q35. A complete product molecule requires 2 chains, an α from chromosome 14 and a β from chromosome 7. In normal health the rearrangement process producing the product of the receptor gene is very similar to that for immunoglobulin gene rearrangements (see Chapter 25). The enzyme Tdt is intimately involved in T-cell rearrangements but is not found in B-cell acute lymphoid leukemia (ALL) or lymphoma and can be used as a distinguishing marker.

Malignant change can occur when genetic defects arise secondary to deletion, mutation or translocation. This can interrupt the normal orderly rearrangement, but what actually initiates the disorganization is not clear in most instances. Accumulating evidence incriminates viruses at least in the pathogenesis of some lymphomas. The products from the retroviruses HTLV-1 and -2 rearrange genes within the host cell, thus stimulating production of interleukin (IL)-2 and its receptor which can activate T-cell proliferation. Clonal or polyclonal proliferation provides the opportunity for a second strike which may be necessary to produce a malignant clone. HTLV-1 is thought to play a role in the genesis of a particular form of adult T-cell leukemia/lymphoma, particularly in Japan. No viral inclusions have yet been found in childhood T-cell NHL.

Much more directly relevant to pediatric practice was the discovery of Epstein–Barr virus (EBV) particles in the nuclei of endemic African BL cells.[2,3] The finding of such viral inclusion and high antibody titers (especially to the viral capsid antigen) to EBV in the vast majority of cases (95%) from tropical regions contrasts with those in temperate regions where the incidence of raised titers and/or viral inclusions is only about 15–20%.[4,5] However, there is increasing evidence of aberrant expression in sporadic cases. In very high incidence regions malaria is endemic and is thought to cause a continuous antigenic stimulus which alters responses to EBV infections which are also endemic (nearly 100% of children have been exposed by age 3 years). EBV infection early in life is thought to enlarge the size of certain pre-B and B-cell populations and maintain them in a proliferative state, thereby rendering them more likely to genetic change. It has alternatively been postulated that EBV produces an immortal cell clone with genetic translocations already present. Since EBV is so endemic in tropical areas, and nearly 90% of adults in Europe have antibodies to EBV as well, EBV alone cannot be the cause of BL.

Repeated infections, especially of malaria (a T-cell suppresser and B-cell mutagen), malnutrition and other cofactors (e.g. the use of phorbol esters as herbal medicine) result in T-cell immunosuppression (reduced CD4:CD8 ratio and decreased number and function of EBV-specific T-cells) and B-cell hyperplasia which can potentiate the effects of EBV infection. A consequent increase in number of EBV genome-positive cells during acute malaria is postulated to increase the chance of genetic changes, including the characteristic translocation involving the long arm of chromosome 8 (region q23–24), usually as part of a t(8;14) (q24;q32) rearrangement, although variants which include t(2;8) (p12;q24) and t(8;22) (q24;q11) are seen in about 15% of cases. The c-myc oncogene lies at the chromosome 8 breakpoint, whilst the immunoglobulin heavy chain locus and κ and λ light chain loci are at 14q32, 2p12 and 22q11, respectively. In all cases, an immunoglobulin gene enhancer is placed close to c-myc and induces its expression. Of great interest has been the finding that the chromosome 8 breakpoint is upstream of c-myc in endemic cases whilst in the sporadic form it occurs within c-myc, or immediately upstream. However, in all forms, the c-myc coding region appears to be left intact so that deregulation of the oncogene rather than mutation seems to be the consequence of the translocation.[6] The myc-encoded protein appears to regulate the expression of target genes required for cell cycle progression through GI into S phase. If it is dysregulated, it leads to progression through the cell cycle and lymphoproliferation. On chromosome 14 the breakpoints involve limited D and J segments, regions prone to physiologic rearrangements during the normal sequence of VDJ recombination. Endemic BL cases usually have low levels of surface immunoglobulin, and sporadic cases have high levels and the cells also secrete immunoglobulin. It is thought that in sporadic cases the translocations are at a later stage of B-cell differentiation. This ever increasing knowledge of the biology of NHL has been applied to the detection of minimal residual disease using polymerase chain reaction techniques to detect specific patterns of immunoglobulin gene rearrangements.

8q24 is a fragile site but what specifically initiates the translocation is not clear. A multiple hit model is postulated for the initiation of BL. Some have speculated that genetic factors might also be involved, since familial clusters of BL have been reported,[7] and genetic factors including inherited mutations of the c-myc oncogene or p53, and the finding of an excess of HLA-DR7 phenotype, raise the possibilities of inherent DNA repair defects or abnormal responsiveness to infection. The intriguing effect of extracts from Euphorbia triucalli (used as a herbal medicine) in inducing c-myc activation[8] further suggests that a complex interaction of environmental and genetic factors is likely. The factors involved in non-endemic cases are far from clear, although EBV still appears critical.

Human immunodeficiency virus (HIV) infection as a result of profound T-helper cell depression predisposes to a variety of tumors, including intermediate- to high-grade B-cell lymphomas, Hodgkin's disease, T-cell NHL and some pre-T and pre-B tumors, especially Kaposi's sarcoma. Some of the resultant lymphomas appear to be polyclonal B-cell proliferations similar to those seen after intense iatrogenic immunosuppression. The characteristic feature of HIV-associated lymphomas is extra-nodal disease, especially of the skin, and a high incidence of EBV positivity, raising the possibility that HIV may predispose to an EBV-driven proliferation.[9]

For T-cell ALL and NHL chromosomal abnormalities are more heterogeneous. About 25% of T-cell ALL cases involve a small deletion of the TAL1 gene on chromosome 1 and this is sometimes associated with a t(1;14) translocation. Also, translocations can involve the locus for the α chain of the T-cell receptor gene on chromosome 14 or for the β chain on chromosome 7.[10] No clear-cut association between these changes and etiological factors has been made but the changes can be used to detect minimal residual disease.

In anaplastic large-cell lymphoma (ALCL) a t(2;5) (p23;q35) translocation has been described.[11] This is found in occasional cases of Hodgkin's disease, and current interest exists in exploring the overlap between these two conditions, and also the association of chromosome 2 anomalies in ALCL with more advanced disease and with a poorer prognosis. To date, no clear etiological link has been made. The translocation produces a fused gene (nucleophosmin, NPM from chromosome 5 and AL kinase gene, ALK from chromosome 2) and a product which is primarily cytoplasmic in location. Its precise function has not been defined.

Genetic factors may be important in NHL development, not just given the occasional familial clustering with BL, but also because a number of inherited or congenital immuno-deficiency syndromes are associated with NHL. These include ataxia telangiectasia (including a number of variants, especially with T-cell malignancies), Wiskott–Aldrich syndrome, Bruton's aggammaglobulinemia, severe combined immunodeficiency (SCID) and IgA deficiency. Post organ transplantation lymphomas representing either monoclonal or polyclonal B-cell proliferation have been referred to already. The X-linked syndrome described by Grierson and Purtillo,[1,2] characterized by undue sensitivity to EBV and leading to uncontrolled EBV proliferation, including hepatitis, encephalopathy, aplasia and malignant lymphomas, has similar features. Other chromosomal or genetic disorders associated with NHL include Klinefelter's syndrome[13] and neurofibromatosis type 1.

Apart from postnatal long-term exposure to phenytoin, which can produce a benign lymphadenopathy, a self-limiting pseudo-lymphoma and, rarely, a true lymphoma, EBV infection for BL and the intense immunosuppression following transplantation or chemotherapy, no other environmental factors have been firmly incriminated in the causation of NHL. Although still the subject of intense investigation, exposure pre- or post-natally to irradiation, chemicals, electromagnetic fields and electricity have not been firmly associated with NHL.

CLASSIFICATION

A confusing array of classifications exists for NHL. For pediatric practice there is a concerted effort to use the Real classification (Revised European American Lymphoma classification), which is an update of the Kiel scheme, incorporating immunophenotyping and dividing NHL into T- and B-cell neoplasms, and further classifying them as of high- or low-grade malignancy (Table 28.1). Virtually all childhood NHL are diffuse and 3 types, namely Burkitt's (42%), T lymphoblastic (20%), and anaplastic large cell (15%), predominate.

Table 28.1 Comparison of Real and Kiel classification schemes for childhood non-Hodgkin's lymphoma.

Kiel	Real
1. Burkitt's	1. Burkitt's (42%)* High-grade B cell Burkitt's like (4%)
2. B lymphoblastic	2. Precursor B lymphoblastic (5%)
3. T lymphoblastic	3. Precursor T lymphoblastic (20%)
4. Centroblastic B immunoblastic	4. Diffuse large B cell (3%) (primary sclerosing mediastinal 0.4%)
5. Pleiomorphic medium and large T cell	5. Peripheral T cell unspecified
6. Large cell anaplastic (Ki-1+)	6. Anaplastic large-cell T or null types (15%)

*Percentages are from a recent review of over 200 cases registered with the UK Children's Cancer Study Group (R Pinkerton and R Carter, Central pathological review of NHL by UKCCSG in UKCCSG Scientific Report, 1997, personal communication).[14] There were in addition 9.2% of cases of indeterminate or non-specific type and 0.4% follicular.

CLINICAL PRESENTATION

Abdominal primary

In Europe, the commonest presentation of high-grade B-cell NHL (Burkitt or non-BL type) is an abdominal mass (30–45% of all NHL cases).[14] There are 2 commonly recognized types. Type 1 are diffuse abdominal tumors with involvement throughout the omentum and mesentery, often including infiltration into the kidney, liver and spleen. With these, bone marrow and central nervous system involvement is common. Only a few cases present with jaw involvement, whereas in African BL this is almost universal, and most frequently involves multiple quadrants, although isolated orbital tumors of the maxillary bone do occur. Abdominal involvement is also present in up to 50% of African patients presenting with jaw primaries. There is a lower incidence of bone marrow involvement in African compared with non-African Burkitt's NHL.

Type 2 are localized tumors of the bowel wall, most commonly in the terminal ileum (thought to arise in Peyer's patches), which can lead to intussusception or bleeding with or without perforation of the bowel. Patients most often present with a right iliac fossa mass and are sometimes thought to have appendicitis or an appendix mass. This type of presentation is much rarer than the rapidly growing diffuse type 1.

Mediastinal primary

Up to two-thirds of patients with precursor T-lymphoblastic NHL and 25–30% of all NHL (T cells and some non-lymphoblastic, large cell and Burkitt's) present with mediastinal masses, with or without pleural effusions. Frequently, there are signs of superior vena caval obstruction with dysphagia, dyspnea and pericardial effusion. Lymphadenopathy is usually confined to the neck and axillae. Abdominal node enlargement is uncommon, but hepatosplenomegaly is common, as is bone marrow involvement ($>50\%$ of cases) and CNS infiltration. These patients are at especially high risk of developing respiratory obstruction and/or distress if general anesthesia is instigated for investigations.

Localized disease

Lymphoid swelling can occur anywhere, but most commonly arises in the head and neck, including Waldeyer's ring and the facial bones (10–20%). Neck nodal tumors apparently have a lower risk of CNS spread. Some 5–10% of tumors arise in nodes or lymphoid tissue at other sites, including pharyngeal masses which are usually of B-cell origin. Rarer sites for primary tumors include bone, skin, thyroid, testis (usually lymphoblastic), orbit, eyelid, kidney (can mimic Wilms' tumor) and epidural space. Bony NHL can be localized or more generalized, and is sometimes associated with hypercalcemia. Lymphoblastic lymphoma can present peripherally with skin and/or bone disease, and these tumors are usually of more mature T-cell phenotype. Subcutaneous lymphoma, often seen in very young children, is usually of precursor B-cell type.

Central nervous system involvement

Primary CNS lymphomas are rare except following organ transplantation, but CNS involvement as secondary spread from disease elsewhere is quite common, particularly in lymphoblastic and advanced Burkitt's NHL. It leads to headache, vomiting, papilloedema, cranial nerve dysfunction and seizures. It is much more common at diagnosis if the bone marrow is also infiltrated, but is occasionally seen in patients with localized disease and those with large-cell histology.

Anaplastic large-cell lymphoma (Ki-1$^+$)

The importance and frequency of this tumor is being increasingly recognized. Formerly, many such tumors were classified as malignant histiocytosis. The most frequent presentation is painful nodal swelling, sometimes with apparent surrounding inflammation or more generalized skin involvement (macules or generalized ichthyosis) and fever. The B symptoms of Hodgkin's disease may be present and may cast doubt on the diagnosis (see below).

DIAGNOSTIC INVESTIGATIONS AND STAGING

Following the taking of a very full history and an extensive clinical examination to define potential tumor extent, the aim of subsequent investigations is to confirm the diagnosis as accurately and as quickly as possible, and to determine the extent of disease so that appropriate therapy is started as soon as possible. All patients should have a preliminary chest X-ray to exclude mediastinal mass and/or pericardial/pleural effusions, and this should certainly be done prior to any anesthetic procedure.

Biopsy

Unless the diagnosis can be made from cytologic examination of tapped pleural fluid or bone marrow, excision biopsy is indicated in the presence of accessible localized disease and if there is peripheral lymphadenopathy associated with a mediastinal mass. If there is truly isolated mediastinal disease, material should be obtained by percutaneous needle or mediastinoscopy. For abdominal primaries, diagnosis should be attempted by cytologic examination of ascitic fluid or by percutaneous needle biopsy. Unless there is an acute abdominal emergency, e.g. gastrointestinal obstruction or intussusception, laparatomy should be avoided wherever possible to avoid the common sequelae of prolonged ileus and even ruptured abdominal wounds. In extensive disease, the most accessible tumor deposits, not necessarily the primary, should be biopsied. All tumor material should be submitted for routine histologic diagnosis, full immunophenotyping profile and cytogenetics. Table 28.2 shows the characteristic diagnostic features which help to distinguish subtypes of NHL.

Bone marrow studies

All patients require the marrow to be examined from at least 2, and preferably 4, sites (ideally from 2 aspirates and 2 trephines). The specimens should be examined cytogenetically and immunologically as well as by routine cytomorphology.

Lumbar puncture

Provided there is no clinical evidence of raised intracranial pressure, cerebrospinal fluid should be examined. If there are signs of raised intracranial pressure, either a CT or MRI scan should be carried out before lumbar puncture to exclude any focal deposit with consequent risk of brain shift.

Imaging

MRI defines nodal and organ masses most effectively, especially for tumors of the head and neck. However, abdominal ultrasonography is often the quickest way to define liver, spleen and kidney involvement, and the extent of abdominal primaries. It can also be carried out without sedation, whereas general anesthesia is frequently required in young children for MRI or CT scanning. In experienced hands ultrasound is very effective for guiding needle biopsies, especially for abdominal masses. Bone scans are only indicated if there is focal bone pain. Although in the past gallium and thallium scans were used to detect occult disease, they

Table 28.2 Characteristic features of main subgroups of non-Hodgkin's lymphoma.

	B cell	Lymphoblastic	Anaplastic large cell
Primary site	Most frequently abdominal primary	Most frequently mediastinal but also nodal	Nodal ± skin
Histology	Burkitt's (small non-cleaved) centroblastic or B-cell immunoblastic	Lymphoblastic	Large cell
Cytomorphology	L3	L1/L2 characteristics (focal capped acid phophatase positivity in T cell)	–
Immunomarkers	Cells display SIg⁺ B cell markers (CD19,22,24+) Tdt negative	CD1–CD8 T-cell markers (SIg⁻ but occas. CyIg⁺) (CD10+ve in precursor B)	CD30 positive
Cytogenetics	t(8;14), t(2;8), t(8;22)	Heterogeneous	t(2;5)

L1, L2, L3 = French–American–British (FAB) classification; SIg = surface immunoglobulin positive; CyIg = cytoplasmic immunoglobulin.

are not specific and require further evaluation before their routine use can be recommended. B-cell lymphomas do take up gallium avidly.

Blood tests

Initial investigation should include a full blood count, liver and renal function studies, serum lactate dehydrogenase levels and urate, calcium, phosphate and urea levels.

Staging

Table 28.3 shows the most commonly used staging system for childhood NHL.[15] All primary mediastinal and diffuse abdominal tumors are considered to be at least Stage III. Spread in NHL, unlike in Hodgkin's disease, is not orderly or contiguous from node to node. Therefore, there is no place for routine staging laparotomy or lymphangiography in childhood NHL.

Prognostic factors

Therapy

With modern aggressive intensive chemotherapy regimens, the overall cure rates are 60–65% for T-cell NHL, 80–85% for B-cell NHL (ranging from 100% for Stage I and II disease, to 60–70% for Stage IV with CNS involvement), and 60% for anaplastic large-cell tumors. Each type requires very specific treatment (see below) and the most significant prognostic factor now appears to be the choice of the right therapy, based on meticulous initial work-up and definition of tumor type. There remains doubt as to the optimal therapy for ALCL, peripheral T-cell lymphoma and even more so for the rare low-grade follicular tumors. The speed of response may be significant, especially in T-cell NHL. Shepherd *et al*[16] reported that for the 25% of patients in full radiologic remission at day 60, 5-year disease-free survival

Table 28.3 St Jude modified staging system for non-Hodgkin's lymphoma.

Stage		Approximate % seen in the UK
I	Single tumor (extranodal) or single anatomic area (nodal). Not mediastinum or abdomen	5
II	Single tumor (extranodal) with regional node involvement. Primary gastrointestinal tumor with or without involvement of associated mesenteric nodes only. On the same side of diaphragm: a) Two or more nodal areas b) Two single (extranodal) tumors with or without regional node involvement	20
III	On both sides of the diaphragm: a) Two single tumors (extranodal) b) Two or more nodal areas. All primary intrathoracic tumors (mediastinal, pleural, thymic); all extensive primary intra-abdominal disease; all primary paraspinal or epidural tumors regardless of other sites	50
IV	Any of the above with initial CNS* or bone marrow involvement (<25%)**	25

*CNS disease = unequivocal blasts >5/mm³ in a cytocentrifuged cerebrospinal fluid specimen ± neurologic deficits, e.g. cranial nerve pulses ± intracerebral nodal deposits.
**Distinction is arbitrarily made at 25% to distinguish between ALL and NHL. This may not be useful for all, e.g. in B-cell NHL there is no difference in outcome between Stage III and IV disease up to a marrow infiltration of 70%.

(DFS) was 84%, compared with only 56% for patients who had some radiologic evidence of residual mediastinal thickening in a UK T-cell NHL study. Patients failing to achieve full remission by 3 months do appear to benefit from high-dose therapy and stem cell rescue.[17]

Staging

In general, the higher the stage the worse the prognosis, but effective therapy is reducing the differential. In T-cell disease, very few relapses occur in Stage I and II tumors, whilst for Stage III 70% and Stage IV 60% 5-year disease free survival is expected. In B-cell NHL, the figures are 95–100% for Stage I and II, and have greatly improved for Stages III and IV. The previously defined adverse prognostic features of extensive abdominal organ involvement, pleural effusions, extra-abdominal disease, poor nutritional status and bulky disease no longer appear significant. The only remaining adverse clinical features in B-cell NHL are the presence of marrow infiltration >70% and CNS-positive disease, but even in the latter more aggressive treatment has increased survival to nearly 70% (see below). Elevated serum lactate dehydrogenase (LDH) levels in Stage III B-cell patients remain an important indicator of poor prognosis.

Site

Stage I patients with orbital or Waldeyer's ring tumors appear to fare worse than those with other localized nodal NHL. Stage II localized abdominal tumors have a better prognosis than a similarly staged nasopharyngeal tumor extending to the skull base.

Anaplastic large-cell lymphomas

Conventional staging is not so useful in these tumors with their extensive skin and nodal disease. Although their prognosis is no worse than that for most other lymphomas, Murphy Stage IV disease is rare. The full significance of fever, weight loss, extent of skin disease and/or parenchymal lung disease is not known. The presence of the classical t(2;5) may carry adverse prognostic significance.

TREATMENT

General principles

Frequently, patients with lymphomas present with poor nutrition, concomitant infection and metabolic problems. Of the latter, spontaneous tumor lysis, especially in Stage IV T- and B-cell disease, is the commonest. The features are hypercalcemia, hyperphosphatemic-hypocalcemia, hyperuricemia and azotemia. When it occurs during therapy, the rapid control of infection, a high fluid intake ($3 \, l/m^2/day$) to induce diuresis, intravenous or oral allopurinol (10 mg/kg/day), careful alkalinization of urine (to maintain urinary pH at about 6.5; above that level phosphate will precipitate) to keep urate and phosphate in solution, aluminium hydroxide or calcium carbonate to lower serum phosphate levels, and slow intravenous or intramuscular magnesium (intravenous calcium tends to be tissue deposited) to reverse any symptomatic tetany, are usually adequate. Maintenance of adequate diuresis is essential, and if necessary frusemide may be required, which, although raising serum urate levels, prevents urate

from being deposited within the renal tubules. However, lysis prior to therapy or at any stage in which the signs of renal failure progress (rapidly rising urea, creatinine and most significantly sustained serum potassium levels >6.5 mEq/l) warrants early instigation of dialysis to facilitate antilymphoma therapy, since the lysis will only really cease when tumor bulk has been reduced.

In the presence of signs of renal failure, it is essential to define causation. Obstructive nephropathy can result from tubular deposition of urate and external tumor compression, but also intrarenal infiltration by tumor and/or hemorrhage, all of which can precipitate renal failure. A tumor compressing the outflow tracks is best treated by transcutaneous pyelostomy, the other problems by dialysis.

Interestingly, the prophylactic use of uricozyme originally reported by Masera et al[18] and used widely in the French Pediatric Oncology Society (SFOP) protocols has reduced the risks of therapeutic lysis, especially for advanced B-cell NHL.[19] The principle of initial low-dose therapy to reduce tumor bulk followed 1 week later by more intensive treatment, pioneered by both the SFOP and German BFM (Berlin–Frankfurt–Münster) groups, appears to help reduce the risks of tumor lysis. Hypercalcemia, although less frequent, and most commonly but not exclusively associated with extensive bony disease, may require long-term therapy with biphosphonates until brought under control.[20]

Provided patients can be acutely supported using nasogastric feeding, malnutrition at diagnosis is not now considered an adverse prognostic feature in European and North American studies, although it may still adversely affect outcome in patients with extensive disease presenting in developing countries.

Prior to the 1970s, surgery and/or radiotherapy were largely unsuccessful in the treatment of NHL, except in truly localized disease. Surgery should, in general, be reserved for biopsy taking and repeat biopsies in the presence of residual masses after intensive therapy, and sometimes the debulking of residual tumor. Extensive initial surgery is strongly contraindicated, especially in mediastinal and extensive abdominal disease. Similarly, radiotherapy probably has a place in the local control of refractory disease, in primary CNS lymphoma and for tumors in unusual primary sites (e.g. testis and bone) but is probably no longer useful for patients who are not CNS positive at diagnosis. Even CNS-positive B-cell NHL may be curable without irradiation (see below).

Wollner et al[21] found that lymphoblastic disease (T and precursor B) responded optimally to an intensive leukemia-type regimen (LSA2L2) and the Children's Cancer Study Group (CCSG)[22] confirmed this for lymphoblastic disease, but also showed that for diffuse undifferentiated lymphoma (especially in extensive abdominal disease), a shorter pulsed cyclophosphamide-based regimen (COMP) produced superior results.[22,23] The likelihood of dissemination in childhood NHL necessitates the need for chemotherapy even in apparently resected localized disease.

Localized non-Hodgkin's lymphoma (Stage I and II)

Localized disease requires less intensive therapy than advanced disease, except for lymphoblastic lymphomas. For low-stage NHL, both the CCSG and Pediatric Oncology Group (POG) have reported short-course therapy (approximately 6 months) using COMP or CHOP protocols to be extremely effective.[24,25]

For Stage I and abdominal Stage II disease, Murphy[15] reported no need for CNS-directed therapy. In the UK, Gerrard et al[26] reported >85% event-free survival (EFS) with short-course pulsed therapy for low-stage B-cell NHL. All groups have attempted to reduce the risks of late cardiotoxicity by limiting or omitting anthracyclines, of infertility by omitting alkylators, or of oncogenesis by limiting exposure to anthracyclines and/or alkylators. Patte et al[27] reported almost 100% cure rates with only 2 pulses of cyclophosphamide-based chemotherapy, and Reiter et al[28] 3 courses for children with fully excised B-cell NHL.

The POG group[25] reported inferior results for lymphoblastic disease, and thus all other collaborative groups have excluded such disease from such short-course chemotherapy protocols, and instead treated them with a longer duration leukemia-type regimen, as they would for non-localized lymphoblastic disease.[28–31] Whether any reduction in intensity can or should be introduced remains unclear (OB Eden and IM Hann. Results of the UKCCSG protocol 9004 for lymphoblastic disease, personal communication).[28,29] Survival for localized T-cell disease with such therapy exceeds 80%, but therapy-related sequelae do occur.

Advanced-stage B-cell lymphomas

With the exception of Stage IV disease with CNS involvement, progressively more intensive protocols building on the COMP/CHOP experience introduced in the 1970s and early 1980s have produced complete remission rates of 85–95%, with 60–65% 5-year EFS for Stage III disease, but only 30–40% at best for Stage IV disease. Those with CNS disease were considered until the mid-1980s to be incurable, but since then the SFOP in a series of studies designated LMB (along with the BFM group, those working at St Jude Research Hospital, Memphis and the UKCCSG) have transformed this view.

The best results remain those reported by the SFOP group.[27] Both the LMB and BFM protocols use initial relatively low-dose cytoreductive therapy, in particular cyclophosphamide, vincristine and prednisolone (COP) before the more intensive induction regimen, which in the case of the LMB protocol consists of high-dose methotrexate, fractionated high-dose cyclophosphamide, vincristine, prednisolone and adriamycin, and this is followed by a consolidation phase using continuous infusion cytarabine. CNS-directed therapy is with high-dose methotrexate and intrathecal methotrexate but not irradiation, except for

those with CNS disease at diagnosis.[19] Since the first LMB study in 1981, EFS has progressively increased, and therapy and duration reduced from 12 to 4–6 months depending on risk stratification.[19,27,32] Identified high-risk groups include those with bone marrow involvement ≥70% (essentially B-ALL) and those with CNS involvement at diagnosis who now receive the most intensive regimen, 8 g/m^2 of systemic methotrexate per dose, along with triple intrathecal therapy and consolidation with continuous infusion high-dose cytarabine and etoposide (CYVE).[27] Those with CNS disease still receive cranial irradiation. The LMB '89 protocol yielded an EFS of 87% in patients with B-ALL without CNS involvement and 81% in those with CNS disease at presentation,[27] which contrasts with only 19% for such patients on the LMB '81 protocol.[32] Inevitably, there is morbidity and some mortality associated with such intensive therapy (in fairness, more in other clinicians' hands than for SFOP participants, who appear to have gained tremendous experience in the management of such patients), and a new combined POG, UKCCSG and SFOP study is addressing the issues of whether the total dose of cyclophosphamide given, duration of therapy or both, can be reduced in those without truly high-risk features.

A similar progressive improvement in EFS was seen with BFM studies (which also stratified patients), especially for Stage IV and B-ALL patients (an improvement from 50 to 80% EFS), and for Stage III patients with raised lactate dehydrogenase (LDH) levels who seem to benefit from an increase in consolidation methotrexate dosage from 0.5 to 5 g/m^2/dose.[33]

The UKCCSG devised a short intensive regimen (MACHO)[34] also using high-dose fractionated cyclophosphamide, high-dose cytarabine and methotrexate for B-ALL and those with Stage III and IV bulky disease, with or without multiorgan involvement. EFS was 73% for Stage III, 50% for Stage IV and 64% for B-cell ALL.[34,35] In the subsequent protocol, UKCCSG 9003, 63 patients with either B-ALL (35) or Stage IV B-cell NHL (28) were treated with a short intensive course based on the French LMB '86 regimen. At a median follow up of 3.1 years, 68% of patients are alive in complete first remission. There was a relapse rate of 16% and a death rate due to toxicity of 11%, with 5 deaths from sepsis and 2 from sepsis with renal failure (A Atra, personal communication). The factors accounting for the slightly inferior UK compared with French results with the same protocol are being tested in a new joint collaborative protocol.

Both the St Jude Pediatric Oncology team and the US Pediatric Oncology Group have used very similar strategic approaches, and have demonstrated the importance of high-dose systemic methotrexate in controlling CNS disease.[36] POG, in their 1986 study, reported a 52% EFS for patients with CNS positivity at diagnosis without using irradiation.[37] The CCSG compared the LMB '89 regimen with a hybrid protocol of their own, and reported 2-year EFS of 80% and 84%, respectively. There was more toxicity in the LMB protocol than their own regimen, which again appears to emphasize the need for experience with the application of any specific protocol, especially in the control of tumor lysis and infection.[38]

Speed of response to initial therapy is of prognostic significance; for example, where there is no tumor reduction following the initial COP in LMB or failure to remit by 3 months, intensification of therapy is indicated.[17] Any residual mass should, however, be biopsied since many are fully necrotic. Relapses in advanced B-cell NHL tend to occur early within the first 1–2 years after diagnosis, and relapses beyond 3 years appear quite rare. Salvage rates are very low.

Advanced-stage non-B-cell NHL

Since the mid-1970s T-cell and precursor B-cell lymphoblastic disease has been treated using sustained, progressively more intensive leukemia-type protocols. Following the initial success of the LSA2L2 protocol for ALL, the BFM group pioneered such therapy with induction, re-induction, 4 courses of high-dose methotrexate as CNS-directed therapy, plus cranial irradiation. The basic protocols have been proven by the test of time; systemic methotrexate dosages have been increased from 0.5 to 5 g/m^2 and the cranial irradiation dose reduced from 18 to 12 Gy. From the BFM '86 study, EFS of 79% ($\pm$ 5%) for 71 patients so treated was reported.[28] Patte et al[29] reported on a modified LSA2L2 protocol in which 10 pulses of 3 g/m^2 of methotrexate infused over 3 hours was used as CNS-directed therapy. EFS was 79% for Stage III (33 patients) and 72% for Stage IV patients (43). CNS control was really quite exceptional. In the UK, a protocol identical to the Medical Research Council ALL protocol, UKALLX, consisting of a standard 4 drug induction, early (week 5) and late (week 20) 6-drug consolidation modules, cranial irradiation (18 Gy) plus 6 intrathecal methotrexate injections, plus 2 years of standard continuing therapy (including 4 weekly pulses of vincristine and prednisolone) has been used. The 4-year EFS for 95 patients with Stage III and IV disease was 65% ($\pm$ 15%).[39] Subsequently, in the protocol 9004, cranial irradiation has been replaced by 3 pulses of high-dose methotrexate (6–8 g/m^2 depending on age), with ongoing intrathecal methotrexate every 3 months during the 2 years of treatment, and in 1995 a third intensification module was introduced at week 35. No increase in CNS relapses was seen in a series of over 100 patients treated on this protocol.[40]

Comparable results have been reported from most unselected series, with single-center studies reporting 5-year EFS of 70–75% and collaborative unselected series 65–70%, with little difference between Stage III and IV patients. The BFM group showed slightly superior results which have not really changed much since its initial breakthrough in 1976.

Failure to remit by day 60 with complete resolution of a mediastinal primary is an adverse prognostic sign.[16] Instigation of more intensive therapy, including high-dose chemotherapy and autologous stem cell rescue, may be justified in the presence of such residual disease. Intriguingly, a finding, which was dismissed earlier, may suggest a useful role for localized mediastinal irradiation. Although incorporated into a modified pulsed LSA2L2-like protocol with overall worse results than now seen, a randomized study performed by the UKCCSG showed significantly improved results in patients who received 15 Gy irradiation to the mediastinum compared with those who did not.[41]

Such mixed modality therapy may now not be justified for all patients given the intensity of chemotherapy. However, in the presence of persistent mediastinal shadowing beyond day 60, further intensification of chemotherapy and/or the local use of irradiation may improve results from the rather stubbornly fixed level of 65–70% now seen. It is important to remember that in lymphoblastic disease, relapses appear to continue to occur up to 5 years from diagnosis. Greater understanding of the cell biology involved in T-cell NHL and ALL may assist in the future application of novel strategies.

Anaplastic large-cell lymphoma

Since clinicians recognized this as an entity, its incidence has progressively risen, but what its adverse prognostic features are and how its variable forms should be treated remains unclear. Indeed, it is not known whether it truly is a single entity or a group of disorders awaiting further classification. Rashes that are very common in this condition may resolve spontaneously,[42] whereas other patients progress rapidly to requiring megatherapy and transplantation.[43] In view of these ambiguities, both sustained leukemia-type regimens, as used for lymphoblastic disease,[44] and B-cell lymphoma protocols have been utilized.[45] Overall, the BFM reported an 81% EFS probability with 3 consecutive protocols.[45] They showed that skin involvement and splenomegaly were adverse features. The UKCCSG has tried to stratify patients on the basis of Murphy staging, using graded B-cell NHL protocols with rather similar results to those reported by BFM. Sandlund et al[46] reported that patients confirmed as CD30-positive fared better than those diagnosed on clinical grounds alone. For ALCL, which appears to be the third largest entity amongst childhood NHL, more needs to be learned about how to stage and prognosticate successfully, and resources need to be pooled internationally so that the group of patients requiring a more intensive approach can be rapidly identified.

Peripheral T-cell lymphomas

Saha et al[31] in a UK series showed that of 28 patients labeled as having peripheral T-cell lymphoma (PTCL), 22% were considered ALCL morphologically, but many more had the classic t(2;5) translocation, and 25 of 27 who were evaluable had CD30 positivity. It would appear that such patients should be treated like those with ALCL.

Other rare forms

There are a small number of CD30-negative PTCL patients for whom the optimal therapy is not known. For large-cell NHL of non-T lineage, standard B-cell protocols such as the LMB '89 regimen seem optimal. Primary mediastinal B-cell NHL is mostly seen in adolescents and young adults, but it mimics T-cell NHL.[47] Bone marrow and CNS involvement are rare. Recommended treatment is as per Stage III B-cell NHL. The possibility that a mediastinal lymphoma may be of B- rather than T-cell origin, and so may not respond to standard lymphoblastic therapy, emphasizes the need in all childhood NHLs for full pathologic confirmation plus immunophenotyping of diagnostic material.

Follicular lymphomas are extremely rare in childhood, but can respond favorably to CHOP-based regimens. As for adults, very late relapse can occur.[48]

NHL following intense immunosuppression

Over the last decade an increasing incidence of lymphoproliferative disorders has been seen in organ-transplant recipients (especially in those receiving high-dose cyclosporin and FK506), and others receiving intense immunosuppression, including patients with a diverse range of diseases (e.g. chronic inflammatory bowel disease). Although some appear to be polyclonal, EBV-driven proliferations which recede with withdrawal of the immunosuppression, others clearly become clonal malignant lymphomas. Almost all appear to be predominantly B-cell disorders. In contrast to Burkitt's lymphoma, the EBV expression patterns in these proliferations consist of a mixture of cells with latency type 1, latency type 2 or cells expressing lytic genes.[49]

In the UK a graded therapeutic response is recommended, starting wherever possible with withdrawal or drastic reduction of the immunosuppressives, followed by weekly pulses of low-dose cyclophosphamide, vincristine and prednisolone if there is no immediate response. If this COP therapy does not produce resolution, then standard intensive B-cell NHL therapy is initiated. Outcome for the true clonal B-cell NHL in these circumstances is poor, and even in the polyclonal responses withdrawal of immunosuppression not infrequently leads to organ rejection (Hann I, UKCCCSG lymphoproliferative disease study (LPD) NHL 9404, 1997, personal communication). Alternative strategies which have been proposed, and to a limited extent activated, include the use of targeted anti-B-cell monoclonal antibodies,[50] and production of cytotoxic T lymphocytes against EBV-infected cells.[51,52] It is too early to know whether these approaches will be more successful.

Indications for high-dose chemotherapy with stem cell support

There now appear to be two clear indications for high-dose therapy:

1. partial remission achieved after intensive induction therapy in either T- or B-cell NHL;
2. those who relapse but respond on reinduction with second-line therapy.[16,17,53,54]

Early relapses tend to show high drug resistance rates, but late relapses, especially after 2 years of therapy for lymphoblastic NHL can be salvaged by high-dose chemotherapy.[40]

Future approaches

For ALL treatment most therapy groups are rapidly substituting systemic methotrexate and/or long courses of intrathecal therapy for cranial irradiation (see Chapter 27). Equi-efficacy and presumed reduced impact on CNS development plus growth are the reasons for this change. For lymphomas without CNS disease at diagnosis, this approach appears to be fully justified in lymphoblastic disease.[40] The SFOP's outstanding results with LMB '86 and '89 (81% EFS for CNS-positive B-cell patients) using high-dose methotrexate, cytarabine and triple intrathecal therapy plus irradiation, has questioned the need for, or at least the widespread use of, cranial irradiation in B-cell NHL also. Reduction of therapy for those with good prognostic features is clearly optimal and is the basis for the SFOP/UKCCCSG/POG B-cell protocol (M Gerrard, FAB LMB '96 protocol for advanced stage B-cell NHL [jointly SFOP/UKCCSG/POG], personal communication). This is a randomized study testing whether graded reduction of either cyclophosphamide dose, in order to reduce the risk of male infertility and possible second tumor formation, or the duration of therapy or both, can be introduced in some patients, particularly those with Stage III B-cell NHL. New prognostic markers may in the future be helpful, but at present, for B-cell disease, elevated LDH plus non-responsiveness after the initial COP therapy or other cytoreductive therapy as per BFM, are the most reliable indicators of poor disease, and a definitive contraindication for reduced therapy.

Specific targeted monoclonal antibody therapy has been utilized in adult high-grade NHL, but not systematically in children. Antisense oligonucleotide therapy has been proposed and tested again in adult tumors,[55] and also *in vitro* in Burkitt's cell lines. McManaway *et al*,[56] using an antisense RNA oligonucleotide sequence, demonstrated a reduction in cell proliferation and in *c-myc* protein synthesis. The method did not work in all B-cell lines. Such targeted therapy looks as if it may have a role in cytoreduction, especially in patients with residual disease. The primatized B-cell-depleting monoclonal antibody IDEC-C2B8 has been approved for trial in adults with non-responsive follicular B-cell NHL. If proven effective, there may be a place for its use in refractory childhood tumors.

HODGKIN'S DISEASE

It is now widely accepted that Hodgkin's disease (HD) is a true malignancy with the mononuclear HD cell and the polynucleated Reed–Sternberg cells representing the malignant cells and derived from immature lymphoid elements. Exciting evidence suggesting an EBV association in some, if not all, childhood HD does not affect this concept of malignancy.

EPIDEMIOLOGY

Age-standardized incidence rates for children (0–15 years) vary considerably around the world, from 0.6/million in Japan to 10.3 in the Middle East, with European rates ranging from 3.3 (Sweden) to 6.9 (Italy). The UK rate is 4.1/million.[57,58] In western industrialized countries, incidence increases with age, whilst in developing countries an earlier onset (even peaking in the first decade) is seen, as well as a much higher relative proportion of mixed cellularity cases.[57,58] Incidence appears to be lower in colder latitudes where nodular sclerosis is more frequent. Genetic factors may be relevant because, for example, within the UK children of south Asian origin have a higher incidence of early onset mixed cellularity disease than those of north European caucasian origin. In the US there is a higher rate for black children under 10 years, but for white children during adolescence. Lymphocyte predominance is more common in black than white children in North America. In northern Europe there is a bimodal pattern with a peak at 15–30 years of age of predominantly nodular sclerotic type, and a second at 45–55 with mixed cellularity and other subtypes predominating. Boys predominate in the first decade (ratio 10:1) but by adolescence there is no sex difference.

ETIOLOGY

Case clusters,[59] patterns of seasonal variation[60] and an increased risk for children living in poor socioeconomic circumstances[57] and amongst large sibships developing HD in early life has long raised the suggestion that HD was of infectious etiology.[61] The bimodal peak seen in north Europe and America strongly resembles the epidemiology of, for example, polio virus. The identification of EBV inclusions, especially in early-onset mixed cellularity subtype[62,63] and in cases from developing countries has fueled speculation of a causative relationship,[64] at least in some circumstances. Rather like Burkitt's lymphoma, other antigens and cofactors may be necessary or are involved, but for at least some cases the response to such viral infection, including genetic rearrangements and initiation of inflammatory and cytokine responses, could explain the mixed pathologic pattern. There have been occasional reports of familial clusters,[65] as well as association with immunodeficiency disorders, sug-

gesting genetic factors may be relevant for some children at least.

CELL BIOLOGY AND PATHOLOGY

The principle malignant cell is considered to be the Reed–Sternberg (R–S) cell, a large multinucleated giant cell, with inclusion-like nucleoli surrounded by a clear halo. The mononuclear cells and the lacunar R–S cell seen especially in nodular sclerosing subtype are also considered to be malignant cells. However, the mere presence of these cells is not diagnostic, since on occasions they can be found in a variety of other conditions, including infectious mononucleosis and graft-versus-host disease. 'Malignant' cells in the midst of a reactive collection of lymphocytes, histiocytes, plasma cells, eosinophils and fibroblasts are the characteristic pattern of HD. Table 28.4 shows the Rye histopathologic classification scheme in universal usage for HD.[66] The categories are determined by the relative proportions of R–S cells, lymphocytes, sclerosis and fibrosis. There is variability in reported series of different proportions of subtypes (Table 28.4), but mixed cellularity is seen much more commonly in younger patients and in those from developing countries.[64,67] Lymphocyte depletion is rare in the UK and north European children, whilst nodular sclerosis and mixed cellularity are seen in roughly equal proportions. Non-random cytogenetic changes have been reported (involving chromosomes 1, 2, 7, 11, 14, 15 and 21) as well as the presence of a t(2;5) translocation in occasional cases. Whether these represent true HD or are ALCL remains unclear.[68]

There does appear to be some correlation between patterns of presentation and histopathology. Mixed cellularity and lymphocyte-depleted forms usually present with more disseminated disease; and nodular sclerosis classically with mediastinal disease in adolescents and lymphocyte predominant disease with focal nodal disease (characteristically in the neck or groin).

CLINICAL PRESENTATION

The commonest presentation is painless cervical lymphadenopathy with or without a mediastinal mass. The cervical nodes quite characteristically fluctuate in size, often over a considerable time, giving long latent periods between first symptom/sign and diagnosis. The presence of certain symptoms (termed 'B' symptoms) confers a less favorable

Table 28.4 Rye histopathologic classification of Hodgkin's disease.

Lymphocyte predominance	(7–14%)*
Nodular Sclerosis	(17–68%)
Mixed Cellularity	(17–68%)
Lymphocyte depletion	(0.5–20%)

*Percentages represent ranges of relative incidence reported by different pathologists in childhood series.

prognosis, and are seen with increasing frequency in more advanced-stage disease. The symptoms of note are: fever, night sweats and loss of 10% or more of body weight over the preceding 6 months, without another clear-cut explanation. Primary disease of the spleen, liver and lung pose particular diagnostic difficulties.

DIAGNOSTIC INVESTIGATIONS AND STAGING

Biopsy

Adequate biopsy from the most accessible, preferably primary, tumor mass is essential. Open rather than needle biopsies are optimal, since reactive surrounding lymphadenopathy can lead to false negativity in HD and the full pattern of cellularity within the tumor needs to be reviewed in order to classify the patient properly. Careful clinical examination to detect nodal disease and organomegaly is essential where a node's involvement would alter the stage of disease and therefore determine appropriate therapy. Confirmation of disease by appropriate imaging and/or biopsy is essential.

Imaging

Especially in the neck, the mere size of nodes is no guarantee of involvement. Mediastinal disease, which is usually clinically silent, is seen in about 60% of children, but this figure rises with age and it should be evaluated using good posterior/anterior and lateral radiographs. CT scanning of the chest is now considered essential to identify nodal, pleural and pulmonary disease, but, as for other diseases, identifies more nodal and pulmonary deposits than previously seen with conventional X-rays. There is a consequent upstaging of patients compared with historic series. MRI scans are being employed increasingly to visualize abdominal organs and nodal disease, but the 'gold' standard imaging for HD at diagnosis remains plain chest radiographs and CT scans of chest and abdomen. Lymphangiography (a technically difficult procedure), once the mainstay of abdominal node detection, is now rarely performed. Ultrasound can be used to monitor nodal, hepatic and splenic shrinkage with therapy. Lymphangiography did enable both size and architecture of nodes to be examined, but MR scanning is probably superior to CT in doing this, and it may be every bit as efficient as lymphangiography and much less invasive. Gallium scanning has its advocates, particularly for mediastinal disease, but it does have a false negativity rate and is only really useful in monitoring response if disease is shown to take up the isotope at diagnosis. There is no doubt that head and neck disease is better defined by MR scanning.

Laparotomy

There now appears to be little or no indication for primary staging laparotomy in children. Once the only truly reliable method of determining subdiaphragmatic disease, and hence in working out appropriate therapy options, especially radiation fields, it is a procedure associated with morbidity (intestinal obstruction) and even mortality (especially the life-long risk of septic death post splenectomy).[69] Where patients have residual disease or recurrence which necessitates such a procedure, especially splenectomy, preoperative vaccination with pneumococcal and *Haemophilus influenzae* vaccines plus life-long prophylactic oral penicillin are essential. Death can occur up to 20 years post-splenectomy from a wide range of infective agents, not just pneumococcus. Thankfully, the use of combined modality therapy, or at least intensive chemotherapy for the majority of patients obviates the need for such primary staging laparatomy, especially as MR scanning and imaging-guided biopsies can be performed if abdominal organ involvement is in doubt. With modern intensive therapy, isolated liver, spleen or other organ relapses are really quite rare.

Bone marrow studies

Bone marrow aspirates (2) and trephines (2) should be performed in all patients. Although bone marrow disease is much more common in advanced disease, an occasional patient with otherwise Stage II disease is found to have marrow infiltration and failure to treat this appropriately leads to early recurrence. Those with B symptoms, an altered blood picture, or the rare bony disease are certainly at higher risk of bone marrow infiltration. MRI is identifying abnormal marrow patterns in an increasing number of cases, but its true significance awaits further evaluation.

Blood tests

Useful laboratory investigations include a full blood count, ESR, viral titers for EBV, CMV, measles, chicken pox and rubella status, and biochemical assessment of renal and liver function. Markers which have been reported to be useful include the non-specific serum copper (elevated levels are a predictor of relapse), IL-2-receptors and CD8 antigen (correlates with advanced disease and B symptoms). However, routine use of any of these is not yet recommended.

Staging

Table 28.5 shows the Ann Arbor staging scheme universally employed in HD.[70] In most reported series low-stage disease (I and II) accounts for 50–70% of cases, while Stage IV is seen in <10% of childhood patients, and Stage III in 20–40%. The variation in percentages reported in different series depends on the methods used in staging, and the rigor of clinical and imaging procedures employed.

Table 28.5 Ann Arbor staging system for Hodgkin's disease.

Stage I	Involvement of 1 lymph node region (I) or a single extra-lymphatic organ or site (IE)
Stage II	Involvement of 2 or more lymph node regions on the same side of the diaphragm (II) or solitary involvement of an extra-lymphatic organ or site and of 1 or more lymph node regions on the same side of the diaphragm (IIE)
Stage III	Involvement of lymph node regions on both sides of the diaphragm (III) which may be accompanied by localized involvement of extra-lymphatic organ or site (IIIE) or by involvement of the spleen (IIIS) or both of the these (IIISE)
Stage IV	Diffuse or disseminated involvement of 1 or more extra-lymphatic organs or tissues with or without associated lymph node enlargement

Prognostic features

Advanced stage in the presence of B symptoms confers adverse prognostic significance. Pathologic subtype used to be more significant in predicting relapse, but with modern aggressive therapy is less so, although patients with the rare lymphocyte-depleted form do fare worse than all other types. Lukes and Butler[66] originally described 2 forms of lymphocyte-predominant type, a diffuse and a nodular form. The latter is a very slowly progressive disease that may with time evolve into a more advanced form of the disease, particularly if not treated.

Lymphopenia is a sign of advanced disease and is consequently a less favorable feature. Neutrophilia and eosinophilia are not thought to be of prognostic significance. An elevated ESR predicts more advanced stage disease, and if found in Stage I disease, unless in the presence of clearly defined and confirmed infection, should lead to a much more extensive search for occult disease. Patients with B symptoms usually have markedly elevated ESR levels. Intensive staging procedures alter the proportions of patients in each stage, pushing about 20% up from Stage I and II to Stage III. If, as in the UK, chemotherapy is used for all except Stage IA patients, precise exclusion of disease elsewhere is only required in Stage I disease. Although clearly the more accurate the definition of disease extent the easier it is to give prognostic advice to patients and their families, the important principle is not to understage the disease.

TREATMENT

Since Kaplan's report in 1970[71] of the effectiveness of 40–44 Gy in curing HD, a number of controversies have dogged the management of childhood disease:

1. If irradiation is to be utilized, how large should the field be and what is the optimal dosage and scheduling?
2. Is chemotherapy as effective, and indeed can it replace, irradiation?
3. Which group of patients requires combined modality therapy?
4. Which combination of drugs is both efficacious and least likely to cause long-term toxicity, either alone or in combination with radiation?

In deciding treatment strategies, therapeutic groups have tried to balance the beneficial and adverse effects of each treatment modality and of individual drug toxicities.

Depending on total dose, fraction size, field and patient's age (the younger the patient, the more likely tissue damage is long-term), neck, mantle and total nodal irradiation will produce compensated or full-blown hypothyroidism,[72] risk of thyroid malignancy,[73] soft tissue thinning, chest and spinal deformities (short clavicles and high spinal kyphosis) and impaired spinal growth.[74] Reactive pleural and pericardial effusions, long-term fibrosis and even restrictive pericarditis have been described, as has an increased risk of coronary artery disease. Chronic radiation enteritis and retroperitoneal fibrosis are reported following abdominal radiation in HD (see below).

Successful chemotherapy regimens from MOPP to ABVD (adriamycin, bleomycin, vinblastine and dacarbazine) carry specific hazards also. Azoospermia is to be expected following the dose of alkylators (mustine, procarbazine, chlorambicil or cyclophosphamide) needed to cure HD.[75] Whether there is a safe alkylator dosage is unclear. MOPP and other derivative regimens appear to have less impact on female fertility, especially in young girls, but loss of follicles may be associated with subsequent premature menopause. The ABVD regimen appears to have much less impact on the gonads, but much greater impact on pulmonary[76] and cardiac function.[77] These risks are compounded by the use of adjuvant radiotherapy and are even seen in hybrid regimens using, for example, 3 cycles of MOPP and 3 of ABVD. Chemotherapy-induced second-tumor induction is a major worry in this disease where long-term survival is over 80%. The Late Effects Study group has reported an actuarial second-tumor risk of 9% at 15 years from diagnosis (two-thirds solid tumors, one-third therapeutically-induced AML).[73] The closest association is between irradiation and alkylators for soft tissue tumors, and with dose of alkylators received for ANLL.[78] Although ABVD was previously reported to be at low risk of inducing such tumors, anthracyclines are increasingly implicated in the causation of leukemia. Consequently, in planning any therapeutic strategy these effects and benefits must be weighed carefully.

Specific treatment

Given the risks of combined modality therapy, attempts have been made to reduce radiation fields to involved areas only, and to reduce the total dose from 40–45 Gy to 20–30 Gy, especially in patients showing good initial response to chemotherapy for Stages I–III disease.[79–81] In addition, the number of courses of chemotherapy given for low-stage disease has been reduced from 6 to 3 cycles of MOPP, along with subsequent involved field irradiation.[79] Similarly, limited cycles of ABVD and local irradiation have been repeatedly demonstrated to be as efficacious as MOPP.[82,83] Donaldson and Link[81] reported a 93% DFS rate for Stage I and II patients treated with short-duration chemotherapy and involved field irradiation. Other regimens have been devised to try to reduce exposure to alkylating agents, including VEBP (vinblastine, etoposide, bleomycin and prednisolone) and VEEP (bleomycin omitted, epirubicin substituted) with varying responses and not always the predicted reduction of late sequelae. Often, one late effect is replaced by another.

Some researchers have attempted to treat the majority of patients with chemotherapy only. Ertem et al[84] recently reported on a series (1985–1995) given COPP or COPP/ABVD alone; over 50% of their patients had advanced disease and 56% mixed cellularity histology. None initially received any radiotherapy. Five-year EFS (total survival) was 92.3% (77.8%) for Stages I and II and 89.5% (67.4%) for Stages III and IV, but all did receive more chemotherapy than is used in the mixed modality regimens. No significant sequelae have been reported but follow-up is still relatively short. The authors emphasize that their series represents good results for mostly high-risk patients with type I HD (i.e. young age and predominantly mixed cellularity). The somewhat superior results reported from the US and north Europe are perhaps more reflective of the disease type than the actual therapy.[83]

Van den Berg et al[85] reported on treatment with 6 cycles of MOPP, with radiotherapy only for patients with bulky disease (nodes >4 cm in diameter), and then from 1984 with 6 courses of ABVD only, and since 1987 with alternating courses of ABVD and MOPP (total of 6). EFS (total survival) was 91% (100%) for those treated with MOPP, 70% (94%) for ABVD only, and 91% (91%) for the hybrid regimen. One patient treated with MOPP developed NHL 10 years from the initial diagnosis of HD but is now in remission, and a girl who relapsed after ABVD was subsequently treated with MOPP (8 cycles) plus total nodal irradiation and developed a myelodysplasia from which she died. Echocardiography has not revealed significant cardiac impairment in their patients, but pulmonary function tests have showed decreased carbon monoxide diffusion in 8 of 17 patients treated with ABVD alone, and 5 of 21 treated with the hybrid regime (bleomycin was given over 6 hours). All boys who received MOPP have severe gonadal damage, whilst in the hybrid regimen 3 of 10 males tested had elevated follicle stimulating or luteinizing hormone levels (in 1 case both). The authors conclude that 6 cycles of ABVD/MOPP without radiotherapy is tolerable and provides good survival. The ABVD/MOPP patients were, however, overwhelmingly of low stage (7 Stage I, 8 Stage II, 2 Stage IIIA) with only 3 Stage IIIB and 1 Stage IVB case.

The UKCCSG recently reported on a series of 369 patients aged 0–16 years treated between 1982 and 1992 using single modality therapy.[86] Patients with Stage IA disease received involved field radiation to a total dose of 35 Gy delivered in 20 fractions. No chemotherapy was given in order to avoid the sequelae of combined modality therapy in these good risk patients. Of the 92 Stage I patients, overall survival was 92%, although progression-free survival (PFS) was 70%, with 28% of patients requiring re-treatment for relapse. Interestingly, the only subgroup where histology appeared to influence relapse rate was mixed cellularity, which showed 48% PFS compared with 77% of the lymphocyte predominant and 80% of the nodular sclerosing subtypes.[86] Histology had no effect in all other stages where chemotherapy was utilized. The UKCCSG still feels that for all but mixed cellularity cases the overall survival figures for Stage IA patients justifies the approach of limited radiotherapy only, since it appears that salvage chemotherapy for these specific patients has a very high rate of success. With this strategy a majority of patients still escape the need for exposure to any gonado-toxic chemotherapy. A number of reports have confirmed that involved field control rates are 99% with dosages in the range of 30–35 Gy and they do not improve with higher dosage.[87,88]

In the UKCCSG study, patients with all other stages of disease received ChlVPP chemotherapy (chlorambucil 6 mg/m^2 orally on days 1–14, vinblastine 6 mg/m^2 intravenously on days 1 and 8; procarbazine 100 mg/m^2 orally on days 1–14, and prednisolone 40 mg/m^2 orally for 14 days). The courses are repeated every 28 days, and the number of cycles delivered ranged from 6 to 10 depending on the speed of remission. Radiotherapy was confined to those with a bulky mediastinal mass (where it exceeded one-third of the maximal chest diameter on plain, posterior/anterior and lateral radiographs). Ten-year PFS (and overall survival rates) were 85% (92%) for Stage II, 73% (84%) for Stage III and 38% (71%) for Stage IV. In this series, contrary to some other reports, most relapses occurred within the first 5 years from diagnosis. The overall survival results are not significantly different from the series reported using limited chemotherapy and involved field radiation, except in Stage IV patients, although EFS for Stage II and III appears to be slightly worse, but it does appear that the majority of relapsing patients with Stages II and III can be salvaged. A careful review of all second tumors has been made on this protocol; there is a 3.4% rate at 10 years (LESG reported 5%) of which 2.7% are leukemic/NHL and 0.7% solid tumors.

Hunger et al[89] reported 68% (standard error ± 13%) DFS (85% ± 10% overall survival) for clinical Stage IV patients given MOPP/ABVD plus involved field radiotherapy, and Oberlin et al[79] reported 62% 6-year DFS for Stage IV patients similarly treated. In the UK series, one-third of patients with Stage IV relapses have died. High-dose chemotherapy with stem cell transplantation (autologous marrow or peripheral stem cells) appears to be indicated for such relapsing patients, but not for most relapses with initially lower stage disease.[90] How many of the advanced-stage patients treated with longer courses of chemotherapy only, as in the UK series, who relapse can really be salvaged is unclear. Schellong et al,[91] in a series of Stage IV patients, reported an 81% EFS using vincristine, prednisolone, procarbazine, adriamycin, cyclophosphamide in the OPPA/ COPP regime, with limited involved field radiation. Following this experience, the International Society of Paediatric Oncology have reproduced the results in a European study, with the total irradiation dose limited to 20 Gy.

Summary

- Stage IA patients appear to be highly curable with involved field irradiation only (dosages 30–35 Gy), but will develop hypothyroidism and some soft tissue thinning of the neck. Chemotherapy can be equally effective, but the number of cycles needed for cure is unclear, and if possible exposure to alkylators should be restricted.
- In *Stages II and IIIA*, both short-course hybrid chemotherapy (3 cycles of MOPP or ChlVPP/AVBD or VEBP) with involved field irradiation (20 Gy), and chemotherapy alone (6 cycles of therapy) can be curative. However, without irradiation more chemotherapy appears to be required, i.e. 6 rather than 3 cycles, and there is probably an increased risk of sterility with therapy including alkylators, or cardiopulmonary dysfunction for those including anthracyclines and/or bleomycin. The long-term safety of the short course of chemotherapy with involved field irradiation has not been fully evaluated.
- For *advanced Stage IIIB and IV* patients, hybrid chemotherapy and limited radiotherapy (20 Gy) appears to be most efficacious, but the total duration of therapy required is not clear. The most favorable results are those reported by Schellong et al.[91]

There remains a need for less toxic chemotherapy regimens, but in a disease with such high survival there is always the danger of delivering reduced toxicity at the price of decreased antitumor efficacy.

LONG-TERM SEQUELAE OF LYMPHOMA THERAPY

Table 28.6 shows some of the potential sequelae of lymphoma therapy. These risks must be taken into consideration for both childhood NHL and HD because of the high overall cure rates now possible.

Late recurrence

Robertson et al[92] demonstrated a falling rate of late deaths from lymphoma since 1970, with only a slight rise in overall therapy-related deaths as intensity of treatment has increased. All but lymphoblastic NHL appears to relapse early, and in general a patient with NHL is deemed to be truly cured if in remission 10 years from diagnosis. HD,

Table 28.6 Potential long-term sequelae of childhood lymphomata.

Late recurrence

Secondary neoplasia

Growth impairment

Endocrine dysfunction

Infertility

Educational and psychologic dysfunction

Other organ toxicity, e.g. cardiac with anthracyclines, pulmonary with bleomycin

Problems with obtaining jobs, insurance and acceptance as adopters

although relapses do appear to occur early with modern therapy, is a rather insidious disease and late relapses are reported.

Second tumors

The overall risk 25 years from diagnosis of developing a second tumor for all children with cancer was reported as 3.7% in a UK population-based study,[93] and 12.1% in a treatment center-based study reported by the Late Effects Study Group,[94] which correspond to 6 and 15 times, respectively, the age-matched general population risk. The highest relative risk is for bone cancer for which exposure of the bone to irradiation in excess of 10 Gy and/or alkylating agents are major contributory factors.[95] This is clearly relevant in the treatment of HD where increasingly strenuous efforts are made to limit total dose of alkylators, especially in the context of mixed modality therapy. Similarly, alkylator exposure is associated with a 5-fold increased risk of developing a therapeutically-induced leukemia t(AL), often with monosomy 5 or 7. The Late Effects Study Group reported a 14-fold increase at 20 years from diagnosis of developing a therapeutically-induced acute leukemia.[96] Hawkins et al[97] reported a 1.4% rate of such leukemias in patients treated for NHL within the first 6 years from diagnosis, compared with only 0.5% for all other tumors. This increased risk appears to be associated with a specific era of treatment when high doses of epipodophyllotoxins were used in schedules not allowing for adequate DNA repair, and with a total dose in excess of 1.2 g/m^2. These second leukemias characteristically have a short latency and are associated with chromosomal translocations involving 11q23 (MLL gene). It is also important to remember that the anthracyclines included in many lymphoma protocols are also topoisomerase II inhibitors and are associated with therapeutically-induced acute leukemia.

Irradiation to the thyroid, especially if compensated hypothyroidism is not treated early, is associated with an increased risk of thyroid cancer.[98] The Late Effects Study Group in a follow-up study of 1380 childhood HD survivors reported an 18-fold overall increase in tumors, principally leukemias, but also a remarkable 75-fold increased risk of young women developing breast cancer at 20 years from diagnosis (17 cases compared with an expected 0.2 cases).[99] It has calculated a 35% risk of such young women developing breast cancer by the age of 40, especially when patients are treated in their teens and with higher total dosages of radiotherapy.

Growth impairment

Any lymphoma patient receiving CNS-directed radiotherapy will suffer the well-documented risk of induced growth hormone insufficiency.[100] Age at treatment and total plus fraction dose of radiation determine the extent of impairment. Modern protocols which omit irradiation probably avoid the risk, but high-dose intensity chemotherapy may have some direct effect on bone growth,[101] although not as great as that from hypothalamic-pituitary axis irradiation.

Endocrine dysfunction

Irradiation to the neck even at very low dosages (0.10 Gy) can induce thyroid dysfunction, initially with a rise in thyroid stimulating hormone and only subsequently a fall in T4.[102] Replacement therapy is almost universally required in HD patients treated with bilateral neck or mantle fields. Although many drugs used for lymphomas, especially alkylating agents, are gonadotoxic, and usually disproportionally affect fertility in boys, they are not steroidogenic (secondary sexual characteristics and potency are preserved). There is much less direct effect of chemotherapy on ovarian function, although follicle numbers may be reduced (inducing premature menopause). Conversely, irradiation, especially total nodal irradiation, has a major effect on ovarian function with a requirement for life-long hormonal replacement.[103]

Fertility

Male long-term survivors exposed to alkylating agents have a very low fertility rate, whilst females do not appear to be as severely affected, but abdominal irradiation affects fertility in both sexes,[104] depending on the dose received by the gonads. As mentioned above, premature menopause is a significant risk for adolescent lymphoma survivors, and is associated with exposure to alkylating agents (9 times the risk) and/or abdominal irradiation (4 times the risk), even in the third decade of life.[105] The prospects for any specific pregnancy are good provided extensive irradiation involving the pelvis (specifically uterine vasculature) has not been required. The original studies performed on mice and sheep to cryopreserve ovarian follicles and testicular tissue are being applied to volunteer teenagers.[106] The risk of cancer occurring in the offspring of childhood leukemia and NHL survivors appears to be very low.[107]

Educational and psychologic functioning

The well recorded impact of cranial irradiation (in dosages of 18–24 Gy) on neuropsychologic functioning includes impairment of attention span and cognitive processing skills.[108] Verbal IQ is frequently well preserved. Age at treatment, and possibly gender, influence the degree of impairment.[108] Current leukemia studies directly comparing function longitudinally between those irradiated and those treated with systemic high-dose methotrexate will help elucidate the impact chemotherapy has on neuropsychologic functioning. Similarly, the impact of intrathecal therapy alone is being assessed (G Vargha-Khadem, B Gibson, OB Eden, Medical Research Council Longitudinal Psychometric Study, 1997, personal communication).

Apart from the physical affects of CNS-directed therapy, patients who do not adjust well to the diagnosis, its treatment and survival have long-term schooling problems (especially attendance) and overall coping problems.

Organ dysfunction

The increasing risk of acute cardiac toxicity with increasing doses of anthracyclines is well recognized, but what is still far from clear is the true long-term risk of more moderate dose exposure. Lipshultz et al,[109] looking at ECG, exercise testing and echocardiograms, showed abnormalities in 65% of patients after a median of 360 mg/m² of doxoribucin. The rate of administration and female gender appear to be independent indicators of higher risk. The authors have reported test abnormalities; in contrast, the reported rate of overt cardiac disease is much lower. Nevertheless, given that survival rates for lymphomas are high, it seems prudent to:

1. Limit total dose of anthracylines wherever possible (the risk of reported abnormality below a cumulative dose of 200 mg/m² appears to be small).
2. Prolong infusion times of anthracyclines, although it appears that for a truly protective effect, infusion times in excess of 72–96 hours are required, and these may be associated with increased mucositis and myelosuppression.
3. Consider the use of cardioprotective agents such as ICRF 187 which has been shown, in a single pediatric study, to give a significantly reduced incidence of sub-clinical cardiotoxicity in patients receiving anthracyclines.[110]

Chest and mediastinal irradiation compounds the cardiotoxicity risk of anthracyclines. Even without chemotherapy, mediastinal irradiation has been reported to be associated with an increased early mortality risk from myocardial infarction (30 times the rate for the general population) amongst HD survivors.[111] These risks appear to be reduced if the total irradiation dose is lowered, and combined modality therapy not involving anthracyclines is used with limited involved field irradiation.

Chest or spinal irradiation in childhood may restrict the

growth of the chest wall and lungs, and subsequently progressive fibrosis may develop. For lymphomas, a much greater risk is associated with the use of bleomycin, particularly for HD. Acute toxicity is associated with high single doses, cumulative dose and exposure to high levels of oxygen.[112] The chronic toxicity of bleomycin is under further investigation. Following ABVD and limited field irradiation, Mefferd et al[77] reported impairment of carbon monoxide diffusion capacity in 6 of 11 HD patients tested, and 40% showed reduced lung volumes. Shaw et al[113] reported impaired lung growth in leukemic patients receiving identical therapy to that used for lymphoblastic lymphomas.

Soft tissue hypoplasia and bony damage from high-dose local irradiation has been mentioned in the context of early HD therapy, and is another reason for the reduction, wherever possible, of total dosages used.

For both HD and NHL, the aim of current worldwide studies is to identify high-risk patients for whom more intensive or novel therapies are required, whilst reducing wherever possible the sequelae of therapy for those with a high chance of cure.

REFERENCES

1. Parkin DM, Stiller CA, Bieber CA, Draper GJ, Terracini B, Young JL (eds). *International Incidence of Childhood Cancer*, IARC Scientific Publication No. 87. Lyon: IARC, 1988

2. Epstein MA, Achong BG, Barr YM. Virus particles in cultured lymphoblasts from Burkitt's lymphoma. *Lancet* 1964; **i**: 702–703

3. Lenoir G, O'Connor G, Olweny CLM (eds). *Burkitt's Lymphoma. A Human Cancer Model*, IARC Scientific Publication No. 60. Lyon: IARC, 1985, pp 165–176

4. Ladjadj Y, Philip T, Lenoir GM et al. Abdominal Burkitt-type lymphoma in Algeria. *Br J Cancer* 1984; **48**: 503–512

5. Gutierrez MI, Bhatia K, Barriga F et al. Molecular epidemiology of Burkitt's lymphoma from South America: differences in breakpoint location and EBV association from tumours in other world regions. *Blood* 1992; **79**: 3261–3266

6. Rabbits T, Boehm T. Structural and functional chimaerism results from chromosomal translocation in lymphoid tumours. *Adv Immunol* 1991; **50**: 119–146

7. Brubaker G, Levin AG, Steel CM et al. Multiple cases of Burkitt's lymphoma and other neoplasms in families in the North Mara District of Tanzania. *Int J Cancer* 1980; **26**: 165–170

8. Aya T, Kinoshita T, Imai S et al. Chromosome translocation and c-MYC activation by Epstein–Barr virus and *Euphorbia tirucalli* in B lymphocytes. *Lancet* 1991; **337**: 1190

9. Hamilton-Dutoit SJ, Rea D, Raphael M et al. Epstein–Barr virus latent gene expression and tumour cell phenotype in acquired immunodeficiency syndrome-related NHL. Correlation of lymphoma phenotype with three distinct patterns of viral latency. *Am J Pathol* 1993; **143**: 1072–1085

10. Hecht F, Morgan R, Gemmill RM et al. Translocations in T-cell leukemia and lymphoma. *N Engl J Med* 1985; **313**: 758

11. Mason DY, Bastard C, Rimokh R et al. CD30-positive large cell lymphomas (Ki-1 lymphomas) are associated with a chromosomal translocation involving 5q34. *Br J Haematol* 1990; **74**: 161–168

12. Grierson H, Purtillo DT. Epstein–Barr virus infections in males with the X-linked lymphoproliferative syndrome. *Ann Intern Med* 1987; **106**: 538–545

13. Attard-Montalto SP, Schuller I, Lastowska MA, Gibbons B, Kingston JE, Eden OB. Non-Hodgkin's lymphoma and Klinefelter syndrome. *Pediatr Hematol Oncol* 1994; **11**: 197–200

14. Murphy SB, Fairclough DL, Hutchison RE, Berard CW. Non-Hodgkin's lymphoma of childhood: an analysis of the histology, staging and response to treatment of 338 cases at a single institution. *J Clin Oncol* 1989; **7**: 186–193

15. Murphy SB. Classification, staging and end results of treatment of childhood non-Hodgkin's lymphoma: dissemination from lymphomas in adults. *Semin Oncol* 1980; **7**: 332–339

16. Shepherd SF, Aherne RP, Pinkerton CR. Childhood T-cell lymphoblastic lymphoma – does early resolution of mediastinal mass predict for final outcome? *Br J Cancer* 1995; **72**: 752–756

17. Philip T, Hartmann O, Biron P et al. High dose therapy and autologous bone marrow transplantation in partial remission after first line induction therapy for diffuse non-Hodgkin's lymphoma. *J Clin Oncol* 1988; **6**: 1118–1124

18. Masera G, Jankovic M, Zurlo MG, Locasciulli A, Rossi M, Underzo C, Recchia M. Urate-oxidase prophylaxis of uric acid-induced renal damage in childhood leukemia. *J Pediatr* 1982; **100**: 152–155

19. Patte C, Philip T, Rodary C et al. High survival rate in advanced stage B cell lymphomas and leukemias without CNS involvement with a short intensive polychemotherapy: results from the French Pediatric Oncology Society of a randomised trial of 216 children. *J Clin Oncol* 1991; **9**: 123–132

20. Leblanc A, Caillaud JM, Hartmann O et al. Hypercalcaemia preferentially occurs in unusual forms of childhood non-Hodgkin's lymphoma, rhabdomyosarcoma and Wilms' tumour. *Cancer* 1984; **54**: 2132–2136

21. Wollner N, Exelby PR, Lieberman PH. Non-Hodgkin's lymphoma in children. A progress report on the original patients treated with the LSA2L2 protocol. *Cancer* 1979; **44**: 1990–1999

22. Anderson JR, Wilson JF, Jenkin DT et al. Childhood non-Hodgkin's lymphoma: results of a randomised therapeutic trial comparing a 4 drug regimen (COMP) to a 10 drug regimen (LSA2L2). *N Engl J Med* 1983; **308**: 559–565

23. Anderson JR, Jenkin RDT, Wilson JF et al. Long term follow up of patients treated with Comp or LSA2L2 therapy for childhood NHL: a report of CCG-551 from the Children's Cancer Study Group. *J Clin Oncol* 1993; **11**: 1024–1032

24. Meadows AT, Sposto R, Jenkin RDT et al. Similar efficacy of 6 and 18 months of therapy with four drugs (COMP) for localised non-Hodgkin's lymphoma of children: a report from the Children's Cancer Study Group. *J Clin Oncol* 1989; **7**: 92–99

25. Hvizdala EV, Berard C, Callihan T et al. Non lymphoblastic lymphoma in children – histology and stage-related response to therapy: A Pediatric Oncology Group Study. *J Clin Oncol* 1991; **9**: 1189–1195

26. Gerrard M, Pinkerton R, Hann I. Excellent outcome for children with localised NHL treated with short duration chemotherapy. Where now with therapy? *Med Ped Oncol* 1990; **18**: 39 (abstract SIOP)

27. Patte C, Michon J, Behrendt H et al. Updated results of the LMB 89 protocol of the SFOP (French Pediatric Oncology Society) for childhood B-cell lymphoma and leukemia (ALL). *Ann Oncol* 1996; **7**: 30 (abstract 96)

28. Reiter A, Schrappe M, Parwaresch R et al. Non-Hodgkin's lymphoma of childhood and adolescence: results of a treatment stratified for biologic subtypes and stage. A report of the Berlin–Frankfurt–Munster Group. *J Clin Oncol* 1995; **13**: 359–372

29. Patte C, Kalifa C, Flamant F et al. Results of the LMT 81 protocol, a modified LSA2L2 protocol with high dose methotrexate, on 84 children with non B-cell lymphoma. *Med Pediatr Oncol* 1992; **20**: 105–113

30. Jenkin RDT, Anderson JR, Chilcote RR et al. The treatment of localised non-Hodgkin's lymphoma in children: a report from the Children's Cancer Study Group. *J Clin Oncol* 1984; **2**: 88–97

31. Saha V, Eden OB, Hann I, Attard-Montalto S, Cotterill S, Carter R.

Primary extra thoracic T-cell non-Hodkgin's lymphoma of childhood. *Leukemia* 1995; **9**: 40–43

32. Patte C, Philip T, Rodary C *et al.* Improved survival rate in children with Stage III and IV B-cell NHL and leukemia using a multi agent chemotherapy regimen: results of a study of 114 children from SFOP. *J Clin Oncol* 1986; **4**: 1219–1229

33. Reiter A, Schrappe M, Henzler D *et al* for the BMF group. Risk group definition, treatment strategy and preliminary results for B-cell neoplasias in trial NHL-BFM90. *Med Pediatr Oncol* 1993; **21**: 550 (abstract SIOP)

34. Hann IM, Eden OB, Barnes J, Pinkerton CR. MACHO chemotherapy for Stage IV B-cell lymphoma and B-ALL of childhood. *Br J Haematol* 1988; **76**: 359–364

35. Pinkerton CR, Hann IM, Eden OB *et al.* Outcome in Stage III non-Hodgkin's lymphoma in children. How much treatment is needed? *Br J Cancer* 1991; **64**: 583–587

36. Murphy SB, Bowman WP, Abromowitch M *et al.* Results of treatment of advanced stage Burkitt's lymphoma and B-cell (Sig+ve) ALL with high dose fractionated cyclophosphamide and co-ordinated high dose methotrexate and cytarabine. *J Clin Oncol* 1986; **4**: 1732–1739

37. Brecher M, Murphy SB, Bowman P, Sullivan MP, Shuster J, Berard C. Results of POG 8617. In: *Proceedings of the American Society of Clinical Oncology*, 1992, p 340 (abstract 1167)

38. Cairo M, Krailo M, Morse M *et al.* Disseminated non-lymphoblastic NHL (DNL NHL) of childhood. *Ann Oncol* 1979; **7**: 29 (abstract 93)

39. Eden OB, Hann I, Imeson J *et al.* Treatment of advanced stage T-cell lymphoblastic lymphoma: results of the United Kingdom Children's Cancer Study Group protocol 8503. *Br J Haematol* 1992; **82**: 310–316

40. Eden OB, Saha V, Hann I *et al.* Results of three consecutive UKCCSG trials for advanced Stage T-cell NHL. *Med Pediatr Oncol* 1993; **21**: 550 (abstract SIOP)

41. Mott MG, Eden OB, Palmer MK. Adjuvant low dose radiation in childhood non-Hodgkin's lymphoma. *Br J Cancer* 1984; **50**: 463–469

42. Paulli M, Berti E, Rosso R *et al.* CD30/Ki-1 positive lymphoproliferative disorders of the skin – clinico-pathological correlation and statistical analysis of 86 cases. *J Clin Oncol* 1995; **13**: 1343–1354

43. Chakravarti V, Kamani NR, Bayever E *et al.* Bone marrow transplantation for childhood Ki positive lymphoma. *J Clin Oncol* 1990; **8**: 657–660

44. Gasparini M, Gianni C, Morandi F *et al.* Large cell anaplastic Ki-1+ lymphoma of children. *Med Pediatr Oncol* 1988; **16**: 406

45. Reiter A, Schrappe M, Tiemann M *et al.* Successful treatment strategy for Ki-1 anaplastic large cell lymphoma of childhood: a prospective analysis of 62 patients enrolled in three consecutive Berlin–Frankfurt–Munster group studies. *J Clin Oncol* 1994; **12**: 899–908

46. Sandlund JT, Pui Ch, Santana VM *et al.* Clinical features and treatment outcome for children with CD3+ large cell non-Hodgkin's lymphoma. *J Clin Oncol* 1994; **12**: 885–898

47. Lazzarino M, Orlandi E, Paulli M *et al.* Primary mediastinal B-cell lymphoma with sclerosis, an aggressive tumor with distinctive clinical and pathological features. *J Clin Oncol* 1993; **11**: 2306–2313

48. Ribeiro PC, Pui CH, Murphy SB *et al.* Childhood malignant non-Hodgkin's lymphoma of uncommon histology. *Leukemia* 1992; **6**: 761–765

49. Oudejans JJ, Jiwa M, van den Brule A *et al.* Detection of heterogeneous Epstein–Barr virus gene expression patterns within individual post transplantation lymphoproliferative disorders. *Am J Pathol* 1995; **147**: 923–233

50. Fischer A, Blanche S, Le Bidois *et al.* Anti B-cell monoclonal antibodies in the treatment of severe B-cell lymphoproliferative syndrome following bone marrow and organ transplantation. *N Engl J Med* 1991; **324**: 1451–1456

51. Papadopoulos EB, Ladanyi M, Emmanuel D *et al.* Infusions of donor leucocytes to treat EBV associated lymphoproliferative disorders after allogeneic bone marrow transplantation. *N Engl J Med* 1994; **330**: 1185–1191

52. Rooney CM, Smith CA, Ng C *et al.* Use of gene modified virus specific T lymphocytes to control EBV related lymphoproliferation. *Lancet* 1995; **345**: 9–13

53. Ebell W, Reiter A, Bettoni da Cunha C *et al.* Busulphan, etoposide and cyclophosphamide (B4/VP76/Cy) or thiotepa (Bu/VP16/TT) as conditioning regimen for BMT in poor risk B-cell neoplasms of childhood: the BFM strategy. *Med Pediatr Oncol* 1993; **21**: 536 (abstract SIOP)

54. Philip T, Hartmann O, Michon J *et al.* Curability of relapsed childhood B-cell NHL following intensive first line therapy. *Blood* 1993; **81**: 2003–2006

55. Webb A, Cunningham D, Cotter F *et al.* BCL-2 antisense therapy in patients with non-Hodgkin's lymphoma. *Lancet* 1997; **349**: 1137–1141

56. McManaway ME, Neckers LM, Loke SL *et al.* Tumour specific inhibition of lymphoma growth by an antisense oligodeoxynucleotide. *Lancet* 1990; **335**: 808–810

57. Guthenson N, Cole P. Epidemiology of Hodgkin's disease in the young. *Int J Cancer* 1977; **19**: 595–604

58. Stiller CA, Parkin DM. International variations in the incidence of childhood lymphoma. *Paediatr Perinat Epidemiol* 1990; **4**: 303–324

59. Alexander FE, Williams J, McKinney PA *et al.* A specialist leukaemia/lymphoma registry in the U.K. Part 2: Clustering of Hodgkin's disease. *Br J Cancer* 1989; **60**: 948–952.

60. Birch JM, Westerbeek R, Blair V, Eden OB, Kelsey A. Seasonal variations in onset of Hodgkin's disease and acute lymphoblastic leukaemia in North West England. *Med Pediatr Oncol* 1997; **29**: 364 (abstract)

61. Guthenson N, Cole P. Childhood social environment and Hodgkin's disease. *N Engl J Med* 1981; **304**: 135–140

62. Herbst H, Niedobitek G, Kneba M *et al.* High incidence of Epstein–Barr virus genomes in Hodgkin's disease. *Am J Pathol* 1990; **137**: 13–18

63. Wright CF, Reid AH, Tsai MM *et al.* Detection of Epstein–Barr virus sequences in Hodgkin's disease by the polymerase chain reaction. *Am J Pathol* 1991; **138**: 393–398

64. Weinreb M, Day PJR, Niggli F *et al.* The role of Epstein–Barr virus in Hodgkin's disease from different geographical areas. *Arch Dis Child* 1996; **74**: 27–31

65. Grufferman S, Cole P, Smith P, Lukes RJ. Hodgkin's disease in siblings. *N Engl J Med* 1979; **300**: 1006–1011

66. Lukes RJ, Butler JJ. The pathology and nomenclature of Hodgkin's disease. *Cancer Res* 1966; **26**: 1063–1068

67. Cavdar AO, Tacoy A, Babacan E *et al.* Hodgkin's disease in Turkish children: a clinical and histopathological analysis. *J Natl Cancer Inst* 1977; **58**: 479–481

68. Orscheschek K, Merz H, Hell J *et al.* Large cell anaplastic lymphoma – specific translocation t(2;5) (p23;q35) in Hodgkin's disease: indication of a common pathogenesis. *Lancet* 1995; **345**: 87–90

69. Donaldson SS, Glatstein E, Vosti KL. Bacterial infection in paediatric Hodgkin's disease: relationship to radiotherapy, chemotherapy and splenectomy. *Cancer* 1978; **41**: 1949–1958

70. Carbone PP, Kaplan HS, Musshof K *et al.* Report of the Committee on Hodgkin's Disease Staging. *Cancer Res* 1971; **31**: 1860–1861

71. Kaplan HS. On the natural history, treatment and prognosis of Hodgkin's disease. In: *Harvey Lectures, 1968–1969.* New York: Academic Press, 1970, pp 251–259

72. Kaplan MM, Garnick MB, Gelber R *et al.* Risk factors for thyroid abnormalities after neck irradiation for childhood cancer. *Am J Med* 1983; **74**: 272–274

73. Meadows A, Obringer A, Marrero O *et al.* Second malignant neoplasms following childhood Hodgkin's disease: treatment and splenectomy as risk factors. *Med Pediatr Oncol* 1989; **17**: 477–484

74. Donaldson SS, Kleeberg P, Cox R. Growth abnormalities with radiation in children with Hodgkin's disease. *Proc Am Soc Clin Oncol* 1988; **7**: 864 (abstract)

75. Aubier F, Flamant F, Brauner R *et al.* Male gonadal function after chemotherapy for solid tumours in childhood. *J Clin Oncol* 1989; **7**: 304–309

76. Cosset JM, Henry-Amar M, Thomas J *et al.* Increased pulmonary

toxicity in the ABVD arm of the EORTC H6-U Trial. *Proc Am Soc Clin Oncol* 1989; **8**: 985 (abstract)

77. Mefford JM, Donaldson SS, Link MP. Pediatric Hodgkin's disease: pulmonary, cardiac and thyroid function following combined modality therapy. *Int J Radiat Oncol* 1979; **16**: 679–685

78. Oberlin O, Bathia S, Robison L, Meadows AT. Second malignant neoplasms after childhood Hodgkin's disease. In: *Proceedings of Third International Symposium on Hodgkin's Lymphoma*, 1995, abstract 65

79. Oberlin O, Boilletot A, Leverger G *et al*. Clinical staging, primary chemotherapy and involved field radiotherapy in childhood Hodgkin's disease. *Eur Paediatr Hematol Oncol* 1985; **2**: 65–70

80. Gehan EA, Sullivan MP, Fuller LM. Report from The Intergroup Hodgkin's Disease in Children. A Study of Stages I and II. *Cancer* 1990; **65**: 1429–1437

81. Donaldson SS, Link MP. Combined modality treatment with low dose radiation for children with Hodgkin's disease. *J Clin Oncol* 1987; **5**: 742–749

82. Fossati-Bellani F, Gasparini M, Kenda A *et al*. Limited field and low dose radiotherapy + ABVD chemotherapy for childhood Hodgkin's disease. In: *Proceedings of 27th International Society of Paediatric Oncology*, Venice, 1985, abstracts 323 and 324.

83. Oberlin O, Leverger G, Paquement H *et al*. Low dose radiation therapy and reduced chemotherapy in childhood Hodgkin's disease: the experience of the French Society of Pediatric Oncology. *J Clin Oncol* 1992; **10**: 1407–1412.

84. Ertem U, Duru F, Dagdemir A, *et al*. Hodgkin's disease in 82 Turkish children diagnosed over a 10 year period: epidemiological, clinical and histopathologic features and prognosis with prolonged chemotherapy. *Pediatr Hematol Oncol* 1997; **14**: 359–366

85. van den Berg H, Zsiros J, Behrendt H. Treatment of childhood Hodgkin's disease without radiotherapy. *Ann Oncol* 1997; **8**: 15–17

86. Shankar AG, Ashley S, Radford M, Barrett A, Wright D, Pinkerton CR. Does histology influence outcome in childhood Hodgkin's disease? Results from the U.K. Children's Cancer Study Group. *J Clin Oncol* 1997; **15**: 2622–2630

87. Hanks G, Kinzie J, Kramer S *et al*. Patterns of care outcome studies: results of the national practice in Hodgkin's disease. *Cancer* 1983; **51**: 569–573

88. Schewe K, Reavis J, Cox JD *et al*. Total dose, fraction size and tumour volume in the local control of Hodgkin's disease. *Int J Radiat Oncol Biol Phys* 1988; **15**: 25–28

89. Hunger SP, Link MP, Donaldson SS. ABVD/MOPP and low dose involved field radiotherapy in pediatric Hodgkin's disease: the Stanford experience. *J Clin Oncol* 1994; **12**: 2160–2166

90. Bessa E, Pacquement H, Hartmann O *et al*. Long term survival of refractory or relapsed Hodgkin's disease treated by high dose chemotherapy (HDC) with haemopoeitic support. *Med Pediatr Oncol* 1993; **21**: 552 (abstract)

91. Schellong G, Hörnig I, Brämswig JH *et al*. Favourable outcome of childhood Stage IV HD with OPPA/COPP chemotherapy and additional radiotherapy. In: *Proceedings of the International Society of Paediatric Oncology*, 29th Meeting, 1987, abstract 132

92. Robertson CM, Hawkins MM, Kingston JL. Late deaths and survival after childhood cancer: implications for cure. *Br J Med* 1994; **309**: 161–166

93. Hawkins MM, Draper GJ, Kingston JE. Incidence of second primary tumours among childhood cancer survivors. *Br J Cancer* 1987; **56**: 339–347

94. Tucker MA, Meadows AT, Boice JD, Hoover RN, Fraumeni JF. Cancer risk following treatment of childhood cancer. In: Boice JD, Fraumeni JF (ed) *Radiation Carcinogenesis: Epidemiology and Biological Significance*. New York: Raven, 1984, pp 211–224.

95. Hawkins MM, Kinnier-Wilson LM, Burton HS *et al*. Radiotherapy, alkylating agents and the risk of bone cancer after childhood cancer. *J Natl Cancer Inst* 1997; **88**: 270–278

96. Tucker MA, Meadows AT, Bosie JD *et al*. Leukemia after therapy with alkylating agents for childhood cancer. *J Natl Cancer Inst* 1987; **78**: 459–464

97. Hawkins MM, Kinnier-Wilson LM, Stovall MA *et al*. Epipodophyllotoxins, alkylating agents and radiation and the risk of secondary leukaemia after childhood cancer. *Br Med J* 1992; **304**: 951–958

98. Ron E, Lubin JH, Shore RE *et al*. Thyroid cancer after exposure to external radiation: a pooled analysis of seven studies. *Radiat Res* 1995; **141**: 259–277

99. Bhatia S, Robison L, Oberlin O *et al*. Breast cancer and other neoplasms after childhood Hodgkin's disease. *N Engl J Med* 1991; **325**: 1330–1336

100. Shalet SM, Clayton PE. Factors influencing the development of irradiation induced growth hormone deficiency. *Hormone Res* 1990; **33**: 99

101. Robson H, Anderson E, Eden OB, Isaksson O, Shalet S. Chemotherapeutic agents used in the treatment of childhood malignancies have direct effects on growth plate chondrocyte proliferation. *J Endocrinol* 1998; **157**: 225–235

102. Constine LS, Donaldson SS, McDougall IR. Thyroid dysfunction after radiotherapy in children with Hodgkin's disease. *Cancer* 1984; **53**: 878–883

103. Shalet SM. Disorders of gonadal function due to radiation and cytotoxic chemotherapy in children. *Adv Intern Med Pediatr* 1989; **58**: 1–21

104. Byrne J, Mulvihill J, Myers MH *et al*. Effects of treatment on fertility in long term survivors of childhood or adolescent cancer. *N Engl J Med* 1987; **317**: 1315–1321

105. Byrne J, Fears TR, Gail MH *et al*. Early menopause in long term survivors of cancer during adolescence. *Am J Obstet Gynecol* 1992; **166**: 788–793

106. Gosden RG, Baird DT, Wade JC, Webb R. Restoration of fertility to oophorectomised sheep by ovarian autografts stored at −196°C. *Hum Reprod* 1994; **9**: 597–603

107. Hawkins MM. Pregnancy outcome and offspring after childhood cancer. *Br Med J* 1994; **309**: 1034

108. Chrisitie D, Leiper AD, Chessells JM *et al*. Intellectual performance after pre-symptomatic cranial radiotherapy for leukaemia: effects of age and sex. *Arch Dis Child* 1995; **73**: 136–140

109. Lipshultz SE, Colan SD, Gelber RD, Perez-Atayde AR, Sallan SE, Sanders SP. Late cardiac effects of doxorubicin therapy for ALL in childhood. *N Engl J Med* 1991; **324**: 808–815

110. Wexler LH, Andrich MP, Venzon D *et al*. Randomised trial of the cardioprotective agent ICRF-187 in pediatric sarcoma patients treated with doxorubicin. *J Clin Oncol* 1996; **14**: 362–372

111. Hancock SL, Donaldson S, Hoppe RT. Cardiac disease following treatment of Hodgkin's disease in childhood and adolescene. *J Clin Oncol* 1993; **11**: 1208–1215

112. Eigen H, Wyszomierski D. Bleomycin lung injury in children. Pathophysiology and guidelines for management. *Am J Pediatr Hematol Oncol* 1985; **7**: 71–78

113. Shaw N, Tweedale PM, Eden OB. Pulmonary function in childhood leukemia survivors. *Med Pediatr Oncol* 1989; **17**: 149–154

Coagulation
disorders

Hemophilia A and B

JEANNE M LUSHER

Hemophilia A and hemophilia B are hereditary bleeding disorders which result from defects in the Factor VIII (FVIII) and Factor IX (FIX) genes, respectively. The defective genes lead to decreased or absent circulating levels of functional FVIII or FIX, thus resulting in excessive and prolonged bleeding. Hemophilia A is the commoner form of hemophilia, accounting for 80–85% of cases, while hemophilia B accounts for 15–20%. The prevalence of hemophilia A is 1/10 000 males, while that of hemophilia B is approximately 1/50 000 males. Hemophilia has a worldwide distribution, and affects all racial groups. The severity of the disease is usually correlated with the degree of FVIII or FIX deficiency, with <0.02 IU/dl being considered severe, 0.02–0.05 IU/dl moderate, and >0.05–0.30 IU/dl as mild. Spontaneous bleeding is usually limited to persons with moderate or severe disease, with mildly affected persons bleeding only after trauma. In a US survey conducted in the early 1970s among 20 297 hemophilia A patients, 12 117 (60%) had severe disease, while 8180 (40%) had moderate disease. In contrast, among 5202 persons with hemophilia B, only 2304 (44%) had severe disease and 2898 (56%) moderate hemophilia.[1]

Normally, both FVIII and FIX circulate in an inactive form. When activated, FIX and FVIII co-operate to cleave and activate the pivotal enzyme, Factor X (FX). Thus together, activated FIX (FIXa) and activated FVIII (FVIIIa) contribute to the proteolytic cascade which controls the conversion of fibrinogen to fibrin. Since hemophilia A and B affect the same part of the coagulation sequence, individuals affected by either type of hemophilia have the same type of bleeding. In fact, hemophilia A and B are clinically indistinguishable. Both affect males almost exclusively, and both are characterized by bleeding into joints and soft tissues.

GENETICS

Both hemophilia A and B are inherited as X-linked recessive disorders, and thus they affect males almost exclusively.

There are, however, a few reports of hemophilia A and B in females, presumably due to extreme lyonization, inheritance of a gene for hemophilia from each parent, or a new mutation.[2] The genes for FVIII and FIX are on the long arm of the X-chromosome, in band Xq28 and band Xq27, respectively.[3]

A large number of mutations in the genes for FVIII and FIX have been found. In approximately one-third of newly diagnosed infants with hemophilia, there is no family history of the disorder, and the hemophilia has resulted from a spontaneous mutation. Many affected families have mutations of independent origin; thus, there is considerable genetic heterogeneity among hemophilia kindreds.[3–5]

The gene encoding FVIII is large and complex. It encompasses 186 kb and 26 exons and represents approximately 0.1% of the human X-chromosome. As technologic advances allowed identification of defects within the FVIII gene of a particular hemophiliac, it became apparent that there were a large variety of point mutations (amino acid substitutions), gene deletions of varying sizes, stop codon abnormalities, frameshift mutations, etc. However, in approximately 45% of severe hemophilia A kindreds, no mutations were found in the expected genomic regions. Relatively recently, it was discovered that these individuals had an 'inversion mutation' (Fig. 29.1). A region of intron 22 of the FVIII gene, which contains FVIII-associated gene A (F8A), also occurs twice more near the Xq telomere. When intrachromosomal homologous recombination occurs between the intron 22 repeat and either of the other 2 (extragenic) copies, an inversion occurs.[3,4,6–8] These inversions originate almost exclusively in male germ cells, due to the monosomic condition of the X-chromosome in males.[9] The inversion mutation can be detected by Southern Blot analysis.[6] Thus, in attempting to identify the precise genetic defect causing hemophilia in a particular kindred (for carrier detection or prenatal diagnosis of other family members), or for study purposes (e.g. correlation of gene defect with inhibitor development), most research laboratories now begin by looking for the inversion mutation by Southern

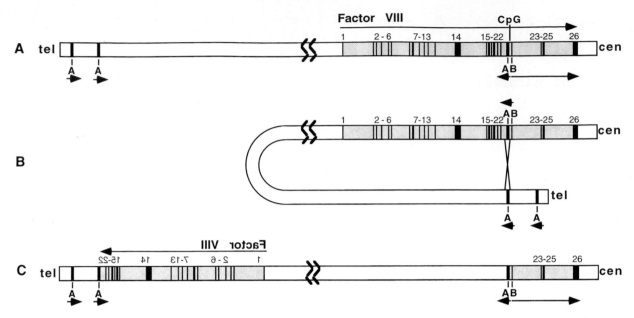

Fig. 29.1 Factor VIII (FVIII) gene and the inversion model. (A) Region of Xq28 that includes the FVIII gene, oriented with the telomere at the left. Three copies of the A gene are indicated, 2 lying upstream of FVIII and 1 inside intron 22. The location of the B transcript is also shown. The arrows indicate the direction of transcription of the FVIII and internal A and B genes. The direction of the upstream A genes is hypothesized to be as shown. (B) Proposed homologous recombination between the intron-22 copy of gene A and 1 of the 2 upstream copies. A cross-over between these 2 identical regions, oriented as shown, would result in an inversion of sequence between the 2 recombined A genes. (C) A recombination could involve either the upstream A genes, but only 1 is presented. The cross-over could occur anywhere in the region of homology which includes the A genes. Reproduced with permission from Ref. 6.

Blot. Only if this is negative does one need to look further for another mutation.

The gene coding for FIX is 33.5 kb in length and located at the boundary between band Xq26 and Xq27 in the distal part of the long arm of the X-chromosome, with 8 exons encoding a mRNA of 1.4 kb. As is the case for hemophilia A, there is considerable genetic heterogeneity among hemophilia B kindreds. Independent mutations occur in >95% of all families with severe or moderate hemophilia B.[10] It has been shown that hemophilia B can be caused by hundreds of different amino acid substitutions. Direct detection of the gene defect allows virtually 100% diagnostic success, with rapid results, and thus can be used for carrier and prenatal detection.

Mutations in the 5′ promoter region can result in the hemophilia B Leiden phenotype. Hemophilia B Leiden is characterized by very low levels of FIX antigen and activity at birth and during early childhood. Levels then rise to >60% following puberty in response to androgens.[11]

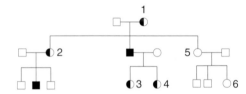

Fig. 29.2 Pedigree of a family with hemophilia. The grandmother, designated 1, is an obligate carrier, as is her daughter (2). Grandaughters 3 and 4 are also obligate carriers, as their father has hemophilia. The females designated as 5 and 6 are possible carriers, and should be offered testing and genetic counseling. (Genetic counseling should, of course, be offered to all family members.)

DIAGNOSIS

AT BIRTH OR PRENATALLY

While a family history is often useful in determining whether a male or female is at risk of having hemophilia or of being a 'carrier' of the hemophilia gene (Fig. 29.2), a negative history for hemophilia does not exclude the diagnosis, due to the high spontaneous mutation rate affecting the FVIII and FIX genes. If there is a family history for hemophilia A or B, and the mother of a male fetus is a known or possible carrier, arrangements can be made to obtain a cord blood sample at the time of delivery. (Since neither FVIII or FIX cross the placenta, the diagnosis can be made at birth.) This can be accomplished by drawing a sample of blood from a vessel on the fetal side of the placenta, placing it immediately into a tube which contains liquid citrate (dilution of blood to citrate is 10:1), and sending it to the laboratory for immediate separation of plasma from red cells and FVIII or FIX assay. The plasma should be frozen at −70°C if not being assayed immediately.

The diagnosis of hemophilia can also be made prenatally from a chorionic villous sample or from cells in the amniotic fluid. Chorionic villus sampling is optimally done at 10–12 weeks' gestation, while amniocentesis is preferably performed after 16 weeks' gestation.[10] These invasive techniques are not without risk to fetus and mother and such risks should be discussed with the parents prior to the procedure.[10] The use of restriction fragment length polymorphisms (RFLPs) (indirect gene analysis) can be informative if the defect in a family is not known. Alternatively, if the mutation causing hemophilia in the family is known, and if direct gene analysis is available, the specific mutation can be looked for. Otherwise, in the case of possible hemophilia A, first the inversion mutation should be looked for by Southern Blot, and only if this is not found would the laboratory proceed to look for another mutation. Direct sequencing of an exon can be done in a few highly specialized laboratories once it has been amplified from genomic DNA with the polymerase chain reaction (PCR) technique.

CARRIER ASSESSMENT

A woman is an 'obligate carrier' of hemophilia if one of the following conditions is met:

- her father has hemophilia;
- she has given birth to 2 or more sons with hemophilia;
- she has given birth to 1 son with hemophilia and there is a well documented family history of hemophilia on the maternal side of her pedigree.

At-risk women who are in families with known hemophilia but who are possible rather than obligate carriers can be investigated by readily available laboratory tests. If the woman's FVIII (or FIX) level is very low, it is reasonably certain that she is a carrier. The ratio of FVIII (or FIX) activity and FVIII (or FIX) antigen in her plasma can also be determined. If she has considerably less FVIII (or FIX) activity than antigen, this indicates that one of her FVIII (or FIX) genes is directing production of an abnormal (and non-functional) form of FVIII (or FIX); i.e. she is a 'carrier' for hemophilia. However, such testing provides only a *probability* of carrier status, and is not helpful in ∼10–15% of cases.

Genotype assessment, by either indirect methods (using RFLPs) or direct gene analysis, is available in highly specialized laboratories only, but is a more accurate method of carrier detection.

Recommendations regarding delivery for carrier females

In a recent survey of US obstetricians and perinatologists, most did not routinely recommend caesarean section for delivery of women who are known carriers of hemophilia.[12] Most surveys have concluded that the risk of serious head bleeding with normal vaginal delivery of hemophilic infants is small, and that delivery of all fetuses known to be at risk of hemophilia by caesarian section would not eliminate the risk.[13,14] However, fetuses at risk of hemophilia should be delivered by the least traumatic method. The use of vacuum extraction should be avoided, as subgaleal hemorrhages and large cephalhematomas can result from this technique.[13–15] Prolonged labor should also be avoided.

CLINICAL MANIFESTATIONS

INFANCY AND EARLY CHILDHOOD (see also Chapter 33)

Since neither FVIII or FIX cross the placenta, a male infant who has inherited a gene for severe (or moderately severe) hemophilia will have no, or very little, FVIII or FIX at birth. As noted above, those born to mothers (particularly primigravidas) who have a long, difficult labor, or vaginal delivery aided by forceps or vacuum extraction may develop large cephalhematomas or even intracranial hemorrhages (ICH).[13–15] In this situation, immediate diagnosis and treatment are crucial. The signs of ICH may be vague, but often include pallor, lethargy, neurologic deficits, unequal pupils, tense fontanel or vomiting. While most cases of delayed recognition and management of ICH in a newborn with severe hemophilia occur when there is no family history (i.e. 1 of the approximately 30% in which a new mutation has occurred), this is not always the case. Some at-risk women have not been tested, do not understand the genetics and their likelihood of having an infant with hemophilia, or fail to tell the obstetrician involved. If neonatal ICH occurs, clotting factor replacement should be instituted immediately. If the type of hemophilia is not known and FVIII and FIX assays cannot be obtained immediately, fresh frozen plasma should be given in a dosage of 10 ml/kg body weight.

If the newborn's mother is a known or possible carrier of hemophilia A or B, but the infant's status is unknown, arrangements should be made to obtain a cord blood sample at the time of delivery (see page 586).

If a newborn is not suspected of having hemophilia and undergoes circumcision, hemorrhage may or may not result (often dependent on the technique used). If it does occur, a prothrombin time, activated partial thromboplastin time (APTT) and FVIII and FIX assays (as well as hemoglobin and hematocrit) should be obtained. In addition to local measures, the missing coagulation factor can be given. Other invasive procedures such as heel sticks, arterial blood sampling, or central line placement may also result in excessive and prolonged bleeding in the neonate with hemophilia.

Beyond the newborn period, most hemophilic infants seldom have bleeding episodes requiring treatment unless accidental injury occurs. Beginning around 11 or 12 months of age, when the child is learning to walk and has frequent falls, or bumps into furniture, acute hemarthroses may occur. Tongue and mouth lacerations may also occur around this time (or even earlier), in young children who are putting objects into their mouth, or are running and falling, often with a spoon or other hard object in their mouth. Soft tissue bruising is also common during the first year of life and beyond, but often is more alarming in appearance than serious, and generally does not require treatment unless quite extensive or in certain locations (e.g. resulting in closing of an eye). If the diagnosis of hemophilia has not been established, neighbors or other acquaintances may suspect the parents of child abuse. Acute hemarthroses in this age group almost always result from trauma. The most commonly affected joints are elbows, knees and ankles; the first episode of joint bleeding may occur from approximately 8 months to 3 years in children with severe hemophilia, and somewhat later in those with moderate or mild hemophilia.[16]

Head injury

Head injury is of particular concern in young children with severe or moderately severe hemophilia, and parents should be advised to call the hemophilia center (or come to the emergency room) if head injury occurs. If the child is on home treatment and the head injury was severe, a dose of clotting factor should be given before coming to the hospital. While a clear-cut history of an observed trivial head bump (as from a fall of small distance and onto a padded surface, with no loss of consciousness and no neurologic abnormalities), may cause no alarm, and does not require treatment, other head bumps may fall into a gray zone. When in doubt as to the severity of the head trauma sustained, even without loss of consciousness or neurologic abnormalities, the physician can 'play it safe' by giving an infusion of clotting factor (aimed at raising the FVIII or FIX level to 0.80–1.00 IU/dl) and then obtaining a computerized tomogram (CT) scan of the head. However, if the head injury is judged to be minor (with a bruise at the site of injury, but no headache, persistent vomiting, drowsiness or neurologic abnormalities), the physician may elect to treat with one or two doses of clotting factor without obtaining imaging studies. In such cases, assuming parental compliance, the child can be sent home with the parents closely observing the child for complaints of headache, recurrent vomiting, lethargy, unsteadiness or neurologic abnormalities. The management of ICH is described below.

In the case of hyperkinetic toddlers, a padded helmet may be prescribed to prevent significant head trauma during accidental falls.

OLDER CHILDREN AND ADOLESCENTS

Joint hemorrhages

In older children and adolescents, injuries due to falls occur less often, and many have learned how to avoid injury leading to joint or other serious bleeding. However, the desire to participate in sports, or risk-taking behavior, may result in recurrent hemarthroses and intramuscular hemorrhage. Repeated joint hemorrhages lead to synovial inflam-

mation, thickening and a vicious cycle of re-bleeding into the joint. In those who have developed these so-called 'target joints', frequent, recurrent bleeding into the joint(s) may occur without trauma.

In addition to assessing the degree of joint swelling, pain and limitation of motion, joints can be assessed by a variety of imaging techniques. These include plain X-ray films, CT scans, ultrasound and magnetic resonance imaging (MRI). The CT scanner produces a series of cross-sectional images of a selected part. Contrast medium can be injected to define blood vessels if indicated. Ultrasound is a very useful technique for assessment of ileopsoas hemorrhage, bleeding into thigh muscles or other abdominal structures; however, it cannot penetrate bone. MRI is expensive, and is often difficult to schedule because demand exceeds available machines. However, MRI provides very good soft tissue pictures, allowing visualization of muscles, tendons, bone and cartilage, synovial thickening and joint effusions (Fig. 29.3). This technique provides the best picture of the actual extent of damage (even early changes) in a joint. Images can be oriented in more than one plane (axial, coronal, etc.), from the same acquisition. The unique capability of MRI is to assess early abnormalities of synovia, soft tissue and cartilage—often well before abnormalities are clinically apparent. MRI is also quite useful in evaluating the brain and spinal cord.

Joint scoring systems have also been developed, and some

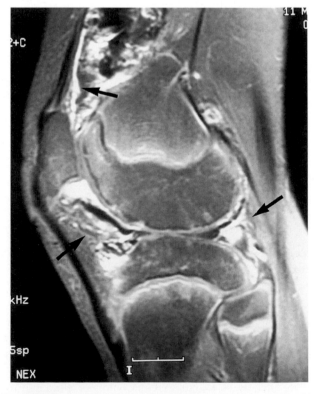

Fig. 29.3 Magnetic resonance imaging (MRI) of knee joint of a 12-year-old boy with severe hemophilia A, saggital view. Note enhancing hypertrophied synovium (arrows). Patella and quadriceps tendon are on left. Kindly provided by Indira Warrier, Children's Hospital of Michigan.

Table 29.1 Radiologic evaluation recommended by the Orthopedic Advisory Committee of the World Federation of Hemophilia.

Type of change	Finding	Score (points)
Osteoporosis	Absent	0
	Present	1
Enlarged epiphysis	Absent	0
	Present	1
Irregular subchondral surface	Absent	0
	Partly involved	1
	Totally involved	2
Narrowing of joint space	Absent	0
	Joint space >1 mm	1
	Joint space ≤1 mm	2
Subchondral cyst formation	Absent	0
	1 cyst	1
	>1 cyst	2
Erosions of joint margins	Absent	0
	Present	1
Gross incongruence of articulating bone ends	Absent	0
	Slight	1
	Pronounced	2
Joint deformity (angulation and/or displacement between articulating bones)	Absent	0
	Slight	1
	Pronounced	2

Possible joint score: 0–13 points per joint.

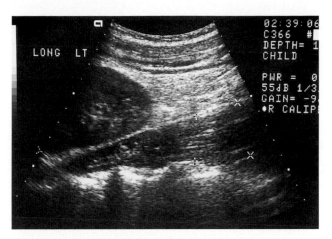

Fig. 29.4 Ultrasound of the left side of the abdomen in a 15-year-old boy with hemophilia, demonstrating ileopsoas hemorrhage. Note echogenicity of ileopsoas muscle (outlined by the two Xs), just below the left kidney. The top of the ultrasound represents the anterior and the bottom, the posterior abdomen. Kindly provided by Indira Warrier, Children's Hospital of Michigan.

of these have proven useful in following the joint status of individuals over time, as well as evaluating groups of individuals being treated with differing dosages of clotting factor, or on prophylactic regimens aimed at preventing joint damage. In 1977, Arnold and Hilgartner[17] designed a 5-grade scale, based on a combination of radiologic and clinical assessments. Completely normal joints are assigned a 0 score. The Pettersson radiologic joint scoring system (Table 29.1) rates each joint (elbows, knees and ankles) on a scale of 0–13 points, with the worst possible score being 78 and the best 0.[18,19] The Pettersson scoring system is currently recommended by The World Federation of Hemophilia (WFH) as it includes radiographic changes which can easily be identified and are not attributable to very recent bleeding. The overall orthopedic joint scoring system, as recommended by WFH, rates each joint on a scale of 0–15 points; the aggregate score for elbows, knees and ankles constitutes the orthopedic joint score and the worst score is 90.[20]

Ileopsoas hemorrhages

In addition to peripheral muscle hemorrhages, adolescents may develop ileopsoas hemorrhages, which may become extensive if not recognized and treated promptly. Signs of ileopsoas bleeding include upward flexion of the thigh, discomfort on passive extension of the thigh, tenderness on palpation of the lower quadrant, and paresthesias just below the inguinal ligament from femoral nerve compression.[21]

With imaging studies (flat plate of the abdomen, ultrasound, pyelogram, CT scan or MRI), an enlarged or even bulging ileopsoas is characteristically seen, with medial displacement of the kidney and ureter. Ultrasound or MRI are the most useful modalities in delineating an ileopsoas hemorrhage (Fig. 29.4). In addition to bed rest, vigorous replacement therapy with clotting factor (every 12 hours, or by continuous infusion to maintain a level of >0.30 IU/dl FVIII or FIX) should be continued for at least a week.

Compartment syndrome

Bleeding into other flexor muscle groups, such as in the forearm or calf, if not promptly treated, can lead to so-called 'compartment syndrome'. Due to the limited space in the compartment in which these muscles are situated, swelling and hemorrhage in the compartment can cause increased pressure, which can result in compression of nerves and blood vessels which travel in the same compartment. Paresthesias or numbness may indicate that nerve compression has occurred. Immediate treatment is indicated. In addition to vigorous clotting factor replacement, fasciotomy may be necessary if vascular supply and nerves are severely compromised.

Intracranial hemorrhage

Traumatic ICH may be subdural, subarachnoid or intracerebral (or a combination of these).[21] An infusion of clotting factor to raise the FVIII or FIX level to at least 0.50 IU/dl should be given immediately if ICH is suspected (prior to imaging studies and neurosurgical consultation). If ICH is documented, FVIII or FIX should be given by continuous infusion, in order to avoid dangerously low trough levels. Following treatment of the acute episode (in general, for approximately 2 weeks), many recommend that prophylactic treatment be given for at least 6 months, in view of the possibility of recurrent ICH even without trauma. For FVIII deficiency, bolus doses of 40 IU/kg (to the nearest vial) should be given every other day, and for FIX deficiency, 50–60 U/kg twice weekly (due to the longer half-life of FIX).

Hematuria

Gross hematuria can result from a blow to the flank, renal calculi or acute glomerulonephritis, or it may be spontaneous and asymptomatic. If other causes are ruled out and it appears that the child or adolescent has painless, spontaneous hematuria, some recommend bed rest and/or a course of corticosteroids (prednisone 1–2 mg/kg/day). The author, however, recommends increased oral fluids only. In most instances, the hematuria clears within 3–4 days. If it does not, a dose or two of clotting factor concentrate (40 IU/kg, to the nearest vial) can be given.

MANAGEMENT

HEMOPHILIA A

Desmopressin

For children and adolescents with mild hemophilia A, bleeding episodes can often be controlled with the synthetic agent, desmopressin (DDAVP; 1-deamino-8-D-arginine vasopressin). The recommended intravenous dosage is 0.3 μg/kg body weight (maximum dose 20 μg).[22] If necessary, doses can be repeated every 12–24 hours. However, it should be noted that many persons with mild hemophilia A exhibit tachyphylaxis (diminishing response) when repeat doses are given at frequent intervals.[23] With an intravenous dose of 0.3 μg/kg, recipients will have an average 3-fold (range 2–12-fold) increase over baseline FVIII levels. The degree of response will be approximately the same if an individual is given desmopressin again at a future time. If the degree of response is insufficient to control or prevent bleeding, a FVIII concentrate should be given (see below).

Side-effects with desmopressin are generally limited to facial flushing and facial warmth. However, the drug is a potent antidiuretic agent and there is a slight risk of hyponatremia, water intoxication and convulsions. This risk can generally be avoided by limiting fluid intake for at least 12 hours after desmopressin, and by not giving hypotonic intravenous fluids post-operatively. Parents of children who are sent home after a dose or two of desmopressin should be advised to restrict the child's fluid intake (for at least 12 hours). Additionally, in view of an increased tendency for fluid balance problems in the very young (and the elderly), desmopressin is not recommended for children under 2 years of age.[24]

Desmopressin can also be used intranasally. For hemostatic purposes, a much larger dose (15 times larger) is needed than for diabetes insipidus. A multi-dose intranasal spray bottle (Stimate nasal spray) includes a metered dose pump which delivers 150 μg/activation of the pump. Most 5-year-old children can be taught to use Stimate nasal spray. The recommended dose is 1 activation of the pump (one nostril) for children, and 2 for adolescents and adults. This form is ideal for home use, and has been used for treatment of bleeding and for prophylaxis before invasive dentistry or contact sports.[24,25]

Clotting factor concentrates

For patients with severe or moderate hemophilia A, clotting factor concentrates should be used. Commercially prepared concentrates have replaced plasma and cryoprecipitate as the treatment of choice in many parts of the world, since they are either produced by recombinant technology, or if plasma-derived, are subjected to viral attenuation and removal processes, and are thus considered safer. A variety of FVIII concentrates are currently available and a recent update describing these (and FIX concentrates) has been prepared by Kasper.[26] While available products, brand names, manufacturers and methods of production vary somewhat from country to country, all human plasma-derived concentrates are now virally attenuated by one or more methods. A listing of products available in the UK was recently published by the UK Haemophilia Centre Directors Organization;[27] and a listing of those licensed and available in the US appears in Table 29.2.[28]

There are currently two available recombinant (r)FVIII concentrates (licensed for use in North America, most European countries, and elsewhere in the early 1990s): Baxter's Recombinate® and Bayer's Kogenate®. Both have undergone extensive clinical trials in persons with hemophilia since 1987–88, and both appear to be effective and safe.[29–32] The main advantage of rFVIII would appear to be viral safety. Both these rFVIII preparations contain human serum albumin, added as a stabilizer unlike newer, as yet unlicensed, rFVIII preparations. These include Bayer's Kogenate SF and Genetics Institute's B-domainless rFVIII preparation (ReFacto®)[33] (which appears to be produced more efficiently than the full-length FVIII molecule).

Available plasma-derived FVIII concentrates vary in purity and in the way in which virus has been removed or inactivated. The scientific debate over whether purer is better has never been settled; however, the higher purity concentrates are more expensive than those of intermediate purity. In addition to extensive screening of all blood and plasmapheresis donors for evidence of infection with human immunodeficiency virus (HIV-1, HIV-2) and hepatitis B and C viruses, plasma-derived clotting factor concentrates are subjected to solvent-detergent treatment and/or pasteurization, vapor treatment, nanofiltration, or dry heating for

Table 29.2 Therapeutic products for hemophilia A and B licensed in the United States (as of March 1998).

Product	Manufacturer	Method of viral depletion or inactivation	Specific activity (IU/mg protein), final product**	Specific activity (IU/mg protein) discounting albumin**	Hepatitis safety studies in humans with this product	Hepatitis safety studies in humans with another product, but similar viral inactivation method
Recombinant Factor VIII products						
Recombinate	Baxter	Immunoaffinity chromatography	1.65–19	>3000	Yes	
Kogenate	Bayer	Immunoaffinity chromatography	8–30	>3000	Yes	
Bioclate	Baxter (distributed by Centeon)	Immunoaffinity chromatography	1.65–19	>3000	Yes	
Helixate	Bayer (distributed by Centeon)	Immunoaffinity chromatography	8–30	>3000	Yes	
Immunoaffinity purified (very high purity) FVIII products derived from human plasma						
Monoclate P	Centeon	1. Immunoaffinity chromatography 2. Pasteurization (60°C, 10 h)	@ 5–10	>3000	Yes	Yes
Hemofil M	Baxter	1. Immunoaffinity chromatography 2. Solvent detergent (TNBP/Triton X-100) 3. Heat (25°C, ≥10 h)	@ 2–11	>3000	Yes	No
Monarc M	Manufactured by Baxter for American Red Cross from American Red Cross-collected plasma	1. Immunoaffinity chromatography 2. Solvent detergent (TNBP/Triton X-100) 3. Heat (25°C, ≥10 h)	@ 2–11	>3000	No	Yes
Intermediate purity and high purity FVIII products derived from human plasma (contain von Willebrand factor)						
Alphanate	Alpha Therapeutics	1. Immunoaffinity chromatography 2. Solvent detergent (tri N-butyl [TNBP] and polysorbate 80) 3. Heat (80°C, 72 h)	@ 8–30	Corrected specific activity of 477	No	Yes
Koate-HP	Bayer	Solvent detergent (TNBP and polysorbate 80)	@ 9–22	50	No	Yes
Humate P	Centeon Pharma (Marberg, Germany)	Pasteurization (60°C, 10 h)				
Porcine FVIII (for use in persons with hemophilia A and FVIII inhibitor with low cross-reactivity to porcine FVIII)						
Hyate C	Speywood Pharmaceuticals (Wrexham, UK)	Pasteurization (60°C, 10 h)				
Recombinant FIX products						
BeneFix	Genetics Institute	1. Affinity chromatography 2. Ultrafiltration	>200		Yes	No
Coagulation FIX products derived from human plasma						
AlphaNine SD	Alpha Therapeutics	1. Dual affinity chromatography 2. Solvent detergent (TNBP and polysorbate 80) 3. Nanofiltration	@ 229 ± 23 (22)		Yes	Yes
Mononine	Centeon	1. Immunoaffinity chromatography 2. Sodium thiocyanate 3. Ultrafiltration	> 160		Yes	No
FIX complex concentrates derived from human plasma						
Konyne 80	Bayer	Dry heat (80°C, 72 h)	@ 1.25		No	Yes
Proplex T	Baxter	Dry heat (68°C, 144 h)	@ 3.9		No	No
Profilnine SD	Alpha Therapeutics	Solvent detergent (TNBP and polysorbate 80)	@ 4.5		No	Yes
Bebulin VH	Immuno (Vienna, Austria) (distributed by Baxter-Immuno)	Vapor heat (10 h, 60°C, 1190 mbar pressure plus 1 h, 80°C, 1375 mbar)	@ 2		Yes	No
Activated FIX complex concentrates derived from human plasma (for use in hemophilia A or B, with inhibitor antibody to FVIII or FIX)						
Autoplex T	Baxter (distributed by Nabi)	Dry heat (68°C,144 h)	@ 5		No	No
FEIBA VH	Immuno (distributed by Baxter-Immuno)	Vapor heat (10 h, 60°C, 1190 mbar plus 1 h, 80°C, 1375 mbar)	@ 0.8		No	Yes

(Continued overleaf)

Table 29.2 (*Continued*).

Product	Manufacturer	US distributor	Formulation	Recommended dosage and administration
Desmopressin formulations useful in disorders of hemostasis				
DDAVP (injection)	Ferring AB (Malmö, Sweden)	Rhone-Poulenc-Rohrer	For parenteral (IV) or SQ use, 4 μg in a 10 ml vial or 15 μg in a 1 ml vial	1. 0.3 μg/kg mixed in 30 ml normal saline solution, infused slowly over 30 min IV 2. 0.4 μg/kg subcutaneously May repeat after 24 hours
Stimate (nasal spray)	Ferring AB	Centeon	Nasal spray, 1.5 mg/ml. The metered dose pump delivers 0.1 ml (150 μg) per actuation. The bottle contains 2.5 ml with spray pump capable of delivering 25 150-μg doses or 12 300-μg doses	In patients weighing <50 kg, one spray in one nostril (delivers 150 μg). For those weighing >50 kg, give one spray in *each nostril* (total dose 300 μg). May repeat after 24 hours

**The degree of product purity is reflected by the specific activity of FVIII (units/mg protein). Since most FVIII concentrates, including recombinant FVIII, have human serum albumin added as a stabilizer, most persons look at the specific activity discounting albumin. Recombinant clotting factor preparations are refered to as 'ultrapure'; immunoaffinity purified products are referred to as 'very high purity' products.

Table 29.3 General dosage guidelines for treatment of bleeding in hemophilia A and B.

Type of bleeding	Desired factor level (IU/dl)	FVIII dose (IU/kg)	FIX dose (IU/kg)	Duration of treatment days	Ancillary treatment
Acute hemarthrosis	0.30–0.50	15–25	30–50	1–2	Non-weight bearing
Intramuscular hemorrhage	0.30–0.50	15–25	30–50	2–5	Non-weight bearing
Tongue, mouth laceration	0.20–0.30	10–15	20–30	1–2	Avoid local trauma (NPO if necessary); antifibrinolytic agent
Persistent* hematuria	0.30–0.50	15–25	30–50	1–2	Increased PO or IV fluids
Ileopsoas or other retroperitoneal bleeding	0.30–0.50	15–25	30–50	3–10	Bed rest
Retropharyngeal bleeding	0.40–0.50	20–25	40–50	3–4	Antifibrinolytic agent
Intracranial hemorrhage	0.80–1.00	40–50	80–100	10–14[+][⊕]	
Surgery	0.80–1.00	40–50	80–100	10–14[+][δ]	

*Painless, spontaneous hematuria usually requires no treatment. Increase fluid intake to maintain renal output.
[+]Continuous infusion is preferable in order to avoid dangerously low trough levels. FVIII or FIX is generally given at a dose of 3–4 IU/kg/h with subsequent doses adjusted according to the circulating plasma level.
[⊕]Following this, 6–12 months of prophylaxis is recommended, in order to prevent recurrent ICH.
[δ]Shorter duration for minor procedures.

long periods. While no process has been shown to kill or remove human parvovirus B19, and while there have been sporadic outbreaks of hepatitis A resulting from certain solvent-detergent-treated FVIII and FIX concentrates,[34,35] commercially available plasma-derived clotting factor concentrates in current use appear to be reasonably safe.

Recommended dosage and dosage schedules are generally based on the severity and type of bleeding episode. While there is no consensus regarding the proper dose to be given for various situations, Table 29.3 provides general guidelines.

HEMOPHILIA B

There is no synthetic equivalent to desmopressin for persons with hemophilia B; thus clotting factor concentrates should be used to treat or prevent bleeding. FIX concentrates fall into three classes:

1. low/intermediate purity plasma-derived concentrates

(FIX complex concentrates, commonly referred to as prothrombin complex concentrates [PCCs]);
2. high purity plasma-derived 'coagulation FIX concentrates';
3. recombinant Factor IX (rFIX).

While PCCs were the mainstay of treatment for persons with hemophilia B for many years, shortly after their introduction reports of thromboembolic complications began to appear.[36,37] Most occurred in immobile postoperative patients (particularly after orthopedic surgical procedures), or following crush injuries or extensive intramuscular hemorrhages, but some did not. Because of the thrombotic risk many physicians postponed planned elective surgery or added heparin to reconstituted PCCs as recommended by the International Committee on Thrombosis & Haemostasis' FVIII and FIX Subcommittee.[38] However, reports of DIC and thromboembolic complications continued to appear, some of which were fatal.[39]

Fortunately, in the early 1990s 'coagulation FIX concentrates' became available.[40,41] In contrast to the PCCs, which contain not only FIX but also Factors II, VII, and X, proteins C and S, and varying amounts of partially activated clotting factors, the coagulation FIX concentrates contain almost exclusively FIX. There have been no reports of thrombotic complications attributable to these high-purity products, which include Mononine® (Centeon, King of Prussia, PA, USA), AlphaNine SD (Alpha Therapeutics, Los Angeles, CA, USA), and Immunine (Immuno AG, Vienna, Austria). The US National Hemophilia Foundation's Medical and Scientific Advisory Council has recommended that a coagulation FIX concentrate be used for persons undergoing surgical procedures, for those with crush injuries, large intramuscular hemorrhages, hepatocellular dysfunction or a history of thrombosis following use of PCC, and for infants.[42]

In February 1997, a rFIX product (BeneFix®; Genetics Institute, Cambridge, MA, USA) was licensed for use in the US and Europe. This recombinant product contains no human or animal proteins. It is produced by a genetically engineered Chinese hamster ovary (CHO) cell line which has been extensively characterized.[43] It should be noted that, in a pre-licensure pharmacokinetic study, recovery was lower for BeneFix® than for high-purity plasma-derived FIX. On average, 1 IU of BeneFix®/kg body weight increased the circulating FIX by 0.8 IU/dl. Thus, it is recommended that a multiplication factor of 1.2 be used in calculating the dose of BeneFix® (i.e. number of FIX units required = body weight [in kg] × desired FIX increase [%] × 1.2). Alternatively, the patient's recovery following a test dose of BeneFix® while not bleeding can be used to calculate the patient's required dose (Package insert, BeneFix®, 1997). This rFIX product appears to be effective and safe in previously untreated as well as previously treated patients with hemophilia B.[44–46]

CONTINOUS INFUSION OF CLOTTING FACTOR CONCENTRATES

Continuous infusion of FVIII-containing products was first described by McMillan *et al* in 1970.[47] While good clinical outcomes were obtained, issues of stability and sterility were not fully addressed.[48] Current improved products, with reliable potency, high purity and stability over many hours, have resulted in increased use of continuous infusion in situations where maintenance of adequate hemostasis for a prolonged period of time is either essential or desirable. Continuous infusion, which avoids the possibility of dangerously low trough levels, is now routinely used in many hemophilia centers intra- and post-operatively, and for treatment of ICH or other very serious bleeding episodes, such as compartment syndrome.[48–52]

In addition to avoiding dangerously low trough levels, continuous infusion reduces the amount of clotting factor required to maintain a certain level, with considerable economic savings. This advantage is thought to result from the optimal saturation produced in most peripheral body compartments when clotting factor is given by continuous infusion.[50]

Continuous infusion of reconstituted but not further diluted FVIII concentrates can be done with a minipump; a small amount of heparin may be used to prevent thrombophlebitis.[48,49]

Ideally, each subject should undergo a pharmacokinetic study before elective surgery to determine the individual's clearance, half-life and recovery of FVIII. If this is done, dosing can be optimal from the start.[49,50] Alternatively, following a bolus dose of 40–50 IU/kg, FVIII can be administered at a rate of 3–4 IU/kg/h, with measurement of the patient's FVIII level and adjustment of the rate accordingly. It should be noted that the *initial* maintenance dose for continuous infusion is often higher than that required a few days following surgery because of the increased clearance of FVIII in the immediate postoperative period.

Using the same principles, FIX concentrates can also be given by continuous infusion.[52]

COST ISSUES

The major cost of hemophilia treatment is the cost of clotting factor. In the 1970s and early 1980s, when only crude or intermediate products were available, FVIII and FIX concentrates in the US cost approximately 8–10 cents/unit. With the introduction of high-purity FVIII concentrates and better screening and viral attenuation methods in the late 1980s, the cost of these products escalated to 65 cents/unit.[53] The 1990s brought increasing purity, additional steps to inactivate or remove viruses, recombinant products, and even higher prices (often > $1/unit, not counting mark-ups by such intermediaries as hospitals and home delivery/home care companies). Many reasons are given for the high cost of modern clotting factor concentrates—research and development costs must be recovered and high-tech operations maintained, including production, quality control, expert personnel and expensive equipment; patents owned by one company but needed by all; royalties; insurance; small market, etc. Nonetheless, if the newer, presumably safer products are to be afforded, costs cannot continue to escalate.[54] Perhaps additional manufacturers, more efficient production (e.g. the B-domainless rFVIII, ReFacto®), or other innovative approaches may bring prices down to levels affordable not only in a few places but ideally throughout the world.

OTHER TREATMENT MODALITIES

Antifibrinolytic agents

Once a clot has formed (as a result of an infusion of FVIII or FIX, or desmopressin), it may be rapidly lysed. This most often occurs in the case of tongue, mouth or oropharyngeal bleeding, as the tissues of the oral cavity are rich in fibrinolytic materials. The 2 available antifibrinolytic drugs are epsilon aminocaproic acid (EACA; trade name Amicar®, Immunex Corp., Seattle, WA, USA), and tranexamic acid (Cyclokapron®, Pharmacia-Upjohn, Bridgewater, NJ, USA). Both are available in oral and parenteral forms. Recommended oral dosage for EACA is 75 mg/kg body weight every 6 hours for 7–10 days, while that for tranexamic acid is 25 mg/kg every 8 hours for 7–10 days. Amicar® tablets and syrup contain 500 mg and 250 mg/dl of aminocaproic acid, respectively. Cyclokapron tablets contain 500 mg of tranexamic acid.

For planned invasive dentistry, an antifibrinolytic agent should be started the evening before and continued for 7–10 days. For other types of oral or oropharyngeal surgery, these agents can be given intravenously (pre- and post-operatively), then changing to the oral form. Following extraction of permanent teeth, some have used an antifibrinolytic agent as a mouthwash as well. Sindet-Pedersen et al[55] recommend the use of a mouthwash consisting of 10% tranexamic acid for injection, diluted with sterile water. It should be stressed, however, that antifibrinolytic agents are useful *adjuncts* to prevent rapid lysis of clots formed following an infusion of FVIII, FIX or desmopressin.

Analgesics

As is true for other underlying bleeding disorders (including von Willebrand disease), drugs which interfere with platelet function should be avoided and in particular, aspirin and all aspirin-containing compounds. Acetaminophen (Tylenol®) is a useful alternative for pain (or fever). Many of the non-steroidal anti-inflammatory drugs (e.g. Indocin: Merck & Co, Inc, West Point, PA, USA; Motrin: Pharmacia & Upjohn, Kalamazoo, MI, USA; Naprosyn, Syntex: Voltarin, Geigy, etc.) also interfere with platelet function, but by a different mechanism from that of aspirin.[56] If chronic, hemophilic arthropathy results in daily aching pain in the ankles or other joints, one of these agents may be tried. Other fairly common side-effects are gastrointestinal (abdominal pain, gastrointestinal bleeding, ulcerations). It should also be noted that most of the non-steroidal anti-inflammatory drugs are not recommended for children below 14 years of age, due to insufficient study in this age group.

Vaccines

Children with hemophilia should receive all of the vaccines recommended for the general childhood population, including hepatitis B vaccine (HBV). The latter is particularly important in view of the hemophilic child's exposure (or potential exposure) to blood products. While all blood and plasmapheresis donors are screened by so-called third-generation screening tests for hepatitis B surface antigen [HBsAg], there is still a very slight risk of acquiring hepatitis B from a blood transfusion. The US National Hemophilia Foundation's Medical & Scientific Advisory Council (MASAC) has also recommended that all persons with hemophilia who are still seronegative to hepatitis A receive the hepatitis A vaccine as well.[57] This vaccine, which is particularly immunogenic, appears to be just as effective when given subcutaneously as intramuscularly. Unfortunately, there are still no vaccines for hepatitis C or HIV-1.

For persons with hemophilia, all vaccines should be given with care, using a small gauge (#25) needle and applying pressure to the site for 2–3 min thereafter.

COMMON INVASIVE PROCEDURES

All invasive procedures such as venipunctures and lumbar punctures should be done with great care. Following venipuncture, pressure should be applied to the site for 5 min. If a diagnostic lumbar puncture is to be done, the infant or child should be given a dose of FVIII (approximately 25–30 IU/kg) or FIX (50–60 IU/kg) prior to the procedure. Whenever feasible, an activated partial thromboplastin time (APTT) and FVIII (or FIX) assay should also be obtained prior to lumbar puncture to ensure that the desired hemostatic effect has been achieved.

COMPLICATIONS OF HEMOPHILIA

Musculoskeletal complications

Joint bleeding is the hallmark of hemophilia. Acute hemarthroses should be treated *immediately* in order to stop the bleeding and to prevent the accumulation of large amounts of blood in the joint space. The latter serves as an irritant to the synovial membrane, resulting in proliferation of vascular synovial tissue into the joint space. When this occurs, even routine activities can lead to trauma to the synovial tissue and a vicious cycle of re-bleeding (target joint bleeding), greater synovial proliferation and thickening, and ultimately erosion of underlying cartilage and bone.[58,59]

It is often difficult for the parents of a young child with hemophilia to recognize when an acute hemarthrosis has started. Often an acute joint bleed is detected only after a parent sees the child limping or observes a very swollen joint. Since immediate treatment—or prophylaxis—is necessary if the development of chronic debilitating joint disease is to be prevented, there has been considerable interest in beginning prophylactic treatment at 1–2 years of age for children with severe hemophilia. Nilsson et al[60,61] in Sweden have had considerable success with this approach over the past 30 years. The goal is to convert severe hemophilia to a milder form of the disease, to prevent spontaneous bleeding and to preserve normal joint function.[60] In view of the demonstrated benefits of this so-called primary prophylaxis in Sweden and other European countries, in early 1994 the US National Hemophilia Foundation's MASAC recommended that prophylaxis be considered optimal care for children with severe hemophilia A and B.[62] Such prophylaxis should begin at an early age, although there is no consensus concerning when this should be. Some recommend beginning prophylaxis after 1–2 episodes of joint bleeding, while others have used a particular age (usually somewhere between 12 and 30 months). There is a rationale for each of these approaches—some children with severe hemophilia do not have their first acute hemarthrosis until 24–30 months of age, and venous access is generally better by that age; however, joint assessment by MRI[63,64] sometimes demonstrates that abnormalities have already occurred even if no hemarthrosis had been recognized clinically. It is also noteworthy that even one severe acute hemarthrosis may lead to synovial hypertrophy, which contributes to the vicious cycle of re-bleeding and inflammation that eventually results in destructive arthritis.[63–65]

The recommended dosage for prophylaxis is 25–40 IU FVIII/kg body weight every other day (or at least 3 times/week), and 25–40 IU FIX/kg, twice weekly (in view of the longer half-life for FIX). While Nilsson's regimen is aimed at keeping trough levels above 1%, others have reported success even when trough levels fall below 1%. Although pharmacokinetics can vary from patient to patient, it is not practical to carry out pharmacokinetic studies in very young children, and this does not appear to be necessary. If at all possible, prophylaxis should be done by venipuncture. If a central venous catheter must be used, the potential complications of central lines should be discussed with the child's family, as well as the need for a surgical procedure to insert the device and education in the use and care of the line, etc.[62] The main complication is line sepsis, necessitating hospitalization, a prolonged course of intravenous antibiotics, and sometimes removal of the line. The rate of complications has been lower with ports (such as Port-a-Cath) than with external central venous catheters (such as Broviac or Hickman catheters), thus most now recommend a port if prophylaxis cannot be done by venipuncture of peripheral veins.

For children or adolescents who already have one or more 'target joints' (with clinical synovitis and frequent bleeding into the joint), prophylaxis will often decrease the frequency of hemarthroses but will not prevent progression of degenerative changes in the joint.

Synovectomy, when indicated, can be done by 1 of 3 approaches:

- open surgical synovectomy,[64]
- arthroscopic synovectomy,[20]
- radionuclide synoviorthesis.[66]

The latter is the least invasive approach, and can be quite successful in preventing re-bleeding in children or adolescents (or adults) who have early chronic synovitis. This procedure, performed by inserting a needle into the joint and injecting a radionuclide ([90]y-yttrium or [32]p-phosphorus), results in ablation of the synovial lining which then does not re-bleed (or does so much less frequently). Radionuclide synoviorthesis is being performed in an increasing number of centers and appears to be safe and often quite effective. While some have done radiosynoviorthesis in children as young as 2 years, most do not adopt this approach in children <6 years of age.

FVIII or FIX inhibitors

Inhibitors to FVIII develop in 25–35% of children with severe hemophilia A, and occasionally in those with moderate hemophilia A. Short-term hepatitis safety studies with new products conducted in the late 1980s revealed a higher than expected number of inhibitors in young children who were being prospectively screened for inhibitors as well as hepatitis markers.[67] This caused concern that the newer, more highly purified FVIII concentrates might be more immunogenic. Thus, in the pre-licensure clinical trials with rFVIII products (Bayer's Kogenate, Baxter's Recombinate and Pharmacia–Upjohn's ReFacto), frequent, prospective monitoring for inhibitors was done over an extended period of time. In clinical trials with each of these rFVIII products, no new inhibitors developed in previously treated patients; however, in previously untreated patients (PUPs), inhibitors were detected in 25–30% after a median of 10–11 exposure days.[31,32,68] In each of these PUP studies, approximately one-half of the inhibitors were low titer (<10 Bethesda units [BU]), and approximately one-third were transient, disappearing within weeks or months despite continued episodic treatment with rFVIII. From these and other studies,[69] it appears that inhibitors develop relatively early in childhood and within the first 50 exposures to FVIII (median 10–11 days).

It also appears that *patient factors* are the major determinants of inhibitor development. Certain abnormalities in the FVIII gene (gene deletions, stop codon abnormalities and frameshift mutations) are associated with a higher likelihood of inhibitor development. Several studies have documented a higher percentage (50%) of inhibitors in black children than in caucasians,[31,32,70] while one survey found a high incidence in Puerto Rican children.[71] As might be expected, there is a higher incidence in brother pairs (i.e. if a boy with hemophilia has a high-titer inhibitor, his hemophilic brother(s) is more likely also to develop a high titer inhibitor).

Two products have proved to be particularly immunogenic. These plasma-derived FVIII products, used only in a few European countries (and no longer marketed), resulted in an unexpectedly high number of inhibitors in patients who had been heavily exposed to other FVIII products in the past. In each instance, the inhibitor disappeared when the patients were changed to another FVIII preparation.[72,73] In view of these observations, many now feel that previously treated patients are more informative than PUPs in detecting unusual immunogenicity of a newly introduced product (as many PUPs develop inhibitors early, with exposure to any form of FVIII, whereas very few heavily treated adults would be expected to develop inhibitors).

Management

In patients with very low titer inhibitors (<5 BU), bleeding can often be controlled with (human) FVIII, in the usual or slightly increased dosage. Some of these low-titer inhibitors will disappear, others remain detectable but low, while yet others become high-titer inhibitors over time.

For higher titer inhibitors, or even those <5 BU if adequate hemostasis cannot be achieved with FVIII, another approach is needed. An attempt can be made to eradicate or suppress the inhibitor by placing the child on an immune tolerance induction (ITI) regimen. Many use large daily doses of FVIII alone, starting with 50–200 IU/kg.[74] If the inhibitor titer becomes undetectable (usually after a few months), and FVIII recovery and half-life are near normal, the dose of FVIII can be decreased and/or the interval between doses increased. A variety of ITI regimens have been developed, some employing lower doses of FVIII given less frequently,[75] and others employing intravenous gamma-globulin and cyclophosphamide in addition to FVIII.[76] Success rates are generally better if the inhibitor concentration is low at the start of ITI. In the author's experience, the likelihood of a good and quick response is enhanced if ITI is begun relatively soon after the development of a problematic inhibitor. The author has had a 75–80% success rate using 50–100 IU FVIII/kg once daily. The International Immune Tolerance Registry and a North American registry are collecting and analyzing data in an attempt to determine which factors determine the degree of success or failure of ITI. Additionally, an international multicenter randomized trial, to begin in 1999, will compare patients treated with low- vs high-dose regimens.

Therapeutic modalities for bleeding in persons with high titer inhibitors include PCC (either standard or activated), porcine FVIII (Hyate:C[®], Speywood Pharmaceuticals, Wrexham, UK) and rFVIIa (NovoSeven[®], Novo-Nordisk, Copenhagen, Denmark). Each of these has advantages and disadvantages.

The PCCs and the purposely activated PCCs (APCC), FEIBA VH[®] and Autoplex-T[®] (Baxter–Immuno and NABI, respectively), have been used for many years. They appear to 'bypass' the need for FVIII and FIX, but their precise mode of action in this regard is still not known with certainty. Large doses must be given (in the order of 75 IU/kg), and there are no laboratory tests for monitoring their effectiveness. They appear to work reasonably well most, but not all, of the time and are generally regarded as being less effective than FVIII in a patient with no inhibitor.[77] Additionally, approximately 15 patients with inhibitors (all young) have developed acute myocardial infarction following repeated infusions of PCC.[78] In view of this, dosage should not exceed 100 IU/kg/dose and giving more than 2 or 3 doses at 12 hour intervals should be avoided if at all possible. If additional treatment is deemed necessary, PCC or APCC should then be given only once daily. Alternatively, where

licensed and available, the patient could be switched to rFVIIa (see below).

Porcine FVIII can be used to treat or prevent bleeding in patients with inhibitors but little or no cross-reacting antibody to porcine FVIII. In patients with inhibitors to FVIII, it is helpful for the coagulation laboratory to run an antiporcine inhibitor assay along with the standard Bethesda assay whenever inhibitor assays are being run. Then, should a child with an inhibitor present with a serious hemorrhage (e.g. ICH, compartment syndrome, large ileopsoas bleed, etc.), it will be known whether Hyate:C[®] is a treatment option. The usual starting dose of Hyate:C[®] is 100 IU/kg, with subsequent doses being determined by the circulating FVIII level. Suboptimal levels on the first day or 2 of treatment should not be considered a treatment failure, as levels often rise by the second or third day.[77]

Side-effects have included transient thrombocytopenia (although this is relatively uncommon), anamnestic rise in antiporcine levels and/or human FVIII inhibitor levels, headache and allergic reactions. Since porcine FVIII is a foreign species protein, there is a risk of anaphylaxis, although this has rarely occurred. Pre-treating the patient with hydrocortisone and avoiding rapid infusion of the product can minimize or prevent allergic reactions.

Recombinant FVIIa (NovoSeven[®]), is licensed for use in Europe and Canada, but (as of September 1998) not in the US. rFVIIa was first used for surgical and postoperative coverage in a Swedish patient with a high-titer inhibitor who underwent open surgical synovectomy in 1988.[79] Hemostasis was reported to be excellent. Subsequently, rFVIIa has been used in clinical trial settings and on a compassionate basis in several hundred patients,[80,81] and appears to be safe and reasonably effective. The recommended dose is 90 μg/kg; if repeat doses are necessary, they should be given at 2–3-hour intervals in view of the short half-life of rFVIIa.[81]

Inhibitors in hemophilia B

Inhibitors occur less often in persons with hemophilia B, with most series reporting a prevalence of 1–3%. As in hemophilia A, most occur in persons with severe hemophilia, and after relatively few exposure days. As noted above, there is considerable heterogeneity in the genetic defects causing hemophilia B, and certain of these defects (large gene deletions, stop codons, frameshift mutations—defects in which there is no gene product) are associated with a higher likelihood of inhibitor development.

For those with high titer, problematic inhibitors, therapeutic options for treatment or prevention of bleeding include PCC, APCC, and (where available) rFVIIa. Dosing with these agents is the same as it would be for patients with FVIII inhibitors. While ITI regimens may be successful in eradicating or suppressing FIX inhibitors, they appear to be less successful (in approximately 50% of patients) as compared to FVIII inhibitors.

A recently recognized complication in children with hemophilia B is the development of anaphylaxis (or severe allergic reactions) in association with inhibitor development. Warrier et al[82] reported clinical and laboratory data on 18 children from the US, Canada and Europe who developed anaphylaxis or anaphylactoid reactions to infused FIX. The median age was 16 months and median number of exposure days was 11. All had large deletions or major derangements in the FIX gene. A variety of FIX products had been used prior to the severe reactions and inhibitor development (crude, intermediate and high-purity plasma-derived FIX concentrates). Subsequently, the author has received reports of at least 12 additional cases. Thus, one should be aware of its potential complication in young children with severe hemophilia B, especially those with certain defects in the FIX gene.[82]

Following desensitization to FIX in some of these children, ITI has been attempted. Not only has the response rate been poor, but 5 children have developed nephrotic syndrome after being on an ITI regimen for 7–8 months.[83] Possible reasons for this are discussed by Ewenstein et al,[83] and the physician should be aware of this potential complication and the poor success rate following the implementation of an ITI regimen.

Acquired inhibitors in non-hemophiliacs

Acquired inhibitors in non-hemophiliacs are usually directed against FVIII. They are quite uncommon in the pediatric age range, occurring mostly in postpartum females[84] or patients with systemic lupus erythematosus (SLE) or other autoimmune disease.[85] Bleeding manifestations include large, expanding ecchymoses following minor trauma or invasive procedures. Coagulation screening tests reveal a prolonged APTT, generally with a normal prothrombin time and platelet count. FVIII assay is low but is not necessarily $<1\%$, and an inhibitor assay is positive. For treatment of bleeding, rFVIII (or human plasma-derived or porcine FVIII concentrate) should by used;[86] if this is ineffective, rFVIIa (90 μg/kg every 2–3 hours) should be tried. Additionally, in an attempt to eradicate or at least suppress the inhibitor, the patient should be started on corticosteroids. While these acquired inhibitors are rarely encountered in the pediatric age group, prompt recognition and treatment may be life-saving. Transplacental transfer of an acquired FVIII inhibitor may also result in life-threatening hemorrhage in the newborn.[87]

Infectious complications of treatment with plasma-derived clotting factor concentrates

Human plasma-derived clotting factor concentrates produced in the late 1960s, 1970s and early 1980s were not treated to destroy blood-borne viruses.[40] While improved methods for donor screening, virucidal treatment[40] and nanofiltration steps were later added, and recombinant clotting factor concentrates are now available (as well as effective vaccines to prevent hepatitis A and B), a very large percentage of persons with hemophilia who received the untreated concentrates became infected with HIV-1[88] and hepatitis viruses, particularly hepatitis C virus (HCV). In North America, the last small cluster of documented HIV-1 seroconversions from clotting factor concentrates was reported in 1987, while some new HCV infections as well as hepatitis A virus (HAV) infections occurred for a few years beyond that time.[34,35] To the author's knowledge, no new cases of HIV-1, HBV, HCV or HAV attributable to clotting factor concentrates *in current use* in North America or Europe have occurred. However, human parvovirus B19 can still be transmitted,[34,35] and there have been numerous withdrawals of plasma-derived products (including intravenous gamma-globulin preparations as well as FVIII and FIX concentrates) because of a donor being found to have Creutzfeld–Jakob Disease (CJD). While there is no proof that CJD can be transmitted by plasma-derived products,[34] the US National Hemophilia Foundation, the Food and Drug Administration (FDA), and other groups have decided that it is safer to avoid the use of these products, at least until more information concerning transmissability by plasma products is available.

In view of the enormous impact of HIV infection on the hemophilia community, in the second half of the 1980s many hemophilia centers sought to establish a close working relationship with infectious disease specialists and/or AIDS clinical trials units. While not successful in all areas, through the interest, energy and determination of many physicians, patients and organizations (such as the US National Hemophilia Foundation), persons with hemophilia who were HIV infected finally gained access to AIDS clinical trials, and often to infectious disease specialists knowledgeable about HIV/AIDS. Among those still surviving, many are now on combination therapy (including protease inhibitors as well as antiviral agents), are receiving prophylaxis to prevent such opportunistic infections as *Pneumocystis carinii* pneumonia, and are having periodic viral load monitoring (HIV RNA determinations).[89] Because of the need to keep up to date on recommendations concerning management of HIV infection, AIDS and HCV infection, the US National Hemophilia Foundation's MASAC currently has 2 members who are infectious disease specialists with a particular interest in AIDS, as well as a very experienced hepatologist.

Surveys of US hemophiliacs who were treated with human plasma-derived clotting factor concentrates prepared in the 1970s and 1980s demonstrated that ~85% were seropositive to HCV. It is now known that HCV is not easily cleared by host defense mechanisms; thus, a persistent infection develops in as many as 85% of those infected with the virus. This inability to clear the virus can lead to the development of chronic liver disease; however, the range of disease states following HCV infection is broad and includes chronic hepatitis, cirrhosis, liver failure and, in a very small percentage of persons, hepatic carcinoma.[90]

Testing for HCV RNA level (viral load) by quantitative assay (either quantitative PCR or branched DNA signal amplification assay), *can* provide accurate and useful information on viral titer. However, there appears to be little or no correlation between disease severity or disease progression and level of HCV RNA. Also, as of 1998, available assays suffer from lack of standardization. Thus, periodic testing is not clinically helpful in managing patients.[90] According to the 1997 National Institutes of Health Consensus Panel, HCV genotyping and tests for HCV RNA levels may provide useful prognostic information regarding response to therapy, but at present are to be considered research tools.[90]

Who should be treated? Since no currently available treatment has proven to be highly effective and safe, treatment is currently recommended for those at greatest risk for progression to cirrhosis (those with persistently elevated alanine aminotransferase [ALT] levels, positive HCV RNA, plus a liver biopsy with portal or bridging fibrosis, inflammation and necrosis). Indication for treatment is more controversial in other patients.[90]

Factors associated with a favorable response to treatment with interferon include HCV genotype 2 or 3,[91] low serum HCV RNA level (< 106 copies/ml), and absence of cirrhosis. Randomized clinical trials have demonstrated that α-interferon benefits some but not all patients with chronic hepatitis C. Generally, when given at a dosage of 3 million units subcutaneously 3 times weekly for 6 months, 40–50% of patients have a biochemical 'end of treatment' response, but only 15–20% have a sustained biochemical response. Slightly fewer have a good virologic response.[92] Twelve-month regimens with interferon have been more successful than 6-month regimens in achieving sustained remissions; thus if interferon alone is used, 12 months would seem preferable. Many patients have side-effects to the drug; however, these are severe in < 2% of patients. Severe side-effects include autoimmune disease, severe depression, seizure disorders, acute cardiac and renal failure, retinopathy, interstitial pulmonary fibrosis, hearing impairment and sepsis. A paradoxical worsening of hepatitis can also occur and has sometimes been fatal.[90]

The disappointing results with interferon have led many to seek new approaches.[93] Recent reports have indicated that ribavirin in combination with α-interferon leads to higher sustained viral response rates (40–50%) than does α-interferon alone. Large-scale trials of the combination are currently being conducted; a multicenter randomized trial comparing α-interferon to the combination therapy in persons with hemophilia began in early 1998.

Co-infection with HCV and HIV-1 accelerates progression to hepatic insufficiency. Eyster *et al*[94] found that among hemophilic men who were co-infected, the cumulative incidence of liver failure was 17% at 10 years after HIV-1 seroconversion. HIV-1 infection probably enhances HCV replication; Eyster *et al*[94] documented an 8-fold increase in HCV RNA levels in HIV-1-infected patients compared to HIV-1-uninfected patients.[94]

Thrombocytopenia

Approximately 25% of HIV-infected hemophilic children have had some degree of thrombocytopenia. If severe, serious spontaneous hemorrhage can occur.[34,95] Zidovudine, or other drugs such as intravenous gammaglobulin, are often helpful in increasing the platelet count.[34,95]

REFERENCES

1. Department of Health and Human Services. *National Heart and Lung Institute Blood Resource Studies. Vol. 2: Pilot Study of Hemophilia Treatment in the U.S.* Washington, D.C.: U.S. Government Printing Office, 1972
2. Lusher JM, McMillan CW. Severe factor FVIII and factor IX deficiency in females. *Am J Med* 1978; **65**: 637–68
3. Giannelli F, Green PM: The molecular basis of haemophilia A and B. *Baillière's Clin Haematol* 1996; **9**: 211–228
4. Green PM, Naylor JA, Giannelli F. The hemophilias. *Adv Genet* 1995; **32**: 99–139
5. Giannelli F, Green PM, Sommer SS *et al*. Haemophilia B: database of point mutations and short additions and deletions. Fifth edition. *Nucleic Acids Res* 1994; **22**: 3534–3546
6. Lakich D, Kazazian HH, Antonarakis SE, Gitschier J. Inversions disrupting the factor VIII gene as a common cause of severe hemophilia A. *Nature Genet* 1993; **5**: 236–241
7. Naylor J, Rinke A, Hassock S, Green PM, Giannelli F. Characteristic mRNA abnormality found in half the patients with severe haemophilia A is due to large DNA inversions. *Hum Mol Genet* 1993; **2**: 1773–1778
8. Naylor JA, Buck D, Green P, Williamson H, Bentley D, Giannelli F. Investigation of the factor VIII intron 22 repeated region (int 22h) and the associated inversion junctions. *Hum Mol Genet* 1995; **4**: 1217–1224
9. Rossiter JP, Young M, Kimberland ML *et al*. Factor VIII gene inversions causing severe hemophilia A originate almost exclusively in male germ cells. *Hum Mol Genet* 1994; **3**: 1035–1039
10. Ljung RCR. Prenatal diagnosis of haemophilia. *Baillière's Clin Haematol* 1996; **9**: 243–257
11. Crossley M, Ludwig M, Stowell KM *et al*. Recovery from hemophilia B Leyden: an androgen-responsive element in the factor IX promoter. *Science* 1992; **257**: 377–379
12. Kulkarni R, Lusher JM, Henry RC, Kallen DJ. Current practices regarding neonatal intracranial hemorrhage and obstetrical care and mode of delivery of pregnant hemophilia carriers: a survey of obstetricians, neonatologists, and hematologists in the United States. *J Ped Hematol Oncol* (in press)
13. Ljung R, Lindgren AC, Petrini P, Tengborn L. Normal vaginal delivery is to be recommended for haemophilia carrier gravidae. *Acta Paediatr* 1994; **83**: 609–611
14. Kadir RA, Economides DL. Obstetric management of carriers of haemophilia. *Haemophilia* 1997; **3**: 81–86
15. Kletzel M, Miller CH, Becton DL, Chadduck WM, Elser JM. Post delivery head bleeding in hemophilic neonates. *Am J Dis Child* 1989; **143**: 1107–1110
16. Onwuzurike N, Warrier I, Lusher JM. Types of bleeding seen in the first 30 months of life in children with severe haemophilia A and B. *Haemophilia* 1996; **2**: 137–140
17. Arnold WD, Hilgartner MW. Hemophilic arthropathy. Current concepts of pathogenesis and management. *J Bone Joint Surg (Am)* 1977; **59**: 287–305
18. Pettersson H, Ahlberg Å, Nilsson IM. A radiologic classification of hemophilic arthropathy. *Clin Orthopaed* 1980; **149**: 153–159

19. Pettersson H. Can joint damage be quantified? *Semin Hematol* 1994; **31 (Suppl 2)**: 1–4

20. Berntorp E. The treatment of hemophilia, including prophylaxis, constant infusion and DDAVP. *Baillière's Clin Haematol* 1996; **9**: 259–271

21. Hanley JP, Ludlam CA. Central and peripheral nervous system bleeding. In: Forbes CD, Aledort LM, Madhok R (eds) *Hemophilia*. London: Chapman and Hall, 1997, pp 87–102

22. Nilsson IM, Lethagen S. Current status of DDAVP formulations and their use. In: Lusher JM, Kessler CM (eds) *Hemophilia and von Willebrand's Disease in the 1990s*. Amsterdam: Elsevier Science Publishers, 1991, pp 443–453

23. Mannucci PM, Bettega D, Cattaneo M. Patterns of development of tachyphylaxis in patients with haemophilia and von Willebrand disease after repeated doses of desmopressin (DDAVP). *Br J Haematol* 1992; **82**: 87–93

24. Lusher JM, Miller E, Wiseman C, Draughn M, Warrier I. Use of a highly concentrated intranasal spray formulation of desmopressin in persons with congenital bleeding disorders. In: Mariani G, Mannucci PM, Cattaneo M (eds) *Desmopressin in Bleeding Disorders*. New York: Plenum Press, 1993, pp 347–353

25. Lethagen S, Ragnarson-Tenvall G. Self-treatment with desmopressin intranasal spray in patients with bleeding disorders. Effects on bleeding symptoms and socio-economic factors. *Am J Hematol* 1993; **66**: 257–260

26. Kasper CK. Registry of clotting factor concentrates. World Fed. Hemophilia, Montreal, 1998

27. United Kingdom Haemophilia Centre Directors Organisation Executive Committee. Guildelines on therapeutic products to treat haemophilia and other hereditary coagulation disorders. *Haemophilia* 1997; **3**: 63–77

28. National Hemophilia Foundation. Medical and Scientific Advisory Council (MASAC). *Recommendations Concerning the Treatment of Hemophilia and Related Bleeding Disorders*. February 22, 1998, Medical Advisory No. 312. New York: The National Hemophilia Foundation, 1998

29. Schwartz RS, Abildgaard CF, Aledort LM et al. Human recombinant DNA-derived antihemophilic factor (factor VIII) in the treatment of hemophilia A. *N Engl J Med* 1990; **323**: 1800–1805

30. White GC II, Courter S, Bray GL, Lee M, Gomperts ED, and the Recombinate Previously Treated Patient Study Group. A multicenter study of recombinant factor VIII (Recombinate®) in previously treated patient with hemophilia A. *Thromb Haemostas* 1997; **77**: 660–667

31. Bray GL, Gomperts ED, Courter S et al. A multicenter study of recombinant factor VIII (Recombinate): safety, efficacy, and inhibitor risk in previously untreated patients with hemophilia A. *Blood* 1994; **83**: 2428–2435

32. Lusher JM, Arkin S, Abildgaard CF, Schwartz RS and Kogenate Previously Untreated Patient Study Group. Recombinant factor VIII for the treatment of previously untreated patients with hemophilia A. *N Engl J Med* 1993; **328**: 453–459

33. Fijnvandraat K, Berntorp E, ten Cate JW et al. Recombinant B-domain deleted F VIII (rFIII-SQ): pharmacokinetics and initial safety aspects in hemophilia A patients. *Thromb Haemostas* 1997; **77**: 298–302

34. Lee CA. Transfusion-transmitted disease. *Baillière's Clin Haematol* 1996; **9**: 369–394

35. Lusher JM, Kessler CM, Laurian Y, Pierce G. Viral contamination of blood products. *Lancet* 1994; **344**: 405–406

36. Kasper CK. Postoperative thromboses in hemophilia B. *N Engl J Med* 1973; **289**: 160

37. White GC II, Lundblad RL, Kingdon HS. Prothrombin complex concentrates: preparation, properties and clinical uses. *Curr Topics Hematol* 1979; **2**: 203–244

38. Menaché D, Roberts HR. Summary report and recommendations of task force members and consultants. *Thromb Haemostas* 1975; **33**: 645–647

39. Lusher JM. Thrombogenicity associated with factor IX complex concentrates. *Semin Hematol* 1991; **28 (Suppl 6)**: 3–4

40. Kasper CK, Lusher JM and Transfusion Practices Committee. Recent evaluation of clotting factor concentrates for hemophilia A and B. *Transfusion* 1993; **33**: 422–434

41. Lusher JM. Factor IX concentrates. In: Forbes CD, Aledort L, Madhok R (eds) *Haemophilia*. London: Chapman and Hall, 1997, pp 203–211

42. National Hemophilia Foundation. Medical and Scientific Advisory Council (MASAC). *Recommendations Regarding the Use of Coagulation Factor IX Products in Persons with Hemophilia B. Medical Bulletin, May 29th*. New York: The National Hemophilia Foundation, 1992

43. Lusher JM. Recombinant clotting factor concentrates. *Baillière's Clin Haematol* 1996; **9**: 291–303

44. White G, Shapiro A, Ragni M et al. Phase I/II pharmacokinetics, safety and efficacy data of recombinant human factor IX in previously treated patients with hemophilia B. *Blood* 1995; **86 (Suppl 1)**: 193A, abstract 761

45. White GC, Lusher JM, Shapiro A, Tubridy K, Courter S. Recombinant factor IX in the treatment of previously treated patients with hemophilia B. *Blood* 1996; **88 (Suppl. 1)**: 327A, abstract 1296

46. Ragni M, White G, Pasi J et al. Dose response relationship of rF IX in the surgical setting. *Blood* 1996; **88 (suppl 1)**: 329A, abstract 1305

47. McMillan CW, Webster WP, Roberts HR, Blythe WB. Continuous infusion of factor VIII in classic hemophilia. *Br J Haematol* 1970; **18**: 659–667

48. Schulman S, Martinowitz U. Design and assessment of clinical trials on continuous infusion. *Blood Coag Fibrinol* 1996; **7 (Suppl 1)**: S7–S9

49. Morfini M, Messori A, Longo G. Factor (F) VIII pharmacokinetics: intermittent versus continuous infusion. *Blood Coag Fibrinol* 1996; **7 (suppl 1)**: S11–S14

50. Goldsmith JC. Rationale and indications for continuous infusion of antihemophilic factor (factor VIII). *Blood Coag Fibrinol* 1996; **7 (Suppl 1)**: S3–S6

51. Martinowitz U, Schulman S, Gitel S et al. Adjusted dose continuous infusion of factor VIII in patients with haemophilia A. *Br J Haematol* 1992; **82**: 729–734

52. Schulman S, Gitel S, Zivelin A et al. The feasibility of using concentrates containing factor IX for continuous infusion. *Haemophilia* 1995; **1**: 103–110

53. Pierce GF, Lusher JM, Brownstein AP, Kessler CM. The use of purified clotting factor concentrates in hemophilia. Influence of viral safety, cost and supply on therapy. *JAMA* 1989; **261**: 3434–3438

54. Bohn RL, Avorn J. Reimbursement for hemophilia care in the United States: current policies and future considerations. *Semin Hematol* 1994; **31 (Suppl 2)**: 26–28

55. Sindet-Pedersen S, Ingerslev J, Ramström G, Blombäck M. Management of oral bleeding in haemophilic patients. *Lancet* 1988; **2**: 566

56. Shattil SJ, Bennett JS. Acquired qualitative platelet disorders due to diseases, drugs and foods. In: Beutler E, Lichtman MA, Coller BS, Kipps TJ (eds) *Williams' Hematology*, 5th edn. New York, McGraw-Hill, 1995, pp 1386–1400

57. National Hemophilia Foundation. Medical and Scientific Advisory Council (MASAC). *Recommendations Regarding Hepatitis A Vaccination in Individuals with Hemophilia and Other Congenital Bleeding Disorders. Medical Bulletin No. 226, April 1995*. New York, The National Hemophilia Foundation, 1995

58. Handelsman JE, Glasser RA. Pathogenesis and treatment of hemophilic arthropathy and deep muscle hemorrhages. In: Kasper CK (ed) *Recent Advances in Hemophilia Care*. New York: Alan R Liss, 1990, pp 199–206

59. Arnold WD, Hilgartner MW. Hemophilic arthropathy: current concepts of pathogenesis and management. *J Bone Joint Surg (Am)* 1977; **59**: 287–305

60. Nilsson IM, Berntorp E, Ljung R, Löfqvist T, Petterson H. Prophylactic treatment of severe hemophilia A and B can prevent joint disability. *Semin Hematol* 1994; **31 (Suppl 2)**: 5–9

61. Petrini P, Lindvall N, Egberg N, Blombäck M. Prophylaxis with factor concentrates in preventing hemophilic arthropathy. *Am J Ped Hematol-Oncol* 199; **12**: 280–287

62. National Hemophilia Foundation. Medical and Scientific Advisory

Council (MASAC). *Recommendations Concerning Prophylaxis. Medical Bulletin No. 193, Chapter Advisory No. 197, 1994.* New York: The National Hemophilia Foundation, 1994

63. Nuss R, Kilcoyne RF, Geraghy S, Wiedel J, Manco-Johnson M. Utility of magnetic resonance imaging for management of hemophilic arthropathy in children. *J Pediatr* 1993; **123**: 388–392

64. Luck JV, Kasper CK. Surgical management of advanced hemophilic arthropathy. An overview of 20 years' experience. *Clin Orthop* 1989; **242**: 60–82

65. Manco-Johnson MJ, Nuss R, Geraghty S, Funk S. A prophylactic program in the United States: experience and issues. *Semin Hematol* 1994; **31 (Suppl 2)**: 10–12

66. Rivard GE. Synoviorthesis with radioactive colloids in hemophiliacs. In: Kasper CK (ed) *Recent Advances in Hemophilia Care.* New York: Alan R. Liss, 1990, pp 215– 229

67. Lusher JM, Salzman P and the Monoclate Study Group. Viral safety and inhibitor development associated with factor VIII ultra-purified from plasma in hemophiliacs previously unexposed to factor VIII concentrates. *Semin Hematol* 1990; **27**: 1–7

68. Lusher JM, Spira J and International r-FVIII SQ Study Group. Safety, efficacy and inhibitor development in previously untreated patients (PUPs) treated exclusively with recombinant B-domain deleted FVIII (rF VIII-SQ): 2.5 study years. *Blood* 1997; **90 (Suppl 1, part 1)**: 599A, abstract 2664

69. Ehrenforth S, Kreuz W, Scharrer I et al. Incidence of factor VIII and factor VIII inhibitors in haemophiliacs. *Lancet* 1992; **339**: 594–598

70. Addiego J, Kasper C, Abildgaard CF et al. Frequency of inhibitor development in haemophiliacs treated with low purity factor VIII. *Lancet* 1993; **342**: 462–464

71. DiMichele D. A U.S. regional survey of factor VIII inhibitors. Presented at the F VIII/F IX Subcommittee meeting. International Society of Thrombosis & Haemostasis, Firenze, June 6, 1997

72. Peerlinck K, Arnout J, Gilles JG, Saint-Remy JM, Vermylen J. A higher than expected incidence of factor VIII inhibitors in multi-transfused haemophilia A patients treated with an intermediate purity pasteurized factor VIII concentrate. *Thromb Haemostas* 1993; **69**: 115–118

73. Peerlinck K, Arnout J, DiGiambattista M et al. Factor VIII inhibitors in previously treated haemophilia A patients with a double virus-inactivated plasma-derived factor VIII concentrate. *Thromb Haemostas* 1997; **77**: 80–86

74. Brettler DB. Inhibitors in congenital haemophilia. *Baillière's Clin Haematol* 1996; **9**: 319–329

75. van Leeuwen EF, Mauser-Bunschoten EP, van Kijken PJ et al. Disappearance of factor VIII:C antibodies in patients with haemophilia A upon frequent administration of factor VIII in intermediate or low dose. *Br J Haematol* 1986; **64**: 291–297

76. Nilsson IM, Berntorp E, Zettervall O. Induction of immune tolerance in patients with hemophilia and antibodies to factor VIII by combined treatment with intravenous IgG, cyclophosphamide, and factor VIII. *N Engl J Med* 1988; **328**: 947–950

77. Lusher JM, Warrier I. The role of prothrombin complex concentrates and factor VIII concentrates (human and porcine) in management of bleeding episodes in inhibitor patients. In: Lusher JM, Kessler CM (eds) *Hemophilia and von Willebrand's Disease in the 1990s.* Amsterdam: Elsevier Science Publishers, 1991, pp 271–277

78. Chavin SI, Siegal DM, Rocco TA Jr, Olson JP. Acute myocardial infarction during treatment with an activated prothrombin complex concentrate in a patient with F VIII deficiency and F VIII inhibitor. *Am J Med* 1988; **85**: 245–249

79. Hedner U, Glazer S, Pingel K et al. Successful use of recombinant factor VIIa in patient with severe haemophilia A during synovectomy. *Lancet* 1988; **2**: 1193

80. Hedner U, Feldstedt M, Glazer S. Recombinant F VIIa in hemophilia treatment. In: Lusher JM, Kessler CM (eds) *Hemophilia and von Willebrand's Disease in the 1990s.* Amsterdam: Elsevier Science Publishers, 1991, pp 283–292

81. Lusher JM, Roberts HR, Hedner U. Recombinant factor VIIa (NovoSeven): summary of world wide clinical experience. *Blood Coag Fibrinol* 1998; **9**: 119–128

82. Warrier I, Ewenstein BM, Koerper MA et al. Factor IX inhibitors and anaphylaxis in hemophilia B. *J Pediatr Hematol Oncol* 1997; **19**: 23–27

83. Ewenstein B, Takemoto C, Warrier I et al. Nephrotic syndrome as a complication of immune tolerance in hemophilia B. *Blood* 1997; **89**: 1115–1116

84. Solymoss S. Postpartum acquired factor VIII inhibitors: results of a survey. *Am J Hematol* 1998; **59**: 1–4

85. Cohen AJ, Kessler CM. Acquired inhibitors. *Baillière's Clin Haematol* 1996; **9**: 331–354

86. Morrison AE, Ludlam CA, Kessler C. Use of porcine factor VIII in the treatment of patients with acquired hemophilia. *Blood* 1993; **81**: 1513

87. Ries M, Wolfel D, Maier-Brandt B. Severe intracranial hemorrhage in a newborn infant with transplacental transfer of an acquired factor VIII:C inhibitor. *J Pediatr* 1995; **127**: 649–650

88. Gored DU, Korea B/L. HIV-1 infection in hemophilia. In: Forces CD, Alert L, Madhok R (eds) *Hemophilia.* London: Chapman and Hall Medical, 1997, pp 275–293

89. Carpenter CCJ, Fischl MA, Hammer SM et al. Consensus statement antiretroviral therapy for HIV infection in 1997. Updated recommendations of the International AIDS Society – USA panel. *JAMA* 1997; **277**: 1962–1969

90. National Institute of Health. *Consensus Development Statement. Management of Hepatitis C.* (March 24–26, 1997). Bethesda: NIH, 1997

91. Kobayashi M, Tanaka E, Sodeyama E et al. The natural course of chronic hepatitis C: a confusion between patients with genotypes 1 and 2 hepatitis C viruses. *Hepatology* 1996; **23**: 695–699

92. Martinot-Peignoux M, Marcellin P, Pouteau M et al. Pretreatment serum hepatitis C virus RNA levels and hepatitis C virus genotype are the main and independent prognostic factors of sustained response to Interferon alfa therapy in chronic hepatitis C. *Hepatology* 1995; **22**: 1050–1056

93. Hoofnagle J, DiBisceglie AM. The treatment of chronic viral hepatitis. *N Engl J Med* 1997; **336**: 347–356

94. Eyster ME, Fried MW, DiBisceglie AM, Goedert JJ. Increasing hepatitis C virus RNA levels in hemophiliacs: relationship to human immunodeficiency virus infection and liver disease. *Blood* 1994; **4**: 1020–1023

95. Ragni MV, Bontempo FA, Myers DJ et al. Hemorrhagic sequelae of immune thrombocytopenic purpura in human immunodeficiency virus infected hemophiliacs. *Blood* 1990; **75**: 1267–1272

von Willebrand disease

DAVID LILLICRAP, JULIE DEAN AND
VICTOR S BLANCHETTE

30

The disorder now recognized to be the commonest inherited bleeding condition, von Willebrand disease (VWD), was originally described by Erik von Willebrand in 1926.[1] He described a severe mucocutaneous bleeding problem in a large family residing in the Åland islands in the Gulf of Bothnia. The propositus was a 5-year-old girl, who later bled to death during her fourth menstrual period. An investigation of this disorder revealed a normal coagulation time, a normal platelet count and a prolonged bleeding time. During the next 4 decades, it was believed that this condition was most likely due to either a vascular defect or to some form of platelet dysfunction. It was not until the 1960s that an abnormality in von Willebrand factor (VWF) was implicated in the pathogenesis of the disorder, and even then, the failure to differentiate VWF from Factor VIII (FVIII) further complicated studies until their eventual definitive separation through genetic cloning in the mid-1980s.[2,3]

DEMOGRAPHICS AND INHERITANCE

Estimates of the prevalence of VWD have varied from ∼1% of the general population[4] to 125 clinically relevant cases/ million. Nevertheless, even in the surveys in which the higher prevalence figures have been obtained, the affected individuals have been documented to have some, albeit mild, clinical evidence of a hemostatic defect.[4] VWD appears to be a disorder that can affect individuals from all ethnic backgrounds, although several localized concentrations of severe disease have been documented in, for example, Israel, Sweden and Iran.

In surveys performed on VWD populations, ∼80% of cases have the mild type 1 form of the disorder; most of the remainder have various type 2 forms of the condition, with types 2A, 2B and 2N comprising the majority of these cases (Table 30.1). The severe type 3 form of the disease is fortunately rare, with a prevalence of ∼1/million.

As more is learnt about the underlying genetic pathogen-

Table 30.1 Classification of von Willebrand disease subtypes based on the 1994 recommendations of the VWD Sub-Committee of the Scientific and Standardization Committee of the International Society of Thrombosis and Haemostasis.

Type 1 VWD: Partial quantitative deficiency of VWF (80%)

Type 2 VWD: Qualitative defects of VWF (15–20%)
   Type 2A VWD: Qualitative variants with decreased platelet-dependent function associated with the absence of high molecular weight multimers
   Type 2B VWD: Qualitative variants with increased affinity for binding glycoprotein Ib
   Type 2M VWD: Qualitative variants with decreased platelet-dependent function associated with a normal distribution of multimers
   Type 2N VWD: Qualitative variants with reduced binding of FVIII

Type 3 VWD: virtual complete absence of VWF (rare)

esis of VWD, the inheritance pattern of the condition continues to be revised. It is believed that most cases of types 1, 2A and 2B disease represent autosomal dominant conditions that exhibit variable phenotypic penetrance and expressivity. In contrast, types 2N and 3 disease are recessive conditions with patients having been documented to be either homozygotes or compound heterozygotes for mutations within the VWF gene.

BIOSYNTHESIS AND FUNCTION

The gene that encodes VWF is located on the short arm of chromosome 12.[3] The VWF gene is a large and complex locus encompassing 175 kb of DNA and comprising 52 exons.[5] Expression of the gene is limited to 2 cell types, vascular endothelial cells[6] and megakaryocytes.[7] The primary translation product of the gene is a pre-pro-VWF protein which has a short amino terminal signal peptide, a ∼100 kDa propeptide that appears to be involved in multimer assembly, and a mature subunit comprised of 2050 amino acid residues. The pro-VWF molecule consists of 4 repeated domains that constitute >90% of the sequence.[8]

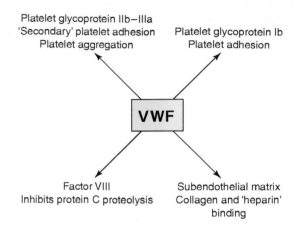

Fig. 30.1 Multiple binding partners for von Willebrand factor (VWF) and functional role of these interactions.

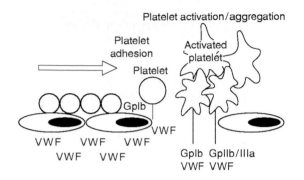

Fig. 30.2 Role of von Willebrand factor (VWF) in mediating the initial events in the hemostatic process. Platelets, rolling along the endothelial cell surface, are tethered to the site of endothelial cell injury through the binding of subendothelial VWF to the glycoprotein (Gp) Ib receptor. The platelets are subsequently activated and the GpIIb-IIIa complex is exposed on the platelet surface. Interaction of VWF with GpIIb-IIIa consolidates the platelet adhesive event and initiates platelet aggregation.

Following translation, the pre-pro-VWF molecule undergoes a series of complex and seemingly essential post-translational modifications. These include signal peptide cleavage, dimerization, glycosylation, sulfation and eventual multimerization and propeptide cleavage in the Golgi. The fully processed protein is then sorted into 1 of 2 pathways involving either constitutive secretion from the cell of synthesis or storage in specialized organelles, the Weibel–Palade bodies of endothelial cells or α-granules of platelets. Following appropriate stimuli, such as thrombin deposition or platelet activation, VWF is released from these storage sites into the plasma, where it circulates with a molecular weight ranging from 600–20 000 kDa depending upon the extent of subunit multimerization.[9]

VWF is a multifunctional adhesive protein that binds to several different ligands in plasma and the subendothelial matrix (Fig. 30.1). Its has 2 major physiologic roles:

- as a carrier protein for the coagulation cofactor FVIII. This has the consequence that low levels of VWF result in correspondingly low levels of FVIII due to its increased proteolytic degradation by activated protein C.[10]
- an essential role in the initial cellular stages of the hemostatic process, platelet adhesion and platelet aggregation (Fig. 30.2). VWF secreted from the basolateral surface of endothelial cells is adherent to the subendothelial matrix and interacts with the platelet receptor glycoprotein (Gp) Ib to initiate platelet adhesion and platelet activation.[11] The GpIIb-IIIa complex is then exposed and VWF plays an additional role in binding to this receptor and facilitating the process of platelet aggregation.[12]

LABORATORY EVALUATION

The laboratory findings of this common bleeding condition are highly variable, ranging from the consequences of the complete absence of VWF in type 3 disease, to minimal alterations in VWF and FVIII levels in patients with type 1 VWD. Indeed, due to the variable penetrance and expressivity of this trait, many individuals may have inherited mutant VWF alleles but fail to manifest any clinical or laboratory abnormalities.

Screening tests

A number of rapid and inexpensive hematologic screening studies should be performed in the initial evaluation of possible VWD. The complete blood count may show evidence of an iron-deficiency anemia due to chronic blood loss and type 2B VWD is often associated with a mild thrombocytopenia. If the plasma VWF level is significantly reduced ($< \sim 0.35$ unit/ml), the correspondingly low level of FVIII may result in a prolonged activated partial thromboplastin time (APTT).

Finally, the bleeding time may be prolonged.[13] However, it is important to note that many patients with proven VWD have normal APTTs and bleeding times and that the results of these screening studies must be interpreted in the context of the patient's clinical history. Although some hematologists no longer use the bleeding time in their diagnostic work-up of potential VWD, its use is probably justified to evaluate the presence of one of the differential diagnoses, platelet dysfunction.

von Willebrand factor—Factor VIII complex

VWF and FVIII circulate in plasma as a bimolecular complex, and the laboratory evaluation of VWD must include tests for both of these proteins. Plasma FVIII coagulant levels are measured using a standard APTT-based assay, utilizing FVIII-deficient plasma. Plasma VWF should be assessed in 2 ways—a quantitative immunologic assay and a functional test that evaluates its platelet-dependent interaction.

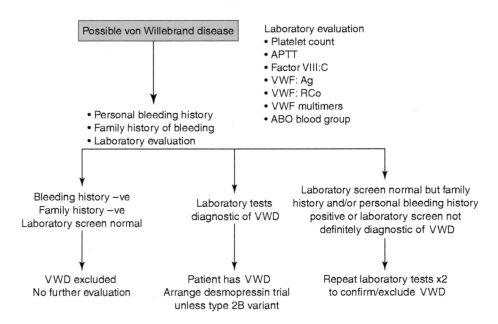

Fig. 30.3 Algorithm for the investigation of patients with possible von Willebrand disease.

The 2 common VWF immunoassays (measuring VWF:Ag) used in clinical laboratories involve either a Laurell rocket immunelectrophoretic assay or an enzyme-linked immunosorbent assay (ELISA). The former protocol is limited by a sensitivity of ~0.10 unit/ml and the tendency to overestimate the levels of VWF in type 2 variants due to the excess of low molecular weight forms of the protein. In comparison, most ELISA assays detect down to 0.01 unit/ml and are unaffected by type 2 variant plasmas.

The functional activity of plasma VWF is usually evaluated by testing its interactive role with platelets. The antibiotic ristocetin induces the binding of VWF to GpIb receptor on platelets and is used in the laboratory to quantify the functional activity of plasma VWF in the ristocetin cofactor assay (VWF:RCo).[14] Ristocetin was withdrawn from clinical use because of its *in vivo* association with thrombocytopenia, presumably due to the clearance of ristocetin-induced platelet aggregates.[15] The other test that utilizes ristocetin is the ristocetin-induced platelet agglutination (RIPA) assay that evaluates the sensitivity of a patient's platelets to low-dose ristocetin. This test is especially useful in

identifying individuals with type 2B VWD in whom the platelet membranes are 'overloaded' with the high-affinity mutant VWF resulting in an increased sensitivity to ristocetin concentrations below 0.6 mg/ml.[16]

The normal plasma level of VWF is ~10 μg/ml, with a wide normal population range of 50–200% of the mean value (0.5–2.0 unit/dl). Several important genetic and environmental influences must be kept in mind when interpreting the results of VWF plasma estimations. The best characterized genetic influence relates to an ABO blood group effect;[17] the FVIII and VWF levels of blood group O individuals are approximately 25% lower than those with blood groups A, B and AB. This has lead to the suggestion that separate blood group O and non-group O normal ranges might enhance the identification of results that are more clearly indicative of pathologically low FVIII and VWF levels (Table 30.2). The major environmental influence on VWF and FVIII levels is their involvement in the acute phase response. The plasma levels of both proteins will increase by 3–5-fold during acute physiologic stress and at times such as the later stages of pregnancy. The plasma levels of these proteins can vary so widely over time from a variety of influences (e.g. hormone levels in women) that at least 2 (and optimally 3) sets of laboratory results should be obtained from patients prior to confirming or refuting the diagnosis of VWD (Fig. 30.3).

The final laboratory evaluation required to characterize VWD involves the assessment of the circulating molecular weight profile of VWF.[18] As mentioned above, VWF circulates in the plasma in the form of a heterogeneous mixture of multimers ranging in size from 600–20 000 kDa. The high molecular weight multimeric forms of the protein are the most effective in mediating the platelet interactive functions of VWF and it is these forms that are absent in some type 2

Table 30.2 Influence of ABO blood group on FVIII and VWF levels: 95% lower confidence limits in 58 children with Group O and non-Group O blood types. Derived from a study of type 1 VWD diagnosis by Dean *et al* at the Hospital for Sick Children in Toronto.

	Group O (unit/ml)	Non-group O (unit/ml)
FVIII:C	0.57	0.80
VWF:Ag	0.37	0.50
VWF:RCo	0.42	0.51

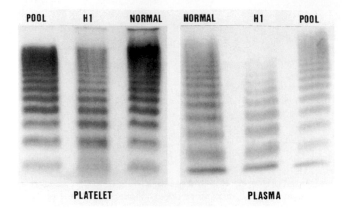

POOL   H1   NORMAL   NORMAL   H1   POOL

PLATELET   PLASMA

Fig. 30.4 Multimer analysis in a patient (H1) with type 2B VWD. While the plasma von Willebrand factor (VWF) from this patient shows a deficit of the highest molecular weight forms of the protein, the platelet multimer pattern is normal. This difference in multimeric composition relates to the enhanced affinity of the mutant VWF for binding to the platelet glycoprotein Ib receptor.

forms of VWD. Two methods have been used to evaluate the molecular weight profile of plasma VWF, an agarose gel 2-dimensional immunoelectrophoresis and the more favored electrophoretic multimer assay (Fig. 30.4). The most recent advances have combined non-radioactive, chemoluminescent detection of VWF multimers with the densitometric analysis of multimer bands in efforts both to simplify and enhance the objectivity of the assay.

CLASSIFICATION

The VWD Sub-Committee of the Scientific and Standardization Committee of the International Society of Throm-

bosis and Haemostasis proposed the currently accepted classification of VWD in 1994 (Table 30.1).[19] This involves 3 major categories:

- *Type 1 disease* comprises ~80% of cases and presents with a partial, mild-moderate quantitative reduction of VWF levels.
- The other quantitative defect, *type 3 disease*, occurs with a frequency of ~1/million and represents a virtual absence of VWF.
- The various *type 2 forms of the disease* involve the synthesis of qualitative mutant forms of the protein that manifest abnormalities in multimerization, platelet and FVIII binding (Fig. 30.5). Type 2 forms of VWD account for ~20% of diagnosed cases.

TYPE 1 VON WILLEBRAND DISEASE

While this is clearly the commonest form of the disease, it is also the most problematic to diagnose with certainty. Plasma levels of VWF (both VWF:Ag and VWF:RCo) and FVIII can range from ~0.05 to ~0.45 unit/ml in this condition and the caveats raised above concerning ABO blood group and acute phase influences, are especially pertinent to the diagnosis of this subtype of VWD. It is important to note that only some patients with this disorder will have abnormal hemostatic screening studies (i.e. prolonged APTT and bleeding times). Recent attempts to clarify the diagnosis of this condition have focused on three factors:

- evidence of a family history of the disease;
- a clinical bleeding history;
- laboratory demonstration of VWF deficiency.

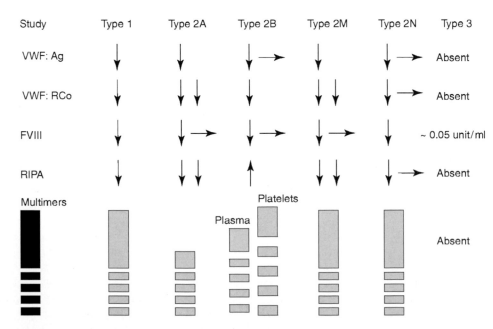

Fig. 30.5 Classification and results of laboratory studies in the common forms of von Willebrand disease (VWD). Rare reports of type 2 variant forms of VWD have appeared, in which the main findings are different abnormalities in the pattern of VWF multimers.

Table 30.3 Clinical definitions of a significant bleeding trait.

Recurrent nose bleeds requiring medical treatment (packing, cautery, desmopressin, etc.) or leading to anemia

Oral cavity bleeding lasting for at least 1 hour, restarting over the next 7 days or requiring medical treatment

Bleeding from skin lacerations lasting for at least 1 hour, restarting over the next 7 days or requiring medical treatment

Prolonged bleeding associated with, or following, dental extraction or other oral surgery

Menorrhagia requiring medical attention or leading to anemia

Spontaneous gastrointestinal bleeding requiring medical treatment or leading to anemia, unexplained by local causes

Prolonged bleeding from other skin or mucous membrane surfaces requiring medical treatment

Without documentation of all 3 of these features, the diagnosis of type 1 VWD is rendered less definitive.

The genetic basis for type 1 VWD remains largely unresolved.[20] The inheritance pattern best fits that of a dominant trait with marked variability of both phenotypic penetrance and expressivity. Very few type 1 VWD mutations have been described on the Internet-accessible VWD Mutation Database (http://mmg2.im.med.umich.edu.) and indeed, it is not at all clear that these mutations occur predominantly at the VWF locus as opposed to loci involved with the post-synthetic processing of the protein.[21]

Patients with type 1 VWD exhibit an increase in mucocutaneous bleeding. The commonest features are nose bleeds, easy bruising, bleeding from trivial cuts and excessive menstrual bleeding. Prolonged and delayed onset bleeding following tooth extractions and oral surgery is also a common feature. Bleeding into soft tissues and joints does not occur unless provoked by trauma. Unfortunately, as with many aspects of this disease, definitive documentation of these clinical characteristics is not always straightforward, and an attempt should be made to enhance the objectivity of these historic details (Table 30.3).

TYPE 3 VON WILLEBRAND DISEASE

Unlike most other forms of the disease (aside from type 2N), the inheritance pattern of type 3 disease best fits that of a recessive condition, with both carriers being asymptomatic. However, some families have been described in which a child with type 3 disease has 1 parent with documented evidence of type 1 VWD, illustrating the heterogeneous nature of the inheritance of this disease subtype and indicating that it is sometimes not a truly recessive trait.

Type 3 patients manifest a clinically severe phenotype. Not only do they exhibit the same mucocutaneous bleeding features seen in type 1 disease (in a more pronounced fashion) but, due to their low levels of plasma FVIII (<0.10 unit/ml), they also experience the joint and soft tissue bleeds seen in hemophilia A patients. In the laboratory, this condition is characterized by prolongation of the APTT and bleeding time, undetectable levels of VWF:Ag and VWF:RCo and FVIII levels below 0.10 unit/ml.

Molecular genetic studies of type 3 patients indicate that many of these subjects have gross deletions and frameshift and nonsense mutations in their VWF genes. In some instances, these mutations are associated with the development of alloantibodies that seriously complicate treatment.[22,23]

TYPE 2 VON WILLEBRAND DISEASE

The current classification divides these qualitative variants into those that affect the platelet-dependent function of VWF and those that reduce binding to FVIII. The clinical features are similar to those seen in type 1 disease.

Type 2A

Type 2A disease is characterized by the presence of VWF that lacks the high and intermediate sized multimers of the protein. This defect appears to result from either the synthesis of proteolytically susceptible multimers or an inherent inability to form the higher molecular weight multimers.[24] This subtype accounts for ~15% of VWD cases in most populations and segregates within families as an autosomal dominant trait.

Type 2A disease can initially be suspected from a disproportionately low VWF:RCo level relative to the VWF:Ag. The FVIII level may be low or normal. Ristocetin-induced platelet agglutination is reduced and the multimer profile will show a loss of intermediate and high molecular weight forms in both the plasma and platelet lysates.

The molecular genetic basis of type 2A VWD has been well characterized, with the majority of mutations being missense changes in the region of the VWF gene encoding the A2 protein domain (Fig. 30.6).[25]

Type 2B

Type 2B VWD represents an interesting 'gain-of-function' mutant form of the disease. In this condition, the mutant form of VWF binds with greater affinity to the GpIb receptor on platelets, resulting in the selective depletion from the plasma of the highest multimeric forms of VWF.[17,26] The increased binding of the mutant VWF to platelets also results in the formation of platelet aggregates and subsequent thrombocytopenia. Thus, type 2B VWD should be considered in the differential diagnosis of inherited forms of thrombocytopenia.

As with type 2A disease, in patients with type 2B VWD, the VWF:RCo will likely be disproportionately low relative to the VWF:Ag, but with this subtype there is increased sensitivity to low-dose ristocetin-induced platelet agglutination. In addition, on multimeric analysis, only the highest

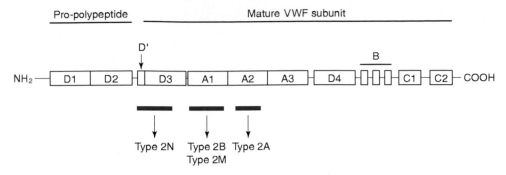

Fig. 30.6 Repeating multi-domain structure of the von Willebrand factor protein. The regions of the protein comprising the pro-polypeptide and mature subunits are indicated at the top of the diagram. Regions of the protein in which the causative mutations for types 2A, 2B, 2M and 2N von Willebrand disease are found are shown at the bottom.

molecular weight forms are absent from the plasma, while in platelets, the multimer pattern is normal (reflecting the increased binding of the mutant VWF to the platelet surface).

Also like type 2A disease, this variant exhibits an autosomal dominant mode of inheritance. The mutations in type 2B disease have been well characterized and represent a variety of different missense mutations in the region of the VWF gene encoding the GpIb binding region of the protein, the A1 domain.[27]

A disorder known as platelet type VWD (PT-VWD) exhibits identical clinical and laboratory features to those of type 2B VWD.[28] This condition is caused by mutations in the GpIb α gene that affect the region of the receptor that binds to VWF.[29] Type 2B VWD and PT-VWD can be differentiated by specialized tests that distinguish enhanced ristocetin-induced binding of VWF to washed patient platelets. Because of the identical nature of the screening laboratory studies in these conditions, their relative frequencies are unknown, although it is assumed that PT-VWD is significantly less prevalent in most populations.

Type 2M

This rare type 2 variant of VWD is characterized by the same disproportionate reduction in VWF:RCo levels relative to VWF:Ag seen in type 2A and 2B disease, but the plasma and platelet multimers are normal and ristocetin-induced platelet agglutination is reduced. In those cases in which the disease-causing mutation has been identified, this has been a missense alteration in the same region of the VWF gene in which the type 2B mutations are localized, the A1 domain.[30]

Type 2N

This VWD subtype represents an important patient population that can be confused for other conditions in which the only laboratory abnormality is a low plasma FVIII level. Unlike the other type 2 forms of VWD, type 2N VWD exhibits a recessive mode of inheritance.

Type 2N disease has been described as an autosomal form of hemophilia A.[31] The bleeding tendency is relatively mild and on laboratory investigation, often the only abnormality is a low FVIII level of between 0.10 and 0.40 unit/ml. The definitive diagnosis of type 2N disease requires one of two strategies,[32] either the demonstration of reduced FVIII binding in a microtiter plate-based assay or the demonstration of the disease causing mutations in the regions of the gene encoding the N-terminal D′ FVIII-binding domain of the protein.

CLINICAL MANAGEMENT

As this is the commonest inherited bleeding condition with a prevalence of up to 1% of the population, physicians of all types are faced with the management of patients with VWD.

It should be evident from the discussion of the laboratory features of the disease and its classification, that one of the most problematic areas of management is the definitive diagnosis of the disorder. While type 3 and type 2 forms of the disorder should be readily identifiable (with access to an experienced coagulation laboratory), the diagnosis of type 1 disease still poses problems.[33] Assigning an incorrect diagnostic label of VWD to a patient can be difficult to revise and may result in confusion and inappropriate management decisions. In addition, the wider implications of this diagnostic label, including its potential social stigma, should be considered before pronouncing any individual to be affected with VWD.

VWD is an inherited disorder and, as such, genetic counseling is appropriate in affected families. However, the variable penetrance and expressivity of the disorder complicate the prediction of phenotypic consequences. Furthermore, the relatively mild nature of the bleeding problems, except in type 3 disease, obviates the need to consider prenatal testing. Although there is no suggestion that infants who have potentially inherited VWD need to be delivered routinely by caesarian section, they should not be subjected to prolonged or complicated (vacuum extraction or mid-cavity forceps) vaginal deliveries.

PROPHYLACTIC AND THERAPEUTIC TREATMENT OF BLEEDING

Adjunctive therapies

In addition to treatments that specifically address the VWF deficit, there are several adjunctive therapies which are effective at reducing blood loss in these patients. The anti-fibrinolytic agents, tranexamic acid and aminocaproic acid, have been used as highly efficacious agents either alone or as complements to desmopressin (DDAVP) and blood component therapy in both prophylactic and therapeutic situations. They should be administered 2 hours prior to an anticipated hemostatic challenge and continued for 7 to 10 days after the challenge. The therapeutic oral doses are 25 mg/kg every 6–8 hours for tranexamic acid and 100–200 mg/kg every 6 hours for aminocaproic acid. Both agents are also available as intravenous preparations and tranexamic acid has also been demonstrated to be effective as a mouth wash.[34] Both drugs are usually well tolerated, aside from occasional mild gastrointestinal upset.

Estrogen therapy has also been shown to be an effective measure in reducing menstrual bleeding and the frequency and magnitude of nose bleeds.

Desmopressin

Desmopressin (DDAVP [1-deamino-8-D-arginine vasopressin]) is a synthetic analog of the antidiuretic hormone vasopressin.[35] Its infusion increases plasma VWF and FVIII levels by 2–8-fold within 1 hour of administration.[36] This effect is presumed to be due to the release of VWF from endothelial cell stores (Weibel–Palade bodies) with the secondary stabilization of additional FVIII. Precisely how this release is achieved is unclear, but the fact that direct exposure of endothelial cells to desmopressin in culture does not result in Weibel–Palade body emptying suggests the involvement of an intermediary molecule in the process.[37]

Desmopressin can be administered by the intravenous, subcutaneous or intranasal route.[38] Peak responses will be achieved within 30 and 90 min with the intravenous and intranasal routes, respectively. The usual parenteral dose is 0.3 μg/kg (to a maximum of 20 μg), infused in 10–50 ml of normal saline over $\sim$20 min. The dose of the highly concentrated intranasal preparation is 150 μg for children under 50 kg and 300 μg for larger children. It should be noted that another intranasal preparation of desmopressin is available for the treatment of diabetes insipidus. However, this is a low concentration compound and does not result in significant increments to the plasma VWF and FVIII levels.

Desmopressin is a safe and generally very effective hemostatic agent. Its only common side-effects are facial flushing, mild headache and minimal changes to the blood pressure and heart rate. All of these can be minimized by increasing the duration of the infusion to $\sim$60 min from the usual $\sim$20 min. The most serious side-effects that can develop are severe hyponatremia and seizures.[39,40] Children <2 years of age are especially prone to this complication and their fluid intake should be reduced to maintenance levels for the 24 hours following desmopressin administration. In addition, with repeated doses of the drug, serial monitoring of the serum sodium should be undertaken.

The other limitation to this agent is the development of tachyphylaxis with repeated administration. When given at repeated intervals of 24 hours or shorter, the magnitude of VWF and FVIII increments achieved often falls to $\sim$70% of that documented with the initial dose.[41] This is presumably related to a partial 'exhaustion' of the endothelial cell stores. The reduced VWF increments obtained with repeated desmopressin infusion is only a relative limitation to its use for several consecutive days and it will often be effective in this clinical setting.

The plasma VWF and FVIII level response should be evaluated in every patient with a therapeutic trial of the agent, preferably prior to the first treatment. This is necessary as not all patients, particularly those with severe type 1 or type 2 VWD, respond adequately to this therapy. Desmopressin can be used as a prophylactic or therapeutic agent in a wide variety of clinical circumstances including the treatment of epistaxis and menstrual bleeding, and prior to dental procedures and minor surgery. Major surgical procedures and life-threatening bleeds should be treated with blood component therapy (see below).

More than 90% of type 1 VWD patients should respond satisfactorily to desmopressin infusion, and for this common form of the disease, the concomitant use of desmopressin and antifibrinolytic therapy should be sufficient for most clinical situations. In contrast, desmopressin has only been reported very rarely to be effective in type 3 patients and should not be considered the treatment of choice for this population. The therapeutic effect of desmopressin in the type 2 variant forms of VWD is variable. Some type 2A patients are very adequately treated and this patient group will be evident from a therapeutic trial infusion. In type 2B patients the situation is more controversial. While infusion of desmopressin consistently results in transient thrombocytopenia in these patients, several investigators have documented an excellent hemostatic effect from this treatment.[42,43] In addition, the theoretical concern of desmopressin-induced thrombosis due to potential platelet aggregate formation has not been documented. Therefore, desmopressin can probably be used safely and with effect in treating or preventing minor bleeding in type 2B patients. Finally, desmopressin has been used in type 2N VWD patients where it has been found to increase both VWF and FVIII levels between 2- and 9-fold.[44] However, due to the fact that the VWF being released is the FVIII-binding mutant, the duration of the FVIII increment is only $\sim$3 hours. This suggests that for type 2N patients, desmopressin should only be used in clinical situations where a brief, transient rise in FVIII is required.

Blood component therapy

Treatment of VWD with blood component transfusion is required for major dental and surgical procedures, following trauma and to treat life-threatening bleeding. Cryoprecipitate, the standard component used for VWD therapy during the 1970s and 1980s, is no longer the material of choice. No effective viral attenuation process has yet been devised for cryoprecipitate and thus the risk of viral transmission has relegated this blood component to a rare alternative therapy in this condition.

The blood components currently used are plasma-derived, intermediate purity FVIII concentrates that have undergone a variety of viral inactivation steps to prevent viral infection.[45,46] The latest, high and ultra-high purity FVIII concentrates, such as the monoclonally purified concentrates and recombinant FVIII, have a very low VWF content and are not useful in this context. Interestingly, although intermediate purity concentrates such as Haemate-P are frequently used with good effect in VWD, none of these materials is licensed for this purpose and their VWF content is often not stated precisely.

Although probably not ideal (nor very logical), most dosing recommendations for treatment of VWD are based on FVIII unit increments. The dose of the intermediate purity concentrate required to elevate plasma FVIII to the required level is calculated in the same way as recommended for hemophilia A (i.e. desired FVIII increment × weight in kg × 0.4) (see Chapter 29). A FVIII level of 1 unit/ml should be the target for major surgery and life-threatening bleeds and 0.5 unit/ml for minor surgical and dental procedures. Plasma FVIII levels can be monitored to assess treatment response and, with a VWF half-life of ~18 hours, repeat infusions should be given every 12–24 hours.

In the rare event that infusion with an intermediate purity concentrate such as Haemate-P is ineffective at stopping bleeding, transfusion with either platelet concentrates[47] or cryoprecipitate has been used as an effective second-line treatment.

Finally, at least 2 recombinant VWF preparations are currently undergoing pre-clinical and limited scale clinical testing. At this stage, it is too early to assess the relative advantages of these compounds.

REFERENCES

1. von Willebrand EA. Hereditar pseudohemofili. *Finska Lakarsallskapets Handl* 1926; **67**: 7–112
2. Sadler JE, Shelton-Inloes BB, Sorace JM, Harlan JM, Titani K, Davie EW. Cloning and characterization of two cDNAs coding for human von Willebrand factor. *Proc Natl Acad Sci USA* 1985; **82**: 6394–6398
3. Ginsburg D, Handin RI, Bonthron DT *et al.* Human von Willebrand factor (VWF): Isolation of complementary DNA (cDNA) clones and chromosomal localization. *Science* 1985; **228**: 1401–1403
4. Rodeghiero F, Castaman G, Dini E. Epidemiological investigation of the prevalence of von Willebrand's disease. *Blood* 1987; **69**: 454–459
5. Mancuso DJ, Tuley EA, Westfield LA *et al.* Structure of the gene for human von Willebrand factor. *J Biol Chem* 1989; **264**: 19514–19527
6. Wagner DD, Marder VJ. Biosynthesis of von Willebrand protein by human endothelial cells: processing steps and their intracellular localization. *J Cell Biol* 1984; **99**: 2123–2130
7. Sporn LA, Chavin SI, Marder VJ, Wagner DD. Biosynthesis of von Willebrand protein by human megakaryocytes. *J Clin Invest* 1985; **76**: 1102–1106
8. Shelton-Inloes B, Titani K, Sadler J. cDNA sequences for human von Willebrand factor reveal five types of repeated domains and five possible protein sequence polymorphisms. *Biochemistry* 1986; **25**: 3164–3171
9. Ruggeri Z, Zimmerman T. The complex multimeric composition of factor VIII/von Willebrand factor. *Blood* 1981; **57**: 1140–1143
10. Koedam JA, Meijers JCM, Sixma JJ, Bouma BN. Inactivation of human factor VIII by activated protein C. Cofactor activity of protein S and protective effect of von Willebrand factor. *J Clin Invest* 1988; **82**: 1236–1243
11. Savage B, Saldivar E, Ruggeri ZM. Initiation of platelet adhesion by arrest onto fibrinogen or translocation on von Willebrand factor. *Cell* 1996; **84**: 289–297
12. Ruggeri ZM. Mechanisms of shear-induced platelet adhesion and aggregation. *Thromb Haemostas* 1993; **70**: 119–123
13. Mannucci PM, Pareti FI, Holmberg L, Nilsson IM, Ruggeri ZM. Studies on the prolonged bleeding time in von Willebrand's disease. *J Lab Clin Med* 1976; **88**: 662–673
14. Howard MA, Firkin BG. Ristocetin – A new tool in the investigation of platelet aggregation. *Thromb Haemostas* 1971; **26**: 362–369
15. Gangarosa EJ, Johnson TR, Ramos HS. Ristocetin-induced thrombocytopenia: site and mechanism of action. *Arch Intern Med* 1960; **105**: 83–89
16. Cooney KA, Lyons SE, Ginsburg D. Functional analysis of a type 2B von Willebrand disease missense mutation: Increased binding of large von Willebrand factor multimers to platelets. *Proc Natl Acad Sci USA* 1992; **89**: 2869–2872
17. Gill JC, Endres-Brooks J, Bauer PJ, Marks WJJ, Montgomery RR. The effect of ABO blood group on the diagnosis of von Willebrand disease. *Blood* 1987; **69**: 1691–1695
18. Hoyer LW, Rizza CR, Tuddenham EGD, Carta CA, Armitage H, Rotblat F. Von Willebrand factor multimer patterns in von Willebrand's disease. *Br J Haematol* 1983; **55**: 493–507
19. Sadler JE. A revised classification of von Willebrand disease. *Thromb Haemostas* 1994; **71**: 520–525
20. Ginsburg D, Bowie EJW. Molecular genetics of von Willebrand disease. *Blood* 1992; **79**: 2507–2519
21. Mohlke KL, Nichols WC, Westrick RJ *et al.* A novel modifier gene for plasma von Willebrand factor level maps to distal mouse chromosome 11. *Proc Natl Acad Sci USA* 1996; **93**: 15352–15357
22. Shelton-Inloes B, Chehab F, Mannucci P, Federici A, Sadler E. Gene deletions correlate with the development of alloantibodies in von Willebrand's disease. *J Clin Invest* 1987; **79**: 1459–1465
23. Ngo K, Glotz Trifard V, Koziol J *et al.* Homozygous and heterozygous deletions of the von Willebrand factor gene in patients and carriers of severe von Willebrand disease. *Proc Natl Acad Sci USA* 1988; **85**: 2753–2757
24. Lyons SE, Bruck ME, Bowie EJW, Ginsburg D. Impaired intracellular transport produced by a subset of type 2A von Willebrand disease mutations. *J Biol Chem* 1992; **267**: 4424–4430
25. Inbal A, Seligsohn U, Kornbrot N *et al.* Characterization of three point mutations causing von Willebrand disease type 2A in five unrelated families. *Thromb Haemostas* 1992; **67**: 618–622
26. Ruggeri ZM, Pareti FI, Mannucci PM, Ciavarella N, Zimmerman TS. Heightened interaction between platelets and factor VIII/von

Willebrand factor in a new subtype of von Willebrand's disease. *N Engl J Med* 1980; **302**: 1047–1051

27. Cooney KA, Nichols WC, Bruck *et al*. The molecular defect in type 2B von Willebrand disease. Identification of four potential missense mutations within the putative GpIb binding domain. *J Clin Invest* 1991; **87**: 1227–1233

28. Miller JL, Castella A. Platelet-type von Willebrand's disease: characterization of a new bleeding disorder. *Blood* 1982; **60**: 790–794

29. Bryckaert MC, Pietu G, Ruan C *et al*. Abnormality of glycoprotein Ib in two cases of "pseudo"-von Willebrand's disease. *J Lab Clin Med* 1985; **106**: 393–400

30. Mancuso DJ, Kroner PA, Christopherson PA, Vokac EA, Gill JC, Montgomery RR. Type 2M: Milwaukee-1 von Willebrand disease: an in-frame deletion in the Cys509-Cys695 loop of the von Willebrand factor A1 domain causes deficient binding of von Willebrand factor to platelets. *Blood* 1996; **88**: 2559–2568

31. Mazurier C. von Willebrand disease masquerading as haemophilia A. *Thromb Haemostas* 1992; **67**: 391–396

32. Nesbitt IM, Goodeve AC, Guilliatt AM, Makris M, Preston FE, Peake IR. Characterisation of type 2N von Willebrand disease using phenotypic and molecular techniques. *Thromb Haemostas* 1996; **75**: 959–964

33. Batlle J, Torea J, Rendal E, Fernandez MF. The problem of diagnosing von Willebrand's disease. *J Intern Med* 1997; **740 (Suppl)**: 121–128

34. Sindet-Pedersen S, Ramstrom G, Bernvil S, Blomback M. Hemostatic effect of tranexamic acid mouthwash in anticoagulant-treated patients undergoing oral surgery. *N Engl J Med* 1989; **320**: 840–843

35. Mannucci PM. Desmopressin: A nontransfusional hemostatic agent. *Annu Rev Med* 1990; **41**: 55–64

36. Rodeghiero F, Castaman G, Di Bona E, Ruggeri M. Consistency of responses to repeated DDAVP infusions in patients with von Willebrand's disease and hemophilia A. *Blood* 1989; **74**: 1997–2000

37. Hashemi S, Tackaberry ES, Palmer DS, Rock G, Ganz PR. DDAVP-induced release of von Willebrand factor from endothelial cells *in vitro*: The effect of plasma and blood cells. *Biochim Biophys Acta Mol Cell Res* 1990; **1052**: 63–70

38. Rose EH, Aledort LM. Nasal spray desmopressin (DDAVP) for mild hemophilia A and von Willebrand disease. *Ann Intern Med* 1991; **114**: 563–568

39. Humphries JE, Siragy H. Significant hyponatremia following DDAVP administration in a healthy adult. *Am J Hematol* 1993; **44**: 12–15

40. Weinstein RE, Bona RD, Altman AJ *et al*. Severe hyponatremia after repeated intravenous administration of desmopressin. *Am J Hematol* 1989; **32**: 258–261

41. Mannucci PM, Bettega D, Cattaneo M. Patterns of development of tachyphylaxis in patients with haemophilia and von Willebrand disease after repeated doses of desmopressin (DDAVP). *Br J Haematol* 1992; **82**: 87–93

42. Fowler WE, Berkowitz LR, Roberts HR. DDAVP for type 2B von Willebrand disease. *Blood* 1989; **74**: 1859–1860

43. Casonato A, Sartori MT, De Marco L, Girolami A. 1-Desamino-8-D-arginine vasopressin (DDAVP) infusion in type 2B von Willebrand's disease: Shortening of bleeding time and induction of a variable pseudothrombocytopenia. *Thromb Haemostas* 1990; **64**: 117–120

44. Mazurier C, Gaucher C, Jorieux S, Goudemand M. Biological effect of desmopressin in eight patients with type 2N (Normandy) von Willebrand disease. *Br J Haematol* 1994; **88**: 849–854

45. Rodeghiero F, Castaman G, Meyer D, Mannucci PM. Replacement therapy with virus-inactivated plasma concentrates in von Willebrand disease. *Vox Sang* 1992; **62**: 193–199

46. Berntorp E, Nilsson IM. Use of a high-purity factor VIII concentrate (Hemate P) in von Willebrand's disease. *Vox Sang* 1989; **56**: 212–217

47. Castillo R, Monteagudo J, Escolar G, Ordinas A, Magallion M, Villar JM. Hemostatic effect of normal platelet transfusion in severe von Willebrand disease patients. *Blood* 1991; **77**: 1901–1905

Rare congenital hemorrhagic disorders

31

VICTOR S BLANCHETTE, JULIE DEAN AND DAVID LILLICRAP

The cessation of bleeding is dependent on the formation of a platelet-fibrin clot at sites of vessel injury. Two key reactions are involved in this process:

- platelet adhesion and aggregation;
- formation of an insoluble fibrin mesh.

Initially, resting ('non-activated') circulating platelets adhere to the site of vessel injury. Under the conditions of flow in small blood vessels, plasma proteins such as von Willebrand factor (VWF) play a key role in this initial step by forming a link between glycoprotein Ib (GpIb) receptors on the surface of platelets and components of the subendothelium such as collagen.[1,2] Platelet adhesion is followed by activation, shape change and aggregation. Fibrinogen plays an important role in this next step by binding to specific receptors such as GpIIb/IIIa on the surface of adjacent activated platelets.[3] Activated platelets provide a source of negatively charged phospholipids essential for

amplification of the coagulation cascade and the formation of an insoluble fibrin clot.

Abnormalities, quantitative and/or qualitative, of key elements required for the formation of a stable, platelet-fibrin clot may result in a clinically significant bleeding disorder. The hemophilias and von Willebrand disease (VWD) are reviewed in Chapters 29 and 30, respectively. This chapter focuses on the rarer congenital bleeding disorders.

COAGULATION CASCADE

The initiation and regulation of the coagulation cascade has been the focus of several excellent reviews.[4–6] A current view of the human blood coagulation system may be summarized as follows (Fig. 31.1): coagulation is initiated at sites of vessel injury when blood is exposed to tissue factor (TF), an integral membrane glycoprotein that is located in

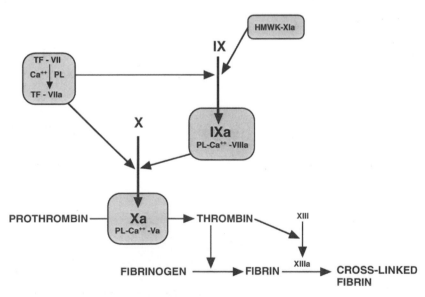

Fig. 31.1 Coagulation cascade. TF = tissue factor; PL = phospholipid; HMWK = high molecular weight kininogen.

subendothelial tissues and which comes into contact with blood only after vascular injury. Once exposed, tissue factor binds tightly to Factor VII (FVII); in the presence of calcium ions and phospholipid, FVII is converted to its active form, FVIIa. The TF-FVIIa complex then activates Factor X (FX) to FXa and Factor IX (FIX) to FIXa. These reactions occur on negatively charged cell membrane surfaces. The initial formation of FXa generates thrombin and triggers activation of platelets and a number of coagulation proteins, such as FXI, FIX, FVIII and FV. The initial stimulus for coagulation is quickly inhibited by the regulator tissue factor pathway inhibitor (TFPI) through the formation of an inactive quaternary FXa-FVIIa-TF complex. The secondary reactions stimulated by the initial generation of thrombin, especially the activation of FIX, are then essential for maintenance of the hemostatic response.

This revised view of the coagulation cascade is consistent with a number of important clinical observations. For example, the fact that severe deficiencies of the contact factors (FXII, prekallikrein, high molecular weight kininogen [HMWK]) are not associated with a clinically significant bleeding disorder is explained by the key role of FVII in initiating coagulation. The role of FIX in maintaining the coagulation response explains why individuals with a severe deficiency of this factor have a clinically significant bleeding disorder. In conditions where the initial quantity of FIXa generated is insufficient, or the processes opposing coagulation such as fibrinolysis, are particularly active, FXIa plays an important role in maintaining hemostasis. This supportive role is consistent with the clinical observation that spontaneous hemorrhage or hemorrhage following surgical procedures is rare in FXI-deficient patients unless the level of FXI is extremely low, whereas bleeding is common when trauma or surgery involves tissues with high fibrinolytic activity such as the oral cavity and urinary tract.

In summary, normal hemostasis is a fine balance between procoagulant and anticoagulant reactions localized on cell surfaces, resulting in initial platelet-fibrin clot formation with cessation of bleeding and later clot dissolution with restoration of an intact endothelial cell surface. Observations in individuals with rare inherited coagulation disorders have contributed significantly to the understanding of the human coagulation system.

DEFICIENCIES OF THE INTRINSIC PATHWAY

CONTACT ACTIVATION SYSTEM

Three proteins are involved in the contact activation pathway:

- Factor XII (Hageman factor);
- prekallikrein (Fletcher factor);

- high molecular weight kininogen (HMWK; Williams–Fitzgerald–Flaujeac factor).

Hereditary deficiencies of these factors have been described.[7–11]

Structure and function

Factor XII (FXII), prekallikrein (PK) and the kininogens are grouped together because they require contact with negatively charged surfaces for activation *in vitro*. Although deficiencies of these factors are characterized by a marked prolongation of the activated partial thromboplastin time (APTT), affected individuals do not have a clinically significant bleeding disorder and recent evidence suggests that the contact system has little to do with the initiation of hemostasis *in vivo*.[12] In the revised view of the contact system (see above), these proteins are, in fact, antithrombotic and profibrinolytic agents. In this context, it is of interest that a number of individuals with congenital deficiencies of FXII, PK and the kininogens, including the index cases, John Hageman and Mayme Williams, experienced significant thrombotic events.[13–18]

The kininogens circulate in plasma in 2 forms: HMWK and low molecular weight kininogen (LMWK). Both are composed of 3 parts: a common N-terminal heavy chain, a bradykinin moiety and unique C-terminal light chains. HMWK contains specific cell-surface binding sites as well as binding sites for PK and FXI (Fig. 31.2); *in vivo* the majority of plasma PK and FXI circulates as bimolecular complexes with HMWK. During activation of the contact system, FXII and PK are converted to their active forms, FXIIa and kallikrein. HMWK acts as a non-enzymatic cofactor for the conversion of prekallikrein to kallikrein, a reaction which occurs on the negatively charged surfaces of endothelial cells (Fig. 31.2). Prekallikrein activation at the cell surface is mediated by an endothelial cell metalloprotease and occurs independently of activated forms of FXII.[19] Once kallikrein is formed, it cleaves HMWK in a sequential manner.[20] The first cleavage step yields a 'nicked' kininogen that has enhanced binding activity for negatively charged

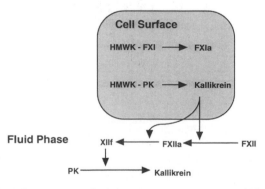

Fig. 31.2 Cell surface and fluid phase contact system reactions. HMWK = high molecular weight kininogen; PK = prekallikrein.

surfaces;[21] the second results in the release of the vasoactive peptide bradykinin; and the third results in stable kinin proteins. FXIIa cleaves HMWK in a manner similar to kallikrein but much more slowly.[22] The net effect of the initial contact reactions is to release bradykinin and kallikrein from the cell surface. Reciprocal activation of the contact system follows. Kallikrein released into the fluid phase reacts with FXII resulting in the formation of FXIIa and Hageman factor fragment (FXIIf). FXIIf retains the catalytic site of FXIIa whilst losing the surface-binding domain and is a potent fluid-phase activator of PK, thus leading to further formation of kallikrein (Fig. 31.2).

Activation of the contact system plays an important role in the pathogenesis of inflammatory disorders such as Gram-negative septicemia and the adult respiratory distress syndrome. Bradykinin, released from the kininogens during activation of the contact system, is a potent vasodilator and also stimulates the formation of prostacyclin (an inhibitor of platelet aggregation) and the release of tissue plasminogen activator. FXIIa and kallikrein stimulate neutrophils and the complement system can be activated by FXII fragments or by plasmin formed by the action of kallikrein on plasminogen.[23,24] *In vitro* kallikrein and FXIIa, FXIIf and FXIa can convert plasminogen to plasmin. The *in vivo* significance of these reactions, however, is unclear because each of these plasminogen activators has twenty-thousandth or lower the plasminogen activity as compared to urokinase.[24]

More important from a physiologic viewpoint may be those antithrombotic and profibrinolytic reactions that result from localization of the contact pathway reactions on negatively charged cell surfaces.[12] Two pathways have been identified. First, the kininogens selectively inhibit α-thrombin-induced platelet activation. Second, activation of prekallikrein bound to HMWK on endothelial cells and platelets results in the activation of prourokinase and an increase in plasminogen activation.[25,26]

The regulators of the contact activation system are the naturally occurring plasma protease inhibitors, C1-inhibitor, α_2-macroglobulin and α_1-antitrypsin. In this regard inhibition of the contact activation enzymes differs from that of the serine proteases in the later stages of the coagulation cascade which are predominantly regulated by antithrombin (AT). C1-inhibitor is the major inhibitor of FXIIa, FXIIf and kallikrein; α_2-macroglobulin also contributes to the inhibition of kallikrein. The predominant inhibitor of FXIa is α_1-antitrypsin.

Inheritance

FXII, prekallikrein, HMWK and LMWK deficiencies are typically inherited as autosomal recessive traits. Affected individuals lack functional activity of these proteins due to quantitative or qualitative defects. Individuals with quantitative defects lack both functional and antigenic material and are designated cross-reacting material negative

(CRM$^-$), whereas those with qualitative defects have cross-reacting material and are designated CRM$^+$.[27,28]

Clinical features

Although some patients with FXII deficiency have experienced menorrhagia and recurrent subarachnoid hemorrhages,[29] it is generally accepted that individuals with deficiencies of FXII, prekallikrein, HMWK and LMWK do not manifest clinically significant bleeding disorders.

Laboratory features

The laboratory abnormality characteristic of the inherited contact factor deficiencies is a marked prolongation of the APTT (Table 31.1). The diagnosis is established by documenting a reduced level of functional FXII, prekallikrein or HMWK and LMWK in the absence of an alternative cause of the deficiency state (Table 31.2).

Treatment

Since individuals with inherited deficiencies of the contact activation pathway do not manifest a significant clinical bleeding disorder, there is no requirement for replacement therapy as a measure either to prevent or treat bleeding.

Table 31.1 Presenting features of index cases with contact factor deficiencies.

| Deficiency | Index case | | Comment |
	Sex	Age (years)	
Hageman factor (Factor XII)[7]	Male	37	Asymptomatic. Prolonged clotting time preoperatively
Fletcher factor (prekallikrein)[8]	Female	11	Asymptomatic. Prolonged clotting time, APTT (250 s) preoperatively
Kininogen			
Williams trait[9]	Female	64	Asymptomatic. Prolonged APTT (171 s) preoperatively
Fitzgerald trait[10]	Male	71	Asymptomatic. Chance discovery of prolonged APTT (>500 s)
Flaujeac trait[11]	Female	50	Asymptomatic. Prolonged APTT (180 s) preoperatively

Table 31.2 Causes of acquired deficiency of contact pathway proteins.

Severe liver disease
  Acute hepatitis
  Cirrhosis

Nephrotic syndrome

Septic shock

Adult respiratory distress syndrome (ARDS)

FACTOR XI DEFICIENCY

FXI deficiency was first described by Rosenthal *et al* in 1953.[30] Three individuals in one family, a 50-year old man and his 2 nieces aged 25 and 29 years, had "shown since childhood only slight to moderate evidences of hemorrhage, marked chiefly by bleeding after tooth extractions." Laboratory findings included prolonged clotting times. The deficient factor, now identified as FXI, was tentatively designated plasma thromboplastin antecedent (PTA).

Structure and function

FXI is a plasma glycoprotein synthesized in the liver and secreted into the plasma where it circulates as a complex with HMWK. Whereas cell-associated HMWK is proteolyzed during the course of prekallikrein activation, resulting in the release of bradykinin from the cell surface, FXIa remains tightly bound to cell-surface HMWK (Fig. 31.2). The major biologic function of FXIa in the coagulation cascade is the conversion of FIX to its active form, FIXa. Formation of FXIa is the result of cleavage of an internal peptide on each of the 2 polypeptide chains of the inactive zymogen, FXI. This cleavage results in the formation of a serine protease composed of 2 N-terminal heavy chains and 2 C-terminal light chains held together by disulfide bonds. Binding sites for HMWK and FIX are located on the heavy chains, and the active or catalytic sites on the light chains.

Inheritance

FXI deficiency is a rare coagulopathy found predominantly, but not exclusively, in Ashkenazi Jews. The disorder is inherited as an autosomal recessive trait. Most cases of FXI deficiency represent a quantitative defect; only a few examples of individuals with a dysfunctional FXI have been described.[31] Homozygotes and heterozygotes are identified by severe or partial deficiency of FXI, respectively; homozygotes generally have FXI coagulant levels of < 15 unit/dl, while heterozygotes have levels > 15 unit/dl but below 70 unit/dl.[31,32]

Four mutations have been reported in FXI-deficient subjects;[33,34] 2 of these mutations, types II and III, account for the majority of the gene defects in Jewish kindreds. Type II, a nonsense mutation, results in the formation of a premature stop codon and the secretion of a truncated molecule that lacks the catalytic site and is probably also unstable. Individuals with the type II defect have very low levels of functional FXI, generally < 1 unit/dl. The type III defect is a mis-sense mutation; homozygotes have FXI levels that are reduced but generally higher than those found in the type II homozygotes (of the order of 10 unit/dl). Type I, a point mutation, and type IV, a 14-bp deletion, are rare causes of FXI deficiency in the Jewish population. Most FXI gene mutations in non-Jewish individuals are as yet undetermined, and types II and III mutations are uncommon.[32]

Table 31.3 Estimated frequencies of homozygous or compound heterozygous and heterozygous Factor XI deficiency in the general Ashkenazi and Iraqi Jewish populations. Modified from Ref. 35.

Category	Genotype	Estimated frequency (%)	Risk
Homozygote/compound heterozygote			
Ashkenazi Jews	II/II	0.047	1/2128
	III/III	0.065	1/1538
	II/III	0.11	1/909
	Combined	0.22	1/450
Iraqi Jews	II/II	0.028	1/3571
Heterozygote			
Ashkenazi Jews	II/-	4.1	1/24
	III/-	4.8	1/21
	Combined	9.0	1/11
Iraqi Jews	II/-	3.3	1/30

Although FXI deficiency is very rare in the general population (< 1/1 000 000), the disorder is more frequent in Jews. Based on DNA studies of 531 Ashkenazi and 509 Iraqi Jews, Shpilberg *et al*[35] have estimated that 1 in 450 Ashkenazi Jews manifest type II, III or compound type II/III homozygosity and 1 in 3571 Iraqi Jews type II homozygosity; estimated frequencies for the homozygous and heterozygous states in these populations are presented in Table 31.3. The absence of the type III mutation in Iraqi Jews and the presence of the type II mutation in both Iraqi and Ashkenazi Jews suggests that this type of mutation may have occurred after divergence of the Ashkenazi Jews from the original gene pool of Iraqi Jews who have lived in isolation in the Middle East since Babylonian times, some 2500 years ago. The Ashkenazi Jews are considered to be a segment of this original pool and descendants of Jews exiled from Israel by the Romans after the destruction of the second temple in 70 AD.

Clinical features

Unlike severe hemophilia A or B, FXI deficiency is generally associated with a mild bleeding disorder that becomes clinically manifest after trauma or surgery, e.g. dental extractions, and only rarely is associated with hemarthroses and muscle hematomas. Chronic epistaxis and menorrhagia may occur, whereas excessive bleeding from small cutaneous lacerations is unusual. Easy bruising is a common symptom. The severity of bleeding in FXI-deficient individuals is variable, and is not determined exclusively by FXI levels.[31]

Homozygotes or compound heterozygotes generally have the lowest levels of circulating coagulant FXI and the most severe injury-related bleeding, whereas heterozygotes are generally asymptomatic. Asakai *et al*[36] observed that surgical procedures involving tissues with high fibrinolytic activity (e.g. tonsillectomy/adenoidectomy, prostatectomy, dental extractions) are frequently associated with excessive bleeding in FXI-deficient patients irrespective of their circulating FXI levels; by contrast, excessive bleeding with major surgery not involving such tissues occurs more commonly in patients with the lowest FXI coagulant levels.

Laboratory features

Patients with congenital FXI deficiency manifest an isolated prolongation of the APTT. Confirmation of the disorder requires demonstration of reduced levels of coagulant FXI and absence of an alternate cause for the laboratory abnormality, e.g. liver disease. Family studies are recommended and may provide additional evidence of an inherited defect.

Treatment

Since spontaneous bleeding is uncommon in patients with FXI deficiency, replacement therapy is necessary only in individuals with a history of clinically significant bleeding or as hemostatic cover for major surgery. When assessing the requirement for replacement therapy, several variables should be taken into consideration, including:

- patient's coagulant FXI level and, if available, his/her FXI genotype;
- personal history of bleeding in the patient and any affected family members;
- type of surgery with specific reference to surgery involving tissues rich in fibrinolytic activity;
- risk of bleeding complications due to the surgical procedure itself.

For high-risk surgical procedures (e.g. neurosurgery, ophthalmic surgery, tonsillectomy/adenoidectomy and surgery of the genitourinary tract) in patients with severe FXI deficiency (defined as a circulating FXI level of <15 unit/dl), or for individuals with a prior history of significant clinical bleeding, pre- and post-operative replacement therapy should be given. Replacement therapy is not man-datory for dental surgery since it has been documented that patients with severe FXI deficiency can safely undergo such surgery under cover of antifibrinolytic therapy (tranexamic acid 25 mg/kg/dose, to a maximum of 1.0 g/dose, 4 times daily, administered from 1 day prior to surgery to 7 days after surgery).[37] Although experience of antifibrinolytic therapy is not available for patients undergoing tonsillectomy and adenoidectomy (an example of surgery involving tissues with increased fibrinolytic activity), it would seem advisable to use such therapy as an adjuvant in this (or similar) situations. The exception is surgery involving the genitourinary tract because of the small but definite risk of provoking unwanted large clot formation with subsequent impairment of urine output. The majority of patients with FXI deficiency do not bleed excessively following delivery. Accordingly, management can be expectant. A similar approach can be taken for FXI heterozygotes who have no history of excessive bleeding but who have not yet undergone a significant hemostatic challenge. A reasonable approach for such patients is replacement of FXI in high-risk situations where any excessive bleeding could cause morbidity or even mortality (e.g. neurosurgery). It should also be borne in mind that any co-existing hemostatic disorders, congenital or acquired, enhance the risk of bleeding, and therefore consideration should be given to correction of these defects in the setting of clinically significant bleeding or when an invasive procedure is planned.[38] Concomitant aspirin use appears to be associated with clinically significant bleeding in some FXI-deficient patients.[39]

Highly purified FXI concentrates prepared from human plasma are available (Table 31.4).[40,41] The product manufactured by the Laboratoire français de Fractionnement et des Biotechnologies is subjected during preparation

Table 31.4 Virus-inactivated Factors XIII, XI, X, VII, II (prothrombin) and fibrinogen concentrates available in Canada (1998).

Factor	Brand name	Company	Source	Virus inactivation
XIII	Fibrogammin®P	Behringwerke AG Marburg, Germany	Human plasma	Heat treated in aqueous solution at 60°C for 10 h (pasteurization)
XI	Factor XI	Bio Products Laboratory, Elstree, UK	Human plasma	Terminal, dry heat treatment at 80°C for 72 h
VII	Factor VII Concentrate (Human) Immuno	Immuno AG, Vienna, Austria	Human plasma	Vapor heated for 10 h at 60°C at 190 mbar and 1 h at 80°C at 375 mbar
II, IX, X	Prothromplex TIM 4	Immuno AG, Vienna, Austria		Vapor heat treatment
Fibrinogen	Fibrinogen Concentrate (Human) Vapor Heated Immuno	Immuno AG, Vienna, Austria	Human plasma	Vapor heated for 10 h at 60°C at 1190 mbar
	Clottagen	Laboratoire français de Fractionnement et des Biotechnologies (LBF), France	Human plasma	Solvent-detergent (tri-n-butyl phosphate [TNBP] and detergent [1% Tween 80])

For a registry of clotting factor concentrates available from other manufacturers consult Kaspar C and Silva M, Registry of clotting factor concentrates. Publication No. 6 prepared for the Factor VIII and IX Subcommittee, Scientific and Standardization Committee, International Society on Thrombosis and Hemostasis 1997/1998, World Federation of Haemophilia, Montreal, Quebec, Canada. (Fax: 514-933-8916. World Wide Web: http://www.wfh.org.)

to both virus elimination (nanofiltration) and inactivation (solvent-detergent) steps. It contains antithrombin III at a final concentration of 2 IU/ml and heparin at 4 IU/ml.[40] The product manufactured by the Bio Products Laboratory (UK) is virus inactivated by terminal, dry heat-treatment at 80°C for 72 hours and contains AT and heparin at a concentration of 10 unit/dl.[41] Bolton-Maggs et al[41] reported the safety and efficacy of the BioProducts FXI concentrate in 30 patients with FXI deficiency: treatment was required for operative procedures on 29 occasions, to cover normal childbirth in 2 cases, and on one occasion for treatment of a suspected knee hemarthrosis. With treatment, all patients achieved normal hemostasis except one individual undergoing coronary artery bypass surgery in whom the treatment with FXI concentrate may have been rendered less effective by massive hemodilution. The mean recovery of the infused FXI concentrate was approximately 91% and the overall half-life 52 ± 22 hours.

A major concern with the use of FXI concentrates is the potential for thrombosis.[42-44] In the report of Bolton-Maggs et al,[43] 4 FXI-deficient patients developed serious thrombotic events associated with FXI concentrate therapy; 3 of the 4 events (2 myocardial infarction, 1 cerebral infarction) were fatal. Although the patients were elderly with other risk factors for thrombosis, and because the administration of FXI concentrate may have contributed to the thrombotic events observed, the authors stated that FXI concentrates should be used with caution in patients with vascular disease. The thrombogenic potential of FXI concentrates was further emphasized by Mannucci et al[44] who described laboratory evidence of intravascular coagulation in 2 FXI-deficient patients following infusion of an FXI concentrate for which no thrombogenic activity had been found in the Wessler model in rabbits at doses of 900–1100 unit/kg of body weight.[45] The investigators concluded that FXI concentrates may be thrombogenic and advocated that they should be used with caution, especially in patients with other risk factors for thrombosis.

The decision to recommend FXI replacement therapy requires careful consideration of both risks and benefits. Currently, virus-inactivated high purity FXI concentrates, if available, are preferred to non-virus inactivated fresh frozen plasma (FFP), providing careful attention is paid to dosage with monitoring of circulating FXI levels. Prior to major surgery in patients with severe FXI deficiency (FXI levels <15 unit/dl), a dose of FXI concentrate should be administered calculated to increase the circulating FXI level to 50–70 unit/dl, and not to exceed 100 unit/dl. A convenient formula to calculate the required dose is:

FXI dose (units)
$$= \frac{[\text{FXI rise required (unit/dl)} \times \text{body weight (kg)}]}{2}$$

The maximum single dose infused should not exceed 30 unit/kg. For post-surgical maintenance, a dose of 10–15 unit/kg

body weight every 2–3 days is usually adequate. Ideally, dosage should be adjusted based on Factor XI assays. Of note, circumcision has been performed on severely deficient FXI patients without excessvie bleeding and dental extractions may be covered with antifibrinolytic therapy alone.[37] The decision concerning replacement therapy in patients with partial FXI deficiency (FXI levels between 15 unit/dl and the lower limit of the normal range) is more difficult. Where there is a clear history of abnormal bleeding in a partially deficient patient with no evidence of other bleeding disorders, e.g. VWD, it is reasonable to use FXI concentrate to cover surgery, especially if the surgery is major (e.g. heart surgery) or in a site particularly prone to fibrinolysis (e.g. tonsillectomy). The FXI dosage guidelines are as described above for patients with severe FXI deficiency. Where there is no helpful history, and depending on the procedure, it is reasonable to proceed with no FXI cover, or with antifibrinolytic therapy alone, but with FXI concentrate available in case excessive bleeding occurs.

Inhibitors (alloantibodies) to FXI deficiency may occasionally occur in severely deficient patients after exposure to plasma products.[46,47] Affected patients may have severe bleeding that cannot be controlled with FXI products but may respond to treatments used to treat patients with inhibitors to Factor VIII or IX, e.g. activated prothrombin complex concentrates, activated FVII (FVIIa).

FACTOR X (STUART–PROWER FACTOR) DEFICIENCY

Factor X deficiency was first reported by Hougie et al in a male patient named Stuart.[48] Independently, and 1 year earlier, Telfer et al had reported a female patient with the surname Prower.[49] It was proposed that this new factor be designated Stuart–Prower factor when experiments showed that mixing plasma from these 2 individuals did not result in mutual correction of the partial thromboplastin time (PTT). The Stuart–Prower factor was later renamed Factor X (FX).

Structure and function

FX is a vitamin K-dependent glycoprotein that is synthesized in the liver. The mature protein is composed of a light chain and a heavy chain that are held together by a single disulfide bond. The light chain of human FX contains the γ-carboxyglutamic acid residues; the heavy chain contains the catalytic domain. The conversion of FX to its active form, FXa, involves the cleavage of a polypeptide from the heavy chain. The reaction is catalyzed by FIXa in the presence of FVIIIa, Ca^{2+} and a negatively charged phospholipid surface, or by FVIIa in the presence of tissue factor. Once formed, FXa catalyzes the conversion of prothrombin to α-thrombin, a reaction that is accelerated in the presence of FVa, Ca^{2+} and phospholipid (Fig. 31.3).

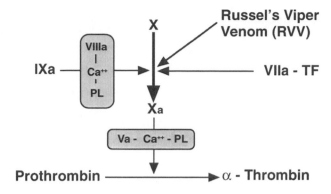

Fig. 31.3 Role of Factor X (FX) in the coagulation cascade. The zymogen FX can be activated to FXa by FIXa (in the presence of FVIIIa, Ca^{2+} and a negatively charged phospholipid [PL] surface), FVIIa complexed to tissue factor (TF) or directly by Russell's viper venom.

Inheritance

FX deficiency is a rare coagulation disorder (incidence $<1/500\,000$ in the general population) that is inherited in an autosomal recessive manner. The molecular genetics of FX deficiency have been summarized,[50] and includes gene deletions, dysfunctional variants and variants that affect synthesis and/or secretion of FX.

Clinical features

Clinical manifestations of FX deficiency vary from a severe bleeding disorder presenting early in life through a very mild bleeding tendency to asymptomatic individuals. Patients with $<1\%$ functional FX activity may experience severe bleeding; individuals with 10% or greater functional activity are only mildly affected. Bleeding sites vary according to the severity of the deficiency. Hemorrhage from the umbilical cord and later hemarthroses, severe epistaxis, menorrhagia, central nervous system hemorrhage and post-operative or post-traumatic hemorrhage have been reported in severely affected patients. Mildly affected patients may experience easy bruising or menorrhagia and occasionally bleed significantly after more severe challenges to the hemostatic system, as with trauma or surgery.

Laboratory features

Characteristic laboratory features of severe congenital FX deficiency include prolongation of the prothrombin time (PT) and APTT. Of note, the PT and APTT may be differentially affected in individuals with dysfunctional FX variants, reflecting the interation of the mutant FX with the FIXa-FVIIIa-Ca^{2+}-phospholipid complex (reflected in the APTT) and the FVIIa-tissue factor complex (reflected in the PT). The Russell's viper venom (RVV) time is a test in which FX is directly cleaved and activated by the venom, and is usually prolonged in patients with severe FX defi-

ciency but may be normal in some variants. The bleeding time is occasionally prolonged in severely affected patients, possibly due to defective FVa-FXa interactions on the platelet surface. For a diagnosis of FX deficiency to be made it is essential that a specific functional assay of FX be performed.

The differentiation of congenital from acquired FX deficiency should include consideration of liver disease and vitamin K deficiency. Another disorder associated with FX deficiency is primary amyloidosis, an association that reflects binding of FX to amyloid fibrils.[51]

Treatment

The need for FX replacement should be guided by the circulating FX level, clinical severity of the hemorrhagic episode, or estimated risk of the hemostatic challenge, e.g. surgery. Generally, a FX level of 10–40% is considered adequate for hemostasis.

Treatment consists of FFP or FX containing prothrombin-complex concentrates (PCCs). Concentrates are currently preferred since commercially available preparations are treated during preparation with methods (e.g. pasteurization, solvent-detergent treatment) known to inactivate lipid-coated viruses (e.g. type I HIV, hepatitis C), whereas FFP does not undergo specific virus inactivation during preparation. It is important to remember, however, that some of the currently available PCCs have been associated with thromboembolic complications and occasional episodes of disseminated intravascular coagulation (DIC). PCCs contain approximately 1 unit of FX/unit of FIX. Because of the risk of thrombosis, it is suggested that FX levels not exceed 50% of normal. If FFP is used, a loading dose of 10–20 ml/kg is recommended. Becasue of the long half-life of FX (24–48 hours), the level of FX can be built up in the circulation by infusion of plasma every 12 hours. The recommended dose is 3–6 ml/kg.

FACTOR V DEFICIENCY

In 1947, Owren described a hemorrhagic disorder due to the absence of a previously unknown coagulation factor.[52] The index case, a woman aged 29 years, had a hemorrhagic diathesis present from early childhood. Clinically, it manifested as skin bleeding, severe and recurrent epistaxis, menorrhagia and possibly an episode of hematuria. The disorder was called parahemophilia and the missing factor was later identified as Factor V (FV), also called accelerator globulin (Ac globulin) or proaccelerin.

Structure and function

FV is a glycoprotein synthesized by hepatocytes and megakaryocytes. It can be converted to its active form, FVa, by FXa, thrombin, meizothrombin (a reaction intermediate formed during prothrombin activation) and Russell's viper

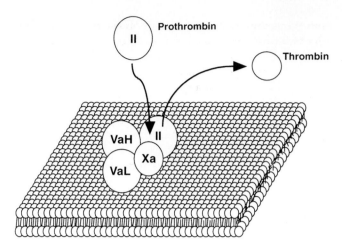

Fig. 31.4 Role of Factor V (FV) in the coagulation cascade. Activated FV (FVa) binds with high affinity to negatively charged phospholipid (PL) surfaces. In the presence of PL, FXa and prothrombin bind to FVa. The interaction of the prothrombinase complex (Va-Xa-Ca^{2+}-PL) with prothrombin leads to the formation of α-thrombin.

venom. Fully activated FVa is a heterodimer consisting of a heavy chain and a light chain that are associated by a single Ca^{2+}. The major biologic role of FV is its participation in prothrombinase assembly on the platelet surface. The prothrombinase complex consists of the serine protease FXa, the non-enzymatic protein cofactor FVa, Ca^{2+} and a negatively charged phospholipid surface. FVa binds with high affinity to negatively charged phospholipids; the binding site for the interaction is located on the light chain of the activated FV molecule (Fig. 31.4). In the presence of phospholipid, FXa binds to both the light and heavy chains of FVa and prothrombin binds to the heavy chain of FVa. Under physiologic conditions FVa accelerates prothrombin activation more than 10 000 fold by:

- increasing the catalytic activity of FXa;
- acting as a receptor that promotes the binding of FXa to negatively charged surfaces;
- promoting the interaction of prothrombin within the prothrombinase complex.

Approximately 20% of the total FV present in healthy individuals is contained in the α-granules of platelets.[53] Following activation of platelets by thrombin, platelet FV is released and converted into FVa which functions as a cofactor in FXa-driven prothrombin activation at the platelet surface. The generation of thrombin at the surface of activated platelets is known to be important in normal hemostasis. Inactivation of FVa is the result of limited proteolysis by activated protein C (APC), a vitamin K-dependent protease formed following activation of the zymogen protein C. The interaction of APC and FVa is stimulated by protein S and inhibited by FXa. FV also acts as a cofactor in the APC-mediated inactivation of FVIIIa, a reaction that is also stimulated by protein S.

Inheritance

FV deficiency is a rare congenital bleeding disorder that is typically inherited as an autosomal recessive trait. The frequency of the disorder is probably < 1/1 000 000 of the general population. Homozygotes have low FV levels and manifest clinically significant bleeding while heterozygotes have FV levels between 30 and 60% and are usually asymptomatic.[54] Both quantitative and qualitative defects have been described.[55] Combined deficiencies of FV and FVIII (or FVII) have been reported.[56]

Clinical features

Individuals with severe congenital FV deficiency and levels below 10% of normal often have hemorrhagic manifestations, although many may be asymptomatic for long periods of time. Common hemorrhagic manifestations include ecchymoses, epistaxis, menorrhagia and excessive postpartum or post-abortion bleeding and bleeding following dental extractions and surgery. Hemarthroses are uncommon even in severely affected patients. Bleeding from the urinary and gastrointestinal tracts and into the central nervous system does occur. The severity of bleeding in FV-deficient patients may correlate more with the amount of platelet-associated FV than with plasma factor.[57]

Laboratory features

Typical laboratory features in FV-deficient patients include prolongation of the PT, APTT and RVV time. The thrombin time is normal. Approximately one-third of patients with hereditary FV deficiency have a prolonged Ivy bleeding time. A definitive diagnosis of FV deficiency requires documentation of a low coagulant FV level using a specific FV assay.

The differential diagnosis of FV deficiency involves exclusion of other causes of the deficiency state, such as severe liver disease and DIC. In these situations other clotting factors will also be decreased, and the clinical picture is usually sufficient to exclude a congenital deficiency. Acquired FV deficiency is sometimes due to the presence of a specific antibody that may be associated with a variety of underlying diseases including infection and malignancy or following the use of topical bovine thrombin. Aminoglycoside antibiotics have also been implicated as a cause of acquired FV deficiency.

Treatment

Hemorrhagic episodes should be treated with FFP and major surgery can be performed under cover of FFP. Generally, the FV level should be raised to 25–30% before surgery, using a loading dose of 20 ml FFP/kg body weight. Maintenance infusion of plasma (3–6 ml/kg every 12 hours) to maintain a minimal level of FV of 10% can then be given since the biologic half-life of transfused FV is of the order of

12 hours with a range of 4.5–36 hours.[58] Platelet transfusions have corrected the bleeding time of patients with inherited FV deficiency for 5–6 days; however, platelet transfusions are not usually indicated for treatment.[59]

DEFICIENCIES OF THE EXTRINSIC PATHWAY

FACTOR VII DEFICIENCY

FVII deficiency was first described by Alexander *et al*.[60] The index case, a 4-year-old girl, had prolonged bleeding from the umbilical cord at birth. Other hemorrhagic symptoms included bruising, epistaxis and recurrent melena.

Structure and function

FVII is a single-chain polypeptide that is synthesized in the liver. Like other vitamin K-dependent proteins, FVII contains γ-carboxyglutamic acid residues located in the Gla domain of the light chain; the heavy chain contains the catalytic domain with the active site residues. Conversion of FVII to its active form, FVIIa, is the result of cleavage of a single peptide bond to yield a 2-chain active enzyme. Activation occurs in the presence of tissue factor, a cell-surface integral protein. FVIIa activates FIX, FX, and by an autocatalytic mechanism, FVII.[61] FVIIa levels are reduced in FIX- but not FVIII-deficient patients, which is consistent with the hypothesis that FIXa is the principal *in vivo* activator of FVII under basal conditions.[62]

Inheritance

FVII deficiency is a very rare coagulation disorder that is inherited in an autosomal recessive manner. Quantitative and qualitative defects have been reported, and affected individuals can be classified as CRM$^-$ (a proportionate reduction in both functional and antigenic FVII activity), CRM$^+$ (FVII antigen is normal whereas the functional activity is reduced) or CRM^{Red} (FVII antigen is reduced but less so than the functional activity).[63,64]

Clinical features

The clinical manifestations of FVII deficiency are variable and the correlation between the circulating FVII coagulant activity and bleeding is often poor. In general, however, those patients with severe deficiency (<1% clotting activity) experience severe hemorrhagic manifestations including easy bruising, epistaxis and menorrhagia. Hemarthroses may occur and gastrointestinal bleeding, hematuria and bleeding into the central nervous system have been reported. Prolonged bleeding following dental extraction is common, although some patients with severe FVII deficiency may tolerate surgery quite well. In some newborn infants bleeding from the umbilical stump has been observed. Patients with mild FVII deficiency (levels >5%) bleed infrequently.[65–67]

Laboratory features

Severe FVII deficiency is characterized by a prolonged PT in the presence of a normal APTT, thrombin time and RVV test. Congenital deficiency must be differentiated from acquired FVII deficiency as may occur in patients with liver disease, vitamin K deficiency secondary to malabsorption or those on oral anticoagulant therapy. On rare occasions, FVII deficiency may be due to circulating inhibitor.

Treatment

A FVII level of >20% is considered hemostatic. Products that may be used to treat Factor VII-deficient individuals include FFP, a prothrombin complex concentrate (containing Factors II, VII, IX and X) and a specific Factor VII concentrate (Table 31.4).[68–76] Where available, a specific virus-inactivated FVII concentrate is preferred to FFP. This recommendation reflects the opinion that a single dose of a virus-inactivated factor concentrate prepared from a very large plasma pool is virally safer than exposure to multiple packs of FFP which have not been virus inactivated.

Replacement therapy for patients with FVII deficiency should be individualized and will depend on the nature and serverity of the coagulation defect, site of bleeding and type of intervention. Experience with a specific FVII concentrate prepared from human plasma (FVII Concentrate [Human] Immuno, vapor heated) has been reported.[69,70,73,75,77,78] The product is virus inactivated using a 2-step vapor-heat process, has an *in vivo* recovery of about 90% and a biologic half-life of 4–6 hours. A plasma level of 10–20% is sufficient to maintain hemostasis; infusion of 1 unit of FVII concentrate/kg of body weight increases the circulating FVII level by approximately 2% (initial infusion) or 2.5% (maintenance therapy). For the treatment of bleeding or as cover for minor surgery, a single dose of FVII concentrate has generally been found to be sufficient. For surgical interventions it is recommended to maintain a plasma level of at least 20% for approximately 8–10 days. The maintenance dose should be given at intervals of 12 hours.

DEFICIENCIES OF THE COMMON PATHWAY

PROTHROMBIN DEFICIENCY

In 1905 Morawitz postulated a central role for a factor 'thromboplastin' that interacted with thrombogen (prothrombin) and calcium to yield thrombin.[79] Thromboplastin was later characterized as a plasma protein now known to be FXa. Hereditary prothrombin deficiency is one of the rarest congenital coagulation defects.

Structure and function

Prothrombin is a vitamin K-dependent glycoprotein that is synthesized in the liver and secreted into the blood. The mature prothrombin molecule is composed of 4 domains: a Gla domain containing γ-carboxyglutamic acid residues, 2 kringle domains and a catalytic region. The γ-carboxyglutamic acid residues allow the protein to bind Ca^{2+} leading to a conformational change that facilitates the binding of prothrombin to negatively charged phospholipids. During blood coagulation prothrombin is converted to thrombin by FXa in the presence of FVa, Ca^{2+} and negatively charged phospholipids present on some cell surfaces, e.g. activated platelets. The overall series of events that leads to the formation of thrombin are shown in Fig. 31.4. Coagulant FV binds to cell surfaces via a membrane-binding site on its C-terminal light chain. The activation of FV by thrombin leaves the light chain embedded in the membrane and the heavy chain non-covalently associated through protein interactions. FXa binds to both the light and heavy chains of FVa; prothrombin binds to the membrane surface through the Gla domain, to FVa through a binding site on 1 of its 2 kringle regions and to the active site of FXa (Fig. 31.4). The initial cleavage of prothrombin gives rise to meizothrombin (an active enzyme deficient in clotting and platelet activating activity). The activation of prothrombin by the prothrombinase complex is 300 000-fold faster than the activation of prothrombin by FXa alone at physiologic concentrations of these proteins.[80]

Inheritance

The mode of inheritance of hypoprothrombinemia appears to be autosomal recessive. Patients who are compound heterozygotes or who are homozygous for the condition may be symptomatic and generally have functional prothrombin levels of <25%. Patients heterozygous for the condition have levels of 50% or greater by both functional and immunologic assays. In addition to quantitative defects, qualitative defects (the dysprothrombinemias) have been described. In dysprothrombinemia the functional assay for prothrombin is usually decreased with the immunologic assay showing near normal levels of prothrombin antigen. The severity of clincial bleeding does not always correlate with the circulating prothrombin level; a patient with a qualitative prothrombin defect and a circulating level of functional prothrombin of 15% experienced no bleeding.[81]

Clinical features

The signs and symptoms of prothrombin deficiency usually vary with the level of functional prothrombin. Patients with prothrombin levels of approximately 50% have no bleeding problems. Patients with lower levels may experience easy bruising, epistaxis, menorrhagia, postpartum bleeding and hemorrhage following surgery or trauma. Hemarthroses are uncommon but have been reported.[82]

Laboratory features

The diagnosis of hypoprothrombinemia or dysprothrombinemia is suggested by the finding of variable prolongation of the PT and PTT and a normal thrombin time. These screening tests are not specific since deficiencies of FV and FX result in the same abnormalities. A definitive diagnosis depends on specific assays for functional and immunologic prothrombin.[83] The differential diagnosis of hypoprothrombinemia and dysprothrombinemia includes liver disease, vitamin K deficiency states and inhibitors to prothrombin (as may occur in patients with systemic lupus erythematosus [SLE]). Studies of family members plus measurement of vitamin K-dependent coagulation factors help to distinguish acquired from inherited prothrombin deficiencies.

Treatment

The treatment of hypoprothrombinemia or dysprothrombinemia depends on the circulating prothrombin level and on the type of bleeding. FFP may be used to treat clinically significant bleeding or as preparation for major surgery. A loading dose of 10–20 ml/kg is suggested followed by 3 ml/kg every 12–24 hours. Since the biologic half-life of prothrombin is about 3 days, the need for replacement therapy is infrequent and should be monitored by specific assays and clinical response. PCCs contain Factors II, VII, IX and X. Advantages of such concentrates include a prolonged shelf-life, ease of administration and the ability to achieve high levels of clotting factors without fluid overload. Importantly, all currently available commercial PCCs are treated during preparation with processes known to inactivate lipid-coated viruses such as the human immunodeficiency type 1 virus and hepatitis C; these preparations are thus preferred to non-virus inactivated preparations such as FFP. The major disadvantage of PCCs is the potential for thrombosis, presumably because of contamination with variable amounts of activated factors such as FXa and FIXa.[84] Because of the risk of thrombosis, the authors recommend that PCCs should not be used in patients with acute liver disease or those with other risk factors for thrombosis such as DIC or AT deficiency. The dose of infused product should not exceed 100 unit/kg, and the frequency of infusion should be adjusted to maintain hemostatic, but not excessive, levels of prothrombin.

FIBRINOGEN DEFICIENCY

Congenital afibrinogenemia was first described in 1920.[85] The normal plasma fibrinogen concentration is 150–350 mg/dl. Afibrinogenemia refers to the total absence of measurable fibrinogen, hypofibrinogenemia to decreased levels of normal fibrinogen and dysfibrinogenemia to the presence of abnormal fibrinogen molecules in the plasma. The first case of a qualitative fibrinogen defect was reported by di Imperato and Deltori in 1958.[86]

Structure and function

Fibrinogen is a dimeric molecule consisting of 3 pairs of polypeptide chains linked by disulfide bonds (Fig. 31.5). The chains are designated α, β and γ, respectively. The key role of fibrinogen in the coagulation system is the formation of fibrin, which together with platelets forms the hemostatic plug. *In vivo* the transformation of fibrinogen to fibrin is catalyzed by thrombin. The first step in this process involves the release of fibrinopeptides A and B with the formation of fibrin monomers; subsequent polymerization leads to the formation of an interconnected network of fibrin fibers. In parallel to these reactions, and key to the stabilization of the fibrin network, is the glutamine-lysine cross-linking of α and γ chains of fibrinogen by the calcium-dependent transglutaminase enzyme, FXIIIa. The cross-linking process renders the fibrin clot mechanically stronger and more resistant to chemical (6 M urea) and enzymatic (plasmin) digestion. The mechanical strength of the fibrin clot is also enhanced by the presence of Ca^{2+}. Fibrinogen is synthesized in the liver prior to its release into the circulation. The synthetic reserve of the liver is large and up to 20-fold increases in production rates have been found in patients with peripheral consumption in fibrinogen. Such observations explain why hypofibrinogenemia due to decreased synthesis is uncommon in liver disease or in most clinical states associated with

increased plasma fibrinogen turnover.[87] Fibrinogen is also present in the α-granules of platelets. The level of platelet fibrinogen may reflect both synthesis in megakaryocytes and uptake from the plasma.[88]

Inheritance

Afibrinogenemia is a rare congenital bleeding disorder that appears to be transmitted as an autosomal recessive trait. Consanguinity is common. Dysfibrinogenemia is generally inherited as an autosomal dominant trait with most cases representing the heterozygous state. Over 200 cases of dysfibrinogenemia have been reported with abnormalities that affect one or more of fibrinogen's known properties including: fibrinopeptide A and B release; fibrin monomer polymerization, fibrin cross-linking by FXIIIa, fibrin binding of thrombin, plasminogen binding, acceleration of tissue plasminogen activator-induced fibrinolysis, acceleration of FXIII activity, wound healing and binding of fibrinogen to platelet GpIIb/IIIa receptors.

Clinical features

Patients with congenital afibrinogenemia suffer from a life-long hemorrhagic diathesis of variable severity. Symptoms are generally present only in patients with fibrinogen levels of <50 mg/dl. Bleeding can be spontaneous and result in ecchymoses, gastrointestinal hemorrhage or hemarthroses. Excessive post-traumatic and surgical bleeding is also common. Intracranial hemorrhage has been reported following forceps delivery and is the severest complication of this congenital bleeding disorder. Menstrual bleeding is often severe and fetal loss due to spontaneous abortion or abruptio placenta is common in pregnant women with very low fibrinogen levels.[90]

Patients with dysfibrinogenemia are often asymptomatic. The bleeding manifestations are usually limited to epistaxis, menorrhagia and mild-to-moderate postoperative bleeding. Individuals with the lowest levels of fibrinogen measured by a functional assay are those most likely to experience significant bleeding. It appears that a basal plasma fibrinogen level of approximately 50 mg/dl is required for hemostasis. Of note, a number of patients with qualitative fibrinogen defects have experienced arterial or venous thromboses, or defective wound healing. These complications are consistent with fibrinolysis and wound healing being dependent on the formation of cross-linked fibrin during blood coagulation. In general, polymerization defects are more frequently associated with thromboses, whereas fibrinopeptide release defects are more common in patients with abnormal bleeding.

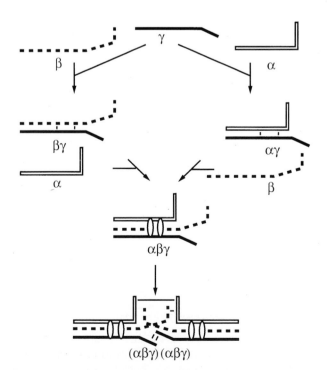

Fig. 31.5 Model for assembly of human fibrinogen. The solid lines represent the dimerizing bonds, and the circles represent the disulfide rings. From Ref. 89.

Laboratory features

The majority of patients with fibrinogen defects manifest some combination of prolonged PT, APTT, thrombin time and reptilase time. Of these tests, the thrombin time is almost always prolonged and the PT is generally more significantly prolonged than the APTT. Only one defect, fibrinogen Oslo I, has been characterized by a shorter than normal thrombin time in plasma, and this defect results in a prothrombotic tendency.[91] The reptilase time, which is based on clotting induced by fibrinopeptide A release, is often more prolonged than the thrombin time in patients with congenital dysfibrinogenemia. Unlike the thrombin time, the reptilase time is not prolonged by heparin and is relatively insensitive to fibrinogen degradation products. Inhibitors of bovine thrombin, a reagent used in laboratory tests, can occur in patients previously exposed to this agent in cardiac surgery; correction of the laboratory abnormalities when tests are performed with human thrombin clarify this situation.[92]

The congenital fibrinogen disorders must be differentiated from the acquired hypodysfibrinogenemias that occur in patients with liver disease or certain malignancies or in those taking drugs such as L-asparaginase. A rare cause of acquired hypofibrinogenemia is the disorder familial hemophagocytic lymphohistiocytosis. The prolonged PT seen in neonates is due to a physiologic fibrinogen variant that results in delayed aggregation of fibrin multimers without causing a bleeding disorder. Acquired inhibitors of fibrin polymerization and fibrin stabilization have been described in patients with SLE,[93] inflammatory bowel disease[94] and following therapy with certain drugs, e.g. isoniazid.[95]

Treatment

Therapy in patients with afibrinogenemia is given to achieve fibrinogen levels that are adequate for hemostasis and wound healing. FFP and cryoprecipitate have been used for replacement therapy.[96,97] Each bag of cryoprecipitate contains 200–300 mg of fibrinogen. In adults, 10 bags of cryoprecipitate raise the circulating level of fibrinogen by 60–80 mg %; the recommended dose in children is 4 bags/10 kg body weight (to a maximum of 10 bags). Since the half-life of fibrinogen is about 3–4 days, replacement is needed only every other day.[98,99] Fibrinogen concentrates prepared from large pools of human plasma are available in some countries and offer the advantage of specific virus inactivation during preparation (Table 31.4). For this reason these preparations, if available, are preferred to non-virus-inactivated FFP and cryoprecipitate as replacement therapy for patients with congenital deficiencies of fibrinogen.[100] One commercially available product (Fibrinogen Concentrate [Human] Vapor Heated Immuno) is virus inactivated during preparation using a 2-step vapor-heat process. The manufacturers recommend that for hypofibrinogenemic patients with massive bleeding or who have undergone surgery or suffered major trauma that the fibrinogen concentration be increased to at least 100 mg/dl. This level should be maintained until complete wound healing has occurred, if necessary by periodic infusion of fibrinogen concentrate. The approximate initial dose to raise the fibrinogen concentration by

100 mg/dl in normal-weight adults is suggested to be 3000–4000 mg. The calculation of maintenance doses should rely on circulating fibrinogen levels obtained on a daily basis. In hypofibrinogenemic patients with lesser hemorrhagic risk, a minimum circulating fibrinogen concentration of 50 mg/dl may be adequate. In most cases minor bleeding may be managed by single infusions. The proposed single dose in adults is 1000 mg; in children 500 mg.

As the correlation between laboratory tests and clinical bleeding is poor for most of the dysfibrinogenemic defects, the individual patient's clinical history should be used to define the need for replacement therapy, taking into consideration the requirement of a basal fibrinogen level of approximately 50 mg/dl to maintain hemostasis.

FACTOR XIII DEFICIENCY

The first case of FXIII deficiency was reported by Duckert *et al* in 1960.[101]

Structure and function

FXIII is a trace component in plasma where it circulates as a tetrameric molecular complex of 2 a and 2 b chains (Fig. 31.6). Free b chains circulate in plasma and FXIII a chains are found intracellularly in megakaryocytes, platelets and monocytes/macrophages. The a chain of FXIII contains both the thrombin cleavage site and a tight calcium-binding site. In the presence of thrombin and calcium, FXIII is converted to its active form, FXIIIa, and the b chain dimer dissociates from the tetrameric complex (Fig. 31.6). The initial reactions in the activation process are accelerated in the presence of fibrinogen or fibrinogen from which fibrinopeptide has been cleaved. The function of the b chain of FXIII is unknown, but it may serve to limit a-chain activation in plasma.

The key function of FXIIIa in the coagulation system is the formation of lysine-glutamine cross-links between the γ and α chains of fibrin. γ-Chain cross-linking yields dimers and

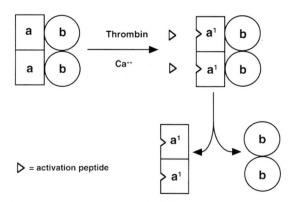

Fig. 31.6 Activation of plasma and platelet Factor XIII. In the presence of thrombin and Ca^{2+} there is cleavage of an activation peptide from the a chain with subsequent conformational change and exposure of the active center cysteine resulting in full enzyme activity. Activation also results in release of b chain dimers.

occurs rapidly; cross-linking of α chains occurs more slowly to yield polymers. γ-Dimer formation may function initially to cement the fibrin gel in place with mechanical strengthening of the clot occurring more gradually due to α-chain cross-linking and polymer formation. An important second action of FXIIIa is the cross-linking of $α_2$-plasmin inhibitor to the α chains of fibrin. When cross-linked to fibrin, $α_2$-plasmin inhibitor forms an active complex with plasmin. This is the primary mechanism for the inhibition of fibrinolysis[102] and fully cross-linked fibrin requires a longer time to be dissolved than does non-cross-linked fibrin or fibrin containing only γ dimers. The physiologic importance of $α_2$-plasmin inhibitor is demonstrated by the fact that patients deficient in the inhibitor have a serious hemorrhagic disorder characterized by delayed bleeding after trauma, a pattern that is similar to that seen in patients with congenital FXIII deficiency.[103] FXIIIa also participates in other physiologically important cross-linking processes: fibrin-fibronectin, fibrin-VWF, VWF-collagen, and fibronectin-collagen. The latter reaction may be important in tissue repair.[104]

Inheritance

FXIII deficiency is a very rare congenital disorder that is inherited as an autosomal recessive trait. There is a high frequency of consanguinity in families with the disorder. Individuals with severe deficiency (homozygotes) are symptomatic whereas heterozygotes are asymptomatic.

Clinical features

The homozygous state results in a moderate-to-severe hemorrhagic disorder. Bleeding from the umbilical stump and delayed and repeated bleeding from superficial wounds are common.[105] Typically, a clot appears to form normally at the wound site which then breaks down 24 hours later and bleeding resumes. This cycle can be repeated many times. A similar scenario is often observed after dental extraction. FXIII-deficient patients also may experience soft tissue and joint hemorrhage after trauma but the spontaneous hemarthroses seen in hemophilia usually do not occur. The most serious form of bleeding is into the central nervous system, and FXIII-deficient patients have a high frequency of intracranial hemorrhage often resulting in death.[106] Women with FXIII deficiency will abort spontaneously if they become pregnant. Full-term pregnancy can be achieved only if the patient is transfused throughout pregnancy.[107,108] Some patients with FXIII deficiency are reported to have severe scar formation from superficial wounds, but this is not true of all cases.

Laboratory features

In the homozygous state, the patient usually has <1% of functional FXIII activity, and the level of immunochemically detectable a protein is correspondingly low; b protein, also measured immunochemically, is present in plasma at approximately the 50% level.[109] Heterozygotes are characterized by partially reduced levels of the a and b proteins; as a group they have approximately 50% of the a protein activity and about 80% the level of the b protein. A variant molecular form of FXIII has been described.[110] One interesting patient with a hemorrhagic history and 2% β subunit activity has been reported.[111] This patient had 24% plasma α-subunit activity and a shortened plasma half-life (3 days); the level of platelet FXIII was normal.

The screening test for FXIII deficiency is the solubility of the patient's recalcified plasma clot in urea or monochloracetic acid. Clots in patients with <1% activity are soluble. This test does not, however, differentiate between heterozygotes and patients with acquired partial deficiency. An unambiguous diagnosis of the disorder among heterozygotes is usually possible with sensitive assays for FXIII and for the a and b protein. In the absence of an inhibitor to FXIII, there is a good correlation between FXIII activity and the immunochemical concentration of the a protein.

Acquired deficiency of FXIII has been reported in association with several diseases including severe liver disease, DIC, inflammatory bowel disease and leukemia; levels of approximately 50% of normal have generally been reported. Acquired inhibitors to FXIII are rare and can result in severe bleeding; reported cases have developed after prolonged therapy with certain drugs (isoniazid, phenytoin, penicillin and procainamide) or transfusions.[106]

Treatment

Bleeding in FXIII deficiency can be treated with plasma or a concentrate containing Factor XIII (Table 31.4). Cryoprecipitate does contain FXIII but in amounts that are not reliable enough to use as replacement therapy. In a number of cases, good results have been obtained by prophylactic infusion of approximately 5 ml/kg of plasma at monthly intervals.[106] Good results have been reported with a placental concentrate of FXIII.[108] A FXIII concentrate prepared from pools of human plasma is available (Fibrogammin P, Behringwerke, Marburg, Germany). The product is virus inactivated by pasteurization (heat treatment in aqueous solution at 60°C for 10 hours) and, if available, is preferred to FFP as replacement therapy for children with congenital FXIII deficiency. The lyophilized material is available in 4 and 20 ml doses containing not less than 250 and 1250 FXIII units, respectively. Pre-operatively, it is recommended that adults receive 40 ml of FXIII intravenously with 8–12 ml on each of the following 5 days or until the wound has healed completely. In the case of severe hemorrhages and extensive hematomas the dose is 8–10 ml daily until bleeding has stopped. For prophylaxis of hemorrhages 8–12 ml should be infused at intervals of 4 weeks with the interval shortened if spontaneous hemorrhages develop. The product insert should always be consulted for specific treatment recommendations.

Treatment of FXIII deficiency is facilitated by the long half-life of FXIII (8–14 days) and by the observation that very low levels (approximately 1%) inhibit bleeding. Because of the risk of intracranial bleeding there is agreement that all injuries to the head should be treated and that children should be treated prophylactically because the probability of intracranial bleeding in children is high.[112,113] Prophylactic therapy may also allow pregnant women successfully to carry fetuses to term.[107,108,114] Dental extractions often lead to significant bleeding in FXIII-deficient patients; thus, prophylactic treatment is justified. The combination of FXIII replacement therapy and anti-fibrinolytic drugs (E-aminocaproic acid or tranexamic acid) has been used with success.[115,116]

SUMMARY

The diagnosis of rare congenital disorders is sometimes delayed as more common conditions are considered. However, as for the more common congenital bleeding disorders, VWD and the hemophilias, the following information is of considerable value in the assessment of any child with a suspected congenital bleeding disorder:

- detailed family history;
- child's personal history of bleeding;
- results of selected coagulation tests.

The information gained from a detailed family history is often useful in the diagnosis and subsequent management of children with rare congenital bleeding disorders. Most of the disorders are inherited in an autosomal recessive manner, although examples of dominant inheritance occur. A bleeding history should be obtained for all family members with particular emphasis on parents, siblings and any affected family members. The criteria used to define abnormal bleeding in the authors' Pediatric Bleeding Disorder Clinic are given in Table 30.3; these are clinically relevant and can be applied reliably by physicians or other trained health-care personnel. A history of abnormal bleeding in the

newborn period should be sought with specific reference to delayed bleeding from the umbilical stump. Parents, or other family members, should be asked to provide information about prolonged bleeding after lacerations, following invasive procedures such as dental extractions or surgery or associated with child birth. The occurrence of hemarthrosis should be noted together with any history of more serious hemorrhage, e.g. bleeding into the central nervous system. Specific inquiry should be made regarding significant mucocutaneous bleeding such as easy bruising, recurrent epistaxis and menorrhagia. Exposure to specific hemostatic agents (e.g. coagulation products) should be recorded as should the effectiveness of therapy. All available coagulation results should be obtained and reviewed. At the conclusion of this part of the evaluation, children may be provisionally classified as family history negative or positive. The next step should be a detailed history and physical examination of the child.

The review of the patient's medical history should include a specific inquiry about systemic disorders such as renal/liver disease, SLE and a detailed current and past medication history. Although the physical examination is often of limited value in the diagnosis of children with rare congenital coagulation disorders, specific attention should be paid to the following:

- presence and extent of mucocutaneous hemorrhages;
- evidence of current or past hemarthroses;
- presence of physical findings that may offer clues about the correct diagnosis in children with abnormal bleeding, e.g. telangiectasias in children with recurrent epistaxis as a manifestation of hereditary hemorrhagic telangiectasia, abnormal scar formation in children with FXIII deficiency.

The final step in the evaluation of children with a suspected congenital bleeding disorder should include screening laboratory testing, including: platelet count and assessment of platelet numbers and morphology on a well stained peripheral blood smear; skin bleeding time; PT; and APTT (Table 31.5). Additional coagulation tests in selected cases include a thrombin time, RVV test, reptilase test, fibrinogen

Table 31.5 Characteristic laboratory findings in rare congenital coagulation disorders.

Deficiency	APTT	PT	Thrombin time	Reptilase time	Russell's viper venom time	Bleeding time	Platelet count
Contact factor deficiencies (XII, XI, prekallikrein, HMWK)	↑	N	N	N	N	N	N
X	↑	↑	N	N	↑	N (occ ↑)	N
V	↑	↑	N	N	↑	N or ↑	N or ↓
VII	N	↑	N	N	N	N	N
Prothrombin	↑	↑	N	N	↑	N	N
Fibrinogen	↑	↑	↑	↑	↑	N	N
XIII	N	N	N	N	N	N	N

N = normal; occ = occasionally.

level and clot solubility in urea. The results of these tests will, in a number of cases, lead to the performance of functional and immunochemical tests of specific coagulation factors. Selective studies in biologic parents and affected family members are often helpful in defining whether a child is normal or affected, and if affected, whether a heterozygote or either a homozygote or double heterozygote. The extent to which the diagnostic work-up should be pursued should be influenced by the family history, child's medical history and history of bleeding, as well as the results of screening laboratory tests. Children who are healthy and who have negative family histories and personal bleeding histories and who are referred because of incidental and often mild abnormalities of screening coagulation tests, e.g. prolongation of the APTT, do not merit extensive laboratory evaluation if repeat testing (including a screen for a non-specific circulating inhibitor and a FVIII or FIX coagulant level in boys with mild prolongation of the APTT) is within normal laboratory limits. Diagnostic criteria for VWD, in particular the common type I variants, are detailed in Chapter 30. Children with a positive history or significant personal history of bleeding warrant more detailed investigation.

The importance of accurate diagnosis in children with suspected congenital bleeding disorders cannot be overemphasized. Once provided with accurate information, physicians can appropriately counsel families about patterns of inheritance, the natural history of the disorder and options for the prevention and treatment of bleeding. Children with rare but severe coagulation disorders should wear a medical alert bracelet, and parents should be counseled that children with severe deficiencies should avoid competitive, contact high-risk sports and should pay particular attention to preventive measures (e.g. regular dental care) and avoidance of medications known adversely to affect hemostasis (e.g. aspirin). Therapeutic options for elective invasive procedures should be discussed; where available, specific factor concentrates that have undergone virus inactivation during preparation (Table 31.4) are preferred to single donor products, e.g. FFP/cryoprecipitate that are not subjected during preparation to specific viral reduction/inactivation steps. Fibrin sealants plus oral antifibrinolytic agents (e.g. tranexamic acid) should be considered in perference to coagulation factor replacement for invasive procedures in the oral cavity (e.g. dental extractions). It is important that parents and dentists be advised about the risk of mandibular blocks in children with severe congenital bleeding disorders. Finally, inappropriate and excessive precautions or prophylactic measures are contraindicated in children with mild defects and a negative personal and/or family history of bleeding. Examples are children with contact factor deficiencies or heterozygotes for other rare coagulation deficiencies. For those disorders where the correlation between the level of the circulating coagulation factor and the extent of clinical bleeding is poor (e.g. FVII and FXI deficiencies), specific advice needs to be given on a case by case basis and after consideration of the family and personal history of bleeding, level of circulating coagulation factor (based on a functional assay) and nature of the hemostatic risk.

Because of the infrequency of the disorders reviewed in this chapter, these clinical situations should be managed by specialist bleeding disorder clinics or after discussion with experts in such clinics.

REFERENCES

1. Girma J-P, Meyer D, Verweij CL, Pannekoek H, Sixma JJ. Structure-function relationship of human von Willebrand factor. *Blood* 1987; **70**: 605–611

2. Ruggeri ZM, Zimmermann TS. von Willebrand factor and von Willebrand disease. *Blood* 1987; **70**: 895–904

3. Bennett JS, Vilaire G, Cines DB. Identification of the fibrinogen receptor on human platelets by photoaffinity labeling. *J Biol Chem* 1982; **257**: 8049–8054

4. Furie B, Furie BC. The molecular basis of blood coagulation. *Cell* 1988; **53**: 505–518

5. Davie EW, Fujikawa K, Kisiel W. The coagulation cascade: initiation, maintenance and regulation. *Biochemistry* 1991; **30**: 10363–10370

6. Davie EW. Biochemical and molecular aspects of the coagulation cascade. *Thromb Haemostas* 1995; **74**: 1–6

7. Ratnoff OD, Colopy JE. A familial hemorrhagic trait associated with a deficiency of a clot-promoting fraction of plasma. *J Clin Invest* 1955; **34**: 602–613

8. Hathaway WE, Belhasen LP, Hathaway HS. Evidence for a new plasma thromboplastin factor I. Case report, coagulation studies and physicochemical properties. *Blood* 1965; **26**: 521–532

9. Colman RW, Bagdasarian A, Talamo RC *et al*. Williams Trait Human kininogen deficiency with diminished levels of plasminogen proactivator and prekallikrein associated with abnormalities of the Hageman factor-dependent pathways. *J Clin Invest* 1975; **56**: 1650–1662

10. Saito H, Ratnoff OD, Waldmann R, Abraham JP. Fitzgerald trait: Deficiency of a hitherto unrecognized agent, Fitzgerald factor, precipitating in surface-mediated reactions of clotting, fibrinolysis, generation of kinins, and the property of diluted plasma enhancing vascular permeability (PF/DIL). *J Clin Invest* 1975; **55**: 1082–1089

11. Lacombe M-J, Varet B, Levy J-P. A hitherto undescribed plasma factor acting at the contact phase of blood coagulation (Flaujeac factor): Case report and coagulation studies. *Blood* 1975; **46**: 761–768

12. Schmaier AH. Contact activation: a revision. *Thromb Haemostas* 1997; **78**: 101–107

13. Ratnoff OD, Busse RJ Jr, Sheon RP. The demise of John Hageman. *N Engl J Med* 1968; **279**: 760–761

14. Currimbhoy Z, Vinciguerra V, Palakavongs P, Kuslansky P, Degnan TJ. Fletcher factor deficiency and myocardial infarction. *Am J Clin Pathol* 1976; **65**: 970–974

15. Dyerberg J, Stoffersen E. Recurrent thrombosis in a patient with factor XII deficiency. *Acta Haematol* 1980; **63**: 278–282

16. Goodnough LT, Saito H, Ratnoff OD. Thrombosis or myocardial infarction in congenital clotting factor abnormalities and chronic thrombocytopenias: a report of 21 patients and a review of 50 previously reported cases. *Medicine* 1983; **62**: 248–255

17. Harris MG, Exner T, Rickard KA, Kronenberg H. Multiple cerebral thrombosis in Fletcher factor (prekallikrein) deficiency: A case report. *Am J Hematol* 1985; **19**: 387–393

18. Colman RW. Contributions of Mayme Williams to the elucidation of the multiple functions of plasma kininogens. *Thomb Haemostas* 1992; **68**: 99–101

19. Molta G, Rojkjaer R, Hasan AAK, Cines DB, Schmaier AN. High molecular weight kininogen regulates prekallikrein assembly and

activation on endothelial cells: a novel mechanism for contact activation. *Blood* 1998; **19**: 516–528

20. Mori K, Nagasawa S. Studies on human high molecular weight (HMW) kininogen. II. Structural change of HMW kininogen by the action of human plasma kallikrein. *J Biochem* 1981; **89**: 1465–1473

21. Scott CF, Silver LD, Schapira M, Colman RW. Cleavage of human high molecular weight kininogen markedly enhances its coagulation activity. Evidence that this molecule exists as a procofactor. *J Clin Invest* 1984; **73**: 954–962

22. Wiggins RC. Kinin release from high molecular weight kininogen by the action of Hageman factor in the absence of kallikrein. *J Biol Chem* 1983; **258**: 8963–8970

23. Ghebrehiwet B, Silverberg M, Kaplan AP. Activation of the classical pathway of complement by Hageman factor fragment. *J Exp Med* 1981; **153**: 665–676

24. Miles LA, Greengard JS, Griffin JH. A comparison of the abilities of plasma kallikrein, β-factor XIIa, factor XIa and urokinase to activate plasminogen. *Thromb Res* 1983; **29**: 407–417

25. Lenich C, Pannell R, Gurewich V. Assembly and activation of the intrinsic fibrinolytic pathway on the surface of human endothelial cells in culture. *Thromb Haemostas* 1995; **74**: 698–703

26. Loza JP, Gurewich V, Johnstone M, Pannell R. Platelet-bound prekallikrein promotes pro-urokinase-induced clot lysis: a mechanism for targetting the factor XII dependent intrinsic pathway of fibrinolysis. *Thromb Haemostas* 1994; **71**: 347–352

27. Saito H, Scott JG, Movat HZ, Scialla SJ. Molecular heterogeneity of Hageman trait (factor XII deficiency): evidence that two of 49 subjects are cross-reacting material positive (CRM$^+$). *J Lab Clin Med* 1979; **94**: 256–265

28. Saito H, Goodnough LT, Soria J, Soria C, Aznar J, España F. Heterogeneity of human prekallikrein deficiency (Fletcher trait): Evidence that five of 18 cases are positive for cross-reacting material. *N Engl J Med* 1981; **305**: 910–914

29. Kovalainen S, Myllylä VV, Tolonen U, Hokkanen E. Recurrent subarachnoid haemorrhages in patient with Hageman factor deficiency. *Lancet* 1979; **i**: 1035–1036

30. Rosenthal RL, Dreskin OH, Rosenthal N. New hemophilia-like disease caused by deficiency of a third plasma thromboplastin factor. *Proc Soc Exp Biol Med* 1953; **82**: 171–174

31. Ragni MV, Sinha D, Seaman F, Lewis JH, Spero JA, Walsh PN. Comparison of bleeding tendency, factor XI coagulant activity, and factor XI antigen in 25 factor XI-deficient kindreds. *Blood* 1985; **65**: 719–724

32. Hancock JF, Wieland K, Pugh RE *et al.* A molecular genetic study of factor XI deficiency. *Blood* 1991; **77**: 1942–1948

33. Asakai R, Chung DW, Ratnoff OD, Davie EW. Factor XI (plasma thromboplastin antecendent) deficiency in Ashkenazi Jews is a bleeding disorder that can result from three types of point mutations. *Proc Natl Acad Sci USA* 1989; **86**: 7667–7671

34. Peretz U, Zivelin A, Usher S, Eichel R, Seligsohn U. Identification of a new mutation in the factor XI gene of an Ashkenazi Jew with severe factor XI deficiency. *Blood* 1993; **82**: 251A

35. Shpilberg O, Peretz H, Zivelin A *et al.* One of the two common mutations causing factor XI deficiency in Ashkenazi Jews (type II) is also prevalent in Iraqi Jews, who represent the ancient gene pool of Jews. *Blood* 1995; **85**: 429–432

36. Asakai R, Chung DW, Davie EW, Seligsohn U. Factor XI deficiency in Ashkenazi Jews in Israel. *N Engl J Med* 1991; **325**: 153–157

37. Berliner S, Horowitz J, Martinowitz U, Brenner B, Seligsohn U. Dental surgery in patients with severe factor XI deficiency without plasma replacement. *Blood Coag Fibrinol* 1992; **3**: 465–474

38. Tavori S, Brenner B, Tatarsky I. The effect of combined factor XI deficiency with von Willebrand factor abnormalities on haemorrhagic diathesis. *Thromb Haemostas* 1990; **63**: 36–38

39. Kitchens CS. Factor XI: a review of its biochemistry and deficiency. *Semin Thromb Hemostas* 1991; **17**: 55–72

40. Burnouf-Radosevich M, Appourchaux P, Huart JJ, Burnouf T. Nanofiltration, a new specific virus elimination method applied to high-purity Factor IX and Factor XI concentrates. *Vox Sang* 1994; **67**: 132–138

41. Bolton-Maggs PHB, Wensley RT, Kernoff PBA *et al.* Production and therapeutic use of a factor XI concentrate from plasma. *Thromb Haemostas* 1992; **67**: 314–319

42. Gitel SN, Varon D, Schulman S, Martinowitz U. Clinical experience with a FXI concentrate: possible side effects. *Thromb Haemostas* 1991; **65**: 1157

43. Bolton-Maggs PHB, Colvin BT, Satchi G, Lee CA, Lucas GS. Thrombogenic potential of factor XI concentrate. *Lancet* 1994; **334**: 748–749

44. Mannucci PM, Bauer KA, Santagostino E *et al.* Activation of the coagulation cascade after infusion of a factor XI concentrate in congenitally deficient patients. *Blood* 1994; **84**: 1314–1319

45. Burnouf-Radosevich M, Burnouf T. A therapeutic, highly purified factor XI concentrate from human plasma. *Transfusion* 1992; **32**: 861–867

46. Stern DM, Nossel HL, Owen J. Acquired antibody to factor XI in a patient with congenital factor XI deficiency. *J Clin Invest* 1982; **69**: 1270–1276

47. Morgan K, Schiffman S, Feinstein D. Acquired factor XI inhibitors in two patients with hereditary factor XI deficiency. *Thromb Haemostas* 1984; **51**: 371–375

48. Hougie C, Barrow EM, Graham JB. Stuart clotting defect I. Segregation of an hereditary hemorrhagic state from the heterogenous group heretofore called "stable factor" (SPCA, proconvertin, factor VII) deficiency. *J Clin Invest* 1957; **36**: 485–496

49. Telfer TP, Denson KW, Wright DR. A 'new' coagulation defect. *Br J Haematol* 1956; **2**: 308–316

50. Cooper DN, Millar DS, Wacey A, Pemberton S, Tuddenham EGD. Inherited factor X deficiency: molecular genetics and pathophysiology. *Thromb Haemostas* 1997; **78**: 161–172

51. Furie B, Voo L, McAdam KPWJ, Furie BC. Mechanism of factor X deficiency in systemic amyloidosis. *N Engl J Med* 1981; **304**: 827–830

52. Owren PA. Parahaemophilia: Haemorrhagic diathesis due to absence of a previously unknown clotting factor. *Lancet* 1947; **i**: 446–448

53. Tracy PB, Eide LL, Bowie EJW, Mann KG. Radioimmunoassay of factor V in human plasma and platelets. *Blood* 1982; **60**: 59–63

54. Mammen EF. Factor V deficiency. *Semin Thromb Hemostas* 1983; **9**: 17–18

55. Chiu HC, Whitaker E, Colman RW. Heterogeneity of human factor V deficiency. Evidence for the existence of antigen-positive variants. *J Clin Invest* 1983; **72**: 493–503

56. Ginsburg D, Nichols WC, Zivelin A, Kaufman RJ, Seligsohn U. Combined factors V and VIII deficiency—the solution. *Haemophilia* 1998; **4**: 677–682

57. Miletich JP, Majerus DW, Majerus PW. Patients with congenital factor V deficiency have decreased factor X_a binding sites on their platelets. *J Clin Invest* 1978; **62**: 824–831

58. Melliger EJ, Duckert F. Major surgery in a subject with factor V deficiency: Cholecystectomy in a parahaemophilic woman and review of the literature. *Thromb Diathesis Haemorr* 1971; **25**: 438–446

59. Borchgrevink CF, Owren PA. The hemostatic effect of normal platelets in hemophilia and factor V deficiency. The importance of clotting factors adsorbed on platelets for normal hemostasis. *Acta Med Scand* 1961; **170**: 375–383

60. Alexander B, Goldstein R, Landwehr G, Cook CD. Congenital SPCA deficiency: a hitherto unrecognized coagulation defect with hemorrhage rectified by serum and serum fractions. *J Clin Invest* 1951; **30**: 596–608

61. Nakagaki T, Foster DC, Berkner KL, Kisiel W. Initiation of the extrinsic pathway of blood coagulation: Evidence for the tissue factor dependent autoactivation of human coagulation factor VII. *Biochemistry* 1991; **30**: 10819–10824

62. Wildgoose P, Nemerson Y, Hansen LL, Nielsen FE, Glazer S,

Hedner U. Measurement of basal levels of factor VIIa in hemophilia A and B patients. *Blood* 1992; **80**: 25–28

63. Mariani G, Mazzucconi MG, Hermans J *et al.* Factor VII deficiency: Immunological characterization of genetic variants and detection of carriers. *Br J Haematol* 1981; **48**: 7–14

64. Triplett DA, Brandt JT, McGann Batard MA, Shaeffer Dixon JL, Fair DS. Hereditary factor VII deficiency: Heterogeneity defined by combined functional and immunochemical analysis. *Blood* 1985; **66**: 1284–1287

65. Marder VJ, Shulman NR. Clinical aspects of congenital factor VII deficiency. *Am J Med* 1964; **37**: 182–194

66. Ragni MV, Lewis JH, Spero JA, Hasiba U. Factor VII deficiency. *Am J Hematol* 1981; **10**: 79–88

67. Mariani G, Mazzucconi MG. Factor VII congenital deficiency. Clinical picture and classfication of the variants. *Hemostasis* 1983; **13**: 169–177

68. Strauss HS. Surgery in patients with congenital factor VII deficiency (congenital hypoproconvertinemia): experience with one case and review of the literature. *Blood* 1965; **25**: 325–334

69. Pollini PTR, Sadum R, Mariani G. Synovectomy of the elbow in a patient with factor VII deficiency (hypoproconvertinemia). *Ital J Orthopod Traumatol* 1977; **3**: 385–389

70. Mariani G, Mannucci PM, Mazzucconi MG, Capitanio A. Treatment of congenital factor VII deficiency with a new concentrate. *Thromb Haemostas* 1978; **39**: 65–72

71. Dike GWR, Griffiths D, Bidwell E, Snape TJ, Rizza CR. A factor VII concentrate for therapeutic use. *Br J Haematol* 1980; **45**: 107–118

72. Greene WB, McMillan CW. Surgery for scoliosis in congenital factor VII deficiency. *Am J Dis Child* 1982; **136**: 411–413

73. Gagliardi C, D'Avino R, Stassano P, Musumeci A, Spampinato N. Open heart surgery with factor VII deficiency. *J Cardiovasc Surg* 1983; **24**: 172–174

74. Kelleher JF Jr, Gomperts E, Davis W, Steingart R, Miller R, Bessette J. Selection of replacement therapy for patients with severe factor VII deficiency. *Am J Pediatr Hematol Oncol* 1986; **8**: 318–323

75. Köhler M, Hellstern P, Pindur G, Wenzel E, von Blohn G. Factor VII half-life after transfusion of a steam-treated prothrombin complex concentrate in a patient with homozygous factor VII deficiency. *Vox Sang* 1989; **56**: 200–201

76. Shapiro A, Abe T, Aledort LM *et al.* Low risk of viral infection after administration of vapor-heated factor VII concentrate or factor IX complex in first-time recipients of blood components. *Transfusion* 1995; **35**: 204–208

77. Cohen LJ, McWilliams NB, Neuberg R *et al.* Prophylaxis and therapy with Factor VII concentrate (Human) Immuno, vapor heated in patients with congenital Factor VII deficiency: A summary of case reports. *Am J Hematol* 1995; **50**: 269–276

78. Brunori A, Greco R, Oddi G, DeBlasio A, Chiappetta F. Successful excision of hemorrhagic cavernous angioma in a patient with severe factor VII deficiency: perioperative treatment with factor VII concentrate. *Neurosurg Rev* 1997; **20**: 67–70

79. Morawitz P. *The Chemistry of Blood Coagulation.* Translated by Hartman RA, Guenther PF. Springfield, IL: Charles C Thomas, 1958

80. Nesheim ME, Taswall JB, Mann KG. The contribution of bovine factor V and factor Va to the activity of prothrombinase. *J Biol Chem* 1979; **254**: 10952–10962

81. Bezeaud A, Drouet L, Soria C, Guillin M-C. Prothrombin Salakta: an abnormal prothrombin characterized by a defect in the active site of thrombin. *Thromb Res* 1984; **34**: 507–518

82. Baudo F, de Cataldo F, Josso F, Silvello L. Hereditary hypothrombinaemia. True deficiency of Factor II. *Acta Haematol* 1972; **47**: 243–249

83. Shapiro SS, Martinez J, Holburn RR. Congenital dysprothrombinemia: an inherited structural disorder of human prothrombin. *J Clin Invest* 1969; **48**: 2251–2259

84. Blatt PM, Lundblad RL, Kingdon HS, McLean G, Roberts HR. Thrombogenic materials in prothrombin complex concentrates. *Ann Intern Med* 1974; **81**: 766–770

85. Raba F, Salomon F. Über faserstoffmangel im Blute bei einem Falle von Hamophilia. *Dtsh Arch Klin Med* 1920; **132**: 240–244

86. di Imperato DC, Deltori AG. Ipofibrinogenemia congenita con fibrinoastenia. *Acta Paediatr Helv* 1958; **4**: 380–399

87. Reeve EB, Franks JJ. Fibrinogen synthesis, distribution and degradation. *Semin Thromb Hemostas* 1974; **1**: 129–183

88. Harrison P, Wilbourn B, Debili N *et al.* Update of plasma fibrinogen into the alpha granules of human megakaryocytes and platelets. *J Clin Invest* 1989; **84**: 1320–1324

89. Huang S, Mulvihill ER, Farrell DH, Chung DW, Davie EW. *J Biol Chem* 1993; **268**: 8925

90. Goodwin TM. Congenital hypofibrinogenemia in pregnancy. *Obstet Gynecol Surv* 1989; **44**: 157–161

91. Thorsen LI, Brosstad F, Solum NO, Stormorken H. Increased binding to ADP-stimulated platelets and aggregation effect of the dysfibrinogen Oslo I as compared with normal fibrinogen. *Scand J Haematol* 1986; **36**: 203–210

92. Lawson JH, Pennell BJ, Olson JD, Mann KG. Isolation and characterization of an acquired antithrombin antibody. *Blood* 1990; **76**: 2249–2257

93. Galanakis DK, Ginzler EM, Fikrig SM. Monoclonal IgG anticoagulants delaying fibrin aggregation in two patients with systemic lupus erythematosus (SLE). *Blood* 1978; **52**: 1037–1046

94. Hoots WK, Carrell NA, Wagner RH, Cooper HA, McDonagh J. A naturally occurring antibody that inhibits fibrin polymerization. *N Engl J Med* 1981; **304**: 857–861

95. Otis PT, Feinstein DI, Rapaport SI, Patch MJ. An acquired inhibitor of fibrin stabilization associated with isoniazid therapy. Clinical and biochemical observations. *Blood* 1974; **44**: 771–781

96. Ness PM, Perkins HA. Cryoprecipitate as a reliable source of fibrinogen replacement. *JAMA* 1979; **241**: 1690–1691

97. McLeod BC, McKenna R, Sassetti RJ. Treatment of von Willebrand's disease and hypofibrinogenemia with single donor cryoprecipitate from plasma exchange donation. *Am J Hematol* 1989; **32**: 112–116

98. Collen D, Tytgat GN, Claeys H, Piessens R. Metabolism and distribution of fibrinogen: fibrinogen turnover in physiological conditions in humans. *Br J Haematol* 1972; **22**: 681–700

99. Rausen AR, Cruchaud A, McMillan CW, Gitlin D. A study of fibrinogen turnover in classical hemophilia and congenital afibrinogenemia. *Blood* 1961; **18**: 710–715

100. Grech H, Majunder G, Lawrie AS, Savidge GF. Pregnancy in congenital afibrinogenaemia: report of a successful case and review of the literature. *Br J Haematol* 1991; **78**: 571–572

101. Duckert F, Jung E, Shmerling DH. A hitherto undescribed congenital hemorrhagic diathesis probably due to fibrin stabilizing factor deficiency. *Thromb Diathesis Hemorrh* 1960; **5**: 179–184

102. Sakata Y, Aoki N. Significance of cross-linking of α2-plasmin inhibitor to fibrin in inhibition of fibrinolysis and in hemostasis. *J Clin Invest* 1982; **69**: 536–542

103. Aoki N, Saito H, Kamiya T, Koie K, Sakata Y, Kobakura M. Congenital deficiency of α2-plasmin inhibitor associated with severe hemorrhagic tendency. *J Clin Invest* 1979; **63**: 877–884

104. Mosher DF, Schad PE, Kleinman HK. Cross-linking of fibronectin to collagen by blood coagulation factor XIIIa. *J Clin Invest* 1979; **64**: 781–787

105. Duckert F. Documentation of the plasma factor XIII deficiency in man. *Ann NY Acad Sci* 1972; **202**: 190–199

106. Lorand L, Losowsky MS, Miloszewski KJM. Human factor XIII: Fibrin stabilizing factor. *Prog Hemostas Thromb* 1980; **5**: 245–290

107. Fisher S, Rikover M, Naor S. Factor 13 deficiency with severe hemorrhagic diathesis. *Blood* 1966; **28**: 34–39

108. Rodeghiero F, Castaman GC, Di Bona E, Ruggeri M, Dini E. Successful pregnancy in a woman with congenital factor XIII deficiency treated with substitutive therapy. Report of a second case. *Blut* 1987; **55**: 45–48

109. Yorifuji H, Anderson K, Lynch GW, Van De Water L, McDonagh J.

B protein of factor XIII: differentiation between free B and complexed B. *Blood* 1988; **72**: 1645–1650

110. Aslam S, Poon MC, Yee VC, Bowen DJ, Standen GR. Factor XIIIA Calgary: a candidate missense mutation (Leu667Pro) in the beta barrel 2 domain of the factor XIIIA subunit. *Br J Haematol* 1995; **91**: 452–457

111. Saito M, Asakura H, Yoshida T *et al*. A familial factor XIII subunit B deficiency. *Br J Haematol* 1990; **74**: 290–294

112. Abbondanzo SL, Gottenberg JE, Lofts RS, McPherson RA. Intracranial hemorrhage in congenital deficiency of factor XIII. *Am J Pediatr Hematol Oncol* 1988; **10**: 65–68

113. Larsen PD, Wallace JW, Frankel LS, Crisp D. Factor XIII deficiency and intracranial hemorrhages in infancy. *Pediatr Neurol* 1990; **6**: 277–278

114. Kobayashi T, Terao T, Kojima T, Takamatsu J, Kamiya T, Saito H. Congenital factor XIII deficiency with treatment of factor XIII concentrate and normal vaginal delivery. *Gynecol Obstet Invest* 1990; **29**: 235–238

115. Colin W, Needleman HL. Medical/dental management of a patient with congenital factor XIII. *Pediatr Dentistry* 1985; **7**: 227–230

116. Suziki H, Kaneda T. Tooth extraction in two patients who had congenital deficiency of factor XIII. *J Oral Maxillofac Surg* 1985; **43**: 221–224

Acquired disorders of hemostasis during childhood

ELIZABETH A CHALMERS AND BRENDA ES GIBSON

DEVELOPMENTAL HEMOSTASIS DURING CHILDHOOD

At birth the term infant's hemostatic system shows significant differences in a number of parameters when compared to adult data.[1] These differences are even more marked in the premature infant and it is generally considered that the hemostatic system at birth is 'physiologically immature' (see Chapter 33).[2] Considerable 'maturation' of the hemostatic system occurs during the first 6 months of life; however, some differences persist throughout childhood and adolescence.[3–6] Recognition of these differences and the availability of normal reference ranges for children is clearly important for accurate diagnosis in this age group. These physiologic differences may also have relevance to the clinical problems observed in children and to the use of therapeutic agents which interact with the hemostatic system.[8]

Published data on normal hemostatic parameters during childhood have until recently been limited and in many situations reference ranges for infants and children have been extrapolated from adult normal ranges. In a prospective cohort study in healthy children undergoing minor elective day surgery, Andrew *et al*[5] performed a comprehensive analysis of coagulation and fibrinolytic parameters across 3 different age ranges and compared the results with normal adult data. This study demonstrated important differences in the mean levels of procoagulant proteins, naturally occurring inhibitors and proteins involved in fibrinolysis. Based on these data, it appears that during childhood mean plasma concentrations of vitamin K-dependent factors (II, VII, IX and X) and the contact factors XI, XII and V are all 15–20% lower than adult values (Table 32.1).[5,7] In contrast, concentrations of fibrinogen, Factor VIII (FVIII) and von Willebrand factor (VWF) are similar to adult values throughout childhood. Of the direct thrombin inhibitors,

antithrombin III (ATIII) is increased by approximately 10% while α_2-macroglobulin (α_2-M) is almost doubled and heparin cofactor II (HC-II) reduced by 10–20% (Table 32.2).[5,7] The other major inhibitory pathway is the protein C/S system and here, while free protein S levels are similar to adult values, mean protein C levels remain significantly reduced even in the 11–16-year age range (Table 32.2).[5,7]

Plasma concentrations of some fibrinolytic proteins are also affected by age and while plasminogen and α_2-antiplasmin (α_2-AP) levels are similar in adults and children, plasminogen activator inhibitor (PAI-1) is increased and tissue plasminogen activator (tPA) decreased so that the overall fibrinolytic capacity appears to be reduced during childhood (Table 32.3).[5,7]

Despite the reduced levels of several procoagulant proteins, the routine screening tests—prothrombin time (PT) and activated partial thromboplastin time (APTT)—are not significantly different in children and adults which reflects the relative insensitivity of these tests to minor changes in procoagulant concentrations (Table 32.1).[5,7] This compares with the bleeding time, which has been reported to be prolonged, particularly during early childhood (Table 32.1).[5,9] The reasons for this prolongation are not well understood but may reflect changes in vessel-wall proteins.

To assess the net effect of these differences on overall hemostasis during childhood, it has been useful to perform *in vitro* studies to examine thrombin regulation and also to look at endogenous markers of coagulation and fibrinolytic activation. The conversion of prothrombin to thrombin is the most important event in the coagulation process and in keeping with the reduced levels of prothrombin during childhood, thrombin generation is reduced by around 20% as compared with adult values.[10] Conversely, the total capacity to inhibit thrombin, as assessed *in vitro* using ^{125}I-thrombin, is increased due to increased binding to α_2-M.[11,12]

Table 32.1 Reference values for coagulation tests in healthy children aged 1 to 16 years compared with adults.

| Coagulation tests | Age | | | |
| | 1–5 years | 6–10 years | 11–16 years | Adult |
	Mean (boundary)	Mean (boundary)	Mean (boundary)	Mean (boundary)
PT (s)	11 (10.6–11.4)	11.1 (10.1–12.1)	11.2 (10.2–12.0)	12 (11.0–14.0)
INR	1.0 (0.96–1.04)	1.01 (0.91–1.11)	1.02 (0.93–1.10)	1.10 (1.0–1.3)
APTT (s)	30 (24–36)	31 (26–36)	32 (26–37)	33 (27–40)
Fibrinogen (g/l)	2.76 (1.70–4.05)	2.79 (1.57–4.0)	3.0 (1.54–4.48)	2.78 (1.56–4.0)
Bleeding time (min)	6 (2.5–10)*	7 (2.5–13)*	5 (3–8)*	4 (1–7)
II (unit/ml)	0.94 (0.71–1.16)*	0.88 (0.67–1.07)*	0.83 (0.61–1.04)*	1.08 (0.70–1.46)
V (unit/ml)	1.03 (0.79–1.27)	0.90 (0.63–1.16)*	0.77 (0.55–0.99)*	1.06 (0.62–1.50)
VII (unit/ml)	0.82 (0.55–1.16)*	0.85 (0.52–1.20)*	0.83 (0.58–1.15)*	1.05 (0.67–1.43)
VIII (unit/ml)	0.90 (0.59–1.42)	0.95 (0.58–1.32)	0.92 (0.53–1.31)	0.99 (0.50–1.49)
VWF (unit/ml)	0.82 (0.60–1.20)	0.95 (0.44–1.44)	1.00 (0.46–1.53)	0.92 (0.50–1.58)
IX (unit/ml)	0.73 (0.47–1.04)*	0.75 (0.63–0.89)*	0.82 (0.59–1.22)*	1.09 (0.55–1.63)
X (unit/ml)	0.88 (0.58–1.16)*	0.75 (0.55–1.01)*	0.79 (0.50–1.17)*	1.06 (0.70–1.52)
XI (unit/ml)	0.97 (0.56–1.50)	0.86 (0.52–1.20)	0.74 (0.50–0.97)*	0.97 (0.67–1.27)
XII (unit/ml)	0.93 (0.64–1.29)	0.92 (0.60–1.40)	0.81 (0.34–1.37)*	1.08 (0.52–1.64)
PK (unit/ml)	0.95 (0.65–1.30)	0.99 (0.66–1.31)	0.99 (0.53–1.45)	1.12 (0.62–1.62)
HMWK (unit/ml)	0.98 (0.64–1.32)	0.93 (0.60–1.30)	0.91 (0.63–1.19)	0.92 (0.50–1.36)
XIIIa (unit/ml)	1.08 (0.72–1.43)*	1.09 (0.65–1.51)*	0.99 (0.57–1.40)	1.05 (0.55–1.55)
XIIIs (unit/ml)	1.13 (0.69–1.56)*	1.16 (0.77–1.54)*	1.02 (0.60–1.43)	0.97 (0.57–1.37)

All factors except fibrinogen are expressed as unit/ml, where pooled plasma contains 1.0 unit/ml. All data are expressed as the mean, followed by the upper and lower boundary encompassing 95% of the population. Between 20 and 50 samples were assayed for each value for each age group. Some measurements were skewed due to a disproportionate number of high values. The lower limit, which excludes the lower 2.5% of the population, is given.
PT = prothrombin time; APTT = activated partial thromboplastin time; VIII = Factor VIII procoagulant; VWF = von Willebrand factor; PK = prekallikrein; HMWK = high molecular weight kininogen.
*Values that are significantly different from adults.
Reproduced with permission from Ref. 5.

Table 32.2 Reference values for the inhibitors of coagulation in healthy children aged 1 to 16 years compared with adults.

| Coagulation inhibitors | Age | | | |
| | 1–5 years | 6–10 years | 11–16 years | Adult |
	Mean (boundary)	Mean (boundary)	Mean (boundary)	Mean (boundary)
ATIII (unit/ml)	1.11 (0.82–1.39)	1.11 (0.90–1.31)	1.05 (0.77–1.32)	1.0 (0.74–1.26)
α_2-M (unit/ml)	1.69 (1.14–2.23)*	1.69 (1.28–2.09)*	1.56 (0.98–2.12)*	0.86 (0.52–1.20)
C_1E-Inh (unit/ml)	1.35 (0.85–1.83)*	1.14 (0.88–1.54)	1.03 (0.68–1.50)	1.0 (0.71–1.31)
α_1-AT (unit/ml)	0.93 (0.39–1.47)	1.00 (0.69–1.30)	1.01 (0.65–1.37)	0.93 (0.55–1.30)
HCII (unit/ml)	0.88 (0.48–1.28)*	0.86 (0.40–1.32)*	0.91 (0.53–1.29)*	1.08 (0.66–1.26)
Protein C (unit/ml)	0.66 (0.40–0.92)*	0.69 (0.45–0.93)*	0.83 (0.55–1.11)*	0.96 (0.64–1.28)
Protein S				
Total (unit/ml)	0.86 (0.54–1.18)	0.78 (0.41–1.14)	0.72 (0.52–0.92)	0.81 (0.60–1.13)
Free (unit/ml)	0.45 (0.21–0.69)	0.42 (0.22–0.62)	0.38 (0.26–0.55)	0.45 (0.27–0.61)

All values are expressed in unit/ml, where for all factors pooled plasma contains 1.0 unit/ml, with the exception of free protein S, which contains a mean of 0.4 unit/ml. All values are given as a mean, followed by the lower and upper boundary encompassing 95% of the population. Between 20 and 30 samples were assayed for each value for each age group. Some measurements were skewed due to a disproportionate number of high values. The lower limits, which exclude the lower 2.5% of the population, are given.
*Values that are significantly different from adults.
Reproduced with permission from Ref. 5.

Analysis of activation markers, which comprise peptides and enzyme complexes liberated with the activation of coagulation and fibrinolysis, e.g. prothrombin fragment $1+2$ ($F1+2$), D-dimers and plasmin-α_2-AP (PAP) complexes, do not show any significant difference when compared with results obtained in young adults.[13,14]

From a clinical viewpoint, despite the reduced levels of certain procoagulant proteins, for any given hemostatic challenge there does not appear to be an increased risk of hemorrhagic problems during childhood. The situation differs in relation to thromboembolic events, where in the context of both inherited and acquired risk factors, the rate of thrombosis appears to be reduced during childhood, suggesting a protective effect.[15,16]

Table 32.3 Reference values for the fibrinolytic system in healthy children aged 1 to 16 years compared with adults.

	Age			
	1–5 years	6–10 years	11–16 years	Adult
	Mean (boundary)	Mean (boundary)	Mean (boundary)	Mean (boundary)
Plasminogen (unit/ml)	0.98 (0.78–1.18)	0.92 (0.75–1.08)	0.86 (0.68–1.03)*	0.99 (0.77–1.22)
tPA (ng/ml)	2.15 (1.0–4.5)*	2.42 (1.0–5.0)*	2.16 (1.0–4.0)*	4.90 (1.40–8.40)
α_2-AP (unit/ml)	1.05 (0.93–1.17)	0.99 (0.89–1.10)	0.98 (0.78–1.18)	1.02 (0.68–1.36)
PAI (unit/ml)	5.42 (1.0–10.0)	6.79 (2.0–12.0)*	6.07 (2.0–10.0)*	3.60 (0–11.0)

For α_2-AP, values are expressed as unit/ml, where pooled plasma contains 1.0 unit/ml. Values for tPA are given as ng/ml. Values for PAI are given as unit/ml, where 1 unit of PAI activity is defined as the amount of PAI that inhibits 1 unit of human single-chain tPA. All values are given as the mean, followed by the lower and upper boundary encompassing 95% of the population (boundary).
*Values that are significantly different from adults.
Reproduced with permission from Ref. 5.

DISSEMINATED INTRAVASCULAR COAGULATION

Disseminated intravascular coagulation (DIC) is a common acquired coagulopathy which in children is almost always acute and related to a generalized disorder. In a recent review, Bick defined DIC as "a systemic thrombohemorrhagic disorder in association with defined clinical situations and laboratory evidence of procoagulant and fibrinolytic activation, inhibitor consumption and evidence of organ damage or failure".[17] This definition encompasses the different aspects of DIC and is as applicable to infants and children as it is to adults.

Etiology

DIC is always a secondary event and in childhood may be precipitated by a number of different disease processes (Table 32.4).[18,19] Infection is the commonest cause in children. Bacterial infections predominate but viruses, systemic fungal infections, malaria and the viral hemorrhagic fevers are also recognized triggers. Many bacterial agents can trigger a consumptive coagulopathy; however, meningococcal meningitis remains one of the most frequent causes of severe DIC in children. The most commonly implicated viremias are varicella, hepatitis and cytomegalovirus. DIC in association with childhood malignancy is relatively uncommon but is very characteristic in acute promyelocytic leukemia and, prior to the use of differentiation therapy, was responsible for much of the morbidity and mortality seen with this condition.[20]

Chronic localized DIC is uncommon in the pediatric age

Table 32.4 Causes of disseminated intravascular coagulation in children.

Infection
Malignancy, e.g. leukemia
Trauma, e.g. burns
Intravascular hemolysis, e.g. ABO incompatible transfusion
Liver disease

group and is almost exclusively documented in association with giant hemangiomas. The Kasabach–Merritt syndrome was initially described in 1940 and has its peak incidence in early infancy.[20] The condition can, however, present later in childhood and although the diagnosis is usually obvious, occult hemangiomas do occur (e.g. spleen and retroperitoneum) and may exist undetected in the presence of a significant coagulopathy.[22,23]

Pathophysiology

These diverse disease processes lead to pathologic activation of the coagulation system via either the contact system, which usually follows endothelial injury, or via the tissue factor pathway following release of tissue factor (see Chapter 31). Once the coagulation system has been activated and DIC triggered, the pathophysiology is basically identical regardless of the underlying etiology.

Following activation, both thrombin and plasmin circulate systematically. Thrombin converts fibrinogen to fibrin monomer which then polymerizes to form cross-linked fibrin. This is associated with the consumption of procoagulant proteins and platelets. Fibrin deposition leads to microvascular and, less frequently, large vessel thrombosis with impaired perfusion and subsequent organ damage. Coagulation inhibitors also become depleted in the face of ongoing thrombin generation.

Circulating plasmin results in the generation of fibrin(ogen) degradation products (FDPs) from fibrin/fibrinogen which interfere with fibrin polymerization and platelet function, leading to hemorrhagic problems. Plasmin, in addition to inactivating coagulation proteins, can activate both the complement and kinin systems which can have wide ranging systemic consequences, including alterations in vascular permeability.[17–19]

Clinical features

Hemorrhage is the most obvious manifestation of DIC. Spontaneous bruising, purpura, oozing from venepuncture sites and bleeding from surgical wounds or sites of trauma are all relatively common, but more serious hemorrhagic problems can also occur. Microvascular and large vessel thrombosis, although clinically more difficult to recognize, are potentially more important as they may eventually lead to irreversible end-organ failure.

Acute infectious purpura fulminans is an uncommon but particularly severe form of DIC in which superficial purpura is followed by the development of bullae and hemorrhagic skin necrosis (Plate 38). The clinical features are indistinguishable from those seen in homozygous protein C and S deficiency (see Chapter 21) and are presumed to be predominantly due to acquired deficiencies of protein C and S.[24–26] The syndrome is most frequently diagnosed in children with meningococcal septicemia but can also follow streptococcal infection and chickenpox.[27] In some cases there may be a co-existing inherited defect as described by Inbal et al[28] in two children who were compound heterozygotes for the Factor V Leiden mutation and protein S deficiency and presented with purpura fulminans triggered by infection.

It is important to note, however, that with modern pediatric intensive care medicine and the use of sensitive screening tests (see below), DIC is often a laboratory diagnosis unaccompanied by clinical manifestation of either hemorrhage or thrombosis.

Laboratory diagnosis

DIC presents a wide clinical spectrum and given its complex pathophysiology can result in quite variable laboratory findings which can present diagnostic difficulties. The diagnosis is based on evidence of both procoagulant and fibrinolytic activation with concomitant inhibitor consumption.[29] In fulminant DIC the diagnosis is usually fairly straightforward and is characterized by prolongation of all the routine coagulation screening tests—PT, APTT and thrombin clotting time (TCT), combined with thrombocytopenia and evidence of increased FDPs. Examination of a peripheral blood film in such cases may also reveal the presence of red cell fragmentation. Although not routinely performed for diagnostic purposes, reduced levels of procoagulant proteins and inhibitors, especially ATIII and protein C, are also present and reflect ongoing consumption.

In milder cases the diagnosis is often less clear and requires careful interpretation of appropriate laboratory investigations. The platelet count is an important predictor of DIC and is reduced in a high proportion of cases. The PT and APTT are less reliable and can be normal in both infants and older children. Prolongation of the TCT, which reflects both reduced fibrinogen and the effect of increased FDPs, again is not always reliable. In the presence of a coagulopathy, measurement of individual procoagulant proteins can be useful in differentiating DIC from other acquired disorders. In particular, FVIII is reduced in DIC but normal or even increased in hepatic disease.

Evidence of increased fibrin degradation is an important component of the diagnosis of DIC. The D-dimer assay is now used routinely in many laboratories to detect the FDPs and appears to be one of the most reliable indicators of DIC. D-dimer is formed following the digestion of cross-linked fibrin by plasmin and is therefore fibrin specific.[30] This compares with the other FDPs, fragments X, Y, D and E, which can be derived from either fibrin or fibrinogen.

An increasing number of sensitive laboratory tests for markers of both thrombin and plasmin generation are now available.[31,32] These include prothrombin fragment $1+2$ (F1+2), fibrinopeptide A and thrombin-antithrombin (TAT) complexes, which provide evidence of thrombin activation, and Bb1-42 and plasmin-α_2-antiplasmin (PAP) which reflect fibrinolytic activity. These assays can provide evidence of ongoing 'biochemical DIC' in the absence of clinical manifestations of DIC and in the presence of normal screening tests. The clinical significance of 'biochemical DIC' remains unclear and the majority of these assays are used only as research tools.

Management

DIC is always a secondary phenomenon and it is therefore logical that the single most important aspect of management, and the only measure of proven efficacy, is treatment of the underlying cause. Virtually all other aspects of management are controversial and there is a clear lack of evidence from randomized controlled clinical trials to indicate how best to utilize the available therapeutic modalities.

Blood product replacement therapy still forms a major component of most treatment strategies. However, the choice of product, the optimal timing of administration and the efficacy of treatment are all unclear. Fresh frozen plasma (FFP), cryoprecipitate and platelets are the most frequently used products. Prothrombin-complex concentrates (PCCs) should be avoided due to the risks of further coagulation activation and thrombosis.[33] Similar concerns have applied to the use of fibrinogen concentrates in the past[34,35] and although there is no good evidence to support this risk with current products, their use in this setting should be carefully monitored. Exchange transfusion is rarely required but can be useful where treatment is limited by problems due to fluid overload.

Replacement therapy is usually reserved for patients with significantly abnormal coagulation profiles associated with clinical signs of bleeding or prior to invasive procedures. FFP is a source of procoagulant proteins and inhibitors and is usually administered in a dose of 10–15 ml/kg. Cryoprecipitate (10 ml/kg) can provide higher concentrations of fibrinogen and FVIII and is particularly useful in the presence of hypofibrinogenemia. There are no randomized clinical trials to define appropriate treatment end points but it is generally agreed that it is reasonable to maintain a platelet count of $>50 \times 10^9/l$ and a fibrinogen concentration of >1 g/l.

Whether more stringent correction of abnormal coagulation parameters improves outcome remains unclear.

Alternatives to blood component replacement therapy in DIC have centered around the use of anticoagulant therapy aimed at down-regulating coagulation activation. Heparin is an important anticoagulant agent which acts via the naturally occurring inhibitor ATIII. In animal models where DIC is triggered by the administration of endotoxins there are data to support the use of both heparin and ATIII concentrates in the treatment of DIC.[36,37] The results of clinical studies in both adults and children have, however, generated conflicting results.[38–40] Some authors have noted improvements both in laboratory and clinical parameters in children following therapy with ATIII concentrates alone or in combination with heparin,[41–43] but these studies have been too small to record reliable conclusions and neither heparin nor ATIII concentrates are currently indicated in the routine management of children with DIC.

More recently, there has been considerable interest in the use of protein C replacement therapy in the management of acute infectious purpura fulminans associated with meningococcal septicemia.[44–46] The rationale for this therapy is based on the similarity between the purpura fulminans observed in patients with homozygous protein C deficiency and that seen in patients with severe meningococcal septic shock (MSS). Acquired protein C deficiency occurs in MSS and it has been suggested that this plays a crucial role in the development of purpura fulminans in this condition. In addition, it has been demonstrated that there is a strong correlation between protein C levels and outcome in MSS, with levels below 10% associated with a high mortality rate.[47] Preliminary studies of protein C replacement therapy in severe MSS appear promising but again a randomized controlled trial is required to prove efficacy.[44–46]

Microvascular thrombosis in MSS is an important cause of end-organ failure and can also necessitate amputation where purpura fulminans results in severe limb ischemia. Impaired fibrinolysis with markedly increased levels of plasminogen activator inhibitor (PAI-1) has been documented in MSS and with this in mind, thrombolytic therapy has been utilized in some cases in an attempt to restore perfusion to pregangrenous limbs.[48–51] There are a small number of reports of the beneficial use of recombinant tPA in this condition; however, such treatments carry the risk of hemorrhagic complications and remain experimental.

Other investigational agents for the treatment of DIC include the alternative anticoagulant agents—low molecular weight heparin (LMWH) and hirudin but there are no data available in the pediatric age group.[52, 53]

VITAMIN K DEFICIENCY

Vitamin K is a fat-soluble vitamin, first identified > 50 years ago by the Danish biochemist Hendrik Dam, who observed bleeding in chicks fed a cholesterol-free diet. Appreciating the significance to the coagulation system, the newly diagnosed fat-soluble vitamin was ascribed the letter K (Koagulation in German).[54] Vitamin K is critical for the post-translational modification of a number of diverse proteins, which have in common γ-carboxyglutamate or 'Gla' residues. In its reduced form, vitamin K is a cofactor for the activation of the microsomal enzyme γ-glutamyl carboxylase, promoting the conversion of protein-bound glutamate residues (Glu) to γ-carboxyglutamate residues (Gla). The presence of Gla residues confers unique physiologic properties for calcium-mediated binding to negatively charged phospholipid surfaces, a requirement for effective hemostasis.[55] In the absence of vitamin K these precursor proteins are functionally inactive and circulate in their decarboxylated form (PIVKA; protein induced by vitamin K absence or antagonism).

Vitamin K-dependent proteins are present in a wide variety of tissues, including plasma (procoagulants—Factors II, VII, IX and X; anticoagulants—protein C and S; protein Z—function unknown), bone (osteocalcin or bone Gla-protein), kidney, lung, testes, spleen and placenta.[56,57] The best characterized are the vitamin K-dependent coagulation factors and osteocalcin. The latter is attracting attention as its importance in calcium homeostasis evolves. Osteocalcin is synthesized by osteoblasts, and although its function remains elusive, it is known that carboxylated osteocalcin binds to the hydroxyapatite matrix of bone.[58] The role of vitamin K in normal bone function is not fully understood. There is currently little evidence for an effect on mature bone but circumstantial evidence that an adequate vitamin K status is necessary for early skeletal development include the bony abnormalities of warfarin embryopathy and a report of similar skeletal changes in a child with congenital deficiency of vitamin K epoxide reductase, a rare autosomal recessive disorder.[59]

Vitamin K exists in two naturally occurring forms. Phylloquinone (vitamin K_1) is the main dietary source of vitamin K and is present predominantly in leafy green vegetables. The menaquinones (vitamin K_2) exist in a number of molecular forms, are restricted in the diet and largely synthesized by intestinal bacteria. In contrast to plasma where phylloquinones predominate, the liver contains substantial concentrations of menaquinones, although little is known of the extent of their intestinal absorption or of their bioavailability.[60–63] Vitamin K after absorption mediated by bile and pancreatic lipases is transported to the liver in chylomicrons and β-lipoproteins, where γ-carboxylation takes place; the system requires O_2, CO_2 and reduced vitamin K. In the process, vitamin K is metabolized to vitamin K-2,3-epoxide from which vitamin K is regenerated (Fig. 32.1). By this means, the vitamin K cycle acts as a salvage pathway for vitamin K.[63] There is some evidence to support the view that vitamin K epoxide reductase and vitamin K quinone reductase activities are carried out by the same enzyme.[64]

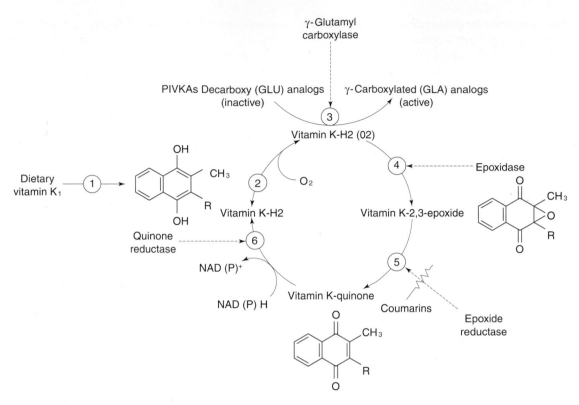

Fig. 32.1 Vitamin K cycle. Step 1: Phylloquninone (vitamin K_1) is reduced by a number of qunione reductases to form vitamin K-H2. Step 2: It is thought that the metabolically active form of vitamin K is an intermediate complex formed from vitamin K-H2, oxygen and the enzyme γ-glutamyl carboxylase. Step 3: The complex then carboxylates multiple glutamic acid residues within the large precursor molecule of the vitamin K-dependent proteins: these non-functional procoagulant proteins are termed PIVKAs. Step 4: The carboxylation step is coupled to the epoxidation of vitamin K-H2 to form K-2,3 epoxide. Step 5: Epoxide reductase converts the epoxide to form vitamin K-quinone. Step 6: Vitamin K-quinone is then reduced further to regenerate K-H2 by means of a reaction driven by NAD(P)H. Reproduced with permission from Ref. 63.

Etiology

Vitamin K deficiency beyond infancy is relatively uncommon and is almost always a secondary event resulting from:

1. inadequate intake or absorption;
2. poor utilization of vitamin K;
3. vitamin K antagonism.

Because of the wide dietary distribution of phylloquinones, after infancy an adequate vitamin K intake generally refers to unsupplemented total parenteral nutrition often combined with the prolonged administration of broad-spectrum antibiotics.[65] Conditions associated with malabsorption are the commonest cause of vitamin K deficiency in the pediatric age group. These include celiac disease, cystic fibrosis, Crohn's disease, biliary atresia and other causes of obstructive jaundice. Vitamin K deficiency secondary to malabsorption from absence of bile salts, either from intrahepatic or extrahepatic biliary obstruction, responds to vitamin K replacement. In contrast, in primary hepatocellular disease, liver parenchymal cells may not be capable of utilizing vitamin K even when present in adequate amounts. However, inadequate bile salt secretion may be a contributing factor and partial improvement may follow vitamin K administration.

The commonest cause of vitamin K antagonism is warfarin therapy, which inhibits vitamin K epoxide reductase resulting in the accumulation of the epoxide metabolite.[63] There is a hepatic NAD(P)H-dependent pathway for vitamin K reduction which is fairly insensitive to warfarin (Fig. 32.1).[67-69] Thus, vitamin K can bypass the enzyme, epoxide reductase, in situations requiring reversal of the warfarin effect. Second- and third-generation cephalosporins can also produce hypoprothrombinemia by inhibiting vitamin K epoxide reductase,[70] but these antibiotics are relatively weak vitamin K antagonists and probably only pose a risk in the presence of co-existing predisposing factors such as malnourishment with compromised vitamin K status.[71,72]

Clinical features

Although laboratory evidence of vitamin K deficiency is quite common in the predisposing conditions described above, clinical bleeding is relatively infrequent and when it occurs it is usually mild to moderate and typified by bruising, oozing from venepuncture sites and, rarely, internal bleeding. The underlying cause can usually be identified from the history and physical examination. In patients with liver disease, impaired synthesis of coagulation factors may co-exist with vitamin K deficiency, increasing the severity of the coagulopathy. At-risk children who require an invasive procedure such as liver or jejunal biopsies should have a coagulation screen prior to the procedure and should receive appropriate vitamin K replacement in the event of a correctable abnormality.

Laboratory diagnosis

FVII and protein C have the shortest half-life of the vitamin K-dependent proteins.[73] FVII is therefore the first of the procoagulants to become deficient, resulting in an isolated prolongation of the PT. Levels of Factors II, IX and X then decline, prolonging the APTT. Both the PT and APTT are corrected by a 1:1 mix with normal plasma. These screening test abnormalities are not specific for vitamin K deficiency and confirmatory tests may be both necessary and helpful in some patients. Specific factor assays may help distinguish isolated vitamin K deficiency from congenital factor deficiency, liver disease or DIC. Measurement of decarboxy-prothrombin (PIVKA II), which is increased in vitamin K deficiency, is a more specific test.[74–76] It is extremely sensitive and able to detect the early subclinical deficiency state. PIVKA II has a long half-life and can be used to diagnose vitamin K deficiency even after vitamin K therapy has normalized the PT. An additional useful test is the Echis prothrombin assay which measures both carboxylated and decarboxylated forms of prothrombin by comparing FII activity in a calcium-dependent system to that in a calcium-independent system (*Echis carinatum*).[77,78] A ratio of FII:Echis II of $\lesssim 0.80$ indicates vitamin K deficiency. Vitamin K can be directly quantified.[61,79,80] Normal serum levels in adults are around 0.5 ng/ml. Vitamin K assays are, however, too time consuming and expensive for routine diagnostic use.

Despite the sophistication of a number of assays for diagnosing vitamin K deficiency, only the PT is known to correlate with the risk of bleeding. The diagnosis of isolated vitamin K deficiency can be confirmed if administration of a therapeutic dose of vitamin K is followed by a fall in the PT, which can occur in as short a period as 30 min if the vitamin is given intravenously.[81,82] However, vitamin K deficiency can complicate other coagulopathies and if there is any doubt about the diagnosis the patient should receive vitamin K in conjunction with any other appropriate treatment.

Treatment

Appropriate treatment of vitamin K deficiency is dictated by the clinical situation. The intramuscular route may result in painful hematoma formation and should be avoided. Intravenous vitamin K should be restricted to those situations where other routes are not feasible, because rarely, severe anaphylaxis may complicate intravenous vitamin K administration even when appropriately diluted and infused

slowly. Subcutaneous administration is safe and effective and is therefore the preferred systemic route. In the presence of normal absorption, oral vitamin K is effective, but correction of the PT is slower than following parenteral administration.

Individuals with no clinical hemorrhage but laboratory evidence of vitamin K deficiency should receive vitamin K subcutaneously or orally if absorption is normal. Patients who are bleeding secondary to vitamin K deficiency and who require rapid correction of their coagulopathy should receive vitamin K parenterally in addition to 10–15 ml/kg FFP which will raise the levels of vitamin K-dependent factors by 0.1–0.2 unit/ml. Virally-inactivated FFP should be used wherever possible. Where only untreated FFP is available, virally inactivated PCCs may offer a safer alternative. In the presence of life-threatening hemorrhage, treatment with PCCs may be appropriate in addition to systemic vitamin K.

Prophylaxis

Vitamin K 1 μg/kg/day is considered an adequate daily requirement.[83] Consideration should be given to the use of vitamin K supplementation in children at high risk of developing deficiency. Vitamin K deficiency generally develops in the setting of an underlying predisposing condition (see above). The risk of developing vitamin K deficiency may be increased by the co-existence of other risk factors such as inadequate nutrition or the prolonged use of broad-spectrum antibiotics. Generally, children receiving total parenteral nutrition are supplemented with vitamin K. There is a surprising paucity in the literature of evidence-based guidelines or indeed recommendations from even small studies. The best researched of the disorders predisposing to vitamin K deficiency is cystic fibrosis, but even here there is no consensus on the need for routine vitamin K supplementation.[84] Studies suggest that vitamin K deficiency is probably unusual in patients with cystic fibrosis not receiving vitamin K supplements, but a negative effect may be masked by the current common use of vitamin K supplements in this patient group.[84] A literature review identified those at greatest risk as those children with:

- severe non-cholestatic or cholestatic liver disease;
- major small bowel resection for intestinal complications;
- pulmonary disease necessitating long-term use of antibiotics;
- pancreatic insufficiency;

and suggested that these categories of patients receive vitamin K prophylaxis until evidence from future studies identifies risk factors.[84] The Consensus Conference of the Cystic Fibrosis Foundation on Nutritional Assessment and Management in Cystic Fibrosis (1990) made dosage recommendations.[85]

HEMOSTATIC COMPLICATIONS OF LIVER DISEASE

HEPATIC FAILURE

Although the underlying disease processes vary, the pathophysiology of abnormal hemostasis in liver disease is similar in neonates, children and adults. Several mechanisms contribute and reflect the important role played by the liver in the maintenance of normal hemostasis.

Pathophysiology

The liver is crucial for the synthesis and clearance of components of both the coagulation and fibrinolytic systems. With the exception of FVIII, von Willebrand factor (VWF), tPA, uPA and PAI, the liver is the sole or predominant site of synthesis for all other hemostatic proteins. Impaired hepatic function therefore results in progressive failure of synthesis which can be further aggravated in some cases by the loss of coagulation proteins into ascitic fluid.[86,87]

The liver is also the site of the post-ribosomal carboxylation of the vitamin K-dependent proteins. In the presence of hepatic impairment, hypocarboxylated proteins may be released due to impaired utilization of vitamin K.[88] Abnormal fibrinogen molecules can also be identified which, like fetal fibrinogen, have an increased content of sialic acid.[89,90]

Failure of the hepatic reticuloendothelial system to clear activated coagulation factors and intermediate complexes, together with local activation due to hepatocellular damage, results in a consumptive coagulopathy which further impairs hemostasis. There is also good evidence that the fibrinolytic system is activated and although primary fibrinolysis secondary to increased levels of tPA may contribute to this, secondary activation in association with DIC appears to be the predominant mechanism.[91]

Thrombocytopenia in liver disease is multifactorial and may reflect increased consumption secondary to DIC as well as pooling due to splenomegaly. Abnormal platelet function due to increased FDPs and other poorly defined mechanims also occurs.[92]

Clinical features

Spontaneous bleeding is relatively uncommon but superficial bruising and hemorrhage in relation to invasive procedures does occur. In more advanced disease with cirrhosis, local bleeding from gastric and esophageal varices can be life-threatening.

In general, the extent to which the hemostatic system is disturbed is directly related to the severity of the hepatocellular damage. In mild-to-moderate hepatic impairment, there may be minimal dysfunction initially. The PT is usually the first screening test to become abnormal with FVII declining first, followed by the other vitamin K-dependent factors. With more extensive damage, the non-vitamin K-dependent factors are also reduced and the APTT becomes prolonged. At this stage the TCT is usually normal and fibrinogen levels may be normal or even increased due to the acute phase response. In advanced disease with liver failure and cirrhosis, a wide spectrum of defects may co-exist. At this stage most of the procoagulants and naturally occurring inhibitors are reduced. The PT and APTT are progressively prolonged, the TCT extends and fibrinogen levels fall. The reptilase time will be abnormal in the presence of dysfibrinogenemia. Fibrinogen degradation products and the molecular markers of activation, e.g. thrombin antithrombin (TAT) complex, are increased reflecting impaired clearance and ongoing DIC. The platelet count is usually reduced and the bleeding time may be prolonged.

Management

Treatment is largely supportive, allowing time for the liver to recover from the underlying insult or less often until transplant surgery can be performed. In the presence of clinical bleeding, replacement therapy should be undertaken with FFP, cryoprecipitate and platelets. Occasionally, where fluid overload is a problem, exchange transfusion has been used. The administration of PCCs should in general be avoided as they can lead to further activation of the coagulation system. Secondary vitamin K deficiency due to cholestasis is common and adequate parenteral vitamin K supplements should be given.

LIVER TRANSPLANT SURGERY

Orthotopic liver transplantation is associated with further imbalances in the hemostatic system which can result in both hemorrhagic and thrombotic problems during the peri- and post-operative period. Children undergoing liver transplantation usually have end-stage liver disease and are therefore likely to have significant preoperative defects. During the procedure, increased primary fibrinolytic activity is characteristic and contributes to blood loss. The first fibrinolytic 'burst' occurs after the liver has been removed, during the anhepatic phase, and the second as the donor liver is being reperfused. At both stages fibrinolysis occurs secondary to massive release of tPA from endothelial cells in association with impaired clearance and low levels of PAI.[93,94] Both the serine protease inhibitor aprotinin and the antifibrinolytic agent epsilon aminocaproic acid, may help to reduce blood loss during surgery.[95,96]

During the postoperative period, usually days 4–10, there is an increased incidence of hepatic artery thrombosis. The incidence varies from 2 to 20% in different series but appears to be higher in children than adults.[97–99] The mechanism is thought to involve a relative delay in the recovery of the naturally occurring inhibitors ATIII, protein C and S, compared with procoagulant proteins, resulting in a transient prothrombotic tendency.[100] Protein C in particular appears to recover slowly, especially in children; in one study protein C levels did not increase above 50% of normal until 1 week after surgery.[99]

HEPATIC VENO-OCCLUSIVE DISEASE

Hepatic veno-occlusive disease (VOD) typically follows high-dose cytoreductive therapy administered in the context of bone marrow transplantation (BMT), but has also been reported in children receiving less intensive chemotherapeutic regimens and very rarely after consumption of pyrrolizidine-containing herbal tea.[101–110]

The incidence of post-transplant VOD is lower in children than in adults; however, figures as high as 22% and 36% have been reported.[111,112] Recognized risk factors include pre-existing liver disease, second transplants and the use of busulphan-containing preparative regimens.[101,113,114] VOD following conventional dose chemotherapy has been reported less frequently and has particularly involved children with Wilms' disease.[105–109] Recently, Bisogno et al[105] documented that 8% of children treated according to the SIOP-9 protocol (dactinomycin, vincristine $\pm$ abdominal radiotherapy) had hepatoxicity consistent with VOD.

The clinical features of VOD include jaundice, right upper quadrant pain, hepatomegaly, weight gain secondary to fluid retention, abdominal distension and ascites. In the context of BMT, the onset of symptoms is usually early and typically problems develop within 3 weeks of transplantation. The diagnosis is largely clinical and both the Seattle and Baltimore transplant groups have defined clinical criteria for the diagnosis of VOD.[102,115] According to the Seattle criteria, 2 of 3 clinical manifestations should be present by day 20 post-BMT—jaundice, painful hepatomegaly, fluid retention.[102]

Histologic features of hepatic VOD, usually documented from autopsy findings including narrowing and fibrosis of the terminal hepatic venules, sublobular veins and centilobular sinusoids with necrosis of zone 3 hepatocytes.[116] The pathogenesis of VOD remains pooly understood but the primary trigger is thought to be damage to the vascular endothelium. This may occur directly or via the actions of cytokines released from macrophages and reticuloendothelial cells and high levels of tumor necrosis factor and interleukin-1 have been recorded in patients with VOD.[117,118] One of the effects of the resulting endothelial cell injury is activation of the coagulation system with the potential development of a local hypercoagulable state.[119–121]

Strategies aimed at the prevention of VOD following BMT have included the use of prostaglandin E_1 (PGE_1), pentoxifylline, ursodeoxycholic acid and heparin.[101] Trials of heparin prophylaxis in adults have yielded conflicting results, with some studies demonstrating a considerable reduction in VOD after both allogeneic and autologous BMT, while others have shown no effect.[101] Studies in children are limited; however, a recent phase II trial of continuous heparin (100 unit/kg/day until day 30 post BMT) found a reduced incidence of moderate and severe VOD compared with historic controls without an increase in major hemorrhagic complications.[122] A randomized controlled trial is required to define the efficacy of this approach.

The management of VOD remains largely supportive with treatment measures aimed at maintaining fluid and electrolyte balance. While this may be adequate in mild-to-moderate VOD, the mortality associated with severe VOD is high and has lead to attempts to modify the clinical course using other agents such as heparin, PGE_1 and recombinant tPA.[123]

The place of thrombolytic therapy with recombinant tPA in children is not yet defined and there are no published randomized studies. A number of case reports have documented a beneficial effect and Leahey and Bunin reported resolution of VOD in 5 of 9 (56%) children treated with a combination of recombinant tPA and heparin, without any major hemorrhagic events.[124–127] This contrasts with results published by Bearman et al[128] in which treatment of 42 adult patients again with a combination of tPA and heparin, at a single center between 1989 and 1995, was successful in only 29% and was associated with a significant risk of life-threatening hemorrhage.

HEMOSTATIC COMPLICATIONS OF RENAL DISEASE

CHRONIC RENAL FAILURE

The commonest form of bleeding in infants and children with end-stage renal failure is mucosal in origin, e.g. gastrointestinal, epistaxis. Less frequently, bleeding following invasive procedures may occur. Although various factors contribute, defective platelet function and heparin therapy for dialysis are the most important causes of impaired hemostasis in uremic patients of all ages.[129,130]

In the absence of heparin, the characteristic findings in children with uremia are a prolonged bleeding time with a normal or mildly reduced platelet count and normal coagulation screening tests. Several mechanims are thought to contribute to platelet dysfunction in renal failure but this remains a poorly defined area with many conflicting results.[129,130]

Abnormal ristocetin-induced platelet aggregation has been described in association with reduced levels of both platelet VWF and the high molecular weight multimers of plasma VWF.[131] In support of this mechanism, it is also known that the administration of cryoprecipitate or desmopressin (DDAVP), both of which increase FVIII and VWF, can transiently shorten the bleeding time.[132,133] Other proposed mechanisms include alterations in both prostaglandin and prostacyclin metabolism, reduced platelet granule content and abnormalities of platelet membrane phospholipids.[129,130] In addition, it has been shown in animal models that there is an association between excess production of the endothelium-derived relaxing factor, nitric oxide, and bleeding in renal failure.[134]

Anemia is also known to contribute and the hematocrit is usually inversely proportional to the bleeding time. This is due to the effect of red blood cells on platelet flow which influences the interaction between platelets and the endothelium. Improving the hematocrit by either transfusion or recombinant erythropoietin can also shorten or even normalize the bleeding time.[135,136]

HEMOLYTIC UREMIC SYNDROME

In the classic form of hemolytic uremic syndrome (HUS) an acute diarrheal illness is followed by the developement of the characteristc triad of microangiopathic hemolytic anemia, acute renal failure and thrombocytopenia (see Chapters 21 and 38). The severity of the syndrome is variable and incomplete forms have been described. Most cases occur sporadically and the majority are due to enterohemorrhagic *Escherichia coli*.[137]

The pathogenesis of HUS is complex but prominent features include toxin-mediated renal endothelial cell and platelet damage.[138,139] The effect on platelets is thought to be mediated via an imbalance between thromboxane A_2, which is increased, and prostaglandin, which is reduced.[140] In addition, total VWF and the VWF high molecular weight multimers are also increased and may enhance platelet activation.

Thrombocytopenia is a consistent finding and is moderate or severe in around 50% of cases. Features of DIC are not prominent, although there is evidence of fibrinolytic activation, which may relate to the release of tPA and PAI from damaged endothelial cells.[141] Treatment remains largely supportive although plasma exchange has been used in high-risk cases.[142]

NEPHROTIC SYNDROME

Thrombotic problems also occur in renal disease and include renal vein thrombosis (see below), thrombosis of the hemodialysis vascular access site and events occurring secondary to nephrotic syndrome.

Proteinuria, hypoalbuminemia and edema are the characteristic features. Primary or minimal change disease is the commonest form seen in childhood and in general carries a good prognosis. The association between thrombosis and the nephrotic syndrome is well recognized in both children and adults. Children with uncontrolled or refractory disease are at particular risk. The frequency of thrombotic events is difficult to predict as figures in different studies vary considerably and range from <5% to >25%.[143] Renal vein thrombosis and pulmonary embolism are the most frequent events.

Several alterations in the hemostatic system may contribute to the development of thrombosis. In general, levels of the procoagulant proteins are increased while the major inhibitor of coagulation, ATIII, is reduced. This is presumed to lead to an imbalance in favor of thrombin generation which is only partially offset by increased levels of the other inhibitors, protein C and α_2-M.[144] Other changes include increased platelet reactivity which again may contribute to thrombosis.[145,146] Data on fibrinolysis conflict with both hyper- and hypo-fibrinolysis having been described.[147]

The management of thrombotic problems in the nephrotic syndrome has been variable but anticoagulants and thrombolytic therapy have been used.[143] Prophylactic anticoagulation should probably be considered in high-risk cases.

CARDIOVASCULAR-RELATED HEMOSTATIC PROBLEMS

CONGENITAL HEART DISEASE

Conflicting data exist regarding the presence and mechanism of coagulation defects in children with congenital heart disease (CHD). The majority have been described in children with cyanotic CHD in association with secondary polycythemia.[147–157] In a study of 41 children, Henriksson et al[150] concluded that hemostatic defects were common in the presence of cyanotic CHD and frequently involved deficiencies of FV and the vitamin K-dependent Factors II, VII, IX and X. The mechanism was postulated to be reduced hepatic synthesis due to hypoxia, as a consequence of high blood viscosity, and there was no evidence of activation of the coagulation system. Other studies suggest that the coagulation system is activated and that low-grade DIC contributes to the observed abnormalities.[151,158]

In contrast, other investigators have demonstrated normal coagulation parameters in cyanotic CHD and it has been suggested that some of the previously documented abnormalities may have been artefactual due to failure to correct *in vitro* for the presence of polycythemia.[155,158] In support of this, a recent prospective study of 22 children with both cyanotic and acyanotic CHD failed to demonstrate any difference in baseline preoperative concentrations of procoagulant proteins and inhibitors when compared with age-related normal ranges.[159] There was, however, an increase in baseline TAT complex levels which has been confirmed in other studies analyzing TAT together with other sensitive markers of coagulation activation.[160,161] This suggests that thrombin generation is increased in at least a proportion of patients but not to such an extent as to result in significant consumption of coagulation proteins.

Mild-to-moderate thrombocytopenia and abnormalities of platelet function have also been recorded in cyanotic CHD but again the mechanisms are poorly understood.[151,154,157,162,163] Coagulation and platelet abnormalities appear less common in acyanotic CHD; however, Gill et al[164] demonstrated loss of high molecular weight multimers of VWF in children with a number of non-cyanotic defects (atrial septal defect, ventricular septal defect and aortic stenosis), which normalized after successful cardiac surgery. Again, the mechanism is unclear but may involve platelet or endothelial cell activation.

A specific coagulopathy is seen in children with Noonan's syndrome, a rare inherited disorder characterized by dysmorphic facies, congenital heart disease, short stature and a bleeding tendency. The condition is thought to be inherited as an autosomal dominant trait and affected individuals have multiple factor deficiencies affecting predominantly the intrinsic coagulation system.[165]

Despite the various hemostatic defects described in the literature, children with CHD rarely have major hemorrhagic problems other than during surgery. They frequently need to undergo corrective cardiac surgery involving cardiopulmonary bypass (CPB) and in some cases multiple procedures may be required.

CARDIOPULMONARY BYPASS SURGERY

Hemorrhage remains an important problem both during and after CPB surgery in children and the etiology is likely to be multifactorial in virtually all cases. Contributing factors include hemodilution of procoagulant proteins, thrombocytopenia and platelet dysfunction, activation of the coagulation and fibrinolytic systems with DIC and iatrogenic anticoagulant effects (Table 32.5). Whereas in adults, platelet dysfunction is through to be the most important factor,[166,167] in children, hemodilution of procoagulant proteins and problems relating to anticoagulant monitoring are probably more important.

In one study, 22 children with CHD undergoing CPB had samples collected for analysis of hemostatic proteins at various time points before, during and after bypass.[159] The very marked effect of hemodilution was demonstrated by a reduction in the concentration of all hemostatic proteins by an average of 56% (range 50–70%) following initiation of CPB. In some cases this resulted in reduction in procoagulant proteins to a level below that generally considered necessary for normal hemostasis. Although there was little further fall in levels during surgery, following completion of bypass the concentrations of certain procoagulants (Factors II, V, VII, IX, XI and XII) remained significantly reduced at 24 hours post procedure. Platelet counts were also significantly reduced post bypass (mean 117×10^9/l; range: $65–172 \times 10^9$/l).

Table 32.5 Causes of bleeding associated with cardiopulmonary bypass.

Preoperative coagulation defects
Hemodilution
Consumption (DIC)
Thrombocytopenia
Platelet dysfunction
Heparin effects

Evidence of increased thrombin generation and increased fibrinolysis are also apparent during CPB and DIC may therefore contribute to hemorrhagic problems.[159,160,168] As well as thrombocytopenia, qualitative platelet defects develop during CPB, resulting in prolongation of the bleeding time independent of the actual platelet count. Platelet dysfunction is thought to be caused by platelet contact with the synthetic surfaces of the bypass circuit and the effects of hypothermia. These functional abnormalities develop soon after the commencement of bypass and are progressive, such that after 2 hours on bypass the bleeding time may exceed 30 min.[169] The effect is, however, transient and normalization is reported after 2–4 hours in adult studies.[169] The nature of the platelet function defect remains controversial and results in keeping with platelet activation, as well as abnormalities of platelet membrane glycoproteins, have been described.[169–172] It has also been suggested that the problem may relate to an *in vivo* shortage of platelet agonists rather than to an actual intrinsic platelet defect.[173]

Anticoagulation with heparin is an important part of the CBP procedure. Current protocols utilize unfractionated heparin monitored using the activated clotting time (ACT) and aim to maintain the ACT above a predefined level (usually >400–450 s). At the end of the bypass procedure, heparin is reversed using protamine sulfate. It is clear, however, that the ACT correlates poorly with actual heparin levels as assessed by anti-Xa assays and this may result in suboptimal anticoagulant control in a significant number of cases.[159,174] The response to heparin may also be affected by the reduction in antithrombin levels which occur during the bypass procedure.[175]

Another less frequently documented complication of heparin therapy in this setting is heparin-induced thrombocytopenia (HIT). Although HIT typically develops 5 or more days after the initiation of heparin therapy, the onset can be more rapid where there has been prior heparin exposure.[176] This typically occurs in children who have had cardiac catheterization performed prior to surgery or in those undergoing a second surgical procedure involving CPB. Paradoxically, patients with HIT are at increased risk of thromboembolic complications which can be arterial or venous and are often life-threatening.[177,178] Patients with HIT who develop thrombotic complications and those with a prior history of HIT who require further anticoagulation have been treated with a variety of agents and recently, Saxon and Leaker[179] reported the successful use of the heparinoid, Orgaran, in a child undergoing repeat CPB.

EXTRACORPOREAL MEMBRANE OXYGENATION

Hemorrhage, particularly intracranial hemorrhage (ICH), is also an important complication of extracorporeal membrane oxygenation (ECMO). This technique allows the transfer of oxygen into blood across a semipermeable membrane and is used in a variety of conditions complicated by severe cardiorespiratory failure.[180–182] Current estimates suggest that ICH occurs with a frequency of around 15% and is an important predictor of long-term outcome.[182] As with CPB, the etiology of bleeding is probably multifactorial with thrombocytopenia, platelet dysfunction, coagulation abnormalities and problems relating to anticoagulant control playing an important part. ICH is more frequent in the neonatal age group which may reflect additional problems relating to immaturity of the hemostatic system as well as problems related to cerebral blood flow (see Chapter 33).[183]

McManus et al[184] examined coagulation factors prior to and following the initiation of ECMO in 19 children, and demonstrated the presence of pre-existing coagulation defects (defined as reduced levels of 2 or more coagulation factors) in 68% of cases pre ECMO. In addition, despite the use of coagulation factors in the circuit prime, which would be expected to compensate at least to some extent for the effect of hemodilution, 53% of patients had similar coagulation abnormalities after the start of ECMO. Four patients (three neonates and one older child) developed ICH and in this subgroup deficiencies in >5 coagulation factors were noted. McManus et al[184] concluded that a high proportion of cases may have significant pre-existing coagulation defects which are inadequately corrected by the circuit prime fluid at the onset of ECMO. This is of particular concern given suggestions that coagulation factors be omitted from the circuit prime and the inconsistencies in the actual products in current use.

Evidence of coagulation activation has also been demonstrated in term infants undergoing ECMO, particularly during the first 24 hours of the procedure and, as with CPB, the ACT shows a poor correlation with actual heparin levels which may increase the risk of both hemorrhagic and thrombotic problems.[185,186]

METABOLIC DISORDERS

GAUCHER'S DISEASE

Gaucher's disease is an inherited (autosomal recessive) condition caused by a deficiency of the enzyme glucocerebrosidase, which results in accumulation of glucocerebroside in cells of the monocyte/macrophage system. Thrombocytopenia due to splenomegaly is frequently observed but in addition various coagulation abnormalities have also been reported, including deficiencies of FIX and FXI and abnormalities of platelet function.[187–189]

Hollak et al[190] performed coagulation studies in 30 patients with type I Gaucher's disease, and reported prolongation of the PT and APTT in 38% and 42%, respectively, and significant deficiencies (<50%) of multiple coagulation factors (XI, XII, VII, X, V and II) in 30–60%. They also documented increased levels of markers of both coagulation

(TAT complex) and fibrinolytic (plasminogen-antiplasmin complex, D-dimer) activation in these patients in keeping with a low-grade consumptive coagulopathy. In a similar study of 9 patients followed up over a 2-year period, the most consistent abnormalities were prolongation of the APTT (55%) and reduced levels of FIX (33%) with variable and inconsistent abnormalities of FVIII and VWF.[191] They also noted increased levels of IgG anticardiolipin antibodies on at least one occasion in 6 patients which has not previously been reported.

Despite the apparent severity of the coagulation abnormality recorded in some patients, clinical bleeding is generally mild and in most cases correlates best with the degree of thrombocytopenia. The pathophysiology of the coagulopathy remains poorly understood but does not appear to reflect impaired synthesis due to hepatic dysfunction. Hollak et al[190] suggested that there may be ongoing low-grade DIC caused by mononuclear cell activation. The spleen has also been implicated in some studies; however, splenectomy is not always associated with resolution of the observed abnormalities. Adsorption of coagulation factors by the accumulated sphingolipid is a likely contributor and some authors have suggested that this may simply occur as an in vitro phenomenon; however, this hypothesis remains unproven.[192] FXI deficiency in some cases may be an independent abnormality as both inherited FXI deficiency and Gaucher's disease are common in Ashkenazi Jews.[193]

The effect of enzyme replacement therapy with alglucerase also appears variable with partial correction of the coagulation disturbance recorded by Hollak et al,[190] while Billet et al[191] did not find any effect.

ACQUIRED INHIBITORS OF COAGULATION

Acquired inhibitors of coagulation can be divided into those which inhibit specific coagulation factors (e.g. VIII and IX), and those which are non-specific and interfere with other aspects of the coagulation cascade (e.g. lupus anticoagulants).

INHIBITORS OF SPECIFIC COAGULATION PROTEINS

Factors VIII and IX inhibitors

Specific inhibitors are a well recognized complication of replacement therapy in the management of the congenital factor deficiencies and are most frequently seen in hemophilia A (see Chapter 29). FVIII and FIX inhibitors in non-hemophiliac children are uncommon but have been reported in a few cases, with some reports documenting the presence of antibodies to both proteins occuring simultaneously in the same patient.[194–200]

In adults, acquired FVIII inhibitors are most commonly

seen in the elderly or in the context of autoimmune conditions, malignancy or following drug ingestion. In children, viral infections are the most commonly reported preceding events, although antibiotic ingestion (penicillin) has also been implicated.[195,199] In other cases, however, these antibodies appear to develop spontaneously.[197,198] The pattern of bleeding is variable with some cases being diagnosed incidentally or in association with only mild-to-moderate bleeding symptoms, while others present with severe life-threatening hemorrhage.

Characterization of these antibodies is limited by their infrequency but most seem to belong to the IgG$_4$ subclass of immunoglobulin.[201] Management of bleeding in children with acquired antibodies to FVIII or FIX is similar to that used for children with hemophilia who develop inhibitors and may involve the administration of high-dose FVIII or FIX, or alternative therapies including porcine FVIII, PCCs or recombinant FVIIa.[202–204] Treatment aimed at the eradication of these antibodies may not always be required as some appear to disappear spontaneously.[196,199] In cases where there are significant hemorrhagic problems, early introduction of immunosuppressive therapy with intravenous immunoglobulin (IVIG) may be beneficial. Steroids and cytotoxic agents, e.g. cyclophosphamide, has also been used successfully in some children with persisting antibodies, but may be associated with significant side-effects.[198,200,201]

von Willebrand factor inhibitors

Acquired inhibitors to VWF are again extremely rare in children but have been reported in association with other autoantibodies and in children with Wilms' tumor.[205–209] In an attempt to document the frequency of acquired VWD in Wilms' tumor, Coppes et al[210] analyzed coagulation parameters in 50 consecutive children with Wilms' tumor at presentation, and documented acquired VWD in 4 of 50 (8%) (type 1 disease = 2, type 3 disease = 2). Recognition of VWD in Wilms' tumor is important as some treatment protocols utilize early surgery and certainly bleeding was recorded as a presenting feature in 3 of the 4 previously documented cases.[204–209]

The mechanism by which VWD develops in Wilms' tumor patients remains poorly defined but it has been suggested that a plasma factor secreted by the tumor binds with VWF and results in premature clearance of VWF.[210] These antibodies usually disappear spontaneously following successful treatment of the tumor; however, in the event of treatment being required, desmopressin (DDAVP) or replacement therapy with factor concentrate containing high molecular weight VWF multimers may be indicated.[208,210]

Factor V inhibitors

Acquired FV inhibitors in children most commonly develop following surgery in which fibrin sealant-containing bovine thrombin has been used to improve hemostasis.[211–214] Only occasionally have they been reported in other situations, typically following major surgery, e.g. a 3-year-old child developed a FV inhibitor following liver transplant.[215,216]

The development of a FV inhibitor following exposure to fibrin sealant is due to the presence of bovine FV in the bovine thrombin component of this preparation. The resulting antibodies have variable cross-reactivity and in most cases have specificity against bovine but not human thrombin and against both bovine and human FV.[212]

These antibodies have most often been seen following the use of a fibrin sealant preparation in cardiac surgery, often for the correction of congenital cardiac defects. The development of a FV inhibitor is characterized by prolongation of both the PT and PTT on routine postoperative coagulation monitoring which may be associated with excess bleeding. While many of these antibodies appear to be transient, it has recently been demonstrated that re-exposure to the same fibrin sealant product during repeat cardiac surgery can result in the reappearance of the antibody despite apparently normal preoperative coagulation screening and can lead to severe hemorrhagic problems.[211]

When treatment is required due to acute bleeding, FFP is the only available source of FV but may result in problems with fluid overload. Alternative strategies inlcude the use of plasmapheresis, high-dose IVIG and recombinant FVIIa.[211,214]

Other inhibitors

Antibodies with specificity against FX, FXI and other contact factors have also been reported and can result in hemorrhagic problems but appear to be extremely rare in the pediatric age group.[217–219]

ANTIPHOSPHOLIPID ANTIBODIES

Antiphospholipid (aPL) antibodies are a heterogeneous group of antibodies which were originally believed to be directed against anionic phospholipids. They can be detected in vitro in solid-phase immunoassays when they are generally termed anticardiolipin (aCL) antibodies or in phospholipid-dependent coagulation tests where the term lupus anticoagulant (LA) is usually applied.

The first aPL antibodies were reported in the early 1950s when it was noted that some individuals had biologically false positive serologic tests for syphilis using the Venereal Disease Research Laboratory (VDRL) test which utilizes the phospholipid cardiolipin as its antigen.[220] These results were obtained in a number of clinical situations but it later became apparent that some cases progressed to develop systemic lupus erythematosus (SLE). A further link with SLE was reported by Conley and Hartmann in 1952 when they reported the presence of an inhibitor to in vitro coagulation (lupus anticoagulant) in two patients with SLE.[221] It was subsequently noted in the 1960s that patients with detectable LAs did not have a bleeding tendency but paradoxically appeared to be at increased risk of thrombo-embolic events.[222] The detection of aPL antibodies was improved by the development in 1983 of the aCL assay which was much more sensitive than the original VDRL test.[223] Using an aCL assay, positive results were documented in a large proportion of patients with SLE, some of whom also had a circulating LA. It was also recognized around this time that there were patients with a positive aPL antibody test, who had an history of thrombosis, recurrent fetal loss or thrombocytopenia but did not have SLE, and this lead to the recognition of primary anti-phospholipid syndrome.[224]

Pathogenesis of thrombosis

The mechanism whereby aPL antibodies result in thrombosis remains poorly understood despite considerable ongoing research in this area. Initially, it was not even clear whether aPL was in fact pathogenic, or whether it occurred as an unrelated epiphenomenon. Recent experiments in animals and prospective clinical trials looking for evidence of coagulation activation in patients with aPL do, however, suggest a role in pathogenesis.[225,226] Progress has also been made in understanding the antigen specificity of these antibodies and it is now clear that aPL antibodies are not primarily directed against phospholipid itself but against proteins bound to phospholipid, which include β_2 glycoprotein 1 and pro-thrombin.[227–229] Beyond this, there is little agreement on the mechanism of action of this heterogeneous group of antibodies but work currently focuses on the protein C system and the platelet/endothelial axis.[225,226]

Laboratory tests

Given the heterogeneity of aPL, it is crucial that patients are tested for the presence of both LA and aCL. Studies have shown that in around 50–60% of cases both tests are positive while in the remainder the results are discordant.

None of the available tests for LA is entirely specific and current guidelines recommend the use of APPT as a screening test combined with a confirmatory test such as a kaolin clotting time (KCT) or a dilute Russell's viper venom time (DRVVT) with a platelet neutralization procedure.[230,231] They also stress the importance of pre-analytical factors in these assays, particularly the avoidance of contaminating phospholipid due to residual platelet material.

Although the system of testing has been adopted by many laboratories, a number of reagent and methodologic variables persists and contributes to inaccuracies in testing. This was demonstrated recently in a UK National External Quality Assessment Scheme, where, although 96% of laboratories demonstrated the presence of a 'strong' LA, >50% failed to recognize a 'weak' LA.[232]

aCL can be detected using either an enzyme-linked immunosorbent assay (ELISA) or a solid-phase radioimmu-noassay.[233] These assays usually determine the presence of both IgG and IgM isotypes. Newer assays aimed at detecting reactivity to β_2-glycoprotein 1 may improve specificity by distinguishing between aCL related to infection and those associated with autoimmune disorders, and are currently being evaluated in this context.[234,235]

Clinical associations

Although there is a considerable body of published data relating to aPL antibodies in adults, there is much less information available in the pediatric age group. aPL antibodies in children often appear transient and in many cases follow a recent viral infection.[236,237] They may be diagnosed on routine coagulation screening and usually resolve within a few weeks. In the vast majority of cases, these transient aPL antibodies appear unassociated with any clinical problems and these children are not usually considered to be at increased risk of thrombosis.

Pediatric SLE is a relatively uncommon disorder accounting for around 10% of cases in most series.[238–240] The association of thromboembolic events with aPL in children with SLE has been documented in a number of case reports and attempts have been made to define the prevalence of aPL antibodies in childhood SLE and their likely clinical significance in this age group.[241–244] Seaman et al[241] studied 29 consecutive patients with SLE diagnosed before 16 years of age and noted aPL (LA, aCL antibodies or false positive VDRL) in 65% of cases. In the group positive for aPL antibodies, 7 patients had a total of 10 thromboembolic events over a period of 4.5 years (deep vein thrombosis 4, stroke 3, pulmonary embolism 1, splenic infarct 1, dural sinus thrombosis 1) as compared with no events in children negative for aPL antibodies. In a similar French collaborative study of 120 children with SLE, 8 children (9%) had a total of 16 thrombotic events (mean follow-up 8.1 years) and 73% had a detectable LA.[244] Thus, aPL antibodies appear to be common in children with SLE and appear to be significantly associated with thromboembolic events.

A number of studies have also examined the prevalence of aPL antibodies in children presenting with thrombosis who do not have SLE. Manco-Johnson et al[245] found aPL antibodies in 19 of 78 (24%) children who presented with thrombosis at a single institution over a 7-year period. Only 5 fulfilled the necessary criteria for a diagnosis of SLE, while the other 14 were classified as having the antiphospholipid syndrome. The association of childhood thrombosis with aPL in the absence of SLE has been recognized in a number of other small case series and, in particular, it has been suggested that there may be a significant association with childhood stroke.[246–250] Children with the antiphospholipid syndrome may also exhibit some of the other clinical features defined in adults with this condition, including chorea, livedo reticularis and thrombocytopenia.[251,252]

With regard to management, standard anticoagulant protocols should be employed in the initial treatment of acute thombotic events in children with aPL antibodies. The subsequent duration and intensity of warfarin therapy and the role, if any, of steroids and immunosuppressive agents in such patients remains uncertain.

Another syndrome which is now fairly well recognized is the association of a lupus anticoagulant with acquired protein S deficiency, resulting in DIC and purpura fulminans following varicella infection.[253–255] Autoantibodies to protein S result in a transient free protein S deficiency, probably as a result of increased clearance of protein S from the circulation. Fragment $1+2$ levels are increased in keeping with DIC. Although most cases involve microvascular thrombosis and purpura fulminans, large vessel thrombosis including DVT and stroke has also been reported. This is a rare condition and the optimal managment strategy is not yet defined. Anticoagulant therapy with heparin has been utilized successfully in some cases but the use of protein S replacement therapy with FFP requires further evaluation to establish a beneficial effect.

Although the vast majority of children with clinically symptomatic aPL have thrombotic events, hemorrhagic problems are occasionally seen in association with the presence of a concomitant autoimmune thrombocytopenia or coagulation factor deficiency. In the latter situation, the so-called hemorrhagic lupus anticoagulant syndrome has most commonly been observed in association with acquired hypoprothrombinemia.[256–262] Typical features of this syndrome include the sudden onset of bleeding symptoms of variable severity in a child with no past history of bleeding problems, who may have had a recent viral infection. Laboratory studies show a prolonged APTT with evidence of a LA and reduced FII levels. The syndrome usually resolves spontaneously within 3 months and does not generally require treatment, although steroids have been given in some cases. In the presence of significant bleeding, the use of PCCs should be considered.

REFERENCES

1. Andrew M, Paes B, Milner R *et al.* Development of the coagulation system in the full term infant. *Blood* 1987; **70**: 165–172
2. Andrew M, Paes B, Milner R *et al.* Development of the human coagulation system in the healthy premature infant. *Blood* 1988; **72**: 1651–1657
3. Nardi M, Karpatkin M. Prothrombin and protein C in early childhood: Normal adult levels are not achieved until the fourth year of life. *J Pediatr* 1986; **109**: 843–845
4. Widdershoven J, Bertina R, Monnens L, van Lier H, de Haan A. Protein C levels in infancy and early childhood: Influence of breast feeding. *Acta Paediatr Scand* 1987; **76**: 7–10
5. Andrew M, Vegh P, Johnston M, Bowker J, Ofosu F, Mitchell L. Maturation of the hematopoietic system during childhood. *Blood* 1988; **80**: 1998–2000
6. van Teunenbroek A, Peters M, Sturk A, Borm JJJ, Beederveld C. Protein C activity and antigen levels in childhood. *Eur J Pediatr* 1990; **149**: 774–778
7. Andrew M, Vegh P, Johnston M, Bowker J, Ofosu F, Mitchell L. Maturation of hemostatic system during childhood. *Blood* 1992; **80**: 1998–2005
8. Andrew M. Developmental hemostasis: Relevance to hemostatic problems during childhood. *Semin Thromb Hemostas* 1995; **21**: 341–356
9. Sanders J, Holtkamp C, Buchanan G. The bleeding time may be longer in children than in adults. *Am J Hematol Oncol* 1990; **12**: 314–318
10. Andrew M, Mitchell L, Vegh P, Ofosu F. Thrombin regulation in children differs from adults in the absence and presence of heparin. *Thomb Haemostas* 1994; **72**: 836–842
11. Mitchell L, Piovella F, Ofosu F, Andrew M. Alpha-2-macroglobulin may provide protection from thomboembolic events in antithrombin III deficient children. *Blood* 1991; **78**: 2299–3304
12. Schmidt B, Mitchell L, Ofosu FA, Andrew M. Alpha-2-macroglobulin is an important progressive inhibitor of thrombin in neonatal and infant plasma. *Thromb Haemostas* 1989; **62**: 1074–1077
13. Ries M, Klinge J, Rauch R. Age related reference values for activation markers of the coagulation and fibrinolytic systems in children. *Thromb Res* 1997; **85**: 341–344
14. Bauer K, Weiss L, Sparrow D, Vokonas P, Rosenberg R. Aging-associated changes in the indices of thrombin generation and protein C activation in humans. *J Clin Invest* 1987; **80**: 1527–1534
15. Andrew M. Developmental hemostasis: Relevance to thromboembolic complications in pediatric patients. *Thromb Haemostas* 1995; **74**: 415–425
16. David M, Andrew M. Venous thromboembolism complications in children: A critical review of the literature. *J Pediatr* 1993; **123**: 337–346
17. Bick RL. Disseminated intravascular coagulation. Objective criteria for diagnosis and management. *Med Clin North Am* 1994; **78**: 511–543
18. Bick RL. Disseminated intravascular coagulation: objective clinical and laboratory diagnois, treatment and assessment of therapeutic response. *Semin Thromb Hemostas* 1996; **22**: 69–88
19. Bick RL. Disseminated intravascular coagulation and related syndromes: a clinical review. *Semin Thromb Hemostas* 1988; **14**: 299–338
20. Tallman MS, Kwaan HD. Reassessing the hemostatic disorder associated with acute promyelocytic leukemia. *Blood* 1992; **79**: 543–553
21. Kasabach HH, Merritt KK. Capillary hemangioma with extensive purpura—report of a case. *Am J Dis Child* 1940; **59**: 1063
22. Hartley RM, Sabio H, Howell CG, Flickinger F, Parrish RA. Successful managment of an infant with a giant hemangioma of the retroperitoneum and Kasabach–Merritt syndrome. *J Pediatr Surg* 1993; **28**: 1356–1357
23. Hoeger PH, Helmke K, Winkler K. Chronic consumption coagulopathy due to an occult splenic haemangioma: Kasabach–Merritt syndrome. *Eur J Pediatr* 1995; **154**: 365–368
24. Fijnvandraat K, Kerkx B, Peters M *et al.* Coagulation activation and tissue necrosis in meningococcal septic shock: severely reduced protein C levels predict a high mortality. *Thromb Haemostas* 1995; **73**: 15–20
25. Leclerc F, Hazelret J, Jude B *et al.* Protein C and S deficiency in severe infectious purpura of children: a collaborative study of 40 cases. *Intensive Care Med* 1992; **18**: 202–205
26. Powars DR, Rogers ZR, Patch MJ, McGhee WG, Francis RB. Purpura fulminans in meningococcemia: association with acquired deficiencies of proteins C and S. *N Engl J Med* 1987; **317**: 571–572
27. Francis RB. Acquired purpura fulminans. *Semin Thromb Hemostas* 1990; **16**: 310–325
28. Inbal A, Kenet G, Zivelin A *et al.* Purpura fulminans induced by disseminated intravascular coagulation following infection in 2 unrelated children with double heterozygosity for factor V Leiden and protein S deficiency. *Thromb Haemostas* 1997; **77**: 1086–1089
29. Chuansumrit A, Hotrakitay S, Hathirat P, Isarangkura P. Disseminated intravascular coagulation in children: diagnosis, management and outcome. *Southeast Asian J Trop Med Pub Health* 1993; **24 (Suppl 1)**: 229–233
30. Francis CW, Marder VJ. A molecular model of plasmin degradation of cross-linked fibrin. *Semin Thromb Hemostas* 1982; **8**: 25–35
31. Bauer KA, Rosenberg RD. Activation markers of coagulation. *Baillière's Clin Haematol* 1994; 7: 523–540
32. Biosclair MD, Ireland H, Lane DA. Assessment of hypercoagulable

states by measurement of activation fragments and peptides. *Blood Rev* 1990; **4**: 25–40

33. Hampton KK, Makris M, Kitchen S, Preston FE. Potential thrombogenicity of heat-treated prothrombin complex concentrates in Haemophilia B. *Blood Coag Fibrinol* 1991; **2**: 637–641

34. Ingram G *et al*. Fatal pulmonary embolus in congenital fibrinopenia. *Acta Haematol* 1966; **35**: 56–62

35. MacKinnon H, Fekete J. Congenital afibrinogenaemia: Vascular changes and multiple thromboses induced infusions and contraceptive medication. *CMAJ* 1971; **4**: 597–599

36. Du Toit HK, Coetzee AR, Chalton DO. Heparin treatment in thrombin induced disseminated intravascular coagulation in the baboon. *Crit Care Med* 1991; **19**: 1195–1200

37. Hauptmann JG, Hassouna HI, Bell TG, Penner JA, Emerson TE. Efficacy of antithrombin III in endotoxin-induced disseminated intravascular coagulation. *Circ Shock* 1988; **25**: 111–122

38. Fourrier F, Chopin C, Huart J, Runge I, Caron C, Goudemand J. Double blind, placebo controlled trial of antithrombin III concentrates in septic shock with disseminated intravascular coagulation. *Chest* 1993; **104**: 882–888

39. Fourrier F, Jourdain M, Tournois A, Caron C, Goudemand J, Chopin C. Coagulation inhibitor substitution during sepsis. *Intensive Care Med* 1995; **21**: S264–S268

40. Lo SS, Hitzig WH, Frick PG. Clinical experience with anticoagulant therapy in the management of disseminated intravascular coagulation in children. *Acta Haematol* 1971; **45**: 1–16

41. Fuse S, Tomita H, Yoshida M, Hori T, Igarashi C, Fujita S. High dose of intravenous antithrombin III without heparin in the treatment of disseminated intravascular coagulation and organ failure in four children. *Am J Hematol* 1996; **53**: 18–21

42. Nowak-Gottl U, Groll A, Kreuz WD *et al*. Treatment of disseminated intravascular coagulation with antithrombin III concentrate in children with verified infection. *Klin Pediatr* 1992; **204**: 134–140

43. Hanada T, Abe T, Takita H. Antithrombin III concentrates for treatment of disseminated intravascular coagulation in children. *Am J Pediatr Hematol Oncol* 1985; **7**: 3–8

44. Smith OP, White B, Vaughan D *et al*. Use of protein C concentrate, heparin and haemodiafiltration in meningococcus induced meningococcal disease. *Lancet* 1997; **350**: 1590–1593

45. Rintala E, Seppala O, Kotilainen P, Rasi V. Protein C in the treatment of coagulopathy in meningococcal disease. *Lancet* 1996; **347**: 1767

46. Rivard GE, David M, Farrell C. Treatment of purpura fulminans in meningococcemia with protein C concentrate. *J Pediatr* 1995; **126**: 646–652

47. Fijnvandraat K, Derkx B, Peters M *et al*. Coagulation activation and tissue necrosis in meningococceal septic shock: Severely reduced protein C levels predict a high mortality. *Thomb Haemostas* 1995; **73**: 15–20

48. Aiuto LT, Barone SR, Cohen PS, Boxer RA. Recombinant tissue plasminogen activator restores perfusion in meningococcal purpura fulminans. *Crit Care Med* 1997; **25**: 1079–1082

49. Zenz W, Muntean W, Zobel G, Grubbauer HM, Gallistl S. Treatment of fulminant meningococcemia with recombinant tissue plasminogen activator. *Thromb Haemostas* 1995; **74**: 802–803

50. Brandtzaeg P, Joo GB, Brusletto B, Kierulf P. Plasminogen activator inhibitor 1 and 2, alpha-2-antiplasmin, plasminogen and endotoxin levels in systemic meningococcal disease. *Thromb Res* 1990; **57**: 271–278

51. Pralong G, Calandra T, Glauser MP *et al*. Plasminogen activator inhibitor 1: a new prognostic marker in septic shock. *Thromb Haemostas* 1989; **61**: 459–462

52. Saito M, Asakura H, Jokahi H *et al*. Recombinant hirudin for the treatment of disseminated intravascular coagulation in patients with haematological malignancy. *Blood Coag Fibrinol* 1995; **6**: 60–64

53. Tazawa S, Ichikawa K, Misawa K *et al*. Effects of low molecular weight heparin on a severely antithrombin III-decreased disseminated

54. Dam H. Cholesterinstoffwëchsel in Hühnereiern und Hühnchen. *Biochem Z* 1929; **215**: 475–492

55. Jackson CM, Nemerson Y. Blood coagulation. *Ann Rev Biochem* 1980; **49**: 765–811

56. Vermeer C. Comparison between hepatic and nonhepatic vitamin K-dependent carboxylase. *Haemostasis* 1986; **16**: 239–245

57. Shearer M. Vitamin K and vitamin K dependent proteins. *Br J Haematol* 1990; **75**: 156–162

58. Shearer MJ. Vitmain K. *Lancet* 1995; **345**: 229–234

59. Pauli M, Lian JB, Mosher DF, Suttie JW. Association of congenital deficiency of multiple vitamin K-dependent coagulation factors and the phenotype of the warfarin embryopathy: clues to the mechanism of teratogenicity of coumarin derivatives. *Am J Hum Genet* 1987; **41**: 566–583

60. Shearer MJ, McCarthy PT, Crampton OE, Mattock MB. The assessment of human vitamin K status from tissue measurements. In: Suttie JW (ed) *Current Advances in Vitamin K Research*. New York: Elsevier, 1988, pp 437–452

61. Uchida K, Komeno T. Relationships between dietary and intestinal vitamin K, clotting factor levels, plasma vitamin K and urinary Gla. In: Suttie JW (ed) *Current Advances in Vitamin K Research*. New York: Elsevier, 1988, pp 477–492

62. McCarthy PT, Shearer MJ, Gau G, Crampton OE, Barkhan P. Vitamin K content of human liver at different ages. *Haemostasis* 1986; **16 (Suppl 5)**: 84–85 (abstract)

63. Thorp JA, Gaston L, Caspers D, Pal ML. Current concepts and controversies in the use of vitamin K. *Drugs* 1995; **49**: 376–387

64. Gardill SL, Suttie JW. Vitamin K epoxide and quinone reductase activities. *Biochem Pharmacol* 1990; **40**: 1055–1061

65. Suttie JW. Vitamin K and human nutrition. *J Am Diet Assoc* 1992; **92**: 585–590

66. Bell RG. Metabolism of vitamin K and prothrombin synthesis: anticoagulants and the vitamin K-epoxide cycle. *Fed Proc* 1978; **37**: 2599–2604

67. Wallin R. Vitamin K antagonism of coumarin anticoagulation: a dehydrogenase pathway in rat liver is responsible for the antagonistic effect. *Biochem J* 1986; **236**: 685–693

68. Wallin R, Patrick SD, Ballard JO. Vitamin K antagonism of coumarin intoxication in the rat. *Thromb Haemostas* 1986; **55**: 235–239

69. Wallin R, Martin LF. Vitamin K-dependent carboxylation and vitamin K metabolism in liver: effects of warfarin. *J Clin Invest* 1985; **76**: 1879–1884

70. Lipsky JJ. Review: antibiotic-associated hypoprothrombinaemia. *J Antimicrob Chemother* 1988; **21**: 281–300

71. Shearer MJ, Bechtold H, Andrassy K *et al*. Mechanism of cephalosporin induced hypoprothrombinemia: relation to cephalosporin side chain, vitamin K metabolism and vitamin K status. *J Clin Pharmacol* 1988; **28**: 88–95

72. Cohen H, Scott SD, Mackie IJ *et al*. The development of hypoprothrombinaemia following antibiotic therapy in malnourished patients with low serum vitamin K levels. *Br J Haematol* 1988; **68**: 63–66

73. Isselbacher KJ, Braumwald E, Petersdorf AG *et al*. *Harrison's Principles of Internal Medicine*, 13th edn. New York: McGraw-Hill, 1994, 1806–1807

74. Motohara K, Kuroki Y, Kan H, Endo F, Matsuda I. Detection of vitamin K deficiency by use of an enzyme-linked immunosorbent assay for circulating abnormal prothrombin. *Pediatr Res* 1985; **19**: 354–357

75. Blanchard RA, Furie BC, Kruger SF, Waneck G, Jorgensen MJ, Furie B. Immunoassays of human prothrombin species which correlate with functional coagulant activities. *J Lab Clin Med* 1983; **101**: 242–255

76. Widdershoven J, van Munster P, De Abreu R *et al*. Four methods compared for measuring des-carboxy-prothrombin (PIVKA II). *Clin Chem* 1987; **33**: 2074–2079

77. Corrigan JJ, Earnst D. Factor II antigen in liver disease and warfarin

induced vitamin K deficiency: correlation with coagulation activity using Echis venom. *Am J Hematol* 1980; **8**: 249

78. Solano C, Cobcroft RG, Scott DC. Prediction of vitamin K response using the Echis time and the Echis prothrombin time ratios. *Thromb Haemostas* 1990; **64**: 353–357

79. De Leenheer AP, Nelis HJ, Lambert WE, Bauwens RM. Chromatography of fat-soluble vitamins in clinical chemistry. *J Chromatogr* 1988; **429**: 3–58

80. Sadowski A, Bacon DS, Hood S et al. The application of methods used for the evaluation of vitamin K nutritional status in human and animal studies. In: Suttie JW (ed) *Current Advances in Vitamin K Research*. New York: Elsevier, 1988, pp 453–463

81. Sutor AH. Vitamin K deficiency bleeding in infants and children. *Semin Thromb Hemostas* 1995; **21**: 317–329

82. Sutor AH, Kunzer W. Time interval between vitamin K administration and effective haemostasis. In: Suzuki S, Hathaway WE, Bonnar J, Sutor AH (eds) *Perinatal Thrombosis and Haemostasis*. Berlin: Springer, 1991, pp 257–262

83. Department of Health. *Report on Health and Social Subjects No 41: Dietary Reference Values for Food Energy and Nutrients for the United Kingdom*. London: HMSO, 1991

84. Durie PR. Vitamin K and the management of patients with cystic fibrosis. *Can Med Assoc J* 1994; **151**: 933–936

85. Ramsey BW, Farrell PM, Pencharz P and the Consensus Committee. Nutritional support and the management in cystic fibrosis. *Am J Clin Nutr* 1992; **55**: 108–116

86. Mammen EF. Coagulation defects in liver disease. *Med Clin North Am* 1994; **78**: 545–554

87. Joist JH. Haemostatic abnormalities in liver disease. In: Coleman RW, Hirsh J (eds) *Hemostasis and Thrombosis*. Philadelphia: JB Lippincott, 1982, pp 861–872

88. Blanchard BA, Furie BC, Jorgensen M et al. Acquired vitamin K dependent carboxylation deficiency in liver disease. *N Engl J Med* 1981; **305**: 242–248

89. Soria J, Soria C, Ryckewaert JJ, Samama M, Thomson JM, Poller L. Study of acquired dysfibrinogenaemia in liver disease. *Thromb Res* 1980; **19**: 29–41

90. Green G, Thomson JM, Dymock JW, Poller L. Abnormal fibrinogen polymerization in liver disease. *Br J Haematol* 1976; **34**: 425–439

91. Permambuco JRB, Langley PG, Hughes RD, Izumi S, Williams R. Activation of the fibrinolytic system in patients with fulminant liver failure. *Hepatology* 1993; **18**: 1350–1356

92. Jaschoneck K, Faul C. Platelets from patients with liver cirrhosis exhibit a defect in von Willebrand factor binding domain. *Gastroenterology* 1993; **31**: 8–10

93. Porte RJ. Coagulation and fibrinolysis in orthoptic liver transplantation. *Semin Thromb Hemostas* 1993; **19**: 191–196

94. Dzik WH, Arkus CF, Jenkins RL, Stump DC. Fibrinolysis during liver transplantation in humans: role of t-PA. *Blood* 1988; **71**: 1090–1095

95. Bechstein WO, Riess H, Blumhardt G et al. Aprotinin in orthotopic liver transplantation. *Semin Thromb Hemostas* 1993; **19**: 262–267

96. Kang Y. Clinical use of synthetic antifibrinolytic agents during liver transplantation. *Semin Thromb Hemostas* 1993; **19**: 258–261

97. Cienfuegos JA, Dominiquez RM, Tanelchoff PJ et al. Surgical complications in the post operative period of liver transplantation in children. *Transplant Proc* 1994; **16**: 1230–1235

98. Krom RAF, Wiesner RH, Rettke SR et al. The first hundred liver transplants at the Mayo Clinic. *Mayo Clin Proc* 1989; **64**: 89–94

99. Harper PL, Edgar PF, Luddington RJ et al. Protein C deficiency and portal thrombosis in liver transplantation in children. *Lancet* 1988; **ii**: 924–927

100. Stahl RL, Duncan A, Hooks MA, Henderson MJ, Millikan WJ, Warren WD. A hypercoagulable state follows orthotopic liver transplantation. *Hepatology* 1990; **12**: 553–558

101. Bearman SI. The syndrome of hepatic veno-occlusive disease after marrow transplantation. *Blood* 1995; **85**: 3005–3020

102. McDonald GB, Hinds MS, Fisher LD et al. Veno-occlusive disease of the liver and multi-organ failure after bone marrow transplantation: a cohort study of 355 patients. *Ann Intern Med* 1993; **118**: 255–267

103. Shulman HM, Hinterberger W. Hepatic veno-occlusive disease liver toxicity syndrome after bone marrow transplantation. *Bone Marrow Transplant* 1992; **10**: 197–214

104. Bearman SI, Appelbaum FR, Buckner CD et al. Regimen-related toxicity in patients undergoing bone marrow transplantation. *J Clin Oncol* 1988; **6**: 1562–1568

105. Bisogno G, de Kraker J, Weirich A et al. Veno-occlusive disease of the liver in children treated for Wilms' tumor. *Med Pediatr Oncol* 1997; **29**: 245–251

106. Ortega JA, Donaldson SS, Ivy SP, Pappo A, Maurer HM. Veno-occlusive disease of the liver after chemotherapy with vincristine, actinomycin D, and cyclophosphamide for the treatment of rhabdomyosarcoma. A report of the Intergroup Rhabdomyosarcoma Study Group. *Cancer* 1997; **79**: 2435–2439

107. Schiavetti A, Matrunola M, Varrasso G, Pasula A, Castello MA. Ultrasound in the management of hepatic veno-occlusive disease in three children treated with dactinomycin and vincristine. *Pediatr Hematol Oncol* 1996; **13**: 521–529

108. Kullendorf CM, Bekassy AN. Hepatic veno-occlusive disease in Wilms' tumor. *Eur J Pediatr Surg* 1996; **6**: 338–340

109. Kanwar VS, Alburquerque ML, Ribeiro RC, Kauffman WM, Furman WL. Veno-occlusive disease of the liver after chemotherapy for rhabdomyosarcoma: case report with a review of the literature. *Med Pediatr Oncol* 1995; **24**: 334–340

110. Sperl W, Stuppner H, Gassner I, Judmaier W, Dietze O, Vogel W. Reversible hepatic veno-occlusive disease in an infant after consumption of pyrrolizidine-containing herbal tea. *Eur J Pediatr* 1995; **154**: 112–116

111. Meresse V, Hartmann O, Vassal G et al. Risk factors for hepatic veno-occlusive disease after high dose busulfan containing regimens followed by autologous bone marrow transplantation: a study in 136 children. *Bone Marrow Transplant* 1992; **10**: 135–141

112. Ozkayank MF, Weinberg K, Kohn D, Sender L, Parckman R, Lenarsky C. Hepatic veno-occlusive disease post bone marrow transplantation in children conditioned with busulfan and cyclophosphamide: incidence, risk factors and clinical outcome. *Bone Marrow Transplant* 1996; **17**: 75–80

113. Rozman C, Carreras E, Qian C et al. Risk factors for hepatic veno-occlusive disease following HLA-identical sibling bone marrow transplants for leukemia. *Bone Marrow Transplant* 1996; **17**: 75–80

114. Vassal G, Koscielny S, Challine D et al. Busulfan disposition and hepatic veno-occlusive disease in children undergoing bone marrow transplantation. *Cancer Chemother Pharmacol* 1996; **37**: 247–253

115. Jones RJ, Lee KSK, Beschorner WE et al. Venoocclusive disease of the liver following bone marrow transplantation. *Transplantation* 1987; **44**: 778–783

116. Shulman HM, McDonald GB, Matthews D et al. An analysis of the hepatic venoocclusive disease and centrilobular hepatic degeneration following bone marrow transplantation. *Gastroenterology* 1980; **79**: 1178–1191

117. Gugliotta L, Catani L, Vianelli N et al. High plasma levels of tumor necrosis factor may be predictive of venoocclusive disease in bone marrow transplantation. *Blood* 1994; **83**: 2385–2386

118. Holler E, Korb HJ, Moller A et al. Increased serum levels of tumor necrosis factor precede major complications of bone marrow transplantation. *Blood* 1990; **75**: 1011–1016

119. Park YD, Yasui M, Yoshimoto T et al. Changes in hemostatic parameters in hepatic veno-occlusive disease following bone marrow transplantation. *Bone Marrow Transplant* 1997; **19**: 915–920

120. Nurnberger W, Kruck H, Mauz-Korholz C, Burdach S, Gobel U. Humoral coagulation and early complications after allogeneic bone marrow transplantation. *Klin Padiatr* 1997; **209**: 209–215

121. Richard S, Siegneur M, Blann A et al. Vascular endothelial lesion in patients undergoing bone marrow transplantation. *Bone Marrow Transplant* 1996; **18**: 955–959

122. Rosenthal J, Sender L, Secola R *et al.* Phase II trial of heparin prophylaxis for veno-occlusive disease of the liver in children undergoing bone marrow transplantation. *Bone Marrow Transplant* 1996; **18**: 185–191

123. Miniero R, Vassallo E, Soldano S *et al.* Management of hepatic veno-occlusive disease (VOD) in pediatric patients: retrospective analysis in 6 AIEOP–BMT (Italian Pediatric Hematology Oncology Association–Bone Marrow Transplantation Group) Centers. *Bone Marrow Transplant* 1996; **18 (Suppl 2)**: 157–159

124. Feldman L, Gabai E, Milovic V, Jaimovich G. Recombinant tissue plasminogen activator (rTPA) for hepatic veno-occlusive disease after allogeneic BMT in a pediatric patient. *Bone Marrow Transplant* 1995; **16**: 727

125. Higashigawa M, Watanabe M, Nishihara H *et al.* Successful treatment of an infant with veno-occlusive disease developed after allogeneic bone marrow transplantation by tissue plasminogen activator, hepain and prostaglandin E1. *Leukemia Res* 1995; **19**: 477–480

126. Patton DF, Harper JL, Wooldridge TN, Gordon BG, Coccia P, Haire WD. Treatment of veno-occlusive disease of the liver with bolus tissue plasminogen activator and continuous infusion antithrombin III concentrate. *Bone Marrow Transplant* 1996; **17**: 443–447

127. Leahey AM, Bunin NJ. Recombinant human tissue plasminogen activator for the treatment of severe hepatic veno-occlusive disease in pediatric bone marrow transplant patients. *Bone Marrow Transplant* 1996; **17**: 1101–1104

128. Bearman SI, Lee JL, Baron AE, McDonald GB. Treatment of hepatic venoocclusive disease with recombinant human tissue plasminogen activator and heparin in 42 marrow transplant patients. *Blood* 1997; **89**: 1501–1506

129. Eberst ME, Berkowitz LR. Hemostasis in renal disease: pathophysiology and management. *Am J Med* 1994; **96**: 168–179

130. Remuzzi G. Bleeding disorders in uremia: pathophysiology and treatment. *Adv Nephrol* 1989; **18**: 171–186

131. Gralnick HR, McKeown LP, Williams SB, Shafer BC, Pierce L. Plasma and platelet von Willebrand factor defects in uremia. *Am J Med* 1988; **85**: 806–810

132. Vigano GL, Mannucci PM, Lattuada A, Harris A, Remuzzi G. Subcutaneous desmopressin (DDAVP) shortens the bleeding time in uremia. *Am J Hematol* 1989; **31**: 32–35

133. Jansen PA, Jubelirer SJ, Weinstein MJ, Deykin D. Treatment of the bleeding tendency in uremia with cryoprecipitate. *N Engl J Med* 1988; **85**: 806–810

134. Remuzzi G, Perico N, Zoja C, Corna D, Macconi D, Vigano G. Role of endothelium-derived nitric oxide in the bleeding tendency of uremia. *J Clin Invest* 1990; **86**: 1768–1771

135. Livio M, Marchesi D, Remuzzi G, Gotti E, Mecca G, de Gaetano G. Uraemia bleeding: role of anaemia and beneficial effect of red cell transfusions. *Lancet* 1982; **ii**: 1013–1015

136. Vigano G, Benigni A, Mendogni D, Mingardi G, Mecca G, Remuzzi G. Recombinant human erythropoietin to correct uremic bleeding. *Am Kidney Dis* 1991; **18**: 44–49

137. Pickering LK, Obrig TG, Stapleton FB. Hemolytic-uremic syndrome and enterohemorrhagic *Escherichi coli*. *J Pediatr Infect Dis* 1994; **13**: 459–476

138. Siegler RL. The hemolytic uremic syndrome. *Pediatr Clin North Am* 1995; **42**: 1505–1529

139. Kaplan BS, Cleary TG, Obrig TG. Recent advances in understanding the pathogenesis of the hemolytic uremic syndrome. *Pediatr Nephrol* 1990; **4**: 279–285

140. Siegler RL. Prostacyclin in the hemolytic uremic syndrome. *J Nephrol* 1993; **6**: 64–69

141. van der Kar NCAJ, van Hinsbergh VWM, Brommer EJP, Monnens LAH. The fibrinolytic system in the hemolytic uremic syndrome: *in vivo* and *in vitro* studies. *Pediatr Res* 1994; **36**: 257–264

142. Gianviti A, Perna A, Caringella A *et al.* Plasma exchange in children with hemolytic uremic syndrome at risk of poor outcome. *Am J Kidney* 1993; **22**: 264–266

143. Andrew M, Brooker LA. Hemostatic complications in renal disorders of the young. *Pediatr Nephrol* 1996; **10**: 88–99

144. Andre E, Voisin PH, Andrew JL *et al.* Hemorheological and hemostatic parameters in children with nephrotic syndrome undergoing steroid therapy. *Nephron* 1994; **68**: 184–191

145. Machleidt C, Mettang T, Starz E, Wever J, Risler T, Kuhlman U. Multifactorial genesis of the enhanced platelet aggregability in patients with nephrotic syndrome. *Kidney Int* 1989; **36**: 1119–1124

146. Walter E, Deppermann D, Andrassy K, Koderrisch J. Platelet hyperaggregability as a consequence of the nephrotic syndrome. *Thromb Res* 1981; **23**: 473–481

147. Du XH, Glass-Greenwalt P, Kani KS. Nephrotic syndrome with renal vein thrombosis: pathogenic importance of alpha-2-antiplasmin inhibitor. *Clin Nephrol* 1985; **24**: 196–191

148. Jootar S, Archararit N, Suvachittanont O. Hemostatic defect in cyanotic and acyanotic congenital heart disease. *J Med Associ Thai* 1988; **71**: 382–387

149. Suarez CR, Menendez CE, Griffin AJ, Ow EP, Walenga M, Fareed J. Cyanotic congenital heart disesae in children: hemostatic disorders and relevance of molecular markers of hemostasis. *Semin Thromb Hemostas* 1984; **10**: 285–289

150. Henriksson P, Varendh G, Lundstrom NR. Haemostatic defects in cyanotic congenital heart disesae. *Br Heart J* 1979; **41**: 23–27

151. Goldschmidt B. Blood coagulation and platelet abnormalities in cyanotic congenital heart disease. *Lancet* 1973; **i**: 607

152. Ihenacho HNC, Breeze GR, Fletcher DJ, Stuart J. Consumption coagulopathy in congenital heart disease. *Lancet* 1973; **i**: 231–234

153. Wedemeyer AL, Edson JR, Krivit W. Coagulation in cyanotic congenital heart disease. *Am J Dis Child* 1972; **124**: 656–660

154. Iolster NJ. Blood coagulation in children with cyanotic congenital heart disease. *Acta Paediatr Scand* 1970; **59**: 551–557

155. Naiman JL. Clotting and bleeding in cyanotic congenital heart disease. *Pediatrics* 1970; **76**: 333–335

156. Ekert H, Gilchrist GS, Stanton R, Hammond D. Hemostasis in cyanotic congenital heart disease. *J Pediatr* 1970; **76**: 221–230

157. Komp DM, Sparrow AW. Polycythemia in cyanotic heart disease—a study of altered coagulation. *J Pediatr* 1970; **76**: 231–236

158. Johnson CA, Abildgaard CF, Schulman I. Absence of coagulation abnormalities in children with cyanotic heart disease. *Lancet* 1968; **ii**: 660–662

159. Chan AKC, Leaker M, Burrows FA *et al.* Coagulation and fibrinolytic profile of paediatric patients undergoing cardiopulmonary bypass. *Thomb Haemostas* 1997; **77**: 270–277

160. Boisclair MD, Lane DA, Philippou H *et al.* Mechanisms of thrombin generation during surgery and cardiopulmonary bypass. *Blood* 1993; **82**: 3350–3357

161. Turner-Gomes S, Lui LB, Saysana N, Dewar L, Williams WG, Ofosu F. Increased thrombin generation in cyanotic congenital heart disease. *Thromb Haemostas* 1997; **78**: P2481

162. Rinder CS, Gaal D, Student LA, Smith BR. Platelet-leukocyte activation and modulation of adhesion receptors in pediatric patients with congenital heart disease undergoing cardiopulmonary bypass. *J Thorac Cardiovasc Surg* 1994; **107**: 280–288

163. Maurer HM, McCue CM, Robertson LW, Haggins JC. Correction of platelet dysfunction and bleeding in cyanotic congenital heart disease by simple red cell volume reduction. *Am J Cardiol* 1975; **35**: 831–835

164. Gill JC, Wilson AD, Endres-Brooks J, Montgomery RR. Loss of the largest von Willebrand factor multimers from the plasma of patients with congenital cardiac defects. *Blood* 1986; **67**: 758–761

165. Sharland M, Patton MA, Talbot S, Chitolie A, Bevan DH. Coagulation factor deficiencies and abnormal bleeding in Noonan's syndrome. *Lancet* 1992; **339**: 19–21

166. Woodman RC, Harker LA. Bleeding associated with cardiopulmonary bypass. *Blood* 1990; **76**: 1680–1697

167. Harker LA. Bleeding after cardiopulmonary bypass. *N Engl J Med* 1986; **314**: 1446–1448

168. Saatvedt K, Lindberg H, Michelen S, Pedersen T, Geiran OR.

Activation of the fibrinolytic, coagulation and plasma kallikrein-kinin systems during and after open heart surgery in children. *Scand J Clin Lab Invest* 1995; **55**: 359–367

169. Harker LA, Malpass TW, Branson HE, Hessel EA, Slitchter SA. Mechanism of abnormal bleeding in patients undergoing cardiopulmonary bypass. Acquired transient platelet dysfunction associated with selective α-granule release. *Blood* 1980; **56**: 824–834

170. Rinder CS, Mathew JP, Rinder HM, Bonan J, Ault KA, Smith BR. Modulation of platelet surface adhesion receptors during cardiopulmonary bypass. *Anesthesiology* 1991; **75**: 563–570

171. George JN, Pickett EB, Saucerman S *et al*. Platelet surface glycoproteins. Studies on resting and activated platelets and platelet membrane microparticle in normal subjects, and observations in patients during adult respiratory distress syndrome and cardiac surgery. *J Clin Invest* 1986; **78**: 340–347

172. Malpass TW, Hanson SR, Savage B, Hessel II EA, Harker LA. Prevention of acquired transient defect in platelet plug formation by infused prostacyclin. *Blood* 1981; **57**: 736–740

173. Kestin AS, Valeri R, Khuri SF *et al*. The platelet function defect in cardiopulmonary bypass. *Blood* 1993; **82**: 107–117

174. Andrew M, MacIntyre B, MacMillan J *et al*. Heparin thearpy during cardiopulmonary bypass in children requires ongoing quality control. *Thromb Haemostas* 1993; **70**: 937–941

175. Hashimoto K, Yamagishi M, Sasaki T, Nakano M, Kurosawa H. Heparin and antithrombin levels during cardiopulmonary bypass: Correlation with subclinical plasma coagulation. *Ann Thorac Surg* 1994; **58**: 799–805

176. Warkentin TE, Kelton JG. A 14 year study of heparin induced thrombocytopenia. *Am J Med* 1996; **101**: 502–507

177. Warkentin TE, Levine MN, Hirsh J *et al*. Heparin-induced thrombocytopenia in patients treated with low-molecular-weight heparin or unfractionated heparin. *N Engl J Med* 1995; **332**: 1330–1335

178. Boshkov LK, Warkentin TE, Hayward CPM, Andrew M, Kelton JG. Heparin induced thrombocytopenia and thombosis: Clinical and laboratory studies. *Br J Haematol* 1993; **84**: 322–328

179. Saxon BR, Leaker M. Heparin induced thrombocytopenia in a young child managed with Orgaran for cardiopulmonary bypass surgery. *Thromb Haemostas* 1997; **78**: P1823

180. Meyer DM, Jessen ME. Results of extracorporeal membrane oxygenation in children with sepsis. The Extracorporeal Life Support Organization. *Ann Thorac Surg* 1997; **63**: 756–761

181. Ichiba S, Bartlett RH. Current status of extracorporeal membrane oxygenation for severe respiratory failure. *Artificial Organs* 1996; **20**: 120–123

182. Tracy TF Jr, DeLosh T, Bartlett RH. Extracorporeal Life Support Organisation 1994. *ASAIO J* 1994; **40**: 1017–1019

183. Graziani LJ, Gringlas M, Baumgart S. Cerebrovascular complications and neurodevelopmental sequelae of neonatal ECMO. *Clin Perinatol* 1997; **24**: 655–675

184. McManus ML, Kevy SV, Bower LK, Hickey PR. Coagulation factor deficiencies during initiation of extracorporeal membrane oxygenation. *Pediatrics* 1995; **126**: 900–904

185. Urlesberer B, Zobel G, Zenz W *et al*. Activation of the clotting system during extracorporeal membrane oxygenation in term infants. *J Pediatr* 1996; **129**: 264–268

186. Green TP, Isham-Schopf B, Steinhorn RH, Smith C, Irmiter RJ. Whole blood activated clotting time in infants during extracorporeal membrane oxygenation. *Crit Care Med* 1990; **18**: 494–498

187. Berrrebi A, Malnick SDH, Vorst EJ, Stein D. High incidence of factor XI deficiency in Gaucher's disease. *Am J Hematol* 1992; **40**: 153–161

188. Humphries JE, Hess CE. Gaucher's disease and acquired coagulopathy. *Am J Hematol* 1994; **45**: 347–353

189. Kelsey H, Christopoulos C, Gray AA, Machin SI. Acquired pseudopseudo Bernard Soulier syndrome complicating Gaucher's disease. *J Clin Pathol* 1994; **47**: 162–165

190. Hollak CEM, Levi M, Berends F, Aerts JMFG, van Oers MHJ. Coagulation abnormalities in type I Gaucher disease are due to low grade activation and can be partially restored by enzyme supplementation therapy. *Br J Haematol* 1997; **96**: 470–476

191. Billet HH, Rizvi S, Sawitsky A. Coagulation abnormalities in patients with Gaucher's disease: Effect of therapy. *Am J Hematol* 1996; **51**: 234–236

192. Boklan BF, Sawitsky A. Factor IX deficiency in Gaucher disease. An *in vitro* phenomenon. *Arch Int Med* 1976; **136**: 489–492

193. Seligsohn U, Zitman D, Many A, Klibansky C. Co-existence of factor XI (plasma thromboplastin antecedent) deficiency and Gaucher's disease. *Isr J Med Sci* 1976; **12**: 1448–1452

194. Stein J, Ratnoff O. An inhibitor of antihemophilic factor (factor VIII) in an eighteen month old nonhemophilic child. *Am J Pediatr Hematol Oncol* 1993; **15**: 346–350

195. Keshara Prasad HS, Bradshaw AE. Circulating inhibitor associated with viral infection. *Acta Haematol* 1990; **84**: 193–194

196. Labbe A, Travade P. Spontaneous disappearance of acquired antifactor III inhibitor after four years in a non-haemophiliac child. *Acta Paediatr Scand* 1985; **74**: 794

197. Labbe A, Dubray C, Bezou MJ, Travade P, Coulet M. Spontaneously acquired factor VIII inhibitor in a non-haemophiliac child. *Acta Paediatr Scand* 1983; **72**: 621–623

198. Nakashima K, Miyahara T, Fujii S, Kaku K, Matsumoto N, Kaneko T. Spontaneously acquired factor VIII inhibitor in a 7-year-old girl. *Acta Haematol* 1982; **68**: 58–62

199. Brodeur GM, O'Neill PJ, Williams JA. Acquired inhibitors of coagulation in non-haemophiliac children. *J Pediatr* 1980; **96**: 439–441

200. Miller K, Neely JE, Krivit W, Edson JR. Spontaneously acquired factor IX inhibitor in a nonhemophiliac child. *J Pediatr* 1978; **93**: 232–234

201. Shapiro SS, Jultin M. Acquired inhibitors to blood coagulation factors. *Semin Thromb Hemostas* 1975; **1**: 336–385

202. Lusher JM, Shapiro SS, Palascak JE, Rao AV, Blatt PM and the Haemophilia Study Group. Efficacy of prothrombin complex concentrates in haemophiliacs with inherited and acquired bleeding disorders. *N Eng J Med* 1980; **303**: 421–425

203. Hedner U, Glazer S, Falch J. Recombinant activated factor VII in the treatment of bleeding episodes in patients with inherited and acquired bleeding disorders. *Transfusion Med Rev* 1993; **7**: 78–83

204. Hay CRM, Lozier JN, Santagostino E *et al*. Porcine factor VIII therapy in patients with congenital hemophilia and inhibitors: efficacy, patient selection and side effects. *Semin Hematol* 1994; **31**: 20–25

205. Igarashi N, Miura M, Kato E *et al*. Acquired von Willebrand's syndrome with lupus-like serology. *Am J Pediatr Hematol Oncol* 1989; **11**: 32–35

206. Han P, Lou L, Wong HB. Wilms' tumour with acquired von Willebrand's disease. *Aust Paediatr J* 1987; **23**: 253–255

207. Bracey AW, Wu AHB, Aceves J *et al*. Platelet dysfunction associated with Wilms' tumor and hyaluronic acid. *Am J Hematol* 1987; **24**: 247–257

208. Scott JP, Montomery RR, Turbergen DG *et al*. Acquired von Willebrand's disease in association with Wilms' tumour: Regression following treatment. *Blood* 1981; **58**: 665–669

209. Noronha PA, Hruby MA, Maurer HS. Acquired von Willebrand disease in a patient with Wilms' tumor. *J Pediatr* 1979; **95**: 997–999

210. Coppes MJ, Zandvoort SWH, Sparling CR, Poon AO, Weitzman S, Blanchette VS. Acquired von Willebrand disease in Wilms' tumor patients. *J Clin Oncol* 1992; **10**: 422–427

211. Muntean W, Zenz W, Edlinger G, Beitzke A. Severe bleeding due to factor V inhibitor after repeated operations using fibrin sealant containing bovine thrombin. *Thromb Haemostas* 1997; **77**: 1223

212. Carroll JF, Moskowitz KA, Edwards NM, Hickey TJ, Rose EA, Budzynski AZ. Immunologic assessment of patients treated with bovine fibrin as a hemostatic agent. *Thromb Haemostas* 1996; **76**: 925–931

213. Israels SJ, Israels ED. Development of antibodies to bovine and human factor V in two children after exposure to topical bovine thrombin. *Am J Pediatr Hematol Oncol* 1994; **16**: 249–254

214. Muntean W, Zenz W, Finding W, Zobel G, Beitzke A. Inhibitor to factor V after exposure to fibrin sealant during cardiac surgery in a two-year-old child. *Acta Paediatr* 1994; **83**: 84–87

215. Gordon B, Haire W, Duggan M, Langnas A, Shaw B. Factor V inhibitor developing after liver transplantation in a 3-year-old child. *Pediatrics* 1991; **88**: 156–159

216. Feinstein DI. Acquired inhibitors of factor V. *Thromb Haemostas* 1978; **39**: 663–674

217. Matsunaga AT, Shafer FE. An acquired inhibitor to factor X in a pediatric patient with extensive burns. *J Pediatr Hematol Oncol* 1996; **18**: 223–226

218. Johnson CA, Schroer RJ, Moore A. Acquired inhibitor to contact activation in an 18-month-old female. *Am J Pediatr Hematol Oncol* 1985; **7**: 191–193

219. Reece E, Clyne L. Spontaneous factor XI inhibitors: seven additional cases and a review of the literature. *Arch Intern Med* 1984; **144**: 525–529

220. Moore JE, Mohr CF. Biologically false positive serologic tests for syphilis. *JAMA* 1952; **150**: 467–473

221. Conley CL, Hartmann RC. Haemorrhagic disorder caused by circulating anticoagulant in patients with disseminated lupus erythematosus. *J Clin Invest* 1952; **31**: 621–622

222. Bowie EJW, Thompson JH, Pascuzzi CA, Owen CA. Thrombosis in systemic erythematosus despite circulating anticoagulant. *J Lab Clin Med* 1963; **62**: 416–430

223. Harris EN, Gharavi AE, Boey ML *et al.* Anticardiolipin antibodies: detection of radioimmunoassay and association with thrombosis in systemic lupus erythematosus. *Lancet* 1983; **ii**: 1211–1214

224. Hughes GRV, Harris EN, Gharavi AE. The anticardiolipin syndrome. *J Rheumatol* 1986; **113**: 486–489

225. Rao LVM. Mechanism of activity of lupus anticoagulants. *Curr Opin Hematol* 1997; **4**: 344–350

226. Triplett DA. Protean clinical presentation of antiphospholipid-protein antibodies (APA). *Thromb Haemostas* 1995; **74**: 329–337

227. Bevers EM, Galli M, Barbui T, Comfurius P, Zwaal RFA. Lupus anticoagulation IgGs (LA) are not directed to phospholipids only, but to a complex of lipid-bound human prothrombin. *Thromb Haemostas* 1991; **66**: 629–632

228. McNeil H, Simpson R *et al.* Antiphospholipid antibodies are directed against a complex antigen that includes a lipid-binding inhibitor of coagulation: 22 glycoprotein I (Apolipoprotein H). *Proc Natl Acad Sci USA* 1990; **87**: 4120–4124

229. Bevers EM, Galli M. Beta 2-glycoprotein I for binding of anti-cardiolipin antibodies to cardiolipin. *Lancet* 1990; **336**: 952–953

230. Exner T, Triplett D *et al.* Guidelines for testing and revised criteria for lupus anticoagulants: SSC Subcommittee for the Standardization of Lupus Anticoagulants. *Thromb Haemostas* 1991; **65**: 320–322

231. Machin SJ, Giddings J, Greaves M *et al.* Guidelines on testing for the lupus anticoagulant. *J Clin Pathol* 1991; **44**: 885–889

232. Jennings I, Kitchen S, Woods TAL, Preston FE, Greaves M. Potentially clinically important inaccuracies in testing for the lupus anti-coagulant: an analysis of results from three surveys of the UK National External Quality Assessment Scheme (NEQAS) for blood coagulation. *Thromb Haemostas* 1997; **77**: 934–937

233. Loizou S, McCrea JD, Rudge AC, Reynolds R, Boyle CC, Harris EN. Measurement of anticardiolipin antibodies by an enzyme linked immunosorbent assay (ELISA): Standardization and quantification of results. *Clin Exp Immunol* 1985; **62**: 738–745

234. Forastiero RR, Martinuzzo ME, Kordich LC, Carreras LO. Reactivity to B₂ glycoprotein I clearly differentiates anticardiolipin antibodies from antiphospholipid syndrome and syphilis. *Thromb Haemostas* 1996; **75**: 717–720

235. Martinuzzo ME, Forastiero RR, Carreras LO. Anti B2 glycoprotein I antibodies: detection and association with thrombosis. *Br J Haematol* 1995; **89**: 691–695

236. Burk CD, Miller L, Handler S, Cohen A. Preoperative history and coagulation screening in children undergoing tonsillectomy. *Pediatrics* 1992; **89**: 691–695

237. Singh AK, Rao KP, Kizer J, Lazarchick J. Lupus anticoagulants in children. *Ann Clin Lab Sci* 1988; **18**: 384–387

238. Klippel JH. Systemic lupus erythematosus: demographics, prognosis, and outcome. *J Rheumatol* 1997; **48**: 67–71

239. Kaufman DB, Laxer RM, Silverman ED, Stein L. Systemic lupus erythematosus in childhood and adolescence—the problem, epidemiology, incidence, susceptibility, genetics and prognosis. *Curr Prob Pediatr* 1986; **16**: 545–625

240. Caeiro F, Michielson FM, Berstein R, Hughes GR, Ansell BM. Systemic lupus erythematosus in childhood. *Ann Rheum Dis* 1981; **40**: 325–331

241. Seaman De, Londino AV, Kwoh CK, Medsger TA, Manzi S. Antiphospholipid antibodies in pediatric systemic lupus erythematosus. *Pediatrics* 1995; **96**: 1040–1045

242. Gattorno M, Buoncompagni A, Molinari AC *et al.* Antiphospholipid antibodies in paediatric systemic lupus erythematosus, juvenile chronic arthritis and overlap syndromes: SLE patients with both lupus anticoagulant and high-titre anticardiolipin antibodies are at risk for clinical manifestations related to the antiphospholipid syndrome. *Br J Rheumatol* 1995; **34**: 873–881

243. Berube C, David M *et al.* The relationship of antiphospholipid antibodies to thromboembolic disease in systemic lupus erythematosus in children: a cross sectional study. *Lupus* 1994; **3**: 360A

244. Montes de Oca MA, Barbron MC, Bletry O *et al.* Thrombosis in systemic erythematosus: a French collaborative study. *Arch Dis Child* 1991; **66**: 713–717

245. Manco-Johnson MJ, Nuss R. Lupus anticoagulant in children with thrombosis. *Am J Hematol* 1995; **48**: 240–243

246. Nuss R, Hays T, Manco-Johnson M. Childhood thrombosis. *Pediatrics* 1995; **96**: 291–294

247. Takanashi J, Sugita K, Miyazato S, Sakao E, Miyamoto H, Niimi H. Antiphospholipid antibody syndrome in childhood strokes. *Pediatr Neurol* 1995; **13**: 323–326

248. Ravelli A, Martini A, Burgio RG, Falcini F, Taccetti G. Antiphospholipid antibody syndrome as a cause of venous thrombosis in childhood. *J Pediatr* 1994; **124**: 831–832

249. Angelini L, Ravelli A, Caporali R, Martini A. Antiphospholipid antibodies in children with idiopathic cerebral ischaemia. *Lancet* 1994; **344**: 1232

250. Olson JC, Konkol RJ, Gill JC, Dobyns WB, Coull BM. Childhood stroke and lupus anticoagulant. *Pediatr Neurol* 1994; **10**: 54–57

251. von Scheven E, Athreya BH, Rose CD, Goldsmith DP, Morton L. Clinical characteristics of the antiphospholipid antibody syndrome in children. *J Pediatr* 1996; **129**: 339–345

252. Falcini F, Taccetti G, Trapani S, Tafi L, Petralli S, Matucci-Cerinic M. Primary antiphospholipid syndrome: a report of two pediatric cases. *J Rheumatol* 1991; **18**: 1085–1087

253. Manco-Johnson MJ, Nuss R, Key N *et al.* Lupus anticoagulant and protein S deficiency in children with postvaricella purpura fulminans or thrombosis. *J Pediatr* 1996; **128**: 319–323

254. Levin M, Eley B, Louis J, Cohen H, Young L, Heyderman R. Postinfectious purpura fulminans caused by an autoantibody against protein S. *J Pediatr* 1995; **127**: 355–363

255. Bodensteiner JB, Hille MR, Riggs JE. Clinical features of vascular thrombosis following varicella. *Arch Pediatr Adolesc Med* 1992; **146**: 100–102

256. Amiral J, Aronis S, Adamtziki E, Garoufi A, Karpathios T. Association of lupus anticoagulant with transient antibodies to prothrombin in a patient with hypoprothrombinemia. *Thromb Res* 1997; **86**: 73–78

257. Becton DL, Stine KC. Transient lupus anticoagulants associated with hemorrhage rather than thrombosis: the hemorrhagic lupus anticoagulant syndrome. *J Pediatr* 1997; **130**: 998–1000

258. Grau E, Real E, Pastor E, Ivorra J, Quecedo E. Prothrombin deficiency and hemorrhage associated with a lupus anticoagulant. *Am J Hematol* 1997; **54**: 85

259. Lee MT, Nardi MA, Hadzi-Nesic J, Karpatkin M. Transient hemorrhagic diathesis associated with an inhibitor of prothrombin with lupus

anticoagulant in a 1 1/2-year-old girl: report of a case and review of the literature. *Am J Hematol* 1996; **51**: 307–314

260. Humphries JE, Acker MN, Pinkston JE, Ruddy S. Transient lupus anticoagulant associated with prothrombin deficiency: unusual cause of bleeding in a 5-year-old girl. *Am J Pediatr Hematol Oncol* 1994; **16**: 372–376

261. Bernini JC, Buchanan GR, Ashcraft J. Hypoprothrombinemia and severe hemorrhage associated with a lupus anticoagulant. *J Pediatr* 1993; **123**: 937–939

262. Jaeger U, Kapiotis S, Pabinger I, Puchhammer E, Kyrle PA, Lechner K. Transient lupus anticoagulant associated with hypoprothrombin-emia and factor XII deficiency following adenovirus infection. *Ann Hematol* 1993; **67**: 95–99

Hemostatic problems in the neonate

33

ELIZABETH A CHALMERS AND BRENDA ES GIBSON

NEONATAL HEMOSTASIS: DEVELOPMENTAL ASPECTS

The hemostatic system in the neonate is generally considered to be immature at birth and this is reflected in the reduced levels of many hemostatic proteins at this time. Although immature, it is a physiologic system which results in few problems for the healthy term infant. The same is not necessarily the case for the sick preterm infant where additional acquired abnormalities may rapidly alter the hemostatic balance resulting in both hemorrhagic and thrombotic problems.

Although in recent years major advances have been made in the understanding of the physiology of normal neonatal hemostasis there are still many issues, particularly with regard to therapy, where data regarding this unique system are lacking.

NORMAL COAGULATION DATA FOR FETUSES AND NEWBORNS

Current understanding of the human hemostatic system allows it to be viewed as a continuum which is profoundly influenced by age. During adult life these effects may be subtle and many are as yet poorly understood. This contrasts sharply with the situation in the fetus and neonate where marked differences have been observed in almost all major coagulation parameters when these are compared with values from older children and adults. These differences necessitate the use of specific normal ranges in this age group. In addition, the coagulation system is very dynamic during the early weeks and months of life and sequential reference ranges are therefore required which can ade-quately reflect the effects of both gestational and postnatal age.

As well as providing important information regarding both physiologic and pathophysiologic processes in the neonate, accurate normal ranges are crucial for both diagnostic and therapeutic purposes. The establishment of reliable ranges was problematic in the past partly due to the sample volumes required for analysis. The introduction of microtechniques in the early 1980s largely resolved this problem by facilitating the analysis of multiple parameters using very small samples.[1]

Despite improved laboratory techniques other problems have persisted and in 1991 the International Society for Thrombosis and Haemostasis (ISTH) Scientific and Stan-dardisation Subcommittee on Neonatal Haemostasis pub-lished a report addressing these issues.[2] It noted that much of the data available in the literature were incomplete and heterogeneous when defined by strict criteria. For example, many studies used cord blood samples which may not be comparable to venous or capillary samples taken from neonates shortly after birth. It has also been noted by various investigators that normal ranges vary widely in neonates, necessitating a relatively large cohort for statistical analysis. The ISTH Subcommittee went on to define guide-lines for future neonatal studies relating to these and other issues which may affect the quality of the data obtained and their subsequent usefulness in clinical practice. These guide-lines deal with the selection of subjects for investigation, sample type, collection and storage, laboratory methodology and data analysis.

Based on the work of several authors, data now exist which provide reference ranges for all the major components of the coagulation system in both term and preterm infants

Table 33.1 Reference values for the components of the fibrinolytic system in healthy full-term infants during the first 6 months of life, compared to those in adults.

Fibrinolytic component	Day 1 mean (boundary)	Day 5 mean (boundary)	Day 30 mean (boundary)	Day 90 mean (boundary)	Day 180 mean (boundary)	Adults mean (boundary)
Plasminogen (unit/ml)	1.95 (1.25–2.65)	2.17 (1.41–2.93)	1.98 (1.26–2.70)	2.48 (1.74–3.22)	3.01 (2.21–3.81)	3.36 (2.48–4.24)
TPA (ng/ml)	9.6 (5.0–18.9)	5.6 (4.0–10.0)[a]	4.1 (1.0–6.0)[a]	2.1 (1.0–5.0)[a]	2.8 (1.0–6.0)[a]	4.9 (1.4–8.4)
α_2-AP (unit/ml)	0.85 (0.55–1.15)	1.00 (0.70–1.30)[a]	1.00 (0.76–1.24)[a]	1.08 (0.76–1.40)[a]	1.11 (0.83–1.39)[a]	1.02 (0.68–1.36)
PAI (unit/ml)	6.4 (2.0–15.1)	2.3 (0.0–8.1)[a]	3.4 (0.0–8.8)[a]	7.2 (1.0–15.3)	8.1 (6.0–13.0)	3.6 (0.0–11.0)

TPA = tissue plasminogen activator; α_2-AP = α_2-antiplasmin; PAI = plasminogen activator inhibitor. For α_2-AP, values are expressed as unit/ml, where pooled plasma contains 1.0 unit/ml. Plasminogen units are those recommended by the Committee on Thrombolytic Agents. Values for TPA are given as ng/ml. Values for PAI are given as unit/ml, where 1 unit of PAI activity is defined as the amount of PAI that inhibits 1 international unit of human single-chain TPA. All values are given as a mean followed by the lower and upper boundary encompassing 95% of the population (boundary).
[a]Values that are indistinguishable from those of the adult.
Reproduced with permission from Ref. 6.

Table 33.2 Reference values for the components of the fibrinolytic system in healthy premature infants during the first 6 months of life, compared to those in adults.

Fibrinolytic component	Day 1 mean (boundary)	Day 5 mean (boundary)	Day 30 mean (boundary)	Day 90 mean (boundary)	Day 180 mean (boundary)	Adults mean (boundary)
Plasminogen (unit/ml)	1.70 (1.12–2.48)[b]	1.91 (1.21–2.61)[b]	1.81 (1.09–2.53)	2.38 (1.58–3.18)	2.75 (1.91–3.59)[b]	3.36 (2.48–4.24)
TPA (ng/ml)	8.48 (3.00–16.70)	3.97 (2.00–6.93)[a]	4.13 (2.00–7.79)[a]	3.31 (2.00–5.07)[a]	3.48 (2.00–5.85)[a]	4.96 (1.46–8.46)
α_2-AP (unit/ml)	0.78 (0.40–1.16)	0.81 (0.49–1.13)[b]	0.89 (0.55–1.23)[b]	1.06 (0.64–1.48)[a]	1.15 (0.77–1.53)	1.02 (0.68–1.36)
PAI (unit/ml)	5.4 (0.0–12.2)[a,b]	2.5 (0.0–7.1)[a]	4.3 (0.0–10.9)[a]	4.8 (1.0–11.8)[a,b]	4.9 (1.0–10.2)[a,b]	3.6 (0.0–11.0)

For explanation of abbreviations see footnote for Table 33.1.
[a]Values that are indistinguishable from those of the adult.
[b]Values that are different from those of the full-term infant.
Reproduced with permission from Ref. 6.

at sequential stages of postnatal development.[3–7] These include ranges for procoagulant proteins, inhibitors of coagulation and proteins involved in the fibrinolytic system (see Tables 6, 31 32 in the Reference values at the front of this book). In the study by Andrew et al,[4] a standard protocol was employed whereby venous blood samples were obtained from healthy full-term infants, all of whom had received 1 mg of intramuscular vitamin K at least 12 hours prior to the first blood sample. Standardized procedures were then followed for the collection, storage and analysis of these samples which were obtained sequentially, at predetermined time points over a 6-month period.

Reference ranges for the commonly used screening tests, prothrombin time (PT), activated partial thromboplastin time (APTT) and thrombin clotting time (TCT) are also published for neonates (see Table 31 in the Reference values at the front of this book).[4] However, in the absence of standardized methods for these screening tests there is inevitably considerable interlaboratory variation and therefore neonatal ranges from individual laboratories should be interpreted in relation to the adult normal range for that laboratory, which should always be quoted for comparison.

The published data for preterm neonates relate to infants born between 30 and 36 weeks' gestation (see Tables 6 and 7 in the Reference values at the front of this book and Tables 33.1 and 33.2).[5] A comparison of the references ranges for term and preterm infants indicates that while many differ-

ences do exist they are relatively small in magnitude, suggesting that this is not a period of particulary rapid development. It has not been possible to establish ranges from an adequate number of healthy premature infants born at <30 weeks' gestation and information relating to this period currently relies on the availability of samples obtained by fetoscopy.

Recently, Reverdiau-Moalic et al[8] published data on 285 healthy fetuses analysed between 19 and 38 weeks' gestation and compared their results with a cohort of normal full-term neonates and an adult control group (Table 33.3). Fetal samples were obtained by direct puncture of the umbilical vein under ultrasound guidance. It is of interest that in the 30–38-week gestation cohort, lower values were observed for the majority of the procoagulant proteins compared with the levels recorded in the study by Andrew et al[4] of preterm infants of equivalent gestation. One possible explanation for this apparent discrepancy is that the birth process itself may affect the coagulation system.

COAGULATION PROTEINS

Procoagulants

Coagulation proteins do not cross the placental barrier but are synthesized in the fetus from around the tenth week of gestation onwards.[9] Both the absolute and relative concentrations of coagulation proteins in the neonate differ from

Table 33.3 Reference values for coagulation screening tests and coagulation factors in fetuses (19–38 weeks' gestation), neonates and adults. Reproduced with permission from Ref. 8.

Parameter	Fetuses (weeks' gestation)			Newborns (n = 60)	Adults (n = 40)
	19–23 (n = 20)	24–29 (n = 22)	30–38 (n = 22)		
PT (s)	32.5 (19–45)	32.2 (19–44)†	22.6 (16–30)†	16.7 (12.0–23.5)*	13.5 (11.4–14.0)
PT (INR)	6.4 (1.7–11.1)	6.2 (2.1–10.6)†	3.0 (1.5–5.0)*	1.7 (0.9–2.7)*	1.1 (0.8–1.2)
APTT (s)	168.8 (83–250)	154.0 (87–210)†	104.8 (76–128)†	44.3 (35–52)*	33.0 (25–39)
TCT (s)	34.2 (24–44)*	26.2 (24–28)	21.4 (17.0–23.3)	20.4 (15.2–25.0)†	14.0 (12–16)
Factor					
I (g/L, Von Clauss)	0.85 (0.57–1.50)	1.12 (0.65–1.65)	1.35 (1.25–1.65)	1.68 (0.95–2.45)†	3.0 (1.78–4.50)
I Ag (g/L)	1.08 (0.75–1.50)	1.93 (1.56–2.40)	1.94 (1.30–2.40)	2.65 (1.68–3.60)†	3.5 (2.50–5.20)
IIc (%)	16.9 (10–24)	19.9 (11–30)*	27.9 (15–50)†	43.5 (27–64)†	98.7 (70–125)
VIIc (%)	27.4 (17–37)	33.8 (18–48)*	45.9 (31–62)	52.5 (28–78)†	101.3 (68–130)
IXc (%)	10.1 (6–14)	9.9 (5–15)	12.3 (5–24)†	31.8 (15–50)†	104.8 (70–142)
Xc (%)	20.5 (14–29)	24.9 (16–35)	28.0 (16–36)†	39.6 (21–65)†	99.2 (75–125)
Vc (%)	32.1 (21–44)	36.8 (25–50)	48.9 (23–70)†	89.9 (50–140)	99.8 (65–140)
VIIIc (%)	34.5 (18–50)	35.5 (20–52)	50.1 (27–78)†	94.3 (38–150)	101.8 (55–170)
XIc (%)	13.2 (8–19)	12.1 (6–22)	14.8 (6–26)†	37.2 (13–62)†	100.2 (70–135)
XIIc (%)	14.9 (6–25)	22.7 (6–40)	25.8 (11–50)†	69.8 (25–105)†	101.4 (65–144)
PK (%)	12.8 (8–19)	15.4 (8–26)	18.1 (8–28)†	35.4 (21–53)†	99.8 (65–135)
HMWK (%)	15.4 (10–22)	19.3 (10–26)	23.6 (12–34)†	38.9 (28–53)†	98.8 (68–135)

Values are the mean, followed in parentheses by the lower and upper boundaries including 95% of the population.
Ag = antigenic value; c = coagulant activity. HMWK = high molecular weight kininogen; PK = prekallikrein.
*P < 0.05.
†P < 0.01.

adult values and are dependent to a varying extent on both the gestational and postnatal age of the infant (see Tables 7 and 31 in the Reference values at the front of this book).

The vitamin K-dependent factors (II, VII, IX and X) are the most extensively studied of all the procoagulant proteins. Mean levels in the term infant are around 50% of normal adult values and are variably reduced further in the premature infant. The postnatal maturation pattern is non-uniform, with Factor VII (FVII) levels reaching the adult range by 5 days, while the other factors increase gradually over the first 6 months of life. Although within the normal adult range, mean levels remain reduced throughout infancy.

The 4 contact factors (XI, XII, prekallikrein [PK] and high molecular weight kininogen [HMWK]) are reduced to around 30–50% of normal at term. HMWK increases rapidly, whereas the other factors show a more gradual increase. Analogous to the the vitamin K-dependent factors, all four are within the adult range at 6 months, but average levels remain lower than comparative adult values.

Factor VIII (FVIII) levels on day 1 are indistinguishable from normal adult values and remain so throughout the neonatal period. von Willebrand factor (VWF) levels are increased at birth and although they decline slightly, remain high compared with adult values until around 3 months of age. The persistent elevation of VWF beyond the immediate postnatal period suggests that its level is more than just a reactive response to the birth process. In addition, VWF, which is made up of a series of multimeric forms of differing molecular weights, is characterized in the neonatal period by an excess of unusually large multimers which are not seen in older children or adults outwith pathologic states.[10,11] These multimers appear to be functionally more active, as indicated by increased platelet aggregation in response to ristocetin.[12]

Mean levels of Factor V (FV) are within the normal adult range at birth and show a further minor increase by day 5. Fibrinogen levels are normal in both term and preterm neonates. A transient increase in fibrinogen is observed at day 5 but thereafter levels are stable throughout the neonatal period. Fetal fibrinogen is not identical to adult fibrinogen, having an increased content of sialic acid, similar to the situation seen in patients with chronic liver disease. The functional significance of fetal fibrinogen is unknown; however, the TCT is normal provided calcium is included in the buffering system.[13] FXIII is 70% of normal at birth and increases to adult levels by day 5.

The knowledge that FVIII levels are normal at birth facilitates the accurate diagnosis of hemophilia A in this age group regardless of severity (see Chapter 29). This is important as hemophilia A is the commonest inherited bleeding disorder to present neonatally. The same is not the case for the commoner forms of von Willebrand disease (VWD) where testing should be delayed until around 6 months of age (see Chapter 30).

Many of the coagulation factors are gestationally dependent and are further reduced in the preterm infant.[5] There is, however, evidence of an accelerated maturation pattern

653

in these infants and levels of coagulation proteins are usually similar by 6 months of age.

Of the commonly used screening tests. The PT is only minimally prolonged in the normal term infant and shortens within the first month of life. This contrasts with the APTT which can be markedly prolonged, particularly in the preterm infant. This is largely due to the reduced levels of contact factors which have a disproportionate effect on APTT compared with reduced levels of FVIII and FIX. The normal range for the APTT is also significantly influenced by the choice of activating reagent.[4] The TCT, as mentioned above, is normal if calcium is added to the buffering system; otherwise it is prolonged, reflecting the effect of fetal fibrinogen.

Inhibitors

The direct inhibitors of thrombin are antithrombin III (ATIII), heparin cofactor II (HCII) and α_2-macroglobulin (α_2-M). ATIII and HCII are around 50% of normal at birth and gradually increase thereafter to reach adult levels by around 3 and 6 months respectively. In contrast, α_2-M is increased at birth and continues to rise postnatally with levels at 6 months which are approximately twice normal adult values.

The indirect inhibitors, protein C and protein S, which are vitamin K dependent, are both reduced to <50% of normal at birth, which parallels the reduction in the vitamin K-dependent procoagulants. Although the concentrations of both proteins increase postnatally, mean protein C concentrations remain significantly reduced during infancy and adult concentrations are not reached until the early teenage years. Protein C, like fibrinogen, circulates in a fetal form characterized by a relative increase in the proportion of single-chain compared with the double-chain form.[14,15] This does not, however, appear to affect the function of the molecule. Protein S in adult plasma is normally present in both free and bound forms, with only the free form being active. The inactive bound form is complexed to the C4b-binding protein. Levels of C4b binding protein are virtually absent in neonatal plasma and protein S therefore circulates entirely in its active free form.[16,17]

Tissue factor pathway inhibitor (TFPI) or extrinsic pathway inhibitor (EPI) has not been as comprehensively investigated as the other naturally occuring coagulation inhibitors. Nevertheless, available data indicate that levels in cord plasma are reduced at birth to around 65% of adult values.[18,19]

EFFECTS ON THROMBIN REGULATION

The results of a number of *in vitro* studies looking at thrombin regulation in neonatal and cord plasma indicate that the capacity of neonatal plasma to generate thrombin is reduced to around 50% of adult values, which is analogous to the situation seen in an adult on therapeutic anticoagulant therapy.[20] In addition, Patel *et al*[21] have demonstrated that even when fibrin is formed, the activity of clot-bound thrombin from cord plasma is reduced compared with that from adult plasma. Both of these effects have been shown to be related to reduced levels of prothrombin.

Thrombin inhibition mediated by the direct thrombin inhibitors (ATIII, HCII and α_2-M) is slower in neonatal plasma, but the overall capacity is similar to that seen in adults.[22] This occurs despite the reduced levels of ATIII which appear to be offset by the increased concentration of α_2-M and increased thrombin binding to HCII.[23-26]

These *in vitro* studies, although providing information on the overall capacity of neonatal plasma either to generate or inhibit thrombin, do not assess the extent to which thrombin generation is actually occuring *in vivo*. This can be quantified *in vivo* by measuring activation peptides, such as prothrombin fragment $1+2$ (F1+2), fibrinopeptide A and thrombin–antithrombin (TAT) complexes which are released at different stages of the coagulation process. Using these activation peptides as markers, it has been possible to demonstrate that the coagulation system is activated in the period immediately following delivery.[22]

FIBRINOLYSIS

The fibrinolytic system in the neonate, as with the coagulation system, can be regarded as physiologically immature with the levels of all major fibrinolytic proteins showing age-dependent variation. The generation of plasmin from plasminogen is the most important step in the fibrinolytic system and is analogous to the generation of thrombin from prothrombin in the coagulation system.

Plasminogen is converted to plasmin by several activators, including tissue plasminogen activator (tPA) and urokinase plasminogen activator (uPA). The inhibitors of the fibrinolytic system include the plasminogen activator inhibitors, of which PAI-1 is the best characterized, and α_2- antiplasmin (α_2-AP) which acts directly on plasmin. α_2-M can also inhibit plasmin but is less important than α_2-AP.

Normal ranges for the major proteins involved in fibrinolysis have been published for both term and preterm infants (see Table 6 in the Reference values at the front of this book and Tables 33.1 and 33.2).[4-6,27] At birth plasminogen levels are around 50% of adult values in the term infant and slightly lower than this in preterm infants. Plasminogen remains reduced throughout the neonatal period, increasing towards normal adult levels by 6 months. Mean α_2-AP levels are around 80% of normal at birth but neonatal and adult ranges do overlap. The levels of both tPA and PAI-1 appear to be transiently increased on day 1 of life in both term and preterm infants. These levels are higher than those documented in cord plasma and it is presumed that both tPA and PAI-1 are released from endothelial cells at the time of delivery.[28]

As well as being reduced at birth, plasminogen is present in a 'fetal' form. Fetal plasminogen has an increased concentration of sialic acid, similar to that found in fetal fibrinogen, and has also been shown to contain increased amounts of mannose. The physiologic significance of these differences from adult plasminogen are unclear. Summaria[29] failed to document any significant difference in the rate of plasmin generation in fetal and adult plasminogen. However, Edelberg et al[30] documented both reduced functional activity and decreased binding to cellular receptors.

Various studies have demonstrated that the fibrinolytic system, like the coagulation system, is transiently activated at birth.[31–34] Although activated, the overall rate of plasmin generation in neonatal plasma is reduced compared to adult values.[28] This is thought largely to relate to the reduced concentration of plasminogen; however, a contribution from a dysfunctional plasminogen molecule, as discussed above, cannot be completely ruled out.

The reduced ability to generate plasmin, theoretically at least, suggests that the neonate may have an impaired ability to lyse thrombi. What part this plays in the overall pathogenesis of thrombotic problems in the neonate is unknown. There are, however, important implications for the use of thrombolytic agents in the neonatal period and it is clear from in vitro studies using fibrin clots derived from cord plasma that there is an impaired response to thrombolysis which again appears to relate to the reduced concentration of plasminogen.[35–37]

Although the precise physiologic consequences of the observed differences in the neonatal coagulation and fibrinolytic systems remain unclear, it is clinically apparent that otherwise healthy neonates do not develop either hemorrhagic or thrombotic problems.

PLATELETS

The platelet count at birth is within the normal range in both the term and preterm infant.[38] The majority of platelet function studies have been performed on cord rather than neonatal platelets and have recorded variable functional defects of uncertain clinical significance. In a study performed on peripheral blood samples from 30 healthy neonates using whole blood flow cytometry, Rajasekhar et al[39] demonstrated reduced reactivity to the agonists thrombin and ADP/epinephrine (adrenaline) in neonatal compared with adult platelets. Again, these results are of unclear clinical significance.

The bleeding time remains the best in vivo assessment of the platelet–vessel wall interaction and special templates are available for use in neonates.[40] Using this device the bleeding time in the neonate is shorter than in adults but using standard techniques may be longer (see Table 36 in the Reference values at the front of this book), which probably reflects increased levels of VWF antigen and activity together with the increased red cell size and hematocrit.

INHERITED DISORDERS OF COAGULATION

The vast majority of bleeding problems seen during the neonatal period are due to acquired disorders of coagulation.[41] It is important to be aware, however, that inherited coagulation disorders can also present at this time.[42] In the absence of a positive family history the diagnosis may go unsuspected and low physiologic levels of many coagulation factors can lead to further difficulties in reaching the correct diagnosis.

HEMOPHILIA A AND B (see also Chapter 29)

Hemophilia A and B are inherited bleeding disorders which result from deficiencies of the procoagulant proteins FVIII and FIX, respectively. They are both inherited as X-linked recessive disorders and together with VWD account for >90% of all inherited bleeding disorders. Current estimates of incidence indicate that 1 in 10 000 males are affected by severe hemophilia A and 1 in 50 000 males by severe hemophilia B.[43] Both FVIII and FIX play a crucial role in the activation of the coagulation cascade and result in clinically indistinguishable bleeding disorders of variable severity. Clinically, it has been useful to classify these disorders according to the measured FVIII:C or FIX:C activity in plasma as:

- severe: <2 unit/dl (in some series <1 unit/dl);
- moderate: 2–5 unit/dl;
- mild: >5 unit/dl.

For the majority of patients, this classification provides a good indication of the likely frequency and severity of bleeding episodes.

Clinical features

The hemophilias are the commonest inherited bleeding disorders to present neonatally.[42] Older studies suggest that bleeding in the neonatal period is a relatively infrequent event. Baehner and Strauss in 1966, reported that <10% of severely affected neonates and <2.5% of those with mild or moderate disease had a clinical event which resulted in a diagnosis being made within the first month of life.[44] More recent studies, however, suggest that these figures may be an underestimate of the true situation. In a cohort of Swedish hemophiliacs diagnosed between 1960 and 1987, 28/140 (20%) were recorded as having abnormal bleeding in the immediate neonatal period (i.e. within 7 days of birth).[45,46] In a similar study from the US, 68.4% of severe hemophiliacs were diagnosed within the first month of life and in almost half of these cases the diagnosis was made after the initiation of appropriate investigations for abnormal bleeding.[47] One possible explanation for the higher incidence of bleeding in the US cohort (33% vs 20%) is the relatively frequent documentation of bleeding following circumcision which is an uncommon procedure at this age in Sweden. The higher incidence of reported bleeding compared with historic studies presumably reflects, at least in part, better recognition of what represents abnormal bleeding in this age group.

Estimates of the frequency of a positive family history in hemophilia vary. Both older and more recent studies report up to 50% of severely affected cases as having a positive family history.[44,47,48] It is a source of concern that both the Swedish and US cohort studies documented a number of cases in which a diagnosis of hemophilia was only made following an episode of bleeding despite the presence of a positive family history. Improvements in questioning and documentation of possible inherited disorders should reduce the incidence of delayed diagnosis in such cases.

The pattern of bleeding observed in neonates tends to differ from that typically seen in older children with hemophilia, where joint and muscle bleeds predominate. Circumcision has already been mentioned and the majority of cases present with bleeding which is iatrogenic in origin. Continued oozing or excessive hematoma formation following venepuncture (Plate 39), heel stab sampling and intramuscular vitamin K have all been observed.[45–47] Umbilical bleeding is relatively uncommon in hemophilia compared with other inherited coagulopathies but is reported. Cephalhematomas (Fig. 33.1), subgaleal hematomas and intracranial hemorrhage (ICH) also occur.[49–52] Less common sites of bleeding include gastrointestinal hemorrhage and intra-abdominal bleeding.[53,54]

Most published papers on ICH are case reports or small case series and the incidence and natural history are therefore poorly defined. Baehner and Strauss reported only 1 of 192 infants with ICH in their study but more recent studies suggest a higher incidence. In all reports, there is a relatively high incidence of residual neurologic deficit.[52] Although a history of birth trauma is not always apparent in hemophiliacs with ICH, current guidelines on the management of known or suspected carriers of hemophilia suggest that if the fetus is male, although vaginal delivery is appropriate, prolonged labor and the use of forceps or vountouse extraction techniques should be avoided.[46,55,56] Fetal scalp electrodes should also be avoided in potentially affected males.

Diagnosis

The diagnosis of hemophilia A is confirmed by finding a reduced level of FVIII activity. FVIII levels are within the normal adult range in both term and preterm infants and it is therefore possible to confirm a diagnosis of hemophilia A in the neonatal period regardless of gestational age and severity. Diagnosing hemophilia B is complicated by the physiologic reduction in FIX during the neonatal period. While this does not preclude the diagnosis of severe (<2 unit/dl) and moderate (2–5 unit/dl) hemophilia B, the diagnosis of mild (>5 unit/dl) cases is problematic due to an overlap with the normal range, and repeat testing when the infant is older is necessary to confirm the diagnosis. Occasionally, the diagnosis can be further confused by the coexistence of an acquired coagulopathy, e.g. disseminated intravascular coagulation (DIC) or vitamin K deficiency.[57]

Management

Neonates requiring treatment should receive replacement therapy with FVIII or FIX concentrates as appropriate. Current UK guidelines recommend recombinant FVIII as the treatment of choice for previously untreated patients with hemophilia A and this will presumably be extended to recombinant FIX concentrate once it is fully licensed.[58] Alternatively, a high purity, plasma-derived product should be used. In the interests of viral safety, the preparation of high-purity concentrates should preferably incorporate two virus inactivation procedures aimed at both lipid-coated and, at least to some extent, non-lipid-coated viruses, e.g. solvent-detergent treatment plus dry heat at 80°C for 72 hours.[59,60] There is little information available on the pharmakokinetics of replacement therapy in neonates and dosing is therefore based on schedules used in older children and adults (see Chapter 29). In keeping with current guidelines, infants likely to receive blood products should be vaccinated against both hepatitis A and B. Appropriate measures should also be taken to reduce the risk of iatrogenic hemorrhage, e.g. vitamin K should be administered orally rather than by intramuscular injection.

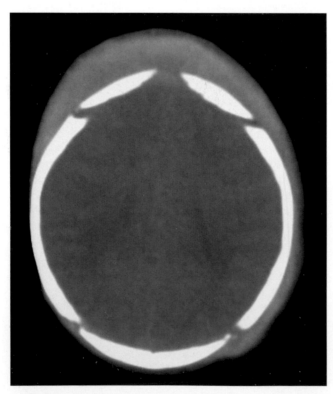

Fig. 33.1 Cephalhematoma in a 2-day-old infant with severe hemophilia A.

VON WILLEBRAND DISEASE (see also Chapter 30)

VWD is the commonest inherited bleeding disorder with an estimated prevalence of 0.8–1.3%.[61,62] It is caused by either a quantitative or qualitative deficiency of von Willebrand Factor (VWF). In most families VWD is inherited as an autosomal dominant disorder and the bleeding tendency is usually mild.[63] VWF is physiologically increased in the neonatal period and high molecular weight multimeric forms are also disproportionately increased at this time.[10]

Clinical features

As the physiologic changes in VWF are presumably protective, bleeding in the neonatal period secondary to VWD is extremely uncommon and is generally restricted to the severe homozygous type 3 disorder in which there is a marked reduction in the levels of both FVIII and VWF. Type 3 disease is rare and accounts for <1% of all patients with VWD. Both superficial bleeding problems and ICH have been reported in affected neonates.[64]

Diagnosis

Type 3 disease is confirmed by recording low levels of both FVIII activity and VWF antigen activity. Most other forms of VWD are masked by physiologically elevated levels of VWF and cannot be diagnosed neonatally other than by molecular analysis.[65] The only other exception to this is type 2B VWD associated with thrombocytopenia, which has been recognized in infancy and should be included in the differential diagnosis of congenital thrombocytopenia.[66]

Management

Treatment of bleeding in type 3 VWD requires the use of a viricidally-treated factor concentrate which contains both FVIII and VWF.[64] Recombinant VWF has been developed but is not widely available.[67,68]

OTHER RARER ABNORMALITIES (see also Chapter 31)

Factors II, V, VII, X and XI are autosomally inherited. The homozygous forms are all relatively rare and consanguinity is often present.[69–74]

Clinical features

Bleeding manifestations have been recorded in the neonatal period for each of these disorders when present in the homozygous state. The pattern of bleeding includes umbilical hemorrhage, bleeding post circumcision, soft tissue hematomas and ICH.[41,71] ICH appears to be particularly common with the severer forms of FVII and FX deficiency. In cases where the Factor VII level is <1 unit/dl, the pattern of bleeding is analogous to that seen in severe hemophilia. In FV deficiency, bleeding manifestations do not always correlate well with the plasma FV level and may depend more on platelet FV levels.[75]

Diagnosis

Plasma levels of Factors II, VII, X and XI are all reduced at term and are further reduced in the preterm infant. Due to an overlap with physiologic values it is not possible to diagnose heterozygotes in the newborn period. Similar problems may exist in some homozygous deficiency states, e.g. homozygous Factors II, X and XI deficiencies are defined by levels of <20, 10 and 15 units/dl, respectively, which are around the lower end of the physiologic range in term infants and within the range for premature neonates.[71]

Management

Treatment of bleeding episodes should be with a specific factor concentrate if available (e.g. FVII and FXI), or with prothrombin-complex concentrate (PCC) (e.g. FII and FX) or fresh frozen plasma (FFP). FXI concentrate and PCC should be used with care in the neonatal period because of the risk of coagulation activation with these products.[76–78] Recombinant FVIIa has recently been used as an alternative to plasma-derived FVII for the treatment of inherited FVII deficiency.[79] In the absence of factor concentrates or where their use is considered inappropriate, consideration should also be given to the use of viricidally-treated FFP if available.[80]

DISORDERS OF FIBRINOGEN (see also Chapter 31)

Congenital abnormalities of fibrinogen are all rare and reflect both quantitative and qualitative defects. They include afibrinogenemia, hypofibrinogenemia and dysfibrinogenemia.[71,81] Both afibrinogenemia and hypofibrinogenemia are usually inherited as autosomal recessive disorders and only the homozygous forms tend to be symptomatic. Afibrinogenemia and the more severe forms of hypofibrinogenemia may present neonatally. Bleeding from the umbilical cord is the most frequently reported problem, but bleeding from other sites also occurs. In both disorders, the PT, APTT and TCT are markedly prolonged. Fibrinogen levels are within the normal adult range at birth. Afibrinogenemia is confirmed by finding undetectable levels of fibrinogen while in hypofibrinogenemia, the levels are usually in the range 20–80 mg/dl. The dysfibrinogenemias are a heterogenous group of disorders most of which are inherited in an autosomal dominant manner. Clinically, they may be asymptomatic or associated with either hemorrhagic or thrombotic problems, but presentation in the neonatal period is uncommon. Functional assays used to confirm the presence of dysfibrinogenemias can be affected by the presence of 'fetal' fibrinogen in newborn infants.[13]

Bleeding episodes requiring treatment should be managed using a viricidally-treated fibrinogen concentrate with the aim of increasing the fibrinogen level to around 100 mg/dl.[41] Fibrinogen has a half-life of 3–5 days which facilitates infrequent dosing. In the absence of fibrinogen concentrate, cryoprecipitate and FFP provide alternative sources of fibrinogen.

HOMOZYGOUS FACTOR XIII DEFICIENCY (see also Chapter 31)

FXIII or fibrin-stabilizing factor is the final enzyme to be activated in the coagulation cascade and is responsible for cross-linking fibrin.[82] Congenital deficiency of FXIII is a rare autosomal recessive disease. The homozygous form was initially described in 1960 and since then only around 200 cases have been reported.[83] The condition results in a moderate-to-severe bleeding disorder associated in some cases with defective wound healing.

Clinical features

Homozygous FXIII deficiency classically presents in the neonatal period with delayed bleeding from the umbilical cord.[84,85] The time to presentation ranges from 1 to 19 days. Although characteristic, this pattern of bleeding is not pathognomic, as around 50% of neonates with afibrinogenemia also present in this way. Bleeding following circumcision and ICH have also been recorded. The risk of ICH is life long and occurs in up to a third of untreated patients.

Diagnosis

FXIII deficiency does not prolong any of the routine screening tests and must be investigated specifically. The urea solubility test is a useful screening test for homozygous deficiency but will not detect heterozygotes. The diagnosis is confirmed by measuring FXIII activity—levels of <1 unit/dl in homozygous cases are easily distinguished from physiologic values. Immunologic assays are useful to subtype the deficiency.

Management

Neonates diagnosed with homozygous FXIII deficiency should be commenced on a prophylactic replacement regimen, preferably using a viricidally-treated FXIII concentrate. A relatively small increase in FXIII to around 3 unit/dl appears to protect against hemorrhage.[86] FXIII has a mean half-life of around 9 days and current regimens utilize a dose of 30 unit/kg administered monthly. If FXIII concentrate is not available, cryoprecipitate or FFP can also be used.

INHERITED THROMBOTIC DISORDERS

ANTITHROMBIN DEFICIENCY

ATIII is a single-chain glycoprotein which is synthesized in the liver and is a member of the serine protease inhibitor (serpin) superfamily.[87] ATIII is one of the direct inhibitors of thrombin but also inhibits most other activated serine proteases involved in the coagulation cascade including Factors Xa, IXa, XIa and XIIa, and is therefore one of the most important regulators of fibrin formation.

The overall prevalence of symptomatic inherited ATIII deficiency in the general population is estimated at between 1:2000 and 1:5000.[88] Type I ATIII deficiency is caused by a quantitative deficiency, whereas type II defects are functional. The latter can affect the reactive site (II RS), heparin binding site (II HBS) or multiple sites (II PE).[89] Clinically, type II HBS defects are associated with a significantly lower incidence of thrombotic problems.[90]

As discussed above, there are important differences in the mechanism of thrombin inhibition in neonatal plasma compared with adults. In neonates, due to differences in the relative proportions of the direct thrombin inhibitors (ATIII, HCII and α_2-M), proportionately more thrombin is inhibited by α_2-M than in adult plasma and there is also a small but significant increase in the relative amount of thrombin bound to HCII.[23,25] It is postulated that these physiologic differences may offer some protection against the effects of ATIII deficiency during the neonatal period.

Clinical features

Homozygous ATIII type II deficiency has been recorded only very rarely and the majority of reports relate to type II HBS defects.[91] Type I defects are probably incompatible with life; one report documented two affected brothers who died within 3 weeks of birth.[92,93]

Homozygous type II HBS defects are uncommon but tend to present early, with a severe thrombotic disorder which may involve arterial as well as venous thrombosis. Most have presented during childhood or adolescence but a neonatal presentation with bilateral deep venous thrombosis and occlusion of the inferior vena cava has been reported.[91]

Heterozygous ATIII deficiency usually presents in the second decade of life but presentation in the neonatal period has been recorded.[94–96] Again, both venous and less frequently arterial thrombotic events can occur. These have tended to involve large vessel thrombosis and purpura fulminans does not appear to be a feature. A precipitating event is not always obvious in these cases; Sanchez et al[97] reported a case of aortic thrombosis in a premature infant which occurred 5 days after birth, which, other than prematurity, was not associated with any clinical risk factors. Jochmans et al[98] reported a similar situation in an apparently healthy term infant who developed multiple thrombotic events, including myocardial infarction and cerebral dural sinus thrombosis during the first few days of life.

Diagnosis

At birth plasma concentrations of ATIII are around 50% of normal adult values and are lower again in premature infants.[4,5] In addition, ATIII may be further reduced in infants who are sick and in the presence of acute thrombosis.[99] Thus, while there should be no difficulty in diagnosing homozygous deficiency states, levels in heterozygotes will overlap with physiologic values. In these cases, sequential measurements and family studies may be crucial in reaching the correct diagnosis. In families at risk of homozygous ATIII deficiency, prenatal diagnosis should be considered if the molecular defect is known.[100]

Management

Treatment of symptomatic neonates with ATIII deficiency includes ATIII replacement and heparin therapy. Replacement therapy should be with a specific ATIII concentrate.[101] Depending upon the site and severity of thrombosis, consideration should be given to the use of thrombolytic therapy. Prophylactic ATIII replacement therapy in heterozygous deficiency during the early neonatal period, particularly in high-risk neonates, has been proposed but given the relatively low risk of thrombosis is unlikely to be justified other than in highly selected cases.

NEONATAL PURPURA FULMINANS (HOMOZYGOUS PROTEIN C AND PROTEIN S DEFICIENCY)

Neonatal purpura fulminans has most frequently been reported in infants with homozygous (or compound heterozygous) protein C deficiency and much less commonly with homozygous protein S deficiency.[102] Both conditions are rare, with the frequency of the former estimated as 1:160 000–1:360 000.[103] The parents of affected infants are often consanguineous.

Protein C is a vitamin K-dependent glycoprotein which is synthesized in the liver and circulates as an inactive zymogen. It is activated by thrombin which occurs most efficiently when thrombin is bound to the endothelial receptor thrombomodulin. Activated protein C (APC) exerts its anticoagulant effect by inactivating FVa and FVIIIa and also has profibrinolytic activity. The free form of protein S (also vitamin K dependent) acts as a cofactor to APC.

Clinical features

Severe homozygous protein C deficiency is associated with undetectable protein C levels and usually presents as a life-threatening disorder in the neonatal period. A less severe form where the level of protein C, although reduced, remains detectable usually presents later.[104]

The onset is usually within the first few days of life and can occur within hours of birth. In a recent series of 9 patients, the mean time to presentation was 3.3 days.[105] The microcirculation is characteristically affected first with the development of purpura fulminans associated with laboratory evidence of disseminated intravascular coagulation (DIC). Cerebral and renal vein thrombosis are also common and can be presenting features. As the condition progresses, widespread thrombotic problems are observed.

The typical skin lesions of purpura fulminans are the result of capillary thrombosis and interstitial hemorrhage. The initial lesions are small ecchymosis affecting mainly the extremities, buttocks, abdomen and scalp, often appearing at sites of pressure or previous trauma, e.g. venepuncture and heel stab sites. Untreated, these lesions gradually enlarge with the development of bullae and purpura, eventually becoming necrotic and gangrenous. Extensive debridement and amputation may be required in advanced cases.

Ocular manifestations are also characteristic and ophthalmologic examination commonly reveals unreactive pupils associated with vitreous or retinal hemorrhage resulting from an initial thrombotic event.[106] It is postulated that, at least in some cases, cerebral and ophthalmic thrombosis may occur as intrauterine events. In infants who survive there is a high incidence of partial or complete blindness, while mental retardation and delayed psychomotor development may follow cerebral events.

Although purpura fulminans is almost always a feature, there are occasional reports of major vessel thrombosis occurring in isolation.[107]

The clinical picture in homozygous protein S deficiency appears to be identical to that seen with protein C deficiency.[108–110]

Diagnosis

In the acute untreated phase, laboratory results are consistent with DIC. There is prolongation of all the routine screening tests (PT, APTT and TCT) with thrombocytopenia, hypofibrinogenemia and increased D-dimers and other markers of coagulation activation. In some cases the blood film shows fragmented red cells in keeping with microangiopathic hemolysis. The definitive diagnosis can be difficult in the neonate. Protein C and S levels are physiologically reduced at birth and are further reduced in the presence of DIC, during which protein C in particular can reach very low levels. The diagnosis is therefore based on finding undetectable protein C (or protein S) activity with heterozygous levels in the parents. Prenatal diagnosis has been reported in families with protein C and S deficiencies where there is a prior history of neonatal purpura fulminans.[111,112]

Management

Although various therapeutic modalities have been attempted, the most important aspect of management in the acute phase appears to be adequate replacement of the deficient inhibitor. There is most experience with protein C replacement. Initially FFP was used as a source of protein C but this has now been largely superseded by a specific protein C factor concentrate, which is the treatment of choice if available. Starting doses of around 40 unit/kg have been used in most cases with subsequent dosing based on protein C recovery data. During the early stages of replacement therapy when active DIC is ongoing, the half-life of the infused protein C may be as short as 2–3 hours, necessitating frequent dosing. Most studies indicate that the half-life improves to around 10 hours once DIC is controlled, which facilitates a single daily treatment.[105,113–115] The optimal protein C level required during replacement is not clearly defined but levels >0.25 unit/ml have been associated with normalization of markers of coagulation activation which can be used to monitor the adequacy of replacement therapy.[116] There is no currently available protein S concentrate and FFP is therefore used for replacement therapy.

The optimal regimen for long-term management remains to be established. Options include long-term replacement therapy and oral anticoagulation. In addition, there is a single case report of the correction of homozygous protein C deficiency following liver transplantation in a child with liver failure.[117]

The majority of cases are treated with oral anticoagulants. During the initiation of treatment replacement therapy must be continued until the International Normalized Ratio (INR) is >3. Most cases seem to require an INR at the upper end of the therapeutic range to prevent recurrent skin necrosis and therefore require careful monitoring. Where possible, dosing should be individualized to identify the minimum dose required to remain symptom free. In the series recently reported by Dreyfus et al,[105] all cases developed intermittent problems requiring temporary or longer term reintroduction of replacement therapy. Similar problems have been reported during the 7-year follow-up of a child with homozygous protein S deficiency who required intermittent replacement with FFP in addition to oral anticoagulants.[109]

ACTIVATED PROTEIN C RESISTANCE

Originally described by Dahlback et al[118] in 1993, APC resistance has recently emerged as an important genetic risk factor for thromboembolic disease. In >90% of cases, APC resistance is due to a single point mutation in the gene for FV (Factor V Leiden). The site of the mutation is a known cleavage site for APC which renders the mutant FVa less sensitive to inactivation by APC leading to a prothrombotic state.

Two recent reports document APC resistance associated with heterozygosity for the Factor V Leiden mutation in neonates presenting with apparently spontaneous thrombotic problems. The first presented within 24 hours of birth with thrombosis of the inferior vena cava which was successfully treated using thrombolysis.[119] The second developed purpura fulminans within 12 hours of birth which resolved following the administration of FFP and did not recur.[120] Why such severe thrombotic problems should have developed in these neonates in the absence of a precipitating cause or co-existing defect is not entirely clear. The Factor V Leiden mutation has a relatively high prevalence in the general population, particularly in northern Europe, and co-existence with other defects is recognized.[121]

Diagnosis is based on the detection of abnormal APC resistance in patient plasma with confirmation from molecular analysis of the Factor V Leiden mutation. The results of molecular analysis are particularly important in neonates for whom only limited coagulation data are available.[122]

ACQUIRED DISORDERS OF COAGULATION

DISSEMINATED INTRAVASCULAR COAGULATION

The term disseminated intravascular coagulation (DIC) is used to describe an acquired thrombohemorrhagic disorder which always occurs as a secondary event to another disease entity. The incidence of DIC is particularly high during the neonatal period, especially in preterm infants.[123]

Etiology

During the neonatal period the events precipitating DIC may differ from those seen in older children (see Chapter 32) reflecting problems arising from birth asphyxia and respiratory distress syndrome (RDS) or disorders of the fetal–placental unit which can lead to the release of tissue factor (Table 33.4).[124] Nevertheless, as in older children, hypotension and sepsis remain important causes of DIC in this age group.

DIC complicated by neonatal purpura fulminans is typically seen in association with homozygous protein C or S deficiency (see above).[102,108] Acquired purpura fulminans secondary to infection, although relatively uncommon in the neonatal period, has been reported in early-onset neonatal group B streptococcal meningitis.[125]

The co-existance of a giant hemangioma with thrombocytopenia and a consumptive coagulopathy was first described in 1940 by Kasabach and Merritt.[126] These hemangiomas usually increase in size and become clinically significant during infancy but can present neonatally.[127,128] A similar syndrome has been recorded antenatally with a variety of other vascular malformations.[129,130]

Table 33.4 Neonatal disseminated intravascular coagulation.

Fetal/neonatal disorders
Hypoxia—acidosis: birth asphyxia, respiratory distress syndrome
Infection: bacterial, viral, fungal, protozoal, parasitic
Necrotizing enterocolitis
Meconium aspiration
Aspiration of amniotic fluid
Brain injury
Hypothermia
Hemolysis
Giant hemangioma (Kasabach–Merritt syndrome)
Homozygous protein C/S deficiency
Malignancy

Maternal/obstetric disorders
Dead twin
Placental abruption
Severe pre-eclampsia

Pathophysiology

This is described in Chapter 32.

Clinical features

The clinical spectrum of neonatal DIC varies greatly with some cases remaining apparently asymptomatic. This reflects the availability of sensitive laboratory tests capable of detecting both the activation of the coagulation and fibrinolytic systems which occur normally following delivery and low-grade compensated DIC. At the other end of the spectrum, fulminant DIC is characterized by bleeding and both microvascular and less often large vessel thrombosis.

Superficial bruising, purpura and iatrogenic bleeding from venepuncture and central line insertion sites are relatively common features. More serious hemorrhagic problems can also occur and both pulmonary and intraventricular hemorrhage in preterm infants may be exacerbated by the presence of thrombocytopenia and an uncompensated coagulopathy. DIC with extensive microvascular thrombosis contributes to end-organ damage which may eventually become irreversible and forms an important, if often poorly recognized, aspect of the syndrome.

Diagnosis

The diagnosis of fulminant neonatal DIC is characterized by prolongation of the routine coagulation screening tests (PT, APTT and TCT), combined with thrombocytopenia and evidence of increased FDPs. Examination of a peripheral blood film may also reveal the presence of red cell fragmentation. Although not routinely performed for diagnostic purposes, reduced levels of procoagulant proteins and inhibitors, especially ATIII and protein C, are also present, reflecting ongoing consumption. Measurement of FV and FVIII levels can be useful in differentiating DIC from other acquired coagulopathies. Thus, in vitamin K deficiency FV should be normal in the face of reduced levels of the vitamin

K-dependent proteins and in hepatic disease FVIII is normal or even increased.

DIC presents a wide clinical spectrum and milder cases can be more difficult to diagnose, particularly in the neonatal period.[131,132] The platelet count is almost universally reduced and has been found to be a useful predictor of coagulopathy in high-risk neonates.[133] The PT and APTT are less reliable and can be normal in both neonates and older children.[132,134] Prolongation of the TCT, which reflects both reduced fibrinogen and the effect of increased FDPs, again is not always prolonged.

Evidence of increased fibrin degradation is an important component of the diagnosis of DIC. The D-dimer assay is now used routinely in many laboratories to detect the products of fibrin degradation. D-dimer is formed following the digestion of cross-linked fibrin by plasmin and is therefore fibrin specific.[135] This compares with the other FDPs, fragments X, Y, D and E, which can be derived from either fibrin or fibrinogen. Raised D-dimer levels should, however, be interpreted with caution in the neonatal period as it is clear from a number of studies that the coagulation system is activated at birth and increased D-dimer levels have been found in both term and preterm infants.[136]

Management

DIC, as discussed above, always occurs as a secondary phenomenon and it is therefore logical that the most important aspect of management is reversal of the underlying disease process. In the critically ill preterm infant in particular this may be difficult to achieve; however, failure to remove the underlying procoagulant stimulus will result in an ongoing coagulopathy. Beyond this there are no clear guidelines on the optimal management of neonatal DIC and a virtual absence of recent randomized controlled trials addressing the available treatment options. Part of the reason for this lies with the heterogeneous nature of the patient population involved which makes such trials difficult to perform.

In current practice blood product replacement therapy remains an important aspect of management and is indicated for the treatment of clinical bleeding in the presence of laboratory confirmation of DIC. FFP (10–15 ml/kg) can improve hemostasis by supplementing reduced procoagulant proteins and is also a source of the naturally occuring inhibitors ATIII, protein C and protein S. Cryoprecipitate (10 ml/kg) contains a higher concentration of FVIII and fibrinogen per unit volume than FFP and is particularly useful in the presence of hypofibrinogenemia. Platelet concentrates (10–15 ml/kg) are also indicated and, although the optimal platelet count to aim for is not defined, it seems reasonable to try to maintain a count of $> 50 \times 10^9/l$. Red cell concentrates are also frequently required and exchange transfusion may be indicated to avoid problems from volume overload. PCCs, although used in the past, are not currently indicated due to the risks of further coagulation activation and thrombosis.

Although the administration of blood products is standard practice in the presence of active bleeding, studies looking at the efficacy of blood product replacement therapy in the overall management of neonatal DIC have yielded conflicting results.[137–141] One controlled study looked at 33 neonates with DIC who were randomized to 1 of 3 treatment arms—exchange transfusion; FFP and platelets; or no therapy directed specifically at the coagulopathy.[140] The results failed to demonstrate any difference in either the resolution of DIC or in survival; however, the numbers in each group were relatively small. Other studies have shown improvement in coagulation profiles and in some cases improved clinical outcome.[137–139,141]

Experimental data exist from animal studies to support the use of both heparin and ATIII concentrates in the treatment of DIC.[142,143] There are, however, only limited data on the use of heparin alone in neonates.[141,144] Gobel et al[144] reported a reduction in the duration of ventilation in a group of neonates with DIC and RDS treated with heparin compared to placebo but the results were not statistically significant and there was no difference in mortality.

ATIII levels are reduced in the neonatal period and are further reduced in the presence of DIC. Since the effectiveness of heparin depends on adequate levels of ATIII it has been postulated that the administration of heparin plus ATIII might be more efficacious than heparin alone. Once again, there are few published data on the use of ATIII with heparin in the pediatric age group, with only one small non-randomized study dealing exclusively with neonates, and this failed to document any major benefit. Therefore, neither heparin nor ATIII, alone or in combination, can be recommended for the routine treatment of neonatal DIC.[145]

VITAMIN K DEFICIENCY

Vitamin K is described in Chapter 32.

Hemorrhagic disease of the newborn

The clinical features of hemorrhagic disease of the newborn (HDN) were first described by Towsend in 1894, but it was only some years later that the link with vitamin K deficiency was established.[146] Levels of the vitamin K-dependent coagulation proteins are already physiologically reduced at birth to around 50% of normal adult values and are functionally inactive in the presence of vitamin K deficiency.[4] In the absence of vitamin K prophylaxis, prothrombin activity has been shown to decrease further on days 2–4 of life.[147]

The tendency of the neonate to become vitamin K deficient is in part due to the limited stores available at birth. The neonate has a very small hepatic reserve of vitamin K, stored almost exclusively as vitamin K_1. Circulating vitamin K levels are low or undetectable at birth with

maternal:cord vitamin K ratios of between 20:1 and 40:1 having been recorded.[148] These findings reflect the limited passage of vitamin K across the placental barrier. The reasons for the apparent protection of the neonate from high levels of vitamin K are not well understood since there is no immediately clear biologic advantage.[149]

The situation is further aggravated by the variable but limited content of vitamin K in breast milk, the small volume intake during the first few days of life and perhaps also by the presence initially of a sterile gut. Vitamin K requirements in the neonate are estimated to be around 1 $\mu g/kg/day$;[150] however, breast milk often contains levels as low as 1–2 $\mu g/l$ with even lower levels in colostrum.[151] This is not the situation in formula-fed infants who achieve significantly higher concentrations of vitamin K by 3–4 days of age and are therefore relatively protected and rarely develop HDN in the absence of other factors.[152]

Clinical features

HDN is generally divided into three forms—early, classical and late. This classification reflects differences not only in the clinical presentation but also in the associated risk factors and prophylactic strategies.[153,154]

Early HDN is the rarest form of the disorder with the onset of bleeding occurring within the first 24 hours of life. The bleeding pattern is variable but can be serious and ICH does occur. This form of HDN is typically, but not exclusively, associated with the ingestion of drugs during pregnancy which can cross the placenta and interfere with vitamin K metabolism. Warfarin, anticonvulsants and the anti-tuberculous drugs rifampicin and isoniazid have all been implicated.[155]

Warfarin is the classic drug which can enter the fetal circulation and cause hemorrhagic problems via reduced carboxylation of vitamin K-dependent proteins. Its use during pregnancy is controversial since in addition to hemorrhagic problems it is also teratogenic with the maximum risk occurring between 6 and 12 weeks' gestation.[156] Despite these problems, it continues to be prescribed for mothers with artificial heart valves, although its use is usually avoided in the first trimester and around the time of delivery.

The risk of HDN following ingestion of anticonvulsant drugs, particularly phenytoin, phenobarbitone and carbamazepine, is poorly defined. Using PIVKA II to assess vitamin K deficiency, Cornelissen et al[157] demonstrated detectable PIVKA II (i.e. vitamin K deficiency) in cord blood from 54% of neonates on anticonvulsant therapy compared with 20% in the control group. The mechanism whereby anticonvulsant drugs cause this problem is not well understood, but is thought to involve the induction of hepatic microsomal oxidase enzymes which result in increased degradation of vitamin K.

Estimates of the frequency of *classical HDN* in the absence of vitamin K prophylaxis vary considerably (0.25–1.7%)

and depend particularly on the method of feeding employed in the study population.[158–162] The condition typically presents between days 2 and 5 with bruising, purpura and gastrointestinal hemorrhage in infants who appear otherwise well. They are almost exclusively breast fed but may have had problems feeding. Bleeding from the umbilicus and mucous membranes is also common, but ICH appears to be relatively infrequent.

Although classical HDN had been recognized for many years, the first reports of *late HDN* were not published until 1967.[163,164] The onset of bleeding occurs after the first week of life, with a peak incidence between 2 and 8 weeks. Recently, it has been suggested that the upper age limit should be extended from 3 to 6 months following the recognition of cases occurring after 15 weeks of age.[165] Unlike classical HDN, ICH is seen in around 50% of cases and is associated with significant morbidity and mortality.

Breast feeding and failure to receive vitamin K at birth are frequently documented risk factors. Late HDN is also seen in association with underlying conditions which result in malabsorption and it can be a presenting feature of cystic fibrosis, celiac disease, α1-antitrypsin deficiency and biliary atresia. In other cases it is thought that transient, mild abnormalities of liver function may contribute to cholestasis and temporarily reduced vitamin K absorption.[166,167]

Again, it has been difficult to estimate the frequency of late HDN in unprotected populations but figures ranging from 4.4/100 000 births in the UK to 72/100 000 in Japan have been published.[168]

Laboratory diagnosis

This is discussed in Chapter 32. The results of factor assays must be interpreted in conjunction with age-adjusted normal ranges.

Vitamin K prophylaxis

Prophylactic strategies differ depending on the type of HND. In an attempt to reduce *early HDN*, guidelines have recently been drafted for the management of pregnant women with epilepsy. In addition to advice regarding the choice of anticonvulsant medication, these suggest the need for both the immediate administration of parenteral vitamin K (1 mg) to the neonate and the use of oral vitamin K (20 mg/day) during the last 4 weeks of pregnancy.[169] The latter recommendation is based on the finding of absent PIVKA II in the cord blood of women who received antenatal oral prophylaxis.[170]

Classical HDN can be effectively prevented by the postnatal administration of a single dose of vitamin K. Various studies have shown that a single oral dose is as effective as parenteral administration.

The prevention of *late HDN* is less straightforward and has been a major source of controversy over the last few years. It was very apparent by the early 1980s that, while a single oral dose of vitamin K provided adequate protection against classical HDN, it did not prevent late HDN.[171] In the study by McNinch and Tripp[172] in 1991, 27 cases of HDN were identified of whom 20 had received no vitamin K prophylaxis and 7 oral prophylaxis. The latter presented significantly later (median 38 days) than those who had not had any prophylaxis (median 13.5 days). The solution to this problem appeared to be the use of a single dose of intramuscular vitamin K at birth which was protective.

In 1992 the safety of this form of prophylaxis was called into question by Golding *et al*'s case-control study reporting an increased incidence of childhood leukemia and cancer following intramuscular vitamin K at birth.[173] Experimental evidence relating vitamin K to mutagenicity was inconclusive and unhelpful.[174,175] Although there were little other data to support these findings, concerns over the potential risks led to conflicting advice. Thus, while the American Academy of Pediatrics recommended the continuation of current policy, the British Paediatric Association recommended that oral vitamin K supplements should be given to newborn infants, with repeated doses for breast-fed infants.[176,177] There followed a general trend in the UK and other parts of Europe towards oral vitamin K prophylaxis but compliance with the triple dose regimen was poor and in 1994 Croucher and Azzopardi[162] reported that >10% of breast-fed infants did not receive the second dose of vitamin K and <40% received a third dose.[178] At the same time, a number of reports documented an increase in the frequency of late HDN.[179–181] Thus, while repeated doses of oral vitamin K may be perceived as being effective and more physiologic than parenteral administration, concerns remain over absorption and compliance with such regimens.[182]

In an attempt to resolve the issue of safety with regard to the use of intramuscular vitamin K, a number of well designed studies have been published which fail to support Golding's original findings of an increased cancer risk and would therefore appear to endorse both the safety and efficacy of this form of prophylaxis.[183–188]

Antenatal administration of vitamin K for the prevention of ICH in premature neonates has also been investigated in a number of studies but there is no evidence of a significant beneficial effect (see also below).[189]

Treatment

In the presence of suspected vitamin K deficiency, the diagnosis can be confirmed by the response to treatment with vitamin K. Following parenteral administration of a 1 mg dose of vitamin K_1, the vitamin K-dependent proteins increase over a few hours. Vitamin K may be administered by slow intravenous injection or subcutaneously; the intramuscular route should *always* be avoided in the presence of a coagulopathy.

In infants who are bleeding and require rapid correction of their coagulopathy, FFP 10–15 ml/kg increases plasma concentrations of vitamin K-dependent proteins by 0.1–0.2

unit/ml and should be administered in addition to vitamin K. In the presence of life-threatening hemorrhage, e.g. ICH, it may only be possible quickly to achieve hemostatic levels of the vitamin K-dependent proteins by the use of PCCs. It should be remembered that most FFP is not currently virus inactivated and, although the relatively low purity factor concentrates are now inactivated against lipid-coated viruses, they carry a risk, albeit small in the uncomplicated setting, of activating the coagulation system with resulting DIC. In addition, with the current move towards treating hemophilia B patients with recombinant and high purity FIX concentrates, PCCs may be less readily available than in the past.

LIVER DISEASE

Although some degree of hepatic impairment is not uncommon in the neonatal period, fulminant hepatic failure is a relatively rare event.[190] Recognized causes of neonatal hepatic failure include viral infections, metabolic disorders, mitochondrial cytopathies, storage disorders and shock.[190] The usual division into acute and chronic liver failure is somewhat arbitrary in the neonate; however, it is recognized that the onset of hepatic dysfunction may occur *in utero* or develop in the perinatal period. Lesser degrees of hepatic impairment may occur in conjunction with sepsis, hypoxia and the use of total parenteral nutrition.

Pathophysiology

The pathophysiology of the coagulopathy in neonatal liver disease is multifactorial but is not significantly different from that seen in older children and adults. Reduced synthesis of procoagulant proteins plays an important role and is further aggravated in the neonatal period by the immaturity of the liver and the physiologically reduced levels of many coagulation proteins. Reduced clearance of activated coagulation factors by the hepatic reticuloendothelial system, activation of fibrinolysis, impaired utilization of vitamin K and thrombocytopenia also contribute.[191–194]

Clinical and laboratory features

The pattern of bleeding is variable and reflects the severity of the coagulopathy. Laboratory features include prolongation of both the PT and APTT and in fulminant hepatic failure, the TCT also becomes prolonged in association with reduced levels of fibrinogen. The main differential diagnosis is vitamin K deficiency and DIC, and specific factor assays and analysis of fibrinogen/fibrin degradation products may be helpful.

Management

Management of the coagulopathy in liver disease is purely supportive. As mentioned above, neonatal liver failure is a relatively infrequent event and there are few published data

on the efficacy of blood product support. In the presence of clinical bleeding, replacement therapy with FFP, cryoprecipitate and platelet concentrates may restore normal hemostasis, at least temporarily. Occasionally, exchange transfusion may be required if there are problems with fluid overload. As in DIC, PCCs should be avoided due to the risks of thrombosis. If there is evidence of cholestasis, the administration of vitamin K supplements may also be helpful.

CARDIOPULMONARY BYPASS

Neonates with congenital heart disease (CHD) who require early corrective surgery involving cardiopulmonary bypass (CPB) are at increased risk of both hemorrhagic and thrombotic complications.[195–198] Excessive bleeding may occur both peri- and post-operatively and is correlated with the duration of the bypass procedure. The actual frequency of significant bleeding is difficult to define and is dependent on the criteria used but is likely to be higher in neonates than in older children.

The pathophysiology of non-surgical post-CPB hemorrhage is complex and several contributing mechanisms are recognized (see Chapter 32).[195,196] Although the mechanisms involved are similar in neonates, children and adults, the relative importance of each is influenced by age, particularly during the neonatal period, when the hemostatic system is physiologically immature.

The presence of a preoperative coagulation defect would be expected to increase the risk of bleeding associated with surgery. In older children there are conflicting reports in the literature regarding the presence of underlying coagulation defects in CHD.[199,200] In cyanotic CHD, some of the previously noted abnormalities may have been artefactual, secondary to polycythemia; however, it is likely that a low-grade consumptive coagulopathy exists in some cases. Abnormalities in acyanotic CHD have also been documented and include the loss of VWF-high molecular weight multimers, which return to normal after surgery.[201] In a recent report, Chan *et al* documented normal procoagulant and inhibitor levels in a group of 22 children (1–15 years) prior to CPB.[202] This contrasts with data from a neonatal study in 1992, in which 53% of infants, aged between 1 and 30 days, had reduced procoagulant levels preoperatively compared with age-matched controls.[203] It was postulated that these abnormalities were due to impaired hepatic maturation secondary to poor organ perfusion or severe cyanosis. It was not, however, possible in this study to predict which neonates were more likely to have a preoperative coagulopathy.

Following the onset of CPB there is a very predictable decrease in the levels of virtually all hemostatic proteins which occurs secondary to hemodilution. Mean plasma concentrations of procoagulant proteins and inhibitors are reduced by around 50% of pre-CPB values.[202,203] There is a similar reduction in the fibrinolytic proteins—plasminogen and α_2-AP. These changes have a significant effect on the regulation of thrombin and *in vitro* studies have demonstrated that the capacity to generate thrombin is also reduced by 50%. This contrasts with the *in vitro* plasma thrombin inhibitory capacity which, despite the reduced inhibitor levels, is relatively spared.[204] It has been suggested that this may be one reason why the risk of hemorrhagic complications post CPB is relatively greater than the risk of thrombosis.

Compared with data from adult studies, the effect of hemodilution in neonates is profound. This reflects the greater degree of dilution in the neonate's circulating blood volume which is estimated to be 5–10 times greater than that seen in an adult. The resulting global reduction in procoagulant proteins combined with the physiologic immaturity of the coagulation system may result in concentrations lower than is generally considered necessary for adequate hemostasis. The situation is further aggravated in the presence of reduced preoperative levels.

In addition to the effects of hemodilution, there is also evidence that both the coagulation and fibrinolytic systems are activated during CPB which may result in a low-grade consumptive coagulopathy. Using prothrombin $F1+2$ and TAT as markers of thrombin generation, studies in both neonates and older children have shown that levels increase during CPB despite the use of heparin.[202,205] Inadequate anticoagulation and tissue damage during surgery are thought to contribute. In support of the latter it has recently been suggested that it is predominantly the extrinsic pathway rather than the contact system which triggers coagulation activation during CPB.[206] tPA and D-dimers are also increased during bypass indicating activation of the fibrinolytic system. In most studies levels fall again postoperatively in keeping with 'fibrinolytic shutdown'.[202,207]

Thrombocytopenia develops at the onset of bypass, again largely due to the effect of hemodilution. Platelet function defects also occur and lead to prolongation of the bleeding time independent of the platelet count. Although contributing to bleeding problems, platelet dysfunction, particularly in neonates, is probably less important than the changes in the coagulation system. This contrasts with the situation in adults where acquired platelet dysfunction is usually the main cause of hemorrhage. The pathophysiology of platelet dysfunction in CBP remains controversial. Partial platelet degranulation and defects of platelet membrane glycoproteins have all been described, while recently it has been suggested that the problem is 'extrinsic' and due to inadequate availability of platelet agonists.[196,208]

Optimal anticoagulation during CPB is crucial to the successful outcome of the procedure. Current protocols use standard heparin, monitored intraoperatively using the activated clotting time (ACT) and reversed by protamine sulfate at the end of the procedure. Inadequate heparinization may cause excess fibrin deposition and consumption of coagulation factors while over anticoagulation increases the risk of bleeding. Despite the importance of anticoagulation,

there are little or no data relating to the use of heparin in neonates undergoing CPB and current regimens are based on data from adult studies.

Current evidence suggests that neonates clear standard heparin faster than adults.[209] In addition, physiologically reduced concentrations of ATIII, which decrease further during bypass due to hemodilution, are likely to impair heparin activity. The use of increased doses of heparin with or without the addition of ATIII supplements might therefore be expected to improve anticoagulation and reduce thrombin generation.[210] It is also clear that use of the ACT to monitor heparin therapy during CPB is unsatisfactory as it is significantly influenced by other factors, particularly hemodilution, and correlates poorly with plasma heparin levels as measured by either antithrombin and anti-FXa assays.[209,211,212]

As well as hemorrhagic problems there is also an increased risk of thrombotic complications following CBP. In a recent survey of 1591 pediatric surgical procedures where bypass was used, the overall incidence of postoperative central venous thrombosis was 1.1%.[198] This figure was 10-fold higher (5.8%) in a subgroup of neonates undergoing cardiac surgery with and without bypass. Overall mortality was increased in the presence of thrombosis. The etiology was considered to be multifactorial with risk factors including the presence of central venous catheters and acquired deficiency of inhibitor proteins. Inherited thrombophilia was also a potential risk factor. Heparin-induced thombocytopenia is a further potential cause of thrombotic problems following CPB, particularly in infants undergoing multiple surgical procedures.[213]

Management of bleeding after CPB is complex and requires careful assessment of the likely causes. Replacement therapy with FFP, cryoprecipitate and platelets may be required to correct hemostatic defects. Adequate reversal of heparin with protamine sulfate is also important. Various measures can also be undertaken in an attempt to prevent excessive blood loss. These include the use of fibrin sealants which can improve local hemostasis during surgery and the serine protease inhibitor aprotinin which has been shown to reduce blood loss and transfusion requirements.[214–218] A number of recent reviews have highlighted considerable variation in the composition of current commercially available fibrin sealants and have emphasized the importance of the inclusion of viral-inactivation procedures in the manufacturing process.[219–221]

INTRAVENTRICULAR HEMORRHAGE

Periventricular-intraventricular hemorrhage (IVH) is the commonest form of intracranial hemorrhage in premature infants. Prior to the use of modern imaging techniques, IVH was thought to be infrequent and associated with a high mortality. Early reports using ultrasound scanning documented a high incidence—up to 40% in infants born at <32 weeks' gestation. More recent studies suggest that this figure has now dropped to around 15–20% which is thought to reflect improvements in neonatal care.[222] Hemorrhagic lesions in most cases originate from the vessels of the germinal matrix and result in periventricular infarction in around 15–20% of cases.

The etiology of IVH is presumed to be multifactorial but remains incompletely understood. Contributing factors include alterations in cerebral blood flow, fragility of the immature germinal matrix vessels, endothelial damage and impaired hemostasis.[223,224] To what extent impaired hemostasis contributes remains unclear. Increasing prematurity and low birth weight are associated with IVH while vaginal delivery, labor prior to cesarean section, intrapartum asphyxia and RDS have all been identified as additional risk factors.[225,226]

Various therapeutic modalities have been utilized including measures aimed at improving cerebral blood flow, cell membrane permeability and hemostasis. The use of prophylactic FFP has been investigated in a number of studies. Beverley et al[227] in 1985 were the first to demonstrate a benefit from prophylactic FFP using ultrasound scanning as the method of assessment. It was not, however, clear from this study whether the reduced incidence of IVH was due to volume expansion or an effect on hemostasis. Other studies have addressed this question by comparing the effect of FPP with other methods of volume expansion and have failed to demonstrate any benefit from either form of therapy.[228,229] These include the recent NNNI Trial group study comparing the administration of FFP, gelatin or glucose in 776 preterm infants (<32 weeks' gestation) in which the outcome at 2 years was used as a measure of efficacy.[230] Other studies looking at prophylactic platelet administration have also failed to demonstrate a beneficial effect.[231]

Antenatal maternal steroid administration appears to be the only measure associated with a reduction in the incidence of IVH and improved survival.[232–236] As well as reducing RDS, antenatal steroids may act by accelerating the maturation of the germinal matrix endothelium.[234] The use of early low-dose indomethacin administered at 6–12 hours post delivery also appears to be beneficial and has been shown to reduce the incidence of severe IVH as assessed by ultrasound.[226,237,238]

ACQUIRED THROMBOTIC PROBLEMS

NEONATAL THROMBOSIS

Within the pediatric age group the peak incidence of thromboembolic complications occurs in neonates and infants <1 year of age.[239–241] Despite this, neonatal thrombosis remains a relatively uncommon event which is reflected in the paucity of good prospective studies.[242] Estimates of the incidence of symptomatic neonatal thromboembolism can be based on recent data published from the Canadian and German registries.[243,244] Schmidt and Andrew[243] reported clinically apparent thrombosis in 2.4/1000 admissions to neonatal intensive care units in Southern Ontario, while Nowak-Gottl et al,[244] using data from a nationwide 2-year prospective survey in Germany, recorded an incidence of 5.1 symptomatic thrombosis/100 000 births. Although under-reporting of cases, particularly in the German study, cannot be completely excluded, these figures at least give some idea of the scale of the problem.

In the Canadian study a total of 97 thrombotic events were recorded of which 60 were venous (renal vein thrombosis = 21; other venous = 39), 33 arterial and 4 mixed. Excluding infants with renal vein thrombosis, the most important risk factor for the development of thrombosis was the presence of an indwelling central line (89% of cases), with systemic infection the second most important factor (29% of cases). The superior and inferior vena cava, right atrium and femoral veins were the commonest sites of venous thrombosis, while the majority of arterial events affected the aorta, femoral and iliac arteries. The sites involved also reflect the vessels most frequently used for catheterization. The clinical sequelae of these events relate to the site and extent of the thrombosis.

A similar distribution of venous and arterial events was recorded in the German study which also confirmed the presence of an indwelling central line as the commonest risk factor. Additional risk factors identified included asphyxia, septicemia, dehydration, maternal diabetes and cardiac disease which clearly reflect the fact that many of these events occur in sick term and preterm infants.[244]

Catheter-related thrombosis

The strong association between neonatal thrombosis and indwelling central lines has been recognized in other studies.[245,246] Many of these events occur in the umbilical artery which is a common site for catheterization due to its size and accessibility. The incidence of clinically overt thrombosis at this site has been estimated at around 1%.[247] However, it is clear from prospective studies using both Doppler scanning and angiography that the incidence of clinically silent thrombosis is considerably higher.[245,246] Similar problems have been documented in the inferior vena cava following catheterization of the femoral vein and in the internal jugular vein following catheterization of this vessel. As with umbilical artery thrombosis, the incidence of clinically apparent thrombosis is relatively low with a much higher incidence on ultrasound scanning.[248,249]

In addition to catheter occlusion, thrombosis in association with an arterial or venous catheter may result in acute problems due to vessel obstruction, e.g. aortic occlusion in association with umbilical catheters or secondary embolic events (Plate 40). Long-term sequelae after symptomatic and asymptomatic thrombotic events are not well defined but may not be inconsiderable and are the subject of ongoing studies.

Non-catheter related events

Spontaneous, non-catheter related, thrombotic events are relatively uncommon in the neonatal period and are largely confined to the renal vein. Other sites at which these have been documented include the aorta, aortic arch and cerebral vessels.[244,250–254]

Renal vein thrombosis

The majority of cases of renal vein thrombosis (RVT) occur during the neonatal period and many present during the first few days of life. In the Canadian registry study, a total of 21 cases were recorded with a median age at diagnosis of 2 days.[243] In addition, it is now clear that in some cases RVT may initially develop antenatally.[255,256] RVT in infancy usually presents with a flank mass together with hematuria, proteinuria and a non-functioning kidney. Thrombocytopenia is also frequently noted. In approximately a quarter of cases, the thrombosis is bilateral with a smaller proportion also extending into the inferior vena cava. In the majority of cases the diagnosis is confirmed on ultrasound.[257]

Although RVT is a well recognized clinical entity, its pathogenesis remains poorly understood. Co-existing disorders which might be anticipated to lead to a hypercoagulable state occur in a significant number of cases and include perinatal asphyxia, dehydration, polycythemia, sepsis, congenital heart disease, nephrotic syndrome and maternal diabetes.

Current management of RVT consists of supportive care only, with heparin and thrombolytic therapy being reserved for cases where thrombosis is extensive or associated with renal failure.[257,258] Optimal management, however, remains to be defined and currently there are no prospective clinical trials assessing outcome after different treatment modalities. Although overall mortality is relatively low in this condition, longer-term follow-up studies suggest that both structural and functional abnormalities of the kidney may not be uncommon.[259,260]

Predisposing factors

The impact of inherited thrombophilic defects on both catheter-related and apparently spontaneous thrombotic events occurring during the neonatal period remains poorly defined. In the German registry, inherited defects were noted in 7/35 (20%) neonates but screening for activated protein C resistance was not available at the time of the study.[244] More recently, APC resistance has been observed in association with neonatal stroke and a small number of case reports have documented underlying thrombophilic defects in association with neonatal thrombosis, including RVT.[261–263] In addition, it has been suggested that acquired deficiencies of protein C and S, particularly in sick preterm infants, may increase the risk of thrombosis.[264] In one study, the lowest protein C levels were recorded in preterm infants

with respiratory distress, infants of diabetic mothers and twin pregnancies.[264] Subsequent thrombosis in this study was inversely correlated with protein C activity, gestational age and RDS, with severe protein C deficiency (<0.1 unit/ml) independently correlating with catheter-related thrombosis.[264–266] Neonatal thrombotic events have also been reported in association with maternal systemic lupus and the antiphospholipid syndrome due to the transplacental passage of IgG anticardiolipin antibodies.[267–270]

Diagnosis

In 1992 the Scientific and Standardisation Subcommittee on Neonatal Hemostasis recommended contrast angiography as the 'gold standard' imaging technique for the confirmation of thrombotic vessel occlusion.[271] This recommendation was based on the absence of good comparative data confirming the diagnostic accuracy of less invasive scanning techniques in the neonatal setting. Despite this recommendation, data from both the Canadian and German registries confirm that Doppler is the most frequently used scanning technique with only 14% of cases in the Canadian study having undergone angiography, while in the German study, 13% had angiography or MRI scanning performed mainly for central nervous system thromobosis.[243,244] It is, however, still recommended that angiography is performed prior to thrombolysis or surgical intervention.

Management

Optimal management strategies for neonatal thrombotic events remain largely undefined and it is generally acknowledged that there is an urgent need for large multicenter studies addressing these issues. Treatment options include supportive care only, anticoagulant therapy (heparin, low molecular weight heparin [LMWH], warfarin), thrombolytic therapy and surgery.

The Canadian registry study noted considerable variation in treatment strategies between individual centers which reflects the inconsistencies which currently exist.[243] Of the 33 infants in this study with arterial events, approximately equal numbers received supportive management, anticoagulation or thrombolysis. In those with venous events (excluding RVT), 46% received anticoagulation, while 23% and 28% respectively received supportive management or thrombolysis. Anticoagulation was almost exclusively with heparin therapy.

In the absence of controlled studies indicating the efficacy of more aggressive therapy, supportive care remains the preferred option for clinically silent thrombosis, which will therefore include the majority of asymptomatic catheter-related events.[271] In the presence of more extensive, clinically apparent thrombosis, standard heparin remains the anticoagulant of choice.[271] Recommended regimens for heparin utilize a loading dose of 50 unit/kg followed by a continuous infusion of 20 unit/kg/h, with laboratory monitoring using an APTT or heparin assay.[271,272]

In practice, dosing schedules vary widely and there is general agreement that regimens extrapolated from adult data are unlikely to be optimal and that a validated therapeutic range for infants is required. This reflects physiologic differences in the neonatal hemostatic system which may alter the activity of certain anticoagulant drugs.[241] Standard heparin acts by binding to antithrombin, leading to accelerated inactivation of several factors including thrombin and FXa, and thus in the presence of reduced levels of antithrombin relative heparin resistance would be predicted. This has been demonstrated in an animal model in which piglets were found to be resistant to the effects of heparin compared to adult pigs.[273] In this study, increasing either the concentration of antithrombin or the dose of heparin reduced this difference. In addition to the mechanism of action, altered pharmakokinetics in the neonate result in quicker heparin clearance as a result of an increased volume of distribution.[274]

In vitro monitoring of heparin therapy is also problematic in the neonate where the APTT is physiologically prolonged and is likely to overestimate the concentration of heparin, while heparin assays (anti-IIa and anti-Xa) result in an underestimate due to the reduced concentration of antithrombin.[275]

LMWH may offer certain advantages over standard heparin for anticoagulation in the neonate. However, there are very few reports of its use in the neonate, although dose finding studies indicate that as with standard heparin dose requirements in the neonate are higher than in older children.[276,277]

In the presence of extensive thrombosis with organ dysfunction or where limb viability is threatened, thrombolytic therapy should be considered. Streptokinase, urokinase and tPA have all been used in neonates but overall experience is relatively limited with published data mainly comprising case reports and small case series.[278–281] In a recent review of thrombolytic therapy in childhood, 21% of those treated were neonates, with congenital heart disease, prematurity and RDS the most frequent underlying problems in this age group.[282] tPA has been used with increasing frequency during the 1990s but again there is considerable variation in practice in terms of the agents used, dose administered and duration of treatment. tPA is usually administered without a loading dose at an infusion rate of between 0.1 and 0.6 mg/kg/h for a period of around 6 hours. Laboratory monitoring should be performed to ensure that a lytic state does occur during the infusion.

As with heparin therapy, the response to thrombolytic agents in the neonate is significantly different from that seen in older children and adults, reflecting physiologic alterations in the hemostatic system.[241] Fibrinolysis is downregulated during the neonatal period and the response to thrombolytic agents impaired due to low concentrations of plasminogen.[35,241] Failure to induce a lytic state as indicated

by a reduction in fibrinogen with a corresponding increase in fibrinogen/fibrin degradation products, may require plasminogen supplementation with FFP. Although the risk of major hemorrhage during thrombolytic therapy is difficult to quantify, it is notable that in the study published by Leaker *et al*[282] there was only one recorded case of neonatal ICH.

NEONATAL THROMBOCYTOPENIA

Data from fetal blood sampling indicate that the fetal platelet count is within the normal adult range from as early as 15–18 weeks' gestation.[283,284] In otherwise healthy term neonates severe thrombocytopenia (platelets $<50 \times 10^9/l$) is an infrequent event. In a large prospective study, platelet counts were determined from $>15\,000$ cord blood samples and in only 19 cases (0.12%) were there $<50 \times 10^9/l$.[285] Six infants in this study had a platelet count of $<20 \times 10^9/l$, all of whom had an underlying diagnosis of neonatal alloimmune thrombocytopenia (NAIT). The incidence of thrombocytopenia in well preterm neonates is slightly higher and it has been estimated that between 2 and 5% of infants have a count of $<100 \times 10^9/l$.[286]

The situation in sick neonates is somewhat different and in this context thrombcytopenia is relatively common. In a 1-year prospective study of 807 infants admitted to a regional neonatal intensive care unit, Castle *et al*[287] documented thrombocytopenia in 22% of cases. Thrombocytopenia was caused by reduced platelet survival and they identified birth asphyxia as an important risk factor. The most serious potential risk associated with neonatal thrombocytopenia is ICH/IVH and it has been shown that in infants weighing <1500 g the incidence of IVH is higher in the presence of co-existing thrombocytopenia.[288]

As with thombocytopenia in other age groups, neonatal thrombocytopenia may relate to inadequate platelet production or a shortened platelet life-span, often due to increased peripheral destruction. During the neonatal period increased platelet destruction is the predominant mechanism although in some cases both mechanisms may apply to a variable extent. A list of the commoner causes of neonatal thrombocytopenia is shown in Table 33.5.

In the initial assessment of a thrombocytopenic neonate it is important to establish whether the infant is well or sick and to take into account both neonatal and maternal factors in addition to any relevant family history.

IMMUNE THROMBOCYTOPENIA

Neonatal alloimmune thrombocytopenia (see also Chapter 21)

NAIT occurs as a result of transplacental passage of maternally derived IgG antibodies directed against paternal anti-

Table 33.5 Causes of neonatal thrombocytopenia.

Increased platelet destruction or reduced life-span
Immune
 Neonatal alloimmune thrombocytopenia
 Neonatal autoimmune thrombocytopenia

Non-immune
 Congenital intrauterine infections (TORCH)
 Maternally-associated disorders (pre-eclampsia, drugs, Rhesus hemolytic
  disease)
 Neonatal sepsis
 Perinatal asphyxia and meconium aspiration
 Respiratory distress syndrome
 Necrotizing enterocolitis
 Neonatal thrombosis
 Hemangiomas
 Hypersplenism

Hereditary thrombocytopenia
 Wiskott–Aldrich syndrome
 Bernard–Soulier syndrome
 May–Hegglin anomaly
 Mediterranean macrothrombocytopenia
 von Willebrand disease (type 2B)

Decreased platelet production
Aplasia/defects of maturation
 Chromosomal abnormalities
 Thrombocytopenia with absent radii (TAR)
 Amegakaryocytic thrombocytopenia
 Fanconi's anemia
 Dyskeratosis congenita

Bone marrow replacement
 Congenital leukemia
 Neuroblastoma
 Histiocytosis

gens on fetal platelets. These antibodies result in immune-mediated platelet destruction leading to fetal thrombocytopenia which may develop *in utero* as early as 20 weeks' gestation. The pathophysiology of the condition is therefore analogous to hemolytic disease of the newborn.

In addition to ABO and HLA Class I antigens, platelets express specific human platelet antigens (HPA, groups 1–5) which represent antigens associated with platelet membrane glycoproteins.[289] In caucasian populations, HPA-1a (previous nomenclature PLA-1) is the commonest human platelet antigen (expressed by almost 98% of the population) and is responsible for the majority of cases of NAIT.[290,291] HPA-5 (Br) and HPA-3 (Bak) are less frequently involved, while in other ethnic groups antigens such as HPA-4 (Yuk/Pen) are more frequently implicated.[292] NAIT has very rarely been reported in association with HLA and ABO alloantibodies.[293]

Recent estimates suggest that the prevalence of clinically significant NAIT is around 1/2000 live births.[290,294] Thus, although around 2.5% of caucasian women are HPA-1a negative and are therefore potentially at risk, platelet antigen incompatibility does not invariably result in alloimmunization and alloimmunization, in turn, does not always result in clinically apparent disease.[295] The immune response in this condition is in part related to the maternal HLA

phenotype, with HLA Dw52a associated with an increased risk of sensitization.[296]

In contrast to the situation in Rhesus hemolytic disease, first pregnancies are affected in around 50% of cases.[290,297] The risk of recurrence in future pregnancies is almost 100% where the father is homozygous for the HPA-1a antigen and 50% in the heterozygous state.[297] Maternal antibodies can cross the placenta from 14 weeks' gestation and fetal thrombocytopenia has been documented as early as 20 weeks' gestation.

In the neonatal period the typical feature of NAIT is moderate-to-severe thrombocytopenia in an otherwise well infant in the absence of any history of maternal thrombocytopenia. The most serious complication ICH which occurs in up to 20% of all cases, with around 10% occurring *in utero*.[298,299] ICH can be clinically silent and it is important that any infant suspected of having NAIT should have a cranial ultrasound scan performed. In addition to ICH, superficial hemorrhage, anemia and gastrointestinal bleeding are also relatively frequent. The risk of bleeding in NAIT is further aggravated by impaired platelet function which occurs as a consequence of antibody blocking the glycoprotein IIb-IIIa complex.[300]

The degree of thrombocytopenia is typically most marked on the first day of life and is followed by a gradual return to normal over a period of around 2–4 weeks. Mortality associated with NAIT is estimated at between 10 and 15%, with the majority of deaths occurring as a consequence of ICH. In addition, neurodevelopmental sequelae in survivors of ICH are frequent and often severe and include cerebral palsy, seizures, hydrocephalus and mental retardation.[301,302]

Laboratory confirmation of NAIT is based on the demonstration of maternal antibody with specificity for paternal antigens. In populations of European origin, rapid typing of maternal platelets for the HPA-1a antigen and screening of maternal serum for evidence of anti-HPA-1a alloantibodies should be undertaken first and will provide confirmation in the majority of cases of NAIT. If these results are negative, platelet phenotping of both parents and screening of maternal serum for alloantibodies against other platelet-specific antigens as well as HLA and ABO antigens should also be performed. Paternal zygosity studies are important for the prediction of recurrent NAIT in future pregnancies.

NAIT is a self-limiting condition; however, until the platelet count recovers, the affected neonate is at significant risk of life-threatening hemorrhage. Once the diagnosis has been confirmed, the most important aspect of management is the rapid administration of compatible, antigen-negative platelets which, in the majority of cases, result in an increase in the platelet count.[303–305] Transfusion of compatible platelets may have to be repeated until the infant's own platelet count recovers.

Where NAIT occurs as an unsuspected event, the infant's mother is a convenient source of compatible platelets since, by definition, she will be negative for the causative antigen.[304] Maternal platelets may be prepared from either a whole blood donation or by platelet pheresis. Regardless of the method of collection, maternal platelets should be plasma depleted (by washing or centrifugation) prior to administration to remove platelet alloantibodies and should also be irradiated to reduce the risk of engraftment of maternal lymphocytes and subsequent graft-versus-host disease.[306–308] It is also recommended that, unless there is extreme clinical urgency, these platelets undergo standard viral screening for HIV and hepatitis B and C prior to use.

Where NAIT is anticipated, which usually occurs following a previously affected pregnancy, antigen-negative platelets should be prepared in advance of delivery either from the mother or from a specifically identified antigen-negative donor. As discussed above, the commonest causative antigen in NAIT is HPA-1a and many larger donor centers now have a registry of known HPA-1a negative donors who can undergo platelet pheresis if required. Very occasionally it may be necessary to use frozen platelets.[309] The only indication for the use of random donor platelets in this condition is life-threatening hemorrhage while awaiting antigen-negative platelets.

While high-dose intravenous immunoglobulin (IVIG) therapy has been shown to be of benefit in increasing the platelet count in NAIT, its effect is usually delayed and is less predictable than that of antigen-negative platelets and should only be used in addition to compatible platelet transfusion.[310,311] IVIG also has the disadvantage of exposing the infant to a pooled blood product and this should be taken into consideration when planning therapy. While IVIG may have a part to play in management, there is no evidence to support the use of corticosteroids.

NAIT, although rare, is potentially life-threatening and prevention is therefore an important aspect of the overall managent of the condition. Screening for HPA-1a phenotypes during pregnancy, which can facilitate the identification of unsuspected cases in a first pregnancy, remains controversial and is not routine practice.[291] Currently, preventive strategies are therefore aimed at reducing the risk of recurrence in future pregnancies following identification of an affected fetus/neonate. There is, however, no consensus on the optimal management strategy.[312] One option is regular maternal IVIG (1 g/kg/week) with or without additional corticosteriods commenced following documentation of fetal thrombocytopenia with subsequent monitoring of the fetal platelet count by percutaneous umbilical blood sampling a few weeks later. Results achieved with this form of therapy are conflicting and it is likely that a significant percentage of cases will not respond adequately.[313–316] The major alternative strategy is cordocentesis with regular platelet transfusion which effectively increases the fetal platelet count but carries a significant risk of procedural complications.[317] To minimize the risks from regular cordocentesis it has been suggested that regular platelet transfusions should be reserved for cases in which medical management with IVIG has been documented to have failed.[312] Avoidance of trauma at the time of delivery is an important aspect of management and early elective delivery by caesarean section is generally advocated.

Neonatal autoimmune thrombocytopenia (see also Chapter 21)

In the presence of maternal autoimmune thrombocytopenia (ITP or other autoimmune conditions), placental transfer of IgG antibodies may result in neonatal thrombocytopenia. The antibodies in this context are directed against antigens common to both maternal and neonatal platelets.

The prevalence of maternal ITP is estimated at between 1 and 5/10 000 pregnancies; however, clinically significant neonatal thrombocytopenia is relatively uncommon.[286] Data from 3 published series which looked at chronic maternal thrombocytopenia recorded significant neonatal thrombocytopenia (platelets $<50 \times 10^9$/l) in 25 of 182 cases (14%) and only 2 (1%) documented cases of ICH.[318]

Unlike NAIT the platelet nadir usually occurs a few days post delivery and bleeding problems *in utero* or at delivery are rare. It should be noted that the count can be normal at birth and fall subsequently, necessitating serial platelet counts. The condition is self-limiting and the count has usually normalized by 2–3 months of age. Where the platelet count is $<50 \times 10^9$/l, treatment options include IVIG and corticosteroids. IVIG 1 g/kg for 2 days is effective in the majority of cases and produces a relatively rapid response.[319,320] The response to platelet transfusion in generally poor and this should only be used in infants with life-threatening hemorrhagic problems.[306]

Management of the fetus in the presence of maternal ITP remains controversial and there is no evidence that any maternal therapy increases the fetal platelet count. In addition, there is no correlation between the maternal and neonatal platelet counts and there is currently no reliable method which can be used to predict the development of clinically significant neonatal thrombocytopenia. Fetal scalp sampling has now been abandoned in most centers due to the risk of bleeding and the high incidence of inaccurate counts.[321] Fetal blood sampling has been advocated by some authors but carries a significant procedural mortality which may be higher in the severely thrombocytopenic fetus and may not be justified by the number of infants at risk.[322] Routine caesarean section for maternal ITP has not been shown to improve fetal outcome and, as the risk of neonatal hemorrhage is low, the route of delivery should be determined primarily by obstetric factors.[323]

NON-IMMUNE THROMBOCYTOPENIA

Thrombocytopenia in the neonatal period is most frequently secondary and non-immune in origin. Especially in sick preterm infants, the etiology is often multifactorial with birth asphyxia, acidosis, RDS, necrotizing enterocolitis and sepsis often co-existing.[287] The underlying mechanism in these cases is thought to relate predominantly to increased platelet destruction due to underlying DIC and thrombocytopenia may occur alone or as part of a generalized coagulopathy.

Fetal congenital infection is also frequently associated with thrombocytopenia (see also Chapters 21 and 38). In addition to increased destruction, reduced platelet production and splenic pooling all contribute to the thrombocytopenia in this situation. In a study looking at the platelet counts of fetuses with known congenital infections, thrombocytopenia was documented in congenital rubella in 20%, toxoplasmosis in 26% and cytomegalovirus (CMV) in 36% of cases.[284] Thrombocytopenia is this study was most marked in cases of CMV infection. In general, however, congenital infections are an uncommon cause of severe ($<20 \times 10^9$/l) thrombocytopenia. HIV infection can also lead to thrombocytopenia but this is an uncommon presentation in the neonatal period.[324]

Rarer causes of thrombocytopenia caused by increased platelet comsumption include giant hemangiomas (Kasabach–Merritt syndrome) and extensive thrombosis.

HEREDITARY THROMBOCYTOPENIA

A number of hereditary syndromes associated with thrombocytopenia may also present in the neonatal period (Table 33.5) (see Chapter 21).

DECREASED PLATELET PRODUCTION

Thrombocytopenia due to decreased platelet production is uncommon, accounting for <5% of all cases of neonatal thrombocytopenia. Nevertheless, in many of these cases thrombocytopenia is severe and affected infants are at risk of serious hemorrhage including ICH.

Chromosomal abnormalities are a well recognized but relatively uncommon cause of neonatal thrombocytopenia.[295] The platelet count is usually only mildly reduced and clinical bleeding is uncommon. The diagnosis is almost always obvious due to the presence of characteristic associated abnormalities. In one study of fetal thrombocytopenia, 43 of 247 cases were due to chromosomal abnormalities.[284] These cases included trisomy 13, 18 and 21, Turner's syndrome and triploidy, of which trisomy 18 was the commonest cause with 26 of 30 (87%) cases affected. In only one infant (triploidy) was a platelet count of under 50×10^9/l recorded. The mechanism of thrombocytopenia is incompletely understood but is thought to involve defects in megakaryocyte maturation.

Two amegakaryocytic syndromes are recognized: thrombocytopenia with absent radii (TAR) and amegakaryocytic thrombocytopenia (AMT). TAR, which is recessively inherited, is characterized by early onset thrombocytopenia which may be severe, together with bilateral hypoplastic or absent radii. In a review of 100 cases, >50% were thrombocytopenic either at birth or within the first week of life, with 38% of affected infants having a platelet count of $<10 \times$

10^9/l.[325] More recently, TAR has been diagnosed prenatally and it is clear that thrombocytopenia does develop *in utero*.[326,327] Although deaths have been reported in infancy, the natural history of the condition is for the thrombocytopenia gradually to resolve with complete or near complete normalization of the platelet count usually occuring during the first few years of life.[325]

Fanconi's anemia is also recessively inherited and typically presents with marrow hypoplasia in association with a variable pattern of co-existing congenital abnormalities.[328] There is increased sensitivity to DNA damage by alkylating agents and ionizing radiation and the diagnosis can be confirmed by performing chromosome breakage studies following exposure to the agent diepoxybutane (DEB). In Fanconi's anemia, although thrombocytopenia is often an early hematologic finding, it usually presents after the neonatal period.

Very rarely, congenital leukemia, neuroblastoma and histiocytosis may present with thrombocytopenia in the neonatal period as a consequence of marrow infiltration.

REFERENCES

1. Johnston M, Zipursky A. Microtechnology for the study of the blood coagulation system in newborn infants. *Can J Med Tech* 1980; **42**: 159–164

2. Hathaway W, Corrigan J. Report of the Scientific and Standardisation Subcommittee on Neonatal Haemostasis: normal coagulation data for fetuses and newborn infants. *Thromb Haemostas* 1991; **65**: 323–325

3. Hathaway WE, Bonnar J. *Hemostatic Disorders of the Pregnant Woman and Newborn Infant*. New York: Elsevier Science Publishing, 1987

4. Andrew M, Paes B, Milner R et al. Development of the coagulation system in the full term infant. *Blood* 1987; **70**: 165–172

5. Andrew M, Paes B, Milner R et al. Development of the coagulation system in the healthy premature infant. *Blood* 1988; **72**: 1651–1657

6. Andrew M, Paes B, Johnston M. Development of the hemostatic system in the neonate and young infant. *Am J Pediatr Hematol Oncol* 1990; **12**: 95–104

7. Corrigan JJ Jr. Normal haemostasis in fetus and newborn. Coagulation. In: Polin RA, Fox WW (eds) *Neonatal and Fetal Medicine. Physiology and Pathophysiology*. Philadelphia: WB Saunders, 1992, pp 1368–1371

8. Reverdiau-Moalic P, Delahousse B, Body G, Bardos P, Leroy J, Gruel Y. Evolution of blood coagulation activators and inhibitors in the healthy human fetus. *Blood* 1996; **88**: 900–906

9. Cade JF, Hirsh J, Martin M. Placental barrier to coagulation factors: its relevance to the coagulation defect at birth and to haemorrhage in the newborn. *Br Med J* 1969; **2**: 281–283

10. Katz JA, Moake JL, McPherson PD et al. Relationship between human development and disappearance of unusually large von Willebrand factor multimers from plasma. *Blood* 1989; **73**: 1851–1858

11. Weinstein MJ, Blanchard R, Moake JL, Vosburgh E, Moise K. Fetal and neonatal von Willebrand (VWF) is unusually large and similar to the VWF in patients with thrombotic thrombocytopenic purpura. *Br J Haematol* 1989; **72**: 68–72

12. Ts'ao CH, Green D, Schultz K. Function and ultrastructure of platelets of neonates: Enhanced ristocetin aggregation of neonatal platelets. *Br J Haematol* 1976; **32**: 225–233

13. Hamulyak K, Nieuwenhuizen W, Devillee PP, Hemker HC. Re-evaluation of some properties of fetal fibrinogen purified from cord blood of normal newborns. *Thromb Res* 1983; **32**: 301–320

14. Greffe BS, Marlar RA, Manco-Johnson M. Neonatal protein C:

671

Molecular composition and distribution in normal term infants. *Thromb Res* 1989; **56**: 91–98

15. Greffe BS, Manco-Johnson MJ, Marlar RA. Molecular forms of human protein C: comparison and distribution in human adult plasma. *Thromb Haemostas* 1989; **62**: 902–905

16. Schwarz HP, Muntean W, Watzke H, Richter B, Griffin JH. Low total protein S antigen but high protein S activity due to decreased C4b-binding protein in neonates. *Blood* 1988; **71**: 562–565

17. Moalic P, Gruel Y, Body G, Foloppe P, Dalahousse B, Leroy J. Levels and plasma distribution of free and C4b-bound protein S in human fetuses and full term newborns. *Thromb Res* 1988; **49**: 471–480

18. Warr TA, Warn-Crammer BJ, Rao LVM, Rapaport SI. Human plasma extrinsic pathway inhibitor activity: Standardisation of assay and evaluation of physiological variables. *Blood* 1989; **74**: 201–206

19. Weissbach G, Harenberg J, Wendisch J, Pargac N, Thomas K. Tissue factor pathway inhibitor in infants and children. *Thromb Res* 1994; **73**: 441–446

20. Andrew M, Schmidt B, Mitchell L, Paes B, Ofosu F. Thrombin generation in newborn plasma is critically dependent on the concentration of prothrombin. *Thromb Haemostas* 1990; **63**: 27–30

21. Patel, P, Weitz J, Brooker LA, Paes B, Mitchell L, Andrew M. Decreased thrombin activity of fibrin clots prepared in cord plasma compared with adult plasma. *Pediatr Res* 1996; **39**: 826–830

22. Andrew M. Developmental hemostasis: relevance to hemostatic problems during childhood. *Semin Thromb Hemostas* 1995; **21**: 341–356

23. Schmidt B, Mitchell L, Ofosu FA, Andrew M. Alpha-2-macroglobulin is an important progressive inhibitor of thrombin in neonatal and infant plasma. *Thromb Haemostas* 1989; **62**: 1074–1077

24. Andrew M, Mitchell L, Berry L *et al*. An anticoagulant dermatan sulfate proteoglycan circulates in the pregnant woman and her fetus. *J Clin Invest* 1992; **89**: 321–326

25. Liu L, Dewar L, Song Y *et al*. Inhibition of thrombin by antithrombin III and heparin cofactor II *in vivo*. *Thromb Haemostas* 1995; **73**: 405–412

26. Ling X, Delorme M, Berry L *et al*. Alpha 2-macroglobulin remains as important as antithrombin III for thrombin regulation in cord plasma in the presence of endothelial cell surfaces. *Pediatr Res* 1995; **37**: 373–378

27. Corrigan J. Neonatal thrombosis and the thrombolytic system. Pathophysiology and therapy. *Am J Pediatr Hematol Oncol* 1988; **10**: 83–91

28. Corrigan JJ, Sluth JJ, Jetter M *et al*. Newborns fibrinolytic mechanism: Components and plasmin generation. *Am J Hematol* 1989; **32**: 273–278

29. Summaria L. Comparison of human normal, full-term, fetal and adult plasminogen by physical and chemical analyses. *Haemostasis* 1989; **19**: 266–273

30. Edelberg JM, Enghild JJ, Pizzo SV, Gonzalez-Gronow M. Neonatal plasminogen displays altered cell surface binding and activation kinetics: Correlation with increased glycosylation of the protein. *J Clin Invest* 1990; **86**: 107–112

31. Suaraz CR, Walenga J, Mangogna LC, Fareed J. Neonatal and maternal fibrinolysis: Activation at time of birth. *Am J Hematol* 1985; **19**: 365–372

32. Kolindewala JK, Das BK, Dube E *et al*. Blood fibrinolytic activity in neonates: Effect of period of gestation, birth weight, anoxia and sepsis. *Ind Pediatr* 1987; **24**: 1029–1033

33. Runnebaum IB, Maurer SM, Daly L *et al*. Inhibitors and activators of fibrinolysis during and after childbirth in maternal and cord blood. *J Pediatr Med* 1989; **17**: 113–119

34. Pinacho A, Paramo JA, Ezcurdia M, Rocha E. Evaluation of the fibrinolytic system in full term neonates. *Int J Clin Lab Res* 1995; **25**: 149–152

35. Andrew M, Brooker L, Leaker M, Paes B, Weitz J. Fibrin clot lysis by thrombolytic agents is impaired in newborns due to a low plasminogen concentration. *Thromb Haemostas* 1992; **68**: 325–330

36. Reis M, Zenker M, Klinge J, Keuper H, Harms D. Age related differences in a clot lysis assay after adding different plasminogen activators in a plasma milieu *in vitro*. *Am J Pediatr Hematol Oncol* 1995; **17**: 260–264

37. Ries M, Klinge J, Rauch R, Keuper H, Harms D. The role of alpha 2-antiplasmin in the inhibition of clot lysis in newborns and adults. *Biol Neonate* 1996; **69**: 298–306

38. Beverly DW, Inwood MJ, Chance GW, Schaus M, O'Keefe B. Normal haemostasis parameters: A study in a well defined unborn population of preterm infants. *Early Hum Dev* 1984; **9**: 249–257

39. Rajasekhar D, Kestin A, Bednarek F, Ellis P, Barnard M, Michelson A. Neonatal platelets are less reactive than adult platelets to physiological agonists in whole blood. *Thromb Haemostas* 1994; **72**: 957–963

40. Andrew M, Paes B, Bowker J, Vegh P. Evaluation of an automated bleeding time device in the newborn. *Am J Hematol* 1990; **35**: 275–277

41. Andrew M, Brooker LA. Blood component therapy in neonatal hemostatic disorders. *Transfusion Med Rev* 1995; **3**: 231–250

42. Smith PS. Congenital coagulation protein deficiencies in the perinatal period. *Semin Perinatol* 1990; **14**: 384–392

43. Levine PH. Clinical manifestations and therapy of hemophilia A and B. In: Coleman RW, Hirsh J, Marder VJ, Salzman EW (eds) *Hemostasis and Thrombosis*, Vol. 6, 2nd edn. Philadelphia: JB Lippincott, 1987, pp 97–111

44. Baehner RL, Strauss HS. Hemophilia in the first year of life. *N Engl J Med* 1966; **275**: 524–528

45. Ljung R, Petrini P, Nilsson IM. Diagnostic symptoms of severe and moderate haemophilia A and B. *Acta Paediatr Scand* 1990; **79**: 196–200

46. Ljung R, Lindgren AC, Petrini P, Tengborn L. Normal vaginal delivery is to be recommended for haemophilia carrier gravidae. *Acta Paediatr* 1994; **83**: 609–611

47. Conway JH, Hilgarter MW. Initial presentations of pediatric hemophiliacs. *Arch Pediatr Adol Med* 1994; **148**: 589–594

48. Schuman I. Pediatric aspects of the mild hemophilias. *Med Clin North Am* 1962; **46**: 93–105

49. Rohyans J, Miser A, Miser J. Subgaleal hemorrhage in infants with hemophilia: report of two cases and review of the literature. *Pediatrics* 1982; **70**: 306–307

50. Olsen TA, Alving BM, Cheshire JL *et al*. Intracerebral and subdural hemorrhage in a neonate with hemophilia. *Am J Pediatr Hematol Oncol* 1985; **7**: 384–387

51. Bray G, Luban N. Hemophilia presenting with intracranial hemorrhage. *Am J Dis Child* 1987; **141**: 1215–1217

52. Yoffe G, Buchanan GR. Intracranial haemorrhage in newborn and young infants with hemophilia. *J Pediatr* 1988; **113**: 333–336

53. Jannoccone G, Pasquino AM. Calcifying splenic hematoma in a hemophilia newborn. *Pediatr Radiol* 1981; **10**: 183–185

54. Reish O, Nachum E, Naor N, Ghoshen J, Merlob P. Hemophilia B in a neonate: unusual early spontaneous gastrointestinal bleeding. *Am J Perinatol* 1994; **11**: 192–193

55. Kletzel M, Miller CH, Becton DL, Chadduck WM, Elser JM. Post delivery head bleeding in hemophilic neonates. Causes and management. *Am J Dis Child* 1989; **143**: 1107–1110

56. Walker ID, Walker JJ, Colvin BT, Letsky EA, Rivers R, Stevens R, on behalf of the Haemostasis and Thrombosis Task Force. Investigation and managment of haemorrhagic disorders in pregnancy. *J Clin Pathol* 1994; **47**: 100–108

57. Schmidt B, Zipursky A. Disseminated intravascular coagulation masking neonatal hemophilia. *J Pediatr* 1986; **109**: 886–888

58. United Kingdom Haemophilia Centre Directors Organisation Executive Committee. Guidelines on therapeutic products to treat haemophilia and other hereditary coagulation disorders. *Haemophilia* 1997; **3**: 63–77

59. Mannucci PM. Viral safety of plasma derived and recombinant products used in the management of haemophilia A and B. *Haemophilia* 1995; **1 (Suppl 1)**: 14–20

60. Ludlam CA. Viral safety of plasma derived factor VIII and XI concentrates. *Blood Coag Fibrinol* 1997; **8 (Suppl 1)**: S19–S23

61. Rodeghiero F, Castaman G, Dini E. Epidemiological investigations of the prevelance of von Willebrand's disease. *Blood* 1987; **69**: 454–457

62. Werner EJ, Emmett H, Tucker E, Giroux D, Schults J, Abshire T.

Prevalence of von Willebrand's disease in children: A multiethnic study. *J Pediatr* 1993; **123**: 893–898

63. Schneppenheim R, Thomas KB, Sutor A. von Willebrand disease in childhood. *Semin Thromb Hemostas* 1995; **21**: 261–275

64. Gazengel C, Fischer A, Schlegel N *et al.* Treatment of type 3 von Willebrand's disease with solvent/detergent treated factor VIII concentrates. *Nouv Rev Fr Hematol* 1988; **30**: 225–227

65. Bignall P, Standen G, Bowen D. Rapid neonatal diagnosis of type 3 von Willebrand's disease by use of the polymerase chain reaction. *Lancet* 1990; **336**: 638–639

66. Donner M, Holmberg L, Nilsson IM. Type IIB von Willebrand's disease with probable autosomal recessive inheritance and presenting as thombocytopenia in infancy. *Br J Haematol* 1987; **66**: 349–354

67. Fischer BE, Schlokat U, Mitterer A *et al.* Structural analysis of recombinant von Willebrand factor produced at industrial scale fermentation of transformed CHO cells co-expressing recombinant furin. *FEBS Lett* 1995; **375**: 259–262

68. Fischer BE, Kramer G, Mitterer A *et al.* Effect of multimerization of human and recombinant von Willebrand factor on platelet aggregation, binding to collagen and binding of coagulation factor VIII. *Thromb Res* 1996; **84**: 55–66

69. Seeler RA. Parahemophilia: Factor V deficiency. *Med Clin North Am* 1972; **56**: 119–125

70. Whitelaw A, Haines M, Bolsover W *et al.* Factor V deficiency and antenatal ventricular hemorrhage. *Arch Dis Child* 1984; **59**: 997–999

71. Girolami A, De Marco L, Dal Bo Zanon R, Patrassi R, Cappellato MG. Rarer quantitative and qualitative abnormalities of coagulation. *Clin Haematol* 1985; **14**: 385–411

72. Bonvini G, Cotta-Ramusino A, Ricciardi G. [Congenital factor V deficiency and intraventricular hemorrhage of prenatal origin] Deficit congenito di fattore V ed emorragia intraventricolare di origine prenatale. *Pediatr Med Chir* 1994; **16**: 93–94

73. Ucsel R, Savasan S, Coban A, Metin F, Can G. Fatal intracranial hemorrhage in a newborn with factor VII deficiency. *Turk J Pediatr* 1996; **38**: 257–260

74. Bolton-Maggs PHB, Hill FGH. The rarer inherited coagulation disorders: a review. *Blood Rev* 1995; **9**: 65–76

75. Cerneca F, Parco S, Simeone R, Bembi B, Giorgi R. A description of two cases of factor V deficiency. *Haemophilia* 1995; **1**: 200–201

76. Hampton KK, Makris M, Kitchen S, Preston FE. Potential thrombogenicity of heat-treated prothrombin complex concentrates in haemophilia B. *Blood Coag Fibrinol* 1991; **2**: 637–641

77. Bolton-Maggs PH. Factor XI deficiency. *Baillière's Clin Haematol* 1996; **9**: 355–368

78. Richards EM, Makris MM, Cooper P, Preston FE. *In vivo* coagulation activation following infusion of highly purified factor XI concentrate. *Br J Haematol* 1997; **96**: 293–297

79. Billio A, Pstcosta N, Rosanelli C *et al.* Successful short-term oral surgery prophylaxis with rFVIIa in severe congenital factor VII deficiency. *Blood Coag Fibrinol* 1997; **8**: 249–250

80. Williamson LM, Allain JP. Virally inactivated fresh frozen plasma. *Vox Sang* 1995; **69**: 159–165

81. Mammen EF. Fibrinogen abnormalities. *Semin Thromb Hemostas* 1983; **9**: 1–9

82. Lorand L, Losowsky MS, Miloszewski KJM. Human factor XIII: Fibrin stabilizing factor. *Prog Haemostas Thromb* 1980; **5**: 245–290

83. Duckert F, Jung E, Shmerling DH. A hitherto undescribed congenital hemorrhagic diathesis probably due to fibrin stabilising factor deficiency. *Thromb Diath Hemorrh* 1960; **5**: 179–182

84. Abbondanzo SL, Gootenberg JE, Lofts RS, McPherson RA. Intracranial hemorrhage in congenital deficiency of factor FXIII. *Am J Pediatr Hematol Oncol* 1988; **10**: 65–68

85. Merchant RH, Agarwal BR, Currimbhoy Z, Pherwani A, Avasthi B. Congenital factor XIII deficiency. *Ind Pediatr* 1992; **29**: 831–836

86. Brackmann HH, Egbring R, Ferster A *et al.* Pharmacokinetics and tolerability of Factor XIII concentrates prepared from human placenta or plasma: a cross over randomised study. *Thromb Haemostas* 1995; **74**: 622–625

87. Lane DA, Caso R. Antithrombin: structure, genomic organization, function and inherited deficiency. In: Tuddenham EGD (ed) The Molecular Biology of Coagulation. *Baillière's Clin Haematol* 1989; **2**: 961

88. Demers C, Ginsberg D, Hirsh J, Henderson P, Blajchman MA. Thrombosis in antithrombin III deficient persons: report of a large kindred and literature review. *Ann Intern Med* 1992; **116**: 754–761

89. Lane DA, Olds RJ, Boisclair M *et al.* Antithrombin III database: First update. *Thromb Haemostas* 1993; **70**: 361–369

90. Finazzi G, Caccia R, Barbui T. Different prevalence of thromboembolism in the subtypes of congenital antithrombin III deficiency: a review of 404 cases. *Thromb Haemostas* 1987; **58**: 1094

91. Chowdury V, Lane DA, Mille B *et al.* Homozygous antithrombin deficiency: Report of two new cases (99 Leu to Phe) associated with venous and arterial thrombosis. *Thromb Haemostas* 1994; **72**: 198–202

92. Hakten M, Deniz U, Ozbay G, Ulutin ON. Two cases of homozygous antithrombin III deficiency in a family with congenital deficiency of AT-III. In: Senzinger H, Vinazzer H (eds) *Thrombosis and Haemorrhagic Disorders: Proceedings of the Sixth International Meeting of the Danubian League against Thrombosis and Haemorrhagic Disorders.* Wurzburg: Schmitt and Meyer GmbH, 1989, pp 177–181

93. Old RJ, Lane DA, Caso R *et al.* Antithrombin III Budapest: a single amino acid substitution (429 Pro to Leu) in a region highly conserved in the serpin superfamily. *Blood* 1992; **79**: 1206–1212

94. Seguin J, Weatherstone K, Nankervis C. Inherited antithrombin III deficiency in the neonate. *Arch Pediatr Adol Med* 1994; **48**: 389–393

95. Peeters S, Vandenplas Y, Jochmans K, Bougatef A, De-Waele M, De-Wolf D. Myocardial infarction in a neonate with antithrombin III deficiency. *Acta Paediatr* 1993; **82**: 610–613

96. Soutar R, Marzinotto V, Andrew M. Overtight nappy precipitating thrombosis in antithrombin III deficiency. *Arch Dis Child* 1993; **69**: 599

97. Sanchez J, Velasco F, Alvarez R, Roman J, Torres A. Aortic thrombosis in a neonate with hereditary antithrombin III deficiency: successful outcome with thrombolytic and replacement therapy. *Acta Paediatr* 1996; **85**: 245–247

98. Jochmans K, Lissens W, Vervoort R, Peeters S, De Waele M, Liebaers I. Antithrombin-Gly 424 Arg: A novel point mutation responsible for Type I antithrombin deficiency and neonatal thrombosis. *Blood* 1994; **83**: 146–151

99. Manco-Johnson MJ. Neonatal antithrombin III deficiency. *Am J Med* 1989; **87 (Suppl 3B)**: 495–525

100. Lane DA, Auberger K, Ireland H, Roscher AA, Thein SL. Prenatal diagnosis in combined antithrombin and factor V gene mutation. *Br J Haematol* 1996; **94**: 753–755

101. Menache D, O'Malley JP, Schorr JB, Wagner B, Williams C. Cooperative Study Group. Evaluation of the safety, recovery, half-life and clinical efficacy of antithrombin (human) in patients with antithrombin III deficiency. *Blood* 1990; **75**: 33–39

102. Marlar RA, Neumann A. Neonatal purpura fulminans due to homozygous protein C or protein S deficiencies. *Semin Thromb Hemostas* 1990; **16**: 299–310

103. Tuddenham EGD, Cooper DN. Protein C and protein C inhibitor. In: Tuddenham EGD, Cooper DN (eds) *The Molecular Genetics of Hemostasis and its Inherited Disorders.* New York: Oxford University Press, 1994, p 149

104. Sharon C, Tirindelli MC, Mannucci PM, Tripodi A, Mariani G. Homozygous protein C deficiency with moderately severe clinical symptoms. *Thromb Res* 1986; **41**: 483–488

105. Dreyfus M, Masterton M, David M *et al.* Replacement therapy with a monoclonal antibody purified protein C concentrate in newborns with severe congenital protein C deficiency. *Semin Thromb Hemostas* 1995; **21**: 371–381

106. Cassels-Brown A, Minford AMB, Chatfield SL, Bradbury JA. Ophthalmic manifestations of neonatal protein C deficiency. *Br J Ophthalmol* 1994; **78**: 486–487

107. Seligsohn U, Berger A, Abend A *et al.* Homozygous protein C

deficiency manifested by massive thrombosis in the newborn. *N Engl J Med* 1984; **310**: 559–562

108. Mahasandana C, Suvvatte V, Chuansumvita A *et al*. Homozygous protein S deficiency in an infant with protein S deficiency. *J Pediatr* 1990; **117**: 750–753

109. Mahasandana C, Veerakul G, Tanphaichitr VS, Opartkiattikul N, Hathaway WE. Homozygous protein S deficiency: 7 year follow-up. *Thromb Haemostas* 1996; **76**: 1122

110. Pegelow CH, Ledford JH, Young JN, Zilleruelo G. Severe protein S deficiency in a newborn. *Pediatrics* 1992; **89**: 674–676

111. Millar DS, Allgrove J, Rodeck C, Kakkar VV, Cooper DN. A homozygous deletion/insertion mutation in the protein C (PROC) gene causing neonatal purpura fulminans: prenatal diagnosis in an at risk pregnancy. *Blood Coag Fibrinol* 1994; **5**: 647–649

112. Formstone CJ, Voke J, Tuddenham EGD *et al*. Prenatal exclusion of severe protein S deficiency by indirect RFLP analysis. *Thromb Haemostas* 1993; **69**: 931

113. Dreyfus M, Magny JF, Bridey F *et al*. Treatment of homozygous protein C deficiency and neonatal purpura fulminans with a purified protein C concentrate. *N Engl J Med* 1991; **325**: 1565–1568

114. Marlar RA, Sills RH, Groncy PK, Montgomery RR, Madden RM. Protein C survival during replacement therapy in homozygous protein C deficiency. *Am J Hematol* 1992; **41**: 24–31

115. Baliga V, Thwaites R, Tillyer ML, Minford A, Parapia L, Allgrove J. Homozygous protein C deficiency—management with protein C concentrate. *Eur J Pediatr* 1995; **154**: 534–538

116. Muller FM, Ehrenthal W, Hafner G, Schranz D. Purpura fulminans in severe congenital protein C deficiency: monitoring of treatment with protein C concentrate. *Eur J Pediatr* 1996; **155**: 20–25

117. Casella JF, Lewis JH, Bontempo FA, Zitelli BJ, Markel H, Starzl TE. Successful treatment of homozygous protein C deficiency by hepatic transplantation. *Lancet* 1988; **i**: 435–438

118. Dahlback B, Carlsson M, Svensson PJ. Familial thrombophilia due to a previously unrecognised mechanism characterised by poor anti-coagulant response to activated protein C. *Proc Natl Acad Sci USA* 1993; **90**: 1004–1009

119. Kodish E, Potter C, Kirschbaum NE, Foster PA. Activated protein C resistance in a neonate with venous thrombosis. *J Pediatr* 1995; **127**: 645–648

120. Pipe SW, Schmaier AH, Nichols WC, Ginsburg D, Bozynski ME, Castle VP. Neonatal purpura fulminans in association with factor V R506Q mutation. *J Pediatr* 1996; **128**: 706–709

121. Brenner B, Zivelin A, Lanir N, Greengard JS, Griffin JH, Seligsohn U. Venous thromboembolism associated with double heterozygosity for R506Q mutation of factor V and for T298M mutation of protein C in a large family of a previously described homozygous protein C-deficient newborn with massive thrombosis. *Blood* 1996; **88**: 877–880

122. Nowak-Gottl U, Koklhase B, Vielaber H, Aschka I, Schneppenheim R, Jurgens H. APC resistance in neonates and infants: adjustment of the APTT based method. *Thromb Res* 1996; **81**: 665–670

123. Dube B, Bhargava V, Dube RK, Das BK, Abrol P, Kolindewala JK. Disseminated intravascular coagulation in the neonatal period. *Ind Pediatr* 1986; **23**: 925–931

124. Schmidt B, Vegh P, Weitz J, Johnston M, Caco C, Roberts R. Thrombin/antithrombin III complex formation in the neonatal respiratory distress syndrome. *Am Rev Respir Dis* 1992; **145**: 767–770

125. Lynn NJ, Pauly TH, Desai NS. Purpura fulminans in three cases of early-onset neonatal group B streptococcal meningitis. *J Perinatol* 1991; **11**: 144–146

126. Kasabach HH, Merritt KK. Capillary hemangioma with extensive purpura—report of a case. *Am J Dis Child* 1940; **59**: 1063

127. Doi O, Takada Y. Kasabach-Merritt syndrome in two neonates. *J Pediatr Surg* 1992; **27**: 1507–1508

128. Chung KC, Weiss SW, Kuzon WM Jr. Multifocal congenital hemangiopericytomas associated with Kasabach–Merritt syndrome. *Br J Plastic Surg* 1995; **48**: 240–242

129. Pierce RN, Dunn L, Knisely AS. Consumptive coagulopathy *in utero* associated with multiple vascular malformations. *Pediatr Pathol* 1992; **12**: 67–71

130. Richards DS, Lutfi E, Mullins D, Sandler DL, Raynor BD. Prenatal diagnosis of fetal disseminated intravascular coagulation associated with umbilical cord arteriovenous malformation. *Obstet Gynecol* 1995; **85**: 860–862

131. Shirahata A, Nakamura T, Yamada K. Diagnosis of DIC in newborn infants. *Bibl Haematol* 1983; **49**: 277–289

132. Schmidt B, Vegh P, Johnston M, Andrew M, Weitz J. Do coagulation screening tests detect increased generation of thrombin and plasmin in sick newborn infants? *Thromb Haemostas* 1993; **69**: 418–421

133. Schmidt BK, Vegh P, Andrew M, Johnston M. Coagulation screening tests in high risk neonates: a prospective cohort study. *Arch Dis Child* 1992; **67**: 1196–1197

134. Chuansumrit A, Hotrakitya S, Hathirat P, Isarangkura P. Disseminated intravascular coagulation in children: diagnosis, management and outcome. *Southeast Asian J Trop Med Pub Health* 1993; **24 (Suppl 1)**: 229–233

135. Francis CW, Marder VJ. A molecular model of plasmin degradation of cross linked fibrin. *Semin Thromb Hemostas* 1982; **8**: 25–35

136. Hudson IRB, Gibson BES, Brownlie J, Holland BM, Turner TL, Webber RW. Increased concentrations of D-Dimers in newborn infants. *Arch Dis Child* 1990; **65**: 383–389

137. Hambleton G, Appleyard W. Controlled trial of fresh frozen plasma in asphyxiated low birth-weight infants. *Arch Dis Child* 1973; **48**: 31–35

138. Turner T, Prowse CV, Prescott RJ, Cash JD. A clinical trial on the early detection and correction of haemostatic defects in selected high-risk neonates. *Br J Haematol* 1981; **47**: 65–75

139. Turner T. Randomized sequential control trial to evaluate effect of purified factor II, VII, IX and X concentrate, cryoprecipitate and platelet concentrate in the management of preterm low birth weight and mature asphyxiated infants with coagulation defects. *Arch Dis Child* 1981; **51**: 810–815

140. Gross SJ, Filston HC, Anderson JC. Controlled study of treatment for disseminated intravascular coagulation in the neonate. *J Pediatr* 1982; **100**: 445–448

141. Yamada K, Shirahata A, Inagaki M, Miyaji Y, Mori N, Horiuchi I. Therapy for DIC in newborn infants. *Bibl Haematol* 1983; **49**: 329–341

142. Hauptmann JG, Hassouna HI, Bell TG, Penner JA, Emerson TE. Efficacy of antithrombin III in endotoxin-induced disseminated intravascular coagulation. *Circ Shock* 1988; **25**: 111–122

143. Du Toit HJ, Coetzee AR, Chalton DO. Heparin treatment in thrombin induced disseminated intravascular coagulation in the baboon. *Crit Care Med* 1991; **19**: 1195–1200

144. Gobel U, von Voss H, Jurgens H *et al*. Efficiency of heparin in the treatment of newborn infants with respiratory distress syndrome and disseminated intravascular coagulation. *Eur J Pediatr* 1980; **133**: 47–49

145. von Kries R, Stannigel H, Gobel U. Anticoagulant therapy by continuous heparin antithrombin III infusion in newborns with disseminated intravascular coagulation. *Eur J Pediatr* 1985; **144**: 191–194

146. Towsend CW. The hemorrhagic disease of the newborn. *Arch Pediatr* 1894; **11**: 559–565

147. Aballi AJ, Lamerens S. Coagulation changes in the neonatal period and in early infancy. *Pediatr Clin North Am* 1962; **9**: 785–817

148. Shearer MJ, Crampton OE, McCarthy PT, Mattock MB. Vitamin K1 in plasma: relationship to vitamin K status. age, pregnancy, diet and disease. *Haemostasis* 1986; **16 (Suppl 5)**: 83

149. Israels LG, Israels ED. Observations on vitamin K deficiency in the fetus and newborn: Has nature made a mistake? *Semin Thromb Hemostas* 1995; **21**: 357–363

150. Food and Nutrition Board, Commission on Life Sciences, National Research Council. *Recommended Dietary Allowances*, edn 10. Washington: National Academy Press, 1988, p 111

151. Greer FR, Marshall S, Cherry J *et al*. Vitamin K status of lactating mothers, human milk and breast feeding infants. *Pediatrics* 1991; **88**: 751–756

152. Widdershoven J, Lambert W, Motohara K *et al*. Plasma concentrations of vitamin K1 and PIVKA-II in bottle fed and breast fed infants with and without vitamin K prophylaxis. *Eur J Pediatr* 1988; **148**: 139–142

153. Sutor AH. Vitamin K deficiency bleeding in infants and children. *Semin Thromb Hemostas* 1995; **21**: 317–329

154. Greer FR. Vitamin K deficiency and hemorrhage in infancy. *Clin Perinatol* 1995; **22**: 759–777

155. Astedt B. Antenatal drugs affecting vitamin K status of the fetus and newborn. *Semin Thromb Hemostas* 1995; **21**: 364–370

156. Ginsberg JS, Hirsh J, Turner DCH, Levine MN, Burrows R. Risks to the fetus of anticoagulant therapy during pregnancy. *Thromb Haemostas* 1989; **61**: 197–203

157. Cornelissen M, Steegers-Theunissen R, Kollee L *et al*. Increased incidence of neonatal vitamin K deficiency resulting from maternal anticonvulsant therapy. *Am J Obstet Gynecol* 1993; **168**: 923–927

158. American Academy of Pediatrics: Committee on Nutrition. Vitamin K compounds and water soluble analogs: use in therapy and prophylaxis in pediatrics. *Pediatrics* 1961; **28**: 501–507

159. Sutherland JM, Glueck HI, Gleser G. Hemorrhagic disease of the neworn. *Am J Dis Child* 1967; **113**: 524–533

160. Keenan WJ, Jewett T, Glueck H. Role of feeding and vitamin K in hypoprothrombinemia of the newborn. *Am J Dis Child* 1971; **121**: 271–277

161. von Kries R, Shearer MJ, Goebel U. Vitamin K in infancy. *Eur J Pediatr* 1988; **147**: 106–112

162. Croucher C, Azzopardi D. Compliance with recommendations for giving vitamin K to newborn infants. *Br Med J* 1994; **308**: 894–895

163. Chan MCK, Boon WH. Late haemorrhagic disease of Singapore infants. *J Singapore Paediatr Soc* 1967; **9**: 72–81

164. Lovric VA, Jones RF. The haemorrhagic syndrome of early childhood. *Aust Ann Med* 1967; **16**: 173–175

165. Sutor AH, Dagres N, Niederhoff. Late form of vitamin K deficiency bleeding in Germany. *Klin Paediatr* 1995; **207**: 89–97

166. von Kries R, Reifenhauser A, Gobel U, McCarthy P, Shearer MJ, Barkhan P. Late onset haemorrhagic disease of the newborn with temporary malabsorption of vitamin K1. *Lancet* 1985; **i**: 1035

167. Matsuda I, Nishiyama S, Motohara K, Endo F, Ogata T, Futagoishi Y. Late neonatal vitamin K deficiency associated with subclinical liver dysfunction in human milk fed infants. *J Pediatr* 1989; **114**: 602–605

168. von Kries R, Hanawa Y. Neonatal vitamin K prophylaxis: Report of the Scientific and Standardization Subcommittee on Perinatal Haemostasis. *Thromb Haemostas* 1993; **69**: 293–295

169. Delgado-Escueta AV, Janz D. Consensus guidelines: preconception counselling, management, and care of the pregnant woman with epilepsy. *Neurology* 1992; **42** (**Suppl 5**): 149–160

170. Cornelissen M, Steegers-Theunissen R, Kollee L *et al*. Supplementation of vitamin K in pregnant women receiving anticonvulsant therapy prevents neonatal vitamin K deficiency. *Am J Obstet Gynecol* 1993; **168**: 884–888

171. Ekelund H. Late haemorrhagic disease in Sweden 1987–89. *Acta Paediatr Scand* 1991; **80**: 966–968

172. McNinch AW, Tripp JH. Haemorrhagic disease of the newborn in the British Isles: Two year prospective study. *Br Med J* 1991; **303**: 1105–1109

173. Golding J, Greenwood R, Birmingham K, Mott M. Childhood cancer, intramuscular vitamin K and pethidine given during labour. *Br Med J* 1992; **305**: 341–346

174. Israels LG, Freisen E, Jansen AH, Israels ED. Vitamin K1 increases sister chromatid exchange *in vitro* in human leucocytes and *in vivo* in fetal sheep cells: a possible role for vitamin K deficiency in the fetus. *Pediatr Res* 1987; **22**: 405–408

175. Cornelissen M, Smeets D, Merkx G, De Abreu R, Kollee L, Monnens L. Analysis of chromosome aberrations and sister chromatid exchanges in peripheral blood lymphocytes of newborns after vitamin K prophylaxis at birth. *Pediatr Res* 1991; **30**: 550–553

176. Vitamin K prophylaxis in infancy. Report of an expert committee. London: British Paediatric Association, 1992

177. Merenstein K, Hathaway WE, Miller RW, Paulson JA, Rowley DL. Controversies concerning vitamin K and the newborn. *Pediatrics* 1993; **91**: 1001–1002

178. Barton JS, Tripp JH, McNinch AW. Neonatal vitamin K prophylaxis in the British Isles: current practice and trends. *Br Med J* 1995; **310**: 632–633

179. von Kries R, Gobel U. Oral vitamin K prophylaxis and late haemorrhagic disease of the newborn. *Lancet* 1994; **343**: 352

180. Barton JS, McNinch AW, Tripp JH. Oral vitamin K prophylaxis and frequency of late vitamin K deficiency bleeding. *Lancet* 1994; **343**: 1168

181. Joubert PH, Stoeckel K. Oral vitamin K in breast fed infants to prevent late haemorrhagic disease of the newborn. *Lancet* 1994; **344**: 484–485

182. Draper G, McNinch A. Vitamin K for neonates: the controversy. *Br Med J* 1994; **308**: 867–868

183. Ekelund H, Finnstrom O, Gunnarskog J, Kallen B, Larsson Y. Administration of vitamin K to newborn infants and childhood cancer. *Br Med J* 1993; **301**: 89–91

184. Klebanoff MA, Read JS, Mills JH, Shiono PH. The risk of childhood cancer after neonatal exposure to vitamin K. *N Engl J Med* 1993; **329**: 905–908

185. Olsen JH, Hertz H, Blinkenberg K, Verder H. Vitamin K regimens and incidence of childhood cancer in Denmark. *Br Med J* 1994; **308**: 895–896

186. Ansell P, Bull D, Roman E. Childhood leukaemia and intramuscular vitamin K: findings from a case-control study. *Br Med J* 1996; **313**: 204–205

187. von Kries R, Gobel U, Hachmeister A, Kaletsch U, Michaelis J. Vitamin K and childhood cancer: a population based case-control study in Lower Saxony, Germany. *Br Med J* 1996; **313**: 199–203

188. Zipursky A. Vitamin K at birth. *Br Med J* 1996; **313**: 179–180

189. Thorp JA, Gaston L, Caspers DR, Pal ML. Current concepts and controversies in the use of vitamin K. *Drugs* 1995; **49**: 376–387

190. Shneider BL. Neonatal liver failure. *Curr Opin Pediatr* 1996; **8**: 495–501

191. Blanchard RA, Furie BC, Jorgensen M *et al*. Acquired vitamin K dependent carboxylation deficiency in liver disease. *N Engl J Med* 1981; **305**: 242–248

192. Joist JH. Hemostatic abnormalities in liver disease. In: Coleman RW, Hirsh J (eds) *Hemostasis and Thrombosis*. Philadelphia: JB Lippincott 1982, pp 861–872

193. Kelly D, Summerfiled J. Hemostasis in liver disease. *Semin Liver Dis* 1987; **7**: 182–191

194. Mammen EF. Coagulation defects in liver disease. *Med Clin North Am* 1994; **78**: 545–554

195. Bick RL. Hemostasis defects associated with cardiac surgery, prosthetic devices, and other extracorporeal circiuts. *Semin Thromb Hemostas* 1985; **11**: 249–280

196. Woodman RC, Harker LA. Bleeding complications associated with cardiopulmonary bypass. *Blood* 1990; **76**: 1680–1697

197. Berman W, Fripp RR, Yabek SM, Wernly J, Corlew S. Great vein and right atrial thrombosis in critically ill infants and children with central venous lines. *Chest* 1991; **99**: 963–967

198. Petaja J, Lundstrom U, Sairanen H, Marttinen E, Griffin JH. Central venous thrombosis after cardiac operations in children. *J Thorac Cardiovasc Surg* 1996; **112**: 883–889

199. Johnson CA, Abildgaard CF, Schulman I. Absence of coagulation abnormalities in children with cyanotic congenital heart disease. *Lancet* 1968; **ii**: 660–662

200. Inenacho HNC, Breeze GR, Fletcher DJ, Stuart J. Consumption coagulopathy in congenital heart disease. *Lancet* 1973; **i**: 231–234

201. Gill JC, Wilson AD, Endres-Brooks J, Montgomery RR. Loss of the largest von Willebrand factor multimers from the plasma of patients with congenital cardiac defects. *Blood* 1986; **67**: 758–761

202. Chan AKC, Leaker M, Burrows FA *et al*. Coagulation and fibrinolytic

profile of paediatric patients undergoing cardiopulmonary bypass. *Thromb Haemostas* 1997; **77**: 270–277

203. Kern FH, Morana NJ, Sears JJ, Hickey PR. Coagulation defects in neonates during cardiopulmonary bypass. *Ann Thorac Surg* 1992; **54**: 541–546

204. Turner-Gomes SO, Mitchell L, Williams WG, Andrew M. Thrombin regulation in congenital heart disease after cardiopulmonary bypass operations. *J Thorac Cardiovasc Surg* 1994; **107**: 562–568

205. Saatvedt K, Lindberg H, Michelsen S, Pedersen T, Geiran OR. Activation of the fibrinolytic, coagulation and plasma kallikrein-kinin systems during and after open heart surgery in children. *Scand J Clin Lab Invest* 1995; **55**: 359–367

206. Boisclair MD, Lane DA, Philippou H *et al.* Mechanisms of thrombin generation during surgery and cardiopulmonary bypass. *Blood* 1993; **82**: 3350–3357

207. Petaja J, Peltola K, Sairanen H *et al.* Fibrinolysis, antithrombin III, and protein C in neonates during cardiac operations. *J Thorac Cardiovasc Surg* 1996; **112**: 665–671

208. Kestin AS, Valeri R, Khuri SF *et al.* The platelet function defect of cardiopulmonary bypass. *Blood* 1993; **82**: 107–117

209. Gruenwald CE, Andrew M, Burrows FA, Williams WG. Cardiopulmonary bypass in the neonate. *Adv Card Surg* 1993; **4**: 137–156

210. Turner-Gomes S, Nitschmann E, Andrew M, Williams WG. Additional heparin affects thrombin generation during cardiopulmonary bypass. *Thromb Haemostas* 1993; **69**: 1167

211. Andrew M, MacIntyre B, MacMillan J *et al.* Heparin therapy during cardiopulmonary bypass in children requires ongoing quality control. *Thromb Haemostas* 1993; **70**: 937–941

212. Gu YJ, Huyzen RJ, van-Oeveren W. Intrinsic pathway-dependent activated clotting time is not reliable for monitoring anticoagulation during cardiopulmonary bypass in neonates. *J Thorac Cardiovasc Surg* 1996; **111**: 677–678

213. Cummins D, Halil O, Amin S. Which patients undergoing cardiopulmonary bypass should be assessed for development of heparin-induced thrombocytopenia? *Thromb Haemostas* 1995; **73**: 890

214. Stark J, de Leval M. Experience with fibrin seal (Tisseel) in operations for congenital heart defects. *Ann Thorac Surg* 1984; **38**: 411–413

215. Hazan E, Pasaoglu I, Demircin M, Bozer AY. The effect of aprotinin (trasylol) on postoperative bleeding in cyanotic congenital heart disease. *Turk J Pediatr* 1991; **33**: 99–109

216. Dietrich W, Mossinger H, Spannagl M *et al.* Hemostatic activation during cardiopulmonary bypass with different aprotinin dosages in pediatric patients having cardiac operations. *J Thorac Cardiovasc Surg* 1993; **105**: 712–720

217. Penkoske PA, Entwistle LM, Marchak BE, Seal RF, Gibb W. Aprotinin in children undergoing repair of congenital heart defects. *Ann Thorac Surg* 1995; **60 (Suppl)**: S529–532

218. Kjaergard HK, Fairbrother JE. Controlled clinical studies of fibrin sealant in cardiothoracic surgery—a review. *Eur J Cardio Thorac Surg* 1996; **10**: 727–733

219. Jackson MR, MacPhee MJ, Drohan WN, Alving BM. Fibrin sealant: current and potential clinical applications. *Blood Coag Fibrinol* 1996; **7**: 737–746

220. Martinowitz U, Spotnitz WD. Fibrin tissue adhesives. *Thromb Haemostas* 1997; **78**: 661–666

221. Radosevich M, Goubran HI, Burnouf T. Fibrin sealant: scientific rationale, production methods, properties, and current clinical use. *Vox Sang* 1997; **72**: 133–143

222. Oh W, Fanaroff AA, Veter J *et al.* Neonatal mortality and morbidity in very low birth weight infants: a seven year trend analysis of the Neonatal Network Data. *Pediatr Res* 1996; **39**: 235

223. Ment LR, Stewart WB, Ardito TA, Madri JA. Germinal matrix microvascular maturation correlates inversely with the risk period for neonatal intraventricular hemorrhage. *Dev Brain Res* 1995; **84**: 142–149

224. Koppe JG. Prevention of brain haemorrhage and ischaemic injury in premature babies. *Lancet* 1996; **348**: 208–209

225. Shankaram S, Bauer CR, Bain R, Wright LL, Zachary J. Prenatal and perinatal risk and protective factors for neonatal intracranial hemorrhage. *Arch Pediatr Adol Med* 1996; **150**: 491–497

226. Vohr B, Ment LR. Intraventricular hemorrhage in the preterm infant. *Early Hum Dev* 1996; **44**: 1–16

227. Beverley DW, Pitts-Tucker TJ, Congdon PJ, Arthur RJ, Tate G. Prevention of intraventricular haemorrhage by fresh frozen plasma. *Arch Dis Child* 1985; **60**: 710–713

228. Wright IMR, Levene MI, Arthur RA, Martinez D. A randomised controlled trial of fresh frozen plasma and volume expansion in very low birth weight and sick preterm infants. *Proceedings of the British Paediatric Association, 67th Annual Meeting.* London: BPA, 1995, p 52

229. Anon. A randomized trial comparing the effect of prophylactic intravenous fresh frozen plasma, gelatin or glucose on early mortality and morbidity in preterm babies. The Northern Neonatal Nursing Initiative [NNNI] Trial Group. *Eur J Pediatr* 1996; **155**: 580–588

230. The NNNI Trial Group. Randomised trial of prophylactic early fresh frozen plasma or gelatin or glucose in preterm babies: outcome at 2 years. *Lancet* 1996; **348**: 229–232

231. Andrew M, Vegh P, Caco C *et al.* A randomized controlled trial of platelet transfusions in thrombocytopenic premature infants. *J Pediatr* 1993; **123**: 285–291

232. Anon. Effect of corticosteroids for fetal maturation on perinatal outcomes. *NIH Consensus Statement* 1994; **12**: 1–24

233. National Institutes of Health Consensus Development Conference Statement. Effects of corticosteroids for fetal maturation on prenatal outcomes. *Am J Obstet Gynecol* 1995; **173**: 246–252

234. Ryan CA, Finer NN. Antenatal corticosteroid therapy to prevent respiratory distress syndrome. *J Pediatr* 1995; **126**: 317–319

235. Wells JT, Ment LR. Prevention of intraventricular hemorrhage in preterm infants. *Early Hum Dev* 1995; **42**: 209–233

236. Ment LR, Oh W, Ehrenkranz RA, Philip AG, Duncan CC, Makuch RW. Antenatal steroids, delivery mode, and intraventricular hemorrhage in preterm infants. *Am J Obstet Gynecol* 1995; **172**: 795–800

237. Ment LR, Oh W, Ehrenkranz RA *et al.* Low-dose indomethacin and prevention of intraventricular hemorrhage: a multicenter randomized trial. *Pediatrics* 1994; **93**: 543–550

238. Ment LR, Vohr B, Oh W *et al.* Neurodevelopmental outcome at 36 months' corrected age of preterm infants in the Multicenter Indomethacin Intraventricular Hemorrhage Prevention Trial. *Pediatrics* 1996; **98**: 714–718

239. David M, Andrew M. Venous thromboembolic complications in children. *J Pediatr* 1993; **123**: 337–346

240. Andrew M, David M, Adams M *et al.* Venous thromboembolic complications (VTE) in children: first analyses of the Canadian Registry of VTE. *Blood* 1994; **83**: 1251–1257

241. Andrew M. Developmental hemostasis: relevance to thromboembolic complications in pediatric patients. *Thromb Haemostas* 1995; **74**: 415–425

242. Roy M, Schmidt B. Neonatal thrombosis: Are we doing the right studies? *Semin Thromb Hemostas* 1995; **21**: 313–316

243. Schmidt B, Andrew M. Neonatal thrombosis: Report of a prospective Canadian and International registry. *Pediatrics* 1995; **96**: 939–943

244. Nowak-Gottl U, von Kries R, Gobel U. Neonatal symptomatic thromboembolism in Germany: two year survey. *Arch Dis Child* 1997; **76**: F163–F167

245. Schmidt B, Zipursky A. Thrombotic disease in newborn infants. *Clin Perinatol* 1984; **11**: 461–488

246. Schmidt B, Andrew M. Neonatal thrombotic disease: Prevention, diagnosis and treatment. *J Pediatr* 1988; **113**: 407–410

247. O'Neill JA, Neblett WW III, Born ML. Management of major thromboembolic complications of umbilical artery catheters. *J Pediatr Surg* 1981; **16**: 972–978

248. Rand T, Kohlhauser C, Popow C *et al.* Sonographic detection of internal jugular vein thrombosis after central venous catheterization in the newborn period. *Pediatr Radiol* 1994; **24**: 577–580

249. Shefler A, Gillis J, Lam A, O'Connell AJ, Schell D, Lammi A. Inferior

vena cava thrombosis as a complication of femoral vein catheterisation. *Arch Dis Child* 1995; **72**: 343–345

250. Mannino FL, Travner DA. Stroke in neonates. *J Pediatr* 1983; **102**: 605–610

251. Hamilton RM, Penkoske PA, Byrne P, Duncan NF. Spontaneous aortic thrombosis in a neonate presenting as coarctation. *Ann Thorac Surg* 1988; **45**: 564–565

252. Barron TF, Gusnard DA, Zimmerman RA, Clancy RR. Cerebral venous thrombosis in neonates and children. *Pediatr Neurol* 1992; **8**: 112–116

253. Evans DJ, Pizer BL, Moghal NE, Joffe HS. Neonatal aortic arch thrombosis. *Arch Dis Child* 1994; **71**: F125–127

254. Kawahira Y, Kishimoto H, Lio M *et al*. Spontaneous aortic thrombosis in a neonate with multiple thrombi in the main branches of the abdominal aorta. *Cardiovasc Surg* 1995; **3**: 219–221

255. Fishman JE, Joseph RC. Renal vein thrombosis *in utero*: duplex sonography in diagnosis and follow-up. *Pediatr Radiol* 1994; **24**: 135–136

256. Wright NB, Blanch G, Walkinshaw S, Pilling DW. Antenatal and neonatal renal vein thrombosis: new ultrasonic features with high frequency transducers. *Pediatr Radiol* 1996; **26**: 686–689

257. Andrew M, Brooker LA. Hemostatic complications in renal disorders of the young. *Pediatr Nephrol* 1996; **10**: 88–99

258. Nuss R, Hays T, Manco-Johnson M. Efficacy and safety of heparin anticoagulation for neonatal renal vein thrombosis. *Am J Pediatr Hematol Oncol* 1994; **16**: 127–131

259. Mocan H, Beattie TJ, Murphy AV. Renal venous thrombosis in infancy: long term follow-up. *Pediatr Nephrol* 1991; **5**: 45–49

260. Keidan I, Lotan D, Gazit G, Boichis H, Reichman B, Linder N. Early neonatal renal venous thrombosis: long-term outcome. *Acta Paediatr* 1994; **83**: 1225–1227

261. Nowak-Gottl U, Strater R, Dubbers A, Oleszuk-Raschke K, Vielhaber H. Ischaemic stroke in infancy and childhood: role of the Arg506 to Gln mutation in the factor V gene. *Blood Coag Fibrinol* 1996; **7**: 684–688

262. Formstone CJ, Hallam PJ, Tuddenham EG *et al*. Severe perinatal thrombosis in double and triple heterozygous offspring of a family segregating two independent protein S mutations and a protein C mutation. *Blood* 1996; **87**: 3731–3737

263. Haffner D, Wuhl E, Zieger B, Grulich-Henn J, Mehls O, Schaefer F. Bilateral renal venous thrombosis in a neonate associated with resistance to activated protein C. *Pediatr Nephrol* 1996; **10**: 737–739

264. Manco-Johnson MJ, Abshire TC, Jacobson LJ, Marlar RA. Severe neonatal protein C deficiency: Prevalence and thrombotic risk. *J Pediatr* 1991; **119**: 793–798

265. Roman J, Valesco F, Fernandez F *et al*. Protein C, protein S and C4b-binding protein in neonatal severe infection and septic shock. *J Perinat Med* 1992; **20**: 111–116

266. MacDonald PD, Gibson BES, Brownlie J, Doig WB, Houston AB. Protein C activity in severely ill newborns with congenital heart disease. *J Perinat Med* 1992; **20**: 421–427

267. Contractor S, Hiatt M, Kosmin M, Kim HC. Neonatal thrombosis with anticardiolipin antibody in baby and mother. *Am J Perinatol* 1992; **9**: 409–410

268. Silver RK, MacGregor SN, Pasternak JF, Neely SE. Fetal stroke associated with maternal anticardiolipin antibodies. *Obstet Gynecol* 1992; **80**: 497–499

269. Tabbutt S, Griswold WR, Ogino MT, Mendoza AE, Allen-JB, Reznik VM. Multiple thromboses in a premature infant associated with maternal phospholipid antibody syndrome. *J Perinatol* 1994; **14**: 66–70

270. Teyssier G, Gautheron V, Absi L, Galambrun C, Ravni C, Lepetit JC. Anticardiolipin antibodies, cerebral ischemia and adrenal hemorrhage in a newborn infant. *Arch Pediatr* 1995; **2**: 1086–1088

271. Schmidt B, Andrew M (for the subcommittee). Report of the Scientific and Standardization Subcommittee on Neonatal Hemostasis: Diagnosis and treatment of neonatal thrombosis. *Thromb Haemostas* 1992; **67**: 381–382

272. McDonald MM, Hathaway WE. Anticoagulant therapy by continuous heparinization in newborn and older infants. *J Pediatr* 1982; **101**: 451–457

273. Schmidt B, Buchanan M, Ofosu F, Brooker L, Hirsh J, Andrew M. Antithrombotic properties of heparin in a neonatal piglet model of thrombin induced thrombosis. *Thromb Haemostas* 1988; **60**: 289–292

274. Andrew M, Ofosu F, Schmidt B, Brooker L, Hirsh J, Bichanan M. Heparin clearance and *ex vivo* recovery in newborn piglets and adult pigs. *Thromb Res* 1988; **52**: 517–527

275. Vieira A, Berry L, Ofosu F, Andrew M. Heparin sensitivity and resistance in the neonate: an explanation. *Thromb Res* 1991; **63**: 85–98

276. Dzumhur SM, Goss DE, Cohen AT. Low molecular weight heparin for venous thrombosis in a neonate. *Lancet* 1995; **346**: 1487

277. Massicotte P, Adams M, Marzinotto V, Brooker LA, Andrew M. Low molecular weight heparin in pediatric patients with thrombotic disease: a dose finding study. *J Pediatr* 1996; **128**: 313–318

278. Dillon PW, Fox PS, Berg CJ, Cardella JF, Krummel TM. Recombinant tissue plasminogen activator for neonatal and pediatric vascular thrombolytic therapy. *J Pediatr Surg* 1993; **28**: 1264–1268

279. Ahluwalia JS, Kelsall AW, Diederich S, Rennie JM. Successful treatment of aortic thrombosis after umbilical catheterization with tissue plasminogen activator. *Acta Paediatr* 1994; **83**: 1215–1217

280. Kothari SS, Varma S, Wasir HS. Thrombolytic therapy in infants and children. *Am Heart J* 1994; **127**: 651–657

281. Wever ML, Liem KD, Geven WB, Tanke RB. Urokinase therapy in neonates with catheter related central venous thrombosis. *Thromb Haemostas* 1995; **73**: 180–185

282. Leaker M, Massocotte P, Brooker LA, Andrew M. Thrombolytic therapy in pediatric patients: A comprehensive review of the literature. *Thromb Haemostas* 1996; **76**: 132–134

283. Forestier F, Daffos F, Galacteros F, Bardakjian J, Rainaut M, Berezard Y. Hematological values of 163 normal fetuses between 18 and 30 weeks gestation. *Pediatr Res* 1986; **20**: 342–346

284. Hohlfeld P, Forestier F, Kaplan C, Tissot JD, Daffos F. Fetal thrombocytopenia: a retrospective survey of 5,194 fetal blood samplings. *Blood* 1994; **84**: 1851–1856

285. Burrows RF, Kelton JG. Fetal thrombocytopenia and its relation to maternal thrombocytopenia. *N Engl J Med* 1993; **329**: 1463–1466

286. George D, Bussel JB. Neonatal thrombocytopenia. *Semin Thromb Hemostas* 1995; **21**: 276–293

287. Castle V, Andrew M, Kelton J, Johnston M, Carter C. Frequency and mechanism of neonatal thrombocytopenia. *J Pediatr* 1986; **108**: 749–755

288. Andrew M, Castle V, Saigal S, Carter C, Kelton KG. Clinical impact of neonatal thrombocytopenia. *J Pediatr* 1987; **110**: 457–464

289. von dem Borne A, Decary F. ICSH/ISBT working party on platelet serology. *Vox Sang* 1990; **58**: 176

290. Mueller-Eckhart C, Kiefel V, Gribert A *et al*. 348 cases of suspected neonatal alloimmune thrombocytopenia. *Lancet* 1989; **i**: 363–366

291. Flug F, Karpatkin M, Karpatkin S. Should all pregnant women be tested for their platelet PLA (Zw, HPA-1) phenotype? *Br J Haematol* 1994; **86**: 1–5

292. Matsui K, Ohsaki E, Goto A, Koresawa M, Kigasawa H, Shibata Y. Perinatal intracranial hemorrhage due to severe neonatal alloimmune thrombocytopenic purpura (NAITP) associated with anti-Yukb (HPA-4a) antibodies. *Brain Dev* 1995; **17**: 352–355

293. Skacel PO, Stacey TE, Tidmarsh CEF *et al*. Maternal alloimmunization to HLA, platelet and granulocyte specific antigens during pregnancy: Its influence on cord blood granulocyte and platelet counts. *Br J Haematol* 1989; **71**: 119–123

294. Blanchette V, Chen L, de Fridberg ZS, Hogan VA, Trudel E, Decary F. Alloimmunisation to the PLA-1 platelet antigen: results of a prospective study. *Br J Haematol* 1990; **74**: 209–215

295. Udom-Rice I, Bussel JB. Fetal and neonatal thrombocytopenia. *Blood Rev* 1995; **9**: 57–64

296. Valentin N, Vergracht A, Bignon JD *et al*. HLA-DRW52a is involved

in alloimmunisation against PLA-1 antigen. *Hum Immunol* 1990; **27**: 73–79

297. Shulman NR, Jordan JV. Platelet immunology. Coleman RW, Hirsh J, Marder VJ, Salzman EW (eds) *Hemostasis and Thrombosis*. Philadelphia: JB Lippincott, 1987, p 477

298. Reznikoff-Etievant MF, Kaplan C, Muller JY, Daffos F, Forestier F. Alloimmune thrombocytopenias, definition of a group at risk: A prospective study. *Curr Stud Hematol Blood Transfusion* 1988; **55**: 119–124

299. Lipitz S, Ryan G, Murphy MF *et al*. Neonatal alloimmune thrombocytopenia due to anti-PLA1 (Anti-HPA-1a): Importance of paternal and fetal platelet typing for assessment of fetal risk. *Prenat Diagn* 1992; **12**: 955–958

300. Kunicki TJ, Beardsley DS. The alloimmune thrombocytopenias: neonatal alloimmune thrombocytopenic purpura and post-transfusion purpura. *Prog Hemostas Thromb* 1989; **9**: 203–232

301. Bonacossa IA, Jocelyn LJ. Alloimmune thrombocytopenia of the newborn: neurodevelopmental sequelae. *Am J Perinatol* 1996; **13**: 211–215

302. Murphy MF, Hambley H, Nicolaides K, Waters AH. Severe fetomaternal alloimmune thrombocytopenia presenting with fetal hydrocephalus. *Prenat Diagn* 1996; **16**: 1152–1155

303. McIntosh S, O'Brien RT, Schwartz AD, Pearson HA. Neonatal isoimmune purpura: Response to platelet infusions. *J Pediatr* 1973; **82**: 1020–1027

304. Vain NE, Bedros AA. Treatment of isoimmune thrombocytopenia of the newborn and transfusion of maternal platelets. *Pediatrics* 1979, **63**: 107–109

305. Blanchette VS, Rand ML. Platelet disorders in newborn infants: Diagnosis and management. *Semin Perinatol* 1997; **21**: 53–62

306. Blanchette VS, Kuhne T, Hume H, Hellmann J. Platelet transfusion therapy in newborn infants. *Transfusion Med Rev* 1995; **3**: 215–230

307. *Standards for Blood Banks and Transfusion Services*, 16th edn. Bethesda, MD: American Association of Blood Banks, 1994

308. BCSH Blood Transfusion Task Force. Guidelines on gamma irradiation of blood components for the prevention of transfusion associated graft versus host disease. *Transfusion Med* 1996; **6**: 261–271

309. McGill M, Mayhaus C, Hoff R *et al*. Frozen maternal platelets for neonatal thrombocytopenia. *Transfusion* 1987; **27**: 347–349

310. Sidiropoulos D, Straume B. The treatment of neonatal isoimmune thrombocytopenia with intravenous immunoglobulin (IgG IV). *Blut* 1984; **48**: 383–386

311. Kaplan C, Morel-Kopp MC, Clemenceau S *et al*. Fetal and neonatal alloimmune thrombocytopenia: Current trends in diagnosis and therapy. *Transfusion Med* 1992; **2**: 265–271

312. Johnson JM, Ryan G, Al-Musa A, Farkas S, Blanchette VS. Prenatal diagnosis and management of neonatal alloimmune thrombocytopenia. *Semin Perinatol* 1997; **21**: 45–52

313. Lynch L, Bussel JB, McFarland JG, Chitkara U, Berkowwitz RL. Antenatal treatment of alloimmune thrombocytopenia. *Obstet Gynecol* 1992; **80**: 67–71

314. Kroll H, Giers G, Bald R *et al*. Intravenous IgG during pregnancy for fetal alloimmune thrombocytopenic purpura. *Thromb Haemost* 1993; **69**: 997, poster 1625

315. Kanhai HH, Porcelijn L, van Zoeren D *et al*. Antenatal care in pregnancies at risk of alloimmune thrombocytopenia: report of 19 cases in 16 families. *Eur J Obstet Gynecol Reprod Biol* 1996; **68**: 67–73

316. Kornfeld I, Wilson RD, Ballem P, Wittmann BK, Farquharson DF. Antenatal invasive and noninvasive management of alloimmune thrombocytopenia. *Fetal Diagn Ther* 1996; **11**: 210–217

317. Murphy MF, Metcalfe P, Waters AH, Ord J, Hambley H, Nicolaides K. Antenatal management of severe fetomaternal thrombocytopenia: HLA incompatibility may affect responses to fetal platelet transfusions. *Blood* 1993; **81**: 2174–2179

318. Bussel JB, Druzin ML, Cines DB, Samuels P. Thrombocytopenia in pregnancy. *Lancet* 1991; **337**: 251

319. Ballin A, Andrew M, Ling E, Perlman M, Blanchette V. High dose intravenous gammaglobulin therapy for neonatal idiopathic autoimmune thrombocytopenia. *J Pediatr* 1988; **112**: 789–792

320. Blanchette V, Andrew M, Perlman M, Ling E, Ballin A. Neonatal autoimmune thrombocytopenia: Role of high-dose intravenous immunoglobulin G therapy. *Blut* 1989; **59**: 139–144

321. Christiaens G, Helmerhorst F. Validity of intrapartum diagnosis of fetal thrombocytopenia. *Am J Obstet Gynecol* 1987; **157**: 864–865

322. Pielet B, Socol M, MacGregor S, Ney J, Dooley S. Cordocentesis: an appraisal of risks. *Am J Obstet Gynecol* 1988; **159**: 1497–1500

323. Cook RL, Miller RC, Katz VL, Cefalo RC. Immune thrombocytopenic purpura in pregnancy: a reappraisal of management. *Obstet Gynecol* 1991; **78**: 567–583

324. Mandelbrot L, Schlienger I, Bongain A *et al*. Thrombocytopenia in pregnant women infected with human immunodeficiency virus: Maternal and neonatal outcome. *Am J Obstet Gynecol* 1994; **171**: 252–257

325. Hedberg VA, Lipton JM. Thrombocytopenia with absent radii. A review of 100 cases. *Am J Pediatr Hematol Oncol* 1988; **10**: 51–64

326. Labrune P, Pons JC, Khalil M *et al*. Antenatal thrombocytopenia in three patients with TAR (thrombocytopenia with absent radii) syndrome. *Prenat Diagn* 1993; **13**: 463–466

327. Weinblatt M, Petrikovsky B, Bialer M, Kochen J, Harper R. Prenatal evaluation and *in utero* platelet transfusion for thrombocytopenia absent radii syndrome. *Prenat Diagn* 1994; **14**: 892–896

328. Joenje H, Mathew C, Gluckman E. Fanconi anaemia research: current status and prospects. *Eur J Cancer* 1995; **31A**: 268–272

Thromboembolic complications

MAUREEN ANDREW AND LU ANN BROOKER

At the turn of the 20th century, thromboembolic disease in pediatric patients is a rapidly increasing, serious problem. The reasons for the emergence of this relatively new problem in children are complex and include:

- the capacity to cure most previously life-threatening disease which then permits the development of new diseases such as thromboembolic events (TEs);
- the necessity for venous and arterial catheters to treat critically ill children;
- the availability of sensitive radiographic tools that can diagnose TEs in unusual locations which were previously undetected;
- the capacity to identify children with congenital pre-thrombotic disorders.

Thromboembolic disease in adults has been recognized for centuries and affects nearly 5% of the population. The frequency and seriousness of TEs in adults led to the development of thromboembolism programs in the 1970s and to an enormous research effort at both the basic and clinical level. In the 1990s, the prevention and treatment of TEs in adults is based on well designed clinical trials that address critical clinical issues. Current studies in adults are directed at the fine tuning of therapies and more cost-effective measures for delivery of comparable care. Unfortunately, there is a paucity of well designed clinical trials in children addressing the issues of prevention and treatment of TEs. The absence of clinical trials reflects the relatively new development of TEs in children, the complexity and diversity of the underlying diseases, and the relatively small numbers of patients which necessitates expensive multicenter, multinational trials to change care. Despite these difficulties, there is an increasing awareness of the problem of TEs in children, and the need to systematically conduct clinical trials that will determine optimal care.

Currently, guidelines for the investigation, prevention and treatment of TEs in children are extrapolated from recommendations for adults with some modifications based upon available information in children.[1] This chapter reviews the available information on the epidemiology of both venous and arterial TEs in children based on Medline searches from 1966 to 1997. The recommendations for the prevention and treatment of TEs in children are based on those for adults, as well as the pediatric literature. All articles are evaluated in a standardized fashion based upon the strengths and weaknesses of study design (Table 34.1).[2] Only results from studies with the strongest designs, in combination with current recommendations for adults, were used as the basis for the recommendations.

In response to the clinical importance of TEs in children, pediatric thromboembolism programs are being developed and are modeled on the highly successful programs for adults. These programs are conducting clinical trials that address critical questions. Within the next 5 years, many of the 'guidelines' for the prevention and treatment of TEs in children will be firm 'recommendations' based upon well designed clinical trials.

VENOUS THROMBOEMBOLIC DISEASE

The incidence of venous thromboembolic disease in children is lower than in adults. The relative infrequency of TEs in children applies to both acquired and congenital prethrombotic states. Newborns, children under 1 year of age and teenagers are at greatest risk of TEs.

CONGENITAL PRETHROMBOTIC DISORDERS

The most frequent congenital prethrombotic disorders are activated protein C resistance (APCR) or Factor V Leiden, the newly described prothrombin mutant (FII 20210A),[3] deficiencies of protein C, protein S, antithrombin (AT) and dysfibrinogenemias. Less frequent congenital prethrombotic disorders are defects within the fibrinolytic system, hyper-homocystinemia, hyperlipidemia and rare platelet defects.

Table 34.1 Levels of evidence and grades of recommendations for therapy. Reproduced with permission from Ref. 2.

Level of evidence	Grade of recommendation
Level I	*Grade A*
Level I	Results come from a single RCT in which the lower limit of the CI for the treatment effect exceeds the minimal clinically important benefit.
Level I+	Results come from a meta-analysis of RCTs in which the treatment effects from individual studies are consistent, and the lower limit of the CI for the treatment effect exceeds the minimal clinically important benefit.
Level I−	Results come from a meta-analysis of RCTs in which the treatment effects from individual studies are widely disparate, but the lower limit of the CI for the treatment effect still exceeds the minimal clinically important benefit.
Level II	*Grade B*
Level II	Results come from a single RCT in which the CI for the treatment effect overlaps the minimal clinically important benefit.
Level II+	Results come from a meta-analysis of RCTs in which the treatment effects from individual studies are consistent and the CI for the treatment effect overlaps the minimal clinically important benefit.
Level II−	Results come from a meta-analysis of RCTs in which the treatment effects from individual studies are widely disparate, and the CI for the treatment effect overlaps the minimal clinically important benefit.
Level III	*Grade C* Results come from non-randomized concurrent cohort studies.
Level IV	*Grade C* Results come from non-randomized historic cohort studies.
Level V	*Grade C* Results come from case series.

RCT = Randomized controlled trial. CI = Confidence interval.

Single gene defects of these disorders usually present following puberty and rarely during childhood.[4-9] In contrast, double gene defects (except for APCR) usually present during childhood, often within hours of birth.[10]

Heterozygote congenital prethrombotic disorders

The incidence of congenital prethrombotic disorders in the general population and estimates of the relative risk they present for TEs are presented in Table 34.2. The commonest congenital prethrombotic disorder is Factor V Leiden, a point mutation in Factor V (R506Q) which was discovered by Dahlback in 1993.[11,12] Factor V Leiden confers resistance of the FVa molecule to degradation by APC.[12] Quantitative and qualitative deficiencies of protein C, protein S and AT are less common than APCR and reflect a variety of molecular defects.[13] The diagnosis of congenital prethrombotic disorders in children, when based on activity assays, must be made using age-related normal values.[14-16] At birth,

physiologic plasma concentrations of protein C, protein S and AT are significantly reduced and are in the range usually seen for heterozygote adults (see Chapter 33).[14-16] Plasma concentrations of protein C remain decreased throughout most of early childhood.[14-16] At birth, fibrinogen circulates in a fetal form, which influences some of the coagulation tests used to diagnose congenital dysfibrinogenemias.[14]

When individuals with a single gene defect for a prethrombotic disorder develop TEs during childhood, a secondary risk factor is usually present.[17] An accurate assessment of the contribution of congenital prethrombotic disorders to TEs during childhood is not available for several reasons. First, the discovery of the most frequent factor, Factor V Leiden, is very recent and most published pediatric studies did not screen for this defect. Secondly, reports on the contribution of congenital prethrombotic disorders to the presence of TEs are often based on referrals to tertiary care pediatric centers, which probably falsely increases the incidence.[18] Thirdly, population-based studies are difficult and expensive in pediatrics. Despite these limitations, some conclusions can be drawn from the pediatric literature. A minimal estimate of the contribution of congenital prethrombotic disorders to children with TEs is 10%[4] with a probable frequency of approximately 25%.[19-22] Although there is agreement on the initial treatment of TEs with anticoagulants, there is a paucity of information on the benefits and safety for long-term prophylaxis versus careful monitoring with intermittent prophylaxis.[2] Treatment of children with a congenital prethrombotic disorder but without a TE, is usually restricted to prophylactic therapy in high-risk acquired conditions (significant immobility, surgery, trauma and others). Anticoagulant options include

Table 34.2 Prevalence of inherited thrombophilic disorders in different populations.

Population	Protein C deficient	Protein S deficient	AT deficient	Factor V:Q[506]
Normal population (%)	0.3	−	0.04	5
Unselected patients with thrombosis (%)	3	1.5	1	20
Patients with thrombosis and suspected thrombophilia (%)	7.9	7.2	5.3	52

heparin, low molecular weight heparin (LMWH) or oral anticoagulants (see below).

Homozygote congenital prethrombotic disorders

The presentation of patients with homozygous congenital prethrombotic disorders depends to some extent on the specific defect and the severity of the deficiency. Newborns with double gene defects for either protein C or S deficiency, and with unmeasurable plasma activities of the affected inhibitor, present within hours of birth with purpura fulminans, cerebral and/or ophthalmic damage which occurred *in utero*, and, on rare occasions, large vessel thrombosis. Purpura fulminans is an acute, lethal syndrome of rapidly progressive hemorrhagic necrosis of the skin due to dermal vascular thrombosis.[23-25] In contrast, patients with double gene defects for either protein C or S deficiency, with measurable plasma activities (usually 0.01–0.2 unit/ml) present during childhood with venous TEs following a minor secondary insult and/or oral anticoagulant-induced skin necrosis.[10] Patients with homozygous Factor V Leiden have an increased risk of thrombosis and usually present in early adult life.[26] However, there is considerable variability in presentation with some patients remaining asymptomatic despite acquired thrombotic risk factors.[27,28]

Initial therapy for purpura fulminans due to homozygous protein C or S deficiency is replacement therapy beginning with 10–20 ml/kg of fresh frozen plasma (FFP) every 8–12 hours.[29-31] Protein C concentrates are available and can be substituted for FFP in doses of 20–60 units/kg when the specific defect is confirmed. Resolution of the clinical lesions from purpura fulminans usually require replacement therapy for 6–8 hours.[32] One approach to long-term therapy is oral anticoagulants alone, or in conjunction with replacement therapy.[10] Unfortunately, the intensity of oral anticoagulant therapy required is usually greater than for the usual treatment of venous TEs because of the imbalance in plasma concentrations between vitamin K-dependent coagulant proteins and either protein C or S. Usually an International Normalized Ratio (INR) between 3.0 and 4.5 is necessary to prevent recurrent purpura fulminans unless concomitant replacement therapy is used.[10] LMWH provides an alternative therapy for homozygous protein C- or S-deficient patients who have detectable plasma concentrations of the deficient protein. LMWH avoids the risk of skin necrosis and reduces the risk of bleeding secondary to oral anticoagulant therapy.[33] The role of LMWH in children with no detectable levels of protein C or S has not been determined and may not be effective. Liver transplantation has also been used to treat patients with undetectable levels of protein C.[34]

ACQUIRED VENOUS THROMBOEMBOLIC COMPLICATIONS

For >95% of children, venous TEs are secondary to serious, underlying disorders.[4] The age distribution shows that infants and teenagers are the pediatric populations at greatest risk for TEs (Fig. 34.1).[4] The age distribution is important because of the relative immaturity of the hemostatic system within the first year of life which influences the response to antithrombotic agents (see Chapter 33). Most children have more than one risk factor for thrombosis. However, the single commonest direct cause for TEs is a central venous line (CVL).[4] Underlying medical conditions include prematurity, cancer, trauma/surgery, congenital heart disease (CHD), systemic lupus erythematosus (SLE) and others (M Andrew, unpublished observations).[4,35-37]

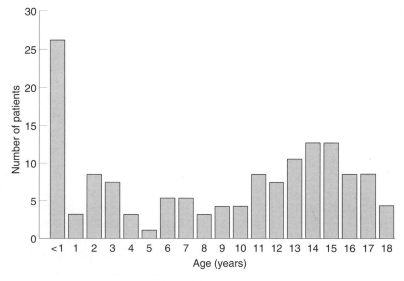

Fig. 34.1 Age distribution of children with a thromboembolic event. Reproduced with permission from Ref. 4.

The clinical presentation of deep vein thrombosis (DVT) consists of pain, discoloration and swelling of the affected extremity, and of pulmonary embolism (PE), shortness of breath, pleuritic chest pain, cyanosis and syncope. In many children the clinical symptoms of DVT and/or PE are subtle and may be initially overlooked.

CVL-related thromboembolic complications

Pediatric populations requiring CVLs can be grouped into those requiring relatively short-term care (i.e. the neonatal and pediatric intensive care settings) and those requiring longer term care (i.e. home total parenteral nutrition [TPN], treatment for cancer or hemodialysis).[38–45] Within each of these groups, another risk factor that influences the incidence of TEs is the solution infused.[37] The clinical presentation of CVL-related TEs is diverse and includes acute symptoms such as 'blocking' of the CVL, swelling and pain of the extremity, headache and/or swelling of the face, persistent sepsis and symptoms of PE. More chronic presentations include the gradual presence of collateral circulation in the skin (Plate 41), and repeated 'problems' with CVL patency. For some children requiring a CVL and who have a CVL-related DVT, low-dose warfarin or LMWH may be helpful until the CVL is removed.

Right atrial thrombosis

A right atrial thrombosis is frequently clinically 'asymptomatic' and identified on a routine echocardiogram in children with CHD, or children receiving cardiotoxic agents for their primary disease (e.g. acute lymphoblastic leukemia). Right atrial thrombosis also seems to occur more frequently in neonates with CVLs.[46,47] Clinically overt symptoms include cardiac failure, CVL malfunction, persistent sepsis and the appearance of a new cardiac murmur.[47–50] Optimal approaches to right atrial thrombosis are uncertain and will probably differ depending upon the patient population. Therapeutic options consist of anticoagulation, thrombolytic therapy and surgery.[47–50]

Renal vein thrombosis

Approximately 80% of all renal vein thromboses (RVT) occur in the first month of life, and usually within the first week of life. Some infants develop RVT *in utero*. The incidence in males and females is similar, and both right and left renal veins are equally affected. Bilateral RVT occurs in approximately one-quarter of patients. The most frequent clinical presentation in newborns consists of hematuria, an enlarged kidney and thrombocytopenia. Acute extensive involvement of the inferior vena cava (IVC) presents with cold, cyanotic and edematous lower extremities. Chronic obstruction of the IVC presents with dilatation of collateral veins over the abdomen and upper thighs. Of the identified etiologies of RVT, perinatal asphyxia,

shock, polycythemia and cyanotic CHD are the most frequent.[51] In older children the common presenting features are hematuria (22%), flank pain (14%), edema (11%) and an enlarged kidney (7%). In these children RVT is most commonly secondary to nephrotic syndrome, burns, dehydration, AT deficiency and SLE.[52] Ultrasound is the diagnostic test of choice as it is easy to perform and sensitive to an enlarged kidney.

Optimal treatment of RVT is unclear. One approach is to use supportive care for unilateral RVT in the absence of uremia and extension into the IVC. Heparin or LMWH are therapeutic options when the RVT is bilateral or the IVC is involved. Thombolytic activity is an option in the presence of bilateral RVT and impending renal failure. The vascular requirements for future kidney transplantation may also influence the decision to use thrombolytic therapy. Although RVT is rarely fatal, the long-term complications have not been adequately studied.

Portal vein thrombosis

In newborns, portal vein thrombosis (PVT) most commonly occurs secondary to umbilical vein catheterization or sepsis,[53,54] and in older children, secondary to liver transplantation, intra-abdominal sepsis, splenectomy, sickle cell anemia and/or antiphospholipid antibodies.[55–62] In approximately 50% of cases an underlying etiology is not identified.[56,63,64] In contrast to adults with PVT secondary to cirrhosis, liver function is usually normal in children.[60] PVT may be partial or complete and the degree of obstruction influences the clinical symptoms.[65] PVT may present acutely, as an acute abdomen, especially in adolescents.[58] More commonly, the clinical presentations due to chronic obstruction are major gastrointestinal bleeding or asymptomatic splenomegaly.[60,63,66] Gastrointestinal bleeding is frequently recurrent.[67]

Radiographic tests that can detect PVT include ultrasound, MRI, angiography and CT scan.[68–71] Within 6–20 days following PVT, a sponge-like mass of collateral vessels forms. This cavernous transformation can extend, resulting in intrahepatic shunting between segmental portal veins, and into the systemic circulation, resulting in portal hypertension.[72] Variceal hemorrhagic complications are an important clinical consequence of portal hypertension secondary to PVT. Less commonly portal hypertension may be associated with fatal pulmonary hypertension.[73]

Therapeutic options are, to some extent, determined by the time from the event and consist of supportive care alone, thrombolysis, antithrombotic agents, balloon thrombectomy, or dilatation and thrombectomy.[74–76] Esophageal varices are usually initially treated with sclerotherapy. Other therapeutic options have included endoscopic variceal ligation[77] and portosystemic shunts. Due to the usually normal liver function, death is often the result of the underlying disorder and not the PVT.[65]

Sinovenous thrombosis

Sinovenous thrombosis in newborns is characterized by thrombosis of the intracranial venous system and frequently presents with seizures, lethargy and/or intermittent hyperexcitability. Heparin therapy is currently recommended for adults based on positive results in one randomized controlled trial.[78] Although there are no controlled studies in newborns, the common pathophysiology and relatively poor prognosis[78-83] suggest that therapy with heparin or LMWH should be considered.[84]

Neonatal venous thromboembolism

Reviews of the literature[85-87] and an international registry of neonatal thrombotic disease[88] provide information on the epidemiology of venous TEs in newborns. They occur in approximately 2.4/1000 admissions to neonatal intensive care units.[88] These infants are usually critically ill with a variety of risk factors for thrombosis including increased blood viscosity, poor deformability of physiologically large red cells, polycythemia, dehydration, and a variety of medical problems that activate the coagulation and fibrinolytic systems. CVLs, placed in umbilical veins or other central locations are responsible for >80% of venous TEs in newborns.[4,37,89] Autopsy studies report that 20–60% of infants who die with a CVL in place have an associated thrombus. Short-term complications from CVL-related TEs include serious organ or limb impairment, PVT, RVT, hepatic necrosis and PE. Potential long-term sequelae of umbilical venous CVLs are PVT with portal hypertension, splenomegaly, gastric and esophageal varices, and hypertension. RVTs are the most frequent form of non-CVL-related TEs in newborns.[88] Spontaneous venous TEs do occur, although rarely, at other sites which include adrenal veins, IVC, portal vein, hepatic veins and the venous system of the brain.[85,87]

DIAGNOSIS

The accurate diagnosis of venous TE events in children is dependent upon the use of objective radiographic tests. The multiple and diverse location of thrombosis, limited mobility of many critically ill patients, and frequency of CVL-related TEs influence the selection of diagnostic tests. The clinical diagnosis of DVT is as non-specific in children as in adults, with only 19% positivity in one retrospective review of venograms performed for clinically suspected DVT.[90] Although non-invasive diagnostic tests for venous TEs in adults have been validated, there are no studies addressing this issue in pediatric patients. Thus, venography remains the 'gold standard' for the diagnosis of most venous TEs in children. Venography (dye injected into a vein in the limb) should not be confused with lineograms (injection of dye into CVLs). Lineograms can locate the tip of CVLs and clots at

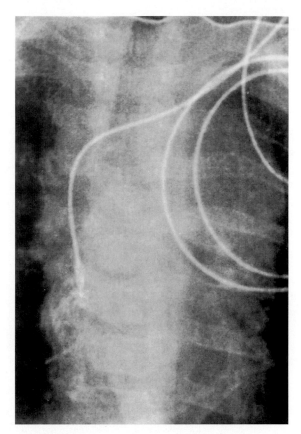

Fig. 34.2 Lineogram showing a clot at the tip of the catheter.

the tip, but cannot detect large vessel thrombosis along the intravascular length of the CVL (Fig. 34.2).

The reported incidences of CVL-related TEs have a wide range and, in large part, reflect the chosen diagnostic test. For example, the incidence of CVL-related TEs in children receiving home TPN ranges from 1 to 70%,[39,91-101] with the lowest frequencies reflecting the clinical diagnosis of superior vena cava (SVC) syndrome and the highest reflecting venographic evidence of thrombosis (Fig. 34.3).[39,98,102-106] For many children, the architecture of the venous system is completely destroyed with extensive, tortuous collaterals providing drainage from the arms and head (Fig. 34.3).

COMPLICATIONS

Acute complications of venous TEs include PE, extension into the heart, end-organ damage and death.[4] Long-term complications include the risk of recurrent TEs, bleeding from the long-term anticoagulants, ruptured collateral varices,[4] loss of venous access and repeated anesthesia/surgery for CVL replacement.

Pulmonary embolism

The clinical presentation of PE in children can be subtle, even asymptomatic, or it can consist of the classical symptoms of dyspnea, tachypnea and associated TEs.[107,108] The

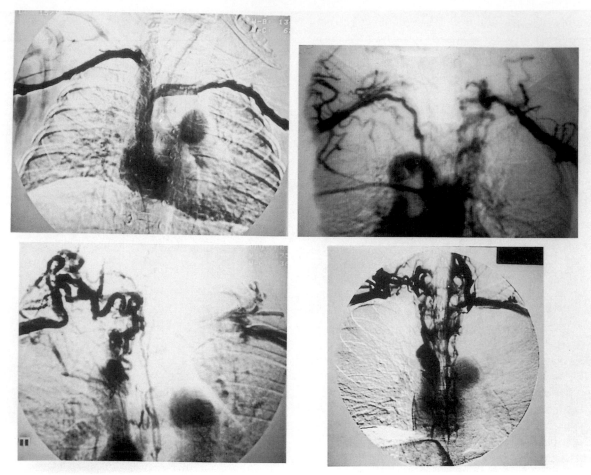

Fig. 34.3 Four panel venography of children with a thromboembolic event. The top left panel shows a normal venogram in a child, and the other three panels show abnormal venograms in three children. Reproduced with permission from Ref. 102.

mortality of PE may be lower in children than in adults, reflecting superior physiologic tolerance to PE in younger patients.[109,110] The diagnosis of PE is usually made with a ventilation/perfusion scan (VQ) or, less commonly, an angiogram.[37] Results of VQ scans can be considered as normal; high probability in the presence of a mismatched segment or multiple mismatched subsegments; and indeterminate when there are matched segmental or subsegmental defects. Low probability V/Q scans have non-segmental perfusion defects or matched V/Q defects. Intermediate scans are those which cannot be categorized as high or low. This group constitutes approximately 70% of clinically driven V/Q scans in adults. An intermediate or indeterminate scan does not exclude PE, as 33% of adults with clinically suspected PE who have intermediate scans do have PE when assessed by the gold standard (pulmonary angiography).[111] PE is probably underdiagnosed in children.[4]

Recurrent thrombotic disease

In a prospective cohort of 405 children with a median follow-up of 2.9 years, the recurrence rate was 8%,[112] which is similar to adults.[113–115] The mean time to recurrence was 6 months (range: 3 months to 5 years). The majority of children (63%) had multiple predisposing risk factors, including the presence of CVLs in 46% of patients.[116] Long-term anticoagulation may be required for some children with recurrent TEs, particularly if ongoing risk factors or a congenital prethrombotic disorder are present.

Post-phlebitic syndrome

Post-phlebitic syndrome (PPS), which is due to persistent damage to venous valves, is characterized by swelling, pain, pigmentation, induration of the skin and ulceration.[117] In adults, symptoms may occur early, or be delayed for as long as 5–10 years after the initial TE. The frequency and severity of PPS are probably related to the extent and recurrence of DVT.[4] The natural history of PPS in children with thromboembolic disease is unknown but is unlikely to be less devastating than for adults. The incidence of PPS in children has been reported in 3 studies and ranges between 10 and 25%.[4,116,117] Further prospective studies are required accurately to determine the incidence and predisposing features for PPS in children. Physiologically, it is feasible that the incidence of PPS in children will exceed that for adults because of the relatively suppressed fibrinolytic system in the young and the number of years that they will be at risk for this complication.[16,118]

Mortality

Although relatively uncommon, death from TE does occur in pediatric patients. In the Canadian registry, 2.2% of children died as a direct result of either TEs due to PE and/or extension of DVT into the heart.[116]

ARTERIAL THROMBOEMBOLIC DISEASE

Successful treatment of serious primary problems in children are paradoxically responsible for arterial TEs which cause considerable morbidity and, in some cases, mortality. Arterial TEs in children can be grouped as either catheter or non-catheter in origin. Arterial catheters are placed for monitoring and providing supportive care to critically ill children. The following sections summarize currently available information, which is largely based on case series or individual case reports.

CATHETER-RELATED ARTERIAL THROMBOEMBOLIC COMPLICATIONS

The commonest forms of arterial catheterization include umbilical artery catheterization (UAC) in newborns, peripheral arterial catheters (PACs) in the intensive care setting and cardiac catheterization (CC) through the femoral artery for diagnostic and therapeutic purposes.

Umbilical artery catheterization

Arterial access in sick newborns is necessary for continuous monitoring of oxygen saturation, blood gas analyses, blood pressure and facilitation of repetitive blood sampling. The umbilical artery is usually chosen because of its relatively large size and easy accessibility. The critical presentation of UAC-related TEs is dependent on the extent of the thrombus, involvement of other arteries, and embolization to distant sites. While some infants are clinically asymptomatic, others present with evidence of severe ischemia to the legs and/or threatened organ function. Based on clinical diagnosis, the reported incidence of UAC-related TEs is approximately 1%.[119] Autopsy studies and angiographic studies report a range of incidences of 3–59%[120] and 10–90%, respectively.[120–125]

The diagnosis of UAC-related TEs is problematic and the choice of radiologic test is responsible to some extent for the variability in the reported incidence of this problem. The reference test for UAC-related TEs is contrast angiography.[85] Unfortunately, transportation of critically ill infants

to the radiology department for angiography is frequently not feasible and bedside ultrasound is the most commonly used diagnostic test.[126] Unfortunately, the sensitivity and specificity of ultrasound for the diagnosis of UAC-related TEs is unknown, with some studies indicating a poor sensitivity.[127] A disturbingly large proportion of aortic TEs (24%) are diagnosed at autopsy.[85]

There are 6 well designed, controlled trials assessing the use of very low dose (3–5 units/h), continous infusion heparin in the prolongation of UAC patency and all reported a consistent benefit (Table 34.3).[128–133] The outcomes assessed were patency, local thrombus and intracranial hemorrhage (ICH), as determined by ultrasound or clinical catheter occlusion. Patency was prolonged in 5 studies[129–133] and continuous heparin was more effective than intermittent heparin flushes.[132] One study with continuous heparin failed to show a reduced incidence of thrombosis, as detected by ultrasound, although catheter occlusion and hypertension were significantly increased in the control arm.[129] Heparin-bonded catheters also reduced the risk of thrombosis.[128] Similarly, the sample size in the one retrospective study that assessed the influence of heparin on ICH was too small to come to any conclusive result.[134] A survey of American neonatal intensive care units reported that 75% use heparin prophylaxis in concentrations between 0.01 and 2.0 units/ml.[135] Therapeutic options for newborns with UAC-related TEs depend on the extent of the thrombus, and compromise of limb or organ. Thrombolytic and anticoagulation therapy are important modalities for clinically significant UAC-related TEs. The outcome of symptomatic UAC-related TEs has been assessed in 7 long-term

Table 34.3 Comparison of outcome for umbilical artery catheterization. Reproduced with permission from Ref. 1.

Reference	Level	Intervention	Number of patients	Outcome Bleeding	Outcome Event (B or TE)
Jackson et al (1987)[128]	II	HB-PU	61	NR	13 TE
		PVC	64	NR	23 TE
Horgan et al (1987)[129]	II	Heparin	59	NR	16 TE
		No heparin	52	NR	18 TE
Rajani et al (1979)[130]	I	Heparin	32	NR	4 B†
		Placebo	30	NR	19 B
David et al (1981)[131]	II	Heparin	26	0*	3 B†
		No heparin	26	0*	15 B
Bosque et al (1986)[132]	II	Heparin (C)	18	NR	0 B†
		Heparin (I)	19	NR	8 B
Horgan et al (1987)[129]	II	Heparin	59	NR	2 B†
		No heparin	52	NR	10 B
Ankola and Atakent (1993)[133]	II	Heparin	15	4 ICH	2 B†
		No heparin	15	5 ICH	11 B

B = Blocked; TE = thromboembolic event; HB-PU = heparin bonded-polyurethane; PVC = polyvinyl chloride; C = continuous; I = intermittent; ICH = intracranial hemorrhage; NR = not reported.
*No hemorrhage; †p = <0.05

studies.[128–133] Symptomatic, acute TE may cause severe organ or limb impairment or death.[136,137] Other morbidity consists of hypertension, impaired renal function, discrepancies in leg length and claudication.

Peripheral arterial catheters

Occlusion of PACs is problematic because of the need to replace them and the potential ischemic insult to the limb involved. The incidence of thrombotic occlusion of PACs in the absence of heparin is influenced by catheter material,[138,139] duration of placement,[139] diameter,[139] length,[140] solution infused,[140] concentration of heparin[141] and arterial site.[139] For these reasons, low-dose heparin therapy is commonly administered locally through arterial catheters as either intermittent flushes or by continuous infusion.[140] Early studies showed that intermittent flushes of heparin do not adequately protect against loss of PAC patency.[139] At least three randomized controlled trials in adults convincingly show a benefit from low-dose infusions of heparin for the patency of PACs.[140,142,143]

Cardiac catheterization

The vast majority of CCs are performed via the femoral artery. The incidence of TEs in the presence of prophylactic heparin therapy is approximately 5%, with young children disproportionately affected.[144–150] Other factors that influence the incidence of CC-related TEs include the ratio of catheter:vessel diameter and balloon dilatation. The incidence of severe arterial complications is diminished by the use of smaller catheters introduced through a femoral artery sheath, and by careful monitoring of distal pulses after catheter removal. The clinical symptoms of TEs following catheterization of the femoral artery include a cold, pale limb with dimished or absent pulses, diminished peripheral perfusion, decreased blood pressure in the affected limb in excess of 10 mmHg compared to the other limb, and diminished skin temperature. Although contrast angiography is probably the most reliable radiographic test, it is rarely practical in the acute situation of arterial thrombosis.

Relatively few trials have focused on the prevention of femoral artery TEs following CC. The most convincing data come from 2 randomized, placebo-controlled trials performed in 1974 by Freed et al.[147,151] The first showed that aspirin had no beneficial influence on the incidence of femoral artery TEs,[151] while the second showed that a bolus heparin dose of 100 units/kg reduced the incidence from 40 to 8%[147] based on the pulse volume index, and the need for surgical embolectomy (p = <0.01). A more recent study by Rao et al[152] reported that approximately 10 units/kg in the flush solution was equivalent to a bolus of 100 units/kg for the prevention of arterial thrombosis. However, 75% of patients were older than 5 years of age which may have influenced the incidence of TEs.[152] Current practice is to administer a heparin bolus of 100–150 units/kg at the time of femoral artery catheterization. If procedures are prolonged, a second heparin bolus is commonly given and an activated whole blood clot time (ACT) is frequently used to monitor hepain therapy.

Unfortunately, femoral artery TEs still occur with an incidence of 3–5%.[146,153,154] Treatment is usually indicated because of the threat of loss of limb or long-term vascular insufficiency resulting in claudication and poor growth with a smaller leg.[155,156] The short-term consequences of a femoral artery TE include threatened viability to the limb, while long-term problems include leg length discrepancies, muscle wasting and claudication.[157] Therapeutic options consist of anticoagulation, thrombolytic therapy and/or embolectomy. Usually, initial therapy consists of anticoagulation with heparin which is effective in approximately 70% of events.[156] If there is no resolution with heparin, thrombolytic therapy is usually initiated as the second-line therapy. Streptokinase, urokinase and tissue plasminogen activator (tPA) have all been used to treat femoral artery TEs in children.[149,156,158] In one study, 85% of femoral artery TEs that failed to resolve on anticoagulant therapy were successfully treated with thrombolytic therapy, with minimal bleeding complications.[156] These patients required, on average, 7 hours of therapy (range: 2–16) with <1% requiring subsequent embolectomy.

NON-CATHETER-RELATED ARTERIAL THROMBOEMBOLIC COMPLICATIONS

Non-catheter-related arterial TEs have congenital and acquired etiologies. *Congenital* etiologies of arterial disease which present during childhood include familial homozygous hypercholesterolemia (FH)[159,160] and hyperhomocystinuria.[161–163] *Acquired* disorders that cause arterial TEs include Takayasu's arteritis,[164–166] occlusion of giant coronary aneurysms secondary to Kawasaki disease,[167–169] occlusion of arteries in transplanted organs,[170–174] acquired heart disease and CHD.[175–177]

Congential prethrombotic disorders

Hyperlipidemia

Hyperlipidemia is a major risk factor for adult atherosclerotic vascular disease and there is considerable evidence that hypercholesterolemic adults have abnormal lipid levels during childhood.[178] The classic hyperlipidemic state associated with myocardial infarction in childhood is homozygous FH.[159,160] This disease is due to absent or defective low density lipoprotein (LDL) receptors leading to increased plasma concentrations of LDL. Inheritance is autosomal dominant with 1/500 of the population being heterozygous and 1/10[6] children being homozygous. Heterozygotes usually do not develop clinical ischemic heart disease until early adult life.[179] However, endothelial dysfunction can be demonstrated in these patients during early childhood.[180,181]

Nearly two-thirds of asymptomatic teenagers with hetero-zygous FH have abnormal cardiac stress thallium scans[182] which correlate with angiographic abnormalities.[183] Homo-zygotes with FH present with markedly increased serum cholesterol levels from birth, cutaneous xanthomata and evidence of coronary artery disease within the first decade of life.[179] Death from acute myocardial infarction has occurred as early as 18 months and survival beyond the third decade is rare.[179,184–187]

Children develop a classic pattern of atherosclerosis involving the aortic root (which leads to aortic stenosis) and coronary artery ostia (which leads to obstruc-tion).[159,185] Distal coronary arteries are often pristine until adult life. Receptor-negative patients have more severe disease than receptor-defective patients.[160] Peripheral atherosclerosis does not usually present during child-hood.[188] Similarly, several retrospective studies have failed to demonstrate a significant role for hyperlipidemia in childhood stroke.[189] Autopsy and radiographic studies have shown that atherosclerosis in the cerebral circulation lags many years behind aortic and coronary artery disease.[190–192] Plasmapheresis and LDL apheresis are the current treatments of choice.[179,193,194] Causes of secondary hyperlipidemia in childhood include poorly controlled insulin-dependent diabetes mellitus, hypothyroidism, hepatic glycogenesis, obstructive liver disease and nephrotic syndrome.[195,196]

Hyperhomocysteinemia

Homocysteine is a sulfur-containing amino acid formed by the demethylation of dietary methionine which is dependent on the cofactors folic acid, vitamin B_6 and vitamin B_{12}. Hyperhomocysteinemia can have both a genetic and a nutritional basis. Genetic cause are cystathionine-B-synthase deficiency[197] and 5,10-methylenetetrahydrofolate reductase deficiency.[198] The recently identified thermolabile variant of methylenetetrahydrofolate reductase, which occurs in 5–30% of the population, causes hyperhomocysteinemia and lower plasma folate concentrations.[199,200] Children classi-cally present wtih a non-progressive encephalopathy, high myopia, lens dislocation, osteoporosis and Marfan's-like habitus. Treatment involves replacement therapy with vitamin B_6 and dietary management.

Nutritional causes of hyperhomocysteinemia may occur in patients with folate deficiency, vitamin B_{12} deficiency and patients with chronic renal failure.[201,202] Hyperhomocystei-nemia is a proven independent risk factor for atherosclerotic vascular disease affecting the coronary, cerebral and periph-eral arteries.[161–163] The mechanim by which homocysteine induces its prethrombotic state reflects an imbalance between procoagulant and anticoagulant properies of the endothelial surface. Homocysteine also promotes vascular smooth muscle cell growth, oxidizes LDL and may adversely affect platelet function. Therapeutically, supplementation with folic acid can reduce plasma concentrations of homo-

cyteine; however, the reduction of vascular disease remains to be proven.[203]

Acquired thrombotic disease

Takayasu's arteritis

Takayasu's arteritis is a rare chronic, idopathic inflamma-tory disease of large arteries predominantly affecting Asian females.[204] Although any artery can be involved, angio-graphic studies show that two-thirds of patients have aortic lesions, with aortic arch, carotid arteries and renal arteries being primarily affected.[205] The clinical presentation is limb or organ ischemia due to gradual stenosis of related arteries.[206] Clinical symptoms reflect the affected arteries.[206,207] Physical findings frequently include a bruit in the involved area.[206] The diagnosis is frequently delayed by several months.[206] Angiography remains the gold standard for the assessment of clinical severity of the disease. Glucocorticoids are the mainstay of medical therapy with at least 60% of patients achieving remission within 1 year of treatment.[204,208] Unfortunately, 50% of patients relapse and additional cytotoxic agents such as methotrexate or cyclophosphamide are required.[204,208] Arterial reconstruction is required for at least one-third of patients.[205–207,209]

Kawasaki disease

Kawasaki disease (mucocutaneous lymph node syndrome) is characterized by fever of >5 days' duration, cervical lym-phadenopathy, bilateral non-exudative conjunctivitis, rash, mucous membrane and peripheral extremity changes, not explained by another disease process.[210,211] Coronary aneur-ysms occur in 20% of children who receive therapy,[212] and can be pervented in most by the early use of high-dose aspirin (80–100 mg/kg/day for up to 14 days)[167–169] and intravenous gamma globulin.[169] A recent meta-analysis of coronary artery aneurysm prevention therapy recom-mended high-dose aspirin and a single large infusion of gamma globulin as the optimal protocol.[213,214] Subsequent use of low-dose aspirin, 3–5 mg/kg/day for 7 weeks or longer, is indicated to prevent coronary aneurysm thrombosis. If giant coronary aneurysms develop, anticoagulation has been recommended;[215] however, the relative benefits of warfarin versus aspirin are unknown. Surgical management is con-sidered in some patients.[216] Myocardial infarction due to thrombosis of a coronary artery aneurysm remains the major cause of death in Kawasaki disease.

Paroxysmal nocturnal hemoglobinuria

Paroxysmal nocturnal hemoglobinuria (PNH) is an acquired disorder of hemopoietic stem cells.[217] A somatic mutation of the phosphatidylinositol glycan class A (PIG A) gene occurs on the X chromosome. To date 84 separate mutations in the PIG A gene, mostly deletion or insertion mutations, have been described in association with PNH.[217] The PIG A gene is involved in the synthesis of the glycosyl phosphatitdylinositol (GPI) anchor, to which many cell surface proteins are attached. Proteins known to be deficient on abnormal PNH cells include complement defense proteins such as decay accelerating factor (DAF, CD55) and membrane inhibitor of reactive lysis (MIRL, CD59); enzymes, e.g. urokinase receptor; and proteins of unknown function such as CD66.[133]

PNH is a rare disease which usually presents in adulthood. Several large studies have reported 12–21% of cases occurring in children.[218,219] The diagnosis is frequently delayed with the mean time to diagnosis being 19 months in both adults and children.[219] There are significant differences in the natural history of PNH in children compared with adults.[219] PNH classically presents with hemoglobinuria, although this presentation is seen in only 15% of children (in contrast to 50% of adults). The commonest presentation in children is bone marrow failure (50% cf 25% of adults). Anemia is commonly associated with macrocytosis in children.[219]

Thrombosis is a major complication of PNH and reported incidence rates are 39% of adults and 31% of children.[219,220] The cumulative incidence increases with duration of follow-up and may be as high as 50% after 15 years.[218] Thrombosis is usually venous and frequently involves the hepatic veins (Budd Chiari syndrome), CNS portal veins and peripheral venous systems.[218–221] Thrombosis is a common cause of death in patients with PNH. Primary prophylactic anticoagulation with warfarin has been recommended, although bleeding complications are frequent.[220] No fibrinolytic or coagulation abnormalities have been documented in PNH, although increased circulating activated platelets are implicated in the thrombotic risk.[222] Median suvival times are approximately 10–15 years in a number of studies.[218–220] Bone marrow transplantation is the only curative treatment and may result in resolution of progressive hepatic venous thrombosis.[223] Spontaneous remissions occur in 15% of patients.[220]

Arterial thrombosis following organ transplantation

Arterial occlusion following organ transplantation is a more frequent problem in children, particularly young infants, compared to older children and adults. Most arterial TEs occur following kidney and liver transplantation.

Kidney transplantation. Following kidney transplantation, renal artery thrombosis (RAT) occurs in 0.2–3.5% of pediatric patients, and presents with primary anuria and/or clinical symptoms of rejection.[224–226] Although multiple factors influence the development of RAT, young donors and small recipients are disproportionately affected, probably reflecting the small size of the vessels and anastomotic techniques.[225,227] Other factors predisposing to thrombosis include surgical technique, preimplantation damage, hypotension or hypoperfusion, prior nephrectomy and rejection.[225] There are no randomized controlled trials assessing prophylactic anticoagulation therapy in children. One large cohort study used prophylactic LMWH at a dose of 0.4 mg/kg bid for 21 days in a case series.[228] Only one child of the 70 developed an arterial thrombosis.[228] Therapeutic options include anticoagulation, thrombolytic therapy and surgical embolectomy.[225] Unfortunately, most therapeutic interventions fail with subsequent renal graft loss and the requirement for another transplantation.

Hepatic artery thrombosis. Hepatic artery thrombosis (HAT), a life-threatening complication, occurs in 3.1–29% of children[229–231] compared to only 1.5% of adults following liver transplantation.[232,233] Similar to renal transplantation, small recipients from young donors are at the greatest risk.[229] The clinical presentation of HAT is delayed, usually until the second week following transplantation.[172,234] The clinical symptoms are frequently subtle, and the clinical course can be indolent. Many centers regularly screen their patients with pulsed Doppler combined with real-time ultrasonography of the liver parenchyma.[235,236] Because false positive and negative results occur, confirmatory tests such as angiography, CT, spiral CT[237] and MRI[172,238] are required. Prophylactic interventions with anticoagulants including heparin, LMWH or aspirin are of unproven benefit. However, the delay in occurrence of HAT and the report of a circulating dermatan sulfate proteoglycan in the first postoperative week, suggest that anticoagulation may be helpful.[239] When HAT occurs, therapeutic options include surgical revascularization procedures,[240,241] thrombolytic therapy,[242] and re-transplantation. Untreated, HAT has a significant mortality.[238,240]

Congenital and acquired heart disease

Mechanical prosthetic heart valves

Cardiac valvular disease occurs as an isolated congenital event, as part of complex CHD, or as a result of treatments for an underlying cardiac disorder. Thrombosis of the valve or embolization to the CNS are both serious complications of mechanical prosthetic heart valves.[175,243–249] Currently, mechanical prosthetic heart valves are usually used in the mitral and aortic position while biologic prosthetic heart valves are used for tricuspid or pulmonary valve replacements in children. Randomized controlled trials in adults with mechanical prosthetic heart valves have clearly delineated the need for oral anticoagulants with an INR of 2.5–3.5.[250–252] Antiplatelet agents have a role if there is more than one valve or a TE has occurred with a therapeutic INR.[253] There are no randomized controlled trials in children, only case series. In the absence of oral anticoagulants, and in the presence of no therapy or antiplatelet agents alone, the incidence of TEs is unacceptably increased in some studies.[254,255] Only oral anticoagulants consistently maintained the incidence of TEs at <5% per patient year, which is similar to that for adults.[254,256–258] With one exception, the rate of major bleeding was <3.5% per patient year. Available data support the recommendation for oral anticoagulation in children with mechanical prosthetic heart valves. Aspirin in combination with oral anticoagulants may be helpful in high-risk patients such as those with prior TEs, atrial fibrillation, a large left atrium and/or multiple mechanical prosthetic heart valves.

Blalock–Taussig shunts

Blalock–Taussig shunts and modifications enhance pulmonary blood flow by redirecting subclavian arterial flow to the pulmonary artery. Gortex grafts are frequently used in 'modified' Blalock–Taussig shunts.[176,259] Since 1980, 624 children with Blalock–Taussig shunts have been reported in several case series and the incidence of thrombotic occlusion ranged from 1 to 17%. Initial treatment with heparin followed by aspirin (1–10 mg/kg/day) is a commonly used prophylactic regimen.[260]

Fontan operation

The principle of the Fontan procedure is the diversion of the systemic venous return directly to the pulmonary arteries, in the setting of single ventricle physiology.[261] This may involve the use of atriopulmonary, total cavopulmonary (lateral tunnel), or extracardiac (constructed with pericardium, Dacron or Gortex) surgical connections. Blood flow through the atria or lateral tunnel may be directed by a polytetrafluoroethylene (PFTE) baffle. TEs, both intracardiac and strokes, remain a major cause of mortality and morbidity following Fontan procedures. Information on TEs following Fontan has been provided by 35 papers and the reported incidences vary with study design and the sensitivity of the diagnostic tests used.[177,261–294] Two cross-sectional studies estimated the point prevalence of intracardiac TE to be 17–20%.[274,290] Approximately 50% of the reported TEs occurred later than 3 months following the procedure. There is no consensus in the literature with regards to specific risk factors. Only one study has assessed routine anticoagulation prophylaxis and reported a TE incidence of 7.4% over short-term follow-up.[268] The optimal prophylactic therapy (warfarin, aspirin) and optimal duration of prophylaxis is unknown. Despite aggressive management, total resolution occurred in only 48% of reported TEs following Fontan procedures and death occurred in 25%.

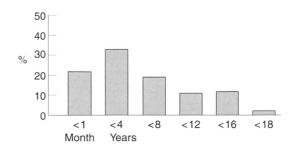

Fig. 34.4 Age distribution of children with ischemic stroke (n = 165).

ISCHEMIC STROKE

Incidence

The advent of CT and MRI has greatly facilitated the diagnosis of stroke in children. Several recent studies show agreement on the incidence of ischemic stroke at 0.63–1.2/100 000 children/year.[295–297] Age has a significant effect with approximately 30% of strokes ocurring in the first month of life (Fig. 34.4).[295] The incidence of stroke in children is paradoxically increasing as children with predisposing diseases, such as prematurity, CHD, sickle cell disease and leukemia, are surviving longer. Although the incidence of ischemic stroke in children is similar to that of brain tumors, there is a paucity of information and absence of therapeutic options validated in controlled clinical trials. Increasing awareness of ischemic stroke will hopefully improve initial therapy directed at decreasing the neurologic devastation from stroke.

Etiology

Approximately one-quarter of children with ischemic stroke have no identifiable etiology.[295] The remaining children have numerous diverse disorders of which embolism from CHD is the single commonest etiology. Recent reports from several countries suggest that congenital prethrombotic disorders including APCR (Factor V Leiden), hyperhomocystinemia, lipoprotein (a), deficiencies of protein C, protein S, AT and plasminogen, the presence of antiphospholipid antibodies and dysfibrinogenemias occur in a minimum of 10% of children with stroke.[298–308]

Clinical presentation

The diagnosis of ischemic infarction is often delayed in children, reflecting the relative rarity of the condition, consideration of other diagnoses, subtlety of symptoms that young patients cannot articulate, and low index of suspicion by pediatricians. The clinical presentation is age related. Infarcts *in utero* often present with pathologic early hand preference late in the first year of life.[8] Neonates present with seizures and lethargy, but rarely with appreciable focal neurologic deficits.[8,309,310] Older children present with hemiparesis with or without seizures.[311–313] Multiple transient ischemic attacks with a varied neurologic presentation are not unusual in older children.[310]

Radiographic features

MRI is the test of choice for detecting ischemic infarction in the brain.[314] Cerebral angiography is still considered the test of choice for visualization of the extra- and intracranial vasculature. Continued refinements in MR angiography (MRA), and studies showing that MRA correlates well with conventional angiography in children with ischemic stroke have made this modality a realistic non-invasive alternative.[315] In all children with idiopathic stroke following MRA, angiography should be strongly considered.[295,309,311,316] CT is still the acute study of choice due to its availability. CT features show low density areas in the large cerebral artery. Distribution is typically wedge-shaped involving the cortex and white matter. Small artery distribution, e.g. lacunar stroke, frequently involves the basal ganglia. A hemorrhagic component may be seen, usually involving the cortex. CT is known to miss small lacunar hemorrhagic components and multiple infarcts.

Outcome

The outcome of children with stroke has been reported in several small case series[295,309,311,316] and in the Canadian Paediatric Ischemic Stroke Registry.[309] Residual neurologic deficits and/or seizures persist in the majority of patients (approximately 66%) while a minority (approximately 22%) fully recover (Fig. 34.5).[295] Recurrence rates as high as 20% have been reported.[316] Long-term follow-up studies are underway and are critically important to the future choices of treatment to be evaluated in clinical trials.

Initial treatment with antithrombotic agents

While there are no large-scale trials assessing the use of either heparin or LMWH in children with ischemic infarcts, studies of these agents for peripheral thrombosis and clinical experience in children with ischemic infarction suggest that they may have a beneficial role. Exciting new results of the

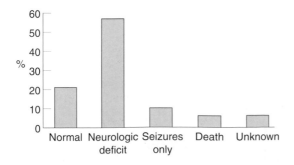

Fig. 34.5 Outcomes in children with arterial ischemic stroke (n = 165).

success of LMWH,[317] and early thrombolytic therapy[318] in adults with ischemic infarction, require urgent evaluation in children in controlled trials. Unfortunately, the delayed diagnosis of ischemic infarction in children may negatively influence the potentially positive response to thrombolytic therapy. Athough thrombolytic therapy has been used in a few pediatric patients, available data are insufficient to comment on its effectiveness.[319–321] The safety profile in children may differ from adults.

ANTITHROMBOTIC AGENTS

Ideally, recommendations for the prevention and treatment of TEs are based on well designed controlled trials. Unfortunately, there are few well designed trials in children and this has resulted in recommendations for adults being extrapolated for children, which is unlikely to be optimal because of the profound age-dependent differences in the hemostatic system, age-dependent pharmacokinetics for some antithrombotic agents, different underlying diseases and different risk of bleeding. The following section summarizes the current information on the use of antithrombotic agents in children. Subsequently, guidelines for antithrombotic treatment in children are provided.

Heparin, LMWH, oral anticoagulants (warfarin), antiplatelet agents (aspirin and others) and thrombolytic agents (streptokinase, urokinase and tPA) are all used in pediatric patients. These agents interact with the endogenous hemostatic system, which differs significantly in the young compared with adults, and this difference probably influences the efficacy and safety of these agents in children.

STANDARD HEPARIN

The activities of heparin can be considered as anticoagulant, which refers to coagulation assays in the laboratory; and antithrombotic, which refers to activities *in vivo*. Both anticoagulant and antithrombotic activities of heparin are mediated by catalysis of the endogenous inhibitor AT, particularly for the coagulation enzymes, thrombin and Factor Xa.[322] The antithrombotic activities of heparin are influenced by plasma concentrations of AT,[323] the capacity to generate thrombin[324] and the pharmacokinetics of heparin.[325] AT levels are decreased during the first weeks of life,[14,326] and in some acquired disease states.[327] Similarly, the capacity to generate thrombin is decreased physiologically during infancy and childhood,[328–330] and in many acquired disease states requiring therapy with heparin.[327] In the presence of heparin, thrombin generation is further delayed and decreased in the young compared to adults.[328,330] Finally, the clearance of heparin is faster in the young, reflecting a larger volume of disribution.[325] Together these observations suggest that optimal dosing of heparin will differ in children from adults.

Results from adult clinical trials suggest that the target therapeutic range for the treatment of DVT/PE in children, is an activated partial thromboplastin time (APTT) that reflects a heparin level of 0.3–0.7 units/ml as measured by an anti-Factor Xa assay.[322] The standardization of APTT results to a heparin concentration is necessary because APTT reagents are not uniform in their response to heparin and may give widely varying results. In pediatric patients, APTT values correctly predict heparin therapy approximately 70% of the time.[331] A nomogram for adjusting heparin therapy in children has been developed (Table 34.4).[331,332] Rapidly achieving therapeutic APTT levels probably reduces the risk of disease extension and recurrence.

The most important complications of heparin therapy are bleeding, osteoporosis and heparin-induced thrombocytopenia (HIT). The incidence of major bleeding, defined as requiring transfusion theapy, or located in the CNS or retroperitoneal space, is infrequent, occuring in <2% of pediatric patients.[331] In the presence of a major bleed, discontinuing heparin is usually sufficient because of the rapid clearance of heparin. Intravenous protamine sulfate neutralizes heparin activity if an immediate effect is required

(Table 34.4). The link between long-term use of heparin and osteoporosis in pregnant women is sufficiently convincing to recommend avoidance of long-term use in children.[333] There have only been 3 case reports of pediatric heparin-induced osteoporosis;[334–336] 2 were on concurrent steroid therapy,[334,336] and 1 on continuous high-dose intravenous heparin for 11 months.[335] Although HIT is rare in pediatric patients,[337–339] unexplained thrombocytopenia requires evaluation for HIT, and if ongoing anticoagulant therapy is required, an alternative anticoagulant is indicated.[337,338,340]

LOW MOLECULAR WEIGHT HEPARIN

The anticoagulant activities of LMWH are also mediated by catalysis of the natural inhibitor AT. LMWHs preferentially inhibit Factor Xa over thrombin due to the decreased capacity to bind both AT and thrombin simultaneously, a necessary step for thrombin inhibition.[341] Decreased plasma concentrations of AT, either physiologically or pathologically, also influence LMWH's anticoagulant activities in children.

LMWHs offer several potential advantages over heparin for anticoagulant therapy in children.[342–348] First, because LMWHs provide a predictable response, minimal monitoring is required which is ideal for pediatric patients.[349] The marked variability in the anticoagulant response to heparin in adults and children necessitates close monitoring.[349] Secondly, LMWHs are at least as effective anticoagulants as heparin. Thirdly, LMWHs are particularly attractive in clinical situations where the use of heparin is problematic, i.e. in patients who require antithrombotic protection but who are particularly vulnerable to bleeding complications. Many children requiring anticoagulant therapy are difficult to manage because of the seriousness of their underlying disorders, increased risk of bleeding, and poor venous access that limits monitoring.[331] Fourthly, LMWH can be administered subcutaneously every 12 hours, eliminating the need for continuous venous access devoted to heparin administration, which is a significant advantage in children. A subcutaneous catheter can further reduce the number of needle punctures for administration of LMWH from 14 to 1 per week.

The pharmacokinetics of two LMWHs, Enoxaparin and Reviparin, have been studied in pediatric patients and both showed a signficant effect of age, with young infants having an accelerated clearance compared to older children.[33,350] Similar to adults, the anticoagulant activities of LMWHs are reflected by an anti-Factor Xa level. For Enoxaparin, a dose of 1.0 mg/kg subcutaneously every 12 hours will achieve a therapeutic anti-Factor Xa level of 0.5–1.0 units/ml for children older than 2 months of age while a dose of 1.5 mg/kg is required for infants <2 months of age.[33] For Reviparin, a dose of 100 units/kg subcutaneously every 12 hours will achieve a therapeutic anti-Factor Xa level of 0.5–1.0 units/ml for children older than 2 months of age while infants have

Table 34.4 Protocol for systemic heparin administration and adjustment for pediatric patients. Reproduced with permission from Ref. 1.

I   Loading dose: heparin 75 unit/kg IV over 10 min
II Initial maintenance dose: 28 unit/kg/h for infants <1 year
III Initial maintenance dose: 20 unit/kg/h for children >1 year
IV Adjust heparin to maintain APTT 60–85 s (assuming this reflects an antifactor Xa level of 0.30–0.70)

APTT (s)	Bolus (unit/kg)	Hold (min)	Rate change (%)	Repeat APTT
<50	50	0	+10	4 h
50–59	0	0	+10	4 h
60–85	0	0	0	Next day
86–95	0	0	−10	4 h
96–120	0	30	−10	4 h
>120	0	60	−15	4 h

V   Obtain blood for APTT 4 h after administration of the heparin loading dose and 4 h after every change in the infusion rate
VI When APTT values are therapeutic, obtain a daily CBC and APTT

Reversal of heparin therapy

Time since last heparin dose (min)	Protamine dose (mg/100 unit heparin received)
<30	1.0
30–60	0.5–0.75
60–120	0.375–0.5
>120	0.25–0.375

Maximum dose of 50 mg
Infusion rate of a 10 mg/ml solution should not exceed 5 mg/min
Hypersensitivity reaction to protamine sulfate may occur in patients with known hypersensitivity reactions to fish or those previously exposed to protamine therapy or protamine-containing insulin

CBC = complete blood count; APTT = activated partial thromboplastin time.

increased requirements at approximately 150 unit/kg.[350] Prophylactic doses of Reviparin have also been studied in children.[350] For children >5 kg, a dose of 30 unit/kg achieves an average anti-Factor Xa level of 20 unit/ml while smaller infants have increased requirements.

Although the need for laboratory monitoring of LMWH in adults is currently controversial, laboratory monitoring of LMWH in children needs to be considered separately from adults for several reasons. First, the pharmacokinetics of LMWHs are age- and/or weight-dependent with enormous differences in requirements in small, growing infants compared to older children and adults. Secondly, LMWH is being used for several months in children in place of oral anticoagulants while the data in adults are primarily from the short-term use of LMWH instead of heparin in the first 5–10 days of treatment. Thirdly, the development of renal compromise and/or an acquired coagulopathy are not unusual in children receiving LMWH. Fourthly, in order for long-term treatment with LMWH to be practical, parents and/or the child must be trained to dilute the LWMH, measure the amount to be injected and administer the LMWH at home. There is the potential for systematic unintentional errors in the preparation of LMWH which would probably be detected by intermittent monitoring.

LMWHs are increasingly being used for 3–6 months to treat venous TEs in children, replacing oral anticoagulants. The reasons for this shift in practice are primarily the difficulty of safely monitoring oral anticoagulants in children due to rapid changes in diet, medications and poor venous access which makes venous blood sampling problematic. The long-term use of LMWHs raises management issues which include the stability of the pharmacokinetics of LMWH when administered to growing children over many months; the effects of long-term LMWH on bone development in growing children; and the safety of long-term LMWH in children with serious primary disorders that are characterized by renal failure, acquired coagulopathies, frequent thrombocytopenia and severe neutropenia.

ORAL ANTICOAGULANTS

Warfarin (4-hydroxycoumarin) is the oral anticoagulant used in North America for children. Warfarin competitively inhibits vitamin K, an essential cofactor for the post-transitional carboxylation of glutamic acid (Gla) residues on specific coagulation proteins (Factors II, VII, IX, X). The Gla residues serve as calcium binding sites which are essential for these coagulation proteins to interact on phospholipid surfaces and for thrombin generation to occur. The prothrombin time (PT) is used to monitor warfarin therapy because it is sensitive to the reduction of Factors II, VII and X.[351,352] Unfortunately, the sensitivity of thromboplastin reagents to low levels of vitamin K-dependent proteins is highly variable.[353–357] Prior to recognition of this problem, patients in North America received excessive amounts of warfarin with unnecessary hemorrhagic side-effects.[358] The

INR corrects for differing sensitivities of PT reagents and is calculated as $(PT[patient]/PT[control])^{ISI}$ where the ISI is the International Sensitivity Index for the reagent.[355–357] Laboratories monitoring warfarin therapy must provide INR values for clinicians to facilitate optimal management. The usual target INR for children with DVT/PE is 2.0–3.0,[102,359] and with mechanical prosthetic valves 2.5–3.5.[359] Patients with their first venous TE are treated for 3–6 months while those with mechanical prosthetic heart valves are treated for life.[4,359]

The dose requirements of warfarin in children are influenced by many parameters including age, diet and concurrent medications.[359] If the baseline INR is normal, a loading dose of 0.2 mg/kg can be used to initiate warfarin therapy.[258,359–362] Maintenance doses for oral anticoagulants are age dependent, with infants having the highest (0.32 mg/kg) and teenagers the lowest (0.09 mg/kg) requirements, similar to adults.[258,351,359–361,363,364] Mechanism(s) responsible for the age dependency of oral anticoagulant doses are not completely clear. Table 34.5 provides a nomogram for loading and monitoring oral anticoagulants in children.[365]

Monitoring warfarin therapy in children is difficult, and requires infrequent INR measurements (often weekly) with appropriate dose adjustments.[359] Alterations in diet, medications, primary disease states, and age contribute to the difficulty of safety resistance (vitamin K supplemented formulae) to warfarin (M Leaker et al, personal communication).[366–371] Children requiring warfarin therapy are usually receiving multiple medications, on both a long-term and intermittent basis, which influences dose requirements.[351] Children <1 year of age and teenagers comprise the two largest populations of patients requiring warfarin.[359] Infants frequently have poor venous access and teenagers are not necessarily compliant with their medication.[372,373] Mechanism(s) for optimizing the safety and efficacy of warfarin in

Table 34.5 Protocol for oral anticoagulation therapy to maintain an International Normalized Ratio (INR) between 2 and 3 for pediatric patients. Reproduced with permission from Ref. 1.

I Day 1: If the baseline INR is 1.0–1.3: dose = 0.2 mg/kg orally

II Loading days 2–4

INR	Action
1.1–1.3	Repeat initial loading dose
1.4–1.9	50% of initial loading dose
2.0–3.0	50% of initial loading dose
3.1–3.5	25% of initial loading dose
>3.5	Hold until INR <3.5 then restart at 50% less than the previous dose

III Maintenance oral anticoagulation dose guidelines:

INR	Action
1.1–1.4	Increase dose by 20%
1.5–1.9	Increase dose by 10%
2.0–3.0	No change
3.1–3.5	Decrease dose by 10%
>3.5	Hold until INR <3.5, then restart at 20% less than previous dose

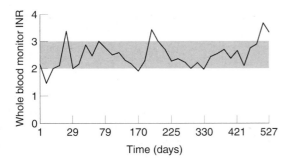

Fig. 34.6 International Normalized Ratio (INR) values for a child in whom a whole blood monitor was used over several years. Reproduced with permission from Ref. 374.

pediatric patients include pediatric anticoagulation clinics,[359] PT/INR monitors used in the clinic and at home,[374] and clinical trials to determine if lower, safer INR ranges are efficacious.

At least 2 whole blood PT/INR monitors have been evaluated in children in the settings of outpatient clinics and at home.[374,375] The correlation between INR values measured by whole blood monitors compared to laboratory values is excellent.[375,376] Fig. 34.6 shows INR values for a child in whom the whole blood monitor was used over several years.[374] Whole blood PT/INR monitors provide one solution to patients with difficult venous access, geographic distance from a laboratory, and a requirement for frequent testing. However, an education program and ongoing close supervision are necessary for safe use of whole blood monitors in children at home.

Bleeding is the main complication of warfarin. Minor bleeding of no clinical consequence occurs in approximately 20%[359] while the risk of serious bleeding is <3.2/100 patient years.[256–258,359,364,373,377–388]

ANTIPLATELET THERAPY

The two most commonly used antiplatelet agents for children are aspirin and dipyridamole. Aspirin acetylates the enzyme cyclo-oxygenase and thereby interferes with the production of thromboxane A_2 and platelet aggregation.[389] Dipyridamole interferes with platelet function by increasing the cellular concentration of adenosine 3′,5′-monophosphate (cyclic AMP). This latter effect is mediated by inhibition of cyclic nucleotide phosphodiesterase and/or by blockade or uptake of adenosine, which acts at A_2 receptors for adenosine to stimulate platelet adenyl cyclase.

Pediatric disorders in which antiplatelet agents are used include cardiac disorders (mechanical prosthetic heart valves, Blalock–Taussig shunts, and endovascular shunts), some cerebrovascular events, Kawasaki disease and others.[363] As adjunctive therapy to oral anticoagulants for mechanical prosthetic heart valves, both aspirin (at doses of 6–20 mg/kg/day)[254,359,364,384,386,390–392] and dipyridamole (2–5 mg/kg/day) have been used.[254,359,364,384,392,393] Major bleeding due to antiplatelet agents is rare in children. The

relatively low doses of aspirin used as antiplatelet therapy seldom cause signficant other side-effects, such as Reye's syndrome, which appear to be dose-dependent.[394–396]

THROMBOLYTIC THERAPY

The three thrombolytic agents used in pediatric patients, streptokinase, urokinase and tPA, all mediate their activities by converting endogenous plasminogen to plasmin. Plasma plasminogen concentrations are reduced physiologically during the first weeks of life[397] and secondarily in many pediatric diseases,[398] thereby reducing the thrombolytic activities of streptokinase, urokinase and tPA (M Leaker *et al*, unpublished observations).[399,400] Supplementation with plasminogen increases the thrombolytic effects of all three agents (M Leaker *et al*, unpublished observations).[400,401] Although there is no therapeutic range for thrombolytic agents, monitoring their activities to ensure that a fibrinogen/fibrinolytic effect is present, is recommended. Commonly used assays are fibrinogen/fibrin degradation products and/or D-dimer.

Thrombolytic therapy is used in low doses to restore catheter patency and in higher systemic doses for arterial TEs, extensive DVT and/or massive PE. Streptokinase should not be used to re-establish catheter patency because of potential allergic reactions with repeated doses. Instillation of 3.0 ml of urokinase (5000 units/ml) for 2–4 hours[96,402–404] or short infusions of low-dose urokinase (150 unit/kg/h) usually restore catheter patency.[96,402–404] Commonly used dose schedules for systemic thrombolytic therapy are summarized in Table 34.6.

Table 34.6 Thrombolytic therapy for pediatric patients. Reproduced with permission from Ref. 1.

Low dose for blocked catheters

	Regimen	Monitoring
Instillation	UK (5000 unit/ml) 1.5–3 ml/lumen 2–4 h	None
Infusion	UK (150 unit/kg/h) per lumen 12–48 h	Fibrinogen, TCT, PT, APTT

Systemic thrombolytic therapy*

	Load	Maintenance	Monitoring
UK	4000 unit/kg	4000 unit/kg/h for 6 h	Fibrinogen, TCT, PT, APTT
SK	4000 unit/kg Max 250 000 units	2000 unit/kg/h for 6 h	Fibrinogen, TCT, PT, APTT
tPA	None	0.5 mg/kg/h for 6 h	Fibrinogen, TCT, PT, APTT

*Start heparin therapy either during, or immediately upon completion of thrombolytic therapy. A loading dose of heparin may be omitted. The length of time for optimal maintenance is uncertain.
Values provided are starting suggestions; some patients may respond to longer or shorter courses of therapy.
UK = urokinase; SK = streptokinase; tPA = tissue plasminogen activator; TCT = thrombin clotting time; PT = prothrombin time; APTT = activated partial thromboplastin time.

TEs due to catheterization, in the form of CCs, CVLs or UACs, account for >80% of children receiving thrombolytic therapy.[398] The literature suggests that partial or complete resolution occurs in the majority of patients.[398] Bleeding is common at local sites, such as recent catheterization sites.[398] Transfusion with packed red blood cells (PRBC) is required in approximately one-quarter of children.[398] Bleeding into the CNS is rare but is of great concern, particularly in newborns.[5] Treatment of mild bleeding secondary to thrombolytic therapy consists of local measures (pressure, topical thrombin preparations), and transfusion of PRBC if necessary. Treatment of major bleeding consists of stopping thrombolytic therapy, replacement of fibrinogen with plasma and/or cryoprecipitate and consideration of an antifibrinolytic agent.

GENERAL RECOMMENDATIONS FOR ANTITHROMBOTIC THERAPY

The following recommendations are reproductions (with permission) of the recommendations from the Fourth ACCP Consensus Conference on Antithrombotic Therapy.[1] The pediatric literature was evaluated according to the level of evidence provided in Table 34.1.

Venous thromboembolism in children

1. Children (>2 months of age) with DVT or PE should be treated with intravenous heparin sufficient to prolong the APTT to a range that corresponds to an anti-Factor Xa level of 0.3–0.7 unit/ml. This grade C recommendation is based on grade A recommendations for adults and 1 level IV study in children.[331]
2. It is recommended that treatment with heparin should be continued for 5–10 days and that oral anticoagulation should be overlapped with heparin for 4–5 days. For many patients heparin and warfarin can be started together and heparin discontinued on day 6 if the PT (INR) is therapeutic. *For massive PE or extensive DVT* a longer period of heparin therapy should be considered. This grade C recommendation is based on grade A recommendations for adults and 1 level IV study in children.[331]
3. LMWH is an accepted form of therapy for DVT/PE in adults and is frequently used in children, despite limited information.[33,405] One approach is to administer LMWH for a minimum of 5 days and overlap LMWH with oral anticoagulation when feasible. The target anti-Factor Xa level is approximately 0.5–1.0 units/ml, 4–6 hours following the previous dose. Further clinical investigation is needed before more definitive recommendations can be made.
4. Long-term anticoagulant therapy should be continued for at least 3 months using oral anticoagulants to prolong the PT to an INR of 2.0–3.0. This grade C recommenda-

tion is based on grade A recommendations for adults; and 1 level IV[359] and 6 level V studies[258,360–364] in children.
5. Either indefinite oral anticoagulant therapy with an INR of 2.0–3.0, low dose anticoagulant therapy (INR <2.0) or close monitoring should be considered for children with first recurrence of a venous TE or a continuing risk factor, such as CVL, AT deficiency, protein C or S deficiency, and lupus anticoagulants in the antiphospholipid antibody syndrome of SLE. This grade C recommendation is based on grade C recommendations for adults and 1 level V study in children.[359]
6. Indefinite oral anticoagulant therapy with an INR of 2.0–3.0 should be considered for children with a second recurrence of venous TEs or a continuing risk factor, such as CVL, AT deficiency, protein C or S deficiency and lupus anticoagulants in the antiphospholipid antibody syndrome or SLE.
7. The use of thrombolytic agents in the treatment of venous TEs continues to be highly individualized. Further clinical investigation is needed before more definitive recommendations can be made.
8. Children with congenital prethrombotic disorders should receive short-term prophylactic anticoagulation in high-risk situations such as immobility, signficant surgery or trauma.

Venous/arterial thromboembolism in newborns

1. The use of anticoagulation therapy in the treatment of newborns with DVT, PE or arterial TEs continues to be highly individualized. Further clinical investigation is needed before more definite recommendations can be made.
2. If short-term anticoagulation therapy is not used, the thrombus should be closely monitored with objective tests and if extending, anticoagulation therapy instituted.
3. If anticoagulation is used, a short course (10–14 days) of intravenous heparin, sufficient to prolong the APTT to the therapeutic range that corresponds to an anti-Factor Xa level of 0.3–0.7 units/ml. The thrombus should be closely monitored with objective tests for evidence of extension of recurrent disease. This grade C recommendation is based on unpublished data.[406] If the thrombus extends following discontinuation of heparin therapy, oral anticoagulation therapy should be considered.
4. The use of thrombolytic agents in the treatment of venous TEs continues to be highly individualized. Further clinical investigation is needed before more definitive recommendations can be made. Supplementation with plasminogen (FFP) may be helpful.[401,406]

Prophylaxis for cardiac catheterization in children and newborns

Newborns and children requiring cardiac catheterization via an artery should be prophylaxed with intravenous heparin in doses of 100–150 units/kg as a bolus. This grade B recommendation is based on 1 level II study in children <10 years of age.[147] Aspirin alone is not recommended (1 level II study).[151]

Mechanical prosthetic heart valves in children

1. It is strongly recommended that children with mechanical prosthetic heart valves receive oral anticoagulation therapy. This grade C recommendation is based on grade C recommendations for adults and 13 level V studies in children.[254,256–258,364,373,382,383,385–388]

2. Levels of oral anticoagulation therapy that prolong the INR to 2.5–3.5 are recommended based on recommendations in adults.[407]

3. Children with mechanical prosthetic heart valves who suffer systemic embolism despite adequate therapy with oral anticoagulation therapy may benefit from the addition of aspirin, 6–20 mg/kg/day (adult level I study).[250] Dipyridamole, 2–5 mg/kg/day, may be used. This recommendation is an extrapolation of a level I study in adults.[250] There is 1 level V study in children.[258]

Biologic prosthetic heart valves in children

Children rarely have biologic prosthetic heart valves. Further clinical investigation is needed before definitive recommendations can be made for this situation. One option is to treat children with biologic prosthetic valves according to adult recommendations.[1]

Kawasaki disease in children

Children with Kawasaki disease should receive intravenous gamma globulin 2 g/kg as a single infusion during the acute phase (up to 14 days) followed by low-dose aspirin (3–5 mg/kg/day) to prevent thrombosis. This recommendation is based on a recent meta-analysis.[214]

Fontan operations

Further clinical investigation is needed before definitive recommendations can be made. One option is initially to treat patients with Fontan procedures with therapeutic amounts of heparin followed by oral anticoagulation therapy to achieve an INR of 2.0–3.0 for 3 months. Patients with fenestrations may benefit from treatment until closure.

Blalock–Taussig shunts

Further clinical investigation is needed before definitive recommendations can be made. One option is initially to treat patients with Blalock–Taussig shunts with therapeutic amounts of heparin, followed by aspirin at doses of 3–5 mg/kg/day indefinitely.

Homozygous protein C- and S-deficient patients

1. It is recommended that newborns with purpura fulminans due to a homozygous deficiency of protein C or S should be treated initially with replacement therapy (either FFP or protein C concentrate) for approximately 6–8 weeks until the skin lesions have healed.

2. Following resolution of the skin lesions, and under the cover of replacement therapy, oral anticoagulation therapy can be introduced with target INR values of approximately 3.0–4.5. Treatment duration with oral anticoagulants is indefinite. Recurrent skin lesions should be treated with replacement therapy of protein C or S.

3. For patients with homozygous protein C and S deficiency but with measurable plasma concentrations, LMWH is a therapeutic option.[409]

PEDIATRIC ANTICOAGULATION PROGRAMS

Emergence of a new field in pediatrics

The emergence of a new medical discipline is often unexpected and without immediate resources or expertise. During the last decade, the development of a new discipline in pediatrics has been witnessed that can be described by the term 'thrombophilia'. Thrombophilia encompasses the diagnosis, prevention and treatment of TEs as well as the use of anticoagulant therapy in other conditions such as CC, cardiopulmonary bypass (CPB), dialysis, extracorporeal membrane oxygenation (ECMO), stents and others. The exponential growth of successful vascular procedures that require anticoagulation, the need to establish expertise within pediatric hematology in the field of thrombophilia, and the lack of well designed clinical trials assessing anticoagulation therapy in these disorders, provide a strong rationale for the formation of Childhood Thrombophilia Programs as a natural component of pediatric hematology/oncology programs.

Models to emulate

One approach to the rapid development of Childhood Thrombophilia Programs is to model on adult thromboembolism programs and pediatric hemophilia programs. In 1991, the Hospital for Sick Children (HSC), Toronto sponsored an institutional Childhood Thrombophilia Program, which is now part of a broader institutional hemostasis program. The HSC Childhood Thrombophilia Program was modeled on the Hamilton Thromboembolism Program for adult patients, established by Dr Jack Hirsh in the 1970s. Its goals were to provide optimal clinical care, education, a training program for physicians and nurses, and advancement of knowledge through both basic and clinical research. A dedicated team of health care professionals was constructed to provide rapidly available consultations, to utilize objective tests to prove or disprove the presence of TEs, to effectively involve the coagulation laboratory in monitoring of antithrombotic agents as well as assessments of prothrombotic disorders, and to provide long-term follow-up when appropriate. An outpatient anticoagulation service was established to optimally monitor anticoagulants, particularly in difficult patients. A full-time nurse practitioner was the key person for the clinical and family educational aspects of the program.

Clinical aspects of the HSC Childhood Thrombophilia Program

Prior to initiating the thrombophilia program, meetings were held with division heads in all subspecialty services to identify conditions in which TEs occurred and antithrombotic therapy was required, either prophylactically or therapeutically. Standardized protocols, developed for heparin, warfarin, antiplatelet therapy and thrombolytic therapy, were approved by institutional regulatory committees and incorporated into the HSC Handbook for residents/fellows. The efficacy/safety of these protocols provided cohort studies that were analyzed and adapted yearly.[4,33,331,410] The inpatient component of the program was incorporated as part of the hematology consult service while the outpatient component revolved around outpatient thrombophiliac clinics.

Outpatient clinics focused on pediatric patients requiring short- or long-term anticoagulation, consultation for acquired or congenital prothrombotic conditions, and long-term follow-up for the morbidity associated with TEs. In addition, children with stroke were followed in a specialized stroke clinic attended by a pediatric neurologist in addition to the physicians and nurse practitioner from the Thrombophilia Program. Standardized data collection forms for anticoagulants, PPS, prothrombotic evaluation, neurologic outcome and other factors were used and analyzed on a regular basis.

A significant proportion of the clinic nurse practitioner's time was spent monitoring oral anticoagulant therapy. Most frequently, children had INR measurements at community laboratories and their results sent directly by a computer link to the nurse co-ordinator on the same day. Dose adjustments of oral anticoagulant therapy were conducted by the nurse practitioner using predefined protocols and with physician backup available at all times.

Educational programs

The nurse co-ordinator developed several educational programs for families. Issues discussed included: the need for anticoagulant therapy, choice of anticoagulant; monitoring with blood tests; symptoms to watch for in case of bleeding or recurrent TEs; and how to access the nurse co-ordinator

during working hours and physician assistance at any time. Specific pamphlets for pediatric patients on heparin, oral anticoagulants, thrombolytic therapy, and mechanical prosthetic heart valves were developed and provided for families. If a whole blood PT/INR monitor was to be used by the parents/patients at home, an indepth educational program was provided which included verbal instruction, written instructions, a practical component and a video. Prior to home use, parents (or in some cases patients) had to demonstrate their ability to successfully use the whole blood PT/INR monitor on at least 3 separate occasions. The nurse co-ordinator remained in close contact with the families, conversing with them after every home test, which was minimally once a week. The family was instructed when to perform the test and to call results to the nurse co-ordinator. If the INR was >4.5 on repeat testing, the child was brought to the hospital for laboratory confirmation of the INR results. For all patients, a calendar for recording daily doses of anticoagulant and laboratory values was given to families and reviewed regularly. For many children, medic-alert bracelets were indicated and families were provided with the necessary forms and information. A specialized educational program was used for the outpatient administration of LMWH. Usually a subcutaneous catheter was placed weekly by the nurse co-ordinator and parents taught to inject LMWH through the catheter twice daily. Some children preferred subcutaneous injections for each dose of LMWH. Discomfort was minimized by the use of a topical anesthetic and a 27-gauge needle.

Analysis of the HSC Thrombophilia Program patient population

The first 350 children attending the HSC Children's Thrombophilia Program were analyzed. The number of active patients receiving anticoagulants for any given month is shown in Fig. 34.7. The indications for antithrombotic therapy are shown in Table 34.7, and illustrate the seriousness and complexity of underlying diseases. The majority of patients required long-term (>6 months) or life-long anticoagulant therapy. The incidence of major hemorrhagic complications was minimal (<1%).[359]

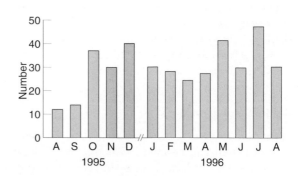

Fig. 34.7 Number of active patients in the HSC Thrombophilia Program receiving anticoagulants for any given month (n = 356).

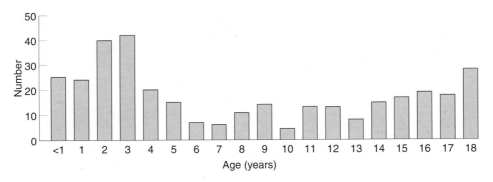

Fig. 34.8 Age distribution of children receiving oral anticoagulants in the HSC Thrombophilia Program.

Table 34.7 Indications for antithrombotic agents in pediatric patients. Reproduced with permission from Ref. 1.

Treatment
  Venous thromboembolic complications
  Arterial thromboembolic complications

Treatment: probable
  Myocardial infarction
  Some forms of stroke

Prophylaxis
  Mechanical prosthetic heart valves
  Biological prosthetic heart valves
  Cardiac catheterization
  Central arterial catheters

Prophylaxis: probable
  Endovascular stents
  Blalock–Taussig shunts
  Fontans
  Central venous catheters
  Atrial fibrillation

Other
  Kawaskai disease
  Cardiopulmonary bypass
  Extracorporeal membrane oxygenation
  Hemodialysis
  Continuous veno-venous hemoperfusion

The International Children's Thrombophilia Network

Following the commencement of HSC's Children's Thrombophilia Program, a national children's thrombophilia program was initiated in Canada. The primary goal was to provide a rapidly available, free, clinical consultative service to the Canadian physicians caring for children with TEs. The tool for achieving this goal was a toll free line (1–800-NO-CLOTS) which was manned 24 hours/day by an hematologist and neurologist. However, within weeks it became apparent that there was an enormous North American interest in the consultative service provided through 1–800-NO-CLOTS. By late 1994, the network (ICTN) was initiated and the 1–800-NO-CLOTS service formally extended to US and non-North American physicians (1–905–573–4795). The ICTN provides an immediate consultation by telephone, protocols and relevant publications from both the pediatric and adult literature. It also established a quarterly newletter, and a package of protocols for antithrombotic therapy, which were regularly updated. All services of the ICTN are provided without cost to physicians and their patients.

CONCLUSIONS

A new disease entity has developed in pediatrics, childhood thrombophilia. The magnitude of the problem and the need for programs focused on the prevention and treatment of childhood thromboembolic disease are now being recognized. Many approaches can be used to deliver excellence in care and, equally important, conduct clinical trials that will optimize care for this relatively new disease. Perhaps ICTN and the somewhat euphemistically named '1–800-NO-CLOTS' are the first steps.

Acknowledgement

This work was supported by a grant-in-aid from the Heart and Stroke Foundation of Canada.

REFERENCES

1. Michelson AD, Bovill E, Andrew M. Antithrombotic therapy in children. *Chest* 1995; **108**: 506S–522S
2. Cook D, Guyatt G, Laupacis A, Sackett D, Goldberg R. Clinical recommendations using levels of evidence for antithrombotic agents. *Chest* 1995; **108 (Suppl)**: 227S–230S
3. Poort SR, Rosendaal FR, Reitsma PH, Bertina RM. A common genetic variation in the 3'-untranslated region of the prothrombin gene is associated with elevated plasma prothrombin levels and an increase in venous thrombosis. *Blood* 1996; **88**: 3698–3703
4. Andrew M, David M, Adams M *et al.* Venous thromboembolic complications (VTE) in children: First analyses of the Canadian Registry of VTE. *Blood* 1994; **83**: 1251–1257
5. Deeg K, Wolfel D, Rupprecht T. Diagnosis of neonatal aortic thrombosis by color coded Doppler sonography. *Pediatr Radiol* 1992; **22**: 62–63
6. Bjarke B, Herin P, Blomback M. Neonatal aortic thrombosis. A possible clinical manifestation of congenital antithrombin III deficiency. *Acta Paediatr Scand* 1974; **63**: 297–301
7. Shapiro ME, Riodvien R, Bauer KA, Salzman EW. Acute aortic

thrombosis in antithrombin III deficiency. *JAMA* 1981; **245**: 1759–1761

8. Mannino FL, Travner DA. Stroke in neonates. *J Pediatr* 1983; **102**: 605–610

9. De Stefano V, Leone G, Ferrelli R *et al.* Severe deep vein thrombosis in a 2 year old child with protein S deficiency. *Thromb Haemostas* 1987; **58**: 1089

10. Andrew M, Brooker L. Blood component therapy in neonatal hemostatic disorders. *Tranfusion Med Rev* 1995; **IX**: 231–250

11. Dahlback B, Hildebrand B. Inherited resistance to activated protein C is corrected by anticoagulant cofactor activity found to be a property of factor V. *Proc Natl Acad Sci USA* 1994; **91**: 1396–1400

12. Sun X, Evatt B, Griffin JH. Blood coagulation Factor Va abnormality associated with resistance to activated protein C in venous thrombophilia. *Blood* 1994; **83**: 3120–3125

13. Koeleman BPC, van Rumpt D, Hamulyak K, Reitsma PH, Bertina RM. Factor V Leiden: An additional risk factor for thrombosis in protein S deficient families. *Thromb Haemostas* 1995; **74**: 580–583

14. Andrew M, Paes B, Milner R *et al.* Development of the human coagulation system in the full-term infant. *Blood* 1987; **70**: 165–172

15. Andrew M, Paes B, Milner R *et al.* Development of the human coagulation system in the healthy premature infant. *Blood* 1988; **72**: 1651–1657

16. Andrew M, Vegh P, Johnston M, Bowker J, Ofosu F, Mitchell L. Maturation of the hemostatic system during childhood. *Blood* 1992; **80**: 1998–2005

17. Grazziano J, Piomelli S, Hilgartner M *et al.* Chelation therapy in beta-thalassemia major II. The role of splenectomy in achieving iron balance. *J Pediatr* 1981; **99**: 695

18. Sifontes MT, Nuss R, Jacobson LJ, Griffin JH, Manco-Johnson MJ. Thrombosis in otherwise well children with the factor V Leiden mutation. *J Pediatr* 1996; **128**: 324–328

19. Andrew M. Developmental hemostasis: Relevance to thromboembolic complications in pediatric patients. *Thromb Haemostas* 1995; **74 (Suppl)**: 415–425

20. Nowak-Gottl U, Koch H, Kohlhase B, Ashka I, Kehrel I, Schneppenheim R. Resistance to activated protein C (APCR) in infants and children with venous or arterial thromboembolism. *Blood* 1995; **86 (Suppl 1)**: 201A

21. Nowak-Gottl U, Koch D, Aschka B *et al.* Resistance to activated protein C (APCR) in children with venous or arterial thromboembolism. *Br J Haematol* 1996; **92**: 992–998

22. Sifontes M, Nuss R, Jacobson L, Griffin J, Manco-Johnson M. Prevalence of activated protein C resistance in children with thrombosis. *Blood* 1995; **86 (Suppl 1)**: 202A

23. Auletta M, Headington J. Purpura fulminans: a cutaneous manifestation of severe protein C deficiency. *Arch Dermatol* 1988; **124**: 1387–1391

24. Adcock D, Brozna J, Marlar R. Proposed classification and pathologic mechanisms of purpura fulminans and skin necrosis. *Semin Thromb Haemostas* 1990; **16**: 333–340

25. Adcock D, Hicks M. Dermatopathology of skin necrosis associated with purpura fulminans. *Semin Thromb Haemostas* 1990; **16**: 283–292

26. Rosendaal FR, Koster T, Vandenbrouke JP, Reitsma PH. High risk of thrombosis in patients homozygous for Factor V Leiden (activated protein C resistance). *Blood* 1995; **85**: 1504–1508

27. Greengard JS, Eichinger S, Griffin JH, Bauer KA. Brief report: variability of thrombosis among homozygous siblings with resistance to activated protein C due to an Arg-Gln mutation in the gene for factor V. *N Engl J Med* 1994; **331**: 1559–1562

28. Samama MM, Trossaert M, Horellou MH, Elalamy I, Conard J. Risk of thrombosis in patients homozygous for factor V Leiden. *Blood* 1995; **86**: 4700–4702

29. Estelles A, Garcia-Plaza I, Dasi A *et al.* Severe inherited protein C deficiency in a newborn infant. *Thromb Haemostas* 1984; **52**: 53–56

30. Marlar R, Montgomery R, Broekmans A. Report on the diagnosis and treatment of homozygous protein C deficiency. Report of the working party on homozygous protein C deficiency of the ISTH – Subcommittee on protein C and protein S. *Thromb Haemostas* 1989; **61**: 529–531

31. Mahasandana C, Suvatte V, Chuansumvita A *et al.* Homozygous protein S deficiency in an infant with purpura fulminans. *J Pediatr* 1990; **117**: 750–753

32. Dreyfus M, Magny J, Bridey F *et al.* Treatment of homozygous protein C deficiency and neonatal prupura fulminans with a purified protein DC concentrate. *N Engl J Med* 1991; **325**: 1565–1568

33. Massicotte P, Adams M, Marzinotto V, Brooker L, Andrew M. Low molecular weight heparin in pediatric patients with thrombotic disease. A dose finding study. *J Pediatr* 1996; **128**: 313–318

34. Marlar R, Montgomery R, Broekmans A, and the working party. Diagnosis and treatment of homozygous protein C deficiency. *J Pediatr* 1989; **114**: 528–534

35. De Stefano V, Leone G, Carolis M *et al.* Antithrombin III in fullterm and preterm newborn infants: Three cases of neonatal diagnosis of AT III congenital defect. *Thromb Haemostas* 1987; **57**: 329–331

36. Mannucci P, Tripodi A, Bertina R. Protein S deficiency associated with 'juvenile' arterial and venous thrombosis. *Thromb Haemostas* 1986; **5**: 440

37. David M, Andrew M. Venous thromboembolism complications in children. A critical review of the literature. *J Pediatr* 1993; **123**: 337–346

38. Ryan JAJ, Abel RM, Abbott WM *et al.* Catheter complications in total parenteral nutrition. A prospective study of 200 consecutive patients. *N Engl J Med* 1974; **290**: 757–761

39. Marzinotto V, Adams M, Pencharz P, Burrows P, Andrew M. Catheter related thrombosis in children receiving home TPN: Incidence, diagnosis, management. *Thromb Haemostas* 1993; **69**: 1079

40. Mollitt DL, Golladay ES. Complications of TPN caterher-induced vena caval thrombosis in children less than one year of age. *J Pediatr Surg* 1983; **18**: 462–467

41. Wakefield A, Cohen Z, Craig M *et al.* Thrombogenicity of total parenteral nutrition solutions: I: Effect on induction of monocyte/macrophage procoagulant activity. *Gastroenterology* 1989; **97**: 1210–1219

42. Wakefield A, Cohen Z, Rosenthal A *et al.* Thrombogenicity of total parenteral nutrition solutions: II. Effect on induction of endothelial cell procoagulant activity. *Gastroenterology* 1989; **97**: 1220–1228

43. Montemurr P, Lattanzio A, Chetta G *et al.* Increased *in vitro* and *in vivo* generation of procoagulant activity (Tissue Factor) by mononuclear phagocytes after intralipid infusion in rabbits. *Blood* 1985; **65**: 1391–1395

44. Franzone AJ, Tucker BL, Brennan LP, Fine FN, Stiles QR. Hemodialysis in children. *Arch Surg* 1971; **102**: 592–593

45. Idris FS, Nikaidok LR, King R, Swenson O. Arteriovenous shunts for hemodialysis in infants and children. *J Pediatr Surg* 1971; **6**: 639–644

46. Chan AKC, Coppes M, Adams M, Andrew M. Right atrial thrombosis in pediatric patients: Analysis of the Canadian Registry of venous thromboembolic complications. *Pediatr Res* 1997; **39**: 154A

47. Ross PJ, Ehrenkranz R, Kleinman CS, Seashore JH. Thrombus associated with central venous catheters in infants and children. *J Pediatr Surg* 1989; **24**: 253–256

48. Berman WJ, Fripp RR, Yabek SM, Wernly J, Corlew S. Great vein and right atrial thrombosis in critically ill infants and children with central venous lines. *Chest* 1991; **99**: 963–967

49. Wacker P, Oberhansli I, Didier D, Bugmann P, Bongard O, Wyss M. Right atrial thrombosis associated with central venous catheters in children with cancer. *Med Pediatr Oncol* 1994; **22**: 55–57

50. Korones DN, Buzzard CJ, Asselin BL, Harris JP. Right atrial thrombi in children with cancer and indwelling catheters. *J Pediatr* 1996; **128**: 841–846

51. Andrew M, Brooker L. Hemostatic complications in renal disorders of the young. *Pediatr Nephrol* 1996; **10**: 88–99

52. Paramo JA, Rifon J, Lloren R, Casares J, Paloma MJ, Rocha E. Intra- and postoperative fibrinolysis in patients undergoing cardiopulmonary bypass surgery. *Haemostasis* 1991; **21**: 58–64

53. Rehan V, Seshia MM. Complications of umbilical vein catheter. *Eur J Pediatr* 1994; **153**: 141

54. Kooiman AM, Kootstra G, Zwierstra RP. Portal hypertension in children due to thrombosis of the portal vein. *Neth J Surg* 1982; **43**: 97–103

55. Brady L, Magilavy D, Black DD. Portal vein thrombosis associated with antiphospholipid antibodies in a child. *J Pediatr Gastroenterol Nutr* 1996; **23**: 470–473

56. Arav-Boger R, Reif S, Bujanover Y. Portal vein thrombosis caused by protein C and protein S deficiency associated with cytomegalovirus infection. *J Pediatr* 1995; **126**: 586–588

57. Skarsgard E, Doski J, Jaksic T *et al.* Thrombosis of the portal venous system after splenectomy for pediatric hematologic disease. *J Pediatr Surg* 1993; **28**: 1109–1112

58. Laishram H, Cramer B, Kennedy R. Idiopathic acute portal vein thrombosis: A case report. *J Pediatr Surg* 1993; **28**: 1106–1108

59. Arnold KE, Char G, Serjeant GR. Portal vein thrombosis in a child with homozygous sickle-cell disease. *West Ind Med J* 1993; **42**: 27–28

60. Wilson KW, Robinson DC, Hacking PM. Portal hypertension in childhood. *Br J Surg* 1969; **56**: 13–22

61. Kowal-Vern A, Radhakrishnan J, Goldman J, Hutchins W, Blank J. Mesenteric and portal vein thrombosis after splenectomy for auto-immune hemolytic anemia. *J Clin Gastroenterol* 1988; **10**: 108–110

62. Harper PL, Luddington RJ, Carrell RW *et al.* Protein C deficiency and portal thrombosis in liver transplantation in children. *Lancet* 1988; **ii**: 924–927

63. Macpherson AIS. Portal hypertension due to extrahepatic portal venous obstruction. *J R Coll Surg (Edin)* 1984; **29**: 4–10

64. Pinkerton JA, Holcomb GW, Foster JH. Portal hypertension in childhood. *Ann Surg* 1972; **175**: 870–886

65. Gollin G, Ward B, Meier GB, Sumpio BE, Gusberg RJ. Central splanchnic venous thrombosis. Often unsuspected, usually uncomplicated. *J Clin Gastroenterol* 1994; **18**: 109–113

66. Koshy A, Bhasin DK, Kapur KK. Bleeding in extrahepatic portal vein obstruction. *Ind J Gastroenterol* 1984; **3**: 13–14

67. Belli L, Puttini M, Marni A. Extrahepatic portal obstruction. *J Cardiovasc Surg* 1980; **21**: 439–448

68. Harkanyi Z, Temesi M, Varga G, Weszelits V. Duplex ultrasonography in portal vein thrombosis. *Surg Endo* 1989; **3**: 79–82

69. Stringer D, Krysl J, Manson D, Babiak C, Daneman A, Liu P. The value of Doppler sonography in the detection of major vessel thrombosis in the neonatal abdomen. *Pediatr Radiol* 1990; **21**: 30–33

70. Levy HM, Newhouse JH. MR imaging of portal vein thrombosis. *AJR* 1988; **151**: 283–286

71. Lee WB, Wong KP. CT demonstration of thrombosis of the portal venous system. *Aust Radiol* 1988; **32**: 360–364

72. De Gaetano AM, Lafortune M, Patriquin H, De Franco A, Aubin B, Paradis K. Cavernous transformation of the portal vein: Patterns of intrahepatic and splanchnic collateral circulation detected with Doppler sonography. *AJR* 1995; **165**: 1151–1155

73. Silver MM, Bohn D, Shawn DH, Shuckette B, Eich G, Rabinovitch M. Association of pulmonary hypertension with congenital portal hypertension in a child. *J Pediatr* 1992; **120**: 321–329

74. Rehan VK, Cronin CM, Bowman JM. Neonatal portal vein thrombosis successfully treated by regional streptokinase infusion. *Eur J Pediatr* 1994; **153**: 456–459

75. Boles ET, Wise WE, Birken G. Extrahepatic portal hypertension in children. *Am J Surg* 1986; **151**: 734–739

76. Dilawari JB, Chawla YK. Spontaneous (natural) splenoadrenorenal shunts in extrahepatic portal venous obstruction: A series of 20 cases. *Gut* 1987; **28**: 1198–1200

77. Karrer FM, Holland RM, Allshouse MJ, Lilly JR. Portal vein thrombosis: Treatment of variceal hemorrhage by endoscopic variceal ligation. *J Pediatr Surg* 1994; **29**: 1149–1151

78. Einhaupl KM, Villringer A, Meister W *et al.* Heparin treatment in sinus venous thrombosis. *Lancet* 1991; **338**: 597–600

79. Barron TF, Gusnard DA, Zimmerman RA, Clancy RR. Cerebral venous thrombosis in neonates and children. *Pediatr Neurol* 1992; **8**: 112–116

80. Govaert P, Achten E, Vanhaesebrouck P. Deep cerebral venous thrombosis in thalamo-ventricular hemorrhage of the term newborn. *Pediatr Radiol* 1992; **22**: 123–127

81. Klowat B, Fahnenstich H, Hansmann M, Keller E, Bartmann P. Konnatale sinusthrombose. *Monatsschr Kinderheilkd* 1996; **144**: 609–612

82. Lee WT, Wang PJ, Young C, Shen YZ. Cerebral venous thrombosis in children. *Acta Paediatr Scand* 1995; **36**: 425–430

83. Einhaupl KM, Masuhr F. Zerebralesinus und venethrombosen therapeutishce umschau. *Therapeutische Umschau* 1996; **53**: 552–558

84. DeVeber G, Andrew M, Adams M *et al.* Treatment of pediatric sinovenous thrombosis with low molecular weight heparin. *Ann Neurol* 1995; **38**: 532 (abstract)

85. Schmidt B, Andrew M. Neonatal thrombotic disease: Prevention, diagnosis and therapy. *J Pediatr* 1988; **113**: 407–410

86. McDonald M, Hathaway W. Neonatal haemorrhage and thrombosis. *Semin Perinatol* 1983; **7**: 213–225

87. Schmidt B, Zipursky A. Thrombotic disease in newborn infants. *Clin Perinatol* 1984; **11**: 461–488

88. Schmidt B, Andrew M. Neonatal thrombosis: Report of a prospective Canadian and International registry. *Pediatrics* 1995; **96**: 939–943

89. Schmidt B, Andrew M. A prospective international registry of neonatal thrombotic diseases. *Pediatr Res* 1994; **35**: 170A

90. Perlmutt L, Fellows KE. Lower extremity deep vein thrombosis in children. *Pediatr Radiol* 1983; **13**: 266–268

91. Stockwell M, Adams M, Andrew M, Cameron G, Pai M. Central venous catheters for out-patient management of malignant disorders. *Arch Dis Child* 1983; **58**: 633–663

92. Pegelow CH, Narvaez M, Toledano SR, Davis J, Oiticica C, Buckner D. Experience with a totally implantable venous device in children. *Am J Dis Child* 1986; **140**: 69–71

93. Shulman RJ, Rahman S, Mahoney D, Pokorny WJ, Bloss R. A totally implanted venous access system used in pediatric patients with cancer. *J Clin Oncol* 1987; **5**: 137–140

94. Bagnall HA, Gomperts E, Atkinson JB. Continuous infusion of low-dose urokinase in the treatment of central venous catheter thrombosis in infants and children. *Pediatrics* 1989; **83**: 963–966

95. Harvey WH, Pick TE, Reed K, Solenberger RI. A prospective evaluation on the Port-a-cath implantable venous access system in chronically ill adults and children. *Surg Gynecol Obstet* 1989; **169**: 495–500

96. Mirro JJ, Rao BN, Stokes DC *et al.* A prospective study of Hickman/Broviac catheters and implantable ports in pediatric oncology patients. *J Clin Oncol* 1989; **7**: 214–222

97. Hockenberry MJ, Schultz W, Bennett B, Bryant R, Falletta JM. Experience with minimal complications in implanted catheters in children. *Am J Pediatr Hematol Oncol* 1989; **11**: 295–299

98. Moore RA, McNicholas KW, Naidech H, Flicker S, Gallagher JD. Clinically silent venous thrombosis following internal and external jugular central venous cannulation in pediatric cardiac patients. *Anesthesiology* 1985; **62**: 640–643

99. Poole MA, Ross MN, Haase GM, Odom LF. Right atrial catheters in pediatric oncology: a patient/parent questionnaire study. *Am J Pediatr Hematol Oncol* 1991; **13**: 152–155

100. Sadiq H, Devaskar S, Keenan W, Weber T. Broviac catheterization in low birth weight infants: Incidence and treatment of associated complications. *Crit Care Med* 1987; **15**: 47–50

101. Mehta S, Connors AFJ, Danish EH, Grisoni E. Incidence of thrombosis during central venous catheterization of newborns. A prospective study. *J Pediatr Surg* 1992; **27**: 18–22

102. Andrew M, Marzinotto VP, Pencharz S *et al.* A cross-sectional study of catheter-related thrombosis in children receiving total parenteral nutrition at home. *J Pediatr* 1995; **126**: 358–363

103. Mulvihill SJ, Fonkalsrud EW. Complications of superior versus inferior vena cava occlusion in infants receiving central total parenteral nutrition. *J Pediatr Surg* 1984; **19**: 752–757

104. Effmann E, Ablow R, Touloukian R, Seashore J. Radiographic aspects of total parenteral nutrition during infancy. *Radiology* 1978; **127**: 195–201

105. Moukarzel A, Azancot-Benisty A, Brun P, Vitoux C, Cezard J, Navarro J. M-mode and two-dimensional echocardiography in the routine follow-up of central venous catheters in children receiving total parenteral nutrition. *J Parent Enteral Nutr* 1991; **15**: 551–555

106. Fonkalsrud EW, Berquist W, Burke M, Ament ME. Long-term hyperalimentation in children through saphenous central venous catheterization. *Am J Surg* 1982; **143**: 209–211

107. Bernstein D, Coupey S, Schonberg S. Pulmonary embolism in adolescents. *Am J Dis Child* 1986; **140**: 667–671

108. Green R, Meyer T, Dunn M, Glassroth J. Pulmonary embolism in younger adults. *Chest* 1992; **101**: 1507–1511

109. Carson J, Kelley M, Duff A *et al.* The clinical course of pulmonary embolism. *N Engl J Med* 1992; **326**: 1240–1245

110. Buck JR, Connors RH, Coon WW, Weintraub WH, Wesley JR. Coran AG. Pulmonary embolism in children. *J Pediatr Surg* 1981: **326**: 1240–1245

111. Prospective Investigation of Pulmonary Embolism Diagnosis (PIOPED). Value of the ventilation/perfusion scan in acute pulmonary embolism. *JAMA* 1990; **263**: 2753–2759

112. Adams M, Monagle P, Ali K *et al.* Long term outcome of paediatric thromboembolic disease: A report from the Canadian Childhood Thrombophilia Registry. *Thromb Haemostas* 1997; **June (Suppl)**: OC-1623 (abstract)

113. Hull R, Rashkob G, Rosenbloom D. Heparin for 5 days as compared with 10 days in the initial treatment of proximal venous thrombosis. *N Engl J Med* 1986; **315**: 1109–1114

114. Hull R, Rashkob G, Hirsh J *et al.* Continuous intravenous heparin compared to intermittent subcutaneous heparin in the initial treatment of proximal vein thrombosis. *N Engl J Med* 1986; **315**: 1109–1114

115. Gallus A, Jackaman J, Tillett J, Mills W, Wycherley A. Safety and efficacy of warfarin started early after submassive venous thrombosis of pulmonary embolism. *Lancet* 1986; **ii**: 1293–1296

116. Adams M, Massicotte MP, Andrew M. Central venous catheter related thrombosis (CVLT) in children. Analysis of the Canadian registry of venous thromboembolism. *Thromb Haemostas* 1997; **(Suppl)**: OC-1619a (abstract)

117. Norotte G, Glorion C, Rigault P *et al.* Complications thromboemboliques en orthopedie pediatrique. Recueil 'multicentrique' de 33 observations. *Chir Pediatr* 1989; **30**: 193–198

118. Siegbahn A, Ruusuvaara L. Age dependence of blood fibrinolytic components and the effects of low-dose oral contraceptives on coagulation and fibinolysis in teenagers. *Thromb Haemostas* 1988; **60**: 361–364

119. O'Neill JA, Neblett WWI, Born ML. Management of major thromboembolic complications of umbilical artery catheters. *J Pediatr Surg* 1981; **16**: 972–978

120. Neal WA, Reynolds JW, Jarvis CW, Williams HJ. Umbilical artery catheterization: demonstration of arterial thrombosis by aortography. *Pediatrics* 1972; **50**: 6–13

121. Goetzman BW, Stadalnik RC, Bogren HG, Blankenship WH, Ikeda R, Thayer J. Thrombotic complications of umbilical artery catheters: a clinical and radiographic study. *Pediatrics* 1975; **56**: 374

122. Olinsky A, Aitken FG, Isdale JM. Thrombus formation after umbilical arterial catheterization: an angiographic study. *S Afr Med* 1975; **49**: 1467–1470

123. Makrohisky ST, Levine R, Blumhagen JB, Wesenberg RL, Simmons SA. Low positioning of umbilical artery catheters increases associated complications in newborn infants. *N Engl J Med* 1978; **299**: 561

124. Saia OS, Rubatelli FF, D'Elia RD *et al.* Clinical and aortographic assessment of the complications of arterial catheterization. *Eur J Obstet* 1987; **128**; 169–179

125. Wesstrom G, Finnstrom O, Stenport G. Umbilical artery catheterization in newborns. I. Thrombosis in relation to catheter type and position. *Acta Paediatr Scand* 1979; **68**: 575–581

126. Barnard D, Hathaway W. Neonatal thrombosis. *Am J Pediatr Hematol Oncol* 1979; **1**: 235–244

127. Vailas G, Brouillette R, Scott J, Shkolnik A, Conway J, Wiringa K. Neontal aortic thrombosis: recent experience. *J Pediatr* 1986; **109**: 101–108

128. Jackson J, Truog W, Watchko J, Mack L, Cyr D, Van Belle G. Efficacy of thromboresistant umbilical artery catheters in reducing aortic thombosis and related complications. *J Pediatr* 1987; **110**: 102–105

129. Horgan M, Bartoletti A, Polonsky S, Peters J, Manning T, Lamont B. Effect of heparin infusates in umbilical arterial catheters on frequency of thrombotic complications. *J Pediatr* 1987; **111**: 774–778

130. Rajani K, Goetzman B, Wennberg R, Turner E, Abildgaard C. Effect of heparinization of fluids infused through an umbilical artery catheter on catheter patency and frequency of complications. *Pediatrics* 1979; **63**: 552–556

131. David R, Merten D, Anderson J, Gross S. Prevention and umbilical artery catheter clots with heparinized infusates. *Dev Pharmacol Therapeutics* 1981; **2**: 117–126

132. Bosque E, Weaver L. Continuous versus intermittent heparin infusion of umbilical artery catheters in the newborn infant. *J Pediatr* 1986; **108**: 141–143

133. Ankola P, Atakent Y. Effect of adding heparin in very low concentration to the infusate to prolong the patency of umbilical artery catheters. *Am J Perinatol* 1993; **10**: 229–232

134. Lesko S, Mitchell A, Eopstein M, Louik C, Gracoia G, Shapiro S. Heparin use a risk factor for intraventricular hemorrhage in low birth weight infants. *N Engl J Med* 1986; **314**: 1156–1160

135. Gilhooly JT, Lindenberg JA, Reynold JW. Survey of umbilical catheter practices. *Clin Res* 1987; **34**: 142A

136. Marsh JL, King W, Barrett C, Fonkalsrud EW. Serious complications after umbilical artery catheterization for neonatal monitoring. *Arch Surg* 1975; **110**: 1203

137. Wigger HJ, Bransilver BR, Blanc WA. Thromboses due to catheterization in infants and children. *J Pediatr* 1970; **76**: 1

138. Hoar PF, Wilson RM, Mangano DT. Heparin bonding reduces thrombogenicity of pulmonary artery catheters. *N Engl J Med* 1980; **305**: 993–995

139. Downs JB, Chapman RL, Hawkins F. Prolonged radial artery catheterization. An evaluation of heparinized catheters and continuous irrigation. *Arch Surg* 1974; **108**: 671–673

140. American Association of Critical Care Nurses. Evaluation of the effects of heparinized and nonheparinized flush solutions on the patency of arterial pressure monitoring lines: The AACN Thunder Project. *Am J Crit Care* 1993; **2**: 3–15

141. Butt W, Shann F, McDonnell G, Hudson I. Effect of heparin concentration and infusion rate on the patency of arterial catheters. *Crit Care Med* 1987; **15**: 230–232

142. Clifton GD, Branson P, Kelly HJ *et al.* Comparison of normal saline and heparin solutions for maintenance of arterial catheter patency. *Heart Lung* 1991; **20**: 115–118

143. Kulkarni M, Elsner C, Ouellet D, Zeldin R. Heparinized saline versus normal saline in maintaining patency of the radial artery catheter. *Can J Surg* 1994; **37**: 37–42

144. McFadden PM, Oschsner JL, Mills N. Management of thrombotic complications of invasive arterial monitoring of the upper extremity. *J Cardiovasc Surg* 1983; **24**: 35–39

145. Mortensson W, Hallbook T, Lundstrom N. Percutaneous catheterization of the femoral vessels in children. II. Thrombotic occlusion of the catheterized artery: Frequency and causes. *Pediatr Radiol* 1975; **4**: 1–9

146. Mortensson W. Angiography of the femoral artery following percutaneous catheterization in infants and children. *Acta Radiol (Diagn)* 1976; **17**: 581–593

147. Freed M, Keane J, Rosenthal A. The use of heparinization to prevent arterial thrombosis after percutaneous cardiac catheterization in children. *Circulation* 1974; **50**: 565–569

148. Vlad P, Hohn A, Lambert EC. Retrograde arterial catheterization of the left heart. *Circulation* 1964; **29**: 787

149. Wessel DL, Keane JF, Fellows KE, Robichaud H, Lock JE. Fibrinolytic therapy for femoral arterial thrombosis after cardiac catheterization in infants and children. *Am J Cardiol* 1986; **58**: 347–351

150. Barlow GH. *Cardiol Young* 1996; **6**: 54–58

151. Freed M, Rosenthal A, Fyler D. Attempts to reduce arterial thrombosis after cardiac catheterization in children: Use of percutaneous technique and aspirin. *Am Heart J* 1974; **87**: 283–286

152. Rao PS, Thapar MK, Rogers JHJ et al. Effect of intraarterial injection of heparin on the complications of percutaneous arterial catheterization in infants and children. *Catheterization Cardiovasc Diagn* 1981; **7**: 235–246

153. Stanger P, Heymann MA, Tarnoff H, Hoffman JI, Rudolph AM. Complications of cardiac catheterization of neonates, infants and children. *Circulation* 1974; **50**: 595–608

154. Hurwitz RA, Franken EA, Girod DA. Angiographic determination of arterial patency after percutaneous catheterization in infants and small children. *Circulation* 1977; **56**: 102–105

155. Mansfield PB, Gozzaniga AB, Litwin SB. Management of arterial injuries related to cardiac catheterization in children and young adults. *Circulation* 1970; **42**: 501–507

156. Ino T, Benson LN, Freedom RM, Barker GA, Zipursky A, Rowe RD. Thrombolytic therapy for femoral artery thrombosis after pediatric cardiac catheterization. *Am Heart J* 1988; **115**: 633–639

157. Kern IB. Management of children with chronic femoral artery ostruction. *Pediatr Surg* 1977; **12**: 83–90

158. Gagnon RM, Goudreau E, Joyal F, Morissette M, Roussin A. The role of intravenous streptokinase in acute arterial occlusions after cardiac catheterization. *Catheterization Cardiovasc Diagn* 1985; **11**: 409–412

159. Haitas B, Baker SG, Meyer TE, Joffe BI, Seftel HC. Natural history and cardiac manifestations of homozygous familial hypercholesterolaemia. *Q J Med New Series* 1990; **76**: 731–740

160. Sprecher DL, Schaefer EJ, Kent KM et al. Cardiovascular features of homozygous familial hypercholesterolemia; Analysis of 16 patients. *Am J Cardiol* 1984; **54**: 20–30

161. Boers GHJ. Heterozygosity of homocystinuria in premature peripheral and cerebral occlusive arterial disease. *N Engl J Med* 1985; **313**: 709–715

162. Genest JJ. Plasma homocysteine levels in men with premature coronary artery disease. *J Am Coll Cardiol* 1990; **16**: 1114–1119

163. Clarke R. Hyperhomocysteinemia: An independent risk factor for vascular disease. *N Engl J Med* 1991; **324**: 1149–1155

164. Hong C, Yun Y, Choi J et al. Takayasu arteritis in Korean children: clinical report of seventy cases. *Heart Vessels* 1992; **7**: 91–96

165. Zheng D, Fan D, Liu L. Takayasu arteritis in China: a report of 530 cases. *Heart Vessels* 1992; **7**: 32–36

166. Wiggelinkhuizen J, Cremin B, Cywes S. Spontaneous recanalization of renal artery stenosis in childhood Takayasu arteritis: A case report. *S Afr Med J* 1980; **57**: 96–98

167. Koren G, Rose V, Lavi S, Rowe R. Probable efficacy of high-dose salicyclates in reducing coronary involvement in Kawasaki disease. *JAMA* 1985; **254**: 767–769

168. Daniels S, Specker P, Capannari TE, Schwartz D, Burke M, Kaplan S. Correlates of coronary artery aneurysm formation in patients with Kawasaki disease. *AJDC* 1987; **141**: 205–207

169. Newburger J, Takahashi M, Burns J et al. The treatment of Kawasaki syndrome with intravenous gamma globulin. *N Engl J Med* 1986; **315**: 341–347

170. Hall T, McDiarmid S, Grant E, Boechat M, Bosulti R. False-negative duplex Doppler studies in children with hepatic artery thrombosis after liver transplantation. *Am J Roentgen* 1990; **154**: 573–575

171. Flint E, Sumkin J, Zajko A, Bowen A. Duplex sonography of hepatic artery thrombosis after liver transplantation. *Am J Roentgen* 1988; **151**: 481–483

172. Lerut J, Gordon R, Tzakis A, Stieber A, Iwatsuk S, Starzl T. The hepatic artery in orthotopic liver transplantation. *Helvet Chir Acta* 1988; **55**: 367–378

173. LeBlanc J, Culham J, Chan K, Patterson M, Tipple M, Sandor G. Treatment of grafts and major vessel thrombosis with low-dose streptokinase in children. *Ann Thorac Surg* 1986; **41**: 630–635

174. Samara E, Voss B, Pederson J. Renal artery thrombosis associated with elevated cyclosporine levels: A case report and review of the literature. *Transplant Proc* 1988; **20**: 119–123

175. Brown J, Dunn J, Spooner E, Kirsh M. Late spontaneous disruption of a procine xenograft mitral valve: Clinical, hemodynamic, echocardiographic and pathologic findings. *J Thorac Cardiovasc Surg* 1978; **75**: 606–611

176. Taussig H. Long-time observations on the Blalock–Taussig operation. IX. Single ventricle (with apex to the left). *Johns Hopkins Med J* 1976; **139**: 69–76

177. du Plessis A, Chang A, Wessel D et al. Cerebrovascular accidents following the Fontan operation. *Pediatr Neurol* 1995; **12**: 230–236

178. Fallat RW, Tsang RC, Glueck CJ. Hypercholesterolemia and hypertriglyceridemia in children. *Prev Med* 1974; **3**: 390–405

179. Goldstein J, Brown M. Familial hypercholesterolemia. In: Stanbury JB (ed) *Metabolic Basis of Inherited Disease*. New York: McGraw Hill, 1989

180. Celermajer DS, Sorenson KE, Gooch VM et al. Non-invasive detection of endothelial dysfunction in children and adults at risk of atherosclerosis. *Lancet* 1992; **340**: 1111–1115

181. Sorenson K. Impairment of endothelium-dependent dilation is an early event in children with familial hypercholesterolemia and is related to the lipoprotein (a) level. *J Clin Invest* 1994; **93**: 50–55

182. Hegele RA, Connelly PW, Cullen-Dean G, Rose V. Elevated plasma lipoprotein(a) associated with abnormal stress thallium scans in children with familial hypercholesterolemia. *Am J Cardiol* 1993; **70**: 1109–1112

183. Mouratidis B. Detection of silent coronary artery disease in adolescents and young adults with familial hypercholesterolemia by single photon emission computed tomography thallium-201 scanning. *Am J Cardiol* 1992; **70**: 1109–1112

184. Goldstein J, Brown M. The LDL receptor defect in familial hypercholesterolemia. *Med Clin North Am* 1982; **66**: 335–362

185. Rose V, Wilson G, Steiner G. Familial hypercholesterolemia: Report of coronary death at age 3 in a homozygous child and prenatal diagnosis in a heterozygous sibling. *J Pediatr* 1982; **100**: 757–759

186. Williams ML. Death of a child as a result of familial hypercholesterolaemia. *Med J Aust* 1989; **150**: 93–94 [Published erratum appears in *Med J Aust* 1989; **150**: 228]

187. Clemens P, Beisiegel U, Steinhagen-Thiessen E. Family study in familial hypercholesterolemia with a receptor-negative homozygous 9 year old boy. *Helv Paediatr Acta* 1986; **41**: 173–182

188. Guarda LA, Borrero JL. Hand and digital ischemia due to arteriosclerosis and thromboembolization in young adults: Pathologic features with cranial correlations. *Med Pathol* 1990; **3**: 654–658

189. Janaki S, Baruah JK, Jayaram SR, Saxena VK, Sharma SH, Tulati MS. Stroke in the young: A four year study, 1968 to 1972. *Stroke* 1975; **6**: 318–320

190. Postiglione A, Nappi A, Brunetti et al. Relative protection from cerebral atherosclerosis of young patients with homozygous familial hypercholesterolemia. *Atherosclerosis* 1991; **90**: 23–30

191. Rubba A, Mercuri M, Faccenda F et al. Premature carotid atherosclerosis: Does it occur in both familial hypercholesterolemia and homocystinuria? Ultrasound assessment of arterial intima-media thickness and blood flow velocity. *Stroke* 1994; **25**: 943–950

192. Mabuchi H. Cause of death in patients with familial hypercholesterolemia. *Atherosclerosis* 1986; **61**: 1–6

193. Hoeg J. Familial hypercholesterolemia. What the zebra can teach us about the horse. *JAMA* 1994; **271**: 543–546

194. Leonard JV, Clarke M, Macartney FJ, Slack J. Progression of atheroma in homozygous familial hypercholesterolemia during regular plasma exchange. *Lancet* 1981; **ii**: 811

195. Haber C, Kwiterovich PO. Dyslipoproteinemia and xanthomatosis. *Pediatr Dermatol* 1984; **1**: 261–280

196. West RJ, Lloyd JK. Hypercholesterolemia in childhood. *Adv Pediatr* 1979; **26**: 1–34

197. Mudd SH, Skovby F, Levy HL *et al.* The natural history of homocysteinuria due to cystathionine b-synthase deficiency. *Am J Hum Genet* 1985; **37**: 1–31

198. Wada Y, Narisawa K, Arakawa T. Infantile type of homocysteinuria with 5,10-methylenetetrahydrofolate reductase deficiency. *Mongr Hum Genet* 1978; **9**: 140–146

199. Jacques PF, Bostom AG, Williams RR *et al.* Relation between folate status, a common mutation in methylenetetrahydrofolate reductase, and plasma homocysteine concentrations. *Circulation* 1996; **93**: 7–9

200. Kluijtmans LA, van den Heuvel LP, Boers GH *et al.* Molecular genetic analysis in mild hyperhomocysteinemia: A common mutation in the methylenetetrahydrofolate reductase gene is a genetic risk factor for cardiovascular disease. *Am J Hum Genet* 1996; **58**: 35–41

201. Selhub J, Jacques PF, Wilson PWF, Rush D, Rosenberg LH. Vitamin status and intake as primary determinants of homocysteinemia in an elderly population. *JAMA* 1993; **270**: 2693–2698

202. Chauveau P, Chadefaux B, Coude M *et al.* Increased plasma homocysteine concentration in patients with chronic renal failure. *Miner Electrol Metab* 1992; **18**: 196

203. Boushey CJ, Beresford SAA, Omenn GS, Motulsky AG. A quantitative assessment of plasma homocysteine as a risk factor for vascular disease: Probable benefits of increasing folic acid intakes. *JAMA* 1995; **274**: 1049–1057

204. Hall S, Barr W, Lie JT. Takayasu arteritis: A study of 32 North American patients. *Medicine* 1985; **64**: 6489–6499

205. Tech PC, Tan LK, Chia BL. Nonspecific aorto-arteritis in Singapore with special reference to hypertension. *Am Heart J* 1978; **95**: 683–695

206. Kohrman MH, Huttenlocher PR, Takayasu's arteritis; A treatable cause of stroke in infancy. *Pediatr Neurol* 1986; **2**: 154–158

207. Lupi-Herrara E, Sanchez-Torres G, Marcushamer J. Takayasu's arteritis: Clinical study of 107 cases. *Am Heart J* 1977; **93**: 94–103

208. Cupps TR, Fauci A. *The Vasculitides.* Philadelphia: WB Saunders, 1981, pp 107–115

209. Gupta SK, Khanna MN, Lahiri TK. Involvement of cardiac valves in Takayasu's arteritis. Report of 7 cases. *Ind Heart J* 1980; **32**: 148–155

210. Dajani AS, Bison AL, Chung KL *et al.* Diagnostic guidelines for Kawasaki disease. *Am J Dis Child* 1990; **144**: 1218–1219

211. Center for Disease Control. Kawasaki disease involvement. *MMWR* 1980; **29**: 61–63

212. Kato H, Koike S, Yokoyama T. Kawasaki disease: Effect of treatment on coronary artery involvement. *Pediatrics* 1979; **63**: 175–179

213. Newburger JW, Takahashi M, Burns JC. The treatment of Kawasaki syndrome with intravenous gamma globulin. *N Engl J Med* 1986; **315**: 341–347

214. Durongpisitkul K, Fururaj VJ, Park JM, Martin CF. The prevention of coronary artery aneurysm in Kawasaki disease: A meta-analysis on the efficacy of aspirin and immunoglobulin treatment. *Pediatrics* 1995; **96**: 1057–1061

215. Gersony WM. Kawasaki disease: Clinical overview. *Cardiol Young* 1991; **1**: 192–195

216. Tatara K, Kusakawa S. Long term prognosis of giant coronary aneurysm in Kawasaki disease: An angiographic study. *J Pediatr* 1987; **111**: 705–710

217. Rosse WF, Ware RE. The molecular basis of paroxysmal nocturnal hemoglobinuria. *Blood* 1995; **86**: 3277–3286

218. Socie G, Mary JY, de Gramont A *et al.* Paroxysmal nocturnal haemoglobinuria: Long term followup and prognostic factors. *Lancet* 1996; **348**: 573–577

219. Ware RE, Rosse WF, Hall SE. Immunophenotypic analysis of reticulocytes in paroxysmal nocturnal hemoglobinuria. *Blood* 1995; **86**: 1586–1589

220. Hillmen P, Lewis SM, Bessler M, Luzzatto L, Dacie JV. Natural history of paroxysmal nocturnal hemoglobinuria. *N Engl J Med* 1995; **333**: 1253–1258

221. Wyatt HA, Mowat AP, Layton M. Paroxysmal nocturnal haemoglobinuria and Budd–Chiari syndrome. *Arch Dis Child* 1995; **72**: 241–242

222. Gralnick HR, Vail M, McKeown LP *et al.* Activated platelets in paroxysmal nocturnal haemoglobinuria. *Br J Haematol* 1995; **91**: 697–702

223. Rosse W. Epidemiology of PNH. *Lancet* 1996; **348**: 560

224. Valdes R, Munoz R, Bracho E, Gordillo G, Velazquez L, Nieto L. Surgical complications of renal transplantation in malnourished children. *Transplant Proc* 1994; **26**: 50–51

225. Harmon WE, Stablein D, Alexander SR, Tejani A. Graft thrombosis in pediatric renal transplant recipients. *Transplantation* 1991; **51**: 406–412

226. Kalicinski P, Kaminski A, Prokural A *et al.* Surgical complications after kidney transplantation in children. *Transplant Proc* 1994; **26**: 42–43

227. Sheldon CA, Churchill BM, McLorie GA, Arbus GS. Evaluation of factors contributing to mortality in pediatric renal transplant recipients. *J Pediatr Surg* 1992; **27**: 629–633

228. Broyer M, Mitsioni A, Gagnadoux MF *et al.* Early failures of kidney transplantation: a study of 70 cases from 801 consecutive grafts performed in children and adolescents. *Adv Nephrol* 1993; **22**: 169

229. Rela M, Muiesan P, Baker A *et al.* Hepatic artery thrombosis after liver transplantation in children under 5 years of age. *Transplantation* 1996; **61**: 1355–1357

230. Jurim O, Csete M, Gelabert HA *et al.* Reduced size grafts: The solution for hepatic artery thrombosis after pediatric liver transplantation. *J Pediatr Surg* 1995; **30**: 533–555

231. Dunn SP, Billmire DF, Falkensein K *et al.* Rejection after pediatric liver transplantation is not the limiting factor to survival. *J Pediatr Surg* 1994; **29**: 1141–1143

232. Drazan K, Shaked A, Olthoff KM *et al.* Etiology and management of symtomatic adult hepatic artery thrombosis after orthotopic liver transplantation (OLT). *Am Surg* 1996; **62**: 237–240

233. Esquivel CO, Jaffee R, Gordon RD, Iwatsuki S, Shaw BW, Starzl TE. Liver rejection and its differentiation from other causes of graft dysfunction. *Semin Liver Dis* 1985; **5**: 369–374

234. Mazzaferro V, Esquivel CO, Makowka L *et al.* Hepatic artery thrombosis after pediatric liver transplantation. A medical or surgical event? *Transplantation* 1980; **47**: 971–977

235. Pariente D, Urvoas E, Riou JY *et al.* Imaging of complications of liver transplantation in children. *Ann Radiologie* 1994; **37**: 372–376

236. Lallier M, St Vil D, Dubois J *et al.* Vascular complications after pediatric liver transplantation. *J Pediatr Surg* 1995; **30**: 1122–1126

237. Legmann P, Costes V, Tudoret L *et al.* Hepatic artery thrombosis after liver transplantation: Diagnosis with spiral CT. *AJR* 1995; **164**: 97–101

238. Sanchez-Bueno F, Robles R, Ramirez P *et al.* Hepatic artery complications after liver transplantation. *Clin Transplant* 1994; **8**: 399–404

239. Andrew M, Mitchell L, Paes B *et al.* An anticoagulant dermatan sulphate proteoglycan circulates in the pregnant woman and her fetus. *J Clin Invest* 1992; **89**: 321–326

240. Yanaga K, Makowka L, Starzl T. Is hepatic artery thrombosis after liver transplantation really a surgical complication? *Transplant Proc* 1989; **21**: 3511–3513

241. Yandza T, Lababidi A, Jaworske W *et al.* Vascular complications of liver transplantation: surgical treatment. *Ann Radiologie* 1994; **37**: 349–355

242. Figueras J, Busquets J, Dominguez J *et al.* Intra-arterial thombolysis in the treatment of acute hepatic artery thrombosis after liver transplantation. *Transplantation* 1995; **59**: 1356–1357

243. Geha A, Laks H, Stansel HJ *et al.* Late failure of porcine valve heterografts in children. *J Thorac Cardiovasc Surg* 1979; **59**: 1356–1357

244. Silver M, Pollock J, Silver M *et al.* Calcification in porcine xenograft valves in children. *Am J Cardiol* 1980; **45**: 685–689

245. Dunn J. Porcine valve durability in children. *Ann Thorac Surg* 1981; **32**: 357–368

246. Williams WG, Pollack JC, Geiss DM, Trusler GA, Fowler RS. Experience with aortic and mitral valve replacement in children. *J Thorac Cardiovasc Surg* 1981; **81**: 326–333

247. Miller D, Stinson E, Oyer P *et al.* The durability of porcine xenograft valves in conduits in children. *Circulation* 1982; **66 (Suppl 1)**: 1172–1185

248. Odell J. Calcification of procine bioprostheses in children. In: Cohn L, Gallucci V (eds) *Cardiac Bioprostheses: Proceedings of the Second International Symposium.* New York: Yorke Medical Books, 1982, p 231

249. Williams D, Danielson G, McGoon D, Puga F, Mair D, Edwards W. Porcine heterograft valve replacement in children. *J Thorac Cardiovasc Surg* 1982; **84**: 446–450

250. Turpie A, Gent M, Laupacis A *et al.* Comparison of aspirin with placebo in patients treated with warfarin after heart valve replacement. *N Engl J Med* 1993; **329**: 524–529

251. Rajah S, Sreeharan N, Joseph A *et al.* Prospective trial of dipyridamole and warfarin in heart valve patients. *Acta Thera (Brussels)* 1980; **6**: 54A

252. Sullivan JM, Harken DE, Gorlin R. Effect of dipyridamole on the incidence of arterial emboli after cardiac valve replacement. *Circulation* 1969; **39–40 (Suppl)**: 149–153

253. Stein PD, Alpert JS, Copeland JG, Dalen JE, Goldman S, Turpie GG. Antithrombotic therapy in patients with mechanical and biological prosthetic heart valves. *Chest* 1995; **108**: 371S–379S

354. Solymar L, Rao PS, Mardini MK, Fawzy ME, Guinn G. Prosthetic valves in children and adolescents. *Am Heart J* 1991; **121**: 557–568

255. Sade R, Ballenger J, Hohn A *et al.* Cardiac valve replacement in children: Comparison of tissue with mechanical prostheses. *J Thorac Cardiovasc Surg* 1979; **78**: 123–127

256. Harada Y, Imai Y, Kurosawa H, Ishihara K, Kawada M, Fukuchi S. Ten-year follow-up after valve replacement with the St Jude Medical prosthesis in children. *J Thorac Cardiovasc Surg* 1990; **100**: 175–180

257. Milano A, Vouhe PR, Baillot-Vernant F *et al.* Late results after left-sided cardiac valve replacement in children. *J Thorac Cardiovasc Surg* 1986; **92**: 218–225

258. Woods A, Vargas J, Berri G, Kreutzer G, Meschengieser S, Lazzari MA. Antithrombotic therapy in children and adolescents. *Thromb Res* 1986; **42**: 289–301

259. Truccone N, Bowman FJ, Malm J, Gersnoy W. Systemic-pulmonary arterial shunts in the first year of life. *Circulation* 1974; **49**: 508–511

260. Tamisier D, Vouhe P, Vernant F, Leca F, Massot C, Neveux J. Modified Blalock–Taussig shunts: Results in infants less than 3 months of age. *Ann Thorac Surg* 1990; **49**: 797–801

261. Gale AW. Modified Fontan operation for univentricular heart and complicated congenital lesions. *J Thorac Cardiovasc Surg* 1979; **78**: 831–838

262. Lam J, Neirotti R, Becker AE, Planche C. Thrombosis after the Fontan procedure: Transoesophageal echocardiography may replace angiocardiography. *J Thorac Cardiovasc Surg* 1994; **108**: 194–195

263. Mahony L. Thrombolytic treatment with streptokinase for late intraatrial thrombosis after modified Fontan procedure. *Am J Cardiol* 1988; **62**: 343–344

264. Mair DD, Rice MJ, Hagler DJ, Puga FJ, McGoon DC, Danileson GK. Outcome of the Fontan procedure in patients with tricuspid atresia. *Circulation* 1985; **72**: 88

265. Matthews K. Cerebral infarction complicating Fontan surgery for cyanotic congenital heart disease. *Pediatr Cardiol* 1986; **7**: 161–166

266. Myers J. A reconsideration of risk factors for the Fontan operation. *Ann Surg* 1990; **211**: 738–744

267. Okita Y, Miki S, Kusuhara K *et al.* Massive systemic venous thrombosis after Fontan operation: report of a case. *Thorac Cardiovasc Surg* 1988; **36**: 335–336

268. Prenger K. Porcine-valved dacron conduits in Fontan procedures. *Ann Thorac Surg* 1988; **46**: 526–530

269. Putnam JB, Lemmer JH, Rocchini AP, Bove EL. Embolectomy for acute pulmonary artery occlusion following Fontan procedure. *Ann Thorac Surg* 1988; **45**: 335–336

270. Rosenthal D. Thromboembolic complications after Fontan operations. *Circulation* 1995; **92**: II-287–II-293

271. Rosenthal D. Thrombosis of the pulmonary artery stump after distal ligation. *J Thorac Cardiovasc Surg* 1995; **110**: 1563–1565

272. Shannon FL, Campbell DN, Clarke DR. Right atrial thrombosis: rare complication of the modified Fontan procedure. *Pediatr Cardiol* 1986; **7**: 209–212

273. Sharratt G, Lacson A, Cornel G, Virmani S. Echocardiography of intracardiac filling defects in infants and children. *Pediatr Cardiol* 1986; **7**: 189–194

274. Stumper O, Sutherland G, Geuskens R, Roelandt J, Bos E, Hess J. Transesophageal echocardiography in evaluation and management after a Fontan procedure. *J Am Coll Cardiol* 1991; **17**: 1152–1160

275. Wilson D. Systemic thromboembolism leading to myocardial infarction and stroke after fenestrated total cavopulmonary connection. *Br Heart J* 1995; **73**: 483–485

276. Kaulitz R. Atrial thrombus after a Fontan operation; Predisposing factors, treatment and prophylaxis. *Cardiol Young* 1997; **7**: 37–43

277. Kreutzer G. An operation for the connection of tricuspid atresia. *J Thorac Cardiovasc Surg* 1973; **66**: 613–621

278. Downing TP. Pulmonary artery thrombosis associated with anomalous pulmonary venous connection: An unusual complication following the modified Fontan procedure. *J Thorac Cardiovasc Surg* 1985; **90**: 441–445

279. Annecchino F. Fontan repair for tricuspid atresia: Experience with 50 consecutive patients. *Ann Thorac Surg* 1988; **45**: 430–436

280. Asante-Korang A. Thrombolysis with tissue type plasminogen activator following cardiac surgery in children. *Int J Cardiol* 1992; **35**: 317–322

281. Cromme-Dijkhuis AH, Hess J, Hahlen K *et al.* Specific sequelae after Fontan operation at mid- and long-term followup. *J Thorac Cardiovasc Surg* 1993; **106**: 1126–1132

282. Cromme-Dijkhuis AH, Henkens CMA, Bijleveld CMA, Hillege HL, Born VJJ, van der Meer J. Coagulation factor abnormalities as possible thrombotic risk factors after Fontan operation. *Lancet* 1990; **336**: 1087–1090

283. Dajee H, Deutsch LS, Benson LN, Perloff JK, Laks H. Thrombolytic therapy for superior vena caval thrombosis following superior vena cava-pulmonary anastomosis. *Ann Thorac Surg* 1984; **38**: 637

284. Danielson G. Invited commentary. *Ann Thorac Surg* 1994; **58**: 1413–1414

285. Day RW, Boyer RS, Tait VF, Ruttenberg HD. Factors associated with stroke following the Fontan procedure. *Pediatr Cardiol* 1995; **16**: 270–275

286. Dobell ARC, Trusler GA, Smallhorn JF, Williams WG. Atrial thrombi after the Fontan operation. *Ann Thorac Surg* 1986; **16**: 270–275

287. Driscoll DJ, Offord KP, Feldt RH, Schaff HV, Puga FJ, Danielson GK. Five to fifteen year follow-up after Fontan operation. *Circulation* 1992; **85**: 469–496

288. Fletcher SE, Case CL, Fyfe DA, Gillette PC. Clinical spectrum of venous thrombi in the Fontan patient. *Am J Cardiol* 1991; **68**: 1721–1722

289. Fontan F, Deville C, Quaegebeur J *et al.* Repair of tricuspid atresia in 100 patients. *J Thorac Cardiovasc Surg* 1983; **85**: 647–660

290. Fyfe DA, Kline CH, Sade RM, Gillette PC. Transesophageal echocardiography detects thrombus formation not identified by transthoracic echocardiography after the Fontan operation. *J Am Coll Cardiol* 1991; **18**: 1733–1737

291. Hedrick M, Elkins RC, Knott-Craig CJ, Razook JD. Successful thrombectomy for thrombosis of the right side of the heart after the Fontan operation. *J Thorac Cardiovasc Surg* 1992; **105**: 297–301

292. Hutto RL, Williams JP, Maertens P, Wilder WM, Williams RS. Cerebellar infarct: late complication of the Fontan procedure? *Pediatr Neurol* 1991; **7**: 161–166

293. Jahangiri M, Ross DB, Redington AN, Lincoln C, Shinebourne EA.

Thromboembolism after the Fontan procedure and its modifications. *Ann Thorac Surg* 1994; **58**: 1409–1414

294. Laks H. Experience with the Fontan procedure. *J Thorac Cardiovasc Surg* 1984; **88**: 939–951

295. deVeber G, Andrew M. Canadian Pediatric Ischemic Stroke Registry. *29th Canadian Congress of Neurological Sciences*, 1994, Abstract

296. Schoenberg B, Mellinger J, Schoenberg D. Cerebrovascular disease in infants and children: A study of incidence, clinical features, and survival. *Neurology* 1978; **28**: 763–768

297. Broderick J, Talbot T, Prenger E, Leach A, Brott T. Stroke in children within a major metropolitan area: The surprising importance of intracerebral hemorrhage. *J Child Neurol* 1993; **8**: 250–255

298. Bonduel M, Torres AF, Pieroni G, Frontroth J, Serviddio RM. Ischemic stroke in children: Diagnosis, treatment and outcome. *Thromb Haemostas* 1997; **Suppl**: PS–353 (abstract)

299. Grandone N, D'Andrea G, d'Addedda M *et al*. Role of factor V Leiden (FV Leiden) and 5,10-methylene-tetrahydrofolate reductase (MTHFR) C>T677 mutations in premature ischemic stroke. *Thromb Haemostas* 1997; **Suppl**: PS–399 (abstract)

300. Iniesta JA, Corral J, Gonzalez-Conejero R, Rivera J, Ferrer F, Vicente V. Factor V (Arg506-Gln) mutation in ischaemic cerebrovascular disease. *Thromb Haemostas* 1997; **Suppl**: PS–400 (abstract)

301. De Luca D, Krekora K, d'Alessio D, Donati MB, Iacoviello L. Multiple cerebral ischemic events in a family homozygous for factor V Arg506 Gln mutation. *Thromb Haemostas* 1997; **Suppl**: PS–402 (abstract)

302. Krekora K, De Lucia D, Papa ML *et al*. Factor V Arg506Gln mutation in juvenile cerebrovascular disease. *Thromb Haemostas* 1997; **Suppl**: PS–403 (abstract)

303. Giordano P, Del Vecchio GC, Labriola P, Sabato KM, De Mattia D. Resistance to activated protein C as an underlying cause of stroke in a thalassemic child. *Thromb Haemostas* 1997; **Suppl**: PS–404 (abstract)

304. Brancaccio V, Orefice G, Iannoccone L, Ames PRJ. Protein C and activated protein C resistance in ischemic stroke. *Thromb Haemostas* 1997; **Suppl**: PS–405 (abstract)

305. Zenz W, Bodo Z. Resistance to activated protein C/factor V Leiden mutation (APCR-F-V-LM) in children with stroke. *Thromb Haemostas* 1997; **Suppl**: PS–408 (abstract)

306. Vielhaber H, Debus O, Findeisen M *et al*. Factor V Leiden, further inhibitors of the protein C anticoagulant pathway and lipoprotein (a) in childhood stroke. *Thromb Haemostas* 1997; **Suppl**: PS–409 (abstract)

307. Ebert W, Schneppenheim R. Perinatal stroke in 4 newborns with FV Leiden. *Thromb Haemostas* 1997; **Suppl**: PS–410 (abstract)

308. Strater R, Albers S, Debus O *et al*. Genetic factors of familial thrombophilia in childhood venous sinus thrombosis. *Thromb Haemostas* 1997; **Suppl**: PS–418 (abstract)

309. Trauner DA, Chase C, Walker P, Wulfeck B. Neurologic profiles of infants and children after perinatal stroke. *Pediatr Neurol* 1993; **9**: 383–386

310. Bouza H, Rutherford M, Acolet D, Pennock JM, Dubowitz LM. Evolution of early hemiplegic signs in full term infants with unilateral brain lesions in the neonatal period: A prospective study. *Neuropediatrics* 1994; **25**: 201–207

311. Lanska M, Lanska D, Horwitz S, Aram D. Presentation, clinical course, and outcome of childhood stroke. *Pediatr Neurol* 1991; **7**: 333–341

312. Trescher W. Ischemic stroke syndromes in childhood. *Pediatr Ann* 1992; **21**: 374–382

313. Roach RS, Riela AR (ed). *Pediatric Cerebrovascular Disorders*. New York: Futura Publishing, 1995

314. Wiznitzer M, Masaryk TJ. Cerebrovascular abnormalities in pediatric stroke: Assessment using parenchymal and angiographic magnetic resonance imaging. *Ann Neurol* 1991; **29**: 585–589

315. Koelfen W, Wentz U, Freund M, Schulze C. Magnetic resonance angiography in 140 neuropediatrics patients. *Pediatr Neurol* 1995; **12**: 31–38

316. Isler W. Stroke in childhood and adolescence. *Eur Neurol* 1984; **23**: 421–424

317. Kay R, Sing Wong K, Ling Yu Y. Low molecular weight heparin for the treatment of acute ischemic stroke. *N Engl J Med* 1995; **333**: 1588–1593

318. The National Institute of Neurological Disorders for Acute Ischemic Stroke. Tissue plasminogen activator for acute ischemic stroke. *N Engl J Med* 1995; **333**: 1581–158

319. Wong VK, LeMesurier J, Franseschini R, Heikali M, Hanson R. Cerebral venous thrombosis as a cause of neonatal seizures. *Pediatr Neurol* 1987; **3**: 235–237

320. Griesemer DA, Theodorou AA, Berg RA, Spera TD. Local fibrinolysis in cerebral venous thrombosis. *Pediatr Neurol* 1994; **10**: 78–80

321. Horowitz M, Purdy P, Unwin H *et al*. Treatment of dural sinus thrombosis using selective catheterization and urokinase. *Ann Neurol* 1995; **38**: 58–67

322. Hirsh J. Heparin. *N Engl J Med* 1991; **324**: 1565–1574

323. Mitchell L, Piovella F, Ofosu F, Andrew M. Alpha-2-macroglobulin may provide protection from thromboembolic events in antithrombin III deficient children. *Blood* 1991; **78**: 2299–2304

324. Wood C, Williams A, McNamara J, Annunziata J, Feorino P, Conway C. Antibody against the human immunodeficiency virus in commercial intravenous gammaglobulin preparations. *Ann Intern Med* 1986; **105**: 536–538

325. Andrew M, Ofosu F, Schmidt B, Brooker L, Hirsh J, Buchanan M. Heparin clearance and *ex vivo* recovery in newborn piglets and adult pigs. *Thromb Res* 1988; **52**: 517–527

326. Andrew M, Paes B, Johnston M. Development of the hemostatic system in the neonate and young infant. *Am J Pediatr Hematol Oncol* 1990; **12**: 95–104

327. Andrew M, Brooker L, Mitchell L. Acquired antithrombin II deficiency secondary to asparaginase therapy in childhood acute lymphoblastic leukemia. *Blood Coag Fibrinol* 1994; **5**: S24–S36

328. Schmidt B, Ofosu F, Mitchell L, Brooker L, Andrew M. Anticoagulant effects of heparin in neonatal plasma. *Pediatr Res* 1989; **25**: 405–408

329. Andrew M, Schmidt B, Mitchell L, Paes B, Ofosu F. Thrombin generation in newborn plasma is critically dependent on the concentration of prothrombin. *Thromb Haemostas* 1990; **63**: 27–30

330. Andrew M, Mitchell L, Vegh P, Ofosu F. Thrombin regulation in children differs from adults in the absence and presence of heparin. *Thromb Haemostas* 1994; **72**: 836–842

331. Andrew M, Marzinotto V, Blanchette V *et al*. Heparin therapy in pediatric patients: A prospective cohort study. *Pediatr Res* 1994; **35**: 78–83

332. Cruickshank M, Levine M, Hirsh J, Roberts R, Siguenza M. A standard heparin nomogram for the management of heparin therapy. *Arch Intern Med* 1991; **151**: 333–337

333. Melissari E, Parker CJ, Wilson NV *et al*. Use of low molecular weight heparin in pregnancy. *Thomb Haemostas* 1992; **68**: 652–656

334. Murphy M. Heparin therapy and bone fractures. *Lancet* 1992; **340**: 1098

335. Sackler JP. Heparin induced osteoporosis. *Br J Radiol* 1973; **46**: 548–550

336. Schuster J. Pathology of osteopathy following heparin therapy. *J Pediatr Surg* 1969; **20**: 410

337. Murdoch I, Beattie R, Silver D. Heparin-induced thrombocytopenia in children. *Acta Pediatr* 1993; **82**: 495–497

338. Spadone D, Clark F, James E, Laster J, Hoch J, Silver D. Heparin-induced thrombocytopenia in the newborn. *J Vasc Surg* 1992; **15**: 306–311

339. Mocan H, Beattie T, Murphy A. Renal venous thrombosis in infancy: long-term follow-up. *Pediatr Nephrol* 1991; **5**: 45–49

340. Honig G, Abildgaard C, Forman E, Gotoff S, Lindley A, Schulman I. Some properties of the anticoagulant factor of aged pooled plasma. *Thromb Diath Haemorrh* 1969; **22**: 151–163

341. Hirsh J, Levine M. Low molecular weight heparin. *Blood* 1992; **79**: 1–17

342. McDonald MM, Hathaway WE. Anticoagulant therapy by continuous heparinization in newborn and older infants. *J Pediatr* 1982; **101**: 451–457

343. Boneu B, Buchanan MR, Caranobe C *et al.* The disappearance of a low molecular weight heparin fraction (CY216) differs from standard heparin in rabbits. *Thromb Res* 1987; **46**: 845–853

344. Andersson L, Barrowcliffe T, Holmer E, Johnson E, Sims G. Anticoagulant properties of heparin fractionated by affinity chromatography on matrix-bound antithrombin III and by gel filtration. *Thromb Res* 1976; **9**: 575–583

345. Johnson E, Kirkwood T, Stirling Y *et al.* Four heparin preparations: anti-Xa potentiating effects of heparin after subcutaneous injection. *Thromb Haemostas* 1976; **35**: 586–591

346. Bergqvist D, Hedner U, Sjorin E, Holmer E. Anticoagulant effects of two types of low molecular weight heparin and administered subcutaneously. *Thromb Res* 1983; **32**: 381–391

347. Carter C, Kelton J, Hirsh J, Cerksus A, Santos A, Gent M. The relationship between the hemorrhagic and antithrombotic properties of a low molecular weight heparin in rabbits. *Blood* 1982; **59**: 1239–1245

348. Ockelford P, Carter C, Cerskus A, Smith C, Hirsh J. Comparison of the *in vivo* hemorrhagic and antithrombotic effects of a low antithrombin III affinity heparin fraction. *Thromb Res* 1982; **27**: 679–690

349. Ofosu FA. *In vitro* and *ex-vivo* activities of CY216: Comparion with other low molecular weight heparins. *Haemostasis* 1990; **20 (Suppl 1)**: 180

350. Massicotte MP, Adams M, Leaker M, Andrew M. A nomogram to establish therapeutic levels of the low molecular weight (LMWH), clivarine in children requiring treatment for venous thromboembolism (VTE). *Thromb Haemostas* 1998 (in press)

351. Hirsh J. Oral anticoagulant drugs. Review article. *N Engl J Med* 1991; **324**: 1865–1875

352. Quick AJ, Grossman AM. Prothrombin concentration in newborns. *Proc Soc Exp Biol Med* 1939; **41**: 227

353. Loeliger E, van den Besselaar A, Lewis S. Reliability and clinical impact of the normalization of the prothrombin times in oral anticoagulant control. *Thromb Haemostas* 1985; **54**: 148–154

354. Roy A, Jaffe N, Djerassi I. Prophylactic platelet transfusions in children with acute leukemia: A dose response study. *Transfusion* 1973; **13**: 283

355. Poller L. Progress in standardization anticoagulation control. *Hematol Rev* 1987; **1**: 225–241

356. Poller L. Laboratory control of oral anticoagulants. *Br Med J* 1987; **294**: 1184

357. International Committee for Standardization in Haematology and International Committee on Thrombosis and Haematosis. ICSH/ICTH Recommendations for reporting prothrombin time in oral anticoagulant control. *Thromb Haemostas* 1985; **53**: 155–156

358. Hirsh J, Poller L, Deykin D, Levine M, Dalen JE. Optimal therapeutic range for oral anticoagulants. *Chest* 1989; **95**: 5S–11S

359. Andrew M, Marzinotto V, Brooker L *et al.* Oral anticoagulant therapy in pediatric patients: A prospective study. *Thromb Haemostas* 1994; **71**: 265–269

360. Carpentieri U, Nghiem QX, Harris LC. Clinical experience with an oral anticoagulant in children. *Arch Dis Child* 1976; **51**: 445–448

361. Doyle JJ, Koren G, Chen MY, Blanchette VS. Anticoagulation with sodium warfarin in children: Effect of a loading regimen. *J Pediatr* 1988; **113**: 1095–1097

362. Evans D, Rowlands M, Poller L. Survey of oral anticoagulant treatment in children. *J Clin Pathol* 1992; **45**: 707–703

363. Hathaway WE. Use of antiplatelet agents in pediatric hypercoagulable states. *Am J Dis Child* 1984; **138**: 301–304

364. Bradley LM, Midgley FM, Watson DC *et al.* Anticoagulation therapy in children with mechanical prosthetic cardiac valves. *Am J Cardiol* 1985; **56**: 533–535

365. Aballi A, de Lamerens S. Coagulation changes in the neonatal period and in early infancy. *Pediatr Clin North Am* 1962; **9**: 785–817

366. Shearer MJ, Barkhan P, Rahim S, Stimmler L. Plasma vitamin K_1 in mothers and their newborn babies. *Lancet* 1982; **ii**: 460–463

367. Greer FR, Mummah-Schendel LL, Marshall S, Suttie JW. Vitamin K_1 (phylloquinone) and Vitamin K_2 (menaquinone) status in newborns during the first week of life. *Pediatrics* 1988; **81**: 137–140

368. Haroon Y, Shearer MJ, Rahim S, Gunn WG, McEnery G, Barkhan P. The content of phylloquinone (vitamin K_1) in human milk, cow's milk and infant formula foods determined by high-performance liquid chromatography. *J Nutr* 1982; **112**: 1105–1117

369. Von Kries R, Shearer MJ, McCarthy PT, Haug M, Hanzer G, Gobel U. Vitamin K_1 content of maternal milk: Influence of the stage of lactation, lipid composition, and vitamin K_1 supplements given to the mother. *Pediatr Res* 1987; **22**: 513–517

370. Andrew M. The hemostatic system in the infant. In: Nathan D, Oski F (eds) *Hematology of Infancy and Childhood*. Philadelphia: WB Saunders, 1992, pp 115–154

371. Davies R, Berman WJ, Wernly J, Kelly H. Warfarin-nafcillin interaction. *J Pediatr* 1991; **118**: 300–303

372. Kumar S, Haigh J, Rhodes L *et al.* Poor compliance is a major factor in unstable outpatient control of anticoagulant therapy. *Thromb Haemostas* 1989; **62**: 729–732

373. Stewart S, Cianciotta D, Alexson C, Manning J. The long-term risk of warfarin sodium therapy and the incidence of thromboembolism in children after prosthetic cardiac valves. *J Thorac Cardiovasc Surg* 1987; **93**: 551–554

374. Massicotte P, Marzinotto V, Vegh P, Adams M, Andrew M. Home monitoring of warfarin therapy in children with a whole blood prothrombin time monitor. *J Pediatr* 1995; **127**: 389–394

375. Becker D, Andrew D, Triplett D. Continued accurate patient prothrombin time self-testing over prolonged duration using the Protime microcoagulation system. *Thromb Haemostas* 1997; **(Suppl)**: PS–2862 (abstract)

376. Marzinotto V, Leaker M, Massicotte MP, Adams M, Andrew M. The evaluation of a whole blood prothrombin time monitor in a pediatric outpatient clinic and home setting. *Thromb Haemostas* 1997; **(Suppl)**: PD–3121 (abstract)

377. Kornblit P, Senderoff J, Davis-Ericksen M, Zenk J. Anticoagulation therapy: Patient management and evaluation of an outpatient clinic. *Nurse Pract* 1990; **15**: 21–32

378. Cortelazzo S, Finazzi G, Viero P *et al.* Thrombotic and hemorrhagic complications in patients with mechanical heart valve prosthesis attending an anticoagulation clinic. *Thromb Haemostas* 1993; **69**: 316–320

379. Petty GW, Lennihan L, Mohr JP *et al.* Complications of long-term anticoagulation. *Ann Neurol* 1988; **23**: 570–574

380. Garabedian-Ruffalo SM, Gray DR, Sax MJ, Ruffalo RL. Retrospective evaluation of a pharmacist-managed warfarin anticoagulation clinic. *Am J Hosp Pharm* 1985; **42**: 304

381. Ellis R, Stephens M, Sharp G. Evaluation of a pharmacy-managed warfarin-monitoring service to coordinate inpatient and outpatient therapy. *Am J Hosp Pharm* 1992; **49**: 387–394

382. Spevak P, Freed M, Castaneda A, Norwood WI, Pollack P. Valve replacement in children less than 5 years of age. *J Am Cardiol* 1986; **8**: 901–908

383. Schaffer MS, Clarke DR, Campbell DN, Madigan CK, Wiggins JW Jr, Wolfe RR. The St Jude Medical cardiac valve and children: Role of anticoagulant therapy. *J Am Coll Cardiol* 1987; **9**: 235–239

384. Rao S, Solymar L, Mardini M, Fawzy M, Guinn G. Anticoagulant therapy in children with prosthetic valves. *Ann Thorac Surg* 1989; **47**: 589–592

385. Schaff H, Danielson G, DiDanato R, Puga F, Mair D, McGoon D. Late results after Starr–Edwards valve replacement in children. *J Thorac Cardiovasc Surg* 1984; **88**: 583–589

386. Borkon AM, Soule L, Reitz BA, Gott VL, Gardner TJ. Five year follow-up after valve replacement with the St Jude Medical valve in infants and children. *Circulation* 1986; **74 (Suppl 1)**: I-110–115

387. Human DG, Joffe HS, Fraser CB, Barnard CN. Mitral valve replacement in children. *J Thorac Cardiovasc Surg* 1982; **83**: 873–877

388. Antunes MJ, Vanderdonck KM, Sussman MJ. Mechanical valve replacement in children and teenagers. *Eur J Cardiothorac Surg* 1989; **3**: 222–228

389. Rajasekhar D, Kestin A, Bednarek F, Ellis P, Barnard M, Michelson A. Neonatal platelets are less reactive than adult platelets to physiological agonists in whole blood. *Thromb Haemostas* 1994; **72**: 957–963

390. Serra A, McNicholas K, Olivier HJ, Boe S, Lemole G. The choice of anticoagulation in pediatric patients with the St Jude Medical valve prosthesis. *J Cardiovasc Surg* 1987; **28**: 588–591

391. McGrath L, Gonzalez-Lavin L, Edlredge W, Colombi M, Restrepo D. Thromboembolic and other events following valve replacement in a pediatric population treated with antiplatelet agents. *Ann Thorac Surg* 1987; **43**: 285–287

392. LeBlanc J, Sett S, Vince D. Antiplatelet therapy in children with left-sided mechanical prostheses. *Eur J Cardiothorac Surg* 1993; **7**: 211–215

393. Goodman-Gilman A, Rall TW, Nies AS, Taylor P (eds). Immunosuppressive agents. In: *The Pharmacological Basis of Therapeutics*, 8th edn. Elmsford: Pergamon Press, 1990, pp 1264–1276

394. Imbach P, Barandun S, d'Apuzzo VA *et al*. High-dose intravenous gammaglobulin for idiopathic thrombocytopenic purpura in childhood. *Lancet* 1981; **i**: 1228–1231

395. Starko K, Ray C, Dominguez L, Stromberg W, Woodall D. Reye's syndrome and salicylate use. *Pediatrics* 1980; **66**: 859–864

396. Makela A, Lang H, Korpela P. Toxic encephalopathy with hyperammonaemia during high-dose salicyclate therapy. *Acta Neurol Scand* 1980; **61**: 146–151

397. Corrigan J, Sluth J, Jeter M, Lox C. Newborn's fibrinolytic mechanism: Components and plasmin generation. *Am J Hematol* 1989; **32**: 273–278

398. Leaker M, Brooker L, Mitchell L, Weitz J, Superina R, Andrew M. Fibrin clot lysis by tissue plasminogen activator (tPA) is impaired in plasma from pediatric patients undergoing orthotopic liver transplantation. *Transplantation* 1995; **60**: 144–147

399. Biggs R. Human blood coagulation. In: Biggs R (ed) *Haemostasis and Thrombosis*. Oxford: Blackwell Scientific Publications, 1972, p 614

400. Leaker M, Superina R, Andrew M. Fibrin clot lysis by tissue plasminogen activator (tPA) is impaired in plasma from pediatric liver transplant patients. *Transplantation* 1995; **60**: 144–147

401. Andrew M, Brooker L, Paes B, Weitz J. Fibrin clot lysis by thrombolytic agents is impaired in newborns due to a low plasminogen concentration. *Thromb Haemostas* 1992; **68**: 325–330

402. Kellam B, Fraze D, Kanarek K. Clot lysis for thrombosed central venous catheters in pediatric patients. *J Perinatol* 1987; **VII**: 242–244

403. Morris J, Occhionero M, Gauderer M *et al*. Totally implantable vascular access devices in cystic fibrosis: A four-year experience with fifty-eight patients. *J Pediatr* 1990; **117**: 82–85

404. Winthrop AL, Wesson DE. Urokinase in the treatment of occluded central venous catheters in children. *J Pediatr Surg* 1984; **19**: 536–538

405. Hyers TM, Hull RD, Weg JC. Antithrombotic therapy for venous thromboembolic disease. *Chest* 1995; **108**: 335S–351S

406. Schmidt B, Andrew M. Report of scientific and standardization subcommittee on neonatal hemostasis: diagnosis and treatment of neonatal thrombosis. *Thromb Haemostas* 1992; **67**: 381–382

407. Stein P, Grandison D, Hua T *et al*. Therapeutic levels of oral anticoagulation with warfarin in patients with mechanical prosthetic heart valves: Review of literature and recommendations based on International Normalized Ratio. *Postgrad Med J* 1994; **70 (Suppl 1)**: S72–S83

408. Turpie A, Gunstensen J, Hirsh J, Nelson H, Gent M. Randomized comparison of two intensities of oral anticoagulant therapy after tissue heart valve replacement. *Lancet* 1988; **i**: 1242–1245

409. Andrew M, Halton J, Massicotte M. Treatment of homozygous Protein C deficiency in two children with low molecular weight heparin (LMWH) therapy. *Thromb Haemostas* 1995; **73**: 939 (abstract 154)

410. Andrew M, deVeber G. *Pediatric Thromboembolism and Stroke Protocols*. Hamilton: BC Decker, 1997

Supportive therapy

Blood components: preparation, indications and administration

HEATHER A HUME

Blood component transfusion is an integral part of the treatment plan of many of the children and adolescents cared for by the pediatrician or the pediatric hematologist/oncologist. Physicians responsible for the transfusion of blood components should have a basic understanding of the components they prescribe, including method of preparation and contents, indications and contraindications for use and the correct storage conditions and procedures for administration. These topics are covered in this chapter. Physicians prescribing blood components should also be knowledgeable about the potential adverse effects of these products including requirements for further modifications of certain components, such as γ-irradiation or the provision of components at low risk for cytomegalovirus (CMV) transmission, to meet special patient needs. These aspects of blood transfusion therapy are addressed in Chapter 36.

BLOOD COMPONENT PREPARATION

Blood components are prepared from blood collected by whole blood (WB) or apheresis donation. WB donations are separated, as required, into red blood cell (RBC), plasma and platelet components by differential centrifugation. Cryoprecipitate may be prepared from a plasma unit as described below. Automated apheresis procedures may be used to collect platelets, granulocytes or plasma. The possibility of obtaining RBCs using apheresis procedures is currently under investigation. Plasma proteins, such as albumin, anti-D, immune serum globulins, intravenous immunoglobulins and concentrated coagulation factors are prepared by more extensive processing of large pools of donor plasma obtained from WB or plasmapheresis donations.

PREPARATION OF COMPONENTS FROM WHOLE BLOOD DONATIONS

WB is collected into sterile blood bags that contain a premeasured amount of anticoagulant/preservative (AP) solution. Standard blood bags contain enough AP solution to collect and store 450 ml WB ($\pm 10\%$). If smaller amounts of WB are to be collected, e.g. in pediatric autologous blood donations, the amount of AP solution must be appropriately adjusted. Two types of AP solutions, namely additive or non-additive, may be used for blood component collection and storage. Using non-additive solutions, the entire amount of the AP solution is present in the primary collection bag, whereas the use of additive solutions consists of collecting WB into the primary bag which contains an anticoagulant solution and adding the constituents necessary for RBC preservation to the RBCs following the separation of the RBCs from the plasma. Because RBCs, platelets, leukocytes and plasma have different specific gravities they can be separated from each other by differential centrifugation. Generally, WB is collected into a primary bag with 1, 2 or 3 satellite bags depending on the components to be prepared. The satellite bags are attached to the primary bag with integral tubing so that components can be prepared in a closed system that maintains sterility. The separation of WB into the most commonly used blood components using

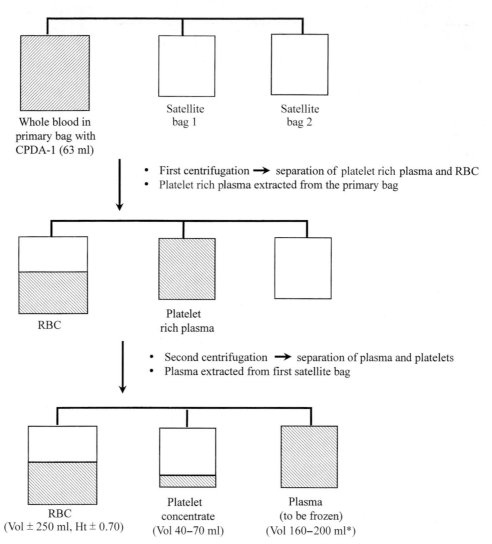

Fig. 35.1 Preparation of blood components from whole blood using the anticoagulant/preservative solution CPDA-1. RBC = red blood cells; Ht = hematocrit; CPDA-1 = citrate-phosphate-dextrose-adenine; Vol = volume. *If a platelet concentrate is not made, the volume of the plasma unit will be proportionally larger.

non-additive or additive solutions is shown in Figs 35.1 and 35.2, respectively.

ANTICOAGULANT/PRESERVATIVE SOLUTIONS

An AP solution must fulfill 3 requirements:

1. prevent coagulation of the stored blood unit;
2. maintain red blood cell viability and function;
3. be non-toxic when re-infused into the recipient.

The only non-additive AP solution in common use is CPDA-1 (citrate–phosphate–dextrose–adenine). Several additive AP solutions are in current use. All AP solutions contain dextrose, which is a source of metabolic energy, adenine to maintain the RBC adenine nucleotide pool and citrate, which as a calcium chelator serves as an anticoagulant. Mannitol which is part of some additive solutions prevents the hemolysis of RBCs which can occur in a plasma-poor medium. The contents of some of the most commonly used AP solutions are shown in Table 35.1.

Red cells undergo physical and biochemical changes during storage at 4°C, which are known collectively as the 'storage lesion'. The volume of red cells does not change significantly but their shape changes from that of discocytes to echinocytes or spheroechinocytes.[1,2] Some of the biochemical changes that occur are shown in Table 35.2.[3,4] The decrease in intraerythrocyte ATP levels is partly but not solely related to a decrease in RBC post-transfusion viability.[5] Intraerythrocyte 2,3-diphosphoglycerate (2,3-DPG) plays a major role in the RBC's capacity to release oxygen to tissues.[6] Nevertheless, the decrease in 2,3-DPG during storage appears to be of little significance in most clinical settings since 2,3-DPG levels of stored RBCs increase (in adults, at least) to >50% of normal within several hours and to normal levels within 24 hours of transfusion.[7] Even in the setting of massive transfusion of stored blood, detrimental effects of the low levels of 2,3-DPG have not been demonstrated in adults, although these observations may not be generalizable to massive transfusions in the neonate, as discussed below.[8] The other biochemical changes also do

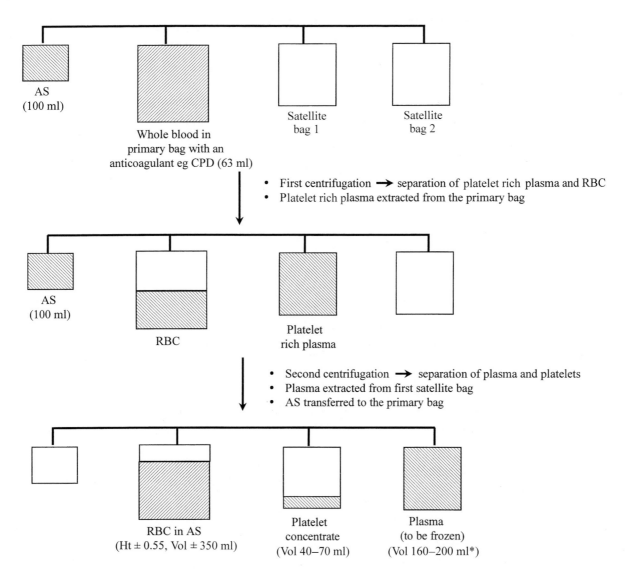

Fig. 35.2 Preparation of blood components from whole blood using an additive solution for RBC preservation. AS = additive solution; RBC = red blood cells; Ht = hematocrit; CPD = citrate-phosphate-dextrose; Vol = volume. *If a platelet concentrate is not made, the volume of the plasma unit will be proportionally larger.

Table 35.1 Contents of selected anticoagulant preservative solutions. Adapted from information supplied by the manufacturers.

Content (g/volume)	CPDA-1 (63 ml)	Adsol system		Nutricel system		SAG-M	
		Primary bag CPD (63 ml)	Additive AS-1 (100 ml)	Primary bag CP2D (63 ml)	Additive AS-3 (100 ml)	Primary bag CPD (63 ml)	Additive
Trisodium citrate	1.66	1.66	—	1.66	0.588	1.66	—
Dextrose	2.01	1.61	2.20	3.22	1.10	1.61	0.820
Citric acid	0.206	0.206	—	0.206	0.042	0.206	—
Monobasic sodium phosphate	0.140	0.140	—	0.140	0.276	0.140	—
Adenine	0.017	—	0.027	—	0.030	—	0.017
Mannitol	—	—	0.75	—	—	—	0.525
Sodium chloride	—	—	0.90	—	0.410	—	0.877
Shelf-life of RBC units (days)*	35		42		42		

*Shelf-life varies from country to country according to licensing authorities.

Table 35.2 Biochemical changes of stored red blood cells. Adapted from Refs 3, 4 and information supplied by the manufacturers.

| Variable | CPDA-1 | | | | AS-1 (Adsol system) | AS-3 (Nutricel system) | SAG-M |
	WB	RBC	WB	RBC	RBC	RBC	RBC
Days of storage	0	0	35	35	42	42	42
Viable cells (24 hours post-transfusion) (%)	100	100	79	71	76	83	>75
pH (measured at 37°C)	7.55	7.60	6.98	6.71	6.6	6.5	7.1
ATP (% of initial value)	100	100	56	45	60	58	–
2,3-DPG (% of initial value)	100	100	<10	<10	<5	<10	<10
Plasma K$^+$ (mmol/l)	5.10	4.20	27.30	78.50	50		–
Plasma Hb (mg/l)	78	82	461	658	N/A	N/A	N/A

WB = whole blood; RBC = red blood cells; Hb = hemoglobin; N/A = not applicable.

not appear to have significant clinical consequences except possibly for massive transfusion in the neonate or young infant (see Chapter 36).[8]

Licensing of AP solutions, including the accepted duration of RBC storage (the 'shelf-life'), depends on the ability of the AP solution to assure 70% recovery of transfused RBCs 24 hours after infusion. RBCs in AP solutions generally have a shelf-life of 42 days, while RBCs stored in CPDA-1 have a shelf-life of 35 days. In addition to a longer shelf-life for RBCs, the advantages of additive solutions are a lower hematocrit in the RBC unit (which facilitates infusion) and the possibility of extracting larger amounts of plasma from the original WB unit. Their one disadvantage is a concern about their safety for large volume transfusions in the neonate (see below).

PREPARATION OF COMPONENTS BY APHERESIS TECHNIQUES

Automated apheresis instruments use computer-controlled technology to draw and anticoagulate blood, separate the blood components either by centrifugation or filtration, collect the desired component, and recombine the remaining components for return to the donor. Automated apheresis procedures are used to separate and collect platelets, granulocytes and plasma. Each apheresis collection can procure larger quantities of 1 of these 3 components than can be extracted from a single whole blood donation. Because RBC loss for the donor is minimal, repeat donations can be performed at more frequent intervals than is permissible for WB donations.

WHOLE BLOOD

DESCRIPTION AND STORAGE

A unit of WB is collected into an AP solution, usually CPDA-1, has a volume of approximately 510 ml (450 ml WB plus

63 ml CPDA-1) and a hematocrit of 0.30–0.40. It must be stored at 1–6°C and, if collected into CPDA-1, has a shelf-life of 35 days. Within 24 hours of collection the platelets as well as the granulocytes in the unit are dysfunctional and several plasma coagulation factors (in particular Factors V and VIII) have fallen to suboptimal levels.[9,10]

INDICATIONS FOR TRANSFUSION

Theoretically, the transfusion of WB could be used in situations such as rapid, massive blood loss, which require the simultaneous restoration of oxygen-carrying capacity and blood volume. However, in most cases, the resuscitation of such patients can be achieved by the use of RBC concentrates and crystalloids or colloid solutions (either albumin or non-blood-derived colloid solutions such as pentastarch). Should plasma coagulation factor replacement become necessary, the levels of coagulation Factors V and VIII in stored WB are rarely sufficient to correct the corresponding deficiencies. Given these considerations, most centers preparing blood components provide little or no WB (except autologous blood) but rather separate WB donations into the more commonly required blood components. As described below, WB <5–7 days old may be used for exchange transfusion in newborn infants.

DOSAGE AND ADMINISTRATION

WB should not be used unless the donor and recipient are ABO-identical (for use in neonates, see below). The volume of transfusion depends on the clinical situation. In an adult, 1 unit of WB will increase the recipient's hemoglobin (Hb) concentration by approximately 1 g/dl. In pediatric patients, a WB transfusion of 8 ml/kg will result in a similar increase. WB must be administered through a blood filter, either a standard 170-μm macroaggregate filter or a microaggregate filter. After an initial slow drip (to allow observation for immediate, severe transfusion reactions), the rate of infusion should be as fast as clinically indicated or tolerated and in all cases must be completed within 4 hours (to avoid bacterial contamination).

RED BLOOD CELLS

DESCRIPTION AND STORAGE

RBC concentrates are prepared from WB donations (Figs 35.1 and 35.2). These concentrates can be further modified for use in specific clinical settings. Characteristics of the various RBC preparations, including their contents and storage conditions, are summarized in Table 35.3.

INDICATIONS FOR TRANSFUSION

Physiologic responses to anemia

Decisions with respect to the need to administer an RBC transfusion to an anemic patient are facilitated by an understanding of the normal physiologic responses to anemia. This subject will therefore be briefly reviewed here. For more detailed discussions of this subject and the original studies summarized in this section readers are referred to the literature.[11–16]

Oxygen availability for the body as a whole (as opposed to regional requirements – see below) usually exceeds resting oxygen requirements by 2–4-fold. For example, in the anesthetized, otherwise normal, healthy adult, oxygen delivery (DO_2) is between 560 and 800 ml/min/m^2, while total body oxygen consumption, on the other hand, is

Table 35.3 Red blood cell components.

Component	Preparation	RBC recovery* (%)	Approximate volume	Hematocrit	Leukocyte count	Storage	Indication for modified component
RBCs in CPDA-1	WB with 200–250 ml of plasma removed	>99	250 ml	0.70–0.75	10^{10}	35 days at 1–6°C	
RBCs in AS	WB with most of the plasma removed and AS 100 ml added	>99	350 ml	0.50–0.60	10^{10}	35–42 days** at 1–6°C	
RBCs, buffy coat poor	WB with most of the plasma and leukocytes removed and AS 100 ml added	90	300 ml	0.60–0.65	10^9	35 days	History of repeated febrile and/or allergic reactions
RBCs, washed	RBCs in AS or CPDA-1 washed then resuspended with USP	80	Variable depending on quantity of USP used for resuspension	Variable depending on quantity of USP used for resuspension	10^8–10^9	24 h at 1–6°C	History of repeated febrile and/or allergic reactions unresponsive to buffy-coat poor or leukodepleted RBCs Prevention of severe allergic reactions or anaphylaxis due to anti-IgA
RBCs, frozen-deglycerolized	RBCs frozen with glyercol (a cryoprotectant); thawed and deglycerolized by washing prior to transfusion. Resuspended in USP	80	Variable depending on quantity of USP used for resuspension	Variable depending on quantity of USP used for resuspension	10^8–10^9	May be stored frozen for up to 10 years (depending on the glycerol concentration) After thawing: storage at 1–6°C for 24 h	Prolonged storage of autologous units or allogeneic units with rare RBC phenotypes
RBCs, leukocyte reduced by filtration	RBCs in CPDA-1 or AS leukodepleted by filtration	>90	CPDA-1: <250 ml AS: <350 ml	CPDA-1: 0.70–0.75 AS: 0.50–0.60	<5 × 10^6	Pre-storage: as for CPDA-1 or AS RBCs Post-storage: for immediate infusion	History of repeated febrile and/or allergic reactions Prevention of HLA alloimmunization and/or CMV transmission

*As compared to WB with 100% of the original RBCs.
**Shelf-life varies from country to country according to licensing authorities.
RBC = red blood cell; CPDA-1 = citrate–phosphate–dextrose–adenine anticoagulant; WB = whole blood; AS = additive solution; USP = 0.9% sodium chloride injection.

maintained near 110 ml/min/m^2. There is therefore, under stable conditions, a significant excess of oxygen delivery over consumption.

DO$_2$ is the product of cardiac output (CO) and the arterial oxygen content (CaO$_2$), i.e. DO$_2$ = CO × CaO$_2$. CaO$_2$ is determined by the Hb concentration and the percent of Hb that is saturated with oxygen. CO is determined by the product of the heart rate and stroke volume (the amount of blood ejected by the ventricule per beat). Tissue hypoxia will occur if DO$_2$ decreases to a level where tissues no longer have enough oxygen to meet metabolic demands. From the above equation, it is apparent that tissue hypoxia may be caused by decreased Hb saturation (hypoxemia), by a decreased RBC mass (anemia) or by cardiac insufficiency. Theoretically, hypoxia could also occur in the presence of adequate DO$_2$ if the tissues are unable to use appropriately the delivered oxygen.

Each of the determinants of DO$_2$ has substantial physiologic reserves. When intravascular volume is stable or increased following the development of anemia (as opposed to hypovolemic anemia and shock), increases in CO have been consistently reported. With progressive reduction in red cell and Hb concentrations, there is an incremental rise in cardiac output which peaks as the Hb approaches 7 g/dl. In adults, the increase in CO is mainly due to an increase in stroke volume (SV). SV is determined by the loading conditions (preload and afterload) of the heart as well as its contractility. A major determinant of preload and afterload is blood viscosity. Blood is most viscous (inherently resistant to flow) at lower flow rates and has its highest viscosity in venules and its lowest in the aorta. Viscosity, independent of flow rate, is primarily a function of red cell concentration. Reduction in the red cell concentration lowers blood viscosity which in turn decreases afterload. Decreased blood viscosity also leads to an increased venous return, i.e. an increased preload. Decreases in blood viscosity appear to play a major role in the increased SV and resulting increase in CO observed in acute normovolemic and chronic anemia in adults. On the other hand, neonates have a very limited capacity to increase SV.[17] Thus increases in CO in neonates are almost entirely due to an increase in heart rate (HR). Cardiovascular responses to normovolemic anemia have been less well studied in children. Three (poorly controlled) pediatric studies gave conflicting results as to whether the increase in CO is mostly a consequence of increased HR or SV.[18–20]

In addition to changes in tissue oxygen delivery, tissue oxygenation may also be increased by an increase in the amount of oxygen released from the hemoglobin transported to the tissues, i.e. tissues may increase oxygen extraction ratios (ER). At an Hb concentration of 15 g/dl, blood carries about 200 ml of oxygen/l. An estimated average of 50 ml/l of oxygen (i.e. an ER of 25%) is taken up in tissue beds. With decreasing Hb concentration, enhanced oxygen extraction may occur in those tissue beds which normally consume a small proportion of the available oxygen. However, in the brain and heart, the ER is 55–70% under basal conditions. To preserve oxygen consumption and aerobic metabolism in the coronary and cerebral vascular beds, regional blood flow must increase proportionally more than the increment in cardiac output. In animals, the onset of coronary lactate production occurs at an Hb concentration below 3.5 g/dl.[21] In a model of coronary stenosis, this anaerobic state occurs at an Hb concentration of 6–7 g/dl.[22]

Tissue oxygenation may also be improved with a rightward shift (to a higher P$_{50}$) of the Hb oxygen dissociation curve. This is achieved through increased red blood cell levels of 2,3-DPG which in turn results in increased off-loading of oxygen to tissues at any given blood oxygen tension (i.e. decreased oxygen affinity). Indeed, the slightly lower Hb levels normally found in childhood are thought to be due to the increased intraerythrocyte 2,3-DPG levels observed in children.[23] Changes in the Hb-oxygen dissociation curve resulting from increases in red cell 2,3-DPG levels take 12–36 hours to occur and are directly proportional to the decreases in Hb levels. Except at very low Hb levels, the resulting reduction in Hb-oxygen affinity facilitates oxygen unloading in the tissues, without hampering Hb-oxygen binding in the lungs. Because of these adaptations, in most types of chronic anemia the decrease in oxygen-carrying capacity is accompanied by a relatively smaller decrease in oxygen availability.

From the above discussion it is apparent that oxygen delivery (DO$_2$) and consumption (VO$_2$) have a biphasic relationship: above a certain threshold DO$_2$, DO$_2$ exceeds VO$_2$ so that VO$_2$ is independent of DO$_2$; below this critical threshold, VO$_2$ is limited by, i.e. dependent upon, DO$_2$. The latter relationship indicates tissue hypoxia. Unfortunately, studies have not identified this critical level of DO$_2$ (and indeed it must vary with different clinical situations) and there are unfortunately no easily obtainable clinical or laboratory measurements to reliably inform physicians exactly when an anemic patient may be approaching a critical DO$_2$ level.

Studies addressing the indications for RBC transfusions in infants and children

A systematic review of the literature addressing allogeneic RBC and plasma transfusions in children has recently been published.[24] The literature search identified only 3 randomized controlled trials of allogeneic RBC blood transfusion therapy in children (excluding studies addressing neonates or very young infants, or patients with thalassemia or sickle cell disease).[25–27] In addition, 4 non-randomized studies addressing the indications for RBC transfusion were identified by the search.[28–31]

In the 1970s, Australian investigators conducted 2 randomized controlled trials of the effect of RBC transfusion on the duration of neutropenia in children with malignancies.[25,26] Patients randomized to receive RBC transfusion to maintain an Hb level of 14–16 g/dl had a significantly quicker rise in neutrophil count, a lower incidence of infection and a lower incidence of interruption to chemotherapy, than patients whose Hb levels were maintained at 12–14 g/dl. However, these studies are of little relevance today: the intensity of chemotherapy has dramatically increased in recent years and the study goals (i.e. decreased duration of neutropenia, etc.) can now be attained, if necessary, through the use of granulocyte colony-stimulating factor (G-CSF).

Two studies, 1 of which was a randomized controlled clinical trial, addressed the issue of blood transfusion in African children with anemia and malaria.[27,28] The investigators of both studies discuss the combined problems in Africa of the frequency in young children of severe anemia associated with malaria, the shortage of blood for transfusion and the high risk of transfusion-transmitted HIV infection. In this setting, it is important to determine if transfusion will in fact decrease mortality. In the randomized controlled trial, 116 children between the ages of 2 months and 6 years with malaria and hematocrit levels between 0.12 and 0.17, but without congestive heart failure or pneumonia, were randomized to receive either treatment for malaria and hookworm alone or in addition a whole blood transfusion.[27] Mean hematocrit at admission was 14.0% in the transfusion group and 14.4% in the no-transfusion group. There was a trend towards more hospital admissions and deaths in the latter group, although the differences were not statistically significant and the 95% confidence intervals were wide (in those with complete follow-up, 2 deaths in the 53 patients in the no-transfusion group and 1 death in the 53 patients in the transfusion group). The authors concluded that a trial with a larger number of patients is necessary to clarify this issue.

The second study was a surveillance study in which data were collected over approximately 12 months on all children under 12 years of age (n = 2433) admitted to a pediatric ward of a Kenyan hospital.[28] Whole blood transfusions were administered according to routine practice and availability. Overall, 29% of patients had severe anemia (Hb level <5 g/dl) and 20% of patients received blood transfusions. Based on laboratory criteria only, children with an Hb level <3.9 g/dl who were transfused had a lower mortality than those who were not, but this finding applied only to children transfused on the day of, or the day after, admission. Based on a combination of laboratory and clinical criteria, children with clinical signs of respiratory distress and Hb levels <4.7 g/dl who were transfused had a lower mortality than those who were not. Among children without respiratory distress there was no association between receipt of blood transfusion and mortality, irrespective of admission Hb level. Based on these observations, the authors recommend, in their setting, that blood transfusions be administered to children with an Hb level <5 g/dl and congestive heart failure or respiratory distress, or to those without clinical complications and an Hb level <3 g/dl. While these studies obviously cannot be generalized to other clinical settings and do not address morbidity associated with severe anemia, they do provide some useful data on children's tolerance for normovolemic anemia.

Two studies addressed the use of RBC transfusions to improve tissue oxygen delivery (DO_2) and consumption (VO_2) in children with septic shock and mild-to-moderate anemia, while the remaining study addressed the relationship between DO_2 and VO_2 in pediatric patients following cardiac bypass surgery.[29–31] No firm conclusions about RBC transfusions in either of these settings can be drawn from the limited information available in these studies.

Thus, despite the large numbers of RBC transfusions administered to children, there is a remarkable paucity of scientific data on which to base RBC transfusion decisions. Recommendations for RBC transfusions in children are, therefore, for the most part based on expert opinion and experience and not on scientific studies.

RBC transfusions for acute blood loss

In the presence of acute hemorrhage it is important to remember that the first priorities are to correct the hypovolemia (with crystalloids and/or colloids) and to attempt to stop the bleeding. In patients with hematologic problems, the latter will often include the need to correct thrombocytopenia and/or deficiencies of coagulation factors, treatment to decrease bleeding from damaged mucosal barriers (e.g. with histamine blockers or antifibrinolytics) and/or reversal of the effects of anticoagulant therapy. In patients with normal or near-normal Hb levels prior to the onset of hemorrhage, RBC transfusions are usually only necessary if the patient remains unstable following volume resuscitation. However, careful ongoing evaluation of children with acute blood loss is essential as the signs of shock may initially be subtle in the child. If acute hemorrhage totals >15% of blood volume, signs of circulatory failure (tachycardia, decrease of intensity of peripheral pulses, delayed capillary refill and cool extremities) will be observed. However, hypotension will not be present until 25–30% or more of the child's blood volume is lost.[32,33] It is also important to realize that in the setting of rapid ongoing hemorrhage with hypovolemia, the Hb concentration may not be an accurate indication of the actual RBC mass.

The classification of hemorrhagic shock in children based on systemic signs is shown in Table 35.4 and guidelines for resuscitation are summarized in Fig. 35.3.[32,33]

RBC transfusions for acute hemolysis

Unlike acute hemorrhage where the patient suffers from both hypovolemia and a decreased RBC mass, patients with acute hemolysis are usually normovolemic. The Hb concentration therefore more accurately reflects RBC mass. The decision to administer an RBC transfusion depends upon a combination of factors, including ongoing clinical evaluation, presence or absence of underlying cardiovascular disease, actual Hb concentration, rate of decrease in Hb

Table 35.4 Classification of hemorrhagic shock in pediatric patients based on systemic signs. Reproduced with permission from Ref. 33.

System	Class I Very mild hemorrhage (<15% TBV loss)	Class II Mild hemorrhage (15–25% TBV loss)	Class III Moderate hemorrhage (26–39% TBV loss)	Class IV Severe hemorrhage (≥40% TBV loss)
Cardiovascular	Heart rate normal or mildy increased	Tachycardia	Significant tachycardia	Severe tachycardia
	Normal pulses	Peripheral pulses may be diminished	Thready peripheral pulses	Thready peripheral pulses
	Normal blood pressure	Normal blood pressure	Hypotension	Significant hypotension
	Normal pH	Normal pH	Metabolic acidosis	Significant acidosis
Respiratory	Rate normal	Tachypnea	Moderate tachypnea	Severe tachypnea
Central nervous system	Slightly anxious	Irritable, confused, combative	Irritable or lethargic, diminished pain response	Coma
Skin	Warm, pink	Cool extremities, mottling	Cool extremities, mottling or pallor	Cold extremities, pallor or cyanosis
	Capillary refill brisk	Delayed capillary refill	Prolonged capillary refill	
Kidneys	Normal urine output	Oliguria, increased specific gravity	Oliguria, increased BUN	Anuria

TBV = total blood volume; BUN = blood urea nitrogen.

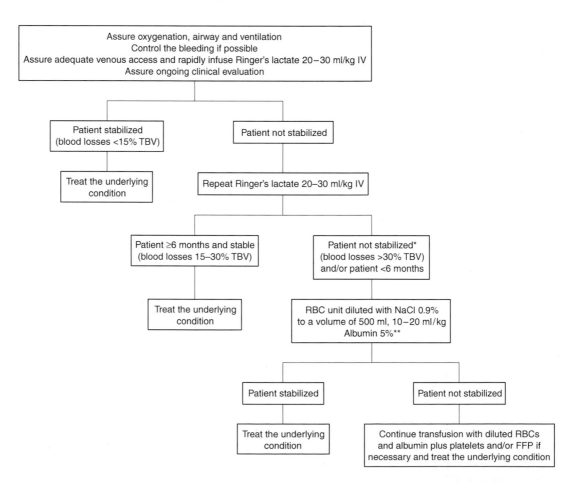

* Patients with significant degrees of anemia prior to acute blood loss will require RBC transfusion support following smaller hemorrhagic losses.
** The use of albumin for fluid resuscitation is controversial (see Refs 34 and 35).

Fig. 35.3 Approach to the treatment of hemorrhagic shock in infants and children. TBV = total blood volume; RBC = red blood cells; FFP = fresh frozen plasma. Adapted and translated from Ref. 32, and reproduced with permission from the publisher.

concentration and possibility of alternate treatments (e.g. corticosteroids for IgG autoimmune hemolytic anemia). The management of a patient with acute severe hemolytic anemia due to the presence of a warm autoantibody presents a particularly difficult challenge to the hematologist. There are two potential problems: the first concerns the provision of appropriate blood should transfusion be necessary and the second the possibility of hemolysis of the transfused blood since most autoantibodies also react with transfused allogeneic RBCs. If the autoantibody is present in the patient's plasma (as well as on the surface of the patient's red cells), it is usually impossible to provide cross-match-compatible blood and, in patients who have been previously transfused or pregnant, the autoantibody may mask the presence of clinically significant alloantibodies. With respect to the second problem, transfused RBCs will have a shortened survival in patients with autoimmune hemolytic anemia but immediate transfusion reactions are rare.[36] If possible, then, in this setting the choice of blood to administer and the decision to administer an RBC transfusion should be made in consultation with a transfusion medicine physician. However, life-saving RBC transfusions should not be withheld from patients with autoantibodies even if such blood is cross-match incompatible.[36]

RBC transfusion for chronic anemia

The majority of patients for whom a pediatric hematologist will consider administering an RBC transfusion have a slowly developing subacute or chronic anemia. In this setting, decisions regarding RBC transfusion rarely need to be taken rapidly. It is therefore possible to consider several factors in the decision to administer an RBC transfusion or series of transfusions and to involve the patient and/or the patient's parents in the decision. Factors to be considered should include:

- presence or absence of symptoms and/or abnormal physical signs and the likelihood that these are due to anemia;
- presence or absence of underlying diseases, particularly cardiac diseases which may decrease the patient's capacity for cardiovascular compensation;
- likely evolution of the underlying disease causing the anemia;
- likely evolution of the anemia and its consequences with or without transfusion in both the short- and long-term;
- possibility of using alternate, safer therapies for the treatment of the anemia.

In general, the above factors are often more important in the decision to administer an RBC transfusion than the Hb concentration *per se*. For example, patients with Diamond–Blackfan anemia unresponsive to corticosteroids are usually placed on a chronic transfusion program with minimum pretransfusion Hb levels of around 7 g/dl in order to maintain growth and an acceptable long-term quality of life while young, otherwise healthy, children with severe iron defi-

ciency anemia may temporarily tolerate Hb levels as low as 4 g/dl provided they are being monitored and iron therapy has been initiated.

RBC transfusions for patients receiving chemotherapy for leukemia or solid tumors are often given according to a predetermined protocol based on Hb level alone. However, there is no scientific basis to this practice, and in the absence of appropriate studies, clinical judgement as to the benefit:risk ratio should be used for these patients too.

The transfusion support of children with sickle cell disease or clinically significant thalassemia syndromes requires several special considerations as discussed below.

RBC transfusions for sickle cell disease

The administration of RBC transfusions in the management and/or prevention of the complications of sickle cell disease (SCD) is so frequent that almost all adult HbSS patients and many HbSC or HbS/β-thalassemia patients have been transfused at least once and often multiple times.[37] RBC transfusions are administered to SCD patients for 2 reasons—to increase oxygen-carrying capacity in the anemic patient and/or to replace the abnormal HbS by normal HbA. Depending on the complication and goal of transfusion, RBC transfusions may be administered as simple transfusions or exchange transfusions, with either being used acutely or in a chronic transfusion program.

Simple RBC transfusions (10–20 ml/kg) are used acutely to treat major splenic sequestration and aplastic or hyperhemolytic crises, as well as other selected complications.[37] In acute splenic sequestration, the spleen rapidly increases in size, leading to sequestration of blood into the spleen. In young children, the splenic sequestration may be sufficiently severe to lead to life-threatening hypovolemic shock. Parvovirus B19 infection in patients with SCD results in temporary aplasia, which may be severe, with hemoglobin levels of 3 g/dl or less.

Transfusions are not indicated for uncomplicated painful (vasoocclusive) crises. However, occasionally an exaggerated hemolysis, associated with an episode of pain, may herald the onset of multiorgan failure syndrome, which appears to respond to RBC transfusion.[37]

The necessity of RBC transfusion prior to surgery in the SCD patient (either simple transfusion to attain a certain total Hb level or exchange transfusion to reduce the HbS level) has been debated in the literature. A large multicenter study comparing the 2 approaches in HbSS or S/β-thalassemia patients has recently been published.[38] There was no difference in perioperative complications between the 2 transfusion strategies. However, transfusion-related complications were twice as common (14%) in the exchange transfusion arm, compared with the simple transfusion arm (7%). These data confirm the safety of using simple transfusions to raise the Hb level to 10 g/dl for common surgical interventions such as tonsillectomy, cholecystectomy, splenectomy and orthopedic procedures in these patients. The role of blood transfusion in SCD patients undergoing very minor procedures (such as myringotomy) or for patients with HbSC disease has not been well studied.

In children with cerebral vascular accidents (CVA) associated with SCD, the administration of regular RBC transfusions to maintain an HbS level below 30% in the first 2 years after the CVA and below 50% thereafter has been shown to prevent recurrent CVAs.[39–41] Moreover, it has recently been shown that a transfusion program can greatly reduce the risk of a first CVA in children with SCD who have abnormal results on transcranial Doppler ultrasonography (a finding associated with CVA in SCD).[42]

RBC transfusions are currently used by most physicians, either acutely or chronically, for a variety of other complications, including acute pulmonary disease (acute chest syndrome), priapism, and leg ulcers. However, their role and the best type (i.e. simple versus exchange transfusion, acute versus chronic transfusions) for these and other complications require further investigation before definitive recommendations can be made.

A major problem in the transfusion support of SCD patients is RBC alloimmunization. The nature and frequency of this problem is discussed in Chapter 36. RBC units for transfusion to SCD patients should be screened for the presence of HbS and transfused only if negative. This will avoid confusion when the goal of transfusion is to decrease the HbS level to a predetermined level and will prevent the use of blood from a donor with undiagnosed HbSC disease.

In vitro, the viscosity of HbS has been shown to increase to potentially clinically significant levels if the hematocrit exceeds 35%.[43] Therefore, when transfusing SCD patients, especially in the presence of high HbS levels, the hematocrit should not be allowed to increase above 35%. Neurologic events, including headache, seizures and CVA, have been described after exchange transfusion in SCD.[44] It has been postulated that some of these events may have been caused by hyperviscosity, although other factors may also have been important in at least some of the patients.

SCD patients in chronic transfusion programs will develop secondary iron overload. The net amount of iron infused can be decreased by using partial exchange transfusion. An algorithm for planning partial manual exchange transfusions in children has been published.[45] Recently, it has been reported that the development of hemachromatosis can be further delayed or even prevented by the use of automated erythrocytopheresis.[46]

RBC transfusions for β-thalassemia

Prior to the introduction of RBC transfusion therapy for β-thalassemia major in the 1950s, β-thalassemia major was an uniformly fatal disease. Initially, children were transfused only to hemoglobin levels of 5–6 g/dl, a level sufficient to ensure survival but insufficient to suppress the exuberant erythroid bone marrow hyperplasia characteristic of this disorder. Consequently, patients survived into their second

decade but developed severe skeletal deformities, osteoporosis and splenomegaly. So-called hypertransfusion regimens, in which endogenous erythroid production is suppressed by maintaining a minimum pre-transfusion hemoglobin level of 9–10 g/dl, were therefore gradually introduced in the 1960s and 1970s, and remain the commonest approach today.[47] During the 1980s, investigators evaluated the possibility of further improving the quality of life of thalassemic patients by introducing a 'supertransfusion' regimen in which the minimum pre-transfusion hemoglobin level was kept entirely within the normal range.[48] However, this regimen led, not surprisingly, to a significant increase in transfusion requirements and has since been abandoned by most physicians caring for thalassemia patients.[47]

Another approach investigated during the 1980s was the possibility of decreasing transfusion exposure and increasing transfusion intervals through the use of young RBCs. These 'neocytes', with an average age of 12–21 days, can be collected by erythrocytapheresis or by fractionation of standard whole blood units using a cell processor. The studies performed in the 1980s reported only modest decreases of 12–16% in transfusion requirements; the use of neocyte transfusions was therefore abandoned.[49,50] More recently, the use of a newly developed neocyte-separation set (Neocel System, Cutter Biological, Berkeley, CA, USA) has been reported.[51,52] Using this system, there is a 15–20% reduction in transfused iron load. Nevertheless, the costs of this system are higher and donor exposure per transfusion episode is approximately doubled.

One of the most difficult decisions facing physicians treating thalassemia patients is the necessity of instituting a chronic RBC transfusion program for patients with thalassemia intermedia and hemoglobin levels of 6–7 g/dl. In addition to the considerations discussed above for patients with chronic anemia, the physician must take into account the fact that non-transfused thalassemia intermedia patients may develop bone deformities due to bone marrow erythroid hyperplasia, and even without RBC transfusions, these patients may develop clinically significant hemochromatosis secondary to the increased intestinal iron absorption induced by their inefficient erythropoiesis.[47] If a transfusion program is embarked upon, the goals of transfusion therapy are the same as those outlined above for thalassemia major patients. The transfusion intervals can usually be longer, although it is often more difficult to completely suppress endogenous erythropoiesis in thalassemia intermedia patients than in thalassemia major patients.

BLOOD GROUP CHOICE, DOSAGE AND ADMINISTRATION

Acceptable choices of ABO blood groups for RBC, plasma and platelet transfusions are shown in Table 35.5. For RBC transfusions, these choices are based on the principle that the recipient plasma must not contain antibodies (antiA/B) corresponding to donor A and/or B antigens. For plasma

Table 35.5 Possible choices of ABO blood groups for red blood cell (RBC), plasma and platelet transfusions.

Recipient blood group	Acceptable ABO group of blood component to be transfused		
	RBCs*	Plasma	Platelets**
O	O	O A, B, AB	O A, B, AB
A	A O	A AB	A AB
B	B O	B AB	B AB
AB	AB A, B, O	AB	AB A

*The choices of ABO blood groups for RBC transfusion may not be appropriate for newborns and infants <4 months of age in whom the potential presence of maternal anti-A/B must also be considered.
**In emergency situations platelets in plasma with A/B antibodies against recipient A/B antigens may be transfused in adults and older children. However, in younger children and infants, platelet units containing antibodies against recipient A and/or B antigens should not be used unless the anti-A/B is of low titer and/or the plasma has been removed.

All pediatric patients who are likely to receive multiple RBC transfusions should have an extended RBC phenotype prior to the first RBC transfusion. In addition to ABO and Rh(D) phenotyping, an extended RBC phenotype usually includes the determination of the other common Rhesus antigens as well as the common antigens of the Kell, Kidd, Duffy and MNSs blood group systems. Patients for whom this should be done include those with congenital or acquired aplastic anemia, sickle cell disease, thalassemia major or intermedia, or other transfusion-dependent congenital anemias and patients undergoing BMT. Knowing a patient's extended RBC phenotype will assist in the identification of irregular RBC antibodies should they develop. In addition, RBC units matched for antigens other than ABO and Rh(D) may be desirable for patients with thalassemia syndromes or sickle cell disease to prevent the development of alloantibodies.[54–60] For sickle cell disease patients in particular, alloimmunization may be a significant and even occasionally a potentially fatal complication. A number of experts therefore recommend providing blood that is phenotypically matched at least for the common Rhesus and Kell antigens and possibly for other blood group antigens.

The quantity of blood administered in simple RBC transfusions depends on the hematocrit of the RBC unit, the pre-transfusion Hb level and the patient's weight. If the Hb level is 5 g/dl or greater, and blood stored in CPDA-1 (hematocrit 0.70–0.75) is used, a transfusion of 10 ml/kg is usually administered. This can be expected to raise the hemoglobin level by approximately 2.5 g/dl. To obtain the same result using blood stored in an additive solution (hematocrit 0.50–0.60), 14 ml/kg needs to be administered.

For patients who weigh <20 kg, the volume of an entire RBC unit is too large to be administered during one

and platelet transfusions, donor plasma must not contain A/B antibodies corresponding to recipient A/B antigens. Patients who are RhD-antigen positive may receive RhD-positive or -negative RBCs; patients who are RhD negative should receive only RhD-negative RBCs. The choice of ABO blood group for RBC as well as platelet and plasma transfusion is more complicated for allogeneic bone marrow transplantation (BMT) patients receiving bone marrow grafts from ABO mismatched donors. Recommended choices of ABO group for blood components for these patients are shown in Fig. 35.4.[53]

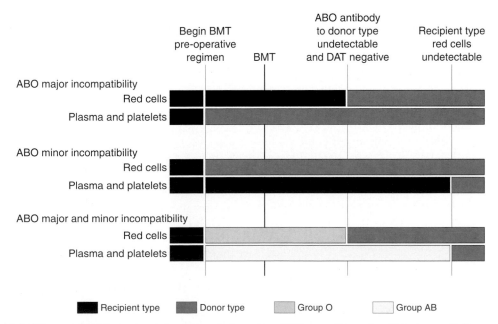

Fig. 35.4 Recommended ABO group of blood components for use in patients receiving ABO-incompatible marrow. Major incompatibility = recipient ABO antibodies to donor ABO antigens; minor incompatibility = donor ABO antibodies to recipient ABO antigens. BMT = bone marrow transplantation; DAT = direct antiglobulin test. Reproduced with permission from Ref. 53.

transfusion. In order to minimize donor exposure, attempts should be made to use the entire unit, either by giving 2 or 3 small transfusions over a 24-hour period if the unit is opened non-sterilely, or by entering the unit using a sterile docking device and transfusing appropriately sized aliquots prior to the unit's original expiry date.

If the anemia has developed slowly and the hemoglobin level is <5 g/dl, it may be necessary to administer RBC transfusions more slowly and/or in smaller quantities to avoid precipitating cardiac failure from circulatory overload. A transfusion regimen for the treatment of children with severe anemia of gradual onset without clinical signs of cardiac decompensation has recently been published.[61] The authors successfully treated 22 such children using RBCs with a hematocrit of 0.70–0.80 at a continuous infusion rate of 2 ml/kg/h until the desired Hb level was achieved. If a severely anemic child has signs of cardiac decompensation, a partial exchange transfusion should be performed. Guidelines for performing partial manual exchange transfusions have been published.[45,62] Alternatively, where available, automated red blood cell exchanges can be performed even in critically ill pediatric patients.[46,63]

RBC units must be administered through a blood filter, either a standard 170-μm macroaggregate filter, a microaggregate filter or a leukoreduction filter. Indications for the use of leukoreduction filters are discussed in Chapter 36. RBC transfusions must be completed within 4 hours from the start of transfusion.

SPECIAL CONSIDERATIONS FOR NEWBORNS

Indications for RBC transfusions

Very low birth weight (VLBW) infants frequently require small volume (10–20 ml/kg) RBC transfusions. In the early 1990s, it was estimated that of the 34 000 infants weighing <1.5 kg born annually in the USA, approximately 80% received RBC transfusions in the first weeks of life.[64] Currently, transfusion practices and/or requirements for VLBW infants appear to be changing: in a recent report from a single institution, the percentage of VLBW infants weighing >1 kg and never receiving an RBC transfusion increased from 17% in 1982 to 64% in 1993. However, >95% of infants weighing 1 kg or less in all years received RBC transfusions.[65]

There are 3 major factors contributing to small volume RBC transfusion requirements in VLBW infants.

1. *The rapid decline in Hb levels that occurs in the first weeks of life.* In the healthy term infant, the mean cord blood Hb level is 16.8 g/dl, rising to 18.4 g/dl in venous blood by 24 hours of life and then gradually decreasing to a mean nadir of 11.5 g/dl (with a lower limit of normal of 9 g/dl) at 2 months of life.[66,67] Because this decline in Hb level occurs in all neonates, and in term infants, at least, is not associated with any adverse events, it is called the physiologic anemia of infancy. In preterm infants Hb levels at birth are slightly lower than those of term infants (14.5 g/dl and 15 g/dl at 28 and 34 weeks' gestation, respectively), and the decline in Hb level occurs earlier and is more pronounced. For example, the hemoglobin concentration drops to approximately 8 g/dl in neonates with birth weights of 1.0–1.5 kg and to 7 g/dl in neonates with birth weights below 1.0 kg.[66,67] Erythropoietin levels in preterm infants at the time of the nadir of hemoglobin levels are lower than those usually found in children or adults with similar hemoglobin levels and therefore probably explain, at least partly, the drop in hemoglobin levels.[64,68] However, whether the erythropoietin levels are appropriately or inappropriately decreased remains unproven. For example, it must be remembered that concomitant with the decrease in absolute hemoglobin levels, the switch from HbF to HbA production is also occurring, so that the change in oxygen-carrying capacity is not so marked as the change in the total Hb level might suggest.

2. *The associated respiratory illnesses often present in these infants.* Early in life VLBW infants are at risk for respiratory distress syndrome which in some may lead to bronchopulmonary dysplasia with continuing requirements for respiratory support. Even relatively stable infants may develop cardiorespiratory irregularities such as apnea and/or bradycardia. The necessity of maintaining hemoglobin values at a predetermined level in infants with these problems is somewhat controversial and has been the subject of several studies and review articles.[69–71]

3. *Phlebotomy losses.* Because of the need for laboratory monitoring of ill neonates and the relatively large volumes of blood required in relation to these tiny infants' total blood volumes, phlebotomy losses contribute significantly to the need for RBC transfusions in VLBW infants.[72]

Guidelines for small volume RBC transfusions for newborns have been published by Canadian, British and American organizations.[73–75] More detailed and somewhat stricter guidelines (Table 35.6) were used without any adverse events relating to anemia in a recent large multicenter USA erythropoietin study.[72]

There are 3 clinical settings in which newborns may require large volume RBC transfusion (exchange transfusion, surgery with cardiopulmonary bypass or during treatment with extracorporeal membrane oxygenation [ECMO]). The mechanics, blood product choice and complications associated with each of these procedures has been thoroughly reviewed.[76]

Practical considerations

RBC units for transfusion to neonates are often chosen exclusively from group O donors, although ABO isogroup (or compatible) units can be used providing the technologists preparing the blood are experienced in the choice of units for

Table 35.6 Indications for small volume red blood cell (RBC) transfusions used in the US Multicenter Erythropoietin Study. Reproduced by permission of *Pediatrics*, vol. 95, page 3, 1995.

Transfuse infants at hematocrit ⩽20%
  (a) if asymptomatic with reticulocytes <100 000/μl

Transfuse infants at hematocrit ⩽30%
  (a) if receiving <35% supplemental hood oxygen
  (b) if on CPAP or mechanical ventilation with mean airway pressure <6 cmH$_2$O
  (c) if significant apnea and bradycardia are noted (>9 episodes in 12 h or 2 episodes in 24 h requiring bag and mask ventilation) while receiving therapeutic doses of methylxanthines
  (d) if heart rate >180 beats/min or respiratory rate >80 breaths/min persists for 24 h
  (e) if weight gain <10 g/day is observed over 4 days while receiving ⩾100 kcal/kg/day
  (f) if undergoing surgery

Transfuse for hematocrit ⩽35%
  (a) if receiving >35% supplemental hood oxygen
  (b) if intubated on CPAP or mechanical ventilation with mean airway pressure ⩾6–8 cmH$_2$O

Do not transfuse
  (a) to replace blood removed for laboratory tests alone
  (b) for low hematocrit alone

CPAP = continuous positive airway pressure by nasal or endotracheal route.

those patients in whom the potential presence of maternal A and/or B antibodies needs to be considered. RBC units stored in any of the currently available storage media, including additive solutions, are suitable for small volume (<20 ml/kg) RBC transfusions.[77,78] Several studies have demonstrated the safety of assigning a fresh (<5 days old) RBC unit to a neonatal patient at the time of his/her first small-volume RBC transfusion and, using a sterile connection device, continuing to use this same unit up to its normal expiry date for subsequent small-volume RBC transfusions.[79–81] Precise descriptions for preparing small-volume RBC aliquots for neonates have been published.[81–83]

In settings of large-volume RBC transfusion, replacement of plasma coagulation factors is often also required so that WB or reconstituted WB, i.e. an RBC unit mixed with a unit of fresh frozen plasma (FFP), is usually used. For WB, or the RBC unit for reconstituted WB, the choice of ABO group is the same as that described above for small volume RBC transfusions. The ABO group of the FFP must also be compatible with the baby's RBCs (see Table 35.5). This may mean that the ABO groups of the RBC unit and the FFP unit are different, e.g. for a group A baby with maternal anti-A in his plasma, a unit of reconstituted WB would be prepared using a group O RBC unit and a group A FFP unit. To limit donor exposure, some experts use group O whole blood in this setting, although group O donors with high anti-A titers have to be excluded.

WB units or RBC units for large volume transfusions should be relatively fresh, i.e. not >5–7 days old. The main reason for this precaution is the high potassium concentration in stored WB or RBC units. While this does not pose a problem in the setting of small volume transfusions (<20 ml/kg) administered slowly (over 3 or 4 hours), the potassium content of stored blood, when administered rapidly and in large volumes, may be lethal for a neonatal patient.[84] It may also be advantageous in the setting of large volume transfusion in neonates to have relatively high 2,3-DPG levels, although this has not been proven. In addition to the issue of potassium content and 2,3-DPG levels, there may be advantage to using very fresh (<48 hours old) WB as opposed to reconstituted WB in neonates and young children undergoing cardiovascular surgery with cardiopulmonary bypass (CPB). In one prospective, controlled study the use of very fresh WB postoperatively resulted in less bleeding in patients younger than 2 years old with complex procedures and, in addition, in neonates a decrease in the rate of re-exploration for bleeding.[85]

A screening test for the presence of a sickling Hb should be performed and found to be negative on RBC or WB units for large-volume transfusions in neonates.[86]

Finally, there are at least theoretical concerns that the constituents of additive solutions may be harmful to newborns if infused in large quantities as could occur with exchange transfusion, CPB surgery or ECMO. In these situations it is recommended that the additive solutions be removed either by washing the RBCs or by centrifuging the unit and removing the supernatant.[77] The packed RBCs are then reconstituted in saline, albumin or FFP as required.

STRATEGIES TO DECREASE RED BLOOD CELL ALLOGENEIC DONOR EXPOSURES

The first and possibly the most important strategy in limiting donor exposure is to administer an RBC blood transfusion only in the presence of an appropriate indication. The risks versus the anticipated benefits should be individually considered for every transfusion a physician orders. A second and equally simple strategy is to ensure the optimum utilization of each blood unit. When transfusing RBC units to very small patients, attempts should be made to use the whole unit (see above). In some situations, described below, allogeneic donor exposure may be avoided or limited using additional, special strategies.

Autologous transfusions

Autologous blood transfusion, i.e. the collection and reinfusion of the patient's own blood, is increasingly used for pediatric surgical patients. Three types of autologous blood transfusion can be used in surgical patients:

1. preoperative blood collection and storage with reinfusion intra-or post-operatively;
2. immediate preoperative phlebotomy (following anesthetic induction) accompanied by normovolemic hemodilution with colloids or crystalloids;
3. intraoperative salvage and reinfusion of shed blood.

721

Guidelines for the use of autologous blood transfusion in the surgical setting have been published.[87–89]

The majority of the published experience with autologous blood transfusion for pediatric patients addresses the use of preoperative autologous blood deposit (PAD). In general for both adults and children, PAD is considered most appropriate for patients predicted to have significant postoperative longevity, who are scheduled to undergo a procedure in which there is a significant likelihood of transfusion and for whom the PAD procedure is likely to be well tolerated.[87–90] A 'significant likelihood of transfusion' has been suggested to be a 10% or greater chance of requiring blood transfusion.[88] Alternatively, a model to predict the need for PAD in individual patients considering both the expected blood loss and minimal tolerable hematocrit has been suggested.[89]

Initially the use of PAD was reported mainly for older pediatric patients, i.e. adolescents, undergoing orthopedic procedures, in particular spinal fusion.[91–93] In this setting, preoperative collection of autologous blood is clearly feasible and efficacious: for example, in one study the use of preoperative blood deposit decreased the need for allogeneic blood transfusion to 11% of patients as compared with 60% in a group of historical controls.[93] Nevertheless, the optimal use of and schedule for PAD is still under study. For example, it has recently been suggested, using a mathematical model, that it may be advantageous, with respect to endogenous erythropoietic response to perform aggressive phlebotomy (e.g. twice weekly for 2 weeks) as long before an intervention as RBC storage conditions permit rather than weekly as is usually done.[89]

There have been a number of published reports describing the use of predeposit autologous blood collections in smaller and younger pediatric patients (with several patients 3 years old or younger and/or weighing as little as 10–12 kg) and in patients undergoing a variety of surgical procedures including open heart surgery, plastic surgery and neurosurgery.[94–98] Autologous blood collection is feasible in these patients but consideration must given to several aspects unique to the pediatric setting. These include both psychologic factors such the creation of an appropriate environment and the need for parental encouragement and commitment to the program, as well as technical considerations such as the use of local anesthesia at the venipuncture site, the use of needles smaller than the standard size (this can be accomplished using a sterile connection device) and the need to adjust the amount of anticoagulant in the collection bag to the amount of blood collected.[91,99] In the published reports, deposit of autologous blood also appears to decrease the requirements for allogeneic blood transfusion in these smaller patients. However, the decision to embark on such a program should be individualized and should include a realistic prediction of whether or not sufficient blood can be collected to avoid the need for allogeneic blood transfusion.

Pediatric patients participating in autologous predeposit programs should receive iron supplementation, beginning if possible at least 3 weeks prior to the first donation and continuing into the postoperative period.

Although the risks of autologous blood transfusion are less than those associated with allogeneic transfusion, autologous blood is not entirely risk-free. Most experts therefore recommend using the same criteria for the transfusion of autologous blood as for allogeneic blood.[15]

The use of acute normovolemic hemodilution and intraoperative red blood cell salvage in adult patients has been extensively reported.[100,101] Studies examining the use of these two modalities in children are beginning to appear.[19,20,102–105] While these approaches to decrease the requirement for allogeneic blood transfusion in pediatric patients will probably prove to be useful in selected patients, their exact roles remain to be defined. More studies are also required to determine the best way to co-ordinate the use of these techniques with the preoperative deposit of autologous blood in pediatric patients undergoing various surgical procedures.

The use of placental blood as a type of autologous blood transfusion for neonates has been investigated. A simple way to administer placental blood at birth is to delay slightly cord clamping.[106–108] A second method, namely the collection, storage and reinfusion of placental blood is obviously considerably more complicated and currently must be considered experimental.[109–111]

Erythropoietin

The efficacy of recombinant human erythropoietin (rHuEpo) for the correction of the anemia of chronic renal failure is now well established in both pediatric and adult patients.[112] The use of rHuEpo for the prevention and/or treatment of non-uremic anemia has been the subject of several studies.[113] In pediatrics, outside of the setting of uremia, the role for rHuEpo has been most extensively studied in preterm infants with anemia of prematurity.[69,114,115] Despite a relatively large number of studies, this indication remains controversial. It is generally agreed that rHuEpo is not indicated for infants with birth weights > 1300 g since they rarely require RBC transfusions.[65,116,117] It also appears unlikely that rHuEpo can avoid the requirement for RBC transfusion in VLBW infants, e.g. those with birth weights < 800 g.[116,117] In infants with birth weights between 800 and 1300 g, rHuEpo administration (in association with relatively large amounts of iron supplementation) does enhance erythropoiesis and in several studies has decreased the number and/or quantity of RBC transfusions. However, these studies have not convincingly shown that donor exposures would in fact be decreased, particularly if alternate strategies (such as sterile aliquotting of an RBC unit and use of the unit up to its usual expiry date) to decrease donor exposures are used.[69]

In adults, the efficacy of rHuEpO therapy in decreasing allogeneic blood exposure in surgical patients, both with and without preoperative autologous blood deposit, has been extensively studied.[113] In general, the perioperative use of rHuEpo appears to be efficacious in patients with low baseline Hb levels who are expected to have large blood losses. Little or no benefit has been found in adults with normal Hb levels. The optimal dosing regimen for rHuEpo in this setting remains to be defined. The role for perioperative rHuEpo administration has not been well studied in pediatric patients.

A number of studies have addressed the potential role for rHuEpo in the treatment of chemotherapy-induced anemia and anemia following BMT,[113,118–124] and suggest that rHuEpo does increase Hb levels and may decrease transfusion requirements in selected patients. However, definitive guidelines for the use of rHuEpo in pediatric oncology or BMT patients have yet to be defined. Although some studies in small numbers of patients have shown encouraging results for the use of rHuEpo in patients with sickle cell anemia or thalassemia intermedia, rHuEpo in these patients must be considered experimental.[125–128] Erythropoietin has been shown to be efficacious in the correction of anemia induced by antiretroviral therapy in HIV-infected children.[129]

Directed donations and limited-exposure blood donor programs

A directed blood donation is one in which an individual, at the request of a patient, or in the case of a child, a parent, donates blood that is reserved specifically for the subsequent transfusion of the requesting patient. When parents wish to be directed donors for their children, or request other family members or friends to do so, it is, presumably, because they believe that blood from such donors is less likely to be a source of transfusion-transmitted diseases than blood from an anonymous volunteer blood donor pool. Whether or not this is in fact true has been a source of controversy in the literature.[130,131] Advocates of directed donations argue that such donors would not consider donating for a loved one if they have known risk factors for transfusion-transmitted diseases. Alternatively, others argue that the absence of confidentiality that this situation entails and/or a strong desire to donate for the given patient may discourage the directed donor from being entirely truthful about his/her eligibility for blood donation.

Studies addressing these questions would involve the follow-up of large numbers of recipients of directed blood donations over a long period of time and consequently are unlikely to be performed. Instead of direct studies, attempts have been made to estimate indirectly the comparative safety of directed and standard donor blood by measuring the frequency of positive infectious disease markers in the 2 donor groups. This approach is, of course, based on the assumption that the risk of an undetected infectious unit is directly related to the frequency of positive infectious markers in the donor population under study. In 3 of 4 studies, there were no statistically significant differences in the results of infectious disease markers in directed donors versus anonymous volunteer donors, while in 1 there was an increased frequency of positive markers among directed donors which could probably be attributed to the relatively larger number of first-time donors.[132–135] From the point of view of transfusion-transmitted viral diseases, directed donors are therefore generally considered neither safer nor less safe than regular volunteer donors.

Apart from the question of safety with respect to the transmission of viral infections, there are additional safety issues to consider when parents give blood for their children. In the case of neonates, blood from biologic mothers poses a potential danger because their plasma may contain HLA antibodies that could react with HLA antigens on the infant's leukocytes and/or platelets. *In utero* the placenta provides a natural barrier to these antibodies that obviously would be bypassed with a blood transfusion. For this reason, it has been suggested that biologic mothers do not provide blood components containing plasma for their neonates and that maternal red cells and platelets be given as washed products.[136]

Biologic fathers may also pose certain difficulties. A father may possess a red cell antigen, not inherited by his infant, to which the mother may have developed an IgG antibody. These antibodies cross the placenta but obviously would cause no harm *in utero*. Most such antibodies are easily detected by routine pre-transfusion testing. However, should such an antibody be directed against an uncommon or private antigen, it may not be detected by routine pre-transfusion testing if this does not include a full antiglobin cross-match.

Another potential risk of parental blood transfusion is chimerism and graft-versus-host disease. For patients of all ages (including adults), all cellular blood components obtained from biologic relatives must be irradiated before transfusion (see Chapter 36).

Finally, as for all allogeneic blood transfusions, there remain the risks related to alloimmunization, allergic reactions and bacterial contamination (see Chapter 36). In addition, as for autologous donations, it is possible that the added complexity of providing directed donations could lead to an increased frequency of errors.[137]

One situation in which directed blood donors may provide an increased level of safety is a limited-donor blood program. For example, a single donor can often provide all the RBC and/or plasma needs of a small pediatric patient ineligible for autologous donation who must undergo elective surgery for which multiple blood units are normally required.[138] Likewise, the RBC transfusion requirements of small pediatric patients with chronic anemia, e.g. Diamond–Blackfan anemia or β-thalassemia major, may be supplied from a small pool of 2–4 donors.[139] While the feasibility and success of such limited-donor programs in decreasing the number of donor exposures in small pediatric patients has been demonstrated, there are no data to support or refute the superiority with respect to safety of these programs over the routine use of unselected but fully tested donor units.

PLASMA

DESCRIPTION AND STORAGE

Plasma for transfusion is prepared from a whole blood donation by separation following centrifugation (see Figs 35.1 and 35.2). Larger volumes of plasma may be collected using automated apheresis techniques. A typical unit of plasma has a volume of 160–250 ml if obtained from a WB donation or 400–600 ml when obtained by plasmapheresis. Immediately following collection from a normal donor, plasma contains approximately 1 unit/ml of each of the coagulation factors as well as normal concentrations of other plasma proteins. Coagulation Factors V and VIII, known as the labile coagulation factors, are not stable in plasma stored at 1–6°C. Plasma frozen within 8 hours of donation contains at least 0.70 unit/ml of Factor VIII and is referred to as fresh frozen plasma (FFP). In plasma frozen 8–72 hours after collection, referred to as frozen plasma (FP), the concentration of coagulation Factors V and VIII may be reduced by as much as 15%.[10] FFP may be stored for 12 months at −18°C or colder. Storage at −30°C or colder is recommended for optimal maintenance of Factor VIII levels.

INDICATIONS AND CONTRAINDICATIONS FOR TRANSFUSION

A recent systematic review of allogeneic transfusions in children or infants >4 months of age identified only 3 controlled trials addressing FFP use in this group: 2 examined the use of FFP for pediatric hemolytic uremic syndrome (HUS) and the other (discussed above) as one of the components of reconstituted WB to replace blood losses following open heart surgery.[24,85,140,141] Thus, as for RBC transfusion, the indications for FFP transfusions in children are most often generalized from observations in adult patients and/or based on expert opinion.

There is broad, general consensus that the appropriate use of FFP is limited almost exclusively to the treatment or prevention of clinically significant bleeding due to a deficiency of one or more plasma coagulation factors.[15,75,142–145] Such situations potentially include the presence of:

1. a diminution of coagulation factors due to treatment with vitamin K antagonists;
2. severe liver disease;
3. disseminated intravascular coagulation (DIC);
4. massive transfusion;
5. isolated congenital coagulation factor deficiencies for which a safer and/or more appropriate product does not exist.

The use of FFP in each of these settings as well as for HUS is discussed below.

In addition, there is a consensus among the experts developing guidelines that FFP is not indicated in the following situations:

1. intravascular volume expansion or repletion (where crystalloids, synthetic colloids or purified human albumin solutions are preferred);
2. correction or prevention of protein malnutrition (where synthetic amino acid solutions are preferred);
3. correction of hypogammaglobulinemia (where purified human immunoglobulin concentrates are preferred);
4. treatment of hemophilia and von Willebrand's disease (where desmopressin [DDAVP] or virus-inactivated plasma-derived or recombinant factor concentrates are preferred);
5. treatment of any other isolated congenital procoagulant or anticoagulant factor deficiency for which a virus-inactivated plasma-derived or recombinant factor concentrate exists;
6. as replacement fluid in therapeutic apheresis procedures for disorders other than thrombotic thrombocytopenic purpura/adult HUS unless proven to be beneficial.

Reversal of warfarin effect

Patients who are anticoagulated with warfarin are deficient in the functional vitamin K-dependent coagulation factors II, VII, IX, X and proteins C and S. Elective reversal of warfarin effect, e.g. prior to elective surgery, can usually be accomplished by stopping warfarin for 72 hours prior to the procedure.[146] Selected patients at high risk of thrombosis may require heparin coverage. More rapid reversal of the warfarin effect may be necessary in the presence of an excessively elevated International Normalized Ratio (INR) or prolonged prothrombin time (PT) and active bleeding or need for an emergency invasive procedure. Depending on the urgency and severity of the clinical situation, warfarin reversal may be attained by stopping or modifying warfarin therapy, by oral or parenteral vitamin K administration, by plasma transfusion or in rare situations by the administration of a virus-inactivated plasma-derived prothrombin complex concentrate. Guidelines for the emergency reversal of the warfarin effect in children developed by the Canadian Children's Thrombophilia Network are listed in Table 35.7.[146]

Severe liver disease

Severe liver disease is associated with multiple abnormalities of hemostasis and coagulation including:

1. deficient biosynthesis of antithrombin III, proteins C and S, plasminogen, antiplasmins and coagulation factors;
2. aberrant biosynthesis of several coagulations factors;
3. accelerated destruction of coagulation factors;

Table 35.7 Canadian Children's Thrombophilia Network: Guidelines for emergency warfarin reversal in children. Reproduced from Ref. 146 with permission.

Vitamin K is the antidote for warfarin. The dose to be administered and concurrent use of fresh frozen plasma (FFP) or a prothrombin complex concentrate (containing Factors II, VII, IX, X) are dependent on the clinical problem. The following are guidelines only.

1. *No bleeding*
   (a) Rapid reversal of warfarin necessary and the patient will require warfarin again in the near future: treat with vitamin K_1 at 0.5–2 mg subcutaneously (not intramuscularly)
   (b) Rapid reversal of warfarin necessary and the patient will not require warfarin again: treat with vitamin K_1 at 2–5 mg subcutaneously (not intramuscularly)

2. *Significant bleeding*
   (a) Significant bleeding that is not life-threatening and will not cause morbidity: treat with vitamin K_1 subcutaneously (not intramuscularly) or intravenously at 0.5–2 mg plus FFP 20 ml/kg*
   (b) Significant bleeding that is life-threatening and will cause morbidity: treat with vitamin K_1 intravenously (5 mg) by slow infusion over 10–20 min because of the risk of anaphylactic shock. Consider giving a prothrombin complex concentrate (containing Factors II, VII, IX, X) at 50 unit/kg intravenously

*Although not recommended by the authors of these guidelines, some experts recommend the use of a virus-inactivated plasma-derived prothrombin complex concentrate rather than FFP in this situation as well as for 2(b).

4. deficient clearance of activated coagulation factors and plasminogen activators;
5. thrombocytopenia and platelet dysfunction;
6. loss or consumption of coagulation factors in ascitic fluid.[147]

Patients with severe liver disease usually have significantly abnormal coagulation studies which raise questions about the need for plasma transfusion. Experts generally agree that patients who are not bleeding or about to undergo an invasive procedure should not receive plasma merely to correct abnormal coagulation tests.[15,142–145] One exception to this may be patients with life-threatening acute fulminant hepatitis and extremely elevated INRs who are awaiting emergency liver transplantation. These patients are sometimes given prophylactic plasma transfusions. However, no studies have specifically addressed this issue and it is difficult to determine whether or not such transfusions actually improve the outcome of this devastating disease.

Three retrospective studies found that patients with liver disease and mild coagulopathy, i.e. a PT 1.5-fold or less than the mean of the normal range (corresponding to an INR of approximately 2.2), did not have excess bleeding with liver biopsy or minor invasive procedures such as paracentesis or thoracentesis.[15,148–150] Most guidelines recommend plasma transfusion prior to invasive procedures or surgery in patients with liver disease and PT levels >1.5-fold normal or an INR >2.2, although there are no studies to support or refute these recommendations.

Disseminated intravascular coagulation

Acute DIC is characterized by the abnormal consumption of coagulation factors and platelets and may lead to thrombocytopenia, hypofibrinogenemia and increased PT, INR and/or activated partial thromboplastin time (APTT) with uncontrollable bleeding from wound and puncture sites. Retrospective and uncontrolled evidence suggests that the transfusion of plasma, along with other blood components, may be useful in limiting hemorrhage, provided aggressive measures are simultaneously undertaken to overcome the triggering disease. Plasma transfusion is generally not recommended in the absence of bleeding or in chronic DIC.

Massive transfusion

Massive transfusion is usually defined as the replacement of a patient's total blood volume with stored blood in < 24 hours. However, even within this definition, the degree and rapidity of blood loss can be quite variable as can the underlying etiologies and associated complications. Thus, assessment of the need for replacement of coagulation factors by FFP transfusion must be individualized. Pathologic hemorrhage in the massively transfused patient is more often caused by dilutional thrombocytopenia than by the depletion of coagulation factors.[142,145]

Past recommendations advocated routine transfusion of plasma (e.g. the administration of 2 units of plasma for every 5 units of red blood cells transfused) to reduce the risk of abnormal bleeding due to coagulation factor depletion during massive transfusion. However, there is no evidence to support the routine or prophylactic administration of plasma in this scenario. Alternatively, should a consumptive disorder accompany the massive blood loss, the use of such predetermined formulae may result in inadequate replacement therapy. Consequently, to the extent that it is possible, blood transfusion therapy in the setting of massive transfusion should be guided by both the ongoing clinical evaluation of the patient and laboratory measurements of hemostasis.

Congenital coagulation factor deficiencies

Plasma has long been used to treat congenital deficiencies of hemostatic or anticoagulant proteins. However, more appropriate alternatives now exist for most of these disorders and, as new treatments are rapidly becoming available, recommendations for treatment are changing frequently. Physicians with special expertise in pediatric hemostasis or thrombosis should supervise the care of children with these disorders and the choice of products for their treatment. These disorders are discussed in detail in Chapters 29–31.

Hemolytic uremic syndrome

Several investigators have studied the use of FFP in the treatment of pediatric HUS.[140,141,151] Experts have reached the consensus that plasma is not indicated for classic childhood HUS, i.e. the syndrome characterized by microangiopathic hemolytic anemia, thrombocytopenia and acute renal failure following diarrhea associated with enterohemorrhagic *Escherichia coli* infection.[152] HUS and thrombotic thrombocytopenia purpura (TTP) may be indistinguishable pathologically, and the clinical manifestations of HUS occasionally approach those of TTP. In the absence of definitive studies, and in light of the adult TTP studies, plasma exchange seems to be a reasonable consideration in treating children with unusually complicated HUS, particularly those with neurologic complications.[153]

SPECIAL CONSIDERATIONS FOR NEWBORNS

The approach to determining the indications for FFP transfusion in the newborn is the same as that for the older patient, i.e. FFP is indicated for the treatment of clinically significant bleeding, or its prevention in the case of an impending invasive procedure, due to a decrease in one or more coagulation factors, where a safer, appropriate, alternative therapy does not exist. In particular, for the neonate as for other patients, FFP is not indicated for the treatment of volume expansion or resuscitation alone. However, the application of this underlying principle to decisions concerning FFP administration may be more difficult in newborns than older patients for a number of reasons. First, it may be difficult to obtain blood specimens of the quality and quantity necessary to obtain reliable laboratory measurements of coagulation parameters in critically ill, tiny preterm infants. Secondly, newborns and infants under 6 months of age have relatively lower levels of the vitamin K-dependent coagulation factors (Factors II, VII, IX, X), as well as the 4 contact factors and the vitamin K-dependent coagulation inhibitors.[154] PT and APTT are correspondingly prolonged. Normal values for coagulant and anticoagulant proteins as well as coagulation tests in healthy, full-term and preterm infants are shown in Tables 35.8 and 35.9, respectively.[154,154a] These values usually reach adult levels by 6 months of age. On the one hand, these differences in the newborn versus the older infant and child may render the correlation of laboratory values to the clinical situation difficult; on the other hand, it is likely that the coagulant and anticoagulant factors that are already relatively low in newborns are more rapidly depleted in situations such as acute hemorrhage or DIC. It may thus be reasonable to administer FFP transfusion relatively sooner in these situations to newborns and infants under 6 months of age than in older infants and children.

In most countries, newborns receive vitamin K prophylactically at birth. Newborns who do not receive vitamin K prophylaxis and who are breast fed may develop the classic form of hemorrhagic disease of newborn (HDN). A late form

Table 35.8 Reference values for coagulation tests in healthy full-term infants during the first 6 months of life. Adapted with permission from Ref. 154.

Test	Day 1 M	Day 1 B	Day 30 M	Day 30 B	Adult M	Adult B
PT (s)	13.0	10.1–15.9*	11.8	10.0–14.3*	12.4	10.8–13.9
INR	1.0	0.53–1.62	0.79	0.53–1.26	0.89	0.64–1.17
APTT (s)	42.9	31.3–54.5	40.4	32.0–55.2	33.5	26.6–40.3
Fibrinogen (g/l)	2.83	1.67–3.99	2.70	1.62–3.78*	2.78	1.56–4.00
V (unit/ml)	0.72	0.34–1.08	0.98	0.62–1.34	1.06	0.62–1.50
VII (unit/ml)	0.66	0.28–10.4	0.90	0.42–1.38	1.05	0.67–1.43
VIII (unit/ml)	1.00	0.50–1.78*	0.91	0.50–1.57*	0.99	0.50–1.49
VWF (unit/ml)	1.53	0.50–2.87	1.28	0.50–2.46	0.92	0.50–1.58
IX (unit/ml)	0.53	0.15–0.91	0.51	0.21–0.81	1.09	0.55–1.63
X (unit/ml)	0.40	0.12–0.68	0.59	0.31–0.87	1.06	0.70–1.52
XI (unit/ml)	0.38	0.10–0.66	0.53	0.27–0.79	0.97	0.67–1.27

PT = prothrombin time; APTT = activated partial thromboplastin time; VIII = Factor VIII procoagulant; VWF = von Willebrand factor; INR = international normalized ratio.
All factors except fibrinogen are expressed as unit/ml, where pooled plasma contains 1.0 unit/ml. All values are expressed as mean (M), followed by the lower and upper boundary encompassing 95% of the population (B).
*Values indistinguishable from those of the adult.

Table 35.9 Reference values for coagulation tests in healthy preterm infants during the first 6 months of life. Adapted with permission from Ref. 134.

Test	Day 1 M	Day 1 B	Day 30 M	Day 30 B	Adult M	Adult B
PT (s)	13.0	10.6–16.2*	11.8	10.0–13.6*	12.4	10.8–13.9
INR	1.0	0.61–1.7	0.79	0.53–1.11	0.89	0.64–1.17
APTT (s)	53.6	27.5–79.4	44.7	26.9–62.5	33.5	26.6–40.3
Fibrinogen (g/l)	2.43	1.50–3.73*	2.54	1.50–4.14*	2.78	1.56–4.00
V (unit/ml)	0.88	0.41–1.48	1.02	0.48–1.56	1.06	0.62–1.50
VII (unit/ml)	0.67	0.21–1.13	0.83	0.21–1.45	1.05	0.67–1.43
VIII (unit/ml)	1.11	0.50–2.13*	1.11	0.50–1.99*	0.99	0.50–1.49
VWF (unit/ml)	1.36	0.78–2.10	1.36	0.66–2.16	0.92	0.50–1.58
IX (unit/ml)	0.35	0.19–0.65	0.44	0.13–0.80	1.09	0.55–1.63
X (unit/ml)	0.41	0.11–0.71	0.56	0.20–0.92	1.06	0.70–1.52
XI (unit/ml)	0.30	0.08–0.52	0.43	0.15–0.71	0.97	0.67–1.27

PT = prothrombin time; APTT = activated partial thromboplastin time; VIII = Factor VIII procoagulant; VWF = von Willebrand factor; INR = international normalized ratio.
All factors except fibrinogen are expressed as unit/ml, where pooled plasma contains 1.0 unit/ml. All values are expressed as mean (M), followed by the lower and upper boundary encompassing 95% of the population (B).
*Values indistinguishable from those of the adult.

of HDN may occur in newborns with a variety of diseases that can compromise the supply of vitamin K (see Chapter 33). The approach to the treatment of these infants is similar to that described above for the reversal of the warfarin effect. Life-threatening bleeding may require FFP treatment or in rare situations treatment with coagulation factor concentrates. The latter should only be used in consultation with a expert in pediatric hemostatic disorders.

Table 35.10 *In vivo* properties of blood clotting factors. Adapted with permission from Ref. 158.

Factor	Plasma concentration required for hemostasis*	Half-life of transfused factor	Recovery in blood (as % of amount transfused)	Stability in liquid plasma and whole blood (4°C storage)
I (fibrinogen)	1.0 g/l	3–6 days	50	Stable
II	0.4 unit/ml	2–5 days	40–80	Stable
V	0.10–0.25 unit/ml	12 hours	80	Unstable***
VII	0.05–0.20 unit/ml	2–6 hours	70–80	Stable
VIII	0.10–0.40 unit/ml	8–12 hours	60–80	Unstable**
IX	0.10–0.40 unit/ml	18–24 hours	40–50	Stable
X	0.10–0.15 unit/ml	2 days	50	Stable
XI	0.15–0.30 unit/ml	3 days	90–100	Stable
XIII	0.01–0.05 unit/ml	6–10 days	5–100	Stable
VWF	0.25–0.50 unit/ml	3–5 hours	—	Unstable

*Upper limit usually refers to surgical hemostasis.
**50% remains at 14 days.
***25% remains at 24 hours.

The use of FFP has been advocated for prevention of periventricular-intraventricular hemorrhage (PVH-IVH) in the preterm infant. A trial carried out in the 1980s demonstrated that FFP administration significantly reduced the risk of IVH as documented by cranial ultrasound.[155] Subsequent studies have not reproduced these results and a recently published study has demonstrated that routine early administration of FFP (or even non-FFP intravascular volume expansion) does not decrease the risk of death or disability in babies born >8 weeks before term.[156,157] Thus current evidence does not support the routine use of prophylactic FFP in preterm infants at risk for PVH-IVH.

In addition to the contraindications for FFP transfusion discussed above, in the newborn FFP should not be used as a fluid for hematocrit adjustment in erythrocyte transfusions nor as a replacement fluid in partial exchange transfusion for the treatment of neonatal hyperviscosity syndrome. As discussed above FFP is used in newborns to prepare reconstituted whole blood where this product is indicated.

DOSAGE AND ADMINISTRATION

Compatibility tests before plasma transfusion are not necessary. Plasma should be ABO compatible with the recipient's RBCs (see Table 35.5). Usually, Rh group need not be considered. However, when large volumes of FFP are given to RhD-negative pediatric patients or women of childbearing age, prevention of RhD immunization by the use of Rh immune globulin should be considered.

FFP may be thawed in a waterbath at 30–37°C; for thawing, the unit should be placed in a watertight protective plastic overwrap or bag to prevent bacterial contamination. Thawing in a waterbath takes 20–30 min. FFP may also be thawed in a microwave specifically designed for this purpose; microwave thawing requires approximately 10 min.

The dose of FFP depends on the clinical situation and the underlying disease process. When FFP is given for coagulation factor replacement, the dose is 10–20 ml/kg. This dose will usually raise the level of coagulation factors by 20% immediately after infusion. Post-transfusion monitoring of the patient's coagulation status (PT, APTT and/or specific coagulation factor assays) is important for optimal treatment. Information on *in vivo* properties of coagulation factors, which may guide plasma transfusion therapy, are summarized in Table 35.10.[158]

PLATELETS

DESCRIPTION AND STORAGE

A platelet concentrate (PC) may be prepared from a WB donation collected into CPDA-1, CPD or CP2D (see Figs 35.1 and 35.2) or by a variety of apheresis procedures in which a single donor donates the equivalent of 4–8 PCs. Platelets collected by apheresis procedures are referred to as apheresis PCs. PCs contain a minimum of 5.5×10^{10} platelets/unit, approximately 50 ml of plasma, trace to 0.5 ml of RBCs and, depending upon the preparation techniques, varying numbers of leukocytes (predominantly monocytes and lymphocytes) up to levels of 10^8/unit. Apheresis PCs contain a minimum of 3×10^{11} platelets, approximately 250–300 ml plasma, trace to 5 ml of RBCs and, depending on the apheresis technique or instrument, 10^6–10^9 leukocytes. PCs and apheresis PCs are stored for up to 5 days at 20–24°C with continuous gentle agitation.

INDICATIONS FOR TRANSFUSION

Decreased platelet production

Decreased platelet production occurs in children with congenital or acquired aplastic anemia, bone marrow infiltration with leukemic or other malignant cells and/or following myeloablative chemotherapy. The majority of studies addressing the indications for platelet transfusions for patients with decreased platelet production have been performed in patients with acute leukemia. It is, however, reasonable to use results of these studies to guide platelet transfusion therapy for the majority of patients with hypoproliferative thrombocytopenia.

Prior to the availability of platelets for transfusion, hemorrhage in patients with leukemia and severe thrombocytopenia was frequently fatal. In a report from the National Cancer Institute in the USA, hemorrhage was considered to have been the major cause of death in 52% of 414 acute leukemic patients studied from 1954 to 1963.[159] With the introduction of plastic blood collection systems in the late 1960s, platelets became available for the treatment of patients with thrombocytopenic bleeding. By the 1980s, deaths due to hemorrhage gradually decreased to the point that only 3% of adults with acute non-lymphoblastic leukemia (ANLL) had lethal hemorrhagic complications.[160]

In the 1970s and 1980s several studies addressed the issue of prophylactic versus therapeutic platelet transfusions for thrombocytopenic patients with acute leukemia.[161–166] These studies demonstrated that platelets given prophylactically do decrease the incidence of significant bleeding episodes in patients with leukemia, but they did not demonstrate a longer survival in patients transfused prophylactically versus those transfused only in the presence of active bleeding. Despite this, several experts began to recommend the use of prophylactic platelet transfusions.[167–170] However, the debate of prophylactic versus therapeutic platelet transfusion therapy continues to be active.[167,171,172] In a survey conducted in 1993 by the American Association of Blood Banks, 70% of 126 institutions treating pediatric hematology/oncology patients reported that the major use of platelets was for prophylaxis, while 20% transfused platelets primarily therapeutically and 10% followed a policy combining both approaches.[173]

For those physicians and institutions who choose to use prophylactic platelet transfusions, the current debate centers around the choice of a platelet count at which routinely to administer platelet concentrates. In the reviews cited above, published in the late 1970s and early 1980s, advocating the use of prophylactic platelet transfusions for leukemic patients, it was often suggested that the platelet count be maintained above $20 \times 10^9/l$. This figure appears to have been derived from a much quoted study by Gaydos et al published in 1962.[174] In this study, the authors tried to determine if there was a threshold platelet level above which bleeding rarely occurred and below which it commonly occurred. They conducted a retrospective review of 92 patients (40 patients were 21 years or older and 52 patients were under 21 years old) with acute leukemia and determined the percent of days with bleeding manifestations at various platelet levels. Gross hemorrhage was visible on <1% of days at all platelet levels $>20 \times 10^9/l$, on 4% of days where platelet counts were $10–20 \times 10^9/l$, on 6% of

days with platelet counts of $5–10 \times 10^9/l$ and increasing to a maximum of 31% of days at platelet counts $<1 \times 10^9/l$. Sixteen of the 92 patients suffered fatal intracranial hemorrhage: 8 were in 'blastic crisis' (not further defined by the authors) and had a median platelet count of $10 \times 10^9/l$; the remaining 8 were not in blastic crisis (7 had a platelet count $<5 \times 10^9/l$, and 1 a platelet count of $5–10 \times 10^9/l$). It must also be remembered that when this study was performed, the platelet inhibitory effects of aspirin were not yet appreciated and many of these patients were probably receiving aspirin. Although the authors concluded that no clear 'threshold' platelet count could be identified, this study has often been cited in the choice of a platelet count of $20 \times 10^9/l$ for prophylactic transfusion.

Recently, the necessity of maintaining a minimum platelet count of $20 \times 10^9/l$ in all patients with malignancies has been questioned. At a Consensus Development Conference addressing platelet transfusion therapy sponsored by the National Institutes of Health in 1986, the panel concluded that patients with severe thrombocytopenia may benefit from prophylactic transfusions but that the commonly used threshold value of $20 \times 10^9/l$ may sometimes be safely lowered.[175] Even more conservative recommendations have recently been published. Slichter, in a review published in 1991, recommended that only patients with platelet counts $<5 \times 10^9/l$ should routinely be given prophylactic platelet transfusions, and for those with platelet counts $>5 \times 10^9/l$ clinical judgement should be used to assess the need for platelet therapy.[176] Beutler likewise suggested abandoning the practice of routinely transfusing patients whenever the platelet count drops below $20 \times 10^9/l$; he, too, suggests that if any level is to be chosen for prophylactic transfusions in a stable patient it should be $5 \times 10^9/l$ with prophylactic transfusions at higher platelet counts being reserved for patients in whom additional risk factors exist.[177]

The rationale for these more conservative recommendations is based on results of older studies as well as more recent ones addressing the safety of lowering threshold levels for prophylactic platelet transfusions. Among the studies cited above addressing the issue of prophylactic versus therapeutic platelet transfusions, 1 was a retrospective review of 70 children with ALL studied during induction and first remission.[165] Platelets were given only for significant bleeding associated with a platelet count below $20 \times 10^9/l$. In this study there were no deaths due to hemorrhage and 84% of patients achieved complete remission without a single platelet transfusion despite the fact that 49% had a platelet count below $20 \times 10^9/l$ at some time during the induction phase. Unfortunately, the actual platelet nadirs were not specified.

More recently, in a retrospective study, the safety of using prophylactic platelet transfusion only for platelet counts below $10 \times 10^9/l$ in patients with ALL and ANLL was reported.[178] In all, 117 episodes of thrombocytopenia (platelet count $<20 \times 10^9/l$) were studied. There were 67 episodes of bleeding of which 85% were minor and 15% major (severe hematuria, hematemesis, melena). There were no intracranial hemorrhages and there was only 1 death due to hemorrhage which occurred in a patient with a platelet count of $5 \times 10^9/l$. All the severe bleeding episodes occurred in patients with decreasing platelet counts and concomitant fever. At platelet counts of $10–20 \times 10^9/l$ versus platelet counts $<10 \times 10^9/l$, patients with ALL had more bleeding episodes than patients with ANLL. In both groups, there were more episodes of bleeding with platelet counts of $10–20 \times 10^9/l$ in leukemia- versus chemotherapy-related thrombocytopenia.

In a second retrospective study, major hemorrhages during hospitalization in 190 patients undergoing BMT were analyzed.[179] In 87 patients transplanted from 1990 to 1991, the $20 \times 10^9/l$ platelet count trigger was used for prophylactic platelet transfusion. In 103 patients transplanted from 1993 to 1994, a more stringent prophylactic policy was adopted: for stable patients, platelets were transfused prophylactically for platelet counts $<10 \times 10^9/l$; when additional platelet consumption factors were present, platelets were transfused for platelet counts $<20 \times 10^9/l$. In the group transfused using the more stringent policy, 12 patients experienced 13 major hemorrhages and 4 died from hemorrhage. In the other group, 12 patients experienced 14 major hemorrhages and 3 died from hemorrhage. Platelet consumption factors were present in 12 of 13 hemorrhages in the former group and in 12 of 14 in the latter group. By contrast, stable patients in both groups experienced fewer hemorrhages (2 of 14 and 1 of 13, respectively).

In a prospective study published in 1991, results were reported of using prophylactic platelet transfusions routinely in 104 patients with newly diagnosed acute leukemia only if the platelet count was $5 \times 10^9/l$ or less.[180] Prophylactic platelet transfusions were administered to patients with platelet counts of $6–10 \times 10^9/l$ in the presence of fresh minor hemorrhagic manifestations or fever and to patients with platelet counts of $11–20 \times 10^9/l$ in the presence of coagulation disorders and/or heparin therapy. Using this prospective protocol, a platelet transfusion was withheld on 69% of days when a morning platelet count was $6–20 \times 10^9/l$. Thirty-one major bleeding episodes occurred in the 104 patients; 3 patients died of complications related to bleeding (1 thrombocytopenic patient with platelet refractoriness, 1 non-thrombocytopenic patient with DIC and heparin therapy, and 1 thrombocytopenic patient with acute pro-myelocytic leukemia and an unrecognized spinal cord hematoma).

While more stringent prophylactic platelet transfusion policies may be appropriate for many patients, 2 groups of leukemic patients appear to be at particularly high risk of fatal hemorrhage during induction chemotherapy, namely those with hyperleukocytosis and/or acute promyelocytic leukemia (ANLL, FAB M3). The German BFM study group reported the causes of early death in 294 children with ANLL.[181] Thirty (10%) died prior to or in the first 12 days of therapy and of these, 12 were due to hemorrhage alone. Of these 12 patients, 8 had leukocyte counts $>100 \times$ $10^9/l$; only 2 had platelet counts $<20 \times 10^9/l$ and 2 had platelet counts between 50 and $100 \times 10^9/l$. The authors noted that several of the hemorrhagic deaths occurred during the period of rapid blast reduction. In patients with acute promyelocytic leukemia, rates of early fatal hemorrhage of 9–26% have been reported.[182] This bleeding tendency is associated with the presence of DIC and fibrinolysis thought to be related to the release of procoagulant substances from the promyelocytic granules.

The incidence of hemorrhage in patients with solid tumors and thrombocytopenia has been addressed in at least 2 reports, although neither specifically studied pediatric patients.[183,184] Based on these studies, the risk factors for hemorrhage in patients with solid tumors are similar to those in leukemic patients, although an additional consideration is the predisposition to hemorrhage associated with local tumor invasion.

In summary, given current data, the use of either therapeutic or prophylactic platelet transfusions for children with hypoproliferative thrombocytopenia can be justified. However, the exclusive use of therapeutic transfusions should be considered only in settings where frequent evaluations by an experienced team of physicians can be carried out and where platelet concentrates, if necessary, can be quickly obtained and administered. Alternatively, for physicians or institutions electing to transfuse platelets prophylactically, consideration should be given to using a threshold platelet count lower than $20 \times 10^9/l$ for routine administration of platelets. Just as the indication for a RBC transfusion should not be determined solely on the basis of an Hb level, the decision to administer a platelet transfusion should also be individualized, taking into account the clinical situation as well as the platelet level.

Prophylactic platelet transfusions are indicated for thrombocytopenic patients undergoing invasive procedures. At least one study suggests that major surgical procedures can be safely performed in leukemic patients at platelet counts of $50 \times 10^9/l$.[185] However, there is little published data concerning appropriate platelet counts for 2 of the commonest invasive procedures that patients with hematologic or other malignancies undergo, namely lumbar puncture and the insertion of permanent indwelling central venous catheters. Bone marrow aspiration and biopsy can be safely performed (with respect to local bleeding) at any platelet level. Suggested guidelines for prophylactic platelet transfusions for pediatric patients with thrombocytopenia due to decreased platelet production are summarized in Table 35.11.[186]

Increased platelet destruction

Patients with thrombocytopenia due to autoimmune thrombocytopenic purpura (AITP) should only be treated with platelet transfusions in the presence of central nervous system or other life-threatening bleeding.[187] Prior to surgical procedures, e.g. splenectomy or caesarian section, the platelet

Table 35.11 Suggested guidelines for prophylactic platelet transfusions in pediatric patients with thrombocytopenia due to decreased platelet production. Reproduced with permission from Ref. 186.

Platelet count $<10 \times 10^9/l$

Platelet count $<20 \times 10^9/l$ and bone marrow infiltration, severe mucositis, DIC, anticoagulation therapy, a platelet count likely to fall below $10 \times 10^9/l$ prior to next possible evaluation, or risk of bleeding due to local tumor invasion

Platelet count $<30–40 \times 10^9/l$ and DIC (e.g. during induction therapy for promyelocytic leukemia), extreme hyperleukocytosis, or prior to lumbar puncture or central venous line insertion

Platelet count $<50–60 \times 10^9/l$ and major surgical intervention

DIC = disseminated intravascular coagulation.

count can usually be raised preoperatively using corticosteroids or intravenous immunoglobins to levels sufficient to assure adequate hemostasis. A variety of conditions other than AITP (e.g. septicemia, trauma, obstetrical complications) may result in platelet consumption that is sufficiently severe to require platelet transfusion. Platelet increment and survival are usually decreased in these patients and a larger number of units administered at more frequent intervals may be necessary.

Massive transfusion

Thrombocytopenia is frequently associated with massive transfusion. Depending on the underlying etiology of the bleeding, the thrombocytopenia may be dilutional from platelet loss through hemorrhage and/or due to platelet consumption. Platelet transfusion therapy should be based on a consideration of several factors including platelet count, an assessment of the role of the thrombocytopenia in the observed bleeding and the estimated hemostatic platelet count necessary for the patient's given clinical situation.

Platelet dysfunction

Platelet dysfunction possibly requiring platelet transfusion is most commonly encountered in 2 situations: patients taking platelet inhibitory drugs and following surgery with cardiopulmonary bypass pump (CBP). Platelet dysfunction due to platelet inhibitory drugs is unlikely to contribute to bleeding if the platelet count is $>50 \times 10^9/l$. Treatment with desmopressin acetate has been shown to prevent bleeding complications in patients who have taken aspirin within 7 days of a surgical intervention.[188,189]

Platelet dysfunction lasting 4–6 hours post-CBP has been well-documented.[190,191] These patients are usually thrombocytopenic, too. Nevertheless, studies have not shown a benefit for the use of prophylactic platelet transfusions for patients undergoing CBP.[192] Platelet transfusions should be reserved for those patients, who following CBP have excessive bleeding thought to be due to platelet function abnormalities and/or thrombocytopenia.[144,145,175]

SPECIAL CONSIDERATIONS FOR NEWBORNS

Newborns should receive platelet transfusions in the same clinical settings as described above for older children. However, since newborns frequently manifest thrombocytopenia and since preterm infants are at risk for PVH-IVH, it is possible that the platelet level at which prophylactic platelet transfusions should be administered to newborns is higher than that recommended for other patients. Responses to a survey conducted by the American Association of Blood Banks in the early 1990s showed that the platelet levels at which prophylactic platelet transfusions were given to neonates varied tremendously: from $<20 \times 10^9/l$ to $>50 \times 10^9/l$ in stable preterm infants and $<20 \times 10^9/l$ to $>80 \times 10^9/l$ in sick preterm infants.[193] Only one prospective randomized study has addressed this issue.[194] Inclusion criteria for the randomized study included a birth weight of 500–1500 g, a gestational age of <33 weeks, and a platelet count of $>50 \times 10^9/$, but $<150 \times 10^9/l$ during the first 72 hours of life. Infants randomized to prophylactic platelet-transfusion therapy received platelet concentrates to maintain the circulating platelet count $>150 \times 10^9/l$. Control infants did not receive an infusion of platelet concentrates unless their platelet count fell below $50 \times 10^9/l$ or they had clinical bleeding. Prophylactic platelet transfusions failed to influence the incidence or extension of IVH. However, control infants with platelet counts $<60 \times 10^9/l$ needed more RBC and FFP transfusions than did infants who received prophylactic platelet transfusions. The investigators concluded that non-bleeding premature infants with platelet counts higher than $60 \times 10^9/l$ should not receive prophylactic platelet transfusions.[194]

Neonates with thrombocytopenia due to maternal platelet alloantibodies require special consideration with respect to the indications for platelet transfusion as described in Chapter 22.

Based on the limited information available, definitive guidelines for platelet transfusions in newborns cannot be made. Suggested guidelines (Table 35.12) have been published.[195]

DOSAGE AND ADMINISTRATION

Platelets possess intrinsic ABH antigens and extrinsically absorbed A and B antigens.[196,197] Nevertheless ABO-incompatible platelets (i.e. platelets with A and/or B antigens given to a donor with a corresponding antibody) are usually clinically effective. However, in some patients, particularly those receiving multiple platelet transfusions, there may be a poorer post-transfusion response than that obtained with ABO-compatible platelets, and some studies have suggested that the transfusion of ABO-incompatible platelets is associated with the development of platelet refractoriness.[198–200] Also, there are reports of acute intravascular hemolysis following the transfusion of platelet concentrates containing ABO antibodies incompatible

Table 35.12 Suggested guidelines for platelet transfusion support of neonates. Adapted with permission from Ref. 195.

Prophylactic platelet transfusions
Stable preterm neonates with platelet counts <30 × 10⁹/l

Stable term neonates with platelet counts <20 × 10⁹/l

Sick preterm neonates with platelet counts <50 × 10⁹/l

Sick term infants with platelet counts <30 × 10⁹/l

Preparation for an invasive procedure, e.g. lumbar puncture or minor surgery in neonates with platelet counts <50 × 10⁹/l, and for major surgery in neonates with platelet counts <100 × 10⁹/l

Platelet transfusions in neonates with clinically significant bleeding
Neonates with platelet counts <50 × 10⁹/l

Neonates with conditions that increase bleeding (e.g. DIC) and platelet counts <100 × 10⁹/l

Neonates with documented significant platelet functional disorders (e.g. Glanzmann thrombasthenia) irrespective of the circulating platelet count

---

DIC = disseminated intravascular coagulation.

with the recipient's RBCs.[201–203] Therefore, it would seem prudent, particularly in small children where the volume of plasma may be relatively large with respect to the patient's total blood volume, to try to use ABO-matched platelets. If these are not available, units with plasma compatible with the recipient's RBCs should be chosen. If this is also not possible, units with low titers of anti-A or -B should be selected or platelets may be volume reduced (see Table 35.5). Testing of PCs for RBC compatibility is not necessary unless red cells are detected by visual inspection.

Platelets do not carry Rh antigens.[204] However, the quantity of RBCs in platelet concentrates is sufficient to induce Rh sensitization even in immunosuppressed cancer patients.[205–207] Rh sensitization caused by platelet transfusions in Rh-negative patients can be prevented by the administration of Rh immunoprophylaxis.[208,209] Thus, if platelets from an Rh-positive donor, or platelets from a donor of unknown Rh phenotype, are given to an Rh-negative recipient, administration of Rh immunoprophylaxis should be considered, especially for female patients. The amount of anti-D immunoglobulin necessary to prevent sensitization depends on the number of contaminating RBCs in the platelet concentrates. A dose of 25 μg (125 IU) of anti-D immunoglobulin will protect against 1 ml of RBCs.[210] If available, it is preferable to use a preparation of anti-D which can be administered intravenously.

A suitable starting platelet dosage that can be expected to raise the platelet level by 50 × 10⁹/l is 1 PC/10 kg body weight. PCs may be pooled before administration or infused individually. An equivalent dose for apheresis platelets is approximately 5 ml/kg. Patients with increased platelet consumption (e.g. with septicemia or DIC) or splenomegaly may require larger amounts of platelets.

PC or apheresis platelets may be volume reduced prior to infusion. However, this extra manipulation leads to platelet loss and if not carefully performed may potentially adversely affect platelet function and/or be a cause of bacterial contamination. Volume reduction should therefore be limited to patients who require severe volume restriction or situations where ABO-incompatible platelets are the only available PCs for a neonate or child.

PCs must be filtered, either using a standard 170-μm filter or a leukoreduction filter. The indications for leukoreduction filters are discussed in Chapter 36. Single PCs or apheresis PCs should be infused as rapidly as clinically tolerated. The transfusion must be completed within 4 hours of beginning the transfusion, or in the case of pooled PCs within 4 hours of pooling.

Many patients requiring platelet transfusions should receive irradiated products only. Indications for irradiation of PCs (and other blood components) are also discussed in Chapter 36.

PLATELET REFRACTORINESS

The response to a platelet transfusion, known as the corrected platelet count increment (CCI), is determined using the following formula which takes into account the recipient's body surface area and number of platelets transfused:

$$CCI = \frac{[(\text{Posttransfusion–pretransfusion}) \text{ platelet count } (\mu l/10^{11})] \times \text{body surface area } (m^2)}{\text{Number of platelets transfused } (\times 10^{11})}$$

In general, a platelet transfusion is considered successful if the CCI is > 7.5 × 10⁹/l (7500 μl/10¹¹) within 10–60 min of a transfusion and > 4.5 × 10⁹/l if measured 18–24 hours after transfusion.

Refractoriness to platelet transfusions is defined as a consistently inadequate response to platelet transfusion, e.g. a CCI of < 5 × 10⁹/l following 2 separate transfusions of an adequate number of platelets. Refractoriness may be due to immune (i.e. the presence in the recipient of HLA or platelet-specific alloantibodies) or non-immune causes. Included among the various non-immune factors reported to be associated with platelet refractoriness are treatment with amphotericin B, vancomycin or ciprofloxacin, fever, splenomegaly, DIC and BMT.[211–214]

The first step in the management of patients who are refractory to random donor platelet transfusions is to assure that ABO-identical platelets are used. Secondly, the use of fresh as opposed to stored platelets may result in increased CCIs, particularly in clinically unstable patients.[215] When HLA alloimmunization is the most likely cause of refractoriness, HLA-matched platelets should be provided.[216] Some centers also use platelet cross-matching to choose platelet units for HLA-alloimmunized patients.[216] The rare patient with platelet-specific alloantibodies should be treated with platelets lacking the corresponding antigen. The use of antifibrinolytic agents such as epsilon-aminocaproic acid may also be helpful in these patients (as well as in

Table 35.13 Guidelines for providing platelet transfusion support for patients refractory to pooled random donor platelets.

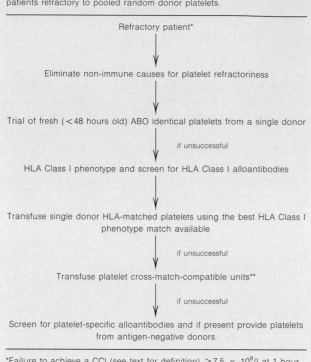

Refractory patient*

↓

Eliminate non-immune causes for platelet refractoriness

↓

Trial of fresh (<48 hours old) ABO identical platelets from a single donor

if unsuccessful

HLA Class I phenotype and screen for HLA Class I alloantibodies

↓

Transfuse single donor HLA-matched platelets using the best HLA Class I phenotype match available

if unsuccessful

Transfuse platelet cross-match-compatible units**

if unsuccessful

Screen for platelet-specific alloantibodies and if present provide platelets from antigen-negative donors

*Failure to achieve a CCI (see text for definition) $\geqslant 7.5 \times 10^9/l$ at 1 hour following an adequate dose (in the non-bleeding patient 1 unit/10 kg, maximum 6 units) of pooled donor platelets on $\geqslant 2$ occasions
**Not all centers use platelet cross-matching techniques while others use them in combination with HLA-phenotyping.[216]

non-refractory patients).[217] Suggested guidelines for platelet support of patients refractory to random donor platelets are outlined in Table 35.13. It is important to remember that some alloimmunized patients may lose their antibodies over time and again become responsive to random donor platelet transfusions.[218,219]

The management of alloimmunized patients who do not respond to the above measures is problematic. It is likely to be of no benefit to administer prophylactic platelet transfusions to such patients. In the presence of clinically significant bleeding, approaches such as the use of larger and/or more frequent platelet transfusions may be attempted. The administration of intravenous immunoglobin may result in improved post-transfusion platelet increments but does not usually increase platelet survival.[220]

GRANULOCYTES

DESCRIPTION AND STORAGE

To assure clinical efficacy, granulocyte concentrates should contain a minimum of 10^{10} polymorphonuclear cells (PMNs)/unit. To obtain this number of PMNs, concentrates are prepared by automated leukapheresis using an erythrocyte sedimenting agent (to enhance the efficacy of separation of granulocytes from erythrocytes) such as hydroxyethyl starch. In addition, donors are usually stimulated with oral corticosteroids prior to collection. The platelet and RBC content varies with the collection method. The plasma volume is 200–400 ml. Recently, there have been reports of leukapheresis collections of $>4 \times 10^{10}$ PMNs/unit following donor stimulation with G-CSF.[221,222] However, the use of G-CSF in normal donors, and the characteristics of granulocyte concentrates following G-CSF stimulation, require further study before this approach can be recommended for routine use.

Granulocytes have also been prepared from single units of fresh WB by separation following centrifugation of the buffy coat (leukocyte) layer. However, the quantity of PMNs obtained (approximately 10^9 leukocytes/unit) is rarely large enough to ensure an efficacious transfusion, even for neonatal patients. There is a recent report of the preparation of granulocytes by pooling buffy coat layers separated from 4–8 units of fresh whole blood. In pediatric patients (ages 2 to 13 years), the mean leukocyte dose transfused was $0.6 \times 10^9/\text{kg}$.[223]

Granulocyte function deteriorates rapidly during storage. Thus, granulocytes should be transfused as soon as possible following collection and should not be given if stored for >24 hours. For the time between collection and infusion, granulocyte concentrates should kept at 20–24°C, with little or no agitation.[224]

INDICATIONS FOR TRANSFUSION

In the 1970s and early 1980s several studies investigating the role for granulocyte transfusions in neutropenic patients were reported. These studies have been recently reviewed.[225] No benefit was found for the prophylactic administration of granulocyte transfusions. Most, although not all, studies demonstrated benefit for their use in neutropenic patients with established infection. However, enthusiasm for granulocyte transfusions generally decreased in the late 1980s, probably for several reasons: granulocyte concentrates are difficult to prepare, cannot be stored and have been associated with severe pulmonary reactions, particularly in patients receiving amphotericin B.[226] Concomitantly, survival from septic episodes began to improve with earlier introduction of antibiotic treatment for septic episodes and the availability of better antibiotics, and more recently GM-CSF and G-CSF. Techniques for preparing granulocytes have improved since the time of the early studies and there have been no recent reports of life-threatening pulmonary toxicity, although physicians administering granulocytes to patients receiving amphotericin B do try to separate the 2 treatments by 10–12 hour intervals. Currently, granulocyte transfusions are reserved for patients with profound neutropenia not expected to recover within a week, or severe forms of congenital neutrophil dysfunction, in whom a severe bacterial infection has been documented and who are clinically deteriorating despite optimal antimicrobial therapy.[225,227] Published information is insufficient to determine the efficacy of granulocyte transfusions in the treatment of fungal infections in neutropenic patients.[228]

SPECIAL CONSIDERATIONS FOR NEWBORNS

Newborns normally have a transient neutrophilia in the first week of life with mean normal absolute neutrophil counts ranging from $11.0 \times 10^9/l$ at birth to $5.5 \times 10^9/l$ at 1 week of life.[229] Septic newborns frequently develop neutropenia, defined in the newborn as an absolute neutrophil count below $3.0 \times 10^9/l$. Between 1981 and 1992, 5 controlled trials of granulocyte transfusions for septic newborns with neutropenia were reported and have recently been reviewed.[230] The data suggest a benefical role for granulocyte transfusion provided an adequate dose is administered. Nevertheless, the use of granulocyte transfusions for neonatal sepsis has not become widespread, possibly because of the difficulty of obtaining granulocytes as rapidly as would be required in this setting. More recently, investigators in the field have begun to study the role of G-CSF in the treatment of neonatal sepsis.[231]

DOSAGE AND ADMINISTRATION

Once the decision to administer granulocyte transfusions has been made, they are administered daily until there is evidence of recovery of peripheral neutrophil counts or clinical evidence of recovery from the infection. To provide granulocyte transfusions daily for several days and to assure both adequate viral testing of donors and/or units and administration of units within 24 hours of collection, special arrangements need to be made with the blood supplier. For neonates and small children, a daily infusion of 1×10^9 PMNs/kg should be given and for larger patients, $2–3 \times 10^{10}$ PMNs. As there is significant RBC contamination, units must be ABO compatible and if possible RhD negative for RhD-negative recipients and must undergo the usual compatibility testing. Patients should be tested for the presence of HLA (and if possible neutrophil) antibodies prior to the first granulocyte transfusion and periodically during a prolonged course of transfusions. Alloimmunization frequently occurs in patients receiving granulocyte transfusions and may render the transfusions ineffective and/or be associated with adverse reactions including respiratory distress.[232] For patients with HLA- and/or granulocyte-specific alloantibodies, only granulocytes from HLA- and/or neutrophil antigen-compatible donors should be used.

Granulocytes must be transfused through a standard 170-μm blood filter. Obviously, a leukoreduction filter must not be used and microaggregate filters are also not recommended.[224] The transfusion is usually administered over 2–3 hours.

CRYOPRECIPITATE

DESCRIPTION AND STORAGE

Cryoprecipitate is the precipitate formed when FFP is thawed at 4°C. The precipitate is then refrozen within 1 hour in 10–15 ml of the donor plasma and stored at -18°C or less for a period of up to 1 year. Cryoprecipitate contains 80–100 units of Factor VIII, 100–250 mg of fibrinogen, 40–60 mg of fibronectin and 40–70% of the von Willebrand factor and 30% of the Factor XIII present in the original unit of plasma.

INDICATIONS FOR TRANSFUSION

The majority of situations in which cryoprecipitate has been used in the past, e.g. to treat hemophilia A and von Willebrand disease, can now be managed with alternative, safer products (see Chapters 29 and 30). Cryoprecipitate has also been used to treat bleeding due to congenital deficiencies of fibrinogen or Factor XIII. Virus-inactivated plasma-derived concentrates are now commercially available for these disorders, although they are not licensed in all countries. If unavailable, cryoprecipitate may be used. Finally, cryoprecipitate was previously used to treat bleeding in patients with uremia. These patients are now treated with dialysis, desmopressin and erythropoietin. Currently, the main indication for cryoprecipitate therapy is to control bleeding due to acquired fibrinogen deficiency, e.g. in severe liver disease, DIC, or certain obstetrical disorders.

DOSAGE AND ADMINISTRATION

Compatibility testing of cryoprecipitate units is unnecessary. However, cryoprecipitate does contain anti-A and -B so the use of ABO-compatible units is preferable. Rh group need not be considered. The number of units of cryoprecipitate required is usually based on the amount necessary to obtain a hemostatic level of fibrinogen, i.e. a fibrinogen level $> 0.8–1.0$ g/l. If the units are carefully pooled this can usually be accomplished by the transfusion of 1 unit/5–10 kg recipient weight.

Cryoprecipitate is prepared for transfusion by thawing at 30–37°C and mixing the thawed precipitate with 10–15 ml of sodium chloride 0.9%, if necessary, according to the amount of plasma in the cryoprecipitate unit. The required number of units is then pooled.

Thawed cryoprecipitate should be stored at room temperature and transfused immediately after thawing or within 6 hours after thawing if used as a source of Factor VIII. All pooled cryoprecipitate units must be used within 4 hours of pooling. Cryoprecipitate must be transfused through a standard 170-μm blood filter and is administered as rapidly as the patient's clinical situation permits. Infusion time should not exceed 4 hours.

ALBUMIN

PREPARATION AND STORAGE

Albumin is derived from pools of donor plasma obtained either from whole blood or from plasmapheresis. It is prepared by the cold alcohol fractionation process (Cohn fractionation) followed by heat treatment at 60°C for 10 hours. Its composition is 96% albumin and 4% other plasma proteins. Albumin is available as a 25% solution in distilled water or as a 5% solution in saline. Plasma protein fraction (PPF) is a similar product except that it is subject to fewer purification steps in the fractionation process. PPF is a 5% protein solution composed of approximately 85% albumin and 15% other plasma proteins. All 3 preparations have a physiologic pH and a sodium content of about 145 mmol/l (145 mEq/l). The 5% solutions are osmotically and oncotically equivalent to plasma, while the 25% solution is osmotically and oncotically 5-fold greater than plasma. These products can be stored for up to 5 years at 2–10°C.

INDICATIONS FOR TRANSFUSION

The indications for the use of albumin (or PPF) are controversial and many transfusion medicine specialists believe this product is overused.[34,233] In particular, controversy remains concerning the use of albumin versus crystalloids or non-blood colloids for intravascular volume expansion.[34,35] Indications, possible indications and contraindications are summarized in Table 35.14. The 25% solution should not be used in dehydrated patients unless it is supplemented by the infusion of crystalloid solutions.

DOSAGE AND ADMINISTRATION

Albumin and PPF do not need to be administered through a filter. Dosage and rate of infusion depend upon the patient's clinical condition. In shock the usual dosage of 5% albumin is 500 ml in adults and 10–20 ml/kg in children.

IMMUNOGLOBULINS

Plasma-derived immunoglobulins are available in 2 forms: intramuscular and intravenous preparations. Intramuscular immunoglublin, commonly known as human immune serum globulin (ISG), is prepared from large pools of donor plasma by cold alcohol fractionation (Cohn fractionation). ISG is 95% IgG with the remaining 5% consisting of other plasma proteins. It is prepared as a sterile solution with a protein concentration of 16.5 g/l. ISG is for intramuscular use; it must not be administered intravenously as it contains aggregated IgG complexes which can activate complement causing adverse reactions if administered intravenously. The commonest use of ISG is for hepatitis A or measles prophylaxis. Several special human immune globulins are available. They are identical to ISG except that they have high titers to an infectious agent or the RhD antigen. The most commonly used preparations are hepatitis B immune globulin and varicella zoster immune globulin for the prevention of hepatitis B and varicella zoster infections, respectively, and RhD immune globulin for the prevention of RhD alloimmunization. An RhD human immune globulin for intravenous injection is also available.

Human ISG may be further treated to prepare intravenous immunoglobin (IVIG), a product virtually free of immunoglobin complexes and therefore safe for intravenous infusion. Several IVIG preparations are commercially available. They differ in their mode of preparation, pH, use of additives, etc., but for practical purposes are generally therapeutically equivalent. Some contain less IgA than others and are therefore preferentially chosen if treating an IgA-deficient patient. IVIG is used as replacement therapy in primary immunodeficiency states and a wide variety of secondary immunodeficiency states. It can also be used as an immunomodulating agent to treat selected patients with autoimmune thrombocytopenic purpura or other autoimmune disorders. The efficacy of IVIG in various clinical settings was assessed in 1990 at a consensus development conference of the National Institutes of Health in the USA and has recently been reviewed.[234,235]

An IVIG preparation with specificity for respiratory syncytial virus (RSV-IGIV) has been developed and studied and was recently approved in the United States for use in the prevention of severe RSV infections in selected patients.[236,237]

Table 35.14 Administration of albumin. Adapted with permission from Ref. 233.

Generally accepted indications
  Following large volume paracentesis
  Nephrotic syndrome resistant to diuretics
  Fluid replacement in therapeutic plasma exchange

Possible indications
  Fluid resuscitation in shock/burns/sepsis
  Cardiopulmonary bypass pump priming
  Neonatal hyperbilirubinemia

Generally accepted contraindications
  Nutritional protein deficiency
  Chronic hypoalbuminemia (e.g. with nephrotic syndrome, cirrhosis or protein-losing enteropathy)
  Simple volume expansion (e.g. surgery or burns)

REFERENCES

1. Haradin AR, Weed RI, Reed CF. Changes in physical properties of stored erythrocytes. Relationship to survival *in vivo*. *Transfusion* 1969; **9**: 229–237

2. Hogman CF, de Verdier CH, Ericson A, Hedlund K, Sandhagen B. Studies on the mechanism of human red cell loss of viability during storage at +4°C *in vitro* I. Cell shape and total adenylate concentration as determinant factors for posttransfusion survival. *Vox Sang* 1985; **48**: 257–268

3. Latham JT, Bove JR, Weirich FL. Chemical and hematologic changes in stored CPDA-1 blood. *Transfusion* 1982; **22**: 158–159

4. Moore GL, Peck CC, Sohmer PR, Zuck TF. Some properties of blood stored in anticoagulant CPDA-1 solution. *Transfusion* 1981; **21**: 135–137

5. Beutler E. Liquid preservation of red cells. In: Rossi EC, Simon TL, Moss GS, Gould SA, (eds) *Principles of Transfusion Medicine*, 2nd edn. Baltimore: Williams and Wilkins, 1996, pp 51–60

6. Benesch R, Benesch RE: The influence of organic phosphates on the oxygenation of hemoglobin. *Fed Proc* 1967; **26**: 673

7. Heaton A, Keegan T, Holme S. *In vivo* regeneration of red cell, 2,3-diphosphoglycerate following transfusion of DPG-depleted AS-1, AS-3, and CPDA-1 red cells. *Br J Haematol* 1989; **71**: 131–136

8. Falchry SM, Messick WJ, Sheldon GF. Metabolic effects of massive transfusion. In: Rossi EC, Simon TL, Moss GS, Gould SA (eds) *Principles of Transfusion Medicine*, 2nd edn. Baltimore, Williams & Wilkins,1996, pp 615–626

9. Baldini M, Costea N, Dameschek W. The viability of stored human platelets. *Blood* 1960; **16**: 1669–1692

10. Rapaport SI, Ames SB, Mikkelsen S. The level of antihemophilic globulin and proaccelerin in fresh and bank blood. *Am J Clin Pathol* 1959; **31**: 297–304

11. Tuman KJ. Tissue oxygen delivery – the physiology of anemia. *Anesthesiol Clin N Am* 1990; **8**: 451–469

12. Adamson JW, Finch CA. Hemoglobin function, oxygen affinity and erythropoietin. *Ann Rev Physiol* 1975; **37**: 351–369

13. Greenburg AG. A physiologic basis for red blood cell transfusion decisions. *Am J Surg* 1995; **170**: 44S–48S

14. Hebert PH, Hu LW, Biro GP. Review of physiologic mechanisms in response to anemia. *Can Med Assoc J* 1997; **156 (Suppl 11)**: S27–40

15. Crosby E, Ferguson D, Hume HA *et al*. Guidelines for red blood cell and plasma transfusion for adults and children. *Can Med Assoc J* 1997; **156 (Suppl 11)**: S1–12

16. Bunn HF. Human hemoglobins: normal and abnormal. In: Nathan DG, Oski FA (eds) *Hematology of Infancy and Childhood*, 5th edn. Philadelphia: WB Saunders, 1997, pp 729–761

17. Dreyer WJ, Fisher DJ. Regulation of cardiac pump function. In: Garson A Jr, Bricker JT, McNamara DG (eds) *The Science and Practice of Pediatric Cardiology*. Philadelphia: Lea & Febiger, 1990, pp 231–243

18. Cropp GJA. Cardiovascular function in children with severe anemia. *Circulation* 1969; **39**: 775–784

19. Martin E, Ott E. Extreme hemodilution in the Harrington procedure. *Bibl Haematol* 1981; **47**: 322–337

20. Fontana J, Welborn L, Mongan P *et al*. Oxygen consumption and cardiovascular function in children during profound intra-operative normovolemic hemodilution. *Anesth Analg* 1995; **80**: 219–225

21. Wilkerson DK, Rosen AL, Sehgal LR *et al*. Limits of cardiac compensation in anemic baboons. *Surgery* 1988; **103**: 665–670

22. Spahn DR, Smith RL, Veronee CD *et al*. Acute isovolemic hemodilution and blood transfusion: effects on regional function and metabolism in myocardium with compromised coronary blood flow. *J Thorac Cardiovasc Surg* 1993; **105**: 694–704

23. Card RT, Brain MC. The "anemia" of childhood: Evidence for a physiologic response to hyperphosphatemia. *N Engl J Med* 1973; **228**: 388–392

24. Hume HA, Kronick JB, Blanchette VB. Review of the literature on allogeneic red blood cells and plasma transfusion in children. *Can Med Assoc J* 1997; **156**: S41–S49

25. Smith PJ, Ekert H. Evidence of stem-cell competition in children with malignant disease. A controlled study of hypertransfusion. *Lancet* 1976; **i**: 776–779

26. Toogood IRG, Ekert H, Smith PJ. Controlled study of hypertrans-

27. fusion during remission induction in childhood acute lymphocytic leukemia. *Lancet* 1978; **i**: 862–864

27. Holzer BR, Egger M, Teuscher R *et al*. Childood anemia in Africa: to transfuse or not transfuse? *Acta Tropica* 1993; **55**: 47–51

28. Lackritz EM, Campbell CC, Ruebush TK *et al*. Effect of blood transfusion on survival among children in a Kenyan hospital. *Lancet* 1992; **340**: 524–528

29. Lucking SE, Williams TM, Chaten FC *et al*. Dependence of oxygen consumption on oxygen delivery in children with hyperdynamic septic shock and low oxygen extraction. *Crit Care Med* 1990; **18**: 1316–1319

30. Mink RB, Pollack MM. Effect of blood transfusion on oxygen consumption in pediatric septic shock. *Crit Care Med* 1990; **18**: 1087–1091

31. Seear M, Wensley D, MacNab A. Oxygen consumption – oxygen delivery relationship in children. *J Pediatr* 1993; **123**: 208–214

32. Guay J, Hume H, Gauthier M, Tremblay P. Choc hémorragique. In: Lacroix J, Gauthier M, Beaufils F (eds) *Urgences et soins intensif pédiatriques*. Montreal: Les Presses de l'Université de Montréal, 1994, pp 73–87

33. Soud T, Pieper P, Hazinski MF. Pediatric trauma. In: Hazinski MF (ed) *Nursing care of the critically ill child*. St. Louis, MO: Mosby Year Book, 1992

34. Margarson MP, Soni N. Serum albumin: touchstone or totem? *Anaesthesia* 1998; **53**: 789–803

35. Cochrane Injuries Group Albumin Reviewers. Human albumin administration in critically ill patients: systematic review of randomised controlled trials. *BMJ* 1998; **317**: 235–240

36. Petz LD. Blood transfusion in acquired hemolytic anemias. In: Petz LD, Swisher SN, Kleinmans, Spence RK, Strauss RG (eds) *Clinical Practice of Transfusion Medicine*, 3rd edn. New York: Churchill Livingstone, 1996, pp 469–499

37. Wayne AS, Kevy SV, Nathan DG. Transfusion management of sickle cell disease. *Blood* 1993; **81**: 1109–1123

38. Vichinsky EP, Haberkern CM, Neumayr L *et al*. A comparison of conservative and aggressive transfusion regimens in the perioperative management of sickle cell disease. *N Engl J Med* 1995; **333**: 206–213

39. Ohene-Frempong K. Stroke in sickle cell disease: demographic, clinical, and therapeutic considerations. *Semin Hematol* 1991; **28**: 213–219

40. Miller ST, Jensen D, Rao SP. Less intensive long-term transfusion therapy for sickle cell anemia and cerebrosvascular accident. *J Pediatr* 1992; **120**: 54–57

41. Cohen AR, Martin MB, Silber JH *et al*. A modified transfusion program for prevention of stroke in sickle cell disease. *Blood* 1992; **79**: 1657–1661

42. Adams RJ, McKie VC, Hsu L *et al*. Prevention of a first stroke by tranfusions in children with sickle cell anemia and abnormal results on transcranial doppler ultrasonography. *N Engl J Med* 1998; **339**: 5–11

43. Jan K, Usami S, Smith JA. Effects of transfusion on the rheological properties of blood in sickle cell anemia. *Transfusion* 1982; **22**: 17–20

44. Rackoff WR, Ohene-Frempong K, Month S *et al*. Neurologic events after partial exchange transfusion for priapism in sickle cell disease. *J Pediatr* 1992; **120**: 882–885

45. Piomelli S, Seaman C, Ackerman K *et al*. Planning an exchange transfusion in patients with sickle cell syndromes. *Am J Pediatr Hematol Oncol* 1990; **12**: 268–276

46. Kim HC, Dugan NP, Silber JH *et al*. Erythrocytapheresis therapy to reduce iron overload in chronically transfused patients with sickle cell disease. *Blood* 1994; **83**: 1136–1142

47. Piomelli S. Management of Cooleys' anemia. *Baillière's Clin Haematol* 1993; **6**: 287–298

48. Propper RD, Button LN, Nathan DG. New approaches to the transfusion management of thalassemia. *Blood* 1980; **55**: 55–60

49. Cohen AR, Schmidt JM, Martin MB *et al*. Clinical trial of young red cell transfusions. *J Pediatr* 1984; **104**: 865–868

50. Marcus RE, Wonke B, Bantock HM *et al*. A prospective trial of young red cells in 48 patients with transfusion-dependent thalassaemia. *Br J Haematol* 1985; **60**: 153–159

51. Collins AF, Gonçalves-Dias C, Haddad S et al. Comparison of a transfusion preparation of newly formed red cells and standard washed red cell transfusions in patients with homozygous β-thalassemia. *Transfusion* 1994; **34**: 517–520

52. Spanos T, Ladis V, Palamidou F *et al*. The impact of neocyte transfusion in the management of thalassaemia. *Vox Sang* 1996; **70**: 217–223

53. McCullough J, Lasky LC, Warkentin PW. Role of the blood bank in bone marrow transplantation. In: McCullough J, Sandler SG (eds) *Advances in immunobiology: blood cell antigens and bone marrow transplantation*. New York, NY: Alan R. Liss, 1984, pp 370–412

54. Rosse WF, Gallagher D, Kinney TR *et al*. Transfusion and alloimmunization in sickle cell disease. *Blood* 1990; **76**: 1431–1437

55. Vichinsky EP, Earles A, Johnson RP *et al*. Alloimmunization in sickle cell anemia and transfusion of racially matched blood. *N Engl J Med* 1990; **332**: 1617–1621

56. Gullis JO, Win N, Dudley JM, Kaye T. Posttransfusion hyperhemolysis in a patient with sickle cell disease: use of steroids and intravenous immunoglobulin to prevent further red cell destruction. *Vox Sang* 1995; **69**: 355–357

57. King KE, Shirey RS, Lankiewicz MW *et al*. Delayed hemolytic transfusion reactions in sickle cell disease; simultaneous destruction of recipient's red cells. *Transfusion* 1997; **37**: 376–381

58. Ambruso DR, Githens JH, Alcorn R *et al*. Experience with donors matched for minor blood group antigens in patients with sickle cell anemia who are receiving chronic transfusion therapy. *Transfusion* 1987; **27**: 94–98

59. Tahhan HR, Holbrook CT, Braddy LR *et al*. Antigen-matched donor blood in the transfusion management of patients with sickle cell disease. *Transfusion* 1994; **34**: 562

60. Michail-Merianou V, Pamphili-Panousopoulou L, Piperi-Lowes L *et al*. Alloimmunization to red cell antigens in thalassemia: comparative study of usual versus better match transfusion programs. *Vox Sang* 1987; **52**: 95–98

61. Jayabose S, Tugal O, Ruddy R *et al*. Transfusion therapy for severe anemia. *Am J Pediatr Hematol Oncol* 1993; **15**: 324–327

62. Berman B. Krieger A, Naiman JL. A new method for calculating volumes of blood required for partial exchange transfusion. *J Pediatr* 1979; **94**: 86–89

63. Fosburg M, Dolan M, Propper R *et al*. Intensive plasma exchange in small and critically ill pediatric patients: Techniques and clinical outcome. *J Clin Apheresis* 1983; **1**: 215–224

64. Strauss RG. Neonatal anemia: pathophysiology and treatment. In: Wilson SM, Levitt JS, Strauss RG (eds) *Improving Transfusion Practice for Pediatric Patients*. Arlington, VA: American Association of Blood Banks, 1991, pp 1–17

65. Widness JA, Seward VJ, Kromer IJ *et al*. Changing patterns of red blood cell transfusion in very low birth weight infants. *J Pediatr* 1996; **129**: 680–687

66. Strauss RG. Red blood cell transfusion practices in the neonate. *Clin Perinatol* 1995; **22**: 641–655

67. Oski FA. Neonatal hematology: the erythrocyte and its disorders. In: Nathan DG, Oski FA (eds) *Hematology of Infancy and Childhood*, 4th edn. Philadelphia, PA: WB Sauders Co, 1993, pp 18–43

68. Keyes WG, Donohue PK, Spivak JL, Jones MD, Oski FA. Assessing the need for transfusion of premature infants and role of hematocrit, clinical signs, and erythropoietin level. *Pediatrics* 1989; **84**: 412–417

69. Hume H, Bard H. Small volume red blood cell transfusions for neonatal patients. *Transfusion Med Rev* 1995; **9**: 187–199

70. Alverson DC. The physiologic impact of anemia in the neonatate. *Clin Perinatol* 1995; **22**: 609–625

71. Hume H. Red blood cell transfusions for preterm infants: The role of evidence-based medicine. *Semin Perinatol* 1997; **21**: 8–19

72. Shannon KM, Keith JF, Mentzer WC *et al*. Recombinant human erythropoietin stimulates erythropoiesis and reduces erythrocyte transfusions in very low birth weight preterm infants. *Pediatrics* 1995; **95**: 1–8

73. Fetus and Newborn Committee of the Canadian Paediatric Society. Guidelines for transfusion of erythrocytes to neonates and premature infants. *Can Med Assoc J* 1992; **147**: 1781–1792

74. Voak D, Cann R, Finney D *et al*. Guidelines for administration of blood products: transfusion of infants and neonates. *Transfusion Med* 1994; **4**: 63–69

75. Stehling L, Luban NLC, Anderson KC *et al*. Guidelines for blood utilization review. *Transfusion* 1994; **34**: 438–448

76. Luban NLC. Massive transfusion in the neonate. *Transfusion Med Rev* 1995; **9**: 200–214

77. Luban NLC, Strauss RG, Hume HA. Commentary on the safety of red cells preserved in extended-storage media for neonatal transfusions. *Transfusion* 1991; **31**: 229–235

78. Goodstein MH, Locke RG, Wlodarczyk D *et al*. Comparisons of two preservation solutions for erythrocyte transfusions in newborn infants. *J Pediatr* 1993; **123**: 783–788

79. Lee DA, Slagle TA, Jackson TM, Evans CS. Reducing blood donor exposures in low birth weight infants by the use of older, unwashed packed red blood cells. *J Pediatr* 1995; **126**: 280–286

80. Liu E, Mannino E, Lane TA. A prospective randomized trial of the safety and efficacy of a limited donor exposure transfusion program for premature neonates. *J Pediatr* 1994; **125**: 92–96

81. Strauss RG, Burmeister LF, Johnson K *et al*. AS-1 red cells for neonatal transfusions: a randomized trial assessing donor exposure and safety. *Transfusion* 1996; **36**: 873–878

82. Chambers LA. Evaluation of a filter-syringe set for preparation of packed cell aliquots for neonatal transfusion. *Am J Clin Pathol* 1995; **104**: 253–257

83. Strauss RG, Villhauer PJ, Cordle DG. A method to collect, store and issue multiple aliquots of packed red blood cells for neonatal transfusions. *Vox Sang* 1995; **68**: 77–81

84. Hall TL, Barnes A, Miller JR *et al*. Neonatal mortality following transfusion of red cells with high plasma potassium levels. *Transfusion* 1993; **33**: 606–609

85. Manno CS, Hedberg KW, Kim HC *et al*. Comparison of the hemostatic effects of fresh whole blood, stored whole blood, and components after open heart surgery in children. *Blood* 1991; **77**: 930–936

86. Murphy RJC, Malhorta C, Sweet AY. Death following an exchange transfusion with hemoglobin SC blood. *J Pediatr* 1980; **96**: 110–112

87. British Committee for Standards in Haematology Blood Transfusion Task Force. Guidelines for autologous donation: Preoperative autologous donation. *Transfusion Med* 1993; **3**: 307–316

88. NHLBI. Transfusion alert: Use of autologous blood. *Transfusion* 1995; **35**: 703–711

89. Goodnough LT, Monk TG, Brecher ME. Autologous blood procurement in the surgical setting: Lessons learned in the last 10 years. *Vox Sang* 1996; **71**: 133–141

90. Etchason J, Petz L, Keeler E *et al*. The cost effectiveness of preoperative autologous blood donations. *N Engl J Med* 1995; **332**: 719–724

91. Thompson HW, Luban NL. Autologous blood transfusion in the pediatric patient. *J Pediat Surg* 1995; **30**: 1406–1411

92. Thomas MJ, Gillon J, Desmond MJ. Consensus conference on autologous transfusion. Preoperative autologous donation. *Transfusion* 1996; **36**: 633–639

93. Moran MM, Kroon D, Tredwell SJ, Wadsworth LD. The role of autologous blood transfusion in adolescents undergoing spinal surgery. *Spine* 1995; **20**: 532–536

94. Tasaki T, Ohto H, Noguchi M, Abe R, Kikuchi S, Hoshino S. Autologous blood donation in elective surgery in children. *Vox Sang* 1994; **66**: 188–193

95. Kemmotsu H, Joe K, Nakamura H, Yamashita M. Predeposited autologous blood transfusion for surgery in infants and children. *J Pediatr Surg* 1995; **30**: 659–661

96. Masuda M, Kawachi Y, Inaba S *et al*. Preoperative autologous blood

donations in pediatric cardiac surgery. *Ann Thorac Surg* 1995; **60**: 1694–1697

97. Mayer MN, deMontalembert M, Audat F *et al*. Autologous blood donation for elective surgery in children weighing 8–25 kg. *Vox Sang* 1996; **70**: 224–228

98. Longatti PL, Paccagnella F, Agostini S *et al*. Autologous hemodonation in the corrective surgery of craniostenosis. *Child Nervous System* 1991; **7**: 40–42

99. *Standards for Blood Banks and Transfusion Services*, 18th edn. Bethesda, MD: American Association of Blood Banks, 1997, p 43

100. Gillon J, Thomas MJG, Desmond MJ. Acute normovolaemic haemo-dilution. *Transfusion* 1996; **36**: 640–643

101. Desmond MJ, Thomas MJG, Gillon J, Fox MA. Perioperative red cell salvage. *Transfusion* 1996; **36**: 644–651

102. Haberkern M, Dangel P. Normovolemic hemodilution and intra-operative autotransfusion in children: experience with 30 cases of spinal fusion. *Eur J Pediatr Surg* 1991; **1**: 30–35

103. Simpson MB, Georgopoulos G, Eilert RE. Intraoperative blood salvage in children and young adults undergoing spinal surgery with predeposited autologous blood: efficacy and cost effectiveness. *J Pediat Ortho* 1993; **13**: 777–780

104. van Interson M, van der Waart FJ, Erdmann W, Trouwborst A. Systemic haemodynamics and oxygenation during haemodilution in children. *Lancet* 1995; **346**: 1127–1129

105. Siller TA, Dickson JH, Erwin WD. Efficacy and cost considerations of intraoperative autologous transfusion in spinal fusion for idiopathic scoliosis with predeposited blood. *Spine* 1996; **21**: 848–852

106. Usher R, Shephard M, Lind J. The blood volume of the newborn infant and placental transfusion. *Acta Paediatr Scand* 1963; **52**: 497–512

107. Yao AC, Lind J, Thasala R, Michelsson K. Placental transfusion in the premature infant with observation on clinical course and outcome. *Acta Paediatr Scand* 1969; **58**: 561–566

108. Kinmond S, Aitchison TC, Holland BM, Jones JG, Turner TL, Wardrop CAJ. Umbilical cord clamping and preterm infants: A randomised trial. *Br Med J* 1993; **306**: 172–175

109. Anderson S, Fangman J, Wager G, Uden D. Retrieval of placental blood from the umbilical vein to determine volume, sterility, and presence of clot formation. *Am J Dis Child* 1992; **146**: 36–39

110. Bifano EM, Dracker RA, Lorah K, Palit A. Collection and 28-day storage of human placental blood. *Pediatr Res* 1994; **36**: 90–94

111. Ballin A, Arbel E, Kenet G *et al*. Autologous umbilical cord blood transfusion. *Arch Dis Child Fetal Neonat* 1995; **73**: F181–183

112. Valderrabano F. Erythropoietin in chronic renal failure. *Kidney Int* 1996; **50**: 1373–1391

113. Cazzola M, Mercuriali F, Brugnara C. Use of recombinant human erythropoietin outside the setting of uremia. *Blood* 1997; **89**: 4248–4267

114. Gallagher PG, Ehrenkranz RA. Erythropoietin therapy for anemia of prematurity. *Clin Perinatol* 1993; **20**: 169–191

115. Doyle JJ. The role of erythropoietin in the anemia of prematurity. *Semin Perinatol* 1997; **21**: 20–7

116. Wilimas JA, Crist WM. Erythropoietin – not yet a standard treatment for anemia of prematurity. *Pediatrics* 1995; **95**: 9–10

117. Strauss RG. Erythropoietin in the pathogenesis and treatment of neonatal anemia. *Transfusion* 1995; **35**: 68–73

118. Spivak JL. Recombinant human erythropoietin and the anemia of cancer. *Blood* 1994; **84**: 997–1004

119. Locatelli F, Zecca M, Beguin Y *et al*. Accelerated erythroid repopula-tion with no stem-cell competition effect in children treated with recombinant human erythropoietin after allogeneic bone marrow transplantation. *Br J Haematol* 1993; **84**: 752–754

120. Ayash LJ, Elias A, Hunt M et al. Recombinant human erythropoietin for the treatment of the anaemia associated with autologous bone marrow transplantation. *Br J Haematol* 1994; **87**: 153–161

121. Henry DH, Abels RI. Recombinant human erythropoietin in the treatment of cancer and chemotherapy-induced anemia: results of double-blind and open-label follow-up studies. *Semin Oncol* 1994; **21**: 21–28

122. Cascinu S, Fedeli A, Del Ferro E *et al*. Recombinant human erythro-poietin treatment in cis-platin-associated anemia: A randomized, double-blind trial with placebo. *J Clin Oncol* 1994; **12**: 1058–1062

123. de Campos E, Radford J, Steward W *et al*. Clinical and in vitro effects of recombinant human erythropoietin in patients receiving intensive chemotherapy for small-cell lung cancer. *J Clin Oncol* 1995; **13**: 1623–1631

124. Wurnig C, Windhager R, Schwameis E et al. Prevention of che-motherapy-induced anemia by the use of erythropoietin in patients with primary malignant bone tumors (a double-blind, randomized, phase III study). *Transfusion* 1996; **36**: 155–159

125. Goldberg MA, Brugnara C, Dover GJ *et al*. Treatment of sickle cell anemia with hydroxyurea and erythropoietin. *N Engl J Med* 1990; **323**: 366–372

126. Rodgers GP, Dover GJ, Uyesaka N *et al*. Augmentation by erythro-poietin of the fetal-hemoglobin response to hydroxyurea in sickle cell disease. *N Engl J Med* 1993; **328**: 73–80

127. Galanello R, Barella S, Turco MP *et al*. Serum erythropoietin and erythropoiesis in high and low-fetal hemoglobin β-thalassemia inter-media patients. *Blood* 1994; **83**: 561–565

128. Olivieri NF, Freedman MH, Perrine SP *et al*. Trial of recombinant human erythropoietin: Three patients with thalassemia intermedia. *Blood* 1992; **80**: 3258–3260

129. Rendo P, Freigerio D, Braie J *et al*. Double-blind multicentric randomized study of recombinant human erythropoietin in HIV + children with anemia treated with antiretrovirals. *Blood* 1996; **88**: 348A

130. Goldfinger D. Directed blood donations: Pro. *Transfusion* 1989; **29**: 70–74

131. Page PL. Directed blood donations: Con. *Transfusion* 1989; **29**: 65–69

132. Grindon AJ. Infectious disease markers in directed donors in the Atlanta region. *Transfusion* 1991; **31**: 872–873

133. Starkey JM, MacPherson JL, Bolgiano DC *et al*. Markers for transfu-sion-transmitted disease in different groups of blood donors. *JAMA* 1989; **262**: 3452–3454

134. Pink J, Thomson A, Wylie B. Infectious disease markers in autologous and directed donations. *Transf Med* 1994; **4**: 135–138

135. Myhre BA, Figueroa PI. Infectious disease markers in various groups of donors. *Ann Clin Laborat Sc* 1995; **25**: 39–43

136. Elbert C, Strauss RG, Barrett F *et al*. Biological mothers may be dangerous blood donors for their neonates. *Acta Haematol* 1991; **85**: 189–191

137. Goldman M, Rémy-Prince S, Trépanier A, Décary F. Autologous donation error rates in Canada. *Transfusion* 1997; **37**: 523–527

138. Strauss RG, Wieland MR, Randels MJ, Koerner TAW. Feasibility and success of a single-donor red cell program for pediatric elective surgery patients. *Transfusion* 1992; **32**: 747

139. Strauss RG, Baarnes A, Blanchette VS *et al*. Directed and limited-exposure blood donations for infants and children. *Transfusion* 1989; **30**: 68–72

140. Loirat C, Sonsino E, Hinglais N *et al*. Treatment of the childhood hemolytic uraemic syndrome with plasma. *Pediatr Nephrol* 1988; **2**: 279–285

141. Rizzoni G, Claris-Appiani A, Edefonti A *et al*. Plasma infusion for hemolytic-uremic syndrome in children: Results of a multicenter controlled trial. *J Pediatr* 1988; **112**: 284–290

142. Consensus Conference. Fresh-frozen plasma: Indications and risks. *JAMA* 1985; **253**: 551–553

143. Contreras M, Ala FA, Greaves M *et al*. Guidelines for the Use of Fresh Frozen Plasma. British Committee for Standards in Haematology, Working Party of the Blood Transfusion Task Force. *Transfusion Med* 1992; **2**: 57–63

144. Development Task Force of the College of American Pathologists. Practice parameter for the use of fresh-frozen plasma, cryoprecipitate, and platelets: Fresh-frozen plasma, cryoprecipitate, and platelets administration practice guidelines. *JAMA* 1994; **271**: 777–781

145. American Society of Anesthesiologists Task Force on Blood Compo-

nent Therapy. Practice guidelines for blood component therapy. *Anesthesiology* 1996; **84**: 732–747

146. Andrew M, deVeber G. *Pediatric Thromboembolism and Stroke Protocols*. BC Decker Inc, Hamilton, 1997, pp 17–18

147. Zalusky R, Furie B. Hematologic complications of liver disease and alcoholism. In: Hoffman R, Benz EJ Jr, Shattil SJ, Furie B, Cohen HJ, Silberstein LE (eds) *Hematology: Basic Principles and Practice*, 2nd edn. New York: Churchill Livingstone, 1995, pp 2096–2103

148. McVay PA, Toy PT. Lack of increased bleeding after paracentesis and thoracentesis in patients with mild coagulation abnormalities. *Transfusion* 1991; **31**: 164–171

149. McVay PA, Toy PT. Lack of increased bleeding after liver biopsy in patients with mild hemostatic abnormalities. *Am J Clin Pathol* 1990; **94**: 747–753

150. Friedman EW, Sussman II. Safety of invasive procedures in patients with the coagulopathy of liver diseases. *Clin Lab Haematol* 1989; **11**:199–204

151. Ogborn MR, Crocker JF, Barnard DR. Plasma therapy for severe hemolytic-uremic syndrome in children in Atlantic Canada. *Can Med Assoc J* 1990; **143**: 1323–1326

152. Frishberg Y, Obrig TG, Kaplan B. Hemolytic uremic syndrome. In: Holliday MA, Barratt TM, Avner ED (eds) *Pediatric Nephrology*, 3rd edn. Baltimore: Williams and Wilkins,1994, pp 871–889

153. Fitzpatrick MM, Walters MDS, Trompeter RS *et al*. Atypical (non-diarrhea-associated) hemolytic-uremic syndrome in childhood. *J Pediatr* 1993; **122**: 532–537

154. Andrew M, Paes B, Milner R *et al*. The development of the human coagulation system in the fullterm infant. *Blood* 1987; **70**: 165–172

154a. Andrew M, Paes B, Milner R *et al*. Development of the coagulation system in the healthy premature infant. *Blood* 1988; **72**: 1651–1657

155. Beverley DW, Pitts-Tucker TJ, Congdon PJ et al. Prevention of intraventricular haemorrhage by fresh frozen plasma. *Arch Dis Child* 1985; **60**: 710–713

156. Tin W, Wariyar U, Hey E. Randomised trial of prophylactic early fresh-frozen plasma or gelatin or glucose in preterm babies: outcome at 2 years. *Lancet* 1996; **348**: 229–232

157. Koppe JG. Prevention of brain haemorrhage and ischaemic injury in premature babies. *Lancet* 1996; **348**: 208–209

158. Lane TA (ed). *Blood Transfusion Therapy: a Physician's Handbook*, 5th edn. Bethesda, MD, American Association of Blood Banks, 1996, p 26

159. Hersh EM, Bodey GP, Nies BA, Freireich EJ. Causes of death in acute leukemia: A ten-year study of 414 patients from 1954–1963. *JAMA* 1965; **193**: 99–103

160. Schiffer CA, Prophylactic platelet transfusion. *Transfusion* 1992; **32**: 295–298

161. Higby DJ, Cohen E, Holland JF, Sinks L. The prophylactic treatment of thrombocytopenic leukemic patients with platelets. A double blind study. *Transfusion* 1974; **14**: 440–446

162. Roy AJ, Jaffe N, Djerassi I. Prophylactic platelet transfusions in children with acute leukemia. A dose response study. *Transfusion* 1973; **13**: 283–290

163. Murphy S, Litwin S, Herring LM *et al*. Indications for platelet transfusion in children with acute leukemia. *Am J Hematol* 1982; **12**: 347–356

164. Solomon J, Bofenkamp T, Fahey JL *et al*. Platelet prophylaxis in acute nonlymphoblastic leukemia. *Lancet* 1978; **1**: 267

165. Ilett SJ, Lilleyman JS. Platelet transfusion requirements of children with newly diagnosed lymphoblastic leukemia. *Acta Hematol* 1979; **62**: 86–89

166. Feusner J. The use of platelet transfusions. *Am J Pediatr Hematol Oncol* 1984; **6**: 255–260

167. Schiffer CA. Some aspects of recent advances in the use of blood cell components. *Br J Haematol* 1978; **39**: 289–284

168. Hoak JC, Koepeke JA. Platelet transfusions. *Clin Haematol* 1976; **5**: 69

169. Kelton JG, Blajchman MA. Platelet transfusions. *Can Med Assoc J* 1979; **121**: 1353–1358

170. Tomasulo PA, Lenes BA. Platelet transfusion therapy. In: Menitove JE, McCarthy LJ (eds) *Hemostatic Disorders and the Blood Bank*. Arlington, VA: American Association of Blood Banks, 1984, pp 63–89

171. Baer MR, Bloomfield CD. Controversies in transfusion medicine. Prophylactic platelet transfusion therapy: pro. *Transfusion* 1992; **32**: 377–380

172. Patten E. Controversies in transfusion medicine. Prophylactic platelet transfusion revisited after 25 years: con. *Transfusion* 1992; **32**: 381–385

173. Pisciotto PT, Benson K, Hume H *et al*. Prophylactic versus therapeutic platelet transfusion practices in hematology and/or oncology patients. *Transfusion* 1995; **35**: 498–502

174. Gaydos LA, Freireich EJ, Mantel N. The quantitative relation between platelet count and hemorrhage in patients with acute leukemia. *N Engl J Med* 1962; **266**: 905–909

175. National Institutes of Health, Consensus Development Conference. Platelet transfusion therapy. *JAMA* 1987; **257**: 1777–1780

176. Slichter SJ. Platelet transfusions a constantly evolving therapy. *Thromb Haemostas* 1991; **66**: 178–188

177. Beutler E. Platelet transfusions: The 20,000/μL trigger. *Blood* 1993; **81**: 1411–1413.

178. Aderka D, Praff G, Santo M, Weinberger A, Pinkhas J. Bleeding due to thrombocytopenia in acute leukemias and reevaluation of the prophylactic platelet transfusion policy. *Am J Med Sci* 1986; **291**: 147–151

179. Gil-Fernandez JJ, Alegre A, Fernandez-Villalta MJ *et al*. Clinical results of a stringent policy on prophylactic platelet transfusion: non-randomized comparative analysis in 190 bone marrow transplant patients from a single institution. *Bone Marrow Transplant* 1996; **18**: 931–935

180. Gmür J, Burger J, Schanz U et al. Safety of stringent prophylactic platelet transfusion policy for patients with acute leukaemia. *Lancet* 1991; **338**: 1223–1226

181. Creutzig U, Ritter J, Budde M *et al*. Early deaths due to hemorrhage and leukostasis in childhood acute myelogenous leukemia. *Cancer* 1987; **60**: 3071–3079

182. Rodeghiero F, Avvisati G, Castaman G et al. Early deaths and anti-hemorrhagic treatment in acute promyelocytic leukemia. A GIMEMA retrospective study in 268 consecutive patients. *Blood* 1990; **75**: 2112–2117

183. Belt RJ, Leite C, Haas CD, Stephens RL. Incidence of hemorrhagic complications in patients with cancer. *JAMA* 1978; **239**: 2571–2574

184. Dutcher JP, Schiffer CA, Aisner J *et al*. Incidence of thrombocytopenia and serious hemorrhage among patients with solid tumors. *Cancer* 1984; **53**: 557–562

185. Bishop JF, Schiffer CA, Aisner J *et al*. Surgery in leukemia: a review of 167 operations on thrombocytopenic patients. *Am J Hematol* 1987; **26**: 147–155

186. Hume H. Transfusion support of children with hematologic and oncologic disorders. In: Petz LD, Swisher SN, Kleinmans, Spence RK, Strauss RG (eds) *Clinical Practice of Transfusion Medicine*, 3rd edn. New York: Churchill Livingstone, 1996, pp 705–732

187. George JN, Woolf SH, Raskob GE *et al*. Idiopathic thrombocytopenic purpura: A practice guideline developed by explicit methods for the American Society of Hematology. *Blood* 1996; **88**: 3–40

188. Flordal PA, Sahlin S. Use of desmopressin to prevent bleeding complications in patients treated with aspirin. *Br J Surg* 1993; **80**: 723–724

189. Sheridan DP, Card RT, Pinilla JC *et al*. Use of desmopressin acetate to reduce blood transfusion requirements during cardiac surgery in patients with acetylsalicylic-acid-induced platelet dysfunction. *Can J Surg* 1994; **37**: 33–36

190. Harker LA, Malpass TW, Branson HE *et al*. Mechanism of abnormal bleeding in patients undergoing cardiopulmonary bypass: acquired transient platelet dysfunction associated with selective α-granule release. *Blood* 1980; **56**: 827–834

191. Buerling-Harbury C, Galvan CA. Acquired decrease in platelet secretory ADP associated with increased postoperative bleeding in post cardiopulmonary bypass patients and in patients with severe valvular heart disease. *Blood* 1978; **52**: 13–23

192. Simon TL, Akl BF, Murphy W. Controlled trial of routine administration of platelet concentrates in cardiopulmonary bypass surgery. *Ann Thorac Surg* 1984; **37**: 359–364

193. Strauss RG, Levy GJ, Sotelo-Avila C. National survey of neonatal transfusion practices: II. Blood component therapy. *Pediatrics* 1993; **91**: 530–536

194. Andrew M, Vegh P, Caco C *et al*. A randomized, controlled trial of platelet transfusion in thrombocytopenic premature infants. *J Pediatr* 1993; **123**: 285–291

195. Blanchette VS, Kühne T, Hume H, Hellmann J. Platelet transfusion therapy in newborn infants. *Transfusion Med Rev* 1995; **9**: 215–230

196. Dunstan RA. The origin of ABH antigens on human platelets. *Blood* 1985; **65**: 615–619

197. Kelton JG, Hamid C, Aker S, Blajchman MA. The amount of blood group A substance on platelets is proportional to the amount in the plasma. *Blood* 1982; **59**: 980–985

198. Brand A, Sintnicolaas K, Claas FHJ, Eernisse JG. ABH antibodies causing platelet transfusion refractoriness. *Transfusion* 1986; **26**: 463–466

199. Lee EJ, Schiffer CA. ABO incompatibility can influence the results of platelet transfusion. Results of a randomized trial. *Transfusion* 1989; **29**: 384–389

200. Carr R, Hutton JL, Jenkins JA, Lucas GF, Amphlett MW. Transfusion of ABO mismatched platelets leads to early platelet refractoriness. *Br J Haematol* 1990; **75**: 408–413

201. Pierce RN, Reich LM, Mayer K. Hemolysis following platelet transfusions from ABO-incompatible donors. *Transfusion* 1985; **25**: 60–62

202. Ferguson DJ. Acute intravascular hemolysis after a platelet transfusion. *Can Med Assoc J* 1988; **138**: 523–524

203. Reis MD, Coovadia AS. Transfusion of ABO-incompatible platelets causing severe hemolytic reaction. *Clin Lab Haematol* 1989; **11**: 237–240

204. Dunstan RA, Simpson MB, Rosse WF. Erythrocyte antigens on human platelets. Absence of the Rhesus, Duffy, Kell, Kidd and Lutheran antigens. *Transfusion* 1984; **24**: 243–246

205. Goldfinger D, McGinnis MH. Rh incompatible platelet transfusion – risks and consequences of sensitizing immunosuppressed patients. *N Engl J Med* 1971; **284**: 942–944

206. McLeod BC, Piehl MR, Sassetti RJ. Alloimmunization to RhD by platelet transfusions in autologous bone marrow transplant recipients. *Vox Sang* 1990; **59**: 185–189

207. Baldwin ML, Ness PM, Scott D *et al*. Alloimmunization to D antigen and HLA in D-negative immunosuppressed oncology patients. *Transfusion* 1988; **28**: 330–333.

208. Heim BU, Bock M, Kold HJ *et al*. Intravenous anti-D gammaglobulin for the prevention of rhesus isoimmunization caused by platelet transfusions in patients with malignant disease. *Vox Sang* 1992; **62**: 165–168

209. Zeiler T, Wittmann G, Zingsem J *et al*. A dose of 100 IU intravenous anti-D gammaglobulin is effective for the prevention of RhD immunisation after RhD-incompatible single donor platelet transfusion. *Vox Sang* 1994; **66**: 243

210. National Blood Transfusion Service Immunoglobulin Working Party: Recommendations for the use of anti-D immunoglobulin. *Prescribers J* 1991; **31**: 137

211. Bishop JK, McGrath K, Wolf MM et al. Clinical factors influencing the efficacy of pooled platelet transfusions. *Blood* 1988; **71**: 383–387

212. Doughty HA, Murphy MF, Telcalfe P *et al*. Relative importance of immune and non-immune causes of platelet refractoriness. *Vox Sang* 1994; **66**: 200–203

213. Alcorta I, Pereira A, Ordinas A. Clinical and laboratory factors associated with platelet transfusion refractoriness: A case-control study. *Br J Haematol* 1996; **93**: 220–224

214. Bock M, Muggenthaler KH, Schmidt U, Heim MU. Influence of antibiotics on posttransfusion platelet increment. *Transfusion* 1996; **36**: 952–954

215. Slichter SJ. Mechanisms and management of platelet refractoriness. In: Nance ST (ed) *Transfusion Medicine in the 1990's*. Arlington, VA: American Association of Blood Bank, 1990: 95–179

216. Engelfriet CP, Reesink HW, Aster RH *et al*. Management of alloimmunized, refractory patients in need of platelet transfusions. *Vox Sang* 1997; **73**: 191–198

217. Shpilberg O, Glumenthal R, Sofer O *et al*. A controlled trial of tranexamic acid therapy for the reduction of bleeding during treatment of acute myeloid leukemia. *Leukemia Lymphoma* 1995; **19**: 141–144

218. Lee EJ, Schiffer CA. Serial measurement of lymphocytotoxic antibody and response to nonmatched platelet transfusions in alloimmunized patients. *Blood* 1987; **70**: 1727–1729

219. Murphy MF, Metcalfe P, Ord J *et al*. Disappearance of HLA and platelet-specific antibodies in acute leukaemia patients alloimmunized by multiple transfusions. *Br J Haematol* 1987; **67**: 255–260

220. Kickler T, Braine HG, Piantadosi S *et al*. A randomized, placebo-controllet trial of intravenous gammaglobulin in alloimmunized thrombocytopenic patients. *Blood* 1990; **75**: 313–316

221. Bensinger WI, Price TH, Dale DC *et al*. The effects of daily recombinant human granulocyte colony-stimulating factor administration on normal granulocyte donors undergoing leukapheresis. *Blood* 1993; **81**: 1883–1888

222. Caspar C, Reinhard A, Burger J *et al*. Effective stimulation of donors for granulocyte transfusions with recombinant methionyl granulocyte-colony stimulating factor. *Blood* 1993; **81**: 2866–2871

223. Saarinen UM, Hovi L, Vilinikka L *et al*. Reemphasis on leukocyte transfuisons: induction of myeloid marrow recovery in critically ill neutropenic children with cancer. *Vox Sang* 1995; **68**: 90–99

224. *Technical Manual*, 12th edn. Bethesda, MD: American Association of Blood Banks, 1996, p 121

225. Strauss RG. Granulocyte transfusion therapy. In: Mintz PD (ed) Transfusion Medicine I. *Hematol Oncol Clin North Am* 1994; **8**: 1159–1166

226. Wright DG, Robichaud KJ, Pizzo PA *et al*. Lethal pulmonary reactions associated with the combined use of amphotericin B and leukocyte transfusions. *N Engl J Med* 1981; **304**: 1185–1189

227. Chanock SJ, Gorlin JB. Granulocyte transfusions. Time for a second look. *Infect Dis Clin North Am* 1996; **10**: 327–343

228. Bhatia S, McCullough J, Perry EH *et al*. Granulocyte transfusions: efficacy in treating fungal infections in neutropenic patients following bone marrow transplantation. *Transfusion* 1994; **34**: 226–232

229. Nathan DG, Oski SH (eds). *Hematology of Infancy and Children*, 5th edn. Philadelphia: WB Saunders, 1997, Appendix 28, p XV

230. Sweetman RW, Cairo MS. Blood component and immunotherapy in neonatal sepsis. *Transfusion Med Rev* 1995; **9**: 251–259

231. Rosenthal J, Healey T, Ellis R *et al*. A two-year follow-up of neonates with presumed sepsis treated with recombinant human granulocyte colony-stimulating factor during the first week of life. *J Pediatr* 1996; **128**: 135–137

232. Stroncek DF, Leonard K, Eiber G *et al*. Alloimmunization after granulocyte transfusions. *Transfusion* 1996; **36**: 1009–1015

233. Hillyer CD, Berkman EM. Transfusion of plasma derivatives: fresh frozen plasma, cryoprecipitate, albumin and immunoglobulin. In: Hoffman R, Benz EJ, Shattil SJ, Furie B, Cohen HJ, Silberstein LE (eds) *Hematology: Basic Principles and Practice*, 2nd edn. New York: Churchill Livingstone, 1995, pp 2011–2019

234. NIH consensus development conference. Intravenous immunoglobulin: Prevention and treatment of disease. *JAMA* 1990; **264**: 3189–3193

235. Stiehn R. Appropriate therapeutic use of immunoglobulin. *Transfusion Med Rev* 1996; **10**: 203–221

236. Meissner HC, Welliver RC, Chartrand SA *et al*. Prevention of respiratory syncytial virus infection in high risk infants: consensus opinion on the role of immunoprophylaxis with respiratory syncytial virus hyperimmune globulin. *Pediatr Infect Dis J* 1996; **15**: 1059–1068

237. Harlsey NA, Abramson JS, Chesney PJ et al. Respiratory syncytial virus immune globulin intravenous: Indications for use. Committee on Infections Diseases 1996 to 1997. *Pediatrics* 1997; **99**: 645–650

Hazards of transfusion

NAOMI LC LUBAN, PATRICIA PISCIOTTA AND CATHERINE MANNO

The hazards of blood and blood product administration are many. They are best considered as those that occur acutely and those with delayed onset. The complications of transfusion therapy may produce significant morbidity and mortality and adverse consequences in the already complicated course of an ill child. This chapter reviews complications of transfusion with particular emphasis on recognition and prevention. Complications of hemophilia and other clotting disorders and the unique serologic complications of bone marrow and hematopoietic stem cell infusion are covered elsewhere in this book.

ACUTE TRANSFUSION REACTIONS

ACUTE HEMOLYTIC TRANSFUSION REACTIONS

Acute hemolytic transfusion reactions (AHTRs) occur most often when ABO-incompatible red blood cells (RBCs) are transfused to a recipient who has preformed antibodies against the major blood group antigens A or B. Due to the absence of preformed anti-A and -B, infants under 4 months of age are not at risk for AHTRs. Hemolytic transfusion reactions can also occur following the passive transfusion of isohemagglutinins found in ABO-incompatible plasma-containing platelet concentrates. The severity of AHTRs is proportional to the rate and volume of transfused incompatible blood. When anti-A and -B binds to the C5–9 component of complement, intravascular RBC lysis occurs. The resultant interleukin (IL) inflammatory response is characterized by the generation of tumor necrosis factor (TNF)-α, IL-8, monocyte chemoattractant protein (MCP)-1, and the anaphylatoxins C3a and C5a, as well as the activation of Hageman factor.[1]

Signs and symptoms of AHTRs include fever, chills, back and chest pain, nausea and shortness of breath. The patient may develop hypotension, vasoconstriction, ischemia and disseminated intravascular coagulation (DIC). Hypotension, microthrombi formation and hemoglobinuria may compromise renal blood flow precipitating acute renal failure.[2]

When an AHTR is suspected, the transfusion must be stopped immediately. A post-transfusion direct antiglobin test (DAT) will demonstrate the presence of antibody on the RBC surface. Life-threatening complications are due to renal injury, DIC and pulmonary involvement. Vital signs should be carefully monitored. Aggressive intravenous hydration is required to maintain intravascular volume and urine output. AHTRs are medical emergencies which are often associated with mortality. Most ABO hemolytic transfusion reactions are a result of misidentifying the intended recipient of a unit of blood and are therefore avoidable.

TRANSFUSION-RELATED ACUTE LUNG INJURY

Transfusion-related acute lung injury (TRALI), a clinical syndrome similar to adult respiratory distress syndrome (ARDS), is characterized by acute respiratory distress occurring 1–6 hours after transfusion of a plasma-containing blood component. TRALI is a serious adverse reaction to transfusion that may be under-recognized in pediatric patients.[3] There is usually fever, hypotension, bilateral pulmonary edema and severe hypoxemia with a normal central venous pressure. Patients with TRALI improve 2–3 days after the onset of symptoms provided aggressive respiratory support has been provided. TRALI has formerly been attributed to white blood cell (WBC) antibodies present in the transfused component which agglutinate with the recipient's WBCs, resulting in pulmonary leukostasis.[4] Recent work has demonstrated that 2 events are required to precipitate TRALI:

- the first may be the patient's underlying condition; groups at risk include patients who have had recent surgery, those with active infection with high concentrations of circulating cytokines, particularly TNF-α, or those who have had massive transfusion;

- the second is the transfusion of biologically active lipids which are present in stored blood components which contribute to WBC activation, endothelial damage and capillary leakage.[4]

ALLERGIC REACTIONS

Allergy to soluble plasma proteins may cause local reactions such as itching and urticaria or systemic symptoms such as bronchospasm or anaphylaxis. The severity of allergic reactions is not dose related; the patient who experiences urticaria during a transfusion will not develop anaphylaxis with continuation of the transfusion. Once established, most patients with allergic reactions respond to oral or parenteral antihistamines. For patients with an history of allergic reactions, pre-treatment with an antihistamine may help prevent recurrence. Washing RBC or platelet concentrates will remove much of the plasma responsible for allergic reactions. Leukoreduction of cellular components will not decrease the incidence of allergic transfusion reactions.

FEBRILE REACTIONS

Fever may be the first sign that a patient is receiving a component which is ABO incompatible or contaminated with bacteria, and such serious consequences must be considered when a patient develops fever during transfusion. A less serious but very common adverse effect seen during transfusion of RBCs, platelets and plasma is the febrile non-hemolytic transfusion reaction (FNHTR).[4-6] The risk for FNHTR is highest following the transfusion of platelets, occurring in 5–30% of transfusions.[7,8] Although the traditional view holds that FNHTRs are due to the interplay of WBCs contained in the components with preformed anti-leukocyte antibodies in the recipient, recent work has demonstrated that bioreactive substances, IL-1β, IL-6, IL-8 and TNF, in the plasma supernatant cause most febrile reactions associated with platelet products. The intensity of the reactions correlates directly with the concentration of IL-1β and IL-6.[8] These reactions may make patients uncomfortable but are rarely associated with more serious problems. The incidence of FNHTRs can be reduced by removing leukocytes at the time of component collection (pre-storage leukoreduction)[5,6,9] or by removing the plasma supernatant of platelets.[8]

MASSIVE TRANSFUSION

Massive transfusion, the replacement of a child's blood volume over a 6-hour period, may be needed for the replacement of massive blood losses due to trauma or coagulation defects.[10] The rapid infusion of large volumes of banked blood is also integral to several life-sustaining pediatric therapies such as extracorporeal membrane oxygenation (ECMO) and exchange transfusion. Certain hazards of massive transfusion are due to the rapid rate of infusion of RBCs which have been stored in a refrigerator in anticoagulant/preservative solution for varying periods of time. Many of these hazards can be anticipated and avoided.

The adverse reactions associated with the rapid infusion of large volumes of cold, stored RBCs are due to the following:

- increased levels of extracellular potassium which develop over the storage period of the RBC unit;
- poor function of the platelets contained in stored RBC components;
- progressively low levels of the intraerythrocytic RBC enzyme, 2,3-diphosphoglycerate (DPG);
- presence of citrate in the anticoagulant/preservative solution;
- metabolic consequences of the rapid infusion of a cold liquid.

STORAGE LESIONS

The storage of RBCs or whole blood in the liquid state results in biochemical derangements which increase with storage time.

- *Hyperkalemia*: Intracellular potassium leaks from the erythrocyte into the extracellular space. After 35 days of storage in citrate-phosphate-dextrose-adenine (CPDA-1),[11] plasma K^+ concentrations reach 27.3 mmol/l on average. Storage in additive solution (AS)-1 results in significantly less potassium leak. The risk of hyperkalaemia is relatively insignificant in the routine administration of small volumes of RBC and whole blood. However, fatal cardiac arrhythmia associated with hyperkalemia during neonatal exchange transfusion[12] and following the rapid intracardiac infusion of old RBCs have been reported.[13] Effective strategies for avoiding hyperkalemia-related arrhythmias during massive transfusion include using RBCs which are <5 days old or washed RBCs.[14] When whole blood is required and hyperkalemia is a concern, units should be <5 days old or reconstituted whole blood can be made by adding fresh frozen plasma (FFP) to washed stored RBCs.
- *Poor platelet function with increased storage time*: The cold storage conditions which are ideal for RBCs are associated with poor *in vivo* platelet survival.[15] The transfusion of large amounts of stored blood causes dilutional thrombocytopenia and does not provide viable platelets to participate in homeostasis. Platelet concentrates rather than whole blood are the preferred source for transfusion to thrombocytopenic, massively transfused patients who are hemorrhaging.
- *Low 2,3-diphosphoglycerate (2,3-DPG) levels*: The levels of intraerythrocytic 2,3-DPG affect the ability of RBCs to release oxygen at a given pH. After 2 weeks of storage, 2,3-DPG levels fall by >50% and reduced levels result in

decreased ability to unload oxygen at the level of the tissues.[16] Although 2,3-DPG levels are gradually restored once red cells are transfused, the repletion of 2,3-DPG is such that even after 8 hours, only one-third of the lost enzyme is regenerated.

ANTICOAGULANT/PRESERVATIVE SOLUTION

The anticoagulant/preservative solution used for whole blood collection contains citrate to bind ionized calcium and prevent coagulation of the donation. Unbound citrate is metabolized to bicarbonate. Massive transfusion of citrated blood components may cause the patient to become hypocalcemic, alkalotic or hypokalemic and these are observed more often in conjunction with plasma transfusion or exchange than with RBC transfusion. Patients with hypocalcemia complain of perioral paresthesia, twitching of the extremities and later, tetany. Children with hepatic or renal insufficiency who become hypocalcemic may develop hypotension or myocardial irritability. Some physicians routinely supplement calcium using 10% calcium gluconate (2 ml/kg), particularly in the context of massive plasma transfusion or plasma exchange. At one author's institution (NLCL), calcium is routinely administered for younger children undergoing plasma exchange or peripheral stem cell collections and those with poor hepatic function because children can rarely warn staff of the signs of citrate toxicity. The dose used is 94 mg of calcium/100 ml of blood processed to a maximum of 2 g administered intravenously at a flow rate no >120 mg/kg/h. When replacing calcium, serum ionized calcium levels should be monitored to avoid over-replacement.

COLD STORAGE CONDITIONS

RBCs are stored in a refrigerator at 4–6°C. The rapid transfusion of components which have been stored in the cold can result in hypothermia and subsequent cardiac arrhythmia/asystole. In adults, hypothermia-induced cardiac arrest is reported in half of those who receive 3 liters or more of refrigerated blood at rates of 50–100 ml/min.[17] In infants, the transfusion of cold blood has been associated with apnea, hypotension and hypoglycemia. Blood warmers, devices which use either wet or dry heat, can raise the temperature of cold-stored RBCs to body temperature. The usefulness of such warmers is limited when large volumes of RBCs are required immediately. Microwave ovens should never be used to warm blood rapidly for transfusion since heating may be inconsistent and may cause *ex vivo* hemolysis.[18]

COAGULOPATHY

Patients who require massive transfusion for treatment of severe hemorrhage are at risk for developing clinical and laboratory evidence of a coagulopathy. Coagulation abnormalities are due to dilution of circulating coagulation factors and platelets, local consumption of coagulation factors and DIC. The development of coagulopathy is strongly associated with the length of time during which a patient has been hypotensive.[19] In the laboratory, the coagulopathy is characterized by thrombocytopenia, hypofibrinogenemia and prolongation of the prothrombin time and partial thromboplastin time. The patient demonstrates microvascular bleeding characterized by oozing from mucosal surfaces, sites of injury and venipuncture sites.[20] Patients with severe tissue injury and profound hypotension are more likely to develop diffuse microvascular bleeding. The development of coagulopathy is strongly associated with mortality.[21] Careful assessment of the patient's clinical course in conjunction with coagulation testing allows the clinician appropriately to support patients with consumptive coagulopathy associated with massive transfusion with platelets, FFP and cryoprecipitate.

BACTERIAL CONTAMINATION

Bacterial contamination of blood and blood products accounted for 4% of transfusion-associated fatalities reported to the US Food and Drug Administration in 1976–1978, and this increased to 10% between 1986 and 1988.[22,23] Severe reactions have been reported most frequently with platelets stored at room temperature but also with refrigerated cellular components, plasma, cryoprecipitate and albumin, in both allogenic and autologous transfusion.[24] Fever, chills, hypotension, oliguria and DIC have been reported. Symptoms suggestive of either hemolytic transfusion reaction or platelet-associated bacteremia include dyspnea and cough. In a review of 5 clinical studies, platelet-associated bacteremia was less severe with a mortality of 26% as compared to RBC-contaminated reactions where a mortality of 71% has been reported.[25] Some septic reactions go unrecognized or unevaluated as patients may be receiving antibiotics for proven or suspected neutropenic sepsis that are cidal to the implicated organisms. Implicated are Gram-positive organisms including coagulase-negative staphylococci, bacillus species, staphylococcus and streptococcus species for platelets. Cold-loving organisms such as *Yersinia enterocolitica*, cryophilic pseudomonads such as *putida* and *fluorescens*, and *enterobacter*, are most commonly identified in RBC contamination.[26] Recently, transfusion-associated babesiosis occurred in 3 of 4 infants in a New York hospital;[26] babesia has the same tick vector as *Borrelia burgdorferi*, the Lyme disease spirochete, which is known to survive in platelets stored at 20°C, RBCs stored at 4°C and FFP stored at −18°C, but has not yet been implicated in a transfusion outbreak.

Estimates of bacterial contamination of blood and blood products vary widely throughout the world. Mean annual incidence figures for the Canadian Red Cross in 1987–1991 were 0.43% for RBC concentrates and 0.35% for platelet concentrates.[24] Higher rates have been reported for platelet concentrates; in Germany, for example, 2.5% of random donor platelet concentrates were found to be contaminated.[28] There are multiple potential sources of blood component contamination, including unrecognized donor bacteremia and inadequate skin decontamination, which in the case of pheresis donors may be from a scarred phlebotomy site. Contamination can also occur secondary to manufacturing issues to do with the bag or apheresis solution used during collection. Pooling of products or contaminated water baths are other sources. The age of the product is also an important variable. Platelets older than 3 days and RBCs older than 21 days are more likely to be contaminated.

Preventive measures to decrease the risks of transfusion-associated bacterial sepsis include extensive donor screening, improved skin decontamination and water bath decontamination. Donor questioning for diarrhea and travel to endemic Lyme Disease areas have been particularly helpful for yersinia and borrelia, respectively. Feasibility studies for pre-transfusion detection using endotoxin, RNA probes or polymerase chain reaction (PCR)-based methods have begun. Chemical or photochemical decontamination using psoralens may hold promise.[29] In 1997, the BACON study was launched. This is a combined effort by the American Association of Blood Banks, American Red Cross and Centers for Disease Control and Armed Forces Blood Program. It will identify and trace patients with confirmed transfusion reactions resulting from bacterial-contaminated blood and blood products.[30]

ADVERSE REACTIONS WITH DELAYED OCCURRENCE

TRANSFUSION-ASSOCIATED ALLOIMMUNIZATION

A delayed complication of transfusion is the development of alloantibodies directed against foreign antigens present on the cellular elements contained in blood components. There are several factors that play a role in the recipient's risk of becoming alloimmunized to erythrocyte, leukocyte or platelet antigens. Immunogenicity and dose of the foreign antigen, and frequency of exposure, as well as the recipient's immune response to an antigenic challenge, are clearly determining factors. The short- and long-term clinical sequelae of alloimmunization will obviously depend on the antigen involved.

ERYTHROCYTE ALLOIMMUNIZATION

RBC alloimmunization may occur when there is a genetic disparity in erythrocyte antigens between donor and recipient. The immunogenicity, or ability of most blood group antigens to stimulate an immune response, is poor. The blood group antigens A and B are by far the most immunogenic. ABO antibodies, however, have been referred to as 'naturally occurring' since they develop without an allogeneic red cell stimulus. ABO antibody production is stimulated by elements that are ubiquitous in nature, such as bacteria which possess substances similar to human A and B antigens.[31] These antibodies (isohemagglutinins) can generally be detected in sera of infants by 3–6 months of age.[32] The Rh system D antigen is the RBC antigen which is considered to be the most immunogenic in terms of antibody production as a result of exposure to foreign RBCs. Approximately 80% of D-negative recipients who receive a single 200 ml transfusion of D-positive red cells develop detectable anti-D antibodies within 2–5 months.[32,33] There has been some evidence that the minimum dose of D-positive red cells necessary for primary immunization is only 0.03 ml.[34] Therefore, it is easy to understand how the small numbers of RBCs present in a D-positive platelet concentrate could be sufficient to immunize a D-negative recipient. The relative immunogenicity or potency of other red cell antigens depends, in part, on the frequency with which the particular alloantibodies are encountered. More than half of the alloantibodies which result from transfusion and pregnancy are Rh antibodies (other than anti-D), with anti-Kell (anti-K) and anti-Duffy (anti-Fy^a) accounting for an additional 40%.[35] Studies have indicated that the relative likelihood of blood-group antibody formation is as follows: D > K > E > Fya > Jka.[32,36]

The rates of immunization vary, with reported frequencies in hospital-based transfused populations ranging from 0.8 to 1.0%.[37] Giblett[38] estimated that, with the exclusion of the D antigen, alloimmunization to RBC antigens is approximately 1% per unit transfused. However, there is evidence that the immune response to blood group antigens is different depending on the patient population and the disease category. Some individuals become immunized after a few transfusions, whereas others rarely become immunized despite repeated transfusions. This variability is not clearly defined and may be due, in part, to the number of transfusions given, the heterogeneity of the donor/recipient population (in terms of expression of RBC antigens), and whether the presence of certain immune response genes, as yet to be determined, influence the response.

Neonates

Despite the frequent need for RBC transfusions, several studies provide evidence that RBC alloimmunization occurs only rarely in neonates transfused during the first 4 months of life. In one study, no unexpected RBC antibodies were detected in 53 premature infants who received a total of 683 RBC transfusions, with at least half being tested 5 months after birth.[39] Ludvigsen et al[40] could detect no antibodies at least 3 weeks after the last transfusion in 90 full-term infants who received a total of 1269 transfusions with an average of 8.9 donor exposures/neonate. Other reports have supported the relative infrequency of alloantibody production directed against RBC antigens in neonates.[41,42] However, accurate transfusion histories could not be determined for all infants in these studies. There have been 3 reports of antibody formation in multiply transfused infants. Two cases involved development of allo-anti-E in infants at age 18 days[43] and 11 weeks,[44] respectively, and the third was an infant who developed anti-K at 12 weeks.[45] The failure of newborns to initiate an immune response to foreign RBC antigens is probably multifactorial, including the immature immune status of the infant and inability of neonatal antigen-presenting cells effectively to prime self T-helper cells. Another contributing factor which may limit lymphocyte activation is the possibility that insufficient numbers of allogeneic lymphocytes are present in components prepared for neonates.[46,47]

Sickle cell anemia

There have been several studies reporting extreme variability in the rates of alloimmunization for patients with sickle cell anemia. Part of the discrepancy can be attributed to whether only clinically significant antibodies were included in the analysis or all antibodies encountered, whether antibody formation as a result of pregnancy versus transfusion was clearly delineated, and finally the population base studied, children versus adults, or both. Reported rates of alloimmunization range from 5.7 to 36%.[48,49] The lower rate was reported in a group of 245 patients who had a median age of 10 years. In the largest prospective study of alloimmunization in patients with sickle cell disease (SCD), 3047 patients were evaluated, of whom 1814 were transfused for an overall rate of RBC alloimmunization of 18.6%.[50] Alloimmunization rates were higher for patients with hemoglobin SS versus hemoglobin SC or sickle-β^+ thalassemia, reflecting fewer numbers of transfusions required for the latter group of patients. Patients transfused at the age of 10 years or under had a lower rate of alloimmunization that those who were first transfused over the age of 10 years (9.6% versus 20.7%, respectively). The majority of the clinically significant antibodies that developed were in the Rh and Kell systems, with 17% of the immunized patients producing 4 or more antibodies. Vichinsky et al[51] found a much higher rate of alloimmunization in chronically transfused black patients with SCD as compared to transfused non-black patients with chronic hemolytic disorders and strongly suggested that the increased risk was related to the transfusion of racially discordant red cells. Luban,[52] reporting a study of 142 children with SCD, found a higher rate of alloimmunization in children of non-American descent versus American-born Afro-Americans, despite similar antigen phenotypes. The former group also developed more antibodies/child (3.17 versus 1.25, respectively). It was postulated that an effect of HLA on specific immune response genes may account for some of these differences. Based on several of these studies, the transfusion practice to reduce the risk of alloimmunization has also been found to vary greatly and includes providing phenotypically matched

red cells for all patients, matching only for those antigens that commonly cause alloimmunization, providing additional antigen matching only for patients who have become immunized,[50–52] and providing antigen-matched blood only for patients who have a high likelihood of going on a chronic transfusion protocol. When antigen-typed red cell products are used prophylactically for sickle cell patients, they are selected to be negative for Rhesus (D, C, E, c, e) and Kell (K, k) depending on the antigen typing of the patient. Additional typing for Kidd (Jk^a, Jk^b), Duffy (Fy^a, Fy^b), the MNS system (M, N, S, s) and Lewis (Le^a, Le^b) may be performed.

The development of autoantibodies in patients with SCD has been reported to occur more often in patients receiving chronic transfusion and in whom alloantibodies have developed.[53] The commonest autoantibodies observed have been cold-reacting antibodies, which although classified as clinically harmless, have caused considerable difficulties in cross-matching. Experimental evidence has shown that auto-immunization may develop after blood transfusion whether or not alloimmunization has occurred.[54]

The clinical outcome of RBC alloimmunization depends on the number and nature of the antibodies produced. Difficulty in finding compatible blood, which may impede the delivery of medical care, and an increased risk of delayed hemolytic transfusion reaction (DHTR), are 2 consequences of alloimmunization. DHTRs in patients with SCD pose additional problems since they may often go unrecognized, i.e. the symptoms can mimic or induce a sickle cell crisis.[55] In a study of 73 patients with SCD, 30% became immunized; however, only 4% developed recognized DHTR.[56] This effect may be attributed in part to a low level of suspicion for DHTR or an inability clinically to separate the symptoms from SCD. A marked drop in hematocrit to levels lower than those prior to transfusion have been observed in some patients with SCD experiencing a DHTR.[57] This extreme decrease in hematocrit may be secondary to hemolysis of donor red cells in conjunction with suppression of erythropoiesis from transfusion. An alternative contribution to the extreme level of anemia may be the destruction of autologous red cells in concert with the transfused antigen-positive red cells, which is referred to as 'bystander hemolysis'.[58] However, the mechanism by which this may occur is not clear.

Thalassemia

The reported incidence of clinically significant antibody production in children transfused for thalassemia has also been variable, ranging from 5.2 to 21.1%.[59,60] A consistent finding in most of these studies, however, is the association between the age at which transfusion is started and the risk of alloimmunization to RBC antigens.[59–61] In one study, patients who received initial transfusions before the age of 3 years were found to have a considerably lower incidence of alloimmunization.[60]

LEUKOCYTE AND PLATELET ALLOIMMUNIZATION

Alloimmunization to leukocyte and platelet antigens may develop in multiply transfused recipients, or as a result of pregnancy or organ transplantation. Class I human leukocyte antigens (HLA-A, HLA-B) are major immunogens and are expressed on all nucleated cells as well as platelets. The Class II antigens have a more limited distribution being found on B lymphocytes, macrophages/monocytes, dendritic cells, activated T cells, endothelial cells and some others. Cells with Class II antigens are capable of presenting antigens to T lymphocytes. Antigen-presenting cells (APCs) express both Class I and II HLA antigens. These cells take up antigen via endocytosis and degrade the antigen. Peptides produced by this process subsequently link to HLA Class II antigens. The resulting complex is then transported to the cell surface for recognition by helper (CD4) lymphocytes and subsequent stimulation of humoral immunity to generate antibodies. In transfusion, donor APCs play a major role in this process. Cellular blood components prepared for transfusion, such as packed RBCs and platelets, contain from 10^8 to 10^9 donor WBC. Studies have indicated that WBC reduction of cellular components to levels generally $<5 \times 10^6$/transfusion can diminish alloimmunization to HLA Class I antigens (Table 36.1).[62,63] Ultraviolet irradiation has been shown to interfere with the function of APCs.[64] Studies evaluating the effectiveness of this technology in reducing alloimmunization to platelet transfusion are ongoing.[65,66]

Alloimmunization to transfused WBC antigens during infancy is rare. Studies have shown either no evidence of HLA antibodies associated with transfusion, whether or not attempts were made to leukocyte-reduce blood components, or transient detection of antibodies.[42,67,68] There is some evidence to suggest that alloantibodies directed against maternal blood cell antigens may develop as a result of intrauterine or perinatal exposure to these antigens.[42] Passive transfer of IgG antibodies against HLA-, platelet- and granulocyte-specific antibodies to the neonate as a result of maternal alloimmunization is known to occur.[69,70]

The rate of HLA alloimmunization in older children and adults has ranged from 18 to over 50%.[71,72] The risk appears to be related to the underlying disease, as well as the chemotherapeutic regimen. In a series of 100 children with malignant disorders (leukemia, lymphoma, Ewing's sarcoma) who were receiving intensive transfusion support, 27% were reported to develop cytotoxic HLA antibodies. Persistence of HLA antibodies, despite continued transfusions, was observed in only 13% of the patients.[73] In contrast to the patients with malignancy, 7 of 8 patients with aplastic anemia developed alloantibodies. The difference in the rate of immunization is most likely due to the immunosuppressive effects of chemotherapy. Unlike HLA antigens, platelet-specific antigens do not appear to be as potent immunogens; however, alloantibodies directed against various platelet antigen systems have been characterized in multitransfused patients.[74]

The clinical manifestation of alloimmunization to leukocyte and platelet antigens can be febrile transfusion reactions, refractoriness to platelet transfusions, post-transfusion purpura (PTP) and TRALI. The latter is usually the result of passive transfusion of HLA-epitope-specific or leukoagglutinins directed against the recipient's antigen which precipitate a chain of reactions that include cytokine release and complement activation. There has been, however, at least one report of a fatal pulmonary reaction in a multitransfused child in whom antibody production was directed against donor leukocytes.[75]

POST-TRANSFUSION PURPURA

Post-transfusion purpura (PTP) is a rare cause of immune thrombocytopenia first recognized by Shulman et al in 1961.[76] This condition is characterized by the development of profound, but self-limiting, thrombocytopenia approximately 5–10 days after a blood transfusion in a recipient who has been previously exposed to platelet antigens through pregnancy or former transfusions. Alloantibodies are produced that destroy not only the transfused platelets, but the patient's own platelets. In the approximately 100 reported

Table 36.1 Blood component filters.

Generation	Pore size (μm)	Filter mechanism	Comment
First	170–260	Screen	Referred to as 'clot' filter Used for all blood and blood components.
Second	20–40	Micropore screen filter	Referred to as 'micro-aggregate' filter Removes 75–90% of WBC Only used for RBCs
Third	N/A	Adhesion, absorption	Referred to as 'leukodepletion' filter Removes 99–99.9% of WBC Used for cellular components including platelets collected by apheresis, platelet pools and RBCs
*Fourth	N/A	Adhesion, absorption, other	Under development

*Multiple manufacturers have variable claims as to degree of WBC removal and subsets of WBC removed by their method.

cases, the most commonly produced platelet antibody has been directed against the specific-platelet antigen HPA-1a (PL^{A1}) located on glycoprotein IIIa (GpIIIa). While other platelet antigens can cause PTP, the relative frequency is extremely low.[77] Although the mechanism of autologous platelet destruction is unclear, several theories have been postulated:

- formation of a foreign antigen-antibody complex that binds to autologous platelets and mediates platelet destruction via a mechanism similar to that observed in drug purpura;[78]
- development of a second antibody with autoimmune specificity that reacts with HPA-1a-negative platelets;[78]
- transfused soluble platelet antigen in the donor plasma absorbs to the recipient's platelets, thereby rendering them reactive with the alloantibody.[79]

PTP is a disease of adults, usually in their late 40s or older, occurring more frequently in females as a result of a previous pregnancy. The youngest patient reported to develop PTP was a 16-year-old female with no previous history of pregnancy.[80] While approximately 3% of the white population is negative for HPA-1a antigen and, therefore, at risk for development of PTP, far fewer than 3% of transfused individuals are affected. Part of the reason for this is that cases that are not clinically apparent may go unrecognized or a specific immune response gene may be necessary to produce anti-HPA-1a. There does appear to be a strong link between the Drw52 allele and the production of anti-HPA-1a alloantibody.[81] Packed RBCs and whole blood have been the components predominantly associated with the precipitation of PTP; however, platelets and plasma transfusion can also trigger the syndrome.[77] Transfusion reactions, generally characterized by chills and fever, have frequently been reported in patients prior to or after the manifestation of PTP. Thrombocytopenia is usually severe, with platelet counts being $<10\,000/\mu l$. The duration of thrombocytopenia in untreated patients ranges from 7 to 48 days. In situations where the patient is not bleeding or at risk of bleeding, careful observation may be all that is necessary. The most feared complication during the period of extreme thrombocytopenia is intracranial hemorrhage. Infusion of high-dose intravenous immunoglobulin has become the first line of therapy; however, this may require 3–4 days for a response. In severe cases of PTP, in the face of active bleeding, HPA-1a-negative platelets may provide transient benefit.[82] The efficacy of corticosteroids and plasma exchange for treatment of PTP has not been well established.

TRANSFUSION-ASSOCIATED GRAFT-VERSUS-HOST DISEASE

Graft-versus-host disease (GVHD) results from the engraftment of immunocompetent donor T lymphocytes into a recipient whose immune system is unable to reject them. It is a common sequela of bone marrow transplantation (BMT), but is also recognized as a rare risk associated with blood transfusion. Early reports of transfusion-associated (TA)-GVHD were recognized in immunocompromised hosts. However, cases have been documented in immunocompetent transfusion recipients.[83]

Several factors play a role in the pathogenesis of TA-GVHD. Kinetic studies of donor leukocyte clearance after allogeneic transfusion have shown rapid clearance over the initial 2 days post transfusion, followed by a transient increase in circulating donor leukocytes at 3–5 days prior to complete clearance by 7–10 days. It has been postulated that the transient increase represents an *in vivo* mixed lymphocyte reaction with activated donor T lymphocytes proliferating in an abortive GVHD.[84] Long-term chimerism (6 months to 1 year), on the other hand, has been observed in trauma patients who were transfused, and this has been postulated to be due to engraftment of stem cells.[85] It has been well recognized that immunocompetent T lymphocytes, capable of a proliferative response, must be present in the initial donor inoculum.

Virtually all cellular blood components have been implicated in reported cases of TA-GVHD. The syndrome has developed after transfusion of whole blood, red blood cells, platelets, fresh (non-frozen) plasma and leukocytes harvested from both normal donors and donors with chronic myelocytic leukemia. The dosage of immunocompetent cells transfused is also important. Based on animal studies, a minimum dose of 1×10^7 cells/kg body weight is necessary to induce a 'runting syndrome' and case studies suggest that a similar threshold is necessary to produce GVHD in man.[86] There have been reports of fatal TA-GVHD, however, occurring in children with severe combined immunodeficiency in which a dose of only 8×10^4 lymphocytes/kg body weight appeared to be transfused.[87] The threshold number of viable cells necessary to produce a graft-versus-host reaction, therefore, may vary depending upon the immune status of the host as well as the antigenic similarity or disparity between donor and recipient. There must be sufficient disparity between donor and host histocompatibility antigens for the host to appear foreign to the donor and, therefore, to be capable of inducing antigenic stimulation. The host, on the other hand, must be incapable of mounting an immunologic reaction against the graft either as a result of an immature or defective cellular immunity or host tolerance of the foreign cells. The latter scenario may occur when there exists donor homozygosity for an HLA haplotype, for which the recipient is haploidentical. In this setting the recipient's lymphocytes see only self-antigens on the donor's cells. However, the homozygous donor cells see non-self antigens on recipient's cells stimulating an alloreaction which can initiate GVHD.[88]

The immune response in GVHD is somewhat complex and is not completely understood. Two basic aspects involve the afferent phase in which recipient tissues stimulate T lymphocytes from the donor which in turn undergoes clonal proliferation and differentiation and the efferent phase in which donor effector cells damage recipient target tissues. The immunologic target is thought to be the host's major histocompatibility complex (MHC) antigens. In TA-GVHD, the recipient's B, T, epithelial and bone marrow stem cells become the main focus of attack. It was initially believed that the effector mechanism was the result of direct cytotoxicity by alloreactive donor T cells. The observation that the phenotype of many of the effector cells infiltrating target tissues was more consistent with natural killer (NK) cells than with mature T lymphocytes suggested a possible role for cytokines in the effector phase of GVHD. In this model, inflammatory cytokines, such as TNF-α and IL-1, released by host tissue damaged by chemotherapy, radiotherapy or infection, result in the increased expression of MHC and other adhesion molecules. This upregulation results in enhanced recognition of donor/recipient differences by alloreactive donor T cells present in the transfused component. The donor T cells then proliferate and secrete cytokines, in particular IL-2. Cytokine release in turn recruits additional donor T cells and macrophages which are induced to secrete IL-1 and TNF-α. In this manner, the creation of a self-amplifying positive feedback loop eventually produces the clinical manifestations of GVHD.[89,90]

GVHD following blood transfusions manifests as an acute syndrome, the onset typically occurring within 4–30 days. The syndrome is characterized by dysfunction of the skin, liver, gastrointestinal tract and bone marrow. The initial clinical manifestations are usually a high fever occurring 8–10 days after the transfusion, followed within 24–48 hours by the appearance of a central maculopapular rash which subsequently spreads to the extremities. In severe cases, the rash may progress to generalized erythroderma and desquamation. Additional clinical findings may include anorexia, nausea, vomiting and watery diarrhea with or without elevated liver enzymes and hyperbilirubinemia. Unlike GVHD following BMT, pancytopenia is a prominent finding in TA-GVHD. This typically results from the ability of the donor cells to recognize the recipient (host) marrow as antigenically foreign, leading to the destruction of stem cells and/or colony forming units. In GVHD associated with BMT, the 'host bone marrow' has been replaced by the donor's bone marrow which, accordingly, is antigenically the same as the reacting donor lymphocytes. The development of bone marrow hypoplasia and aplasia associated with TA-GVHD places the patient at increased risk for hemorrhage or overwhelming infection. The duration of TA-GVHD is short with the majority of patients dying within a few days to weeks (median time 21 days from onset), usually as a complication of marrow failure.[91] While immunosuppressive therapies such as prednisone, cyclosporine and antithymocyte globulin have been used to treat GVHD associated with BMT, this approach has not been effective for TA-GVHD which is nearly uniformly fatal. A review of the clinical manifestation of TA-GVHD in neonates has shown that infants present later (median time of onset 28 days) with a slightly prolonged course. However, they have a similarly high rate of mortality.[92]

Diagnosis of TA-GVHD is usually based on the clinical presentation in conjunction with histologic findings on skin biopsy and supportive evidence of persistence of donor lymphocytes by cytogenetic, HLA or DNA analyses. Since there are several other clinical entities that may mimic TA-GVHD, including viral syndromes and drug reactions, it becomes important to make the correct diagnoses and to have an appreciation of those patients who are at greatest risk for TA-GVHD.

TA-GVHD has been reported in patients with several different clinical conditions. It has been difficult, however, to assess the risk of TA-GVHD for any particular group of patients for several reasons. First, the diagnosis may be difficult to make in the situation where there is a critically ill, multiply-transfused patient with infectious as well as other complications. Usually only severe cases are recognized, often only after death. Mild cases may go unrecognized or be mistaken for a viral infection or drug reaction, both of which may present with similar symptoms. Secondly, since the development of TA-GVHD depends on several variables, including the number of viable T lymphocytes transfused, the extent of immune suppression in the patient, and the degree of HLA sharing between donor and recipient, each transfusion episode presents its own spectrum of risk. To assess the risk in any patient group, the number of blood components a particular category of patients will receive during the course of treatment must be taken into account. Finally, due to the high mortality rate, there are no prospective studies evaluating the risk of developing TA-GVHD in susceptible groups of patients.

Until recently, patients developing TA-GVHD all shared either a congenital or acquired deficiency of cell-mediated immunity, which is one of the major risk factors. The first reported cases occurred in children with immunodeficiency syndromes involving a T-cell defect.[93] Infants known either to have or who are suspected of having a congenital deficiency of T-cell function, including DiGeorge's syndrome, Wiskott–Aldrich syndrome, severe combined immunodeficiency syndrome, reticular dysgenesis and purine nucleoside phosphorylase deficiency, are at risk. Infants with humoral immunodeficiency (B cell), however, are not. Another group of infants who appear to be at risk are those who receive intrauterine transfusions (IUT) and subsequently exchange transfusion. It has been postulated that the lymphocytes in the IUT may induce a state of nonspecific tolerance through exhaustion of fetal immune defenses which then, with subsequent exchange transfusion, results in GVHD. Other occurrences of TA-GVHD in the neonatal setting are assumed to be related to the relative immunologic immaturity of the premature infant combined with transfusion of large volumes of fresh blood, such as may occur with exchange transfusion. Transfusion of maternal components, as occurs in the setting of neonatal alloimmune thrombocytopenia, has been associated with TA-GVHD.

Table 36.2 Indications for use of irradiated blood/blood components in neonatal/pediatric patients.

Infants/fetus <4 months of age
  Fetus received *in utero* transfusion
  Premature infants and those of low birth weight (<1200 g)
  Known or suspected congenital cellular immunodeficiency
  Congenital leukemia, malignancy undergoing chemotherapy
  Infant undergoing exchange transfusion for Rh hemolytic disease with/
  without history of intrauterine transfusion
  Recipient of familial blood or HLA-matched cellular products

Children >4 months of age
  Known or suspected congenital cellular immunodeficiency
  Malignancy (hematologic/solid tumor) undergoing chemotherapy/
  radiotherapy
  Recipient of solid organ or stem cell transplantation
  Recipient of familial blood or HLA-matched cellular products

Patients for whom risk is not well established to support irradiation
  Infants >1200 g in NICU setting but without history as described above
  All children undergoing open-heart procedures, including ECMO
  Any child with a conal-truncal heart defect until congenital T-cell
  immunodeficiency is ruled out
  HIV infection

A transfusion from blood relatives or unrelated donors who share HLA haplotypes with the recipient is a risk factor whether in the setting of transfusion to a neonate, older child or adult with or without immunoincompetence. The risk of TA-GVHD in premature infants, with no other identifiable risk factors, as a result of routine small volume transfusion is rare (Table 36.2).[94]

TA-GVHD has been reported in patients with hematologic malignancies and solid tumors, who have received cytotoxic chemotherapy, radiation treatment or both.[95] Once again, the overall risk is difficult to assess, especially as therapeutic approaches to various malignancies become more intensive. The strong association, however, between Hodgkin's disease of any stage and the development of TA-GVHD is believed to be the result of the intrinsic T-cell defects known to occur with this disease.[96] Reports of TA-GVHD in association with ablative chemotherapy and autologous BMT for solid tumors have also been reported.[95] The doses of chemotherapy given render these patients severely immunocompromised. In this setting it is important to remember that components transfused during harvesting of either bone marrow or peripheral blood stem cells, which is actually prior to ablative therapy, may also potentially be implicated in the development of TA-GVHD. Viable allogeneic T lymphocytes contaminating the harvested component may be reinfused to the recipient, with the recipient's own stem cells, at a time when the recipient is aplastic and immunosuppressed.

There have been various clinical settings in which TA-GVHD has been reported to occur in patients presumed to be immunocompetent. While in a few cases no risk factors could be identified, the majority have been associated with transfusion of relatively fresh blood from an HLA-homozygous donor to a recipient who is an heterozygote for the

donor's HLA haplotype. This is more likely to occur with transfusions from blood relatives; however, it has been reported to occur with unrelated donor transfusion.[97] Cardiac surgery has been the clinical setting for most of the reported cases; however, once again this has occurred in association with the use of relatively fresh blood from either family donors or in the context of donor/recipient haplotype sharing. The frequency of blood being transfused from an unrelated donor homozygous for an HLA haplotype for which the recipient is heterozygous depends on the HLA homogeneity of the population.[92,98]

No reports of patients with AIDS developing TA-GVHD have been published. An explanation for this apparent paradox, i.e. why such an immunosuppressed group should not show signs of GVHD, is lacking. It has been suggested that in AIDS patients the donor T lymphocytes may also become infected with HIV and thus are rendered unable to initiate the GVHD syndrome. There also have been no reported cases of TA-GVHD developing in patients with aplastic anemia other than in the setting of BMT.

Table 36.2 reviews the indications for the use of irradiated blood and blood products utilized at the facility of one of the authors (NLCL). To ensure that all oncology patients receive irradiated products whether they are receiving bone marrow transplantation, stem cell rescue or experimental immunomodulatory therapy, patients receive irradiated blood and blood products when they begin chemotherapy. The authors are aware that a few institutions are providing irradiated blood/blood products for all infants and children in an effort to avoid missing an undiagnosed cellular immunodeficiency patient.

Since the treatment of TA-GVHD is almost always ineffective, efforts have been made to prevent and minimize the risk by reducing or inactivating transfused donor lymphocytes. The methods available in blood banks physically to remove T lymphocytes through washing or filtration do not provide effective prophylaxis against TA-GVHD. Current leukocyte-reduction filters, which can achieve a 3-log reduction in leukocyte content of components, cannot guarantee removal of sufficient lymphocytes to prevent TA-GVHD. Inactivation of transfused lymphocytes by γ-irradiation of blood components remains the most effective method for inhibiting lymphocyte blast transformation and mitotic activity and hence the prevention of TA-GVHD. The current recommended dose of irradiation is 25 Gy to the midplane of the component with a minimum of 15 Gy to any other region of the component. The effects of this dose on platelet and granulocyte viability are not clinically significant. However, long-term 4°C storage of irradiated red cells results in increased levels of potassium.[99] This may be of clinical concern if large volumes of blood need to be infused over a short period of time into patients who may be susceptible to the development of hyperkalemia, such as premature infants and patients with severe renal impairment.

TRANSFUSION-ASSOCIATED IMMUNE MODULATION

Blood transfusion has been known to alter immune function since the observation in the 1970s of improved renal allograft survival in transfused patients. While this proved to be of beneficial effect, concern has developed over the immuno-suppressive effects of transfusion and the potential clinical consequences, including increased rate of solid tumor recurrence and postoperative bacterial sepsis.[100] The mechanism of the immunosuppressive effect of transfusion is poorly understood. The role of the cellular elements of components versus plasma is also not clearly delineated. Several changes in T-cell subpopulations have been reported in multitransfused patients, including a reversal in the CD4/CD8 ratio and an increased number of HLA-DR-activated lymphocytes.[101,102] Similar findings have not been observed in infants receiving washed, irradiated red cells.[47] Other immunologic alterations observed either in animal or human studies have included decreased NK cell activity, decreased lymphocyte responses to mitogens, and decreased cytotoxic T-cell number and anergy to intradermal antigens.[100–102] There have been several retrospective and prospective studies evaluating the relationship between transfusion and the immune system but the clinical significance of this remains controversial.[103,104]

TRANSFUSION TRANSMITTED INFECTIONS

Advances in blood donor screening have supported the concept that a zero-risk blood supply may be possible in the future. While the application of a large number of serological tests and more stringent donor questioning have certainly aided the ability to screen out donors, risks still remain. Screening in the US includes testing for hepatitis B and C, HIV 1 and 2, HTLV-I and -II, syphilis and, in some donors, cytomegalovirus (CMV). Newer assays that measure viral antigen rather than antibody response are being promulgated to identify donors who are infective. HIV p24 antigen testing, for example, was added in 1996 to decrease HIV window cases. The high sensitivity of these assays has decreased the window period of infectivity.[105] Molecular assays based on viral protein using polymerase chain reaction (multiplex PCR) are undergoing feasibility trials. Despite improvements in the questioning of donors, donors may still not be truthful about high-risk behaviors in which they engage.[106,107] New and emerging transfusion-transmitted diseases, such as Chagas disease and Creutzfeld–Jacob disease, continue to challenge transfusionists and recipients of blood and blood products.

The current estimates of the risk of transfusion transmitted viral infections has been made possible through the Retroviral Epidemiology Donor Study. In this study, rates of seroconversion of large numbers of donors are combined with estimates of the probability that blood was donated during a window period when donor testing would have been negative. Using data from 2 300 000 allogeneic blood transfusions where all donor screening was passed, the risk of transmission in the US is: 1 in 493 000 for HIV; 1 in 641 000 for HTLV1; 1 in 103 000 for HCV; and 1 in 63 000 for HBV.[104]

Hepatitis C virus

Hepatitis C virus (HCV) is a single-stranded RNA virus belonging to the Flaviviridae family. It can be transmitted by cellular and non-cellular blood and blood products, including intravenous immunoglobulin. The most notable characteristic of HCV is its persistence in host hepatocytes. Studies have found that 90% of post-transfusion non A, non B hepatitis is caused by HCV.[108] Long-term follow-up (by the National Institutes of Health) of patients with post-transfusion hepatitis, showed that approximately 70% of HCV-infected individuals develop chronic hepatitis.[109] The mechanism of persistence is probably due to the virus's ability to rapidly mutate under immune pressure and to co-exist as multiple mutants. These mutants have been termed 'quasi-species' and they provide an excellent mechanism for the virus to escape the immune response.[110] In addition, HCV can persist in the liver in a dormant state by down-regulating its replication to protect itself from immune clearance. While there is an adequate humoral response to HCV, the neutralizing antibodies which develop rapidly become ineffective against emerging strains.[111]

First-generation screening tests for HCV were used in 1990 and were targeted against the c100–3 antigen. Second-generation screening assays were introduced in 1992 and were directed against multiple epitopes: c100–3 antigen, core protein designated c22–3 and an NS3 protein designated c33c; antibodies to the latter 2 epitopes appear earlier than anti-c100–3. Of HCV-infected individuals, 80% will develop specific antibody by 15 weeks from exposure and 100% by 6 months;[109] in the majority of individuals, anti-HCV antibodies persist for very long periods. Since the licensing of second-generation assays in March 1995, the incidence of transfusion-associated HCV has declined from 5% in 1989 to <1%.[109]

Acute post-transfusion hepatitis C infection is, in the majority of patients, asymptomatic and anicteric. The significance of infection with HCV lies in the virus's propensity for persistent indolent infection. In both community-acquired and transfusion-associated HCV, the frequency of chronic hepatitis exceeds 60% and that of persistent infection may exceed 90%.[108,112] Of those with chronic hepatitis, two-thirds develop chronic active hepatitis, cirrhosis, and/or hepatocellular carcinoma (HCC). At least 20% of HCV-infected patients develop cirrhosis within two decades, and the risk for development of HCC is 1–5% after 20 years.[113] Once cirrhosis is established, the rate of development of HCC increases by 1–4%/year.[114] Patients with chronic HCV hepatitis can also present with a variety of extrahepatic manifestations thought to be of immunologic origin, including arthritis, lichen planus, glomerulonephritis, keratoconjunctivitis sicca and mixed cryoglobulinemia.[114]

HCV infection in children can be divided into that acquired pre- or peri-natally or through transfusion of blood and blood products. Transmission of HCV from mother to infant has been documented, but the risk of transmission is unclear; estimates range from 0 to 10%.[115–117] Palomba et al[116] found HCV antibodies in 9.2% of 108 infants born to HIV-1-infected mothers and followed prospectively, which confirms that the mother's HIV status favors HCV transmission. None of the infected infants recovered from HCV infection and all progressed toward chronic hepatitis. This persistence is particularly ominous because of the natural history of HCV infection.

The majority of data concerning HCV infection in children comes from studies on multiply transfused hematology and oncology patients diagnosed prior to implementation of HCV screening. In children treated for malignancy, the prevalence of HCV varies from 17 to 40% depending on the geographic area.[118–120] In an Italian study, Cesaro et al[120] found that 117 of 658 children who completed treatment for pediatric malignancy were HCV positive. Among these, 91 (77.8%) had received at least one blood transfusion and chronic liver disease was found in 92 (78.6%). Fifty-one patients underwent a liver biopsy and 1 of 37 (2.7%) anti-HCV-positive only patients was found to have cirrhosis as compared with 3 of the 14 (21.5%) HBV-HCV co-infected patients. No hepatic failure or hepatocellular carcinoma was noted after a 14-year follow-up period of these patients. Another study by Ni et al[121] in Japan analyzed data from 61 children, most of whom had transfusion-dependent thalassemia, who were followed for 4 years. Twenty-six were HCV infected and of these 24 had elevated ALT, while only 10 of 34 non-infected patients had evidence of liver dysfunction. Six patients from each group had a liver biopsy. Five HCV-positive patients had evidence of portal fibrosis compared with 2 of the negative group. All specimens from both groups had evidence of hemochromatosis; iron overload is a known confounder of hepatic fibrosis and HCC development in adults. These data suggest that chronic HCV infection may produce more severe liver damage in transfusion-dependent children than in those with malignancy.

Current treatment of HCV consists of interferon-α2b, 3 million units 3 times weekly for 6 or 12 months. The sustained biochemical remission rate is approximately 20%, as about 50% of initial responders relapse after cessation of treatment with interferon.[114] Also, it has been found that patients with lower serum titers of HCV-RNA tend to have a more favorable response to therapy. Current consensus among hepatologists is that patients with chronic active hepatitis or active cirrhosis on liver biopsy with compensated liver disease should be treated. The controversy lies in whether to treat HCV carriers with mild disease; most treat only if there is biopsy-proven active disease.[114] Studies testing the efficacy of combination drugs including ribavirin and interferon have not yet been performed in children. Given that HCV is a chronic disease with significant morbidity and mortality, early intervention has significant appeal. Particularly in children, in whom abnormal pathology is seen early in the disease, studies for recipients of HCV-positive blood units should, therefore, target neonatal and pediatric transfusion recipients.

Hepatitis G virus

Hepatitis G virus (HGV), and its strain variant GBV-C, are recently discovered human Flaviviruses. HGV/GBV-C is transmitted by transfusion of blood products and is found in 1–2% of eligible volunteer US blood donors.[122,123] Currently, HGV/GBV-C can be detected by RNA PCR and by an antibody to the envelope region E2 of the virus. Anti-E2 is a recovery-phase antibody that is detectable only when HGV/GBV-C RNA has been cleared.[123–125] Studies have shown that the exposure rate among volunteer blood donors is 3–6-fold the rate of viremia. In high-risk groups such as hemophiliacs and IV drug users, the rate of exposure may be as high as 80–90% with a viremia rate of 15–20%.[126–128] This large difference between exposure rates and active infection rates suggests that most of the HGV/GBV-C carriers eventually clear the virus.[124,125] In the NIH prospective transfusion study, Alter et al[129] found HGV/GBV-C RNA in 23% of patients with transfusion-associated non-A, non-B, and non-C hepatitis. However, there was a dissociation between the subjects' ALT levels and the HGV/GBV-C RNA levels. This casts doubt on the causality of hepatitis by this agent and raises the possibility that it may be an innocent bystander. Among HCV-infected individuals, 10–20% are co-infected with HGV/GBV-C. Many studies have shown that HGV/GBV-C has no impact on the clinical course of HCV infection.[130,131] Also, response to interferon is identical in patients infected with HGV/GBV-C and HCV and in those infected with HCV alone.

There is evidence of HGV/GBV-C viremia in children, but the available literature on the subject is small. Vertical transmission from mother to infant has been demonstrated and preliminary data suggest persistent infection in those children without clinical or biochemical evidence of hepatitis.[132,133] HGV/GBV-C RNA has also been detected in multiply transfused children with chronic hepatitis B and C infection and persisted after interferon-α therapy.[134–136]

Despite the absence of a practical screening assay, a debate has already ensued as to whether donor screening for HGB/GBV-C should be routinely implemented when it is developed. The paradox underlying the debate is that although HGV is easily transmittable by transfusion of blood products and is capable of causing persistent infection, it has not been clearly associated with disease.[126,137,138] Current data do not show that HGV resides in hepatocytes or that it replicates in the liver. Thus, the designation 'hepatitis' virus may have been premature. More research is needed to evaluate the demographic and clinical characteristics of HGV/GBV-C infection.

Human immunodeficiency virus

Transfusion-transmitted HIV, from either clotting factor concentrate or blood and blood products, has brought the inherent mortality risk from transfusion to the clinician, patient and lay public. No other transfusion-transmitted disease has generated as much fear in the minds of patients and as much action on the part of regulatory agencies and manufacturers of plasma-derived products.

Several studies of adults receiving blood and blood products demonstrated a peak in infection for individuals transfused in 1984. Clinical presentation occurred several years later, supporting a long incubation period.[139] The NHLBI-sponsored, multicenter Transfusion Safety Study (TSS) traced individuals who received known infected blood units over time. About 90% of the recipients seroconverted, while the other 10% remained PCR and viral culture-confirmed uninfected. Variables associated with infectivity included the level of donor viremia at the time of donation, duration of refrigerator storage and type of blood component transfused.[140] Blood product manipulations that reduce WBC number (leukoreduction) or free virus (washing) were thought to affect inoculum and therefore infectivity.[140]

While there are several published cases and small cohort studies, only 2 studies have reported large numbers of children infected by transfusion. Jones et al[142] reported on 212 cases reported to the CDC from 1981 to 1987. The median age at HIV diagnosis was 4 years with a range of 0.3–12.8 years. The median survival was 13.7 months, longer than the reported adult survival of 5.6 months. Of interest, 71% of cases were transfused in the first year of life. AIDS-associated illnesses were similar to those reported for perinatal transmission, except that there was less lymphoid interstitial pneumonitis and more encephalopathy. In a cohort study of infants transfused in Los Angeles, a high HIV risk area of the US, from 1980 to March 1987, 443 were traced and tested. Thirty-three had antibody to HIV and no other risk factor except for transfusion; 14 had unrecognized HIV infection and were identified through this lookback study. Estimates on the time interval from date of infection (birth) to date of HIV-related symptoms was on average 63 months (5.25 years) with a range of 3–95 months.[143]

The authors' studies involving transfused neonates and older children in an urban area demonstrate children presenting symptom free as late as 9.5 years post-transfusion.[144] It is therefore recommended that parents of adolescents and pre-adolescents who present with positive HIV screenings tests be questioned about transfusion occurring before the introduction of HIV testing. Medical record reviews may be needed, as many families are unaware that transfusion was a routine part of neonatal supportive care. HIV-infected children from areas of the world where blood is purchased from commercial donors or where HIV testing is not routinely performed will probably continue to present as transfusion-associated cases.

Cytomegalovirus

Cytomegalovirus is a ubiquitous virus of the herpes family that is harbored in WBCs. A significant proportion of blood donors (30–70%) are CMV seropositive, although there are regional differences that may in part be due to different donor demographics such as age, sex, race and socio-economic status. Older age, female sex and lower socio-economic status predispose to higher seroprevalence rates. Despite studies confirming that seropositive donors can transmit CMV to seronegative recipients, few have been able to document viremia in blood donors. This has led to the concept that both actively infected as well as latently infected donors can transmit CMV.[145]

Three types of CMV infections are seen in the transfusion recipient: primary infection and two kinds of secondary infection, reactivation and reinfection. Primary infection occurs in a seronegative recipient of blood from a donor who is actively or latently infected. Patients are frequently symptomatic with a mononucleosis-like syndrome that is heterophile-negative. Viremia, viruria, an IgM-specific and then IgG-specific anti-CMV antibody response can be demonstrated. Reactivation occurs when a CMV-seropositive recipient is transfused with blood from either a CMV-seropositive or -seronegative donor. The donor leukocytes trigger an allograft reaction that reactivates the recipient's latent CMV. An IgG antibody titer rise and viral shedding may be found. Most of these infections are asymptomatic, except in an immunocompromised host. Re- or co-infection occurs in a CMV-seropositive recipient of blood with a strain of CMV that differs from the strain that initially infected the recipient. An IgM and IgG response as well as viral shedding may be seen. The only way to distinguish reinfection from co-infection is to use molecular markers, wherein multiple strains of CMV may be identified in the co-infected recipient.

There is a wide clinical spectrum associated with post-transfusion CMV. CMV infection may be asymptomatic and discovered only because of serial serologic tests, or it may produce significant morbidity and mortality.[146] Certain select patient groups are at risk for the pneumonia, cytopenias, hepatitis, graft rejection, unexplained fever, and increased risk of bacterial and fungal infections associated with post-transfusion CMV. These groups include certain neonates, specifically those < 1250 g who are seronegative and who require large amounts of blood (> 50 ml), bone marrow and solid-organ transplant recipients, infants who receive intrauterine transfusions and other severely immunocompromised individuals. Other immunocompromised patients, whether seronegative or seropositive, do not appear to be at increased risk for mortality and morbidity from CMV. At the time of writing, no studies have addressed the need for specialized CMV-attenuated products for either seronegative or seropositive patients with HIV infection and practices clearly vary among hospitals.[147]

The use of IgG-seronegative blood is considered to be the

Table 36.3 Recommendations of AABB on use of CMV safe blood.

Category*	Clinical circumstance	CMV-seronegative blood (unmodified)	Leukocyte-reduced (LR) blood (CMV-unscreened)
I	CMV- + ve patient	Not indicated	Not indicated
	CMV- − ve patient	Not indicated	Not indicated
II	CMV- + ve patient	Not indicated	Use of LR blood to prevent viral reactivation awaits further research
	CMV- − ve patient	Either CMV-seronegative blood or LR blood is indicated	Either CMV-seronegative blood or LR blood is indicated
III	CMV- + ve recipient	Not indicated	Not indicated
	CMV- − ve recipient of CMV-organ donor	Either CMV-seronegative blood or LR blood is indicated	Either CMV-seronegative blood or LR blood is indicated
IV	CMV- + ve recipient	Not indicated	Use of LR blood to prevent viral reactivation awaits further research
	CMV- − ve recipient of CMV- + ve donor	Either CMV-seronegative blood or LR blood is indicated	Either CMV-seronegative blood or LR blood is indicated
V	CMV- + ve recipient	Either CMV-seronegative blood or LR blood is indicated	Either CMV-seronegative blood or LR blood is indicated
	CMV- − ve recipient	Either CMV-seronegative blood or LR blood is indicated	LR blood may be slightly preferred to CMV-seronegative blood (passive CMV immunoglobulin)

*Category I patients: General hospital patients and general surgery patients (including cardiac surgery); patients receiving chemotherapy that is not intended to produce severe neutropenia (adjuvant therapy for breast cancer, treatment of chronic lymphocytic leukemia, etc.); patients receiving corticosteroids (patients with immune thrombocytopenic purpura, collagen vascular diseases, etc.); full-term infants.
Category II patients: Patients receiving chemotherapy that is intended to produce severe neutropenia (leukemia, lymphoma, etc.); pregnant patients; HIV-infected individuals.
Category III patients: Solid-organ allograft patients who do not require massive transfusion support.
Category IV patients: Patients receiving allogeneic and autologous hematopoietic progenitor cell transplants.
Category V patients: Low birth weight (<1200 g) premature infants.
Source: American Association of Blood Banks. *Association Bulletin 97-2*, April 1997.

gold standard, despite the fact that most IgG-seropositive units are not infectious. Depending on the donor demographics in an area, such products are sometimes difficult to obtain. Donors with IgM-specific CMV antibody may transmit CMV more readily, as they are more likely to have acute viral infection and replication.[148] IgG antibody assays, however, are not well standardized. Hence, several different methods have been used to prevent or ameliorate post-transfusion CMV. Because the virus is probably harbored in WBCs, manipulations that can reduce or attenuate leukocyte cell number should reduce the risk of transmission. These methods include washing, freezing followed by washing, and filtration.[149] Lower rates of CMV infection have been seen in open-heart and neonatal patients receiving washed red blood cells. Frozen deglycerolized RBCs, regardless of serostatus, are effective in preventing CMV in neonates and patients on dialysis. The recently developed third-generation leukocyte-depletion filters have been shown to be effective in preventing primary CMV infection in neonates, in adult patients with hematologic malignancies, and in patients post BMT.[145]

Based on a study by Bowden *et al*,[150] which suggests equivalence between CMV seronegative and leukoreduced products, no >5 × 10^6 WBCs should remain in the product to abrogate CMV transmission in at-risk populations. This study, its design and outcome have been debated widely.[151] It should be noted that of 250 patients who received filtered blood and blood products, 6 developed CMV disease, including 5 cases of fatal pneumonia. Of the 252 patients receiving seronegative blood and blood products, 4 developed CMV disease, but none was fatal. No subsequent studies using other manufacturers' filters or pre-storage-leukodepleted products have been performed to validate equivalencies.

Some oncologists argue that patients who may undergo BMT regardless of marrow donor serology should have blood and blood products manipulated to prevent reactivation of CMV or reinfection. There have been no studies that support this practice, although theoretically infection with CMV and clinical manifestations of newly acquired diseases may be significant. Several studies have demonstrated high failure rates for bedside leukodepletion filters. More routine use of pre-storage leukodepletion filters that have undergone stringent quality control checks in the setting of blood centers and transfusion services adhering to good manufacturing practices, may well provide an acceptable product that does not depend on donor serostatus. The transfusion of stringently quality controlled leukoreduced products, regardless of serostatus, may be considered equivalent to CMV-seronegative products by some clinicians.

Cesium or γ-irradiation of blood to inhibit DNA replication will not prevent CMV infection. Many patients undergoing chemotherapy with or without transplantation receive irradiated blood for prevention of GVHD. Similarly, many patients who receive blood that is CMV seronegative or mechanically leukodepleted, receive CMV hyperimmune globulin or intravenous immunoglobulin with variable titers of CMV antibody and, in addition, may be receiving

Table 36.4 Prevention of some transfusion complications by leukocyte removal.

Established indications	Threshold level of WBC reduction to prevent the reaction
Febrile nonhemolytic transfusion reaction	5×10^8
Alloimmunization to Class I HLA antigens	$<5 \times 10^6$
Infectious disease transmission by leukocytes	Unknown and dependent on virus in question. Plasma viremia may transmit disease, despite leukodepletion. See text
Graft versus host disease	Unknown. Gamma irradiation should be used
TRALI	Passive transfer of antibody in plasma will not be attenuated by leukocyte removal

FFP for coagulopathies. They receive these plasma products to attenuate the development of graft-induced CMV or nosocomial acquisition of CMV. It may be very difficult to assess the serostatus of these individuals because of passive acquisition of CMV antibody. Tests for CMV early antigen, CMV PCR or molecular markers will be necessary to establish post-transfusion CMV in these patients.

At one author's institution (NLCL), all newly diagnosed oncology patients have their CMV serostatus evaluated on their first pre-transfusion specimen. Their serostatus and diagnosis then determines the nature of the restrictions they are placed on, based on an algorithm. This algorithm provides CMV-seronegative blood and blood products to seronegative recipients who are on a protocol that may result in either transplant or stem cell rescue. CMV-seronegative patients are provided with leukodepleted products to reduce febrile reactions and as a surrogate for CMV-seronegative products. Other patients who have low risk for transplantation or rescue, regardless of serostatus, receive untested, non-leukodepleted, irradiated products unless their clinical circumstance changes or they develop a febrile non-hemolytic transfusion reaction. The algorithm is modified yearly after review of the current adult and pediatric literature with oncology staff. The algorithm developed by the American Association of Blood Banks (AABB) is shown in Table 36.3. Each institution should select their own algorithm based on a review of the literature.

REFERENCES

1. Davenport RD, Streiter RM, Kunkel SL. Red cell ABO incompatibility and production of tumor necrosis factor-alpha. *Br J Haematol* 1991; **78**: 540–544
2. Capon SM, Goldfinger D. Acute hemolytic transfusion reaction, a paradigm of the systemic inflammatory response: new insights into pathophysiology and treatment. *Transfusion* 1995; **35**: 513–520
3. Popovsky MA, Chaplin HC, Moore SB. Transfusion-related acute lung injury: a neglected serious complication of hemotherapy. *Transfusion* 1992: **32**; 589–592
4. Silliman CC, Paterson AJ, Dickey WO *et al*. The association of biologically active lipids with the development of transfusion-related acute lung injury: a retrospective study. *Transfusion* 1997; **37**: 719–726
5. Aye MT, Palmer DS, Giulivi A, Hashemi S. Effect of filtration of platelet concentrates on the accumulation of cytokines and platelet release factors during storage. *Transfusion* 1995; **35**: 117–124
6. Shanwell A, Kristiansson M, Remberger M, Ringden O. Generation of cytokines in red cell concentrates during storage is prevented by prestorage white cell reduction. *Transfusion* 1997; **37**: 678–684
7. Heddle NM, Kelton JG. Febrile nonhemolytic transfusion reaction. In: Popovsky MA (ed) *Transfusion Reactions*. Bethesda: AABB Press, 1996, p 48
8. Heddle NM, Klama L, Singer J *et al*. The role of the plasma from platelet concentrates in transfusion reactions. *N Engl J Med* 1994; **33**: 625–628
9. Federowicz I, Barrett BB, Andersen JW, Urashima M, Popovsky MA, Anderson KC. Characterization of reactions after transfusion of cellular blood components that are white cell reduced before storage. *Transfusion* 1996; **36**: 21–28
10. Kevy SV. Red cell transfusion. In: Nathan DG, Oski FA (eds) *Hematology of Infancy and Childhood*, 4th edn. Philadelphia: WB Saunders, 1993, pp 1769–1780
11. Walker RH (ed). *Technical Manual*, 12th edn. Bethesda: American Association of Blood Banks, 1996
12. Scanlon JW, Krakaur R. Hyperkalemia following exchange transfusion. *J Pediatr* 1984; **105**: 321–324
13. Hall TL, Barnes A, Miller JR, Bethencourt DM, Nestor L. Neonatal mortality following transfusion of red cells with high plasma potassium levels. *Transfusion* 1993; **33**: 606–609
14. Blanchette VS, Grey E, Hardie MJ *et al*. Hyperkalemia following exchange transfusion: Risk eliminated by washing red cell concentrates. *J Pediatr* 1993; **123**: 285–288
15. Murphy S, Gardner FH. Platelet preservation: Effect of storage temperature on maintenance of platelet viability – Deleterious effect of refrigerated storage. *N Engl J Med* 1969; **280**: 1094–1099
16. Beutler E, Meul A, Wood LA. Depletion and regeneration of 2,3-diphosphoglyceric acid in stored red blood cells. *Transfusion* 1969; **9**: 109–114
17. Boyan CP, Howland WS. Cardiac arrest and temperature of blood bank blood. *N Engl J Med* 1963; **183**: 58–60
18. Staples PJ, Griner PF. Extracorporeal hemolysis of blood in a microwave blood warmer. *N Engl J Med* 1971; **285**: 317–319
19. Harke H, Rahman S. Haemostatic disorders in massive transfusion. *Bibl Haematol* 1980; **46**: 213–224
20. Harrison SR, Sawyer PR. Special issues in transfusion medicine. *Clin Lab Med* 1992; **12**: 743–757
21. Phillips TF, Soulier G, Wilson RF. Outcome of massive transfusion exceeding two blood volumes in trauma and emergency surgery. *J Trauma* 1987; **27**: 903–910
22. Honig CK, Bove Jr. Transfusion-associated fatalities: Review of Bureau of Biologics reports 1976–1978. *Transfusion* 1980; **20**: 653–661
23. Sazama K. Reports of 355 transfusion-associated deaths: 1976 through 1985. *Transfusion* 1990; **30**: 583–590
24. Blajchman MA, Ali AM. Bacteria in the blood supply: An overlooked issue in transfusion medicine. In: Nance SJ (ed) *Blood Safety: Current Challenges*. Bethesda, MD: American Association of Blood Banks, 1992, pp 213–228
25. Goldman M, Blajchman M. Bacterial contamination. In: Popousky M

(ed) *Transfusion Reactions*. Bethesda, MD: American Association of Blood Banks, 1996, pp 126–158

26. Wagner SJ, Moroff G, Katz AJ, Friedman LI. Comparison of bacteria growth in single and pooled platelet concentrates after deliberate inoculation and storage. *Transfusion* 1995; **35**: 298–302

27. *Blood Weekly* 1997; **May 5**: 3–4

28. Illert WE, Sänger W, Weise W. Bacterial contamination of single-donor blood components. *Transfusion Med* 1995; **51**: 57–61

29. Lin L, Londe H, Janda JM *et al*. Photochemical inactivation of pathogenic bacteria in human platelet concentrates. *Blood* 1994; **83**: 2698–2706

30. Communicable Diseases Center. Year long estimation of the frequency of bacterial contamination of blood products in the United States. *Fed Register* 1997; **62**: 22952–22955

31. Springer GF, Horton RE. Blood group isoantibody stimulation in man by feeding blood group-active bacteria. *J Clin Invest* 1969; **48**: 1280–1291

32. Mollison PL, Engelfriet CP, Contreras M. Transfusion in oligaemia. In: *Blood Transfusion in Clinical Medicine*. Oxford: Blackwell Scientific Publications, 1993, pp 161–162

33. Urbaniak SJ, Robertson AE. A successful program for immunizing Rh-negative volunteers for anti-D production using frozen/thawed blood. *Transfusion* 1981; **21**: 64–69

34. Jakobowicz R, Williams L, Silberman F. Immunization of Rh negative volunteers by repeated injections of very small amounts of Rh positive blood. *Vox Sang* 1972; **23**: 376–381

35. Grove-Rasmussen M, Huggins CE. Selected types of frozen blood for patients with multiple blood group antibodies. *Transfusion* 1973; **13**: 124–129

36. Issitt PD. *Applied Blood Group Serology*, 3rd edn. Miami: Montgomery Scientific, 1985, pp 9–42

37. Walker RH, Lin D-T, Hartrick MB. Alloimmunization following blood transfusion. *Arch Pathol Lab Med* 1989; **113**: 254–261

38. Giblett ER. A critique of the theoretical hazard of inter- vs. intra-racial transfusion. *Transfusion* 1961; **1**: 233–238

39. Floss AM, Strauss RG, Goeken N, Knox L. Multiple transfusions fail to provoke antibodies against blood cell antigens in human infants. *Transfusion* 1986; **26**: 419–422

40. Ludvigsen CW Jr, Swanson JL, Thompson TR, McCullough J. The failure of neonates to form red blood cell alloantibodies in response to multiple transfusions. *Am J Clin Pathol* 1987; **87**: 250–251

41. Pass MA, Johnson JD, Shulman IA *et al*. Evaluation of a walking-donor blood transfusion program in an intensive care nursery. *J Pediatr* 1976; **89**: 646–651

42. Rawls WE, Wong CL, Blajchman M *et al*. Neonatal cytomegalovirus infections: the relative role of neonatal blood transfusion and maternal exposure. *Clin Invest Med* 1984; **7**: 13–19

43. Smith MR, Storey CG. Allo-anti-E in an 18-day-old infant (letter). *Transfusion* 1984; **24**: 540

44. DePalma L, Criss VR, Roseff SD, Luban NLC. Presence of the red cell alloantibody anti-E in an 11-week-old infant. *Transfusion* 1992; **32**: 177–179

45. Nurse GT. Directed donation and the developing world (letter). *Transfusion* 1993; **33**: 90

46. Holman P, Blajchman MA, Heddle N. Noninfectious adverse effects of blood transfusion in the neonate. *Transfusion Med Rev* 1995; **9**: 277–287

47. DePalma L, Duncan B, Chan MM, Luban NLC. The neonatal immune response to washed and irradiated red cells: lack of evidence of lymphocyte activation. *Transfusion* 1991; **31**: 737–742

48. Sarnaik S, Schornack J, Lusher JM. The incidence of development of irregular red cell antibodies in patients with sickle cell anemia. *Transfusion* 1986; **26**: 249–252

49. Orlina AR, Unger PJ, Koshy M. Post-transfusion alloimmunization in patients with sickle cell disease. *Am J Hematol* 1978; **5**: 101–106

50. Rosse WF, Gallagher D, Kinney TR *et al*. Transfusion and alloimmunization in sickle cell disease. *Blood* 1990; **76**: 1431–1437

51. Vichinsky EP, Earles A, Johnson RP *et al*. Alloimmunization in sickle cell anemia and transfusion of racially unmatched blood. *N Engl J Med* 1990; **322**: 1617–1621

52. Luban NLC. Variability in rates of alloimmunization in different groups of children with sickle cell disease: Effect of ethnic background. *Am J Pediatr Hematol Oncol* 1989; **11**: 314–319

53. Ambruso DR, Githens JH, Alcorn R *et al*. Experience with donors matched for minor blood group antigens in patients with sickle cell anemia who are receiving chronic transfusion therapy. *Transfusion* 1987; **27**: 94–98

54. Petz L, Garratty G. *Acquired Immune Hemolytic Anemias*. New York: Churchill Livingstone, 1980, pp 318–337

55. Diamond WJ, Brown FL, Bitterman P, Klein HG, Davey RJ, Winslow RM. Delayed hemolytic transfusion reaction presenting as sickle-cell crisis. *Ann Intern Med* 1980; **93**: 231–233

56. Cox JV, Steane E, Cunningham G, Frenkel P. Risk of alloimmunization and delayed hemolytic transfusion reactions in patients with sickle cell disease. *Arch Int Med* 1988; **148**: 2485–2489

57. Petz LD, Calhoun L, Shulman IA, Johnson C, Herron RM. The sickle cell hemolytic transfusion reaction syndrome. *Transfusion* 1997; **37**: 382–392

58. Sirchia G, Zanella A, Parravicini A, Morelati F, Rebulla P, Masera G. Red cell alloantibodies in thalassemia major. Results of an Italian cooperative study. *Transfusion* 1985; **25**: 110–112

59. Spanos Th, Karageorga M, Ladis V, Peristeri J, Hatziliami A, Kattamis Ch. Red cell alloantibodies in patients with thalassemia. *Vox Sang* 1990; **58**: 50–55

60. Michail-Merianou V, Pamphili-Panousopoulou L, Piperi-Lowes L, Pelegrinis E, Karaklis A. Alloimmunization to red cell antigens in thalassemia: Comparative study of usual versus better-match transfusion programmes. *Vox Sang* 1987; **52**: 95–98

61. King KE, Lankiewicz MW, Young-Ramsaran J, Ness PM. Delayed hemolytic transfusion reactions in sickle cell disease: simultaneous destruction of recipients' red cells. *Transfusion* 1997; **37**: 376–381

62. Lane TA, Anderson KC, Goodnough LT *et al*. Leukocyte reduction in blood component therapy. *Ann Intern Med* 1992; **117**: 151–162

63. Sirchia G, Rebulla P. Evidence-based medicine: the case for white cell reduction. *Transfusion* 1997; **37**: 543–549

64. Deeg HJ, Sigaroudinia M. Ultraviolet B-induced loss of HLA Class II antigen expression on lymphocytes is dose, time, and locus dependent. *Exp Hematol* 1990; **18**: 916–919

65. Andreu G, Boccaccio C, Klaren J *et al*. The role of UV radiation in the prevention of human leukocyte antigen alloimmunization. *Transfusion Med Rev* 1992; **6**: 212–224

66. Blundell EL, Pamphilon DH, Fraser ID *et al*. A prospective, randomized study of the use of platelet concentrates irradiated with ultraviolet-B light in patients with hematologic malignancy. *Transfusion* 1996; **36**: 296–302

67. Strauss RG. Selection of white cell-reduced blood components for transfusions during early infancy. *Transfusion* 1993; **33**: 352–357

68. Bedford-Russell AR, Rivers RPA, Davey N. The development of anti-HLA antibodies in multiply transfused preterm infants. *Arch Dis Child* 1993; **68**: 49–51

69. Skacel PO, Stacey TE, Tidmarsh CEF, Contreras M. Maternal alloimmunization to HLA, platelet and granulocyte-specific antigens during pregnancy: its influence on cord blood granulocyte and platelet counts. *Br J Haematol* 1989; **71**: 119–123

70. Elbert C, Strauss RG, Barrett F, Goeken NE, Pittner B, Cordle D. Biological mothers may be dangerous blood donors for their neonates. *Acta Haematol* 1991; **85**: 189–191

71. Godeau B, Fromont P, Seror T, Duedari N, Bierling P. Platelet alloimmunization after multiple transfusions: A prospective study of 50 patients. *Br J Haematol* 1992; **81**: 395–400

72. Howard JE, Perkins HA. The natural history of alloimmunization to platelets. *Transfusion* 1978; **818**: 496–503

73. Holohan TV, Terasaki PI, Deisseroth AB. Suppression of transfusion-related alloimmunization in intensively treated cancer patients. *Blood* 1981; **58**: 122–128

74. Kickler T, Kennedy SD, Braine HG. Alloimmunization to platelet-specific antigens on glycoproteins IIb-IIIa and Ib/IX in multiply transfused thrombocytopenic patients. *Transfusion* 1990; **30**: 622–625

75. Wolf CFW, Canale VC. Fatal pulmonary hypersensitivity reaction to HLA incompatible blood transfusion: report of a case and review of the literature. *Transfusion* 1976; **16**: 135–140

76. Shulman NR, Aster RH, Leitner A, Hiller MC. Immunoreactions involving platelets. V. Post-transfusion purpura due to a complement fixing antibody against a genetically controlled platelet antigen. A proposed mechanism for thrombocytopenia and its relevance in autoimmunity. *J Clin Invest* 1961; **40**: 1597–1620

77. McFarland JG. Posttransfusion Purpura. In: Popovsky MA (ed) *Transfusion Reactions.* Bethesda, MD: AABB Press, 1996, pp 205–229

78. Morrison FS, Mollison PL. Post transfusion purpura. *N Engl J Med* 1966; **275**: 243–248

79. Kickler TS, Ness PM, Herman JH, Bell WR. Studies on the pathophysiology of post-transfusion purpura. *Blood* 1986; **68**: 347–350

80. Chapman JF, Murphy MF, Berney SI *et al.* Post-transfusion purpura associated with anti-Baka and anti-PlA2 platelet antibodies and delayed haemolytic transfusion reaction. *Vox Sang* 1987; **52**: 313–317

81. Valentin N, Vergrcht A, Bignon J *et al.* HLA-Dw52a is involved in alloimmunization against PlA1 antigen. *Hum Immunol* 1990; **27**: 73–79

82. Brecher ME, Moore SB, Letendre L. Posttransfusion purpura: the therapeutic value of PlA1-negative platelets. *Transfusion* 1990; **30**: 433–435

83. Ohto H, Anderson KC. Survey of transfusion-associated graft-versus-host disease in immuno-competent recipients. *Transfusion Med Rev* 1996; **10**: 31–43

84. Lee TH, Donegan E, Slichter S, Busch MP. Transient increase in circulating donor leukocytes after allogeneic transfusions in immuno-competent recipients compatible with donor cell proliferation. *Blood* 1995; **85**: 1207–1214

85. Lee TH, Ohto H, Paglieroni T, Holland PV, Busch MP. Survival kinetics of specific donor leukocyte subsets in transfused immunocompetent patients. *Transfusion* 1996; **36**: 45S

86. Bekkum van DW, Vos O. Immunological aspects of homo- and heterologous bone marrow transplantation in irradiated mice. *J Cell Comp Physiol* 1957; **50**: 139–156

87. Rubinstein A, Radl J, Cottier H. Unusual combined immunodeficiency syndrome exhibiting kappa-IgD paraproteinemia, residual gut immunity and graft versus host reaction after plasma infusion. *Acta Pediatr Scand* 1973; **62**: 365–372

88. Wagner FF, Flegel WA. Transfusion associated graft-versus-host disease: risk due to homozygous HLA haplotypes. *Transfusion* 1995; **35**: 284–291

89. Antin JG, Ferrara JLM. Cytokine dysregulation and acute graft-versus-host disease. *Blood* 1992; **80**: 2964–2968

90. Vogelsang GB, Hess AD. Graft-versus-host disease: new directions for a persistent problem. *Blood* 1994; **84**: 2061–2067

91. Linden JV, Pisciotto PT. Transfusion-associated graft-versus-host disease and blood irradiation. *Transfusion Med Rev* 1992; **11**: 116–123

92. Ohto H, Anderson KC. Posttransfusion graft-versus-host disease in Japanese newborns. *Transfusion* 1996; **36**: 117–123

93. Hathaway WE, Brangle RW, Nelson TL, Roeckel IE. Aplastic anemia and alymphocytosis in an infant with hypogammaglobulinemia: Graft-versus-host reaction? *J Pediatr* 1966; **68**: 713–722

94. Sanders MR, Graeber JE. Posttransfusion-graft-versus-host disease in infancy. *J Pediatr* 1990; **117**: 159–163

95. Greenbaum BH. Transfusion-associated graft-versus-host disease: Historical perspectives, incidence, and current use of irradiated blood products. *J Clin Oncol* 1991; **9**: 1889–1902

96. Anderson KC, Weinstein HJ. Transfusion-associated graft-versus-host disease. *N Engl J Med* 1990; **323**: 315–321

97. Shivdasani RA, Haluska FG, Dock NL *et al.* Graft-versus-host disease associated with transfusion of blood from unrelated HLA-homozygous donors. *N Engl J Med* 1993; **328**: 766–770

98. Ohto H, Yasuda H, Noguchi M, Abe R. Risk of transfusion-associated graft-versus-host disease as a result of directed donations from relatives. *Transfusion* 1992; **32**: 691–693

99. Davey RJ. The effect of irradiation on blood components. In: Baldwin ML, Jeffries L (eds) *Irradiation of Blood Components.* Bethesda, MD: American Association of Blood Banks, 1992, pp 51–62

100. Blumberg N, Heal JM. Transfusion and recipient immune function. *Arch Pathol Lab Med* 1989; **113**: 246–253

101. Gascon P, Zoumbos NC, Young NS. Immunologic abnormalities in patients receiving multiple blood transfusions. *Ann Intern Med* 1984; **100**: 173–177

102. Kaplan J, Sarnaik S, Gitlin J, Lusher J. Diminished helper/suppressor lymphocyte ratios and natural killer activity in recipients of repeated blood transfusions. *Blood* 1984; **64**: 308–310

103. Blajchman MA. Allogeneic blood transfusions, immunomodulation, and postoperative bacterial infection: do we have the answers yet? *Transfusion* 1997; **37**: 121–125

104. Vamvakas ED. Perioperative blood transfusion and cancer recurrence: meta-analysis for explanation. *Transfusion* 1995; **35**: 760–768

105. Schreiber GB, Busch MP, Kleinman SH *et al.* The risk of transfusion-transmitted viral infections. *N Engl J Med* 1996; **334**: 1685–1690

106. Williams AE, Thomson RA, Schreiber GB *et al.* Estimates of infectious disease risk factors in US blood donors. *JAMA* 1997; **277**: 967–972

107. Conry-Cantilena C, Van Raden M, Gibble J *et al.* Routes of infection, viremia, and liver disease in blood donors found to have hepatitis C virus infection. *N Engl J Med* 1996; **334**: 1691–1696

108. Alter HJ. Posttransfusion hepatitis in the United States. In: Nishioka K *et al* (eds). *Viral hepatitis and liver disease.* Proceedings of the 8th International Symposium on Viral Hepatitis, Tokyo 1993. New York: Springer-Verlag, 1994, pp 551–553

109. Alter HJ. To C or not to C: These are the questions. *Blood* 1995; **85**: 1681–1695

110. Ogata NR, Alter HJ, Miller RH *et al.* Nucleotide sequence and mutation rate of the H strain of hepatitis C virus. *Proc Natl Acad Sci USA* 1991; **88**: 3392–3396

111. Shimitzu YK, Yoshikura H, Hijikata M *et al.* Neutralizing antibodies against hepatitis C virus and the emergence of neutralization escape mutant viruses. *J Virol* 1994; **68**: 1494–1500

112. Alter MJ, Margolis HS, Krawczynski K *et al.* The natural history of community-acquired hepatitis C in the United States. The sentinel counties chronic non-A, non-B hepatitis study team. *N Engl J Med* 1992; **327**: 1899–1905

113. Tong MJ, El-Farra NS, Reikes AR *et al.* Clinical outcomes after transfusion-associated hepatitis C. *N Engl J Med* 1995; **332**: 1463–1466

114. Management of Hepatitis C. *NIH Consensus Statement 1997* March 24–26; 15(13) (in press)

115. Kelly DA. Hepatitis C infection after blood product transfusion. *Arch Dis Child* 1996; **75**: 363–365

116. Palomba E, Manzini P, Fiammengo P *et al.* Natural history of perinatal hepatitis C virus infection. *Commun Infect Dis* 1996; **23**: 47–50

117. Ohto H, Terazawa S, Sasaki N *et al.* Transmission of hepatitis C from mothers to infants. *N Engl J Med* 1994; **330**: 744–750

118. Monteleone PM, Andrzejewski C, Kelleher JF. Prevalence of antibodies to hepatitis C virus in transfused children with cancer. *Am J Pediatr Hematol Oncol* 1994; **16**: 309–313

119. Neilson JR, Harrison P, Skidmore SJ, *et al.* Chronic hepatitis C in long term survivors of haematological malignancy treated in a single center. *J Clin Pathol* 1996; **49**: 230–233

120. Cesaro S, Petris MG, Rossetti F, *et al.* Chronic hepatitis C infection after treatment for pediatric malignancy. *Blood* 1997; **90**: 1315–1320

121. Ni Y, Chang M, Lin K *et al.* Hepatitis C viral infection in thalassemic children: Clinical and molecular studies. *Pediatr Res* 1996; **39**: 323–328

122. Alter H, Nakatsuji Y, Melpolder J *et al.* The incidence of transfusion-associated hepatitis G virus and its relation to liver disease. *N Engl J Med* 1997; **336**: 747–754

123. Tacke M, Kiyosawa K, Stark K *et al.* Detection of antibodies to a putative hepatitis G virus envelope protein. *Lancet* 1997; **349**: 318–320

124. Schleuter V, Schmolke S, Stark K *et al*. Reverse transcription-PCR detection of hepatitis G virus. *J Clin Microbiol* 1996; **34**: 2660–2664

125. Dille BJ, Surowy TK, Guitierrez RA *et al*. An ELISA for detection of antibodies to the E2 protein of GB virus C. *J Infect Dis* 1997; **175**: 458–461

126. Alter HJ. G-pers creepers, where'd you get those papers? A reassessment of the literature on the hepatitis G virus. *Transfusion* 1997; **37**: 569–572

127. Stark K, Bienzle U, Hess G *et al*. Detection of the hepatitis G virus genome among injecting drug users, homosexual and bisexual men, and blood donors. *J Infect Dis* 1996; **174**: 1320–1323

128. Roth W, Waschk D, Marx S *et al*. Prevalence of hepatitis G virus and its strain variant, the GB agent in blood donations and their transmission to recipients. *Transfusion* 1997; **37**: 651–656

129. Alter HJ, Nakatsuji Y, Melpolder J *et al*. The incidence of transfusion-associated hepatitis G virus infection and its relation to liver disease. *N Engl J Med* 1997; **336**: 747–754

130. Alter M, Gallagher M, Morris T *et al*. Acute non A-E hepatitis in the United States and the role of hepatitis G infection. *N Engl J Med* 1997; **336**: 741–746

131. Bralet MP, Roudot-Throval F, Pawlotsky JM *et al*. Histopathologic impact of GB virus C infection on chronic hepatitis C. *Gastroenterology* 1997; **112**: 188–192

132. Feucht H, Zollner B, Polywka S *et al*. Vertical transmission of hepatitis G. *Lancet* 1996; **347**: 615–616

133. Fischler B, Lara C, Chen M *et al*. Genetic evidence for mother-to-infant transmission of hepatitis G virus. *J Infect Dis* 1997; **176**: 281–285

134. Neilson J, Harrison P, Milligan DW *et al*. Hepatitis G virus in long-term survivors of haematological malignancy. *Lancet* 1996; **347**: 1632–1633

135. Kudo T, Morishima T, Tsuzuki *et al*. Hepatitis G virus in immuno-suppressed paediatric allograft recipients. *Lancet* 1996; **348**: 751

136. Lopez-Alcorocho JM, Millan A, Garcia-Trevijano ER *et al*. Detection of hepatitis GB virus type C RNA in serum and liver of children with chronic viral hepatitis B and C. *Hepatology* 1997; **25**: 1258–1260

137. Kew MC, Kissianides C. HGV: hepatitis G virus or harmless G virus? *Lancet* 1996; **348 (Suppl II)**: 10

138. Kao JH, Chen PJ, Wang JT *et al*. Blood-bank screening for hepatitis G. *Lancet* 1997; **349**: 207

139. Busch MD, Young MJ, Simpson SM *et al*. Risk of human immunodeficiency virus transmission by blood transfusion prior to implementation of HIV antibody screening in the San Francisco Bay area. *Transfusion* 1991; **31**: 4–11

140. Kleinman SH, Niland JC, Azen SP *et al*. Prevalence of antibodies to human immunodeficiency virus type: among blood donors prior to screening: the Transfusion Safety Study/NHLBI donor repository *Transfusion* 1989; **29**: 572–580

141. Rawal BD, Busch MP, Endoow R *et al*. Reduction of human immunodeficiency virus-infected cells from donor blood by leukocyte filtration. *Transfusion* 1989; **26**: 460–462

142. Jones DS, Byers RH, Bush TJ, Oxtoby MJ, Rogers MF. Epidemiology of Transfusion-Associated Acquired Immunodeficiency Syndrome in children in the United States, 1981 through 1989. *Pediatrics* 1993; **89**: 123–127

143. Lieb LE, Mundy TM, Goldfinger D *et al*. Unrecognized human immunodeficiency virus type 1 infection in a cohort of transfused neonates: a retrospective investigation. *Pediatrics* 1995; **95**: 717–721

144. Wayne C, Cornell M, O'Donnell R, Caldwell B, Luban NLC. Seroprevalence of HIV in a tranfused pediatric cardiac cohort in a high prevalence area. *Transfusion* 1993; **33**: 544

145. Gunter KC, Luban NLC. Transfusion transmitted cytomegalovirus In Rossi EC, Simm TL, Moss GS, Gould SA (eds) *Principles of Transfusion Medicine*. Baltimore: Williams & Wilkins, 1996, pp 717–733

146. Sayers MH, Anderson KC, Goodnough LT *et al*. Reducing the risk for transfusion-transmitted cytomegalovirus. *Ann Intern Med* 1992; **116**: 55–62

147. Popovsky MA, Benson K, Glassman AB *et al*. Transfusion Practices in human immunodeficiency virus infected patients. *Transfusion* 1995; **35**: 612–616

148. Lamberson HV, McMillan JA, Weiner LB *et al*. Prevention of transfusion-associated cytomeglalovirus (CMV) infection in neonates by screening donors for IgM to CMV. *J Infect Dis* 1988; **157**: 820–823

149. Przepiorka D, LeParc GF, Werch J, Lictiger B. Prevention of transfusion-associated cytomegalovirus infection: Practice parameter. *Am J Clin Path* 1996; **106**: 163–169

150. Bowden RA, Slichter SJ, Sayers M *et al*. A comparison of filtered leukocyte-reduced and cytomegalovirus (CMV) seronegative blood products for the prevention of transfusion-associated CMV infection after marrow transplant. *Blood* 1995; **86**: 3598–3603

151. Landaw EM, Kanter M, Petz LD. Safety of filtered leukocyte-reduced blood products for prevention of transfusion-associated cytomegalovirus infection (letter). *Blood* 1996; **87**: 4910

152. Ledent E, Berlin G. Factors influencing white cell removal from red cell concentrates by filtration. *Transfusion* 1976; **36**: 714–718

153. American Association of Blood Banks. *AABB Association Bulletin*, #97.2. April 23, 1997

Management of infection in children with bone marrow failure

IAN M HANN

The development of new and often more successful regimens of treatment for childhood blood and malignant diseases has usually been associated with a panoply of infectious problems. In recent years these successes have often, in the absence of new effective drugs, been achieved by pushing the dosages and frequency of administration of conventional drugs beyond previous limits. Such dosage intensification can only proceed with improvements in supportive care in much the same way that heroic surgery requires advances in anesthesiology and intensive care methods. This chapter is not intended to deal with every possible infection or clinical manifestation of such, but rather to be a practical current guide to the management of infection. The last few years have seen major improvements in the development of hematopoietic growth factors, new antifungal agents, new antibiotics and new ways to use aminoglycosides. Attempts are being made to identify good and poor risk factors for outcome of infection in order to facilitate shorter courses of antimicrobial agents. In addition, the special needs of children are being recognized in view of the restricted use of quinolones in this age group and the different organisms and types of infection that they experience.

INFECTIONS IN NEUTROPENIC CHILDREN

Comparison with adults

There are several recent large reviews of children with serious infections and neutropenia. The largest compared 759 children with 2321 adults admitted to 4 European Organization for Research into the Treatment of Cancer (EORTC) International Antimicrobial Therapy Group (IATG) trials.[1] This is the ideal way to look at patterns of infection and to determine whether risk factors predicting outcome can be identified. Children tended to have lower risk disease with regard to outcome of infection compared

with adults, despite common enrolment criteria within the EORTC centers, i.e. fever and neutropenia. Not surprisingly, the children had acute myeloid leukemia (AML) less frequently and acute lymphoblastic leukemia (ALL) more often, and proportionately more children were undergoing intensive therapy for solid tumors. On average, the diagnostic groups more frequently seen in children are more likely to respond to antimicrobial therapy, presumably because their blood counts recover more rapidly and reliably. The children had more upper respiratory and fewer lower respiratory sites of infection. The incidence of bacteremia in these febrile neutropenic children was similar to that in the adults (22% versus 24%), but pyrexia of unknown origin was commoner in the younger patients (49% versus 38% in adults) due to a lower incidence of clinically documented infections including pneumonias. The pattern of organisms causing bacteremia was also different, children experiencing more streptococcal species in blood cultures, whilst adults had more staphylococcal species. Most importantly, it was shown for the first time that the outcome in febrile neutropenic children was better with an overall success rate for the initial empirical regimen of 66% versus 59% in adults and a lower mortality of 3% versus 10%. Mortality rate from infection was only 1% in children compared with 4% in adults and time to deferevescence of temperature was shorter in the younger age group (median of 3 versus 4 days).

Bone marrow transplant patients

One of the dramatic changes in practice over the last few years has been the introduction of non-matched or non-sibling allogeneic bone marrow transplants. Previously, such procedures were associated with an unacceptably high risk of rejection, graft-versus-host disease (GVHD) and infection. However, this picture has changed and a review from Minneapolis has looked at the pattern of late infection in these children.[2] The period after 7 weeks from the day of transplant was examined because the development of unrelated donor-bone marrow transplant (UD-BMT) has been associated with delayed infection problems, which is at least in part related to the prolonged immunosuppression (including high-dose steroids) and more frequent and severe GVHD. One hundred and fifty-one matched sibling donor (MSD) BMT procedures were compared with 98 UD-BMT; 85% of UD-BMT children developed late infections compared with 68% in the MSD group. Two-thirds of infections occurred within the first 6 months and few after the first year, but UD-BMT patients were at risk for longer. About half of the infections were bacterial, evenly split between Gram-negative and -positive organisms. Slightly more than one-third were viral and of these a third were due to cytomegalovirus (CMV), with the remainder due to herpes simplex (HSV), varicella zoster (VZV), respiratory syncytial virus (RSV) and influenza viruses. Eleven percent were due to fungi; in the UD-BMT group, half were due to candida and a quarter to aspergillus.

Children on antileukemic therapy

Over the last decade, treatment for AML has become much more intensive and survival has dramatically improved. Patients with AML have frequent infections and are at risk of overwhelming Gram-negative bacteremia and serious systemic fungal infections. Children with ALL have a better prognosis overall and fewer serious infections. However, it is all the more tragic when an eminently curable child dies of an infection induced principally by the antileukemic therapy. A recent review from the UK Acute Lymphoblastic Leukaemia (UKALL) trials run by the Medical Research Council serves as a good contemporary review of the problem.[3] Between 1985 and 1990, 1612 children were entered into the UKALL X trial. Thirty-eight (2.3%) died during the first 4 induction weeks; 31 died from infections of which 19 were due to bacteria, 9 fungi and 3 unknown infection. Gram-negative bacteria accounted for 12 cases, 7 being Gram positive, 4 aspergillus, 4 candida and 1 mucor infection. Thus, the message is that Gram-negative cover (which the author believes should include an aminoglycoside as well as another agent [vide infra]), as well as Gram-positive cover in a broad-spectrum empirical antibiotic regimen given immediately to these febrile neutropenic patients, remains essential. Also, the physician must remain wary of deep-seated fungal infections, especially aspergillus affecting the lower and upper airways (including the paranasal sinuses) and candida involving the liver and spleen. The use of empirical amphotericin therapy must also be continued for patients who remain febrile after 3 or 4 days of broad-spectrum antibiotic therapy.

The UKALL X study also looked at those patients who entered and remained in complete remission after the induction month. There were 53 deaths in these patients (3.3%); 37 (70%) were due to infection (11 bacterial [4 Gram-positive, 3 Gram-negative and 4 presumed but not microbiologically documented], 7 to fungal infection [2 aspergillus, 3 candida and 2 unconfirmed] and 3 to *Pneumocystis carinii* pneumonia). There were also 16 viral infections due to: measles (5 cases), HSV (2), VZV (2), RSV (2), CMV (1), mumps (1) and 2 pneumonias and 1 encephalitis of unknown cause. These results indicate that prophylaxis with co-trimoxazole against pneumocystis pneumonia must be considered (see below), and the vaccination of all contacts against measles encouraged. The question of VZV vaccination remains controversial and is discussed below.

RISK FACTORS AND PROGNOSTIC FACTORS WITH REGARD TO OUTCOME OF INFECTION

The UKALL X study showed clearly that children with Down's syndrome and also girls with ALL are at increased risk of fatal infection. In addition, as is well known, fatal infections occurred more frequently in those patients with very high risk ALL who received an allogeneic BMT in first remission. There have been a number of other studies which have sought to predict who might be susceptible to serious infections and also, amongst those with fever, who will prove to have bacteremia.[4-6] The aim of these studies was to try to predict who can safely receive attenuated courses of antibiotics or even be treated at home or on experimental monotherapy antibiotic protocols.

The EORTC study looked at 759 children in 4 antibiotic trials and showed that high temperature, prolonged neutropenia prior to fever and shock were prognostic indicators for the presence of bacteremia (which carries a relatively poor prognosis).[1] It has been known for many years that length and severity of neutropenia are consistent features of a poorer outcome.[7] However, it must be remembered that the level of neutrophils may be an indicator correlated with other defects leading to susceptibility and impaired response to infection. For example, monocyte and splenic function is impaired in these children and such defects are probably of major importance in dealing with fungal infection, especially following BMT and total body irradiation.[8]

Three other studies have looked at small groups of children with neutropenia. A study from North Carolina included 276 episodes of fever and neutropenia and found that children with leukemia had more episodes of infection than those with solid tumors undergoing intensive therapy.[4] They also found that, as with many previous studies in adults, patients with severe neutropenia ($<0.2 \times 10^9$/l) had more of the higher risk types of infections with fungi, Gram-negative bacteremia and infection with multiple organisms. A study of 150 febrile episodes in 72 neutropenic children from Indianapolis[5] showed for the first time that low monocyte levels ($<0.1 \times 10^9$/l) predicted a poorer outcome, suggesting again that there is not just the problem of low neutrophils. They also confirmed the adverse prognostic importance of high temperature ($>39°C$). Finally, a study from New York[6] examined 500 episodes of fever in this situation. As in the EORTC study, shock at presentation was an important poor risk feature and again the most important adverse prognostic variable was persistent neutropenia ($<0.1 \times 10^9$/l) after 48 hours of antimicrobial treatment. The authors conclude that patients whose neutrophil counts begin to recover at 48 hours can be discharged for outpatient therapy. This is a potentially important development which could lead to more cost-effective therapy out of hospital, but it needs to be verified in prospective studies.

In conclusion, patients with high temperature and persistent neutropenia and also those with hypovolemic shock are at highest risk of serious infection and these tend to be children with leukemia, especially those with AML and following BMT.

PROPHYLAXIS

Having defined the groups of patients who are susceptible to severe infection, it is of course logical to consider preventing such events. In fact this has proved to be a great deal more difficult than was ever envisaged. One of the overriding problems has been the difficulty of organizing large randomized trials. In this area, placebo-controlled and double-blind studies are undoubtedly the ideal because there is little evidence, with few exceptions, that anything works and the end points are open to observer prejudice, e.g. the institution of therapeutic courses of antibiotics. In addition, it has not been possible to perform trials of prophylaxis with quinolone antibiotics which are active in preventing Gram-negative infections in adults but which may carry a risk of arthropathy in children.[9]

MOUTH CARE AND ORAL NON-ABSORBABLE ANTIBIOTICS

These maneuvers are best considered together because that is what the patient is expected to do. In real life, all mouth care and oral non-absorbable antibiotic (ONA) regimens are extremely difficult to manage in children. Although there have been many vogues for prevention of infection with ONA,[10,11] the regimens are usually very unpalatable, may cause diarrhea and compliance is almost impossible without psychologic disturbance in children. It is not surprising therefore that evidence that such regimens are effective in preventing infection in young patients is lacking. With regard to mouth care, there is no doubt that this modality of therapy is important and certainly improves the tolerability of therapy,[10] although which mouth washes should be used is unclear, with evidence that chlorhexidine causes discomfort, taste change and teeth staining.[11] Ideally, all patients should have regular dental checks in order to reduce the risk of infections, gum problems and mucositis.

FUNGAL INFECTIONS

The increasing prevalence of fungal infection, allied to the rising use of unrelated BMT and very intensive therapy for diseases like AML, is one of the greatest challenges in antileukemic therapy. Treatment of these infections is difficult, often involves unacceptable costs and toxicity and is frequently unsuccessful. Therefore, this is a situation that demands prevention but this has met with only limited success. The use of high efficiency air filter systems has undoubtedly reduced the risk of aspergillus infection in high-risk patients.[12] Avoidance of other high-risk factors such as prolonged courses of high-dose steroids in susceptible patients (e.g. BMT patients with GVHD) is desirable where feasible. Susceptible patients should be nursed in air-filtered rooms wherever possible and avoid contact with spores from compost heaps and food with a high spore content, such as pepper.

Three main oral drug prophylaxis regimens have been tried. The original schedules contained frequent high-dose polyenes (nystatin and oral amphotericin) and these are still widely used, although the evidence for their efficacy is limited and they are often not well tolerated by children. More recently, a large multicenter trial in 502 children showed that once daily oral fluconazole prophylaxis was more effective than the polyenes in preventing oropharyngeal candidiasis.[13] This drug is palatable and the once daily usage is a major bonus; however, it should only be used in patients with a high risk of candida infection, because of the danger of emergence of resistant strains, e.g. *Candida cruzei*, and because it will probably not prevent infection with other fungi such as aspergillus. The other imidazole, intraconazole, may have greater efficacy in also preventing aspergillus infections and is currently being evaluated. A different approach has been to use nasal amphotericin prophylaxis.[14] Most trials have been small or non-randomized, but have purported to show a reduction in serious aspergillus infection. Some are difficult to interpret because of concomitant use of other agents such as intravenous amphotericin.[14] Neither the use of sprays nor intravenous amphotericin or intravenous lipid amphotericin preparations have been adequately evaluated and thus have not entered routine practice.

PNEUMOCYSTIS CARINII INFECTION

It has been known for 20 years that this infection, with an organism now believed to be a fungus, can be prevented by co-trimoxazole prophylaxis. What has been more uncertain is whether this antibiotic can prevent other infections.[15] In general, the prophylactic effect against bacterial infections is at best a weak one and thus co-trimoxazole is now used almost exclusively to prevent pneumocystis infection. Reactions to it are very uncommon and other antibiotics and maneuvers, such as the use of inhaled pentamidine, have a much shorter track record and may be more toxic and less effective. Patients at highest risk of pneumocystis pneumonia are those undergoing allogeneic BMT, infants receiving intensive protocols for ALL and other patients following induction therapy for ALL. Pentamidine inhalations are usually reserved for children who do not tolerate co-trimoxazole and are at very high risk of infection, e.g. previous pneumocystis pneumonia, infant lymphoblastic leukemia and allogeneic BMT.

ANTIVIRAL PROPHYLAXIS

As stated above, the most important preventive measure against viral infection is vaccination. Where vaccines are live or live attenuated as with measles, the conventional policy is to rely upon herd immunity and vaccination of siblings and other child contacts. There is a continuing controversy over the prevention of VZV infections which rarely cause fatal infections now that intravenous acyclovir can cure most infections and prompt use of zoster immune globulin (ZIG) following contact can prevent most serious episodes. However, the risk of infection is still quite high with an approximate risk of 4.6/100 patient years in children undergoing continuation therapy for ALL.[16] The problem with vaccination is that the treatment schedule has to be interrupted for several weeks and mild skin reactions are relatively common. Currently, this is an unresolved issue, although cost–benefit analysis indicates that vaccination is likely to be safe and to reduce the need for painful intramuscular ZIG injections.

Several studies have shown that herpes simplex infections can be prevented in patients undergoing BMT procedures and treatment for leukemia.[17] As a consequence, most BMT patients are given oral acyclovir prophylaxis during the period of neutropenia. Longer periods of prophylaxis for a number of months may prevent some VZV infections but the risk period is long and there is clearly a problem with diminishing returns. In childhood, herpes simplex infections are uncommon other than in BMT patients and it is usually not considered justified to use acyclovir prophylactically when there will be a long period of relatively low risk and the possibility of allowing the development of resistant viral strains. CMV infection is not prevented to any clinically significant extent by oral acyclovir prophylaxis but a recently published policy which shows promise is high-dose intravenous acyclovir followed by pre-emptive therapy (based on positive blood tests for CMV viremia or bronchoalveolar lavage) with ganciclovir.[18] In view of the fact that CMV infection is a serious problem following allogeneic BMT, various prophylactic measures have been attempted, including vaccination.[19] The introduction of CMV antibody-negative blood products and leukocyte-depletion filters has probably significantly reduced the risk of infection, although there is no definite proof of this. The use of intravenous hyperimmune globulin has also been associated with a reduced risk of infection.

INDWELLING VENOUS CATHETER SEPSIS

It is always assumed, although rarely proven, that many infections occurring in the modern era are caused or exacerbated by the now ubiquitous indwelling intravenous catheters. Thus, it would be good to prevent such infections. It is often forgotten that by far the most important means of preventing infection in any situation is by very careful handwashing. This is particularly true when handling intravenous catheters and it is everyone's experience that problems with infection increase when there is inadequate or over-pressurized nursing. The use of other measures is less scientific and often cumbersome, psychologically damaging and ineffective. Face masks are only valuable for short high-risk procedures. Head and shoe covering is of no proven value but wearing aprons is of value when moving from patient to patient. Parents can stay with their children unless they have a transmissible infection and do not need to wear protective garments unless carrying out high-risk procedures such as catheter manipulations.

The value of continuous staff and family education regarding aseptic techniques in handling catheters was shown serendipitously in a well-designed trial.[20] Children with central venous catheters were entered into a placebo-controlled double-blind study of adding broad-spectrum antibiotics to the flush solution. By doing the trial, as is often the case, the authors heightened awareness of the problem and reduced the incidence of infection to a level which made it impossible to assess the effectiveness or otherwise of the antibiotic flush. Their conclusion is to be commended: "staff education is essential and probably the most effective factor in preventing catheter-related sepsis". It should be added that educating the parents is just as important. There are no other proven effective methodologies, although it is likely that it is important to have a surgeon within each unit who is responsible for carefully and continuously monitoring the infectious complications and surgical procedures.

PLANNED PROGRESSIVE ANTIMICROBIAL THERAPY

ANTIBIOTICS

Over the last 25 years since early empirical antibiotic therapy first came into routine practice, there have been a multitude of attempts to modify the protocols.[21] Clinicians who are not microbiologists nor infectious disease specialists can be forgiven if they are totally confused by the number of very small trials of new antibiotics carried out in very heterogeneous groups of patients. Such trials are really of no value because they stand no chance of reaching secure conclusions. Fortunately, the EORTC IATG has led the way in large multicenter trials whereby the number of patient entries meets statistical criteria for meaningful end-points. Several recent important advances have been made with this approach, including the demonstration that single daily dosing of an aminoglycoside (amikacin given with ceftriaxone in this trial)[22] was as effective as multiple daily dosing of an aminoglycoside (with ceftazidime). Subsequently, there has been a deluge of papers about once daily aminoglycoside therapy which have been subjected to the newly reinvented specialty of evidence-based medicine.[23–25] The conclusion of all these studies has been that once daily aminoglycosides have a lower risk of nephrotoxicity, probably equivalent risk of ototoxicity and equivalent or possibly superior efficacy. There has not been a vast published experience in children, but where this has been examined, the above statements hold up.[26] The utility of measuring serum concentrations remains controversial and there is currently no good evidence to support the measurement of peak concentrations when using single daily dosing. However, trough level monitoring is of value although it is uncertain as to whether this should be done at 8 or 24 hours after the previous dose. Overall, it has been stated that, "once daily dosing of aminoglycosides should become the routine way these drugs are administered in clinical practice".[25]

Another contentious issue has been whether or not the use of an aminoglycoside could be omitted and instead monotherapy could be used with a drug such as ceftazidime. The largest study of this problem investigated the possibility of dropping the aminoglycoside after 3 days in combination with ceftazidime.[27] This approach was adopted as a 'halfway house' because of the potential damage of single agent therapy in high-risk neutropenic patients. Gram-negative bacteremia occurred in 129 of 872 evaluable patients and the success rate with short courses of amikacin was 48% versus 81% for the longer courses (p = 0.002). Among patients with neutrophils of <0.001 × 10^9/l, the response rate was only 6% with the short course of amikacin and long course of ceftazidime and 50% with prolonged amikacin and cetazidime. The conclusion is that, where Gram-negative bacteremia is a risk, it is not justified to drop the aminoglycoside nor to give very short courses, although recent evidence suggests that once daily dosing with a carbapenem such as meropenem may be justified in low risk patients.

When choosing which antibiotic combination to use empirically for fever and neutropenia, it is absolutely essential to know about the local flora and fauna. Close liaison with microbiologists and infectious disease specialists is never more important than when making these decisions. One major consideration, for example, would be the existence of multi-resistant organisms within an individual institution. Thus, the recommendations below must not be regarded as being cast in stone, must be regularly reviewed and should be adapted to local circumstances. It is not the only possible approach but is based on the larger available studies (Fig. 37.1). The principle involved is that the regimen must have excellent Gram-negative cover and efficacy, with a broad spectrum of cover against other organisms. Piperacillin-tazobactam was chosen on the basis of a study of 858 febrile

episodes in neutropenic patients.[28] Although cutaneous reactions were more frequently associated with piperacillin-tazobactam, these were relatively mild and this antibiotic with amikacin was superior to amikacin plus ceftazidime with regard to overall efficacy, faster time to resolution of fever and better efficacy in bacteremia (50% versus 35% for ceftazidime). Thus, the empirical regimen suggested in Fig. 37.1 is once daily aminoglycoside plus pip-tazobactam. In fact, there is little evidence with regard to the choice of aminoglycoside and the choice should rest on an assessment of local circumstances.

The proposed planned progressive approach to therapy suggested in Fig. 37.1 contains a number of other controversial features. An assessment on day 2 or 3 is valuable because this is the stage at which blood culture results become available. If Gram-positive organisms are grown and the patient is responding, then it is reasonable to continue with the empirical regimen because in the EORTC studies such a policy was associated with a good outcome. However, the addition of vancomycin or teicoplanin at this stage for a microbiologically proven Gram-positive infection is an alternative approach. This does not mean that all patients with an inflamed central venous catheter exit site should be treated with an additional Gram-positive agent because there is only a poor correlation between this frequent clinical finding and the existence of serious Gram-positive infections.

MANAGEMENT OF UNRESPONSIVE FEVER AND ANTIFUNGAL THERAPY

Children with persistent severe neutropenia frequently do not respond to a wide variety of antimicrobial agents. It must, however, be remembered that the mortality in this situation is very low and defervescence often occurs only when the blood counts begin to recover and probably irrespective of what therapy is given. Thus, a panic-stricken approach to the problem is entirely unjustified, especially when it involves multiple agents which are potentially toxic, not efficacious and antagonistic. For example, the use of metronidazole should be reserved for high-risk situations, e.g. children with real perineal problems or gastrointestinal fistulae, because anaerobic infections are otherwise very rare in this situation. There is no justification for using this drug for every patient with diarrhea, sinusitis or oral mucositis. The most important point is regularly to repeat blood cultures and to look carefully clinically and with chest X-rays for specific infections. One important point is to look for disseminated candidiasis in patients with splenomegaly (abdominal sonar) and for aspergillosis in patients with rhinosinusitis and those with suggestive X-ray changes and/or pleuritic pain, when CT scanning is most sensitive.

The empirical use of amphotericin after 72–96 hours in patients who are persistently febrile and neutropenic is a valuable approach.[29] Other empirical approaches such as the use of intravenous fluconazole and liposomal amphotericin have been tried.[30,31] However, the numbers in the

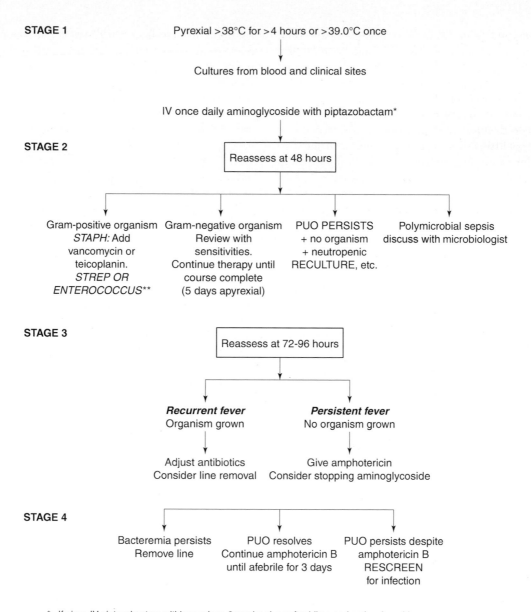

STAGE 1   Pyrexial >38°C for >4 hours or >39.0°C once

Cultures from blood and clinical sites

IV once daily aminoglycoside with piptazobactam*

STAGE 2   Reassess at 48 hours

Gram-positive organism	Gram-negative organism	PUO PERSISTS	Polymicrobial sepsis
STAPH: Add vancomycin or teicoplanin. *STREP OR ENTEROCOCCUS***	Review with sensitivities. Continue therapy until course complete (5 days apyrexial)	+ no organism + neutropenic RECULTURE, etc.	discuss with microbiologist

STAGE 3   Reassess at 72-96 hours

Recurrent fever
Organism grown

Persistent fever
No organism grown

Adjust antibiotics
Consider line removal

Give amphotericin
Consider stopping aminoglycoside

STAGE 4

Bacteremia persists
Remove line

PUO resolves
Continue amphotericin B
until afebrile for 3 days

PUO persists despite
amphotericin B
RESCREEN
for infection

*   If given IV piptazobactam within previous 2 weeks give ceftazidime and aminoglycoside.
     If ceftazidime-resistant organisms or ceftazidime within previous 2 weeks, give ciprofloxacin + aminoglycoside first.
** If on piptazobactam and aminoglycoside, review with sensitivities. If on ceftazidime or ciprofloxacin + aminoglycoside add vancomycin or teicoplanin as in *Staph.* regimen.

Fig. 37.1 Planned progressive approach to infection in severely neutropenic children.

studies are not large enough to be sure of equivalent efficacy. Both fluconazole and liposomal amphotericin are significantly less toxic but there is a problem with the emergence or resistant organisms such as *Candida cruzei* when using fluconazole and with cost with the liposomal preparation. In a recent trial, 134 adults and 204 children were randomized to receive Amphotericin B or AmBisome 1 mg/kg/day or AmBisome 3 mg/kg/day. In both AmBisome arms there was a 2–6-fold reduction in the incidence of drug-related toxicity and severe side-effects occurred in only 1% of AmBisome patients versus 12% of those treated with Amphotericin B. Nephrotoxicity occurred in 1.4% of the liposomal-treated patients and in 23% of those on the conventional drug.[31]

For many years, Amphotericin B (Amph B) has remained the gold standard and there is now a great need to assess the efficacy of the new lipid-based compounds Abelcet, Amphocil and AmBisome. These 3 formulations differ significantly in composition and pharmacokinetics from each other and all 3 have lower nephrotoxicity than Amphotericin B, with Amphocil showing the highest level of acute reactions and AmBisome the lowest rate.[32] Subsequent studies have also shown that the liposomal preparation AmBisome is associated with a lower rate of subsequent proven systemic infection than conventional Amphotericin B. The approximate dosage of these compounds for prophylactic and therapeutic use is uncertain, but some studies have shown that dosages can be increased and patients with deep-seated mycoses not responding to Amph B have responded to the lipid preparation.[33] However, the practice of putting Amph B into fat emulsion should be discontinued because they do not mix.[34] In conclusion, the lipid formulations is usually restricted to patients with renal dysfunction or severe hypokalemia and those with deep-seated fungal infection not responding very promptly to Amph B. The use of monocyte/macrophage growth factors to treat fungal infection is addressed below.

VIRAL INFECTIONS AND INTERSTITIAL PNEUMONIA

Most viral infections occur at times when patients are not neutropenic and thus this subject is not dealt with in great detail here. The only very effective antiviral agent is acyclovir which is an active agent for herpes simplex and VZV infections. There is no really effective treatment for measles, pneumonia or encephalitis, although various drugs such as interferons and ribavirin have been tried, along with intravenous immunoglobulin. CMV infection does occasionally occur in neutropenic children, sometimes with hepatitis or gastroenterologic problems, but usually with an interstitial pneumonia (Fig. 37.2). The management of pneumonia is tricky and there is again a temptation to indulge in polypharmacy. Fig. 37.2 provides a suggested plan of action and there are some additional points which are worth making. First, it is most important to institute a thorough diagnostic search at an early stage. Secondly, with the proposed approach, it is now very rarely necessary

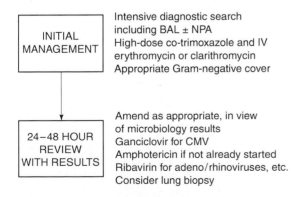

CAUSES
- *Pneumocystis carinii*
- cytomegalovirus
- measles (usually *no* preceding rash)
- varicella-zoster (rare)
- fungal infections
- mycoplasma; Legionella
- common respiratory viruses: influenza, parainfluenza, adenovirus, RSV

INITIAL MANAGEMENT → Intensive diagnostic search including BAL ± NPA
High-dose co-trimoxazole and IV erythromycin or clarithromycin
Appropriate Gram-negative cover

24–48 HOUR REVIEW WITH RESULTS → Amend as appropriate, in view of microbiology results
Ganciclovir for CMV
Amphotericin if not already started
Ribavirin for adeno/rhinoviruses, etc.
Consider lung biopsy

Fig. 37.2 Management plan for interstitial pneumonia. BAL = bronchoalveolar lavage; NPA = nasopharyngeal aspirate; CMV = cytomegalovirus; RSV = respiratory syncytial virus.

to proceed to lung biopsy with the risk of bleeding, pneumothorax, etc., because the patients usually respond to therapy or there is an answer from less invasive tests. Finally, *Pneumocystis carinii* pneumonia will often respond to high dosages of co-trimoxazole with or without pentamidine. Non-responders usually respond to steroid therapy and, if not, moribund patients have been rescued by surfactant therapy.

HEMATOPOIETIC GROWTH FACTORS

Very few good clinical studies have been carried out with these new agents and these have been recently reviewed.[35] It can be said that granulocyte colony-stimulating factor (G-CSF) reduces the duration of neutropenia and probably leads to a reduced number of febrile days and days on antibiotics in adults and children undergoing BMT for non-myeloid disorders. Their safety in children with myeloid disorders, i.e. mainly AML, is largely unproven. Their efficacy in other situations, e.g. the primary treatment of infection in neutropenic patients and in the prevention of infection in other high-risk groups such as patients receiving intensive ALL protocols, is also unproven. A number of trials are allegedly underway and currently it is probably reasonable to reserve G-CSF therapy for patients who would previously have been given granulocyte-rich transfusions. The latter have been abandoned in most centers because of their dubious efficacy, infection transmission risk and the associated severe logistic difficulties.

As previously stated, there is some evidence that macrophage CSF (M-CSF) may assist the response of severe systemic fungal infection to amphotericin.[36–38] This may be useful prophylactically or in patients who have failed to respond to amphotericin and its lipid formulations. This activity could be related to augmentation of the antifungal activity of monocytes, macrophages and neutrophils exposed to M-CSF and GM-CSF. In view of the life-threatening nature of these infections, this is a potentially important development and it is to be hoped that randomized trials in patients with systemic infections will be completed shortly.

FUTURE DEVELOPMENTS

A number of new antibiotics have been developed which have shown initial promise in small trials in neutropenic patients. Imipenem, a broad-spectrum agent, is superior to aztreonam whose activity is restricted to Gram-negative organisms.[39] It has activity against other organisms which produce β-lactamases which hydrolyze third-generation cephalosporins such as ceftazidime. However, methicillin-resistant staphylococci and *Enterococcus faecium* are resistant to imipenem and other organisms such as *Pseudomonas aeruginosa* may increasingly become so. Meropenem[40] is a similar carbapenem β-lactam antibiotic and is as effective as imipenem and is equally expensive. It has signficant advantages over imipenem (better activity and less toxicity in meningitis) and will probably replace it in hospital formularies. Larger trials in neutropenic patients are warranted and for now it should be reserved for the treatment of defined resistant infection.

It is also hoped that pharmaceutical companies will come up with an answer to vancomycin-resistant enterococci because the macrolide antibiotics represent the last line of defense against methicillin-resistant *Staphylococcus aureus* and β-lactam-resistant enterococci.[41] It is probably only a matter of time before these defenses are more seriously breached. In fact, the main defense line is the human mucosal barrier and the evidence of progressive agents is at last on the horizon with the production of keratinocyte-derived growth factors. The ensuing years will hopefully see the completion of trials looking at a variety of 'networked' cytokines, including mucosal protective agents, G- and GM-CSF and thrombopoietin. It should be an exciting era.

Initial plans to produce safer central venous catheters with, for example, integral permanently bonded antiseptic agents are underway. The general hope that most infections in neutropenic patients could be prevented has not been realized but this and other developments may lead the way so long as the temptation to side-step the need for large randomized trials is avoided.

CONCLUSIONS

Clinicians can be forgiven for looking askance at the apparent cornucopia of antimicrobial agents which have been produced over recent years. What are the best agents, when should they be used, and why do they still fail? The fact is that there is still a lot to learn and there is a desperate need for better agents, e.g. to prevent the development of invasive fungal infections. The suggestions made above for a planned progressive approach to the management of infections is an attempt to adopt a rational, calm and hopefully scientific approach to the problem.

REFERENCES

1. Hann IM, Viscoli C, Paesmans M, Gaya H, Glauser M. Comparison of outcome from febrile neutropenic episodes in children and adults: results from four EORTC studies. *Br J Haematol* 1997; **99**: 580–588
2. Ochs L, Shu XO, Miller J *et al*. Late infections after allogeneic bone marrow transplantation: comparison of incidence in related and unrelated donor transplant recipients. *Blood* 1995; **86**: 3979–3986
3. Wheeler K, Chessells JM, Bailey CC, Richards SM. Treatment-related deaths during induction and in first remission in acute lymphoblastic leukaemia: MRC UKALL X. *Arch Dis Child* 1996; **74**: 101–197
4. Jones GR, Konsler GK, Pusek SN. Infection risks in febrile, neutropenic children and adolescents. *Pediatr Hematol Oncol* 1996; **13**: 217–229
5. Rackoff WR, Gonin R, Robinson C, Kreissman SG, Breitfeld PP. Predicting the risk of bacteremia in children with fever and neutropenia. *J Clin Oncol* 1996; **14**: 919–924
6. Lucas KG, Brown AE, Armstron D, Chapman D, Heller G. The identification of febrile, neutropenic children with neoplastic disease at low risk for bacteremia and complications of sepsis. *Cancer* 1996; **77**: 791–798
7. Klastersky J. Empiric treatment of infections in neutropenic patients with cancer. *Rev Infect Dis* 1983; **5 (Suppl)**: S21–S23
8. McCarthy J, Redmond HP, Duggan SM *et al*. Characterisation of the defects in murine peritoneal macrophage function in the early post splenectomy period. *J Immunol* 1995; **155**: 387–396
9. Alfaham M, Holt ME, Goodchild MC. Arthropathy in a patient with cystic fibrosis taking ciprofloxacin. *Br Med J* 1987; **296**: 699
10. Carl W. Oral complications of local and systemic cancer treatment (part two). Mucositis in bone marrow transplantation and hypoptyalism. *Topics Supportive Care Oncol* 1995; **17**: 8–10
11. Foote RL, Lopinzi CL, Frank AR *et al*. Randomized trial of a chlorhexidime mouthwash for alleviation of radiation-induced mucositis. *J Clin Oncol* 1994; **12**: 2630–2633
12. O'Donnell MR, Schmidt GM, Tegtmeier BR *et al*. Prediction of systemic fungal infection in allogeneic marrow recipients: impact of amphotericin prophylaxis in high risk patients. *J Clin Oncol* 1992; **12**: 827–834
13. Ninane J, Multicentre Group. Multicentre study of fluconazole versus oral polyenes in the prevention of fungal infection in children with haematological or oncological malignancies. *Eur J Clin Microbiol* 1994; **13**: 330–337
14. Trigg M, Morgan D, Burus T *et al*. Successful program to prevent aspergillus infection in children undergoing marrow transplantation: use of nasal amphotericin. *Bone Marrow Transplant* 1997; **19**: 43–47
15. EORTC International Antimicrobial Therapy Project Group. Trimethoprim-sulphamethoxazole in the prevention of infection in neutropenic patients. *J Infect Dis* 1984; **150**: 372–379
16. Buda K, Tubergen DG, Levin MJ. The frequency and consequences of varicella exposure and varicella infection in children receiving maintenance therapy for acute lymphoblastic leukemia. *J Pediatr Hematol Oncol* 1996; **18**: 106–112
17. Hann IM, Prentice HG, Blacklock HA *et al*. Acyclovir prophylaxis against herpes virus infections in severely immunocompromised patients: randomised double blind trial. *Br Med J* 1983; **287**: 384–388
18. Prentice HG, Kho P. Clinical strategies for the management of cytomegalovirus infection and disease in allogeneic BMT. *Bone Marrow Transplant* 1997; **19**: 135–142
19. Sullivan KM, Kopecky KJ, Jocom J *et al*. Immunomodulatory and antimicrobial efficacy of intravenous immunoglobulin in bone marrow transplantation. *N Engl J Med* 1990; **323**: 705–712
20. Daghistani D, Horn M, Rodrigquez Z, Schoenike S, Toledano S. Prevention of indwelling central venous catheter sepsis. *Med Pediatr Oncol* 1996; **26**: 405–408
21. Gaya H, Fenelon LE. Planned progressive therapy: logical sequence of management of infection in the neutropenic patient. In: Jenkins GT, Williams JD (eds) *Infection and Haematology*. Oxford: Butterworth–Heinemann, 1994, pp 145–163
22. EORTC International Antimicrobial Therapy Group. Efficacy and toxicity of single daily doses of amikacin and cetriaxone versus multiple daily doses of amikacin and ceftazidime for infection in patients with cancer and granulocytopenia. *Ann Intern Med* 1993; **119**: 584–593
23. Hatala R, Dink T, Cook DJ. Meta-analysis: A single daily dose of aminoglycosides is as effective as multiple daily dosing. *J Evidence Based Med Therapeut* 1996; **145**
24. Barza M, Ioannidis JPA, Cappelleri JC, Lan J. Meta-analysis: A single daily dose of aminoglycosides is as effective as multiple daily dosing with less nephrotoxicity. *J Evidence Based Med Therapeut* 1996; **144**

25. Barza M, Ioannidis JPA, Cappelleri JC, Lan J. Single or multiple daily doses of aminoglycosides: a meta-analysis. *Br Med J* 1996; **312**: 338–345

26. Viscoli C, Dudley M, Ferrea G *et al.* Serum concentrations and safety of single daily dosing of amikacin in children undergoing bone marrow transplantation. *J Antimicrob Chemother* 1991; **27**: 113–120

27. EORTC International Antimicrobial Therapy Cooperative Group. Ceftazidime compared with a short or long course of amikacin for empirical therapy of Gram-negative bacteremia in cancer patients with granulocytopenia. *N Engl J Med* 1987; **317**: 1692–1698

28. Cometta A, Zinner S, deBock R *et al.* Piperacillin-tazobactam plus amikacin versus ceftazidime plus amikacin as empiric therapy for fever in granulocytopenic patients with cancer. *Antimicrob Agents Chemother* 1995; **39**: 445–452

29. EORTC International Antimicrobial Therapy Cooperative Group. Empiric antifungal therapy in febrile granulocytopenic patients. *Am J Med* 1989; **86**: 668–672

30. Viscoli C, Castagnola E, Van Lint MT *et al.* Fluconazole versus amphotericin B as empirical antifungal therapy of unexplained fever in granulocytopenic cancer patients. *Eur J Cancer* 1996; **32A**: 814–820

31. Prentice HG, Hann IM, Herbrecht R *et al.* A randomized comparison of liposomal versus conventional amphotericin B for the treatment of PUO in neutropenic patients. *Br J Haematol* 1997 (in press)

32. Leenders ACAP, de Marie S. The use of lipid formulations of amphotericin B for systemic fungal infections. *Leukaemia* 1996; **10**: 1570–1575

33. Mills W, Chopra R, Linch DC, Goldstone AH. Liposomal amphotericin in the treatment of fungal infections in neutropenic patients. A single centre experience of 133 episodes in 116 patients. *Br J Haematol* 1994; **86**: 754–760

34. Trissel LA. Amphotericin B does not mix with fat emulsion. *Am J Health System Pharm* 1995; **52**: 1463–1464

35. Hann IM. Haemopoietic growth factors and childhood cancer—Review. *Eur J Cancer* 1995; **31A**: 1476–1478

36. Roilides E, Sein T, Holmes A *et al.* Effects of macrophage colony-stimulating factor on antifungal activity of mononuclear phagocytes against Aspergillus fumigatus. *J Infect Dis* 1995; **172**: 1028–1034

37. Capetti A, Bonfanti P, Magui C, Milazzo F. Employment of recombinant human GM-CSF in oesophageal candidiasis in AIDS patients. *AIDS* 1995; **9**: 1378–1379

38. Peters BG, Adkins DR, Harrison BR *et al.* Antifungal effecs of yeast-derived rhu-GM-CSF in patients receiving high-dose chemotherapy given with or without autologous stem cell transplantation: a retrospective analysis. *Bone Marrow Transplant* 1996: **18**: 93–102

38. Read I, Whimbey EE, Rolston KVI *et al.* A comparison of aztreonam plus vancomycin and imipenem plus vancomycin as initial therapy for febrile neutropenic cancer patients. *Cancer* 1996; **77**: 1386–1394

40. Anon. Meropenem—An advantageous antibiotic? *Drugs Therap Bull* 1996; **34**: 53–55

41. Rowe PM. Preparing for battle against vancomycin resistance. *Lancet* 1996; **347**: 252

Hematologic effects of systemic disease

Hematologic effects of systemic disease and toxins

JOHN S LILLEYMAN

Many disorders are not primarily blood diseases but they do have important hematologic effects. These effects may be sufficiently striking for initial referral to a hematologist, or a laboratory worker may recognize abnormalities in blood or marrow leading to a diagnosis. Many of the conditions are covered in other chapters: disturbances of hemostasis are described in Chapter 32; storage disorders are described in Chapter 40, and abnormalities produced by non-hemopoietic malignant disease form the basis of Chapter 39. The remaining disorders, however, do not fit easily elsewhere and, together with the hematologic effects of toxins and drugs, form the miscellany contained in this chapter.

ANEMIA OF CHRONIC DISEASE

The 'anemia of chronic disease' is a diagnosis of exclusion. It is a relatively common phenomenon associated with a wide range of disorders both in children and adults, and is most frequently encountered in malignancy, connective tissue diseases and chronic infections.[1] Generally, the anemia is mild, 2–3 g/dl below the lower normal limit for a given individual, of slow onset with normochromic normocytic red cells, and is associated with a normal or low reticulocyte count. It is characterized by a low serum iron, iron-binding capacity and transferrin saturation, but normal or raised serum ferritin and no shortage of stainable reticuloendothelial iron in bone marrow particles. Hypochromia and microcytosis are seen, but less commonly than is generally supposed unless co-existent true iron deficiency is present (as it not uncommonly is in children). The recent introduction of serum transferrin receptor measurements has further helped to tease apart the anemia of iron deficiency and chronic disease as high values are seen in the former but not the latter.[2]

The anemia is multifactorial. There is an element of shortened red cell survival, although the reason for this is not fully understood. It may be due to hemophagocytosis.[1] There is also a defective marrow response to anemia, with only a 1–2-fold increase in erythropoiesis rather than the normal 6–8-fold response. This is not associated with an endogenous deficiency of erythropoietin (EPO), or defective release of the cytokine. It appears to be due to an erythropoietic inhibitory role played by other cytokines such as the acute-phase reactants interleukin (IL)-1 and tumor necrosis factor (TNF) derived from macrophages. These compounds may mediate their effect by stimulating the production of interferons from marrow stromal cells and T lymphocytes.[3,4]

A third component of the problem is impaired release of iron from reticuloendothelial cells for use in the marrow, again possibly cytokine mediated,[4] but the anemia of chronic disease cannot be attributed simply to iron-deficient erythropoiesis.[5] Iron absorption from the gut remains normal or low. Compounding factors include bleeding, nutritional deficiencies and drug-induced red cell changes, and it is important to explore any easily correctable component of anemia in any child simply assumed to have a low hemoglobin through chronic disease. The response to pharmacologic doses of EPO is variable but if the endogenous concentration is <500 unit/l it can occasionally be clinically worthwhile, particularly where the anemia is severe enough to warrant transfusion support.[6,7]

RENAL DISEASE

Anemia of chronic renal disease

Basically a variant of the anemia of chronic disease, the low hemoglobin seen in children with chronic renal failure is more severe than that of other chronic inflammatory disorders due to the compounding factor of secondary EPO deficiency from damage to the cells producing the cytokine. In such circumstances, treatment with recombinant EPO is highly effective and beneficial if given with care. It is expensive, however, and it is important to explore other correctable components of the anemia before using it. Iron stores may be reduced, for example, and failure to respond to EPO should provoke a search for compounding problems before dose escalation is considered.[8] It is interesting that the mild bleeding tendency commonly seen in chronic renal failure can be improved after correction of the anemia by EPO.[9]

Hemolytic uremic syndrome

Hemolytic uremic syndrome (HUS) is a combination of a microangiopathic hemolytic anemia, thrombocytopenia and acute renal failure. The thrombocytopenia is not associated with a consumption coagulopathy, and tests of coagulation are usually normal or only mildly deranged. The platelet count may be modestly or profoundly reduced. Platelet survival is shortened, and platelet-aggregating activity has been found in the plasma of some affected children.[10] The disease occurs sporadically and in epidemics, and the majority of children have a prodromal illness of abdominal pain and bloody diarrhea.

The epidemic form of HUS is associated with infection by enteropathogenic Gram-negative bacteria, usually *Escherichia coli* serotype O157:H7, which produce exotoxins similar to those produced by *Shigella dysenterie* type 1 and collectively referred to as Shiga toxins. These toxins bind to cell receptors, identified as ceramide trihexoside, which are expressed to varying degrees in different tissues (being particularly prevalent in infant glomerular endothelial cells).[11]

Most infants eventually recover without sequelae. Overall, mortality is 5% and long-term severe morbidity is around 10%.[12] Older children have a greater chance of progressing to end-stage renal failure, and have a higher incidence of atypical HUS (that without prodromal diarrhea). It is more serious and has other distinguishing features including normal urine output, gross proteinuria, hypertension, a relapsing course and more severe changes on renal biopsy.[13]

Treatment is supportive with the addition of fresh frozen plasma (FFP) infusions or plasma exchange for severe cases. Platelet transfusions are seldom indicated except occasionally to cover the surgical insertion of dialysis catheters. As the mechanism producing the thrombocytopenia is *in vivo* aggregation, there are theoretical grounds for keeping such transfusions to a minimum to avoid further microvascular thrombosis.

Thrombotic thrombocytopenic purpura

Also known as Moschcowitz's syndrome (after the first author to describe the disease in the early 1920s), this is a syndrome of undetermined cause chiefly affecting young adults. It is characterized by a pentad of features which include:

- thrombocytopenia;
- microangiopathic hemolytic anemia;
- neurologic disturbances;
- renal dysfunction;
- fever.

There is no evidence that the disorder observed occasionally in children differs from that encountered in adults.[14] The pentad described above is the same as the triad for HUS with the addition of two features – fever and neurologic disturbances. It is probable that TTP and HUS (at least the sporadic and atypical type of the latter, see above) represent a similar pathological process with TTP being the more serious multisystem form of the disorder. The clinical course of TTP is variable, but the disease is serious with a high mortality if untreated. Two-thirds of patients die within 3 months.[14] The problem can wax and wane, with some patients pursuing a chronic relapsing course.[15]

The majority of patients respond to empirical plasma exchange with FFP.[16] Based on the rationale that von Willebrand multimers may be involved in the pathogenesis of the disorder, some patients failing to respond have subsequently improved if cryosupernatant (i.e. plasma with cryoprecipitate removed) is used rather than whole plasma.[17]

LIVER DISEASE

Cirrhosis

Chronic liver disease of any type can be associated with the clinically important disturbances of hemostasis described in Chapter 32. Cirrhosis is also commonly associated with anemia that may be multifactorial or simply the anemia of chronic disease (see above). Compounding factors may be blood loss from esophageal varices, poor iron absorption, and hypersplenism from congestive splenomegaly.

Wilson's disease (hemolytic anemia)

Wilson's disease is a recessive inborn error of metabolism with defective biliary excretion of copper which accumulates in body tissues and causes damage to the liver, brain, kidney and cornea. It presents in the middle years of childhood with insidious evidence of dysfunction of one or more of these organ systems.[18] Occasionally, it can present as a symptomatic non-immune hemolytic anemia, the cause of which may be obscure unless Kayser–Fleischer rings are sought by slit-lamp ophthalmoscopy. The red cell changes are minimal and unspecific, and the exact mechanism of the hemolysis is unclear, although it is presumably some manifestation of copper toxicity (see below).

Reye's syndrome

This is an incompletely understood syndrome of acute encephalopathy and fatty liver degeneration that typically follows a few days after apparent resolution of an unremarkable febrile viral infection. It has been linked to the use of aspirin as an antipyretic, and for this reason the drug is not recommended for children, particularly those with influenza or varicella. Hematologic changes are those of acute hepatic disruption (chiefly disturbances of coagulation with occasional disseminated consumption and thrombocytopenia). Jaundice is absent. Given adequate supportive therapy most children recover, but death from cerebral edema or progressive encephalopathy can occur.

ENDOCRINE DISORDERS

Thyroid disease

Hypothyroidism is associated with mild or (occasionally) moderate anemia which is normochromic and mildly macrocytic. In addition, there may be small numbers of irregularly contracted cells.[19] Red cell survival is normal. Hyperthyroidism conversely is associated with an increase in red cell mass, although hemoglobin concentration is usually normal. Numerous effects of thyroid hormone on red cell metabolism, platelet function and coagulation have been described but these are seldom of clinical importance.

Adrenal insufficiency

This gives rise to a mild normochromic anemia and is associated with eosinophilia and neutropenia. The anemia may be paradoxically exacerbated with the start of replacement therapy as the reduced plasma volume increases promptly out of step with red cell mass.

Pituitary insufficiency

Anemia associated with hypofunction of the pituitary is partly due to target endocrine organ failure but is probably mostly due to growth hormone deficiency which affects erythropoiesis directly. The effect of growth hormone on developing red cells is mediated by its paracrine growth-promoting mediator, insulin-like growth factor 1 (IGF-1)[20] and the blood concentrations of IGF-1 and IGF binding protein-3 directly correlate with hemoglobin measurements in short children.[21]

HEART DISEASE

Cyanotic congenital heart disease

Some children with secondary polycythaemia due to cyanotic congenital heart disease (CCHD) are prone to vaso-occlusive disease, but paradoxically some become thrombocytopenic and may bleed excessively if subjected to corrective surgery. The cause of the thrombocytopenia is not well established, and there is debate about the presence or otherwise of disseminated intravascular coagulation (DIC) in such patients.

Wedemeyer et al[22] studied 33 unselected children with CCHD, 12 of whom had a platelet count $<150 \times 10^9/1$, and 4 below $100 \times 10^9/1$. The severity of the thrombocytopenia was directly related to the hematocrit. All those over 70% had thrombocytopenia associated with a variety of abnormalities in clotting factor concentrations, although the authors concluded that none had DIC. Ihenacho et al[23] studied another 55 children with broadly similar results, but felt their findings were consistent with low-grade DIC, adding the observation that in 3 of 5 patients the platelet count rose after heparin therapy. A later study of autologous platelet survival in CCHD[24] found that those with the highest hematocrits had the shortest survival, but that short survival did not correlate with abnormal coagulation tests, and there was little evidence of DIC.

Naiman[25] reviewed the hemostatic problems of CCHD without reaching a conclusion, although he pointed out the technical pitfalls of an uncorrected anticoagulant:plasma ratio in polycythemic children when performing clotting factor assays. He recommended avoiding heparin therapy and suggested conservative management of the hemostatic defects by venesection and replacement of volume by FFP. The value of this procedure was endorsed in a later small study where reduction of the hematocrit resulted in correction of platelet aggregation defects and bleeding tendency.[26]

LUNG DISEASE

Pulmonary hemosiderosis

This term describes a number of rare childhood disorders where repeated intra-alveolar micro-hemorrhages result in pulmonary dysfunction, hemoptysis and hemosiderin-laden macrophages being lost to the external environment through the gut by swallowing. A major feature is therefore anemia due to iron deficiency. There are primary and secondary causes, with the former being more common in children. Apart from a primary idiopathic type, there is also a variant associated with hypersensitivity to cows' milk and one that occurs with a progressive glomerulonephritis (Goodpasture's syndrome).

Loeffler's syndrome

This is not a distinct clinical entity and probably represents an unusual allergic manifestation to a variety of antigens. It is characterized by transient widespread pulmonary infiltrates seen on X-ray in association with a high eosinophil count. In the absence of an identifiable allergen (such as migrating parasites), the condition usually resolves after a few days or weeks. It is distinct from the rare hypereosinophilic syndrome which is a chronic disorder of unknown cause involving higher counts (up to $100 \times 10^9/l$) and which may damage other organs, notably the heart.[27]

SKIN DISEASE

Mast cell disease

Mast cells remain something of an enigma. They are now thought to be more closely related to monocytes and macrophages than to basophils. Mast cell disease or mastocytosis is a collective term for a group of disorders where abnormal accumulations of such cells occur in the dermis (cutaneous mastocytosis) or internal organs (systemic mastocytosis). The systemic form of the disease is rare in childhood, and malignant evolution to true mast cell leukemia is essentially confined to adults.[28,29]

In childhood mast cell disease is commonest in infants under 2 years. It usually presents either as a solitary cutaneous mastocytoma or, more commonly, as urticaria pigmentosa. Solitary lesions may be present at birth or arise during early infancy. They can arise anywhere but are most frequent on the wrist, neck or trunk. They are palpable, pink or yellow plaque-like eruptions of variable size from millimetres to centimetres. They have an orange-peel appearance and may be hyperpigmented. They usually involute spontaneously during early childhood.

Urticaria pigmentosa is the more common manifestation of mast cell disease and is usually acquired in infancy. Initially, lesions are bullous or urticarial and wax and wane at the same site until they become fixed and pigmented like the solitary lesions described above. They may be sparse or numerous and are most frequently distributed symmetrically on the abdomen, trunk and limbs. The condition spontaneously resolves by adulthood in the majority of patients. Mast cell disease can present as bullous eruptions or there may be diffuse skin involvement. Involvement beyond the skin is unusual in children; bone lesions are the commonest but marrow involvement is rare.[30]

Mast cells in these disorders commonly produce histamine which causes itching and hypersecretion of gastric acid. Skin lesions flare if stroked, and dermographism is common between lesions. Mast cells also produce heparin like compounds which rarely can lead to disturbed coagulation and bleeding.[31] Symptoms from histamine release tend to abate before the mast cell infiltrates disappear. Treatment is symptomatic with H_1 and H_2 antihistamines.[32]

CONNECTIVE TISSUE DISORDERS

Although all connective tissue disorders may have the features of anemia of chronic disease described above, other more specific hematologic features also arise.

Systemic onset juvenile rheumatoid arthritis

True iron deficiency frequently complicates the picture as a result of gastrointestinal blood loss from analgesics (particularly salicylates) and steroid ingestion, although the response to oral iron is blunted, possibly due to high circulating concentrations of IL-6. Parenteral iron has been recommended in children whose circulating transferrin receptor concentration is increased.[33] As well as anemia, a modest secondary thrombocytosis is not uncommon, and a neutrophilia is observed in flare-up of the disease and needs to be differentiated from secondary bacterial infections.

Of children with juvenile rheumatoid arthritis, 20% have splenomegaly, although not necessarily the triad of rheumatoid arthritis, splenomegaly and neutropenia described by Felty. Neutropenia may result from hypersplenism alone, or be immune-mediated with detectable anti-neutrophil IgG antibodies. It does not always resolve after splenectomy. There is evidence in some patients for a granulocyte maturation arrest, with low levels of granulocyte colony-stimulating factor activity.

Systemic lupus erythematosus

Many hematologic changes in addition to anemia of chronic disease have been described in systemic lupus erythematosus (SLE). Autoantibodies to red cells, neutrophils or (most commonly) platelets result in peripheral destruction, reflected by cytopenias and increased marrow precursors. The disease can present as an immune cytopenia, mimicking chronic immune thrombocytic purpura (ITP), although the serology may be different, with lupus-associated antiplatelet antibodies more commonly fixing complement.[34] As might be anticipated, thrombocytopenic babies can be born to mothers with SLE as they can to mothers with ITP if maternal antiplatelet antibodies cross the placenta. Therapy for SLE-associated thrombocytopenia is as for chronic ITP, and the problem tends to respond to steroids along with other manifestations of the disease. There is evidence that splenectomy is less likely to be successful than in 'true' ITP[35] and severe refractory cases are difficult to manage. The presence or otherwise of thrombocytopenia has no prognostic importance in terms of other manifestations and progress of the SLE.[36]

SLE may also be the cause of marrow aplasia, or selective

granulocyte aplasia. Lymphopenia, with abnormalities of T-cell function proportional to disease activity, is common. Circulating antiphospholipid antibodies ('lupus anticoagulants'), seen in other conditions as well as SLE, are discussed in Chapter 32.

Polyarteritis nodosa

Microangiopathic hemolytic anemia is sometimes seen in this rare childhood disorder in association with renal disease or hypertensive crises. Eosinophilia is also prominent.

Wegener's granulomatosis

This presumed autoimmune disorder is rare in childhood. It presents with fever, cough, hemoptysis, epistaxis, nasal discharge, nodular pulmonary infiltrates and renal failure as the result of widespread necrotizing granulomatous inflammation and vasculitis. Hematologic features variably include normochromic, normocytic anemia, red cell fragmentation typical of microangiopathic hemolytic anemia, leukocytosis with neutrophilia and eosinophilia, and a secondary thrombocytosis. The frequency of disease relapse can be reduced by co-trimoxazole, although the drug's mechanism (and the pathogenesis of the disease) is unknown.[37]

INFECTIONS

The hematologic response to infection depends on the type of invading organism and the state of health of the patient prior to becoming infected. Serious or overwhelming infections can be associated with profound disturbances of hemostasis and DIC. Acute bacterial infections produce a neutrophilia, except where sepsis is overwhelming or in preterm neonates where a paradoxical neutropenia is common. An increase in the number of immature neutrophils (band or stab cells) is also seen, and the ratio of band cell:mature forms is a more reliable indicator of sepsis in the neonate than the absolute neutrophil count.[38]

Subacute or chronic bacterial sepsis (such as that due to salmonella, brucella and tuberculosis) tends to increase the number of monocytes. Virus infections can produce a transient neutrophilia as part of an acute phase response, and subsequently, if they produce hematologic changes, tend to cause disturbances in the number and/or morphology of lymphocytes. Parasites, if they penetrate tissues, cause an eosinophilia. Infections with many different organisms can occasionally provoke inappropriate hemophagocytosis (so-called infection-associated hemophagocytic syndrome [IAHS]; see Chapter 17). Specific organisms and infections of particular hematologic importance are considered in more detail below.

Epstein–Barr virus

Epstein–Barr virus (EBV) was first described in 1964 as a herpes-like isolate from patients with the African epidemic form of Burkitt's lymphoma. The chance observation that a laboratory worker exposed to the virus developed infectious mononucleosis (IM) and subsequently produced antibodies to EBV led to an epidemiologic study of undergraduates at Yale University which confirmed that EBV was causally associated with this form of 'glandular fever'.[39] The virus preferentially infects B lymphocytes that express CD21 on their surface, but it can also bind to (and infect) other tissues such as nasopharyngeal epithelial cells.[40] It achieves latency in B cells.

The virus has several antigenic determinants that can be identified serologically. The clinically important ones are the viral capsid antigen (VCA), early antigens (EA, D and R subtypes), membrane antigen (MA) and nuclear antigen (NA or EBNA). Following infection, IgM antibodies to VCA and EA (D) rise temporarily and later IgG antibodies to VCA, MA, NA and other antigens appear and persist for life. The detection of IgM VCA is the best evidence of recent or current infection but may be missed since it is present for only a short time during the onset and acute phase of the disease. Conversely the detection of IgG anti-NA is the most reliable indicator of past infection.[41] Persisting active infection associated with malignant disease (Burkitt's lymphoma or nasopharyngeal carcinoma) can give rise to high and rising titers of antibodies to EA (D) and EA (R), respectively.

EBV infection in some individuals with cellular immune deficiency states can give rise to uncontrolled lymphoproliferative disorders. X-linked lymphoproliferative disease (Purtilo's or Duncan's syndrome) is a rare inherited inability to combat EBV infection where patients may die of progressive disease occasionally associated with a virus-induced hemophagocytic syndrome.[42] They also suffer from marrow aplasia, hypogammaglobulinemia and lymphomas. Those on aggressive immunosuppresive therapy following solid organ transplants, recipients of allogeneic marrow grafts and patients with HIV infection can all develop polyclonal proliferation of B lymphocytes that carry the EBV genome and which in some instances progresses to a fatal clonal lymphoma. In marrow transplant patients, the problem usually involves donor-derived lymphocytes and occurs in recipients of mismatched T-cell-depleted marrow after treatment with T-cell antibodies for graft-versus-host disease. A later form of the disease may arise from host cells.[43]

Infectious mononucleosis

EBV is ubiquitous and in the underdeveloped world primary infection occurs in 90% of children usually without symptoms.[44] In the developed world, however, 50% of individuals will pass through childhood without being infected. As adolescents or young adults primary exposure may manifest as acute infectious mononucleosis (IM) in about half of those infected.[45] Classical IM can occur in infants and young children,[46] but is unusual before puberty. An intermediate disorder of mild sore throat with a few atypical lymphocytes and fever is not exceptional in the middle years of childhood and may be associated with typical heterophile antibodies (see below) as well as seroconversion to EBV.

Symptoms and signs. In the typical syndrome, initial symptoms vary in severity and are non-specific, including fatigue, malaise, fever, anorexia and occasional nausea and vomiting. After a few days, a sore throat develops with or without swelling in the neck. Fever is almost invariable and persistent. A tonsillar exudate may be present. Lymphadenopathy is usual and is the reason for the term 'glandular fever'. It can involve all groups of nodes or chiefly those of the head and neck. Splenomegaly is found in around 75% of patients and hepatomegaly in 25%. The impression of hepatitis may be strengthened by mild clinical jaundice in 5–10%. Rarely, there may be a generalized rash. The incidence of rash approaches 100% in patients given ampicillin, a strange, induced allergy that is almost pathognomonic for the disease. The same applies to the now more commonly used analogous antibiotic, amoxycillin.

Typical changes in the blood count include an initial neutrophilia followed by the characteristic atypical lymphocytes appearing after 5–7 days. These usually comprise over 25% of the total lymphocytes (commonly >50%) in contrast to the 'EBV negative' IM-like syndromes. The morphology of the lymphocytes is variable but can be alarming, leading to Damashek's classical observation that IM is an acute self-limiting leukemia. The cells are chiefly uninfected reactive oligoclonal CD8$^+$ T cells. The massive expansion of a few clones of such cells may be an important part of the primary response to the virus and is necessary for its control.[47]

Diagnosis. The diagnosis is made by the typical hematology together with specific EBV serology as noted above. A widely used and reliable near-patient screening test detects heterophile red cell agglutinins, a feature of classical 'glandular fever' noted by Paul and Bunnell in the 1930s. Unlike naturally occurring heterophile antibodies, the agglutinins seen in IM are not absorbed by guinea pig kidney. They are absorbed by ox red cells, and agglutinate sheep and horse red cells. These features are exploited in the popular 'monospot' test of Lee and Davidshon, where sera are exposed to either guinea pig kidney or beef red cell stroma before being assessed for their potential to agglutinate horse red cells. Heterophile antibodies appear around the same time as the atypical lymphocytosis, or shortly thereafter, and peak around 2 weeks. They can persist for several months. They are not specific, and can occasionally arise in disorders other than IM, including acute leukemia.

Differential diagnosis. There is seldom much difficulty in diagnosing the typical disease in adolescents. Problems can arise if the monospot test is negative, or if the clinical picture is complicated or atypical, particularly in a younger child. Disorders most commonly confused with IM are toxoplasmosis and cytomegalovirus infections, but in these infections atypical lymphocytes are less numerous. Less commonly, hepatitis A, brucellosis, lymphoma or leukemia may also be mistaken for IM.

Clinical course and complications. Immunocompetent children will recover completely without sequelae, although there has long been a belief that the infection predisposes to an extended chronic fatigue syndrome. Recent studies support this belief.[48] Rare deaths do occur during the acute phase due to spontaneous rupture of a rapidly enlarging spleen.[49] There are other serious complications. IM occasionally involves the central nervous system to produce meningoencephalomyelitis or a Guillain–Barré syndrome,[50] and aplastic anemia has been anecdotally described.[51]

Immune-mediated cytopenias can arise during the course of the disease. Increased cold agglutinins with a positive direct antiglobulin test occur in the majority of patients, but clinically important hemolysis is unusual. The antibodies most frequently are anti-i, or less commonly anti-I or anti-N.[52] Thrombocytopenia also occurs, but very low platelet counts producing symptoms arise in <1% of patients.[53]

Treatment. There has long been debate about the use of steroids, and latterly the role of acyclovir has been questioned. Whether either alters the course of uncomplicated cases is doubtful, and a recent randomized double-blind placebo controlled study suggested that giving both together for 10 days does not alter the duration or severity of clinical symptoms or the development of EBV-specific cellular immunity. There was some evidence, however, that oropharyngeal virus shedding is inhibited during the treatment period.[54]

The use of steroids for symptomatic thrombocytopenia or severe hemolysis is commonplace and at least does not appear to be harmful. As both problems normally recover quickly with or without therapy, any benefit is difficult to assess. High-dose immunoglobulin has also been used.[55]

Parvovirus B19

Human parvovirus was discovered fortuitously in 1975 and is now recognized as the cause of erythema infectiosum (Fifth disease), the most frequently encountered manifestation of infection in childhood. Many infections go unnoticed or undiagnosed. The virus is probably most often transmitted by droplets,[56] but it may enter the body through other routes including contaminated blood products from which it is difficult to remove.[57] It has caused abortion of severely affected fetuses and also gives rise to arthritis and arthralgia in children.[56]

It is of interest to hematologists because the widespread small DNA virus has a peculiar predilection for rapidly growing cells, particularly red cell precursors in the bone marrow. Its preference for red cell precursors may be because it uses the P antigen as a receptor,[58] but it can also affect other cell lines to a lesser extent. It is now well recognized as the agent responsible for aplastic crises in patients with chronic hemolytic states such as hereditary spherocytosis,[56] and can also occasionally cause symptomatic pancytopenia in otherwise healthy children.[59] It can produce prolonged pancytopenia in children with deficient immunity[60] and this phenomenon is also not infrequently seen in children on chemotherapy for leukemia,[61] suggesting that normal immunity is necessary for virus control. There is no specific treatment.

Human immunodeficiency virus

HIV infection in children is covered in detail in Chapter 25. The direct hematologic (as opposed to the immunologic) effects of the virus can briefly be summarized as cytopenias due either to a direct effect on marrow stem cells resulting in decreased production or as a consequence of autoantibodies to blood cellular elements.[62,63]

Anemia in HIV-infected children is commonly due to many factors other than the virus. A recent study in Abidjan, where the prevalence of HIV infection in unselected children admitted to hospital is 8.2%, showed that the most frequent reason for admission in such patients was malnutrition; malaria can also co-exist.[64] The virus can, however, produce an autoimmune hemolytic state and also cause reticulocytopenia.[62]

ITP is a common manifestation of HIV infection and can be the first sign of infection in otherwise apparently well children.[65] It can therefore be mistaken for simple ITP (see Chapter 22), although careful examination of the HIV child will usually identify lymphadenopathy or hepatosplenomegaly and wholesale HIV screening of all thrombocytopenic children is probably hard to justify. Neutropenia is not uncommon and may be immune mediated, but may also be compounded by reduced production due to zidovudine therapy or co-trimoxazole. Immunoglobulin replacement therapy may help if repeated bacterial infections become a clinical problem.[63]

Lymphomas and other HIV-associated malignancies arise less frequently in children than adults, although this picture may change as children live longer and the number with HIV infection increases.[66]

TORCH INFECTIONS

This is a miscellaneous group of congenital infections, including TOxoplasma, Rubella, Cytomegalovirus (CMV), Herpes simplex (HSV), and syphilis. While they are all very different diseases, the collective acronym is justified by certain common features; they can all cause neonatal anemia, thrombocytopenia (see also Chapter 21) and hepatosplenomegaly.

Toxoplasmosis

This is caused by an ubiquitous coccidian protozoan, *Toxoplasma gondii*, and can be congenital or acquired later in childhood. It is the congenital form that gives rise to hematologic problems. If a susceptible woman acquires infection during pregnancy (which may well be asymptomatic), there is around a 30% chance that she will transmit the infection to the fetus if she is not treated. Of infected fetuses, 60% will be asymptomatic, but 20% will be severely affected.[67,68] They may be stillborn, premature, or born at term; they may be clearly ill at birth, or become so over a few days. They may have lymphadenopathy, hepatosplenomegaly, jaundice and petechiae with profound thrombocytopenia, although such low platelet counts will only arise in 1–2% of infected newborns (5–10% of those severely affected). Anemia is more common. Nearly all have chorioretinitis and many will have intracerebral calcification. Those asymptomatic at birth may well develop chorioretinitis, mental handicap or other neurologic disability in later childhood. For this reason, all infected newborns should be treated irrespective of symptoms.

Rubella

Pregnant mothers who develop rubella in their first trimester have a high chance (90%) of infecting their fetus, but this figure falls in the second trimester to 50% and to 35% in the third. The earlier in pregnancy the fetus becomes infected, the worse the degree of organ damage. Babies infected at any stage can subsequently carry the virus for long periods of time. Of those severely affected, two-thirds will be of low birth weight and have hepatosplenomegaly. Petechiae and profound thrombocytopenia arise in 20–50%. A very low platelet count is indicative of a poor outlook and arises in particularly severely affected infants with multiple manifestations.[69] Many other organ systems are involved, including the lungs, heart and liver. Cataracts are the most characteristic lesion but may not be seen in the neonatal period. Infected infants without symptoms in the newborn period are at high risk of subsequent deafness, congenital heart disease, mental handicap, cataracts or glaucoma.

Herpes simplex

HSV infection in the neonate is most commonly acquired at the time of birth or shortly afterwards due to the presence of active maternal infection. Of the two types, HSV 1 and 2, most neonates are infected with type 2, which is associated with genital infection, rather than type 1, the oral strain.[70] A small proportion of babies have true congenital infection and, although this is also most commonly due to HSV type 2, their clinical picture is quite different from natally or postnatally acquired disease. Many will have a vesicular rash and severe CNS involvement. Postnatal HSV infection presents more like bacterial sepsis with lethargy, poor temperature control, vomiting and respiratory distress.[69] The hepatosplenomegaly, anemia and thrombocytopenia seen in other TORCH infections is least evident in HSV disease.

Cytomegalovirus

CMV is a member of the herpes virus family and consists of several strains; an individual can have more than one CMV infection. The organism is ubiquitous. The peak ages for primary acquired infection are infancy and adolescence/early adulthood. Congenital infection occurs as a consequence of primary infection of the mother during pregnancy or reactivation of latent infection. Because of the latter possibility, mothers can infect more than one baby.[71] Severity of disease correlates with gestational age at transfer (the later the better).[72] Around 90% of infected babies are asymptomatic in the neonatal period, but those born to mothers with primary as opposed to reactivated infection are more likely to be clinically affected.[73] Congenital CMV is typically associated with hepatosplenomegaly, jaundice, anemia and thrombocytopenic purpura. The CNS is also a target with chorioretinitis (indistinguishable from that due to toxoplasmosis—see above), microcephaly and cerebral calcifications. The outlook for neonates with clinically symptomatic and severe CMV infection is historically depressing as up to 30% have perished and up to 90% of the survivors have had late CNS sequelae.[74] Whether therapy with ganciclovir will improve these figures is not clear.[75] The major late effects of congenital CMV infection are mental handicap and deafness.

Neonates can also acquire CMV during birth from maternal genital contamination or later in the neonatal intensive care unit through infected blood products. Full-term babies are usually asymptomatic in such circumstances, but low birth weight infants (<2000 g) are vulnerable to either event. Natal infection echoes congenital infection but is much less severe. Transfusion-transmitted disease is more serious and is associated with hepatosplenomegaly and an atypical lymphocytosis. It mimics sepsis and has a significant mortality.[76]

Syphilis

Congenital syphilis is now rarely seen in the western world, but still occurs, particularly in poor socioeconomic groups and drug abusers.[77] It should not be forgotten in the differential diagnosis of an infant with TORCH infection symptoms and signs. The problem occurs where mothers have untreated primary or secondary syphilis while pregnant or shortly before conceiving. Around half of infected fetuses do not survive, around 75% being stillborn and the remainder dying as neonates.[77] The survivors have a wide spectrum of manifestations affecting chiefly skeleton, liver, spleen, skin and blood. Hematologic abnormalities include anemia compounded by hemolysis (the direct antiglobulin test is negative), leukopenia and thrombocytopenia.[78] Paroxysmal cold hemoglobinuria is an unusual late manifestation of congenital or tertiary syphilis. In children it is much more frequently associated with viral infections (see Chapter 10).

Bordetella pertussis

This organism causes pertussis or whooping cough, a highly infectious disease chiefly affecting infants and young children and now controlled in the developed world (but not eliminated) by immunization. It is of interest to hematologists because it is characteristically (but not invariably) associated with a striking lymphocytosis ($>25 \times 10^9$/l) in the early stages of infection, which, although the cells are mature, can occasionally lead the inexperienced microscopist to suspect leukemia. The phenomenon lasts until the convalescent phase of the disease (up to 6 weeks).

Kawasaki disease

First described in 1967,[79] this disease is presumed by many to be infective in origin, but no organism has been identified. It is also known descriptively as the 'mucocutaneous lymph node syndrome'. It is an acute multisystem vasculitic disorder that occurs chiefly in infants and young children. Its clinical importance is that, if untreated, it has a significant mortality from coronary artery vasculitic occlusion or rupture of coronary artery microaneurysms. Treatment is based on the use of aspirin and intravenous immunoglobulin.[80] A curious hematologic feature, apart from the usual impressive neutrophilia and acute-phase response seen during the acute stage of the disease (up to 4 weeks), is a secondary thrombocytosis. This commonly arises during the second week of the illness and may persist into the subacute and convalescent phase with counts well in excess of 1000×10^9/l being commonplace. It is probably mediated by some thrombopoietic cytokine. The author has seen 3 children where the diagnosis was made retrospectively based on a high platelet count in association with the characteristic peeling desquamation of the fingers and toes.

Acute infectious lymphocytosis

Described in 1968,[81] this is a rare but benign self-limiting childhood condition associated with low-grade fever and diarrhea and which has the hallmark of a very high lymphocyte count of the order of 50×10^9/l. The lymphocytes are unremarkable and are mainly CD4$^+$ T cells.[82] The condition resolves in 2–3 weeks without treatment. It is probably due to a Coxsackie virus.[83]

Bartonellosis

Confined to the mountain valleys of the Andes in Peru, Ecuador and Colombia, the small Gram-negative bacillus *Bartonella bacilliformis* can be injected by a bite from an infected local sand fly. The organism multiplies in the vascular endothelium and then enters the blood stream to parasitize red cells and destroy them. The consequent, sometimes fatal, syndrome of severe hemolytic anemia with fever is called Oroya fever. At that stage, the organism can be easily seen in red cells using a Giemsa stain. Later in the course of the disease, the organisms leave the blood stream and subsequently cutaneous and internal hemangiomatous lesions may appear. These vary in size, although some may be large enough to require surgical excision. Such lesions can harbor the bacillus on a long-term basis. The organism is sensitive to many antibiotics including penicillin and chloramphenicol.[84]

Another species of Bartonella, *B. hensele*, is now known to be the cause of cat scratch fever. This is an uncommon but ubiquitous disorder chiefly affecting children and caused by cats, as the name suggests. It is associated with regional lymphadenitis, usually with signs of inflammation, and may be confused with tularemia or tuberculosis. An associated idiosyncratic thrombocytopenia has been described.[85] Rarely, the liver may show granulomatous lesions.[86] There are no specific peripheral blood features and the course is generally benign.

Tuberculosis

Childhood tuberculosis is an increasing problem with the emergence of multidrug resistance and HIV co-infection. Traditional factors such as poverty and overcrowding are still as important in the developed world as in poorer countries.[87] Most confirmed cases of *Mycobacterium tuberculosis* infection in children are asymptomatic and are discovered on contact tracing. Extrapulmonary disease is present in 25% of infant cases, and most commonly manifests as cervical lymphadenopathy. Later presentations include chronic mastoiditis, meningitis, renal disease, or fever of unknown origin.[88] Hematologic changes in cryptic disseminated tuberculosis have been described, including reactions mimicking chronic myeloid leukemia, secondary myelosclerosis, monocytosis and pancytopenia,[89] but these are uncommon in childhood.

Mantoux tests need to be interpreted carefully, taking into account the clinical and social circumstances of the child and his vaccination history. In addition to traditional culture, laboratory diagnosis can be made using DNA probes or nucleic acid detection using polymerase chain reaction (PCR) amplification. For susceptible micro-organisms, a combination of isoniazid, rifampicin and pyrazinamide can be used, but where multidrug-resistance is present the addition of drugs such as ciprofloxacin, clarithromycin or meropenem may be needed.[88]

Lyme disease

Transmitted by Ixodid ticks and due to a spirochete of the genus Borrelia discovered in 1982,[90] Lyme disease is a triphasic illness starting with erythema migrans at the site of the tick bite and progressing to involve the brain and meninges, myocardium, and eventually large joints. During the acute phase it can be associated with generalized lymphadenopathy. The organism is sensitive to tetracycline. Borreliae of other species transmitted by lice or ticks cause classical relapsing fever, an illness characterized by bouts of fever and myalgia and commonly associated with hepatosplenomegaly. Erythromycin is the treatment of choice for children.

Leptospirosis (Weil's disease)

Leptospirosis is caused by spirochetes of the genus Leptospira of which the best known is *L. icterohemorrhagiae*. Rodents are the most important reservoir but many species of mammal can be infected and transmit the disease, including dogs. The organism is picked up by contact with body fluids or tissues of infected animals. Human-to-human transmission is rare. Many mild cases may go undiagnosed and 90% of infections do not produce jaundice or abnormal bleeding. The picture is of fever and myalgia with a variety of skin rashes progressing in some cases to meningitis and encephalitis. Associated physical signs include lymphadenopathy and hepatosplenomegaly. Classical Weil's disease is a life-threatening illness characterized by the additional presence of jaundice and renal failure together with a severe bleeding tendency. The coagulopathy is complex and can be at least partly corrected by vitamin K. Thrombocytopenia is not always present, suggesting that DIC is not invariable.[91] Penicillin is effective against the infecting organism.[92]

Tularemia

This is an acute bacterial infection caused by the Gram-negative organism *Francisella tularensis*. It is primarily a disease of animals and humans become infected by contact with them or contaminated water. Tick bites can also transmit the disease, but human-to-human transmission has not been described. The commonest manifestation of infection is lymphadenitis local to the site of entry. This can be the oropharynx including the tonsils. More seriously, the gut or lungs can be involved. There is no characteristic blood picture but the clinical features may mimic glandular fever. The treatment of choice is streptomycin.[93]

PARASITES

Malaria

Malaria is a febrile disease caused by the invasion and reproduction of protozoan parasites of the genus Plasmodium in erythrocytes. It affects about 250 million people and kills between 1 and 2 million children each year.[94] The definitive host is the mosquito, with man serving as the intermediate host. The parasite's sexual cycle (sporogony) occurs in the mosquito, with the asexual cycle (schizogony) in man. Sporozoites enter the human circulation through the bite of an infected mosquito, and migrate to the liver, where schizogony occurs. Metacryptozoites are released into the circulation, red cells are penetrated, and trophozoites form. Division and maturation of trophozoites into schizonts occurs within the red cell, with eventual release of merozoites into the circulation, and reinfection of other red cells. In *P. ovale*, *vivax* and *malariae* infections, some merozoites return to the liver, and a new exoerythrocytic cycle is set up, providing a reservoir of dormant organisms that can cause recurrent episodes of fever over many years. *P. falciparum* does not have an exoerythrocytic cycle. Some trophozoites do not divide, but form male and female gametocytes (micro- and macro-gametocytes). No further development occurs in man, but if a mosquito is infected, the sexual cycle will restart.

Diagnosis

Malaria is diagnosed by examination of the peripheral blood. Precise species identification may be impossible if only one parasite stage is seen, and it should be remembered that infection with more than one species is not uncommon. Examination of a thick film, stained with Giemsa or Leishman, allows a relatively large volume of blood to be examined, and parasites should be identified, even if scanty. Parasites can also be seen on May–Grunwald–Giemsa (MGG) staining of thin films (Fig. 38.1), but Giemsa or Leishman staining makes the morphologic features much clearer, and aids species identification. Fluorescent micro-

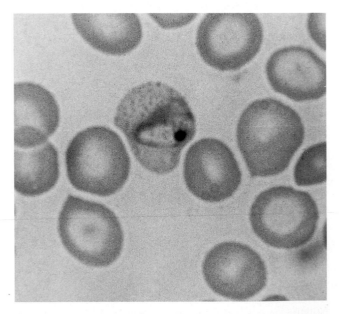

Fig. 38.1 Ring trophozoite of *Plasmodium vivax* in a thin blood film stained with May–Grünwald–Giemsa. The cell cytoplasm shows Schuffner's dots, pink red granules not seen with all species of Plasmodia.

scopy at low power is a further useful test, as malaria parasites fluoresce intensely with acridine orange. A parasite count/100 red cells is a useful guide to disease severity, 4% being a severe infection likely to be associated with serious complications. The morphology of the parasites can be seen in an atlas of hematology.[95]

Epidemiology

Malaria poses a threat to around half of the world's population. Four species of Plasmodium invade humans. *P. falciparum* and *vivax* are the commonest and are widely distributed in Central and South America, Africa and south-east Asia. *P. malariae* is found in Africa and south-east Asia, and *P. ovale* is largely confined to Africa. Most deaths are due to *P. falciparum* and occur in the non-immune and children under 5 years old.[96]

Clinical features

Acute infections cause anemia which is multifactorial.[97] Parasitization of the red cells distorts the cell membrane and causes altered permeability with increased osmotic fragility. Intracellular parasite metabolism alters the negative charge normally found on the red cell surface. During passage through the spleen, damaged red cells are either removed, or 'pitted' to remove parasites, leaving microspherocytes. Autoimmune destruction is also described, an IgG antibody forming against the parasite. The resulting immune complex attaches non-specifically to red cells, complement is activated, and cell destruction occurs. A positive direct antiglobulin test due to IgG is found in 50% of patients with *P. falciparum* malaria.

P. falciparum is occasionally associated with a particularly severe form of acute intravascular hemolysis and acute tubular necrosis called Blackwater fever. It also causes cerebral malaria characterized by delirium, coma, hyperpyrexia and convulsions. The pathology is small vessel occlusion with parasitized red cells with associated intravascular fibrin and perivascular hemorrhage. Similar changes can occur in other organs. Patients dying of malaria have massive hypertrophy of their reticuloendothelial tissue with abundant parasites and erythrocytes in macrophages.

Thrombocytopenia without DIC is a common feature of malaria and is known to be immune mediated.[98] Malaria antigens are released from lysed red cells, and bind to specific sites on the platelet membrane. IgG antimalarial antibody then bonds to the platelet-bound malaria antigen, and the IgG-platelet-parasite complex is removed in the reticuloendothelial system.

Immunity and resistance

The distribution of certain genetic disorders parallels the distribution of malaria that existed before WHO eradication programs. The heterozygous states for sickle cell anemia, thalassemia and glucose-6-phosphate dehydrogenase (G6PD) deficiency appear to confer some protection, particularly against cerebral malaria in infancy and early childhood. This protection has resulted in a high incidence of these genes in malaria areas. It has also been noted that the absence of Duffy blood group antigens is much higher in blacks (>70%) than in caucasians (<5%), and that the majority of blacks are resistant to *P. vivax* infection. The connection was made by Miller *et al*,[99] who found that the Duffy antigen is required by the parasite for penetration of the red cell. *P. falciparum* does not need the Duffy antigen but has been found to bind to glycophorin A or B on the red cell surface. Red cells lacking glycophorin A and B cannot be penetrated by the parasite, suggesting that a specific antibody blocking these receptors could be a therapeutic approach for the future.

How sickle cell disease or thalassemia might protect against malaria is not understood. Recently, in a southwestern Pacific island it was noticed that there is a higher incidence of *P. vivax* malaria and splenomegaly in children with α-thalassemia than in normal children. It is suggested that α-thalassemia might increase susceptibility to the benign *P. vivax* malaria which might, in turn, act as a natural vaccine inducing some limited cross-species protection against the more lethal *P. falciparum*.[100]

Treatment

The treatment of malaria has changed over the last few years due to declining drug sensitivity of *P. falciparum*. The benign malarias (*P. vivax*, *malariae* and *ovale*) are still largely sensitive to chloroquine which clears the peripheral blood effectively, but a further 2-week course of primaquine is needed to eradicate liver parasites. The therapy of *P. falciparum* is more complicated and depends on the sensitivity pattern in the area where the infection was acquired. If resistance to chloroquine and sulfadoxine-pyrimethamine is suspected, alternative agents include mefloquine, halofantrine, artesunate and artemether. The latter drugs were developed in China and are not widely available. There is concern that if resistance in *P. falciparum* continues to develop at the present rate, then malaria may become untreatable in parts of southeast Asia by the millennium.[94] Prevention is difficult and attempts at vaccination have generally not been successful, although insecticide-impregnated bed nets have reduced morbidity in parts of Africa.[101]

Babesiosis

Babesiosis is a protozoan disease caused by several species from the genus Babesia that colonize erythrocytes. It has many clinical features similar to malaria. It is relatively common in animals but rare in humans and only a handful of cases have been described in children.[102] It is a zoonotic disease transmitted by Ixodid ticks (the same organism that

transmits Lyme disease (see above). The ticks indiscriminately feed on deer, rodents and humans. Babesiosis ranges from being asymptomatic to causing fulminating disease and death. The clinical picture is fever, myalgia and arthalgia, together with mild heptosplenomegaly and hemolysis. Risk factors include prior splenectomy.[102] The diagnosis is made serologically or by identification of the organism in thick or thin blood films. The morphology is similar to the ring forms of *P. falciparum* and the two are sometimes confused, but schizonts and gametocytes are not seen. Standard antimalarial therapy is largely ineffective and current alternatives include a combination of clindamycin and quinine[103] or pentamidine and co-trimoxazole.[104]

Leishmaniasis

The protozoal species Leishmania causes a variety of diseases producing cutaneous, mucocutaneous or visceral involvement. Visceral leishmaniasis is known as kala-azar, meaning 'black skin' and referring to the skin hyperpigmentation sometimes seen in chronic cases. The distribution of the disease is worldwide and includes Central and South America, Asia, Mediterranean regions of Europe and North Africa, sub-Saharan Africa and the Middle East. The female sandfly (Phlebotomous sp) is the vector, with the dog serving as an important reservoir of infection. In the Mediterranean type, infants and young children are affected, with 80% of patients in Malta being under 5 years of age. In contrast, in Asia the disease affects mainly older children and adults.[105]

Presenting with progressive splenomegaly, pancytopenia and fever, children with visceral leishmaniasis in Northern Europe often have delayed diagnosis while a search is made for malignant disease or a histiocytic syndrome, particularly if there are relatively few parasites to be seen. The long incubation period means that the importance of long past overseas travel may be overlooked.[106] A case reported in Austria[107] had no known travel to an endemic area, suggesting that the infection had resulted from an imported infected sandfly, but the problem is most often seen in infants who have been on holiday to the Mediterranean.

Clinical and laboratory findings

The incubation period depends *inter alia* on the number of protozoa inoculated and varies from 2 weeks to 9 years after exposure, but most cases appear within 3–24 months. The onset may be insidious. Usually there is a 2–3-week history of increasing malaise and lethargy, poor feeding, fever and pallor. Clinical findings are of intermittent fever, massive splenomegaly with a lesser degree of hepatomegaly, and anemia. Failure to thrive and edema from hypoalbuminemia are seen, but lymphadenopathy is not a feature. The peripheral blood changes include anemia, neutropenia (in 70–75%) and thrombocytopenia (in 50–60%). The bone marrow is usually hypercellular with or without an excess of macrophages that may or may not display intracellular parasites and hemophagocytosis; 10% of children will show coagulation disturbances.[108] Untreated, the disease fluctuates with slow progression, and most patients die within 2 years.

The differential diagnosis includes a range of infections, particularly viral (congenital and acquired), subacute endocarditis, typhoid fever, tuberculosis, syphilis, brucellosis, or other tropical diseases such as malaria or schistosomiasis. Malignant disorders, particularly lympho- or myelo-proliferative disease, and storage disorders (Gaucher's and Niemann–Pick disease) should also be excluded. Histiocyte disorders should be considered. Leishmaniasis has been described as a trigger infection for the 'infection-associated hemophagocytic syndrome' (IAHS) (see Chapter 17).[109]

Diagnosis

The diagnosis is made by finding oval Leishman–Donovan (L–D) bodies, the amastigote stage of Leishmania, in and around cells of the reticuloendothelial system from samples obtained by bone marrow or splenic aspirate (Fig. 38.2). The organism multiplies by fission, is released by cell rupture, and is then taken up by other reticuloendothelial cells. The parasite burden may be high, with numerous macrophages stuffed with L–D bodies seen, but often a prolonged search may be required to identify only a few organisms and some may be lying free outside cells. Bone marrow is visibly involved in over 50% of cases. Splenic aspirate is more likely to be diagnostic, but can be a hazardous procedure, and should not be done lightly if platelet counts are $<50 \times 10^9/l$ or coagulation abnormalities exist. Marrow or splenic aspirates can be cultured for Leishmania, using special culture techniques, and antibody may be detected by complement fixation, ELISA, and immunofluorescent antibody tests. Antibody titers may be negative early in the course of the disease, and should not exclude the diagnosis in a clinically typical case with a history of travel to an endemic area.

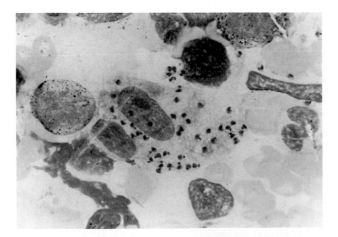

Fig. 38.2 Amastigotes of *Leishmania donovani* lying in and around a macrophage in the bone marrow from a child with the Mediterranean infantile form of visceral Leishmaniasis.

Treatment

Treatment with pentavalent antimony has been available for the last 40 years. The classical therapy is sodium stibogluconate given intravenously at a dose of 20–25 mg/kg/day for 3 weeks. Response is prompt, with fever disappearing and correction of hematologic abnormalities in the first few days of therapy. Return of hepatosplenomegaly to normal is usually rapid, as relatively little fibrosis develops in response to the infection. Follow-up is essential, as a clinical response can be followed by recurrence of symptoms a few months later. Drug-resistance has been reported in the Mediterranean area and in South America.

Latterly there has been a swing towards the use of amphotericin B.[110] The liposomal preparation of this drug may be particularly effective as it is less toxic and liposomes are taken up by macrophages and so may provide an effective drug delivery system to parasites in the same cell.[106]

Hookworm

Worldwide, hookworms are a major cause of anemia. Two species infest man, *Ancylostoma duodenale* and *Necator americanus*. They are most prevalent in the tropical and subtropical zones. *A. duodenale* is found in the Mediterranean region, North Africa and the west coast of South America, whereas *N. americanus* dominates in the western hemisphere, most of Africa, southern Asia, some Pacific islands and parts of Australia.

The parasite larvae are found in warm, moist soil contaminated by human feces. They penetrate exposed skin, typically through the soles of bare feet causing irritation, and migrate through the circulation to the right side of the heart, escaping from the pulmonary capillaries (causing an eosinophilic reaction) to crawl up the airway and down the esophagus. They mature in the small intestine and attach with their mouthparts to the mucosa. They suck blood, with each adult *A. duodenale* consuming some 0.2 ml/day and the smaller *N. americanus* consuming 0.02 ml. In heavy infestations there may be an acute reaction as the worms reach the intestine, characterized by pain, diarrhea, nausea and anorexia. This settles. Untreated, the worms can live from 4 to 8 years, and heavily infested children may present with profound iron-deficiency anemia (with hemoglobin concentrations as low as 2 g/dl) and hypoproteinemia due to loss of plasma.[111] Eosinophilia is almost invariable.

The diagnosis is made by finding worm eggs in feces (Fig. 38.3). Treatment is by de-worming with pyrantel pamoate or mebendazole. The latter is more effective against *A. duodenale*, but the 2 parasites cannot be distinguished on the morphology of their eggs. From larval penetration to the development of mature worms takes around 6 weeks. Children moving from endemic areas to temperate climates may be thought to have simple dietary iron lack. Eosinophilia should prompt careful stool examination.

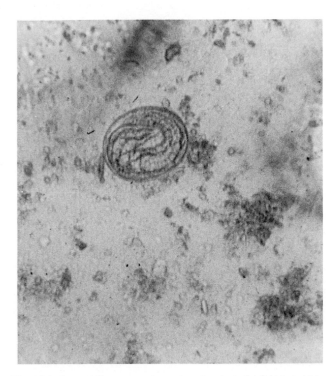

Fig. 38.3 Ovum of *Necator americanus* from the stool of a Pakistani child presenting with profound iron deficiency.

Tapeworm

Tapeworms are of interest to hematologists because of the peculiar voracity of the fish tapeworm, *Diphyllobothrium latum*, for vitamin B_{12}. The worm is ubiquitous and is acquired by eating uncooked freshwater fish. It is prevalent in cultures where people like raw or lightly salted fish or fish roes such as the Baltic states, Japan, South America, Scandinavia, Switzerland and the lake regions of Italy, and can arise in young children. Megaloblastic anemia due to secondary B_{12} deficiency is virtually confined to Finland, and it seems that strains of the worm found elsewhere may not have such an affinity for the vitamin. Host factors may also play a part.[112]

Filariasis

Filarial worms infect 200 million people between the two tropics. Six species infect humans, the commonest being *Wuchereria bancrofti*, *Loa loa* and *Onchocerca volvulus*. They are all spread by insect vectors (mosquitoes or other biting flies) and the adult worms invade the lymphatics (causing lymphoedema), skin, connective tissue or blood. Onchocerciasis also causes blindness as the parasite invades the eye. The injected adult worms mate, and the young larvae invade the bloodstream where the insect vectors collect them to complete the life cycle. The time from an infective bite to microfilarie appearing in the blood can be up to 6 months.

The diagnosis is based on identification of the microfilarial larvae in the bloodstream or (where there are cutaneous lesions) from a skin biopsy. There is a circadian periodicity in the appearance of large numbers of larvae in the peripheral blood, and specimens need to be collected at the appropriate time. Treatment is based on the drugs diethylcarbamazine or ivermectin. Allergic reactions to released worm antigens may limit the way chemotherapy can be given.[111]

Trypanosomiasis

There are two major types of trypanosome-mediated disease in humans, Chagas' disease, or American trypanosomiasis, and African sleeping sickness, or African trypanosomiasis.

Chagas' disease

This is a major health problem in South America and can be found from Mexico to Chile and Argentina. It is caused by *Trypanosoma cruzi*, a spindle-shaped protozoan organism transmitted by blood-sucking reduviid bugs of the genus triatoma. These bugs live in the cracks of primitive dwellings, but are more frequently found in forests. They infect wild animals and domestic pets. The organism is not transmitted directly by inoculation through a bite but from exposing mucous membranes or abraded skin to infected insect feces.

The organisms initially invade macrophages and reproduce by forming large numbers of amastigotes which are released and invade new cells, initially in the relevant regional lymph nodes. The acute infection is associated with dissemination and the invasion of many tissues with subsequent cellular destruction and inflammation. The disease has 3 phases; acute, latent and chronic. The acute phase is manifest in children as lymphadenopathy, hepatosplenomegaly, vomiting, diarrhea and meningeal irritation, together with evidence of acute myocarditis; 5–10% of patients will die at this stage, either of acute myocarditis or (more commonly in young infants) of meningoencephalitis. On recovery the latent phase ensues and can last for over 10 years before chronic symptoms emerge, although some individuals may never show clinical problems. The commonest chronic manifestation is cardiomyopathy and heart failure. Megacolon can also occur due to destruction of the ganglion cells of the myenteric plexus.

Chagas' disease is diagnosed by demonstration of the parasite in blood during its acute phase (Fig. 38.4). The organism can also be seen in liver biopsy, splenic puncture or bone marrow aspirate. In chronic or apparently negative cases, attempts to infect animals from the patient, either directly or by a deliberately fed reduviid bug, may help. There is no uniformly effective treatment. Nifurtimox or benznidazole may help during the acute stage but are of little value in chronic disease. Both are toxic.[113] Chronic disease may be improved with itraconazole and allopurinol.[114]

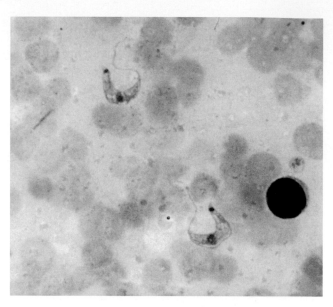

Fig. 38.4 *Trypanosoma cruzi.* Trypomastigotes in thick blood film from a Brazilian child with Chagas' disease.

African sleeping sickness

This is confined to the African subcontinent and is caused by 2 different trypanosomes, both carried by species of the tsetse fly. Gambian sleeping sickness is caused by *T. brucei gambiense*, is more chronic and evolves slowly. The Rhodesian form is due to *T. brucei rhodesiense*, and is more acute, running a course of weeks or months. Both are fatal if untreated.

The onset is marked by bouts of fever that may be mistaken for malaria. Cervical lymphadenopathy may be present. Central nervous system invasion can be subtle, beginning with personality change or other psychiatric disturbance. Dementia ensues leading to coma and eventual death. Early diagnosis can be difficult in children, and usually is only made after the onset of lassitude, seizures or psychomotor retardation.

The definitive diagnosis can only be made by finding trypanosomes in blood and bone marrow smears or in the cerebrospinal fluid. Concentration techniques such as spun buffy coat examination may be needed, or culture through animal inoculation. Treatment for the early stages of the disease can be successful using difluoromethylornithine, suramin or pentamidine. Chronic advanced disease may respond to melarsoprol.[113]

NUTRITIONAL DISORDERS

Hematinic deficiencies are described in Chapters 6 and 8, but brief consideration is given here to protein-calorie malnutrition, scurvy and anorexia nervosa, all of which can produce hematologic abnormalities.

Protein-calorie malnutrition

This all-embracing term covers:

- malnutrition due to protein deficiency in the presence of adequate carbohydrate calorie intake (kwashiorkor);
- simple calorie deficiency (marasmus);
- as commonly occurs, a combination of the two.

While primarily a problem of underdeveloped countries, malnutrition can also arise in children of strict vegetarians and can complicate some chronic diseases such as renal failure, malignancy and serious intestinal disorders.

Anemia is usual in children with severe protein deficiency. Uncomplicated, it is usually mild, normochromic and normocytic and appears to be due to reduced cell production despite adequate erythropoietin drive.[115] Frequently, concomitant iron or folate deficiency will complicate the picture. Protein-calorie malnutrition also predisposes children to infection which is in part due to impaired leukocyte function.[116]

Scurvy

Scurvy (vitamin C deficiency) is rare, but is occasionally seen in children between the ages of 6 months and 2 years due to poor dietary intake and where fruit juices are boiled. Those affected become irritable and dislike being handled. The legs become tender and this can result in pseudoparalysis where the child lies in a frog-like pose. Purple spongy swellings appear around erupted teeth. Petechial, subperiosteal, orbital or subdural hemorrhages may arise, together with hematuria or melena. Mild anemia is common, probably due to extravasation of blood. The bleeding tendency is due to loss of vascular integrity with collagen deficiency.

Anorexia nervosa

Anorexia nervosa produces hematologic changes in its more advanced stages. As might be expected, these are similar to those seen in severe malnutrition and include macrocytosis,[117] mild anemia, neutropenia and thrombocytopenia. There is a predisposition to infection associated with neutropenia and the lower ranges of body mass index.[118] The marrow undergoes gelatinous change and occasionally can become severely hypoplastic.[119] Small numbers of irregularly contracted erythrocytes are seen, similar to those of hypothyroidism, possibly reflecting a disturbance in the composition of membrane lipids.[120]

POISONING AND INJURY

Lead

Lead is a metal that humans do not need. There is no 'normal' amount in the body, and to speak of 'normal' concentrations of blood lead is to reflect on the level of contamination that prevails in the population studied. Lead can be ingested or inhaled from a variety of sources including car exhaust fumes, canned foods, water pipes, lead toys and paint dust or flakes. Young children, with their hand-to-mouth habits, are especially prone to oral intoxication from lead paint which is found most frequently in old and dilapidated houses occupied by overcrowded poor families. Coincident iron deficiency may predispose to lead poisoning by being associated with pica and by increasing the absorption of lead.[121]

Lead binds to proteins, modifies their tertiary structure, and inactivates their enzymatic properties. It has a predilection for mitochondrial enzymes and interferes with heme synthesis because, amongst other things, it strongly inhibits δ-aminolevulinic acid dehydratase[122] and ferrochetolase, 2 rate-limiting enzymes. Heme synthesis is important not only for erythropoiesis but for basic cellular respiration through the mitochondrial cytochrome system and this may in part explain some of the other effects of lead toxicity, particularly those on the central nervous system.

One of the most striking hematologic features of lead intoxication is basophilic stippling of erythrocytes. This is due to deposition of ribosomal DNA and mitochondrial fragments. An explanation may be found in the inhibition by lead of the activity of pyrimidine-5'-nucleotidase,[123] an enzyme responsible for degrading redundant nucleic acids and which, if genetically deficient, produces a hemolytic anemia with similarly striking basophilic stippling.

The anemia seen in lead poisoning is frequently due to associated iron deficiency, at least in large part,[124] and it is iron lack rather than lead toxicity that produces microcytosis and a low hemoglobin. Lead produces basophilic stippling and ring sideroblasts in the marrow but seldom a clinically important drop in hemoglobin concentration. Lead also binds to red cell membranes and affects electrolyte transfer, producing a modest shortening in erythrocyte survival which can be easily compensated. Deficient heme synthesis produces an accumulation and excess excretion of heme intermediates and this is the basis of some screening tests for lead intoxication, but red cell zinc protoporphyrin concentration may not be a sensitive indicator of lead concentration in the absence of iron deficiency.[124]

The definition of lead poisoning is somewhat arbitrary. Blood lead concentrations below 50 μg/l will probably not produce the hematologic signs described, but much lower levels (<20 μg/dl) can cause adverse effects on neuropsychologic function and what constitutes a 'safe' concentration is still a matter of debate.[125] Prevalent 'normal' values in different populations vary from 3 μg for children living in the clean air of the Himalayan highlands to 10 μg/dl or more for children in urban and rural communities of Cape Province in South Africa.[126]

Nitrites, aniline dyes, nitrobenzene and azo compounds

Such substances can all cause methemoglobinemia, and if the concentration of methemoglobin reaches 20% or more, therapy with methylene blue or exchange transfusion may necessary.

Sodium chlorate

Commonly used as a weedkiller, sodium chlorate is a powerful oxidizing substance and causes acute intravascular hemolysis and renal failure if ingested; 30 g is a fatal dose in adults.

Copper

Intoxication with copper sulfate can lead to hemolysis and renal failure in addition to vomiting, diarrhea and abdominal pain.[127] A similar picture can arise with the use of a copper sulfate dressing for burns and following copper contamination of hemodialysis units. The underlying mechanism of hemolysis may be similar to that seen in Wilson's disease (see above).

Burns

Extensive burns can cause spherocytosis, osmotic lysis of red cells and anemia. In severely burned patients, up to 30% of the red cell mass may be destroyed.

Trauma

Major tissue damage can liberate thromboplastic material into the circulation and the coagulation cascade can be triggered by this and by complement activation, giving rise to a consumption coagulopathy. Wounds infected with *Clostridium perfringens* can give rise to severe intravascular hemolysis with spherocytosis due to toxins liberated by the organism.

HEMATOLOGIC SIDE-EFFECTS OF DRUGS

Myelosuppression affecting all cell lines is a dose-dependent side-effect of many antineoplastic agents (see Chapters 19 and 27). Idiosyncratic marrow failure (aplasia) can also occur as an aberrant response to non-cytotoxic drugs such as chloramphenicol and butazone (see Chapter 2).

Drugs can also reduce the numbers of circulating blood cells through short survival, either by an immune-mediated effect or through direct damage. Neutropenia is covered in Chapter 16. Drug-induced immune hemolytic anemia is discussed in Chapter 10 and red cell damage from oxidant drugs in Chapter 14.

Drug-induced thrombocytopenia is most commonly seen as a result of antineoplastic drug suppression of cell production, but drugs can also shorten platelet survival by immune-mediated destruction or by causing direct activation and aggregation of circulating platelets, as occurred with the antibiotic ristocetin and some early non-human clotting factor concentrates. These agents have now been withdrawn from use.

Mild thrombocytopenia of the direct activation type is still occasionally seen during the infusion of antilymphocyte (or antithymocyte) globulin (currently used as immunosuppressive therapy for aplastic anemia, graft-versus-host disease and transplant rejection episodes),[128] and a more serious problem arises in a few recipients of heparin (see below). Much more commonly, drugs promote premature destruction of platelets by direct immune-mediated destruction. They do this in 1 of 3 currently understood ways:

1. by forming soluble drug–antibody immune complexes which attach themselves loosely to the surface of the platelet, fix complement and so lead to cell destruction;
2. by attaching themselves firmly to the cell surface and acting as a hapten;
3. by provoking the production of antibodies that cross-react with cell-surface antigens, thus creating a true autoimmune thrombocytopenia.[129]

From a practical point of view, the distinction between the 3 mechanisms only becomes important in terms of how long the problem lasts after withdrawal of the offending agent, being slowest in the third.

The diagnosis of drug-induced immune-mediated thrombocytopenia is seldom easy. It rests on the exclusion of other causes of a low platelet count observed while the patient is taking the agent in question, and which resolves only after its withdrawal. Direct *in vitro* laboratory confirmation is seldom feasible, although demonstration of drug-dependent binding of IgG to platelets can be attempted.[130] The most likely source of confusion is the occurrence of ITP (see Chapter 22) while a child is receiving innocent drugs for a coincidental reason.

The list of candidate drugs capable of causing immune-mediated thrombocytopenia is long,[129] but in practice the majority of problems are due to only a few agents (Table 38.1). Probably the single most important compound causing ITP in children is sodium valproate. In a prospective study of 45 children, one-third had a measurable fall in their platelet count and 1 reached a nadir of $35 \times 10^9/l$.[131] Bleeding problems have been described and appear to be due to a reduction in platelet numbers rather than drug-induced functional defects.[132] Whether the thrombocytopenia is always or wholly immune-mediated is not clear. Defective platelet production through myelosuppression has been described.[133]

Other frequently or increasingly used agents worthy of special mention are rifampicin[134] and co-trimoxazole.[135]

Table 38.1 Commonly used drugs in pediatric practice occasionally causing immune-mediated thrombocytopenia.

Sodium valproate[131]
Phenytoin[140]
Carbamazepine[141]
Co-trimoxazole[135]
Rifampicin[134]
Acetozolamide[142]
Cimetidine[136]
Aspirin[143]
Heparin[138]

There are, of course, other drugs occasionally used in children which have been implicated as causes of thrombocytopenia. The classical examples of quinidine, quinine, gold, sulfa compounds and non-steroidal anti-inflammatory agents are well known[129] and there are many more. It should be assumed that any drug is capable of producing an immune-mediated thrombocytopenia when a low platelet count occurs in a child for no other obvious reason. All should resolve within days or weeks after stopping the offending drug, with odd exceptions such as gold compounds. These produce thrombocytopenia of the type whereby true autoantibodies are stimulated (and which should not be confused with the irreversible aplastic anemia also associated with their use), and which takes longer than that caused by other drugs to resolve after withdrawal of the drug because gold is very slowly excreted from the body.[136]

Heparin-induced thrombocytopenia

Heparin is not as frequently used in pediatrics as in adult medicine due to the lower incidence of thromboembolic disease. It is used, however, and all patients on intensive care invariably receive small but significant amounts from indwelling catheters and arterial lines.

Low platelet counts can arise in as many as 5% of heparin recipients and may occur more frequently with bovine than porcine material.[138] The thrombocytopenia produced by the drug is of 2 types: one is immediate, usually mild, and not immune mediated; the other is severe, arises after 8–10 days, and is associated with a paradoxical arterial and venous thromboembolism. This second type, both more common and more serious, is due to an antibody against a heparin/platelet factor 4 complex which activates platelets and can cause major vascular occlusion.[138] Although rare, this complication of heparin therapy is so devastating that all who use the drug should be aware of it. If necessary, it is possible to confirm the diagnosis of heparin-dependent thrombocytopenia using an *in vitro* test assessing the effect of patients' sera on the release of serotonin from normal platelets in the presence of heparin.[139]

REFERENCES

1. Lee G. The anaemia of chronic disease. *Semin Hematol* 1983; **20**: 61–80
2. Cook J. Iron deficiency anaemia. *Baillière's Clin Haematol* 1994; **7**: 787–804
3. Krantz S. Pathogenesis and treatment of the anemia of chronic disease. *Am J Med Sci* 1994; **307**: 353–359
4. Means RJ. Pathogenesis of the anemia of chronic disease. *Stem Cell* 1995; **13**: 32–37
5. Cavill I, Ricketts C, Napier J. Erythropoiesis in the anaemia of chronic disease. *Scand J Haematol* 1977; **19**: 509–512
6. Means RJ. Clinical application of recombinant erythropoietin in the anemia of chronic disease. *Hematol Oncol Clin North Am* 1994; **8**: 933–944
7. Krantz S. Erythropoietin and the anemia of chronic disease. *Nephrol Dial Transplant* 1995; **10 (Suppl 2)**: 10–17
8. MacDougall I, Hutton R, Cavill I. Treating renal anaemia with recombinant human erythropoietin: practical guidelines and a clinical algorithm. *Br Med J* 1990; **300**: 655–659
9. Moia M, Mannucci P, Vizzotto L, Casati S, Cattaneo M, Ponticelli C. Improvement in the haemostatic defect of uraemia after treatment with recombinant human erythropoietin. *Lancet* 1987; **ii**: 1227–1229
10. Monnens L, van de Meer W, Langenhuysen C, van Munster P, van Oustrom C. Platelet aggregating factor in the epidemic form of haemolytic–uraemic syndrome of childhood. *Clin Nephrol* 1985; **15**: 14–17
11. Rondeau E, Peraldi M-N. *Escherichia coli* and the hemolytic uremic syndrome. *N Engl J Med* 1996; **355**: 660–662
12. Siegler R. The hemolytic uremic syndrome. *Pediatr Clin North Am* 1995; **42**: 1505–1529
13. Renaud C, Niaudet P, Gagnadoux M, Broyer M, Habib R. Haemolytic uraemic syndrome: prognostic factors in children over 3 years of age. *Paediatr Nephrol* 1995; **9**: 24–29
14. Sills R. Thrombotic thrombocytopenic purpura: 1. Pathophysiology and clinical manifestations. *Am J Pediatr Hematol Oncol* 1984; **6**: 425–430
15. Upshaw J. Congenital deficiency of a factor in normal plasma that reverses microangiopathic hemolysis and thrombocytopenia. *N Engl J Med* 1978; **298**: 1350–1352
16. Rock G, Shumak K, Buskard N *et al*. Comparison of plasma exchange with plasma infusion in the treatment of thrombotic thrombocytopenic purpura. *N Engl J Med* 1991; **325**: 393–397
17. Rock G, Shumak K, Sutton D *et al*. Cryosupernatant as replacement fluid for plasma exchange in thrombotic thrombocytopenic purpura. *Br J Haematol* 1996; **94**: 383–386
18. Mowat A. *Liver Disorders in Childhood*, 3rd edn. Oxford: Butterworth–Heinemann, 1994
19. Wardrop C, Huthinson H. Red cell shape in hypothyroidism. *Lancet* 1969; **ii**: 1243
20. Merchav S, Tatarsky I, Hochberg Z. Enhancement of erythropoiesis *in vitro* by human growth hormone is mediated by insulin-like growth factor 1. *Br J Haematol* 1988; **70**: 267–71
21. Vihervuori E, Virtanen M, Koistinen R, Seppala M, Siimes M. Hemoglobin level is linked to growth-hormone dependent proteins in short children. *Blood* 1996; **87**: 2075–2081
22. Wedemeyer A, Edson R, Krivit W. Coagulation in cyanotic congenital heart disease. *Am J Dis Child* 1972; **124**: 656–660
23. Ihenacho H, Breeze G, Fletcher D, Stuart J. Consumption coagulopathy in congenital heart disease. *Lancet* 1973; **i**: 231–234
24. Waldman J, Czapek E, Paul M, Schwartz A, Levin D, Schindler S. Shortened platelet survival in cyanotic heart disease. *J Pediatr* 1975; **87**: 77–79
25. Naiman J. Clotting and bleeding in cyanotic congenital heart disease. *J Pediatr* 1970; **76**: 333–335
26. Maurer H, McCue C, Robertson L, Haggins J. Correction of platelet dysfunction and bleeding in cyanotic congenital heart disease by simple red cell volume reduction. *Am J Cardiol* 1975; **35**: 831–835
27. Weller P, Bubley G. The idiopathic hypereosinophilic syndrome. *Blood* 1994: **83**: 2759–2779
28. Kettelhut B, Metcalfe D. Pediatric mastocytosis. *Ann Allergy* 1994; **73**: 197–202
29. Valent P. Biology, classification and treatment of human mastocytosis. *Wien Klin Wochenschr* 1996; **108**: 385–397
30. Azana J, Torrelo A, Mediero I, Zambrano A. Urticaria pigmentosa: a review of 67 pediatric cases. *Pediatr Dermatol* 1994; **11**: 102–106
31. Smith T, Welch T, Allen J, Sondheimer J. Cutaneous mastocytosis with bleeding: probable heparin effect. *Cutis* 1987; **39**: 241–244
32. Kettelhut B, Metcalfe D. Pediatric mastocytosis. *J Invest Dermatol* 1991; **96**: 15S–18S
33. Cazzola M, Ponchio L, de-Benedetti F *et al*. Defective iron supply for erythropoiesis and adequate endogenous erythropoietin production in the anemia associated with systemic-onset juvenile chronic arthritis. *Blood* 1996; **87**: 4824–4830
34. Dixon R, Rosse W, Ebbert L. Quantiative determination of antibody in idiopathic thrombocytopenic purpura. *N Engl J Med* 1975; **292**: 230–236
35. Hall S, McCormick J, Griepp P, Michet C, McKenna C. Splenectomy does not cure the thrombocytopenia of systemic lupus erythematosus. *Ann Intern Med* 1985; **102**: 325–328
36. Miller M, Urowitz M, Gladman D. The significance of thrombocytopenia in systemic lupus erythematosus. *Arthritis Rheumatol* 1983; **26**: 1181–1186
37. Stegeman C, Tervaert J, de Jong P, Kallenberg C. Trimethoprim-sulfamethoxazole (co-trimoxazole) for the prevention of relapses of Wegener's granulomatosis. *N Engl J Med* 1996; **335**: 16–20
38. Zipursky A, Palko J, Milner R *et al*. The hematology of bacterial infections in premature infants. Pediatrics 1976; **57**: 839–853
39. Evans AS, Niederman JC, McCollum RW. Seroepidemiologic studies of infectious mononucleosis with EB virus. *N Engl J Med* 1968; **279**: 1121–1127
40. Hutt-Fletcher L. Epstein Barr virus tissue tropism: a major determinant of immunopathogenesis. *Springer Semin Immunopathol* 1991; **13**: 117–131
41. Henle W, Henle GE, Horwitz CA. Epstein–Barr virus specific diagnostic tests in infectious mononucleosis. *Hum Pathol* 1974; **5**: 551–565
42. Purtilo DT. X-linked lymphoproliferative disease (XLP) as a model of Epstein–Barr virus-induced immunopathology. *Springer Semin Immunopathol* 1991; **13**: 181–197
43. Gratama J. Epstein–Barr virus infections in bone marrow transplant recipients. In: Forman S, Blume K, Thomas E (eds) *Bone Marrow Transplantation*. Boston: Blackwell Scientific Publications, 1994
44. Venkitaraman AR, Lenoir GM, John TJ. The seroepidemiology of infection due to Epstein–Barr virus in southern India. *J Med Virol* 1985; **15**: 11–16
45. Lai PK, Mackay-Scollay EM, Alpers MP. Epidemiological studies of Epstein–Barr herpes virus infection in Western Australia. *J Hyg Lond* 1975; **74**: 329–337
46. Schaller R, Counselman F. Infectious mononucleosis in young children. *Am J Emerg Med* 1995; **13**: 438–440
47. Callan M, Steven N, Krausa P *et al*. Large clonal expansions of CD8+ T cells in acute infectious mononucleosis. *Nature Med* 1996; **2**: 906–911
48. White P, Thomas J, Amess J, Grover S, Kangro H, Clare A. The existence of a fatigue syndrome after glandular fever. *Psychol Med* 1995; **25**: 907–916
49. Sakulsky SB, Wallace RB, Silverstein MN, Dockerty MB. Ruptured spleen in infectious mononucleosis. *Arch Surg* 1967; **94**: 349–352
50. Silverstein A, Steinberg G, Nathanson M. Nervous system involvement in infectious mononucleosis. The heralding and/or major manifestation. *Arch Neurol* 1972; **26**: 353–358
51. Lazarus KH, Baehner RL. Aplastic anemia complicating infectious mononucleosis: a case report and review of the literature. *Pediatrics* 1981; **67**: 907–910
52. Bowman HS, Marsh WL, Schumacher HR, Oyen R, Reihart J. Auto

anti-N immunohemolytic anemia in infectious mononucleosis. *Am J Clin Pathol* 1974; **61**: 465–472

53. Sharp A. Platelets, bleeding and haemostasis in infectious mononucleosis. In: Carter R, Penman H (eds) *Infectious Mononucleosis.* Oxford: Blackwell Scientific, 1969

54. Tynell E, Aurelius E, Brandell A *et al.* Acyclovir and prednisolone treatment of acute infectious mononucleosis: a multicenter, double-blind, placebo-controlled study. *J Infect Dis* 1996; **174**: 324–331

55. Duncombe A, Amos R, Metcalfe P, Pearson T. Intravenous immunoglobulin therapy in thrombocytopenic infectious mononucleosis. *Clin Lab Haematol* 1989; **11**: 11–15

56. Goldfarb J. Parvovirus infection in children. *Adv Pediatr Infect Dis* 1989; **4**: 211–222

57. Mortimer P, Luban N, Kelleher J, Cohen B. Transmission of serum parvovirus-like virus by clotting factor concentrates. *Lancet* 1983; **ii**: 482–484

58. Brown K, Anderson S, Young N. Erythrocyte P antigen: cellular receptor for B19 parvovirus. *Science* 1993; **262**: 114–117

59. van Horn D, Mortimer P, Young N *et al.* Human parvovirus-associated red cell aplasia in the absence of underlying haemolytic anemia. *Am J Pediatr Hematol Oncol* 1986; **8**: 235–239

60. Kurtzman G, Ozawa K, Cohen B, Hanson G, Oseas R, Young N. Chronic bone marrow failure due to persistent B19 parvovirus infection. *N Engl J Med* 1987; **317**: 287–294

61. Mihal V, Dusek J, Hajduch M, Cohen B, Fingerova H, Vesely J. Transient aplastic crisis in a leukemic child caused by parvovirus B19 infection. *Pediatr Hematol Oncol* 1996; **13**: 173–177

62. Zon L, Groopman J. Hematologic manifestations of the human immunodeficiency virus. *Semin Hematol* 1988; **25**: 208–218

63. Hilgartner M. Hematologic manifestations in HIV-infected children. *J Pediatr* 1991; **119**: S47–S49.

64. Vetter KM, Djomond G, Zadi F *et al.* Clinical spectrum of human immunodeficiency virus disease in children in a West African city. Project RETRO-CI. *Pediatr Infect Dis J* 1996; **15**: 438–442

65. Ellaurie M, Burns E, Bernstein L *et al.* Thrombocytopenia and human immunodeficiency virus in children. *Pediatrics* 1988; **82**: 905–908

66. Hanson C, Shearer W. Pediatric HIV infection and AIDS. In: Feigin R, Cherry J (eds) *Textbook of Pediatric Infectious Diseases,* 3rd edn. Philadelphia: WB Saunders, 1992, pp 990–1011

67. Desmonts G, Couvreur J. Congenital toxoplasmosis. A prospective study of 378 pregnancies. *N Engl J Med* 1974; **290**: 1110–1116

68. Desmonts G, Couvreur J. Congenital toxoplasmosis. Prospective study of the outcome of pregnancy in 542 women with toxoplasmosis acquired during pregnancy. *Ann Pediatr Paris* 1984; **31**: 805–809

69. Overall J. Viral infection of the fetus and neonate. In: Feigin R, Cherry J (eds) *Textbook of Pediatric Infectious Diseases,* 3rd edn. Philadelphia: WB Saunders, 1992, pp 924–959

70. Corey L, Spear PG. Infections with herpes simplex viruses (1). *N Engl J Med* 1986; **314**: 686–691

71. Stagno S, Reynolds DW, Huang ES, Thames SD, Smith RJ, Alford CA. Congenital cytomegalovirus infection. *N Engl J Med* 1977; **296**: 1254–1258

72. Stagno S, Pass RF, Cloud G *et al.* Primary cytomegalovirus infection in pregnancy. Incidence, transmission to fetus, and clinical outcome. *JAMA* 1986; **256**: 1904–1908

73. Preece PM, Pearl KN, Peckham CS. Congenital cytomegalovirus infection. *Arch Dis Child* 1984; **59**: 1120–1126

74. Pass RF, Stagno S, Myers GJ, Alford CA. Outcome of symptomatic congenital cytomegalovirus infection: results of long-term longitudinal follow-up. *Pediatrics* 1980; **66**: 758–762

75. Demmler GJ. Infectious Diseases Society of America and Centers for Disease Control. Summary of a workshop on surveillance for congenital cytomegalovirus disease. *Rev Infect Dis* 1991; **13**: 315–329

76. Adler SP, Chandrika T, Lawrence L, Baggett J. Cytomegalovirus infections in neonates acquired by blood transfusions. *Pediatr Infect Dis* 1983; **2**: 114–118

77. Ricci J, Fojaco R, O'Sullivan M. Congenital syphilis: the University of Miami/Jackson Memorial Medical Center experience 1986–1988. *Obstet Gynecol* 1989; **74**: 687–693

78. Gutman L. Syphilis. In: Feigin R, Cherry J (eds) *Textbook of Pediatric Infectious Diseases,* 3rd edn. Philadelphia: WB Saunders, 1992, pp 552–563

79. Kawasaki T. Acute febrile mucocutaneous syndrome with lymphoid involvement with specific desquamation of the fingers and toes in children. *Areugi* 1967; **16**: 178–222

80. Samuel J, OSullivan J. Kawasaki disease. *Br J Hosp Med* 1996; **55**: 9–14

81. Horwitz M, Moore G. Acute infectious lymphocytosis: an etiologic and epidemiologic study of an outbreak. *N Engl J Med* 1968; **279**: 399–404

82. Bertotto A, Arcangeli CDF, Spinozzi F *et al.* Acute infectious lymphocytosis: phenotype of the proliferating cell. *Acta Paediatr Scand* 1985; **74**: 633–635

83. Grose C, Horwitz M. Characterization of an enterovirus associated with acute infectious lymphocytosis. *J Gen Virol* 1976; **30**: 347–355

84. Stechenberg B. Bartonellosis. In: Feigin R, Cherry J (eds) *Textbook of Pediatric Infectious Diseases,* 3rd edn. Philadelphia: WB Saunders, 1992, pp 1056–1058

85. Billo O, Wolff J. Thrombocytopenic purpura due to cat scratch disease. *JAMA* 1960; **174**: 1824–1826

86. Lamps L, Gray G, Scott M. The histologic spectrum of hepatic cat scratch disease. A series of six cases with confirmed *Bartonella henselae* infection. *Am J Surg Pathol* 1996; **20**: 1253–1259

87. Drucker E, Alcabes P, Bosworth W, Sckell B. Childhood tuberculosis in the Bronx, New York. *Lancet* 1994; **343**: 1482–1485

88. Jacobs R, Starke J. Tuberculosis in children. *Med Clin North Am* 1993; **77**: 1335–1351

89. Glasser R, Walker R, Herion J. The significance of hematologic abnormalities in patients with tuberculosis. *Arch Intern Med* 1970; **125**: 691–695

90. Burgdorfer W, Barbour A, Hayes S *et al.* Lyme disease – a tick borne spirochetosis? *Science* 1982; **216**: 1317–1319

91. Feigin R, Anderson D. Leptospirosis. In: Feigin R, Cherry J (eds) *Textbook of Pediatric Infectious Diseases,* 3rd edn. Philadelphia: WB Saunders, 1992, pp 1167–1180

92. Watt G, Padre L, Tuazon M *et al.* Placebo controlled trial of intravenous penicillin for severe and late leptospirosis. *Lancet* 1988; **i**: 433–435

93. Yow M. Tularaemia. In: Feigin R, Cherry J (eds) *Textbook of Pediatric Infectious Diseases,* 3rd edn. Philadelphia: WB Saunders, 1992, pp 1316–1321

94. White N. The treatment of malaria. *N Engl J Med* 1996; **335**: 800–805

95. Hann I, Lake B, Lilleyman J, Pritchard J. *Colour Atlas of Paediatric Haematology.* Oxford: Oxford University Press, 1996

96. Gilles H. Malaria: an overview. *J Infect* 1989; **18**: 11–23

97. Woodruff A, Ansdell V, Pettitt L. Cause of anaemia in malaria. *Lancet* 1979; **i**: 1055–1057

98. Kelton J, Keystone J, Moore J *et al.* Immune mediated thrombocytopenia of malaria. *J Clin Invest* 1983; **71**: 832–836

99. Miller L, Mason S, Clyde D, McGinniss M. The resistance factor to *Plasmodium vivax* in blacks. *N Engl J Med* 1976; **295**: 302–304

100. Williams T, Maitland K, Bennett S *et al.* High incidence of malaria in alpha-thalassaemic children. *Nature* 1996; **383**: 522–525

101. Newton C. Falciparum malaria in children. *Curr Opin Pediatr* 1996; **8**: 16–20

102. Krause P. Babesiosis. In: Feigin R, Cherry J (eds) *Textbook of Pediatric Infectious Diseases,* 3rd edn. Philadelphia: WB Saunders, 1992, pp 2010–2016

103. Wittner M, Rowin K, Tanowitz H *et al.* Successful chemotherapy of transfusion babesiosis. *Ann Intern Med* 1982; **96**: 601–604

104. Raoult D, Soulayrol L, Toga B *et al.* Babesiosis, pentamidine and co-trimoxazole. *Ann Intern Med* 1987; **107**: 944

105. Maegraith B. Leishmaniasis. In: Maegraith B (ed) *Clinical Tropical Diseases.* Oxford: Blackwell, 1984

106. Smith O, Hann I, Cox C, Novelli V. Visceral leishmaniasis: rapid response to AmBisome treatment. *Arch Dis Child* 1995; **73**: 157–159

107. Kollaritsch S, Emminger W, Zaunschirm A, Aspock H. Suspected autochthonous kala-azar in Austria. *Lancet* 1989; **i**: 901–902

108. al-Jurayyan N, al-Nasser M, al-Fawaz I *et al.* The hematological manifestations of visceral leishmaniasis in infancy and childhood. *J Trop Pediatr* 1995; **41**: 143–148

109. Mantzer Y, Behar A, Beeri E, Gunders A, Hershko C. Systemic leishmaniasis mimicking malignant histiocytosis. *Cancer* 1979; **43**: 398–402

110. Mishra M, Biswas U, Jha A, Khan A. Amphotericin versus sodium stibogluoconate in first line treatment of Indian kala-azar. *Lancet* 1994; **334**: 1599–1600

111. Katz M. Nemathelminthes. In: Feigin R, Cherry J (eds) *Textbook of Pediatric Infectious Diseases*, 3rd edn. Philadelphia: WB Saunders, 1992, pp 2078–2088

112. Turner J. Cestodes. In: Feigin R, Cherry J (eds) *Textbook of Pediatric Infectious Diseases*, 3rd edn. Philadelphia: WB Saunders, 1992, pp 2098–2112

113. Wittner M. Trypanosomiasis. In: Feigin R, Cherry J (eds) *Textbook of Pediatric Infectious Diseases*. Philadelphia: WB Saunders, 1992, pp 2070–2078

114. Apt W, Aguilera X, Arribada A *et al.* Treatment of chronic human Chagas' disease with itraconazole and allopurinol. Preliminary report. *Rev Med Child* 1994; **122**: 420–427

115. Fondu R, Haga P, Halvorsen S. The regulation of erythropoiesis in protein-calorie malnutrition. *Br J Haematol* 1978; **38**: 29–36

116. Selvaraj R, Bhat K. Metabolic and bactericidal activities in leukocytes in protein-calorie malnutrition. *Am J Clin Nutr* 1972; **25**: 166–174

117. Keenan WJ. Macrocytosis as an indicator of human disease. *J Am Board Fam Pract* 1989; **2**: 252–256

118. Devuyst O, Lambert M, Rodhain J, Lefebvre C, Coche E. Haematological changes and infectious complications in anorexia nervosa. *Q J Med* 1993; **86**: 791–799

119. Bailly D, Lambin I, Garzon G, Parquet P. Bone marrow hypoplasia in anorexia nervosa: a case report. *Int J Eat Disord* 1994; **16**: 97–100

120. Mant M, Faragher B. The haematology of anorexia nervosa. *Br J Haematol* 1972; **23**: 737–749

121. Watson W, Hume R, Moore M. Oral absorption of lead and iron. *Lancet* 1980; **ii**: 236–237

122. Hernberg S, Nikkanen J. Enzyme inhibition by lead under normal urban conditions. *Lancet* 1970; **i**: 63–64

123. Paglia D, Valentine W, Dahlgren J. Effects of low-level lead exposure on pyrimidine-5'-nucleotidase and other erythrocyte enzymes. Possible role of pyrimidine-5'-nucleotidase in the pathogenesis of lead-induced anemia. *J Clin Invest* 1975; **56**: 1164–1169

124. Clark M, Royal J, Seeler R. Interaction of iron deficiency and lead and the hematologic findings in children with severe lead poisoning. *Pediatrics* 1988; **81**: 247–254

125. Piomelli S. Childhood lead poisoning in the '90s. *Pediatrics* 1994; **93**: 508–510

126. Nriagu J, Blankson B, Ocran K. Childhood lead poisoning in Africa: a growing public health problem. *Sci Total Environ* 1996; **181**: 93–100

127. Walsh F, Crosson F, Bayley M, McReynolds J, Pearson B. Acute copper intoxication. Pathophysiology and therapy with a case report. *Am J Dis Child* 1977; **131**: 149–151

128. Champlin R, Ho W, Gale RP. Antithymocyte globulin treatment in patients with aplastic anemia. *N Engl J Med* 1983; **308**: 113–118

129. Meischer PA, Graf J. Drug-induced thrombocytopenia. *Clin Haematol* 1980; **9**: 505–51

130. Hackett T, Kelton J G, Powers P. Drug induced platelet destruction. *Semin Thromb Hemostas* 1982; **8**: 116–137

131. Barr RD, Copeland SA, Stockwell ML, Morris N, Kelton JC. Valproic acid and immune thrombocytopenia. Arch Dis Child 1982; **57**: 681–684

132. Winfield DA, Benton P, Espir ML, Arthur LJH. Sodium valproate and thrombocytopenia. *Br Med J* 1976; **2**: 981

133. Ganick DJ, Sunder T, Finley JL. Severe hematologic toxicity of valproic acid: a report of four patients. *Am J Pediatr Hematol Oncol* 1990; **12**: 80–85

134. Blajchman MA, Lowry RC, Pettit JE, Stradling P. Rifampicin-induced immune thrombocytopenia. Br Med J 1970; **3**: 24–26

135. Claas FHJ, van der Meer JWM, Langerak J. Immunological effect of co-trimoxazole on platelets. Br Med J 1979; **2**: 898–899

136. Kelton J G, Meltzer D, Moore J *et al.* Drug-induced thrombocytopenia is associated with increased binding of IgG to platelets both *in vivo* and *in vitro*. *Blood* 1981; **58**: 524–529

137. King DJ, Kelton JG. Heparin-associated thrombocytopenia. *Ann Intern Med* 1984; **100**: 535–540

138. Warkentin TE, Kelton JG. A 14 year study of heparin-induced thrombocytopenia. *Am J Med* 1996; **101**: 502–507

139. Sheridan D, Carter C, Kelton JG. A diagnostic test for heparin-induced thrombocytopenia. *Blood* 1986; **67**: 27–30

140. Weintraub RM, Pechet L, Alexander B. Rapid diagnosis of drug-induced thrombocytopenic purpura. *JAMA* 1962; **180**: 528–532

141. Pearce J, Ron MA. Thrombocytopenia after carbamazepine. *Lancet* 1968; **ii**: 223

142. Bertino J R, Rodman T, Myerson R. Thrombocytopenia and renal lesions associated with acetazoleamide (Diamox) therapy. *Arch Intern Med* 1957; **99**: 1006–1008

143. Niewig H O, Bouma H G, DeVries K, Janz A. Haematological side effects of some antirheumatic drugs. *Ann Rheum Dis* 1963; **22**: 440–443

Hematologic effects of non-hemopoietic tumors

MM REID

A pediatric hematologist has an important role in providing diagnostic help and support in the investigation and management of children with cancer. An enormous range of hematologic abnormalities affecting peripheral blood and bone marrow, some directly caused by the presence of a tumor within the tissue, some secondary to the effects of the tumor and others to treatment, are encountered by those involved in their management. Many are obscure and of interest only to the hematology laboratory because they are of no known practical value to the clinician. This whole arena is sparsely documented in the literature, except as incidental details in individual case reports. The range, scale and significance of many of these abnormalities remain almost within the realm of folk lore: 'everyday' experiences are handed down by word of mouth from hematologist to hematologist and, to some extent, oncologist to oncologist, and the two groups do not always hand down similar information about the same phenomena. This chapter concentrates on the common abnormalities of blood and bone marrow which are not directly caused by treatment and also highlights some characteristic and other less common features of infiltrated bone marrow.

PERIPHERAL BLOOD

Anemia, erythrocytosis, leukopenia, leukocytosis, thrombocytopenia, thrombocytosis, microangiopathic hemolysis and rouleaux have all been seen at presentation in children with cancer. No single pattern is restricted to any particular form of cancer. It would be possible to construct a list of peripheral blood disturbances for each type of cancer but this would be a largely sterile exercise. However, it is worth highlighting some of the typical peripheral blood patterns and pointing out where personal experience is at variance with orthodox views.

ANEMIA OF CHRONIC DISORDER (ANEMIA OF SYSTEMIC DISEASE)

The anemia may be mild or severe and is often a concern to the treating physician. Characteristic features include red blood cells that are normochromic and microcytic with normal or raised serum ferritin, low serum iron and rouleaux resulting in a raised erythrocyte sedimentation rate—an unfavored investigation in many pediatric oncology centers. The anemia is probably caused by the complex interaction of a variety of cytokines produced in response to the presence of a tumor. It may be associated with some degree of reactive thrombocytosis. In most children with cancer anemia is not primarily due to marrow infiltration or bleeding. Even in those with disseminated disease, bone marrow infiltration is not the sole (or even, necessarily, the prime) cause of anemia. Concomitant iron deficiency is difficult to exclude by laboratory tests, and assessment of reponse to oral iron therapy is impractical in most children with cancer.

It is easier to appreciate the importance of anemia of chronic disorders if cancers which have not infiltrated the marrow are considered. Wilms' tumor and hepatoblastoma stand out in this regard. Although both erythrocytosis and anemia are said to be features, albeit rare ones, of Wilms' tumor,[1] the typical pattern is of mild or moderate anemia. In the last 19 consecutive children with Wilms' tumor seen at the author's hospital, the average hemoglobin was 10.4 g/dl (range: 6.1–14 g/dl). The average mean corpuscular volume (MCV) was 74 fl (range: 64–91 fl). Ferritin levels were only measured in those with an MCV of $\leqslant 70$ fl and were normal or raised in all 5 cases. It was not possible to estimate what contribution bleeding from the renal tract may have made to the usually mild anemia. The regular finding of raised ferritin levels in such children has led the author to abandon this investigation of microcytosis in children presenting with cancer unless it is required by specific management protocols for other reasons. In 6 children with hepatoblastoma (median age 8 months; range: 1 month–7 years), the average hemoglobin was 10.1 g/dl (range: 5.5–

15.6 g/dl) and MCV 71.4 fl (range: 61–79 fl). These two diseases are associated, in the author's experience, with the most strikingly microcytic anemia of any non-hemopoietic childhood cancer; the regularity with which it occurs rivals Hodgkin's disease. To illustrate this, blood counts at presentation from the last 29 consecutive patients with Hodgkin's disease seen in the author's hospital were studied. One was a child, aged 8 years, whose MCV was 70 fl. The other 28 ranged in age from 17 to 58 years. Fourteen had an MCV <80 fl (mean 75; range: 66–79 fl). The remaining 14 had a mean MCV of 84 fl (range: 80–92 fl).

Although anemia of chronic disorder does occur in neuroblastoma, such frequent or marked microcytosis is less common in patients from the author's hospital. The sole child with neuroblastoma and marked microcytosis (MCV <70 fl) among the last 28 cases with widely disseminated disease had β-thalassemia trait. These examples of discrepancy between textbook descriptions of classical features and routine experience suggest that the 'classical' picture may have been inordinately influenced by individual cases with 'exciting' hematologic features; erythrocytosis, occasionally seen in Wilms' tumor, is a rare condition in childhood and thus worthy of reporting while microcytosis is commonplace and of less interest.

REACTIVE THROMBOCYTOSIS

A variety of stimuli and diseases can sometimes produce dramatically high platelet counts in children,[2] in some of whom elevated interleukin (IL)-6 levels may be a contributory factor.[3,4] Rebound during cancer treatment is one of the common causes, but thrombocytosis is not thought to be particularly common at presentation.[2] To some extent the frequency of thrombocytosis depends on its definition (see Chapter 23). Patients with Wilms' tumor and hepatoblastoma provide a useful source of information about platelet counts. The average platelet count in our group of patients with Wilms' tumor was 398 × 10⁹/l (range: 91–885, 4 children with counts >500 × 10⁹/l) and in hepatoblastoma 860 × 10⁹/l (range: 641–1149 × 10⁹/l). Similar platelet counts may be found in some children with localized neuroblastoma, rhabdomyosarcoma, Ewing's tumor and other cancers. Perhaps more surprising is the average platelet count of 244 × 10⁹/l (range: 49–839 × 10⁹/l) for the last 28 cases of neuroblastoma with *infiltrated* bone marrow seen in the author's hospital, of whom 5 had elevated counts and of which 3 were between 400 and 500 × 10⁹/l. Both sets of observations, in Wilms' tumor, hepatoblastoma and disseminated neuroblastoma, suggest that other factors may influence the platelet count rather more than the presence (or absence) of marrow infiltration.

NEUTROPHILIA AND NEUTROPENIA

There is an even less consistent pattern in neutrophil counts at presentation. Moderate reactive neutrophilia seems to be as common as mild neutropenia, even in children with infiltrated marrows. Beyond awareness of potential infective risks, there is little of practical importance in the neutrophil count in most cases.

MICROANGIOPATHIC HEMOLYSIS

Microangiopathic hemolytic anemia, manifest by red cell fragmentation with perhaps a degree of thrombocytopenia and either with or without derangements in coagulation, has been seen in a wide range of cancers. Acute promyelocytic leukemia is the most infamous cause of disseminated intravascular coagulation (DIC) in childhood cancer. However, among the non-hemopoietic tumors no single type stands out. Minor red cell fragmentation or poikilocytosis is so common and non-specific that it is of little value as a diagnostic pointer or in alerting hematologists (or clinicians) to a clinically important coagulopathy.

LEUKOERYTHOBLASTIC PICTURE

The presence of circulating nucleated red blood cells and myelocytes immediately raises the possibility of bone marrow infiltration but this peripheral blood picture is not generally as striking in children as in adults with disseminated cancer. Leukoerythroblastic pictures may be associated with pancytopenia, isolated cytopenias and normal or raised white cell counts. A case can be made for examining the bone marrow in any child with such a picture at diagnosis, even if this is not one of the recommended initial investigations for the tumor, whatever the rest of the blood count indicates. However, it is a poor diagnostic aid and should not be used to help discriminate between leukemia and non-hemopoietic cancer in cases where the initial differential diagnosis is broad; it is the bone marrow appearances which matter. The author has been impressed with the frequency of a leukoerythroblastic picture in Burkitt's lymphoma and striking leukoerythroblastosis may occur in non-malignant conditions such as infection or hemolytic anemia.

CIRCULATING TUMOR CELLS

Most hematologists working in children's cancer centers will have seen occasional primitive, blast-like cells in the blood of children with disseminated neuroblastoma or other small round cell cancers. It is usually impossible to determine the nature of these cells; they could as easily be tumor as immature hemopoietic cells released as part of a leukoerythroblastic reaction, as far as a morphologist is concerned.

Neuroblastoma,[5] medulloblastoma[6] and rhabdomyosarcoma[7] have all been mistaken for acute leukemia because of peripheral blood abnormalities and, in the case of the cited example of rhabdomyosarcoma, cerebrospinal fluid (CSF) and pleural fluid involvement. Such reports are sometimes used as examples of 'circulating tumor cells'. Highlighting these rare cases may give an unrealistic impression of the typical child with cancer for at least two reasons. First, they are extremely rare. Secondly, closer inspection of these 3 published cases shows that very small numbers of circulating 'blasts' ($0.03–0.12 \times 10^9/l$) were found, there were no distinctive features which could help distinguish between non-hemopoietic cells and normal or malignant hemopoietic precursors, and the striking blood abnormality was simply a leukoerythroblastic reaction. In none of these cases did the authors claim that the circulating blasts were necessarily tumor cells. One other striking case, also of rhabdomyosarcoma, has been described,[8] in whom 37% of the total white cell count of $4.4 \times 10^9/l$ were blasts. The circulating blasts were not described, but the primitive cells in the marrow sounded typical of alveolar rhabdomyoblasts. If indeed the circulating cells were non-hemopoietic, this case may well be unique, but there is no convincing evidence to support the phenomenon of morphologically detectable circulating tumor cells in children with non-hemopoietic cancer. The syndrome of carcinocythemia in which clumps of tumor cells may be found in the blood seems to be more common in adults and may reflect tumor emboli rather than recirculating tumor cells. It is difficult to imagine such clumps freely passing through both pulmonary and peripheral capillary beds to return to venous blood.

More modern techniques such as immunocytochemical stains[9] or molecular studies to detect the tyrosine hydroxylase gene in neuroblastoma[10,11] or EWS/FLI1 and EWS/ERG hybrid genes in Ewing's tumor and primitive neuroectodermal tumor (PNET)[12] have demonstrated that tumor cells do indeed circulate in the blood of many children with small round cell tumors, albeit in numbers far below the level at which most microscopists could regularly expect to detect and recognize them. This is hardly surprising, bearing in mind the frequency of widespread dissemination at presentation in some of these cancers. More important issues than the ability merely to detect and recognize circulating tumor cells, by whatever technology, need to be faced. Does such 'minimal' tumor detected in a bone marrow aspirate indicate the presence of micrometastases or simply circulating tumor cells present in the 'contaminating' blood in the aspirate? What bearing does detection of such cells in blood (or bone marrow) have on outcome and should the therapeutic approach to some tumors of apparently identical clinical stage be changed based on such tests? These issues are beyond the scope of routine hematologic investigation and may, over the next decade, add a new dimension to the examination of the peripheral blood (and bone marrow) of many children with cancer.

BONE MARROW

For many hematologists the most important compartment is the bone marrow, and this is no less true in the investigation

of children with cancer. From early studies,[13,14] experience of the pattern of metastases and relapse has grown and has indicated those tumors in which there is a sufficiently high incidence of dissemination to warrant routine examination of the bone marrow at diagnosis. In most centers attention has focused on the small round cell tumors: neuroblastoma, Ewing's tumor, PNET, and rhabdomyosarcoma. Countless published studies of varying size have attempted to measure the likely incidence of infiltration at presentation. Most should be regarded with some caution; accuracy of the primary diagnosis has steadily improved over the past 30 years and there has been little uniformity in published series in the enthusiasm or criteria for adequacy of bone marrow examination. It is only within the last 10 years that the routine practice of obtaining marrow from more than one site, and by both aspirate and trephine biopsy, has gained wider acceptance. The role of monitoring progress in treatment by attempting to measure the response of bone marrow metastases is still in its infancy. Apart from unique clinical circumstances, routine monitoring of bone marrow is virtually restricted to neuroblastoma, for which internationally agreed criteria for staging and assessment of response have been developed.[15,16]

This section deals in the main with the appearances of infiltrated bone marrow and draws on both the scanty published data and personal experience. In contrast to the discussion of the peripheral blood changes, there is enough information about some tumors to make their individual consideration worthwhile.

NEUROBLASTOMA

Neuroblastoma is the commonest malignant infiltrate of bone marrow of children after leukemia. In most cases its detection and correct identification present few problems; there is usually a strong clinical suspicion of the correct diagnosis and a simple diagnostic test allows the detection of high levels of catecholamine metabolites in over 90% of patients with neuroblastoma. The simplicity of this test and its general reliability have probably contributed to the lack of vigor with which hematologists have studied the tumor cells. This apparent lack of interest contrasts sharply with the enthusiasm for examining, describing, classifying, and investigating the blasts of leukemia. Despite the frequency with which neuroblastoma is seen by hematologists (who see more cytologic preparations of this tumor than any other pathologists), only sporadic descriptions, as opposed to studies of frequency of infiltration, existed until Mills and Bird[17] described the 'variability of the microscopic pattern of marrow infiltration,' having studied both bone marrow aspirate smears and trephine biopsies from 48 new cases.

Cytology

Superficially, individual neuroblasts often resemble lymphoblasts, and occasionally they may also have a few vacuoles. Provided the marrow smear is carefully examined under low power, this illusion soon fades. Hematologists should resist the temptation to move too quickly to oil immersion, high power lenses. Three patterns were recognized: 'clumps', 'clumps and rosettes' and a 'pseudoleukemic' pattern. While recognizing the validity and importance of these 3 patterns, the author has found that none is mutually exclusive within an individual case, particularly if marrow aspirates are obtained from more than one site. Neuroblasts have a tendency to adhere so strongly to each other that in the process of aspirating the marrow, which is often difficult to achieve, cells are often ripped apart from each other and from the tumor stroma and/or the reactive marrow fibrous tissue. This leaves numerous bare nuclei and often large amounts of cytoplasmic or stromal debris over the surface of the smear, as well as producing the more familiar clumps, doublets and intact single cells.

Mills and Bird[17] often found ball-like clumps, some with a central lumen, resembling rosettes. Others failed to find significant numbers of rosettes[18] but one study showed that, provided the smears were examined carefully, rosettes were present in the majority of cases,[19] and large numbers of these structures were virtually diagnostic of neuroblastoma. In the author's hospital, bone marrow smears are made at the bedside from freshly aspirated bone marrow. The practice of putting aspirated bone marrow into EDTA and making cytologic preparations later may introduce other artifacts and should not, if possible, be relied on as the sole or routine method of handling aspirated bone marrow.

The partially fibrillar nature of the center of the rosettes strongly resembles earlier descriptions of neuroblastoma cytoplasm,[20] and their centers also stain strongly with UJ13A,[19] a monoclonal antibody to the neural cell adhesion molecule (NCAM) which reacts strongly with most neuroblastomas.[21] Although syncytia have often been described, it remains possible that they too are artifacts. Careful examination of rosettes on smears suggests that filamentous extensions of neuroblast cytoplasm extend into the centers of the rosettes which may also contain secreted substances; together they may give the impression of multinucleate cells. Examples of some cytologic features of neuroblastoma which cannot be found with ease in many atlases of hematology are shown in Plates 42 and 43.

Bone marrow histology

Mills and Bird[17] also provided the first satisfactory descriptions and illustrations of the histologic features of neuroblastoma in the bone marrow, highlighting the prominent reticulin fibrosis. The range of appearances they described was confirmed shortly after in a larger study.[22]

From these two studies it is clear that the term 'small round cell tumor', when used to describe neuroblastoma within the bone marrow, can be very misleading. Tumor cells ranging in size from that of a lymphoblast to that of a megakaryocyte can be found, with variable amounts of fibrotic stroma. In some biopsies, fibrosis with few easily identifiable tumor cells predominates. In others, almost monomorphous sheets of tumor cells can be found. Both extremes can occur in different biopsies taken at the same time from the same patient. Occasionally, clear-cut differentiation to ganglion cells is obvious. The classic rosettes in histologic sections of the primary tumor in neuroblastoma are less often found in sections of the marrow than apparently similar structures on aspirate smears. This may reflect some degree of crush artifact in relatively small pieces of tissue or some effect of the tissue (i.e. bone marrow) in which the metastases have developed. It also begs the question that rosettes in aspirated bone marrow represent a cytologic manifestation of the classic rosette found in histologic preparations.

The extent of infiltration may vary between two simultaneous biopsies from different sites; in one there may be complete replacement of hemopoietic tissue, and in the other no evidence of tumor or a single, small, well circumscribed cellular nodule. There is often marked discrepancy between the apparent tumor load inferred from the aspirate and biopsy appearances. Such variations highlight the patchy, non-uniform distribution of metastases within bone marrow and the naïveté of attempting to quantify infiltration of marrow as a simple percentage of aspirated cells. Typical patterns of bone marrow histology are shown in Plates 44–48.

Despite studies carried out over 25 years ago,[23] it is only quite recently that pediatric oncologists and hematologists have come to accept that single aspirates are inadequate for staging.[18,24,25] This growing appreciation has culminated in internationally agreed criteria for both staging and assessing response to treatment[15,16] which recommend at least 2 aspirates and 2 trephine biopsies from 2 separate sites as part of the initial staging and also on each occasion that full re-assessment of response is carried out. The exception to this general advice is that trephine biopsy, as opposed to aspirate, is recognized as being technically difficult in infants aged <6 months; it could then remain an optional investigation. Some guide is also given about the size of biopsy core which operators should aim to obtain: 1 cm of marrow, as opposed to bone or cartilage. Further experience has shown that many centers within the European Neuroblastoma Study Group often fail to obtain interpretable cores of bone marrow of even half this size.[26] The reasons for this failure are complex and probably include a combination of lack of suitable training and supervision of junior doctors, a striking lack of involvement of hematologists in the procedure in some centers and, perhaps, the size of the patients. Despite the documented frequency of 'inadequate' samples, one recent estimate of marrow involvement within some European centers showed that only 10% of children with stage 4 disease at presentation have no 'conventionally' detectable tumor at presentation.[27]

Monitoring effects of treatment: restaging

Once treatment has started it is difficult to find tumor cells in aspirated marrow, even from children with previously heavy infiltration. The trephine biopsy assumes even greater importance. There has only been one attempt to describe the range of histologic abnormalities in bone marrow of treated children.[22] Four main patterns emerged:

1. marrow without abnormal architecture, infiltrate or fibrous stroma, albeit often very hypocellular;
2. marrow with similar features but with a pathologic increase in reticulin;
3. marrow with distorted architecture, increased fibrous stroma and abnormal although not frankly malignant mononuclear cells;
4. marrow with an obvious infiltrate of malignant cells.

This grading of bone marrow histology was offered as an alternative to the simple 'yes or no' reports apparently demanded by clinicians who, perhaps understandably, tend to equate the absence of clearly malignant cells with 'normal marrow'. Whether such a grading system will prove to be clinically important remains to be seen. However, it was clear from the material examined in this study that histologic patterns identical to the post-treatment fibrotic picture could be found in children with infiltrated bone marrow who had not yet received any treatment. One small study[28] showed that the massive reticulin fibrosis and distorted architecture (grade 3 appearances), which often persisted after treatment, was most unlikely to be caused by the trauma of earlier biopsies. It also contrasted the persistence of abnormal fibrous tissue in treated neuroblastoma with the speed of resolution of fibrosis in B-precursor acute lymphoblastic leukemia. The hypothesis that such persisting fibrosis implies failure to eradicate all tumor from the bone marrow has not yet been effectively tested. The combination of fibrosis, unidentifiable mononuclear cells and, occasionally, ganglion-like cells also raises the possibility that differentiation may be taking place. Whether some of these cells can revert to aggressive neuroblastoma also remains unknown.

Alternative techniques

Accurate staging is most problematic in apparently limited stage disease (stages 1–3) and those rare children with stage 4 disease but without obvious marrow involvement. Simple morphology is, by definition, inadequate. There have been numerous studies of the potential ability of immunologic tests to detect occult neuroblastoma in bone marrow,[25, 29–35] and even short-term culture experiments which reveal the product of clonogenic neuroblastoma cells as 'spheroids' of tumor cells.[36] Panels or mixtures of antibodies seem popular but the results are often conflicting and no study has convincingly demonstrated the superiority of immunologic tests over properly executed, conventional tests. The arguments against replacing conventional techniques with immuno-

logic studies have been summarized elsewhere.[37] In the author's hospital neither immunocytochemical stains of bone marrow aspirates[32] nor immunohistologic stains of sections of frozen or formalin-fixed tissue[33] matched careful examination of the routinely processed bone marrow biopsies. In the author's experience, expertly carried out immunologic tests might well be superior to superficially or hurriedly examined smears or sections of bone marrow because the staining reaction draws the eye to positive cells.

One common theme of many of the studies has been the potentially complementary role of immunologic studies. However, factors such as expense, technical complexity, immense practical difficulties in examining frozen sections of bone marrow and caveats about specificity of antibodies have limited their incorporation into the 'routine' battery of investigations offered by most centers. It seems probable that if an individual center's pathologists/hematologists become familiar with the practical limitations of 1 or 2 antibodies and the methodology involved (immunofluorescence, immunoalkaline phosphatase, immunoperoxidase, alkaline phosphatase/antialkaline phosphatase techniques), they may be useful additions to a laboratory's repertoire of investigations.

In the author's hospital there are particular reservations about immunofluorescent tests on cell suspensions because of the microscopist's inability to identify the nature of individual fluorescing cells. NCAM-positive osteoblasts[31–33] are a recurring problem, particularly in hypocellular marrow aspirates after treatment has started. These immunologic tests also have drawbacks in terms of diagnosis, apart from excluding leukemia or lymphoma. In the author's experience, NCAM may be expressed by Ewing's tumor, PNET, rhabdomyosarcoma, medulloblastoma, retinoblastoma and pinealblastoma, and neurone-specific enolase (NSE; sometimes cynically called 'never specific ever') by most of the neural-origin tumors.

One further caveat concerns the use of antibodies against hemopoietic malignancies; some laboratories think it useful to use antibodies against CD10, CD19 or terminal transferase (TdT) to 'exclude' acute lymphoblastic leukemia but encounter problems when they find surprisingly high numbers of positive cells. Elevated numbers of what are almost certainly reactive, non-malignant B precursors are found in a variety of non-leukemic disorders among which are a range of small round cell tumors.[38] The author has also seen this phenomenon in neuroblastoma and concludes that the use of these antibodies usually causes more confusion than it solves. Examples of some immunologic tests on infiltrated bone marrow aspirates and trephine biopsies are shown in Plates 49–53.

Technology continues to move on. Molecular detection of the tyrosine hydroxylase gene, thought to be 'specific' for neuroblastoma, is now being reported.[10,11] Very small numbers of putative neuroblasts ($1/10^5$ or 10^6 hemopoietic cells) can be detected in aspirated bone marrow by this method. Such technology remains the province of the molecular biology rather than the hematology laboratory. Some molecular techniques such as fluorescent *in situ* hybridization (FISH) can be applied directly to bone marrow aspirates to detect chromosomal or genetic features of neuroblasts which are known to be of prognostic significance: amplification of *N-myc*, deletions of chromosome 1p and hyperdiploidy can all be demonstrated in intact tumor cells on infiltrated native bone marrow smears.[39] It is still too early to know what impact such techniques will have on staging and re-assessment but it seems likely that the FISH technology could in due course produce results which might directly affect management at the outset.

RHABDOMYOSARCOMA

This is the commonest soft tissue sarcoma of childhood. Marrow infiltration at presentation is thought to occur in 25–30% of cases.[14,40] Many have been thought to be embryonal rhabdomyosarcoma. Such figures should be viewed with caution. Diagnostic criteria for rhabdomyosarcoma have improved over the past 25 years.

Disseminated alveolar rhabdomyosarcoma has in the past often been misdiagnosed as lymphoma or other forms of cancer. Etcubanas *et al*[41] from St Jude Children's Hospital reported 10 cases of disseminated rhabdomyosarcoma with occult primary tumors, all of whom had initially been diagnosed as having leukemia, lymphoma, neuroblastoma or other unknown non-hemopoietic tumor. From their report it seems that rhabdomyosarcoma may be the commonest cause of disseminated non-hemopoietic cancer of children and adolescents in whom the primary tumor is hard to find, apart from occasional cases of neuroblastoma in whom it may also be difficult to distinguish between some metastatic lesions and the primary; however, in neuroblastoma the diagnosis is usually easy to confirm by detection of elevated urinary catecholamine metabolites and there is no reason to believe that the histologic features of, for example, large intra-abdominal metastatic masses differ from those of the primary itself.

Cytology

Etcubanas *et al*'s[41] description of the cytologic features in a series of 10 patients is a valuable reference source for hematologists. In several cases the tumor had alveolar features. Three cases clearly did not have this subtype. The cytologic features described closely resembled those found in a study from the author's hospital.[42] Tumor invasion in the author's series was extensive and superficially resembled leukemia. There was a tendency for the cells to clump, but not as prominently as in neuroblastoma, Ewing's tumor or PNET. Mutlinuclearity was common and several had giant cells with up to 10 nuclei/cell. Vacuolation of cytoplasm was prominent, often peripherally placed in a rim of cytoplasm which stained darker than the main body of cytoplasm. Vacuoles often coalesced into elongated lakes. There was

striking periodic acid-Schiff (PAS) positivity which often corresponded with the position of the vacuoles. Tumor cells which had ingested other tumor cells, red cells or erythroblasts could often be found. This last feature has also been observed in the author's hospital in some cases of Ewing's tumor as well as in histiocytic malignancy, monocytic leukemia and breast cancer, and therefore it is not specific for rhabdomyosarcoma. Nonetheless, this combination of cytologic features is characteristic of rhabdomyosarcoma and should suggest the correct diagnosis. The author also found the primary tumor difficult to detect in 3 cases and undetectable in 1. It is of interest that all the cases of disseminated rhabdomyosarcoma seen by the author were determined to be of the alveolar variant (see below). No case of bone marrow infiltration at presentation in other subtypes of rhabdomyosarcoma has yet been recognized in the author's center. Examples of characteristic cytologic features of alveolar rhabdomyosarcoma are shown in Plates 54 and 55.

Bone marrow histology

Despite the frequency with which rhabdomyosarcoma infiltrates bone marrow, no adequate descriptions of the bone marrow histologic features had appeared until the author's study was reported.[42] In part this reflects past underuse of bone marrow trephine biopsy in the staging and investigation of children with cancer. There are descriptions of alveolar patterns in metastases to other tissues,[43] so it came as little surprise that such patterns could also be found in the bone marrow metastases. However, the importance lies in the fact that the alveolar pattern is so characteristic that, once recognized, the correct diagnosis may be made even in children in whom no primary tumor can be found. Supportive evidence may also be found in the almost universal expression of desmin by the tumor cells and by detecting the translocation t(2;13). All 7 cases in the author's study with this alveolar pattern had desmin-positive tumor cells. The 2q + marker chromosome was found in 3 cases, in 1 of whom the complete translocation was found. Examples of characteristic histologic features are shown in Plates 56 and 57.

While the author's study revealed an overall rate of marrow infiltration similar to those reported elsewhere, it was striking that none of the cases had anything other than alveolar patterns of bone marrow histology. It is difficult to reconcile the high rate of exclusively alveolar-type marrow infiltration in the author's series with reports from some other centers in which embryonal rhabdomyosarcoma seems to feature strongly. For example, Ruymann *et al*[40] reported that 12 of 30 cases with bone marrow infiltration had the embryonal subtype. If this rate is representative, at least 1 case of embryonal rhabdomyosarcoma might have been expected to be found in the author's series. In part this discrepancy may reflect the relatively small number of published cases investigated by both aspirates and trephine biopsies and the small number of cases examined in the author's hospital. However, there remains some suspicion about the accuracy of diagnosis of the primary tumor in past series, particularly now that mixed alveolar/embryonal and 'solid' alveolar types of rhabdomyosarcoma are being described.[44,45] It is also impossible to estimate the number of cases of disseminated alveolar rhabdomyosarcoma which have been misdiagnosed as some other form of malignancy. Further experience of trephine biopsies and more uniform diagnostic criteria within the entire field of small round cell cancers is needed to build up an accurate picture of the frequency of bone marrow dissemination in rhabdomyosarcoma.

EWING'S TUMOR AND PRIMITIVE NEUROECTODERMAL TUMOR

The Ewing's family of tumors comprises classic Ewing's tumor, primitive neuroectodermal tumor of bone, soft tissue Ewing's and Askin tumor of the chest wall. The subject is well reviewed by Roessner and Jürgens.[46] Considerable interest has arisen because of the presence of a unifying feature, the translocation t(11;22) and its rarer variant t(21;22). These translocations result in hybrid genes comprised of elements of the EWS gene on chromosome 22 and FLI1 on 11 or ERG on 21. Hybrid transcripts when detected seem to be of major diagnostic value,[12] but more experience of their diagnostic specificity is needed; such hybrids may yet be reported in some cases of non-Ewing's tumor. Their value to staging and monitoring progress have not yet been studied adequately. In this family of tumors, as in neuroblastoma, technical advances are progressing faster than the ability to mount the studies which might answer an increasing range of clinically important questions. Indeed, there is still room for improvement in deciding which are the most important questions to ask. Even if the questions are limited to initial staging, morphologic examination of bone marrow remains, for the time being, the standard approach, the responsibility of hematologists/pathologists and the closest to a gold standard against which newer technologies must be compared.

The bone marrow is infiltrated in approximately 22% of cases.[47] Over half of those with bone marrow infiltration have evidence of metastases elsewhere. Studies emphasize the focal nature of bone marrow metastases and, as in neuroblastoma, highlight the need for examination of more than 1 site with both aspirates and biopsies. The author's experience of the bone marrow appearances in disseminated disease is limited, but a similar proportion of infiltrated marrows has been found. In one 5-year period, 2 aspirates and 2 biopsies in 13 children with Ewing's tumor were examined: 8 never had morphologic evidence of infiltration; 5 had tumor within the bone marrow at some stage of their disease—3 at diagnosis and 2 at relapse. Of the 3 with infiltrated marrow at diagnosis, 1 had tumor in both smears and biopsies, 1 had detectable tumor in an aspirate smear but not the biopsy from the same site (the other being clear of tumor in both samples), and 1 in the biopsy but not the

aspirate smear from the iliac crest opposite the primary tumor.

In general, tumor infiltration as judged crudely from aspirate and biopsy core appearances was less extensive than in neuroblastoma. The cells were approximately the same size as neuroblasts, and were occasionally prominently vacuolated with a pattern much more akin to that seen in Burkitt's lymphoma than either neuroblastoma (in which prominent vacuolation is unusual) or rhabdomyosarcoma. The tendency to form clumps or smaller aggregates was similar to that of neuroblastoma. The author also found occasional rosettes in 3 cases.[19] The PAS reaction is often positive in Ewing's cells but has not been as dramatic as in those cases of rhabdomyosarcoma studied by the author. Occasional tumor cells which contained ingested cellular material could be found but this was less striking than in rhabdomyosarcoma. Histologic features of the biopsy have been relatively non-specific, beyond strongly suggesting a non-hemopoietic tumor because of the patchy nature of the deposits and the reticulin pattern. Unlike rhabdomyosarcoma, desmin positivity is unknown in the author's experience.

PNET is even rarer than Ewing's sarcoma and hematologists/pathologists in any single center will rarely see this tumor infiltrating bone marrow. In the 3 cases the author has seen, the tumor cells clumped more avidly than either neuroblasts or Ewing's cells. Vacuolation was striking, again resembling or exceeding that observed in Ewing's tumor. The author has not seen enough cases to recognize any characteristic features of bone marrow histology. Although rosette formation is a classic feature of the primary tumor in PNET of bone, it was not present in either aspirate smears or bone marrow trephine biopsies in the 3 cases but the author has too little experience to know whether this is no more than a chance observation. The author has not diagnosed bone marrow infiltration in any case of soft tissue Ewing's tumor or Askin tumor. Examples of infiltrated bone marrow are shown in Plates 58–61.

Immunocytochemical stains have thus far been disappointing as an aid to diagnosis, apart from detecting the apparent lack of desmin positivity. There is some expression of NCAM in well over half of these 'neural' tumors. One antigen, MIC2 protein, is said to be expressed in the great majority of Ewing's family tumors,[48] but increasing experience is already suggesting that there may be some questions about both its specificity and sensitivity. It is possible that molecular techniques for the Ewing's family hybrid genes will be more useful, at least in centers with the appropriate technical expertise at hand, but further experience is needed before this can be judged. It is still not clear how pediatric oncologists will use the information gained from such investigations.[49] As with the molecular approach to diagnosis of poor prognosis neuroblastoma, the arena for such techniques is moving away from the conventional hematology department; however, it would be premature to replace conventional approaches by more technically exciting and currently fashionable methods of tumor detection. Their complexity and expense make them unappealing to all but a few highly specialized centers in wealthy countries.

OTHER TUMORS

There can scarcely be a cancer of childhood which has not been found to infiltrate bone marrow at some stage of the disease. No single center will ever see enough to obtain a comprehensive and reliable 'in house' background of experience. Instead, occasional examples in atlases of hematology, the handing down of knowledge from hematologist to hematologist and the opinions of other experienced microscopists must be relied upon.

Among those cancers rarely involving bone marrow, the author has seen examples of osteosarcoma, retinoblastoma and medulloblastoma. Only classic osteosarcoma stands out in the author's experience as worthy of particular mention to hematologists. The morphologic features of widespread disseminated osteosarcoma in a trephine biopsy were virtually diagnostic in their own right: tumor cells embedded in a matrix of osteoid and almost impossible to aspirate. The few aspirated cells obtained were strongly positive for alkaline phosphatase. The tumor cells appeared to be too firmly embedded in osteoid for trephine 'touch' or 'roll' preparations to provide significant numbers of cells for detailed cytologic assessment. Plate 62 shows the characteristic histologic features.

Only 1 case each of medulloblastoma and retinoblastoma (Plate 63) involving the bone marrow have been seen in the author's hospital, in both of whom tumor infiltration was found at relapse. In the case of medulloblastoma, there was a ventriculo-peritoneal shunt which may have allowed systemic dissemination to occur more easily when the tumor relapsed. There were no distinguishing features in either of these cases beyond their uniform tendency to form clumps on the smear and patchy infiltrates in the bone marrow trephine biopsy, which allowed them to be easily differentiated from leukemia or non-Hodgkin's lymphoma. As in many other small round cell tumors, antibodies against NCAM and NSE may be useful in differentiating them from leukemia or lymphoma but they will not reliably distinguish between various members of this group.

OTHER TISSUES

Samples of tissue other than blood or bone marrow are often examined in hematology laboratories. They include CSF, pleural effusions, ascites and joint fluid. Local arrangements for examining such tissues vary, but hematology laboratories in most cancer centers have developed some expertise in examining CSF because of its relatively frequent involvement in leukemia and lymphoma. The technology needed for accurate cell counting (familiarity with hemocytometers for 'low' count infiltration, availability of blood cell counters for 'high' counts) and cell identification (making cytospin preparations, cell surface marking by flow cytometry or immunocytochemistry, and routine cytochemistry) mean the hematology laboratory is often asked to examine these fluids.

Many hematologists have therefore acquired considerable expertise in examining Romanowsky-stained cytospin preparations and have learned to make allowances for the peculiar, 'flattening' artifact of the cytocentrifuge, and the frighteningly 'malignant' appearance of perfectly normal non-hemopoietic cells present in, for example, pleural fluid or ascites. Such cells are usually mesothelial lining cells or reactive macrophages. It is the mesothelial cells that look most worrying to hematologists. In the author's experience, pleural or ascitic fluid infiltrated with lymphoblasts or Burkitt cells seldom cause a major problem, usually because such cells predominate and it is easy to ignore the presence of occasional mesothelial cells. In any case, the author always supplements morphologic assessment with immunophenotypic analysis to confirm the B-precursor or T-cell lineage of the infiltrate in the case of lymphoblastic lymphoma and B-cell lineage in the case of Burkitt's lymphoma. Cytogenetic analysis can also provide convincing evidence of the diagnosis. However, problems in correctly identifying mesothelial cells are more likely to arise if non-hemopoietic malignant infiltration is suspected, not least because the number of malignant cells in effusions or ascites in such cases is often much lower than in cases of lymphoblastic or Burkitt's lymphoma, and mesothelial cells are thus relatively more prominent. In such cases there may also be a scattering of lymphoid cells. Immunophenotypic analysis of these lymphoid cells is unhelpful and, at worst, confusing. Most will be T cells and no evidence of clonality (or otherwise) can be obtained from the immunophenotype. Molecular studies to show polyclonal T-cell infiltrates may not be readily available in many centers and may take too long to be immediately helpful to clinicians. In this situation, morphologic expertise is of great importance.

In doubtful cases, consultation with an experienced cytopathologist is beneficial to both hematologist and patient. Cytologists are professional observers of non-hemopoietic tumor cells while hematologists often have much less experience and a more restricted repertoire of useful monoclonal antibodies at their disposal. Co-operation across specialties may prevent embarrassing, and more importantly, clinically misleading reports.

During the last 10 years the author has seen examples of metastatic neuroblastoma, pinealblastoma (Plates 64–66) and medulloblastoma in CSF, and rhabdomyosarcoma in pleural fluid. Brain tumors and retinoblastoma are well known to involve the CSF. In the case of retinoblastoma, CSF involvement is so rare at presentation (<1% of low-stage cases) that routine CSF examination could probably be stopped.[50] If extra-global progression is found after enucleation, or other signs or symptoms of central nervous system involvement are present, both bone marrow and CSF examination should be carried out.

Apart from the hallmark of non-hemopoietic tumor, the tendency towards clumping, and the pattern of vacuolation in the single case of rhabdomyosarcoma in pleural fluid, the author has not seen any characteristic cytologic features that distinguish between many of these other small round cell tumors. The single case of pinealblastoma contained cells which could confidently be said not to resemble neuroblastoma or leukemia, but it is not known if the appearances were unique to this case or typical of the condition. All the small round cell tumors found to be infiltrating pleural fluid or CSF expressed NCAM.

CONCLUSIONS

There are few descriptions of peripheral blood, bone marrow and other body fluid abnormalities in children with non-hemopoietic cancer. Also, there are too few histopathologists who confer closely with hematologists and vice versa. There is no shortage of attempts to measure the frequency with which any given tumor may have involved the bone marrow (or CSF or other body fluid) but such studies are of limited practical help to hematologists. Much of this chapter reflects personal experience but what strikes one observer may be unimpressive to another. Because of the rarity of many of these cancers, one center will never attain enough experience to provide a truly rounded picture; the paucity of personal experience in many areas revealed in this chapter attests to this. Unless there is more uniformity in diagnostic and investigative standards, any single center's experience may provide a curiously and unintentionally distorted view. This chapter may, however, stimulate some to record their experiences systematically. The results of such efforts should help future hematologists, pediatric oncologists and their patients.

Acknowledgement

The author thanks Professor AJ Malcolm for numerous discussions about the histologic features of infiltrated bone marrow in children with cancer, Dr JT Kemshead for donating UJ13A and Professors AW Craft and ADJ Pearson for encouraging him to look carefully at and record his experience of bone marrow appearances in their patients.

REFERENCES

1. Altman AJ. Management of malignant solid tumors. In: Nathan DG, Oski FA (eds) *Hematology of Infancy and Childhood*, 4th edn. Philadelphia: WB Saunders, 1992, p 1384
2. Vora AJ, Lilleyman JS. Secondary thrombocytosis. *Arch Dis Child* 1993; **68**: 88–90
3. Frenkel EP. Southwestern internal medicine conference; the clinical spectrum of thrombocytosis and thrombocythemia. *Am J Med Sci* 1991; **301**: 69–80
4. De Benedetti F, Martini A. Secondary thrombocytosis. *Arch Dis Child* 1993; **69**: 170–171
5. Christenson WN, Ultmann JE, Mohos SC. Disseminated neuroblastoma in an adult presenting the picture of thrombocytopenic purpura. *Blood* 1956; **11**: 273–278
6. Pollack ER, Miller HJ, Vye MV. Medulloblastoma presenting as leukemia. *Am J Clin Pathol* 1981; **76**: 98–103
7. Nunez C, Abboud SL, Lemon NC, Kemp JA. Ovarian rhabdomyosarcoma presenting as leukemia. *Cancer* 1983; **52**: 297–300
8. Fitzmaurice RJ, Johnson PAE, Liu Yin JA, Freemont AJ. Rhabdomyosarcoma presenting as 'acute leukaemia'. *Histopathology* 1991; **18**: 173–175
9. Moss TJ, Sanders DG, Lasky LC, Bostrom B. Contamination of peripheral blood stem cell harvests by circulating neuroblastoma cells. *Blood* 1990; **76**: 1879–1883
10. Miyajima Y, Kato K, Numata S, Kudo K, Horibe K. Detection of neuroblastoma cells in bone marrow and peripheral blood by the reverse transcriptase-polymerase chain reaction for tyrosine hydroxylase mRNA. *Cancer* 1995; **75**: 2757–2761
11. Burchill SA, Bradbury FM, Selby P, Lewis IJ. Early clinical evaluation of neuroblastoma cell detection by reverse transcriptase-polymerase chain reaction (RT-PCR) for tyrosine hydroxylase m-RNA. *Eur J Cancer* 1995; **31A**: 553–556
12. Delattre O, Zucman J, Melot T *et al.* The Ewing family of tumors—a subgroup of small-round-cell tumors defined by specific chimeric transcripts. *N Engl J Med* 1994; **331**: 294–299
13. Delta BG, Pinkel D. Bone marrow aspiration in children with malignant tumors. *J Pediatr* 1964; **64**: 542–546
14. Finklestein JZ, Ekert H, Isaacs H Jr, Higgins G. Bone marrow metastases in children with solid tumors. *Am J Dis Child* 1970; **119**: 49–52
15. Brodeur GM, Seeger RC, Barrett A *et al.* International criteria for diagnosis, staging and response to treatment in patients with neuroblastoma. *J Clin Oncol* 1988; **6**:1874–1881
16. Brodeur GM, Pritchard J, Berthold F *et al.* Revisions of the international criteria for neuroblastoma diagnosis, staging and response to treatment. *J Clin Oncol* 1993; **11**: 1466–1477
17. Mills AE, Bird AR. Bone marrow changes in neuroblastoma. *Pediatr Pathol* 1986; **5**: 225–234
18. Franklin IM, Pritchard J. Detection of bone marrow invasion by neuroblastoma is improved by sampling at two sites with both aspirates and trephine biopsies. *J Clin Pathol* 1983; **36**: 1215–1218
19. Smith SR, Reid MM. Neuroblastoma rosettes in aspirated bone marrow. *Br J Haematol* 1994; **88**: 445–447
20. Head DR, Kennedy PS, Goyette RE. Metastatic neuroblastoma in bone marrow aspirate smear. *Am J Clin Pathol* 1979; **72**: 1008–1011
21. Kemshead JT, Clayton J, Patel K. Monoclonal antibodies used for the diagnosis of the small round cell tumors of childhood. In: Kemshead JT (ed) *Pediatric Tumors: Immunological and Molecular Markers.* Boca Raton: CRC Press, 1989, pp 31–45
22. Reid MM, Hamilton PJ. Histology of neuroblastoma involving bone marrow: the problem of detecting residual tumour after initiation of chemotherapy. *Br J Haematol* 1988; **69**: 487–490
23. Savage RS, Hoffman GC, Shaker K. Diagnostic problems involved in detection of metastatic neoplasms by bone-marrow aspirate compared with needle biopsy. *Am J Clin Pathol* 1978; **70**: 623–627
24. Bostrom B, Nesbit ME Jr, Brunning RD. The value of bone marrow trephine biopsy in the diagnosis of metastatic neuroblastoma. *Am J Pediatr Hematol Oncol* 1985; **7**: 303–305
25. Favrot MC, Frappaz D, Maritaz O *et al.* Histological, cytological and immunological analyses are complementary for the detection of neuroblastoma cells in bone marrow. *Br J Cancer* 1986; **54**: 637–641
26. Reid MM, Roald B. Adequacy of bone marrow trephine biopsy specimens in children. *J Clin Pathol* 1996; **49**: 226–229

27. Reid MM, Pearson ADJ. Bone-marrow infiltration in neuroblastoma. *Lancet* 1991; **337**: 681–682

28. Turner GE, Reid MM. What is marrow fibrosis after treatment of neuroblastoma? *J Clin Pathol* 1993; **46**: 61–63

29. Beck D, Maritaz O, Gross N *et al*. Immunocytochemical detection of neuroblastoma cells infiltrating clinical bone marrow samples. *Eur J Pediatr* 1988; **147**: 609–612

30. Rogers DW, Treleaven JG, Kemshead JT, Pritchard J. Monoclonal antibodies for detecting bone marrow invasion by neuroblastoma. *J Clin Pathol* 1989; **42**: 422–426

31. Oppedal BR, Storm-Mathisen I, Kemshead JT, Brandtzaeg P. Bone marrow examination in neuroblastoma patients: a morphologic, immunocytochemical, and immunohistochemical study. *Hum Pathol* 1989; **20**: 800–805

32. Carey PJ, Thomas L, Buckle G, Reid MM. Immunocytochemical examination of bone marrow in disseminated neuroblastoma. *J Clin Pathol* 1990; **43**: 9–12

33. Reid MM, Malcolm AJ, McGuckin AG. Immunohistochemical detection of neuroblastoma in frozen sections of bone marrow trephine biopsy specimens. *J Clin Pathol* 1990; **43**: 334–336

34. Reid MM, Wallis JP, McGuckin AG, Pearson ADJ, Malcolm AJ. Routine histological compared with immunohistological examination of bone marrow trephine biopsy specimens in disseminated neuroblastoma. *J Clin Pathol* 1991; **44**: 483–486

35. Moss TJ, Reynolds CP, Sather HN, Romansky SG, Hammond GD, Seeger RC. Prognostic value of immunocytologic detection of bone marrow metastases in neuroblastoma. *N Engl J Med* 1991; **324**: 219–226

36. Adams JA, Kelsy AM, Carr TF, Stevens RF, Morris-Jones P. Detection of bone marrow metastases in neuroblastoma using a short term tissue culture technique. *J Clin Pathol* 1992; **45**: 424–426

37. Reid MM. Detection of bone marrow infiltration by neuroblastoma in clinical practice: how far have we come? *Eur J Cancer* 1994; **30A**: 134–135

38. Longacre TA, Foucar K, Crago S *et al*. Hematogones: a multiparameter analysis of bone marrow precursor cells. *Blood* 1989; **73**: 543–552

39. Taylor CPF, McGuckin AG, Bown NP *et al*. Rapid detection of prognostic genetic factors in neuroblastoma using fluorescence *in situ* hybridisation on tumour imprints and bone marrow smears. *Br J Cancer* 1994; **64**: 445–451

40. Ruymann FB, Newton WA Jr, Ragab AH, Donaldson MH, Foulkes M. Bone marrow metastases at diagnosis in children and adolescents with rhabdomyosarcoma. A report from the intergroup rhabdomyosarcoma study. *Cancer* 1984; **53**: 368–373

41. Etcubanas E, Peiper S, Stass S, Green A. Rhabdomyosarcoma, presenting as disseminated malignancy from an unknown primary site: a retrospective study of ten pediatric cases. *Med Pediatr Oncol* 1989; **17**: 39–44

42. Reid MM, Saunders PWG, Bown N *et al*. Alveolar rhabdomyosarcoma infiltrating bone marrow at presentation: the value to diagnosis of bone marrow trephine biopsy specimens. *J Clin Pathol* 1992; **45**: 759–762

43. Enzinger FM, Weiss SM. *Soft Tissue Tumors*, 3rd edn. St Louis: C Mosby, 1995, pp 539–578

44. Tsokos M, Webber BL, Parham DM *et al*. Rhabdomyosarcoma. A new classification scheme related to prognosis. *Arch Pathol Lab Med* 1992; **116**: 847–855

45. Yule SM, Bown N, Malcolm AJ, Reid MM, Pearson ADJ. Solid alveolar rhabdomyosarcoma with a t(2;13). *Cancer Genet Cytogenet* 1995; **80**: 107–109

46. Roessner A, Jürgens H. Round cell tumors of bone. *Pathol Res Pract* 1993; **189**: 1111–1136

47. Oberlin O, Bayle C, Hartmann O, Terrier-Lacombe MJ, Lemerle J. Incidence of bone marrow involvement in Ewing's sarcoma: value of extensive investigation of the bone marrow. *Med Pediatr Oncol* 1995; **24**: 343–346

48. Ambros IM, Ambros PF, Strehl S, Kovar H, Gadner H, Salzer-Kuntschik M. MIC2 is a specific marker for Ewing's sarcoma and peripheral primitive neuroectodermal tumors. *Cancer* 1991; **67**: 1886–1893

49. Kretshmar CS. Ewing's sarcoma and the "peanut" tumors. *N Engl J Med* 1994; **331**: 325–327

50. Pratt CB, Meyer D, Chenaille P, Crom DB. The use of bone marrow aspirations and lumbar punctures at the time of diagnosis of retinoblastoma. *J Clin Oncol* 1989; **7**: 140–143

Storage disorders

BRIAN D LAKE

The metabolic storage disorders present difficult diagnostic problems, not only for the clinician but also for the laboratory-based diagnostic service. Many of the disorders appear similar clinically and require careful clinical histories to be taken by those who may have rarely, if ever, seen the condition before. It is easy to send a blood sample to an experienced laboratory and to have a wide range of enzyme assays performed, but this is not an economic approach to diagnosis. Also, this approach will take some time to produce an answer and the laboratory may well be a supraregional center dealing with many samples from a wide area. To facilitate the diagnosis and indicate the direction the biochemical tests should take, some simple morphologic studies can be undertaken. Great Ormond Street has for many years studied blood and bone marrow samples from patients with defined disorders and as a result of this experience can guide the biochemists, so that the definitive assay can be performed rather than the whole screen. In addition to the storage disorders involving the lysosomal system, a small number of conditions have characteristic abnormalities which can be found in a peripheral film or bone marrow aspirate.

While it may appear easy to detect the presence of vacuolation of lymphocytes, it is the author's experience that most hematologists fail to find any but the most obvious examples. In the preparation of the standard peripheral film, the abnormal lymphocytes, either because of their size or density or a combination of both, are drawn preferentially to the trails of the film. This area is usually ignored because the cells may be distorted and are less well spread. However, it is here that vacuolated lymphocytes are most abundant. Any of the standard staining methods are suitable, as long as the nucleus and cytoplasm are both defined. Some workers advocate the use of buffy coat preparations, but this is unnecessary in the search for vacuolated lymphocytes, since if they are not visible by light microscopy using a $\times 25$ objective, they are unlikely to be found by electron microscopy. Ultrastructural examination is necessary in a few conditions where specific inclusions

can only be detected by electron microscopy. The clinical input is most important to guide the most appropriate type of examination.

In additon to the standard morphologic staining method, it is sometimes helpful to stain for glycogen, neutral lipid or evidence of acidic mucopolysaccharide deposition. Some methods for the detection of enzyme activity are occasionally helpful, but many are not sufficiently specific or sensitive. Examination by polarization microscopy, particularly of bone marrow aspirates in storage disorders, gives additional information.

The clinical, biochemical, molecular and morphologic details of the lysosomal and metabolic disorders covered in this chapter are decribed in depth by Scriver et al.[1] Further hematologic details are to be found in Smith[2] and are also illustrated in Hann et al.[3]

BLOOD FILMS

Lymphocyte vacuolation, when present and when looked for in the right place, is always very clear with sharply delineated vacuoles in the cytoplasm of a variable percentage of lymphocytes. The occasional very small single vacuole in the cytoplasm of a lymphocyte is not significant. Similarly, if the vacuole is not clearly defined and it is not clear whether it is a vacuole or not, then it is not a vacuole within the meaning of the term. There are two main categories of lymphocytic vacuolation:

- few small vacuoles in many lymphocytes;
- many larger vacuoles in many lymphocytes.

In a few disorders the vacuolation may involve only a small proportion of lymphocytes. While examining the lymphocyte population, it is also important to look at the neutrophils and eosinophils for evidence that might help in the diagnosis of metabolic disease.

It is worth mentioning that in blood films prepared from

anticoagulated blood there will almost inevitably be monocytes with cytoplasmic vacuoles. The 'normal' vacuoles found in monocytes are usually less well defined and more irregular than the specific vacuolation of the storage disorders. Similarly, the clear, well defined vacuoles in lymphoblasts found in acute lymphoblastic leukemia (ALL; FAB type L3 mainly), while appearing to simulate a storage disorder, should not be a problem of interpretation if this is done in the clinical context. A common perception is that the mucopolysaccharidoses have lymphocytic vacuolation, but vacuolation is not found and the presence of vacuoles excludes the mucopolysaccharidoses (with the exception of Morquio type B).

VACUOLATED LYMPHOCYTES AND LYMPHOCYTE INCLUSIONS

Few small vacuoles in many lymphocytes (Table 40.1)

In this group there are a small number (1–6) of small discrete vacuoles in a large proportion of lymphocytes. The diagnosis will include Pompe's disease, Wolman's disease and Niemann–Pick disease type A. Staining to demonstrate glycogen (celloidinized periodic acid-Schiff [PAS]), will define *Pompe's disease* and all the vacuoles will be filled with strongly PAS-positive glycogen. In the infantile form, in which there is gross hypotonia and marked cardiomegaly, almost all the lymphocytes contain the discrete deposits of glycogen which may also appear, artefactually, to be within the nucleus. In the older patient and adults with acid maltase deficiency, a smaller percentage of lymphocytes is affected. In the author's experience, all cases of acid maltase deficiency can be detected in this way and it gives no false positive or negative results. It should be noted that B lymphocytes in older normal subjects may have a 'wreath' of PAS-positive droplets encircling the nucleus and in some these deposits can be quite marked and the cells appear to be vacuolated in routine stains. In the adult and teenage populations, these cells are known as Mott cells. The PAS-positive deposits represent the glycoprotein moiety of the immunoglobulin secreted by the B cells.

In *Wolman's disease* (acid esterase/acid lipase deficiency), a situation similar to that in Pompe's disease occurs (Plate 67).

The severe infantile form has a large proportion of lymphocytes containing the small vacuoles which stain for neutral lipid with Oil Red O or Sudan black after fixation in an aqueous formalin fixative. Fixation is done to permeabilize the cells and allow the dye to enter, and without fixation a much smaller proportion of lymphocytes contains demonstrable sudanophilic lipid. The older childhood and adult cases of acid esterase deficiency (cholesteryl ester storage disease) have a lower but still significant proportion of lymphocytes with vacuoles.

In *Niemann–Pick disease type A* (acute infantile) there is no demonstrable sudanophilic lipid or glycogen but the vacuoles are similar to but less frequent than those in Pompe's disease. Electron microscopy is necessary to show the membranous contents of the vacuoles. No vacuolation is found in the later onset type B, while in Niemann–Pick disease type C, the lymphocytes may be coarsely vacuolated in occasional cases.

Many large vacuoles in many lymphocytes (Table 40.2)

This group contains the majority of lysosomal storage disorders in which lymphocytic vacuolation is seen. There are many large bold discrete vacuoles in a large proportion of lymphocytes in the trails of films (Plate 68). Without a clinical summary it is impossible to give a diagnosis, but given an adequate history it is usually possible to give guidance for further investigation. In the presence of striking lymphocyte vacuolation, it is not only the lymphocytes that need to be examined, and a careful search for eosinophils and their granules (see below) is also necessary. In addition to the numerous large vacuoles, some lymphocytes may be filled with small discrete vacuoles and others may contain only several large bold vacuoles. These appearances are quite different from those found in the disorders listed in Table 40.1.

In fucosidosis, mucolipidosis III, Salla disease (non-infantile sialic acid storage disease) and aspartylglucosaminuria, the lymphocytic vacuoles may be small and involve a small proportion of lymphocytes or may be quite prominent in many lymphocytes. Examination of the trails of the blood film is always rewarding in these conditions.

Table 40.1 Storage disorders with few small vacuoles in many cells.

Pompe's disease and all forms of acid maltase deficiency (vacuoles contain glycogen)

Wolman's disease and all forms of acid esterase deficiency (vacuoles contatin sudanophilic lipid)

Niemann–Pick disease type A (acid sphingomyelinase deficiency) (electron microscopy is needed to show contents)

Table 40.2 Storage disorders with many large vacuoles in many lymphocytes.

G_{M1}-gangliosidosis type 1 (β-galactosidase deficiency)
I-cell disease (mucolipidosis II)
Infantile sialic acid storage disease
Sialidosis (α-neuraminidase deficiency, dysmorphic type)
Galactosialidosis
Mannosidosis (α-mannosidase deficiency)
Classic juvenile Batten's disease
Morquio disease type B (β-galactosidase deficiency)

Colour plates

SECTION 6 COAGULATION DISORDERS

Chapter 32 Acquired disorders of hemostasis during childhood

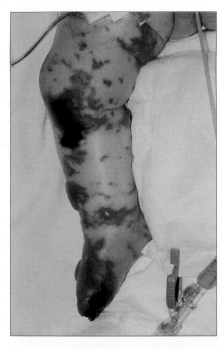

Plate 38 Acquired purpura fulminans in a child with menigococcal septicemia.

Chapter 33 Hemostatic problems in the neonate

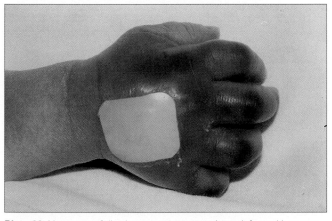

Plate 39 Hematoma following a venepuncture in an infant with severe hemophilia A.

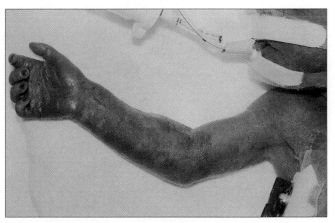

Plate 40 Ischemic arm following a catheter-related thrombosis.

1

Colour plates

Chapter 34 Thromboembolic complications

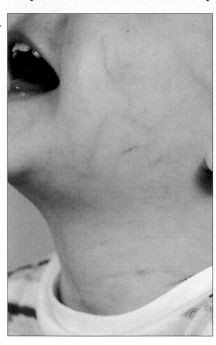

Plate 41 Collateral circulation in a child with a thromboembolic event.

SECTION 8 HEMATOLOGIC EFFECTS OF SYSTEMIC DISEASE

Chapter 39 Hematologic effects of non-hematopoietic tumors

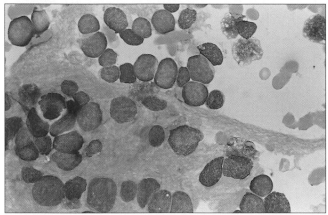

Plate 42 Fibrillar nature of neuroblastoma cytoplasm and/or an admixture of neurofibrils and other secreted 'ground substance' material. Such material may well have been the centre of a rosette (see Plate 50). These appearances sometimes, usually erroneously, give the impression of a syncytium. (Leishman stain.)

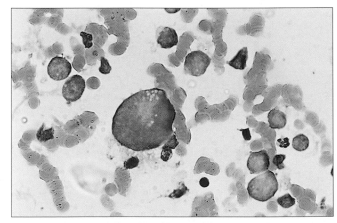

Plate 43 'Giant' neuroblastoma cell in aspirated bone marrow. In more thickly spread areas of a marrow smear such cells may be mistaken for young megakaryocytes. (Leishman stain.)

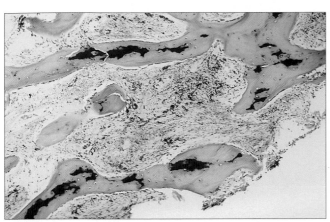

Plate 44 Low power view of trephine biopsy section of marrow replaced with neuroblastoma, showing prominent fibrosis. (Giemsa stain.)

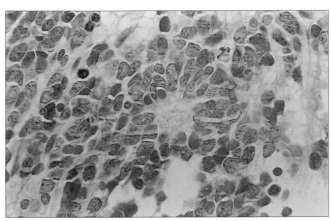

Plate 45 High power view of section of trephine biopsy showing a classical Homer Wright rosette. (Hematoxylin and eosin stains.)

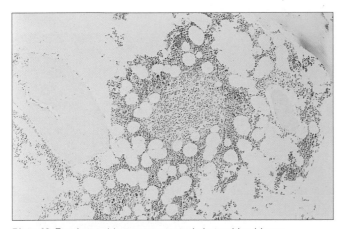

Plate 46 Focal neuroblastoma metastasis in trephine biopsy. (Hematoxylin and eosin stains.)

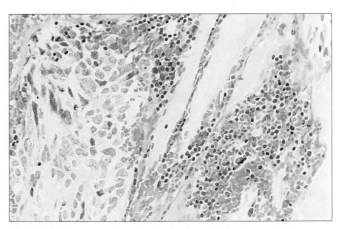

Plate 47 High power view showing large neuroblastoma cells in a focal metastasis, contrasted with normal hemopoietic tissue in the same field. (Giemsa stain.)

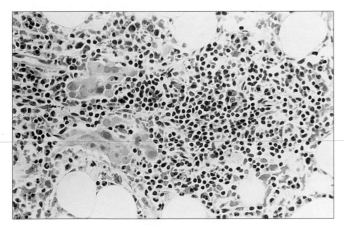

Plate 48 Neuroblastoma cells about the size of small megakaryocytes, showing some differentiation, with associated lymphocytic infiltrate. These cells should not be mistaken for megakaryocytes but in cases of doubt are never periodic acid-Schiff (PAS) positive. (Hematoxylin and eosin stains.)

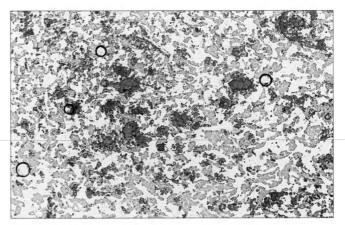

Plate 49 Low power view of bone marrow heavily infiltrated with neuroblastoma, showing clumps and rosettes staining for neural cell adhesion molecule (NCAM). (Immunoalkaline phosphatase stain.)

Colour plates

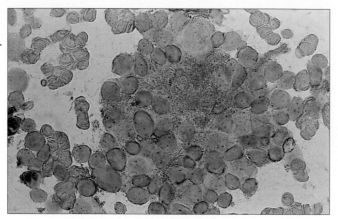

Plate 50 High power view of neuroblastoma rosette showing fibrillar pattern of neural cell adhesion molecule (NCAM)-positive material. (Immunoalkaline phosphatase stain.)

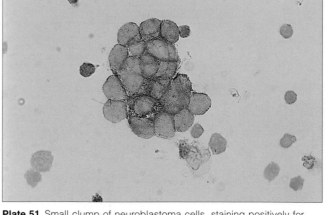

Plate 51 Small clump of neuroblastoma cells, staining positively for neural cell adhesion molecule (NCAM). This was the only clump of tumor cells in one bone marrow aspirate smear. They are clearly morphologically distinct from osteoblasts. (Immunoalkaline phosphatase stain.)

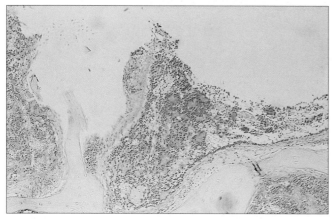

Plate 52 Homer Wright rosettes in trephine biopsy staining positively for neurone-specific enolase. (Immunoperoxidase stain.)

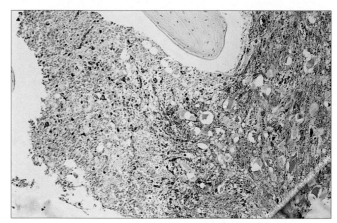

Plate 53 Ganglion cells in sections of a vertebra obtained post mortem, staining positively for neurone-specific enolase (NSE). They are the size of megakaryocytes. There has been some shrinkage of the ganglion cells, giving rise to the impression of smaller cells within large lacunae. Note large amounts of NSE-positive 'stroma'. (Immunoperoxidase stain.)

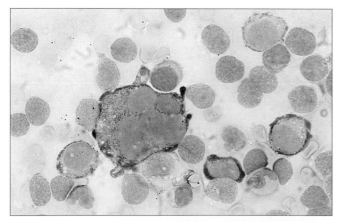

Plate 54 Alveolar rhabdomyosarcoma cells in bone marrow aspirate. There are many coalesced lakes of periodic acid-Schiff (PAS)-positive material, most of which are peripherally placed. (PAS stain.)

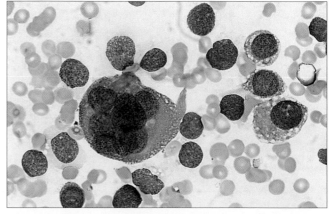

Plate 55 Alveolar rhabdomyosarcoma in bone marrow aspirate. Giant multinucleate rhabdomyoblast, the cytologic counterpart of the wreath-like cell found in histologic sections (see Plate 57), and other smaller mononuclear tumor cells are seen. (Leishman stain.)

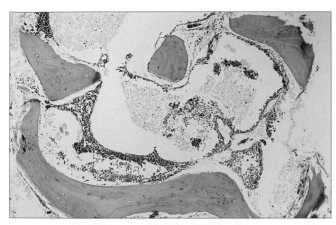

Plate 56 Trephine biopsy of bone marrow infiltrated with alveolar rhabdomyosarcoma, showing adherence of tumor cells to the alveolar 'lining' with loss of central cohesion between tumor cells. (Giemsa stain.)

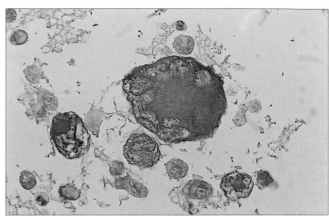

Plate 57 Giant multinucleate rhabdomyoblast with 'wreath-like' arrangement of nuclei in a trephine biopsy, staining positively for desmin. (Immunoperoxidase stain.)

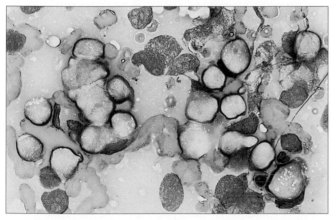

Plate 58 Typical Ewing's tumor cells in aspirated bone marrow. There is more vacuolation than is usually found in neuroblastoma. The periodic acid-Schiff (PAS) stain is often positive in Ewing's cells, but the peripheral vacuolation usually found in rhabdomyosarcoma is not present. (Leishman stain.)

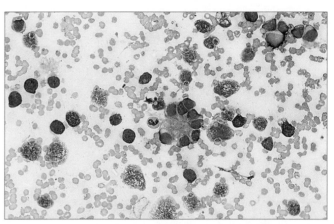

Plate 59 Vestigial rosette in aspirated bone marrow infiltrated with Ewing's sarcoma. This cytologic feature is indistinguishable from neuroblastoma, but rosettes are much less frequently found in aspirated bone marrow in this disease. (Leishman stain.)

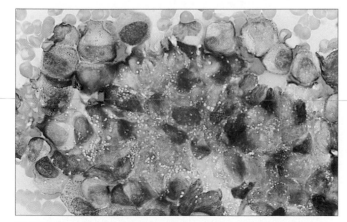

Plate 60 Marked vacuolation in a tightly adherent clump of primitive neuroectodermal tumor (PNET) cells. Such prominent vacuolation is rare in neuroblastoma. See also Plate 61. (Leishman stain.)

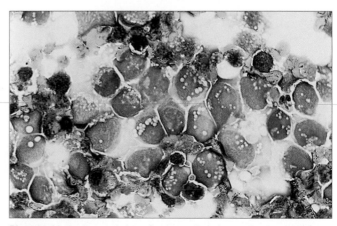

Plate 61 Marked vacuolation of tumor cells in less adherent primitive neuroectodermal (PNET) cells. This is a different patient from Plate 60. (Leishman stain.)

5

Colour plates

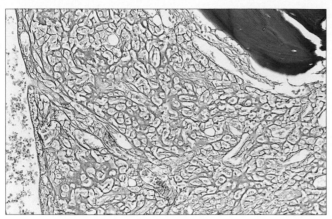

Plate 62 Low power view of trephine biopsy of bone marrow infiltrated with osteosarcoma. Sliver staining highlights the osteoid, with tumor cells sitting in lacunae. The osteoid nature of the material is inferred, not proven, because the specimen was routinely decalcified prior to sectioning.

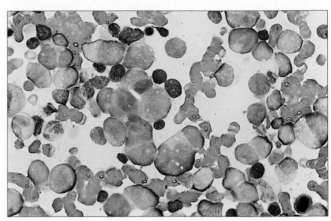

Plate 63 Retinoblastoma cells in aspirated bone marrow. Only the clinical context allows the microscopist to distinguish between this diagnosis and some other small round cell tumors. (Leishman stain.)

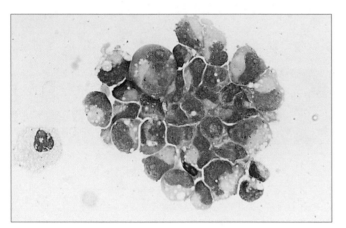

Plate 64 Cytospin preparation of cerebrospinal fluid (CSF) showing a clump of pinealblastoma cells. The cells are clearly not hemopoietic tissue, nor do they resemble neuroblastoma (see Plate 66) or medulloblastoma. (Leishman stain.)

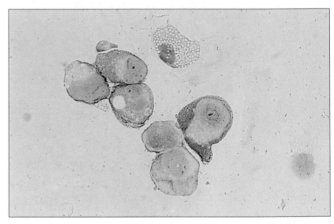

Plate 65 Cytospin of cerebrospinal fluid (CSF) showing pinealblastoma cells expressing neural cell adhesion molecule (NCAM). (Immunoalkaline phosphatase stain.)

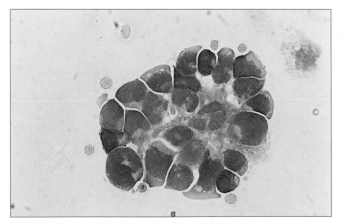

Plate 66 Cytospin of cerebrospinal fluid (CSF) showing a clump of neuroblastoma cells at relapse after allogeneic bone marrow transplant. (Leishman stain.)

Chapter 40 Storage disorders

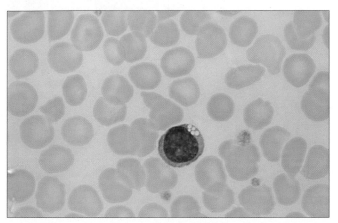

Plate 67 Blood film stained with the May-Grünwald-Giemsa method showing a few small discrete vacuoles in the cytoplasm of a lymphocyte from a patient with Wolman's disease. These vacuoles contain neutral fat. A similar appearance is seen in Pompe's disease (glycogen storage disease type II) but in this case the vacuoles contain glycogen.

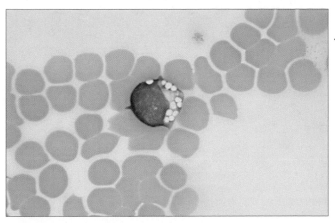

Plate 68 Blood film stained with the May-Grünwald-Giemsa method showing many large bold vacuoles in a lymphocyte from a patient with classic juvenile Batten's disease (juvenile neuronal ceroid lipofuscinosis). This appearance is also seen in many other storage disorders (see Table 40.2) and the clinical setting is an important factor in the interpretation.

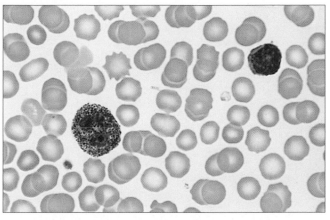

Plate 69 Blood film stained with the May-Grünwald-Giemsa method from a patient with mucopolysaccharidosis type VI (Maroteaux-Lamy) showing Alder granulation in a neutrophil. Alder granulation is also found in mucosulfatidosis and in β-glucuronidase deficiency.

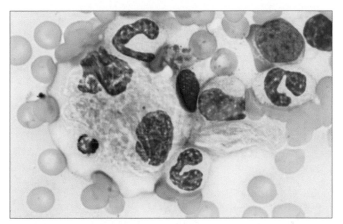

Plate 70 Bone marrow aspirate from a patient with Gaucher's disease showing the Gaucher cell morphology which may not always be stripy and may be palely stained.

Colour plates

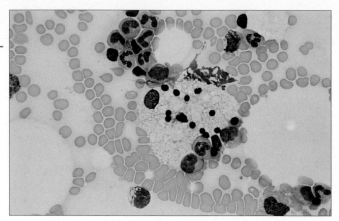

Plate 71 Bone marow aspirate from a patient with Niemann-Pick disease type C. The storage cell contains vacuoles of variable size and in addition has engulfed several normoblasts, a feature which is always prominent in this disorder and is rarely seen in other storage conditions.

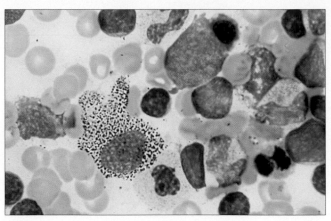

Plate 72 Bone marrow aspirate from a patient with mucopolysaccharidosis type III (San Filippo), showing one of the 'reticulum' cells containing fine to coarse basophilic granules. These cells are more prominent around marrow fragments, and are found in most of the mucopolysaccharidoses.

Other lymphocyte inclusions

The mucopolysaccharidoses do not display lymphocyte vacuolation (except Morquio B) but do have a proportion of abnormal lymphocytes. These are mainly of two types:

- Gasser cells in which there are vacuoles with a basophilic inclusion;
- lymphocytes with 1–2 coarse basophilic granules which are different from the fine granules seen in some normal lymphocytes.

Gasser cells are not specific to any one of the mucopolysaccharidoses and can occur in any of them. The lymphocytes with coarse basophilic vacuoles are more prominent in SanFilippo syndrome (probably in all 4 types of mucopolysaccharidosis [MPS] type III), accounting for between 10 and 40% of the total number of lymphocytes, and may be present in large numbers in Hunter's syndrome (MPS type II) but are barely detectable in Hurler's or Scheie's syndrome (MPS type I). The basophilic inclusions are metachromatic when stained with the toluidine blue method described by Muir et al,[4] and are best quantified by examination under an oil immersion objective and counting 100 lymphocytes. In β-glucuronidase deficiency (MPS type VII), the lymphocytes have coarse basophilic inclusions and display striking Alder granulation of neutrophils.

NEUTROPHIL ABNORMALITIES

Alder granulation (occasionally known as Reilly granules or Alder–Reilly bodies) is seen in neutrophils and resembles toxic granulation, but differs from it in color, being more lilac-rose than brown. In addition, there are no other changes in toxicity and all neutrophils contain Alder granulation. The granulation may be quite coarse, particularly in β-glucuronidase deficiency. Alder granulation occurs in three conditions:

- Maroteaux–Lamy syndrome (MPS type IV; Plate 69);
- multiple sulfatase deficiency (Austin disease);
- β-glucuronidase deficiency (MPS type VII, Sly disease);

and is reputed to be present in some spiders, toads and snakes. A mild and less constant Alder granulation has been noted in infantile sialic acid storage disease.[2] In Morquio syndrome (MPS IV), the neutrophils may contain a few coarse azurophil granules, but these may be difficult to appreciate. Abnormal neutrophil vacuolation (apart from that associated with toxicity) is seen in neutral lipid storage disease where it is known as Jordans' anomaly. Vacuolation is also found in eosinophils (more prominent than usual), but not in lymphocytes. The vacuoles are filled with neutral lipid and stain with the sudanophil dyes Oil Red O and Sudan black after aqueous formalin fixation. Electron microscopy of the buffy coat also reveals occasional lipid droplets in platelets. Neutral storage disease is a multisystem disorder affecting liver, skin, intestine and muscle. The skin component of the disease presents as an ichthyosis and screening of all patients with an ichthyosis for Jordans' anomaly is a valuable diagnostic procedure.

Infrequent neutrophil vacuolation affecting a small number of neutrophils may be found in some cases of Wolman's disease.

Neutrophil inclusions staining pale gray-blue may be seen in Chédiak–Higashi syndrome, but the neutrophil count in this disorder may be extremely low and consequently the inclusions, similar in appearance to Döhle bodies or the May-Hegglin anomaly, are sometimes difficult to find. Lymphocytes in Chédiak–Higashi syndrome may occasionally contain a single large eosinophilic/reddish inclusion.

EOSINOPHIL ABNORMALITIES

Abnormal eosinophils are seen in multiple sulfatase deficiency, β-galactosidase deficiency and infantile sialic acid storage disease. The granules are usually larger, grayish-blue and sparse in the eosinophils and are recognizable by the bilobed appearance of the nuclei. Normal eosinophils are only rarely encountered. Occasionally, the granules appear just to be coarser than normal and fewer in number per cell. They are always encountered accompanied by either Alder granulation or prominent lymphocytic vacuolation. In Chédiak–Higashi syndrome the eosinophil granules may be larger and prominent. Bone marrow samples are better for this diagnosis.

MACROPHAGE ABNORMALITIES

Very rarely, occasional foamy macrophages may be detected in peripheral blood films in Wolman's disease, G_{M1}-gangliosidosis and galactosialidosis.

BUFFY COAT PREPARATIONS

In a number of conditions, no morphologic features are visible by light microscopy and examination by electron microscopy is necessary. The method of buffy coat preparation is critical for success, and the method given below is applicable for the study of lymphocytes, neutrophils and platelets.

1. Use anticoagulated blood (EDTA is preferable); 0.5–2 ml is adequate.
2. Select a centrifuge tube (tall and narrow) of such a size that the blood sample just fills the tube. This will ensure that the buffy coat is as thick as possible and not thinly spread over a large area.
3. Centrifuge at maximum speed in a bench centrifuge for 5–10 min.
4. Gently remove the upper plasma layer using a pasteur pipette without disturbing the buffy coat layer. Remove as much plasma as possible.
5. Gently add a glutaraldehyde-based electron microscopy

fixative, again without disturbing the buffy coat. Remove the fixative after 2–3 min and replace with fresh fixative. Leave for 15–30 min.

6. Using a sharpened orange stick or histologic seeker needle, gently loosen the edges of the buffy coat from the sides of the tube. Lift out the whole intact button of buffy coat with a small spatula, and place it in fresh fixative.

7. After an appropriate and convenient time in fixative, select blocks taken vertically through the buffy coat for processing through secondary osmium tetroxide fixation, dehydration and infiltration with the resin of choice for electron microscopy.

This procedure gives consistent results and any section contains all the cellular constituents from platelets through to lymphocytes, neutrophils and a thin layer of red cells. The success of the method derives from the presence, between all the cells, of plasma albumin which is cross-linked by the glutaraldehyde fixative and holds the buffy coat intact during processing.

Batten's disease

Examination by electron microscopy is necessary to find the inclusions characteristic of those in the infantile, late infantile and early juvenile types of Batten's disease.[5] While this is not the main diagnostic route, it has its place in the investigation of Batten's disease where the clinical index of suspicion is very high and in the screening of younger siblings. It is also useful where there are no facilities or expertise for the laboratory diagnosis of Batten's disease in a referring hospital. A blood sample sent by post to arrive within 24 hours is adequate, or the buffy coat in fixative can be sent by post.

Late infantile Batten's disease (CLN 2)

The inclusions in lymphocytes consist of curvilinear bodies of variable size in around 20% of lymphocytes in any one ultrathin section.

Infantile Batten's disease (CLN 1)

Granular osmiophilic deposits (GRODs) are present in 10–20% of lymphocytes. Identical findings are present in the lymphocytes of patients with 'juvenile Batten's disease with GROD'. These latter patients do not have vacuolated lymphocytes and electron microscopy is necessary to aid the differentiation between the 'juvenile' forms.

Early juvenile Batten's disease (CLN 6)

This is also known as variant late infantile presenting Batten's disease. These patients may have discrete fingerprint bodies in a small proportion (about 2–5%) of lymphocytes. Several different genotypes are represented within this group and at least one is said to have no abnormal inclusions.

NON-IMMUNE HYDROPS

Many of the lysosomal storage disorders can present *in utero* as fetal hydrops or ascites detected at routine ultrasound scanning. In this situation, a sample of fetal blood is taken for screening for parvovirus and other more common causes of fetal hydrops. The changes found in blood films of term and older children with the storage disorders mentioned above are present in the fetus[6] and examination of a blood film from the sample usually excludes a storage disease or less frequently indicates that the cause of the hydrops is due to a storage disease.

BONE MARROW SAMPLES

The investigation of a patient who presents with hepatosplenomegaly or isolated splenomegaly usually includes examination of a bone marrow sample to clarify the cause of the enlarged spleen. Such an examination differentiates between storage disorders, malignancy and infection. Absence of storage cells in an adequate sample will exclude any visceral storage disease. The abnormal storage cells will generally be present in profusion and single cells should be regarded with suspicion only. The normal adipose or fat cell should not be mistaken for a storage cell. Some storage disorders have fewer cells, but the cells present will still be in sufficient numbers for significance. The findings should always be interpreted in the light of the clinical history. The diagnosis of a storage disease always requires confirmation by the appropriate biochemical assay since there will be genetic and treatment implications. Most of the conditions have little or no effect on the normal hematologic parameters, except in Gaucher's disease type I (adult, non-neuropathic) and Niemann–Pick disease type B where there may be low platelet and white cell counts due to hypersplenism.

For the evaluation of storage cells and other morphologic abnormalities, a bone marrow aspirate gives much more information than histologic sections prepared from a trephine sample. While most hematologic evaluations are best conducted on films made directly from the needle, storage disease evaluation benefits from films made from anticoagulated (EDTA) marrow samples. The advantages are that the cells are well spread and more readily recognized, retain their lipid, carbohydrate and enzyme content in contrast with the trephine sections where lipids and some carbohydrates have been removed and the enzyme activity is inhibited by the fixation and decalcification processes. Anticoagulated samples can also be used for the preparation of a marrow buffy coat for electron microscopy as described above for blood samples.

A small number of special stains are useful for the examination of marrow films in the evaluation of storage disorders. Apart from a general stain for morphology (any that is normally used in the routine laboratory will be adequate), a PAS reaction for carbohydrate components, a lipid stain (Oil Red O or Sudan black) after fixation in formalin and a reaction for acid phosphatase activity are the most useful methods. Fixation in formalin produces a cloud of denatured hemoglobin over the film, which, if not washed away with more formalin, settles on the slide and masks the cellular detail. Note that the lipid method with Oil Red O or Sudan black is different from that commonly used in hematology and fixation must be aqueous to preserve the lipid components. In addition, an alchoholic basic fuchsin stain, the ferric hematoxylin method for sphingomyelin, and examination in polarized light may be useful on occasions. The acid phosphatase reaction serves to identify storage cells very readily since very few cells in normal marrow display activity, and those that do so have a discrete fine particulate pattern (megakaryocytes) or strong activity within slender processes (normal histiocytes). Storage cells are always strongly stained, and cells which display hemophagocytosis are also clearly shown. Survey of the film with a ×10 objective reveals any storage cells or evidence of hemophagocytosis.

TYPES OF STORAGE CELL

In storage disorders there are in general two main types of storage cell:

- Gaucher or Gaucher-like;
- foamy and vacuolated.

The *classic Gaucher cell* is stained palely in Giemsa-type stains, has a pale gray-blue appearance and when examined under ×40 to ×100 objectives the rather loose stripy nature of the storage bodies can be seen (Plate 70). This appearance has been likened to crumpled tissue paper. Not all cells are as distinctive as those shown in the textbooks and some appear more vacuolated than striped. Gaucher cells are weakly PAS positive, have a very pale gray stripy appearance with Sudan black and show strong acid phosphatase activity (tartrate stable). They may contain a little iron and generally are not birefringent. In G_{M1}-gangliosidosis type 2 (but not type 1) cells which superficially resemble Gaucher cells are found. They differ in that their cytoplasm is more compact and in Giemsa-type stains has a much more distinctive blue (sky blue) color in contrast to the pale gray-blue of Gaucher cells. They are also more strongly PAS positive. The *pseudo-Gaucher cell* of adult type chronic granulocytic leukemia, thalassemia major, Shwachman's syndrome and some patients who have systemic atypical mycobacteria infection is usually sparsely distributed and more strongly stained with PAS. They may also be birefringent. Their presence is probably related to rapid turnover of cells causing overload of normal histiocytes. In this situation a range of appearances and ingested material in various states of digestion may be seen, which serves to distinguish pseudo-storage from real storage where there is uniformity in the appearance of storage cells.

Table 40.3 Storage disorders with foamy or vacuolated storage type cells in marrow.

G_{M1}-gangliosidosis type 1
Mannosidosis
Wolman's disease
Cholesteryl ester storage disease
Niemann–Pick disease type A
Niemann–Pick disease type B
Niemann–Pick disease type C
Infantile sialic acid storage disease
Sialidosis type 1
Galactosialidosis
Fucosidosis
Mucopolysaccharidosis (all types)
Fabry's disease
Farber's disease (acid ceramidase deficiency)
Cystinosis
Hyperlipoproteinemias (all types) including Tangier disease

Foamy cells occur in a large number of conditions and the appearance should be interpreted in the light of the clinical situation. Table 40.3 lists conditions in which foamy or vacuolated cells occur.

Full descriptions of the cells in each of these disorders are not given as color photomicrographs have been reproduced elsewhere.[2,3] General comments which outline some of the features helpful in the differential diagnosis of the various disorders are given below.

Niemann–Pick diseases

The more classic foamy cell as a hallmark of a storage disease is found in many conditions and the interpretation of the morphology should always be made in the knowledge of the clinical situation. With a little care and a few additional staining methods, several conditions can be distinguished and differentiated from each other. The foamy cells in *Niemann–Pick disease type A* have cytoplasmic vacuoles which are generally uniform in each cell, and there are only rarely any other cellular inclusions present. The cells are birefringent (white) in the native state and after staining with Sudan black have a reddish birefringence, which indicates an organized lamellar structure to the inclusions and is not specific to the sphingomyelin storage. The cells are positive with the ferric hematoxylin method after alkaline hydrolysis which is specific for sphingomyelin. Similar cells are also observed among the more striking sea-blue histiocytes present in *Niemann–Pick disease type B*.

In *Niemann–Pick disease type C* the storage cells are characterized by cytoplasmic vacuoles of varying size and shape within any one cell, often accompanied by ingested white cells and particularly by normoblasts (Plate 71). The vacuoles are best described as ragged. The cells are not birefringent and do not stain with Sudan black. The contents of the vacuoles are PAS-positive and appear diffusely granular. Occasional sea-blue histiocytes may be present in older patients. Niemann–Pick disease type C is a condition in which the biochemistry is not understood and the clinical presentation varies widely from severe neonatal hepatitis to isolated asymptomatic splenomegaly in childhood or adult life, to psychotic disturbance with splenomegaly in adult life or even to a movement disorder with dementia but no clinical splenomegaly. From complementation studies it is apparent that there are at least two genotypes. It is important to note that in the carrier (heterozygous) state of Niemann–Pick disease type C there will be a number of cells in the marrow identical to those of the disease itself, and carrier testing should only be attempted by the biochemical route.

Sea-blue histiocytes

This term is used to describe macrophages which are filled with *numerous* coarse granules staining blue with Giemsa-type stains. It is mistakenly used for cells which have a few dark blue granules (probably iron) in a foamy cytoplasm. There is no syndrome of the sea-blue histiocyte and the cases initially described by Silverstein *et al*[7] were of a variety of different disorders. He included in the description of the cells those that were foamy without any trace of blue and this is where confusion has occurred. Profuse real sea-blue histiocytes occur primarily in Niemann–Pick disease type B in the older patient. Their presence in large numbers should alert the observer to search for the foamy cells which always accompany the sea-blue cells in Niemann–Pick disease type B (adult, non-neurologic). Occasional sea-blue histiocytes are also present in the marrow of Niemann–Pick disease type C. The sea-blue histiocytes represent cells in which the stored material is in the form of lipofuscin (or ceroid) and has the characteristics of autofluorescence, stable sudanophilia and a positive PAS reaction. They appear to increase with the age of the patient, thus a few might be seen in older Niemann–Pick type A patients, and with increasing age the sea-blue cells become more frequent in Niemann–Pick type C. Sea-blue histiocytes also occur in Fabry's disease, Hermansky–Pudlak syndrome and lethicin-cholesterol acyl transferase (LCAT) deficiency.

G_{M1}-gangliosidosis type 1

The cells are foamy with comparatively neat discrete vacuoles of varying size, are not birefringent and do not stain with lipid stains or PAS. No inclusions are found. In addition to the foamy cells, the marrow contains coarsely vacuolated lymphocytes and the eosinophil granulocytes have abnormal granules. In contrast, *G_{M1}-gangliosidosis type 2* has cells which are sky-blue and compactly stripy in Giemsa stains (see above). *Galactosialidosis* has an appearance similar to that in G_{M1}-gangliosidosis type 1, but has in addition foamy cells which show some ingested red and white cells. In *infantile sialic acid storage disease* the foamy cells often contain ingested red cells among the vacuoles.

Wolman's and cholesteryl storage diseases

In these conditions the foamy cells are intensely sudanophilic with both Oil Red O and Sudan black. Fewer cells are found in cholesteryl ester storage disease and are less distinctive.

Mannosidosis, fucosidosis and sialidosis

The foamy cells in mannosidosis vary from those packed with small discrete uniform vacuoles to cells with vacuoles of widely different sizes. In addition to the foamy cells, the plasma cells are strikingly vacuolated, as they are also in fucosidosis. The contents of the cells in both mannosidosis and fucosidosis are quite water soluble and fail to stain with PAS, although in fucosidosis there may be strong granular staining in some cells. Marked hemophagocytosis can be a feature of some foamy cells in fucosidosis. In sialidosis type 1 (normosomatic type, cherry red spot–myoclonus syndrome), the foamy cells are intensely PAS positive.

Mucopolysaccharidoses

It is not usually necessary to investigate these disorders by examination of the bone marrow since the clinical presentation will have prompted analysis of the urine for mucopolysaccharides and glycoconjugates, as well as the examination of a peripheral blood film for vacuolated lymphocytes. In the rare instance of some patients with SanFilippo syndrome who do not show dysmorphic features, the bone marrow displays collections of histiocytes with the cytoplasm containing fine vacuoles in which fine or coarse basophilic granules are present (Plate 72). These cells are referred to as Gasser-type reticulum cells by Smith.[2] The cells are distinguished from basophils by the vacuolation which separates the granules. These reticulum cells which display metachromasia with toluidine blue may occur singly or in syncytia close to or within the marrow fragments in the film. All MPSs show similar cells. Vacuolation of plasma cells in which the vacuoles contain basophilic inclusions (Buhot cells) can also be present in the MPSs. Osteoblasts may show vacuolation and metachromatic inclusions. Alder granulation will be evident and quite dramatic in the granulocytic series in Maroteaux–Lamy syndrome (MPS VI).

Cystinosis

Bone marrow aspirates contain macrophages filled with cystine crystals; however, in the spreading of the film the cells are often disrupted and the crystals dispersed. Cystine is usually regarded as insoluble but the solubility is finite and the aqueous staining solutions are sufficient to dissolve much of the cystine present and leave a few crystals with a rounded outline in contrast to the neat rectangular and hexagonal habit seen in films stained with alcoholic basic fuchsin. The best way to detect cystine crystals in suspected cases of cystinosis is to take one drop of anticoagulated marrow, place it on a slide, add a cover slip and allow the marrow to spread under the weight of the coverslip. Observe in polarized light. With this technique the macrophages remain intact and the crystals are in no danger of dissolving. There are very rare reports of cystine crystals being observed in a blood film but even with the help of electron microscopy the search for cystine crystals in peripheral blood samples is not a viable diagnostic route. The diagnosis of cystinosis is mainly made by biochemical assay of the cystine content of white cells and marrow samples are now rarely examined.

Hyperlipoproteinemias

The hyperlipoproteinemias may present with hepatosplenomegaly in childhood and the marrow contains foamy cells which can be mistaken for storage cells, particularly those of Niemann–Pick diseases A and B.

Hemophagocytosis

Occasional foamy cells displaying hemophagocytosis can be found in all marrows, particularly if an acid phosphatase reaction is used. These cells have no significance. Where there is marked hemophagocytosis, the diagnoses of Langerhans cell histiocytosis, infection-associated lymphohistiocytosis or Griscelli syndrome[8] are possibilities.

REFERENCES

1. Scriver CR, Beaudet AL, Valle D, Sly WS (eds). *The Metabolic and Molecular Bases of Inherited Disease*, 7th edn. New York: McGraw-Hill, 1995
2. Smith H. *Diagnosis in Pediatric Hematology*. New York: Churchill Livingstone, 1996
3. Hann IM, Lake BD, Lilleyman JL, Pritchard J. *Colour Atlas of Paediatric Haematology*, 3rd edn. Oxford, Oxford University Press, 1996
4. Muir H, Mittwoch U, Bitter T. The diagnostic value of isolated muccopolysaccharide and of lymphocytic inclusion in gargoylism. *Arch Dis Child* 1963; **38**: 358
5. Lake BD. Lysosomal and peroxisomal disorders. In: Graham DI, Lantos PL (eds) *Greenfield's Neuropathology*. London: Edward Arnold, 1997, Chapter 11
6. Lake BD. Histopathological investigation of prenatal tissue samples. In: Reed GB, Claireaux AE, Cockburn F (eds) *Diseases of the Fetus and Newborn*, 2nd edn. London: Chapman and Hall, 1995, Chapter 70
7. Silverstein MH, Ellefson RD, Ahern EJ. The syndrome of sea-blue histiocytes. *N Engl J Med* 1970; **282**: 1–4
8. Gogus S, Topcu M, Kucukali T *et al*. Griscelli syndrome. Report of 3 cases. *Pediatr Pathol Lab Med* 1995; **15**: 309–319

Index

Page numbers in **bold** refer to major discussions in the text, those in *italic* refer to figures or tables.